NEUROPSYCHIATRY

NEUROPSYCHIATRY

Editors

Barry S. Fogel, M.D.

Professor of Psychiatry and Human Behavior
Associate Director, Center for Gerontology and Health Care Research
Brown University School of Medicine
Providence, Rhode Island
Medical Director for Psychiatry
Eleanor Slater Hospital
Cranston, Rhode Island

Randolph B. Schiffer, M.D.

Professor of Neurology, Psychiatry, and Environmental Medicine
University of Rochester School of Medicine and Dentistry
Rochester, New York

Associate editor

Stephen M. Rao, Ph.D., A.B.P.P

Professor of Neurology
Co-Director, Section of Neuropsychology
Medical College of Wisconsin
Milwaukee, Wisconsin

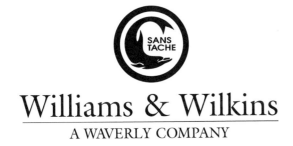

Williams & Wilkins

A WAVERLY COMPANY

BALTIMORE • PHILADELPHIA • LONDON • PARIS • BANGKOK
BUENOS AIRES • HONG KONG • MUNICH • SYDNEY • TOKYO • WROCLAW

1996

Managing Editor: Katey Millet
Production Coordinator: Danielle Santucci
Typesetter: Graphic World, Inc.
Printer: Maple Press
Binder: Maple Press

351 West Camden Street
Baltimore, Maryland 21201-2436   USA

Rose Tree Corporate Center
1400 North Providence Road
Building II, Suite 5025
Media, Pennsylvania 19063-2043   USA

Accurate indications, adverse reactions, and dosage schedules for drugs are provided in this book, but it is possible that they may change. The reader is urged to review the package information data of the manufacturers of the medications mentioned.

Printed in the United States of America

ISBN 0-683-03305-0

The Publishers have made every effort to trace the copyright holders for borrowed material. If they have inadvertently overlooked any, they will be pleased to make the necessary arrangements at the first opportunity.

96 97 98 99
1   2   3   4   5   6   7   8   9   10

Reprints of chapters may be purchased from Williams & Wilkins in quantities of 100 or more. Call Isabella Wise in the Special Sales Department, (800) 358-3583.

FOREWORD

A hundred years ago, the disciplinary activities and interests of neurology, psychiatry, and neuropathology could hardly be distinguished, either by the clinical pursuits of their practitioners or the way those who chose one or the other field diagnosed and attempted to treat patients. Few persons nowadays know that Alzheimer, who first described the morphology of the disease that bears his name, was a psychiatrist as well as a neuropathologist. Freud himself was initially a child neurologist and only later committed his life to the study of the subconscious-preconscious mind and how it might influence human behavior. Along with Jung and Adler, Freud and his followers provided psychological theories and therapeutics that led psychiatry forward into a psychological revolution, and away from the neurobiological explanation of behavior. Neurology marched deliberately forward, superimposing technological advances on meticulous clinical observations in order to identify and classify the signs, symptoms, and neuropathology of structural disorders affecting the central and peripheral nervous systems. There were struggles for theoretical and clinical territory, and for status. As Pearce Bailey, the first director of the National Institute of Neurological Diseases and Blindness put it (1951), "At the end of the nineteenth century, a psychiatrist almost had to be a neurologist to be respectable."

Gradually, however, a gulf of mutual disinterest arose between the anatomically grounded basis of neurological thinking and the psychological preoccupation of many psychiatrists. This shift peaked just after World War II, over 50 years ago. The separation of interests largely reflected the huge demand for psychiatric counseling for the many persons who became psychologically devastated by the disastrous political and material damage created by the war. Psychiatrists were learning how to talk with their patients and how to soothe their suffering. Meanwhile, neurology, with its demanding emphasis on physical causes and provable treatments at that time, was viewed by a large proportion of the public and medical profession as a rather arcane discipline. Although meticulously accurate in clinical diagnosis, its leaders seemed bereft of specific treatment for any neurological disease except epilepsy. Its practitioners were seen as by-and-large not very interested in patient care.

During the late 1940s, several things halted the interdisciplinary drift and began to set the pattern by which psychiatry and neurology would eventually close ranks in the medical battle against brain disease. Neurology and psychiatry had been militarily unified into the category of neuropsychiatry during World War I, and the designation was continued during World War II. After the war stopped, however, the large number of neurologically damaged veterans not only forced an immediate need for neurologists, but emphasized the principle that for neurology to survive it must become a therapeutic specialty as well as a diagnostic one. By the late 1940s, military needs had greatly improved neurophysiological instrumentation and had stimulated the advent of antibiotics capable of treating neurological infections. The development of the Kety-Schmidt cerebral blood flow technique, first introduced in 1948, whetted the appetite of neurologists and psychiatrists alike to know about brain mechanisms in neurological and psychiatric illness. Probably most important of all the stimuli bringing psychiatry and neurology together, however, was the rapid discovery of new psychoactive and soma-active drugs. Once and for all, the effects of these agents demonstrated not only that a large proportion of psychiatric illnesses have their biologically specific origins in abnormal brain mechanisms, but also that many of the aches and pains that neurologists attempt to treat are due to psychophysiological disturbances that can be explained in biological terms. Always bonded by their common efforts to understand the brain but sometimes treating each other as estranged relatives, the disciplines of neurology and psychiatry now find themselves addressing with similar scientific questions, using similar approaches to treatment and even more importantly, applying similar scientific techniques to the analysis of their problems. If not representing a revolution in the way that neurologists and psychiatrists face the problems of brain disease, this certainly represents an enormous change from the barriers that divided the two specialties only a few years ago.

Neuropsychiatry helps to strengthen the common features of the disciplines. A review of its contents illustrates the remarkable breadth of the topic. Similarly, a review of its authors and their backgrounds illustrates how greatly the fields of neurology, psychiatry, and neuropsychology already have joined forces to define, solve, and treat disturbances of the mind and behavior. In this textbook, we hear from prominent experts in the neurosciences as well as from published neuropsychiatric researchers. Many of the chapters suggest great progress in dealing with their topics. Others reflect how readily one can obtain clinical and scientific material about certain behavioral problems, but also how difficult it is to link the results of science into a testable, mechanistically governed, and treatable process. Still other aspects of the mind-brain mystery remain almost entirely clinically descriptive, offering invitations to all readers to explore the basic pathogenesis and develop rational treatments of the still poorly understood disorders.

Having had an opportunity to review *Neuropsychiatry,* I regard it as an original and indispensable single resource volume for every practicing neurologist and psychiatrist, which will be equally valuable for many academicians as well.

Of one thing I am sure: this volume will catalyze much future thinking on this subject. Undoubtedly, many subsequent editions of this text will follow.

Fred Plum, M.D.
New York, 1995

PREFACE

Since the renascence of neuropsychiatry began in the 1970s, several books have been published that have surveyed the field. *Neuropsychiatry* aims to cover new ground in three ways: by offering a deeper treatment of many neuropsychiatric issues than that provided by introductory texts, by including the work of more neurologists, and by combining British and American perspectives. Our hope is these features will engage the interest of a broader range of clinicians and scientists.

Neuropsychiatry comprises the scientific study and medical treatment of the psychiatric aspects of neurologic diseases, and an approach to psychiatric disorders that emphasizes the role of brain dysfunction. During the past decade, neuropsychiatry has grown and developed with extraordinary vigor, both as a subspecialty and as an aspect of mainstream psychiatry. Widely-disseminated work has been done on dementia and on schizophrenia, and on depressive phenomena in patients with gross brain disease. Nonetheless, we believe it remains true as of 1995 that in daily practice, general neurologists do not approach their patients' mental and behavioral problems rigorously, nor are

most general psychiatrists knowledgeable about such common neuropsychiatric problems as frontal lobe syndromes and partial epilepsy. For years to come, specialists in neuropsychiatry, neuropsychology, and behavioral neurology will have a major role not only in diagnosis and treating neuropsychiatric disorders, but also in raising consciousness of the field and its concerns among general neurologists and psychiatrists.

In *Neuropsychiatry,* we have tried to pull together much of the existing scientific basis of neuropsychiatry. We hope it will serve as a reference text and clinical guide for readers from various disciplines, including neurology, psychiatry, and neuropsychology. In presenting this comprehensive view of contemporary neuropsychiatry, we aim to improve the current care of patients with neuropsychiatric disorders, and to inspire investigators to turn their attention to the many unresolved questions in the field.

Barry S. Fogel, M.D.
Randolph B. Schiffer, M.D.
Stephen M. Rao, Ph.D.

ACKNOWLEDGMENTS

The editors acknowledge with deep gratitude the thousands of hours of effort spent by our contributors in preparing their contributions to this volume. Special thanks are due also to Michael G. Fisher for encouraging this project and helping us refine our conception through his thoughtful questions. Katey Millet and David Retford, our editors at Williams & Wilkins, kept us going through the many delays we encountered in completing this ambitious project. We also thank our staff, with special gratitude to Nancy Malloy and Rita St. Pierre.

CONTRIBUTORS

John R. Absher, M.D.
Assistant Professor of Neurology
Associate in Psychiatry and
 Biobehavioral Medicine
Bowman Gray School of Medicine
Winston-Salem, North Carolina

Robert Ader, Ph.D., M.D.
George L. Engel Professor of
 Psychosocial Medicine
Director, Center for Psycho-
 neuroimmunology Research
University of Rochester School
 of Medicine and Dentistry
Rochester, New York

**Michael J. Aminoff, M.D.,
F.R.C.P.**
Professor of Neurology
University of California, San
 Francisco, School of Medicine
San Francisco, California

David M. Bear, M.D.
Professor of Psychiatry
University of Massachusetts Medical
 School
Chairman, Department of Psychiatry
The Medical Center of Central
 Massachusetts
Worcester, Massachusetts

Denise L. Bellinger, Ph.D.
Assistant Professor of Neurobiology
 and Anatomy
University of Rochester School of
 Medicine and Dentistry
Rochester, New York

D. Frank Benson, M.D.
Professor of Neurology, Emeritus
University of California,
 Los Angeles, School of Medicine
Los Angeles, California

Dawn Bowers, Ph.D.
Associate Professor of Neurology
 and Clinical and Health
 Psychology
University of Florida College of
 Medicine
Gainesville, Florida

J. Douglas Bremner, M.D.
Assistant Professor of Psychiatry
Yale University School of Medicine
New Haven, Connecticut
Research Scientist
National Center for Post Traumatic
 Stress Disorder
Veterans Administration Medical
 Center
West Haven, Connecticut

David Caplan, M.D., Ph.D.
Associate Professor of Neurology
Harvard Medical School
Neuropsychology Laboratory
Massachusetts General Hospital
Boston, Massachusetts

Dennis S. Charney, M.D.
Professor of Psychiatry
Associate Chairman for Research
Yale University School of
 Medicine
New Haven, Connecticut
Chief, Psychiatry Service
Veterans Administration Medical
 Center
West Haven, Connecticut

Nicholas Cohen, Ph.D.
Professor of Microbiology,
 Immunology and Psychiatry
University of Rochester School
 of Medicine and Dentistry
Rochester, New York

Peggy Compton, R.N., Ph.D.
Assistant Clinical Professor of
 Acute Care Nursing
University of California,
 Los Angeles School of Nursing
Research Scientist
The Los Angeles Addiction
 Treatment Research Center
Los Angeles, California

Yeates Conwell, M.D.
Associate Professor of Psychiatry and
 Oncology
Director, Laboratory of Suicide
 Studies
University of Rochester School of
 Medicine and Dentistry
Rochester, New York

Jody Corey-Bloom, M.D., Ph.D.
Assistant Professor of Neurology
University of California, San Diego,
 School of Medicine
Attending Neurologist
Veterans Administration Medical
 Center
San Diego, California

Dean C. Delis, Ph.D., A.B.P.P.
Professor of Psychiatry
University of California, San Diego
 School of Medicine
Director, Psychological Assessment
 Unit
Veterans Administration Medical
 Center
San Diego, California

**Beatriz M. DeMoranville,
M.D.**
Clinical Instructor in Medicine
Brown University School of Medicine
Chief, Endocrinology Section
Veterans Administration Medical
 Center
Providence, Rhode Island

Orrin Devinsky, M.D.
Professor of Neurology
New York University School of
  Medicine
Chief, Department of Neurology
Hospital for Joint Diseases
Orthopaedic Institute
Director, NYU-HJD Comprehensive
  Epilepsy Center
New York, New York

**George H. Dooneief, M.D.,
M.P.H.**
Assistant Professor of Neurology
College of Physicians and Surgeons
  of Columbia University
Assistant Attending Neurologist
Columbia-Presbyterian Medical
  Center
New York, New York

Maureen P. Dymek
Doctoral Candidate in Clinical
  Psychiatry
University of Alabama at
  Birmingham
Birmingham, Alabama

David Faust, Ph.D.
Professor of Psychology
University of Rhode Island
Kingston, Rhode Island

Deborah Fein, Ph.D.
Professor of Psychology
University of Connecticut School
  of Medicine
Storrs, Connecticut

Robert G. Feldman, M.D.
Professor and Chairman
Department of Neurology
Boston University School of
  Medicine
Boston, Massachusetts

David L. Felten, M.D., Ph.D.
Kilian J. and Caroline F. Schmitt
  Professor and Chair
Depatment of Neurobiology and
  Anatomy
University of Rochester School
  of Medicine and Dentistry
Rochester, New York

Howard L. Fields, M.D., Ph.D.
Professor of Neurology, Physiology
  and Psychiatry
University of California,
  San Francisco
San Francisco, California

Christopher M. Filley, M.D.
Associate Professor of Neurology
  and Psychiatry
Director, Behavioral Neurology
  Section
University of Colorado School
  of Medicine
Denver, Colorado

**David A. Fishbain, M.D.,
F.A.P.A.**
Professor of Psychiatry and
  Neurological Surgery
University of Miami School
  of Medicine
Miami, Florida
Comprehensive Pain and
  Rehabilitation Center
South Shore Hospital and
  Medical Center
Miami Beach, Florida

Barry S. Fogel, M.D.
Professor of Psychiatry and
  Human Behavior
Associate Director, Center for
  Gerontology and Health Care
  Research
Brown University School of Medicine
Providence, Rhode Island
Medical Director for Psychiatry
Eleanor Slater Hospital
Cranston, Rhode Island

Joachim M. Fuster, M.D., Ph.D.
Professor of Psychiatry
University of California, Los
  Angeles, School of Medicine
Los Angeles, California

Douglas Galasko, M.D.
Assistant Professor of Neuroscience
University of California, San Diego
  School of Medicine
Staff Physician in Neurology
Veterans Administration Medical
  Center
San Diego, California

Angela Genge, M.D.
Neurologist
Department of Neurology
Montreal Neurological Hospital
Montreal, Quebec, Canada

Andrew W. Goddard, M.D.
Assistant Professor of Psychiatry
Yale University School of Medicine
New Haven, Connecticut

D. Gregory Gorman, M.D.
Associate Clinical Professor of
  Neurology
University of New Mexico School
  of Medicine
Neurobehavioral Program
Department of Neurology
Lovelace Medical Center
Albuquerque, New Mexico

Jordan Grafman, Ph.D.
Chief, Cognitive Neuroscience
  Section
Medical Neurology Branch
National Institute of Neurological
  Disorders and Stroke
National Institutes of Health
Bethesda, Maryland

Eric Granholm, Ph.D.
Assistant Professor of Psychiatry
University of California, San Diego
  School of Medicine
Staff Psychologist
Veterans Administration Medical
  Center
San Diego, California

Steven J. Grant, M.D.
Senior Staff Fellow
Intramural Research Program
National Institute on Drug Abuse
National Institutes of Health
Bethesda, Maryland

Lee Anne Green, M.A.
Doctoral Candidate in Clinical
  Psychology
Research Assistant in Psychology
University of Connecticut
Storrs, Connecticut

Kenneth M. Heilman, M.D.
The James E. Rooks Jr. Professor
of Neurology
University of Florida College of
Medicine
Staff Neurologist
Veterans Administration Medical
Center
Gainesville, Florida

Robin E. Henderson, Ph.D.
Assistant Professor of Orthopedics
(Rehabilitation Medicine) and
Psychiatry
University of Rochester School
of Medicine and Dentistry
Monroe Community Hospital
Rochester, New York

Ivor Jackson, M.D.
Professor of Medicine
Chief, Division of Endocrinology
Brown University School of
Medicine
Director, Division of Endocrinology
Rhode Island Hospital
Providence, Rhode Island

Dilip V. Jeste, M.D.
Professor of Psychiatry and
Neuroscience
University of California, San Diego
School of Medicine
Director, Geriatric Psychiatry
Clinical Research Center
Veterans Administration Medical
Center
San Diego, California

Stephen Joy, M.A.
Doctoral Candidate in Clinical
Psychology
University of Connecticut
Storrs, Connecticut
Instructor in Psychology
Albertus Magnus College
New Haven, Connecticut

Daniel K. Kido, M.D.
Professor of Radiology
Chief, Neuroradiology Section
Mallinckrodt Institute of Radiology
Washington University School
of Medicine
St. Louis, Missouri

*Michael D. Kopelman, Ph.D.,
F.R.C.Psych*
Reader in Neuropsychiatry
Neuropsychiatry and Memory
Disorders Clinic
United Medical and Dental Schools
of Guy's and St. Thomas's
Hospitals
St. Thomas Campus
London, United Kingdom

Walter Ling, M.D.
Professor and Chief, Substance
Abuse Program
University of California, Los
Angeles, School of Medicine
Director, Los Angeles Addiction
Treatment Research Center
Associate Chief of Psychiatry for
Substance Abuse
West Los Angeles Veterans
Administration Medical Center
Los Angeles, California

Edythe D. London, Ph.D.
Adjunct Associate Professor of
Pharmacology and Experimental
Therapeutics
University of Maryland School of
Medicine
Associate Professor of Radiology
Johns Hopkins School of Medicine
Baltimore, Maryland
Chief, Neuroimaging and Drug
Action Section
National Institute on Drug Abuse
National Institutes of Health
Bethesda, Maryland

John A. Lucas, Ph.D.
Assistant Professor of Psychiatry
Mayo Medical School
Rochester, Minnesota
Senior Associate Consultant
Mayo Clinic Jacksonville
Jacksonville, Florida

Kelley S. Madden, Ph.D.
Scientist in Neurobiology and
Anatomy
University of Rochester School
of Medicine and Dentistry
Rochester, New York

*Karen S. Marder, M.D.,
M.P.H.*
Assistant Professor of Neurology
College of Physicians and Surgeons
of Columbia University
New York, New York

Robert J. Morecraft, Ph.D.
Assistant Professor of Anatomy
and Structural Biology
University of South Dakota School
of Medicine
Sioux Falls, South Dakota

Michael J. Morgan, Ph.D.
Lecturer in Psychology
University of Wales, Swansea
Singleton Park, Swansea, United
Kingdom

Jonathan Mueller, M.D.
Associate Clinical Professor of
Psychiatry
University of California, San
Francisco School of Medicine
Director, San Francisco
Neuropsychiatric Associates
San Francisco, California

Linda M. Nagy, M.D.
Assistant Professor of Psychiatry
Yale University School of Medicine
New Haven, Connecticut
Research Director, Outpatient
Division
National Center for Post Traumatic
Stress Disorder
Veterans Administration Medical
Center
West Haven, Connecticut

John B. Penney, Jr., M.D.
Professor of Neurology
Harvard Medical School
Neurologist
Massachusetts General Hospital
Boston, Massachusetts

Susan P. Proctor, D.Sc.
Research Assistant Professor of
Neurology and Environmental
Health
Boston University Schools of
Medicine and Public Health
Boston, Massachusetts

Henry J. Ralston III, M.D.
Professor of Anatomy
W.M. Keck Foundation Center for
  Integrative Neuroscience
University of California, San
  Francisco, School of Medicine
San Francisco, California

**Stephen M. Rao, Ph.D.,
A.B.P.P.**
Professor of Neurology
Co-Director, Section of
  Neuropsychology
Medical College of Wisconsin
Milwaukee, Wisconsin

John Ratey, M.D.
Assistant Professor of Psychiatry
Harvard Medical School
Boston, Massachusetts

Richard Rawson, Ph.D.
Executive Director, Matrix Center
Deputy Director
Matrix/University of California,
  Los Angeles Alcoholism and
  Addiction Medicine Services
Los Angeles, California

Alison Reeve, M.D.
Assistant Professor of Psychiatry and
  Neurology
Mental Health Programs
The University of New Mexico
School of Medicine
Albuquerque, New Mexico

Howard A. Ring, M.D.
Senior Lecturer in Psychiatry
London Hospital Medical College
Honorary Senior Lecturer
Institute of Neurology, Queen
  Square
London, United Kingdom

Lynn C. Robertson, Ph.D.
Professor of Neurology and
  Psychiatry
University of California, Davis
School of Medicine
Davis, California
Research Career Scientist
Veterans Administration Medical
  Center
Martinez, California

**Mary M. Robertson, M.B.ChB,
M.D., D.P.M., F.R.C.Psych**
Reader in Neuropsychiatry
University College London Medical
  School
Consultant Neuropsychiatrist
National Hospital for Neurology
  and Neurosurgery
London, United Kingdom

Robert G. Robinson, M.D.
Professor and Chairman
Department of Psychiatry
University of Iowa College of
  Medicine
Iowa City, Iowa

Maria A. Ron, M.Phil, Ph.D.
Professor of Neuropsychiatry and
  Consultant Psychiatrist
The Institute of Neurology
National Hospital for Neurology and
  Neurosurgery
London, United Kingdom

Andres Salazar, M.D.
Professor of Neurology
Uniformed Services University of the
  Health Sciences
Director, Defense and Veterans Head
  Injury Program
Walter Reed Army Medical Center
Washington, DC

Stephen P. Salloway, M.D.
Assistant Professor of Clinical
  Neurosciences and Psychiatry and
  Human Behavior
Brown University School of Medicine
Director of Neurology
Butler Hospital
Providence, Rhode Island

Mary Sano, Ph.D.
Assistant Professor of Neurology
College of Physicians and Surgeons
  of Columbia University
New York, New York

Ghislaine Savard, M.D.
Assistant Professor of Neurology and
  Psychiatry
McGill University
Attending Psychiatrist
Montreal Neurological Hospital and
  Institute
Montreal, Quebec, Canada

Jeffrey L. Saver, M.D.
Assistant Professor of Clinical
  Neurology
University of California, Los
  Angeles, School of Medicine
Attending Neurologist
University of California, Los
  Angeles Center for Health
  Sciences
Los Angeles, California

Randall T. Schapiro, M.D.
Clinical Professor of Neurology
University of Minnesota Medical
  School
Medical Director of Rehabilitation
The Fairview MS Center
Fairview Riverside Medical Center
Minneapolis, Minnesota

Randolph B. Schiffer, M.D.
Professor of Neurology, Psychiatry,
  and Environmental Medicine
University of Rochester School of
  Medicine and Dentistry
Rochester, New York

Bettina Schmitz, M.D.
Psychiatrische Klinik und Poliklinik
Klinikum Benjamin Franklin
Free University
Berlin, Germany

**Robert Taylor Segraves, M.D.,
Ph.D.**
Professor of Psychiatry
Case Western Reserve University
Interim Director, Department of
  Psychiatry
MetroHealth Medical Center
Cleveland, Ohio

Katerina Semendeferi, Ph.D.
Postdoctoral Associate in Neurology
  and Anatomy
University of Iowa
Iowa City, Iowa

Yvette I. Sheline, M.D.
Assistant Professor of Psychiatry
  and Radiology
Washington University School
  of Medicine
St. Louis, Missouri

Steven M. Southwick, M.D.
Associate Professor of Psychiatry
Yale University School of Medicine
New Haven, Connecticut
Director, National Center for Post
   Traumatic Stress Disorder
Clinical Neurosciences Division
Veterans Administration Medical
   Center
West Haven, Connecticut

James F. Toole, M.D.
Teagle Professor of Neurology
Professor of Public Health Sciences
Director, Stroke Center
Bowman Gray School of Medicine
Winston-Salem, North Carolina

Javier I. Travella, M.D.
Research Fellow, Department of
   Psychiatry
University of Iowa College of
   Medicine
Iowa City, Iowa

**Michael R. Trimble, M.D.,
F.R.C.P., F.R.C.Psych**
Professor of Behavioral Neurology
University Department of Clinical
   Neurology
Institute of Neurology
Queen Square, London, United
   Kingdom

Gary J. Tucker, M.D.
Professor and Chairman, Department
   of Psychiatry and Behavioral
   Sciences
University of Washington School of
   Medicine
Seattle, Washington

Gary W. Van Hoesen, Ph.D.
Professor of Anatomy and
   Neurology
University of Iowa College of
   Medicine
Iowa City, Iowa

Stanley Walens, Ph.D.
Research Associate, Department of
   Psychiatry
University of California, San Diego
   School of Medicine
San Diego, California

Lynn Waterhouse, Ph.D.
Director, Child Behavior Study
Trenton State College
Trenton, New Jersey

Charles E. Wells, M.D.
Clinical Professor of Psychiatry
   and Neurology
Vanderbilt University School of
   Medicine
Nashville, Tennessee

Donald R. Wesson, M.D.
Medical Director and Scientific
   Director
MPI Treatment Services
Summit Medical Center
Oakland, California

**Roberta F. White, Ph.D.,
A.B.P.P.**
Professor of Neurology
   (Neuropsychology) and
   Environmental Health
Boston University School of
   Medicine and School of Public
   Health
Director, Clinical Neuro-
   psychology
Research Director, Boston
   Environmental Hazards
   Center
Department of Veterans Affairs
   Medical Center
Boston, Massachusetts

**Peter J. Whitehouse, M.D.,
Ph.D.**
Professor of Neurology
Case Western Reserve University
Director, Alzheimer Center
University Hospitals of Cleveland
Cleveland, Ohio

Tony M. Wong, Ph.D.
Assistant Professor of Physical
   Medicine and Rehabilitation
University of Rochester School of
   Medicine and Dentistry
Director of Neuropsychiatry
Brain Injury Rehabilitation Program
St. Mary's Hospital
Rochester, New York

**Jessica Yakeley, M.A.,
M.B.B.Chir., M.R.C.P.**
Registrar in Psychiatry
Maudsley Hospital and Institute of
   Psychiatry
London, United Kingdom

Rachel Yehuda, Ph.D.
Assistant Professor of Psychiatry
Yale University School of Medicine
New Haven, Connecticut
Scientific Director, National Center
   Post Traumatic Stress Disorder
Veterans Administration Medical
   Center
West Haven, Connecticut

Stephen R. Zukin, M.D.
Professor of Psychiatry and
   Neuroscience
Albert Einstein College of Medicine
   of Yeshiva University
Bronx, New York
Director, Division of Clinical and
   Services Research
National Institute on Drug Abuse
National Institutes of Health
Rockville, Maryland

CONTENTS

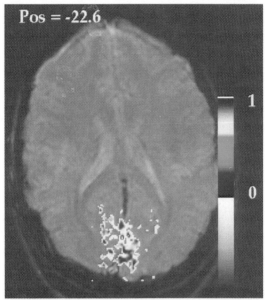

Figure 4-15

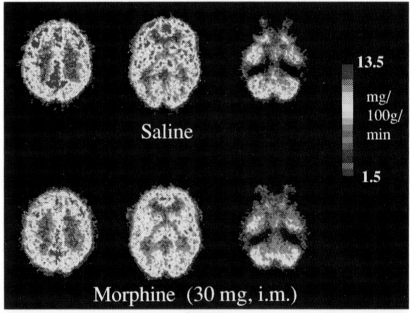

Figure 29-5

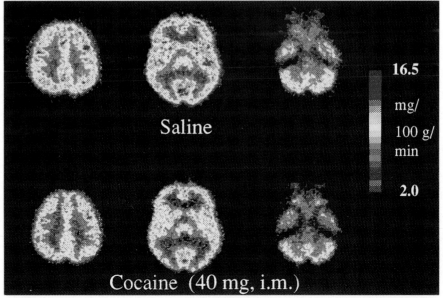

Figure 29-6

1

EVOLUTION OF NEUROPSYCHIATRIC IDEAS IN THE UNITED STATES AND UNITED KINGDOM—1800–2000

Randolph B. Schiffer and Barry S. Fogel

There has always been a creative tension in science and medicine between psychological and neurological theories of behavior, and certain remarkable similarities exist in the way in which different times have addressed this issue. This chapter is about the recent history of neuropsychiatric ideas in the United Kingdom and the United States. It is worth reminding ourselves that ideas about the neurological basis of behavior have existed for a considerable time and have changed dramatically in response to political, cultural, and scientific developments.

The current practice of neuropsychiatry can be described as a subspecialty either of more traditional psychiatry or of neurology. Neuropsychiatric practice encompasses two Janus-like realms of care delivery in the clinical neurosciences: the diagnosis and treatment of psychiatric disorders from the perspective of their neurological bases, and the clinical care of neurological patients with concomitant mood or behavior disturbance. Neuropsychiatry also includes a research endeavor, which seeks to advance knowledge concerning the neural basis of both normal behavior and psychopathology. The search for boundaries of this specialty has been the subject of several editorials (1–5). We are especially indebted to the thoughtful comments provided by Professor W.A. Lishman (6).

There is a certain neuropsychiatric perspective on each psychiatric or neurological disorder. Yet for some diseases neuropsychiatric insights are of much greater heuristic value than are others. Neuropsychiatric perspectives continually evolve in the face of new research. Other subspecialty disciplines contribute complementary approaches for care and understanding of illness. Such subspecialties include at least behavioral neurology, "biological" psychiatry (psychopharmacology), neuropsychology, medical (consultation-liaison) psychiatry, and perhaps others. Sharp boundaries do not exist among these subspecialties because all seek to understand behavior as partly shaped by brain function. At present, neuropsychiatry may be the broadest of such endeavors.

PREMODERN ERA

In the summer of 1453, Henry VI became suddenly ill at the Royal Lodge of Clarendon (7). The immediate cause was said to have been a great fright. For a year and a half he was "without natural sense." He seemed unable to administer the government. He had a loss of time sense and of memory. He had "hardly any control over his limbs." He could not walk or keep his head up, and he remained usually in a slumped position. When his two-month-old son, Edward, was presented for blessing, only a fleeting glance could be elicited. Henry was treated by many physicians using a number of physically based treatments according to humoral logic:

1. Electuaries, potions, waters, syrups, and confections;
2. Unguents and wax ointments;
3. Laxatives, clysters, and suppositories;
4. Head-shaving, head purges, applications of heat to the scalp on the theory that some of the brain's waste products were excreted through the scalp;
5. Gargles to shift the catarrhal fluids;
6. Baths, poultices, plasters, and embrocations;
7. Bloodletting.

By Christmas 1454 the king had returned to his premorbid state of health.

In this sequence of diagnostic and therapeutic interventions for a royal pique, we hear wafts of a primitive, galenic neuropsychiatry antedating both psychiatry and neurology as they are presently known. Galen himself does not seem to have distinguished diseases of the soul from those of the body (8). He felt that mental processes derived from the brain, and that such mental processes could be disturbed by the circulation of abnormal humors. Included in Galen's treatises were humoral descriptions of such disorders as melancholia, invoking bilious and vaporous influences upon the brain (9). Black bile in particular was felt to cause some forms of madness when it rose to the brain and adversely affected the hollow spaces within. Late 19th century psychiatric theories of autointoxication and 20th century theories of endocrine dysregulation in psychiatric disorders may not be so very far removed from such views. Of course it is not possible to extrapolate from an applied regal neuropsychiatry to the common person or common practice in Britain during premodern times. Still, the application of medical treatments to a mental and behavioral condition is notable in this account. Moreover, the physicians who attended Henry VI seem to have been general physicians who did not treat the king's malady as if it were categorically different from other more obviously physical diseases. Notions of psychiatry and psychology as specialties apart from general medicine did not yet exist.

The belief that madness was a proper province of medicine may not have been quite so widespread in the American colonies. Supernatural and religious news of the mentally disturbed were stronger in the Puritan colonies across the ocean (10). Satan was felt to have the power of witchcraft and possession, but also the power to drive or tempt a person into madness (11). Moral transgression could also be seen as a precipitant for madness. Satanic temptation and moral transgression views were considerably more widespread than was the idea of possession by the devil, if for no other reason than that the latter required an inquisition, a witch hunt, and similar activities which, at best, must have been burdensome for the authorities. Treatments in these early colonial times were primarily family and community based. The acutely disturbed were sometimes jailed, but they were more likely to be remanded for custody to their family or to a foster family. Prayer and fasting were considered therapeutic, and church congregations could be enlisted to help. It would not be until the end of the 18th century that medical remedies for madness began to appear in contemporary records, and physicians were regarded as agents of authority in its management.

FIRST NEUROPSYCHIATRIC PERIOD (1800–1900)

Toward the end of the 18th century, liberal forces of great strength swept the Western world. It was a time of cultural change not to be equaled perhaps until the 1960s. The French and American revolutions occurred, monarchies weakened and toppled, and democracies were founded. Intellectual and cultural changes of a less cataclysmic nature were also occurring. Silk stockings and wigs for men disappeared. Primogeniture and reverence for the aged weakened (12). Along with these changes, a more neurological view of madness began to develop.

It would be wrong to say that a single neuropsychiatric theory emerged during these years, or even that a single intellectual movement was at work. There was a series of shifts in the way physicians viewed and treated behavioral disturbances, which were associated with various social and scientific developments. Medicine itself was struggling to find a place for rationalism within its own discourse. As

it did, neurology and psychiatry were very close or indistinguishable.

At the close of the 18th century, medicine generally lacked the therapeutic and diagnostic organization of the disease concept. Vague notions of functional interrelationships between mental and physical states dominated diagnostic thinking, so that a distracted mind could be understood as curdling the stomach, or a dyspeptic stomach as agitating the mind (13). The body of a sick individual was also understood as dynamically interrelated with environmental forces, which could be either ameliorative or destructive. The therapeutics of the premodern era had remained fairly simply somatic. This would soon change with the advent of certain psychosocially-based treatments early in the 19th century, and nothing in the medical theoretic of the time would prove averse to such changes.

Social forces associated with the industrial revolution exerted pressures for change in the medical therapeutics of the insane. In earlier times, obviously disturbed individuals had been cared for by families or local communities. However, with the increasing population growth, immigration, and urbanization of the early 19th century, new systems were needed. Movements to segregate and quarantine the insane poor developed. In England a number of public subscription hospitals were founded in provincial towns during the 18th century, and the insane poor often were included with more general medical patients (14). In the United States, the more locally based almshouses for the poor were an alternative location for some mentally disturbed individuals. In the 19th century, however, larger lunatic hospitals began to be located in more rural environments with the new therapeutic intention of providing the patients with amusement, exercise, and healthier employment.

In Great Britain, Wynne's Act of 1808 enabled each county to build its own insane asylum so that the impoverished mentally ill might have an alternative to jail (15). In the United States as well, psychiatry coalesced as a medical specialty around such hospitals for the insane, which were filled with both chronic and acute patients (16).

There was a wealth of neurology among these psychiatric patients, and a therapeutic neuropsychiatry existed to the extent that all patients were treated in the same place and by the same physicians. The therapeutics themselves were quite primitive and prescientific, emphasizing bloodletting, purgatives, emetics, and a variety of drugs available for medical conditions at the time including niter, peruvian bark, opium, digitalis, and camphor (10). Some actual descriptions of therapy from a Boston almshouse in the period 1807–1808 appear in letters from the physician John Gorham to Benjamin Vaughan of Philadelphia (17):

A 35-year-old blacksmith was admitted for insanity after an attack of pneumonia. He was turbulent, ungovernable, and inflicted wounds on various parts of his body. June 30: "Ordered 150 drops of tincture of opium immediately and 50 drops to be repeated every half hour till he became quiet and drowsy." Afterward he slept and was better.

A man was insane for several months with religious preoccupations. He was bled; a blister was applied to his neck; a cathartic given; he was confined in a straight waistcoat. More opium was administered. He jumped out a window in a suicide attempt. Later, "a complete inactivity of the mental powers" ensued. "He seemed to have exchanged the state of active mania only for the quietude of ideotism." He was employed in the open air and gradually recovered over five months.

In some of the asylums, more psychological therapeutics ("moral therapy") were being introduced which were in many cases kind, humane, and probably effective. These therapeutics had originated with asylum-based reforms in France under Esquirol and Pinel, but found support from William Tuke and John Conolly in England. The principles of the therapy included a reeducation of the patient in a humanistic environment, usually in a rural setting. Kindness and courtesy on the part of staff were also emphasized. Amariah Brigham, one of the original 13 founders of the Association of Medical Superintendents of American Institutions for the Insane (the forerunner of the American Psychiatric Association), defined moral therapy as the removal of the insane from home and former associates, combined with manual labor and the establishment of regular habits (18). There is evidence from vignettes such as those above as well as from discharge statistics that a substantial number of patients improved under these therapies and were discharged from the asylums.

There is no doubt that theoretic neuropsychiatry also existed during this period in which the asylums were establishing themselves as the dominant treatment venue for individuals with disturbed behavior. In the United States, Benjamin Rush (Fig 1.1) published a psychiatric textbook in 1812, *Medical Inquiries and Observations Upon the Diseases of the Mind.* In it, he expounded an interactionist view of the causation of mental disease. He felt that excessive congestion of the blood vessels of the brain was the proximate cause of brain inflammation and behavioral disturbance. He considered that physiological disturbance of the body or brain could produce mental disturbance, but that upsetting mental events could also react with causal effect upon the brain, disturbing its vasculature (19). He suggested that patients could benefit by recording their memories and experiences, thus demonstrating a certain therapeutic balance between the somatic and the psychological (20), and perhaps providing a hint of sensitivity to the future importance of the life historical narrative in psychotherapeutic work.

One can understand a certain galenic neuropsychiatry in Rush's views. There are echoes of ancient themes in the image of excess blood rising to clog and inflame the brain, with presages of neurally based behavioral theories to come. Rush's ideas were, of course, prescientific in the sense that they did not derive from empirical experiments. However, his theories had clear therapeutic implications, which would set them apart from the neurobehaviorism of the latter 19th century. Bloodletting made

sense for psychiatric patients, but so did the "moral therapies" which may have been efficacious. We can understand Rush as a man poised in time between ancient speculation and the beginning of an era in which medicine would come to be defined as partly science.

Toward the middle of the 19th century, the neurobehavioral side of the neuropsychiatric equation began to deepen. There were several motivating forces of this change including theories of morbid heredity from France (21) and neurobehavioral theories from Germany. Social upheavals related to industrialization were also occurring, changing attitudes toward the mentally ill in the direction of callousness and indifference. The time-intensive moral therapies may have come to seem less appropriate. It is clear in retrospect that neurology was emerging as a medical specialty, and as its identity first coalesced, many neurologists claimed large areas of psychiatric practice for their own.

In the United States, the Civil War provided defining experiences for two men who would shape American neurology. Silas Weir Mitchell (Fig 1.2) worked at the Turner's Lane Military Hospital in Philadelphia, where he became especially fascinated by peripheral nerve injuries among the veterans (22). He published a book during the war, *Gunshot Wounds and Other Injuries of Nerves* (1864), which became widely known and focused attention upon neurological disease. After the war, he wrote and spoke

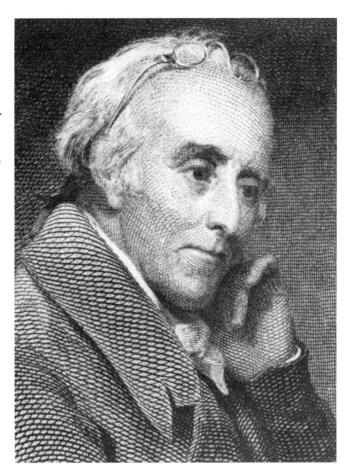

Figure 1.1. Benjamin Rush.

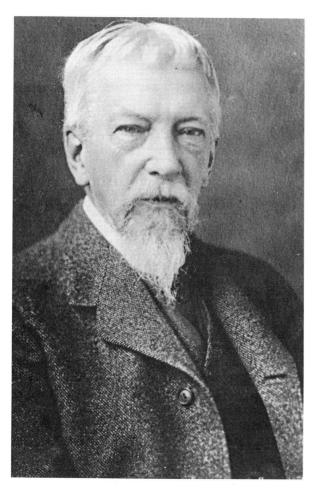

Figure 1.2. Silas Weir Mitchell.

vague neuropsychiatric symptoms, quite reminiscent of today's "chronic fatigue syndrome": insomnia, fatigue, headache, dyspepsia, and depression. Beard promulgated a neurometaphoric pathophysiology for the syndrome, with neurons becoming exhausted and worn out by the fast pace of late 19th century life. As he put it, "The bustle of urban life coupled with a peculiarity of climate . . . conspired to deprive the professional classes . . . of their reserve nerve force" (23). He felt that a predisposing heredity was also a relevant causative factor, and that the disease was sex-modulated and more common among women. The therapy of neurasthenia included a mix of modalities including rest cures, diets, hydrotherapy, electrotherapy (not *electroconvulsive* therapy), and drugs such as strychnine. Beard's view of the appropriate therapy for neurasthenia also included a process of reeducating the patient about adaptation to the stress of modern life. Although most neurologists opposed overt psychotherapies, the neurologist-based therapies of neurasthenia established a model of successive ambulatory visits during which a learning process was facilitated between patient and physician. This surely helped to modify and strengthen physician-patient relationships.

Later writers on neurasthenia elaborated diagnostic schemes that included subtypes, such as the "lithemic" subtype described by Roberts Batholow, which was felt to be due to an unspecified autointoxication (23). Hammond himself elaborated a theory of "cerebral hyperaemia" to diagnose large numbers of patients complaining of headache, dizziness, noises in the ears, lapses of memory, transitory illusions or delusions, heaviness of limbs, and insomnia (24). Gowers even devoted 10 pages in his 1888 book, *Manual of Diseases of the Nervous System,* to neurobehavorial disorders caused by cerebral hyperaemia. Hammond's diagnostics with such patients were quite technical, emphasizing the use of the ophthalmoscope, aesthesiometer, aural speculum, thermoelectric differential calorimeter, and other gadgets.

The story of neurasthenia is one of a failed attempt by the new neurology to diagnose and treat neurotic mental illness. The theories had a certain elegance, compelling to both physicians and patients. The problem seems to have been that these theories were not therapeutically useful because they were too radically neurological.

The new leaders of neurology promulgated a very reductionistic view of mental symptoms (24). Hammond, for example, said in 1871 that "the modern science of psychology is neither more nor less than the science of mind considered as a physical function" (25). Such views set them apart from the institutional psychiatrists and fostered conflicts between the specialties. Inflammatory papers and diatribes against asylum psychiatrists appeared, such as E.C. Spitzka's 1878 paper presented before the New York Neurological Society, "The Study of Insanity Considered as a Branch of Neurology, and the Relations of the General Medical Body to this Branch" (26). Perhaps the culmination of this conflict occurred when Dr. Mitchell addressed the

extensively about the need to study diseases of the nervous system. It is ironic that the peripheral nervous system appears to be of historical importance in the history of neuropsychiatry!

William Alexander Hammond (Fig. 1.3) served as Surgeon General during the early years of the Civil War, before Secretary of War Stanton fired him in 1863 (he was subsequently vindicated of any wrongdoing in a post-war courtmartial). After the war he was appointed lecturer in neurology and psychiatry at the College of Physicians and Surgeons in New York, and he published the first American textbook of neurology in 1871, *A Treatise on Diseases of the Nervous System.* This book went through seven editions over the subsequent 10 years and had a defining impact upon the emerging medical specialty.

In these post-Civil War years, neurology and psychiatry were taught together in the medical schools, and the early practitioners of neurology practiced both specialties. At the first annual meeting of the American Neurological Association in 1875, papers on neurasthenia were read along with papers on peripheral neurology.

Neurasthenia was a peculiarly American neuropsychiatric diagnosis that emerged during the late 19th century (23). The term was coined by George M. Beard, a New York neurologist, in 1869. The syndrome included a variety of

50th annual meeting of the American Medico-Psychological Association, the association of asylum psychiatrists that was the more immediate forerunner of today's American Psychiatric Association (27). In this address he attacked the alienists once again for their lack of neuroscientific research, as well as for their isolation from general medicine.

The neurologists did not prevail in their battle for control of the asylums and of psychiatric disease in general. That is, in political and economic terms they did not prevail to the extent that the major "business" of inpatient psychiatric care remained with the alienists. This was not because of any particular creativity or dynamism on the part of the asylum psychiatrists. The therapeutic enthusiasm of some of the earlier founders of institutional psychiatry had long since waned, and it is more likely that the alienists merely continued to do what they had always done—segregate and control the psychotic and chronically mentally ill, relying primarily upon various occupational and milieu therapies. Indeed, the asylum system in a stagnated form persisted until well into the 20th century, within living memory of some psychiatrists. John Romano has provided a reminiscence of his first experience with an asylum in the early 1930s (18):

> Most persons did not seem to change much except, we thought, for the worse when they became excited or assaultive. Few were discharged and even fewer ran away. The mortality rate was high, as many old persons died of lobar pneumonia, bronchopneumonia, cerebral vascular disease, and pyelonephritis. We saw no harshness or cruelty but were deeply impressed with the ambience of monotony, apathy, and anonymity and with the fact that so many patients seemed to have been abandoned. Each large ward was overcrowded and manifestly understaffed for all personnel. As there was no semblance of a treatment program, the setting was purely custodial.

The psychiatrists remained in control of these inpatient settings, perhaps because the neurobehaviorism of the time offered no useful alternative therapeutics for the psychotic, demented, or elderly mental patient. Ironically, the ambulatory carriage trade in psychiatry belonged more to the early neurologists and to their theories of neuronal fatigue and brain hyperaemia. Perhaps the neurological elegance of such theories, then as now, proved overwhelmingly attractive to middle class patients with stress-related syndromes. The growth success of the institutional psychiatric system, however, was creating pressures that would ultimately shift more psychiatric attention outward from the asylums into the more middle-class ambulatory environment. As the century moved into its second half, more and more psychiatric patients became consolidated in the state hospitals (28). The institutions became overcrowded, and as the county asylums decreased in number, the distinction between acute and chronic patients was lost. The belief that insanity was *curable,* which had been zealously held by the founders of the asylum movement, began to weaken. These environments were becoming less attractive to young psychiatrists for the establishment of their careers.

The neuropsychiatric conflicts in the United States occurred partly in response to powerful neuroscientific developments that transpired in Europe during the second half of the 19th century. From the German laboratories of Fritsch and Hitzig and from the clinical observations of Broca at Le Salpetrière came early localizationist theories of neuropsychiatric function (29). In England these localizationist ideas found powerful allies among the brilliant neurologists at the National Hospital for Nervous Disease in London. Here, in the years between 1870 and the turn of the century, researchers including John Hughlings Jackson (Fig. 1.4), David Ferrier, William Gowers, and Victor Horsley worked to compile evidence that sensory, motor, and other functions were controlled by discrete anatomic centers and systems within the brain (30).

Jackson was appointed assistant physician to the National Hospital in 1862 (29). He co-founded the first British neurology journal, *Brain,* and worked tirelessly to develop a theory by which neurological function was understood as generated by localizable, hierarchical brain structures developing in response to evolutionary pressures. These views led him and his group toward a very neurological, reductionistic view of mental function. As Jackson put it:

> Are we to believe that the hemisphere is built on a plan fundamentally different from that of the motor tract? What can an "idea," say of a ball, be, except a process representing certain impressions of surface and particular muscular adjustments? What is recollection, but a revivification of such processes which, in the past, have become part of the

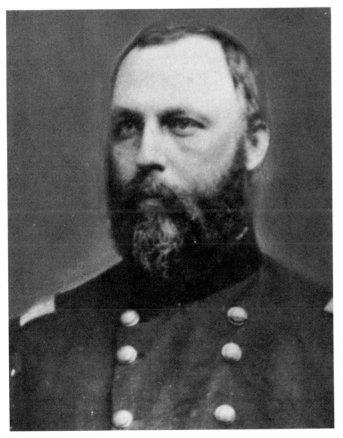

Figure 1.3. William Alexander Hammond.

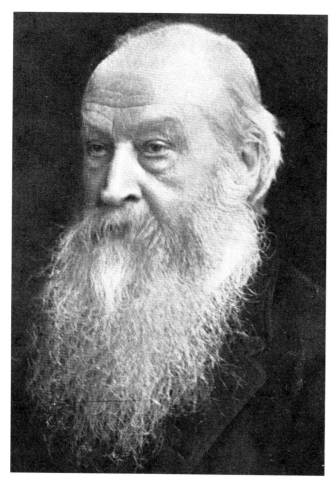

Figure 1.4. John Hughlings Jackson.

organism itself? What is delirium, except the disorderly revival of sensory-motor processes perceived in the past: What is a mistake in a word, but a wrong movement, a chorea? . . . Surely the conclusion is irresistible, that "mental" symptoms from disease of the hemisphere are fundamentally like hemiplegia, chorea, and convulsion. (29, p. 206)

Freud would soon have something quite different to say about what the significance of word mistakes might be.

English psychiatry at this time could scarcely compete with the neurolocalizationists' new theories. One can sense the impact of these ideas upon psychiatry in the writings of Henry Maudsley. Maudsley was at the peak of his career during these same years, between 1870 and 1900 (30). In 1870 he was elected president of the Medico-Psychological Association. By this time he had already served as joint editor of the *Journal of Mental Science,* physician at the West London Hospital, lecturer on insanity at St. Mary's Hospital, and professor of medical jurisprudence at University College, London. He had already written one psychiatric textbook, and in 1874 he wrote in another, capturing the feel of the neuroscientific optimism at that time as it might apply to psychiatry:

> It is not our business, it is not in our power, to explain psychologically the origin and nature of any of the depraved instincts manifested in typical cases of insanity . . . it is

sufficient to establish their existence as facts of observation, and to set forth the pathological conditions under which they are produced; they are facts of pathology, which should be observed and classified like other phenomena of disease . . . The explanation, when it comes, will come not from the mental, but from the physical side—from the study of the neurosis, not from the analysis of the psychosis. (31)

There were other clear effects of the new neuroscience upon psychiatric thought during these years. In Bucknell and Tuke's textbook, *Manual of Psychological Medicine,* it was urged that psychiatric nosologies should be reformulated to conform with neurological advances in cerebral localization (32).

One credible version of the origin of the term "neuropsychiatry" is that it emerged during these times from the political tension between the new neurological movement and established psychiatry during the First World War. In 1917 the National Committee for Mental Hygiene (NCMH) in the United States was organizing psychiatric units for base hospitals in France. According to Frankwood E. Williams, a former medical director of NCMH, the neurologists were reluctant to join such units because of the stigma of association with psychiatrists. The term "neuropsychiatry" offered a political solution (33):

> In renaming the unit neuro-psychiatric unit, it was neither Dr. Bailey's idea, I am sure, and not mine, nor Dr. Salmon's, when he was later consulted, nor anyone else's, so far as I know, that we were naming a specialty in medicine. The name grew not out of a medical need but a political one. The term had only political significance to those of us who used it first in the war work or in connection with the war work. I do not think that any of us felt that it represented anything that existed at the time in medicine, or had any idea that its use would continue after the war.

ERA OF PSYCHODYNAMICS (1900–1960)

> "Utter Rubbish"
> "Preposterous"
> "Nothing but Sex"
> "Filthy"
> "Vile"
>
> —Remarks of a senior British psychiatrist upon hearing his first lecture on Freudian Theory (34)

In March 1915, W.H.B. Stoddart delivered the Morison Lectures at the Royal College of Physicians of Edinburgh. These lectures were subsequently printed and circulated in a volume entitled *The New Psychiatry* (35). In these lectures he reviewed the principles of the emerging psychoanalytic theory, including notions of the unconscious mind, psychic determination, sexual drives, and symptom mechanisms such as displacement and condensation. He also reviewed the therapeutic techniques implied by this theory, including active listening and interpretation. He reviewed his personal experience with such techniques and indicated that they were especially effective in cases of hysteria, obsessive-compulsive disorders, and neurasthenia. He added the telling statement that, "it is the commonest complaint of neurotic patients that they are not understood, but in the psycho-analyst they have found a man who listens sympathetically." (35, p. 44)

In retrospect, it is difficult to exaggerate the revolutionary impact of psychoanalytic ideas upon the prevailing neurobehaviorism. Although the therapeutic use of passion in curing disease had appeared in the writings of certain ancient physicians (36), there was little of psychology left in late 19th century neuropsychiatry.

Psychoanalysis provided for the first time a coherent psychological theory by which mental illness could be understood. Moreover, such a theory provided a therapeutic course of action for the physician which was for the first time understandably connected with a theoretic context. The neurobehaviorism of the late 19th century could not match this. The psychodynamic therapies in Britain soon received additional support from their apparent effectiveness in a psychogenic wartime disorder, shell shock.

In the United States, psychoanalytic ideas gained an even more rapid and unqualified acceptance. There are probably several reasons for this. An important figure in the facilitation of this process was Adolf Meyer (Fig. 1.5) , who was unquestionably the dominant intellectual figure in American psychiatry during the early years of the 20th century. Meyer had come from Switzerland and had participated in neuropathological and neurological research. He emigrated to the U.S. and in the early 1890s was appointed pathologist at the Illinois Eastern Asylum in Kankekee. He began to work with psychiatric patients and to consider the importance of environmental influences upon mental illness (37). In 1895 he became pathologist to the Worcester Lunatic Asylum, and in 1913 he became head of the new Henry Phipps Clinic at Johns Hopkins University. From this position he would substantially influence a generation of leaders in psychiatric practice and theory.

When Meyer joined what is now the American Psychiatric Association in 1893, it changed its name from "The Association of Hospital Superintendents" to the "American Medico-Psychological Association," modeling its title upon the British association and presaging new developments that would lead beyond asylum psychiatry. Meyer himself was evolving his interests in the life history and psychology of the individual patient — issues that were not relevant to localizationist neurology. As he later put it, "My own preoccupation becomes the individual patient examined and discussed in staff meeting and considered as an experiment of nature, with special attention to the modifiable factors, and followed to an adjustment or, in case of death, to autopsy and beyond autopsy, with a study of reaction sets and the factors at work" (38). His developing psychobiological assessment of mental illness did not discount biological and genetic factors, but the emphasis upon life experience and dynamic psychological adjustments (the "ergasias" of meyerian theory) provided a background that made psychoanalytic ideas sound much less shocking than in Europe (39).

As mentioned previously, two other developmental themes in the United States facilitated the acceptance of a radically individualistic psychology. The neurologists, in their treatments of neurasthenia, had contributed to the strengthening of the physician-patient relationship through their emphasis upon reeducation. In addition, the social "success" of the state institutions in establishing hegemony over the delivery of psychiatric inpatient care contained within it an unanticipated vulnerability. Therapy in these environments began to appear to be futile (33). The proportion of chronic patients in these institutions grew steadily into the early years of the 20th century. The numbers of untreatable elderly patients also grew. Psychiatrists who preferred to see therapeutic results grew restive in such an environment. Psychodynamic psychiatry offered above all else an optimistic, therapeutic orientation toward patients, both theoretically and technically. Its ideas provided an attractive alternative to inpatient psychiatry with its focus on chronic conditions with poor prognoses.

Prior to World War II the new dynamic psychiatry grew slowly and did not produce a metamorphosis in clinical practice. Wartime experiences with stress casualties had a telling impact upon the next generation of psychiatrists, however. Many returned from their experiences convinced of the importance of experience over biology in the causation of mental illness. The National Mental Health Act of 1946 funded a major expansion of research and training in psychiatry, with an emphasis on dynamic and social models of illness.

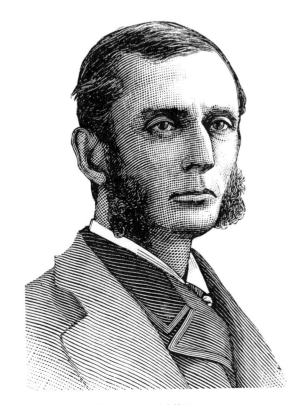

Figure 1.5. Adolf Meyer.

By 1960 more than half of those who chaired departments of psychiatry in the United States held membership in psychoanalytic societies (40).

DECLINE OF PSYCHOANALYSIS AND REEMERGENCE OF NEUROPSYCHIATRY

With a little effort, certain warnings for the future of psychoanalysis can be found in the very first issue of *The Psychoanalytic Review*. These were some of the titles that appeared in that 1913–1914 issue (41):

"The Wildsbuch Crucified Saint," by T. Schroeder
"The Matron of Ephesus, An Investigation of the Meaning of the Fable of the Faithless Widow," by O. Rank
"Remarks on a Case with Griselda Phantasies," by J.J. Putman
"The Grandfather Complex," by S. Ferenczi
"A Little Human Rooster," by S. Ferenczi
"Eroticism of the Posteriors," by J. Sadger

There is a certain absurdity in some of these titles, an impression perhaps destined to trigger a critique of the field. Skeptical impressions were held by many at the time, and one appears in this very issue of the *Review*, "The Pragmatic Advantage of Freudo-Analysis," by K. Dunlap (42). In the midst of such a seminal issue of the *Psychoanalytic Review*, Dunlap complains about the fantastical quality of some of the speculation going on around him:

> There is absolutely nothing in the universe which may not readily be made into a sexual symbol . . . all natural and artificial objects can be turned into Freudian symbols. We may explain by Freudian principles why trees have their roots in the ground; why we write with pens; why we put a quart of wine into a bottle instead of hanging it on a hook like a ham, and so on. (42)

Dunlap was also aware of the propensity of some psychoanalytic theorists to make ad hominem retorts. He adds at the end of his piece, "I may add that I have already been told that this paper is an interesting revelation of my own complexes."

Even in a simple chapter, there can be no simple story of the scientific and intellectual threads that gradually undermined the analytic hegemony of the first half of the 20th century. For one thing, Freud himself was alive until 1939, and he was also internationally known as a *neurologist* (43). Freud had first used the term "agnosia." He had written lucidly about aphasia and stroke in children, and he had described the juvenile form of ceroid lipofuscinosis. He retained certain neurological ideas about the substrate of psychodynamic forces, as described in his *Project for a Scientific Psychology*.

There were also models of behavioral disturbances extant during these years which were incontrovertibly *neurological* in their basis. For example, from 1917 to the early 1930s there was a prolonged epidemic of encephalitis lethargica (44). This (presumably) viral encephalitis left some patients with sequelae characterized by ocular palsies, parkinsonism, and hypersomnolence, but also with more psychiatric sequelae including hyperactivity, personality change, psychosis, and obsessive-compulsive behavior. Many observers could not help but see hints of a neuropsychiatry to come in such a disease.

Biological treatments for psychiatric disease were also being developed during these early decades of the 20th century. It would be a mistake to assume that "biological psychiatry" in the therapeutic sense was strictly a product of the 1960s. Von Jauregg began his fever investigations in 1887 and continued them, using various agents, until turning to benign tertian malaria in 1917 (45). In small, controlled trials of this agent in conjunction with arsphenamine, he demonstrated efficacy in some patients suffering from general paresis. For this first effective biological treatment of a psychiatric disorder, Von Jauregg was later to be awarded the Nobel Prize in medicine, the only psychiatrist to be so recognized.

Other biological therapies for psychiatric disease were developed during the second quarter of this century. Sakel applied insulin as a "shock treatment" for patients with schizophrenia in 1934–1935 (46). In 1934, Von Meduna was developing other modes of convulsive therapy for schizophrenics, first using injected camphor, and later an intravenous agent, pentamethylenetetrazole (47). In 1938, Cerletti and Bini induced convulsions electrically (48). Psychosurgery was also under development during these years. In 1935 the surgeon Almida Lima, under the direction of Moniz, injected alcohol into the white matter of the anterior aspects of the frontal lobes of a psychotic and depressed woman (49). Several modifications of such operations came into widespread use in the United States and the United Kingdom during the 1940s. By midcentury a sudden cascade of psychopharmacological discoveries began:

1949   Cade's report of the antimanic effect of lithium salts
1952   Discovery of chlorpromazine by Delay and Deniker
1954   Discovery of the antipsychotic properties of reserpine
1957   Discovery of the antidepressant properties of iproniazid and imipramine
1960   Introduction of chlordiazepoxide

The impact of these and subsequent psychopharmacologic discoveries upon the development of neuropsychiatry may not have been as fundamental as is often imagined, however. Stuart Yudofsky has argued that early psychopharmacology imparted a superficial simplicity to the neurological side of neuropsychiatry (50). Armed with these new tools, psychiatrists could prescribe a therapy without having to develop a "feel" for the complexity of the targeted neurobiological processes.

Behavioral neurology presented an extremely important contrast during this time of the reawakening of neuropsychiatry. The persistent, pioneering writings and clinical observations of Norman Geschwind (Fig. 1.6) and later of his pupils dramatically changed the way certain behavioral disturbances were viewed, imparting a radical and compelling neurological reductionism reminiscent of the previous century (51). When he described the disconnection syndromes in 1965, American clinicians began to think for the first time since the 19th century in terms of a neuroanatomy of behavior (52). Certain unexplained behavioral observations such as the apraxias could now be understood in terms of structural or functional cerebral hemispheric asymmetries. Other discoveries, (or "rediscoveries," as Geschwind himself would have called them) followed: the existence of structural brain asymmetries, the temporal lobe epilepsy syndromes, the aphasias, the dyslexias. They engendered a cornucopia of hypotheses for investigation by future investigators (53, 54). A neuroanatomy of behavior was being developed, and psychiatry was in danger of being left out. There was even a neurological model for unconscious intentions and conflicts in the behaviors of corpus callosum-sectioned patients studied by Sperry and his colleagues (55).

By midcentury a paradigm shift of great consequence was beginning in the way psychiatrists viewed their patients. They were beginning to see the major psychiatric syndromes as determined in part by enduring neurological systems of high variability and sensitivity. Discerning clinicians gradually came to see things differently. C.M. Anderson described this phenomenon within herself in 1952, as she described how her views of the psychogenetic aspects of schizophrenia had changed (56):

> There was a time when I would have given an opinion regarding the etiology of schizophrenia with a certain degree of assurance and inner conviction. I would have placed the responsibility at the door of the parent, who, no matter how much he or particularly she appeared to be giving love and acceptance to the child, actually was rejecting of him under the surface . . . This outstanding modification in my conceptual thinking concerning schizophrenia would be in seeing the development of these reactions as determined not by a rather ambiguous rejection-behavior on the part of the mother, or other significant person but as a failure in interpersonal relations brought about primarily by a very specific type of organic brain deficit in the child.

The second era of neuropsychiatry was beginning, and we are presently in the midst of it. The chapters that follow provide, we hope, a cross-sectional view of neuropsychiatric research and expert practice as it exists at the end of the 20th century.

References

1. Yudofsky SC, Hales RE. The reemergence of neuropsychiatry: definition and direction. J Neuropsychiatry Clin Neurosci 1989;1:1–6.
2. Yudofsky SC, Hales RE. When patients ask . . . what is neuropsychiatry? J Neuropsychiatry Clin Neurosci 1989;1:362–365.
3. Fogel BS, Schiffer RB. Defining neuropsychiatry: professional activities and opinions of psychiatrist-neurologists with dual certification. J Neuropsychiatry Clin Neurosci 1989;1:173–175.
4. Fogel BS. Localization in neuropsychiatry. J Neuropsychiatry Clin Neurosci 1990;2:361–362.
5. Caine ED, Joynt RJ. Neuropsychiatry—Again. Arch Neurol 1986;43: 325–327.
6. Lishman WA. What is neuropsychiatry? J Neurol Neurosurg Psychiatry 1992;55:983–985.
7. Clarke B. Mental disorder in earlier Britain. Cardiff: University of Wales Press, 1975.
8. Siegel RE. Galen: on psychology, psychopathology, and function and diseases of the nervous system. Basel: S. Karger, 1973.
9. Ellenberger HF. Psychiatry from ancient to modern times. In: Arieti S, ed. American handbook of psychiatry. 2nd ed. New York: Basic Books, 1974:3–27.
10. Brand J.L. Neurology and psychiatry. In: Numbers RL, ed. The education of American physicians, Berkeley: University of California Press, 1980:226–249.
11. Jimenez MA. Changing faces of madness. Hanover: University Press of New England, 1987.
12. Fischer DH. Growing old in America. New York: Oxford University Press, 1977.
13. Rosenberg CE. The therapeutic revolution: medicine, meaning, and social change in nineteenth century America. Perspect Biol Med 1977;20:485–506.
14. Allederidge P. Hospitals, madhouses and asylums: cycles in the care of the insane. Br J Psychiatry 1979;134:321–334.
15. Thomson DG. Presidential address, annual meeting of the Medico-Psychological Association of Great Britain and Ireland. Br Med J 1914;Sept:474–475.
16. Bynum WF. The nervous patient in eighteenth and nineteenth century Britain: the psychiatric origin of British neurology. In: Bynum WF, Porter R, Sheperd M, eds. The anatomy of madness: essays in the history of psychiatry, Vol I, People and Ideas, Tavistock Publications, 1985:89–102.

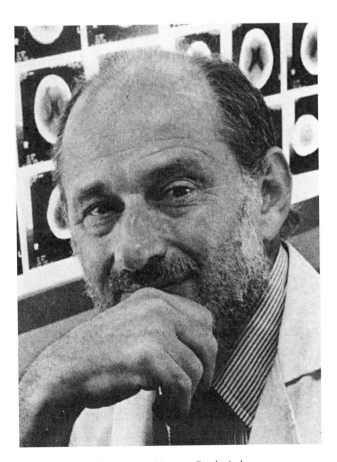

Figure 1.6. Norman Geschwind.

17. Quen JH. Early nineteenth-century observations on the insane in the Boston Almshouse. J History Med Allied Sci 1968;23:80–85.
18. Romano JR. Boundaries. Bull Rochester Psychiatr Cent Staff 1991; 9:2-3.
19. Brand JL. Neurology and psychiatry. In: Numbers RL, ed. The education of American physicians: historical essays. Berkeley: University of California Press, 1980:226–249.
20. Lebensohn ZM. American psychiatry – retrospect and prospect. Med Ann Dist Columbia 1962;31:379–392.
21. Dowbiggin I. Degeneration and hereditarianism in French mental medicine 1840–90: psychiatric theory as ideological adaptation. In: Bynum WF, Porter R, Shepherd M, eds. The anatomy of madness, essays in the history of psychiatry. Volume III. The Asylum and its Psychiatry. London: Routledge, 1988:188–232.
22. Russell NDeJ. A history of American neurology. New York: Raven Press, 1982.
23. Gosling FG. Neurasthenia in Pennsylvania: a persepective on the origins of American psychotherapy, 1870–1910. J History Med Allied Sci 1985;40:188–206.
24. Bluestein BE. A hollow square of psychological science: American neurologists and psychiatrists in conflict. In: Scull A, ed. Madhouses, mad-doctors, and madmen. The social history of psychiatry in the Victorian era. Philadelphia: University of Pennsylvania Press, 1981: 241–270.
25. Unsigned review of John P. Gray. The dependence of insanity on physical disease, Utica, NY: Utica Asylum Press, 1871, in J Psychol Med 1871;5:576.
26. Spitzka EC. Reform in the scientific study of psychiatry. J Nerv Ment Dis 1878;5:200–229.
27. Mitchell SW. Address before the fiftieth annual meeting of the American Medico-Psychological Association. J Nerv Ment Dis 1894; 21:413–437.
28. Dowbiggin I. "Midnight clerks and daily drudges": hospital psychiatry in New York State, 1870–1905. J History Med Allied Sci 1992;47: 130–152.
29. Young RM. Mind, brain, and adaptation in the nineteenth century. Oxford: Clarendon Press, 1970.
30. Turner T. Henry Maudsley – psychiatrist, philosopher and entrepreneur. Psychol Med 1988;18:551–574.
31. Maudsley H. Responsibility in mental disease. 2nd ed. London: Kegan Paul, 1874:154.
32. Clark MJ. The rejection of psychological approaches to mental disorder in late nineteenth century British psychiatry. In: Scull A, ed. Madhouses, mad-doctors, and madmen. The social history of psychiatry in the Victorian era. Philadelphia: University of Pennsylvania Press, 1981:271–312.
33. Grob GN. The forging of mental health policy in America: World War II to new frontier. J History Med Allied Sci 1987;42:410-446.
34. Pines M. The development of the psychodynamic movement. In: Berrios GE, Freeman H, eds. 150 years of British psychiatry, 1841–1991. Royal College of Psychiatrists, 1991:206–231.
35. Stoddart WHB. The new psychiatry. London: Bailliere, Tindall and Cox, 1915.
36. Jackson SW. The use of the passions in psychological healing. J History Med Allied Sci 1990;45:150–175.
37. Gelder M. Adolph Meyer and his influence on British psychiatry. In: Berrios GE, Freeman H, eds. 150 years of British psychiatry 1841–1991. London: Royal College of Psychiatrists, 1991:419–435.
38. Meyer A. Presidential address: thirty five years of psychiatry in the United States and our present outlook. Am J Psychiatry 1928;8:1–31.
39. Lidz T. Adolf Meyer and the development of American psychiatry. Am J Psychiatry 1966;123:320–331.
40. Eisenberg L. Mindlessness and brainlessness in psychiatry. Br J Psychiatry 1986;148:497–508.
41. 1913–1914;1:I. White WA, Jelliffe SE, eds. Psychoanal Rev. White WA, Jelliffe SE (eds). Psychoanalytic Review 1913-1914; Volume I, Number 1.
42. Dunlap K. The pragmatic advantage of Freudo-analysis. Psychoanal Rev 1913;1:149–152.
43. Pribram KH. The neuropsychology of Sigmund Freud. In: Experimental foundations of clinical psychology. Bachrach AJ, ed. New York: Basic Books, 1962:442–468.
44. Ward CD. Encephalitis lethargica and the development of neuropsychiatry. Psychiatr Clin North Am 1986;9:215–224.
45. Kiloh LG, Smith JS, Johnson GF. Physical treatments in psychiatry. Melbourne: Blackwell Scientific Publications, 1988.
46. Sakel M. Zur methodik der hypoglykamiere – handlung von psychosen. Wien Klin Wochenschr 1936;49:1278–1282.
47. Von Meduna L. General discussion of the cardiazol therapy. Am J Psychiatry 1938;94(May suppl):40–50.
48. Cerletti U, Bini L. L'elletroshock. Arch Gen Neurol Psychiatr Psicoanal 1938;19:266–268.
49. Moniz E. Tentatives operatoires ans le traitement de certaines psychoses. Paris: Masson, 1936.
50. Yudofsky S. Psychoanalysis, psychopharmacology, and the influence of neuropsychiatry. J Neuropsychiatry Clin Neurosci 1991;3:1–5.
51. M-Marsel Mesulam. Principles of behavioral neurology. Philadelphia: F.A. Davis, 1985.
52. Geschwind N, Kaplan E. A human cerebral disconnexion syndrome: a preliminary report. Neurology 1962:12:675–685.
53. Geschwind N, Galaburda AM. Cerebral lateralization, biological mechanisms, associations, and pathology: I. A hypothesis and a program for research. Arch Neurol 1985;42:428–459.
54. Geschwind N. Cerebral lateralization, biological mechanisms, associations, and pathology: II. A hypothesis and a program for research. Arch Neurol 1985;42:521–552.
55. Elliott FA. Historical perspective on neurobehavior. Psychiatr Clin North Am 1986;9:225–239.
56. Anderson CM. Organic factors predisposing to schizophrenia. Nerv Child 1952;10:36–42.

2

NEUROPSYCHIATRIC EXAMINATION

Jonathan Mueller and Barry S. Fogel

The neuropsychiatric examination is a specialized evaluation that comprises a complete psychiatric evaluation, a neurological history and examination, detailed assessment of cognitive mental status, and the integration of findings to form inferences about altered brain function and its relationship to changes in mood, thinking, or behavior. Its points of departure are the adult psychiatric evaluation, as described in the American Psychiatric Association Practice Guideline for the Psychiatric Evaluation of Adults (1), the neurological examination, as described comprehensively by DeJong (2), and the neurobehavioral mental status examination, as described by Strub and Black (3), Trzepacz and Baker (4), and Weintraub and Mesulam (5). This chapter surveys the components of the neuropsychiatric examination, emphasizing parts that are virtually always done, and mentioning points that regularly have been of clinical value to the authors. A comprehensive discussion of examination techniques is beyond the scope of this chapter; readers unfamiliar with the references cited are encouraged to consult them.

DISTINCTIVE FEATURES OF THE NEUROPSYCHIATRIC APPROACH

Neuropsychiatric examination, like conventional psychiatric evaluation, aims to identify both subjective and objective dimensions of patients' mental disorders. The assessment is sensitive to sociocultural context and to issues of the patient's psychological development (1). Likewise, the examination is designed to identify and localize regional or systemic deficits in brain function. The following points of emphasis and difference are characteristic of the neuropsychiatric examination, may distinguish it from conventional psychiatric and neurological assessments:

1. Strong consideration is given to the possibility that the history given by the patient may be affected by brain dysfunction. Independent confirmation or amplification of historical details using collateral sources of information is considered in every case.

2. When mental symptoms are described, precise description of the core psychopathology takes precedence over organization of the patient's symptoms into standard psychiatric syndromes and disorders. The possibility is kept in mind that the patient may have a recognized psychiatric syndrome whose symptomatic expression is modified by brain dysfunction, or a recognized neurobehavioral syndrome whose symptomatic expression is modified by psychological defense mechanisms or by sociocultural influences (6).

3. Specific neurobehavioral syndromes are considered:
   a. frontal system dysfunction, including apathetic, disinhibited, and dysexecutive syndromes;
   b. temporal lobe dysfunction, including general and specific amnestic disorders, and the personality disturbances associated with temporolimbic epilepsy;
   c. basal ganglia dysfunction, especially the combination of movement disorder with subcortical-type cognitive impairment;
   d. dementia syndromes;
   e. various forms of aphasia, alexia, agraphia, agnosia, apraxia, and amusia;
   f. disturbances of paralinguistic communication; and
   g. denial, anosognosia, and impaired insight.

In addition to identifying these syndromes when they are present in their entirety, partial expressions of the neurobehavioral syndromes are considered as dimensions of illness. Examples include the dimension of impaired insight in patients with dementia (7) or schizophrenia (8), and the dimension of impaired executive function in patients recovering from traumatic brain injury (TBI) (9, 10).

4. Neurological and mental status examination include specialized or intensive components when the history identifies a potential area of brain dysfunction not routinely tested in detail. For example, a patient whose history suggested a visual agnosia would be asked to describe complex scenes, would be given a formal test of naming to confrontation, and would receive detailed visual field mapping using a small test object. Or, a patient suspected of impaired paralinguistic communication would have formal tests of receptive and expressive prosody, and would be asked to describe what emotions were represented on the faces of people in drawings or photographs.

5. Psychiatric history and mental status data are regarded as potentially localizing neurological findings, to be com-

bined with traditional neurological data to support inferences about regional or systemic brain dysfunction. Thus, a late-onset major depressive syndrome would be combined with observations of impaired executive cognitive function, hyperactive reflexes, and impaired fine motor coordination to support a hypothesis of vascular dementia due to diffuse subcortical ischemia or multiple subcortical strokes. Or, a disinhibited state would be combined with an observation of hyposmia to support the hypothesis of an orbitofrontal lesion. The importance of performing the neurological examination with the patient's history in mind is underscored by a recent study of interobserver variation in the evaluation of neurological signs in 202 consecutive neurological inpatients (11). Without knowledge of the case history, two senior neurologists attained κ coefficients of only 0.40–0.67 on such basic neurological signs as anisocoria, jerky eye movements, the finger-to-nose test, the knee jerk, and the extensor plantar reflex. Reliabilities were substantially better when examiners knew the patient's history.

6. The synthesis of observations is inclusive, and usually does not attempt traditional "organic versus functional" distinctions. Based on the history and examination, hypotheses are developed regarding how regional brain dysfunction, psychological development, genetics, sociocultural factors, current environment, and individual psychology combine to produce the presenting mental status and behavior (12, 13). Proximate causes of behavioral changes are identified, as are potentially remediable factors that contribute to the problem. Not infrequently, what causes a particular problem is not what can be most readily changed. For example, a frontal lobe injury may cause problematic behavior by making an individual much more responsive to the immediate environment. An environmental change may be the most feasible way to correct the behavior (14).

7. The process of conducting the examination frequently is circular and iterative, rather than linear. If, for example, the examiner develops a suspicion of impaired memory or cognition while eliciting the patient's history, formal testing to estimate the severity of the impairment may follow rapidly, to prevent the examiner from spending excessive time eliciting a history that may be grossly inaccurate. Or, if a patient unexpectedly fails several "frontal lobe" tests during formal cognitive examination, the examiner may return to the history and inquire further about incidents of impulsiveness or poor planning, past TBI, and subtle academic difficulties during school or college.

With this background in mind, we present a survey of the mental status examination, the interpretation of the mental status examination, and the neurological examination of the neuropsychiatric patient.

MENTAL STATUS EXAMINATION

PATIENT PRESENTATION

Level of Consciousness

In the state of alert wakefulness, patients respond promptly and appropriately to auditory, visual, and tactile stimulation. When a patient's level of alertness or capacity for interaction fluctuates, the examiner should describe the quality of interactions as precisely as possible. The degree of arousal or level of consciousness is evaluated by examining the patient's spontaneous behavior and responsiveness to environmental stimuli. When noxious stimulation fails to elicit either verbal or motor responses, the patient is said to be "comatose."

Patients who respond only to vigorous and repeated stimulation are described as "stuporous." Whenever a disturbance in the level of consciousness exists, it must be realized that associated attentional problems will color the patient's response to much of the mental status examination. Responses may be superficial and random. In this situation, a patient's cognitive performance will reflect less than his or her full abilities, and, therefore, will need to be reassessed when the patient is more alert.

Depth of stupor or coma, especially in the traumatic context, can be quantified with the Glasgow Coma Scale (GCS). Developed by Jennett and Bond (14a), the GCS quantifies reactivity to verbal and physical stimulation in terms of a 15-point scale, subdivided into eye-opening (score: 1–4), motor responses (score: 1–6), and verbal responses (score: 1–5). On this scale, a score of 3 represents deep coma, while 15 represents alert wakefulness.

The Glasgow Coma Scale on presentation is unfortunately of little value in quantitating the severity of mild or very mild brain injury. Such patients score 13–15 on presentation, and the vast majority of those who are conscious will score 15. For these patients, the duration of posttraumatic amnesia (PTA) is the most useful quantitative measure of injury severity. PTA begins with the loss of consciousness and ends when a full, coherent stream of consciousness has been regained. If memory testing on a conscious patient with recent brain trauma shows markedly impaired attention and short-term memory, the patient is still within the period of PTA.

Appearance

The examiner notes the patient's height, body type, posture, hygiene, clothing, and gross evidence of health or illness. Does the patient appear healthy, or pale, ashen, or gray? Are there stigmata of alcoholism, such as palmar erythema, facial flushing, spider angiomata, or jaundice? Does the appearance suggest an endocrine disorder such as Cushing's disease, or the use of exogenous steroids (moon facies and "buffalo hump")? Facial asymmetry, pupillary asymmetry, or discrepancy in the size of a patient's hands may be observed before the formal neurological examination begins.

Attitude

Patients adopt a variety of attitudes toward physicians, ranging from arrogant evasiveness on the one hand to deferential cooperation on the other. Some patients are forthcoming with information, while others need to be urged repeatedly to provide information. The quality of the interaction between the physician and the patient determines to a large extent the quality and quantity of information that the patient will provide. It may also provide evidence of personality traits that can modify the symptomatic presentation of brain dysfunction.

Behavior

Patients move in qualitatively different ways, depending on whether pathology lies at the level of the basal ganglia, cerebellum, pyramidal system, or lower motor neuron. Dysfunction of the basal ganglia is suggested by movements that are rapid, jerky, tic-like, or choreiform (i.e., hyperkinesis), or impoverished in frequency and amplitude (i.e., hypokinesis), "Psychomotor retardation," a phrase that is often used to describe the sluggish thought and motor activity of patients with depressive syndromes, is not specific for mood disorders. Patients with parkinsonism, stuporous conditions, and drug toxicity may also move and think slowly. When patients make unusual or sudden movements, it is helpful to note the context in which they occur and, if possible, identify the provoking stimuli—either physical or psychological. Anxiety may manifest as repetitive tapping of the feet, turning of the head, or any other number of stereotyped movements, but it may be difficult to distinguish anxiety-induced restlessness from drug-induced akathisia. Patients taking dopamine-blocking drugs can show any combination of parkinsonian phenomena and dyskinesia or dystonia (15). Adventitious movements of the mouth, tongue, face, eyes, or neck, suggesting dystonia or dyskinesia, often are best observed when the patient is walking or carrying out intentional movements.

In patients who are mute, it is helpful to determine whether they mirror the movements of the examiner ("echopraxia"). "Waxy flexibility" or catalepsy refers to a condition in which a patient's limbs remain in unnatural postures once the examiner places them there. Clinicians should also note whether patients who are mute respond in any fashion to discussion of highly charged personal items, such as the physical or mental condition of friends and family. It is also important to decide whether an "unresponsive" patient is actually better described as negativistic (e.g., averts gaze consistently from the examiner or forcibly resists passive movement of the limbs). Such observations will help the examiner distinguish among causes of catatonia.

When approaching any form of repetitive movement, the examiner should attempt to determine, whether the movement is of neocortical origin (a habit or perseverative goal-directed behavior), limbic origin (a compulsion or stereotypy), or basal ganglia origin (a tic, tremor, or dyskinesia). Purposefulness suggests movements of cortical origin; association with a specific emotional state implies involvement of limbic cortex. Patients may elaborate tics into apparently purposeful movements to disguise their nature. The patient may be conscious of doing so, but such awareness is variable, and usually absent when the movement disorder is associated with dementia.

Speech

Spontaneous speech can be characterized in terms of its flow, volume, pressure, rhythm and intonation. Prosody, the emotional coloring of speech, is a manifestation of affect. Alteration in prosody can reflect either a change in affect or dysfunction of mechanisms of affective expression. Thus, loss of emotional coloring in speech can occur in a range of disorders, including major depression, degenerative illnesses affecting the basal ganglia, drug-induced akinesia, damage to the right frontal lobe, or Broca-type aphasia secondary to left frontal damage (16). Both the patient and caregivers should be asked whether any change has been noted in the patient's style of speaking.

Disturbances of speech as a motor act, as distinguished from language disorders, are called "dysarthrias" (2). Dysarthria can be spastic, flaccid, ataxic, hypokinetic, or hyperkinetic. In practice, however, distinctions among types of dysarthria are somewhat difficult to make because patients often suffer from mixed dysarthrias that are characterized, for instance, by both spastic and ataxic features.

Stammering and stuttering are types of speech disorders that can be either developmental or acquired. The developmental forms do not imply gross brain pathology.

Affect

This term refers to the outward display of emotion, which may or may not correspond to internal or felt emotion (mood). Significant discrepancies between inner emotion and outward affect occur frequently in patients with brain diseases affecting the frontal lobes or their connections. Affective states can be altered by brain diseases involving the right hemisphere. Pseudobulbar palsy refers to a state in which upper motor neuron regulation of the brainstem nuclei subserving emotional expression is disrupted. Such patients may complain of excessive and sometimes even explosive affective display in response to trivial emotional stimuli. They may describe "emotional incontinence," either sobbing uncontrollably when feeling only somewhat sad, or laughing in a grotesquely loud and disinhibited fashion in response to something that may strike them as only mildly amusing. Occasionally such patients become tearful when finding something humorous. At other times they may complain of laughing when they experience sadness.

Affect and thought content (as expressed verbally) normally are congruous; marked discrepancy suggests mental illness, or anatomical or physiological disconnection of limbic areas associated with emotion from the neocortical and brainstem areas associated with emotional expression. Patients with schizophrenia or with bilateral frontal lobe damage may smile strangely when discussing suicide, or discuss feelings of extreme agitation with little or no facial expression. In addition to the appropriateness of affect to content of thought, the examiner pays particular attention to the range, intensity, and lability of affect. Emotion is reflected not just in facial expression but also in shifts of posture, gesticulation, flow, and "coloring" of speech.

COGNITIVE STATUS

Orientation

This is assessed with reference to name, place, and time. Orientation to personal identity usually is preserved even in the face of extensive gross brain disease. Important exceptions include postictal and postconcussive confusional states, and aphasic disorders such as pure word deafness that make orientation to name impossible to verify. The most common reason for a nonaphasic patient to show disorientation to name or personal identity is a dissociative disorder. Disorientation to person also can be malingered. Orientation to location may be assessed through inquiry as to the city, type of building, address, name of building (if any) and further with reference to the floor and/or office number. Loss of orientation to location may be seen in a variety of contexts, most commonly in confusional states, dementing processes, and amnestic disorders—all of which prevent patients from updating themselves on their current location (i.e., remembering transitions from one place to another). Patients with visual-perceptual problems may also be unable to utilize visual cues to orient themselves. Patients with aphasia may be unable to state where they are, yet indicate correct orientation to place through their behavior. Patients with the syndrome of dominant angular gyrus damage characteristically show this pattern.

Reduplicative paramnesia refers to a condition in which patients mistakenly identify one object, person or place for another. Such individuals may fail to modify their false beliefs even in light of overwhelming evidence to the contrary. For instance, a patient at the San Francisco VA Hospital insisted that he was at the Fresno VA Hospital, even after being shown the Pacific Ocean from his hospital window. He insisted that the Fresno VA, which is located inland, had been moved to the coast. Reduplicative paramnesia implies bilateral brain dysfunction.

Orientation to time is assessed with reference to year, month, date, day, and time of day. When patients give an inaccurate response, it is important to record their precise response rather than simply note that their answer was incorrect. Grossly inaccurate dates in patients who are not acutely confused suggest a long-standing amnestic disorder. Among confused patients, greater inaccuracy in stating the date and time is associated with more severe confusion. As confusional states resolve, answers to questions about orientation become increasingly close to the present date and time.

Patients who fail to correctly state the present location or date sometimes do so because they have had no opportunity to orient themselves. For example, a patient who was transported from one hospital to another while comatose might not have had the chance to ask someone where he or she was, or might assume he or she was in the place where he or she was last conscious. To fully assess orientation in such patients, they should be told the correct location, date, and time. After several minutes have passed, they should be asked again if they now know their present place and time.

Attention

Attention span is most typically assessed by asking the patient to repeat a string of digits given at a rate of one per second. In presenting a digit string, it is important to avoid any grouping of the numbers that makes the task easier. Most healthy individuals can repeat a six-digit string. It is important to test the upper and lower limits of a patient's attention span. Patients who are unable to repeat five or six digits should be presented a series of shorter digit strings (beginning with two or three digits and increasing in length) to determine how long a sequence the individual can retain. On the other hand, patients who easily repeat a six-digit sequence should be requested to repeat progressively longer sequences until they are unable to do so accurately.

Any impairment in attention as measured by digit span has very important consequences for the interpretation of the rest of the cognitive assessment. If patients are not able to repeat five or six digits, they are likely to have difficulty with a wide range of mental status tests because of inability to attend to them sufficiently. This will likely be reflected in "global" impairment on cognitive assessment. Disorders of attention are the hallmark of confusional states (either quiet confusional states or agitated confusional states—sometimes referred to as delirium). Confusional states most commonly occur in the context of toxic, infectious, and metabolic encephalopathy and usually respond to treatment of the causative medical condition. Patients with preexisting dementia syndromes are at particular risk for the development of superimposed confusional states (sometimes called "beclouded dementia") in response to a wide variety of problems such as drug toxicity, pulmonary and urinary tract infections, anesthesia, and sleep deprivation.

A second important measure of attention is the patient's ability to register the list of words presented for the standard verbal memory task. After the patient has been given a list of words, he or she is asked to repeat them immediately. This allows the examiner to establish that the patient has in fact registered the words. If the patient does not register all the words, additional presentations are made, and the number of trials required to register the list of words is recorded. Registration is impaired by attentional problems. Hearing loss and aphasia must be excluded before attributing poor registration of the items to inattention. Auditory perception problems are sometimes detected by the examiner when the patient attempts to repeat the words given for the memory task and distorts one or more of the words.

Although digit span is a convenient quantitative bedside test of attention, the ability to repeat digit sequences does not imply that a patient possesses the capacity to appropriately sustain, direct, and shift attention over time, when faced with competing stimuli and one or more tasks to be completed. Tests that provide a broader view of attentional capacities include (*a*) the Digit-Symbol Test; (*b*) cancellation tasks (a page covered with letters or digits is presented to the patient, who is asked to strike out a particular digit or letter whenever it occurs); (*c*) trails, or the Trail-Making Test

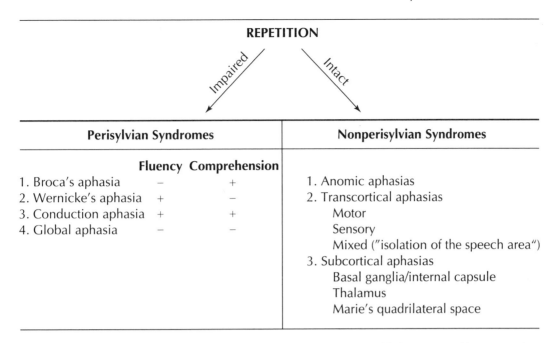

Figure 2.1. Classification of aphasic syndromes. (From Mueller J, Flynn FG, Fields HL. Brain and behavior. In: Goldman HH (ed) Review of general psychiatry, 4th ed. E Norwalk, CT: Appleton & Lange, 1995:58)

(the patient's task is to convert in sequence a set of numbers, or of letters alternating with numbers); *(d)* the Stroop Test, in which the patient begins by naming several different colors and then is asked to identify the color of the ink in which each of a list of color names is printed and then to name the color of the ink in which the names of different colors are printed, where the names do not correspond to the color of the ink; and *(e)* Corsi's Block Tapping Test, in which a series of numbered blocks arrayed on a board, are tapped in a sequence which the patient is asked to imitate.

These supplementary tests of attention overlap with frontal lobe tests, because they attempt to characterize the manner in which patients shift attention among a variety of stimuli and modify their strategies in response to changing criteria or environmental demands. Basic attention and concentration, as tested by digit span, represent a kind of elementary skill or ability, the intactness of which is a precondition for the meaningful testing of many specific cognitive areas. The capacity for sustained and distributed attention, as tested by the procedures listed above, is a complex capacity closely related to an individual's thought process and capacity for abstraction and problem solving.

Language

Any disruption in the patient's ability to speak fluently, to comprehend, to repeat, or to name, is likely to have significant consequences in terms of cognitive performance and interpersonal relations. Careful delineation of any linguistic deficits is therefore crucial. Distinguishing primary language disturbance from memory disturbance is particularly important. The etiologies of amnestic and aphasic disturbances are different, as are treatment approaches.

In contrast to disorders of speech such as mutism and dysarthria, where writing is preserved, disorders of language represent central problems in the reception and manipulation of linguistic symbols. Disturbances of writing usually parallel those of spoken language in aphasic conditions. Figure 2.1 enables clinicians to rapidly classify an aphasia by assessing fluency, comprehension, and repetition. More detailed consideration of language disorders in neuropsychiatry is provided in Chapter 31 of this book.

Adequate assessment of language entails consideration of: *(a)* fluency, *(b)* comprehension, *(c)* repetition, *(d)* naming, *(e)* reading, *(f)* writing, and *(g)* spelling.

Fluency (Spontaneous Speech)

This refers to the rate, rhythm, and degree of effort in producing spontaneous speech. An alternative way to assess fluency is to request that a patient describe a physical scene (such as the Cookie Theft Picture from the Boston Diagnostic Aphasia Examination) (17). The advantage of using a visual stimulus is that the examiner quickly becomes familiar with the range of possible responses and learns to note hesitations or circumlocutions. In describing spontaneous speech, the examiner records word-finding pauses and paraphasic errors (substitution of inappropriate syllables or entire words). Although test batteries such as the Boston Diagnostic Aphasia Examination provide quantitative scoring of the degree of fluency, most neurologists and psychiatrists describe speech in all-or-nothing terms as either fluent or nonfluent."

Comprehension

Problems with hearing and comprehension may initially be unappreciated in patients with gross cognitive deficits.

Such unappreciated disturbances in comprehension may lead caregivers to conclude that a patient is uncooperative, negativistic, or inattentive, or that the patient's memory is poor. Even subtle comprehension disturbance can significantly constrain the patient's capacity to interact with other people. Because the capacity to repeat can be preserved in some patients with impaired comprehension, comprehension should be tested separately from repetition. In fact, any tendency on the part of the patient to consistently echo or repeat what others say should raise the question of a comprehension disturbance. Such individuals may be thought of as attempting to "run the tape by" one more time in order to extract as much information as possible.

A common method of assessing comprehension is to have the patient perform one-, two-, or three-step tasks. Individuals who correctly perform three-step tasks may be considered to have intact comprehension. Patients who are able to correctly perform one- or two-step, but not three-step tasks, are likely to have difficulties in interactions with hospital staff and others. Careful documentation of such inability to comprehend multi-step instructions will, therefore, prove to be of great value to hospital staff and family members. Simplifying verbal interactions with such patients may prevent a range of misunderstandings and frustrations.

With patients who have impaired upper extremity function or who may have apraxia, other means of assessing comprehension are needed. One approach is to offer a series of questions that can be answered with yes-or-no responses. If the latter approach is utilized, a series of questions of increasing difficulty must be asked, because a patient who does not understand a question still has a 50% chance of correctly answering a yes-or-no question. Correct answers to five consecutive yes-or-no questions could occur by chance alone in only 3% of cases.

Repetition

Repetition is impaired by all four of the major aphasic disorders that result from damage to the perisylvian speech areas of the dominant hemisphere: Broca's, Wernicke's, conduction aphasia, and global aphasia (Fig. 2.1). Thus, any patient who can accurately repeat phrases of significant length either has no language disorder or has one of the nonperisylvian aphasias: anomic, subcortical, or transcortical (Fig. 2.1). As mentioned previously, repetition can be dissociated from comprehension, and patients who are able to repeat well are often mistakenly assumed to comprehend. Repetition can be assessed for single words, short phrases, and lengthy sentences. Patients with receptive aphasias, particularly those with damage to Wernicke's area, often make paraphasic errors when attempting to repeat longer phrases. Paraphasias may involve substitution of wholly inappropriate words (verbal paraphasias), or of individual syllables (phonemic or literal paraphasias). Demonstration of paraphasic errors on a repetition task provides convincing evidence that a patient does, in fact, suffer from a language

disturbance. One example of a series of phrases and sentences of increasing difficulty to repeat is provided below:

A. Out the window.
B. He swam across the lake.
C. The winding road went to the village.
D. He left the latch open.
E. The honeycomb drew a swarm of bees.
F. No ifs, ands, or buts.
G. The beginning movement revealed the composer's intention.

Naming

The vast majority of patients with aphasic disorders have word-finding difficulty (dysnomia). Therefore, patients with bizarre speech can be initially screened for aphasia by being asked to name objects. A simple object to use for this task is a pen, whose point, cap, and clip the patient is asked to name. If the pen and its parts are successfully named, it can be inferred that the patient does not suffer from an aphasic disorder of sufficient severity to account for bizarre or incoherent spontaneous speech. (However, milder yet significant anemia is not ruled out.)

Although aphasia typically includes word-finding difficulty, word-finding difficulty can be caused by other conditions. Word-finding difficulties may occur in metabolic encephalopathies, or as a side effect of psychotropic medication. Physical exhaustion, sleep deprivation, extreme anxiety, and depression may also occasionally produce word-finding difficulties. Thus, whenever dysnomia is detected, it is important to establish whether there also exists any other disturbance of language — namely, problems with fluency, comprehension, repetition, reading, writing, or spelling. Naming performance can be tested using booklets of line drawings of common objects, or using actual objects at hand at the bedside. These latter items might include a watch, the band, the stem, the crystal, the face, and the hands.

Reading

All individuals with aphasic disorders are very likely to have reading problems. Clinicians who wish to familiarize themselves with a variety of reading disturbances are referred to the monograph by Benson, *Aphasia, Alexia and Agraphia* (18) and to standard neuropsychological texts (17, 19). For the purposes of this chapter, it suffices to indicate that damage to the left-inferior parietal lobule produces a syndrome known as alexia with agraphia, whereas damage to the left-occipital cortex produces a syndrome of pure alexia (alexia without agraphia).

Patients may be asked to read individual words, sentences, or paragraphs of varying difficulty. It is important to realize that reading aloud is different from reading for comprehension. The fact that a patient can read a passage aloud does not indicate that he or she is able to understand it, much less remember it. Patients who complain of problems with reading more often have problems with recall of written material rather than with the actual reading of the individual words.

Writing

All individuals with true aphasic disorders will exhibit disturbances in both speech and writing. Because it may be difficult for examiners to transcribe the speech of aphasic individuals, it is helpful to obtain samples of the patient's writing. Sentences, either written to dictation or following a theme suggested by the examiner, are requested. The patient's signature or brief conventional phrases such as "I'm fine," are of little value. Writing samples are invaluable for documenting paraphasic errors. They also serve as a kind of snapshot of the aphasic disturbance. Serial writing samples can be used to document the resolution of aphasia following a transient ischemic attack, migraine headache, or postictal confusional period.

Spelling

Orthographic errors are common following insults that produce aphasia. It is important, however, for the clinician to establish that the patient's current difficulties with spelling represent change from an established baseline. Patients should be asked about a personal or family history of dyslexia, as well as any remedial classes or special instruction they received for difficulties with writing during their school years.

Memory

Neuropsychiatrists should be familiar with a broad spectrum of psychogenic as well as neurogenic memory disorders (see Chapter 17). Nonmalingered psychogenic amnesia, a dissociative phenomenon, occurs when an individual is faced with overwhelming feelings: the memory of the provoking situation or thought is repressed from conscious awareness. Patients with nonmalingered psychogenic amnesia may recall memories in response to suggestion, in surroundings that they consider safe, under hypnosis, or in response to sodium amytal. Still other individuals experience return of repressed memories in the form of intrusive images or recurring nightmares. A hallmark of psychogenic amnesia is that the material forgotten relates to personal events, but typically spares historical, public, and nonpersonal information from the same period. Clinicians should also realize that patients in intense states of psychotic agitation, whether due to depression, mania or schizophrenia, may fail to lay down a consecutive series of memories regarding events in their environment, or their interactions with others. Circumscribed gaps in autobiographical memory in such individuals may reflect a failure of registration rather than a true problem with memory.

In patients whose memory disturbance is secondary to gross brain dysfunction, a distinction is made between isolated memory disturbance (pure amnestic syndrome) and a more widespread disturbance of intellectual function that includes impaired memory (either a dementia syndrome or a confusional state). Among the causes of pure memory disorders are hypoxic events and thiamine deficiency secondary to chronic alcohol consumption and malnutrition.

Short-term verbal memory is typically assessed at the bedside by asking a patient to recall a list of four words. The examiner must establish that the patient actually registers the words initially; otherwise it is impossible to distinguish a memory disturbance from an attentional problem. It is helpful for the examiner to employ a graded approach in the assessment of memory. If, for instance, 3 points are given for each word recalled spontaneously, 2 points for a word recalled after a category prompt, and 1 point if the word is chosen from a list of three or four alternatives, then one has a 12-point range. This is superior to simply recording the number of words recalled, since it offers qualitative data on any memory problem. Its greater detail also enables the clinician to form a clearer opinion of the progression (or remission) of any memory disturbance when the patient is reexamined on another occasion.

Assessment of memory is a crucial element in all neuropsychological evaluations; thus, it is not surprising that a large number of tests for verbal memory have been developed. Among the more popular are the Logical Memory Paragraphs from the Wechsler Memory Scale (20). In this test, patients are read two paragraphs, each containing 25 idea units, and are asked to repeat as much of the two stories as possible. Following a 30- or 60-minute interval, patients are again asked to repeat whatever they recall from each of the two stories. This allows the examiner to look at the decay of memory over time. Another popular test is the Rey Auditory Verbal Learning Test (AVLT) (21). The Rey AVLT consists of a list of 15 words that are read to the patient five times. Following each reading, the patient is asked to recall as many words as possible. This test allows the examiner to look at the patient's learning curve when confronted with a "supraspan" list of words. After the five trials, a second list of 15 words is read and the patient is again asked to recall as many words as possible. Following this "interference" trial, the patient is asked to recall as many words as possible from the original list. Finally, the patient is read a list of 30 words, half of which were on the first list. He or she is asked to say "yes" following each word that appeared on the initial list. A test such as the Rey AVLT, or the slightly different Selective Reminding Task of Buschke (22), or the California Verbal Learning Test (23), provides a great deal of information about a patient's: (a) mnemonic strategies; (b) "learning curve;" (c) decay of memory traces following an interference task; and (d) capacity for recognition of material not recalled. Bedside use of one of these more demanding memory tests is helpful when the patient's history suggests memory impairment, but four of four items are successfully recalled.

A second type of memory testing is that which assesses visuospatial recall. The examiner may place several objects around the patient's room at the start of the interview, and after 5, 10, or 15 minutes, inquire how many objects were hidden, what they were, and where they were placed. Another approach is to ask a patient to study a drawn or printed figure and then reproduce it shortly afterward. The Rey-Osterrieth Complex Figure is a line drawing patients may be asked to copy (21). Delayed recall of the Rey Figure is a challenging test of the patient's ability to recall visuospatial information. Because there is tremendous variation in the population regarding visuospatial memory, examiners need to be extremely cautious in interpreting poor performance on the Rey figure alone as evidence of an acquired deficit. When figure drawings are used to test memory, the patient should also be asked to copy the figure directly to exclude constructional apraxia or visuoperceptual problems as a cause for failure.

Remote memory, which refers to a patient's recall of past events, may be difficult unless the examiner is familiar with the patient's biography. An alternate way of exploring remote memory is to ask the patient about famous people or historical events. Patients with dementia or with amnesia due to acquired brain disease, may accurately recall events from the distant past but not from the more immediate past. Absence of such a temporal gradient should always raise the possibility of a psychogenic memory disturbance. Patients with major depression, for instance, may find all memory tasks equally difficult. Delirious patients may find it difficult to recall either remote or recent information.

Visuospatial Skills

Visuospatial skills usually are assessed by paper-and-pencil drawing exercises. Patients are asked to draw circles, triangles, and three-dimensional cubes, a person, a bicycle, a house, or the face of a clock with the hands placed at a particular time. The clock drawing in particular has established value as a screening test for dementia (24–26). However, highly intelligent patients can use left-hemisphere strategies to plan and draw an acceptable clock face. Line-cancellation and line-direction tests are more sensitive and more specific tests of visuospatial skills.

Visuospatial skills can be disrupted because of perceptual problems, including visual field cuts due to damage to the retina, optic nerve, optic chiasm, optic tract, lateral geniculate body, optic radiations, or calcarine cortex. It is important that limitations of visual acuity be detected and that sensory-perceptual deficits be ruled out before the examiner ascribes any visuospatial deficit to "higher cortical" dysfunction. Cerebral of visuospatial problems include damage to the visual association cortex in the parietal and temporal lobes.

In addition to drawing tasks, patients may be asked to manipulate either tokens or three-dimensional blocks to make a series of designs of increasing complexity. The examiner records the time required to complete each design.

As with visual memory, other visuospatial functions vary greatly among persons without brain damage. Therefore, before concluding that a patient has an acquired visuospatial disability, it is essential to estimate the patient's baseline skills.

The classic syndromes of visuospatial disability are those associated with parietal lobe damage, particularly that of the nondominant hemisphere. The drawings of these individuals often omit major elements of the figure being copied, with particular difficulty manifested with the left side of the drawing. On the other hand, damage to the dominant parietal lobe may produce some difficulty reproducing some aspects of figures, but the deficits tend to be less coarse and may be confined to difficulty with accurate depiction of the inner details of complex figures.

It should be noted that most techniques for assessing visuospatial skills rely on motor activity of the patient. An alternative approach is to ask an individual to identify a particular geometric figure among a series of figures oriented in different planes. Such tasks require mental manipulation of figures without physical effort. They may be useful, therefore, in examining individuals who have difficulty using their upper extremities.

Calculations

Patients are asked to perform mental computations. The speed and ease with which they perform these tasks is noted. The examiner who asks these questions should be aware that many questions that are presented as measures of computational capacity in fact represent remote recall of arithmetical tables learned as a student in elementary school. Some examiners give patients practical questions, such as the following one: "If you went to the store with a dollar bill and bought three items for five cents, and four items for two cents, how much change would you receive?"

Though such questions resemble real-life situations, they cannot be viewed as purely arithmetical questions because they also test the patient's ability to recall a sequence of steps. Problems with attention, language comprehension, or memory may, therefore, lead to apparent "arithmetical" errors.

Another common arithmetical task to request from patients is the "serial 7s" task: start with 100, subtract 7 from it, and continue to subtract 7 from each answer, working one's way downward. There are several problems with this task. For many individuals, serial 7s is more a test of sustained concentration than of arithmetical ability per se. Also, different examiners respond differently to patients' errors (some correct and redirect the patient with each error, while others do not). Different examiners request the patient to continue all the way down to 2, while others stop in the 60s or 50s. Finally, few examiners record the actual time for completion, or specify the precise number of errors made. Thus, "serial 7s" is far from a standardized test. This makes it hard to know how to interpret the statement that "performance of serial 7s was intact."

Damage to the inferior parietal lobule of the dominant hemisphere may produce a constellation of cognitive difficulties known as the Gerstmann syndrome. This consists of the following tetrad of findings: acalculia, agraphia, right-left confusion, and finger agnosia. Damage to this region, however, seldom produces a pure Gerstmann syndrome. Some degree of language difficulty, usually a receptive aphasia with word-finding difficulty, typically accompanies damage to the left inferior parietal lobule.

Reasoning

The capacity to reason may be examined in several ways. Practical judgment, appreciation of abstract similarities, and interpretations of proverbs have all been utilized. The examiner should be aware, however, that the "practical judgment" that a patient appears to exercise in a hypothetical situation may not carry over into a real-life situation. This is particularly true in cases of frontal lobe dysfunction. Thus, caution must be exercised in inferring the patient's real world behavior from performance on paper-and-pencil tests or verbal responses to abstract questions. Indeed, it is always problematic to extrapolate from artificial settings, where a range of provocations and environmental cues may not exist, to real-life behavior.

THOUGHT

Allowing patients to speak in a nondirected and open-ended fashion enables the examiner to observe both the style of a patient's thought and the recurring themes. Although neuropsychiatrists rarely adhere to a psychoanalytic model, it is important that they allow patients to speak freely for a period of time without having their thoughts excessively shaped by directed questions.

Process

The organization, coherence, and style of a patient's thought processes are noted. The examiner records a patient's capacity to respond to questions in a focused and coherent fashion, noting any tendencies toward "circumstantiality" (in which excessive and digressive details are given) or "tangentiality" (responses that veer off from the question without returning to it). The nature of a patient's associative processes in response to questions will be reflected both in the degree to which relevant information is organized and the manner in which historical information is conveyed. Patients with manic conditions may speak in a rapid, pressured manner, evincing a looseness of association that prevents them from communicating in a straightforward, economical fashion. "Flight of ideas" refers to a pattern in which the patient leaps from one idea to another on the basis of idiosyncratic associations. Some manic individuals may make "clang" associations, in which the sound of a word, or its rhyming with another word, serves as the basis for shifting from one topic to another. At the other end of the spectrum, patients with psychomotor retardation appear to have a poverty of thought and lack bridging associations from one idea to the next. Similar slowing may be seen in brain diseases affecting the frontal lobe or basal ganglia, as well as in major depressive disorder. The term "Witzelsucht" refers to a facetious punning style exhibited by some patients with frontal lobe disinhibition. This jocularity resembles the playful quality of some hypomanic patients.

Content

The themes or subject matter of a patient's conversation is recorded. Traumatized patients may have recurring intrusive preoccupations with sounds, images, or feelings associated with the trauma. Psychotic individuals may be preoccupied with recurring hallucinations. Other themes of a patient's thought may be anger, guilt, diminished self-esteem, desire for closeness, or fear of intimacy. Discrepancy between thought content and feeling states should be noted. The most striking dissociations between the two are seen in schizophrenic individuals and in pseudobulbar palsy, but lesser discrepancies are common in right-hemisphere and frontal lobe disorders.

Insight

Patients vary tremendously with regard to their awareness of, and degree of concern about, problems in their life. Many patients with hypomanic or manic conditions enjoy the acceleration of their thought process, the diminished need for sleep, and the sense of heightened energy. Such individuals tend to lose touch with the needs and feelings of those around them, and are reluctant to hear the concerns or criticism expressed by family members or business associates, much less take antimanic medications from physicians. On the other hand, many patients who are depressed are unaware that they suffer from a depressive disorder, and the idea of seeking help does not occur to them. With lesions involving the parietal lobe of the right hemisphere, patients may be unaware of, or deny or minimize problems involving the contralateral hemibody.

Babinski coined the term "anosognosia" to describe the striking lack of awareness that he observed in patients whose right-hemisphere strokes were associated with left hemiplegia. Critchley's book, *The Parietal Lobe* (28), describes a wide range of neglect syndromes. Prigatano and Schachter (29) offer a more contemporary treatment of awareness of deficits after brain injury. Patients with Wernicke's aphasia usually are unaware of (agnostic for) their language deficits at the onset of the deficit. Speech therapy with such individuals cannot progress until the patient becomes aware of the problem. Patients with amnestic syndromes typically are less concerned about their memory disturbance than others around them, largely because they are unable to remember that they forget. Patients with dementia may or may not have insight into their loss of intellect. In Alzheimer's disease, those with early loss of insight may have greater right-hemisphere involvement (30).

To approach issues of denial and insight, clinicians should inquire of patients whether they are aware of problems with strength, sensation, or intellectual functioning. After the examiner has established that the patient is aware of a deficit, he or she may then proceed to determine what is most bothersome about the deficit, and in what situations it creates difficulties. A related series of questions to ask is, "To what degree do your deficits:

1. affect those around you?
2. limit your ability to work (or deal with household tasks)?
3. affect your ability to socialize?
4. impair your ability to drive a vehicle safely?"

These questions parallel a four-question test for awareness of dementia developed by Ott and Fogel (7).

If a patient shows no awareness of an apparent problem, the patient may be asked directly whether the apparent deficit has created any problems for the patient in relation to his family or employer. Awareness of a problem does not imply that the patient will be able to modify behavior based on that awareness. Antisocial patients and individuals with frontal lobe syndromes, for instance, may speak clearly about their awareness of society's regulations, or the feelings of their spouse, but then behave in a fashion that seems to ignore both. Patients with borderline personality disorders may acquire, through years of therapy and reading about their condition, a sophisticated knowledge of their own psychodynamics. This knowledge does not ensure that they will acquire the capacity to modify rageful behavior or a tendency to split the world into "good" and "bad" individuals.

Mood

While affect refers to the outward display of felt inner emotion, mood refers to the state of inner emotionality. In general, mood may be thought of as an internal emotional climate. For many individuals, mood states last for days or weeks, whereas in others, including rapidly cycling bipolar patients, borderline personalities, normal adolescents, and persons with limbic epilepsy, mood may fluctuate rapidly and dramatically.

In exploring a patient's depression, the examiner should inquire into the presence of neurovegetative signs such as sleep disturbance, appetite disturbance, constipation, and poor concentration. The pattern of mood throughout the day should be explored. A diurnal mood swing is typical of major depressive disorder, the morning typically being the most difficult time of the day for most depressed patients. Thoughts of suicide should be explored, with particular attention paid to the means of suicide patients consider employing. Patients with impaired verbal capacity can be evaluated using a visual analogue scale, with a happy face at one end and a sad face at the other (31).

Feelings of anxiety can occur in many different guises. Heart palpitations, diaphoresis, shortness of breath, dizziness, and feelings of impending doom may all reflect an underlying anxiety or panic disorder. Knowledge of the situations in which anxiety arises and awareness of particular triggers will help the examiner understand the patient's subjective experiences.

INTERPRETATION OF THE MENTAL STATUS EXAMINATION

The interpretation of mental status examination findings must avoid false-positive assessments of brain dysfunction or psychopathology (overinterpretation) or false-negative assessments (underinterpretation). Accuracy of diagnosis of cognitive deficits can be improved by confirming suspected deficits with additional tests that approach the same function using a different task. In a recent evaluation of methods of screening for mild dementia in the community, it was found that pairs of tests performed better than any single test (32). Similarly, accuracy of diagnosis of psychopathological syndromes can be improved by eliciting clusters of associated symptoms.

A number of specific ideas to enhance the interpretation of mental status examination findings are discussed in the pages that follow.

Time Factor

The mental status examination looks at a patient's mental "state" at a *particular time*. Many factors, such as anxiety, insomnia, exhaustion, and medications can affect patients' mental states and, therefore, their test performance. To determine whether impaired performance at one time reflects an enduring deficit, the examiner may need to repeat portions of the mental status examination at different times after the initial evaluation. Ideally, the clinician seeks to determine the *range* (both the zenith and the nadir) of a patient's cognitive capacity. The examination of a dementia patient at 10 A.M. may show only moderate deficits in memory and reasoning, while the examination at 10 P.M. may reveal hallucinations and disorientation, or even frank delirium. For patients who are suspected of having a progressive dementing illness, assessment of cognition at different times over the course of several months or years may be required. Such serial testing should allow for practice effects, and alternate forms of formal tests should be used when feasible. Alternate word lists for testing naming and memory are readily available.

Psychometric Properties of Tests

Clinicians should always be aware of the psychometric properties of the test they employ.

False Negatives

It is not uncommon for a patient with superior premorbid intelligence to have significant decrements in intellectual functioning, but still perform within the normal range on cognitive screening tests designed to detect major impairments. The absence of impairment on an insensitive instrument does not imply that such a patient has no intellectual problem. The assessment of suspected cognitive decline in a patient with superior premorbid function usually requires both formal neuropsychological assessment and efforts to quantitate premorbid functions. This can be aided by obtaining records of performance on intelligence tests and school entrance examinations such as the SAT, GMAT, LSAT, GRE, and MCAT, and grades from high school, college, or graduate school. In the nonaphasic patient, the vocabulary portion of the Wechsler Adult Intelligence Scale (WAIS) (33) can be used as the basis of an estimate of premorbid intellectual capacities.

Many of the briefer bedside instruments for cognitive assessment, such as the Mini-Mental State Examination (MMSE) (34) and the Cognitive Capacity Screening Examination (CCSE) (35) approach cognition as univariate (i.e., global) and have such low cutoff scores for the diagnosis of "organicity" that impairment must be very significant before a "hit" or detection occurs. This leads to false negatives in patients with restricted deficits, particularly of right-hemisphere or frontal lobe functions. Tests that cover right-hemisphere and executive functions and that use disjunctive rather than summary scoring, avoid this problem. Two examples of such tests are the High Sensitivity Cognitive Screen of Faust and Fogel (36) and the Neurobehavioral Cognitive Status Examination (37). Both of these tests yield a multidimensional "report card" of patients' cognitive abilities in several domains.

False Positives

False-positive assessments of cognitive decline tend to occur in two situations: when educational limitations or cultural factors are not taken into account, and when long-standing, stable learning disabilities are misinterpreted as more recently acquired deficits. Restricted difficulties with spatial orientation, sentence structure, or arithmetic, for instance, commonly reflect learning disabilities that may not have been previously defined.

The diagnosis of a learning disability is particularly likely to be missed or delayed if the patient has dropped out of school without any formal evaluation of academic difficulties, or if the patient had above average intelligence and was able to pass courses despite difficulties. Directly asking the patient whether there were special areas of difficulty in school, regardless of the grades obtained, may yield clues. Examples of schoolwork or narrative evaluations by teachers sometimes are available.

FRONTAL LOBE LESIONS

Frontal lobe lesions are compatible with normal performance in many areas of higher intellectual functioning. To assess frontal lobe deficits, it is necessary to employ tests that allow one to examine a patient's capacity for sustaining and shifting attention, for self-monitoring, and for responding to challenges in the face of shifting environmental cues and contingencies. Because examiners often perform their assessment in a structured environment and provide patients with explicit instructions as to how to proceed on tests, they actually create an artificial world where the examiner "takes over the role of the patient's frontal lobes." When patients with frontal lobe damage are observed outside the test situation, their real-life behavior often differs considerably from their verbal responses to hypothetical situations. A

classic case of a frontal polar lesion reported by Eslinger and Damasio illustrates the potential for severe behavioral disinhibition with normal results on standard neuropsychological tests of "frontal" cognitive functions (38).

MEDICATIONS

Medications taken at the time of cognitive assessment or even a few days earlier, can affect cognitive performance. Among the list of medications that can affect cognition are: digitalis, lithium, antidepressants, antiepileptic drugs, neuroleptics, antianxiety agents, sedatives, and analgesics. Medication-related cognitive deficits usually involve attentional mechanisms. Impaired performance in one or more areas of "higher cortical function" in a medicated patient should be interpreted conservatively if attentional tests such as digit span or letter cancellation show deficits.

NEUROLOGICAL EXAMINATION

Problems with hearing, vision, or touch can lower test performance. Unless such perceptual or sensory impairments are noted, poor performance or low scores can be falsely construed as evidence of "higher" cognitive problems. In a similar vein, disturbances in motor function (weakness, tremor, or incoordination) may also affect performance. Thus, test results cannot be properly interpreted with knowledge of the clinical neurological examination.

LEVEL OF CONSCIOUSNESS

Whenever a patient is less than fully alert, and particularly when the level of consciousness fluctuates (secondary to physical exhaustion, sleep deprivation, narcolepsy, postictal states, etc.), cognitive test results must be interpreted conservatively. Ideally, areas of deficit are reexamined when the patient is more alert.

ATTENTION AND CONCENTRATION DEFICITS

Problems with attention or concentration can impair performance on a number of higher intellectual tasks. The distinction between attention-related problems on the one hand and true problems with specific cortical functions is an important element of all cognitive assessment.

LANGUAGE IMPAIRMENT

Any impairment of language, such as word-finding difficulty or comprehension, may impair performance on other parts of the mental status examination, such as verbal memory, judgment, or thought process assessment, which are evaluated through verbal communication.

OVERALL PATTERN OF COGNITIVE DEFICITS

The overall pattern of cognitive deficits provides the greatest insight into the patient's condition. For example, impairment in verbal memory has a different significance when associated with disorientation and intact attention, than with impairment in digit span. The former combination suggests an organic amnestic syndrome, while the latter suggests a primary disorder of attention.

TIME REQUIRED TO COMPLETE TESTS

The time taken to complete cognitive tests provides information complementary to the accuracy with which they are completed. Patients may be able to successfully complete cognitive tasks given sufficient time, but may be unable to do them in the time usually allocated to the task. Patients with bradyphrenia due to basal ganglia diseases offer some of the most striking examples, but the same phenomenon of trading off speed for accuracy can be seen with cortical lesions. For example, a patient with right-parietal damage may be able to draw a clock slowly but accurately using an entirely verbal plan of action.

Performances that are accurate but unusually slow should be distinguished from those that are accurate and of normal speed; the former do not represent normal performance. On the other hand, when patients cannot do a task within a normal time allowance, they should be offered the chance to do it more slowly, to help determine whether their cognitive deficit is absolute or relative.

Some of the effects of medication on cognitive testing, both positive and negative, are mediated by medication effects on cognitive and motor speed. Stimulants sometimes enable better performances; sedatives frequently impair performance. When a patient's performance is already slower than normal, further slowing may lead to complete failure.

DESCRIPTIVE AND DIAGNOSTIC TERMINOLOGY

Finally, descriptive and diagnostic terminology should be carefully distinguished. For example, "cognitive impairment" or "a dementia syndrome" describe a mental status finding; "dementia" or "Alzheimer's Disease" imply neuropathology.

MEDICAL HISTORY

Systematic consideration of the medical history and a thorough review of systems reassure patients that they are being seen by a physician who appreciates the interplay between physical illness and mental distress. The medical history of neuropsychiatric patients may provide clues to the underlying cause of changes in their mental status or behavior. Furthermore, comprehensive history taking serves to build a collaborative relationship between the clinician and the patient.

The earliest events that influence central nervous system (CNS) development occur in utero. These include physical injury to the mother during pregnancy, consumption of teratogenic medications, or exposure to substances to which the mother is addicted, such as alcohol, heroin, nicotine, or cocaine. The possibility of birth-related problems such as prematurity, low birth weight, perinatal asphyxia and ABO

incompatibility should be explored. Patients themselves are often unaware of major prenatal and natal events. Thus, review of documentation from previous medical records and history obtained from siblings, parents, or other relatives are helpful.

Early childhood illnesses may cause enduring effects on the brain or other major organ systems. Major medical illnesses in a child, its sibling, or other members of the family may also be of psychological significance by occasioning prolonged and possibly traumatic separation of the child and parents. It can also cause parents to focus their time and attention on the ill child, with resultant problems in attachment, or self-esteem for the physically healthy siblings. Developmental delays in standing, walking, or talking should be recorded. Surgical procedures, regardless of the age at which they are performed, have special importance as events during which control of the body is relinquished to medical personnel.

All current medications and dosage schedules should be listed, along with past and present consumption of alcohol and other substances. When patients themselves are unable to give complete medication histories, vigorous pursuit of data from other sources is worthwhile.

GENERAL PHYSICAL EXAMINATION

General Observations

Meticulous observation of the patient's general appearance is a high-yield activity with the neuropsychiatric patient population and sometimes must substitute for part of the formal examination when the patient is uncooperative. The presence of a physical illness may not require detailed examination, but may instead be provided by clues of subtle facial asymmetry, a butterfly rash over the cheeks, slowness of movements, or difficulty relaxing a grip. Detection of a relevant and previously unnoticed physical sign may afford the physician unexpected leverage in developing a relationship with the patient or the patient's caregivers.

Vital Signs

Vital signs should be recorded before medications are started or changed. Measurements of pulse and blood pressure should be taken in both the supine and standing positions, because autonomic disorders, endocrine diseases, and drug effects are prevalent in the neuropsychiatric population.

Tachycardia may reflect anxiety, pain, hyperthyroidism, heart failure, or ingestion of either adrenergic agonists or anticholinergic substances. Some arrhythmias, especially paroxysmal atrial tachycardia, produce marked anxiety. Bradycardia is common in patients with anorexia nervosa.

Hypertension places patients at increased risk for stroke. The finding of significant hypertension increases the suspicion of occult stroke as a cause of behavioral or cognitive change.

Hypothermia is a potentially dangerous complication of

neuroleptic use in older people. Hyperpyrexia may reflect infection anywhere in the body (including the CNS), atropine poisoning, toxicity due to dopamine-blocking agents ("neuroleptic malignant syndrome"), or the hypermetabolic state of delirium tremens.

Although hyperventilation may arise in the context of stress disorders, anxiety states, or panic attacks, it may also reflect metabolic acidosis with a compensatory respiratory drive. Central respiratory drive can be diminished by barbiturates, benzodiazepines, alcohol, or lesions that compress the brainstem.

NEUROLOGICAL EXAMINATION

The neurological examination often is regarded as more "objective" than the mental status examination. However, it is subject to substantial interobserver variation (11). Although reliability is improved by general neurological training, the two most potent ways to increase reliability are to conduct the examination with the patient's history in mind (39), and to have specific training on the assessment of the specific neurological signs to be evaluated. For example, neurologists familiar with dystonia show much higher inter-rater reliability in the assessment of dystonia than general neurologists with no special interest in movement disorders (40).

Even when measures are taken to increase reliability, the neurological examination is of limited sensitivity, and may be normal even in the presence of gross brain disease. Stein et al. (41) studied the relationship of CT scan findings and neurological assessments in 686 patients with mild head injury, of whom 127 had intracranial lesions and 38 required surgery. Of the 127 patients with intracranial lesions, 19 had normal neurological examinations; nine of these required surgery. Similar concerns about the limits of the neurological examination have been raised concerning the assessment of peripheral nerve disease. Electrical studies can establish the presence of clinically significant peripheral polyneuropathy before unequivocal signs can be demonstrated on bedside sensory examination (42). Adaptation of causal bedside testing, such as the use of precisely weighted needles for testing of pinprick sensation (43), have been proposed as a partial solution to this problem. In general, quantification of findings on motor and sensory examinations holds some promise for enhancing reliability and accuracy (44).

Furthermore, the detail with which the examination is done varies according to clinical circumstances. Precise mapping of visual fields differs from doing confrontation fields with wiggling fingers; one would not expect the latter to detect a paracentral scotoma, or even necessarily a subtle upper quadrant field cut. When conducting the examination, the detailed attention given to each part should be in accord with the diagnostic hypotheses that have evolved by that point in the clinical encounter. The examiner should not hesitate to return to earlier parts of the examination, such as mental status or visual fields, if later findings change the likelihood and probable location of a focal neurological deficit.

Cranial Nerves

CRANIAL NERVE I

The tendency of many internists as well as some neurologists to omit testing of the olfactory nerves is unfortunate and should not be emulated by neuropsychiatrists. Disturbance of the sense of smell may occur in a wide variety of neurological disorders. Shearing of the olfactory filaments as they traverse the cribiform plate occurs frequently with closed head injury and can take place without loss of consciousness. Typically such patients strike the frontal or occipital portions of their head, but changes in olfactory function can also occur when the skull is struck elsewhere. Complete anosmia should be distinguished from partial loss of olfactory capacity (hyposmia). Alteration in olfactory ability may lead to changes in sexual behavior, appetite, or food preference. When olfactory loss is associated with orbital frontal injury, patients may show disinhibition and inappropriate social behavior.

Meningioma of the olfactory groove can cause unilateral anosmia. Olfactory hallucinations may occur not only in temporal lobe epilepsy associated with uncal scarring, but also may be seen in schizophrenia, in migraine, and as a deafferentation phenomenon following damage to the peripheral elements of the olfactory network. Whereas some patients are unaware of their olfactory loss and may not appear concerned even when a clear olfactory deficit is documented, other individuals complain bitterly of their loss of olfactory perception.

The olfactory nerves should be assessed with substances such as vanilla or coffee that do not irritate the trigeminal nerves. "Scratch-and-sniff" cards are available for systematic, validated olfactory screening using standardized stimuli.

CRANIAL NERVE II

Examination of the optic nerve entails examination of the optic fundus (retina), visual fields, visual acuity, and the pupil. Funduscopic examination allows consideration of the retinal vascularity and the optic disc. Visual acuity can be assessed with a pocket screener or a wall chart. It is important to indicate whether acuity is assessed with patients wearing corrective lenses or glasses. In the absence of corrective lenses, a pinhole can be used to correct for refractive errors. Visual fields can be tested with small red and white objects on the tip of a pointer; cotton swabs on long sticks will serve at the bedside if standard test objects are not at hand. Each eye is examined independently. Pupillary reactivity to direct and consensual light is recorded, as is the near reflex (accommodation and convergence).

CRANIAL NERVES III, IV, AND VI

Extraocular motility is examined by observing the patient's upward, downward, lateral, and angular gaze. The examiner looks closely for nystagmus, diplopia, or limitation of gaze in any direction.

CRANIAL NERVE V

Facial sensation over each of the three branches of the trigeminal nerve is tested with light touch and pinprick, and each side compared to the other. The corneal reflex (afferent limb via cranial nerve V, efferent limb via cranial nerve VII) should be tested with a wisp of cotton. Its absence can be the sole evidence of trigeminal nerve dysfunction; its presence is evidence against facial anesthesia.

CRANIAL NERVE VII

Evidence of facial asymmetry is noted both at rest and during facial expression. In peripheral facial nerve lesions, the entire hemiface is involved, whereas in a central lesion, the forehead is spared. Central lesions involving the right face may also be associated with aphasia. Temporal lobe lesions can produce symmretry on spontaneous emotional expression with intact facial movements to commands.

CRANIAL NERVE VIII

Is there sensorineural or conductive hearing loss? High-frequency hearing loss (presbyacusias) is common in the elderly. Hearing may be assessed at the bedside with whispering, tuning forks, or, ideally, an audioscope. The examiner also performs the Weber test in which a 512 Hz tuning fork is placed on the vertex and the patient asked whether the sound is heard equally well in both ears. In conductive hearing loss, the sound will be louder on the defective side. In sensorineurol hearing loss, the sound will be greater on the less impaired side. Finally, bone conduction is compared with air conduction by placing the base of the vibrating tuning first on the mastoid process behind the ear and asking the patient to compare the strength of that sound with the sound of the tuning fork in the air. In conductive hearing loss, bone conduction is greater than air conduction.

The vestibular component of cranial nerve VIII may be tested with the Nylen-Barany maneuver, which stimulates the vestibular apparatus. The patient is initially seated and then moved rapidly into a supine posture with head tilted 45° backward below the level of the table, and 45° degrees to the left. The patient resumes the seated posture, and the maneuver is repeated, moving the head backward and 45° to the right. The examiner notes whether nystagmus or symptoms of vertigo are produced by this maneuver, and compares the intensity and duration of nystagmus with turning of the head toward the left and the right sides.

CRANIAL NERVES IX AND X

The afferent limb of the gag reflex is via cranial nerve IX and efferent limb via cranial nerve X. Patients with upper motor neuron palsy may have an overly brisk reflex, with excessive coughing, while patients with lower motor neuron palsy may have a diminished or absent gag reflex, leading to increased risk of aspiration. Swallowing is a complex act that can be impaired even if the gag reflex is intact. Timed swallowing of liquid is a sensitive bedside test for dysphagia (45). A rate of less than 10 ml/second is strongly associated with objective demonstration of dysphagia on cineesophogram.

CRANIAL NERVE XI

Function of the accessory nerve is tested by palpation of the sternocleidomastoid muscle as the patient turns his or her head to the left and right alternately while being opposed by the hand of the examiner. Weakness of the *left* sternocleidomastoid impairs head turning to the *right,* and vice versa. This point is occasionally useful in identifying weakness due to (hysterical) conversion. Shrugging or elevation of the shoulders is accomplished through activation of the trapezius muscle. The examiner requests the patient to elevate his or her shoulders, while palpating the involved muscle.

CRANIAL NERVE XII

The patient is asked to protrude the tongue and move it from side to side. In unilateral paralysis of cranial nerve XII, the tongue will be observed to deviate toward the side of the weakness.

Motor Examination

Muscle mass is observed for any asymmetry of bulk and for any focal atrophy due to peripheral lesions or disuse.

MUSCLE TONE

Muscle tone is tested by passively moving the patient's limb. The examiner compares tone in both extremities and notes the presence or absence of increased tone. Increased tone may be characterized as having a "jackknife" quality typical of upper motor neuron disease; paratonic (a ratchet-like, intermittent tone seen in frontal lobe disease), cogwheeling (parkinsonian), or negativistic (the rigid resistance of catatonia). Absence or flaccidity of muscle tone is indicative of lower motor neuron disease, and decreased tone is associated with cerebellar lesions. Tone varies considerably among normal individuals.

MUSCLE STRENGTH

Muscle strength is graded from 0–5, where 0 = no movement, 1 = trace movement, 2 = movement with gravity in a horizontal plane, 3 = movement against gravity, 4 = movement against gravity and against applied force, and 5 = normal strength. The examiner compares left versus right, proximal versus distal, and upper versus lower extremity strength.

REFLEXES

Reflexes are graded from 0–4, with 2 being average. Briskness of reflexes varies in healthy normal individuals, and areflexia that is not asymmetrical and is not associated with weakness or other motor or sensory problems is not necessarily pathological. In individuals who are anxious, consuming benzodiazepines, or withdrawing from alcohol, reflexes may be diffusely increased. Asymmetry between reflexes and discrepancy between reflexes in upper and lower extremities can have localizing significance.

Pathological reflexes: In a normal adult, stimulation of the plantar surface of the foot produces either no response or plantar flexion (a down-going toe). In individuals with upper motor neuron pathology (i.e., a pyramidal tract lesion), the great toe may dorsiflex (i.e., extend) and the toes fan out. An upgoing toe with or without fanning of the other toes is referred to as a Babinski sign. The Babinski sign in an adult usually implies structural disease of the CNS, or a toxic-metabolic encephalopathy.

There are a number of "primitive" reflexes that may be seen in infants during the first year of life. Reappearance of these reflexes (i.e., grasp, suck, snout, root) suggest frontal lobe disorders. However, the occurrance of primitive reflexes in elderly persons is of relatively low diagnostic specificity.

COORDINATION

Coordination (cerebellar) testing consists of finger-nose-finger, heel-knee-shin, and rapid alternating movements. Weakness can interfere with coordination testing. Spasticity can cause clumsiness, but not the dysmetria typical of cerebellar lesions.

STATION

Is the patient able to stand comfortably with feet together? Is there evidence of swaying when the patient is asked to close his or her eyes (positive Romberg sign)? Can the patient stand on one foot?

GAIT

The examiner should observe several components in a patient's gait: How wide is the stride? How broad-based is the gait? Are movements made in a shuffling, tentative fashion? Is there a foot-drop with a "steppage" gait? Is turning done smoothly or "en bloc"? Is there asymmetry of arm-swing? The time taken to walk a fixed distance can be used as a quantitative measure of a patient's gait.

ABNORMAL MOVEMENTS

Is there a paucity or an excess of movements (hypokinesia vs. hyperkinesia)? Are there spontaneous dyskinesias (such as those of Huntington's disease or tardive dyskinesia)? Is there a tremor visible at rest (parkinsonian tremor), postural tremor (familial or essential tremor), or tremor that appears only with intention (cerebellar tremor)?

Myoclonic jerks may involve a single limb or the entire body. Fasciculations (movements of small muscle groups) can be seen in amyotrophic lateral sclerosis (ALS) and in nerve-root lesions.

SOFT SIGNS

The neurological and psychiatric literature has been inconsistent as to whether the traditional neurological examination is of assistance in the evaluation of learning difficulties. Several pediatric neurologists have attempted to refine the neurological examination by asking patients to repetitively perform certain tasks such as jumping on one foot and noting the nature of difficulties seen over specific periods of time.

In contrast to "subtle" signs of neurological abnormalities, such as reflex asymmetries or equivocal Babinski signs, "soft" signs are unlikely to imply lateralized pathology, and more often reflect developmental immaturity of the CNS.

"Soft neurological signs" include:

1. *Fine motor incoordination:* awkwardness at such tasks as handwriting, finger-nose-finger and finger pursuit in the absence of frank cerebellar dysmetria;
2. *Dysrhythmia:* a lack of smooth transitions between different motor tasks.
3. *Mirror movements:* the contralateral overflow of motor activity in homologous muscle groups.
4. *Synkinesis:* ipsilateral overflow of extraneous associated movements when the patient is asked to perform an activity involving a specific set of muscle groups.

Both mirror movements and synkinesis can be elicited by asking the patient to perform activities involving discrete muscle groups: (*a*) tap one foot; (*b*) alternately tap heel and toe; (*c*) pat one's thigh; (*d*) flip-flop one hand on one's thigh; (*e*) tap one's thumb and index finger repeatedly; (*f*) successively touch one's index, middle, ring, and little fingers to one's thumb.

Mirror movements and synkinesis may be seen as a failure to inhibit or suppress movements in larger or distant muscle groups while attempting to perform a discrete task.

The reliability of rating of soft signs can be enhanced by having a standard routine for eliciting the signs, such as having the patient do movements *a–f*, just listed, 10 times in succession on the right, and then on the left. Timing the sets of 10 with a stopwatch can give further useful information about lateralized differences in speed of performance.

Soft signs, while not consistently correlated with anatomical brain abnormalities on imaging, have been shown to have predictive or discriminant validity in particular clinical situations. For example, Gupta et al. (46) found soft signs in 23% of schizophrenic patients who had never received neuroleptics, but in 46% of those receiving neuroleptics. Aronowitz (47) found left-sided soft signs were more prevalent in adolescents with conduct disorder and attention deficit hyperactivity disorder than in those with conduct disorder alone. Gurvits et al. (48) found medication-free veterans with posttraumatic stress disorder (PTSD) had more soft signs than non-PTSD controls, and that those with more soft signs showed more abnormalities on neuropsychological testing. Schizophrenic patients with more soft signs are more likely to develop tardive dyskinesia when treated with neuroleptics (49).

Sensation

The examiner tests primary sensory perception by examining the patient's awareness of pinprick, light touch, position, and vibration. Parietal sensory testing consists of examining a patient's capacity to recognize numbers or letters written on the palm or on the sole of the foot (50) while the patient is not looking (graphesthesia); the ability to recognize an object from manipulating or palpating it (stereognosis); and the ability to detect sensory stimuli applied at the same time in different anatomical regions (double-simultaneous stimulation). It is meaningless to test for parietal deficits in a region of significant primary sensory loss.

The Neurological Examination of Patients Suspected of Hysteria, Malingering, and Other Psychogenic Disorders

Individuals who exaggerate their neurological deficits, whether for conscious or unconscious reasons, prove a particular challenge to neuropsychiatrists. The distinction between "psychogenic" and "organic" sources of functional disability is one of the tasks that neurologists are frequently asked to perform. DeJong's encyclopedic text, *The Neurologic Examination (2),* devotes 18 pages to signs that may be seen in patients with hysteria, malingering, and other psychogenic conditions. Although the detection of nonorganic findings on a neurological examination raises strong questions of psychological factors, the presence of these findings cannot be used as proof that the entirety of a patient's presentation is feigned, hysterical, or psychological in origin.

Motor Examination

Inconsistency of motor performance is typical of psychogenic illness. On testing of strength, the examiner may discover that a patient exerts effort but only for a brief period. Other individuals fail to exert a full effort. When this occurs, the examiner should establish whether pain is a factor, and determine whether the patient is able, even for a brief period, to give a maximal effort.

When asked to turn the head first to one side, then the other, the patient with hysterical hemiplegia may mount less effort in turning his or her head toward the allegedly weak side. If the examiner palpates the contralateral sternocleidomastoid muscle, he or she will feel the lack of tension (i.e., effort) on turning toward the allegedly paretic side.

The Hoover sign may also be helpful in cases of individuals with either hysterical hemiplegia or hysterical monoplegia. The patient is asked to lie supine and then raise first the strong leg, then the weak leg. As the patient pushes up with the intact leg, the examiner offers resistance to this raising, while at the same time positioning his hand beneath the heel of the allegedly paretic leg. If both legs are in fact intact, the examiner can feel downward pressure from the allegedly paretic leg as the patient attempts to raise the intact leg against the resistance of the examiner. The examiner next places his or her hand beneath the heel of the intact leg and requests the patient to lift the allegedly paretic limb against resistance. Failure to exert an effort to raise the allegedly paretic limb may be detected by the absence of downward pressure in the intact leg.

Patients who present with neurologically based weakness have reflexes that are increased with pyramidal tract lesions or decreased with lower motor neuron lesions. Examiners may test cooperation by palpating both agonist and antagonist muscle groups. For instance, when asked to extend the knee, there should be some increase in muscle tone within the quadriceps accompanied by relaxation within the hamstrings. If the hamstrings tighten and the quadriceps remain flaccid, this is inconsistent with full cooperation. In cases of hysterical hemiplegia, some patients may, in response to an unanticipated noxious stimulus, move the allegedly paretic limb.

Sensory Examination

When patients complain of sensory deficits, the pattern of their alleged alteration in sensation should be noted. Nondermatomal distributions may be claimed for alleged sensory loss. Patients who claim anesthesia may be instructed to respond with a "yes" when they feel a pinprick and a "no" when they do not feel it. If a patient responds "no" when an allegedly anesthetic region is touched, he or she demonstrates perception of the stimulus. If a patient complains of blindness, any reaction to visual threat (blinking and/or head aversion) should be noted, as should pupillary reaction to light.

Sensory complaints that split the midline in a precise fashion tend to be of nonorganic origin, particularly when they involve both the face and trunk. Lesions of the ventral posteromedial (VPM) and ventral posterolateral (VPL) nuclei of the thalamus, however, may cause sensory disturbances that affect both the trunk and extremities.

CONCLUSION

In recent years, psychometric studies of the neurological and mental status examinations, and studies correlating brain imaging with clinical assessment, have offered clinicians a lesson in humility. The artistry of the best clinician will be less reliable than a standardized rating scale, and the reflex hammer will be no match for an MRI in establishing the presence of a structural lesion of the CNS. However, far from indicating the obsolescence of the neuropsychiatric examination, these developments have clarified its roles:

1. To identify disturbances of brain *function;*
2. To determine the functional consequences of structural lesions;

3. To establish the experiential and phenomenological significance of abnormalities of brain function;
4. To develop diagnostic hypotheses;
5. To determine the need for investigation with imaging, electrophysiological, or psychometric studies;
6. To focus the application of technology-intensive studies if they are needed; and
7. To enable interpretation of their findings.

The combination of "psychiatric" mental status assessment, cognitive evaluation, and traditional neurological examination is the most comprehensive and therefore sensitive means for identifying probable brain dysfunction, or determining functional consequences of a known structural lesion. It offers the clinician the opportunity to discern patterns of deficit that cross several domains of brain function (e.g., cognitive, motor, emotional). Such patterns form a sound basis for diagnostic inferences.

Moreover, the routine conduct of neuropsychiatric examinations gradually alters the clinician's perception of certain diseases as essentially neuropsychiatric rather than as purely neurological or psychiatric. The neurologist who systematically inquires about emotion and cognition in patients with multiple sclerosis (MS) will discover that mental changes are a major source of impairment for many MS patients, even though paralysis may be more obvious. The psychiatrist who systematically performs cognitive and neurological examinations on patients with schizophrenia will discover that truly normal cognition is rare, and that poor cognition, minor neurological abnormalities, and intolerance of neuroleptics go together. Such discoveries alter the clinician's approach to the patient, in the direction of better understanding, greater empathy, and more comprehensive care.

References

1. American Psychiatric Association Work Group on Practice Guidelines for the Psychiatric Evaluation of Adults. Practice guidelines for the psychiatric evaluation of adults. Am J Psychiatry 1995; 152(11)(supplement):65-80.
2. DeJong R. The neurologic examination. 4th ed. New York: Harper & Row, 1979.
3. Strub RL, Black FW. The mental status examination in neurology. 3rd ed. Philadelphia: FA Davis, 1993.
4. Trzepacz PT, Baker RW. The psychiatric mental status examination. New York: Oxford University Press, 1993.
5. Weintraub S, Mesulam M-M. Mental state assessment of young and elderly adults in behavioral neurology. In: Mesulam M-M. Principles of behavioral neurology. Philadelphia: FA Davis, 1985:71–124.
6. Lishman WA. Physiogenesis and psychogenesis in the "post-concussional syndrome." Br J Psychiatry 1988;133:460–469.
7. Ott B, Fogel B. Measurement of depression in dementia: self vs. clinician rating. International Journal of Geriatriac Psychiatry 1993; 7:899–904.
8. Michalakeas A, Skoutas C, Charalambous A, et al. Insight in schizophrenia and mood disorders and its relation to psychopathology. Acta Pyschiatr Scand 1994;90:46–49.
9. Sohlberg MM, Mateer CA, Stuss DT. Contemporary approaches to the management of executive control dysfunction. Journal of Head Trauma and Rehabilitation 1993;8:45–58.
10. McAllister TW. Neuropsychiatric sequelae of head injuries. Psychiatr Clin North America 1992;15:395–413.
11. Hansen, Sindrup SH, Christensen PB, et al. Interobserver variation in the evaluation of neurological signs: observer dependent factors. Acta Neurol Scand 1994;90:145–149.
12. Fogel B, Ratey JJ. A neuropsychiatric approach to personality and behavior. In: Ratey JJ, ed. Neuropsychiatry of personality disorders. Cambridge, MA: Blackwell Science, 1995:1–16.
13. Weinstein CS, Seidman LJ, Feldman JJ, Ratey JJ. Neurocognitive disorders in psychiatry: a case example of diagnostic and treatment dilemmas. Psychiatry 1991;54:65–75.
14. Campbell JJ, Duffy JD, Salloway SP. Treatment strategies for patients with dysexecutive syndromes. Journal of Neuropsychiatry and clinical Neuroscience 1994;6:411–418.
14a. Jennett B, Bond M. Assessment of outcome after severe brain damage. A practical scale. The Lancet, i, 480-48-1, 1975.
15. Gardos G, Cole JO. Drug-induced parkinsonism and concomitant tardive dyskinesia. In: Joseph AB, Young RR, eds. Movement disorders in neurology and neuropsychiatry. Boston: Blackwell Scientific Publications, 1992:61–66.
16. Heilman KM, Bowers D, Valenstein E. Emotional disorders associated with neurological diseases. In: Heilman KM, Valenstein E, eds. Clinical neuropsychology. 3rd ed. New York: Oxford University Press, 1993:461–498.
17. Lezak M. Verbal functions and language skills. In Neuropsychological assessment. 3rd ed. New York: Oxford University Press. 1995:523–558.
18. Benson DF. Aphasia, alexia, and agraphia. New York: Churchill Livingstone, 1979.
19. Friedman R, Ween JE, Albert ML. Alexia. In: Heilman KM, Valenstein E, eds. Clinical neuropsychology. New York: Oxford University Press, 1993:37–62.
20. Wechsler D. Wechsler Memory Scale-Revised manual. San Antonio: The Psychological Corporation, 1987.
21. Lezak M. Memory I: Tests. In Neuropsychological assessement. 3rd ed. New York: Oxford University Press, 1995:429–498.
22. Buschke H, Fuld PA. Evaluation of storage, retention, and retrieval in disordered memory and learning. Neurology 1974;11:1019–1025.
23. Delis DC, Kramer JH, Kaplan E, Ober BA. California Verbal Learning Test: Adult Version. San Antonio: The Psychological Corporation, 1987.
24. Watson YI, Arfken CL, Birge SJ. Clock completion: an objective screening test for dementia. J Am Geriatr Soc 1993;41:1235–1240.
25. Shulman KI, Gold DP, Cohen CA, Zucchero CA. Clock-drawing and dementia in the community: a longitudinal study. International Journal of Geriatric Psychiatry 1993;8:487–496.
26. Pan GD, Stern Y, Sano M, Mayeux R. Clock-drawing in neurological disorders. Behavioral Neurology 1989;2:39–48.
27. Ishiai S, Sugishita, Ichikawa T, et al. Clock-drawing test and unilateral spatial neglect. Neurology 1993;43:106–110.
28. Critchley M. The parietal lobes. London: Hafner, 1953.
29. Prigatano GP, Schachter DL. Awareness of deficit after brain injury. New York: Oxford University Press, 1991.
30. Ott B, Noto R, Fogel BS. Insight and apathy in Alzheimer's disease: correlation with SPECT. Journal of Neuropsychiatry and Clinical Neuroscience, in press.
31. Stern RA, Bachman DL. Depressive symptoms following stroke. Am J Psychiatry 1991;148:351–356.
32. Hooijer C, Jonker C, Lindeboom J. Cases of mild dementia in the community: improving efficacy of case finding by concurrent use of pairs of screening tests. International Journal of Geriatric Psychiatry 1993;8:561–564.
33. Wechsler D. Wechster Adult Intelligence Scale-Revised Manual. New York: The Psychological Corporation, 1981.
34. Folstein M, Folstein S, McHugh PR. Mini-Mental State: A practical method for grading the cognitive state of the patient for the clinician. J Psychiatr Res 1975;12:189–198.
35. Jacobs JW, Bernard MR, Delgado A, Strain JJ. Screening for organic

mental syndromes in the medically ill. Ann Intern Med 1977;
86:40–47.

36. Faust D, Fogel BS. The development and initial validation of a sensitive
bedside cognitive screening test. J Nerv Ment Dis 1989;177:25–31.

37. Kiernan RJ, Mueller J, Langston JW, VanDyke C. The neurobehavioral
cognitive status examination. I. A brief but quantitative approach to
cognitive status testing. Ann Intern Med 1987;15:481–486.

38. Eslinger PJ, Damasio AR. Severe disturbance of higher cognition after
bilateral frontal lobe ablation. Neurology 1985;35:1731–1741.

39. Vogel HP. Influence of additional information on interrater reliability
in the neurologic examination. Neurology 1992;42:2076–2081.

40. Defazio G, Lepore V, Abbruzzese G, et al. Reliability among
neurologists in the severity assessment of blepharospasm and oromandibular dystonia: a multicenter study. Mov Disord 1994;9:616–621.

41. Stein SC, Spettell C, Young G, Ross SE. Limitations of neurological
assessment in mild head injury. Brain Inj 1993;7:425–430.

42. Bell-Krotoski J, Weinstein J, Weinstein C. Testing sensibility, including
touch-pressure, two-point discrimination, point localization, and
vibration. J Hand Ther 1993;6:114–123.

43. Chan AW, MacFarlane IA, Bowsher D, Campbell JA. Weighted needle
pinprick sensory thresholds: a simple test of sensory function in
diabetic peripheral neuropathy. J Neurol Neurosurg Psychiatry 1992;
55:56–59.

44. Wade DT. Measurement in neurologic rehabilitation. Curr Opin
Neurol 1993;6:778–784.

45. Nathadwarawala KM, Nicklin J, Wiles CM. A timed test of swallowing
capacity for neurological patients. J Neurol Neurosurg Psychiatry
1992;55:822–825.

46. Gupta S, Andreasen NC, Arndt S, et al. Neurological soft signs in
neuroleptic-naive and neuroleptic-treated schizophrenia patients and in
normal comparison subjects. Am J Psychiatry 1995;152:191–196.

47. Aronowitz B, Liebowitz MR, Hollander E, et al. Neuropsychiatric and
neuropsychological findings in conduct disorder and attention-deficit
hyperactivity disorder. Journal of Neuropsychiatry and Clinical Neurosciences 1995;6:245–249.

48. Gurvits TV, Lasko NB, Schachter SC, et al. Neurological status of
Vietnam veterans with chronic post-traumatic stress disorder. Journal
of Neuropsychiatry and Clinical Neurosciences 1993;5:183–188.

49. King DJ, Wilson A, Cooper SJ, Waddinton JL. The clinical correlates
of neurological soft signs in chronic schizophrenia. Br J Psychiatry
1991;158:770–775.

50. Richards P, Persinger MA. Toe graphesthesia as a discriminator of
brain impairment: the outstanding feet for neuropsychology. Percept
Mot Skills 1992;74;1027–1030.

3

NEUROPSYCHOLOGICAL ASSESSMENT

Stephen M. Rao

This chapter describes the clinical neuropsychological examination and its role in the management of individuals with presumed or verified brain dysfunction. Although the study of brain-behavior relationships has a rich history, extending from the 19th century revelations of Broca and Wernicke, the field of human neuropsychology has only recently evolved (1). Using psychological tests to study brain dysfunction took hold in the decades following World War II, with the pioneering experimental studies of focal brain damage by Hans-Lukas Teuber, Brenda Milner, Alexander Luria, Arthur Benton, Henry Hècaen, and Ward Halstead. These psychological investigations, based on accidents of nature (strokes and tumors), warfare (penetrating head wounds), and surgery (cortical excision of epileptic foci), provided important new insights regarding cerebral localization and lateralization. These early studies formed the basis for the scientific field of human neuropsychology.

As a scientific endeavor, human neuropsychology has grown exponentially along with all other areas of neuroscience research during the past two decades. The emphasis in human neuropsychology has broadened to include individuals with more diffuse brain damage (closed head injury, Alzheimer's disease, AIDS, demyelinating disease). The field has also turned its attention to traditional psychiatric disorders, such as schizophrenia and affective disorders. At the same time, validation of the lesion models of localization can be achieved through comparison with an unprecedented variety of sophisticated brain imaging technologies used to extract structural and functional information from the intact human brain. Results derived from these techniques, e.g., computerized tomography (CT), structural and functional magnetic resonance imaging (MRI), positron emission (PET), single proton emission computed tomography (SPECT), magnetoencephalography, event-related potentials, are not only providing concurrent validation of existing models, but are also generating new ideas about brain functional organization. In addition, human neuropsychological models and techniques have become increasingly more sophisticated with the emergence of cognitive neuropsychology as a scientific discipline. These new paradigms are theory-driven components of cognitive systems, such as attention, memory, and language, in ways that more closely match the distributed neural networks of the human brain.

Clinical neuropsychology as a professional specialty is a fairly recent development, originating in the 1970s. Whereas human neuropsychology is multidisciplinary, involving specialists in experimental, cognitive, and clinical psychology, neurology, psychiatry, linguistics, speech pathology, and neuroscience, clinical neuropsychology is typically practiced by clinical psychologists, who are charged with applying the scientific knowledge derived from human neuropsychological research to the evaluation and treatment of individuals suspected of brain dysfunction. (At the end of this chapter I describe the training, qualifications, and credentialing of clinical neuropsychologists.) The purpose of this chapter, therefore, is to provide an overview of the field of clinical neuropsychological practice. For more detailed discussions of the points raised in this chapter, the reader is referred to textbooks pertaining to clinical neuropsychology (2) or to the scientific field of human neuropsychology (3).

Because of space limitations, this chapter focuses on the assessment of adults. The tests and assessment issues involved in pediatric clinical neuropsychology are sufficiently different that this area could not be covered here in detail. Likewise, this chapter emphasizes the assessment of acquired rather than developmental brain disorders (attention deficit hyperactivity disorder, learning disabilities). Finally, this chapter focuses on assessment, not treatment of neurobehavioral disorders. Several comprehensive textbooks have recently been published that address issues associated with cognitive and behavioral interventions (4–7).

INDICATIONS FOR NEUROPSYCHOLOGICAL ASSESSMENT

The reasons for performing a clinical neuropsychological assessment have broadened over the years. During the 1950s and 1960s, evaluations were frequently performed to address a single question: is the patient experiencing symptoms of "organicity?" In response, clinical psychologists relied on conventional testing instruments, such as the Wechsler intelligence scales, the Bender-Gestalt figure copying test, or personality tests like the Minnesota Multiphasic Personality

Inventory (MMPI) and the Rorschach Inkblot Test. With the proliferation of more specialized neuropsychological procedures, such as the Halstead-Reitan battery in the 1960s, clinicians began to broaden their role and started to vie with the neurological examination and diagnostic procedures of the period (e.g., electroencephalogram, pneumoencephalogram) for localizing lesions within the cerebral hemispheres. With the advent of more sophisticated brain imaging techniques, such as CT in the late 1970s and MRI in the mid-1980s, localization of lesions with neuropsychological testing became less important. Some neuropsychologists began to wonder whether these technological advances would, in fact, eliminate the need for psychological testing of organic brain syndromes.

Subsequent studies have shown the limitations of structural brain imaging in predicting the type and extent of behavioral change in dementing and traumatic brain disorders (8). The emphasis of neuropsychological assessment shifted from lesion localization to a more comprehensive characterization of the patient's cognitive and emotional status. Thus, the more frequently asked referral question is no longer, "Where is the lesion?," but rather "What are the nature and severity of the cognitive and emotional symptoms in this patient with a glioma in the right temporal lobe?"

The applications for neuropsychological testing have widened considerably in recent years. Neuropsychological testing has been used to establish baseline measures to monitor changes in time associated with progressive cerebral diseases (neoplasms, demyelinating, and dementing conditions) or the recovery from acute brain disorders (traumatic head injury, stroke). Neuropsychological testing has also been used as an outcome measure in clinical efficacy trials involving surgical, pharmacological, and behavioral interventions. Examples include both medically oriented treatments (e.g., drug trials, revascularization, tissue excision, shunts) designed to treat specific symptoms or monitor side effects, and psychological treatments (e.g., language or cognitive retraining) oriented to improving various aspects of neurobehavioral functioning. While practical problems do arise in exposing subjects to repeated neuropsychological testing (see discussion of practice effects below), such testing can be a useful adjunct to the neurological examination, brain imaging, and other biologically oriented outcome measures. Neuropsychological testing has the advantage of providing information that may be useful in predicting changes in quality of life, e.g., employment and social adjustment. Furthermore, improvements in brain structure or physiology may be viewed with some skepticism if there is no measurable behavioral change, particularly in the context of a managed health care environment.

In the forensic area, neuropsychological testing has become an important component of civil and criminal cases involving individuals with suspected acquired brain damage. In personal injury lawsuits, the most common of which arise from motor vehicle accidents, neuropsychological testing is frequently the only objective method for describing the neurobehavioral sequelae associated with mild closed head injuries, where CT and MRI may show little if any observable signs of brain damage (8). Testing can also be helpful in establishing whether such individuals are competent to make judgments regarding their medical management, personal finances, and their ability to drive. In criminal cases, neuropsychological assessments have provided assistance in determining if an individual is competent to stand trial or in determining whether a person is not guilty by reason of insanity secondary to acute or chronic brain dysfunction.

Finally, neuropsychological testing can be applied to determine the cognitive and affective status of the patient for formulation and design of rehabilitation and remedial interventions. By defining a patient's strengths and weaknesses, neuropsychological testing also can be useful for educational and vocational planning. Family members and caretakers can experience considerable emotional turmoil in trying to adjust to the neurobehavioral changes of the patient (9) and may require education or psychotherapeutic intervention. Neuropsychological assessment can provide valuable information to family members as they try to cope with the cognitive and emotional changes associated with brain dysfunction. Such an assessment can determine the patient's level of insight and awareness and define his or her readiness and appropriateness for psychotherapy.

NEUROPSYCHOLOGICAL ASSESSMENT APPROACHES

In light of the diverse origins of human neuropsychology and the ever-expanding scientific literature in this field, it is not surprising that there are different philosophies regarding how to conduct a clinical neuropsychological examination. In the developing years of clinical neuropsychology, many clinicians favored a fixed or standard battery of neuropsychological tests, such as the Halstead-Reitan Test Battery (10) or the Luria-Nebraska Battery (11). The standard battery typically takes 3–8 hours to administer and provides a comprehensive assessment of cognitive, perceptual, linguistic, and sensory-motor skills. Normative standards have been generated in healthy individuals, and a large body of research comparing the performance of various patient groups on these batteries has been published (11, 12). The clinical assessment is noninteractive in that the clinician rarely changes the assessment procedures in light of the referring questions or the patient's clinical status. While most clinicians who adapt a battery approach integrate test data with results from a comprehensive psychosocial interview of the patient and family members and from pertinent medical, school, and legal records, others view the test battery as a laboratory procedure that should stand on its own and will interpret results in a "blinded" fashion, i.e. without knowledge of these other sources of clinical information.

The standard battery approach, however, has been criticized on a number of grounds (13, 14). Batteries may not be as comprehensive as their developers had hoped. For example, most clinicians typically supplement the Halstead-

Reitan battery with more comprehensive measures of recent memory. Giving the same procedures to all patients may not be cost-effective when the referral question could be addressed with a shorter examination. The identical battery of tests may not be suitable for all patient groups. For example, the Halstead-Reitan battery consists of several tests that require upper extremity speed and dexterity. The interpretation of such tests in patients who also have brainstem, cerebellar, or spinal cord lesions may be invalid or misleading. Blinded interpretation of test data may be a useful academic exercise but may unnecessarily lead to numerous interpretive errors and result in over- or under-diagnosis of brain dysfunction. Finally, the emphasis in the battery approach is to interpret test scores. This quantitative approach may miss some of the rich qualitative features of the patient's performance, such as errors created by hemi-spatial neglect, motor perseveration, or confabulation.

An alternative approach, advocated initially by Luria (15) and described by Lezak (2), calls for greater flexibility in the selection of neuropsychological tests. The test battery is specifically tailored to the referral question and is influenced by the interview and prior medical and psychosocial records. Thus, an obviously aphasic patient with a CT scan-verified left hemisphere stroke may receive a more comprehensive language assessment than a patient with no obvious signs of aphasia in spontaneous conversation. The testing approach is hypothesis driven and highly interactive. The clinical neuropsychologist may include additional tests based on the performance of the patient on earlier testing to evaluate a specific hypothesis regarding the nature of a cognitive deficit. This testing philosophy also emphasizes a qualitative analysis of test performance, as best exemplified by the Boston process approach (16).

The primary disadvantages of the flexible approach are, in fact, most of the advantages of the fixed battery. A flexible battery may miss an area of neuropsychological impairment that a more comprehensive, fixed battery would detect. The flexible approach relies more heavily on clinical experience and knowledge of the examiner with regard to the testing procedures being used. Finally, clinical research involving group studies of various patient populations is hindered because the same testing procedures are not used across patient groups. As an alternative, several scientific commit-tees have advocated the use of specific test batteries tailored to a particular disease, such as multiple sclerosis (17) or human immunodeficiency virus infection (18). In most cases, most clinical neuropsychologists who advocate a flexible approach give their patients a core battery of tests that provide a brief screen of a wide range of neuropsycho-logical functions, which is then supplemented by further testing, depending on the outcome of the screening battery.

METHODS OF INTERPRETATION

Neuropsychological assessment typically involves an in-tegration of interview data, medical and school records when available, and neuropsychological test data. Determination of the presence, type, and degree of brain dysfunction is based on several inferential methods. The most common methods include measurement of the patient's level of performance, the appearance of pathognomonic signs for brain dysfunction, testing for lateralized brain dysfunction, and a profile analysis that is consistent with known pathology.

Level of Performance

The most common method for inferring brain impair-ment from neuropsychological testing is based on a deficit model (2). This model assumes that cognitive impairment has occurred when a discrepancy is observed between the patient's level of test performance and his or her estimated ability level prior to the onset of brain dysfunction. This method also assumes that the patient's premorbid ability level can be accurately predicted. Rarely, however, does the clinical neuropsychologist have available information re-garding the patient's premorbid cognitive ability level at the time of assessment. School records, when available, may yield pertinent data, such as group-administered intellectual and academic achievement test scores. Such information may indicate an individual's level of functioning relative to a local or national normative standard prior to the onset of brain dysfunction. However, group-administered tests may not provide a measure of optimal ability. Tests of intelligence may also be negatively affected by the presence of a learning disability.

More commonly, the patient's highest level of functioning is inferred indirectly through demographic data or from the current testing session. Several investigators have generated regression formulas from the standardization sample for the Wechsler intelligence scales for calculating premorbid intel-ligence from demographic variables, i.e., sex, age, race, education, occupational status, and region of the country (19–21). Because these predictor sets have less than perfect correlations with intelligence, the estimated IQs generated from these regression equations tend to underestimate deviation from the mean that is most apparent in cases at the extremes of the normal distribution.

An alternative method is to use the patient's current level of performance on tests that are less sensitive to brain dysfunction. Lezak (2) advocated a method whereby the patient's highest performance score on a test battery is used as an estimate of premorbid ability. More recently, clinicians have advocated the use of specialized tests of premorbid intellectual ability. One such test is the National Adult Reading Test (NART) (22, 23). This test assumes that the ability to read words aloud is retained in the presence of cognitive decline. Recent studies have shown, however, that although the NART may provide a reasonably accurate estimate of premorbid ability in mild dementing conditions, NART scores drop significantly with more severe forms of dementia (24). Furthermore, Wiens et al. (25) found that the correlation between the NART-estimated IQ and the Wechsler Full-Scale IQ was relatively low ($r = .46$), result-ing in lower premorbid estimates in the high IQ group and higher estimates in the low IQ group. One is left with the impression that only in circumstances where the neuropathological process does not affect the neural circuitry critical to the "hold" function might this strategy of estimation of premorbid function be useful or appropriate.

Besides the inherent limitations of inferring decline from a level of functioning that is imperfectly predicted, this approach also assumes that the patient's premorbid level of intellectual functioning will be uniform across a wide range of cognitive domains. Intercorrelations between measures of intelligence, attention, memory, and visuospatial abilities are less than perfect in healthy adults. Individuals with a developmental learning disability will be difficult to detect using such premorbid estimation models.

Pathognomonic Signs

An additional method of inferring cognitive decline is based on detection of qualitative changes that are characteristic of specific types of brain dysfunction, particularly in the acute state. Such changes have an extremely low base rate in the normal population. Examples would include the appearance of left-sided neglect, motor perseverations, confabulation, and paraphasic speech. In Figure 3.1, a patient with a midline frontal lobe lesion with a deep extension involving the basal ganglia was asked to copy a design consisting of three connected half-circles. The reproduction demonstrates the inability of the patient to voluntarily stop a motor program after it has begun.

Laterality

The third inferential method involves testing of abilities that imply dysfunction in one cerebral hemisphere relative to the other. Most neuropsychological examinations include measurements of upper extremity motor strength, speed, and coordination as a means of comparing right and left body sides. Assessments of visual, auditory, and tactile perceptual asymmetries are performed for similar purposes. Clinicians also test more complex perceptual and memory processes with verbal and visual test stimuli as a means of inferring lateralized dysfunction. Thus, it is not uncommon to compare a patient's recall of a story (as derived from the Logical Memory subtest of the Wechsler Memory Scale—Revised [WMS-R]) to their recall of a complex geometric design (from the Visual Reproduction subtest of the WMS-R) to determine if there may be selective involvement of the left or right medial temporal lobe, respectively (26).

Profile Analysis

This interpretive approach posits that a neurobehavioral syndrome will demonstrate a fairly specific pattern or profile of deficits on a comprehensive neuropsychological test battery (2). It is assumed that there is consistency in the expression of cognitive functions within an individual. When test scores are converted to a similar metric (standard scores, T scores, percentiles) and plotted, one can readily observe a patient's strengths and weaknesses. A good

example of this approach is employed in the Boston Diagnostic Aphasia Examination (27) in which different test profiles are believed to be indicative of a specific aphasic syndrome (e.g., Broca's vs. Wernicke's vs. anomic aphasia).

ISSUES AFFECTING INTERPRETATION OF NEUROPSYCHOLOGICAL TESTING

Numerous factors can influence or modify the interpretation of neuropsychological testing. In this section, some of the more relevant factors are discussed, including issues pertaining to test reliability and validity, the adequacy of normative standards, motivational factors, the influence of affective disorders and medication effects, the validity of specific neuropsychological tests in patients with sensorimotor dysfunction, the problems of interpretation created by practice effects with repeated testing, and fatigue effects with extended neuropsychological testing.

Test Reliability and Validity

An important issue in psychometric testing is the ability of a test to demonstrate adequate levels of reliability. Reliability can be assessed by examining a test's consistency

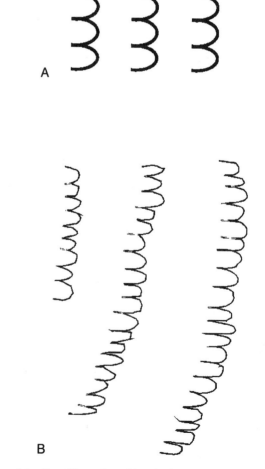

Figure 3.1. Repetitive series writing. **A.** The patient is asked to copy these line drawings. **B.** The patient's copy demonstrates an inability to suppress a motor program once started.

over time or its internal consistency (do all test items assess the same psychological construct?). Whereas tests with high levels of reliability may be insensitive in detecting brain dysfunction, the converse is not true: unreliable measures cannot be valid measures of brain dysfunction.

An important question for all neuropsychological instruments is whether the test is capable of discriminating between healthy individuals and patients with presumed brain dysfunction (test validity). An increasingly important question pertains to whether a test can also discriminate between various groups with brain damage (e.g., frontal lobe degeneration vs. Alzheimer's disease). Whereas a test may demonstrate a statistically significant group difference based on mean scores, one may also ask whether the instrument has *clinical* utility, i.e., can the test be used in making discriminations on a case-by-case basis?

Some neuropsychological tests are allegedly sensitive to brain disruption in a specific brain region (e.g., the frontal lobes). The double dissociation method is a common method for validating such claims. This validation method typically involves two focal lesion groups and two test instruments. According to this procedure, if patients with a lesion in brain region X are impaired on test A but not on test B, and patients with a lesion in region Y are impaired on test B but not on test A, it is assumed that the two tests are selectively sensitive to disruption of each of the separate brain regions. As an example, Heindel and colleagues (28) have shown that patients exhibiting a subcortical dementia from Huntington's disease were impaired on implicit memory measures involving perceptuomotor learning, but performed normally on priming tasks. In contrast, the cortical dementia associated with Alzheimer's disease was found to disrupt priming but not perceptuomotor learning.

Finally, test validity can also involve an evaluation to determine if the neuropsychological test measures the psychological construct (e.g., recent memory) it is purported to evaluate. Factor analysis studies performed on tests of the same construct (e.g., concept formation) can indicate whether they are redundant (i.e., load on a single factor) or tap different constructs. One method for assessing construct validity is to use the multitrait-multimethod approach developed by Campbell and Fiske (29). In this approach, three or more cognitive domains (e.g., recent memory, attention, conceptual reasoning) would be assessed by at least three neuropsychological tests per domain. Tests that use different methods to measure the same cognitive domain should correlate at a higher level than tests that use the same method but test different cognitive domains. This method can be used to establish both convergent and discriminant validity.

Normative Standards

Estimates of cognitive decline require the use of normative data to determine the ranking of the patient's test performance relative to an appropriate peer group. Neuropsychological tests are frequently influenced by age, education, race, socioeconomic status, and, less frequently, sex (30). The effects of these demographic factors can be complex and nonuniform either across or within cognitive domains. For example, numerous studies have demonstrated a reliable age decrement in memory tests that require spontaneous or cued recall of previously presented material (31). In contrast, age differences are much less pronounced when memory is assessed using recognition tasks, which require the subject to discriminate between previously presented information and new material. Presumably, recall tasks require more self-initiated and effortful processing than recognition tasks (32); furthermore, recognition tests also have a large degree of environmental support (i.e., cues) that is absent in recall tests.

The ideal neuropsychological test, therefore, has normative data derived from a large (preferably nationwide), stratified, and randomized standardization sample. Few neuropsychological tests approach this ideal, and in some cases the "norms" are based on a small control sample ($n < 30$) reported in a clinical investigation. Although some neuropsychological tests have well-documented manuals available from the test publishers, other tests in the public domain have norms that are available on a less formal basis. Several textbooks provide norms for the latter tests (2, 12, 33, 34).

Motivational Factors

The outcome of neuropsychological testing can be influenced by the degree of cooperation and effort put forth by the patient. The validity of neuropsychological test performance has recently been called into question in patients seeking financial compensation for injuries (35, 36). Precise prevalence estimates of malingering on neuropsychological testing are unknown, although preliminary data from personal injury and workers' compensation cases suggest rates of 47–64% (36). To compound this issue, several investigations have found that neuropsychologists were unable to discriminate between neuropsychological test protocols of patients without financial incentives from subjects asked by the investigators to simulate cognitive deficits (37, 38). It should be noted that the neuropsychologists in these studies were blinded to interview data and medical records.

In recent years, neuropsychologists have tried to improve the accuracy of detecting malingering by applying specialized testing procedures. In her textbook, Lezak (2) advocated the use of Rey's (1964) 15-Item Memory Test. For this test, the patient is presented 15 items on a sheet of paper and asked to reproduce the items from memory after a 10-second exposure interval (see Fig. 3.2). The instructions emphasize the large number of items to be recalled. The actual amount of information required to correctly recall items in this array, however, is small and within span memory. In fact, a majority of patients with brain impairments are capable of recalling at least two of the rows in the correct order. Figure 3.2B demonstrates the performance of a suspected malingerer. Although this test has been criticized for having low

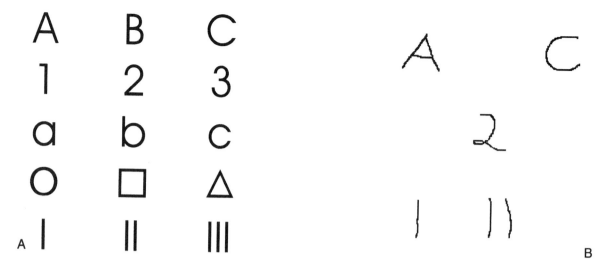

Figure 3.2.   15-Item Test. **A.** The patient is shown this design for 10 seconds. The design is removed and the patient is given a blank piece of paper and asked to draw the design from memory. **B.** This drawing is from a patient suspected of malingering.

sensitivity (4–22%) (36), a recent study (39), using a cutoff score of less than two correct rows, yielded acceptable sensitivity and specificity values in the 47–64% and 96–97% ranges, respectively, in discriminating patients with neurological impairments from subjects instructed to feign memory impairment.

An alternative method for assessing malingering, referred to as symptom-validity testing (40), involves a two-choice, multi-trial sensory or memory testing format where the chance of obtaining a correct response is typically 50%. Malingerers are expected to perform below chance levels as determined from the binomial probability for wrong responses. Thus, a subject who obtains only 10% correct is felt to be feigning impairment. One such technique, the Portland Digit Recognition Test (41), consists of a forced-choice measure of recognition memory. Numerous studies have examined the sensitivity and specificity of this test. Using the below-chance criterion, low sensitivity rates (less than 35% of simulators) have been achieved (36). Cutoff scores that are less restrictive (90% correct), however, have produced higher sensitivity rates for detection of feigned memory loss without lowering specificity rates (42).

Affective Disorders

Patients with major affective disorders may exhibit potentially reversible cognitive decline on neuropsychological testing. Weingartner and his colleagues (43) have proposed a central motivational hypothesis to account for the memory disorders observed on neuropsychological testing in depressed patients. According to this hypothesis, depressed patients will perform poorly on tests requiring high degrees of mental effort, such as on free recall tests, but perform normally on memory tests that are more automatic and requiring less effort, as in recognition testing formats or incidental learning tasks. Using an incidental memory task as a modification of the Digit Symbol subtest of the WAIS-R, Hart and colleagues (44) were able to successfully classify

elderly patients under neuropsychological evaluation to differentiate Alzheimer's disease from pseudodementia.

Some investigators view the effects of major depression as not simply a complication in interpreting neuropsychological testing. Evidence has accumulated that some patients with major affective disorders may be experiencing a form of subcortical dementia, which may have correlates with changes on structural and functional neuroimaging (45). There also appears to be an interaction between age and depressive mood state and cognitive decline (46). Finally, there is some evidence that the cognitive decline is not reversed with treatment of depression (47). Thus, it is often difficult to determine whether depression is a normal psychological reaction to chronic physical illness or part of a specific neurobehavioral syndrome associated with brain dysfunction (48).

Medication Effects

A variety of prescription medications can have an impact on cognitive functioning and thereby alter the interpretation of neuropsychological testing (for a review, see Weingartner et al. [49, 50]). Examples of such drug classes include: antidepressants with significant anticholinergic side effects (e.g., amitriptyline), anticonvulsants (particularly phenobarbital), anxiolytics (particularly the benzodiazepines), and the antipsychotic agents. In addition, various drugs of abuse (alcohol, stimulants, cocaine, heroine, cannabinol, and nicotine to mention a few) can have short- and long-term effects on cognitive test performance. Typically, these effects are most often observed on measures of attention, memory, information processing speed, and fine motor dexterity.

Sensorimotor Dysfunction

Many neuropsychological tests that assess higher cognitive functions make the assumption that patients have adequate primary sensory and motor functions to perform the task. Many neurological and nonneurological conditions produce sensorimotor impairment from disease or trauma, with the greatest impact occurring outside the cerebral hemispheres. For example, patients with severe rheumatoid arthritis will perform worse on the performance subtests of the WAIS-R because of an inability to manipulate the test stimuli in a speeded fashion. Patients with multiple sclerosis will experience visual and tactile sensory loss or motor impairment from white matter lesions, affecting the optic nerve, brainstem, spinal cord, or cerebellum. Such lesions should have little or no effect on cognitive processes, but can reduce performance scores on cognitive tests, particularly those that demand motor speed/dexterity or fine visual acuity (51). Despite these obvious limitations, it is not unusual for inexperienced neuropsychological clinicians to administer an extensive test battery to patients with sensorimotor deficits and attempt to infer cognitive impairment.

Several methods are available to address these interpretive problems. Clinicians knowledgeable of the nature of the primary sensorimotor deficit will attempt to select neuropsychological tests that provide unambiguous test findings. As an example, paper and pencil tests may be avoided in favor of tests that require a vocal response. When information regarding the speed of cognitive processing is required, tests that use the identical motor response across a range of conditions varying in cognitive complexity can provide useful information. For example, subtracting timed scores on Trails A from Trails B, tests of visual search and sequencing of different levels of cognitive difficulty, may be a more valid approach than comparing each test score separately to normative standards.

Practice Effects

As noted previously, neuropsychological testing has been used to monitor changes in a patient's status over time or as an outcome variable to evaluate various forms of treatment interventions. Several studies (52–58) have demonstrated that repeated neuropsychological testing results in improvements in test scores in both normal and brain-damaged populations. Practice effects, as they have come to be known, can present challenges in test interpretation. For example, a patient may obtain an identical score on a test administered 6 months apart. From this data, it is unclear whether the patient's status is unchanged or if a deterioration occurred that was canceled out by an improvement associated with practice.

Why practice effects occur is unclear. Some clinicians have assumed that practice effects result from the explicit and conscious recollection of the identical test stimuli. If this is the case, it might follow that practice effects will be minimized after longer retest intervals (greater than 1 year) due to normal forgetting from long-term memory. Furthermore, practice effects could be eliminated over shorter intervals by constructing alternate test forms of equivalent difficulty. Unfortunately, most of the studies just cited used brief retest intervals and did not use alternate, equivalent test forms. In a recently completed study (59), both assumptions have been shown to be incorrect. Practice effects were demonstrated after a 3-year retest period in the majority of test scores derived from a lengthy neuropsychological test battery. Additionally, alternate equivalent test forms, administered in counterbalanced fashion, did not appear to eliminate the effect. These data suggest that practice effects do not entirely result from the explicit recall of identical test stimuli, but occur as a function of learning how to take a test. This type of procedural or implicit memory may be more resistant to decay over time than explicit memory.

To address the problem of practice effects, manuals for neuropsychological tests might also include retest norms for various follow-up periods. In group treatment studies that use neuropsychological outcome measures, it is highly recommended that a yoked control group be incorporated into the experimental design. This control group would be administered the identical battery of neuropsychological tests at the same time intervals as the group of interest. In this way, standardized corrections of test scores could be accomplished at each test period and a genuine change in test performance could be appreciated.

Fatigue Effects and Duration of Testing

A common complaint about neuropsychological testing is the length of testing, which for fixed batteries like the Halstead-Reitan battery can extend over a 6–8 hour period. Patients frequently experience fatigue and reduced motivation at the end of a lengthy testing session. These effects may potentially influence the validity of such tests. To counteract this problem, most neuropsychologists administer tests that are most likely to be influenced by fatigue (e.g., attention and memory) at the beginning of the test session.

A related question concerns the need for extended testing to perform a reliable, valid, and clinically meaningful assessment. This issue is becoming more important in an era where cost containment of medical and psychological procedures is being carefully scrutinized. Clinical neuropsychologists who adopt a flexible approach to testing tend to tailor the amount of testing to answer the referral questions, while also taking into consideration the capacity of the patient to tolerate an extended examination. Thus, it may not make a great deal of sense to subject an elderly patient in the middle to late stages of Alzheimer's disease to an extended examination when the referral question is a relatively simple one, i.e., to determine if the patient has deteriorated cognitively from the previous evaluation 6 months ago.

On the other hand, the same patient presenting at an earlier stage of the illness may display symptoms of mild memory loss in the context of a clinical depression. An evaluation at this stage of the disease is more complicated because the cognitive deficits may be subtle or confined to a single domain, such as memory. Furthermore, more complicated questions arise regarding the patient's capacity to work, drive, and make financial decisions. The outcome of this neuropsychological evaluation may assist in determining whether the patient has a potentially treatable disorder (depression) or a progressive dementing illness. Thus, the length of neuropsychological testing will likely increase with the complexity of the referral question and the associated risk of making errors in interpretation.

Several investigators have developed screening examinations for quickly assessing cognitive functions at the bedside (60). The most commonly used screening instrument, the Mini-Mental State Examination (MMSE) (61), is brief (5–10 minutes), can be administered by a health care professional without psychological training, and yields a single score that minimizes interpretative skills. Unfortunately, the MMSE is insensitive to most of the milder forms of cognitive dysfunction or to dementing disorders affecting primarily subcortical structures (62). The Mattis Dementia Rating Scale (63) addresses many of the criticisms of the MMSE, but takes longer to administer and requires greater psychological expertise to administer and interpret.

SPECIFIC NEUROPSYCHOLOGICAL TESTING PROCEDURES

This section describes the neurobehavioral areas typically assessed in a neuropsychological examination. Standardized tests most commonly used by neuropsychologists in clinical practice are described here. In addition, newly developed standardized tests are described along with occasional experimental measures that hold promise as clinical assessment tools, but have not as yet been standardized.

Intelligence

Neuropsychological assessments typically begin with a measurement of intellectual functioning. The most common test used in clinical practice is the Wechsler Adult Intelligence Scale-Revised (WAIS-R) (64), which consists of six verbal and five performance subtests. Three intelligence quotients, a Full-Scale, Verbal, and Performance IQ, are derived. A major advantage of this test is its large, stratified, normative database, which corrects for age differences. Comparisons of tested IQ values with premorbid IQ estimates (from demographic variables or tests like the NART, as noted earlier) can be achieved to obtain a gross measure of the degree of cognitive deterioration. A major disadvantage of this test is that it was designed to provide a measure of an individual's general ability levels. Consequently, performance on each subtest is influenced by multiple cognitive operations. A low score on a subtest like Block Design may result from deficits in focused or lateralized attention, general planning and organizational skills, visuospatial perception, constructional abilities, psychomotor slowing, or primary sensorimotor impairment. Thus, while the intelligence measures may be sensitive, they lack specificity for understanding the reasons why an individual may perform in an impaired fashion. Recent attempts to modify the examination process to extract the qualitative features of the patient's test performance (65)

may address this limitation to some degree, although most clinicians will continue to supplement the WAIS-R with more specific neuropsychological tests.

In addition to comparing estimated versus actual IQ test scores, clinicians will frequently examine various patterns of test performance. One such method is to compare the Verbal and Performance IQ scores as a measure of lateralized brain dysfunction. Whereas low Verbal relative to Performance IQ scores are suggestive of left hemisphere damage, the opposite pattern (low Performance relative to Verbal IQ) is thought to be indicative of right hemisphere damage. Group studies of patients with lateralized lesions generally support this test pattern (66), although the effect is attenuated in females (67) and in patients with more chronic lesions (66). Still, it is easy to find clinical examples of patients who are misdiagnosed by this index (e.g., patients with subcortical pathology, nondominant parietal lobe lesions). It should be noted that Verbal-Performance IQ differences by as much as 15 points can occur in 20% of college-educated, healthy individuals (68). Caution should therefore be exercised in interpreting this index, unless there is a large Verbal-Performance IQ discrepancy (>21 points).

Another method of interpretation involves an analysis of inter-subtest scatter. Individual subtests of the WAIS-R are standardized with a mean of 10, a standard deviation of 3, and a range from 1 to 19. Scatter analysis is achieved by comparing the highest and lowest scores of the 11 subtests. An implicit assumption is that the highest scores reflect premorbid skill levels, whereas the lowest scores are indicative of brain dysfunction. Matarazzo et al. (69) have shown that scatter is common in the WAIS-R standardization sample. Typically, a scatter of at least 9–12 points, depending on the Full-Scale IQ level, is necessary to be clinically significant (defined as less than the 5th percentile).

A final method of interpretation involves an examination of intra-subtest scatter. Most of the subtests of the WAIS-R are composed of items that become progressively more difficult. It is assumed that healthy individuals will begin to fail portions of the test abruptly as they approach the upper end of their ability level. In contrast, patients with brain damage, particularly those of high premorbid ability, may pass difficult items at the end of the subtest, but fail easy items at the beginning. Several investigators (70, 71) have developed various indices of intra-subtest scatter and have shown that it may be useful in discriminating some types of brain dysfunction.

As noted before, results from the WAIS-R Performance subtests may be of questionable validity in some patient groups due to the emphasis on upper extremity motor speed. Patients with cervical spinal cord injuries or rheumatoid arthritis, for example, may achieve lower than expected IQ scores because they were unable to obtain "bonus" points for rapidly manipulating the test stimuli. As an alternative, some clinicians will generate a nonverbal IQ from administering the Raven's Standard Progressive Matrices (72), which has been shown to be sensitive to various forms of brain damage (2).

Conceptual Reasoning and Executive Functions

Neuropsychological assessments have traditionally included measurement of nonverbal, abstract thinking or concept formation. The two most common tasks used in this regard are the Wisconsin Card Sorting Test (WCST) (73, 74) and the Category Test (75). The WCST, in particular, is used by over 70% of practicing neuropsychologists (76). Both measures are sensitive to cerebral dysfunction in neurological (77–82) and psychiatric (78, 83–85) disorders. The WCST is viewed as a measure particularly sensitive to focal frontal lobe dysfunction. Several studies have found a greater number of WCST perseverative errors in patients with frontal lobe lesions than those with nonfrontal lesions (79, 86, 87), although this relationship has not been uniformly observed (88, 89).

Error scores on the WCST and the Category Test are correlated on a statistical basis, but share only 12–30% of the common test variance. A recent study by Perrine (90) suggests that the two tests may emphasize different concept formation operations. Specifically, the WCST may be related to the identification of stimulus attributes, whereas the Category Test involves a greater degree of rule learning. Not surprisingly, therefore, the Category Test has a stronger correlation with the Wechsler Full-Scale IQ than the WCST (80) and is more likely to be influenced by premorbid intellectual ability.

Conceptual reasoning may be subsumed under a broader category of cognitive operations, commonly referred to as executive functions. Executive functions reflect the "ability to spontaneously generate efficient strategies when relying on self-directed and task-specific planning" (91). According to Shallic and Burgess (92), executive or supervisory functions involve planning or decision making that requires error-correction or troubleshooting, resulting in the performance of novel sequences of actions that overcome strong habitual responses. The frontal lobes are assumed to be the critical structures involved in the performance of executive functions. Clinically, patients with executive disorders exhibit perseveration (an inability to stop a sequence of actions once begun), a loss of initiative or intention to act, an inability to generate plans, a tendency to act impulsively, and problems incorporating feedback in modifying their behavior.

A wide variety of tasks have been used to tap this diverse cluster of cognitive abilities. Some, like the Tower of Hanoi or the Tower of London (93, 94), require patients to rearrange blocks from an initial position into a goal position in a minimum number of moves. Verbal (95) and design (96) fluency tasks assess the ability of the patient to spontaneously generate items consistent with established rules. The Porteus Maze Test (97) assesses the patient's ability to trace the correct path through a maze. Copying repetitive line drawings (multiple loops; see Fig. 3.1) or recurrent series writing *("mnomnomno")* can be used to assess motor perseveration (15). Finally, executive functions can involve the ability to plan, follow, arrange, or recall the temporal order or sequence of events. Frontal lobe patients,

for example, may experience problems in judging which of two stimuli was presented more recently, but have little or no impairment on recognition testing in which the patient must discriminate whether a stimulus was or was not presented previously (98). Tasks that require patients to generate a script (99) that describes the sequence of events they would perform, for example, in getting ready for work in the morning or selecting and attending a restaurant, may prove useful in understanding the executive deficits of patients and may also provide useful information for developing meaningful rehabilitation strategies.

Executive functions are also associated with the patient's ability to evaluate the accuracy of their own performance. Some patients with brain damage, particularly those with severe impairment, show little or no awareness of deficits (i.e., anosognosia), despite profound cognitive deficits (100). Patients can be particularly impaired in rating their memory ability. This ability, referred to as metamemory, can be assessed by asking patients to rate their confidence in recalling or recognizing previously-presented material. Such testing can be performed in conjunction with standardized memory testing.

Attention

Attention is frequently impaired in neurological disorders and may be the primary area of cognitive dysfunction in psychiatric disorders, like schizophrenia (101). Attention can be segregated into focal, sustained, and divided processes (102). Focused attention refers to the process of searching for, and locating target stimuli. Sustained attention, sometimes used interchangeably with the term vigilance, refers to the monitoring of target stimuli over an extended duration of time. Divided attention refers to the ability to perform two tasks simultaneously. Most neuropsychological tests of attention used in clinical practice assess one or more of these attentional components.

Some attentional measures emphasize speed of information processing. Slowing frequently occurs in patients with symptoms of a subcortical dementia (103). One of the commonly used tests in clinical practice, the Trail Making Test (10), requires the patient to "connect the dots" using a paper and pencil format. Two forms are administered: Trails A involves a simple numerical series, while Trails B alternates between a numerical and alphabetical series. Although norms are available for time to completion for each form, a pure measure of mental processing speed with increasing task complexity can be achieved by subtracting Trails A from B, since the same motor response is used for both conditions. The Stroop Test (104) also has multiple forms of increasing complexity. Unlike the Trails Test, which examines primarily focused and divided attention (alternation of two series), the Stroop Test assesses the patient's vulnerability to interference effects (focused attention). In the simpler (control) conditions of this test, patients are timed while either reading a list of color word names printed in black or while reading the color name to a series of identical nonverbal stimuli printed in various colors. In the interference condition, a series of color words is printed in colors different from what the word represents (e.g., the word "blue" is printed in the color green). The patient is asked to name the color the word is printed in rather than read the word. Healthy subjects typically take longer to complete the interference task than the control tasks. Norms are available for assessing abnormally long interference effects in patient populations (33). Another sensitive test of mental processing speed with excellent norms and allowing either an oral or written test format is the Symbol Digit Modalities Test (105).

Although reaction time tasks take longer to administer, some clinicians prefer them to distinguish mental from motor processing speed. One method involves comparing reaction times from simple (one-choice) versus complex (multi-choice) stimulus presentations. The same motor response is required for all conditions, enabling a subtraction of the simple from complex reaction times. Similarly, the Sternberg paradigm (106) has been used to demonstrate slowing of mental processing in patients with substantial motor impairment, i.e., Parkinson's disease (107) and multiple sclerosis (108). For this task, the patient must hold

a digit sequence of varying length (1 to 5 digits) in working memory and decide whether a single probe digit presented on a computer screen matches one of the numbers in memory. Most individuals achieve better than 95% correct on this task. Reaction times, however, increase linearly with the number of digits held in memory. Abnormal slowing is demonstrated by a steeper slope than in healthy individuals.

Other attentional measures emphasize accuracy of performance, such as the Paced Auditory Serial Addition Test (109). This demanding test requires the patient to add consecutive single-digit numbers presented at rates ranging from about one every second to one every 3 seconds. The test does not require a cumulative tally, but rather addition of the current digit with the immediately preceding digit. This test has been particularly sensitive to the subtle attentional problems observed in patients with mild head injury (109) and multiple sclerosis (62).

Finally, some attentional tasks have been designed to assess unilateral spatial neglect. Two of the more common include the Letter Cancellation (110) and Line Bisection (111) tasks. For the Cancellation tasks, the patient must

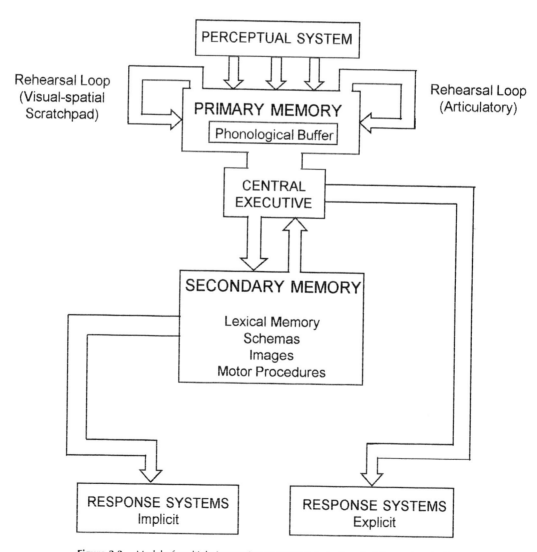

Figure 3.3. Model of multiple interacting memory systems (see text for explanation).

cross out with a pencil specified letters (e.g., C's and E's) from an array of letters presented on a piece of paper. The number of omissions and commissions, as well as the total time to completion, are recorded for this task. The Line Bisection task requires the patient to mark the middle of 20 horizontally arranged lines that are centered in the left, right, or center of the page. Deviation from the true center of the lines is recorded. Patients with left-sided hemineglect will typically make more omission errors on the left side of the stimulus array than on the right on the Letter Cancellation task or will mark the center of the line to the right of midline on the Line Bisection task.

Memory

The theoretical and empirical underpinnings of assessing memory impairment are described in detail in Chapter 18. Briefly, one view of memory (112) posits that information flows "linearly" from sensory input to a limited-capacity store, referred to as primary (short-term) memory (see Fig. 3.3). Primary memory is defined as the information processing system dedicated to the temporary storage of information. Information held in primary memory is lost to conscious awareness if not immediately rehearsed. This system is hypothesized to include postperceptual storage of information, rehearsal mechanisms required to reactivate information for greater processing, and consolidation processes. Each part of this memory system has capacity and speed of processing constraints. Clinically, this system can be assessed by using tasks that measure the amount of information that can be briefly held in short-term store, such as the Digit Span subtest of the WAIS-R, or the rate of forgetting from short-term storage using the Brown-Peterson task (113, 114). More experimental procedures, developed by Baddeley and colleagues (115), have examined the effects of a parallel task load upon temporary storage and rehearsal mechanisms in short-term store (referred to as working memory), although such tasks have not as yet been applied routinely to clinical assessment.

Secondary (long-term) memory represents a larger-capacity, more permanent store of newly acquired information that has been consolidated from primary memory. Both recent and remote personal information and historical events are considered part of secondary memory. The preponderance of published memory studies typically evaluate secondary memory impairment. Tasks that assess secondary memory typically ask the patient to recall or recognize units of information that exceed the capacity of primary memory (i.e., at least 8 or 9 units). The importance of the distinction between span and supraspan stimulus presentations is illustrated by the "memory cliff" associated with increasing the number of digits beyond the patients maximal digit capacity (116). The most commonly employed secondary memory tasks used in clinical practice involve the immediate and delayed (typically 30–60 minutes) recall of a paragraph-length story, such as the Logical Memory subtest of the Wechsler Memory Scale-Revised (117). The delayed recall score enables the examiner to assess the rate of forgetting from secondary memory.

Secondary memory can also be evaluated by examining word list learning on multitrial stimulus presentations. Capacity for learning with repeated stimulus presentations can be assessed with such free recall tasks. In addition, delayed free recall, cued recall, and recognition memory are also typically assessed. Recognition memory tests are useful for examining the relative contributions of encoding/storage versus retrieval failure to secondary memory impairment. It is assumed that if a patient is unable to spontaneously recall an item of information, but can successfully discriminate this item in a list combining old and new information, then the item must have entered into long-term storage. Hence the patient's deficits occur primarily in gaining access to information in long-term store. The most common list-learning tests used in clinical practice include the Rey Auditory-Verbal Learning Test (118), the California Verbal Learning Test (119), and the Buschke Selective Reminding Test (120). The Selective Reminding Test has the advantage of differentiating words recalled from primary vs. secondary memory (121). The California Verbal Learning Test also assesses the patient's ability to use semantic clustering to aid encoding.

Since the early discovery by Milner and colleagues (26) that right temporal lobectomy produces a selective *visuospatial* memory impairment, whereas a left temporal lobectomy results in a memory loss for *verbal* material, most clinical neuropsychologists assess nonverbal as well as verbal memory. The most commonly used tests of nonverbal memory are the Benton Visual Retention Test (122), the Visual Reproduction subtests of the Wechsler Memory Scale—Revised, and the Rey-Osterrieth Complex Figure Test (118). These tests require the patient to copy from memory a previously presented geometric design and have excellent norms, but may be invalid in patients with a constructional apraxia or in patients with primary motor impairment, such as ataxia or hemiplegia. As an alternative, we have adapted Barbizet and Cany's (123) 7/24 Spatial Recall Test for clinical practice (118, 124). This task requires the patient to reproduce a design generated with seven checkers presented on a 6 × 4 checkerboard. The structure of the checkerboard reduces the perceptual demands of the test. In addition, this test can be administered to motor-impaired patients with the capability of pointing to the appropriate squares and having the examiner place the checkers. A more demanding variation of the 7/24 test, called the Visual Spatial Learning Test, has also recently been developed (125).

All of the secondary memory tasks used in these studies were designed to measure the patient's conscious and explicit recollection of factual material. Recent studies have suggested that there is an alternate memory system in which learning is expressed implicitly (126). On implicit memory tasks, such as motor skill acquisition (e.g., pursuit rotor task) or priming (e.g., stem-completion task), patients with global amnesia have been found to perform normally (127, 128).

As noted previously, an interesting double dissociation has been noted in two dementing conditions: patients with Huntington's disease exhibit deficits in motor skill learning (129) but have normal priming (128), while patients with Alzheimer's disease have the opposite pattern of deficits, abnormal priming (130), and intact motor skill learning (129). While of considerable theoretical interest, experimental tests of implicit memory have not been routinely administered in clinical assessments.

Language

Aphasia is a common symptom of focal dominant hemisphere lesions as well as diffuse cerebral dysfunction. The assessment of aphasia typically involves an evaluation of spontaneous speech, repetition, comprehension, naming, reading, and writing. Several comprehensive aphasia batteries have been developed over the years, including the Boston Diagnostic Aphasia Examination (27), Western Aphasia Battery (131), Multilingual Aphasia Examination (132), Illinois Test of Psycholinguistic Ability (133), and the Porch Index of Communicative Ability (134). Reitan's Aphasia Screening Test (135) provides a less thorough language assessment, but can be administered rapidly. More specific language tasks include the Token Test (136) to assess verbal comprehension of commands of increasing difficulty, the Boston Naming Test (137) to assess the ability to name pictured objects, and the Peabody Picture Vocabulary Test—Revised (138) to assess auditory comprehension of picture names. As mentioned in a previous section, the Controlled Oral Word Association Test (95) (also known as the Word Fluency or F-A-S test), which assesses spontaneous generation of words beginning with a given letter within a limited amount of time, is impaired in nonaphasic patients with left frontal lobe lesions (139).

Perception

An assessment of higher perceptual processes is commonly included in a comprehensive neuropsychological evaluation. Agnosia is classically defined as a failure to recognize a percept that cannot be accounted for by defects in elementary sensory function. The correct interpretation of perceptual tasks, therefore, cannot be made unless more primary sensory data are collected using screening tests of visual, auditory, tactile, and olfactory function either during the neuropsychological examination (e.g., visual field assessment through bedside confrontation, two-point tactile stimulation) or from specialized diagnostic procedures performed by other specialties (e.g., formal perimetric visual field testing, audiometric testing). Double simultaneous stimulation can frequently identify patients experiencing a mild, residual neglect that may not be observed during unilateral presentations.

The most common tests for assessing visuospatial perception include the Benton Facial Recognition Test (95), Benton Line Orientation Test (95), Hidden Figures Test (140), and Hooper Visual Organization Test (141). The first three of these tests use a recognition format, and the fourth examines visual organization processes by having patients name fragmented objects. The Halstead-Reitan Battery (10) contains several tests of tactile perception, including the Finger Localization Test, Tactile Form Perception (stereognosis), Fingertip Number-Writing Perception, and the Tactual Performance Test. Two tests from the Halstead-Reitan Battery, the Seashore Rhythm Test and the Speech-Sounds Perception Test, are also used to assess auditory perception, although the diagnostic validity of these tests has recently been called into question (142). The dichotic listening task is used routinely in several medical centers. In this task, different speech or nonverbal auditory stimuli are presented simultaneously to both ears (143). Unilateral brain damage (144) or lesions involving the corpus callosum (145) may be inferred if a large deviation from the normal right ear accuracy advantage for speech sounds is observed. Smell perception can also be assessed using bedside techniques (146).

Praxis and Motor Dexterity

Apraxia is a disorder of skilled movements that cannot be accounted for by primary motor dysfunction (diminished strength, speed, and coordination), sensory loss, impaired language comprehension, or inattention to commands. Lesion (147) and functional imaging (148) studies point to the motor association cortex (premotor and supplementary motor areas) and the parietal cortex, particularly of the left hemisphere, as critical brain structures in performing skilled movements. Testing for apraxia involves an assessment of the motor system at the highest level of programming. Specialized screening batteries have been developed for assessing limb apraxia (149, 150); these batteries require the production of gestures to command and/or imitation.

Constructional apraxia is frequently associated with parietal lobe lesions, although it can also occur with frontal lesions. Clinical assessments consist of asking patients to copy designs from a two- or three-dimensional model or to spontaneously generate common objects, such as a house, a clock, or a daisy. More commonly used tests include the Bender Gestalt Test (151), the copy forms of the Rey-Osterrieth Complex Figure and the Benton Visual Retention Test, the Block Design subtest of the Wechsler intelligence tests, and the Benton Test of Three-Dimensional Constructional Praxis (95).

To determine the integrity of *primary* motor functions, neuropsychological assessments also include tests of strength, speed, and coordination involving the upper extremities. Tests derived from the Halstead-Reitan Battery (10) can be used to assess motor strength (Hand Dynamometer Test), speed (Finger Tapping Test), and coordination (Grooved Pegboard Test). The Purdue Pegboard Test (2) is also used to measure motor coordination. In addition to these three tests, the Wisconsin Motor Battery (34) also includes measures of maze coordination and static steadiness. Such tests can provide useful information regarding the absolute level of performance as well as the degree of lateralized impairment.

Academic Achievement

A common complaint of patients is an impairment in their ability to read, spell, or calculate as well as they had prior to the onset of brain damage. Although academic achievement tests have been developed specifically for assessing developmental learning disorders, they can also be useful in evaluating and understanding acquired cognitive deficits in the academic skill areas. The most commonly used tests in neuropsychological assessments include the Woodcock-Johnson Psycho-Educational Battery—Revised (152) and the Wide Range Achievement Test—3 (153).

Personality and Socioadaptive Functions

Personality change is one of the most common and debilitating symptoms associated with acquired brain disorders (9, 154, 155). Such changes can occur as a direct result of the brain damage or disease, a psychological reaction to experiencing a chronic injury/disease, premorbid personality characteristics, or a combination of these factors. Common interpersonal problems resulting directly from brain dysfunction include loss of impulse control, insensitivity, emotional lability, irritability, loss of self-awareness, lack of initiative, euphoria, and an inability to profit from experience. Patients with brain damage can also experience emotional reactions to their disability, including anger, anxiety, denial, dependency, repression, and depression. The development of psychometric instruments for assessing personality change in neurological disorders has lagged behind the development of instruments for assessing cognition.

One of the most common techniques for assessing personality involves patient self-ratings. The Minnesota Multiphasic Personality Inventory (MMPI), which has been recently restandardized (156), is frequently used in the evaluation of personality and emotional status in neurological patients. More specialized tests for depression, such as the Beck Depression Inventory (157) and the Zung Depression Scale (158), and for anxiety, such as the State-Trait Anxiety Inventory (159), are also employed. Several problems can occur, however, when interpreting these scales in populations with brain damage, since these tests were standardized on psychiatric populations. For example, numerous items on these scales (the MMPI in particular) assess valid symptoms of neurological or systemic diseases (17, 160), thereby giving inflated estimates of psychopathology in patients with neurological problems. Self-rating scales may also lack validity in patients who experience gross changes in personal insight and self-awareness (4).

An alternative method of assessing personality change is

to use relative ratings, which can also be compared to self-reported symptoms. One such instrument, the Katz Adjustment Scale (161), has been used with success in evaluating interpersonal problems of patients with neurological deficits from the perspective of a close relative or friend. Such information can be invaluable for developing a psychological intervention program. Finally, standardized instruments developed from structured psychiatric interviews (see Chapter 2) of the patient can provide useful information about the patient's socioadaptive capabilities and can also be applied to treatment planning.

NEUROPSYCHOLOGICAL ASSESSMENT OF NEUROBEHAVIORAL DISORDERS

Over the past 20 years countless neuropsychological studies have been conducted relating to a wide range of neurological and neuropsychiatric disorders. A detailed discussion of the applications of neuropsychological assessment to specific disorders is beyond the scope of this chapter. The reader is referred to recent integrative reviews of the neuropsychological research in cerebrovascular disease—some in this textbook (Chapter 37; 162), head injury (Chapter 39; 163, 164), Alzheimer's disease (Chapter 36; 165), Parkinson's disease (166) and other basal ganglia disorders (Chapter 36), Huntington's disease (165), multiple sclerosis (167) and other white matter disorders (168), progrssive supranuclear palsy (169), amnesic disorders (170), neoplasms (165), neurotoxic disorders (171), alcohol and drug abuse, epilepsy (172), human immunodeficiency virus infection (173), schizophrenia (174), affective disorders (48), and anxiety disorders.

QUALIFICATIONS TO PRACTICE CLINICAL NEUROPSYCHOLOGY

The practice of clinical neuropsychology is fairly new in the health care delivery system. Prior to 1980, training in neuropsychology was limited to a few doctoral programs and clinical internships. It was not uncommon for clinical psychologists in clinical practice to take brief workshops on neuropsychological assessment and, without a comprehensive knowledge of the behavioral neurosciences or clinical neurology, begin assessing patients with neuropsychological test procedures. Recognizing the need to identify qualified neuropsychological practitioners, the American Board of Professional Psychology in 1983, in conjunction with the newly formed American Board of Clinical Neuropsychology (175), identified clinical neuropsychology as a specialty area and developed an examination process to evaluate the training, knowledge, and skills of psychologists specializing in neuropsychology. At present, there are over 200 board-certified clinical neuropsychologists in North America.

The training of clinical neuropsychologists has also expanded rapidly in recent years. At a recent survey, there were 26 doctoral training programs, 39 predoctoral internships, and 48 postdoctoral fellowship programs providing specialty training in neuropsychology (176). In 1987, a task force sponsored by the International Neuropsychological Society (INS) and the neuropsychology division of the American Psychological Association (APA) developed guidelines for education and training at the doctoral, internship, and postdoctoral level (177). To evaluate and accredit postdoctoral training programs and to determine if these programs are meeting the INS/APA guidelines, the Association of Postdoctoral Programs in Clinical Neuropsychology was recently formed (178). The work of such committees is necessary to ensure that the clinical neuropsychological assessment is conducted by highly qualified, trained, and competent professionals. In this way, the consumers, i.e., the patient, family members, referring physicians, mental health professionals, teachers, and attorneys, can be assured of the highest quality of neuropsychological services.

Acknowledgments

The author appreciates the critical suggestions of this chapter provided by T.A. Hammeke and S.J. Swanson.

References

1. Benton A. Evolution of a clinical specialty. Clinical Neuropsychologist 1987;1:5–8.
2. Lezak MD. Neuropsychological assessment. 3rd ed. New York: Oxford University Press, 1995.
3. Kolb B, Whishaw IQ. Fundamentals of human neuropsychology. New York: W.H. Freeman & Co., 1990.
4. Prigatano GP, Schacter DL. Awareness of deficits after brain injury: clinical and theoretical issues. New York: Oxford University Press, 1992.
5. Meier MJ, Benton AL, Diller LD. Neuropsychological rehabilitation. New York: Guilford Press, 1987.
6. Wilson BA. Rehabilitation of memory. New York: Guilford Press, 1987.
7. Sohlberg MM, Mateer CA. Introduction to cognitive rehabilitation: theory and practice. New York: Guilford Publications, 1989.
8. Charletta DA, Bennett DA, Wilson RS. Computed tomography and magnetic resonance imaging. In: Parks RW, Zec RF, Wilson RS, eds. Neuropsychology of Alzheimer's disease and other dementias. New York: Oxford University Press, 1993:534–561.
9. Lezak MD. Living with the characterologically altered brain injured patient. J Clin Psychiatry 1978;39:592–598.
10. Reitan RM, Davison LA. Clinical neuropsychology: current status and applications. New York: John Wiley & Sons, 1974.
11. Golden CJ, Hammeke TA, Purisch AD. Luria-Nebraska Neuropsychological Battery. Los Angeles: Western Psychological Services, 1976.
12. Heaton RK, Grant I, Matthews CG. Comprehensive norms for an expanded Halstead-Reitan Battery: demographic corrections, research findings, and clinical applications. Odessa, FL: Psychological Assessment Resources, 1991.
13. Delis DC, Kaplan E. Hazards of a standardized neuropsychological test with low content validity: comment on the Luria-Nebraska Neuropsychological Battery. J Consult Clin Psychol 1983;51:396–398.
14. Delis DC, Kaplan E. The assessment of aphasia with the Luria-Nebraska Neuropsychological Battery: a case critique. J Consult Clin Psychol 1982;50:32–39.
15. Luria AR. Higher cortical functions in man. New York: Basic Books, 1966.
16. Milberg WP, Hebben N, Kaplan E. The Boston process approach to neuropsychological assessment. In: Grant I, Adams KM, eds. Neuropsychological assessment of neuropsychiatric disorders. New York: Oxford University Press, 1986:65–86.
17. Peyser JM, Rao SM, LaRocca NG, Kaplan E. Guidelines for neuropsychological research in multiple sclerosis. Arch Neurol 1990;47:94–97.
18. Butters N, Grant I, Haxby J, et al. Assessment of AIDS-related cognitive changes: recommendations of the NIMH workshop on neuropsychological assessment approaches. J Clin Exp Neuropsychol 1990;12:963–978.
19. Wilson RS, Rosenbaum G, Brown G, Rourke D, Whitman D, Grisell J. An index of premorbid intelligence. J Consult Clin Psychol 1978;46:1554–1555.
20. Barona A, Reynolds CR, Chastain R. A demographically based index of premorbid intelligence for the WAIS-R. J Consult Clin Psychol 1984;52:885–887.
21. Barona A, Chastain R. An improved estimate of premorbid IQ for blacks and whites on the WAIS-R. Int J Clin Neuropsychol 1986;8:169–172.
22. Nelson HE. National Adult Reading Test (NART): test manual. Windsor, UK: NFER Nelson, 1982.
23. Nelson HE, O'Connell A. Dementia: the estimation of pre-morbid intelligence levels using the new adult reading test. Cortex 1978;14:234–244.
24. Stebbins GT, Wilson RS, Gilley DW, Bernard BA, Fox JH. Use of the National Adult Reading Test to estimate premorbid IQ in dementia. Clinical Neuropsychologist 1990;4:18–24.
25. Wiens AN, Bryan JE, Crossen JR. Estimating WAIS-R FSIQ from the National Adult Reading Test—Revised in normal subjects. Clinical Neuropsychologist 1993;7:70–84.
26. Milner B. Hemisphere specialization: scope and limits. In: Schmitt FO, Worden FG, eds. The Neurosciences Third Study Program. Cambridge, MA: MIT Press, 1974:75–89.
27. Goodglass H, Kaplan E. The assessment of aphasia and related disorders. Philadelphia: Lea & Febiger, 1983.
28. Heindel WC, Salmon DP, Shults CW, Walicke PA, Butters N. Neuropsychological evidence for multiple implicit memory systems: a comparison of Alzheimer's, Huntington's, and Parkinson's disease patients. J Neurosci 1989;9:582–587.
29. Campbell DT, Fiske DW. Convergent and discriminant validation by the multitrait-multimethod matrix. Psychol Bull 1959;56:81–105.
30. Heaton RK, Grant I, Matthews CG. Differences in neuropsychological test performance associated with age, education, and sex. In: Grant I, Adams KM, eds. Neuropsychological assessment of neuropsychiatric disorders. New York: Oxford University Press, 1986:100–120.
31. Craik FIM, McDowd JM. Age differences in recall and recognition. J Exp Psychol [Learn Mem Cogn] 1987;13:474–479.
32. Hasher L, Zacks RT. Automatic and effortful processes in memory. J Exp Psychol [Gen] 1979;108:356–388.
33. Spreen O, Strauss E. A compendium of neuropsychological tests: administration, norms, and commentary. New York: Oxford University Press, 1991.
34. Beardsley JV, Matthews CG, Cleeland CS, Harley JP. Experimental T-score norms on the Wisconsin Neuropsychological Test Battery. Madison, WI: University of Wisconsin Center for Health Science, 1978.
35. Dorward J, Posthuma A. Validity limits of forensic neuropsychological testing. Am J Foren Psychol 1993;11:17–26.
36. Rogers R, Harrell EH, Liff CD. Feigning neuropsychological impairment: a critical review of methodological and clinical considerations. Clin Psychol Rev 1993;13:255–274.
37. Heaton RK, Smith HH, Lehman RA, Vogt AT. Prospects for faking believable deficits on neuropsychological testing. J Consult Clin Psychol 1978;46:892–900.
38. Faust D, Hart K, Guilmette TJ, Arkes HR. Pediatric malingering: the

capacity of children to fake believable deficits on neuropsychological testing. J Consult Clin Psychol 1988;56:578–582.

39. Arnett PA, Hammeke TA, Schwartz L. Quantitative and qualitative performance on Rey's 15-Item Test in neurological patients and dissimulators. Clinical Neuropsychologist (in press).

40. Pankratz L. Symptom validity testing and symptom retraining: Procedures for the assessment and treatment of functional sensory deficits. J Consult Clin Psychol 1979;47:409–410.

41. Binder LM. Assessment of malingering after mild head trauma with the Portland Digit Recognition Test. J Clin Exp Neuropsychol 1993;15:170–182.

42. Guilmette TJ, Hart KJ, Giuliano AJ. Malingering detection: The use of a forced-choice method in identifying organic versus simulated memory impairment. Clinical Neuropsychologist 1993;7:59–69.

43. Weingartner H. Automatic and effort-demanding cognitive processes in depression. In: Poon LW, ed. Handbook for clinical memory assessment of older adults. Washington, DC: American Psychological Association, 1986:218–225.

44. Hart RP, Kwentus JA, Wade JB, Hamer RM. Digit symbol performance in mild dementia and depression. J Consult Clin Psychol 1987;55:236–238.

45. Massman PJ, Delis DC, Butters N, Dupont RM, Gillin JC. The subcortical dysfunction hypothesis of memory deficits in depression: neuropsychological validation in a subgroup of patients. J Clin Exp Neuropsychol 1992;14:687–706.

46. King DA, Caine ED, Cox C. Influence of depression and age on selected cognitive functions. Clinical Neuropsychologist 1993;7:443–453.

47. Sackeim HA, Freeman J, McElhiney M, Coleman E, Prudic J, Devanand DP. Effects of major depression on estimates of intelligence. J Clin Exp Neuropsychol 1992;14:268–288.

48. Starkstein SE, Robinson RG. Depression in neurologic disease. Baltimore: Johns Hopkins University Press, 1993.

49. Wolkowitz OM, Tinklenberg JR, Weingartner H. A psychopharmacological perspective of cognitive functions. II. Specific pharmacologic agents. Neuropsychobiology 1985;14:133–156.

50. Wolkowitz OM, Tinklenberg JR, Weingartner H. A psychopharmacological perspective of cognitive functions. I. Theoretical overview and methodological considerations. Neuropsychobiology 1985;14:88–96.

51. Kempen JH, Kritchevsky M, Feldman ST. Effect of visual impairment on neuropsychological test performance. J Clin Exp Neuropsychol 1994;16:223–231.

52. Casey JE, Ferguson GG, Kimura D, Hachinski VC. Neuropsychological improvement versus practice effect following unilateral carotid endarterectomy in patients without stroke. J Clin Exp Neuropsychol 1989;11:461–470.

53. Dodrill CB, Troupin AS. Effects of repeated administrations of a comprehensive neuropsychological battery among chronic epileptics. J Nerv Ment Dis 1975;161:185–190.

54. Duke R, Bloor B, Nugent R, Majzoub H. Changes in performance on WAIS, Trail Making Test and Finger Tapping Test associated with carotid artery surgery. Percept Mot Skills 1968;26:399–404.

55. McCaffrey RJ, Ortega A, Orsillo SM, Nelles WB, Haase RF. Practice effects in repeated neuropsychological assessments. Clinical Neuropsychologist 1992;6:32–42.

56. Putnam SH, Adams KM, Schneider AM. One-day test-retest reliability of neuropsychological tests in a personal injury case. Psychol Assess [J Consult Clin Psychol] 1992;4:312–316.

57. Ryan JJ, Paolo AM, Brungardt TM. WAIS-R test-retest stability in normal persons 75 years and older. Clinical Neuropsychologist 1992;6:3–8.

58. Ryan JJ, Georgemiller RJ, Geisser ME, Randall DM. Test-retest stability of the WAIS-R in a clinical sample. J Clin Psychol 1985;41:552–556.

59. Anderson BL, Rao SM, Bernardin LJ, Luchetta T. Long term practice effects in neuropsychological testing. Clinical Neuropsychologist, in press.

60. Nelson A, Fogel BS, Faust D. Bedside cognitive screening instruments. J Nerv Ment Dis 1986;174:73–83.

61. Folstein MF, Folstein SE, McHugh PR. Mini-Mental State: A practical method for grading the cognitive state of patients for the clinician. J Psychiatr Res 1975;12:189–198.

62. Rao SM, Leo GJ, Bernardin L, Unverzagt F. Cognitive dysfunction in multiple sclerosis: I. Frequency, patterns, and prediction. Neurology 1991;41:685–691.

63. Mattis S. Mental status examination for organic mental syndrome in the elderly patient. In: Bellak L, Karasu TB, eds. Geriatric psychiatry. New York: Grune & Stratton, 1976:88–105.

64. Wechsler D. Manual for the Wechsler Adult Intelligence Scale–Revised. New York: Psychological Corporation, 1981.

65. Kaplan E, Fein D, Morris R, Delis DC. WAIS-R as a neuropsychological instrument. New York: Psychological Corporation, 1991.

66. Matarazzo JD. Wechsler's measurement and appraisal of adult intelligence. 5th ed. New York: Oxford University Press, 1972.

67. Inglis J, Lawson JS. Sex differences in the effects of unilateral brain damage on intelligence. Science 1981;212:693–695.

68. Bornstein RA, Suga L, Prifitera A. Incidence of Verbal IQ-Performance IQ discrepencies at various levels of education. J Clin Psychol 1987;43:387–389.

69. Matarazzo JD, Daniel MH, Prifitera A, Herman DO. Inter-subtest scatter in the WAIS-R standardization sample. J Clin Psychol 1988;44:940–949.

70. Mittenberg W, Hammeke TA, Rao SM. Intrasubtest scatter on the WAIS-R as a pathognomonic sign of brain injury. Psychol Assess [J Consult Clin Psychol] 1989;1:273–276.

71. Hallenbeck CE, Fink SL, Grossman JS. Measurement of intellectual inefficiency. Psychology Reports 1965;17:339–349.

72. Raven JC. Guide to the standard progressive matrices. London: H.K. Lewis, 1960.

73. Grant DA, Berg EA. A behavioral analysis of degree of reinforcement and ease of shifting to new responses in a Weigl-type card-sorting problem. J Exp Psychol 1948;38:404–411.

74. Heaton RK, Chelune GJ, Talley JL, Kay GG, Curtiss G. Wisconsin Card Sorting Test manual: revised and expanded. Odessa, FL: Psychological Assessment Resources, 1993.

75. Halstead WC. Brain and intelligence: a quantitative study of the frontal lobes. Chicago: University of Chicago Press, 1947.

76. Butler M, Retzlaff P, Vanderploeg R. Neuropsychological test usage. Professional Psychology: Research and Practice 1991;22:510–512.

77. Corrigan JD, Agresti AA, Hinkeldey NS. Psychometric characteristics of the Category Test: replication and extension. J Clin Psychol 1987;43:368–376.

78. Crockett D, Bilsker D, Hurwitz T, Kozak J. Clinical utility of three measures of frontal lobe dysfunction in neuropsychiatric samples. Int J Neurosci 1986;30:241–248.

79. Milner B. Effects of different brain lesions on card sorting. Arch Neurol 1963;9:90–100.

80. Pendleton MG, Heaton RK. A comparison of the Wisconsin Card Sorting Test and the Category Test. J Clin Psychol 1982;38:392–396.

81. Rao SM, Hammeke TA, Speech TJ. Wisconsin Card Sorting Test performance in relapsing-remitting and chronic-progressive multiple sclerosis. J Consult Clin Psychol 1987;55:263–265.

82. Teuber HL, Battersby WS, Bender MB. Performance of complex visual tasks after cerebral lesions. J Nerv Ment Dis 1951;114:413–429.

83. Fey ET. The performance of young schizophrenics and young normals on the Wisconsin Card Sorting Test. J Consult Psychol 1951;15:311–319.

84. Goldberg TE, Kelsoe JR, Weinberger DR, Pliskin NH, Kirwin PD, Berman KF. Performance of schizophrenic patients on putative neuropsychological tests of frontal lobe function. Int J Neurosci 1988;42:51–58.

85. Stuss DT, Benson DF, Kaplan EF, et al. The involvement of the orbitofrontal cerebrum in cognitive tasks. Neuropsychologia 1983;21:235–248.

86. Arnett PA, Rao SM, Bernardin L, Grafman J, Yetkin FZ, Lobeck L. Relationship between frontal lobe lesions and Wisconsin Card Sorting Test performance in patients with multiple sclerosis. Neurology 1994;44:420–425.

87. Robinson AL, Heaton RK, Lehman RAW, Stilson DW. The utility of the Wisconsin Card Sorting Test in detecting and localizing frontal lobe lesions. J Consult Clin Psychol 1980;48:605–614.

88. Anderson SW, Damasio H, Jones RD, Tranel D. Wisconsin Card Sorting Test performance as a measure of frontal lobe damage. J Clin Exp Neuropsychol 1991;13:909–922.

89. Mountain MA, Snow WG. Wisconsin Card Sorting Test as a measure of frontal pathology: a review. Clinical Neuropsychologist 1993;7:108–118.

90. Perrine K. Differential aspects of conceptual processing in the Category Test and Wisconsin Card Sorting Test. J Clin Exp Neuropsychol 1993;15:461–473.

91. Bondi MW, Kaszniak AW, Bayles KA, Vance KT. Contributions of frontal system dysfunction to memory and perceptual abilities in Parkinson's disease. Neuropsychology 1993;7:89–102.

92. Shallice T, Burgess P. Higher-order cognitive impairments and frontal lobe lesions in man. In: Levin HS, Eisenberg HM, Benton AL, eds. Frontal lobe function and dysfunction. New York: Oxford University Press, 1991:125–138.

93. Lezak MD. The problem of assessing executive functions. Int J Psychol 1982;17:281–297.

94. Lezak MD. Newer contributions to the neuropsychological assessment of executive functions. Journal of Head Trauma Rehabilitation 1993;8:24–31.

95. Benton AL, Hamsher Kd, Varney NR, Spreen O. Contributions to neuropsychological assessment: a clinical manual. New York: Oxford University Press, 1983.

96. Jones-Gottman M, Milner B. Design fluency: the invention of nonsense drawings after focal cortical lesions. Neuropsychologia 1977;15:653–674.

97. Porteus SD. Porteus Maze Test: fifty years' application. Palo Alto, CA: Pacific Books, 1965.

98. Shimamura AP, Janowsky JS, Squire LR. Memory for the temporal order of events in patients with frontal lobe lesions and patients with amnesia. Neuropsychologia 1990;28:803–813.

99. Grafman J, Thompson K, Weingartner H, Martinez R, Lawlor BA, Sunderland T. Script generation as an indicator of knowledge representation in patients with Alzheimer's disease. Brain Lang 1991;40:344–358.

100. McGlynn SM, Schacter DL. Unawareness of deficits in neuropsychological syndromes. J Clin Exp Neuropsychol 1989;11:143–205.

101. Weinberger DR. Schizophrenia and the frontal lobes. Trends Neurosci 1988;11:367–370.

102. Posner MI, Boies SJ. Components of attention. Psychol Rev 1971;78:391–408.

103. Cummings JL. Subcortical dementia. New York: Oxford University Press, 1990.

104. Stroop JR. Studies of interference in serial verbal reactions. J Exp Psychol 1935;18:643–662.

105. Smith A. Symbol Digit Modalities Test. Manual. Los Angeles: Western Psychological Services, 1973.

106. Sternberg S. Memory scanning: mental processes revealed by reaction-time experiments. American Scientist 1969;57:421–457.

107. Wilson RS, Kaszniak AW, Klawans HL, Garron DC. High speed memory scanning in parkinsonism. Cortex 1980;16:67–72.

108. Rao SM, St. Aubin-Faubert P, Leo GJ. Information processing speed in patients with multiple sclerosis. J Clin Exp Neuropsychol 1989;11:471–477.

109. Gronwall DMA. Paced auditory serial-addition task: a measure of recovery from concussion. Percept Mot Skills 1977;44:367–373.

110. Diller L, Ben-Yishay Y, Gertsman LJ, Goodkin R, Gordon W, Weinberg J. Studies in cognition and rehabilitation in hemiplegia. New York: New York University Medical Center Institute of Rehabilitation Medicine, 1974.

111. Schenkenberg T, Bradford DC, Ajax ET. Line bisection and unilateral visual neglect in patients with neurologic impairment. Neurology 1980;30:509–517.

112. Waugh NC, Norman DA. Primary memory. Psychol Rev 1965;72:89–104.

113. Brown J. Some tests of the decay theory of immediate memory. Q J Exp Psychol 1958;10:12–21.

114. Peterson LR, Peterson MJ. Short-term retention of individual verbal items. J Exp Psychol 1959;58:193–198.

115. Baddeley A. Working memory. Oxford: Clarendon Press, 1986.

116. Drachman DA, Zaks MS. The "memory cliff" beyond span in immediate recall. Psychol Reports 1967;21:105–112.

117. Wechsler D. Wechsler Memory Scale-Revised. New York: Psychological Corporation, 1987.

118. Rey A. L'examen clinique en psychologie. Paris: Presses Universitaires de France, 1964.

119. Delis DC, Kramer JH, Kaplan E, Ober BA. California Verbal Learning Test, research edition. Manual. New York: Psychological Corporation, 1987.

120. Buschke H. Selective reminding for analysis of memory and learning. Journal of Verbal Learning and Verbal Behavior 1973;12:543–550.

121. Buschke H, Fuld PA. Evaluating storage, retention, and retrieval in disordered memory and learning. Neurology 1974;24:1019–1025.

122. Benton AL. Revised Visual Retention Test. New York: Psychological Corporation, 1974.

123. Barbizet J, Cany E. Clinical and psychometrical study of a patient with memory disturbances. Int J Neurol 1968;7:44–54.

124. Rao SM, Hammeke TA, McQuillen MP, Khatri BO, Lloyd D. Memory disturbance in chronic progressive multiple sclerosis. Arch Neurol 1984;41:625–631.

125. Malec JF, Ivnik RJ, Hinkeldey NS. Visual Spatial Learning Test. Psychol Assess [J Consult Clin Psychol] 1991;3:82–88.

126. Schacter DL. Priming and multiple memory systems: perceptual mechanisms of implicit memory. J Cogn Neurosci 1992;4:244–256.

127. Corkin S. Acquisition of a motor skill after bilateral medial temporal-lobe excision. Neuropsychologia 1968;6:255–264.

128. Shimamura AP, Salmon DP, Squire LR, Butters N. Memory dysfunction and word priming in dementia and amnesia. Behav Neurosci 1987;101:347–351.

129. Heindel WC, Butters N, Salmon DP. Impaired learning of a motor skill in patients with Huntington's disease. Behav Neurosci 1988;102:141–147.

130. Salmon DP, Shimamura AP, Butters N, Smith S. Lexical and semantic priming deficits in patients with Alzheimer's disease. J Clin Exp Neuropsychol 1988;10:477–494.

131. Kertesz A. Western Aphasia Battery. London, Ont.: University of Western Ontario, 1980.

132. Benton AL, Hamsher Kd. Multilingual aphasia examination. Iowa City: University of Iowa, 1976.

133. Kirk SA, McCarthy J, Kirk W. The Illinois Test of Psycholinguistic Ability. rev. ed. Urbana, IL: Illinois University Press, 1968.

134. Porch B. The Porch Index of Communicative Ability, vol. 2: administration and scoring. Palo Alto, CA: Consulting Psychologists Press, 1971.

135. Reitan RM. Aphasia and sensory-perceptual deficits in adults. Tucson, AZ: Reitan Neuropsychology Laboratory, 1984.

136. De Renzi E, Vignolo L. The Token Test: a sensitive test to detect receptive disturbances in aphasics. Brain 1962;85:665–678.

137. Kaplan EF, Goodglass H, Weintraub S. The Boston Naming Test. Philadelphia: Lea & Febiger, 1983.

138. Dunn LM, Dunn LN. Peabody Picture Vocabulary Test—Revised Manual. Circle Pines, MN: American Guidance Service, 1981.

139. Benton AL. Differential behavioral effects in frontal lobe disease. Neuropsychologia 1968;6:53–60.

140. Talland GA. Deranged memory. New York: Academic Press, 1965.

141. Hooper HE. The Hooper Visual Organization Test manual. Los Angeles: Western Psychological Services, 1958.

142. Sherer M, Parsons OA, Nixon SJ, Adams RL. Clinical validity of the Speech-Sounds Perception Test and the Seashore Rhythm Test. J Clin Exp Neuropsychol 1991;13:741–751.

143. Kimura D. Functional asymmetry of the brain in dichotic listening. Cortex 1967;3:163–178.

144. Berlin CI, Lowe-Bell SS, Jannetta PJ, Kline DG. Central auditory deficits after temporal lobectomy. Arch Otolaryngol 1972;96:4–10.

145. Rao SM, Bernardin L, Leo GJ, Ellington L, Ryan SB, Burg LS. Cerebral disconnection in multiple sclerosis: relationship to atrophy of the corpus callosum. Arch Neurol 1989;46:918–920.

146. Doty RL. Smell Identification Test administration manual. Haddonfield, NJ: Sensonics, Inc, 1983.

147. Haaland KY, Yeo RA. Neuropsychological function and neuroanatomic aspects of complex motor control. In: Bigler ED, Yeo RA, Turkheimer E, eds. Neuropsychological function and brain imaging. New York: Plenum Publishing Corp. 1989:219–243.

148. Rao SM, Binder JR, Bandettini PA, et al. Functional magnetic resonance imaging of complex human movements. Neurology 1993;43:2311–2318.

149. Haaland KY, Flaherty D. The different types of limb apraxia errors made by patients with left vs. right hemisphere damage. Brain Cogn 1984;3:370–384.

150. Poizner H, Mack L, Verfallie M, Gonzalez Rothi LJ, Heilman KM. Three-dimensional computergraphic analysis of apraxia. Brain 1990;113:85–101.

151. Hutt ML. The Hutt adaptation of the Bender-Gestalt test. 3rd ed. New York: Grune & Stratton, 1977.

152. Woodcock RW, Mather N. Woodcock-Johnson Psycho-Educational Battery—Revised. Allen, Texas: DLM Teaching Resources, 1989.

153. Wilkinson GS. WRAT3: Administration manual. Wilmington, DE: Wide Range, Inc., 1993.

154. Crosson B. Treatment of interpersonal deficits for head-trauma patients in inpatient rehabilitation settings. Clinical Neuropsychologist 1987;1:335–352.

155. Levin HS, Benton AL, Grossman RG. Neurobehavioral consequences of closed head injury. New York: Oxford University Press, 1982.

156. Butcher JN, Dahlstrom WG, Graham JR, Tellegen AM, Kaemmer B. MMPI-2: Manual for administration and scoring. Minneapolis: University of Minnesota Press, 1989.

157. Beck AT, Ward CH, Mendelson M, Mock J, Erbaugh J. An inventory for measuring depression. Arch Gen Psychiatry 1961;41:561–571.

158. Zung WK. A self-rating depression scale. Arch Gen Psychiatry 1965;12:63–70.

159. Spielberger CD, Gorsuch RL, Lushene RE. STAI manual for the State-Trait Anxiety Inventory. Palo Alto, CA: Consulting Psychologists Press Inc, 1970.

160. Alfano DP, Finlayson MAJ, Stearns GM, Nellson PM. The MMPI and neurologic dysfunction: profile configuration and analysis. Clinical Neuropsychologist 1990;4:69–79.

161. Katz MM, Lyerly SB. Methods of measuring adjustment and behavior in the community: I. Rationale, description, discriminative validity, and scale development. Psychological Reports 1963;13:503–535.

162. Bornstein RA, Brown GG. Neurobehavioral aspects of cerebrovascular disease. New York: Oxford University Press, 1991.

163. Levin HS, Grafman J, Eisenberg HM. Neurobehavioral recovery from head injury. New York: Oxford University Press, 1987.

164. Levin HS, Eisenberg HM, Benton AL. Mild head injury. New York: Oxford University Press, 1989.

165. Parks RW, Zec RF, Wilson RS. Neuropsychology of Alzheimer's disease and other dementias. New York: Oxford University Press, 1993.

166. Huber SJ, Cummings JL. Parkinson's disease: neurobehavioral aspects. New York: Oxford University Press, 1992.

167. Rao SM. Neurobehavioral aspects of multiple sclerosis. New York: Oxford University Press, 1990.

168. Rao SM. White matter dementias. In: Parks RW, Zec RF, Wilson RS, eds. Neuropsychology of Alzheimer's disease and other dementias. New York: Oxford University Press, 1993:438–456.

169. Litvan I, Agid Y. Progressive supranuclear palsy: clinical and research approaches. New York: Oxford University Press, 1992.

170. Squire LR, Butters N. Neuropsychology of memory. 2nd ed. New York: Guilford Press, 1992.

171. Hartman DE. Neuropsychological toxicology: identification and assessment of human neurotoxic syndromes. New York: Pergamon Press, 1988.

172. Hermann BP, Whitman S. Behavioral and personality correlates of epilepsy: a review, methodological critique, and conceptual model. Psychol Bull 1984;95:451–497.

173. Grant I and Martin A. Neuropsychology of HIV infection. New York: Oxford University Press, 1994.

174. Weinberger DR, Berman KF, Daniel DG. Prefrontal cortex dysfunction in schizophrenia. In: Levin HS, Eisenberg HM, Benton AL, eds. Frontal lobe function and dysfunction. New York: Oxford University Press, 1991:275–287.

175. Bieliauskas LA, Matthews CG. American Board of Clinical Neuropsychology: policies and procedures. Clinical Neuropsychologist 1987;1:21–28.

176. Cripe LI. Listing of training programs in clinical neuropsychology—1993. Clinical Neuropsychologist 1993;7:371–419.

177. Report of the INS-Division 40 Task Force on Education, Accreditation, and Credentialing. Clinical Neuropsychologist 1987;1:29–34.

178. Hammeke TA. The Association of Postdoctoral Programs in Clinical Neuropsychology (APPCN). Clinical Neuropsychologist 1993;7:197–204.

4

NEUROIMAGING FOR NEUROPSYCHIATRY

Daniel K. Kido and Yvette I. Sheline

The purpose of noninvasive neuroradiologic imaging techniques such as computed tomography (CT) and magnetic resonance (MR) imaging is to display lesions of the central nervous system in patients with corresponding signs and symptoms. In patients with essentially normal scans a variety of linear, planar, and more recently volumetric measurements of the brain as well as the corresponding cerebrospinal fluid spaces have been performed to detect subtle atrophic changes. The purpose of this chapter is to demonstrate how the brain can be segmented into lobes by identifying key sulci and fissures and thus to facilitate the correlation of neurologic changes with specific locations within those lobes. We will begin by demonstrating how sulci and fissures present in images of the whole brain can be used to segment it into lobes. In turn, we will show how whole brain information about sulci and fissures can be applied to individual MR and CT slices in order to segment them into lobes. Finally, we will review how MR and CT images should be requested from a radiologist if they are to be studied in detail.

MR ANATOMY OF THE CEREBRAL HEMISPHERES

Surface Anatomy of the Cerebral Hemispheres

Two-dimensional (2D) images of the lateral, medial, and superior surfaces of whole brains are familiar to all physicians. However, relating information about gyri and sulci from the whole brain to specific axial CT and MR scans is difficult because these techniques slice the brain into less familiar planes. This difficulty is most evident on MR scans taken in the axial and sagittal planes. In an attempt to overcome this barrier we will take a set of sagittal MR scans and reconstruct them into a set of 2D textbook-type whole brain images (Figs. 4.1–4.3) and review the major sulci and fissures on these images which can be used to segment the brain into lobes. These images of the whole brain were obtained using a software program called VOXEL-MAN (Siemens, Erlangen, Germany). Similar whole brain images can be produced from MR scans by using programs such as Analyze (Mayo Foundation for Medical Education and

Research, Rochester, MN) and 3D VIEWNIX (Medical Image Processing Group, Philadelphia, PA). Later, in the asymmetry section, these whole brain images will be transformed into 2D surface maps to allow comparison between each side of the brain. In the section of this chapter on sectional anatomy, the information regarding the location of sulci and fissures on whole brain, which follows, will be applied to individual axial, coronal, or sagittal scans of the brain to demonstrate how these slices can be segmented into lobes by using internal landmarks.

LATERAL SURFACE OF THE CEREBRAL HEMISPHERES (WHOLE BRAIN)

The most prominent surface marking on the lateral surface of the reformatted whole brain is a deep horizontal depression (sylvian fissure) about two-thirds of the way between the top and the bottom of the image (1). The sylvian fissure separates the frontal lobe and anterior portion of the parietal lobe from the anterior two-thirds of the temporal lobe (Fig. 4.1*A*). The sylvian fissure terminates posteriorly in the supramarginal gyrus of the inferior parietal lobule (Fig. 4.4). The superior temporal sulcus, which is located just below the sylvian fissure, terminates posteriorly behind the supramarginal gyrus in the angular gyrus. Figure 4.1 corresponds roughly to the sagittal MR scan in Fig. 4.4.

The middle cerebral artery divides within the sylvian fissure into a superior and inferior division in approximately 80% of individuals (2, 3). The superior division always supplies the lateral surface of the frontal lobe and the most anterior portion of the parietal lobe (somatosensory cortex); damage to it in the dominant hemisphere results in motor or expressive (Broca's) aphasia as well as contralateral motor weakness or paralysis (Fig. 4.1*B*). The inferior division supplies most of the superior and middle temporal gyri; damage to it results in receptive (Wernicke's) aphasia. When the superior division is dominant, it supplies the remainder of the lateral surface of the parietal and occipital lobes; if the inferior division is dominant, it supplies these areas (2, 3).

Superior to the posterior portion of the sylvian fissure is another horizontal sulcus, the intraparietal sulcus. It is

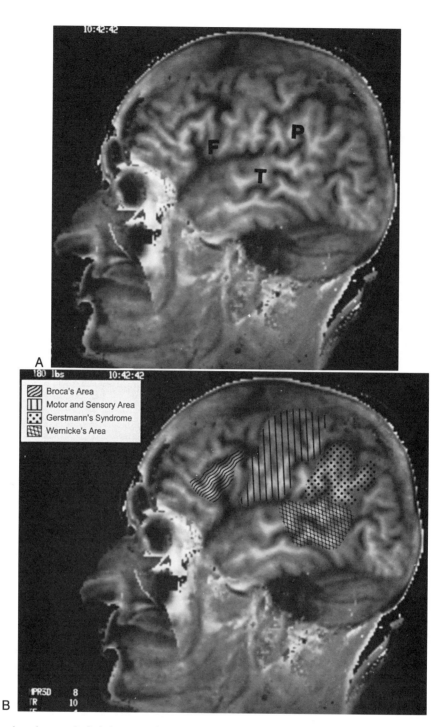

Figure 4.1. Lateral view of a reformatted whole brain. **A.** The sylvian fissure separates the frontal *(F)* and parietal *(P)* lobes from the temporal *(T)* lobe. The sagittal scan in Figure 4.4 corresponds roughly to this image. **B.** Broca's area *(wavy lines)*. Motor and sensory cortex *(vertical lines)*. Wernicke's area *(cross-hatches)*. Inferior parietal lobule *(small circles)*.

located above both the supramarginal and angular gyri and separates these gyri from the superior portion of the parietal lobe. This area of the brain is supplied by the posterior parietal artery, which may be a branch of either the superior or inferior division of the middle cerebral artery. Lesions to this area of this brain in the dominant hemisphere may result in Gerstmann's syndrome: digital agnosia, impaired ability to calculate and write, and right-left disorientation (Fig. 4.1*B*).

Superior to the most anterior position of the sylvian fissure is another horizontal sulcus, the superior frontal sulcus. This sulcus can be followed posteriorly until it terminates in the vertically oriented precentral sulcus. This relationship exists in approximately 90% of individuals (4). This is seen clearly on a view of the whole brain which has been rotated to view the superior-lateral surface of the brain (Fig. 4.2). Coincidentally, the central sulcus is located behind and parallel to the precentral sulcus. The primary

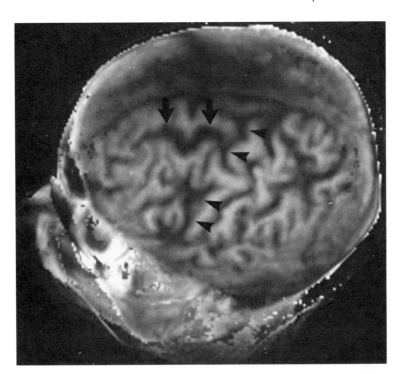

Figure 4.2. Oblique view of a reformatted whole brain midway between Figures 4.1 and 4.4. The superior frontal sulcus *(arrows)* and the precentral sulcus *(arrowheads)* are identified.

motor gyrus (precentral) is located between the precentral and central sulci.

MEDIAL SURFACE OF THE CEREBRAL HEMISPHERES

The posterior boundary of the somatosensory cortex, on the medial surface of each hemisphere, is formed by the marginal ramus of the cingulate sulcus (Fig. 4.5). The marginal ramus is formed when the cingulate sulcus terminates above the body of the corpus callosum and divides into the horizontally directed subparietal sulcus and the coronally oriented marginal ramus of the cingulate sulcus. The cingulate sulcus forms an arch around the corpus callosum.

The marginal ramus not only forms the posterior border of the somatosensory cortex (the paracentral lobule) but also the anterior border of the precuneus. The precuneus is the medial surface of the parietal lobe, posterior to the sensory cortex. The inferior surface of the precuneus is outlined by the horizontally oriented extension of the cingulate sulcus while its posterior border is formed by the parieto-occipital fissure (Fig. 4.5). The parieto-occipital fissure in turn forms the anterior border of the cuneus (i.e., occipital lobe). The parieto-occipital fissure joins the more inferiorly located calcarine sulcus behind the splenium of the corpus callosum.

SUPERIOR SURFACE OF THE CEREBRAL HEMISPHERE (WHOLE BRAIN)

The boundary between the frontal and parietal lobes can be located by following the sagittally oriented superior frontal sulcus posteriorly until it terminates in the coronally directed precentral gyrus (Fig. 4.3). This junction is either "L" or "V" shaped. In fewer than 10% of individuals, the superior frontal sulci continue backward to the central sulcus

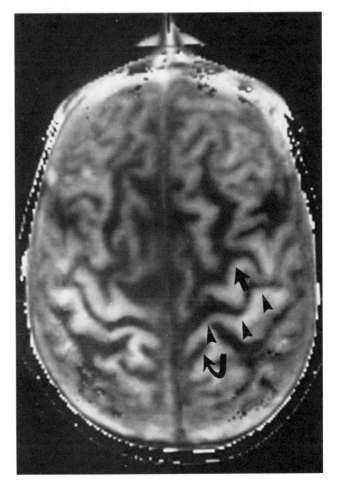

Figure 4.3. Superior surface of a reformatted brain. The junction between the left superior frontal and precentral sulcus is identified by an *arrow*. Central sulcus *(arrowheads)*. Marginal ramus of the cingulate sulcus *(curved arrow)*. The axial vertex scan in Figure 4.6 corresponds roughly to this image.

(Fig. 4.3). Regardless, the frontal lobe can be segmented from the parietal lobe because the central sulcus can be positively identified by comparing the gray matter of the motor cortex which is twice as thick as that of the somatosensory cortex.

Sulci on the superior surface of the whole brain can be used to relate gyri and sulci on the lateral surface of the brain with those on the medial surface. Some of these can also be used to segment the frontal lobe from the parietal lobe and the parietal lobe from the occipital lobe. The marginal ramus of the cingulate sulcus, which is seen clearly on the medial surface, extends for a short distance over the vertex of the brain and is always located at or anterior to the postcentral sulcus but posterior to the central sulci (Fig. 4.3). The right and left marginal rami are frequently not located adjacent to each other and this reflects one of many normal asymmetries present in the brain. The anterior border of the paracentral lobule is related to the precentral sulci, but is much less prominent and more inconsistent in its position than is the marginal ramus.

Sectional Anatomy

AXIAL

The description of sulci and fissures in the previous section on the whole brain can be used to divide individual axial scans into lobes (segments). Four axial scans will be described in detail to illustrate how these axial scans can be segmented. Axial sections close to the vertex can be almost directly correlated to the superior view of the whole brain. Thus, information regarding sulci in the frontal lobe can be used to segment axial slices above the lateral ventricle into a frontal and a parietal lobe. On an axial slice close to the vertex, the superior frontal sulcus can be traced backward to its junction with the precentral sulcus as it can be on the whole brain images (Fig. 4.6). In turn, the central sulcus is located just behind the precentral sulcus. The superior frontal sulcus is sagittally oriented whereas the precentral and central sulci are coronally oriented. The central sulcus is identifiable because gray matter in the motor cortex is two times the thickness of gray matter in the sensory cortex. Unfortunately, the thickness of the gray matter could not be

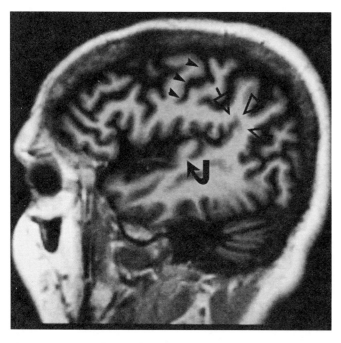

Figure 4.4. Saggital scan through the sylvian fissure. Central sulcus *(arrowheads)*. Heschl's gyrus *(curved arrow)*. The supramarginal gyrus *(open arrows)* is located around the termination of the sylvian fissure.

Figure 4.5. Sagittal section through the medial surface of a brain. A *horizontal line* is drawn through the bicommissural plane. A *small vertical line* is located just behind the anterior commissure. Posterior commissure *(arrow)*. Marginal ramus of the cingulate sulcus *(curved arrow)*. Parieto-occipital fissure *(open arrow)*. Calcarine sulcus *(arrowheads)*.

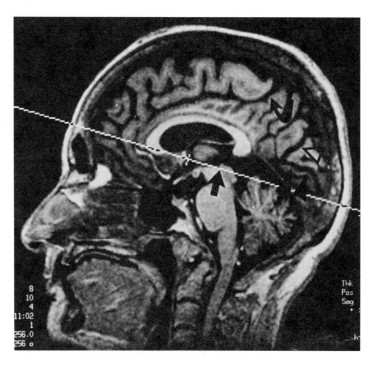

reproduced in the photographs of the axial scans. The full course of the central sulcus can be identified by tracing the central sulcus from slice to slice until it terminates just above the sylvian fissure.

On a slightly more inferior slice through the centrum ovale, the parieto-occipital fissure is located on either side of the interhemispheric fissure behind the marginal ramus of the cingulate sulcus (Fig. 4.7). By extending a horizontal line from the parieto-occipital fissure to the lateral surface of the brain, the parietal lobe can be arbitrarily segmented from the occipital lobe.

Further inferiorly, on an axial slice through the posterior portion of the sylvian fissure, the frontal and parietal lobes can be separated from the temporal lobe by identifying Heschl's gyrus on the superior surface of the temporal lobe. Identifying Heschl's gyrus on the superior surface of the temporal lobe permits separation of the temporal lobe from the more superiorly located frontal and parietal lobes (Fig. 4.8). Heschl's gyrus is located approximately at the junction between the middle third and the posterior third of the sylvian fissure and differs from other gyri by being oblique instead of perpendicular to the surface of the brain. This plane is also important because it contains the inferior portion of the subcortical nuclei of the basal ganglia as well as the thalamus. These structures will be described in the section on deep nuclei.

Another method of identifying sulci and gyri as well as deep nuclei is to localize them stereotactically. This is done by identifying the anterior and posterior commissures (bicommissural plane) on a midline sagittal MR slice and then obtaining a series of axial scans parallel to it (Fig. 4.5). Next, structures on a particular axial scan can be identified by deciding how many millimeters the scan is located above or below the bicommissural plane and then comparing that particular MR scan with the corresponding anatomically labeled axial drawing in the stereotactic atlas (5).

The first two slices described previously, close to the vertex and through the centrum ovale, which were used to separate the frontal from the parietal lobes, are located 55 and 45 mm above the bicommissural plane (Figs. 4.6 and 4.7). The third scan, through the posterior border of the sylvian fissure, is located 10–15 mm above the bicommissural plane (Fig. 4.8). The fourth axial scan, through the middle temporal gyrus (bicommissural plane), is the reference scan (Fig. 4.9). Axial scans below this level contain both the hippocampus and the amygdala. The amygdala will be described in the section on deep nuclei. The hippocampus will be described in the coronal section. The scan through the bicommissural plane also contains the midbrain and its substantia nigra which is best seen on T2-weighted images because of the paramagnetic material they contain (Fig. 4.9).

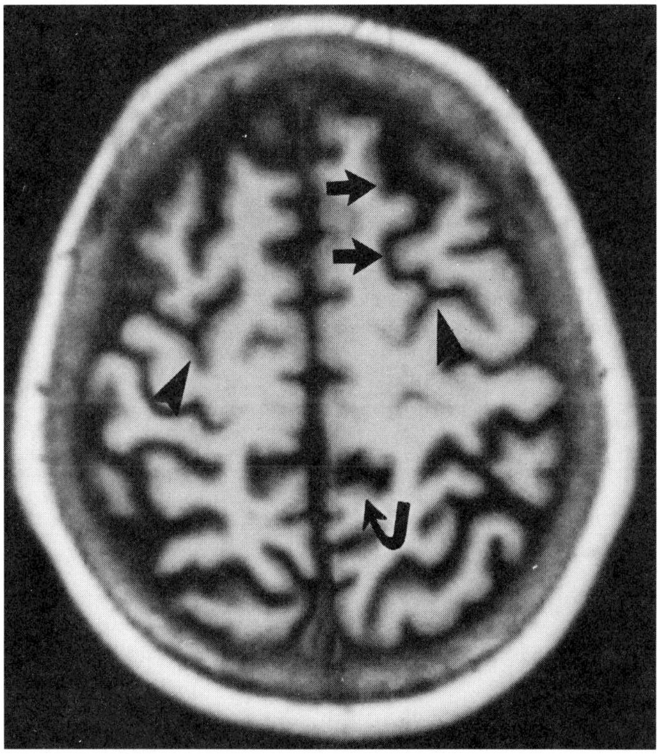

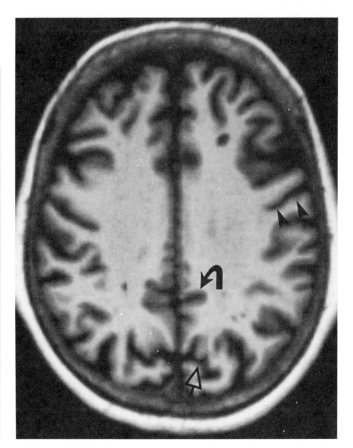

Figure 4.6. Vertex scan (axial). The left superior frontal sulcus *(arrow)* is better visualized than the right. However, the junction between the superior frontal and precentral sulcus *(arrowheads)* can be identified bilaterally. Marginal ramus of the cingulate sulcus *(curved arrow)*.

Figure 4.7. Centrum ovale scan (axial). The marginal ramus of the cingulate sulcus *(curved arrow)* and parieto-occipital fissure *(open arrow)* are located on either side of the interhemispheric fissure. Central sulcus *(arrowheads)*.

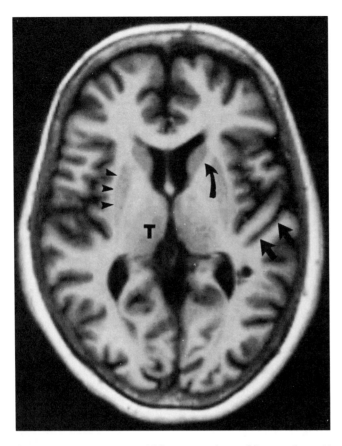

Figure 4.8. Superior temporal lobe scan (axial). Heschl's gyrus *(arrows)* is located within the sylvian fissure. Head of caudate nucleus *(curved arrow)*. Putamen *(arrowheads)*. Thalamus *(T)*.

the posterior commissure runs just behind the posterior border of the paracentral lobule.

The paramedian sections also clearly demonstrate the third ventricle and the structures associated with it. The anterior commissure is located at the superior end of the lamina terminalis at its junction with the rostrum of the corpus callosum. The anterior commissure is thus located anterior to the foramen of Monro and the columns of the fornix. The posterior commissure is located in front of and beneath the pineal body. Superior to the roof of the third ventricle and frontal horns of the lateral ventricle is the corpus callosum. The cingulate gyrus arches around the periphery of the corpus callosum.

Approximately 25–30 mm lateral to the midline is located the long axis of the hippocampus (Fig. 4.10). Identifying the long axis of the hippocampus is important if accurate comparisons are to be made between the two hippocampi in patients with problems such as memory deficits or temporal lobe seizures, since the MR scans need to be performed perpendicular to the long axis for accurate measurement. The anterior portion of the hippocampus is slightly larger than the rest of the structure. Further laterally on sagittal images through the sylvian fissure ($\geq$40 mm from the midline), both the motor and somatosensory cortices are contained within the borders of the vertical lines drawn perpendicular to the anterior and posterior commissures (Fig. 4.4). The sagittal scan through the sylvian fissure is similar to the lateral view of the whole brain in Figure 4.1.

Some of the structures in the basal ganglia, present on scans through the posterior border of the sylvian fissure, are connected to the substantia nigra in the midbrain (bicommissural plane slice) through the striatonigral tract (6). The caudate nucleus and putamen (striatum) receive most of their input from the neocortex, the output from these nuclei occurs via the striatonigral tract to the substantia nigra in the midbrain or to the globus pallidus. In Huntington's disease the synthesis of γ-aminobutyric acid (GABA) is greatly reduced in the striatum along with its transport along the striatonigral tract. In contrast, in Parkinson's disease the synthesis of dopamine as well as its transport along the nigrostriatal fibers is greatly reduced. Thus, in contrast to patients with Parkinson's disease, striatal dopamine may be normal in patients with Huntington's disease.

SAGITTAL

The lobar boundaries described in a previous section (Medial Surface of the Cerebral Hemispheres) are visible in the midline sagittal section. In the midline, a vertical line perpendicular to the anterior commissure runs just behind the anterior border of the paracentral lobule (Fig. 4.5). Further inferiorly beneath the bicommissural plane the vertical line runs just behind the anterior wall of the third ventricle (lamina terminalis). A vertical line perpendicular to

CORONAL

Coronal scans between the anterior and posterior commissures show the central sulcus. The inferior end of the central sulcus is located close to the bottom of the coronal scan taken through the anterior commissure, while the superior end is located close to the top of the coronal scan taken through the posterior commissure (Fig. 4.11). Thus, as sections progress posteriorly from the anterior to the posterior commissure, the motor cortex moves progressively superiorly from the sylvian fissure to the vertex of the brain.

Coronal images through the anterior commissure but inferior to the bicommissural plane contain the tip of the amygdala (Fig. 4.11*A*), which extends posteriorly for approximately 1 cm. Coronal images through the posterior commissure, again inferior to the bicommissural plane, contain the posterior portion of the body of the hippocampus where it begins to diverge (Fig. 4.11*B*). The hippocampus is easiest to examine just anterior to the plane through the posterior commissure since it has not begun to diverge or become redundant as it is at its tip (pes hippocampus) (Fig. 4.12). Decrease in hippocampal volume is frequently present in patients who have Alzheimer's disease (7). In patients with schizophrenia this decrease in size occurs particularly on the left where there is associated decrease in size of the amygdala and parahippocampal gyri (8, 9). Atrophy as well as gliosis have been reported in some patients with psychomotor seizures. Recently, a right-sided

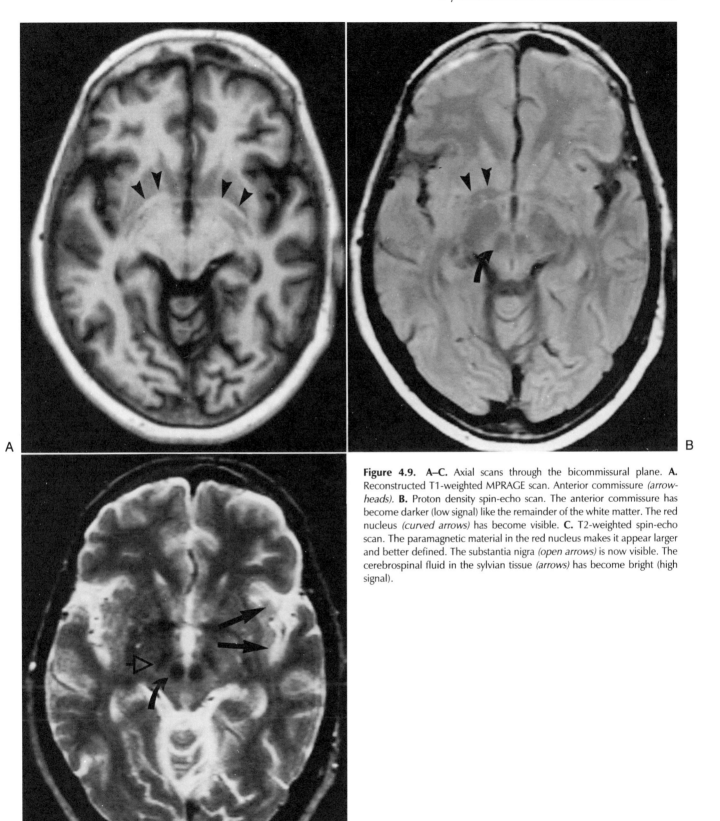

Figure 4.9. A–C. Axial scans through the bicommissural plane. **A.** Reconstructed T1-weighted MPRAGE scan. Anterior commissure *(arrowheads)*. **B.** Proton density spin-echo scan. The anterior commissure has become darker (low signal) like the remainder of the white matter. The red nucleus *(curved arrows)* has become visible. **C.** T2-weighted spin-echo scan. The paramagnetic material in the red nucleus makes it appear larger and better defined. The substantia nigra *(open arrows)* is now visible. The cerebrospinal fluid in the sylvian tissue *(arrows)* has become bright (high signal).

hippocampal volume decrease has been reported in patients with posttraumatic stress disorder (10).

The hippocampus can be located on coronal scans by following the medial surface of the temporal lobe (parahip-

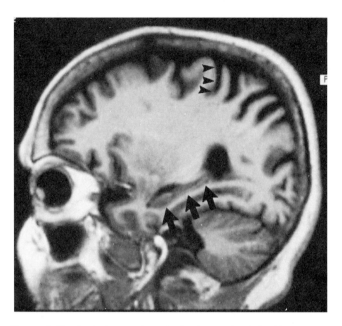

Figure 4.10. Sagittal scan through the long axis of the hippocampus *(arrows)*. Central sulcus *(arrowheads)*.

pocampal gyrus) superiorly until it meets the hippocampal sulcus. The portion of parahippocampal gyrus which forms the inferior lip of hippocampal sulcus is called the subiculum (Fig. 4.12). The superior lip is the dentate gyrus. The subiculum is separated from the dentate gyrus located above it by the hippocampal sulcus. The subiculum continues superiorly and medially in a reverse "C" configuration as the hippocampal formation (Ammon's horn). The subiculum and dentate gyrus differ from the rest of the cortex by having only three layers instead of six. Superior and lateral to the hippocampal formation is the alveus which contains efferent fibers from the hippocampal region. The outflow fibers from the alveus (fimbria) form a bump along the superior medial border of the temporal lobe. The fimbria merges posteriorly with the fornix.

White Matter

The white matter deep to the gyri on the axial vertex and centrum ovale sections can also be used to locate the precentral and postcentral gyri; this is an alternate way of separating the frontal and parietal lobes. The white matter medullary pattern can be divided into the following six divisions from anterior to posterior: superior frontal gyrus, middle frontal gyrus, precentral gyrus, postcentral gyrus, inferior parietal lobule, and superior parietal lobule (Fig. 4.7) (11). On the vertex view, the middle frontal gyrus and

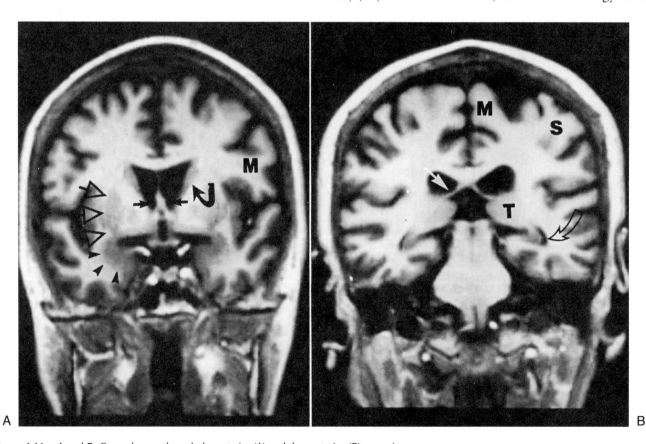

Figure 4.11. **A** and **B.** Coronal scans through the anterior **(A)** and the posterior **(B)** commissures.
Precentral gyrus *(M)*; postcentral gyrus *(S)*; amygdala *(arrowheads)*; fornix *(arrows)*; head of caudate nucleus *(curved arrow)*; putamen *(open arrows)*; thalamus *(T)*; hippocampus *(open curved arrow)* medial to the temporal horn.

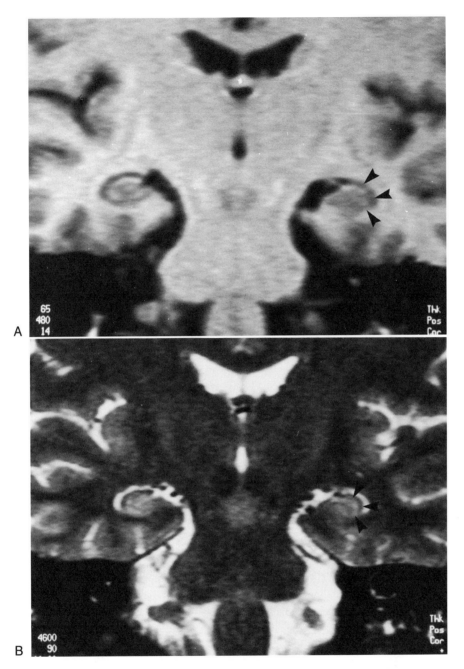

Figure 4.12. High resolution coronal image of the hippocampus *(arrowheads)* taken between the anterior and posterior commissures. **A.** T1-weighted gradient-echo image. TR480/TE14, matrix = 144/512, FOV = 24 × 18 cm, slice thickness = 4 mm, FA 65°, 8 spin-echo acq. **B.** T2-weighted fast spin-echo image taken in a plane corresponding to **A.** TR460/TE90, matrix = 192 × 512, FOV = 26 × 20 cm, slice thickness = 4 mm, 4 spin-echo acq (continued).

inferior parietal lobule may not always be visible, whereas the remaining four divisions are always present (Fig. 4.6). This method of identifying the central sulcus is especially useful in sections through the lower edge of the centrum ovale where the central sulcus is more shallow and thus more difficult to identify and in young children where gyri and sulci may be difficult to identify.

The corpus callosum is the main interhemispheric commissure and connects the white matter, which was described in the previous paragraph. The corpus callosum is divided into four sections from anterior to posterior: the genu, which connects the frontal lobes; the body, which connects the motor and somatosensory cortices as well as the temporal lobes; and the splenium, which connects the occipital lobes (Fig. 4.13). The fourth division is the rostrum which connects the genu to the lamina terminalis. The shape of the splenium may vary by gender; it has been reported to be more bulbous in females (12). Linear measurements have been made throughout the genu, body, and splenium of the corpus callosum in the sagittal plane. The average width of the genu is 7.9 mm, the body 3.5 mm, and the splenium 8.4 mm (13). Measurements greater than 13 mm in either

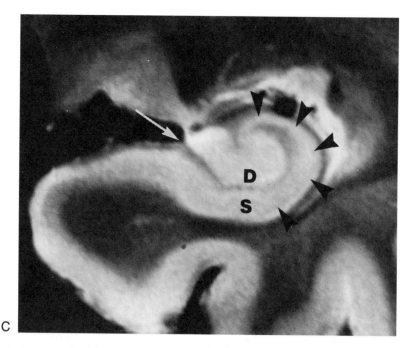

Figure 4.12 (continued). **C.** Proton density image of a brain specimen (fixed in formaldehyde) through roughly the corresponding left hippocampus. The subiculum *(S)* and dentate *(D)* gyri can be separated from each other by the hippocampal fissure *(arrow)*. Hippocampal formation *(arrowheads)*. TR1500/TE 19, matrix = 256 × 512, slice thickness = 2 mm, 7 acq.

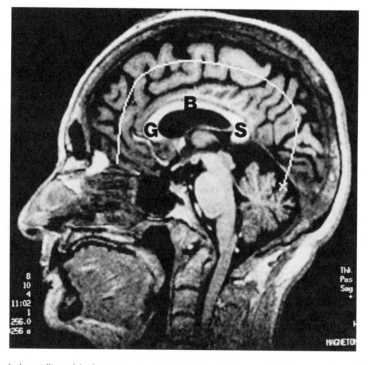

Figure 4.13. Sagittal section through the midline of the brain (same as Fig. 4.5). The *white curved line* between the surface of skull and the corpus callosum is the plane along which Fig. 4.14 has been reconstructed. Genu *(G)*; body *(B)*; and splenium *(S)* of the corpus callosum.

the genu or splenium are considered to be abnormally large (14).

Several smaller interhemispheric commissures exist on the bicommissural plane: the anterior commissure connects the olfactory bulbs and the inferior and middle temporal gyri; the posterior commissure connects the thalami and some structures in the midbrain (Fig. 4.5). The most unusual interhemispheric connection is the fornix. The body of the fornix is located just beneath the body of the corpus callosum. Interhemispheric commissural fibers cross the midline to connect the bodies of the fornix (Fig. 4.11B). The medial part of the body of the fornix is connected to the corpus callosum close to the midline and the lateral part to the superior surface of the thalamus. The body of the fornix in this region thus forms part of the floor of the lateral ventricles. The anterior extension of the fornix (columns of the fornix) descends just anterior to the foramen of Monro and connects it to the mammillary bodies (15, 16) (Fig. 4.11*A*). The posterior-inferior extension of fornix, called the crus of the fornix, connects the body of the fornix to the fimbria. The crus of the fornix is present on the coronal images taken behind the posterior commissure.

White matter hyperintensities (unidentified bright objects (UBOs), leuko-araiosis) occur frequently in middle aged and older adults but should be regarded as abnormal in individuals younger than 45 years (17, 18). These focal hyperintensities are present on proton and T2-weighted images but not on T1-weighted images. Although the significance of these lesions is unknown, their frequency and severity seems to increase in individuals with cardiovascular risk factors and cerebrovascular symptoms. Gerard and Weisberg reported that patients with cardiovascular risk factors have four times the incidence of white matter hyperintensities (19). Furthermore, individuals with both cerebrovascular risk factors and cerebral symptoms have a 10 times higher incidence of white matter hyperintensities. Similar lesions can also be seen in individuals with multiple sclerosis, radiation necrosis, vasculitis, or multiple infarcts. White matter lesions have been reported in higher numbers of psychiatric patients compared with normal controls (20), and particularly in older patients with depression (21, 22).

Deep (Subcortical) Nuclei

The high contrast that MR provides between gray and white matter permits direct visualization of many deep nuclei. In the axial plane through the posterior sylvian fissure, the subcortical nuclei in the basal ganglia (caudate nucleus, putamen, and globus pallidus) as well as the thalamus are imaged (Fig. 4.8). The caudate nucleus can be separated from the putamen and globus pallidus because of the intervening "V"-shaped internal capsule (white matter). The caudate nucleus is located medial to the anterior limb of the internal capsule, and the thalamus is located medial to the posterior limb of the internal capsule. In contrast, the putamen and globus pallidus lie lateral to the internal capsule. The putamen, which is located lateral to the globus pallidus, can also be differentiated from the globus pallidus by the amount of paramagnetic material it contains (23). The globus pallidus contains more paramagnetic material than the putamen, thus on T2-weighted images it appears darker. The width of the caudate nucleus has been measured on axial scans (24). Widths less than 9 mm suggest that there is atrophy, as in Huntington's disease. Similarly, putamen widths less than 10 mm indicate that they may also be atrophic. Volumetric measurements should be able to more accurately detect atrophy in these structures (25).

Although the nuclei in the basal ganglia are primarily associated with the extrapyramidal system, they are also important to intellectual function. Dysfunction of these nuclei, as reflected in their atrophy or the abnormal deposition of paramagnetic material, may result in slowing of mental processes, in coordination, inability to solve complex problems, and memory failure, as seen in patients with Parkinson's disease and Huntington's disease (26, 27). Cognitive impairment of this nature has led to the concept of subcortical dementia (dementia without aphasia and apraxia) (28).

The thalamus extends anteriorly from the interventricular foramen posteriorly to the posterior commissure (Fig. 4.8). Laterally it is bordered by the posterior limb of the internal capsule and medially by the third ventricle. The myelinated fibers (internal medullary lamina) which subdivide the thalamus into an anterior, a medial, and a lateral group are not currently visible by MR imaging. Lesions in the posterior portion of the lateral nucleus can result in contralateral hemianesthesia, transient hemiparesis, chorea-thetosis, and pain as well as mild hemiataxia and astereognosis (Dejerine-Roussy syndrome) (29). Neuropsychological dysfunction is common in the presence of lesions affecting the anterior subdivision, whereas a change in consciousness, amnesia, and even confabulation can result from a lesion in the dorsomedial group (29, 30).

The amygdala, another subcortical gray matter collection, is located in the temporal lobe just below the bicommissural plane (Fig. 4.11*A*). The amygdala is located superior and medial to the tip of the temporal horn and just lateral to the uncus. It is a large oval mass that is difficult to measure because its lateral borders merge into the adjacent white matter. The amygdala is important because it is a key structure in the limbic system associated with emotional control (31).

Lateral Ventricles

The lateral ventricles are divided from anterior to posterior into the frontal horns, body (cella media), atrium (trigone), and occipital horns. The temporal horns are connected to the body of the lateral ventricles and occipital horns by the atria. These structures have been measured in a variety of ways to determine indirectly when cerebral atrophy exists. Ventricular casts of the lateral ventricles indicate that the ventricular volume is approximately 16 mL (32, 33), whereas the volume of the third ventricle is less than 2.0 mL. Ventricular volumes greater than 30 mL suggest that there is generalized cerebral atrophy. The size of the ventricular system has been related to the brain by an index termed the ventricular-brain ratio (VBR). Enlargement of the ventricles has been demonstrated in schizophrenic patients both in CT studies (34) and in MR imaging studies (35). Most studies have found ventricular enlargement to occur early in the course of schizophrenia (36) and have found the degree of enlargement to correlate with severity of symptoms (37, 38). Some studies have also found an increase in the VBR in patients with depression (39), particularly in late-life depression (40), when there may be an association with dementing illnesses. Evidence for ventricular enlargement in bipolar illness is less conclusive (41).

Enlargement of the width of the frontal horns (> 3.5 cm) reflects loss of brain parenchyma in the frontal lobes. This measurement has been refined by relating it to the maximum width of either the brain or the cranial cavity (range 0.16–0.29) (32, 42, 43). Maximum frontal horn ratios greater than 40% or less than 18% suggest abnormal ventricles (44). Enlargement of the maximum width of the cella media of the lateral ventricles reflects loss of brain tissue in the paracentral lobule, precentral gyrus, and postcentral gyrus. The maximum width of the cella media has been related to the width of the cranium (cella media ratio = 0.29) (45). Measurements of the atria and occipital horns are difficult to reproduce because of their variability.

CEREBRAL ASYMMETRIES

Although the descriptions of the sulci, deep nuclei, and ventricles in this chapter depend on their symmetry, most of them are slightly asymmetric. The most obvious asymmetries are related to the frontal and occipital poles. The right frontal pole, in right-handed individuals, usually extends further forward and is slightly broader than the left (46). In contrast, the left occipital pole extends further back and is broader when compared to the right. The posterior position of the left occipital pole is associated with a more posterior location of the corresponding occipital horn as suggested by the frequent posterior position of the choroid plexus, in the left trigone. The normal asymmetry associated with the frontal and occipital poles is also reflected in the sulci (4). On CT and MR scans taken close to the vertex, the left central sulcus is slightly posterior to the right. The left central sulcus is also longer than the right. Some of these relationships can be studied on 2D surface maps of the brain's surface which can be reconstructed from a three-dimensional (3D) data set of the brain (Fig. 4.14).

The width of the hemisphere is also asymmetric, with the right being slightly larger than the left in right-handed individuals. This asymmetry is reflected in the frequent location of the pineal gland slightly to the left of midline (47). In contrast, the left lateral ventricle is slightly larger than the right (32).

The left sylvian fissure is longer than the right (48). Furthermore, the posterior point of the left sylvian fissure (sylvian point) is lower than the right due to the left parietal operculum growing further inferiorly on the left in right-handed individuals (49). The inferior portion of the left postcentral gyrus is wider on the left when compared to the right (48, 50). The superior surface of the left temporal gyrus is narrower than the right, and the planum temporale (length of the superior fissure behind Heschl's gyrus) is longer on the left (51, 52). Fissures are more frequent on the superior surface of the left temporal lobe (50). Reversal of the left-right temporal lobe asymmetry occurs in some schizophrenic persons (53).

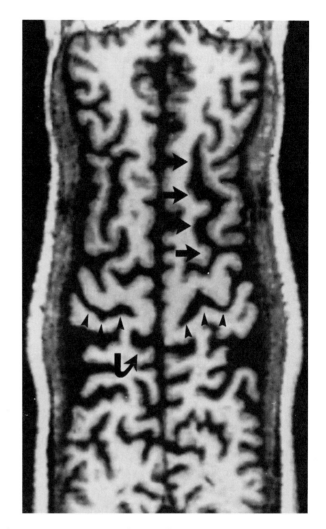

Figure 4.14. Reconstructed 2D surface map of the brain. The superior portion of the orbits is at the upper end of the figure. The marginal rami of the cingulate sulcus *(curved arrow)* are on different planes. The width of the left superior frontal *(arrows)* gyrus is different from the corresponding gyrus on the right. The central sulcus *(arrowheads)* differs in contour from side to side.

MR BACKGROUND TO ANALYZE BRAIN ANATOMY

Almost all of the illustrations in this chapter were obtained from a single T-weighted, gradient-echo, 3D (MPRAGE) sequence which took 11 minutes to acquire. The patient was a 70-year-old female whose scans demonstrated some minor abnormalities. The exceptions to the 3D images are Figure 4.9, *B* and *C*, and Figure 4.12. Figure 4.9, *B* and *C* is a set of routine spin-echo proton density and T2-weighted scans taken of the 70-year-old patient. Figure 4.12 consists of scans taken of a separate individual, and a specimen to demonstrate how high resolution images of small structures can be obtained. The scanning parameters of the high resolution images are listed in the illustration.

The MPRAGE images were obtained in the sagittal plane at 1.3-mm intervals. The axial and coronal images were reconstructed from these sagittal images at a thickness of 4.0 mm. In contrast, most 2D MR images are currently being obtained at a thickness of 5 mm. The axial and coronal 2D images in our illustrations thus contain approximately 20% less signal than they might have had had they been reconstructed at 5 mm, whereas the sagittal midline images (Figs. 4.5 and 4.13) contain approximately 75% less signal. The 4 mm and 1.3 mm thick images were used in this chapter to show the robustness of this technique. The T1 MPRAGE sequence is especially good at differentiating gray from white matter. Unfortunately, the gray-white matter difference was difficult to reproduce in the illustrations.

Figure 4.9, *B* and *C*, consists of a standard spin-echo proton and T2-weighted sequence which took approximately 6 minutes to acquire. When the T2-weighted sequence is compared with the corresponding gradient-echo T1 MPRAGE sequence the CSF is bright, whereas it is dark on the T1 and proton sequence. On the proton density image CSF can be made to be either bright or dark, depending on the chosen parameters. In addition, on the T2-weighted image the gray matter is brighter whereas the white matter is darker; on the corresponding T1-weighted sequence the opposite is true. Images similar to T2 and proton density weighted images can be obtained with gradient-echo and fast spin-echo sequences.

Figure 4.12 consists of high resolution T1- and T2-weighted coronal images. The T1 gradient-echo image (Fig. 4.12*A*) took 9.2 minutes to acquire. In contrast, a routine T1 spin-echo scan would only take 2 minutes to perform. The longer acquisition time was designed in an attempt to more clearly demonstrate the hippocampal formation. The T2 turbo (fast) spin-echo image (Fig. 4.11*B*) was also designed to maximize image quality and took 10 minutes to acquire. Figure 4.12*C* is an MR scan of a brain specimen taken in a 1.5 T large-bore scanner using a 5 cm circular small animal coil and demonstrates how well a clinical MR scanner can image the hippocampal formation provided that there are no limits in time or motion. The scan (Fig. 4.12*C*) took 1 hour to acquire.

3D reconstructions present in Figures 4.1–4.3 utilized a Siemens software called VOXEL-MAN. The "surface of interest" was shifted 2–3 voxels deep to avoid the scalp signal and 10 voxels beneath this depth were integrated for the 3D reconstruction. The structures beneath the surface are thus visualized. A 2D surface map of the cortex was also reconstructed in the axial plane from the 3D MPRAGE images (Fig. 4.14). The plane of reconstruction is outlined on the sagittal image in Figure 4.13. The 2D surface map allows easy comparison of gyri and sulci in the left and right hemispheres.

FUNCTIONAL IMAGING

Nuclear Studies

Functional studies that examine regional cerebral blood flow (RCBF) and cerebral metabolism have been helpful in identifying patients with psychiatric illnesses. Positron emission tomography (PET) has been used to study cerebral glucose metabolism following the injection of [^{18}F] fluoro-2-deoxy-D-glucose (FDG). RCBF has been studied by PET following the injection of oxygen$^-$15. Similar information has been obtained with single photon emission computed tomography (SPECT) following the injection of ^{123}I and ^{99}Tc tracers.

Functional studies are helpful in differentiating the various forms of dementia (54). Patients with Alzheimer's disease, the most common dementing illness, have temporal-parietal cortex hypometabolism which is correlated with behavioral deficits and clinical course, demonstrated in PET (55) and SPECT (56) studies. In contrast, patients with Pick's disease have predominantly frontal hypometabolism, and patients with Huntington's disease and Parkinson's disease have striatal hypometabolism (57), although depressed Parkinson patients also may have frontal hypometabolism (58). Another characteristic that can be used to distinguish the dementias is the presence of focal changes. Multi-infarct dementia can be distinguished from Alzheimer's disease by the presence of asymmetric, scattered perfusion defects (59).

Other psychiatric disorders also show regional changes in metabolism relative to normal controls. Schizophrenic patients, for example, have often been shown to have frontal hypometabolism (60). Although this was initially thought to be confounded by neuroleptic treatment effects (61), subsequent investigations in never-medicated schizophrenic patients indicated a difference in metabolic rate independent of medication exposure (62). In addition, decreases in striatal perfusion (63) and increases in medial temporal lobe perfusion (64) have been demonstrated. Depressed patients with both unipolar major depression and bipolar patients in the depressed or mixed state have also demonstrated frontal hypometabolism (65, 66). When bipolar depressed patients become manic, this metabolic rate increases. Depressed patients appear also to have increased limbic metabolism as well as frontal hypometabolism (67, 68), perhaps reflecting the involvement of the functional circuit in which these structures are encompassed (69).

MR

In addition to detailed information about brain anatomy, MR can now provide information about brain function. Neuronal activity that induces small changes in brain microvasculature can be detected with the appropriate imaging sequences and hardware. It is believed that the most common functional technique (blood oxygen level dependent effect) relies on a difference in the amount of paramagnetic oxyhemoglobin in the microvasculature at the activated site which in turn leads to a change in T2 signal intensity. Studies measure signal difference between task performance and resting state. To date it has only been possible to detect large changes in brain activity, such as those induced in the primary visual cortex by photic stimulation or in the primary motor cortex by hand or finger squeeze (70) (Fig. 4.15). Other studies are also being

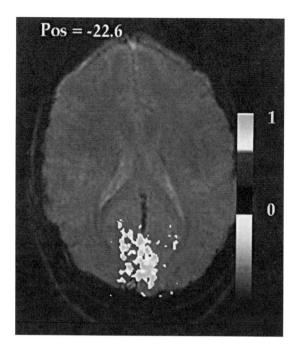

Figure 4.15. Functional MR changes in the occipital lobe during visual stimulation.

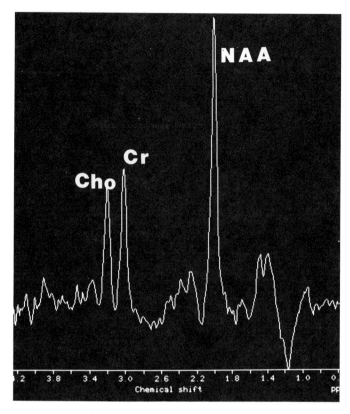

Figure 4.16. Normal proton spectroscopy. Cho = choline; Cr = creatine/phosphocreatine; NAA = *N*-acetylaspartate.

performed to study the brain's response to auditory and sensory stimulation (71). In functional MR imaging experiments, just as in PET or SPECT, the observed changes occur with a latency of several seconds, reflecting a time delay between the neuronal activity and the measured MR response. MR changes are thus a derivative of net neuronal activity rather than a direct measure of neuronal activity which operates in the millisecond range.

The new imaging techniques and equipment used to obtain functional MR images have also been used to study cerebral blood flow (perfusion) and blood volume (72, 73) noninvasively. Determining the reserve in these parameters, through the administration of acetazolamide, could be helpful in evaluating patients with stroke as well as dementia (74). Cerebral blood flow and volume can also be examined following injection of several MR imaging contrast agents by dynamically studying the susceptibility effect of these agents as they pass through the brain (75–77). The advantage of using a contrast agent is that it can potentially produce greater signal changes than can the noncontrast techniques. Unfortunately, however, because the contrast agent must be injected, such experiments can be repeated only a limited number of times. Diffusion weighted MR imaging has been used to examine regional shifts in water content following brain injury and cerebral ischemia (78–80). To date there are no published accounts of diffusion weighted imaging being performed in patients with psychiatric illnesses.

MR spectroscopy (MRS) is a technique that can be used to quantify biochemical differences in specific brain regions since the different chemical forms of an element create peaks at characteristic frequencies. Proton MRS measures neurons through the *N*-acetylaspartate (NAA) peak (Fig. 4.16).

Additional resonances that are frequently observed at 1.5 T include glutamine/glutamate (Glu/Glx), creatine/phosphocreatine (Cr), choline, (Cho), and myoinositol (myo-Ins). Under pathologic conditions, lactate may also be detected. Phosphorus MRS measures the energy metabolites phosphocreatine (PCr), inorganic phosphate (Pi), adenosine triphosphate (ATP), as well as phosphomonoesters (AMP) and phosphodiesters (ADP). Like functional MR imaging the strength of MRS is its noninvasive nature with no known side effects. The major limitation of MRS performed at the relatively low field strength used in clinical scanners is the poor separation between the metabolite peaks and poor signal-to-noise ratio compared with those obtained with high field strength laboratory instruments.

The number of MRS studies being performed on neuropsychiatric patients is increasing. Schizophrenic patients have been found to have a decrease in phosphomonoesters (AMP) in the frontal lobes, presumably reflecting alterations in cell membrane phospholipid metabolism (81–83). Changes in AMP and ADP have also been reported in patients with dementia of the Alzheimer's type (DAT) (84, 85), and in HIV-positive dementia patients (86, 87).

In proton MRS the NAA peak is believed to be an index of neuronal health; a decrease in the NAA/Cr ratio indicates either neuronal dysfunction or its loss within a volume. A decrease in the NAA/Cr ratio has been observed in demented patients with Alzheimer's disease and in HIV-positive patients with dementia (88–91). In Alzheimer's disease the decrease occurs initially in the temporal lobes and then generally throughout the entire brain (92). In schizophrenic patients a decrease in the NAA/Cr ratio has been observed in the temporal and frontal lobes (93–95). Patients with major depression have demonstrated elevated choline peaks in the brain (96). Similar changes have been demonstrated in the basal ganglia of not only depressed patients but in those with bipolar disorder in the depressed state (97, 98). The pharmacokinetics of psychotropic agents can be investigated in vivo using ^{19}F MRS (99). The naturally occurring lithium isotope ^7Li is MRS sensitive and can be used to compare serum and brain lithium (100).

References

1. Gado M, Hanaway J, Frank R. Functional anatomy of the cerebral cortex by computed tomography. J Comput Assist Tomogr 1979; 3:1–19.
2. Altemus, LR, Roberson GH, Fisher CM, Pessin M. Embolic occlusion of the superior and inferior divisions of the middle cerebral artery with angiographic-clinical correlation. Am J Roentgenol 1976;126:576–581.
3. Gibo H, Carver CC, Rhoton AL, Len Koy C, Mitchell RJ. Microsurgical anatomy of middle cerebral artery. J Neurosurg 1981;54:151–159.
4. Kido DK, LeMay M, Levinson AW, Benson WE. Computed tomographic localization of the precentral gyrus. Radiology 1980; 135:373–377.
5. Talairach J, Tournoux P. Co-planar stereotaxic atlas of the human brain. New York: Thieme Medical Publishers, 1988.
6. Haber SN. Neurotransmitters in the human and nonhuman primate basal ganglia. Hum Neurobiol 1986;5:159–168.
7. Seab JP, Jagust WJ, Wong STS, Roos MS, Reed BR, Budinger TF. Quantitative NMR measurements of hippocampal atrophy in Alzheimer's Disease. Magn Reson Med 1988;8:200–208.
8. Dauphinais ID, DeLisi LE, Crow TJ, et al. Reduction in temporal lobe size in siblings with schizophrenia: a magnetic resonance imaging study. Psychiatry Res 1990;35:137–147.
9. Rossi A, Stratta P, Mancini F, et al. Magnetic resonance imaging findings of amygdala-anterior hippocampus shrinkage in male patients with schizophrenia. Psychiatry Res 1994:52:43–53.
10. Bremner J, Randall P, Scott T, et al. MRI-based measurement of hippocampal volumes in patients with combat-related post traumatic stress disorder. Am J Psychiatry 1995; 152:973–981.
11. Iwasaki S, Nakagawa H, Fukusumi A, et al. Identification of pre- and postcentral gyri on CT and MR images on the basis of the medullary pattern of cerebral white matter. Radiology 1991;179: 207–213.
12. Reinarz SJ, Coffman CE, Smoker WRK, Godersky JC. MR imaging of the corpus callosum: normal and pathologic findings and correlation with CT. AJNR 1988;9:649–656.
13. Rakic P, Yakovlev PI. Development of the corpus callosum and cavum septi in man. J Comp Neurol 1968;132:45–72.
14. McLeod N, Williams JP, Machen B, Lum GB. Normal and abnormal morphology of the corpus callosum. Neurology 1987;37:1240–1242.
15. Mark LP, Daniels DL, Naidich TP. The fornix. AJNR 1993;14: 1355–1358.
16. Curnes JT, Burger PC, Djang WT, Boyko OB. MR imaging of compact white matter pathways. AJNR 1988;9:1061–1068.
17. Hunt AL, Orrison WW, Yeo RA, et al. Clinical significance of MRI white matter lesions in the elderly. Neurology 1989;39:1470–1474.
18. Hendrie HC, Farlow MR, Austrom MG, Edwards MK, Williams MA. Foci of increased T2 signal intensity on brain MR scans of healthy elderly subjects. AJNR 1989;10:703–707.
19. Gerard G, Weisberg LA. MRI periventricular lesions in adults. Neurology 1986;36:998–1001.
20. Deicken RF, Reus VI, Manfredi L, Wolkowitz OM. MRI deep white matter hyperintensity in a psychiatric population. Soc Biol Psychiatry 1991;29:918–922.
21. Guze BH, Szuba MP. Leukoencephalopathy and major depression: a preliminary report. Psychiatry Res Neuroimaging 1992;45:169–175.
22. Brown FW, Lewine RJ, Hudgins PA, Risch SC. White matter hyperintensity signals in psychiatric and nonpsychiatric subjects. Am J Psychiatry 1992;149:620–625.
23. Drayer B, Burger P, Darwin R, Riederer S, Herfkens R, Johnson GA. MRI of brain iron. AJR 1986;147:103–110.
24. Kido DK, Shoulson I, Manzione JV, Harnish PP. Direct caudate nucleus and putamen measurements in patients with Huntington's Disease: a high field strength MR study. Neuroradiology 1991; 336(suppl):604–606.
25. Aylward EH, Schwartz J, Machlin S, Pearlson G. Bicaudate ratio as a measure of caudate volume on MR images. AJNR 1991;12:1217–1222.
26. Barbeau A. Parkinson's disease: clinical features and etiopathology. In: Vinken PJ, Bruyn GW, Klawans HL, eds. Handbook of Clinical Neurology, vol 5 (No. 49): extrapyramidal disorders. New York: Elsevier, 1986.
27. Bamford KA, Caine ED, Kido DK, Plassche WM, Shoulson I. Clinical-pathologic correlation in Huntington's disease: a neuropsychological and computed tomography study. Neurology 1989;39: 796–801.
28. McHugh PR. The basal ganglia: the region, the integration of its systems and implications for psychiatry and neurology. In: Franks AJ, Ironside JW, Mindham RHS, et al, eds. Function and dysfunction in the basal ganglia. Manchester, England: Manchester University, 1990.
29. Bogousslavsky J, Regli F, Uske A. Thalamic infarcts: clinical syndromes, etiology, and prognosis. Neurology 1988;38:837–848.
30. Stuss DT, Guberman A, Nelson R, Larochelle S. The neuropsychology of paramedian thalamic infarction. Brain Cogn 1988;8:348–378.
31. Aggleton J. The contribution of the amygdala to normal and abnormal emotional states. TINS 1993;16:328–333.
32. Last RJ, Thompsett DH. Casts of cerebral ventricles. Br J Surg 1953;40:525–542.
33. Bull JWD. The volume of the cerebral ventricles—The Robert Wartenberg Memorial Lecture. Neurology 1961;11:1–9.
34. Van Horn JD, McManus IC. Ventricular enlargement in schizophrenia—a meta-analysis of studies of the ventricle:brain ratio (VBR). Br J Psychiatry 1992;160:687–697.
35. Zipursky RB, Marsh L, Lim KO, et al. Volumetric MRI assessment of temporal lobe structures in schizophrenia. Biol Psychiatry 1994; 35:501–516.
36. Turner SW, Toone BK, Brett-Jones JR. Computerized tomography scan changes in early schizophrenia: preliminary findings. Psychol Med 1986;16:219–225.
37. DeGreef G, Ashtari M, Bogerts B, et al. Volumes of ventricular system subdivisions measured from Magnetic Resonance Images in first-episode schizophrenic patients. Arch Gen Psychiatry 1992;49: 531–537.
38. Shenton ME, Kikinis R, Jolesz FA, et al. Abnormalities of the left temporal lobe and thought disorder in schizophrenia. N Engl J Med 1992;327:604–612.
39. Jeste DV, Lohr JB, Goodwin FK. Neuroanatomical studies of major affective disorders. Br J Psychiatry 1988;153:444–459.
40. Alexopolos GS, Young RC, Shindledecker RD. Brain computed tomography findings in geriatric depression and primary degenerative dementia. Biol Psychiatry 1992;31:591–599.
41. Andreasen NC, Swayze V II, Faum M, Alliger R, Cohen G. Ventricular abnormalities in affective disorder: clinical and demographic correlates. Am J Psychiatry 1990;147:893–900.
42. Evans WA, Jr. An encephalographic ratio for estimating the size of the cerebral ventricles; further experience with serial observations. Am J Dis Child 1942;64:820–830.

43. Davidoff LM, Dyke CG. The normal pneumoencephalogram. Philadelphia: Lea & Febiger, 1951.
44. Hahn FJY, Rim K. Frontal ventricular dimensions on normal computed tomography. AJR 1976;126:593–596.
45. Soininen H, Puranen M, Riekkinen PJ. Computer tomography findings in senile dementia and normal aging. J Neurol Neurosurg Psychiatry 1982;45:50–54.
46. LeMay M, Kido DK. Asymmetries of the cerebral hemispheres on computed tomograms. J Comput Assist Tomogr 1978;2:471–476.
47. LeMay M. Morphological cerebral asymmetries of modern man, fossil man, and nonhuman primate. Ann NY Acad Sci 1976;280:349–366.
48. Cunningham DJ. Contribution to the surface anatomy of the cerebral hemispheres. Dublin: Royal Irish Academy, 1892.
49. LeMay M, Culebras A. Human brain—morphologic differences in the hemispheres demonstrable by carotid arteriography. N Engl J Med 1972;287:168–170.
50. Connolly CJ. External morphology of the primate brain. Springfield, IL: Charles C Thomas, 1950.
51. Hyde JB, Akesson EJ, Berinstein E. Assymetrial growth of the superior temporal gyri in man. Experientia 1973;29:1131.
52. Geschwind N, Levitsky W. Human brain: left-right assymmetries in temporal speech region. Science 1968;161:186–187.
53. Johnstone EC, Cowens DG, Crow TJ, et al. Temporal lobe structure as determined by nuclear magnetic resonance in schizophrenia and bipolar affective disorder. J Neurol Neurosurg Psychiatry 1989;52:736–741.
54. Phelps ME, Mazziotta JC, Huang SC. Study of cerebral function with positron computed tomography. J Cereb Blood Flow Metab 1982;2:113–162.
55. Haxby JV, Grady CL, Duara R, Schlageter N, Berg G, Rapoport SI. Neocortical metabolic abnormalities precede nonmemory cognitive defects in early Alzheimer's-type dementia. Arch Neurol 1986;43:882–885.
56. Pearlson GD, Harris GJ, Powere RE, et al. Quantitative changes in medical temporal volume, regional cerebral blood flow, and cognition in Alzheimer's disease. Arch Gen Psychiatry 1992;49:402–408.
57. Kuhl DE, Metter EJ, Reige WH, Markham CH. Patterns of cerebral glucose utilization in Parkinson's disease and Huntington's disease. Ann Neurol 1984;15(suppl):119–125.
58. Mayberg HS, Starkstein SE, Sadzot B, et al. Selective hypometabolism in the inferior frontal lobe in depressed patients with Parkinson's disease. Ann Neurol 1990;28:57–64.
59. Kuhl DE, Metter EJ. Patterns of cerebral glucose utilization in depression, multiple infarct dementia, and Alzheimer's disease. Res Publ Assoc Res Nerv Ment Dis 1985;63:211–226.
60. Weinberger DR, Berman KF, Illowsky BP. Physiological dysfunction of dorsolateral prefrontal cortex in schizophrenia. Arch Gen Psychiatry 1988;45:609–615.
61. DeLisi LE, Holcomb HH, Cohen RM, et al. Positron emission tomography in schizophrenic patients with and without neuroleptic medication. J Cereb Blood Flow Metab 1985;5:201–206.
62. Buchsbaum MS, Haier RJ, Potkin SG, et al. Frontostriatal disorder of cerebral metabolism in never-medicated schizophrenics. Arch Gen Psychiatry 1992;49:935–942.
63. Carlsson M, Carlsson A. Schizophrenia: a subcortical neurotransmitter imbalance syndrome? Schizophr Bull 1990;16:425–432.
64. Friston KJ, Liddle PF, Frith CD, Hirsch SR, Frackowiak RSJ. The left medial temporal region and schizophrenia. Brain 1992;115:367–382.
65. Buchsbaum MS, WU J, DeLisi LE, et al. Frontal cortex and basal ganglia metabolic rates assessed by positron emission tomography with [^{18}F]2-deoxyglucose in affective illness. J Affect Disord 1986;10:137–152.
66. Baxter LR, Schwartz JM, Phelps ME, et al. Reduction of prefontal cortex glucose metabolism common to three types of depression. Arch Gen Psychiatry 1989;46:243–250.
67. Drevets WC, Videen TO, Price JL, Preskorn SH, Carmichael ST, Raichle ME. A functional anatomical study of unipolar depression. J Neurosci 1992;12:3628–3641.
68. Wu JC, Cristian Gillin J, Buchsbaum MS, Hershey T, Hohnson C, Bunney WE. Effect of sleep deprivation on brain metabolism of depressed patients. Am J Psychiatry 1992;149:538–543.
69. Swerdlow NR, Koob GF. Dopamine, schizophrenia, mania and depression: toward a unified hypothesis of cortico-striato-pallido-thalamic function. Behav Brain Sci 1987;10:197–245.
70. Kwong KK, Belliveau JW, Chesler DH, et al. Dynamic magnetic resonance imaging of human brain activity during primary sensory stimulation. Proc Natl Acad Sci USA 1992;89:5675–5679.
71. Ogawa S, Tank DW, Menon R, et al. Intrinsic signal changes accompanying sensory stimulation: functional brain mapping with magnetic imaging. Proc Natl Acad Sci USA 1992;89:5951–5955.
72. Rosen BR, Belliveau JW, Vevea JM, Brady TJ. Perfusion imaging with NMR contrast agents. Magn Reson Med 1990;14:249–265.
73. Rosen BR, Belliveau JW, Buchbinder BR, et al. Contrast agents and cerebral hemodynamics. Magn Reson Med 1991;19:285–292.
74. Graham GD, Zhong J, Petroff OAC, Constable RT, Gore JC, Prichard JW. Magnetic resonance image monitoring of changes in cerebral perfusion induced by acetazolamide and hypercarbia in the rat. Stroke 1994;25:270.
75. Belliveau JW, Rosen BR, Kantor HL, et al. Functional cerebral imaging by susceptibility-contrast NMR. Magn Reson Med 1990;14:538–546.
76. Perman WH, Gado MH, Larson KB, Perlmutter J. Simultaneous MR acquisition of arterial and brain signal-time curves. Magn Reson Med 1992;28:74–83.
77. Rosen BR, Belliveau JW, Aronen HJ, et al. Susceptibility contrast imaging of cerebral blood volume: human experience. Magn Reson Med 1991;22:293–299.
78. Chien D, Kwong KK, Gress DR, Buonanno FS, Buxton RB, Rosen BR. MR diffusion imaging of cerebral infarction in humans. AJNR 1992;13:1097–1102.
79. Moseley ME, Cohen Y, Kucharczyk J, et al. Diffusion-weighted MR imaging of anistropic water diffusion in cat central nervous system. Radiology 1990;176:439–445.
80. Moseley ME, Cohen Y, Mintorovitch J, et al. Early detection of regional cerebral ischemia in cats: comparison of diffusion- and T2-weighted MRI and spectroscopy. Magn Reson Med, 1990;14:330–346.
81. Pettegrew JW, Keshavan MS, Panchalingam K, et al. Alterations in brain high-energy phosphate and membrane phospholipid metabolism in first-episode, drug-naive schizophrenics. Arch Gen Psychiatry 1991;48:563–568.
82. Kato T, Shiorii T, Murashita J, Hamakawa H, Inubushi T, Takahashi S. Phase-encoded ^{31}P-MRS of the frontal lobes in patients with schizophrenia (abstr). Proc Soc Magn Reson 1994;602.
83. Williamson P, Drost D, Stanley J, Carr T, Morrison S, Merskey H. Localized phosphorus 31 magnetic resonance spectroscopy in chronic schizophrenic patients and normal controls. Arch Gen Psychiatry 1991;48:578.
84. Pettegrew JW, Panchalingam K, Moossy J, Maritnez J, Rao G, Boller F: Correlation of phosphorus-31 magnetic resonance spectroscopy and morphological findings in Alzheimer's disease. Arch Neurol 1988; 45:1093–1096.
85. Brown GG, Levine SR, Gorell JM, et al. In vivo phosphorus NMR profiles of Alzheimer's disease and multiple subcortical infarct dementia. Neurology 1989;39:1423–1427.
86. Deicken R, Hubesch B, Jensen P, et al. Alterations in brain phosphate metabolite concentrations in patients with HIV infection. Arch Neurol 1990;48:203–209.
87. Whaley R, Hall C, Kwock L. MRI and P-31 MRS of HIV-positive individuals (abstr). Proc Soc Magn Reson Med 1991;1:10.
88. Menon DK, Baudouin CJ, Tomlinson D, Hoyle C. Proton MR spectroscopy and imaging of the brain in AIDS: evidence of neuronal loss in regions that appear normal with imaging. J Comput Assist Tomogr 1990;14:882–885.

89. Jarvik JG, Lenkinski RE, Grossman RI, Gomori JM, Schnall MD, Frank I: Proton MR spectroscopy of HIV-infected patients: characterization of abnormalities with imaging and clinical correlation. Radiology 1993;186:739–744.

90. Meyerhoff DJ, Mackay S, Bachman L, et al. Reduced brain N-acetylaspartate suggests neuronal loss in cognitively impaired human immunodeficiency virus-seropositive individuals: in vivo ^{1}H magnetic resonance spectroscopic imaging. Neurology 1993;43: 509–515.

91. Chong WK, Sweeney B, Wilkinson ID, et al. Proton spectroscopy of the brain in HIV infection: correlation with clinical, immunologic, and MR imaging findings. Radiology 1993;188:119–124.

92. Ide M, Naruse S, Furuya S, et al. [1]H-CSI study of the Alzheimer disease—comparison between the the early stage and the late stage (abstr). Proc Soc Magn Reson 1994;599.

93. Moore CM, Redmond OM, Buckley P, et al. In vivo proton NMR spectroscopy (STEAM) in patients with schizophrenia (abstr). Proc Soc Magn Reson Med, 1992;1933.

94. Yurgelun-Todd DA, Renshaw PF, Waternaux CM, Gruber SA, Cohen BM. [1]H spectroscopy of the temporal lobes in schizophrenic and bipolar patients (abstr). Proc Soc Magn Reson Med 1993;1539.

95. Choe B, Kim K, Shu T, Shinn K, Lee C, In-ho P, Lenkinski RE. Alterations of proton metabolites in drug-naive, chronic schizophrenia by MRS (abstr). Proc Soc Magn Reson 1994;603.

96. Charles HC, Lazeyras F, Krishnan RKK, Boyko O, Payne M, Moore D. Brain choline in depression: in vivo detection of potential pharmacodynamic effects of antidepressant therapy using hydrogen localized spectroscopy med. Proc Soc Magn Reson (abstr) 1992;757.

97. Renshaw PF, Stoll AL, Rothschild A, et al. Proton MRS studies of the basal ganglia in major depression: side and treatment effects (abstr). Proc Soc Magn Reson med 1993;433.

98. Kato T, Hamakawa H, Shioiri T, Murashita J, Inubushi T, Takahashi S. Proton MRS of the basal ganglia in patients with bipolar disorder (abstr). Proc Soc Magn Reson 1994;605.

99. Durst P, Schuff N, Crocq MA, Mokrani MC, Macher JP. Noninvasive in vivo detection of a fluorinated neuroleptic in the human brain by ^{19}F nuclear magnetic resonance spectroscopy. Psychiatry Res Neuroimaging 1990;35:107–114.

100. Komoroski RA, Newton JEO, Walker E, Cardwell D. In vivo MR spectroscopy of lithium-7 in humans. Magn Reson Med 1990;15: 347–356.

5

CLINICAL NEUROPHYSIOLOGY IN NEUROPSYCHIATRY

Alison Reeve

Developments in technology are particularly exciting when they can be used to increase understanding of our human experiences. Tools that operate within the time frame of neuronal events have the greatest usefulness for this purpose because the brain is the source and repository for sensory and intellectual experience, attribution of meaning, and integration of memory.

The common technique at our disposal involves recording electrical events. This is done by electroencephalography (EEG) and magnetoencephalography (MEG). The discussion that follows reviews some basic aspects of these technologies and their application to neuropsychiatry. EEG and MEG are particularly meaningful techniques because they collect information in millisecond time range that can be linked to brain function (or dysfunction).

Clearly, there is still much to learn in this field of neurophysiology. EEG findings are notorious for their frequent nonspecificity. Part of the reason for an apparent lack of specificity in findings lies in the organization of the brain (with replication of functions, multiple representations, plasticity of neurons and of function). Disappointment over early hopes for the diagnostic specificity of EEG may have led to an underestimation of the strength of the technique. Neuropsychiatric applications of EEG & MEG deserve intensive study. EEG and MEG are tools that have much to tell us about brain function and have the advantage of being noninvasive.

NEUROPHYSIOLOGICAL MEASUREMENTS

Electroencephalography

Electroencephalography (EEG) is a standardized, seemingly straightforward method of recording the electrical activity of the brain at the scalp. The field was founded by Hans Berger in the 1920s. As discussed more fully in later sections of this chapter, the clinical EEG is both a useful and, at times, misleading source of information about the brain.

Definition. The EEG measures a summation of electrical activity, as recorded as a difference in electrical potential between two active recording electrodes. It is not a direct measure of brain electrical activity. Rather, brain activity is measured indirectly as a difference between electrical potentials received at two recording electrodes. The choice of placement of electrodes, and the properties of material between the source (the brain) and the electrodes affect the type, the intensity, and the specificity of the activity measured.

Factors that influence EEG record. Sources that can alter the electrical signal include: skull, scalp, sweat, metal, and poor physical contact of the electrode with the scalp. Electrode paste has properties that increase conductance of electrical signal through it. Because of this, it is important that the area of paste not be significantly larger than the recording electrode, or else there will be some loss of regional specificity around that electrode. These different factors are all contributors to resistance that must be minimized at the recording electrode. Of course, sources of resistance within the scalp such as the thickness of the skull, scar tissue in the meninges, blood, fresh or coagulated, are factors that usually cannot be controlled. Every effort has to be made in the laboratory setting to minimize the confounding factors that *can* be controlled, by assuring clean electrodes, little to minimal oil on the scalp surface (by cleaning with an abrasive agent), a discrete area of conductive gel, and minimal to no movement of the electrode from its contact with the scalp.

The electrical signal of the neurons of the brain is relatively weak. Therefore, the signal coming from the electrode must be amplified. The electromechanical properties of amplifiers vary greatly. It is important that the configuration of the amplifier be designed to maximize the type of recording one is trying to obtain. Amplifiers are used to increase the voltage difference between the input to that of the output. They are characterized in terms of sensitivity and gain.

Sensitivity is reflected as the ratio of the input voltage to the output pen deflections in the standard EEG recording. A typical ratio is seven microvolts (μV)/mm. A higher numerical value for sensitivity reflects less amplification, i.e., a sensitivity of 10 indicates 10 μV/mm. EEG machines have an array of amplifiers set up to allow individual sensitivity adjustment for each channel, or general adjustment for all channels.

Gain is the ratio of the voltage obtained at the output of the amplifier to the voltage applied at the input. Often described in terms of volts (V) and microvolts (μV), gain is sometimes expressed in terms of decibels (dB) or 20 times the logarithm in base 10 of the gain. For example, a gain of 10 equals 20 dB; a gain of 1,000,000 equals 120 dB. In clinical EEG, sensitivity is usually used to describe the amplification because the gain is not directly measured from the output of the amplifier.

Electrical signals coming through a recording channel have a characteristic frequency. The band width of the signal is defined by the frequency range within which the signal is contained. Some information will be lost if the frequency range of the recording channels is narrower than the frequency range of the EEG signal. Likewise, extraneous information will be included if the frequency range of the recording channels is wider than the band width of the EEG signal. Different types of filters are used to maximize the EEG signal and minimize noise and signals of non-cerebral origin. In practice, EEG recording channels can have high-pass, low-pass, or band-pass filters. High-pass filters are designed to let higher frequencies pass through and to block lower frequencies, such as those below 1 Hz. Low-pass filters are designed to let low-frequency activity through and to filter highfrequency activity. Band-pass filters are designed around a range of frequency to filter on both the high and low ends of the frequency spectrum. Most filters are designed to have the signal drop off gradually, to minimize the artifacts that can be seen with an abrupt attenuation of signal outside the chosen range.

Many filters induce a phase difference between the output and input signals. This phase difference can create a time difference between different tracings. The choice of filters will affect the recording achieved. When the output is to a paper record, the timing of signals may be critical in interpretation of the clinical data. In a computerized EEG data collection system, it may be more important to allow more "noise" through if necessary to preserve phase relationships.

Montage and reference electrodes.   Recordings over the head are usually done following the international 10–20 system. This localizes the electrodes proportionately (10% and 20% spacings) between certain landmarks–inion, nasion, and preauricular points (Fig. 5.1). By convention, the electrodes over the left side of the head are numbered odd, and those on the right side of the head are even. Z stands for zero or midline. The letters of the electrode placement reflect relative position over the head; in other words, Fp (frontopolar), F (frontal), C (central), P (parietal), T (temporal), O

(occipital), A (auricular), M (mastoid). The number of electrodes that are applied varies depending on the montage (series or patterns in which the electrodes are connected to each other), the population being studied, the type of activity considered important to detect, and the number of channels/amplifiers available. The American EEG Society recommends that the full 21 electrodes of the 10–20 system be used and that a record be obtained in both bipolar and referential montages. They recommend that electrode connections for each channel be indicated at the beginning of each montage and that over the course of the record, bipolar recordings be made in both longitudinal and transverse directions (i.e., front-to-back and left-to-right). Standard clinical laboratories may have from 8–32 channel EEG machines with which to make recordings. The number of montages recorded will be different depending on the number of channels available to make a simultaneous recording.

The montages used in EEG are of two general types. The first is referential, the second bipolar. A common form of referential montage is to have a series of electrodes attached to the same common reference, often the earlobe or mastoid. The printout can then be alternated between left and right, which aids the detection of hemispheric asymmetry. To maximize the ability to detect subtle differences, the left-temporal electrodes may be referenced to the right ear or mastoid and vice versa for the right side. Another form of commonly used reference is that of the linked ears. It was thought that this would make a neutral reference; however, the ear lobe tends to be very easily "contaminated" by electrical activity of the heart. One attempt to avoid this difficulty involves putting one electrode over the right sternoclavicular junction and another on the spine of the first thoracic vertebrae. These two electrodes are connected together through a 20,000 Ω-variable resistor that can change in its resistance such that the electrocardiogram is cancelled or essentially cancelled (1). A different type reference is a common average reference, created by a computerized analysis system, after the recording is completed. These various attempts to make a "neutral reference" must always be carefully checked for artifacts. In addition, it is important that the details by which the reference was chosen are carefully documented.

Bipolar montages are particularly useful to compare the polarity of signals, and to detect the so-called phase reversal that occurs around an area of high amplitude signal change. To be useful, bipolar montages should cover relatively large areas of the head so that interpretation of the direction (or polarity) can be made in a reasonable manner. There is a general rule that higher voltages are seen as the interelectrode distance increases. This is particularly noticeable when an activity is noted on a bipolar montage and the montage is switched to a reference montage. The voltage may be so much larger after the switch that the sensitivity of the record needs to be decreased.

The clinical report on the actual paper tracing should document that the mechanical instrumentation is intact

INTERNATIONAL 10-20 SYSTEM FOR ELECTRODE PLACEMENT

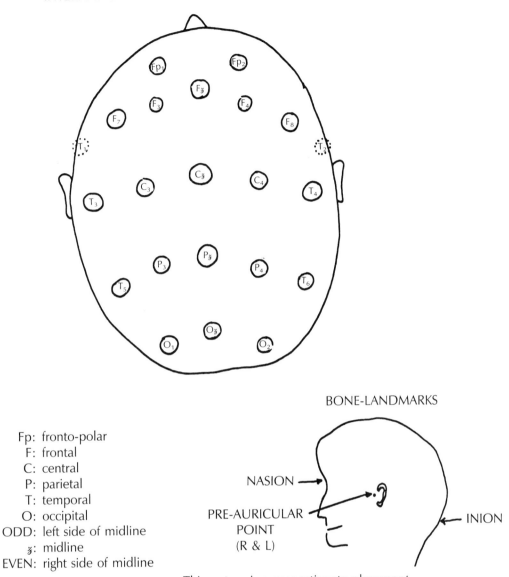

BONE-LANDMARKS

Fp: fronto-polar
F: frontal
C: central
P: parietal
T: temporal
O: occipital
ODD: left side of midline
ℨ: midline
EVEN: right side of midline

NASION
PRE-AURICULAR
POINT
(R & L)
INION

This system is a proportionate placement
of electrodes (at 10% and 20% increments)
between anterior-posterior/right-left landmarks.

Figure 5.1.   International 10–20 system of electrode placement.

(Table 5.1). In other words, the calibration signal should show up in proper alignment across all channels, the voltage of that signal should be consistent across all channels, and the tracing should show little or no variation in deflections when not connected to a biological substrate. This is necessary so that changes in wave forms can be attributed to the brain and the conditions under which the recordings were made, rather than to the electrical/mechanical properties of the instrumentation. The paper speed of recording should be noted, along with the specific montage used and the activity that the patient is undertaking while the recording is being made. The duration of each montage can be deduced by knowing the paper speed. There should be several montages; there should be a period of certain kinds of activation such as hyperventilation (for 3 minutes at least); and photostimulation. Other types of stimulation can be done depending on the condition. For example, a patient who experiences seizure-like symptoms during reading should be asked to read; or conversely, a person who exhibits specific behaviors hearing music, or some other specific activity, should be exposed, if possible, to the provocative stimulus. The technician should change the montages to maximize views of any abnormalities seen in the EEG. Standard frequency activities are listed in Table 5.2. The disorders or states which particularly elicit a frequency are not exclusive but rather characteristic for a frequency type.

Table 5.1. Variables in EEG Data

Artifacts
 muscle tension and movement
 mechanical
 electrical
 drug effects
Reactivity
 awake/asleep
 drug effects
 level of consciousness
Interpretation
 state of subject
 human vs. computer
 clinical factors
 subject age

Alternate electrode placements. Electrode placement other than that of the 10–20 system can make the information provided by the EEG record much more useful for specific studies. One limitation in using an elastic cap that has electrodes fixed in relation to each other and can be stretched over the person's head is that when an abnormality is discovered or a particular area of the head is of interest for study, it is very difficult to add more electrodes. The closer the spacing of electrodes, the more the specific information can be obtained regarding a region of interest. However, the signal must be large enough for it to be resolved or focal enough so that the electrodes can differentiate the activity over the region. In some laboratories (2), 128 channel recordings are not uncommon. The argument is that increasing spatial information will permit better resolution of any particular activity. This becomes an important factor when considering neuropsychiatric disorders and diagnoses. Usually, the routine EEG reports no abnormalities or diffuse abnormalities that are nonspecific for any behavioral disturbances. The resolution that can be obtained by very close spacing of electrodes and careful analysis of the record may begin to provide the kind of specificity of information that clinicians working with neuropsychiatric disorders would like to have. There may be some loss of information as more electrodes are placed over a specific region, because the amplitude of the signal is lower. If the signal/noise ratio is too low, the desired improvement in spatial resolution cannot be attained.

Telemetry. The type of disorder one is trying to study will influence the recording strategy. Intermittent, infrequent activity is the most difficult to catch. At times, correlating behaviors of the patients with changes in EEG activity is essential. Simultaneous video recording with EEG recording is one way to differentiate clinical and electrical events that are occurring in relation to one another from events that are occurring completely independently from each other. The video camera can be directed to encompass whole body activity or to focus on certain areas of interest. Portable systems allow the equipment to be set up in any hospital room and can be used with scalp electrodes or implanted electrodes, and with cabled or radio-transmitted connections to amplifiers. This technique often is used to demonstrate pseudoseizure activity. However, pseudoseizure activity may involve so much muscle artifact in the EEG that an occasional true seizure may be obscured. The clinical history and careful observation of the actual behaviors (direct observation and/or video) carry as much weight as the EEG abnormality in making the diagnosis of pseudoseizures.

Other forms of telemetry are useful for long-term monitoring of EEG activity during normal daily routines for a patient. Here, the video aspect is not so important. The purpose of these recordings is to obtain long-term records of infrequently occurring activity (such as sharp waves or spikes). Patients are asked to keep a diary of their activity, especially noting any sensory changes that occur and the time of day and duration of symptoms. Patients who are candidates for surgical removal of an epileptic focus need to be carefully assessed for the stability of the focus and the degree of disability it is producing.

EEG that has been collected over hours to days can be analyzed by computer to yield a summary of frequency and amplitude patterns over small chunks of time (e.g., 2, 4, or 10 seconds). If there is an area of interest, one can return to the original (expanded) dataset to read the activity more carefully. During certain procedures, such as during carotid endarterectomy, on-line analysis of EEG activity in 2-second bits can provide immediate and clearly visible change in brain activity to the surgical team. Immediate feedback about decrements in brain activity can guide the vigor of the procedure and help to improve outcome for the patient.

Sleep studies. Sleep monitoring is of two types. The first, obtained frequently during routine EEG, is brief, often drug-induced, and may not require any special adaptation of technique. The second is to monitor through all phases and types of sleep, usually over a period longer than 8 hours. Again, maintaining adequate electrode-to-head contact is essential. This may be done by an electrode cap, needle electrodes, or implanted (cortical or depth) electrodes, and some form of cable-to-transmitter box arrangement, rather than direct connection to amplifiers. A lot of movement occurs during sleep, and one does not want the patient wrapped up in wires, or disconnecting the electrodes. Evaluation for sleep apnea and other respiratory compromise require monitoring oxygenation, heart rate, and peripheral muscle tone, in addition to brain activity. Disorders of excessive daytime drowsiness are important to evaluate because of the associated psychological malfunction they produce. For example, average sleep latency as measured during the Multiple Sleep Latency Test (MSLT) of less than 5 minutes is a sign of pathological drowsiness and correlates with poor work performance because of the intrusion of sleep episodes into the wakeful state.

Standards for interpretation. Over the decades, the paper presentation of the EEG record has become more standardized. Usually, this tracing is read by the naked eye. This leads to an emphasis on recognition of familiar patterns and deviation from those patterns. It difficult for an encephalographer to quantitate the distribution of power in adjacent frequency bands, record, to differentiate minor interhemi-

Table 5.2. EEG Frequency Band and Its Characteristics

Name	Frequency	Location	Factors
β	13–25 Hz	frontal	increased by benzodiazepines and barbiturates
α	8–12 Hz	occipital	awake, resting state with eyes closed (meditative); does not slow appreciably with increased age
θ	5–8 Hz	central	awake, task oriented; may be generalized in drowsiness
δ	1–4 Hz	frontal and central	generalized in deep sleep; seen in encephalopathy, coma, and toxic states

EEG FREQUENCY EXAMPLES

A.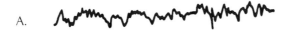

B.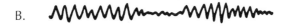

C.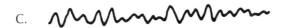

D.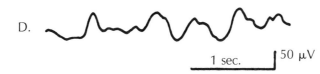

1 sec.   50 μV

A. Beta: 20-25 Hz.;   B. Alpha: 9-10 Hz.;
C. Theta: 5-6 Hz.;   D. Delta: 2-2.5 Hz.

spheric and intrahemispheric differences, and to subtract eye movement artifacts from frontal lead potentials. Notwithstanding, the paper record, interpreted by an experienced EEG reader, permits an expert comparison of the patient's EEG with the hundreds of others seen previously, enabling rejection of subtle artifacts recognizable by a trained eye.

The advent of computerized topographic mapping of the EEG has made analysis of the record much easier in many ways. It has also allowed people who were not familiar with many variants of a normal recording to attempt to rely on a computer-based algorithm for deciding whether or not an activity is normal or abnormal. The advantage of computerized, quantitative EEG is that the display can be rearranged easily, after the recording session is over. Information can be gleaned from the record months and years after the recording session. Areas of activity can be highlighted, with gray scales or color scales, to make it easy to see temporal and regional changes in the record. There are many different programs written—some for dedicated systems and some that run on a personal computer (PC). In general, those that run on the PC and are geared for research purposes have greater flexibility, and those that are designed to be

run in a clinical setting have more "canned" programs. One difficulty and major drawback of computerized EEG and the subsequent topographic mapping is the necessity that the recording be of high quality at the time that it is made. For example, one must be cautious in interpreting slow activity over the frontal regions if there is significant eye movement at the time of the reading. Eye movement can be detected in leads as far posterior as central area. Fortunately, many programs now provide algorithms for distinguishing eye movement potentials from cerebral activity and eliminating it from the record electronically by subtraction.

Understanding the sources of the EEG. The electrical potential at any specific point in the brain is the sum of potentials generated by underlying cellular activity. Biochemical activity at the cellular level generates ionic currents that create the electrical potentials and currents. The electrical and magnetic field associated with these potentials and currents follow well-known physical laws. For EEG, the field potential of a group or population of neurons reflects the sum of the contributions of a collection of individual neurons. Asynchronous and/or irregular firing of neurons cannot be accurately detected by EEG electrodes distant from the source. Therefore, the scalp EEG reflects activity from regularly arranged neuronal sources, firing in more or less synchronous patterns. The contribution from radially and tangentially oriented currents is equally appreciated at the EEG electrode. The pyramidal neurons of layers IV and V of the cortex often are activated synchronously, producing brain activity measured at the scalp.

An electrical event recorded at the cortex will seem to be of shorter duration than that same event recorded at the scalp. This is because a moving dipole observed from a greater distance can be recorded for a longer period of time than when seen from nearby. Another factor that influences recordings obtained at the scalp is the conduction of electrical activity by the different layers between the neuronal population and the scalp. One of the difficulties with solving for the source of electrical activity, as it is recorded in the EEG, is to correctly account for the (conductive) inhomogeneities of the different layers. Mathematical models exist that account for concentric spheres of different conductive properties. In addition, research studies are comparing the mathematical solutions to actual recordings of skull, scalp, meninges, and fluid in the same subject (usually animal). Values for the conductivities do not agree thus far because differences in the conditions under which recordings were made, and differences between species. A difficulty inherent in finding the sole solution to the question of which group of cells or what sequence of activities originated the electrical recording obtained in an EEG is that there may be no unique solution to this problem (named the inverse problem). Many different combinations of activity can result in a similar or even the same EEG pattern. One way to reduce the number of potential sources is to solve the problem for an equivalent current dipole (ECD) of activity in the brain. Thus, when we speak of solving for dipole localization, we are actually talking about an abstract representation of brain activity occurring within a defined region.

There are a number of programs written that deal with this problem of dipole localization. As with MEG, which is more fully discussed later, it is quite difficult to distinguish between multiple dipoles occurring relatively superficially versus a single, deeper source, or large focal events versus simultaneous diffuse small events. The EEG, by providing information about multiple sources of activity in several different montages, may permit deductions about the underlying source of activity. Large contiguous areas of activity as opposed to many discrete areas that are near to each other, however, are difficult to distinguish from each other unless a great number of electrodes placed over the scalp (2). Another factor that is accounted for only with difficulty in dipole localization algorithms is that of activity having different time constants. In other words, closely superimposed sources with different rates of onset and offset of electrical signal can be very confusing to distinguish from each other. They tend to blur into one source. Different algorithms for dipole localization use different approaches. Some make assumptions regarding what activity is "background" at all electrodes and what other activity represents "true" activity of interest. Others make assumptions about the timing or orientation of the EEG signal of interest.

Magnetoencephalography

Definition. The electrical activity of the brain, as all electrical activity, generates magnetic fields. For a long time the magnetic fields of the brain could not be detected because of the lack of sufficiently sensitive instrumentation. Compared with the earth's magnetic field, the brain's magnetic field's roughly one billion times weaker. Unlike the EEG, which is affected by the attenuation of electrical potential by the boundaries between brain and scalp as well as the inherent properties within those boundaries, the magnetoencephalogram (MEG) records a magnetic field of brain and surrounding tissues in a region of constant magnetic permeability. Specific dipole activity within the brain produces measurable perturbations in the magnetic field. The magnetic field is affected by the strength, direction, and location of the electrical source. To begin to deduce the equivalent source for the recorded magnetic field, some properties of biomagnetism must be kept in mind.

Biomagnetic properties. Every electrical current generates an associated magnetic field, following what is commonly called "the right hand rule." If the thumb of a person's right hand indicates the direction of electrical current flow, the curl of the fingers indicates the direction of flux of the magnetic field around that current (Fig. 5.2). All electrical currents in the brain can be modeled as the sum of their tangential and radial components. The interaction of cerebral magnetic fields within a certain geometrical configuration causes the radial components of the bioelectrical sources to be virtually invisible in the MEG. Thus, the fields recorded in MEG are those from the tangential components of electrical signals. This at once simplifies and complicates the information recorded in the MEG. A limited number of solutions (though many) can be found to account for the magnetic field that is generated.

It is possible to detect the weak magnetic field of brain activity because of the advent of superconducting quantum interference devices (SQUID). As the name implies, the SQUID must be bathed in a super-cooled environment, usually helium. The SQUID is a component of a gradiometer, a device intended to differentiate nearby magnetic fields from those that are farther away, and therefore more invariant. The gradiometers can be arranged with different numbers of coils and with different shapes of the coils. Each configuration enhances the recording of a specific phenomenon: weak magnetic fields; activities that are located close together; or activities that occur in a plane versus a curved surface. New configurations are continually being developed. Placing many channels in close proximity to each other has the advantage of increasing the sensitivity to the signal and the disadvantage of "cross-talk" between the channels because of being housed so closely. Physical limitations on how small the components can be made and the biophysical properties of the instrumentation also place constraints on the spacing of SQUIDs from each other and their geometri-

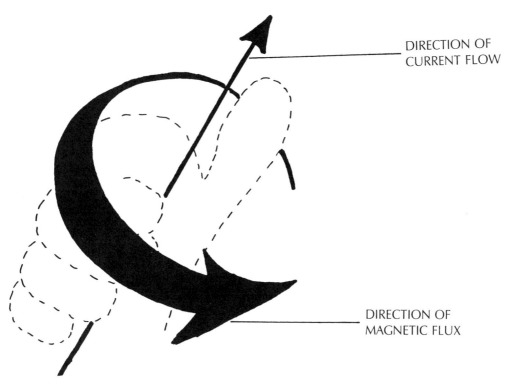

Figure 5.2. The "right hand rule" of magnetic flux around electrical current.

cal array. The goal for human studies is to achieve a reliable means by which to record over the entire head simultaneously.

Instrumentation. The earliest human MEG was collected with single channel instruments. At the time of this writing, there are 40 commercially-available systems with up to 40 channels. Some systems are designed to detect fields on a convex surface, others on a planar surface. A 137-channel system is in production, and another 100- to 150-channel system full-head is in the design stage. High temperature superconducting metals will allow the development of smaller gradiometers. As research develops in the near future, the cost of components can be expected to decrease dramatically. Some systems are designed to allow two 7-channel systems to record orthogonally to each other. Although this provides more information with regard to the site being studied, it does not solve the problem of recording over only part of the head.

The dilemma of recording at different locations and putting this information together is that the field maps for brain activity are often broader than a single channel or even a 7-channel MEG system. When pieces of recorded information, that are not recorded simultaneously are put together for a composite map as if representing simultaneous activity, assumptions are made about the temporal relationship of all the data. The logistical problems have been relatively great, and questionable assumptions have been made frequently when time has passed between successive recordings, the state of the individual's brain may not be the same. To truly compare the field strength arising simultaneously at different channels, composite maps should not be made. In the case of evoked responses, where repetitive stimuli are given (presumably producing similar conditions), there is evidence to support composite rendering of the evoked field. However, one can never remove the variable influence that progression of time may have on the recorded signal and on the state of the individual being recorded.

Artifact and noise reduction. In addition to the magnetometer design, placing the instrument inside a specially designed room assists in reducing background "noise." Two sheets of mu metal arranged at roughly 8 inches apart provide a major source of deflection of nearby strong magnetic fields by dispersing them within the metal sheets. Every 2–3 years, shielded rooms should be degaussed. A shielded room, usually located within a laboratory environment, is the chamber in which the recordings are made. Significant advances have been occurring to improve patient comfort and tolerance of the procedures. Because the magnetometers are usually suspended from the ceiling or have other forms of limitations of their movement, the subject must be able to assume certain positions. Most of the current instrumentation continues to contain liquid helium to maintain the supercooled temperature, therefore, tilting of the magnetometer can be done only partially. Most laboratories have either chairs or a supportive bed for subjects to be lying on comfortably with the neck supported. It is important that there be adequate support for the subject so that the strain of keeping still does not cause unnecessary muscle artifact. It is also customary that there be some form of communication—e.g., video monitoring and radio link—between the room and the operators outside the shielded room. This is both to reassure the subject and to provide a means of communication.

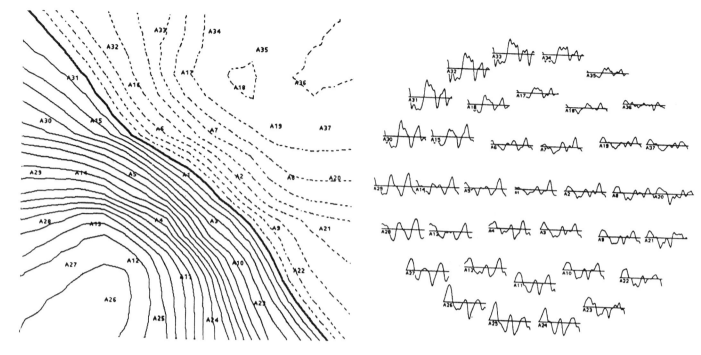

Figure 5.3. Sample magnetic field map and waveforms.

Even with all these precautions, there are many sources of magnetic field artifact. Many can be prevented if carefully sought before study is begun. The most common include metal objects on the subject, including dental fillings. Obviously, the teeth cannot be removed. However, undergarments with metal portions in them, shoes with metal shanks, belt buckles, watches, and anything else with metal content must always be removed. Additionally, it is often helpful to degauss the subject. This is especially true if simultaneous EEG electrodes are being applied. Extraneous sources of electromagnetic fields sometimes include equipment for particular studies that is brought into the shielded room, a bad electrode, or metal fragments inside the head. The cardiac pulse can also disturb both MEG and the EEG when it is of an extreme polarity, or the subject is tall and thin. Rarely does the respiratory effort or the cardiac pulse disturb the recording to the point that it causes the body to shift in a rhythmic manner. When this does happen, repositioning the person may help. As with the EEG, all attempts to remove sources of artifact, including mechanical problems (EEG equipment, a bad MEG channel or too low a level of helium) must be made before the recording is in progress.

Clinical application.   Unlike EEG, MEG is not considered a routinely reimbursable clinical test. In the United States, reimbursements are starting to be made for some presurgical evoked field studies. It is likely that in the near future certain other clinical examinations related to epilepsy will also be reimbursed. For other disorders, MEG is likely to remain a research procedure rather than a clinical test for several more years. At present, there are no uniform standards of practice or predetermined clinical indications for obtaining a MEG.

Perhaps because of the tradition of EEG, or to make it more similar to what people expected for brain activity, the MEG is often presented as a series of wave forms. This is a useful means of presenting the data because it allows an analysis of field activity (ingoing/outgoing or positive/negative) over time (Fig. 5.3). It is, however, somewhat misleading in that one is looking at magnetic fields and not electrical current. Also, the line of wave forms cannot be assumed to be coming from a single source.

The wave form can be displayed for multiple channels recorded at the same time, or from one channel, either sequentially or superimposed on itself over time. Superimposition of a single channel's wave forms, such as in an evoked field response, can help to distinguish the stability of the response over time. Superimposition of multiple channels recorded at the same time can help to readily identify an area of simultaneous maximum and minimum field, i.e., a dipolar field. Another way to present magnetic field data is to use contour mapping. The relative field strength is plotted in concentric circles, with the zero line identified between the two directions of flux. Areas of neuronal activity that are fairly widely distributed may at times present with simple dipolar maps, or may present a series of convoluted stronger and weaker areas of magnetic flux. These maps resemble topographical survey maps. A surface rendition of this sort usually does not convey much meaningful information. Either picking the areas of perceived maximal activity, or changing the plane in which one is presenting the field map will allow the reader to get more specific information from this contour. Each of these different approaches will help to determine which part of the magnetic field is the area of interest. (Because this is all activity related to the brain, it is potentially all interesting. However, one generally is seeking to learn about a specific region or a specific function.) In evoked responses, for example, the assumption has often been that a single dipole is responsible for the dipolar magnetic field recorded. When more elaborate contours appear, questions are then raised as to whether or not there has been a clear-cut evoked response, whether other factors are entering into the recording, or whether the stimulus has elicited multiple superimposed responses.

Magnetic field data require selective filtering in a manner similar to EEG data. Filter band widths are often similar as for EEG; 60 Hz activity is also a problem. Often spontaneous activity or certain types of evoked responses are of relatively weak amplitude. Appropriately chosen filters can improve the signal-to-noise ratio.

The clinical report of MEG resembles a research report. It includes the conditions under which the data were collected, the ways in which the data were analyzed, including filter settings and the relevant variation in state of the individual during the testing period. Generally, the data will be spoken of in terms of the location of the equivalent current dipole (or dipoles) deemed responsible for the activity recorded. It is assumed that an MRI has been obtained with the same set of reference landmarks. At least three, if not five, external landmark points should be identified that are common to the MEG and the MRI. Data analysis, even using the most automated programs, takes at least as long as the recording session, to up to five times the duration of a recording session. This represents a significant investment of both computer and personnel time.

The inverse problem. Solving the inverse problem is a particular challenge in MEG because it is virtually impossible to prove the source for the magnetic field. Any validating technique uses other technology. The most straightforward and most frequently used algorithms at present solve for single ECDs. Although this is often appropriate when the table is confirming an epileptic focus, the algorithms tend to force the data into dipolar pattern, possibly ignoring other relevant data. If there is insufficient field strength to warrant a single dipole, the algorithm(s) will fail to identify any potential ECD.

Recently, visual evoked field studies have been analyzed in a way that allows for more than one dipole contributing to the field map. This complicates the mathematical solution because of the need to impose some arbitrary constraints on the number of dipoles or the amount to which the dipoles can move over time (3). Multiple ECDs have the advantage that when a field map is constructed based on the solution, the resulting theoretical magnetic field map looks more like the empirically recorded evoked field map. In addition, multiple ECDs make sense when one considers the associative functions that must occur in the brain, even under fairly simple conditions, such as responses evoked by simple stimuli. Depending on where these dipoles are located, i.e., in a gyrus, on a gyrus, or in a sulcus, the effect of their activity, the time course, and the associated magnetic field will vary and contribute differentially to the evoked field.

Interpolation. In MEG, as in EEG, there is a need to extrapolate or interpolate between points of data collection. The interpretation of the magnetic field between individual channel recordings is less affected, generally, by the spatial separation of those channels than is the electrical potential difference between electrodes in EEG. However, one iterative program type, called minimum norm localization, relies on determining local changes in magnetic field strength or direction. The difficulty for this program to solve for a single dipole, or even multiple dipoles, is that a local norm may be identified that does not represent the largest change in field polarity of the entire data set that one is analyzing. This is particularly true if the magnetic field is not a simple, clean dipolar pattern, but has multiple areas of different directions of flux. Other techniques of extrapolation are based on comparing the coherence of channels to each other (4). This latter analysis is of particular interest for analysis of neuropsychiatric disorders not likely to be associated with gross brain disease. Processing difficulties or abnormal connections of circuits of neurons can be detected using spatial filtering techniques that assess sequences of changes in activity.

Electroencephalography and Magnetoencephalography: Comparison

These two neurophysiological imaging techniques for brain activity are very different from each other. Perhaps the best analogy to other imaging techniques is positron emission tomography (PET) versus single photon emission computed tomography (SPECT), which measure metabolic activity and cerebral blood flow, respectively, although both are influenced by activity of radioligands, binding, and delivery and retention of radioligands to brain areas. The MEG and EEG record activity from the same substrate, yet are primarily recording different aspects or components of that activity (Table 5.3). When MEG was first being introduced into clinical laboratories, it was touted as being much superior to EEG. Actually, MEG is better seen as different rather than superior to EEG at present. One major advantage of MEG is that it records the *absolute* magnetic field at one location in space. As discussed earlier, the EEG always requires a "reference" that must be considered when the data are analyzed. Another advantage of MEG is that the instrument can be put into position over the subject's head rather quickly, and thus, when time is critical, may provide the relevant study in a timely manner.

EEG has an advantage over MEG in that, using at least the international 10–20 system of electrodes, recording is made over the entire scalp simultaneously. Most MEG, whether single, 7-, or 37-channel systems, do not cover the entire head. Often, to obtain full field maps around each extremum of the magnetic field, the magnetometer must be repositioned several times. This leads to the potential for the state of the subject, drug effects, or other variables to change over time and contribute to a variability in the record. Until whole-headset MEG is available, this will be a major limitation.

Table 5.3. Comparison of EEG and MEG

Variable	EEG	MEG
Time domain	milliseconds	milliseconds
Physical sources of artifact	scalp; bone; fluids; poor electrode contact	nonphysiological magnetic fields and electrical currents
Records directly	electrical activity	magnetic fields
Direction of recorded dipoles	all that come to electrode	tangential
Cost	+ +	+ + + + +
Established clinical standards	yes	no

Limitations. A challenge for both techniques is to differentiate multiple superficial sources of activity that are occurring simultaneously or nearly simultaneously from those that are a combination of superficial and deeper sources with close temporal relationships to each other. With MEG, this is possible by careful analysis and multiple forward iterative solutions, being calculated to account for the varying contributions to the magnetic field. In some ways, this is an easier task with MEG because one is analyzing an *absolute* field rather than a difference between two electrodes. For the EEG, it is difficult to be certain that the apparent contribution to the recorded potential or difference in potential over several electrodes is coming from sources close to the recording electrodes and not from the reference electrode.

Cost factors. Like other relatively new brain imaging techniques, MEG is expensive. Proper shielding, instrumentation, the need for cooling to the temperature of liquid helium, and maintenance of software on large computers all contribute to an equipment cost of over $2,000,000. At present, however, EEG is much cheaper to install, fairly inexpensive to maintain, and has the benefit of portability and compactness. Therefore, it is especially useful in situations where money and space are major obstacles. The advent of adequate EEG analysis programs for personal computers has increased the information that can be obtained from the EEG. This fact needs to be appreciated when reviews and original articles written before the mid- to late 1980s are read. There is a large and established literature that had enormous hopes that the EEG would "see the brain working," but these hopes were dashed by the lack of specificity between subjects and disease states. The advent of new analysis paradigms is permitting more sophisticated questions to be asked.

Applications of the technologies. Both these neurophysiological tools have the capability of collecting data from neuronal activity in real time. Both, however, require extensive manipulation and analysis of data after they are collected. The technological advances accompanying MEG have greatly benefitted the entire field of EEG. The next several decades will bring significant new information from both these technologies to bear on specific neuropsychiatric disorders.

Among the challenges when studying diseases and dis-eased states is the choice of appropriate controls. Some researchers have attempted to study groups of patients with disorders such as schizophrenia, manic depression, and obsessive-compulsive disorder. Although doing a resting-state analysis on each one of these subgroups is a laudable proposition, one would *not* expect there to be readily apparent abnormalities when compared with a similar number of normal control subjects. There are several reasons for this. First, the prevalence of these illnesses is low, and the normal population shows substantial variability. A substantial number of normal controls must be studied before one can say with reasonable certainty what normative findings are.

Second, most subjects who join these studies on an outpatient basis represent the less severe forms of the illness under study, since they are competent to participate in the research and are able to understand and cooperate with the protocols.

Third, there are many variables that need to be carefully controlled and accounted for in all neurophysiological studies. Both MEG and EEG will be affected by medications and drugs, chronicity of illness, age, time of day and level of arousal, as well as by specific diseases. It is also known that certain drugs given to an individual with a need for the drug will have a different effect from a drug given to someone for whom such a need does not exist. It is a well documented fact that high levels of antihistaminic drugs may be well tolerated and beneficial to those with allergies or pruritis, while the normal subject ingesting a much lower dose may be immediately sedated. Therefore, claims about drug effects on the EEG should be considered with due regard to the clinical state of the individual receiving the drugs.

The current trend is to combine EEG and MEG for clinical research studies. There are several advantages for this approach. First, it compares directly the results on individual subjects at the same point in time. Therefore, changes in attendance state, drug effects, disease effects, and time will affect both the MEG and EEG equally. Second, it allows for direct comparison and cross-validation of results from both MEG and EEG. Third, simultaneous EEG and MEG analysis has promoted the development of paradigms in both fields for better models to account for equivalent current dipoles, for explanation of field and potential patterns, and gradually for more user-friendly software for all of these analyses.

IDEALIZED EVOKED POTENTIAL
(an averaged response)

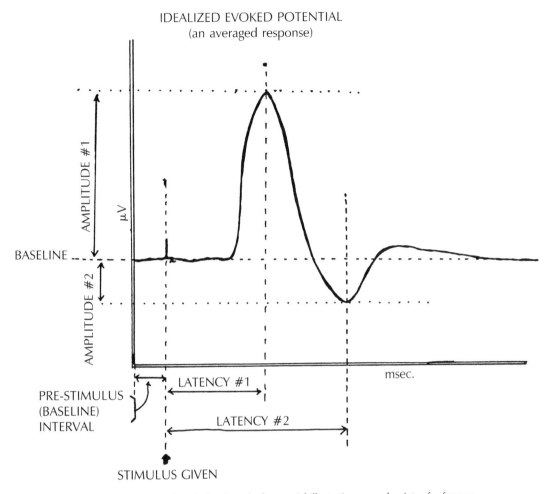

Figure 5.4. Sample (idealized) evoked potential illustrating general points of reference.

Evoked Potentials and Fields

The evoked response in either EEG or MEG is the activity linked to a specific stimulus, as distinguished from background activity. Multiple presentations of the stimulus are given and the activity is summed and averaged. Better noise cancellation can be obtained with more repetitions of the stimulus, but signal can be last as the brain habituates to a repeated stimulus. When the evoked responses under study are due to cortical activity, the ability for any brain to adapt to the stimulus is great.

The summation (averaging) period in an evoked response study usually is selected to start just before the stimulus and to continue for some time longer than the response being studied (Fig. 5.4). The number of repetitions for cortical evoked responses is usually somewhere between 50–200; for subcortical responses, between 1000–4000 repetitions.

Sensory modality. Traditional evoked responses have used three sensory modalities, visual, somatosensory, and auditory. There are standardized norms for early responses, middle, and late responses. In the visual domain, there are several standardized types of stimuli that are used for eliciting these responses (checkerboard, flash, central versus

peripheral field). Somatosensory potentials can be evoked by a painful stimulus that is generally an electric shock just above threshold and sufficient to cause a muscle twitch, e.g., a thumb twitch. Auditory stimuli include broad-band clicks presented in rapid succession for brainstem-evoked responses or series of tone pips or more complicated sound presentations for later cortical responses.

Considerable research effort has focused on potential charges associated with various cognitive tasks. Sometimes these tasks are cross-modal, involving auditory and visual stimuli presented simultaneously. Sometimes these can differ within a category, such as variations in visual stimuli between color stimuli and written word stimuli that do not correspond to the color, or visual stimuli of words which sound similar if they were spoken but some of which are nonsense and similar variations. Tasks that require mental manipulation, i.e., retention in short-term memory and recall, or processing two types of information simultaneously, simultaneously stimulate different regions of the brain and can help differentiate processes occurring in connected brain regions.

Timing. The rate of stimulus presentation in each

domain is critical for producing a maximal response. For example, when auditory tones are presented at rates faster than one per second, the amplitude of the response is significantly decreased. If, on the other hand, the interstimulus interval is closer to 4 or 6 seconds, various components associated with the early cortical response can begin to be isolated. Therefore, there is a large difference in approach between a clinical EEG laboratory that is running evoked responses for neurological testing or presurgical/intraoperative testing and a research laboratory geared toward understanding what areas of the brain are being activated by different stimuli. If the study is being done to understand the contribution to an abnormal finding or abnormal sensation for a given individual, the stimulus should be designed in all aspects of presentation to most nearly replicate that which the subject indicates produces the abnormal response.

For the same reason, the quality of the stimulus, the instrumentation used to generate it, and the specific timing characteristics must all be documented in any publication so that repeat studies can be done. Subtle differences between different types of equipment can produce minor differences in the stimulus, particularly in visual and auditory systems, such that the response may either be enhanced or reduced and therefore not replicate previous findings. When in doubt, it is best to call the investigator who first reported the finding that one is trying to replicate.

Brainstem auditory evoked potentials are a sensitive test of CNS myelination and of acquired demyelination. The interpeak latency from peak 1–5 is a sensitive measure of the degree of myelination. In newborns it is considerably longer and shortens with increasing age, plateauing at about 3 years of life. In a recent study by Brivio et al. (5), it was found that males at age 3 had a somewhat longer interpeak latency than females, perhaps due to hormonal and dimensional effects summating. There was little between-ear difference.

Findings of Questionable Significance

A number of findings are seen in EEG, particularly clinical EEGs, that are of questionable significance. Incidental sharp waves, spikes, slow waves, exaggerated transitional phenomena (e.g., excessive post-hyperventilation high-voltage activity), and low-grade dysrhythmia can all occur without diagnostic specificity. It is noteworthy that patients with neuropsychiatric disorders appear to have a greater incidence of these types of findings in a setting where there are no clearly distinct accompanying behavioral changes. Although no electroencephalographer will be willing to ascribe a specific meaning of such findings, they should not be dismissed. First, it is imperative to ascertain whether the pattern in a particular patient is caused by medication. Second, when behavior changes or the patient's medication class is changed, a repeat EEG can be compared to the initial EEG. Third, some EEG findings suggest a physiologic correlate of the patient's symptoms. For example, if a person is complaining of feeling especially sensitive to exercise or being in a small space (indirectly inducing some hyperven-

tilation) and the EEG is hyperreactive to hyperventilation, then one might understand the patient's neurologic symptoms as being due to an altered brain response, somewhat atypical in nature, to the environmental stimulus.

The caveat to this discussion is that these same incidental findings can occasionally be seen in normals who are asymptomatic. The challenge is to determine whether there is meaning to any disruption in the well-modulated EEG. If one is inclined to ignore this finding in a normal, how much can be made of the same finding in someone who has a neuropsychiatric illness, without a clearly defined behavioral abnormality?

NEUROPHYSIOLOGICAL MEASURES IN NEUROPSYCHIATRIC DISORDERS

Schizophrenia

Many studies of patients with psychoses, including schizophrenia, were made with EEG. During the first decades of EEG technology, it was hoped that this measurement of brain function would yield an immediate demonstration of the etiology of the severe and disturbing symptoms. When a direct, evident abnormality was not forthcoming, clinicians lost interest in the technique. "Nonspecific" dysrhythmia and slow waves were frequently reported, without lateralization. Although the clinical picture appeared dramatic, the paper EEG record, recorded in a quiet setting, was not sensitive enough to characterize the differences of brain function underlying the behaviors observed. Until the last decade, there has been widespread consensus among psychiatrists and neurologists that the EEG was essentially useless for the detection of clinically-relevent abnormalities in patients with schizophrenia, apart from demonstrating seizure foci in patients with psychosis and epilepsy. The quantification inherent in evoked responses, with the requirement to repeat stimuli until a significant signal to noise ratio is achieved, and the development of computerized recording systems slowly began to change both what was being measured and what questions that were asked.

A skeptical view of the usefulness of EEG (and consequently MEG) to understanding diseases such as schizophrenia is at once realistic and unrealistic. It is true that there are no immediate, definitive answers from these technologies to the search regarding the etiology of schizophrenia. On the other hand, no other techniques can as reliably and repeatedly measure brain function in real time. A study of two patients who experienced transitory hallucinations reported observable differences in MEG auditory evoked responses between the nonhallucinating and hallucinating states (6). During the normal periods they recorded a prominent N100m wave that peaked between 73–94 msec. During the hallucinating period, the N100m was narrower in distribution (92–98 msec), and the response was dampened in several of the 24 channels. The equivalent dipole explained 90% of the variance of the magnetic field in the normal condition, but only 73% of the variance during hallucinations. The source locations of the two equivalent dipoles were only 1 cm apart and in supratemporal auditory cortex, which is consistent with the findings for normal subjects in a similar task. Interestingly, the authors reported no diminution in amplitude of response.

This study has several important design features. It uses two cooperative subjects who could accurately report the onset and offset of symptoms, and who could tolerate repeat studies. The subjects were used as their own controls. During normal periods and abnormal periods, the latency values for their N100m were within a range distribution for normal subjects. The data from the subjects were compared to data from normals in whom binaural tones were administered with and without unilateral masking noise. Similar effects on the N100m were found, suggesting that functioning neuronal substrate could be manipulated to produce abnormality of evoked response. The authors were careful not to make claims about the etiology for the symptoms (only one patient clearly met criteria for schizophrenia) but to address the likelihood that "a distorted interplay between auditory associative areas and the limbic structures, rather than with a malfunction of the primary auditory cortex itself"(6, p. 257) could produce alterations in measurements of auditory cortex functioning.

Evoked potentials show many group tendencies for acute and chronic schizophrenia. Somatosensory responses tend to have higher overall amplitude before 100 msec, but lower amplitude after 100 msec. The distribution of P30 and N60 responses were found to be more posterior in patients with schizophrenia than for normals, depressed, or nonpsychotic subjects (7, 8). The amplitude of auditory responses is usually lower after 50 msec than in normal controls, with average latency often being shorter.

Many components of auditory evoked responses, especially at 100 msec, are influenced by attention. In much of the literature before 1980, and even since, the level of attention of patients with schizophrenia was not well controlled or documented. Thus, we cannot be sure whether the lower amplitude of averaged responses is due to variation in latencies, increase in random background activity, variation in arousal or attention to a task, or from an inherent inability to activate as large a group of neurons or to elicit as large a response. Visual evoked responses tend to have somewhat *greater* amplitude for patients with chronic schizophrenia than normals, with less after-rhythm. The P300, in both auditory and visual domains, tends to have low amplitude and be less responsive to uncertainty in the stimulus presentation. A significant temporal (latency) variability was not demonstrated by Roth et al. (9), but other studies have shown a greater spread of latencies in individual trials making up the average response in patients with schizophrenia compared with normal controls.

A study by Faux et al. (10) emphasizes the lack of effect of antipsychotic medications on evoked potential findings in schizophrenia. These investigators repeated a study of the auditory P300 event-related potential on 14 neuroleptic-

withdrawn male subjects with schizophrenia and 14 healthy male controls. The patients were drug-free with a range of 14–71 days. The ERPs were recorded using linked-ear reference with an auditory "odd-ball" paradigm. Attention was monitored by having the subject stare at a fixation point and press a button when hearing a high-pitched infrequent tone. EEG was measured using 28 electrodes, incorporating the 10–20 system and eight interpolated electrodes. The P300 mean amplitude was measured as the mean voltage between 300–400 msec during the attentive condition. They also computed a latency-adjusted P300 mean amplitude for the schizophrenic subgroup in order to adjust for latency delays. In the normal group, the P300 amplitude was largest in the midline with symmetrically reduced amplitudes and lateral positions. The schizophrenic group showed amplitude reduction overall, with a greater right P300 component amplitude than left-sided amplitude.

When comparing group differences, the normals showed consistent amplitude overall, or a slightly left greater than right, in contrast to the schizophrenic group, which showed a distinct left smaller than right amplitude pattern. The intent of this study was to show that medication did not exert the effect in the patient group. A serious caveat is that a large range of drug-free duration was included in this study. Because the group as a whole showed very close grouping, with little spread, of the amplitude size, quite possibly, the duration of the drug-free state was sufficient to remove any drug effects on the findings. The authors suggest that perhaps the decreased amplitude of the left P300 may be related to left temporal lobe abnormalities in schizophrenia. Their previous studies demonstrated an association with left sylvian fissure enlargement on CT scans. Other studies have showed decreased temporal lobe tissue on MRI. The researchers note that they have not done within-subject comparisons on and off neuroleptic medication, nor have they controlled for the duration of neuroleptic exposure. The authors thus identify an electrophysiological finding that correlates to previously reported anatomical findings. They also support the conclusion that neuroleptic medication per se does not influence the measure of the P300 asymmetry found in schizophrenia (10).

Another hypothesis to explain the symptoms of schizophrenia is that of impaired filtering of sensory information, or altered sensory gating. Using paired auditory clicks, presented 1 second apart, with 5–8 seconds between pairs (ISI), Adler et al. (11a) and Waldo et al. (11b) demonstrated that normal subjects and their relatives have a reduced amplitude of response (P50) to the second click. Patients with schizophrenia have no reduction in their response to the second click; their first-degree relatives are between the patients and normals in size of response to the second click. Although this finding was thought to be idiosyncratic to their laboratory at first, it has been replicated by independent labs (12). The idea is that schizophrenia impairs the ability of the individual to dampen an automatic processing response (at 40–50 msec, signals are thought to be arriving at primary auditory cortex) when there is no new information contained in the signal.

Sleep recordings reveal persistent abnormality of sleep structure in treated and untreated patients with schizophrenia (13). Although delayed sleep onset, more arousals, and more early morning awakening are present in never-treated, untreated, and treated patients, these findings are not specific for schizophrenia. Rather, they most likely contribute to impaired arousal, excessive daytime sleepiness during the day, and a tendency to be disorganized. It is likely that sleep disturbance reflects the altered balance of several neurotransmitters (cholinergic, dopaminergic, serontonergic, noradrenergic systems all have been implicated in sleep disorders). Shortened REM latency (prominent with previously treated patients) is associated with severity of negative symptoms, consistent with a hypothesis of increased cholinergic activity that contributes to both (14).

The issue of medication effects on patients with schizophrenia is a complicated one. Antipsychotic medications have been shown to cause intermittent slow waves of large amplitude (EEG) over central and frontal regions. These patterns may have contributed to some interpretations of records as low-grade dysrhythmia. On the other hand, patients who have not been taking antipsychotic medications or have never been exposed to antipsychotic medications have also been found to have nonspecific changes in the EEG. It is difficult to assess the direct effect of antipsychotics because in normal controls this type of medication tends to rapidly induce sedation. At low dosage it does not cause gross changes in EEG pattern to visual inspection.

In an attempt to open the effect of the antipsychotic haloperidol on processing of sensory information, Malaspina et al. (15) gave amphetamine (.3mg/kg) to normals who were subsequently given 2 mg haloperidol intramuscularly and then were studied with a standard continuous performance task (CPT) and auditory conditioning testing (C-T) (to elicit paired p50). Amphetamine improved performance on CPT, and haloperidol caused a larger decrement in performance than when given alone. Sensory gating on C-T was increased by amphetamine (second p50 was even smaller or absent than in drug-free condition); this effect was eliminated by haloperidol. Haloperidol alone reduced both first and second responses (p50) to the paired stimuli. By contrast, in patients with schizophrenia, neuroleptic treatment can *improve* performance on CPT and *increase* sensory gating in C-T paradigms. These results suggest that there may be very different effects of haloperidol on EEG and EPs in acute and chronic treatment; that the effects of haloperidol in normals are quite different from those in patients with psychotic illnesses; and that the state of the individual (e.g., amphetamine, drug-free, resting, or task-oriented) may be important influences on the effects of a neuroleptic.

Another class of drug frequently administered to patients with schizophrenia is benzodiazepines. Known to increase fast (β) activity, benzodiazepines can confound the interpretation of fast activity in patients with schizophrenia. The increased left-sided β reported from a study of schizophrenic patients not taking benzodiazepines (16) is intriguing for the possible contribution this may have to nonspecific abnormalities of EEG.

When considering explanations for the symptoms of schizophrenia (impaired attention, auditory and visual hallucinations, impaired reality testing, disinhibited behaviors, disorganization of thought and action, poor ability to change mode of operation with new information), one tends to look at the functioning of primary and association cortex of frontal and temporal lobes. Abnormalities of ventricular volume, temporal lobe size, blood flow, and metabolism have been reported for schizophrenia. MEG and EEG provide a means of testing these areas of brain in real time, if appropriate study paradigms are used. Reite et al. (17) reported loss of normal asymmetry of equivalent dipoles for N100m in male patients with schizophrenia compared to male normals. In our laboratory we have found that the latency of the N100m in patients with schizophrenia is not reproducible. Single-trial analysis of 100 trials shows great variation in areas of cortex contributing to the waveforms.

Future studies need to concentrate on combining region-specific tasks during EEG and MEG measurements. The standard clinical EEG will continue to be useful as a screening tool to make sure a treatable, definable organic etiology is not causing the impairments in function (e.g., tumor, seizure disorder). Pharmaco-MEG and EEG can be expected to become more sophisticated and to provide meaningful information about rapidity of response to different classes of drugs, predicting individuals who will respond to specific classes of drugs. The EEG and MEG in combination will be most useful as tools to develop understanding of sequential processing of information during periods of exacerbation and remission.

Parkinson's Disease

Typically in Parkinson's disease (PD), the EEG remains normal in the early stages of the disease. Certain evoked potentials may be abnormal. For example, audiospinal facilitation is significantly reduced in amplitude during the 75–150 msec period after conditioning stimulation using the soleus H-reflex test. This is improved by treatment with levodopa (L-dopa), but not by anticholinergic agents. This represents an example of dysfunction of the reticular nuclei in PD (18). A related study by Beckley et al. (19) examined the interaction between motor response and cognitive set using EMG to look at long-latency postural reflexes in patients with PD compared with normal controls and young normals. Patients with PD had postural long-latency reflexes of lower amplitude and slower onset, especially with unpredictable testing conditions. Young normals and older healthy subjects were able to scale long-latency responses under both predictable and unpredictable conditions to anticipate the degree of perturbation encountered. Patients with PD were unable to anticipate the need for modifying the effort in the long-latency response. This defective modulation may be affected by abnormal frontal influence on the basal ganglia through the caudate. These results correlate with studies that show that PD often causes difficulty with complex motor tasks involving shifts in cognitive set. Response latencies were not affected by whether there was a predictable or unpredictable perturbation amplitude. They were consistent with previous findings that the latencies are programmed from minimal sensory information, unlike the response amplitude.

Patients with parkinsonism and dementia have been studied by Chen et al. (20) using clinical EEG. With the presence of dementia, the earliest EEG abnormality was slowing of the α-rhythm to below 7 Hz. In the last 2½ years of life, three-quarters of the patients studied had diffuse bilateral synchronous bursts of 5–7 Hz waves of 30–50 μV-amplitude. The EEG rhythm slowed to 4–5 Hz with interspersed asynchronous irregular waves at 3–4 Hz, with progressive diminution of amplitude and reactivity. These sometimes were localized over temporal lobes. There were no clear epileptiform discharges, and sleep records were generally normal. Sleep spindles were rare and lasted for a shorter duration. There was no correlation with extrapyramidal signs, i.e., patients who had marked rigidity, akinesia, but no dementia had only moderate changes in the EEG that were not specific. Tremors had no obvious relationship with the EEG. All patients with severe dementia had early abnormal EEGs.

To better understand the role of the reticular formation in motor control in PD patients, Nakashima et al. (21) evaluated the effects of sound on the blink reflex. They paired sound stimulation with the electrically elicited blink reflex. The blink reflex, which was measured by EMG, was conditioned by sound stimulation that was not loud enough to produce a blink response by itself. They varied the condition of time between the conditioning sound and the electrical stimulus to the supraorbital nerve. In control subjects, sound stimulation facilitated the first component of the blink reflex. In PD subject rigidity in the neck positively correlated with the degree of *suppression* of the *second* component when there was 500 msec interval between the conditioning sound and electrical stimulation. The durations and amplitudes of the first and second components of the electrically elicited blink reflex were the same in both normal and in PD subjects, suggesting that the reflex pathway components were normal in the PD patients. The authors' test paradigm differentiated between the function reflex arc itself and the function of facilitory and inhibitory interneurons, as modulated by basal ganglia in parkinsonism.

Epilepsy

EEG is widely used to document the existence of seizures or the presence of a focal electrical abnormality that is causing behavioral disturbances. For partial seizures, EEG has limited sensitivity because the seizure events do not occur continuously (the EEG will can be normal interic-

tally), and because the electrical activity may not be generated in or near the cortical surface (not all activity from depth will be recorded by the scalp EEG). The clinical history of alterations in behavior, perception, and cognition may support a diagnosis of partial seizures even when the EEG is normal.

tj;6The degree of inaccuracy of localization from the traditional noninvasive EEG is highlighted in a study by Salanova et al. (22), which compared interictal and intraictal scalp EEG and subdural electrocortigram recordings. The patients whom they studied all had frontal lobe seizures. A significant proportion of patients (seven of 12) had no interictal sharp waves on scalp EEG. However, these same patients had significant interictal seizure activity on the subdural electrode array recordings. In addition, those who had a localizing scalp EEG often had larger epileptogenic zones on the subdural electrode recordings.

Although some studies are being carried out to compare EEG and MEG of temporal spike localization (Ebersole, personal communication, 1993 [23]), extensive comparisons between MEG, scalp EEG, and subdural electrocortigrams need to be done to establish the most valid procedure for localizing epileptic foci. The textbook by Niedermeyer and Lopes de Silva comprehensively reviews the present state of the field [24].)

Pseudoseizure

Differentiation of seizure from "pseudoseizure" is often a requested use of the clinical EEG. Video monitoring of the onset of behavioral changes with the EEG is one of the best methods for documenting either absence or presence of electrical activity accounting for the patient's behavior. There are occasionally times when true epileptiform activity is missed because of motor activity, especially of the head musculature. Recording can be done with cortical and depth electrodes as well, which increases the likelihood of capturing an active source. Mesial temporal lobe foci are the most difficult to document accurately and can cause many unusual sensory complaints and behaviors.

When a diagnosis of pseudoseizure is made with relative confidence, it usually is not beneficial to the clinician to directly "confront" the patient with proof that seizures are not epileptic. Behaviors of dyscontrol, such as pseudoseizures, are indicators and expressions of psychological difficulty that the person has found no other way to express or to understand. It is particularly common to have both true seizures and pseudoseizures intermixed. Illness behavior(s) are learned over time and serve as a form of adaptation to an alteration in general function. It is important to directly express to the patient that illness behavior can be understood and changed, but is not often responsive to medications. This should be discussed from the beginning of any evaluation for seizure. The least helpful to the epileptologist or to the patient is to leave these "psychiatric spasms" as a discard diagnosis at the end of a long and grueling evaluation. There is the added caution that a small number of patients who appear to have only psychological etiology for their disorder will develop over the subsequent 5–10 years a definite neurological disorder (aneurysm, tumor, inflammation, etc.). This is an additional reason for repeated examinations over time.

Depression

The literature on EEG in depression is confusing to evaluate because a broad range of symptoms and severity have been lumped under the label "depression". In this area, EEG sleep studies have been the most consistent with one another. Biological markers of abnormalities of sleep are found in people prone to this disorder compared with controls. Krieg et al. (25) found that subjects who are at high risk for depressive disorder but did not yet meet the American Psychiatric Association's Diagnostic and Statistical Manual (DSM) criteria had decreased sleep efficacy and decreased amount of slow-wave sleep during the second non-REM period. The high-risk group also had twice the number of awakenings during the night than the controls. Of 20 subjects at high risk for developing a depressive disorder, the EEG in four of these subjects was found to have alterations characteristic of major depression (in general, these are considered to be decreased sleep efficiency, prolonged sleep-onset latency, frequent spontaneous awakenings, early-morning awakening, reduced amounts of slow-wave sleep with a slight increase in REM sleep and, often, shortened latency to the first REM period).

The group at high risk also showed greater overall variability in sleep parameters compared with the normal controls.

Studies of EEG in depression have employed various data reduction techniques. Dierks (26) described an attempt to use fast Fourier transformation (FFT) within a narrow band width (1–30 Hz), followed by equivalency dipole source localization for various frequencies. The five depressed subjects in his study showed more superficial and more anterior localization of the equivalent current dipoles (ECD) than age-matched medication-free patients with schizophrenia or normal controls. The ECD localizations were intriguing for there being differences between diagnostic groups, raising the question of whether there are different actual generators for EEG in each group. With such a low number of subjects, it would be difficult to generalize to all patients with depressive symptoms. In their study the α-equivalent sources were more superficial and anterior in the people with depression. This finding is significant because as a person moves from wakefulness to the early stages of sleep in stage 1, the α generators appear to move more anterior and temporally (27).

One wonders if in depression, a person is more ready to make this stage shift, or if this localization reflects an abnormality in sleep regulation as part of the dysfunction of depression. Using a combination of MEG and EEG, Lu et al. (28) demonstrated the various contributions from MEG and EEG in determining equivalents for localizations

for various components in the sleep EEG. The temporal localization of α tends to be more resistant to changes or decreases in vigilance than the occipital generators (29, 30). What contribution depressive disorder and its attendant neurotransmitter defects may have to the abnormalities reflected in EEG and MEG is difficult to separate from the effects it may have by disruption of sleep and wakefulness patterns overall. If the increase in the amount of α activity during depressive phases is actually reflecting a change in arousal state that has not been observed clinically, then previously reported results would need to be revised to identify changes in state of arousal-somnolence rather than of mood. Compared with normals, patients with depression often show increases in δ and θ activity over the right-posterior temporal regions and bilaterally increased β activity over the frontal areas (31). Many studies have shown both power and coherence changes found in many frequency bands over both hemispheres under different stimulation conditions, not always in the same direction, not always consistently, but differing from normal controls (32). Nagakubo et al. (33) attempted to differentiate epileptic subjects from patients with schizophrenia and depression and normal controls on the basis of EEG patterns. These researchers analyzed spikes, sharps, and irregular β patterns (either single small sharp waves or persistent irregular β patterns). To their disappointment, they discovered that those with epilepsy, depression, and schizophrenia had approximately the same rate of irregular β patterns (about 11–14%), compared with 4% in healthy controls. The prevalence of spikes and sharp waves in the epileptic group was significantly higher (35%) compared with either of the psychiatric disorders (4–5%).

There may be a correlation with increased somatic complaints in persons who demonstrate an irregular β pattern. This finding emphasizes the idea that rather than attempting to focus on the primary psychiatric disorder, the EEG (or MEG) may be more useful as a diagnostic tool in its own right, not to prove or disprove a clinical diagnosis, but to suggest treatment possibilities (responsiveness to antiepileptic drugs) or patterns of symptoms (i.e., somatization). The increased amount of irregular β was not attributable to drugs and was more common in patients over 40 than in younger patients.

In their attempt to understand different animal models of depression, Ehlers et al. (34), used a rat model to look at the effect of gender and social isolation on the EEG. Female rats had increases in slow-wave sleep during non-REM periods. Both male and female rats show increases in θ activity in the first 30 minutes after isolation is terminated, which then normalizes (θ activity is correlated with motor activity in rats).

In normal women, higher-power density in frequencies below 11 Hz (particularly δ) has been observed during non-REM sleep. Women had 50% greater values than men for power density in this range (35). Increased amounts of stage 4 slow-wave sleep in normal older women compared with male subjects has been reported by Webb (36) and Reynolds et al. (37).

One of the intriguing questions raised by the just-cited studies is the relationship between specific frequencies seen in the EEG and the level of activity of the individual. In rats, there is a clear correlation; in humans, it is more difficult to accurately identify a specific activity, because, for example, theta is not directly correlated with movement. However, often in typical unipolar depression, subjects are reporting that it is difficult to get themselves motivated, to complete tasks, and to be mobile. The increased amount of slower-frequency activity in the EEG may be related to this depressed state. In attempting to understand how various abnormalities may be reflected or represented in the EEG, it is interesting to note that one study reports decreased size of caudate nuclei on MR images in patients with depression (38). The authors speculate that there may be some parallels to the prevalence of depressive symptoms in Huntington's disease, which is known to have decreased caudate nucleus size. They draw on the studies from animals that show that caudate nuclei are functionally and anatomically related to prefrontal cortex, and comment on changes in complex social behavior, decreased initiation of activities, and decreased ability to solve problems when the caudate nuclei are damaged. Krishnan et al. (38) were unable to obtain baseline scans prior to the onset of symptoms as within-subject controls for these individuals. However, decreased metabolic functioning has been shown by PET in patients with depressed mood, and correlated with changes in mood following stroke (39–45). Differentially, subjects with seasonal affective disorder (SAD) were found to have abnormal prefrontal and parietal cortex regional activation by PET compared with normal controls, and different from patients with major depressive disorder (45). Subjects who received light therapy showed improved and increased function in occipital cortex compared to normals.

These regions of the brain have also been studied by various evoked potential paradigms, because of their role in maintaining sustained attention. An example of this is the study on selective attention by Burkhart and Thomas (46). Using the selective attention paradigm of Hilliard (slightly adapted), they studied subjects who had moderate depression and did not meet the criteria for major depressive disorder and were not taking any antidepressant medication. They were principally looking at the Nd, or negative difference wave, which is the difference in the evoked potential response between the attended and the ignored stimuli. Overall, there seemed to be a larger response in the control group compared with the depressed group, regardless of attentional condition. There were no significant differences between groups in terms of accuracy of response or type of response.

The results did not show any definitive differences in selective attention between the depressed and control subjects. As they noted, the attentional changes that can be seen with mild to moderate levels of depression are more likely to be evident with affectively-toned stimuli and less

likely to be present when there are neutral stimuli such as auditory tones presented in their study. This supports a behavioral study done by Mushman (46a), which showed that depressed subjects could recall essentially the same *amount* of information that normal controls could, but the *nature* of the information was different. They selectively recalled negatively toned material better. This suggests that a simple "objective measure of selective attention" may not be specific enough to differentiate depressive disorder and/or major depression even from normal controls or from other neuropsychiatric disorders, because it is not designed specifically enough for the characteristics being investigated.

Pharmaco-EEG and Pharmaco-MEG

The EEG and MEG can be useful tools in the measurement of drug effects on brain function. What is most clear from all research to date is that there is a lack of drug-specific characteristic findings (EEG/MEG) for all individuals under all conditions. Evoked potentials can provide a mechanism by which aspects of the drug can be highlighted differentially. For example, lithium highlights the early components of the evoked potential compared with antidepressants or neuroleptics or other medications. A review of the recent literature can be read in Hegerl (47). Sannita (48) has also reviewed the history and use of quantitative EEG in human neuropharmacology. This is an important article because it reviews only studies in humans (Table 5.4), whereas much pharmaco-EEG has been done in animals. Animals are always used in testing new drug development to indicate effects on the brain in an "objective manner." The purposes of performing pharmaco-EEG are summarized as follows:

1. To study drugs of abuse;
2. To classify psychoactive compounds;
3. To attempt to predict the therapeutic indications for, or responses to, certain classes of drugs;
4. To develop bioavailability and pharmacodynamic correlations,
5. To attempt to classify subgroups of psychiatric patients; and
6. To predict responders to certain types of treatment.

One must be cautious in extrapolating pharmaco-EEG and pharmaco-MEG findings based on small doses of a certain compound in normal controls. For example, 1 or 5 mg of haloperidol in a drug-free normal human control produces a different response than it would a person with chronic schizophrenia who has been taking 40 mg of haloperidol daily. Notwithstanding, certain categories of drug produce predictable responses; for example, benzodiazepines increase fast activity (β). Under certain conditions, there appears to be a decrease in synchronization which can appear as varying lateralization within certain frequency bands. Perhaps the best approach is to combine resting state and some form of activation condition specific to both the disease state being studied and

Table 5.4ᵃ. Effect of Psychoactive Substances on EEG Frequencies

	delta	theta	α	β
Benzodiazepines	↓			↑
Antipsychotics	↑	↑		
Tricyclics	↑			(↑)
Opioids	↑		↑	
Phenobarbitol	↑		↓	(↑)
Methylphenidate				↓
Nicotine			↓	
Alcohol			↑	

ᵃAdapted from Sannita (ref. 48).

to the presumed mechanism of action for the class of drug being studied.

Violence

There is an increased rate of neurological impairment in patients who are persistently violent compared with those who are transiently violent or nonviolent. In one study of EEG between three groups of inpatients, some of whom were persistently violent, some transiently violent, or those who were nonviolent, there was no significant differentiation between groups by the presence of an abnormal EEG. Abnormality was defined by the presence of increased amounts of θ or δ activity, sharp-wave asymmetry, a temporal lobe focus, an abnormal response to hyperventilation, or persistent low voltage (49). Neurological abnormalities differentiated the three groups most clearly; however, the neurological deficits were subtle, diffuse or multifocal deficits. The EEG (visually inspected) did not differentiate between the groups. In another study of violent psychiatric in patients, Convit et al. (50) found significant lateralization in the centrotemporal region on computerized EEG spectral analysis. The greater the violence, the greater the amount of δ power over the left hemisphere compared with the right. Williams (51) found increased amounts of slow activity over frontotemporal areas in habitually aggressive offenders. The patients studied by Convit included 15 who were schizophrenic, five with mood disorders, and one with personality disorder. δ Activity was positively correlated with violence variables, whereas α activity was negatively related to violence variables. These were not affected by medication (neuroleptic) effects. The authors plan to control for the relatively large proportion of patients with schizophrenia in their population by repeating a study with violent and nonviolent age-matched patients with schizophrenia of both sexes.

A review of reports linking abnormal brain waves and violent behavior has been done by Volavka (52), which shows the difficulty in generalizing from an individual case to all violent persons or all persons with certain patterns in the EEG. After epilepsy is removed as a cause for participating in a poorly organized violent act, there does not seem to be a good EEG predictor of either the severity or persistence of violent acts.

Aging and Dementia

One of the difficulties in identifying characteristic abnormalities or patterns of both normal and abnormal aging processes is that the clinical diagnoses for both these conditions have not been well defined for many years. In the last decade enormous efforts have been made to develop more consistent clinical standards for the diagnosis and measurement of age-associated changes in behavior. In reporting on preliminary results from the Kunzs-Holmen project in Stockholm, Sweden, Jorm et al. (53) report that one of the primary differentiating factors to separate Alzheimer's type dementia (AD)-cases from other dementias and nondemented subjects was of a "disturbed behavior" factor. As they note, this is not currently a requirement to meet criteria for primary degenerative dementia of the Alzheimer type. Three other factors differentiate the dementing process: (a) the presence of cognitive impairment, (b) cerebral vascular disease, and (c) depressive symptoms. Additionally, Black et al. (54), highlight the importance of knowing the premorbid cognitive capacities and educational background of individuals in order to adequately evaluate a dementing process. They emphasize the heritability and persistence of cognitive functions such as semantic processing. Previous studies (55) had indicated that spatial abilities were most heritable, followed in order by vocabulary, word fluency, speed in arithmetic, and reasoning.

AD of mild to moderate severity is reported to produce increased slowing in the EEG. Martin-Loeches (56) reported significantly more slow activity in 20 AD patients compared to normal controls. The slow activity was found over primarily frontal and midline recording locations, especially in the δ and θ bands (in 0–2 Hz and 4–6 Hz range). This is consistent with the cortical damage theory of AD. Significantly, there was no slowing in the α frequency for the control group (9 Hz). In another study, there was slowing of the peak frequency (in one patient there was no peak detectible) with an increased ratio of θ to α power. Correlation with SPECT scan showed a significant association between the temporoparietal cerebellar ratio (T-P/C) on the SPECT scan and the peak frequencies reported from the EEG leads. However, no left-right asymmetry was reported (57). They noted that local slowing of the EEG paralleled local decreased blood flow and that the decline of peak frequency was highly correlated with severity of dementia. The patients could be differentiated on a severity scale. Those who had normal EEG peak frequencies and normal SPECT scans had a shorter duration of disease than patients with normal EEGs but abnormal SPECT scans, who in turn had a shorter duration than those with both abnormal EEG peaks and abnormal SPECT scans. Thus, their data suggest that blood flow changes may be a more sensitive measure of a dementing process than EEG changes.

Brenner et al. (58, 59), in two studies analyzed EEG from patients with AD, patients with major depression and healthy controls to differentiate the various effects of aging that could be measured electrophysiologically. Compared to controls, dementia patients showed a shift to slower frequencies, significant increase in θ activity, increase in a θ-β difference, increase in α_1, and decreases in overall mean frequency and decreases in β_1 and β_2. Depressed patients differed from demented patients in that they had more α_2 activity with less δ and θ activity. Depressed patients had decreases in mean frequency and β_1 and β_2 compared with controls, however. The increased θ-β ratio difference in AD compared with normal controls is due to both an increase in θ activity and a decrease in β_1 and β_2 activity, whereas in depression, the difference is due to a decrease in β_1 and β_2 activity without an increase in θ activity. Thus, EEG measures could be used in a discriminant analysis to differentiate groups. Their analyses showed that while not 100% predictive, they were able to separate out the groups.

In a study of computerized spectral analysis versus visual EEG analysis, they found that three of 61 controls were misclassified; however, generalized mild or moderately abnormal EEGs correctly classified 20 of 25 AD patients. Using a δ plus θ percentage score, they identified 17 of the 35 demented patients with no misclassification. Of the 17 patients, 11 had a moderately generalized abnormal EEG. Six of them had either a normal EEG or mild generalized or focal abnormalities. All of those who were identified by a combined δ and θ activity percentage had a lower Folstein Mini Mental Status Exam (MMSE) score than those who were misidentified. As shown previously, the severity of intellectual impairment correlated with the abnormalities on visual inspection of EEG and on spectral data. Duffy et al. (60) and Princhep et al. (61) have reported that maximal group differences between controls and patients were in frontal and temporal regions.

The visual evoked responses to checkerboard pattern-reversal stimulation shows a curvilinear relationship between P100 latency and age over the life span. The shortest latency occurs during middle adulthood, with increasing latencies found at ages over 60. Tobimatsu et al. (62) reported that the differential age effect on the P100 latency caused by changes in contrast depended on the check size of the stimuli as well. In general, as the pattern contrast decreased, P100 latency was prolonged and the amplitude decreased. There have been several reports of reduced contrast sensitivity with increasing age over age 40–50 years. Other groups have found that the evoked potential latency of elderly subjects became comparable to younger subjects when the stimulus contrast was increased to an appropriate degree (having accommodated for physical changes to the lens and eyeball that accompany increasing age). A number of hypotheses have been proposed to explain changes in visual function with increased age, including decreased conduction velocity of the optic nerve and visual pathways, degeneration of retinal ganglion cells, changes in neurotransmitter function and increased synaptic delay, and neuronal loss in the lateral geniculate and striate cortex. In primates there are two major retinogeniculate visual pathways—the magnocellular and the parvocellular. The magnocellular system has high luminous contrast sensitivity and excellent temporal frequency resolution, while the parvocellular system shows color selectivity, low-contrast sensitivity, and low temporal resolution. The authors concluded that modification of visual evoked responses by changes in luminance, contrast, and stimulus size can be strong. Their data support the validity of a hypothesis that aging may differentially influence separate channels of the human visual system.

In an auditory task with the same patients, the response time was fastest when the stimulus was longest; i.e., 320 msec cues elicited faster responses than 2 msec cues. Between these stimulus durations, there were auditory responses whose duration followed in a linear relationship. The subjects had to correctly identify the difference between two tones and then, sequentially, at progressive levels of difficulty, the difference between two tones in different places in a room. There was a significant decrease of accuracy and speed of response as the stimulus cue was shortened and location was requested in the response. When there was a delay between the stimulus cue and the response, patients who had a history of alcoholism performed much worse than normal elderly subjects. There was a significant increase in extraneous responses when there was a 5-second delay rather than no delay, whether or not a correct response was given. Korsakoff syndrome patients were the most severely affected by short visual exposure durations and had the most clearly progressive decline in response, with prolonged delay between stimulus cue and response in both auditory and visual dimensions. However, visual cues were much worse than auditory. Patients who had a significant history of alcoholism without Korsakoff's syndrome were more impaired than normal aged controls. These data provide further support for a disorder of orbitofrontal regions of the cortex, particularly in Korsakoff's syndrome.

Mental Retardation/Down Syndrome

This heterogeneous group of disorders certainly has a wide clinical spectrum, from mild to very severe intellectual deficits. There is little in the EEG or MEG that can specifically diagnose the etiology for a particular type of mental retardation. Generally, the EEG shows diffuse patterns of slowing and, at times, dysrhythmia similar to a dementia pattern, usually with preserved α rhythm. Depending on the severity of the illness, there is a range in abnormal findings from mild retardation with relatively well-organized EEG, to severe retardation, with disorganization of the EEG and large slow waves, sometimes associated with spikes.

EEG abnormalities consistent with a diagnosis of dementia were seen in patients over the age of 35 who had epilepsy and Down syndrome. Patients under the age of 35 with or without epilepsy showed no EEG abnormalities. Most patients with seizures had partial seizure onset that became generalized. The prevalence of epilepsy in adults with Down syndrome was 9.4% (63) and increased with age (46% in patients who were over age 50). The age of onset, if late, was associated with poorer outcome and clinical signs and symptoms of dementia.

Diagnosis is complicated by the fact that in more severe cases of retardation there are often concomitant disorders such as epilepsy, drug intoxication, and movement disorders. In a recent article, Elliott and Weeks (64) attempted to explain how an underlying disorder may affect brain specialization, which could account for some of the information processing deficiencies and/or peculiarities associated with Down syndrome. They proposed a model of using a verbal-motor impairment index and dichotic listening tests related to verbal and nonverbal measures of intellectual functioning. The results indicated that persons with Down syndrome had a slight tendency for left ear advantage for speech sounds. Under verbal testing and instruction, patients with Down syndrome had more difficulty in preserving the order of responses, and they produced more irrelevant responses. They calculated the difference between each subject's performance on visual tasks in an apraxia battery and their scores on a verbal apraxia battery. They hypothesized that people with Down syndrome may have trouble performing movements on the basis of verbal information, because right-hemisphere speech perception systems appear to be functionally isolated from left-hemisphere systems of movement, planning, and execution. Thus, the greater the difficulty between understanding verbal cues and instructions and being able to carry out organized behavior based on those instructions either in testing or in passive daily living, the greater the separation of these two hemispheric functions. This made them wonder if the tendency for the right hemisphere to develop receptive language functions interferes with the more typical right-hemisphere visual and spatial functions. This study represents an attempt to integrate neuropsychological studies, clinical observations, and behavioral observations with evoked potential models, to infer relative strengths and weaknesses of brain function specific to a disorder.

Stroke

EEG and MEG can be useful in the evaluation of recovery from stroke. While imaging techniques such as CT and MRI permit assessing lesion size, neither technique measures which tissue remains functional or has the potential to recover function. Physiological measures can assist in the assessment of recovery and in quantifying the degree of alteration in normal function that has resulted from the stroke—such as motor function, sleep patterns, and alerting or sensory perceptual changes.

Neurological examination combined with EEG (mapping) permits localization of the lesion and compares favorably to CT scan in the same patients, according to Lukacher et al. (65). To better understand the mechanism of damage during stroke, several experimental models have been used, including lesioned animals and carotid artery clamping in both humans and animals. Patient candidates for endarterectomy have been studied pre- and intraoperatively with EEG to assess the risk of developing intra- or postoperative strokes. Jansen et al. (66) found that EEG changes indicating poorer neuronal function along with information about rate of blood flow from transcranial doppler ultrasonography gave immediate and accurate feedback to the surgeon as to the state of perfusion to the brain. This feedback allowed them to reduce the rate of intraoperative stroke. This was confirmation of a study of 375 patients by Facco et al. (67). Another group, Fava et al (68), used EEG and sensory evoked potentials (SEPs) to determine which subjects should receive shunting during the endarterectomy. When SEPs were severely depressed (P25 latency and amplitude), an intraoperative shunt was placed. On the other hand, Redekop and Ferguson (69) found that risk of intraoperative stroke was correlated with major EEG changes, but not with amount of carotid occlusion or other risk factors. In their view, shunting is not a useful technique to alter risk of intraoperative stroke.

The dilemma of which technique to use for assessment of clinical damage was partly addressed in a study comparing EEG, EEG mapping, and CT of 70 patients with completed strokes (70). EEG mapping provided more information on lateralization of deficit than routine EEG. EEG mapping also provided lateralization information in 12 patients with negative CT findings and in 21 patients with negative routine EEG. Kappelle et al. (71) reported a high correlation between computerized EEG focal abnormalities and lacunar infarct location (by head CT).

Accuracy of detection of intraoperative ischemia was greater when power spectrum was used rather than alteration of spectral edge frequency (72). This study was relevant for the few electrodes used, covering only central-parietal regions bilaterally, yet providing useful diagnostic assessment.

Milandre et al. (73) reported that the incidence of post-stroke epilepsy was greater with hemorrhagic stroke. A follow-up EEG after several weeks increased the specificity

EEG abnormalities which showed only focal or diffuse slowing in 63% of records initially. Gras et al. (74) reported that periodic lateralized epileptiform discharges (PLEDs) correlated with ischemic stroke in older persons.

Sleep function, as might be expected, is altered in stroke. As acute cerebral changes resolve, there is a shorter time to onset of sleep and to first REM period. Domzal et al. (75) studied patients 4 weeks after stroke and found a higher proportion of stage 1 non-REM sleep in patients with right-sided middle cerebral artery stroke. Hachinski et al. (76) studied one patient, a 70-year-old woman, in whom they were able to obtain pre- and postinfarct sleep EEG records. In the immediate postinfarct state, slow activity increased on the side of the infarct, REM was not recorded at all until day 3, and sleep spindles almost disappeared. One year later, there remained persistant δ activity over the unaffected hemisphere, with other aspects of sleep recording having normalized over both hemispheres.

To better understand mechanisms by which stroke can be aggravated, peri-infarct depolarizations were induced in a rat model of stroke. Rats were subjected to 3 hours of middle cerebral artery occlusion (77), and the size of the infarct volume was measured. Repeat depolarizations resulted in increased infarct volume, progressive increase in DC shift duration, EEG amplitude recovery time, and EEG δ power. Stimulation of cerebellar fastigial nucleus increased cerebral blood flow but not metabolism, and was found to reduce (in rats) the extent of infarct in neocortex and enhance recovery of EEG amplitude in the ischemic cortex (78).

EEG has been recorded in some cases of transient ischemic attacks, usually after resolution of the episode (because of the short duration of symptoms in most patients). Rapid dysrhythmia and diffuse temporal (right or left) θ activity were reported by Constantinovici et al. (86) in one retrospective study of transient global amnesia. The variability of time after onset of symptoms and variation in extent of clinical symptoms were two major factors limiting the ability to generalize the findings from this study to predictions about recovery response. Still, it serves as an example of information about brain function that could be routinely studied.

These recent data suggest that EEG and possibly MEG can be used to assess the volume of brain at nite during an ischemic episode, and thereby provide a means for evaluating the efficacy of neuroprotective strategies. At present, neuropsychologic tests have their greatest utility in cases of clinical stroke with discrepant findings or anatomic brain imaging.

Traumatic Brain Injury (TBI)

The physical examination and anatomic imaging studies (e.g. CT) are the most relevant sources of information in the immediate postinjury period. More subtle and persistent deficits of cognitive function can be difficult to evaluate. The challenge to the patient and the clinician is to differentiate between psychiatric illness, embellishment or malingering, and integrative difficulties (sensory, cognitive, motor).

Somatosensory evoked potentials (SSEPs) have been reported to be useful predictors of good recovery in patients who were in coma due to TBI (80). Eight patients (out of 29) with bilaterally absent N20 responses died, whereas 14 of 20 with normal SSEPs had good outcomes.

Seizures are a frequent sequela of TBI, either from scarring or from an excitatory lesion. As with other sources for seizure, patients with TBI may have psychogenic seizures. The risk of treating pseudoseizures with antiepileptic drugs is to impede cognitive processes even further, while reinforcing the sick role. Self-control relaxation paradigms can be effective treatments for psychogenic seizures and for some types of true partial seizures. Conder and Zasler (81) reported that an aphasic brain-injured patient responded well to an individualized self-control paradigm with improved responsiveness to antiepileptic drug(s) (AED) as well as decrease in pseudoseizures. The EEG was useful in making the differential diagnosis between the two types of seizure behavior (as discussed previously).

EEG is often used in the intensive care unit to monitor the stability of patients in the acute postinjury phase of illness. Because of the limitations of space and demands for other equipment, EEG has often been limited to single-channel recording. Even a single channel can provide documentation of paroxysmal events, general arousal and particularly change in arousal, and drug effects (82). Limitations include the lack of regional specificity and the relatively small chance of noting changes distant from the electrode site.

Sports often cause brain trauma. Of particular note is boxing, which has been studied using EEG. Dementia pugilistica (83) is a traumatic encephalopathy. Critchley (84) found increased frequency of EEG abnormalities in boxers who had this encephalopathy, though he found no correlation between the degree of encephalopathy and abnormalities of the EEG. Repeated fights in short periods of time do not give the brain sufficient time to recover from the trauma. Immediately (15–30 minutes) after a fight, the EEG shows diminished amplitude and slowed irregular θ activity (85). In older fighters these differences due to the fight are not as readily seen. This allows one to speculate as to whether the brain has become more resilient to blunt trauma or, more likely, that the effects of aging and repeated injury have damaged the brain to a degree that acute change is not as likely to stand out against the chronically-slower background activity. It should be noted that the presence of a normal EEG does not exclude either the existence of encephalopathy or its development.

Pain

The coherence of the EEG can be affected by pain. Specific SSEP values can be altered by chronic pain, with longer latencies the usual finding. Arkhipova et al. (86) reported on patients studied with EEG before and after surgery for deafferentation chronic pain. EEG improvement after surgery included increased inter- and intrahemispheric coherence, a broader distribution of frequencies at rest, decreased bilateral synchronous θ activity, a shorter P220–P300 (SSEP) and more readily detectable visual evoked responses (VEPs).

EEG is a useful tool in animal models of pain and the effect of pain eradication. It provides an objective measure of brain responses that can be correlated with an animal's activity and behavior. Van Praag et al. (87) demonstrated that the excitatory effects of opiates (injections of morphine into neonatal rats) do not occur until the third week of life in a developing rat. EEG spikes can be produced by increasing doses of morphine during the second week of life, but these spikes are not reversible by opiate antagonists. It is not until the third week that the effects of morphine begin to mimic the effects in adults. In this example, electrophysiology is used to objectively monitor brain activity and to provide an assessment of treatment effects.

Nonsteroidal anti-inflammatory drugs are used commonly for the control of pain. Bromm et al. (88) measured the effects of acetaminophen and antipyrine on pain perception, on evoked potentials, and on resting EEG in healthy volunteers in a placebo-controlled, double-blind crossover study, using 20 msec electrical pulses as the noxious stimulus. Both drugs reduced pain perception by 6%, reduced stimulus-induced δ power in the EEG by 21%, and did not alter AEPs or reaction times. In the resting EEG, acetaminophen enhanced power in the θ range; antipyrine depressed α frequency. It would be worthwhile to determine if people who experience little to no relief of pain from these drugs have the same physiological responses as the subjects of this study.

Another group attempted to differentiate elicited muscle pain from memory of pain (89). The authors injected normal saline or hypertonic saline (5%) to produce a painful stimulus, and later evoked a memory of the stimulus by suggestion. Increased β_1 and β_2 over bilateral temporal regions were recorded, although some contamination from facial muscles cannot be ruled out. The increased power density in the β range was not different between the actual pain and imagined pain conditions.

A related measure of behavioral disturbance due to pain is sleep disturbance. Rheumatoid arthritis is a chronic disease associated with chronic pain, especially during flares of illness. Sleep disturbance (90) is a factor in increased perception of fatigue and increased pain.

Migraine

The etiology of migraine headache is thought to differ from that of tension headache. Prevalent theories include an electrophysiological spreading depression, and vascular contraction and dilatation as causal factors in both the production of aura and subsequent painful headache. Researchers have used EEG extensively to attempt to better characterize the brain activity during migraine and to attempt to identify people who are prone to having migraine headache. The data

are intriguing and suggest there may be more different etiologies, or more differing final pathways, than the single diagnostic category would lead one to expect (91, 92).

There are frequent cases of mixed headache—migraine and tension. When tension headache is prominent, one would expect muscle artifact to obscure many, if not all, of the findings discussed in the following pages.

Basilar migraine is characterized by symptoms referable to dysfunction of the brainstem. EEG studies (93–95) show increased δ activity, generalized, which resolves after symptoms subsided. Both prior to attacks and afterwards, the EEG is normal. In cases where symptoms have a slightly longer duration, the EEG can provide useful confirmation of transient alteration in brain function. One unusual case documented burst-suppression and frontal intermittent rhythmic delta activity (FIRDA) in the EEG during coma, which recurred due to basilar artery migraine (96). Transient occipital spike-wave complexes during basilar migraine attacks have been recorded by Morimoto et al. (97) and by De Romanis et al. (98). This latter group followed seven children who outgrew the basilar migraines; follow-up EEGs were normal. Childhood cyclic vomiting has been attributed varying etiologies, including epilepsy, migraine, and a somatoform disorder. Quantitative EEG has shown, in at least one case of cyclic vomiting, δ activity during the episodes that resolved with termination of the vomiting (99). Demonstration of transient EEG abnormalty was important to making the diagnosis of migraine.

A number of studies have tried to differentiate classic migraine from common migraine, with conflicting results. Corona et al. (100) postulate that EEG abnormalities may indicate a lower ischemic threshold. They found a much higher incidence of abnormalities during headache (93% vs. 38%) in the migraineurs with aura compared to those without aura. Children with migraine with aura have an increased θ-α ratio in posterior temporal and occipital areas as compared to those without aura, with tension headache, or normal age-matched controls (101). Migraine is more frequently associated with a lateralized decreased α power during an attack than tension headache (102). Topographic EEG may assist in distinguishing migraine from tension headache episodes in the same individual, especially in children, who may have greater difficulty expressing the difference in words. Routine EEG and topographic EEG were studied in young adults with common migraine, those with classic migraine, and those without headaches (normal controls) (103). The routine EEGs revealed minor nonspecific slowing in 10–15% of subjects in each group. Topographic EEG showed lower peak α power, lower α reactivity, and slightly faster peak α frequency (in the eyes closed state) in the patient group with history of classic migraine. The differences between the three groups were relatively small and could not be used to a priori distinguish those with migraine from those without migraine. Facchetti et al. (104) reported increased asymmetry of α power (42%) and peak frequency (55%) over posterior regions and increased θ and δ activity over temporal regions bilaterally (65%) in patients with migraine compared to normal controls.

Another study of children with migraines reported changes in the topographic EEG map during the course of an attack (105). α Power was decreased over the occipital area contralateral to the hemifield affected by visual aura. This was followed by increase in δ power over the frontal electrodes, and then, during the headache, increased δ power in posterior temporal and occipital areas. All abnormalities resolved with resolution of the headache. Symmetric frontal δ activity was recorded by Fuller et al. (106) in an elderly man during migraine with a time-limited psychosis (formed visual hallucinations, delusions, reduplicative paramnesia). EEG showed reduced activity over one hemisphere during an episode of abdominal migraine, thereby assisting in establishing the etiology for the symptom of abdominal pain in a 10-year old boy (107).

Soriani et al. (108) reported one case of a boy, aged 8, who had auras without headache. EEG during the episodes revealed diffuse continuous β activity. As the authors point out, recognizing this condition as not being due to a drug-induced confusional state is important.

Migraine is sometimes associated with epilepsy, most often of complex partial type. Increased background slow activity is particularly seen in patients with epilepsy and classic migraine (109). Marks and Ehrenberg (110) studied 395 patients with seizures, 13 of whom had migraine aura immediately preceding their seizures. Distinctive EEG changes occurred during the aura in two patients and could be distinguished from partial seizure activity. Five patients had lateralized epileptiform discharges in close temporal relation to migraine attacks. Six patients who did not achieve good seizure control with antiepileptic drugs had improved seizure control with the combination of treatments directed at migraine and seizure.

De Romanis et al. (111) recorded occipital spike-wave complexes occurring only during migraine attacks in 13 children who also had seizures. Wilder-Smith and Nirkko (112) were able to distinguish between focal epilepsy and migraine by the combination of EEG and Doppler sonography. They reported one case with episodes of visual symptoms who had nonspecific generalized changes in the EEG and showed increased blood flow velocity with a latency of a few seconds only in the posterior cerebral arteries. The pattern was consistent with autoregulatory hyperperfusion in response to increased neuronal activity.

The role of sleep and fatigue in the worsening of migraine attack frequency is unclear. Drake et al. (113) studied nocturnal sleep in 10 patients with common migraine, 10 patients with tension headache, and 10 patients with chronic tension-vascular headache. The migraine group had mild increases in REM and REM latency. The tension group had reduced sleep efficiency, increased movements and awakenings, and decreased slow wave sleep without change in REM. The mixed group had decreased sleep, decreased slow-wave sleep, decreased REM and REM latency. These changes suggest that chronic headache may be worsened by chronically poor sleep and have some overlap with depressive disorders.

The causation of both the aura and painful headache remain controversial. MEG studies have shown slow current shifts associated with auras (personal communications) that could support both a primary neuronal or a primary vascular/ischemic etiology. Some would argue that abnormalities shown in blood flow, by SPECT, support a vascular dysfunction (114, 115). It remains difficult to reliably duplicate the clinical picture in a laboratory setting because of the brevity of most auras.

Evoked potential measurements as a diagnostic tool for migraine has not been particularly useful. Visual evoked responses during the interictal period, for example, would not be expected to be delayed. The extreme photosensitivity usually present during the headache attack precludes valid testing. van Dijk et al. (116) measured background activity using power-spectral analysis in eight unmedicated migraineurs between attacks and found higher α and β power in the patient group than in age-matched controls.

One innovative application of EEG to clinical treatment was reported by Good et al. (117). Twenty children with clinically diagnosed migraine were asked to wear either rose-tinted or blue-tinted glasses for 4 months. The group that wore rose-tinted glasses had a reduction in mean migraine frequency of 6.2–1.6 per month and showed a concomitant reduction in visually evoked β activity. The group wearing blue-tinted glasses had a transient improvement in headache at 1 month, which was not sustained.

In routine evaluation of chronic headache, clinical judgment will continue to be most useful. Morill et al. (118) found that the very low rate of nonspecific abnormalities in routine EEG and the low rate of abnormalities found in CT increased in specificity only when tests were ordered in response to an abnormal clinical examination. While EEG has been of some value in the study of migraine, MEG will not be a useful diagnostic tool in migraine until a full head configuration is available.

Multiple Sclerosis

Multiple sclerosis (MS) affects the myelination of axon, slowing their conduction. EEG and MEG show diffuse or focal patterns of slowing, depending on the area affected and severity of disease. Early in the course of illness abnormal findings will return to normative values during remission. Impaired mental function can be associated with generalized slowing and, more rarely, epileptiform discharges (119). Periodic lateralized epileptiform discharges (PLED) have also been reported (120).

Brainstem auditory evoked potentials (BAEPs) are frequently abnormal. Prologation of the I-V peak interval indicates brainstem dysfunction. In contrast to patients with metabolic encephalopathy, patients with MS typically have a normal wave I. BAEP is most useful in patients who have a history consistent with MS and do not have clinically evident brainstem lesion(s).

Abnormal SSEPs are reported in most patients with MS (121). The most frequently ordered, confirmatory test for MS, is the VEP during an initial episode of acute onset of loss of visual acuity. Waveforms are prolonged overall, and at specific latencies corresponding to sites of demyelinating plaques. Brau and Ulrich (122) reported improved visuomotor tracking performance and increased absolute α power during periods of remission compared to periods of exacerbation in 23 patients with MS. However, repeated SSEPs do not correlate with the course of the disease (123,124). Topographic or quantitative EEG allows for more sensitive monitoring of changes in the CNS, and alterations in EPs by this method have been found to correlate with changes in clinical state.

Not infrequently patients with MS will develop seizure disorders due to lesions that have inflammatory processes and myelin breakdown products within them (125). If it is a smaller lesion, and transient, the EEG abnormalities resolve in the same time course as the flare. Unresolving lesions tend to be associated with continuing seizure(s). The prevalence of seizure in 2,353 cases of MS was 1.7% (126), although these researchers did not find any correlation between seizure frequency and MS severity.

As more is learned about brain function, it becomes clear that there are times when focal lesions can cause disturbance(s) elsewhere in the brain. Rudkowska et al. (127) reviewed EEGs that showed paroxysmal changes in patients with MS. The patients all had clinical findings consistent with brainstem lesions that could be responsible for the paroxysmal EEG activity. VEP N100 latency was slightly slower, and the amplitude of the P100/N120 complex was slightly larger in these 12 patients compared with matched MS controls who did not have paroxysmal activity in the EEG.

Complicated cases of MS reveal both the usefulness and limitations of electrophysiology to localize disturbances within the brain. Periodic synchronous discharges were reported in a 12-year-old girl with MS (128). This EEG pattern is more frequently identified with subacute sclerosing panencephalitis. An example of the limits of EEG specify is a case report of nonspecific diffuse θ activity in a 53-year-old woman, with a 6-year history of MS (129). CSF, MRI, and other imaging techniques were used to confirm the diagnosis and to evaluate her state of health during a very complicated course with multiple pneumonias. Autopsy revealed continuous cystic lesions along the lateral ventricles from the frontal tips of the anterior horns to posterior and temporal horns of the lateral ventricles. There were also more classic demyelinated lesions in the white matter, brainstem, cerebellum, and spinal cord.

Autism

Childhood disorders are difficult to diagnose because the body and brain are (usually) growing and changing all the time. The developmental disorders, including autism, pervasive developmental disorder, and Asperger's syndrome do not have pathognomonic EEG/MEG findings. Minor generalized EEG abnormalities are not uncommon but are made more compelling by their association with a family history significant for affective disorder (130). In another group

of children with autism, Rothenberger (131) found that the power spectrum of the EEG could reflect the degree of "change" or "non-change" in children as he followed them longitudinally. In a review of pineal gland function and maturation of α rhythm, Sandyk (132) suggests that disorders of cerebral maturation, such as autism, may be related to disturbance of pineal melatonin function in early life. This hypothesis implies a differential influence of the pineal maturation of the left hemisphere, perhaps accounting for lefthemisphere vulnerability to cerebral insult.

Ciesielski and colleagues (133) demonstrated the importance of using complementary paradigms to assess more subtle deficits. In their study of high-functioning autistic adults (meeting criteria for pervasive developmental disorder) compared with normal age-matched controls, divided attention tasks showed deficits in the patient group. This was shown by lack of normal modulation of the slow negative wave (P3b) during final decision-making about target selection. The study provides support for the idea that people with autism may process information differently than normals.

Acquired Immunodeficiency Disorder/Human Immunodeficiency Virus

Electrophysiology can be an important component in the evaluation of the effects of HIV in the CNS, since anatomical imaging techniques are not sensitive enough to follow disease progression in many cases. Noninvasive EEG measures, from resting state coherence and power spectrum analysis to specific EPs are being administered to patients who have the virus, without full-blown clinical disease. As the research continues, one can expect more specific knowledge about the progression of the disease in the CNS (134). The utility of EEG and MEG will be the characterization, in real time, of brain function in people who have changes in cognition or motor performance without gross neurological defects. Therefore, hemispheric asymmetries, variation in latencies or amplitudes of evoked potentials, and changes in coherence are likely to be the most sensitive and specific measures of alteration in brain functioning.

Other Neuropsychiatric Disorders

Somatosensory evoked potentials/fields (SEP/SEF) can be a useful diagnostic tool when there is a focal lesion. The amplitude of response will generally be larger over the side or site of the lesion. For example, Furlong et al. (135) describe a case of a 75-year-old man with a highly cellular, poorly differentiated metastatic tumor located in the area of the right central sulcus and slightly displacing the prefrontal gyrus anteriorly. There was a significant interhemispheric difference in SEPs. The patient had presented with a history of paresthesia and occasional involuntary movements of the left thumb and index finger. On examination there was some loss of joint position sense and 2-point discrimination in the left hand, with diminished stereognosis. During the period of recording, no involuntary movement or EEG epileptiform activity was recorded. Somatosensory evoked potentials were obtained for both the right- and left-wrist stimulation. This resulted in augmentation of the right-hemisphere P22 component with relative attenuation of all other right-hemisphere components. The P22-M31 complex represented a "giant" potential relative to a comparison control group, associated with an interhemispheric amplitude asymmetry of greater than 50%. The P22 and M31 components had a discrete locus of positivity and negativity maxima over C3, C4 electrodes for the respective sides (135). Other latencies were not grossly different between the hemispheres or from standard controls. This suggests that the P22 and M31 complexes arise from central and prefrontal regions.

Children and adolescents with mitochondrial encephalomyopathies have slowing of the α rhythm and epileptiform discharges on EEG (136). Repeat recordings in one study did not show a fluctuating pattern. Physiological techniques helped to provide assessment of the degree of variability in the state of the brain in these young patients.

Walter et al. (137) studied the topographical organization of sensorimotor cortex by matching results of MEG, PET, and MRI. Although this procedure is very labor-intensive at present, the likelihood is that in the future it will become much easier to accomplish. Simultaneous physiological measurements with accurate anatomical localization and metabolic measurements enable encephalographers to better determine the significance of regional findings in EEG or MEG.

CONCLUSIONS

The field of electro- and magnetoencephalography is evolving rapidly. Rather than overwhelm the reader with minutiae of the differences and similarities of the two techniques, the emphasis has been on fundamentals of each technique and applications that are applicable to the study of neuropsychiatric disorders. There is a long-standing realization among users of these physiological techniques that individualized applications are relevant (138) and further our understanding of the expression of disorders in the brain (139).

Although specific findings in certain disorders have been identified, the greatest importance of EEG and MEG may remain as techniques for recording brain *function*. Integration of source modeling with other anatomically-based imaging studies will support the validity of these physiological measurements. The particular value of EEG/MEG to the neuropsychiatrist is that it remains directly tied to neuronal function, normal and abnormal, without reliance on uptake of labeled substances such as are required by metabolic or blood flow measures. With the development of whole-head MEG systems, we are entering a decade in which noninvasive study of brain function is becoming a reality. The reader is encouraged to integrate the findings from a variety of technical approaches to brain study. The information

collated from different types of studies (i.e., anatomical imaging, functional measures with varying time courses from milliseconds to hours) will increase our appreciation of normal and disordered brain function.

Focused application to clinical and research questions will be the most rewarding approaches to the use of EEG or MEG. In this manner there can be continued refinement of our understanding of the complex interactions that characterize the communication between neurons in the brain. As with early hopes in EEG studies, the likelihood that a single, readily identifiable pattern of activity (EEG or MEG) will characterize any neuropsychiatric disorder is almost nil. In most disorders, we are considering difficulties that wax and wane, can vary in their response to pharmacological treatment, and are affected by the state of the individual (e.g., stressed/not stressed). Careful study of physiological changes (aided by developing technology) that fluctuate in meaningful patterns from minute to minute, even from millisecond to millisecond, are needed to develop understanding of CNS function in neuropsychiatric disorders.

References

1. Stephenson WA, Goetz FA. Balanced non-cephalic reference electrode. Electroencephalogr Clin Neurophysiol 1951;3:237–240.
2. Gevins A. High resolution EEG (Review). Brain Topogr 1993;5: 321–325.
3. Supek S, Aine CJ. Simulation studies of multiple dipole neuromagnetic source localization model order and limits of source resolution. IEEE Trans Biomed Eng 1993;40:529–540.
4. Robinson SE. Theory and properties of lead field synthesis analysis. In: Williamson SJ, Hoke M, Stroink G, A Kotani M, eds. New York: Plenum, Advances in Biomagnetism 1989:599–602.
5. Brivio L, Grasso R, Salvaggio A, Principi N. Brain Stem auditory evoked potentials (BAEPs): maturation of interpeak latency I-V (IPL I-V) in the first years of life. Electroencephalogr Clin Neurophysiol 1993;88:28–31.
6. Tiihonen J, Hari R, Naukkarinen H, Rimon R, Jousmaki V, Kajola M. Modified activity of the human auditory cortex during auditory hallucinations. Am J Psychiatry 1992;149:255–257.
7. Shagass C, Roemer RA, Straumanis JJ, Amadeo M. Temporal variability of somatosensory, visual and auditory evoked potentials in schizophrenia. Arch Gen Psychiatry 1979;36:1341–1351.
8. Shagass C, Roemer RA, Straumorris JJ, Amadeo M. Topography of sensory evoked potentials in depressive disorders. Biol Psychiatry 1980;15:183–207.
9. Roth WT, Pfefferbaum A, Horvath TB, Berger PA, Kopell, BS. P3 reduction in auditory evoked potentials of schizophrenics. Electroencephalogr Clin Neurophysiol 1980;49:497–505.
10. Faux SF, McCarley RW, Nestor PG, et al. P300 topographic asymmetries are present in unmedicated schizophrenics. Electroencephalogr Clin Neurophysiol 1993;88:32–41.
11a. Adler LE, Waldo MC, Freedman, R. Neurophysiologic studies of sensory gating in schizophrenia: comparison of auditory and visual responses. Biol Psychiatry 1985;20:1284–1296.
11b. Waldo MC, Adler LE, Freedman, R. Defects in auditory sensory gating and their apparent compensation in relatives of schizophrenics. Schizophr Res 1988;1:19–24.
12. Braff DL, Grillon C, Geyer MA. Gating and habituation of the startle reflex in schizophrenic patients. Arch Gen Psychiatry 1992;49: 206–215.
13. Tandon R, Shipley JE, Taylor S, et al. Electroencephalographic sleep

abnormalities in schizophrenia. Relationship to positive/negative symptoms and prior neuroleptic treatment. Arch Gen Psychiatry 1992;49:185–194.

14. Tandon R, Shipley JE, Taylor S, Greden JF. Sleep abnormalities in schizophrenia: cholinergic contribution. Clin Neuropharmacol 1992; 15:294A–295A.

15. Malaspina D, Maclin E, Cornblatt B, et al. Stimulant/Haldol study of SPEM, CPT and P50 in normals. APA Annual Meeting, San Francisco, 1989.

16. Karson CN, Coppola R, Morihisa JM, Weinberger DR. Computed electroencephalographic activity mapping in schizophrenia: The resting state reconsidered. Arch Gen Psychiatry 1987; 44:514–517.

17. Reite M, Teale P, Goldstein L, Whalen J, Linnville S. Late auditory magnetic sources may differ in the left hemisphere of schizophrenic patients. Arch Gen Psychiatry 1989;46:565–572.

18. Delwaide PJ, Pepih JL, Maertens de Noordhout A. The audiospinal reaction in parkinsonian patients reflects functional changes in reticular nuclei. Ann Neurol 1993;33:63–69.

19. Beckley DJ, Bloem BR, Remler MP. Impaired scaling of long latency postural reflexes in patients with Parkinson's disease. Electroencephalogr Clin Neurophysiol 1993;89:22–28.

20. Chen K, Abrams BM, Brody JA. Serial EEGs of patients with Parkinsonism-dementia syndrome of Guam. Electroencephalog Clin Neurophysiol 1968;25:380–385.

21. Nakashima K, Shimoyama R, Yokoyama Y, Takahashi K. Auditory effects on the electrically elicited blink reflex in patients with Parkinson's disease. Electroencephalogr Clin Neurophysiol 1993;89: 108–112.

22. Salanova V, Morris HH, Van Ness PC, Lüden H, Dinner D, Wyllie E. Comparison of scalp electroencephalogram with subdural electrocorticogram recordings and functional mapping on frontal lobe epilepsy. Arch Neurol 1993;50:294–299.

23. Ebersole JS. Non-invasive localization of the epileptogenic focus by EEG dipole modeling [Review]. Acta Neurol Scand 1994;152 (Suppl):20–28.

24. *Electroencephalography: basic principle, clinical applications, and related fields.* E. Niedermeyer, F. Lopes de Silva, eds. Baltimore: Urban & Schwarzenberg, 1987.

25. Krieg JC, Lauer CJ, Hermle L, von Bardeleben U, Pollmacher T, Holsboer F. Psychometric, polysomnographic, and neuroendocrine measures in subjects at high risk for psychiatric disorders: preliminary results. Neuropsychobiology 1990;23:57–67.

26. Dierks T. Equivalent EEG sources determined by FFT approximation in healthy subjects, schizophrenic and depressive patients. Brain Topography 1992;4:207–213.

27. Zeitlhofer J, Anderer P, Obergottsberger S, et al. Topographic mapping of EEG during sleep. Brain Topog 1993;6:123–129.

28. Lu ST, Kajola M, Joutsiniemi SL, Knuutila J, Hari R. Generator sites of spontaneous MEG activity during sleep. Electromyogr Clin Neurophysiol 1992;82:182–196.

29. Wang G, Takigawa M. A non-linear method for estimating the alpha generators from an EEG over the scalp. Frontiers Medic Biolog Engineer 1992;4:169–179.

30. Tiihonen J, Hari R, Kajola M, Karhu J, Ahlfors S, Tissari S. Magnetoencephalographic 10-Hz rhythm from the human auditory cortex. Neurosci Lett 1991;129:303–305.

31. Schatzberg AF, et al. Topographic mapping in depressed patients. In: Duffy FH, ed. Topographic mapping of brain electrical activity. Boston: Butterworths, 1986.

32. Williamson PC, Kaye H. EEG mapping applications in psychiatric disorders. Can J Psychiatry 1989;34:680–686.

33. Nagakubo S, Kumagai N, Kameyama T, et al. Diagnostic reliability and significance of irregular beta patterns. Jpn J Psychiatry Neurol 1991;45:631–640.

34. Ehlers CL, Kaneko WM, Owens MJ, Nemeroff CB. Effects of gender and social isolation on electroencephalogram and neuroendocrine parameters in rats. Biol Psychiatry 1993;33:358–366.

35. Dijk DJ, Beersma DG, Bloem GM. Sex differences in the sleep EEG of young adults: visual scoring and spectral analysis. Sleep 1989;12: 500–507.

36. Webb WB. The measurement and characteristics of sleep in older persons. Neurobiol Aging 1982;3:311–319.

37. Reynolds CF, Kupfer DJ, Hoch CC, Stack JA, Houck, PR, Berman, SR. Sleep deprivation in healthy elderly men and women: Effects on mood and on sleep during recovery. Sleep 1986;9:492–501.

38. Krishnan KRR, McDonald WM, Escalona R, et al. Magnetic resonance imaging of the caudate nuclei in depression. Arch Gen Psychiatry 1992;49:553–557.

39. Buchsbaum MS, Wu J, Delisi LE, et al. Frontal cortex and basal ganglia metabolic rates assessed by position emission tomography with [18F]-2-deoxyglucose in affective illness. J Affect Disord 1986;10:137–152.

40. Baxter LR, Phelps ME, Mazziotta, JC, et al. Central metabolic rates for glucose in mood disorders. Arch Gen Psychiatry 1985;42: 441–447.

41. Mendez MF, Adams NL, Lewandoski KS. Neurobehavioral changes associated with caudate lesions. Neurology 1989;39:349–354.

42. Starkstein SE, Robinson RG, Price TR. Comparison of cortical and subcortical lesions in the production of poststroke mood disorders. Brain 1987;110:1045–1059.

43. Krishnan KRR, Figiel GS, Ellinwood EH. Neurobehavioral changes with caudate lesions. Neurology 1989;39:1410–1411.

44. Figiel GS, Krishnan KRR, Doraiswamy PM, Rao VP, Nemeroff CB, Boyko OB. Subcortical hyperintensities on brain magnetic resonance imaging: a comparison of late-onset and early onset elderly depressed patients. Neurobiol Aging 1991;26:245–247.

45. Cohen RM, Gross M, Nordahl TE, et al. Preliminary data on the metabolic brain pattern of patients with winter seasonal affective disorder. Arch Gen Psychiatry 1992;49:545–552.

46. Burkhart MA, Thomas DG. Event-related potential measures of attention in moderately depressed subjects. Electromyogr Clin Neurophysiol 1993;88:42–50.

46a. Goldstein G, NcCue M, Rogers J, Nussbaum PD. Diagnostic differences in memory test based predictions of functional capacity in the elderly. Neuropsychol Rehab 1992;2:307–317.

47. Hegerl U. Psychopharmaka und Kortikale Evozierte Potentiale. Fortschr Neurol Psychiatry 1989;57:267–280.

48. Sannita WG. Quantitative EGG in human neuropharmacology. Acta Neurol 1990;12:389–409.

49. Krakowski MI, Convit A, Jaeger J, et al. Inpatient violence. J Psychiatr Res 1989;23:57–64.

50. Convit A, Czobor P, Volavka J. Lateralized abnormality in the EEG of persistently violent psychiatric inpatients. Biol Psychiatry 1991; 30:363–370.

51. Williams D. Neural factors related to habitual aggression—consideration of differences between those habitual aggressives and others who have committed cribes of violence. Brain 1969;92: 503–520.

52. Volavka J. Aggression, electroencephalography, and evoked potentials: a critical review. Neuropsychiatry Neuropsychol Behav Neurol 1990;3:249–259.

53. Jorm AF, Fratiglioni L, Winblad B. Differential diagnosis in dementia. Principal components analysis of clinical data from a population survey. Arch Neurol 1993;50:73–77.

54. Kurita A, Blass JP, Nolan, KA, Black RS, Thaler HT. Relationship between cognitive status and behavioral symptoms in Alzheimer's disease and mixed dementia. J Amer Geriatr Society 1993;41: 732–736.

55. DeFries JC, Vandenberg SG, McClearn GE. Genetics of specific cognitive abilities. Annu Rev Genet 1976;10:179–207.

56. Martin-Loeches M, Gil, Rubia FJ. Two-Hz-wide EEG bands in Alzheimer's disease. Biol Psychiatry 1993;33:153–159.

57. Kwa VIH, Weinstein HC, Posthumus Meyjes EF, et al. Spectral analysis of the EEG and 99m-Tc-HMPAO SPECT-Scan in Alzheimer's disease. Biol Psychiatry 1993;33:100–107.

58. Brenner RP, Ulrich RF, Spiker DG, et al. Computerized EEG spectral analysis in elderly normal, demented and depressed subjects. Electroencephalogr Clin Neurophysiol 1986;64:483–492.

59. Brenner RP, Reynolds CF, III, Ulrich RF. Diagnostic efficacy of computerized spectral versus visual EEG analysis in elderly normal, demented and depressed subjects. Electroencephalogr Clin Neurophysiol 1988;69:110–117.

60. Duffy FH, Albert MS, McAnulty G. Brain electrical activity in patients with presenile and senile dementia of the Alzheimer type. Ann Neurol 1984;16:439–448.

61. Prichep LS, John ER, Ferris SH, Reisberg B, et al. Quantitative EEG correlates of cognitive deterioration in the elderly. Neurobiol Aging 1994;15:85–90.

62. Tobimatsu S, Kurita-Tashima S, Nakayama-Hiromatsu M, Akazawa K, Kato M. Age-related changes in pattern visual evoked potentials and differential effects of luminance, contrast and check size. Electroencephalogr Clin Neurophysiol 1993;88:12–19.

63. McVicker RW, Shanks OE, McClelland RJ. Prevalence and associated features of epilepsy in adults with Down's syndrome. Brit J Psychiatry 1994;163:117.

64. Elliott D, Weeks DJ. Cerebral specialization for speech perception and movement organization in adults with Down's syndrome. Cortex 1993;29:103–113.

65. Lukacher GI, Strelets VB, Marsakova GD, Golikova Z. [A comparison of the results of topographic EEG mapping with the data from a neurological examination and computed tomography of the brain]. [Russian]. Zhurnal Nevropatologii i Psikhiatrii Imeni S - S - Korsakova 1994;94:26–30.

66. Jansen C, Moll FL, Vermeulen FE, et al. Continuous transcranial Doppler ultrasonography and electroencephalography during carotid endarterectomy: a multinodal monitoring system to detect intraoperative ischemia. Ann Vasc Surg 1993;7:95–101.

67. Facco E, Deriu GP, Dona B, et al. EEG monitoring of carotid endarterectomy with routine patch-graft angioplasty: an experience in a large series. Neurophysiol Clin 1992;6:437–446.

68. Fava E, Bortolani E, Ducati A, Schieppati M. Role of SEP in identifying patients requiring temporary shunt during carotid endarterectomy. Electroencephalogr Clin Neurophysiol 1992;84:426–432.

69. Redekop G, Ferguson G. Correlation of contralateral stenosis and intraoperative electroencephalogram change with risk of stroke during carotid endarterectomy. Neurosurgery 1992;30:191–194.

70. Logar C. [The place of EEG mapping in cerebral ischemia]. [German]. EEG-EMG Zeitschrift fur Elektroenzephalographie Elektromyographie und Verwandte Gebiete 1990;21:161–162.

71. Kappelle LJ, van Huffelen AC, van Gijn J. Is the EEG really normal in lacunar stroke? J Neurol Neurosurg Psychiatry 1990;53:63–66.

72. Hanowell LH, Soriano S, Bennett HL. EEG power changes are more sensitive than spectral edge frequency variation for detection of cerebral ischemia during carotid artery surgery: a prospective assessment of processed EEG monitoring. J Cardiothorac Vasc Anest 1992;6:292–294.

73. Milandre L, Broca P, Sambuc R, Khalil R. [Epileptic crisis during and after cerebrovascular diseases. A clinical analysis of 78 cases]. [French]. Rev Neurol 1992;148:767–772.

74. Gras P, Grosmaire E, Soichot P, Giroud M, Dumas R. [EEG periodic lateralized activities associated with ischemic cerebro-vascular strokes: physiopathologic significance and localizing value]. [French]. Neurophysiol Clin 1991;21:293–299.

75. Domzal T, Malowidzka-Serwinska M, Mroz K. [Electrophysiological pattern of sleep after stroke]. [Polish]. Neurologia i Neurochirurgia Polska 1994;28:27–34.

76. Hachinski VC, Mamelak M, Norris JW. Clinical recovery and sleep architecture degradation. Can J Neurol Sci 1990;17:332–335.

77. Mies G, Iijima T, Hossmann KA. Correlation between peri-infarct DC shifts and ischaemic neuronal damage in rat. Neuroreport 1993;4:709–711.

78. Zhang F, Iadecola C. Stimulation of the fastigial nucleus enhances EEG recovery and reduces tissue damage after focal cerebral ischemia. J Cereb Blood Flow Metabo 1992;12:962–970.

79. Constantinovici A, Radutoiu E, Osanu M, Moldovan M, Niculescu M. [Transient global amnesia (a study of 30 cases)]. [Rumanian]. Revista de Medicina-Interna, Neurologie, Psihiatrie, Neurochirurgie, Dermato-Venerologie-Neurologie, Psihiatrie, Neurochirurgie 1990;35:61–68.

80. Hume AL, Cant BR. Central somatosensory conduction after head injury. Ann Neurol 1981;10:411–419.

81. Conder RL and Zasler ND. Psychogenic seizures in brain injury: Diagnosis treatment and case study. Brain Inj 1990;4:391–397.

82. Tasker RC, Boyd SG, Harden A, Matthew DJ. The cerebral function analyzing monitor in pediatric medical intensive care: applications and limitations. Intensive Care Medicine 1990;16:60–68.

83. Millspaugh JA. Dementia pugilistica. U S Naval Military Bulletin 1937;35:297–303.

84. Critchley M. Medical aspects of boxing, particularly from a neurological standpoint. Br Med J 1957;5015:357–362.

85. Pampus F, Grote W. [Electroencephalographic and clinical findings in boxers and their significance in the pathophysiology of traumatic brain disorders]. [German]. Arch Psychiatr 1956;194:152–178.

86. Arkhipova NA, Shevelev IN, Grokhovskii NP. [The spatial organization of bioelectrical activity during the treatment of the chronic pain syndrome]. [Russian]. Zhurnal Vysshei Nervnoi Deyatelnosti Imeni i P Pavlova 1993;43:730–737.

87. Van Praag H. Falcon M, Guendelman D, Fenk H. The development of analgesic pro- and anti-convulsant opiate effects in the rat [Review]. Annali Dell Lurtituto Superiore di Sanita 1993;29:419–429.

88. Bromm B, Forth W, Richter E, Scharein E. Effects of acetaminophen and antipyrine on non-inflammatory pain, and EEG activity. Pain 1992;50:213–221.

89. Veerasarn P, Stohler CS. The effect of experimental muscle pain on the background electrical brain activity. Pain 1992;49:349–360.

90. Crosby LJ. Factors which contribute to fatigue associated with rheumatoid arthritis. J Adv Nurs 1991;16:974–981.

91. Schoenen J. [Electrophysiologic investigations in migraine]. [French]. Pathol Biol 1992;40:293–304.

92. Sand T. EEG in migraine: a review of the literature. Funct Neurol 1991;6:7–22.

93. Muellbacher W, Mamoli B. Prolonged impaired consciousness in basilar artery migraine. Headache 1994;34:282–285.

94. Passier PE, Vredeveld JW, de Krom MC. Basilar migraine with severe EEG abnormalities. Headache 1994;34:56–58.

95. Ganji S, Hellman S, Stagg S, Furlow J. Episodic coma due to acute basilar artery migraine: correlation of EEG and brainstem auditory evoked potential patterns. Clinical Electroencephalog 1993;24:44–48.

96. Frequin ST, Linssen WH, Pasman JW, Hommes OR, Merx HL. Recurrent prolonged coma due to basilar artery migraine. A case report. Headache 1991;31:75–81.

97. Morimoto Y, Nakajima S, Nishioka R, Nakamura H. [Basilar artery migraine with transient MRI and EEG abnormalities]. [Japanese]. Rinsho Shinkeigaku [Clinical Neurology] 1993;33:61–67.

98. De Romanis F, Buzzi MG, Assenza S, Brusa L, Cerbo R. Basilar migraine with electroencephalographic findings of occipital spike-wave complexes: a long-term study in seven children. Cephalalgia 1993;13:192–196.

99. Jernigan SA, Ware LM. Reversible quantitative EEG changes in a case of cyclic vomiting: evidence for migraine equivalent. Dev Med Child Neurol 1991;33:80–85.

100. Corona T, Otero-Siliceo E, Reyes Baez B, Rivera Nava C, Garcia P. [Electroencephalographic alterations in patients with migraine with and without aura.] [Spanish]. Neurologia 1994;9:81–84.

101. Valdizan JR, Andreu C, Almarcegui C, Olivito A. Quantitative EEG in children with headache. Headache 1994;34:53–55.

102. Pothmann R. Topographic EEG mapping in childhood headaches. Cephalalgia 1993;13:57–58.

103. Neufeld MY, Treves TA, Korczyn AD. EEG and topographic frequency analysis in common and classic migraine. Headache 1991;31:232–236.
104. Facchetti D, Marsile C, Faggi L, Donati E, Kokodoko A, Poloni M. Cerebral mapping in subjects suffering from migraine with aura. Cephalalgia 1990;10:279–284.
105. Seri S, Cerquiglini A, Guidetti V. Computerized EEG topography in childhood migraine between and during attacks. Cephalalgia 1993;13:53–56.
106. Fuller GN, Marshall A, Flint J, Lewis S, Wise RJ. Migraine madness: recurrent psychosis after migraine. Journal Neurol, Neurosurg Psychiatry 1993;56:416–418.
107. Sangermani R, Pirovano S, Vaccari R, Gibelli M, Rossi A. [Abdominal migraine simulating acute abdomen]. [Italian]. Pediatria Medica e Chirurgica 1992;14:163–165.
108. Soriani S, Scarpa P, Faggioli R, De Carlo L, Voghenzi A. Uncommon EEG pattern in an 8-year-old boy with recurrent migraine aura without headache. Headache 1993;33:509–511.
109. Farkas V, Kohlheb O, Benninger C, Matthis P. Comparison of the EEG background activity of epileptic children and children with migraine. Epilepsy Res 1992;6:199–205.
110. Marks DA, Ehrenberg BL. Migraine-related seizures in adults with epilepsy, with EEG correlation. Neurology 1993;43:2476–2483.
111. De Romanis F, Buzzi MG, Cerbo R, Feliciani M, Assenza S, Agnoli A. Migraine and epilepsy with infantile onset and electroencephalographic findings of occipital spike-wave complexes. Headache 1991;31:378–383.
112. Wilder-Smith E, Nirkko AC. Contribution of concurrent Doppler and EEG in differentiating occipital epileptic discharges from migraine. Neurology 1991;41:2005–2007.
113. Drake ME, Pakalnis A, Andrews JM, Bogner JE. Nocturnal sleep recording with cassette EEG in chronic headaches. Headache 1990;30:600–603.
114. Olsen TS, Friberg L, Lassen NA. [Migraine aura —vascular or neuronal disease?]. [Danish]. Ugeskrift for Laeger 1990;152:1507–1509.
115. Tomaiolo S, Stiglich F, Bonomo F, et al. [SPECT with 99m-TC HM PAO in the study of classical hemicrania]. [Italian]. Radiol Med (Torino) 1991;81:537–541.
116. van Dijk JG, Dorresteijn M, Haan J, Ferrari MD. Visual evoked potentials and background EEG activity in migraine. Headache 1991;31:392–395.
117. Good PA, Taylor RH, Mortimer MJ. The use of tinted glasses in childhood migraine. Headache 1991;31:533–536.
118. Morill B. Neurological evaluation of chronic headache patients: is laboratory testing always necessary? Biofeedback and Self Regul 1990;15:27–35.
119. Lević ZM. Electroencephalographic studies in multiple sclerosis. Specific changes in benign multiple sclerosis. Electroencephalogr Clin Neurophysiol 1978;44:471–478.
120. Awerbuch GI, Verma NP. Periodic lateralized epileptiform discharged from a patient with definite multiple sclerosis. Clin Electroencephalogr 1987;18:38–40.
121. Chiappa KH. Pattern shift visual brainstem auditory and short-latency somatosensory evoked potentials in multiple sclerosis [Review]. Neurology 1980;30:110–123.
122. Brau H, Ulrich G. Electroencephalographic vigilance dynamics in multiple sclerosis during an acute episode and after remission. Eur Arch Psychiatry Clin Neurosci 1990;239:320–324.
123. Aminoff MJ, Davis SL, Panitch HS. Serial evoked potential studies in patients with definite multiple sclerosis. Clinical relevance. Arch Neurol 1984;41:1197–1202.
124. Matthews WB, Small JG. Serial recordings of visual and somatosensory evoked potentials in multiple sclerosis. J Neurol Sci 1979;40:11–21.
125. Thompson AJ, Kermode AG, Moseley IF, MacManus DG, McDonald WI. Seizures due to multiple sclerosis: seven patients with MRI correlations. J Neurol, Neurosurg Psychiatry 1993;56:1317–1320.
126. Ghezzi A, Montanini R, Basso PF, Zaffaroni M, Massimo E, Cazzullo CL. Epilepsy in multiple sclerosis. Eur Neurol 1990;30:218–223.
127. Rudkowska A, Gruszka E, Serwacka B, Ejma M, Bilinska M. [Paroxysmal EEG changes in patients with multiple sclerosis]. [Polish]. Neurologia i Neurochirurgia Polska 1992;26:466–472.
128. Tsuda M, Miyazaki M, Tanaka Y, Kuzuhara S. [A case report of childhood multiple sclerosis with periodic synchronous discharge on EEG]. [Japanese]. No to Hattatsu 1991;23:612–616.
129. Miura H, Mukoyama M, Kamei N. [An autopsy case of multiple sclerosis with bilateral continuous cystic lesions along lateral ventricles and caudate-callosal angles (Wetterwinkel)]. [Japanese]. No To Shinkei - Brain and Nerve 1991;43:1087–1091.
130. DeLong R, Nohria C. Psychiatric family history and neurological disease in autistic spectrum disorders. Dev Med Child Neurol 1994;36:441–448.
131. Rothenberger A. [Research on autism. Different aspects of changes observed during the development period]. [French]. Encephale 1992;18:217–223.
132. Sandyk R. Alpha rhythm and the pineal gland. International J Neurosci 1992;63:221–227.
133. Ciesielski KT, Knight JE, Prince RJ, Harris RJ, Handmaker, SD. Event-related potentials in cross-modal divided attention in autism. Neuropsychologia 1995;33:225–246.
134. Syndulko K, Singer EJ, Nogales-Gaete J, Conrad A, Schmid P. Laboratory evaluations in HIV-1-associated cognitive/motor complex. Psychiatr Clin North Am 1994;17:91–123.
135. Furlong PL, Wimalaratna S, Harding GFA. Augmented P22-N31 SEP component in a patient with a unilateral space occupying lesion. Electromyogr Clin Neurophysiol 1993;88:72–76.
136. Tulinius MH, Hagne I. EEG findings in children and adolescents with mitochondrial encephalomyopathies: a study of 25 cases. Brain Dev 1991;13:167–173.
137. Walter H, Kristeva R, Knorr U. Individual somatotopy of primary sensorimotor cortex revealed by intermodal matching of MEG, PET, MRI. Brain Topogr 1992;5:83–87.
138. Myslobodsky MS, Coppola R, Weinberger DR. EEG laterality in the era of structural brain imaging. Brain Topogr 1991;3:381–390.
139. Reite M. Advances in the study of mental illness. Adv Neurol 1990;54:207–222.

6

AUTONOMIC NERVOUS SYSTEM

Michael J. Aminoff

The autonomic nervous system is concerned primarily with the innervation of various internal organs, the maintenance of the internal environment, and the regulation of processes that are not usually considered to be under voluntary control. It is traditionally divided into the sympathetic and parasympathetic systems, which have seemingly opposing activities, ensuring the harmonious integration of different functions. The autonomic nervous system is also instrumental in generating the physical responses to emotional stimuli that characterize certain aspects of behavior. Thus, the cardiovascular changes accompanying anger (i.e., an increase in heart rate and blood pressure) or embarrassment (i.e., a cutaneous vasodilation or "blush") depend on autonomic activity. Similarly, the dry mouth of excitement, the excessive sweating that occurs with anxiety, the urinary incontinence associated with intense fear, and the "wide-eyed" appearance of surprise all depend on autonomic activity. Such autonomic responses have to be integrated with any somatic responses necessitated by the emotional stimulus, such as offensive or predatory maneuvers occasioned by anger, or defensive behavior elicited by fear.

ANATOMY OF THE AUTONOMIC NERVOUS SYSTEM

Autonomic Efferent Pathway

The efferent autonomic pathways consist of two neurons, one of which has its nerve cell body in the central nervous system (CNS)—the preganglionic neuron—and the other with its perikaryon situated peripherally—the postganglionic neuron. The preganglionic neurons of the *parasympathetic system* are located intracranially and sacrally (Fig. 6.1). The neurons of the cranial division are located in the brainstem adjacent to the somatic efferent nuclei of the third, seventh, ninth, and tenth cranial nerves. More specifically, parasympathetic fibers destined for the third nerve arise from the Edinger-Westphal and anteromedian nuclei, those for the seventh nerve from the superior salivatory nucleus, those for the ninth nerve in the inferior salivatory nucleus, and those for the tenth nerve in the dorsal motor nucleus of the vagus and the nucleus ambiguus. In the sacral cord,

preganglionic parasympathetic neurons are grouped laterally and medially in the intermediate gray matter of the cord between the anterior and posterior horns.

Axons of these neurons extend as far as, or close to, the organs to be innervated before synapsing with postganglionic cells in distinct ganglia or more diffuse intramural plexuses in the target organs. For example, parasympathetic fibers pass in the third (oculomotor) nerve to the ciliary ganglion in the orbit, from which postganglionic fibers pass in the short ciliary nerves to the ciliary muscle and sphincter of the iris. The course of parasympathetic fibers traveling in the facial nerve (to the lacrimal and certain salivary glands, and mucosal glands in the nose) and glossopharyngeal nerve (to the parotid gland) is documented in standard texts, but its importance mandates further comment concerning the vagus nerve. Preganglionic parasympathetic fibers arise from the dorsal motor nucleus of the vagus and nucleus ambiguus and pass toward their target organs, where they end in ganglia or plexuses related to the heart, pharynx, esophagus, and abdominal viscera. Parasympathetic fibers to the heart travel through the superior, middle, and inferior cardiac nerves to terminate on cells in the cardiac plexus, especially around the origin of the aorta and pulmonary artery and along the coronary arteries. The vagus nerves pass through the diaphragm to supply the stomach and contribute to the celiac plexus from which fibers pass (with sympathetic fibers in the peri-arterial plexuses) to the abdominal viscera.

The preganglionic parasympathetic sacral fibers pass with the anterior sacral roots (S2–S4) and eventually form the nervi erigentes or pelvic nerves on each side of the rectum, synapsing with postganglionic neurons in the walls of the bladder, rectum, and genitalia.

In the *sympathetic system,* the small, preganglionic efferent neurons are located in the thoracic and upper two lumbar segments of the spinal cord. Their axons leave the cord in the anterior roots and pass via the white rami communicantes (Fig. 6.2) to the sympathetic trunk, a chain of paravertebral ganglia situated on either side of the vertebral column, and interconnected by longitudinally arranged nerve fibers. In addition, there are transverse connections below the level of the fifth lumbar vertebra. Postganglionic sympathetic neurons are found in the paravertebral ganglia and also in the

Figure 6.1. Diagrammatic representation of the parasympathetic nervous system.

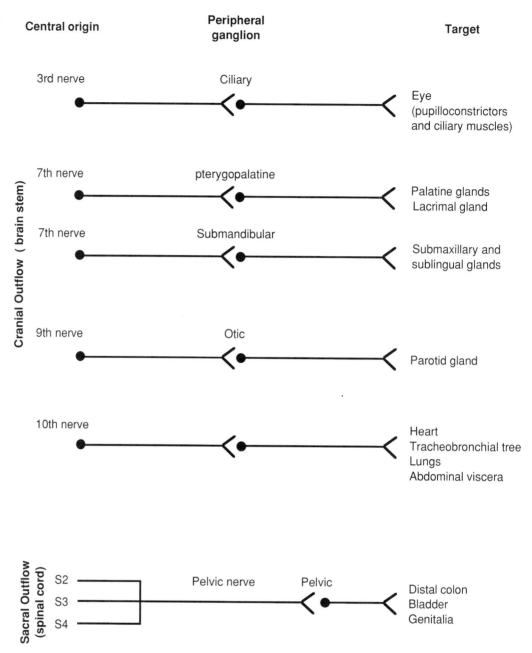

Central origin   Peripheral ganglion   Target

prevertebral ganglia that are situated more peripherally (Fig. 6.3). The precise anatomy of the sympathetic trunk and its contained ganglia varies in different individuals, but certain generalizations can be made.

There are three cervical ganglia: the superior (at the level of the upper two cervical vertebrae), middle (at the sixth cervical vertebra) and inferior ganglia (behind the subclavian artery). The inferior cervical ganglion is often fused with the first thoracic ganglion to form the stellate ganglion. An intermediate ganglion may be present between the middle and inferior ganglia. The ansa subclavia goes around the subclavian artery to join the intermediate with the inferior ganglion. The superior cervical ganglion sends postganglionic fibers to the upper four cervical spinal nerves and branches to the vagal and glossopharyngeal ganglia, hypoglossal nerve, carotid body, jugular bulb, cardiac plexus,

periarterial plexus about the carotid arteries, and certain salivary and facial sweat glands. The middle cervical ganglion has a major cardiac branch and also supplies the fifth and sixth cervical nerves, thyroid and parathyroid glands, esophagus, and trachea. The stellate ganglion supplies the lower cervical and first thoracic spinal nerves and contributes to the cardiac plexus and various perivascular plexuses, especially about the vertebral artery. Preganglionic fibers destined for the upper limb arise in the upper thoracic cord and ascend in the sympathetic trunk to synapse in the stellate ganglion, whence postganglionic fibers pass to the brachial plexus.

In the thoracic and lumbar regions there is generally one ganglion for each segment, and in the sacral region there is usually a total of four or five ganglia; in addition, a single (unpaired) coccygeal ganglion is frequently present. Sympathetic ganglion cells are typically present along the gray rami communicantes (discussed below) as well as in the ganglia themselves.

The unmyelinated axons of the postganglionic sympathetic neurons in the paravertebral and prevertebral ganglia pass to the skin, muscles, and organs they innervate. They either return to the spinal nerves as gray rami communicantes or pass along the major arteries as perivascular plexuses of nerve fibers. These perivascular plexuses are exemplified by the fibers that accompany the internal carotid artery and its branches to supply various cranial structures or join certain cranial nerves. Fibers from the stellate ganglion may pass with the subclavian artery to the upper limb or in the gray rami communicantes to the lower cervical nerves. The superior, middle, and inferior cardiac nerves arise from postganglionic neurons in the cervical ganglia and form the cardiac plexus, which also contains postganglionic sympathetic fibers from the upper thoracic ganglia and parasympathetic fibers from the vagus nerve. Nerves to the coronary vessels are given off from this plexus.

Postganglionic sympathetic fibers pass from various prevertebral abdominal ganglia (including the celiac) with aortic branches to form autonomic plexuses that also contain parasympathetic fibers related to the viscera, and with the gonadal and iliac arteries to supply eventually the pelvic organs. Although the intermediolateral cell columns of the spinal cord are restricted to the thoracic and upper two lumbar segments, all regions of the body are supplied by sympathetic fibers. This is because some preganglionic sympathetic fibers pass without interruption through the nearest sympathetic ganglia to ascend or descend to ganglia at other levels in the sympathetic trunk before synapsing, or exit without synapsing to relay in the prevertebral (preaortic) ganglia, i.e., the celiac, aorticorenal, superior mesenteric, and inferior mesenteric ganglia.

Several different types of postganglionic sympathetic fibers can be distinguished, depending on their target organ, and these—in turn—may have different physiological characteristics. The postganglionic sympathetic fibers to the skin, for example, consist of vasomotor and sudomotor fibers, with different conduction velocities (1).

Afferent Fibers

Afferent fibers are important in permitting autonomic reflex activity, but their precise pathways have been defined less clearly than those taken by efferent fibers.

The afferent pathway subserving the pupillary reflex response to light originates in the retina, whence information concerning luminance passes to the pretectum via fibers in the optic tract. From there, neurons project to the pupilloconstrictor neurons in the Edinger-Westphal nucleus. Afferent fibers from the cornea and the nasal and oropharyngeal mucosa pass in the trigeminal nerve to the trigeminal nuclei and nucleus tractus solitarius in the brainstem; stimulation of these afferent fibers elicits lacrimal, nasal, and oral secretions by brainstem reflexes.

Afferent fibers from baroreceptors in the carotid sinus and aortic arch are carried in branches of the ninth (glossopharyngeal) and tenth (vagus) nerves, respectively. Cell bodies for the fibers in the ninth nerve lie in its inferior ganglion and for the tenth nerve in the nodose ganglion. Cardiac afferent fibers transmit impulses from mechanoreceptors or chemoreceptors about the openings of the great veins, in the walls of the atria and interatrial septum, and in the walls of the ventricles, atrioventricular valves, and aorta. They pass in the vagus and in sympathetic nerves. The vagus nerve also contains afferent fibers from the tracheobronchial tree and abdominal viscera

Figure 6.2. Sympathetic pathways from the cord.

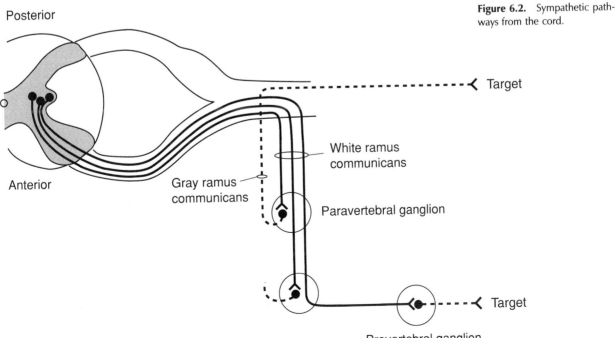

Posterior

Anterior

Target

Gray ramus communicans

White ramus communicans

Paravertebral ganglion

Target

Prevertebral ganglion

Figure 6.3. Diagrammatic representation of the efferent sympathetic nervous system.

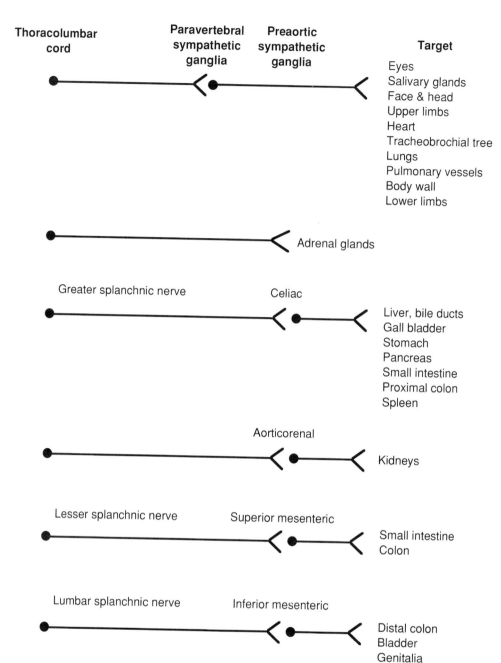

that pass, via the nodose ganglion, to the nucleus tractus solitarius.

Visceral afferent fibers arise in the S2–S4 dorsal root ganglia and are involved in anorectal and urogenital reflex activity.

Sensory neurons associated with the sympathetic system are in the dorsal root ganglia. Afferent information is derived from both the sympathetic ganglia and the peripheral target organs, and is transmitted to the dorsal horn of the spinal cord (2).

Central Autonomic Structures

The autonomic nervous system is represented at many different levels of the CNS, including the *cortex* of the superior frontal gyrus, and areas 4 and 6 of the cerebral cortex (3). Cerebral pathology may lead to disturbances of cardiovascular, pilomotor, sudomotor, or gastric function. For more than a century it has been known that cortical lesions or stimulation may influence the heart, respiratory rate, and blood pressure. The anterior cingulate cortex is involved in the control of bladder and bowels, and loss of sphincter function accompanies bilateral cingulate lesions. The temporal lobe and amygdala also have autonomic functions. This probably accounts for the autonomic accompaniments of certain complex partial seizures (4). There are profuse connections between those parts of the cerebral cortex involved in autonomic activity and other CNS regions having autonomic functions, but the specific pathways mediating this activity are unknown.

The *hypothalamus* seems to be a major (direct or indirect) relay station for autonomic pathways from the spinal cord, brainstem, and hippocampus, and is connected with the premotor frontal cortex. There are also rich efferent connections (direct or indirect) with autonomic neurons in the spinal cord and a close association between the hypothalamus and hypophysis. The anterior hypothalamic or preoptic area contains temperature-sensitive neurons that respond to either heat or cold. This area has a major role in integrating thermal inputs from different sources. Hypothalamic stimulation influences cardiovascular, pilomotor, and thermoregulatory function. For example, with electrical stimulation of the hypothalamus in cats anesthetized with chloralose, there is an increase in heart rate and mean arterial blood pressure and inhibition of cardiac and vasomotor components of baroreceptor reflexes (5, 6). The hypothalamic region also influences feeding behavior; hypothalamic pathology leads to either hyperphagia and obesity or aphagia and weight loss, depending on the precise site of the lesion.

The *cerebellum* has profound influences on autonomic function. Thus, Bradley et al. (7) have noted that electrical or chemical activation of a localized region of the posterior vermis may markedly influence vagal and sympathetic activity, leading in turn to changes in heart rate, arterial blood pressure, regional blood flow, and renal sympathetic nerve discharge. Other studies have revealed that the posterior vermis of the cerebellum (including the uvula) is essential for the acquisition of classically conditioned bradycardias; vermian lesions lead to severe attenuation of bradycardic responses to simple conditioning situations without altering resting heart rate and unconditioned heart rate orienting responses to a tone stimulus (8). The cerebellum also influences respiratory activity, but it is not clear whether it influences gastrointestinal function and sphincter control.

There are major, often reciprocal, connections between certain *pontine nuclei* and lower brainstem (medullary), forebrain, and hypothalamic structures that are also concerned with cardiovascular and respiratory control (9). The pontine regions influencing cardiovascular control connect with the *nucleus tractus solitarius,* which is the site of termination of afferent fibers from the arterial baroreceptors and chemoreceptors (Fig. 6.4), and the gastrointestinal system (10). Bilateral lesions of the nucleus tractus solitarius at the level of the obex in rats abolishes baroreceptor reflexes and results in an elevation in blood pressure without change in heart rate (11). The nucleus tractus solitarius is also influenced by—and itself influences—neocortical regions and forebrain, diencephalic, and rostral brainstem nuclei. It is situated in the dorsomedial portion of the medulla and connects with the dorsal nucleus of the vagus and neurons in the lateral region of the reticular formation that project via the bulbospinal pathway to the spinal cord, thereby influencing the cardiovascular system (Fig. 6.4). Through connections with the dorsal motor nucleus of the vagus, the nucleus tractus solitarius also influences gastrointestinal motility and secretions (12).

The brainstem has important influences on ventilation.

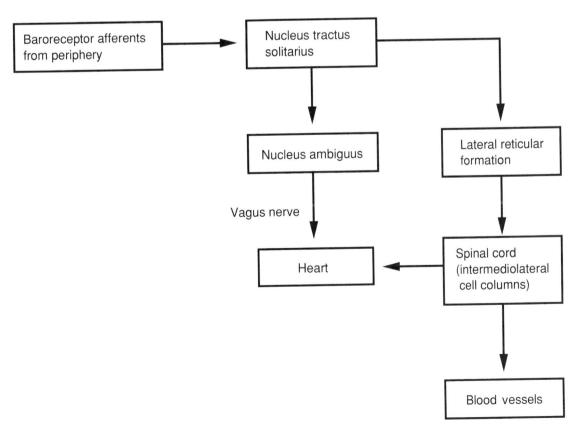

Figure 6.4.   Baroreceptor reflex regulation of the circulation.

Neuronal activity related to respiration occurs in discrete regions of the upper pons, and electrical stimulation of these regions leads to change in the ventilatory phase (13). Brainstem transection below the level of the so-called pontine pneumotaxic center in vagotomized animals produces apneustic ventilation, with prolonged end-inspiratory pauses (14). In the medulla, a dorsal respiratory group of neurons has been identified in part of the nucleus tractus solitarius; these are active during inspiration and receive vagal pulmonary afferents. A ventral respiratory group of neurons has also been identified within the nucleus ambiguus and nucleus retroambigualis and contains cells that are active in inspiration or expiration (15). Fibers from these respiratory neurons in the medulla pass to the contralateral motor neurons, whose axons constitute the phrenic and intercostal nerves.

Descending pathways conduct impulses from the brainstem to the preganglionic sympathetic neurons in the intermediolateral cell columns in the thoracic and upper lumbar regions of the cord. These cells have the staining characteristics of motor neurons. Their number diminishes with age at a rate of about 8% per decade (16). The axons of these cells exit with the anterior nerve roots as preganglionic sympathetic fibers passing to adjacent ganglia. Descending spinal pathways also connect with the parasympathetic outflow in the cranial and sacral regions. The spinal autonomic fibers are small in diameter and are probably most profuse in the lateral funiculi, but their precise pathway is unknown.

NEUROTRANSMITTER AND NEUROMODULATORS

The major postganglionic neurotransmitter of the sympathetic system is *norepinephrine,* which is transported along postganglionic fibers to their terminals, where it is stored in dense-core vesicles until released. There are two types of adrenergic receptors—the so-called α and β receptors—and subclasses within these two broad categories. Plasma norepinephrine levels normally increase markedly with change from recumbency to an upright posture, reflecting an increase in sympathetic activity. *Epinephrine* is released from the adrenal medulla and has important effects on cardiovascular function as well as other responses to stress. In a rare disorder characterized by deficiency of dopamine β-hydroxylase, sympathetic dysfunction results from inability to synthesize norepinephrine (and epinephrine). In this disorder, dopamine, not norepinephrine, is released from adrenergic nerve terminals.

Acetylcholine is the main peripheral neurotransmitter in the parasympathetic system, but it is also released from preganglionic sympathetic fibers and at postganglionic sympathetic nerve terminals to the sweat glands and certain blood vessels in the skeletal muscles, as well as from fibers supplying the adrenal medulla. Numerous central pathways are cholinergic. Cholinergic receptors are divided into muscarinic receptors (e.g., in CNS neurons, skeletal post-

ganglionic sympathetic neurons, and smooth and cardiac muscle), and nicotinic receptors (autonomic ganglia, skeletal neuromuscular junctions, and spinal cord). There are at least three different muscarinic and nicotinic receptors. *Serotonin* is probably important also as a neurotransmitter in central autonomic pathways.

Neuropeptides are present in autonomic neurons and may function as co-transmitters or modulators of neurotransmission, but their precise role has yet to be clarified. Neuropeptide Y is present in a variety of sympathetic, parasympathetic, and enteric neurons; it is contained, for example, in many nonadrenergic vasomotor neurons in the sympathetic ganglia. Opioid (and other) peptides are similarly widespread in peripheral autonomic neurons and may coexist with neuropeptide Y in the same nerve cells (17). Various neuropeptides also seem to function as co-transmitters at the nerve terminals of sudomotor fibers (18). The neurons in the intermediate cell columns are apparently influenced by several different neuropeptides. For example, immunoreactivity to substance P exists in several of the projections to these columns, immunoreactivity to somatostatin occurs in the intermediolateral cell columns and in sacral preganglionic parasympathetic neurons, and vasoactive intestinal polypeptide occurs in a number of different autonomic (and somatic) neurons including cells in the cord, hypothalamus, and sympathetic ganglia (19). Numerous peptides are involved in the regulation of cardiovascular function in concert with the autonomic nervous system. Thus, the release of atrial natriuretic factor, a peptide with diuretic and vasodilating properties, depends on atrial distension, but seems to be modulated by the sympathetic system (20).

Recent studies have shown that during development the environment into which the axon of a sympathetic neuron grows affects the phenotype of the cell. Thus, cholinergic sympathetic sudomotor neurons in rats initially are noradrenergic and acquire their cholinergic properties only after contact with their target sweat glands in the postnatal period by a mechanism that is unclear (21). The neuropeptide phenotype of sympathetic neurons is also influenced by environmental factors (17). Recent studies of vasomotor neurons projecting to different levels of the vascular bed in the skin of the ears and paws of guinea pigs have shown differences in immunoreactivity to various peptides, implying remarkable specificity among nerve cells supplying targets of similar type (17). Thus, neuropeptide Y is present in sympathetic noradrenergic neurons innervating large distributing arteries, whereas neurons supplying the smallest cutaneous arterioles contain prodynorphin-derived peptides but not neuropeptide Y; neurons innervating the rest of the vasculature contain prodynorphin-derived peptides and neuropeptide Y (17).

Nerve growth factor and other neurotrophic factors may suppress built-in self-destruction programs as well as stimulating growth (22–24). Certain rats are prone to hereditary hypertension, and their superior cervical ganglia contain fewer neurons and many more axonal terminals containing substance P than control animals (25, 26). These changes are prevented by neonatal treatment with nerve growth factor (27).

AUTONOMIC INNERVATION AND REGULATION OF VARIOUS STRUCTURES

In this section, further details of the autonomic innervation of specific structures are provided. In addition, certain clinical deficits resulting from disturbed autonomic regulation are considered.

Heart and Blood Vessels

Vasomotor tone and peripheral resistance are determined primarily by the sympathetic nervous system. The sympathetic outflow to different regions and structures (such as the skin and muscle) is regulated separately. Postganglionic sympathetic fibers pass mainly with the somatic nerves to the distant peripheral blood vessels and from the celiac and other abdominal ganglia to the splanchnic vascular bed.

The main action of the sympathetic nervous system on blood vessels is constrictive and is induced by norepinephrine. The existence and importance of sympathetic vasodilator fibers is less clear, and vasodilation in limb vessels probably relates to axon reflexes, antidromic conduction, or—most importantly—reduced sympathetic activity. Peripheral nerve lesions may disrupt vasoconstrictor fibers, thereby leading to erythema and an increased cutaneous temperature in an appropriate distribution in the limbs. Microelectrode studies in humans have shown that baroreceptor activity has a major influence on impulse traffic in sympathetic fibers to muscle, whereas brief mental stress has very little effect (1). By contrast, sympathetic (vasoconstrictor) activity in human cutaneous nerves is increased by emotional and mental stress. Some of the blood vessels in muscle are probably also supplied by sympathetic cholinergic vasodilator fibers. Vasodilator cholinergic fibers are present in the parasympathetic supply to the cranial, pelvic, and visceral blood vessels.

A tachycardia results from sympathetic stimulation of fibers (derived from T1 to T4) to the heart, and a bradycardia follows parasympathetic (vagal) stimulation.

The baroreceptor reflexes are important in the control of the heart and blood pressure (Fig. 6.4). Arterial high-pressure baroreceptors are located primarily in the aortic arch (and send their afferent fibers in branches of the vagus nerve) and carotid sinus (branches of the glossopharyngeal nerve). The wall of the carotid sinus is characterized by more elastic tissue and less muscle than the wall of the adjacent vessel. The baroreceptor endings are located in the adventitia and are stimulated by mechanical deformation of the vessel wall. Their sensitivity may be influenced by the sympathetic nerves that terminate in the carotid sinus.

Direct recordings from sympathetic efferent vasomotor fibers to blood vessels in the skin or muscles reveal that bursts of impulses occur rhythmically, time-locked to the pulse and often to the respiratory cycle. This rhythmic sympathetic activity is virtually eliminated below the level of complete cord transection, indicating its dependence on supraspinal mechanisms. Sympathetic efferent activity can be inhibited by an increase in blood pressure in the carotid sinus and aortic arch. The baroreceptor reflexes elicited by this increased pressure also cause slowing of the heart, which is mediated primarily through the vagus nerve. In contrast, hypotension leads to a tachycardia by inhibition of vagal activity, as well as to peripheral vasoconstriction from increased sympathetic activity.

Change in posture from a recumbent to erect position leads to pooling of blood in the legs and lower abdomen. This may lead to a slight fall in systolic blood pressure, with little or no fall in the diastolic pressure. The reduced systolic pressure leads to activation of the baroreceptor reflexes so that vasoconstriction occurs in the periphery, and there is an increase in rate and contractile force of the heart. Intraneural recordings in humans have shown that the response to postural head-up tilt and to the Valsalva maneuver consists of an increase in sympathetic activity in vasomotor nerves to muscle but not skin.

Assumption of the upright posture also leads to a reduction in hepatic blood flow, and there is increasing evidence that regulation of the splanchnic vasculature is important in maintaining the blood pressure. Other regulatory mechanisms to permit hemodynamic adjustments during postural changes include constriction of the capacitance (venous) beds and activation of the renin-angiotensin system.

The initiation of spontaneous physical activity is accompanied by a central command that arises above the level of the pons and influences cardiovascular and respiratory centers in the brainstem or elsewhere, leading to an immediate increase in cardiac and respiratory rates and blood pressure (28). The motor cortex is not essential for this purpose, and feedback mechanisms are not required for the genesis of respiratory and circulatory changes during exercise (28). There may also be a cholinergically mediated vasodilation in certain muscles (29, 30).

The CNS plays an important integrative role in regulating cardiovascular function. Inputs to various brainstem "centers" arise not only in the periphery, but also from other CNS structures. Neurogenic hypertension may result from lesions at different sites within the CNS, such as the hypothalamus. With brainstem lesions, such as bilateral lesions of the nucleus tractus solitarius, hypertension results from an increase in vasomotor tone and total peripheral resistance (31), but other factors—such as elevated plasma vasopressin levels—probably contribute as well (32). Posterior fossa tumors may cause hypertension (33), and compression or ischemia of the dorsal medullary reticular formation from either intrinsic pathology or increased intracranial pressure (Cushing response) may lead to hypertension, bradycardia, and apnea. By contrast, lesions of the ventrolateral medulla or rostral transection of the spinal cord lead to profound resting or postural hypotension in animals. Humans with brainstem tumors (34), syringobulbia (35), or spinal transection (36) also exhibit major disturbances of blood pressure regulation.

Ventilation and Bronchial Function

The importance of certain medullary and pontine centers in the regulation of ventilation was noted earlier. The medullary respiratory neurons are influenced by peripheral (carotid sinus and aortic body) and central (medullary) chemoreceptors and by more rostral regions. Spinal transection in the upper cervical region interrupts the descending influence from the brainstem and abolishes all rhythmic ventilatory movements. Integration of various inputs to respiratory motor neurons, e.g., from the forebrain, also occurs at a spinal (segmental) level. The forebrain's influence on ventilation is evident from the changes that can be exerted volitionally, as during breath-holding, and from the apnea that sometimes occurs during seizures (37). In animals, electrical stimulation of the uncus, fornix, and amygdala, and of certain cortical areas (anterior cingulate, anterior insular, inferior medial temporal, and posterior lateral frontal cortex) has an inhibitory effect on ventilation (38).

Sleep apnea—the impairment of automatic but not volitional ventilatory movements—may be central, obstructive, or mixed in type. Central sleep apnea is usually idiopathic but may result from unilateral or bilateral medullary infarction (39) or other brainstem pathology (40). Central pathology, such as syringobulbia (41) and olivopontocerebellar atrophy (40), may also cause obstructive sleep apnea. Sleep apnea sometimes occurs in patients with the dysautonomia of multisystem atrophy, who may also have hypopnea and laryngeal stridor. Iatrogenic sleep apnea has followed bilateral cervical tractotomy for pain (42).

Neuromuscular disorders can impair ventilation, necessitating supportive measures, as exemplified by certain cases of poliomyelitis, amyotrophic lateral sclerosis, Guillain-Barré syndrome, and myasthenia gravis.

Bronchodilation results from sympathetic stimulation, whereas vagal stimulation leads to constriction of the bronchioles and may increase bronchial secretions.

Eyes, Pupils, and Lacrimal Glands

The sympathetic control of the pupil depends on an uncrossed three-neuron pathway. Axons descend from hypothalamic neurons to the intermediolateral cell column of the cord at the level of the first thoracic segment. Preganglionic sympathetic neurons project from there to the superior cervical ganglion. The adrenergic sympathetic postganglionic fibers to the pupil arise from the superior cervical ganglion, proceed adjacent to the internal carotid artery to the cavernous sinus, and then pass to the orbit to supply the dilator muscle of the pupil. Parasympathetic fibers to the pupil travel with the third nerve from the mesencephalic Edinger-Westphal nucleus to the ciliary ganglion in the orbit, from which cholinergic postganglionic fibers pass in the short ciliary nerves to the pupillary constrictor and ciliary muscle (accommodation).

Stimulation of the parasympathetic fibers (or application of pilocarpine) leads to pupillary constriction and contrac-

tion of the ciliary muscle; mydriasis occurs in response to atropine or with a complete third nerve palsy. Degeneration of the ciliary ganglion or a postganglionic parasympathetic lesion is responsible for the tonic pupil of Adie; the pupil is large and reacts only sluggishly to light and accommodation. The abnormality is usually unilateral, and it may be associated with absent tendon reflexes or with segmental anhidrosis (Ross syndrome). As a result of denervation supersensitivity, the pupil constricts in response to instillation of 0.125% pilocarpine or 2.5% methacholine, which has no effect on normal pupils.

Argyll Robertson pupils have come to be regarded as a hallmark of neurosyphilis, but they also occur in other disorders such as encephalitis, multiple sclerosis, and diabetes. They are small, irregular, unequal pupils that are unresponsive to light but reactive to convergence and accommodation. The responsible pathology probably involves the rostral midbrain.

Stimulation of sympathetic fibers causes pupillary dilation, while sympathetic lesions cause a small pupil, often associated with ptosis, enophthalmos, and anhidrosis (Horner's syndrome). This may result from preganglionic or postganglionic (superior cervical ganglion) lesions, and thus occurs, for example, with lateral medullary infarcts, cervical cord lesions, carotid artery thrombosis, pulmonary apical or mediastinal tumors, and injuries to the neck.

The lacrimal glands produce tears. The main gland receives parasympathetic innervation that arises in the pontine tegmentum and passes with the nervus intermedius to join the seventh cranial nerve as it enters the internal auditory meatus. The parasympathetic fibers eventually emerge as the greater superficial petrosal nerve and pass to the sphenopalatine ganglion before reaching the lacrimal glands, where they stimulate the production of tears.

Bladder

Bladder function is regulated by several different parts of the CNS, including the frontal cortex, basal ganglia, and lower brainstem. Lesions of the anterior frontal lobes are notorious for causing disturbances of micturition (43, 44). There may be urinary incontinence, voluntary micturition in inappropriate circumstances, or both. Less frequently, urinary hesitancy or retention occurs with frontal lesions (43). In patients with hydrocephalus, the enlarged ventricles may stretch or distort corticobulbar fibers, leading to incontinence. It thus appears that descending fibers from the frontal lobe have a regulatory effect on micturition. Frequency, urgency, and urgency incontinence are common in patients with basal ganglia dysfunction resulting from Parkinson's disease. Hesitancy and difficulty of micturition occur less often. Detrusor hyperreflexia and abnormal cystometric findings are common in parkinsonism (45), regardless of whether there are any symptoms of bladder dysfunction. Experimental studies in animals suggest that various pontomedullary regions (46) are also involved in regulating the bladder, but evidence in humans is lacking.

The cerebral influences on micturition (and defecation) are exerted through pathways traversing the spinal cord. With lesions interrupting afferent pathways in the cord, the normal sensation of bladder fullness is lost; the bladder becomes overdistended and overflow incontinence occurs. In addition, bladder emptying will occur reflexly if the influence of the supraspinal control mechanisms is lost, and detrusor-sphincter dyssynergia occurs. The pattern of voiding after complete traumatic myelopathy depends on the site of the lesion. With spinal lesions above the conus, urinary retention occurs in the acute phase and is then followed by reflex voiding that is initiated by various stimuli and is incomplete. With lesions of the conus medullaris (or cauda equina), by contrast, there is urinary retention. In patients with incomplete cord lesions above the conus, such as cervical spondylotic myelopathy, urinary frequency, urgency, and urgency incontinence are common, and cystometry reveals detrusor hyperreflexia.

The bladder is supplied by both sympathetic and parasympathetic fibers, while the external sphincter receives a somatic innervation. Parasympathetic preganglionic fibers originate from the S2–S4 segments of the cord, passing with the anterior roots and then in the pelvic nerves to form a diffuse network over the bladder, where they synapse with postganglionic cells innervating the bladder and urethra. The external urinary sphincter and penis/clitoris are supplied by pudendal (somatic) fibers arising from the sacral plexus. Afferent fibers responsible for reflex bladder contraction pass with the parasympathetic nerves to enter the spinal cord through the posterior S2–S4 roots. Sympathetic preganglionic efferent fibers arise from the intermediolateral column of the spinal cord and pass through the sympathetic ganglia and splanchnic nerves to the hypogastric plexus. Postganglionic fibers arise from cells in this plexus or the vesical plexus and supply the bladder muscle. The role of the sympathetic efferent system in regulating micturition is unclear.

Urinary incontinence results from disruption of somatic afferent and efferent fibers to the external urinary sphincter, as by tumors, trauma, spinal stenosis, and diabetic polyradiculopathy. Selective damage to the neurons supplying the external sphincter occurs in the Shy-Drager syndrome or multisystem atrophy (47).

Many elderly patients have urinary incontinence without evidence of any underlying neurological disorder. In some instances the incontinence occurs only at times of stress to the control system, as with coughing. Recent studies relate this to damage that has previously occurred to the striated pelvic floor sphincter muscles or their nerve supply, e.g., during childbirth (47). In other instances, incontinence occurs during confusional states or in circumstances when voluntary control of sphincter function is reduced.

Gastrointestinal Tract

Parasympathetic fibers to the organs associated with digestion are secretory; they also cause increased gastrointestinal peristalsis and relaxation of sphincters. Conversely, sympathetic stimulation reduces peristalsis and secretion and increases sphincter tone. The anteromedial frontal lobes are involved in the regulation of defecation. Lesions in this region may lead to fecal incontinence (43).

Intramural plexuses (Auerbach's plexus in the external muscular coat, Meissner's submucosal plexus, and other ill-defined neuronal networks) are important for the regulation of gastrointestinal motility and secretions (48, 49). This so-called enteric nervous system is regulated, in turn, by the sympathetic and parasympathetic systems, the former primarily via the celiac and mesenteric ganglia, the latter via the vagus and sacral (S2–S4) spinal nerves. Functionally complete circuits within the enteric nervous systems permit integrated motor and reflex responses to occur regardless of parasympathetic input. Such responses can, however, be modulated by vagal and sympathetic activity.

Dysphagia may occur for many different reasons, such as structural abnormalities or neuromuscular disorders (e.g., progressive bulbar palsy, brainstem stroke, or bulbar poliomyelitis). In some patients, however, it relates to a failure of the esophageal sphincter to relax (as in achalasia) or impaired esophageal peristalsis. Gastroparesis leads to a sense of postprandial fullness, discomfort, and vomiting, and is a common feature of certain dysautonomias, especially diabetic autonomic neuropathy. Somewhat similar symptoms may result from intestinal pseudoobstruction, such as sometimes occurs in amyloidosis. Constipation is a very common and rather nonspecific symptom, and its etiology is frequently multifactorial. In Parkinson's disease, for example, it may relate to antiparkinsonian medication, bradykinesia, reduced gastrointestinal motility (perhaps related to involvement of the dorsal motor nucleus of the vagus), or pelvic floor dysfunction; primary involvement of the enteric nervous system may also have a role (50). Traumatic myelopathy leads to paralytic ileus and fecal incontinence in the acute phase; after this period the defecatory reflexes recover, but there is loss of voluntary control of defecation and an inability to strain.

There are many causes of fecal incontinence, but in general the neurological ones are similar to those discussed earlier as causing disturbances of bladder function. Both pure autonomic failure and the Shy-Drager syndrome may lead to constipation, fecal incontinence, and impaired gastrointestinal motility.

Sexual Function

The hypothalamus and limbic regions have an important role in sexual arousal. Electrical stimulation of various hypothalamic areas causes erection, whereas lesions in these regions—and especially of the medial preoptic-anterior hypothalamic area—suppress sexual behavior (51). Bilateral temporal lobectomy in monkeys (52) and humans (53) leads to an increase in sexual activity as well as other behavioral changes, and a similar clinical picture may occur clinically with other encephalopathies (54). Gautier-Smith (55) concluded that lesions of the amygdala correlated best with the sexual disturbance.

Descending pathways traverse the midbrain, lower brainstem, and lateral columns of the cord to the thoracolumbar and sacral regions. Spinal cord lesions may have profound effects on sexual function, depending on the extent and level of the lesion. Many patients with complete cervical lesions have reflex erections, but the pleasurable experience of orgasm is abolished. With more caudal lesions, erectile and ejaculatory failure are common.

The thoracolumbar sympathetic supply to the sexual organs has a complex and variable course. Some preganglionic sympathetic fibers synapse with postganglionic fibers in the sympathetic chain, whereas others pass through to reach the inferior mesenteric and superior hypogastric plexuses where they synapse with postganglionic fibers that reach the pelvic organs via the hypogastric nerves, pelvic plexus, and cavernous nerves. Other sympathetic fibers reach the pelvic plexus with the parasympathetic nerves, and some travel in the pudendal nerves. Preganglionic parasympathetic (sacral) fibers form the pelvic nerves, which join the pelvic plexus. Both sympathetic and parasympathetic pathways are probably involved in arousal and orgasm (55). Lesions of the sacral nerve roots and pelvic nerves lead to erectile failure in men and failure of arousal in women.

The sympathetic and parasympathetic fibers innervate the blood vessels of various pelvic structures, erectile tissues in the penis and clitoris, and smooth muscle of the vagina, uterus, prostate, and seminal vesicles. The mechanisms involved in erection are complex and poorly understood. Cavernosal tissue becomes engorged because of increased blood flow resulting from dilation of cavernosal and helicine arteries. This engorgement leads to compression of emissary veins, and venous drainage is therefore reduced. Detumescence results from contraction of the helicine arteries and the trabecular walls of the lacunar spaces of cavernosal tissue. Blood inflow is thus reduced, and decompression of veins leads to increased drainage. The sympathetic nervous system is primarily responsible for emission. The smooth muscle of the epididymis, vas deferens, seminal vesicles, and prostate contracts, as also does the sphincter at the bladder neck to prevent retrograde ejaculation. Ejaculation (i.e., rhythmic seminal transport along, and expulsion from, the urethra) and orgasm are mediated primarily by pudendal somatic efferent and afferent fibers respectively. The neuropharmacological basis of these events is unclear, but erection probably involves vasoactive intestinal polypeptide and endothelium-derived releasing factor, which are activated by the parasympathetic system (51). Neurological mechanisms of sexual function, and their clinical assessment, are discussed in detail by Seagraves in Chapter 32 of this volume.

Thermoregulation and Sweating

Descending fibers from the hypothalamic preoptic area pass through the ipsilateral brainstem to the cells in the intermediolateral columns of the spinal cord. Preganglionic axons from these neurons pass through the white rami communicantes to the sympathetic ganglia, from which postganglionic cholinergic fibers emerge to join the peripheral nerves and ultimately to innervate the eccrine sweat glands. Several neuropeptides are found in the nerve terminals related to these glands and may function as co-transmitters (18). Thermoregulatory sweating occurs following a rise in central temperature that activates the preoptic hypothalamic area, but thermal receptors in other regions of the CNS and in the skin are probably involved as well. Sweating may occur in response to emotion in certain regions, such as the axillae, from apocrine glands. Palmar and pedal sweating also occurs in the absence of heat and is enhanced by emotional stress.

Excessive sweating, or hyperhidrosis, may occur as a generalized phenomenon with exercise, infections, or certain metabolic disorders such as thyrotoxicosis, pheochromocytoma, or carcinoid syndrome. It also occurs with brainstem (pontine) ischemia. The most common cause, however, probably is anxiety. In essential hyperhidrosis no specific cause can be found. Localized or regional hyperhidrosis may occur in association with lesions of the cord or peripheral nerves, or as a result of sweat gland abnormalities.

Anhidrosis or hypohidrosis occurs distally in some patients with polyneuropathy and in a more restricted territory with discrete peripheral nerve or root involvement. Segmental anhidrosis occurring in association with Adie's tonic pupils is labeled Ross syndrome. Anhidrosis sometimes occurs in dermatological disorders or with a widespread distribution as a consequence of neuroleptic, anticholinergic, or tricyclic antidepressant drugs. Generalized or patchy anhidrosis is a feature of pure autonomic failure and of central dysautonomias such as Shy-Drager syndrome and may occur with hypothalamic or posterior fossa tumors, syringomyelia or syringobulbia, multiple sclerosis, and other diffuse brainstem lesions. In Wallenberg's syndrome and other unilateral brainstem lesions, there is ipsilateral hypohidrosis rather than anhidrosis. Chronic idiopathic anhidrosis is characterized by a disturbance of thermoregulatory sweating without evidence of more extensive autonomic involvement except for occasional pupillary abnormalities (56). Patients with this uncommon disorder are intolerant of heat and become hot, flushed, weak, and dyspneic, but do not sweat, with activity or when the ambient temperature is high.

CLINICAL EVALUATION OF AUTONOMIC FUNCTION

A variety of noninvasive tests of autonomic function has been developed to test the integrity of parasympathetic (vagal) fibers to the heart and the sympathetic vasomotor and sudomotor fibers. Such tests can be used to evaluate the autonomic nervous system in patients with symptoms suggestive of dysautonomia. The aim is to determine the presence and severity of any autonomic disturbance and the site of the underlying lesion. These studies can also be used to determine the functional integrity of the unmyelinated

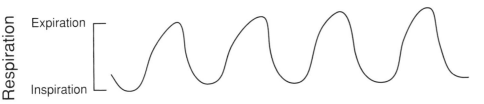

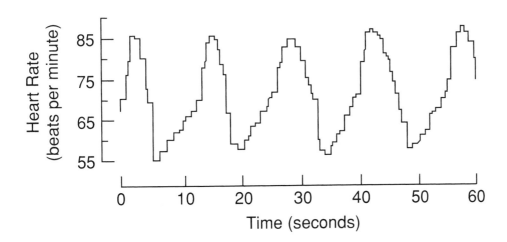

Figure 6.5. Variation in heart rate with deep breathing in a normal subject.

and small myelinated fibers that comprise the peripheral component of the autonomic nervous system in patients with small-fiber peripheral neuropathies.

Heart Rate and Blood Pressure Responses

Measurement of the heart rate response to *deep breathing* is a noninvasive, sensitive, quantitative test that is simple to perform and provides a reliable index of the afferent and efferent parasympathetic (vagal) innervation of the heart. A tachycardia normally occurs during inspiration because of a reduction in cardiac vagal activity (Fig. 6.5). For clinical purposes an electrocardiograph is used to record the R-R intervals continuously over 60 seconds in the recumbent patient. After a 5-minute rest period, the patient takes six deep breaths over 1 minute. The difference between the longest and shortest R-R intervals is noted. The variation of heart rate with respiration is age-dependent (57), but is normally at least 15 beats per minute; values of less than 10 are clearly abnormal (58). In addition, an expiratory: inspiratory (E:I) ratio is calculated from the ratio of the mean of the maximum R-R intervals during expiration to the mean of the minimum R-R intervals during inspiration. This ratio also declines with advancing age.

The heart rate response to *standing* is another useful, simple, noninvasive test of vagal function. Upon standing from the recumbent position, there is an initial tachycardia followed by a bradycardia that begins after about 20 seconds and stabilizes after about the 30th heartbeat. For clinical purposes, the R-R interval of the ECG can be

measured during the performance of the maneuver, and the ratio of the R-R interval at the 30th beat to the 15th beat is determined (59). This "30:15" ratio depends on vagal function and is age-dependent (57), but in young adults it normally exceeds 1.04.

The heart rate responses to *passive head-up tilt* can also be measured after the patient has remained supine for 10 minutes. There is normally an increase of between 10 and 30 beats per minute, reflecting a change in both sympathetic and parasympathetic activity, with 60° head-up tilt. The systolic and diastolic blood pressures usually fall slightly, but this does not exceed 20 and 10 mm Hg, respectively, in normal subjects. Recent studies have emphasized the value of maintaining the head-up tilt for up to 60 minutes, particularly in patients in whom vasodepressor syncope is suspected (60).

The cardiovascular responses to sustained handgrip (30% of maximum for 5 minutes) have also been used as a means of assessing adrenergic function. The sustained muscle contraction produces a rise in heart rate and blood pressure. The diastolic pressure normally rises by at least 15 mm Hg, when the last value recorded before release of the handgrip is compared to the mean value obtained in the 3 minutes before commencing the maneuver. The test, however, is of limited sensitivity and specificity.

The *Valsalva maneuver,* in which the subject performs a forced expiration against a closed glottis, provides important information concerning the integrity of cardiovascular innervation. For clinical purposes, an ECG machine or heart rate monitor can be used to record the heart rate responses

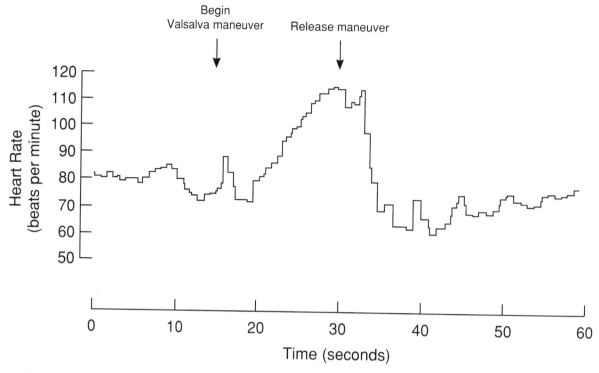

Figure 6.6. Response to the Valsalva maneuver, recorded with a heart rate monitor in a normal subject. There is a tachycardia during the forced expiratory maneuver and a compensatory bradycardia when the maneuver is released.

(Fig. 6.6). The recumbent subject makes a sustained expiration that is sufficient to maintain a column of mercury at 40 mm for 15 seconds by blowing into a mouthpiece with a calibrated air leak. A Valsalva ratio can then be determined from the shortest interbeat interval (or fastest heart rate) generated during the forced expiration divided into the longest interbeat interval (slowest rate) that occurs following it. This reflects both sympathetic and vagal function. Ewing and associates (61) have arbitrarily defined a value of 1.1 or less as abnormal and 1.21 or greater as normal, but the ratio is age-dependent; in subjects younger than 40 years, the Valsalva ratio normally exceeds 1.4.

The Valsalva response was originally studied using an intraarterial cannula to record the blood pressure as well as the heart rate (Fig. 6.7). This can now be determined noninvasively using a photoplethysmographic recording device (Finapres) that also permits beat-to-beat variation in blood pressure during the maneuver to be determined. The response to Valsalva's maneuver is traditionally divided into four phases. In phase I there is a transient increase in blood pressure as the increase in intrathoracic pressure is transmitted to the great vessels. In phase II the blood pressure falls due to a reduced cardiac output (resulting from the decline in venous return). This is associated with a tachycardia caused by diminished vagal activity. The decline in blood pressure is arrested within about 5 seconds and then reversed as increased sympathetic activity increases the peripheral resistance. With release of the forced expiratory maneuver, there is a transient decline in blood pressure due to pooling of blood and expansion of the pulmonary vascular bed with

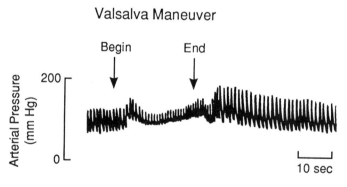

Figure 6.7. Response to the Valsalva maneuver, recorded with an intra-arterial needle in a normal subject.

the reduced intrathoracic pressure (phase III), following which the blood pressure overshoots its original baseline value as cardiac output returns to normal while the tachycardia and peripheral vasoconstriction persist (phase IV). This overshoot of the blood pressure leads in turn to a compensatory bradycardia. Dysautonomic patients typically show a continuous and excessive decline in blood pressure in phase II and no overshoot in phase IV (Fig. 6.8).

Startle (as by a sudden loud noise) or *mental stress* (induced, for example, by attempting to perform the serial-sevens test despite constant distraction) normally leads to an increase in heart rate and blood pressure. In the *cold pressor test,* immersion of one hand in cold (4°C) water normally produces an increase in systolic pressure of 15 mm Hg within 1 minute. Abnormalities of these responses imply a lesion centrally or in sympathetic efferent pathways. Normal responses in patients with an abnormal response to the Valsalva maneuver suggest an afferent baroreceptor lesion.

Tests of Cutaneous Vasomotor Function

Cutaneous blood flow can be studied by plethysmography or a laser Doppler flow meter. The vasomotor responses to various stimuli are evaluated as a measure of adrenergic function. For convenience, digital blood flow is recorded for clinical purposes.

A sudden inspiratory gasp normally produces a digital vasoconstriction as a spinal reflex (Fig. 6.9). The response is lost or impaired in patients with a cord lesion or a disturbance of sympathetic efferent pathways, such as in peripheral neuropathies (62, 63). A cold stimulus (ice-cold water at 4°C) to the opposite hand also produces a reflex vasoconstriction, as does mental stress.

Sweat Tests

The thermoregulatory sweat test is a highly sensitive test in which the body temperature is raised by 1°C by exposure of the subject to radiant heat from a heat cradle. The presence and distribution of sweating is determined by a change in color of an indicator powder placed on the skin. Abnormalities may reflect pre- or postganglionic lesions.

The quantitative sudomotor axon reflex test (QSART) is a test of postganglionic sudomotor sympathetic function (64). Axon terminals are activated by iontophoresed acetylcholine; the resulting impulses travel antidromically to a branching point and then orthodromically down another branch of the axon to its terminals, where they release acetylcholine, which generates a sweat response. The sudomotor responses elicited are measured quantitatively. The test is highly sensitive and specific and yields reproducible results. Normal findings are obtained in preganglionic disorders.

The sympathetic skin response is another means of evaluating sudomotor function. It depends on the electrical activity arising from sweat glands and adjacent tissues either spontaneously or in response to certain stimuli. For clinical purposes, electrical stimulation of a mixed or cutaneous nerve is used to elicit a response from the palms of the hands and soles of the feet, and the resulting change in voltage is measured from the skin surface (65). Though easy to perform, the sympathetic skin response is of uncertain specificity, is not quantitative, and habituates. Accordingly, it can reliably be considered as abnormal only when it is absent.

Plasma Catecholamine Levels and Norepinephrine Infusion

The resting plasma norepinephrine level provides an index of sympathetic activity. It is diminished in disorders with postganglionic (as opposed to preganglionic) pathology. The plasma norepinephrine level normally increases with change in posture from recumbent to standing, and this postural response may be markedly attenuated or absent with pre- or postganglionic lesions.

Another approach is to measure the blood pressure changes that occur with intravenous infusion of norepinephrine at different dosage rates up to 20 μg per minute (66). To increase the systolic pressure to 40 mm Hg above baseline, normal subjects require infusion at a rate of 15 to 20 μg per minute, whereas patients with the Shy-Drager syndrome require 5 to 10 μg per minute and those with primary autonomic failure less than 2.5 μg per minute (66).

Bladder and Gastrointestinal Function

Bladder function is assessed by several methods. These include determination of the volume of residual urine after attempted voiding, which is normally less than 100 cc. Cystometry is an important investigative approach in which the bladder is filled with water or radiological contrast medium, or inflated with carbon dioxide via a self-retaining catheter, and the relationship between intravesical pressure and volume is determined. Bladder filling is normally first appreciated at volumes of 100 to 200 cc, and the desire to void increases as filling continues. Impaired sensation may reflect peripheral or central pathology. In the normal subject, vesical pressure does not increase by more than 10 cm H_2O until maximum capacity (generally between 300 and 600 cc) is reached. Detrusor hyperreflexia is found in patients with central (cerebral or spinal) disturbances of micturition, and detrusor areflexia (i.e., an absence of detrusor reflex contractions during cystometry) occurs in patients with peripheral (root or nerve) pathology. It is also helpful to measure urinary flow, and in particular the mean and maximal flow rates, duration and pattern of flow, and volume voided. The technique is helpful in distinguishing between flow disturbances from obstruction and abnormal detrusor activity.

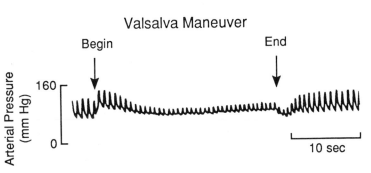

Figure 6.8. Abnormal, intra-arterially recorded response to the Valsalva maneuver in a patient with Shy-Drager syndrome.

Valsalva Maneuver

Begin

End

Arterial Pressure (mm Hg)

160

0

10 sec

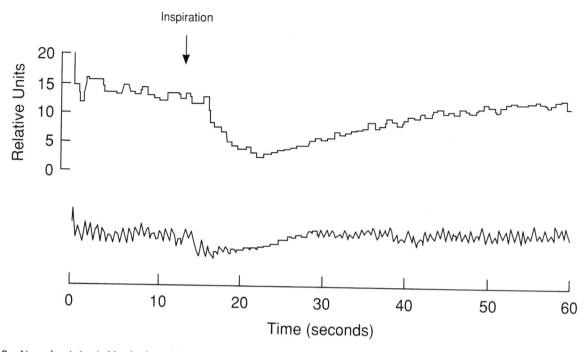

Figure 6.9.   Normal variation in blood volume following a deep inspiration, recorded photoplethysmographically by an infrared emitter and detector on the pad of the index finger. The *bottom trace* represents the sensor output after amplification by the photoplethysmographic module of a computerized autonomic testing system and is a function of the absolute blood volume in the finger. Each peak represents a heartbeat, and the amplitude of each wave reflects blood volume in the area about the sensor. The apparent shift of the DC signal component results from the long time constant required to prevent loss of signal information. The *upper trace* shows the relative voltage, representing the amplitude of each pulse. Following the deep inspiration there is a reduction in digital blood flow (i.e., reduced amplitude of the waveforms in the lower trace and a corresponding decline in the upper trace).

Radiological studies are important in evaluating gastrointestinal function and especially in excluding mechanical causes of symptoms such as dysphagia, delayed gastric emptying, intestinal pseudoobstruction, or intractable constipation. Fluoroscopy and studies of colonic transit time may also be helpful. Catheter probes connected to a pressure transducer can be used to measure anorectal pressure. In the region of the anal sphincter, resting pressure reflects internal anal sphincter tone. Activity in the external anal sphincter muscle is reflected by the pressure recorded on voluntary contraction. Rectal distension with a balloon causes reflex relaxation of the internal anal sphincter. This rectoanal reflex depends on intramural nerves (67) and is absent in Hirschsprung's disease.

Sphincter Electromyography and Evoked Potential Studies

Denervation of the urethral and anal sphincters may result from cell loss in Onuf's nucleus in the sacral cord or from pathology situated more distally. Needle electromyography permits recognition of abnormal motor unit action potentials in the sphincteric muscles in patients with dysautonomia and thereby helps to localize the lesion. With pyramidal lesions, volitional control of sphincter function is impaired, and the urethral striated sphincter muscle fails to relax during detrusor contraction (detrusor-sphincter dyssynergia).

The cerebral potentials elicited by electrical stimulation in the anorectum, at the neck or trigone of the bladder, or of the pudendal nerve (dorsal nerve of the penis or clitoris) and pelvic urethral nerve are easy to record. The utility of such evoked potential studies, which are somewhat uncomfortable, in the investigation of patients with impotence or a disturbance of voiding or defecation is unclear.

Pharmacological Evaluation of Pupillary Reactivity

Anticholinergic (parasympatholytic) agents applied topically cause pupillary dilation, as do sympathomimetic agents. Conversely, parasympathomimetic or sympatholytic agents cause pupillary constriction.

Pilocarpine and methylcholine are cholinergic (parasympathomimetic) agents. In patients with parasympathetic denervation, very weak solutions of pilocarpine (e.g., 0.125%) will cause pupillary constriction because of denervation supersensitivity. A dilated pupil that is unresponsive to instilled cholinergic agents probably reflects sympathetic overactivity.

Sympathomimetic agents will cause dilation of denervated pupils at concentrations that are ineffective on normal pupils. For example, 1% phenylephrine hydrochloride will produce dilation of the pupil in Horner's syndrome because of denervation supersensitivity. Cocaine hydrochloride (4%) can also be instilled into the conjunctival sac and normally causes pupillary dilation by sympathetic activation. In Horner's syndrome resulting from peripheral sympathetic denervation, this effect of cocaine is lost.

CLINICAL FEATURES OF DYSAUTONOMIA

The clinical features of dysautonomia vary in different patients and depend in part upon the nature of the underlying disorder, as does the existence and nature of any somatic neurological manifestations. For example, dysautonomia occurring in diabetics may be associated with symptoms and signs suggestive of a peripheral neuropathy, whereas parkinsonism, cerebellar dysfunction, a pyramidal disturbance, or some combination of these abnormalities occurs in patients with central disorders of autonomic function (such as the Shy-Drager syndrome).

Impotence and loss of libido are common presenting features in men with dysautonomia, and are often mistakenly attributed to psychogenic factors until other autonomic disturbances develop. Ejaculation may also be impaired. When retrograde ejaculation occurs, patients feel as if they have ejaculated but little is produced; the subsequently voided urine is found to be discolored and to contain spermatozoa. Abnormalities of micturition are another common early symptom, and in men may be attributed to prostatic hypertrophy.

The most disabling symptom of autonomic dysfunction is usually postural hypotension. A feeling of impending loss of consciousness occurs on standing or walking, and the patient may ultimately fall to the ground unconscious, unless symptoms are aborted by sitting or lying down. Unlike a typical syncopal episode, there is no preceding sweating. Symptomatic postural hypotension is more likely to occur in the early part of the day, postprandially, with activity, or in hot weather, because of the cardiovascular and hemodynamic alterations that occur in these circumstances.

An impairment or loss of thermoregulatory sweating is common and may be life-threatening in hot climates. The distribution of any anhidrosis may suggest the site of pathology. For example, impaired sweating distally in the extremities suggests an underlying peripheral neuropathy, whereas a more generalized disturbance of sweating, with involvement of the trunk, implies a central lesion.

Disturbances of bladder or bowel regulation are especially distressing. Urinary urgency, frequency, and nocturia may occur, and there may be urgency incontinence. In other instances, an atonic bladder leads to overflow incontinence. Cystometry clarifies the nature of the bladder disturbance and thereby indicates the appropriate therapeutic approach. Intractable constipation, intermittent diarrhea, or an alternation between constipation and diarrhea also occurs. Rectal incontinence during episodes of diarrhea is particularly troublesome. Nausea, postprandial fullness, and severe vomiting may reflect gastroparesis.

Visual blurring and dryness of the eyes are sometimes troublesome, and there may be a variety of pupillary abnormalities in patients with dysautonomia. The effect of lesions affecting the parasympathetic innervation (i.e., the third cranial nerve) or the sympathetic system (causing a Horner's syndrome) has already been described.

Disturbances of breathing may consist of inspiratory gasps or cluster breathing in patients with the Shy-Drager syndrome of autonomic failure. Occasional patients experience central sleep apnea. Laryngeal stridor may also occur.

SELECTED CAUSES OF DYSAUTONOMIA

Acute Peripheral Pathology

There are many causes of autonomic dysfunction. Neuropathies are among the most important causes. Acute involvement of peripheral autonomic fibers may occur in several contexts. First, a pure autonomic neuropathy may occur acutely or subacutely, either as an idiopathic or postviral disorder or a paraneoplastic syndrome, with diffuse, generalized sympathetic and parasympathetic dysfunction (68–70). Examination typically reveals significant postural hypotension, a fixed heart rate, anhidrosis, xerostomia, dry eyes, a distended bladder, and dilated unresponsive pupils. There is often no motor or sensory deficit, but minor sensory abnormalities are sometimes evident, especially an impairment of those sensory modalities mediated by small fibers (pain and temperature appreciation). Recovery occurs gradually, and may be incomplete. The dysautonomia is sometimes confined to the cholinergic system (71), in which case postural hypotension does not occur.

Autonomic dysfunction is common in patients with a peripheral neuropathy but is usually overshadowed by the coexisting motor and sensory deficits. In the Guillain-Barré syndrome, however, autonomic disturbances may be life-threatening (72–74). There may be severe hypotension, paroxysmal hypertension, or extreme fluctuations in blood pressure; disturbances of cardiac rhythm, regional anhidrosis or hyperhidrosis, pupillary abnormalities, gastroparesis, constipation, urinary retention, and urinary or fecal incontinence also occur. The cause of the paroxysmal hypertension is unclear, but denervation supersensitivity to circulating catecholamines or denervation of baroreceptors may be responsible.

Autonomic dysfunction, resulting from a disturbance of cholinergic mechanisms, is a feature of botulism. Constipation, urinary retention, dryness of the eyes, anhidrosis, and xerostomia present the most common evidence of such dysfunction. Disorders of autonomic, especially cholinergic, function are well described in Lambert-Eaton myasthenic syndrome (75).

A number of iatrogenic neuropathies may be associated with autonomic involvement, such as those related to amiodarone, perhexiline maleate, cis-platinum, or vincristine. Dysautonomia also follows exposure to acrylamide, organic solvents, and Vacor (a rodenticide).

Chronic Peripheral Pathology

The most common cause of dysautonomia in developed countries is probably diabetes. Diabetic autonomic neuropathy may occur in isolation or in association with any of the neuromuscular complications of diabetes, especially a symmetrical sensory or sensorimotor polyneuropathy, entrapment neuropathy, mononeuropathy multiplex, polyradiculopathy, or plexopathy. Postural hypotension, abnormal cardiovagal function, and impaired distal thermoregulatory sweating are typically found; impotence, gastroparesis, constipation, fecal incontinence (often in association with diarrhea), and bladder disturbances are not uncommon (76, 77).

Autonomic disturbances also occur in patients with the neuropathy of chronic renal failure (78), leprosy (79), vitamin B_{12} deficiency (80), and various connective tissue diseases (81). Indeed, a chronic autonomic disturbance may occur with any polyneuropathy, but especially a neuropathy involving small fibers. Axonal neuropathies are more likely to be associated with autonomic disturbances than are demyelinating neuropathies.

Chagas's disease occurs mainly in patients from South or Central America, is due to infection with the protozoan *Trypanosoma cruzi,* and is especially likely to cause a chronic dysautonomia. Cholinergic dysfunction predominates, with involvement of the heart and gastrointestinal system. Cardiomegaly and cardiac conduction defects are frequent, and there may be distention of parts of the gastrointestinal tract, especially the esophagus, duodenum, and colon. Postural hypotension, abnormal cardiovascular reflexes (82–84), and reduced plasma norepinephrine levels (85) may be found.

Autonomic dysfunction is an early cause of symptoms in either sporadic systemic amyloid neuropathy or familial amyloidosis. Postural hypotension is common and disabling (86, 87). Abnormalities of gastrointestinal motility reflect infiltration of the enteric plexuses. Anhidrosis is common, as is impotence in men. Somatic neurological deficits typically consist of impaired pain and temperature appreciation due to an underlying axonal neuropathy, with deposition of amyloid. Examination of autonomic function reveals marked postural hypotension, abnormal heart rate responses to deep inspiration and to the Valsalva maneuver, widely impaired thermoregulatory sweating, and impaired peripheral vasomotor responses to such maneuvers as deep inspiration.

A variety of hereditary disorders are associated with autonomic failure. Familial dysautonomia (Riley-Day syndrome) is a recessively inherited neuropathy that begins in infancy with disturbances of thermoregulation, lacrimation, blood pressure regulation, and gastrointestinal function. Repeated episodes of pneumonia are typical. Somatic involvement is manifest by impaired pain and temperature appreciation, weakness, poor sucking, depressed tendon reflexes, and arthropathy. Several other types of hereditary sensory and autonomic neuropathy have been described (88).

Autonomic dysfunction sometimes occurs in hereditary motor and sensory neuropathy type I or type II and is manifest especially by pupillary changes, impaired vasomotor regulation of the distal blood vessels, and occasionally by impaired cardiovascular reflexes (89, 90). Minor abnormalities of dubious clinical relevance have also been reported in myotonic dystrophy (89).

Dopamine β-hydroxylase deficiency is a rare disorder affecting central and peripheral adrenergic neurons that was described earlier in this chapter. It leads to postural hypotension and a variety of other symptoms. Improvement occurs with administration of dihydroxyphenylserine, which is converted endogenously to norepinephrine (91).

Central Dysautonomias

Autonomic manifestations are a feature of many different disorders of the CNS. Seizures, for example, may have autonomic accompaniments, especially when they arise from limbic and paralimbic structures. The most common clinical evidence of autonomic involvement during seizures is a sinus tachycardia, but a variety of other cardiac manifestations may occur ictally, including atypical anginal pain, bradycardias, conduction defects, sinus arrest, tachyarrhythmias, and atrial fibrillation (92). Another common, possibly dysautonomic, feature of seizures—especially complex partial attacks arising from the temporal lobe—is a curious feeling of discomfort that ascends from the epigastrium, accompanied sometimes by nausea. Pupillary dilatation, respiratory arrest, other changes in respiratory rate or pattern, blood pressure changes, cutaneous vasodilation or vasoconstriction, piloerection (93), and vomiting (94) are other autonomic accompaniments of seizures, especially those arising from the temporal lobe. When vomiting occurs as a seizure phenomenon, patients are typically unaware of vomiting, and other ictal phenomena are associated (94).

Lesions of the *mesial frontal lobe,* especially the cingulate gyrus, may produce disturbances of sphincter function, with urinary incontinence, fecal incontinence, or both. *Hydrocephalus* sometimes leads to a similar effect, presumably because of distortion and stretch of corticobulbar fibers.

Hypothalamic pathology may affect temperature regulation, mainly leading to hypothermia. This may be the basis of the hypothermia that is sometimes associated with episodic hyperhidrosis and agenesis of the corpus callosum (95, 96). In other instances, episodic hyperthermia occurs after head injury or with hypothalamic pathology or acute hydrocephalus (97), and may be associated with tachycardia, hyperpnea, transient hypertension, cutaneous vasoconstriction or vasodilation, pupillary changes, and increased muscle tone. Hypothalamic pathology such as infarction occasionally leads to an ipsilateral Horner's syndrome (98). Pathological involvement of the anterior hypothalamus may affect circadian rhythms (99).

Diseases of the *basal ganglia* are also accompanied by autonomic dysfunction. In patients with *Parkinson's disease,* many symptoms (such as disturbances of sweating, postural dizziness, and sphincter dysfunction) suggest autonomic involvement. However, the cardiovascular reflexes are generally normal, although there may be increased sensitivity to infused catacholamines. This finding may suggest a subtle disturbance of autonomic function due to a central rather than a peripheral lesion (100, 101). In some patients there seems to be a disturbance in "set" of the baroreceptor reflexes without disruption of their integrity (100, 102). Autonomic symptoms also occur in other extrapyramidal disorders. Some patients with *progressive supranuclear palsy* have postural hypotension, but this does not usually exceed the postural change sometimes encountered in normal subjects (103, 104). In *Huntington's disease,* there may be sphincter disturbances, abnormalities of swallowing and respiration, hyperhidrosis, sialorrhea, polyuria, polydipsia, and hypogenitalism (101). Pathological changes in this disorder involve the caudate nuclei, and these structures have been implicated in the regulation of blood pressure during change in posture. Aminoff and Gross (105) investigated 11 patients with Huntington's disease and found no abnormality of either resting blood pressure or baroreceptor reflex responses; there was nevertheless a significantly greater fall in blood pressure on 60° head-up tilt compared to controls, implying that suprabulbar structures including the caudate nuclei may indeed influence postural vasoregulatory mechanisms without affecting baroreceptor reflexes.

Autonomic hyperactivity (with tachycardia, hypertension, hyperhidrosis, and hyperthermia) is a major feature of *fatal familial insomnia,* where it is conjoined with intractable insomnia and motor abnormalities including myoclonus, ataxia, and pyramidal deficits. The disorder is associated with pathology involving the anterior ventral and dorsomedial nuclei of the thalamus (106).

Tumors, ischemia, or degenerative disorders affecting the *brainstem* or *cerebellum* may lead to postural hypotension (34, 107) or, less commonly, to hypertension (33). In some cases the blood pressure abnormality precedes development of other neurological deficits, and its cause may pass unrecognized unless the CNS is imaged. Blood pressure regulation may be impaired in Wernicke's encephalopathy due to central or peripheral pathology (108, 109).

The *Shy-Drager syndrome* (or multisystem atrophy) is a condition in which marked autonomic dysfunction occurs in association with a somatic neurological deficit characterized primarily by parkinsonian features, but also by cerebellar signs, pyramidal deficits, and sometimes lower motor neuron involvement (110). It can therefore be distinguished by its neurological accompaniments from the syndrome of primary (or pure) autonomic failure, in which the autonomic dysfunction occurs in isolation. The Shy-Drager syndrome may simulate classic Parkinson's disease, but the existence of more widespread neurological deficits and an impairment of baroreceptor reflexes distinguish it from the latter disorder. The disorder tends to pursue a progressive course, and many patients are dead within 5 years of the diagnosis being established. The dysautonomia results primarily from a loss of sympathetic cells in the intermediolateral cell columns of the spinal cord, and there may also be pathological changes in the dorsal nucleus of the vagus, nucleus tractus solitarius, and locus ceruleus in the brainstem. Dysautonomia may occur in patients with olivopontocerebellar atrophy (OPCA) or striatonigral degeneration; these disorders probably reflect different manifestations of multisystem atrophy (111).

Complete lesions of the *spinal cord,* as by trauma, have major effects on autonomic function. After transection of the cervical cord, reflex function returns to the isolated spinal segment after a variable period (usually a few weeks), but cerebral regulation of autonomic activity is lost. With lesions above T6, the resting blood pressure is reduced and there is marked orthostatic hypotension, with an overshoot of the blood pressure on resumption of a recumbent posture (36). Changes in cardiac rate still occur with change in posture, so that on head-up tilt the heart rate increases; this is because the influence of the vagus nerve on the heart is preserved. There may be disturbances of temperature regulations because of an inability to sweat or alter vasomotor function below the level of the lesion. Bladder, bowel, and sexual function are markedly impaired, as discussed earlier. Autonomic dysreflexia is sometimes a major management problem in these patients. Visceral, muscle, or cutaneous stimulation below the level of the lesion leads to reflex sympathetic and parasympathetic excitation, with consequent activity in a number of organs supplied by the autonomic nervous system. A marked and rapid elevation of the blood pressure may lead to intracranial hemorrhage. Stroke volume and cardiac output also increase. Cutaneous vasodilation and sweating sometimes occur above the level of the lesion, but the mechanism of this is unclear.

Cardiac arrhythmias, neurogenic hypertension, and acute pulmonary edema may occur in patients with acute intracranial pathology such as subarachnoid hemorrhage or increased intracranial pressure, and sometimes lead to sudden death. They probably relate to excessive sympathetic activity.

Old Age

Many subjects over 70 years of age have a postural drop in systolic pressure of 20 mm Hg or more on standing (112). There may be alterations in baroreceptor sensitivity with age, and reduction in the elasticity of blood vessels and of adrenoreceptor sensitivity may also account for the postural drop in blood pressure (113). Syncope is a common problem in the elderly and often occurs for unclear reasons (114).

TREATMENT OF DYSAUTONOMIA

The treatment of the various manifestations of autonomic dysfunction is beyond the scope of this chapter. For further information, the reader is referred to other sources (115, 116).

References

1. Wallin BG, Elam M. Microneurography and autonomic dysfunction. In: Low PA, ed. Clinical autonomic disorders. Boston: Little, Brown & Co, 1993:243–252.
2. Loewy AD. Anatomy of the autonomic nervous system: an overview. In: Loewy AD, Spyer KM, eds. Central regulation of autonomic functions. New York: Oxford University Press, 1990:3–16.
3. Cechetto DF, Saper CB. Role of the cerebral cortex in autonomic function. In: Loewy AD, Spyer KM, eds. Central regulation of autonomic functions. New York: Oxford University Press, 1990:208–223.

4. Wannamaker BB. Autonomic nervous system and epilepsy. Epilepsia 1985;26(suppl 1):S31–S39.
5. Hilton SM. Inhibition of baroreceptor reflexes on hypothalamic stimulation. J Physiol 1963;165:56P–57P.
6. McAllen RM. Inhibition of the baroreceptor input to the medulla by stimulation of the hypothalamic defence area. J Physiol 1976;257: 45P–46P.
7. Bradley DJ, Ghelarducci B, Paton JFR, Spyer KM. The cardiovascular responses elicited from the posterior cerebellar cortex in the anaesthetized and decerebrate rabbit. J Physiol 1987;383:537–550.
8. Supple WF, Leaton RN. Cerebellar vermis: essential for classically conditioned bradycardia in the rat. Brain Res 1990;509:17–23.
9. Spyer KM. Physiology of the autonomic nervous system: CNS control of the cardiovascular system. Curr Opin Neurol Neurosurg 1991;4:528–532.
10. Loewy AD. Central autonomic pathways. In: Loewy AD, Spyer KM, eds. Central regulation of autonomic functions. New York: Oxford University Press, 1990:88–103.
11. Doba N, Reis DJ. Acute fulminating neurogenic hypertension produced by brainstem lesions in the rat. Circ Res 1973;32:584–593.
12. Barron KD, Chokroverty S. Anatomy of the autonomic nervous system: brain and brainstem. In: Low PA, ed. Clinical autonomic disorders. Boston: Little, Brown & Co, 1993:3–15.
13. Mitchell RA, Berger AJ. Neural regulation of respiration. In: Hornbein TF, ed. Regulation of breathing, part I. New York: Marcel Dekker, 1981:541–620.
14. Lumsden T. Observations on the respiratory centres in the cat. J Physiol 1923;57:153–160.
15. Berger AJ, Mitchell RA, Severinghaus JW. Regulation of respiration. N Engl J Med 1977;297:92–97, 138–143, and 194–201 (three parts).
16. Low PA, Okazaki H, Dyck PJ. Splanchnic preganglionic neurons in man: I. Morphometry of preganglionic cytons. Acta Neuropathol (Berl) 1977;40:55–61.
17. Gibbins IL, Morris JL. Sympathetic noradrenergic neurons containing dynorphin but not neuropeptide Y innervate small cutaneous blood vessels of guinea-pigs. J Auton Nerv Syst 1990;29: 137–149.
18. Tainio H, Vaalasti A, Rechardt L. The distribution of substance P-, CGRP-, galanin-, and ANP-like immunoreactive nerves in human sweat glands. Histochem J 1987;19:375–380.
19. Harati Y. Anatomy of the spinal and peripheral autonomic nervous system. In: Low PA, ed. Clinical autonomic disorders. Boston: Little, Brown & Co, 1993:17–37.
20. Pettersson A, Ricksten S-E, Towle AC, Hedner J, Hedner T. Effect of blood volume expansion and sympathetic denervation on plasma levels of atrial natriuretic factor (ANF) in the rat. Acta Physiol Scand 1985;124:309–311.
21. Schotzinger RJ, Landis SC. Acquisition of cholinergic and peptidergic properties by sympathetic innervation of rat sweat glands requires interaction with normal target. Neuron 1990;5:91–100.
22. Bell C. Anatomical aspects of growth and ageing in the autonomic nervous system. Curr Opin Neurol Neurosurg 1991;4:524–527.
23. Scott SA, Davies AM. Inhibition of protein synthesis prevents cell death in sensory and parasympathetic neurons deprived of neurotrophic factors in vitro. J Neurobiol 1990;21:630–638.
24. Chang JY, Martin DP, Johnson EM. Interferon suppresses sympathetic neuronal cell death caused by nerve growth factor deprivation. J Neurochem 1990;55:436–445.
25. Gurusinghe CJ, Bell C. Substance P immunoreactivity in the superior cervical ganglia of normotensive and genetically hypertensive rats. J Auton Nerv Syst 1989;27:249–256.
26. Gurusinghe CJ, Harris PJ, Abbott DF, Bell C. Neuropeptide Y in rat sympathetic neurons is altered by genetic hypertension and by age. Hypertension 1990;16:63–71.
27. Messina A, Bell C. Are genetically hypertensive rats deficient in nerve growth factor? Neuroreport 1991;2:45–48.
28. Eldridge FL, Millhorn DE, Kiley JP, Waldrop TG. Stimulation by central command of locomotion, respiration and circulation during exercise. Respir Physiol 1985;59:313–337.
29. Duprez DA, Essandoh LK, Vanhoutte PM, Shepherd JT. Vascular responses in forearm and calf to contralateral static exercises. J Appl Physiol 1989;66:669–674.
30. Sanders JS, Mark AL, Ferguson DW. Evidence for cholinergically mediated vasodilation at the beginning of isometric exercise in humans. Circulation 1989;79:815–824.
31. Doba N, Reis DJ. Role of central and peripheral adrenergic mechanisms in neurogenic hypertension produced by brainstem lesions in rat. Circ Res 1974;34:293–301.
32. Sved AF, Imaizumi T, Talman WT, Reis DJ. Vasopressin contributes to hypertension caused by nucleus tractus solitarius lesions. Hypertension 1985;7:262–267.
33. Reis DJ, Doba N. Hypertension as a localizing sign of mass lesions of brainstem. N Engl J Med 1972;287:1355–1356.
34. Hsu CY, Hogan EL, Wingfield W, et al. Orthostatic hypotension with brain stem tumors. Neurology 1984;34:1137–1143.
35. Aminoff MJ, Wilcox CS: Autonomic dysfunction in syringomyelia. Postgrad Med J 1972;48:113–115.
36. Mathias CJ, Frankel HL. Cardiovascular control in spinal man. Annu Rev Physiol 1988;50:577–592.
37. Plum F. Neurological integration of behavioural and metabolic control of breathing. In: Porter R, ed. Breathing: Hering-Breuer centenary symposium. London: Churchill, 1970:159–175.
38. Kaada BR. Somato-motor, autonomic and electrocorticographic responses to electrical stimulation of "rhinencephalic" and other structures in primates, cat and dog. Acta Physiol Scand 1951; 24(suppl):83.
39. Levin BE, Margolis G. Acute failure of automatic respirations secondary to a unilateral brainstem infarct. Ann Neurol 1977;1: 583–586.
40. Adelman S, Dinner DS, Goren H, Little J, Nickerson P. Obstructive sleep apnea in association with posterior fossa neurologic disease. Arch Neurol 1984;41:509–510.
41. Haponik EF, Givens D, Angelo J. Syringobulbia-myelia with obstructive sleep apnea. Neurology 1983;33:1046–1049.
42. Tranmer BI, Tucker WS, Bilbao JM. Sleep apnea following percutaneous cervical cordotomy. Can J Neurol Sci 1987;14:262–267.
43. Andrew J, Nathan PW. Lesions of the anterior frontal lobes and disturbances of micturition and defaecation. Brain 1964;87: 233–262.
44. Maurice-Williams RS. Micturition symptoms in frontal tumours. J Neurol Neurosurg Psychiatry 1974;37:431–436.
45. Murnaghan GF. Neurogenic disorders of the bladder in parkinsonism. Br J Urol 1961;33:403–409.
46. Holstege G, Tan J. Supraspinal control of motoneurons innervating the striated muscles of the pelvic floor including urethral and anal sphincters in the cat. Brain 1987;110:1323–1344.
47. Swash M, Mathers S. Sphincter disorders and the nervous system. In: Aminoff MJ, ed. Neurology and general medicine. New York: Churchill Livingstone, 1989:449–470.
48. Wood JD. Enteric neurophysiology. Am J Physiol 1984;247:G585–G598.
49. Furness JB, Bornstein JC, Smith TK. The normal structure of gastrointestinal innervation. J Gastroenterol Hepatol 1990;1:1–9.
50. Kupsky WJ, Grimes MM, Sweeting J, Bertsch R, Cote LJ. Parkinson's disease and megacolon: concentric hyaline inclusions (Lewy bodies) in enteric ganglion cells. Neurology 1987;37:1253–1255.
51. Steward JD. Autonomic regulation of sexual function. In: Low PA, ed. Clinical autonomic disorders. Boston: Little, Brown & Co, 1993: 117–123.
52. Klüver H, Bucy PC. "Psychic blindness" and other symptoms following bilateral temporal lobectomy in Rhesus monkeys. Am J Physiol 1937;119:352–353.
53. Terzian H, Ore GD. Syndrome of Klüver and Bucy reproduced in man by bilateral removal of the temporal lobes. Neurology 1955;5: 373–380.

54. Lilly R, Cummings JL, Benson DF, Frankel M. The human Klüver-Bucy syndrome. Neurology 1983;33:1141–1145.

55. Gautier-Smith PC. Sexual dysfunction and the nervous system. In: Aminoff MJ, ed. Neurology and general medicine. New York: Churchill Livingstone, 1989:471–486.

56. Low PA, Fealey RD, Sheps SG, Su WPD, Trautmann JC, Kuntz NL. Chronic idiopathic anhidrosis. Ann Neurol 1985;18:344–348.

57. Vita G, Princi P, Calabro R, Toscano A, Manna L, Messina C. Cardiovascular reflex tests: assessment of age-adjusted normal range. J Neurol Sci 1986;75:263–274.

58. Watkins PJ, MacKay JD. Cardiac denervation in diabetic neuropathy. Ann Intern Med 1980;92(part 2):304–307.

59. Ewing DJ, Campbell IW, Clarke BF. Assessment of cardiovascular effects in diabetic autonomic neuropathy and prognostic implications. Ann Intern Med 1980;92(part 2):308–311.

60. Low PA. Laboratory evaluation of autonomic failure. In: Low PA, ed. Clinical autonomic disorders. Boston: Little, Brown & Co, 1993: 169–195.

61. Ewing DJ, Campbell IW, Burt AA, Clarke BF. Vascular reflexes in diabetic autonomic neuropathy. Lancet 1973;2:1354–1356.

62. Aminoff MJ. Involvement of peripheral vasomotor fibres in carpal tunnel syndrome. J Neurol Neurosurg Psychiatry 1979;42: 649–655.

63. Aminoff MJ. Peripheral sympathetic function in patients with a polyneuropathy. J Neurol Sci 1980;44:213–219.

64. Low PA, Caskey PE, Tuck RR, Fealey RD, Dyck PJ. Quantitative sudomotor axon reflex test in normal and neuropathic subjects. Ann Neurol 1983;14:573–580.

65. Shahani BT, Halperin JJ, Boulu P, Cohen J. Sympathetic skin response—a method of assessing unmyelinated axon dysfunction in peripheral neuropathies. J Neurol Neurosurg Psychiatry 1984;47: 536–542.

66. Polinsky RJ. Multiple system atrophy: clinical aspects, pathophysiology, and treatment. Neurol Clin 1984;2:487–498.

67. Lubowski DZ, Nicholls RJ, Swash M, Jordan MJ. Neural control of internal anal sphincter function. Br J Surg 1987;74:668–670.

68. Chiappa KH, Young RR. A case of paracarcinomatous pandysautonomia. Neurology 1973;23:423.

69. Young RR, Asbury AK, Corbett JL, Adams RD. Pure pandysautonomia with recovery. Description and discussion of diagnostic criteria. Brain 1975;98:613–636.

70. Low PA, Dyck PJ, Lambert EH, et al. Acute panautonomic neuropathy. Ann Neurol 1983;13:412–417.

71. Hopkins A, Neville B, Bannister R. Autonomic neuropathy of acute onset. Lancet 1974;1:769–771.

72. Birchfield RI, Shaw CM. Postural hypotension in the Guillain-Barré syndrome. Arch Neurol 1964;10:149–157.

73. Lichtenfeld P. Autonomic dysfunction in the Guillain-Barré syndrome. Am J Med 1971;50:772–780.

74. Tuck RR, McLeod JG. Autonomic dysfunction in Guillain-Barré syndrome. J Neurol Neurosurg Psychiatry 1981;44:983–990.

75. Khurana RK, Koski CL, Mayer RF. Autonomic dysfunction in Lambert-Eaton myasthenic syndrome. J Neurol Sci 1988;85: 77–86.

76. Clarke BF, Ewing DJ, Campbell IW. Diabetic autonomic neuropathy. Diabetologia 1979;17:195–212.

77. Ewing DJ, Campbell IW, Clarke BF. The natural history of diabetic autonomic neuropathy. Q J Med 1980;49:95–108.

78. Naik RB, Mathias CJ, Wilson CA, Reid JL, Warren DJ. Cardiovascular and autonomic reflexes in haemodialysis patients. Clin Sci 1981;60:165–170.

79. Kyriakidis MK, Noutsis CG, Robinson-Kyriakidis CA, et al. Autonomic neuropathy in leprosy. Int J Lepr 1983;51:331–335.

80. McCombe PA, McLeod JG. The peripheral neuropathy of vitamin B$_{12}$ deficiency. J Neurol Sci 1984;66:117–126.

81. McLeod JG. Autonomic dysfunction in peripheral nerve disease. J Clin Neurophysiol 1993;10:51–60.

82. Manco JC, Gallo L Jr, Godoy RA, Fernandes RG, Amorim DS. Degeneration of the cardiac nerves in Chagas' disease. Further studies. Circulation 1969;40:879–885.

83. Gallo L Jr, Marin Neto JA, Manço JC, Rassi A, Amorim DS. Abnormal heart rate responses during exercise in patients with Chagas' disease. Cardiology 1975;60:147–162.

84. Sousa ACS, Marin Neto JA, Maciel BC, Gallo L, Amorim DS. Cardiac parasympathetic impairment in gastrointestinal Chagas' disease (letter). Lancet 1987;1:985.

85. Iosa D, DeQuattro V, Lee DD-P, Elkayam U, Palmero H. Plasma norepinephrine in Chagas' cardioneuromyopathy: a marker of progressive dysautonomia. Am Heart J 1989;117:882–887.

86. Kyle RA, Greipp PR. Amyloidosis: clinical and laboratory features in 229 cases. Mayo Clin Proc 1983;58:665–683.

87. Kyle RA, Kottke BA, Schirger A. Orthostatic hypotension as a clue to primary systemic amyloidosis. Circulation 1966;34:883–888.

88. Dyck PJ. Neuronal atrophy and degeneration predominantly affecting peripheral sensory and autonomic neurons. In: Dyck PJ, Thomas PK, Griffin JW, Low PA, Poduslo JF, eds. Peripheral neuropathy, 3rd ed. Philadelphia: WB Saunders, 1993:1065–1093.

89. Bird TD, Reenan AM, Pfeifer M. Autonomic nervous system function in genetic neuromuscular disorders. Arch Neurol 1984;41:43–46.

90. Brooks AP. Abnormal vascular reflexes in Charcot-Marie-Tooth disease. J Neurol Neurosurg Psychiatry 1980;43:348–350.

91. Biaggioni I, Goldstein DS, Atkinson T, Robertson D. Dopamine-β-hydroxylase deficiency in humans. Neurology 1990;40:370–373.

92. Devinsky O, Price BH, Cohen SI. Cardiac manifestations of complex partial seizures. Am J Med 1986;80:195–202.

93. Green JB. Pilomotor seizures. Neurology 1984;34:837–839.

94. Kramer RE, Lüders H, Goldstick LP, et al. Ictus emeticus: an electroclinical analysis. Neurology 1988;38:1048–1052.

95. LeWitt PA, Newman RP, Greenberg HS, Rocher LL, Calne DB, Ehrenkranz JRL. Episodic hyperhidrosis, hypothermia, and agenesis of corpus callosum. Neurology 1983;33:1122–1129.

96. LeWitt P. Hyperhidrosis and hypothermia responsive to oxybutynin. Neurology 1988;38:506–507.

97. Erickson TC. Neurogenic hyperthermia. (A clinical syndrome and its treatment.) Brain 1939;62:172–190.

98. Stone WM, de Toledo J, Romanul FCA. Horner's syndrome due to hypothalamic infarction. Arch Neurol 1985;43:199–200.

99. Schwartz WJ, Busis NA, Hedley-Whyte ET. A discrete lesion of ventral hypothalamus and optic chiasm that disturbed the daily temperature rhythm. J Neurol 1986;233:1–4.

100. Aminoff MJ, Wilcox CS. Assessment of autonomic function in patients with a parkinsonian syndrome. Br Med J 1971;4:80–84.

101. Aminoff MJ. Other extrapyramidal disorders. In: Low PA, ed. Clinical autonomic disorders. Boston: Little, Brown & Co, 1993: 527–535.

102. Gross M, Bannister R, Godwin-Austen R. Orthostatic hypotension in Parkinson's disease. Lancet 1972;1:174–176.

103. Sandroni P, Ahlskog JE, Fealey RD, Low PA. Autonomic involvement in extrapyramidal and cerebellar disorders. Clin Auton Res 1991;1:147–155.

104. Gutrecht JA. Autonomic cardiovascular reflexes in progressive supranuclear palsy. J Auton Nerv Syst 1992;39:29–36.

105. Aminoff MJ, Gross M. Vasoregulatory activity in patients with Huntington's chorea. J Neurol Sci 1974;21:33–38.

106. Manetto V, Medori R, Cortelli P, et al. Fatal familial insomnia: clinical and pathologic study of five new cases. Neurology 1992;42: 312–319.

107. Thomas JE, Schirger A, Love JG, Hoffman DL. Orthostatic hypotension as the presenting sign in craniopharyngioma. Neurology 1961;11:418–423.

108. Birchfield RI. Postural hypotension in Wernicke's disease. Am J Med 1964;36:404–414.

109. Cravioto H, Korein J, Silberman J. Wernicke's encephalopathy. Arch Neurol 1961;4:510–519.

110. Shy GM, Drager GA. A neurological syndrome associated with orthostatic hypotension. Arch Neurol 1960;3:511–527.

111. Oppenheimer D. Neuropathology and neurochemistry of autonomic failure. In: Bannister R, ed. Autonomic failure. 2nd ed. Oxford: Oxford University Press, 1988:451–463.

112. Johnson RH, Smith AC, Spalding JMK, Wollner L. Effect of posture on blood-pressure in elderly patients. Lancet 1965;1:731–733.

113. Aminoff MJ. Postural hypotension. In: Aminoff MJ, ed. Neurology and general medicine. New York: Churchill Livingstone, 1989: 123–143.

114. Lipsitz LA. Syncope in the elderly. Ann Intern Med 1983;99: 92–105.

115. McLeod JG, Tuck RR. Disorders of the autonomic nervous system. Part 2: investigation and treatment. Ann Neurol 1987;21: 519–529.

116. Low PA, ed. Clinical autonomic disorders. Boston: Little, Brown & Co, 1993.

7

Functional Neuroanatomy of the Limbic System and Prefrontal Cortex

Gary W. Van Hoesen, Robert J. Morecraft, and Katerina Semendeferi

The limbic system concept was coined by MacLean (1) near the midpoint of this century to reintroduce and reemphasize the seminal thinking of Papez (2) on the neuroanatomical correlates of emotion and to integrate his deductions with advances from both the clinic and the laboratory. This led to a larger "circuit for emotion" in neuroanatomical terms and a somewhat more multifaceted one in functional terms. A scant 5 years later, memory function was added to the functional correlates (3) because acquiring new information and learning rely critically on an intact Papez's circuit. MacLean's efforts, along with Brodal's influential review (4) a few years earlier, laid to rest the "small brain" or rhinencephalon concept of limbic lobe function, relegating olfactory sensation to its appropriate place as only one of several sensory inputs to the limbic system.

Although slightly obscured by anatomical detail, the backbone of Papez's circuit deals with the rather simple anatomical notion of how the cerebral cortex (and, by definition all sensory systems) influences the hypothalamus (the building up of the "emotive process") and how the latter influences the cerebral cortex ("psychic coloring"). He was successful in elaborating one facet of these relationships, but the full panorama was not appreciated until the past four decades with the advent of newer experimental neuroanatomical methodology and a major effort by neuroanatomists. These have led to an expanded conception of the limbic system both in neuroanatomical and functional terms. Although confusing because the term "system" implies unity of function, the core of the concept is the limbic system as the mediator of two-way communication between the cerebral cortex and the external world, and the hypothalamus and the internal world of the organism. Behavior in general, whether it be the consequence of autonomic, endocrine, or somatic effects, is governed by this interplay of the external and internal worlds. Thus, a multifunctional limbic system should be expected (5).

The term prefrontal cortex is attributed to Sir Richard Owen (6). It refers to that cortex anterior to the electrically excitable motor cortex. This is a large area of cortex in the human and nonhuman primate brain and includes a large dorsolateral sector, orbital sector, and medial sector. The latter typically includes the anterior cortices of the cingulate gyrus, which wrap around the genu of the corpus callosum and follow its rostrum ventrally and posteriorly.

There have been many conceptualizations of prefrontal cortical function, ranging from the most lofty domains of behavior to those dealing with more fundamental matters such as emotion, motivation, social behavior, and inhibition. Recent studies have linked it to working memory (7) and decision making (8). The former refers to the ordering of behavior, or the manner in which time is bridged neurally to enable completion of a sequence of intended acts or tasks. The latter function, decision-making behavior, complements working memory in critical ways and involves an assessment of somatic markers (9) that impart reason and reality to choices of behavior. Some patients with frontal lobe damage have preserved intellect, analytical abilities, social consciousness, and sensory awareness, but lack the ability to make accurate predictions about the outcome of decisions on their own well-being. The apparent overlap between functional correlates of the prefrontal cortices and limbic system is of great interest and a matter of active inquiry in neuropsychiatric research (10).

Our goal in this chapter is to examine recent neuroanatomical findings regarding the major parts of the limbic system and the prefrontal cortices and new concepts that emerge from them. We close with a consideration of degenerative diseases that affect these parts of the brain, evolutionary issues, and the implications that these and functional neuroanatomy have for neuropsychiatric disorders.

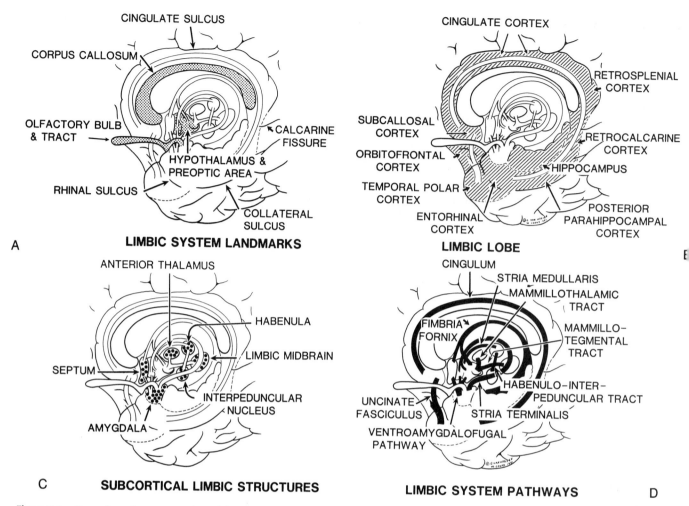

Figure 7.1. Four schematic representations of the medial surface of the cerebral hemisphere depicting the anatomical components of the limbic system. **A,** The relevant landmarks. **B,** The limbic lobe or cortical components. **C,** Subcortical limbic structures (the nucleus basalis of Meynert and the diagonal bands of Broca, both of which contain cholinergic neurons, are not shown). **D,** Interconnecting limbic system pathways. From Damasio and Van Hoesen, 1983, Guilford Press, with permission.

LIMBIC SYSTEM

Anatomical structures included under the term limbic system have diverse locations in the cerebral hemisphere and occupy parts of the telencephalon, diencephalon, and mesencephalon. In general, they are the so-called "conservative" parts of the brain—those found in a wide range of mammals and to some extent vertebrates in general. The cortical parts comprise what are frequently termed the "older" parts of the cerebral cortex, those parts of the cerebral cortex common to many species that form the edge or "limbus" of the cerebral cortex (11). Care has to be taken in the use of terms such as "older" and "conservative". They are best reserved for discussions relating to phylogeny, since, limbic system structures have evolved like all other parts of the cerebral hemisphere, and have assumed functional roles specific to the adaptations of a given species. Although a general core of behaviors may unite diverse species, species-specific functions may be more impressive. However, these may be mediated neurally by structures that resemble each other across species.

A useful way of dealing with the complex anatomy of the limbic system is shown in Figures 7.1, which divides the term into four conceptual units: landmarks, cortical components, subcortical structures, and interconnecting pathways. The cortical structures of the limbic system are well demarcated on the medial surface of the hemisphere by the cingulate sulcus dorsally and the collateral sulcus ventrally (Fig. 7.1A). Bridging areas such as the subcallosal gyrus, the posterior orbital, anterior insular, temporal polar, and perirhinal cortices connect the cingulate and parahippocampal gyri rostrally, while the retrosplenial and retrocalcarine cortices provide a bridge caudally. Altogether, they form the classic "limbus" in the sense of Broca's original intent (Fig. 7.1B). The areas differ widely in cytoarchitecture and include Brodmann's areas 23–29, 35, 36, and 38. None is a true isocortical area. Rather, they fall under the categories of periallocortex and proisocortex of Sanides's terminology, or when combined, the mesocortices of Filimonoff, which are intermediate in structure between the allocortices and the isocortices (5).

The subcortical structures included in the limbic system

(Fig. 7.1C) vary widely among authors and are scattered throughout many parts of the hemisphere. However, it seems appropriate to include the amygdala, septum, nucleus basalis of Meynert, anterior thalamus, habenula complex, interpeduncular nucleus, and some additional limbic mid-brain areas. A structural criterion common to this list relates to the fact that all are connected among themselves as well as with the hypothalamus. Additionally, as noted later, many of these nuclei receive direct cortical projections from one or more parts of the limbic lobe.

The final units of the limbic system are the interconnecting pathways (Fig. 7.1D), those within the limbic lobe, those that connect limbic lobe areas with subcortical limbic structures, those that connect subcortical limbic structures to each other, and lastly, those that connect elements of the limbic system to the hypothalamus. These include such pathways as the cingulum, uncinate fasciculus, fimbria-fornix, stria terminalis, ventroamygdalofugal pathway, mam-millothalamic tract, mammillotegmental tract, stria med-ullaris, and habenulointerpeduncular pathway.

All aspects of this extensive topic of neuroanatomy are not reviewed here. Instead, we deal with it selectively, with an emphasis on new concepts and on the relationship of the limbic system to the frontal lobe.

Cingulate Gyrus

The cingulate gyrus is the major dorsal part of the limbic lobe on the medial wall of the cerebral hemisphere, and forms the upper half of the cortical ring of gray matter (Fig. 7.2). Its main portion is located dorsal to the corpus callosum and callosal sulcus and ventral to the cingulate sulcus, although it extends into the depths of the latter. Its anterior part coincides with Brodmann's area 24 and its posterior part with area 23 (12–14). The cingulate gyrus continues anteriorly and arches ventrally, around the genu of

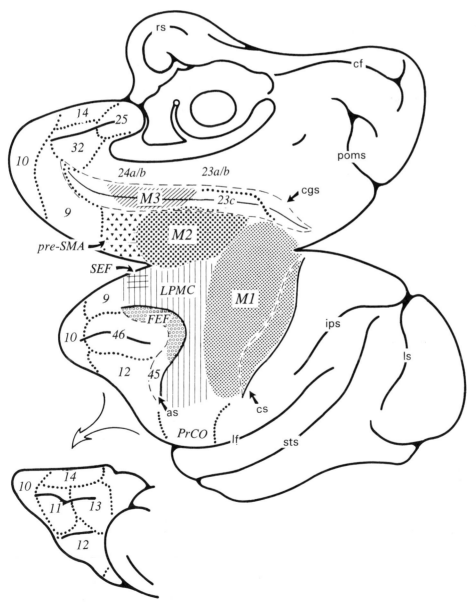

Figure 7.2. Medial, lateral, and orbital views of the rhesus monkey cerebral hemisphere depicting the functional parts of the frontal lobe, Brodmann and Walker's cytoarchitectural fields, and the cingulate gyrus. Note the three motor representations, M1, M2, and M3, the lateral premotor cortex (LPMC) and the frontal and supplementary eye fields (FEF and SEF). M1 is synonymous with the term primary motor cortex and Brodmann's area 4. M2 is synonymous with the supplementary motor cortex and medial area 6. It, along with the LPMC, corresponds to Brodmann's lateral area 6. The supplementary motor cortex is separated from prefrontal area 9 by a presupplementary motor cortex (pre-SMA). M3 is synonymous with the cingulate motor area and lies in the fundus and lower bank of cingulate sulcus. It corresponds to Brodmann's area 24 and particularly area 24c. Area 23c is also thought to be a component of the cingulate motor area. All other (unhatched) fields correspond to prefrontal association areas or to anterior and medial parts of the limbic lobe adjacent to or within the frontal lobe. (Abbreviations: *as* = arcuate sulcus; *cf* = calcarine fissure; *cgs* = cingulate sulcus; *cs* = central sulcus; *ips* = intra-parietal sulcus; *lf* = lateral fissure; *ls* = lunate sulcus; *poms* = parieto-occipital medial sulcus; *rs* = rhinal sulcus.)

Figure 7.3. The somatic topography of the primary and supplementary motor cortices is shown on a partial flattened view of the monkey hemisphere. The opposing convex lines in the center of the illustration represent the true dorsal convexity of the superior frontal lobule such that the lateral surface extends inverted toward the top of the page, and the medial surface of the hemisphere extends upright toward the bottom of the page. The projections of cingulate motor areas 24c or M3 and 23c with the somatic topography of the supplementary and primary motor cortices are shown. Note that the face area (FA) forelimb (FL) and hindlimb (HL) of 24c or M3 projects the appropriate representations of the other motor maps. Area 23c seems to lack a face representation, but forelimb (FL) and hindlimb (HL) parts are in register. Both areas 24c and 23c contribute to the corticospinal projection (Abbreviations: *cgs* = cingulate sulcus, *ilas* = inferior limb of arcuate sulcus, *ps* = principal sulcus).

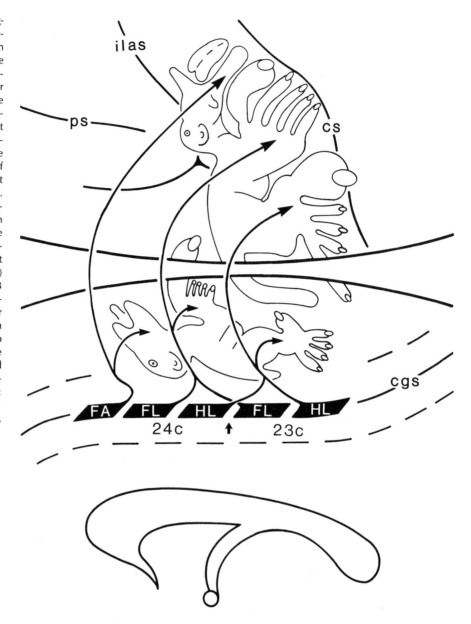

the corpus callosum. This ventral extension forms area 25. Posteriorly, the cingulate gyrus arches ventrally, around the splenium of the corpus callosum. Most of this ventral extension is designated as area 23 except for cortex buried in the callosal sulcus, which is referred to as retrosplenial cortex (areas 29 and 30). The most ventral part of this posterior continuation is called the isthmus of the cingulate gyrus and ends at the level of the calcarine sulcus. Buried within the gyrus is a prominent interconnecting white matter pathway known as the cingulum bundle. The cingulum bundle follows the curvature of the cingulate gyrus, and some of its axons form the longest corticocortical association connections in the cerebral hemisphere. Along its length, axons enter and exit to interconnect the cingulate cortex with a multiple cortical and subcortical targets, including the basal ganglia and thalamus.

The various subsectors of the cingulate cortex, and in particular, areas 24 and 23, are coupled anatomically by a vast and organized set of intracingulate connections (15–17). The cingulate gyrus also is connected to the frontal lobe, parietal lobe, occipital lobe, temporal lobe, other parts of the limbic lobe, as well as to the insula (15, 18, 19–30). In general, both the anterior and posterior divisions of the cingulate gyrus are connected with the prefrontal, orbitofrontal, posterior parietal, posterior parahippocampal, perirhinal, entorhinal and lateral temporal cortices as well as the presubicular and subicular/CA1 parts of the hippocampal formation. Topographic differences in these connections occur. For instance, more anterior levels of the orbitofrontal cortex are linked primarily to area 23, while more posterior levels are linked to area 24. The superior and inferior parietal lobules are both connected with area 23, while the parietal connection with area 24 is less strong and involves primarily the inferior parietal lobule. With respect to the parahippocampal region, medial levels are linked primarily to area 24, whereas lateral levels are linked to area 23.

Other connections are known to target only the anterior cingulate region, which underscores the cytoarchitectural distinction of this more anterior "agranular" part of the cingulate gyrus (areas 24, 25, and 32) from the more posterior "granular" part of the cingulate gyrus (area 23). For example, frontal area 32, temporal polar area 38, and the amygdala are connected with only the anterior cingulate gyrus. This unique set of projections would suggest that neural events taking place in the anterior cingulate gyrus are different in part, from those occurring posteriorly. However, because area 24 and 23 are strongly interconnected, it is likely that projections to the anterior cingulate gyrus influence the posterior cingulate gyrus.

Like the different patterns of connectivity that distinguish the anterior from posterior parts of the cingulate gyrus, the dorsal part of the cingulate gyrus (subdivision c) differs on a connectional basis from the more ventral parts of the cingulate gyrus (subdivisions a and b). For example, input from the prefrontal and limbic cortices more heavily target cingulate cortex located on the surface of the gyrus (areas 24a, 24b, 23a, and 23b) than cingulate cortex lining the lower bank of the cingulate sulcus (areas 24c and 23c). The subicular/CA1 sector of the hippocampal formation projects only to the more ventrally located cingulate areas (areas 24a,

23a, and 25). Areas 24c and 23c, which form the dorsal part of the cingulate gyrus, are located in the depths of the cingulate sulcus and are the only parts of the cingulate gyrus connected with the primary motor cortex (M1) (Fig. 7.3). Similarly, areas 24c and 23c are strongly interconnected with the supplementary motor cortex (M2), while fewer cells in area 24b project to M2. Area 24C is the only part of the cingulate gyrus connected with the ventral part of the lateral premotor cortex and area prostriata of the retrocalcarine region. Likewise, area 23c appears to be the only part of the cingulate gyrus connected with the adjacent primary somatosensory cortex (areas 1 and 2).

Based on the anatomical observations just summarized, several conclusions can be drawn. First, the vast network of intracingulate connections, and in particular, those linking area 24 with area 23, provide multifaceted avenues for information exchange between anterior and posterior parts of the cingulate gyrus. Second, widespread parts of the cingulate gyrus are linked to multimodal and limbic cortices. Multimodal sources would include prefrontal, rostral orbitofrontal, posterior parietal, and lateral temporal cortices. Limbic sources include posterior orbitofrontal, temporopolar, posterior parahippocampal, perirhinal, and entorhinal cortices (Fig. 7.4). Thus, highly processed and abstract

Convergence of Limbic Inputs to Area 24c

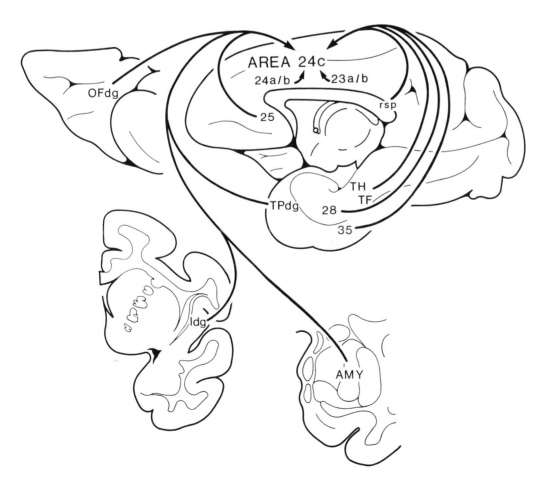

Figure 7.4. Schematic representation of the convergence of limbic system inputs to area 24c or M3. Note the extensive input from other parts of the limbic lobe as well as the amygdala (AMY) (Other abbreviations: *Idg* = insular dysgranular cortex; *Ofdg* = orbitofrontal dysgranular cortex; *rsp* = retrosplenial cortex; and *Tpdg* = temporopolar dysgranular cortex).

information from neocortical association areas, and perhaps, emotionally and motivationally relevant information from limbic sources, can influence a wide variety of cingulate subsectors. Third, cingulocortical connections appear to be made throughout much of the cingulate gyrus. Direct motor cortex interactions appear to occur through cingulate cortex lining the depths of the cingulate sulcus (areas 24c and 23c), and direct somatosensory cortex interactions occur through area 23c.

SUMMARY AND FUNCTIONAL CONSIDERATIONS

Although the cingulate gyrus does not contain areas that specifically subserve a primary modality, selected parts of it may be involved in regulating the fundamental outcome of specific complex behaviors. For example, lesions of the posterior cingulate gyrus alter an animal's ability to navigate appropriately in its environment despite receiving extended training to accomplish a learned task (31). Therefore, posterior cingulate cortex may be an essential component of spatially-guided orientation.

Available data suggest that the anterior cingulate gyrus may be implicated in the expression of affectively-triggered movements related to painful stimuli (32). For example, units here respond selectively to a variety of noxious stimuli. In line with this observation, it has been demonstrated that the anterior cingulate cortex may mediate vocal expressions that reflect the internal state of the animal. For example, stimulation of the anterior cingulate gyrus evokes simple vocalizations, whereas lesions placed rostral to the peri-aqueductal gray matter, which apparently disrupt the cin-guloperiaqueductal projection, abolish the response. It is well known that the periaqueductal gray matter has a role in brainstem pain mechanisms and vocalization.

The anterior cingulate cortex has been implicated in the production of other forms of vocal expression that are linked to emotional expression. The separation cry, produced by primates for maintaining contact with a distant group of individuals, and induced by separating a mother from her offspring, is adversely affected following ablation of the anterior subcallosal region of the cingulate gyrus (33). A different form of emotion-related vocalization, namely that of laughter, may also be mediated by the anterior cingulate gyrus (34). Based upon observations of patients with epileptic seizures, Arroyo and colleagues suggested that the anterior cingulate gyrus is involved in generating the motor act of laughter and basal temporal cortex with the development of laughter's emotional content. It seems that regardless of the emotional phenomena expressed, the anterior cingulate gyrus plays an important role in developing the associated motor response. It would also appear from the common engagement of the head and neck region in these responses, that brainstem centers mediating the operation of structures such as the larynx, tongue, and muscles of facial expression, are heavily influenced by ongoing activity in the anterior cingulate gyrus.

The anterior cingulate gyrus may also regulate autonomic responses because its stimulation evokes pupillary dilation, piloerection, altered heart rate, and changes in blood pressure (35–38). Specifically, these are elicited from the cortex located below the genu of the corpus callosum, or Brodmann's area 25. These physiological findings, coupled with the underlying neuroanatomical circuitry described for this part of the cingulate gyrus, has led to the suggestion that this part of the cingulate gyrus serves as a "visceral motor cortex" (39).

In addition to autonomic responses, electrical stimulation of the anterior cingulate gyrus in humans (40) and nonhuman primates (35, 36) also gives rise to complex forms of somatic movement. Although surface stimulation studies conducted over 50 years ago had noted the potential influence of the primate cingulate gyrus on somatomotor mechanisms, more recent physiological (41–43) and anatomical (13, 18, 27, 28, 44–46) studies have been able to pinpoint a cingulate motor region and identify within this region an organized somatotopy (Fig. 7.3). The cingulate motor cortex lies in the depths of the cingulate sulcus and corresponds cytoarchitectonically to areas 24c and 23c. In area 24c of the monkey, the face representation is anterior to the forelimb representation, which in turn, is anterior to the hindlimb representation. Utilizing neuroimaging techniques, Paus and colleagues have demonstrated that the somatotopic organization in the human anterior cingulate cortex is consistent with the reported somatotopy in the monkey anterior cingulate cortex (47). Their observations also indicated that the anterior cingulate gyrus mediates the execution of appropriate motor responses and suppresses inappropriate ones. Based upon the suggestive physiological and anatomical data collected in nonhuman primates, as well as the suggestion that area 24 may be the developmental progenitor of the isocortical motor fields M1 and M2 (48), area 24c may be conceptualized as an M3 in the scheme of cortical motor representation (28) (Fig. 7.5). Like the more traditional isocortical motor areas (M1 and M2), modern tract tracing techniques employed in monkeys show that M3 and area 23c give rise to a host of projections that target various motor centers positioned at all parts of the neuraxis. For example, M3 and area 23c give rise to somatotopically organized projections that target the primary and supplementary motor cortices (Fig. 7.3). Therefore, M1, M2, M3, and area 23c are highly interconnected at the cortical level. From a subcortical standpoint, the same motor centers targeted by M1 and M2 are targeted by M3. For example, area M3 projects heavily to the ventrolateral part of the putamen, medial and dorsal parts of the parvocellular red nucleus, ventromedial part of the pontine nuclei, and the intermediate zone of the cervical enlargement of the spinal cord (17, 27, 44, 49–51). Judging from detailed comparisons of the descending projections arising from M1 and M2, those from M3 target different and similar parts of the basal ganglia, red nucleus, and pontine gray matter, as well as spinal cord (50, 51). Therefore, the highly interconnected motor cortices seem to also be characterized by an overlap in their corticofugal projection zones. As noted before, the

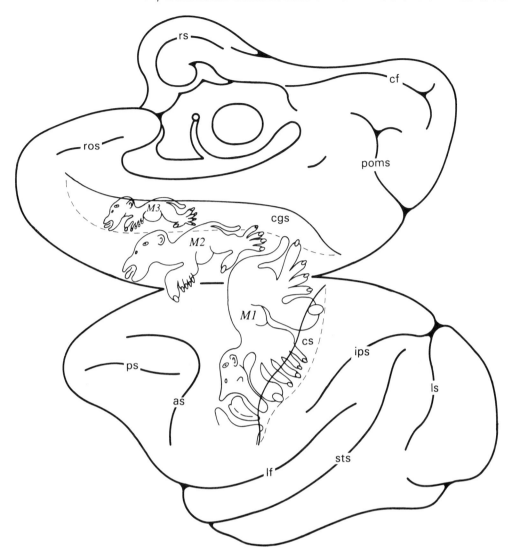

Figure 7.5. Schematic representation of the three motor representations (M1, M2, and M3) found in the agranular cortex of the frontal lobe. As discussed in the text, M3 is the major entry point for both limbic and prefrontal input to motor cortex that gives rise to corticospinal projections (Abbreviations: *as* = arcuate sulcus; *cf* = calcarine fissure; *cgs* = cingulate sulcus; *ips* = intraparietal sulcus; *lf* = lateral fissure; *ls* = lunate sulcus; *poms* = parieto-occipital medial sulcus; *ps* = principal sulcus; *ros* = rostral sulcus; *rs* = rhinal sulcus, *sts* = superior temporal sulcus).

cortical inputs to the cingulate motor cortex are unique when compared with those targeting M2 and M1 in that the cingulate motor cortex receives strong and widespread inputs from the prefrontal cortex and limbic lobes (29, 52–54). From the perspective of motor cortex organization, the powerful and direct input from prefrontal cortex, limbic lobe, and amygdala serve in part, as a distinguishing element of M3.

Hippocampal Formation and Parahippocampal Gyrus

The hippocampal formation is comprised of three allocortical areas: *(a)* the pyramids that form the CA zones of the hippocampus (CA1, CA2, CA3); *(b)* the dentate gyrus, including the CA4 polymorph neurons that are found in its hilum; and *(c)* the various subicular cortices (55–59). The latter includes the subiculum proper, a true allocortical zone,

and two periallocortical zones, the presubiculum and parasubiculum. The latter are multilayered and are associated closely with the hippocampal formation. They have continuity with the subiculum in their deep layers. Because they are multilayered periallocortical areas related to the entorhinal cortex of the parahippocampal gyrus, it is appropriate to include them with this part of the ventromedial temporal lobe. In short, they form the medial boundary of the parahippocampal gyrus, intervening between the entorhinal cortex and the subiculum proper of the hippocampal formation.

Cajal (60, 61) published many seminal observations on the cytoarchitecture, fiberarchitecture, and connections of the hippocampal formation using descriptive methods such as the Golgi technique. His work led to a conceptualization of the hippocampal formation that persisted for many decades. It is only in recent years (56) that these findings have been embellished using newer experimental methods

(Fig. 7.6). The major input to the hippocampal formation was thought to arrive via two conspicuous white-matter pathways, the fimbria-fornix system and what Cajal termed the temporoammonic or perforant pathway. Axons from these were observed to end on the pyramidal cells of the hippocampus and the granule cells of the dentate gyrus. A two-part sequential series of intrinsic connections was also demonstrated. The first part is a large projection from the dentate gyrus granule cells to the proximal part of the apical dendrites of the CA3 pyramidal cells. This system sends no axons outside of the hippocampal formation and is known as the mossy fiber system. The second part is known as the Schaffer collateral system. It arises from the axons of CA3

pyramids and terminates on the basal and apical dendrites of the adjacent CA1 pyramids.

The view that emerged from these studies of hippocampal connectivity held that input would arrive via the fimbria-fornix and perforant pathway and activate the pyramidal neurons directly, or indirectly, via the dentate gyrus and intrinsic pathways. Pyramidal axons entered the alveus and the fimbria-fornix system and conveyed hippocampal output to subcortical structures. There are no errors in this anatomy, and indeed, nearly all aspects of Cajal's careful research observations have been verified. However, both he and his student, Lorente de Nó, failed to fully document an important extension of the intrinsic circuitry of the hippo-

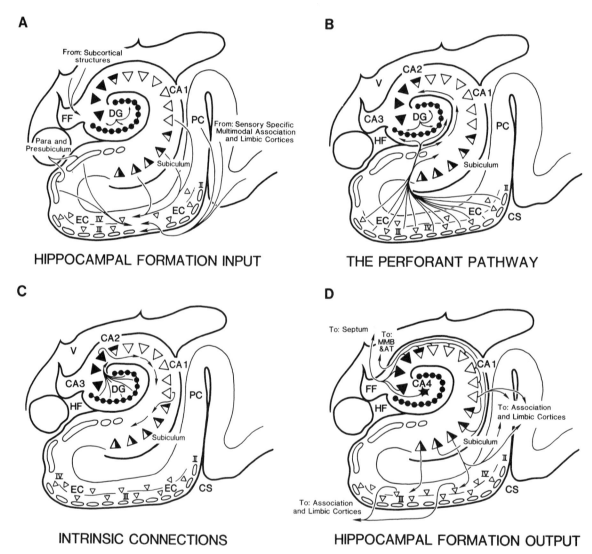

Figure 7.6. Cross-sections of the ventromedial temporal lobe showing the major connection of the entorhinal *(EC)* and perirhinal cortices *(PC)* and the hippocampal formation. **A,** Entorhinal input from neighboring cortical areas, the subiculum, and from the sensory-specific and multimodal association areas and the limbic lobe. Subcortical input directly to the hippocampal formation arrives via the fimbria-fornix *(FF)*. **B,** The origin and course of the major output pathway of the EC, the perforant pathway. Note its strong distribution to the pyramidal neurons of the subiculum, hippocampus *(CA1–CA3)* and dentate gyrus *(DG)*. **C,** The major intrinsic connections of the hippocampal formation. Note in particular the *DG* projections to the CA3 pyramids, CA3 pyramid projections to CA1 pyramids, and CA2 pyramid projections to the subiculum. **D,** The major output projections of the hippocampal formation and the EC. Note that all hippocampal formation pyramidal neurons project to the anterior thalamus (AT) and mamillary bodies (MMB). However, these neurons give rise to output projections to the association and limbic cortices. Direct projection to the deep layers of the EC and their projections to the same areas provide the anatomical basis for a powerful hippocampal influence on other cortical areas. (Other abbreviations: *cs* = collateral sulcus, *hf* = hippocampal fissure, *v* = inferior horn of the lateral ventricle.)

ENTORHINAL CORTICAL
AFFERENT CONNECTIONS

ENTORHINAL CORTICAL
EFFERENT CONNECTIONS

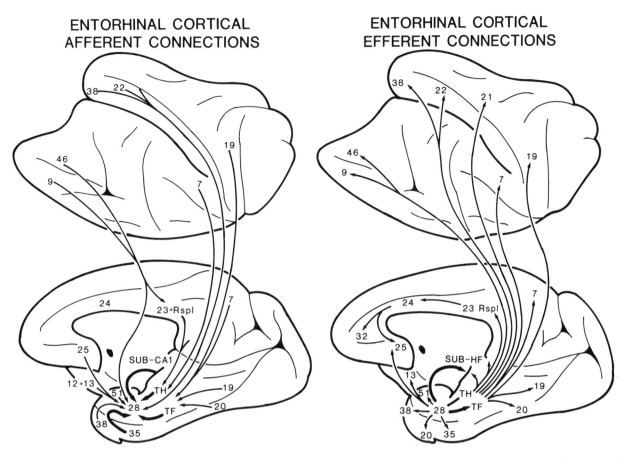

Figure 7.7.   The major afferent or input and efferent or output connections of the entorhinal (Brodmann's area 28) and posterior parahippocampal (area TF and FH) cortices are summarized on lateral (inverted) and medial (upright) views of the rhesus monkey hemisphere. Note the convergence of afferents to this part of ventromedial temporal lobe and the divergence of efferents from it back to the association and limbic cortices. These link the hippocampal formation to the association and limbic cortices in a bi-directional manner.

campal formation, namely, CA1 projections to the adjacent subicular cortices (62, 63). It is now known that the neurons that form the subiculum, and not the hippocampal pyramids per se, are responsible for a large amount of hippocampal formation output and nearly all of its diversity with regard to influencing other brain areas (64–66). For example, the axons of CA3 pyramids project mainly to the septum, although they also give rise to major intrinsic and commissural inter- and intrahippocampal projections. With the exception of commissural projections, this is somewhat true for CA1 pyramidal neurons as well. However, the neurons that form the subicular cortices, and to a lesser extent those of the CA1 zone, have extensive extrinsic projections that divide hippocampal output into major components; one to a variety of cortical areas and another to a variety of subcortical structures such as the basal forebrain, amygdala, thalamus, and hypothalamus (64, 66–68). Thus, hippocampal output is disseminated much more widely than previously thought, and importantly, projects not to only subcortical areas, but to cortical ones as well. The latter are thought to be the neural basis of whether information is stored or remembered (56).

Another feature of hippocampal anatomy not described by early anatomists concerns the issue of afferent input, and,

in particular, the input to the entorhinal cortex. Early investigators saw axons entering the entorhinal cortex, but use of the Golgi method precluded ascertaining their origin. This meant that the input to the major source of afferents to the hippocampal formation was left uncharacterized. It has been shown in recent studies that the entorhinal cortex receives powerful projections from many cortical areas (Figs. 7.7 and 7.8) in the temporal lobe (69–76) and from subcortical structures, such as the amygdala and midline thalamus (77–79). It is important to note that amygdaloid input to the entorhinal cortex is derived from amygdaloid nuclei that receive both limbic cortical input as well as input from association cortices located in both the frontal and temporal lobes (80–84). Additionally, these same nuclei receive direct or indirect hypothalamic (84) and basal forebrain input (85, 86). Thus, input to the entorhinal cortex is extensive. It arises largely from the cortices that form the limbic lobe, the amygdala, and the midline thalamus. In terms of cortex, proisocortical areas such as the perirhinal, posterior parahippocampal, cingulate, temporal polar, and posterior orbitofrontal cortices, and periallocortical areas such as the retrosplenial, presubicular, and parasubicular cortices are the major contributors. These transitional cortical areas, interposed between the allocortex and neocortex, receive major

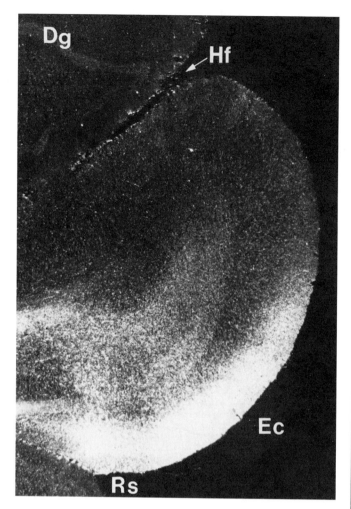

Figure 7.8. A dark-field photomicrograph of the entorhinal cortex *(EC)* in a rhesus monkey experiment where tritiated amino acids were injected into the posterior parahippocampal cortex to label axons and their terminals. White areas indicate the location of terminal labeling. Note the dense band of labeling in the superficial layer of the EC, indicating that the posterior parahippocampal area projects powerfully to the EC. (Other abbreviations: *Dg* = dentate gyrus, *HF* = hippocampal fissure, *Rs* = rhinal sulcus.)

projections from both sensory-specific and multimodal association cortices. Thus, the entorhinal cortices receive a digest or abstract of the sensory output generated by subcortical and cortical areas, that includes both interoceptive and exteroceptive information. Like a censor and archivist, it seems to determine whether this is good for the organism or not, worthy of storage, or to be left to decay.

SUMMARY AND FUNCTIONAL CONSIDERATIONS

The hippocampal formation is the focal point for major forebrain neural systems that are interconnected with the sensory-specific association cortices and the multimodal association cortices. These are widespread systems that involve much of the cortical mantle. As mentioned, the cortices that form the limbic lobe in general, and the amygdala and posterior parahippocampal area in particular, receive input from the various association cortices and either project directly to the hippocampal formation or first to the entorhinal cortex,

which then project to the hippocampal formation. The most compact part of this latter system, the perforant pathway, is the major output system of the entorhinal cortex (Fig. 7.9). It mediates a powerful excitatory input to the hippocampal formation that culminates in extrinsic output to the septum via the fimbria-fornix or intrinsic output to the subicular cortices. These latter areas then project to several basal forebrain areas, including the amygdala, various diencephalic nuclei, and many parts of the limbic lobe and association cortex. Thus, hippocampal output is disseminated widely by the subicular and CA1 pyramids of the hippocampal formation (Figs. 7.7, 7.10, and 7.11).

Amygdaloid Complex

As mentioned previously, several amygdaloid nuclei receive inputs from the cerebral cortex (Fig. 7.12) and from

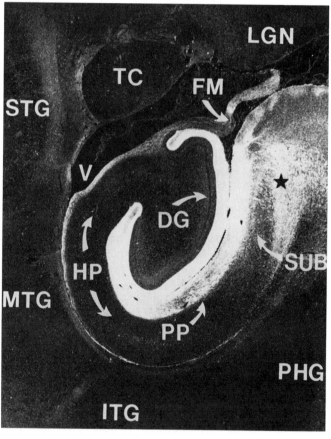

Figure 7.9. A dark-field photomicrograph of the hippocampal formation in a rhesus monkey experiment where tritiated amino acids were injected into the entorhinal cortex to label perforant pathway axons and their terminals. White areas indicate the location of terminal labeling. Note the dense terminal labeling in the subiculum (Sub) CA1, CA3, and dentate gyrus (Dg) molecular layers, indicating a powerful linkage between the entorhinal cortex and hippocampal formation. The perforant pathway is one of the largest projections of the cerebral cortex and the major avenue by which the limbic and association cortices influence the hippocampal formation. (Other abbreviations: *Tc* = tail lf caudate nucleus, *V* = ventricle, *ITG* = inferior temporal gyrus, *MTG* = middle temporal gyrus, *STG* = Superior temporal gyrus, *HP* = Hippocampus, *PHG* = parahippocampal gyrus, *LGN* = Lateral geniculate nucleus, *PP* = perforant pathway.)

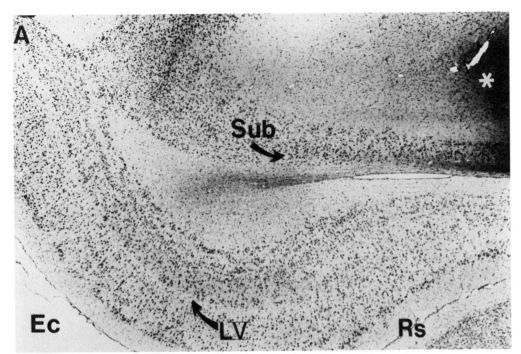

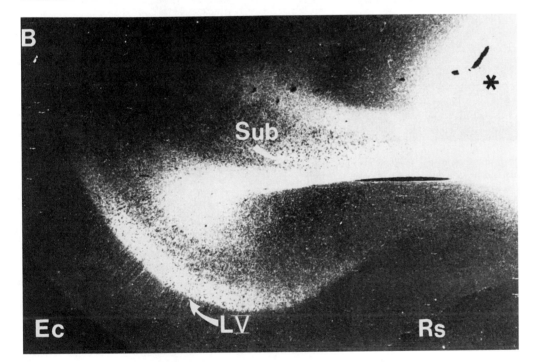

Figure 7.10. A, Nissl-stained bright-field photograph of the anterior subiculum *(Sub)* and the entorhinal cortex *(EC)* in a rhesus monkey. The dark area (marked with an *asterisk*) shows where tritiated amino acids are injected into the subiculum *(Sub)*. B, The same microscopic field shown in A, but with dark-field viewing conditions. Note the dense subicular projection to layer V of the EC. This direct projection from the hippocampal formation to the cortex is one of many cortical projections that arise from the subiculum and CA1 parts of the hippocampal formation. (Other abbreviations: *Lv* = lateral ventricle, *Rs* = rhinal sulcus.)

a host of subcortical structures of both diencephalic and mesencephalic origin. The latter includes such structures as the hypothalamus, periaqueductal gray matter, peripeduncular nucleus, ventral tegmental area, supramammillary nucleus, and midline thalamic nuclei (84, 85, 87).

Unlike the hippocampal formation, whose input is derived largely from limbic lobe areas that receive input from the association cortices, many association areas project directly to the amygdala without relays in the limbic lobe. For example, the visual association cortices of the lateral temporal neocortex send direct projections to the lateral amygdaloid nucleus and to the dorsal part of the laterobasal

amygdaloid nucleus (80–82, 88, 89). Some investigators have shown also that the auditory association cortex of the superior temporal gyrus also projects directly to the lateral amygdaloid nucleus. Input related to somatic sensation also converges on this nucleus from the insular cortex (90).

Although neocortical input from association cortices constitutes a major source of input to the lateral amygdaloid nucleus, it is erroneous to characterize all corticoamygdaloid input as derived from the neocortex. Indeed, the proisocortices, periallocortices, and allocortices make a large contribution (83). For example, the medial half of the lateral nucleus receives input from the insular, temporal polar, and

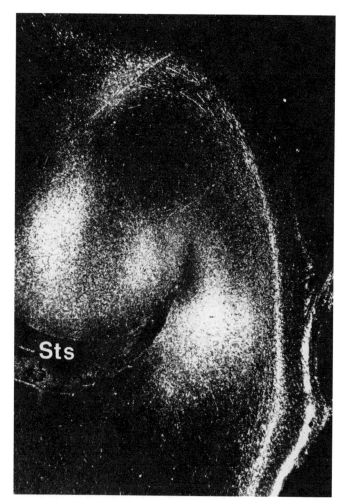

Figure 7.11. A dark-field photomicrograph showing terminal labeling in the depths of the superior temporal sulcus (Sts) in a rhesus monkey experiment where labeled amino acids were injected into the cortex of the posterior parahippocampal gyrus. The latter receives a strong hippocampal output and projects in turn to association areas in all other lobes.

example, it receives input from the lateral temporal isocortex, the temporal polar, orbitofrontal, and insular proisocortex, the entorhinal periallocortex, and the periamygdaloid and primary olfactory allocortex (83). The superficial nuclei of the amygdala, such as the medial nucleus and the various cortical nuclei, receive input largely from allocortical regions, such as the subicular and periamygdaloid cortices and olfactory piriform cortex.

Until quite recently, it was believed that the major input and output relationships of the amygdala were with the hypothalamus. Such connections are strong (84) but the diversity of amygdaloid output is far more extensive than appreciated previously. For example, the lateral nucleus and some components of the basal complex project strongly to the entorhinal cortex (91), to several association areas, and even to the primary visual cortex (92). Additionally, the basal amygdaloid complex has strong reciprocal interconnections with the subiculum, the major source of hippocampal output

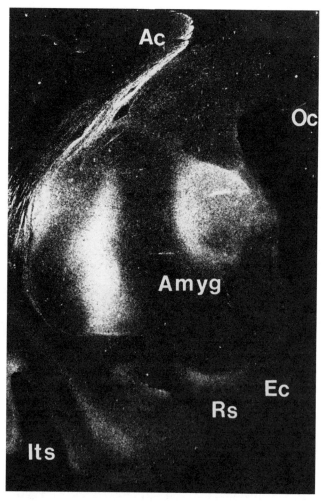

Figure 7.12. A dark-field photomicrograph of the amygdala *(Amyg)* and entorhinal cortex (Ec) showing terminal labeling in a rhesus monkey experiment where labeled amino acids were injected into the cortex of the temporal pole. The amygdaloid terminal labeling is primary over the medial part of the lateral nucleus and over the accessory basal nucleus (other abbreviations: *Ac* = anterior commissure, *Its* = inferior temporal sulcus, *Oc* = optic chiasm, *Rs* = rhinal sulcus).

orbitofrontal cortices, and all parts of the limbic lobe (Fig. 7.12). The basal complex of the amygdala, consisting of the laterobasal, accessory basal, and mediobasal nuclei, receives cortical projections derived almost exclusively from the proisocortices and the periallocortices. The accessory basal nucleus, for example, receives strong projections from the temporal polar cortex, the insular cortex, the medial frontal cortex, and to some extent, the orbitofrontal cortex. The mediobasal nucleus is not well characterized in terms of input, but receives projections from the perirhinal and subicular cortices (66). The laterobasal nucleus receives input from many of the cortical areas just listed, but additionally, is characterized by having input from the anterior cingulate cortex. The subiculum and entorhinal cortices also project to part of the basal amygdaloid complex. These nuclei collectively form the basal complex, the largest mass of the amygdala, and thus, limbic lobe input must be regarded as the major source of cortical input.

The central amygdaloid nucleus is unusual in the sense that it receives input derived from all types of cortex. For

(66, 91, 93, 94). From these studies, it is clear that the amygdala is very much interrelated with the hippocampal formation in anatomical terms and that these two temporal neighbors undoubtedly influence each other to a great degree.

Nonhypothalamic subcortical projections arise from several amygdaloid nuclei and link the structure with many parts of the neuraxis. Of special interest are powerful projections to parts of the basal forebrain, including the nucleus basalis of Meynert (95). Additional nonhypothalamic subcortical projections course to the dorsomedial thalamic nucleus (96–98) and to several autonomic centers in the brainstem (95, 99).

Among the more surprising aspects of amygdaloid anatomy described recently is that this structure has strong projections to many parts of the temporal association, insular, and frontal cortices (90, 94, 96, 97, 100–102). In the frontal lobe, these projections end on parts of the isocortices that form the frontal granular cortex, the frontal agranular cortex, and the cingulate, medial frontal, and posterior orbitofrontal proisocortices. Powerful projections from the basal complex of the amygdala to the neostriatum and ventral striatum also have been described (103).

SUMMARY AND FUNCTIONAL CONSIDERATIONS

From a neural systems viewpoint, the amygdala must be considered from a broader perspective than its classically-described interrelationships with the hypothalamus and olfactory system. For example, the amygdala has powerful direct interconnections with much of the anterior cortex of the limbic lobe and with neocortical areas of the frontal, temporal, and even occipital lobes. Additional smaller projections have been reported to terminate in the premotor cortices and limbic lobe area 24, both of which project directly to the supplementary motor cortex. Moreover, projections to the cingulate motor area, and especially M3, provide a means for it to influence corticospinal axons. Additional projections connect the amygdala with the neostriatum and ventral striatum, involving it in basal ganglia circuitry. Certain amygdaloid nuclei also project strongly to the nucleus basalis of Meynert, whose axons provide a powerful cholinergic input to the cortex. Descending amygdaloid projections from the central amygdaloid nucleus also provide input to autonomic centers in the brainstem. Although much of the input to the amygdala, particularly from subcortical areas, cannot be characterized well in functional terms, this is not the case for amygdaloid output. Overall, it can be concluded that amygdaloid output is directed toward the origin of what may be termed effector systems that influence motor, endocrine, and autonomic areas along the full extent of the neuraxis. Thus, it is very much unlike the hippocampal formation, whose output to such areas is either less strong or more indirect, and instead shifted more toward the association cortices. A persuasive argument could be made that the amygdala more greatly influences overt behavior, while the hippocampus more greatly influences more covert aspects of behavior such as cognition and memory.

Nucleus Basalis of Meynert

The neurons that form the nucleus basalis of Meynert have attracted substantial attention because they project to the cerebral cortex (104–108) and they are affected frequently in Alzheimer's disease (AD) (109). Such projections had been suggested in earlier ablation experiments, but the magnitude of this projection was not appreciated. It is now clear that probably all of the nucleus basalis of Meynert projects to the cortex and all parts of it. These findings are intriguing, but they assume added significance with the demonstration that the majority of these neurons contain cholinergic enzymes, and, in fact, provide the major source of cholinergic input to the cortex (107, 110). Thus, they mirror the cholinergic projections of their counterparts in the diagonal band nuclei and medial septum that project to the allocortices of the hippocampal formation.

The neurons forming the nucleus basalis are large, hyperchromatic, multipolar, and fusiform-shaped cells that lie among the ascending and descending limbic, hypothalamic, and brainstem pathways that course through the basal forebrain. Part of the nucleus is found within the substantia innominata, but cholinergic neurons span the anterior-posterior expanse of the ventral surface of the hemisphere all the way from the septum anteriorly to the midbrain posteriorly. They also have a lateral extension that follows the course of the anterior commissure into the temporal lobe (106, 110). Scattered acetylcholinesterase and choline acetyltransferase-positive neurons are also found within the internal and external medullary lamina of the globus pallidus, in the lateral hypothalamus, and in the dorsal parts of various amygdaloid nuclei. Calling this a "nucleus" somewhat stretches the imagination, although the common cholinergic nature of its neurons somewhat salvages the term.

The output of the nucleus basalis to the cortex has been well characterized in the rat and monkey. These studies reveal that a rigid topography exists with regard to where in the cortical mantle they end (108, 110–112). Additionally, it has been demonstrated recently that the nucleus basalis projects to the basal complex of the amygdala (85, 86). Importantly, it is also known that this nucleus projects to the reticular nucleus of the thalamus (113–116). This places the nucleus basalis in a position to influence the cortex directly as well as indirectly, because the reticular nucleus governs thalamic transmission via intrinsic thalamic connections (117). However, beyond these observations, little else is known about the efferent connections of the nucleus basalis of Meynert, and there remains a fundamental need for further study of this in experimental neuroanatomy. Suggestive evidence was provided in early studies that nucleus basalis axons project at least as far caudally as the midbrain (105).

The input to the nucleus basalis of Meynert is better understood. In terms of cortex, it has been shown that it receives projections from only a small percentage of the cortical areas to which it sends axons (118). These include such areas as the olfactory, orbitofrontal, anterior insular, temporal polar, entorhinal, and medial temporal cortices— all components of the limbic lobe. Subcortical projections to the nucleus basalis arise from the septum, nucleus accumbens, hypothalamus, amygdala, preoptic nucleus, and from the peripeduncular nucleus of the midbrain (106, 119–121).

SUMMARY AND FUNCTIONAL CONSIDERATIONS

With regard to neural systems, it is reasonable to believe that the nucleus basalis of Meynert is a key structure. For example, the widespread projections to the cortex and the fact that acetylcholine serves as the transmitter for these projections are of fundamental importance. These neurons are much like serotonergic neurons in the raphe complex, noradrenergic neurons in the locus ceruleus, and dopaminergic neurons in the ventral tegmental area with similar cortical projections. Like these neurons, many of their projections are not reciprocated by projections from the cortex their axons innervate. The input to nucleus basalis neurons seems topographically organized and rather specific. At least two investigations have reported afferent input that seemingly "picks out" the clusters of nucleus basalis neurons. Some of these originate in the amygdala and may provide a highly specific, albeit indirect, manner for this structure to exert its influence on widespread parts of the cortical mantle. These projections arise from amygdaloid nuclei that receive intrinsic amygdaloid projections, suggesting that, at least in so far as the amygdala is concerned, its output to the nucleus basalis reflects output deriving from much of the structure. In this context, it should not be overlooked that the subiculum of the hippocampal formation projects both to the basal complex of the amygdala and to other basal forebrain areas that project to the nucleus basalis. Thus, a highly synthesized output from the hippocampal formation would seem plausible. On these grounds, and on the basis of its direct limbic cortical input, it can be concluded that the major input to the nucleus basalis originates with the entire limbic system as a whole. Interestingly, the nucleus basalis of Meynert is not influenced directly by the major part of the cortex to which it projects. It is only influenced indirectly, after the whole sequence of corticocortical connections is retraced.

Finally, the nucleus basalis of Meynert receives projections from the hypothalamus. These need further study, but provide a structural basis by which the internal state of the organism can indirectly influence both the motor and the sensory cortices and influence the manner by which the organism interacts with its environment. Many well-documented behavioral observations suggesting such influences have not had strong anatomical backing in the past. In this regard, however, it should be noted that several limbic structures, notably the amygdala and hippocampal formation, receive hypothalamic projections and project back to the cortex. Thus, the nucleus basalis of Meynert is not unique in this sense.

Dorsomedial and Midline Thalamic Nuclei

The dorsomedial thalamic nucleus is known to play a role in many behaviors in humans, including visuospatial processing, attention, and memory. Contributing roles have also been argued for aphasia, dementia, and temporal disorientation when the nucleus is diseased or damaged. Some authors attribute damage to this nucleus as the pathological basis for the debilitating cognitive changes that occur in the alcoholic Korsakoff syndrome (122). Evidence from penetrating wounds (123) and thalamic infarcts (124) support this contention. The literature regarding prefrontal lobotomy also applies here, because one would think that this surgery would cause extensive retrograde cell changes in the dorsomedial thalamic nucleus. However, only a subset of the behavioral changes listed earlier was reported in individuals having this surgical procedure, and proportedly, these were confined largely to the realm of personality changes.

The dorsomedial thalamic nucleus is a large midline association nucleus having powerful interconnections with the prefrontal granular association cortex (125–127). From a cytoarchitectural viewpoint, it is a complex composed of several subdivisions. These form partially concentric areas around the third ventricle. In general terms, they have topographically organized reciprocal connections with the prefrontal cortex in the monkey (125–129). For example, the most medial subdivision of the dorsomedial nucleus projects to and receives projections from the posterior orbital, anterior cingulate, and medial frontal cortex. A more lateral subdivision projects to and receives projections from the prefrontal association cortex dorsal and ventral to the principal sulcus and the anteriormost parts of the orbitofrontal cortex. The most lateral subdivision of the dorsomedial nucleus sends projections to and receives projections from the periarcuate cortex in the anterior bank of the arcuate sulcus.

With the exception of its prefrontal cortex connections, the neural systems of the dorsomedial nucleus are understood poorly. In fact, known input and output relationships with other structures are decidedly sparse in comparison with other nuclei of the thalamus and even other association nuclei, such as the pulvinar nuclei.

Some evidence, however, is accumulating that enables at least a partial characterization of this structure. For example, early ablation-degeneration experiments identified another cortical projection to this large nucleus from the lateral temporal cortex (80). Additional evidence suggests that certain cortical areas of the limbic lobe, such as the anterior cingulate cortex, have connections with the dorsomedial nucleus (130). This is of some interest because this part of the cingulate cortex (Brodmann's area 24) contributes axons to the corticospinal pathway directly to the supplementary and primary motor cortices.

A direct input from the amygdala to the dorsomedial nucleus has been known for several years. Recent tracing experiments buttress and extend these findings (77, 97, 98). These axons arise from the basal complex of the amygdala and terminate in the more medial parts of the dorsomedial nucleus. The mediobasal nucleus seems to be the primary focus for this projection, although other basal nuclei (laterobasal and accessory basal) appear to contribute as well. These axons course largely via the ventroamygdalofugal pathway and the inferior thalamic peduncle. Curiously, the temporal cortical projections to the dorsomedial nucleus and those that arise from the amygdala are not reciprocated by thalamocortical or thalamoamygdaloid projections. Additional input from the ventral pallidum, substantia nigra, septum, superior colliculus, and hypothalamus have been reported.

SUMMARY AND FUNCTIONAL CONSIDERATIONS

Overall, the neural systems involving the dorsomedial thalamic nucleus are not well known. The position of this nucleus ventral to two large fiber systems, the fimbria-fornix and corpus callosum, its encasement within the internal medullary lamina of the thalamus, and the fact that the mammillothalamic tract traverses its ventral parts, have discouraged experimental study. Investigators' attention has focused primarily on the amygdalothalamic and temporothalamic projections. These link the dorsomedial nucleus with temporal structures known to play a role in memory. For example, the lateral temporal cortex has been characterized as playing a mnemonic role in certain perceptual learning tasks. Also, the mediobasal amygdaloid nucleus, which contributes strongly to the amygdalothalamic projection, is a direct recipient of subicular output from the hippocampal formation. Finally, recent anatomical findings reveal that the frontal association cortices that receive powerful input from the dorsomedial nucleus themselves receive projections from the hippocampal formation and project to the cortex around the rhinal sulcus, which, in turn, projects directly to the subiculum.

The findings themselves may be sufficient to implicate the dorsomedial thalamic nucleus in at least some aspects of memory and many other behaviors. However, caution must be exercised when making clinicopathologic inferences involving this nucleus. Several midline nuclei of the thalamus project directly to the hippocampal formation, entorhinal cortices, and amygdala. These include the nucleus reuniens, the paracentral nucleus, and the thalamic paraventricular nucleus. These are likely to be involved in hemorrhagic and nonhemorrhagic infarcts to the midline thalamus, and to be damaged penetrating wounds that involve the thalamus. They also are likely to be damaged in patients with alcoholic Korsakoffs syndrome. At present, an association of midline thalamic damage with memory impairments and behavioral changes is known, but the role of specific thalamic nuclei remains to be evaluated by further study.

PREFRONTAL CORTEX

The frontal lobe lies anterior to the central sulcus and can be divided into two major parts, a caudal part containing the electrophysiologically "excitable" motor cortices and a rostral part containing the prefrontal association cortex (Fig. 7.2). The motor cortices include the primary (M1 or area 4), supplementary (M2 or area 6m), and lateral premotor cortices (LPMC or areas 6D and 6V) (131–135). All are characterized as agranular cortex, attesting to the fact that their internal granular layer, or layer IV, is not conspicuous. It is well known that M1 plays a critical role in activating and facilitating independent body movements. On the other hand, M2 seems more involved with whole body movements and internally generated movements that are integrated in orderly fashion. Significant modulation of neuronal activity in the lateral premotor cortex, and, in particular, the ventral part of lateral area 6, has been shown to be coupled with stimulus-triggered (visual and somatosensory cued) motor responses and during the execution of purposeful movements such as grasping and/or bringing the hand to the mouth.

Also included as part of the motor cortices are the frontal eye field (FEF or area 8), supplementary eye field (SEF or area F6) and presupplementary motor area (pre-SMA) (Fig. 7.2) The FEF and SEF are located on the lateral surface of the hemisphere (136–138). The FEF is located anterior to the midportion of lateral premotor cortex and has a dysgranular cytoarchitecture. This refers to the fact that FEF is characterized by a poorly defined or incipient, internal granular layer IV. The SEF appears to be a subfield within area 6D. The rostral part of area 6D of the lateral premotor cortex has also been shown to be dysgranular (139). Both the FEF and SEF regulate contralateral saccadic eye movements. The pre-SMA is located on the medial wall of the hemisphere (140), rostral to M2, and corresponds to Walker's area 8B (141). Neurons in this field modulate their activity prior to and during movement.

The prefrontal cortex lies rostral to the motor-related cortices and extends to the frontal pole (Fig. 7.2). On the medial surface, the prefrontal cortex lies anterior to the medial component of motor cortex as well as the anterior part of cingulate gyrus. The primate prefrontal cortex is subdivided commonly on broad, anatomical grounds. Its major partitions include ventrolateral, dorsolateral, medial, and orbitofrontal regions. In the monkey, the principal sulcus is located on the lateral surface of the hemisphere, and its depths form the boundary between the ventrolateral and dorsolateral regions of prefrontal cortex. As named, the medial region of the prefrontal cortex is located on the medial surface of the hemisphere. Finally, the orbitofrontal region of the prefrontal cortex lies in the anterior cranial fossa above the bony orbit and forms the basal, or ventral, surface of the frontal lobe.

A large portion of the prefrontal cortex is classified cytoarchitecturally as granular cortex and has six well-differentiated layers, including a prominent external granular layer II and internal granular layer IV (142, 143). However, differences in layers II and IV as well as the other cortical laminae serve as a basis for partitioning the frontal granular cortex into several subfields. They are designated numeri-

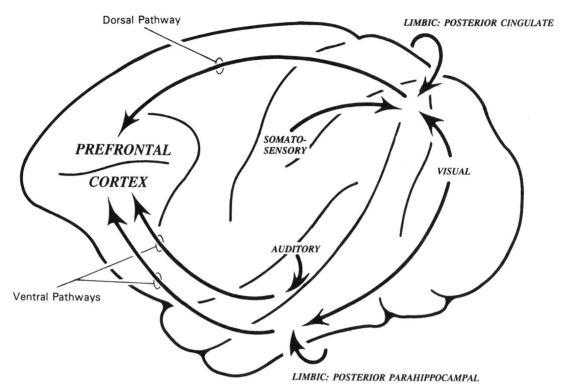

Figure 7.13. Some of the major cortical association input to the prefrontal cortex is depicted on a lateral view of the monkey cerebral hemisphere. Note the dorsal pathway from the inferior parietal gyrus and dorsal peristriate area carrying cingulate information and the ventral pathways carrying auditory, visual and posterior parahippocampal information. These provide cortical information from all of the other lobes, including the limbic lobe.

cally, according to Brodmann and others. The prefrontal cortex includes areas: 45, 12, 46, 10 and 9 laterally, 9, 10 and 32 medially; and 12, 13, 11, 10 and 14 ventrally (Fig. 7.2). Many of these areas have recently been redefined and further subdivided.

Cortex on the orbitofrontal surface lobe can also be subdivided on cytoarchitectural criteria into a caudal agranular sector, an anterior granular sector, and a transitional dysgranular sector between them (142, 144, 145). From this perspective, general trends and distinguishing features of major orbitofrontal organization are clearly recognizable. For example, agranular and dysgranular components are located caudally on the orbitofrontal surface and are strongly connected with the limbic cortices, amygdala, and midline nuclei of the thalamus. In contrast, the granular component is situated rostrally on the orbitofrontal surface. This cortex is linked strongly to isocortical association areas and association nuclei of the thalamus. As expected, these unique patterns of neural interconnections would differentially influence activity and events processed in rostral versus caudal parts of the orbitofrontal cortex. Lesions rarely affect small parts of the orbitofrontal surface, and thus are correlated with more global behavioral changes and not specific impairments. For example, posterior lesions disrupt limbic and medial temporal connections and lead to changes in emotional and social behavior, as well as in autonomic regulation. More anterior lesions disrupt association inputs and affect more complex behaviors.

Cortical Association Connections of Prefrontal Cortex

In addition to its obvious role in motor behavior, frontal lobe function has long been associated with a variety of higher-order behaviors and cognitive processes. Some of the more notable ones include working memory, motor planning, developing and implementing long-term strategies; decision making, and problem solving (146–153). When considering the higher-order functions mediated by the prefrontal cortex, the finding that prefrontal cortex is linked directly to a constellation of cortical association areas should not be surprising. Indeed, the prefrontal cortex is well known for its widespread corticocortical connections with distal parts of the cerebral cortex, specifically including primary association and multimodal association cortices (Fig. 7.13).

Primary association cortex is committed functionally to the early processing of sensory data, conveyed by the neurons of an adjacent primary sensory area. Primary association cortex operates in a more integrative fashion than primary sensory area. In contrast, multimodal association cortex is not committed to processing information related to one modality, but rather integrates highly transformed information, whose source can be traced back to multiple, sensory modalities. Although the traditional dogma suggests that multimodal association cortex represents the end stages of cortical processing, it is becoming more clear that information flowing in the reverse direction, i.e. directed from multimodal association back to the primary association areas, may initiate and synchronize neural elements that are responsible for forming selective preceptions (154).

The prefrontal cortex is linked to sensory association and multimodal association cortices of the parietal lobe (areas 7a, 7b, and 7m) and temporal lobe (areas V4t, MT, and MST) as well as sensory association cortices of the anterior part of the occipital lobe (area V3) (22, 24, 26, 88, 144, 155, 156). It has been shown in the monkey that the posterior part of the inferior parietal lobule (area 7a), anterior part of the occipital lobe, and the medial parietal lobule (area 7m) are reciprocally connected with the dorsolateral and sulcal principalis regions of the prefrontal cortex. Anatomical and behavioral investigations conducted over the past three decades have led to the conclusion that long association pathways, reciprocally linking posterior parietal cortex and prefrontal cortex, are particularly important for the appropriate execution of visually guided movements. Presumably, somatosensory and visual inputs converge on posterior part of the inferior parietal lobule, and information related to spatial orientation and motion analysis is conveyed to the dorsolateral prefrontal cortex (Fig. 7.13) (157, 158). Therefore, the dorsolateral part of the prefrontal cortex is thought to process information concerned with understanding *where* an object is in space. It is also known that the more rostral part of the inferior parietal lobule (area 7b) and ventrolateral part of the temporal lobe project to the ventrolateral part of the prefrontal cortex. Specifically, the projection from the ventrolateral part of temporal lobe is thought to carry information dealing with form and object recognition. Therefore, it has been suggested that the ventral pathway may constitute a processing stream that addresses *what* an object represents in the extrapersonal environment. The prefrontal cortex is also influenced by other parts of the temporal lobe through a subcomponent of the ventral pathway, whose origin arises from the rostral part of the superior temporal gyrus as well from the temporal pole. This projection probably represents an important source of auditory input to the ventrolateral part of the prefrontal cortex.

In addition to the long association pathways linking the prefrontal cortex with the parietal, occipital, and temporal lobes, short association pathways interlock the various parts of the prefrontal cortex with one another in an organized fashion (142). The less-differentiated (in terms of cytoarchitectonic lamination) agranular and dysgranular cortices, located posteriorly on the basal and medial surface of the prefrontal cortex, give rise to widespread *intrinsic* prefrontal connections. In contrast, the more differentiated isocortical granular areas, which are situated anteriorly and laterally, are characterized by more limited *intrinsic* connections; they account instead for a large component of the frontal lobe's widespread *extrinsic* prefrontal connections.

Cortical Limbic Connections of the Prefrontal Cortex

The strong structural relation between prefrontal cortex and association cortex has played a dominant role in shaping our views on prefrontal organization and function. However, it is important not to neglect the structural interaction between the prefrontal cortex and limbic lobe, which is also very strong. There are many direct connections between the limbic lobe and the prefrontal cortex. Limbic projections to the prefrontal cortex arise from diverse and widespread parts of the limbic lobe, including the cingulate, orbitofrontal, temporopolar, perirhinal, entorhinal, posterior parahippocampal and the insular cortices (20, 21, 26, 30, 70, 74, 76, 159, 160). Although the lateral prefrontal cortex is a target for some of these connections, the bulk of this anatomical interrelationship is established with the posterior orbitofrontal and medial prefrontal regions.

As outlined previously, the prefrontal cortex maintains a highly organized anatomical affiliation with the cingulate gyrus. The more anterior dorsolateral prefrontal cortex is connected with the posterior cingulate cortex (area 23), while the posterior dorsolateral prefrontal cortex is more strongly linked to the anterior cingulate gyrus. Similarly, the anterior orbitofrontal cortex is connected to area 23 and the posterior part is connected to area 24.

Early studies that relied on the Marchi technique to trace neural connections failed to recognize a strong connection between the frontal and temporal lobes. However, use of more sensitive tracing techniques enabled investigators to demonstrate that fibers forming a subcomponent of the uncinate fasciculus, as well as the extreme capsule, interconnect the frontal and temporal lobes in a strong and highly specific fashion. The strongest links with the limbic portion of temporal lobe involve the posterior orbitofrontal cortex and medial prefrontal cortex, followed by the lateral prefrontal cortex.

Although a precise topography has yet to be determined, a number of other areas in the temporal portion of the limbic lobe are connected to the prefrontal cortex. They include the temporal pole (area 38), perirhinal (area 35), entorhinal (area 28), posterior parahippocampal (areas TH and TF), presubicular, and subicular cortices. All but the subicular connection have been shown to be reciprocal. The subiculum of the hippocampal formation projects to the posterior part of the orbitofrontal cortex and send some afferents to the dorsolateral part of the prefrontal cortex. A particularly heavy component of this projection terminates in the posterior part of the gyrus rectus, on the orbitofrontal surface. Hippocampal output is known to be mediated heavily by the subiculum and to some extent the CA1 sector of the hippocampal formation. Thus, subicular/CA1 output represents a direct hippocampal influence on the prefrontal cortex.

All parts of the prefrontal cortex are reciprocally connected with the insula, and a distinct anatomical relationship between cortex forming the orbitofrontal surface and the insula has been demonstrated. The agranular part of the orbitofrontal cortex is preferentially linked to the agranular part of the insula. In terms of topography, this translates into distinct connections between the posterior orbitofrontal cortex and the anterior insula. Likewise, granular orbitofrontal cortex is preferentially linked to granular insula.

Anterior parts of the insula receive direct input from the gustatory and olfactory cortex, and the posterior parts receive input from primary somatosensory and auditory areas. This suggests that the insula may be a common site of *direct* convergence of all nonvisual sensory afferents. This is remarkable because integration of multimodal sensory information occurs elsewhere in the brain *after* a polysynaptic relay through sensory association cortex to multimodal cortex. All parts of the insula appear to receive input from sensory association and multimodal association cortices. The diversity of projections to the insula implies that prefrontal input from the insula may either be as little as one synapse away from a primary sensory area, or may be highly processed.

Amygdala projections to prefrontal cortex arise primarily from the basolateral and accessory basal nuclei, and to a lesser extent from cortical and lateral nuclei (92, 144, 161). The strongest amygdalofrontal projection ends in the posterior part (agranular and dysgranular sectors) of the orbitofrontal cortex. Another strong projection terminates in the medial prefrontal cortices (areas 14, 25, and 32). Projections to isocortical areas on the lateral convexity (areas 9, 10, 45, and 46) are less strong. As mentioned previously, the amygdala is the recipient of a wide variety of cortical inputs from allocortical, periallocortical, proisocortical, and isocortical association areas. The latter includes converging input from both auditory and visual association areas as well as multimodal association cortices. Therefore, there is reason to believe that amygdala output directed toward the prefrontal cortices is influenced by a variety of neural systems related to the interplay of both the internal and external environments of the organism.

Motor Cortex Connections with Prefrontal Cortex

It is well known that the prefrontal corticofugal axons are not directed to cranial nerve nuclei or the spinal cord. However, since the latter part of the 19th century, it has been appreciated that prefrontal cortex plays a special and important role in guiding the outcome of voluntary motor behavior. How this is accomplished anatomically has been an enigma for many years. The view that emerged from classic studies suggested that corticospinal neurons in M1 were influenced by prefrontal input through an indirect series of connections passing through lateral area 6, or premotor cortex (88, 155). However, the discovery that cortex located outside the primary motor cortex, including the lateral premotor cortex, supplementary motor cortex, and cingulate motor cortex, contained corticospinal neurons, suggested otherwise (46, 162–164).

As summarized in Figure 7.14, more recent efforts have shown clearly that the prefrontal cortex projects directly to parts of the motor cortices, giving rise to the corticospinal axons (29, 52, 53). In the lateral premotor cortex, only the very rostral parts of areas 6D and 6V that contain corticospinal neurons receive prefrontal input, with area 6V being the primary link. Prefrontal input to M2 converges on the rostral part of M2 that contains the face area and less so on corticospinal output zones that subserve the arm. Thus, the more rostral parts of the lateral premotor cortex and supplementary motor cortex receive prefrontal input. However, the cingulate motor cortex (M3 or area 24c) and area 23c has also been shown to receive strong prefrontal input that converges on parts of these cortices that rise to corticospinal axons. Thus, recent work implies that several anatomically distinct sources of corticospinal axons are directly influenced by prefrontal output. Moreover the ventral part of M1 receives input from the caudal part of the ventrolateral operculum of the prefrontal cortex. The target of this projection resides outside the M1-corticospinal projection zone, and may correspond to the face representation. In many nonhuman primate models, the frontal eye field has been shown to give rise to projections that innervate midbrain centers regulating ocular motor behavior. Although no corticospinal projections arise from the frontal eye field, it does receive strong prefrontal input.

Subcortical Connections of Prefrontal Cortex

The corticostriate projection from the prefrontal cortex is substantial. It is directed toward targets in the caudate nucleus and, to a much lesser extent, the putamen (24, 165–167). Because a portion of the outflow of the basal ganglia is directed to the thalamus and eventually back to all parts of the frontal lobe, the corticostriate projection represents initial stages of a sequential pathway by which prefrontal cortex can influence a wide variety of neural systems.

The corticothalamic projection is one of the most studied corticofugal pathways leaving from the prefrontal cortex (126, 127, 168–171). The work of Akert (125) and Nauta (168) demonstrated that the mediodorsal thalamic nucleus is connected to all parts of the prefrontal cortex in the primate, including the granular sectors located anteriorly and laterally, as well as dysgranular and agranular sectors located medially and ventrally (the posterior orbitofrontal cortex). The medial part of the magnocellular division of the mediodorsal nucleus was found to be connected primarily with the orbital surface of the prefrontal cortex and the lateral part (parvocellular division) with the lateral surface of the prefrontal cortex. Anatomical findings and functional observations have since combined to suggest that the prefrontal cortex can be viewed as having at least four major subdivisions. They include dorsolateral, ventrolateral, medial, and orbitofrontal divisions, with each having its own unique thalamic projection pattern. Although the strong reciprocal anatomical relationship between the mediodorsal nucleus and prefrontal cortex is often emphasized, like all other cortical areas, numerous thalamic nuclei are linked to this brain region. They include the midline, ventral anterior, intralaminar, anterior medial and pulvinar nuclei.

Several important brainstem projections from prefrontal cortex have been identified that may play a role in motor control (24, 172, 173). Corticotectal projections have been

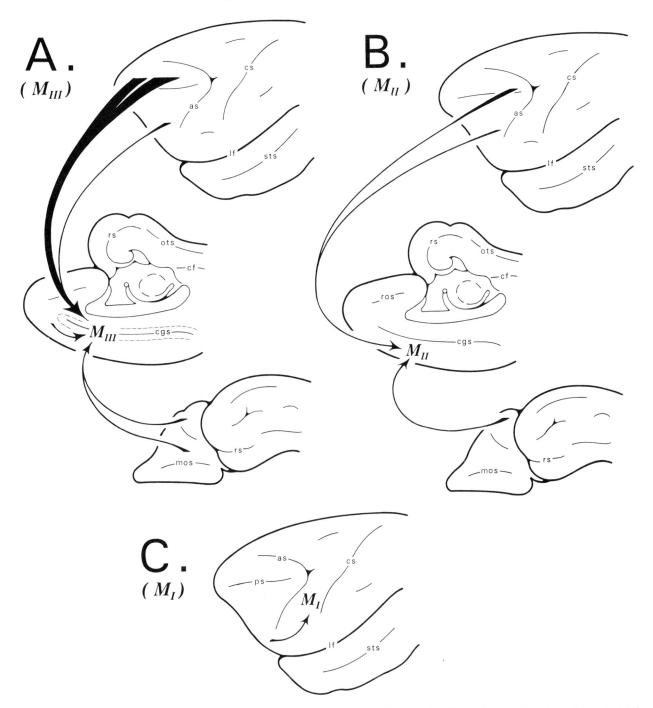

Figure 7.14.   The diversity and strength of prefrontal input to M3 **(A)**, M2 **(B)**, and M1 **(C)**. Note, that M3 receives dorsolateral, medial, and orbitofrontal projections. M2 or supplementary motor cortex receives some direct prefrontal input, but M1 or primary motor cortex receives virtually no direct prefrontal cortex input. (Abbreviations: sulcus labeling is the same as for Fig. 7.5, except for the additions of *cs* = central sulcus, *mos* = medial orbital sulcus, and *ots* = occipitotemporal sulcus.)

demonstrated to arise from the dorsolateral-principalis region in the monkey and terminate in the intermediate and deep layers of the superior colliculus. Such projections are likely candidates for influencing behaviors linked to eye movement, particularly those ocular motor tasks requiring on-line, or working memory, to order and issue an appropriate set of behavioral commands. Projections from prefrontal cortex to the pontine reticular formation have also been reported. This projection appears to be distributed over

the paramedian portion reticular formation, an area corresponding in location to the central superior nucleus.

The prefrontal cortex also gives rise to a strong corticopontine projection that ends in the medial part of the basilar pontine gray matter (173, 174). This projection is a major component of the corticopontocerebellar system. Transneuronal labeling techniques have shown that cerebellar as well as pallidal neurons are labeled following injections of herpes simplex virus type 1 into the dorsolateral prefrontal cortex

Figure 7.15. Lateral **(A)** and medial **(B)** views of the cerebral hemisphere at end-stage Alzheimer's disease after a long duration of illness (13 years) in an 83-year-old female. Note, the pronounced atrophic changes in the prefrontal, parietal, and temporal association cortices, but the relative preservation of the pre- and postcentral gyri on either side of the central sulcus (the latter is marked by the *arrow* in both photographs). The *asterisk* in **B** marks the location of the entorhinal cortex.

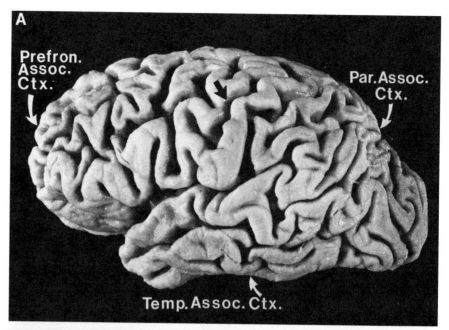

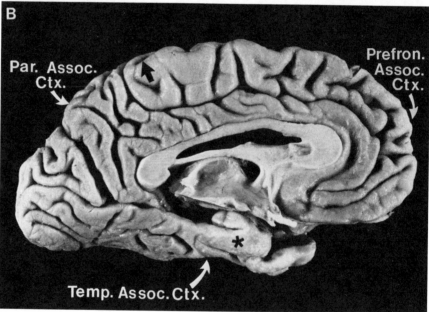

(175). This indicates that thalamocortical input to the prefrontal cortex is influenced by both basal ganglia as well as cerebellar circuits. If the basal ganglia and cerebellar loops are organized in parallel, it is likely that corticopontine projection from the prefrontal cortex is involved with the cerebellothalamocortical pathway that converges back onto the prefrontal cortex.

The prefrontal cortex is connected to several small but important brainstem nuclei that synthesize and transmit selective neurotransmitters to widespread parts of the prefrontal cortex. It has been suggested that these projections may play an important role in regulating global as well as discrete behavioral states (176, 177). For example, as discussed previously, the nucleus basalis of Meynert gives rise to cholinergic projections that innervate all parts of the

prefrontal cortex. The ventral tegmental area, dorsal raphe nucleus, and locus ceruleus also belong to pharmacologically distinct classes of subcortical nuclei, and like the nucleus basalis, also project to all parts of the prefrontal cortex. The ventral tegmental area (VTA) is a dopaminergic mesencephalic nucleus located ventral and caudal to the red nucleus. The dorsal raphe nucleus (DR) is situated in the midbrain and pons, immediately ventral to the periaqueductal gray matter and consists of serotonergic neurons. Finally, neurons of the locus ceruleus (LC) give rise to norepinephrine projections. There are several notable and interesting exceptions regarding the issue of reciprocity when considering the pharmacologically specific subcortical nuclei. For example, the nucleus basalis appears to project to all the cerebral cortex, including the prefrontal cortex, but receives input from only the limbic lobe. From the standpoint of the frontal lobe, this would include the posterior parts of the orbitofrontal cortex and medial prefrontal cortex. Also, unlike the rest of the cerebral cortex, which probably does not send projections back to the VTA, DR, and LC, the dorsolateral and medial parts of the prefrontal cortex have been found to send a reciprocal subcortical efferent projection to these brainstem centers (178). Therefore, the selective reciprocity of these connections gives distinct parts of the prefrontal cortex feedback control over their own monoaminergic and cholinergic innervation as well as influencing innervation that distributes to widespread parts of the cerebral cortex.

SUMMARY AND CONCLUSIONS

The widespread extent of prefrontal cortex connections underlies the complex functions subserved by it. The diverse set of associative connections converging on prefrontal cortex indicate that transformed and integrated information, associated with multiple sensory modalities, shape the outcome of prefrontal-guided behaviors. The anatomical interaction between prefrontal and limbic cortices may affect the motivational state and emotional tone or temperament of prefrontal behaviors in addition to involving memory features, such as the storage and retrieval of information.

Moreover, the prefrontal cortex gives rise to a host of descending projections that contribute to the corticostriate, corticothalamic, corticotectal, corticoreticular, and cortico-pontine pathways. Information directed away from the prefrontal cortex through nonreciprocating projections, such as the corticostriate and corticopontine projections, eventually converges back on the prefrontal cortex only after coursing through a sequential and parallel set of subcortical circuits or "loops." Others, such as the corticothalamic projections, being heavily reciprocated, allow for direct interaction between prefrontal and discrete subcortical diencephalic nuclei. Finally, chemically-specific subcortical projections from cholinergic and monoaminergic sources to all parts of the prefrontal cortex may globally and perhaps homogeneously affect the operation of cortical states associated with arousal, attention, motivation, and learning. Likewise, projections from selected parts of the prefrontal cortex to the monoaminergic and cholinergic centers suggest that prefrontal cortex may modulate its own afferent neurochemical innervation.

Degenerative Diseases Affecting the Prefrontal Cortex and Limbic System

It has been recognized for many years (179) that the limbic system and, to some degree, the frontal lobes are the preferred targets for particular disease mechanisms. For example, this is the case for degenerative diseases such as AD and Pick's disease (180, 181) as well as schizophrenia (182–184). Several of the viral encephalitides also some-what selectively attack these brain areas (185–187). Why

this is the case, and why the parietal and occipital lobes as well as numerous subcortical brain areas are not targeted as greatly is an open question of fundamental importance. AD has been well-characterized in terms of topographical neuropathology and neuroanatomy (Fig. 7.15): the limbic system and temporal lobe (Fig. 7.16) are damaged disproportionately in this disorder (188, 189). The frontal lobe always contains pathology, but its involvement is moderate and may not be heavily damaged until closer to the end stage of the disease (190). Neurofibrillary tangles occur first in the cortex of the limbic lobe and only later in the illness do they involve the association areas. The perirhinal and entorhinal cortices (Figs. 7.16 and 7.17) are first affected (190–192), followed closely by the temporal polar cortex (193). Curiously, the entorhinal and cingulate cortices are altered in

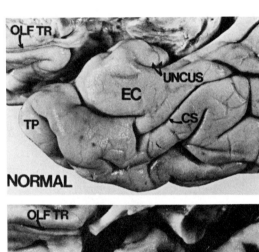

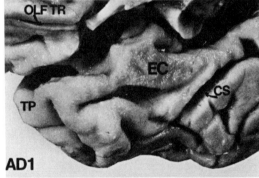

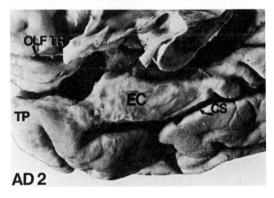

Figure 7.16. Three views of the ventromedial temporal area focusing on the entorhinal cortex *(EC)*. The top photo is from a normal nondemented elderly donor (age 76 years). The bottom two photos (AD1 and AD2) are from pathologically confirmed Alzheimer's disease donors (ages 71 and 79). Note the atrophic pitted appearance of the EC (other abbreviations: *cs* = collateral sulcus, *OLF TR* = olfactory tracts, *TP* = temporal pole).

Figure 7.17. A cross-section through the EC in Alzheimer's disease stained with the fluorochrome thioflavin S to reveal neurofibrillary tangles. Note that the neurons of layers II and V are heavily invested with this form of pathology. The former link the hippocampal formation to the cortex, whereas the latter receive hippocampal output and project to the cerebral cortex. The disease-related pathology of Alzheimer's disease thereby disconnects the hippocampal formation from the cerebral cortex.

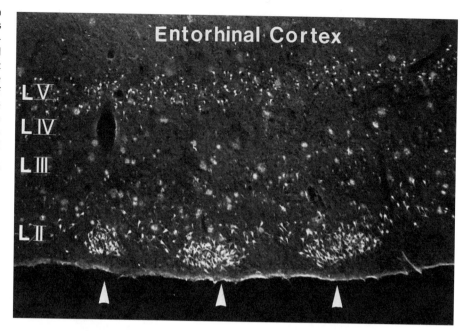

Figure 7.18. A medial view of the cerebral hemisphere from a donor with pathologically confirmed Pick's disease. The arrow marks the medial tip of the central sulcus, and the asterisk marks the location of the entorhinal cortex. Note the marked atrophy of the prefrontal association and the temporal association cortices compared with the preservation of the parietal association cortices. Neuron loss, gliosis, and occasional Pick's bodies were observed in the former areas.

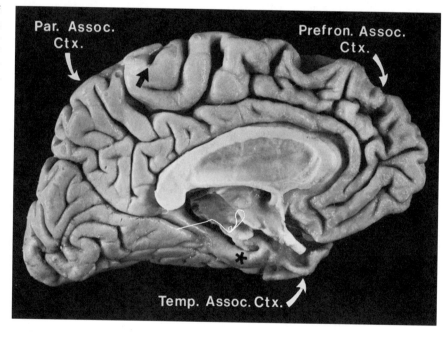

some schizophrenics (189, 194, 195), and the prefrontal and the temporal polar cortices are frequently atrophic in Pick's disease (Fig. 7.18) (193). Although there are neuroanatomical and some behavioral similarities between these three disorders, their overall profile is not isomorphic, and the pathological picture is quite disimilar. In AD, for example, changes in memory and cognition are correlated with neurofibrillary tangles, while in Pick's disease, they are associated with cell loss and cytoplasmic inclusion bodies. In schizophrenia, more subtle cell or gray matter loss occurs in the temporal lobe (196) and anterior cingulate gyrus (195), but laminar alterations in cytoarchitecture hint also of a preexisting developmental disorder in the genesis or sculpting of the cortex (194).

For many of the neural systems and connections of the limbic system and frontal lobe described previously, the projection neurons that give rise to association axons reside in layer III of the cerebral cortex and to some extent in layer V. A subset of layer III also mediates callosal connections, and various subsets of layer V give rise to corticofugal axons that course to subcortical targets. In both AD and Pick's disease, these larger projection neurons of layers III and V are targeted for pathology, whether it be neurofibrillary tangles in the former case (198) or cell loss and cytoplasmic inclusion bodies in the latter case. Thus, although the etiology of cortical neuronal death is different in both diseases, the outcome can be somewhat similar because corticocortical connections are destroyed.

Less information is available on this issue with regard to schizophrenia, but a strong possibility exists that some of the clinical signs of this disorder reflect a disconnection (183). The "frontal-like" signs of certain psychiatric diseases may be due to subtle cortical neuroanatomical changes elsewhere yielding behavior that is more a manifestation of frontal lobe deafferentation than the direct result of diffuse and subtle lesions in the areas that provide afferent input to the frontal lobes. AD, Pick's disease, schizophrenia, and other disorders characterized by changes in behavior, all affect cortical association systems that supply input to the frontal lobes. They share some clinical features with lobar atrophy of the frontal cortex (197–199), where the pathological change involves not an afferent or input to the frontal cortex coming from elsewhere, but the efferent or projection neurons of the frontal lobe itself. If the major degenerative disorders serve in any way as a model for the seemingly more subtle developmental disorders of schizophrenia, (200, 201), the entire cerebral cortex will have to be screened carefully because of the extensive limbic and association connections of the frontal lobe (202).

CONTEMPORARY ISSUES REGARDING THE EVOLUTION OF THE FRONTAL LOBE

Historical Observations and Biases

The frontal lobes were in all likelihood first associated with higher mental functions by the Greeks, who represented some gods, demigods, poets, and artists with large foreheads in their sculptures and paintings (6). Anatomical records and illustrations that originated in classical antiquity have been traced by way of Byzantium to both the Medieval West and East (203), and the association between large frontal lobes and special cognitive abilities accompanied them.

During the Renaissance, clinical observations began to emerge, suggesting a special role of the frontal lobes for the human intellect. Studies included frontal lobe injuries in soldiers and cases of patients with brain tumors (6). Also, comparative studies between human and animal brains attracted the attention of many anatomists like Willis and, later, Tiedemann and Owen (203).

In the late 18th century, physiognomists devised the first anthropometric measures associating mental characteristics with physical features. Larger facial angles caught their fancy, and more fully developed foreheads were attributed more to whites than blacks and an increase in the facial angle was found when apes and humans were compared in the "natural chain of being" (6).

Phrenology and craniometry were both introduced in the 19th century. Supporters of the former believed in the notion that distinct functional units in the cerebrum correlated with cranial surface features, while supporters of craniometry saw a strong association between brain size and intellectual capacities (204). Higher functions especially were associated with a presumably larger frontal lobe in humans, while smaller frontal lobes present in monkeys and dogs represented rudimentary forms of intellect (6). Gall's phrenological system included eight organs in the frontal lobe that set humans apart from animals. These included poetic talent, kindness and moral sense, faculty to imitate, and religion (205).

Burdach in the 1820s (6) supported the idea that the frontal region is more developed in humans than in other mammals and therefore it logically had to be involved in intellectual functions. In keeping with the racist ideology of the mid 19th century, Huschke declared the Caucasian race the "frontal race." Gratiolet stated that it is the frontal lobes that distinguish humans from other animals (6).

Reports of actual measurements that compare the size of the frontal lobes in humans and other mammals were absent from the 19th century literature, but the support of the idea linking unique human intellectual capacities with large frontal lobes was abundant and persisted throughout the next century. Bianchi (206) stated that intellect appeared to be correlated with the growth of the prefrontal cortex and that the progression is clear from cats to dogs to monkeys and to humans. A notable exception was Monakow (6), who disputed the link on the basis of the large frontal lobes that he identified in the horse brain (which he estimated to be 30% of the cortical volume).

With the turn of this century, actual measurements started being performed on comparative material. For example, Brodmann performed measurements on parts of the human and nonhuman primate cortex (207). The surface area of the neocortex, the prefrontal cortex (regio frontalis), and the frontal lobe (lobus frontalis) were estimated for the human, chimpanzee, gibbon, and macaque, along with a few other monkeys and prosimians. The size of the surface area for the entire *frontal lobe* was reported to be 36.3% for the human, 30.5% for the chimpanzee, and 21.4% for the gibbon. The size of the *prefrontal cortex* relative to total neocortical size was reported to be 29% for the human, 16.9% for the chimpanzee, 11.3% for the gibbon, and 11.3% for the macaque (the other primates ranging from 11.3–7.2%).

Leboucq (208) found that the volume of the frontal lobe in the human is 38.3% (surface, 36.5%), 39% in the chimpanzee (surface, 37%), and 30% in the macaque (surface, 30.4%).

Tilney (209) estimated the surface area of the frontal lobe in relationship to the "neopallium" to be: 47% for the human, 33% for the chimpanzee, and 32% for the gorilla. Combining these results and his studies of hominid endocasts, he also concluded: "A distinguishing metrical feature in the development of the human brain is the consistent gain in length and height from *Pithecanthropus erectus* to *Homo sapiens*. The gain in length is to be ascribed largely to frontal increments."

Weil (210) measured the surface of endocranial casts and favored the idea of an enlarged human frontal lobe. He concluded that "the frontal part of the cap of the casts, which was limited by a line perpendicular to the horizontal base line at the intersecting point of frontal and temporal lobes, is best developed in the specimen of living races which were investigated. Measured in percentages of the total surface of the cap, this part, in the specimen of living races, is from 28 to 31; in the casts of the other prehistoric men, from 21 to 25; and in the casts of the four anthropoids that were investigated, from 17 to 20 per cent" (210). It should be noted that his measurements included only the external cortical surface and not that buried within the sulci. Additionally, as he himself admitted, "naturally, the subdivisions which were introduced for comparative purposes of the cast do not indicate which parts of the brain were compared" (210). Furthermore, Holloway reported that Weil's measurements were criticized by Weidenreich (211), who was an expert in endocasts and who instead suggested a relative increase in the size of the parietal and temporal lobes.

In summary, the historical record reveals that sources of information regarding the size of the frontal lobe are available. One consists of the promotions of the phrenologists of the last century, who suggested that the human frontal lobe is associated with high mental functions, and is larger in humans than in other primates.

The second source of information consists of a few studies from the first half of the 20th century that involved measurements of the size of the frontal lobes on hominid and hominoid endocasts (209, 210). These supported the idea of an enlarged human frontal lobe, but their accuracy has been criticized by other researchers.

The last source of information comes from surface and volume measurements on human and nonhuman primate brain specimens, also performed in the beginning of this century. These studies were few in number and their methods varied considerably (207–209). Some suggested that the human frontal lobe is relatively larger, and some supported a similar relative size in humans and apes. Figure 7.19 illustrates the relative size of the prefrontal regions in four primate species.

FUNCTIONAL OBSERVATIONS

The idea that frontal lobe function and personality characteristics might be related had already emerged during the last century, when Harlow reported on his famous patient Phineas Gage, the so-called "crowbar case" (5). Gage underwent major personality changes after partial damage in his frontal lobes (153) and, in Harlow's words, "was no longer Gage" after the accident.

Early in this century it became clear that an association indeed exists between frontal lobe function and aspects of emotional behavior. At the International Neurological Congress in London in the summer of 1935, great interest was generated in the presentation of the results of frontal lobe extirpation in two chimpanzees, Becky and Lucy (212, 213).

After bilateral prefrontal cortex removal, Becky and Lucy's behavior changed strikingly. They did not show their usual excitement, but rather knelt quietly before the cage or

ambled around. Whenever they would make a mistake when choosing between an empty or reforced cup, they showed no emotional disturbance, but quietly awaited the next trial. "They merely continued to play quietly and did not pick over their fur . . . It was as if the animals had joined the happiness cult of the Elder Micheaux, and had placed their burdens in the hands of Lord" (214).

Egaz Moniz, a Portuguese neurosurgeon participating in the congress, commented to Dr. Fulton and Dr. Jacobsen that, "if after frontal lobe removal, an animal no longer tends to develop an experimental neurosis and no longer has temper tantrums when frustrated, why would this not be an ideal operation for human beings suffering from persistent anxiety states?" (213). Within a year of that meeting, his now famous monograph on frontal leucotomy was published (215, 216), describing the neurosurgical procedure he used on psychotic patients and its outcome, which involved an improvement in the anxiety symptoms in many of his patients.

Brickner (5) described patient *A* who was disciplined, organized, and motivated prior to developing a tumor in the frontal lobes and undergoing its removal, but became socially uninhibited, not concerned with his profession, or the planning of his daily routine and future responsibilities.

Ackerly and Benton (217) reported on another patient who also suffered a bilateral frontal lobe defect of major proportions, but maintained most aspects of his average intelligence level. Because aspects of his personality were damaged, the authors suggested that the concept of "primary social defect" might best characterize his symptoms.

Thus, a mutual reinforcement pervaded the literature combining myth, mismeasurement, and emerging clinical observations to preserve the primacy of the frontal lobes in humans for both intellect and emotional stability.

Modern Forms of Frontal Lobe Measurement

In the second half of this century more serious studies emerged on the issue of the size of the frontal lobes. Blinkov and Glezer (218) estimated the surface area of the "frontal region" (prefrontal cortex) and of the precentral region (areas 4 and 6) in relation to total surface of the hemisphere to be: 32.8% in the human, 22.1% in the chimpanzee, 21.3% in the orangutan, and 21.2% in the gibbon.

Von Bonin (219) plotted Brodmann's figures on the surface of the frontal lobes and concluded that "they illustrate a very simple case of relative growth, and that man has precisely the frontal lobe which he deserves by virtue of the overall size of his brain." Holloway (211) emphasized that "the measurements which are most direct, that directly measure cortical area or volume rather than endocasts, give little basis for accepting relative increase." Also, Clarke and Dewhurst (203) concluded that "this association between the frontal lobe and highest intellectual capacity must finally be abandoned."

Despite the aforementioned criticisms, the long-

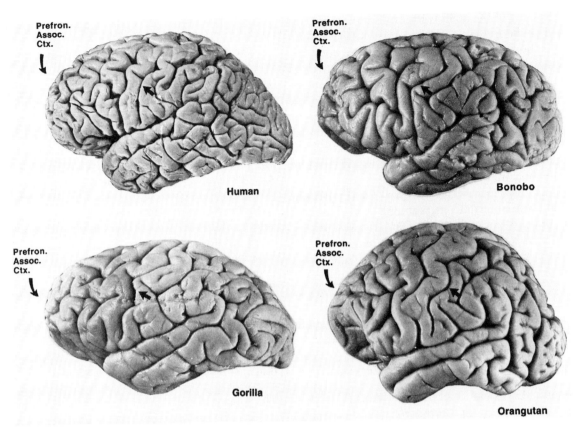

Figure 7.19. Lateral views of cerebral hemisphere for the human, bonobo (pygmy chimpanzee), gorilla, and orangutan. The arrow indicates the central sulcus in each species. Recent volumetric comparisons indicate that the human brain contains the largest frontal lobe among hominids in terms of absolute size, but with regard to relative size, it is no larger than that of the great apes.

cherished notion of an association between a large frontal lobe and high mental capacities persisted and is still the "common wisdom" promoted in textbooks and teaching as well as research rationale. Notable caution by Passingham (220) and Armstrong (221) pointed out that conflicting data existed and more studies are necessary.

Recent comparative studies of the human and ape frontal lobes have addressed the issue of size of specific cortical areas and their internal organization (222), as well as the issue of the volume and cortical surface of the hominoid frontal lobe and its subdivisions (223, 224) using modern imaging and quantitative techniques.

In a cytoarchitectonic study of the hominoid prefrontal cortex, the frontal pole region (area 10) and the posterior parts of the orbitofrontal cortex (area 13) were analyzed in the human, chimpanzee, bonobo, gorilla, orangutan, and gibbon, as well as in the well-studied rhesus monkey. The presence, qualitative appearance (based on Gallyas cell stains), aspects of the internal organization (relative size of cortical layers, neuropil space, and neuronal numbers), as well as total volumes were investigated for the two areas across species.

It was found that area 13 is present in all hominoids in the posterior parts of the orbitofrontal cortex. It is a small cortical area, particularly in the human and the bonobo brains. Its internal organization is similar among humans

and apes. The infragranular layers are larger than the supragranular layers in all species, and the neuropil space (reflecting possibly dendritic and postsynaptic space) is larger in the supragranular layers and smaller in the infragranular layers across species.

Area 13 is part of the limbic lobe and cortical parts of the limbic system. It is involved in emotional reactions, inhibitory mechanisms, decision making, and social behavior. Area 13 is thus viewed as a conservative feature of brain evolution that provides a function common in all hominoids. The results suggest that it was part of the ancestral hominoid and hominid brain.

Area 10 forms the hominoid frontal pole and is larger than area 13 in all species. Its structural features present slight variations among hominoids, with the gorilla frontal pole having the most distinct ones. In contrast to area 13, the internal organization of area 10 is more species-specific. Area 10 is part of the prefrontal association cortex involved in cognition, planning of future actions, and the undertaking of initiatives. It is here suggested that its relative size increased considerably during hominid evolution after the hominids' divergence from the line leading to modern African apes.

In additional studies, the volume and cortical surface of the frontal lobe and its subdivisions were investigated, using three-dimensional reconstructed images from MR scans of human and ape brains. It has been observed that although the whole volume of the brain is largest in the human, the relative size of the frontal lobes in relation to the brain is similar across hominids. Human frontal lobes are not larger than expected on the basis of the ape data, and the human and chimpanzee frontal lobe have similar relative values. Also, the proportions accorded to the volume of the dorsolateral, mesial, and orbital frontal lobe sectors are similar across species. However, a remarkable difference exists in the proportion of white matter in the sector of the frontal lobes anterior to the basal ganglia, which indeed is largest in the human.

Thus, the anatomical correlates for the remarkable cognitive and behavioral differences among primates should probably not be sought at the level of large cortical sectors. It is possible that differentiation of cortical areas within each sector of the frontal lobe, along with interconnectivity among them and between them, as well as cortical areas in other lobes, are the key to the neural correlates of complex human capacities. Moreover, structural differences should also be sought in other cortical areas that coevolved with the frontal lobe, such as the temporal and parietal cortices.

SUMMARY AND FUNCTIONAL CONSIDERATIONS

More modern cytoarchitectural and volumetric analyses of frontal lobe evolution are inconsistent with the assumptions and dogma that have accrued historically. Humans undoubtedly have the largest frontal lobe in absolute terms, outstripping our extant ape kin. But we have larger brains in general, and the part devoted to frontal lobe is not significantly different between apes and humans in relative terms. To paraphrase von Bonin and Bailey, we have about what we deserve. However, the picture is much more complicated than this. For example, there is the suggestion that among hominids the pie is sliced differentially to meet species-specific adaptations. Although the general cytoarchitectural plan is similar, some cell fields may be more elaborate than others, and, in fact, may be so at the expense of others. Humans, for example, have a highly differentiated frontal pole (area 10), whereas a comparable area in the gorilla is difficult to find. The largely solitary orangutan appears to have a less elaborate orbitofrontal area, which is thought to be the neural substrate for social behavior.

In short, the human frontal lobe may be unique, not so much for quantity of frontal lobe, but instead, for other reasons relating to its internal structure and convectivity. We share with our ape relatives many basic behaviors, a tendency to be social, to band together in units, to be intelligent, and to manipulate our environment. But, we may be set apart by a greater balance to deal frontally with other parts of our neuraxis and the events provoked in these areas by our environment. In this regard, it is of great interest to find that white-matter volume of the prefrontal cortices is, in fact, the one anatomical variable that distinguishes humans from apes. Indeed, this is the neural substrate that governs the balance and precision of neural systems' communication. In essence, we are better wired.

CONCLUSIONS

The neural systems of the limbic system and frontal lobes have been studied extensively for over a century. The results attest to a continually evolving experimental neuroanatomy, where progressively better methods have supplanted earlier and less informative ones, or ones that had very restrictive application such as the Golgi method. Despite the neuroanatomical complexity of these brain areas, the skeleton, or the common wisdom that has survived is largely accurate. For example, Papez's original circuit has been found to have few flaws; Cajal's early descriptions of hippocampal and limbic lobe circuitry remain intact and the descriptions of extensive interconnections of the frontal lobe with other association areas and the limbic system are truer than ever. It seems that what has changed the most has been an appreciation for the degree of interaction between structures. These findings have provided fresh insights. In the case of more recent research, the strength and topography of connections between the limbic system and the association cortices has been one of the major payoffs of better methodology. Structures such as the amygdala, cingulate cortex, and hippocampal formation are now known to have extensive and widespread connections with the association cortices. These occur directly rather than via the pathways of Papez's circuit. For example, both the amygdala and hippocampal formation project strongly to parts of the prefrontal cortex, and the amygdala has output to the occipital lobe and to cingulate cortex neurons that give rise to corticospinal projections. The entorhinal cortex conveys cortical association input to the hippocampal formation and, after receiving hippocampal output, projects back strongly to association areas. Among the truly new findings, the nucleus basalis of Meynert projections to all of the cerebral cortex link the hypothalamus to the cortex and provide a manner for the basal forebrain to have widespread cholinergic influence on the cortical mantle. Its projections to the reticular nucleus of the thalamus also establish a morphological basis for it to influence thalamic output before it relays to the cortex. Direct amygdaloid projections to the dorsomedial thalamic nucleus provide a manner for this temporal limbic structure to influence not only the orbital and medial prefrontal cortices, but the extensive dorsolateral prefrontal cortices as well. Lastly, and of critical importance, direct projections from cingulate area M3 to the spinal cord provides an unambiguous manner for the limbic system to influence somatic effectors and behavior, and the extensive prefrontal cortex output to this area gives this cortex more direct influence on lower motor neurons than previously appreciated.

Thus, refined and augmented older findings, and truly new neuroanatomical findings, insure the generation of fruitful hypotheses regarding neural networks that might explain behavior. Furthermore, they provide a richer description of normality against which neurological and psychiatric diseases affecting the limbic system and frontal cortex can be assessed.

References

1. MacLean P. Some psychiatric implications of physiological studies on frontotemporal portion of limbic system (visceral brain). Electroencephalogr Clin Neurophysiol 1952;4:407–418.
2. Papez JW. A proposed mechanism of emotion. Arch Neurol Psychiatry 1937;38:725–743.
3. Scoville WB, Milner B. Loss of recent memory after bilateral hippocampal lesions. J Neurol Neurosurg Psychiatry 1957;20:11–21.
4. Brodal A. The hippocampus and the sense of smell. A review. Brain 1947;70:179–222.
5. Damasio AR, Van Hoesen GW. Emotional disturbances associated with focal lesions of the limbic frontal lobe. In: Heilman KM, Satz P, eds. Neuropsychology of human emotion. New York: Guilford Press, 1983:85–108.
6. Finger S. Origins of neuroscience: a history of explorations into brain function. New York: Oxford University Press, 1994.
7. Goldman-Rakic PS. Working memory dysfunction in schizophrenia. J Neuropsychiatry 1994;6:348–357.
8. Eslinger PJ, Damasio AR. Severe disturbance of higher cognition after bilateral frontal lobe ablation: patient EVR. Neurology 1985;35:1731–1741.
9. Damasio AR. Descartes' error. New York: Grosset and Putnam Publishers, 1994.
10. Weinberger DR, Aloia MS, Goldberg TE, Berman KF. The frontal lobes and schizophrenia. J Neuropsychiatry 1994;6:419–427.
11. Van Hoesen GW, Alheid GF, Heimer L. Major brain structures. In: Kaplan HI, Sadock BJ, eds. Comprehensive textbook of psychiatry. 5th ed. Baltimore: Williams & Wilkins, 1989:5–26.
12. Brodmann K. Beitrage zur histologischen localisation der grosshirnrinde. III. Mitteilung: die rindenfelder der niederen. J Psych Neurol 1905;4:177–266.
13. Braak H. A primitive gigantopyramidal field buried in the depth of the cingulate sulcus of the human brain. Brain Res 1976;109:219–233.
14. Vogt BA, Pandya DN, Rosene DL. Cingulate cortex of the rhesus monkey: I. Cytoarchitecture and thalamic afferents. J Comp Neurol 1987;262:256–270.
15. Baleydier C, Mauguiere F. The duality of the cingulate gyrus in monkey. Neuroanatomical study and functional hypotheses. Brain 1980;103:525–554.
16. Vogt BA, Pandya DN. Cingulate cortex of rhesus monkey: II. Cortical afferents. J Comp Neurol 1987;262:271–289.
17. Van Hoesen GW, Morecraft RJ, Vogt BA. Connections of the monkey cingulate cortex. In: Vogt BA, Gabriel M, eds. Neurobiology of the cingulate cortex and limbic thalamus: a comprehensive handbook. Boston: Birkhauser, 1993:249–284.
18. Muakkassa KF, Strick PL. Frontal lobe inputs to primate motor cortex: evidence for four somatotopically organized "premotor" areas. Brain Res 1979;177:176–182.
19. Pandya DN, Van Hoesen GW, Mesulam M-M. Efferent connections of the cingulate gyrus in the rhesus monkey. Exp Brain Res 1981;42:319–330.
20. Mesulam M-M, Mufson EJ. Insula of the old world monkey. III. Efferent cortical output and comments on function. J Comp Neurol 1982;212:38–52.
21. Mufson EJ, Mesulam M-M. Insula of the old world monkey. II: Afferent cortical input and comments on the claustrum. J Comp Neurol 1982;212:23–37.
22. Petrides M, Pandya DN. Projections to the frontal cortex from the posterior parietal region in the rhesus monkey. J Comp Neurol 1984;228:105–116.
23. Vogt BA, Pandya DN. Cingulate cortex of rhesus monkey: II. Cortical afferents. J Comp Neurol 1987;262:271–289.
24. Selemon LD, Goldman-Rakic PS. Common cortical and subcortical targets of the dorsolateral prefrontal and posterior parietal cortices in the rhesus monkey: evidence for a distributed neural network subserving spatially guided behavior. J Neurosci 1988;8:4049–4068.
25. Vogt BA, Barbas H. Structure and connections of the cingulate vocalization region in the rhesus monkey. In: Newmann JD, ed. The physiological control of mammalian vocalization. New York: Plenum Press, 1988;203–225.
26. Cavada CC, Goldman-Rakic PS. Posterior parietal cortex in rhesus monkey. I: Parcellation of areas based on distinctive limbic and sensory corticocortical connections. J Comp Neurol 1989;287:393–421.
27. Morecraft RJ. The cortical and subcortical efferent and afferent connections of a proposed cingulate motor cortex and its topographical relationship to the primary and supplementary motor cortices of the rhesus monkey. The University of Iowa, Iowa City, IA 1989;1-297 thesis.
28. Morecraft RJ, Van Hoesen GW. Cingulate input to the primary and supplementary motor cortices in the rhesus monkey: evidence for somatotopy in areas 24c and 23c. J Comp Neurol 1992;322:471–489.
29. Morecraft RJ, Van Hoesen GW. Frontal granular cortex input to the cingulate (M3), supplementary (M2) and primary (M1) motor cortices in the rhesus monkey. J Comp Neurol 1993;337:669–688.
30. Morecraft RJ, Geula C, Mesulam M-M. Architecture of connectivity within a cingulo-fronto-parietal neurocognitive network for directed attention. Arch Neurol 1993;50:279–284.
31. Sutherland RJ, Whishaw IQ, Kolb B. Contributions of cingulate cortex to two forms of spatial learning and memory. J Neurosci 1988;8:1863–1872.
32. Sikes RW, Vogt BA. Nociceptive neurons in area 24 of the rabbit cingulate cortex. J Neurophysiol 1992;68:1720–1732.
33. MacLean PD, Newman JD. Role of midline frontolimbic cortex in the production of the isolation call of squirrel monkeys. Brain Res 1988;45:111–123.
34. Arroyo A, Lesser RA, Gordon B, et al. Mirth, laughter and gelastic seizures. Brain 1993;116:757–780.
35. Smith WK. The functional significance of the rostral cingular cortex as revealed by its responses to electrical excitation. J Neurophysiol 1945;8:241–259.
36. Ward AA. The cingular gyrus: area 24. J Neurophysiol 1948;11:13–23.
37. Kaada BR, Pribram KH, Epstein JA. Respiratory and vascular response in monkeys from temporal pole, insula, orbital surface and cingulate gyrus. J Neurophysiol 1949;12:348–356.
38. Neafsey EJ. Prefrontal autonomic control in the rat: anatomical and electrophysiological observations. Prog Brain Res 1990;85:147–166.
39. Neafsey EJ, Terreberry RR, Hurley KM, et al. Anterior cingulate cortex in rodents: connections, visceral control functions, and implications for emotion. In: Vogt BA, Gabriel M, eds. Neurobiology of the cingulate cortex and limbic thalamus: a comprehensive handbook. Boston: Birkhauser, 1993;206–223.
40. Talairach J, Bancaud J, Geier S, et al. The cingulate gyrus and human behavior. Electroencephagr Clin Neurophysiol 1973;34:45–52.
41. Mitz AR, Wise SP. The somatotopic organization of the supplementary motor area: intracortical microstimulation mapping. J Neurosci 1987;7:1010–1021.
42. Luppino G, Matelli M, Camarda RM, et al. Multiple representations of body movement in mesial area 6 and the adjacent cingulate cortex: an intracortical microstimulation study in the macaque monkey. J Comp Neurol 1991;311:463–482.
43. Shima K, Aya K, Mushiake H, et al. Two movement-related foci in the primate cingulate cortex observed in signal-triggered and self-paced forelimb movements. J Neurophysiol 1991;65:188–202.
44. Hutchins KD, Martino AM, Strick PL. Corticospinal projections from the medial wall of the hemisphere. Exp Brain Res 1988;71:667–672.
45. Morecraft RJ, Van Hoesen GW. Somatotopical organization of cingulate projections to the primary and supplementary motor cortices in the old-world monkey. Society for Neuroscience Abstracts 1988;14:820.
46. Dum RP, Strick PL. The origin of corticospinal projections from the premotor areas in the frontal lobe. J Neurosci 1991;11:667–689.

47. Paus T, Petrides M., Evans AC., et al. Role of the human anterior cingulate cortex in the control of oculomotor, manual, and speech responses: a positron emission tomography study. J Neurophysiol 1993;70:453–469.

48. Sanides F. Comparative architectonics of the neocortex of mammals and their evolutionary interpretation. Ann N Y Acad Sci 1969;167:404–423.

49. Humphrey DR, Gold R, Reed DJ. Sizes, laminar and topographic origins of cortical projections to the major divisions of the red nucleus in the monk. J Comp Neurol 1984;225:75–94.

50. Morecraft RJ, Van Hoesen GW. Descending projections to the basal ganglia, red nucleus and pontine nuclei from the cingulate motor cortex (M3 or area 24c) in the rhesus monkey. Society for Neuroscience Abstracts 1994;20:986.

51. Morecraft RJ, Keifer J, Saoi DJ. The corticospinal projection from the cingulate motor cortex (M3 or area 24c) to the cervical enlargement in rhesus monkey. Soc Neurosci Abst, 1995; in press.

52. Bates JF, Goldman-Rakic PS. Prefrontal connections of medial motor areas in the rhesus monkey. J Comp Neurol 1993;336:211–228.

53. Lu MT, Preston JB, Strick PL. Interconnections between the prefrontal cortex and the premotor areas in the frontal lobe. J Comp Neurol 1994;341:375–392.

54. Morecraft RJ, Van Hoesen GW. Convergence of limbic input to the cingulate motor cortex in rhesus monkey. J Comp Neurol, 1996; in press.

55. Blackstad TW. Commissural connections of the hippocampal region in the rat, with special reference to their mode of termination. J Comp Neurol 1956;105:417–537.

56. Van Hoesen GW. The parahippocampal gyrus: new observations regarding its cortical connections in the monkey. Trends Neurosci 1982;5:345–350.

57. Rosene DL, Van Hoesen GW. The hippocampal formation of the primate brain: a review of some comparative aspects of cytoarchitecture and connections. In: Jones EG, Peters A, ed. Cerebral cortex. Further aspects of cortical function, including hippocampus, vol. 6. New York: Plenum Press, 1987:345–456.

58. Duvernoy HM. The human hippocampus. An atlas of applied anatomy. München, Bergmann, 1988:1–66.

59. Amaral DG, Insausti R. The hippocampal formation. In: Paxinos G, ed. The human nervous system. New York: Academic Press, 1990.

60. Cajal Ramón y S. Studies on the cerebral cortex. Chicago: Year Book, 1955:1–174.

61. Cajal Ramón y S. The structure of Ammon's horn. Translated by Kraft LM. Springfield: Charles C Thomas, 1968:78.

62. Hjorth-Simonsen A. Some intrinsic connections of the hippocampus in the rat: an experimental analysis. J Comp Neurol 1973;147:145–162.

63. Andersen P, Bland BH, Dudar JD. Organization of the hippocampal output. Exp Brain Res 1973;17:152–168.

64. Swanson LW, Cowan WM. Hippocampo-hypothalamic connections: origin in subicular cortex, not Ammon's horn. Science 1975;189:303–304.

65. Meibach RC, Siegel A. The origin of fornix fibers which project to the mammillary bodies of the rat: a horseradish peroxidase study. Brain Res 1975;88:518–522.

66. Rosene DL, Van Hoesen GW. Hippocampal efferents reach widespread areas of the cerebral cortex and amygdala in the rhesus monkey. Science 1977;198:315–317.

67. Swanson LW, Wyss JM, Cowan WM. An autoradiographic study of the organization of intrahippocampal association pathways in the rat. J Comp Neurol 1978;181:681–716.

68. Sorenson KE, Shipley MT. Projections from the subiculum to the deep layers of the ipsilateral presubicular and entorhinal cortices in the guinea pig. J Comp Neurol 1979;188:313–334.

69. Van Hoesen GW, Pandya DN, Butters N. Cortical afferents to the entorhinal cortex of the rhesus monkey. Science 1972;175:1471–1473.

70. Van Hoesen GW, Pandya DN. Some connections of the entorhinal (area 28) and perirhinal (area 35) cortices of the rhesus monkey. II. Efferent connections. Brain Res 1975;95:39–59.

71. Shipley MT. The topographic and laminar organization of the presubiculum's projection to the ipsi- and contralateral entorhinal cortex in the guinea pig. J Comp Neurol 1975;160:127–146.

72. Van Hoesen GW, Rosene DL, Mesulam M-M. Subicular input from temporal cortex in the rhesus monkey. Science 1979;205:608–610.

73. Amaral DG, Insausti R, Cowan WM. Evidence for a direct projection from the superior temporal gyrus to the entorhinal cortex in the monkey. Brain Res 1983;275:263–277.

74. Insausti R, Amaral DG, Cowen WM. The entorhinal cortex of the monkey: II. Cortical afferents. J Comp Neurol 1987;264:356–395.

75. Witter MP. Organization of the entorhinal–hippocampal system: a review of current anatomical data. Hippocampus 1993;3:33–44.

76. Suzuki WA, Amaral DG. Topographic organization of the reciprocal connections between the monkey entorhinal cortex and the perirhinal and parahippocampal cortices. J Neurosci Methods 1994;14:1856–1877.

77. Krettek JE, Price JL. Projections from the amygdala to the perirhinal and entorhinal cortices and the subiculum. Brain Res 1974;71:150–154.

78. Herkenham M. The connections of the nucleus reuniens thalami: evidence for a direct thalamo-hippocampal pathway in the rat. J Comp Neurol 1978;177:589–610.

79. Amaral DG, Cowan WM. Subcortical afferents to the hippocampal formation in the monkey. J Comp Neurol 1980;189:573–591.

80. Whitlock DG, Nauta WJH. Subcortical projections from the temporal neocortex in Macaca mulatta. J Comp Neurol 1956;106:183–212.

81. Herzog AG, Van Hoesen GW. Temporal neocortical afferent connections to the amygdala in the rhesus monkey. Brain Res 1976;115:57–69.

82. Turner BH, Mishkin M, Knapp M. Organization of the amygdalopetal projections from modality-specific cortical association areas in the monkey. J Comp Neurol 1980;191:515–543.

83. Van Hoesen GW. The different distribution, diversity and sprouting of cortical projections to the amygdala in the rhesus monkey. In: Ben Ari Y, ed. The amygdaloid complex. New York: Elsevier, 1981:77–90.

84. Amaral DG, Veazey RB, Cowan WM. Some observations on hypothalamo-amygdaloid connections in the monkey. Brain Res 1982;252:13–27.

85. Aggleton JP, Burton MJ, Passingham RE. Cortical and subcortical afferents to the amygdala of the rhesus monkey (Macaca mulatta). Brain Res 1980;190:347–368.

86. Woolf NJ, Butcher LL. Cholinergic projections to the basolateral amygdala: a combined Evans blue and acetylcholinesterase analysis. Brain Res Bull 1982;8:751–763.

87. Mehler WR. Subcortical afferent connections of the amygdala in the monkey. J Comp Neurol 1980;190:733–762.

88. Jones EG, Powell TPS. An anatomical study of converging sensory pathways within the cerebral cortex of the monkey. Brain 1970;93:793–820.

89. Klinger J, Gloor P. The connections of the amygdala and of the anterior temporal cortex in the human brain. J Comp Neurol 1960;115:333–369.

90. Mufson EJ, Mesulam M-M, Pandya DN. Insular interconnections with the amygdala in the rhesus monkey. Neuroscience 1981;6:1231–1248.

91. Krettek JE, Price JL. Projections from the amygdaloid complex and adjacent olfactory structures to the entorhinal cortex and to the subiculum in the rat and cat. J Comp Neurol 1977;172:723–752.

92. Amaral DG, Price JL. Amygdalo-cortical projections in the monkey (Macaca fascicularis). J Comp Neurol 1984;230:465–496.

93. Saunders RC, Rosene DL. A comparison of the efferents of the amygdala and the hippocampal formation in the rhesus monkey: I. Convergence in the entorhinal, prorhinal and perirhinal cortices. J Comp Neurol 1988;271:153–184.

94. Saunders RC, Rosene DL, Van Hoesen GW. Comparison of the afferents of the amygdala and hippocampal formation in the rhesus monkey: II. Reciprocal and non-reciprocal connections. J Comp Neurol 1988;271:185–207.

95. Price JL, Amaral DG. An autoradiographic study of the projections of the central nucleus of the monkey amygdala. J Neurosci 1982;1:1242–1259.

96. Nauta WJH. Fibre degeneration following lesions of the amygdaloid complex in the monkey. J Anat 1961;95:515–531.

97. Porrino LJ, Crane AM, Goldman-Rakic PS. Direct and indirect pathways from the amygdala to the frontal lobe in rhesus monkeys. J Comp Neurol 1981;198:121–136.

98. Aggleton JP, Mishkin M. Projections of the amygdala to the thalamus in the cynomolgus monkey. J Comp Neurol 1984;222:56–68.

99. Hopkins DA, Holstege G. Amygdaloid projections to the mesencephalon, pons and medulla oblongata in the cat. Exp Brain Res 1978;32:529–547.

100. Jacobson S, Trojanowski JQ. Amygdaloid projections to prefrontal granular cortex in rhesus monkey demonstrated with horseradish peroxidase. Brain Res 1975;100:132–139.

101. Krettek JE, Price JL. Projections from the amygdaloid complex and adjacent olfactory structures to the entorhinal cortex and to the subiculum in the rat and cat. J Comp Neurol 1977;172:723–752.

102. Avendano C, Price JL, Amaral DG. Evidence for an amygdaloid projection to premotor cortex but not to motor cortex in the monkey. Brain Res 1983;264:111–117.

103. Kelley AE, Domesick VB, Nauta WJH. The amygdalostriatal projection in the rat—an anatomical study by anterograde and retrograde tracing methods. Neuroscience 1982;7:615–630.

104. Kievit J, Kuypers HGJM. Basal forebrain and hypothalamic connections to the frontal and parietal cortex in the rhesus monkey. Science 1975;187:660–662.

105. Divac I. Magnocellular nuclei of the basal forebrain project to neocortex, brain stem and olfactory bulb: review of some functional correlates. Brain Res 1975;93:385–398.

106. Jones EG, Burton H, Saper CB, Swanson LW. Midbrain, diencephalic and cortical relationships of the basal nucleus of Meynert and associated structures in primates. J Comp Neurol 1976;167:385–420.

107. Mesulam M-M, Van Hoesen GW. Acetylcholinesterase containing basal forebrain neurons in the rhesus monkey project to neocortex. Brain Res 1976;109:152–157.

108. Pearson RCA, Gather KC, Bridal P, Power TPS. The projection of the basal nucleus of Meynert upon the neocortex in the monkey. Brain Res 1983;259:132–136.

109. Whitehouse PJ, Price DL, Clark AW, Coyle JT, De Long MR. Alzheimer disease: evidence for selective loss of cholinergic neurons in the nucleus basalis. Ann Neurol 1981;10:122–126.

110. Mesulam M-M, Mufson EJ, Levey AI, Wainer BH. Cholinergic innervation of cortex by the basal forebrain: cytochemistry and cortical connections of the septal area, diagonal band nuclei, nucleus basalis (subsantia innominata), and hypothalamus in the rhesus monkey. J Comp Neurol 1983;214:170–197.

111. Wenk H, Bigl V, Meyer V. Cholinergic projections from magnocellular nuclei of the basal forebrain to cortical areas in rats. Brain Res Rev 1980;2:295–316.

112. Fibiger HC. The organization and some projections of cholinergic neurons of the mammalian forebrain. Brain Res Rev 1982;4:327–388.

113. Levey AI, Hallanger AE, Wainer BH. Cholinergic nucleus basalis neurons may influence the cortex via the thalamus. Neurosci Lett 1987;74:7–13.

114. Buzsaki G, Bickford RG, Ponomareff G, Thal LJ, Mandel R, Gage FH. Nucleus basalis and thalamic control of neocortical activity in the freely moving rat. J Neurosci 1988;8:4007–4026.

115. Asanuma C. Axonal arborizations of a magnocellular basal nucleus input and their relation to the neurons in the thalamic reticular nucleus of rats. Proc Natl Acad Sci USA 1989;86:4746–4750.

116. Tourtellotte WG, Van Hoesen GW, Hyman BT, Tikoo RK, Damasio AR. Alz-50 immunoreactivity in the thalamic reticular nucleus in Alzheimer's disease. Brain Res 1989;515:227–234.

117. Jones EG. Some aspects of the organization of the thalamic reticular complex. J Comp Neurol 1975;162:285–308.

118. Mesulam M-M, Mufson EJ. Neural inputs into the nucleus basalis of the substantia innominata in the rhesus monkey. Brain Res 1984;107:253–274.

119. Nauta WJH, Haymaker W. Hypothalamic nuclear and fiber connections. In: Haymaker W, Anderson E, Nauta WJH, eds. The hypothalamus. Springfield, IL: Charles C. Thomas 1969:136–209.

120. Saper CB, Swanson LW, Cowan WM. Some afferent connections of the rostral hypothalamus in the squirrel monkey (saimiri sciureus) cat. J Comp Neurol 1979;184:205–242.

121. Price JL, Amaral DG. An autoradiographic study of the projections of the central nucleus of the monkey amygdala. J Neurosci 1981;1:1242–1259.

122. Victor M, Adams RD, Collins GH. The Wernicke-Korsakoff syndrome. Philadelphia: FA Davis, 1971:1–206.

123. Squire LR, Moore RY. Dorsal thalamic lesion in a noted case of chronic memory dysfunction. Ann Neurol 1979; 6:505–506.

124. Graff-Radford NR, Eslinger PJ, Damasio AR, Yamada T. Nonhemorrhagic infarction of the thalamus: behavioral, anatomical and physiological correlates. Neurology 1984;34:14–23.

125. Akert K. Comparative anatomy of the frontal cortex and thalamocortical connections. In: Warren JM, Akert K, eds. The frontal granular cortex and behavior. New York: McGraw-Hill, 1964:372–396.

126. Goldman-Rakic PS, Porrino LJ. The primate medial dorsal (MD) nucleus and its projection to the frontal lobe. J Comp Neurol 1985;242:535–560.

127. Ray JP, Price JL. The organization of projections from the mediodorsal nucleus of the thalamus to orbital and medial prefrontal cortex in macaque monkeys. J Comp Neurol 1993;337:1–31.

128. Tobias TJ. Afferents to prefrontal cortex from the thalamic mediodorsal nucleus in the rhesus monkey. Brain Res 1975;83:191–212.

129. Tanaka D. Thalamic projections of the dorso-medial prefrontal cortex in the rhesus monkey (Macaca mulatta). Brain Res 1976;110:21–38.

130. Arikuni T, Sakai M, Kubota K. Columnar aggregation of prefrontal and anterior cingulate cortical cells projecting to the thalamic mediodorsal nucleus in the monkey. J Comp Neurol 1983;220:116–125.

131. Penfield W, Welch K. The supplementary motor area of the cerebral cortex: a clinical and experimental study. Arch Neurol Psychiatry 1951;66:289–317.

132. Woolsey CN, Settlage PH, Meyer DR, Sencer W, Hamuy TP, Travis AM. Patterns of localization in precentral and "supplementary" motor areas and their relation to the concept of a premotor area. Res Publ Assoc Res Nerv Ment Dis 1952;30:238–264.

133. Barbas H, Pandya DN. Architecture and frontal cortical connections of the premotor cortex (area 6) in the rhesus monkey. J Comp Neurol 1987;256:211–228.

134. Mitz AR, Wise SP. The somatotopic organization of the supplementary motor area: intracortical microstimulation mapping. J Neurosci 1987;7:1010–1021.

135. Rizzolatti G, Camarda R, Fogassi L, et al. Functional organization of inferior area 6 in the macaque monkey II. Area F5 and the control of distal movements. Exp Brain Res 1988;71:491.

136. Wurtz RH, Mohler CW. Enhancement of visual responses in the monkey striate cortex and frontal eye fields. J Neurophysiol 1976;39:766–772.

137. Schlage J, Schlag-Rey M. Evidence for a supplementary eye field. J Neurophysiol 1987;57:179–200.

138. Huerta MF, Krubitzer LA, Kaas JH. Frontal eye field as defined by intracortical microstimulation in squirrel monkeys, owl monkeys and macaque monkeys: II. Cortical connections. J Comp Neurol 1987;265:332–361.

139. Di Pellegrino G, Wise SP. A neurophysiological comparison of three

distinct regions of the primate frontal lobe. Brain 1991;114: 951–978.

140. Luppino G, Matelli M, Camarda RM, Rizzolatti G. Corticocortical connections of area F3 (SMA-proper) and area F6 (pre-SMA) in the macaque monkey. J Comp Neurol 1993;338:114–140.

141. Walker AE. A cytoarchitectural study of the prefrontal area in the macaque monkey. J Comp Neurol 1940;262:256–270.

142. Barbas H, Pandya DN. Architecture and intrinsic connections of the prefrontal cortex in the rhesus monkey. J Comp Neurol 1989;286: 353–375.

143. Preuss TM, Goldman-Rakic PS. Myelo- and cytoarchitecture of the granular frontal cortex and surrounding regions in the strepsirhine primate galago and the anthropoid primate macaca. J Comp Neurol 1991;310:429–474.

144. Morecraft RJ, Geula C, Mesulam M-M. Cytoarchitecture and neural afferents of orbitofrontal cortex in the brain of the monkey. J Comp Neurol 1992;323:341–358.

145. Carmichael ST, Price JL. Architectonic subdivision of the orbital and medial prefrontal cortex in the Macaque monkey. J Comp Neurol 1994;346:366–402.

146. Harlow JM. Recovery from the passage of an iron bar through the head. Mass Med Soc Pub 1868;2:327–346.

147. Geschwind N. Disconnexion syndromes in animals and man. I. Brain 1965;88:237–294.

148. Roland PE, Friberg L. Localization of cortical areas activated by thinking. J Neurophysiol 1985;53:1219–1243.

149. Goldman-Rakic PS. Circuitry of prefrontal cortex and regulation of behavior by representational memory. In: Mountcastle VB, Plum F, eds. Handbook of physiology. The nervous system. Bethesda: American Physiological Society, 1987;5:373–417.

150. Fuster JM. The prefrontal cortex. Anatomy, physiology and neuropsychiatry of the frontal lobe. 2nd edition. New York: Raven Press, 1989.

151. Freund H-J. Abnormalities of motor behavior after cortical lesions in humans. In: Mountcastle VB, Plum F, eds. Handbook of physiology. the nervous system, vol. 5. Bethesda: American Physiological Society 1990;763–810.

152. Mesulam M-M. Large-scale neurocognitive networks and distributed processing for attention, language, and memory. Ann Neurol 1990;28:597–613.

153. Damasio H, Grabowski T, Frank R, Galaburda AM, Damsio AR. The return of Phineas Gage: clues about the brain from the skull of a famous patient. Science 1994;264:1102–1105.

154. Damasio AR. The time-locked multiregional retroactivation: a systems level proposal for the neural substrates of recall and recognition. Cognition 1989;33:25.

155. Pandya DN, Kuypers HGJM. Cortico-cortical connections in the rhesus monkey. Brain Res 1969;13:13–36.

156. Felleman DJ, Van Essen DC. Distributed hierarchical processing in the primate cerebral cortex. Cereb Cortex 1991;1:1–47.

157. Ungerleider LG, Mishkin M. Two cortical visual systems: In: Ingle DG, Goodale MA, Mansfield RJQ, eds. Analysis of visual behavior. Cambridge, MA: MIT Press, 1992;549–586.

158. Wilson FAW, Scalaidhe SPO, Goldman-Rakic PS. Dissociation of object and spatial processing domains in primate prefrontal cortex. Science 1993;260:1955.

159. Goldman-Rakic, PS, Selemon LD, Schwartz ML. Dual pathways connecting the dorsolateral prefrontal cortex with the hippocampal formation and parahippocampal cortex in the rhesus monkey. Neuroscience 1984;12:719–743.

160. Moran MA, Mufson EJ, Mesulam M-M. Neural input into the temporopolar cortex of the rhesus monkey. J Comp Neurol 1987; 256:88–103.

161. Barbas H, De Olmos J. Projections from the amygdala to basoventral and mediodorsal prefrontal regions in the rhesus monkey. J Comp Neurol 1990;300:549–571.

162. Biber MP, Kneisley LW, LaVail JH. Cortical neurons projecting to the cervical and lumbar enlargements of the spinal cord in young adult rhesus monkeys. Exp Neurol 1978;59:492–508.

163. Murray EA, Coulter JD. Organization of corticospinal neurons in the monkey. J Comp Neurol 1981;195:339–365.

164. He SQ, Dum RP, Strick PL. Topographic organization of corticospinal projections from the frontal lobe: motor areas on the lateral surface of the hemisphere. J Neurosci 1993;13:952–980.

165. Goldman PS, Nauta WJH. An intricately patterned prefronto-caudate projection in the rhesus monkey. J Comp Neurol 1977;171: 369–386.

166. Yeterian EH, Van Hoesen GW. Cortico-striate projections in the rhesus monkey: the organization of certain cortico-caudate connections. Brain Res 1978;139:43–63.

167. Yeterian EH, Pandya DN. Prefrontostriatal connections in relation to cortical architectonic organization in rhesus monkeys. J Comp Neurol 1991;312:43–67.

168. Nauta WJH. Neural associations of the frontal cortex. Acta Neurobiol Exp 1972;32:125–140.

169. Kievit J, Kuypers HGJM. Organization of the thalamo-cortical connexions to the frontal lobe in the rhesus monkey. Exp Brain Res 1977;29:299–322.

170. Barbas H, Haswell-Henion TH, Dermon CR. Diverse thalamic projections to the prefrontal cortex in the rhesus monkey. J Comp Neurol 1991;313:65–94.

171. Yeterian EH, Pandya DN. Corticothalamic connections of paralimbic regions in the rhesus monkey. J Comp Neurol 1988;269:130–146.

172. Goldman PS, Nauta WJH. Autoradiographic demonstration of a projection from prefrontal association cortex to the superior colliculus in the rhesus monkey. Brain Res 1976;116:145–149.

173. Leichnetz GR. The prefrontal cortico-oculomotor trajectories in the monkey. J Neurol Sci 1981;49:387–396.

174. Brodal P. The corticopontine projection in the rhesus monkey: origin and principles of organization. Brain 1978;101:251–283.

175. Middleton FA, Strick PL. Anatomical evidence for cerebellar and basal ganglia involvement in higher cognitive function. Science 1994;266:458–461.

176. Aston-Jones G, Ennis M, Pieribone VA, et al. The brain nucleus locus coeruleus: restricted afferent control of a broad efferent network. Science 1986;234:734–737.

177. Mesulam M-M. Asymmetry of neural feedback in the organization of behavioral states. Science 1987;237:537–538 (Letter).

178. Arnsten AFT, Goldman-Rakic PS. Selective prefrontal cortical projections to the region of the locus coeruleus and raphe nuclei in the rhesus monkey. Brain Res 1984;306:9–18.

179. Corsellis JAN. The limbic areas in Alzheimer's disease and in other conditions associated with dementia. In: Wolstenhome GEW, O'Connor M, eds. London: Churchill Livingstone, 1970:37–45.

180. Brun A, Gustafson L. Distribution of cerebral degeneration in Alzheimer's disease. Arch Psychiatr Nervenk 1976;223:15–33.

181. Schoene WC. Degenerative diseases of the central nervous system. In: Davis RL, Robertson DM, eds. Textbook of neuropathology. Baltimore: Williams & Wilkins, 1985;788–823.

182. Berman KF, Weinberger DR. The prefrontal cortex in schizophrenia and other neuropsychiatric diseases: in vivo physiological correlates of cognitive deficits. Prog Brain Res 1990;85:521–537.

183. Weinberger DR. A connectionist approach to the prefrontal cortex. J Neuropsychiatry 1993;241–253.

184. Weinberger DR, Aloia MS, Goldberg TE, Berman KF. The frontal lobes and schizophrenia. J Neuropsychiatry 1994;6:419–427.

185. Damasio AR, Van Hoesen GW. The limbic system and the localisation of herpes simplex encephalitis. J Neurol Neurosurg Psychiatry 1985;48:297–301.

186. Sutton RC, Lipper MH, Brashear HR. Limbic encephalitis occurring in association with Alzheimer's disease. J Neurol Neurosurg Psychiatry 1993;56;808–811.

187. Khan N, Wieser HG. Limbic encephalitis: a case report. Epilepsy Res 1994;17:175–181.

188. Hyman BT, Van Hoesen GW, Damasio AR, Barnes CL. Alzheimer's disease: cell specific pathology isolates the hippocampal formation. Science 1984;225:1168–1170.

189. Arnold SE, Hyman BT, Van Hoesen GW, Damasio AR. Cytoarchitectural abnormalities of the entorhinal cortex in schizophrenia. Arch Gen Psychiatry 1991;48:625–632.

190. Braak H, Braak E. Neuropathological stageing of Alzheimer-related changes. Acta Neuropathol (Berl) 1991;82:239–259.

191. Van Hoesen GW, Hyman BT, Damasio AR. Entorhinal cortex pathology in Alzheimer's disease. Hippocampus 1991;1:1–8.

192. Van Hoesen GW, Solodkin A. Some modular features of temporal cortex in humans as revealed by pathological changes in Alzheimer's disease. Cerebral Cortex 1993;3:465–475.

193. Arnold SE, Hyman BT, Van Hoesen GW. Neuropathologic changes of the temporal pole in Alzheimer's disease and Pick's disease. Arch Neurol 1994;51:145–150.

194. Jakob H, Beckmann H. Prenatal developmental disturbances in the limbic allocortex in schizophrenics. J Neural Transm 1986;65:303–326.

195. Benes FM, McSparren J, Bird ED, SanGiovanni JP, Vincent SL. Deficits in small interneurons in prefrontal and cingulate cortices of schizophrenic and schizoaffective patients. Arch Gen Psychiatry 1991;48:996–1001.

196. Suddath RL, Casanova MF, Goldberg TE, Daniel DG, Kelsoe JR, Weinberger DR. Temporal lobe pathology in schizophrenia: a quantitative magnetic resonance imaging study. Am J Psychiatry 1989;146:464–472.

197. Baldwin B, Förstl H. "Pick's Disease" – 101 years on still there, but in need of reform. Br J Psychiatry 1993;163:100–104.

198. Pickering-Brown SM, Siddons M, Mann DMA, Owen F, Neary D, Snowden JS. Apolipoprotein E allelic frequencies in patients with lobar atrophy. Neurosci Lett 1995;188:205–207.

199. Brun A, England B, Gustafson L, et al. Clinical and neuropathological criteria for fronto-temporal dementia. J Neurol Neurosurg Psychiatry 1994;57:416–418.

200. Akbarian S, Bunney WE, Potkin SG, et al. Altered distribution of nicotinamide-adenine dinucleotide phosphate-diaphorase cells in frontal lobe of schizophrenics implies disturbances of cortical development. Arch Gen Psychiatry 1993;50:169–177.

201. Akbarian S, Viñuela A, Kim JJ, Potkin SG, Bunney WE, Jones EG. Distorted distribution of nicotinamide-adenine dinucleotide phosphate-diaphorase neurons in temporal lobe of schizophrenics implies anomalous cortical development. Arch Gen Psychiatry 1993;50:178–187.

202. Goldman-Rakic PS. Cellular and circuit basis of working memory in prefrontal cortex of nonhuman primates. Prog Brain Res 1990;85:325–336.

203. Clarke E, Dewhurst K. An illustrated history of brain function. University of California Press, 1972.

204. Gould SJ. The mismeasure of man. W. W. Norton, 1981.

205. Zola-Morgan S. Localization of brain function: the legacy of Franz Joseph Gall (1758–1828). In: Cowan WM, Shooter EM, Stevens CF, Thompson RF, eds. Ann Rev Neurosci 1995;18:359–384.

206. Bianchi L. The mechanism of the brain and the functions of the frontal lobes. Edinburgh: Churchill Livingstone, 1922.

207. Brodmann K. Neue ergebnisse uber die vergleichende histologische Lokalisation der Grobhirnrinde mit besonderer Berücksichtigung des Stirnhirns. Anat Anz 1912;41:157–216.

208. Leboucq G. Le rapport poids-surface dans le cerveau des singes. In: Collin R, ed. Comptes rendus de l'association des anatomistes. Bull Assoc Anat (Nancy) 1928;2:268–273.

209. Tilney F. The brain from ape to man. New York: Paul B. Hoeber, Inc., 1928.

210. Weil A. Measurements of cerebral and cerebellar surfaces. Am J Phys Anthropol 1929;13:69–90.

211. Holloway RL. The evolution of the primate brain. Some aspects of quantitative relations. Brain Res 1968;7:121–172.

212. Jacobsen CF, Wolfe JB, Jackson TA. An experimental analysis of the functions of the frontal association areas in primates. J Nerv Ment Dis 1935;82:1–14.

213. Fulton JF. Physiological basis of frontal lobotomy. Acta Med Scandi (Suppl) 1947;196:617–625.

214. Jacobsen CF. A study of cerebral function in learning: the frontal lobes. J Comp Neurol 1931;52:271–340.

215. Moniz E. Tentatives opératoires dans le traitement de certaines psychoses. Paris: Masson, 1936.

216. Moniz E. Prefrontal leucotomy in the treatment of mental disorders. Am J Psychiatry 1937;93:1379–1385.

217. Ackerly SS, Benton AL. Report of case of bilateral frontal lobe defect. In: Fulton JF, Aring CD, Wortis SB, eds. The frontal lobes. Baltimore: Williams & Wilkins, 1948;479–504.

218. Blinkov SM, Glezer II. Das zentralnervensystem in Zahlen and Tabellen. Jena: Fischer, 1968.

219. Von Bonin G. The frontal lobe of primates: cytoarchitectural studies. Baltimore: Williams & Wilkins, 1948;67–83.

220. Passingham RE. Anatomical differences between the neocortex of man and other primates. Brain Behav Evol 1973;7:337–359.

221. Armstrong E. Evolution of the brain. In: Paxinos G, ed. The human nervous system. New York: Academic Press, 1990;1–16.

222. Semendeferi K. Evolution of the hominoid prefrontal cortex: a quantitative and image analysis of areas 13 and 10. Ph.D. thesis, University of Iowa, 1994 (unpublished).

223. Semendeferi K, Damasio H, Van Hoesen GW. Evolution of the frontal lobes: an MRI study on apes and humans. Society for Neurosciences 1994;20:1415.

8

NEUROCHEMICAL NEUROANATOMY

John B. Penney, Jr.

The human brain is the most complex organized structure known to exist. In addition to the billions of nerve cells with their trillions of synapses, there are dozens of neurotransmitters and neuromodulators. These transmitters, along with their receptors and second messenger systems, make the brain's chemistry unique. This chapter first reviews the synaptic organization that makes neurotransmission possible. It continues with a review of the anatomical distribution of these transmitters, modulators, and their receptors. Finally, the distributions of second messenger systems are briefly described. The numerous other compounds unique to brain are omitted from this chapter. These include some compounds with distinct regional distribution such as growth factors and others such as neurofilament proteins, ion channel proteins in axons, and specific glial markers that are without special regional localization. This review is based on secondary sources, which are cited at the end of the chapter.

SYNAPTIC ORGANIZATION AND NOMENCLATURE

Except for the gases, whose mechanisms of action as neuronal messengers are entirely different, all neurotransmitters require a number of specialized structures at the synapse in order to convey a message from one neuron to another (Fig. 8.1).

Within the presynaptic terminal are the enzymes necessary for synthesis of the neurotransmitter. An exception to this rule is the peptides, which are synthesized on ribosomes in the neuronal cell body and then transported down the axon to the terminal. Terminals typically have several mitochondria to supply energy. Adjacent to the presynaptic membrane are a number of "synaptic vesicles" in which the neurotransmitter is stored. Several "vesicular transporters" have been described. These are proteins that transport the neurotransmitter into the storage vesicle. Vesicular transporters are specific for the neurotransmitter that is being stored.

Along the presynaptic membranes itself, there are a number of specialized molecules. There are also release points to which the synaptic vesicles bind. Once bound, the vesicles fuse with the membrane and release neurotransmitter. There are also high-affinity "neuronal transporters" that

remove the neurotransmitter from the synaptic cleft. These transporters serve two purposes: (*a*) they terminate the action of the most neurotransmitters by removing them from the synaptic cleft; and (*b*) they spare the presynaptic cell the work of resynthesizing the neurotransmitter by providing a pre-made source of the chemical. Neuronal transporters are different proteins from the vesicular transporters. Most of the known neurotransporters are in a single family of proteins. Members of this family transport neurotransmitters across the cell membrane by transporting a sodium and, frequently, a chloride ion along with each molecule of transmitter. The family includes the transporters for GABA, norepinephrine, dopamine, serotonin, glycine, adenosine, and proline. These transporters all share a similar structure having 12 membrane spanning regions (Fig. 8.2). However, three transporters for glutamate that have significant differences from the other family of transporters have been cloned. Instead of transporting a glutamate molecule with a sodium and a chloride ion, the glutamate is transported along with two sodium ions while one potassium ion and one hydroxyl ion are countertransported during the process. The glutamate transporters have a different structure as well with either eight (or possibly 10) transmembrane regions rather than the 12 transmembrane regions found in the main family of neurotransmitter transporters.

There may also be "presynaptic receptors" located on the presynaptic terminal's membrane. These molecules bind neurotransmitters but do not transport them into the terminal. Instead, binding of the transmitter stimulates the receptor to modulate the activity of the terminal through one of two mechanisms. Presynaptic receptors can influence neurotransmitter release by being coupled to ion channels that change the presynaptic terminal's membrane potential. Since neurotransmitter release is governed by the amount of membrane depolarization that occurs when the impulse that has been conducted along the axon reaches the terminal, depolarizing the presynaptic terminal decreases neurotransmitter release while hyperpolarizing it increases release. Alternatively, presynaptic receptors may be coupled via second messengers to either change the rate of neurotransmitter synthesis or to modulate it. *Autoreceptors* bind the neurotransmitter that the pre-

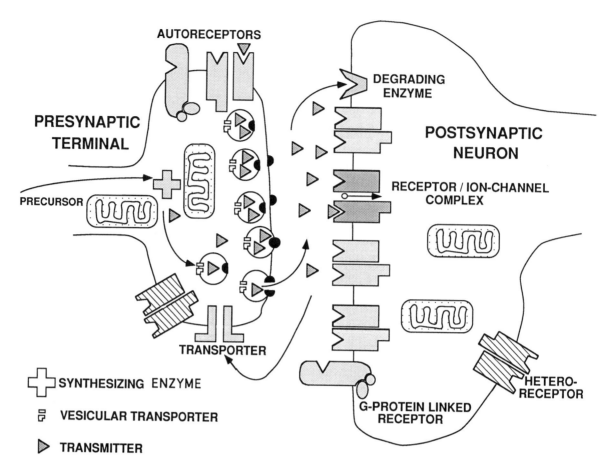

AUTORECEPTORS

PRESYNAPTIC
TERMINAL

DEGRADING
ENZYME

POSTSYNAPTIC
NEURON

PRECURSOR

RECEPTOR / ION-CHANNEL
COMPLEX

TRANSPORTER

G-PROTEIN LINKED
RECEPTOR

HETERO-
RECEPTOR

SYNTHESIZING ENZYME

VESICULAR TRANSPORTER

TRANSMITTER

Figure 8.1. Schematic drawing of the fate of neurotransmitters in synaptic transmission. In the presynaptic terminal the transmitter is synthesized from a precursor, transported into storage vesicles by a vesicular transporter, and released into the synaptic cleft by depolarization of the presynaptic terminal. Once released the transmitter diffuses into the synaptic cleft, where it can interact with receptors that have sites to which it can bind. Receptors can be either on the postsynaptic or the presynaptic cell. Autoreceptors on the presynaptic terminal regulate transmitter synthesis and release. Receptors on the postsynaptic membrane initiate changes in the postsynaptic cell that are the ultimate result of transmission at the synapse. Heteroreceptors (receptors for other neurotransmitters.) may also regulate synaptic activity. Receptors may be either of the ligand-gated ion channel or the G-protein-coupled type. Ligand-gated ion channels open on binding the transmitter to permit passage of ions through the cell's plasma membrane. (One channel is shown being opened and passing an ion on the postsynaptic cell.) G-protein-coupled receptors initiate second messenger cascades within the cells on which they reside. Regardless of whether or not the transmitter binds to a receptor, it eventually is removed from the synapse either by being metabolized by a degrading enzyme so that it is no longer active or by being transported back into the presynaptic terminal by a high-affinity transporter.

synaptic terminal is releasing. *Heteroreceptors* bind other neurotransmitters.

In the synaptic cleft itself are enzymes that degrade the neurotransmitter after it has been released from the presynaptic terminal. These enzymes are particularly important for terminating the actions of acetylcholine and the peptides.

The postsynaptic membrane is studded with a high density of neurotransmitter receptors. Binding of the neurotransmitter to its postsynaptic receptor, except for the gases, starts the postsynaptic cell's response to the transmitter. Receptors are either linked to ion channels that open to initiate the cell's response or are linked to guanosine triphosphate binding proteins (G proteins) which, in turn, activate second messenger systems within the postsynaptic cell. Numerous types of receptor may be located at a single synapse.

The ion channel-linked receptors are made up of multiple subunits, usually five, that are coded by different genes. Each

subunit has four (or, possibly, five) membrane spanning regions with the amino terminal end of the protein being extracellular (Fig. 8.2). The neurotransmitter binds to a site on this portion of the protein, although not all subunits necessarily have binding sites. The second membrane spanning portions of the subunits form the walls of the ion channel. Specific amino acids in this region determine which ions are allowed to pass through the channel. The second intracytoplasmic loop usually contains regions such as phosphorylation sites where the activity of the receptor can be regulated.

G-protein-linked receptors typically have seven membrane spanning regions (Fig. 8.2). The amino terminal end is extracellular. Neurotransmitter appears to bind to sites within the membrane, typically to the third and fifth membrane spanning regions. The third intracellular loop contains most of the regulatory regions. The G protein is coupled to the second and third intracytoplasmic loops along

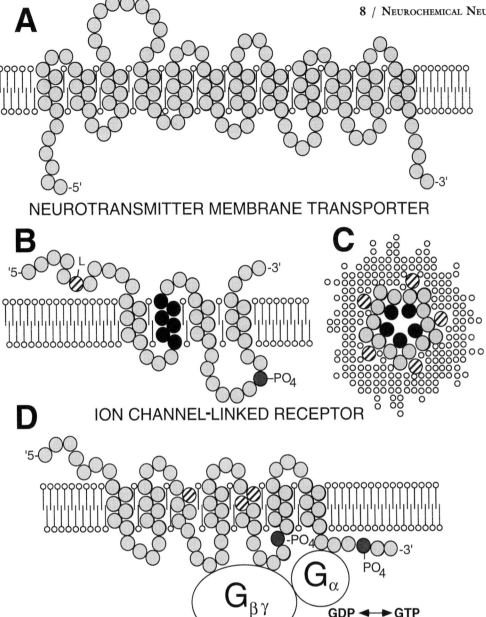

A

NEUROTRANSMITTER MEMBRANE TRANSPORTER

B

ION CHANNEL-LINKED RECEPTOR

C

D

GDP ⟷ GTP

G-PROTEIN-LINKED RECEPTOR

Figure 8.2. Schematic drawing of the presumed shapes of the proteins that bind to neurotransmitters and are inserted in the synaptic membrane. The proteins are shown as a chain of circles that are a simplified representation of the protein's amino acid that make up sequence running from the amino (5′) to the carboxy (3′) terminal. In reality, all the proteins depicted have several times as many amino acids as are shown in these schematics. **A.** Cross-section of a member of the family of high-affinity transporters of neurotransmitters that includes the GABA, norepinephrine, dopamine, and serotonin transporters. These proteins remove transmitters from the synaptic cleft by transporting them into the presynaptic terminal along with sodium and chloride ions. These transporters are thought to have 12 membrane-spanning regions with long 5′ and 3′ intracytoplasmic ends. The second extracellular loop is also thought to be longer than the other loops. The transmitter-binding portions of these transporters and the spot at which the transmitter passes through the membrane remain unknown. **B.** Cross-section of the presumed structure of one of the peptides that make up the ligand-gated ion channel type of neurotransmitter. Each peptide probably has four membrane-spanning regions, with the 5′ end of the peptide on the extracellular side of the membrane. The portion of the peptide chain that binds the transmitter (*striped*) is in the 5′ extracellular end. Regulatory phosphorylation sites (*stippled*) are typically on the second intracytoplasmic loop. The second transmembrane segment is shown in black because this is the region believed to line the ion channel itself. **C.** Depiction of a face-on view of how five peptide chains are thought to fit together to make a functional ion channel. The 5 membrane-spanning regions form the walls of the ion channel, with the ligand-binding regions on the outside of the membrane. Usually two molecules of neurotransmitter are required to bind to the receptor in order to cause the allosteric change that opens the ion channel. **D.** Typical G-protein-coupled receptor. These receptors have seven membrane-spanning regions, with the transmitter-binding region located on the third, fifth, and possibly more membrane-spanning regions. Phosphorylation sites are located on the third intracytoplasmic loop and the 3′ end of the peptide. The G-protein complex is thought to bind to the second and third intracytoplasmic loops and the 3′ end of the receptor. Somehow binding of neurotransmitter to the transmembrane regions of the receptor induces an allosteric change in the G protein's α subunit so that it binds guanosine triphosphate (GTP) with higher affinity than guanosine diphosphate (GDP). Once GTP binds to the α subunit, the subunit dissociates from the β and γ subunits and diffuses into the cell, where it can stimulate or inhibit specific second messenger systems. The ultimate action induced in the cell is determined by the α subunit. However, each receptor subtype will bind only one type of G-protein α-subunit.

with the carboxyterminal region. Neurotransmitter binding to the outside of the receptor changes the α subunit of the G protein from a guanosine diphosphate (GDP) to a guanosine triphosphate (GTP)-preferring form. Once the α subunit has bound to GTP, it splits from the receptor and the β and γ subunits of the G proteins. The α subunit then diffuses through the cell or along the membrane to a second messenger-activating protein such as adenylate cyclase, the enzyme that forms cyclic AMP, or phospholipase C, the enzyme that initiates the phosphatidylinositol cycle. Binding of the α subunit to the second messenger-activating protein reduces the GTP to GDP and activates the second messenger cascade.

There are at least six different kinds of G proteins that are characterized by different α subunits. G_s α subunits activate adenylate cyclase (and thus cyclic AMP) and calcium channels. Several G_i proteins inhibit the activity of adenylate cyclase and activate phospholipase C, phospholipase A2, and potassium channels. G_o subunits appear to be involved in modulating the activity of voltage-sensitive calcium channels and phospholipase C. G_{olf} is located in the neurons in the nasal mucosa, where it appears to amplify the signal received from the olfactory receptors. G_t proteins are the "transducins" that serve as a receptor mechanism for the opsins. A sixth class of G proteins, the $G_{z/x}$ proteins have been cloned, but their function is not known.

The effect that activation of the receptor has on the postsynaptic neuron is highly dependent on the synapse's location on the postsynaptic neuron. Ion channel-linked receptors located on the neuronal soma near the axon hillock (where the cell's action potential is generated) will strongly influence the hillock's membrane potential and thus whether or not an action potential will be generated. Ion channel-linked receptors on the spines of distant dendrites will have almost no effect on the membrane's potential at the axon hillock. The effects of G-protein-linked receptors are not so limited by their location since they activate second messenger cascades.

NEUROTRANSMITTERS AND MODULATORS

The neurotransmitters and neuromodulators fall into several categories. The first is the amino acids. These compounds are responsible for rapid synaptic activity at the vast majority (>90%) of synapses in the brain. Amino acid pathways tend to go from one specific spot in the nervous system to another specific spot. The second category comprises the amines, acetylcholine, and adenosine. These compounds largely act through second messenger systems. The axon terminals of neurons that use this class of transmitter tend to be more widely distributed than those of the amino acids. The third major class is the peptides. Like the amines, these neuromodulators act through second messenger systems, but the axon terminals of peptide neurons tend to have a more limited distribution than those of the amines. The fourth, and newly discovered class of neurotransmitters, is the gases. The gases seem to be used

in local circuit neurons rather than in long projection pathways.

Many neurons use more than one type of molecule as a neurotransmitter or modulator. Peptides are often used by cells that also use an amino acid, amine, or gas. This enables neurons to give signals of differing durations. Whether all the neurotransmitters/modulators contained in a neuron are released at every synapse remains unknown. Thus, it is possible that neurons can release one neurotransmitter at some of its terminals and another at other terminals. Alternatively, while every neurotransmitter that a neuron possesses may be released at every synapse, the postsynaptic cell may not be sensitive to all the transmitters released. This concept is consistent with the finding that the distribution of receptors, particularly peptide receptors, often does not match the distribution of presynaptic terminals containing that transmitter. It has been hypothesized that the transmitters released at a synapse where there are no receptors for them may diffuse away to distant places, contributing to a general neuropeptide milieu reflecting the total ongoing peptidergic activity in the brain. This hypothesis remains highly controversial. All that is known with certainty is that the distribution of neurotransmitters and their receptors do not always match.

The rest of this section of the chapter describes the distribution of neurotransmitter pathways and their receptors. The distributions are presented in a series of schematic drawings showing the neurotransmitter-specific pathways and the densities of their receptors in a variety of brain regions. The names of these regions are shown on the accompanying figure (Fig. 8.3). In the subsequent figures the neurotransmitter specific pathways and densities of receptors are shown. The densities shown are based on available human and animal reports. Where the density of a receptor in a region has not been reported, the author has made an estimate of the density based on the known distribution in similar regions.

Amino Acid Neurotransmitters

Amino acids are the neurotransmitters used by the vast majority of neurons for rapid (millisecond timescale) intracellular communication. Well in excess of 90% of neurons use an amino acid for neurotransmission. Frequently, cells that use an amino acid will also use an amine or a peptide. The amino acids used for excitatory neurotransmission are glutamic acid and, possibly, aspartic acid. The inhibitory amino acids are glycine, γ-aminobutyric acid (GABA), and possibly taurine and proline. Taurine and proline will not be discussed further.

GLUTAMIC ACID

Glutamic acid (glutamate) is by far the most important excitatory neurotransmitter in vertebrate brains. Its actions are so ubiquitous that, at first, investigators thought that glutamate's ability to excite neurons must be a nonspecific

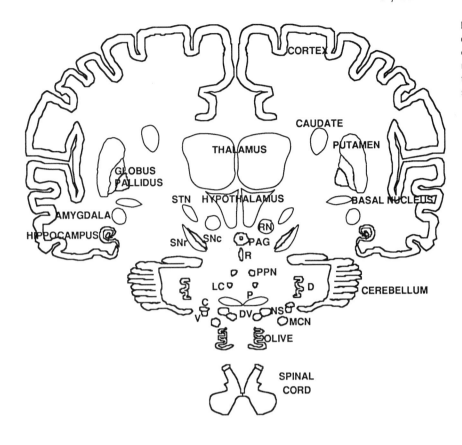

Figure 8.3. Key to the subsequent neurotransmitter and receptor distribution figures. The names of various structures in the brain are provided here. The subsequent figures are all schematic drawings that show the current concept of the distribution of a neurotransmitter and/or its receptors. The loci of transmitter-specific neurons are shown as filled circles with their pathways shown as lines projecting from the neurons. The density of receptors is shown as cross-hatching of the various regions. Where the density of a receptor in human brain is unclear, the author has estimated the density from reports of other species and from measurements from similar structures. Abbreviations: *C,* cochlear nucleus; *D,* dentate nucleus of cerebellum; *DV,* dorsal motor nucleus of the vagus nerve; *LC,* locus ceruleus; *MCN,* somatic motor cranial nerve nuclei; *NS,* nucleus of the solitary tract; *P,* pontine nuclei; *PAG,* periaqueductal grey; *PPN,* pedunculopontine nucleus; *R,* raphe nuclei; *RN,* red nucleus; *SNc,* substantia nigra pars compacta; *SNr,* substantia nigra pars reticulata; *STN,* subthalamic nucleus; *V,* vestibular nuclei.

artifact rather than a true neurotransmitter action because all neurons tested responded to glutamate's excitatory effects.

Glutamate is used in the neuron's ordinary metabolism so that only about 25% of the glutamate in the central nervous system is in the neurotransmitter pool. While much of the neurotransmitter glutamate may come from the ordinary metabolic pool, there are also enzymes present at some excitatory synapses that can synthesize glutamate. These are aspartic acid aminotransferase and glutaminase.

Glutamate that is released at the synapse is handled in several different ways. There are several types of high-affinity uptake molecules that transport glutamate back into the presynaptic terminal. Glutamate that diffuses away from the synaptic cleft is usually transported into the glia (astrocytes) that surround the synapse. There the glutamate is converted to glutamine. This astrocytic glutamine is thought to be transported to the neuronal presynaptic terminal, where it is converted back into glutamate.

At present, there are no drugs that affect the glutamate-synthesizing enzymes, or the glutamate transporters. Glutamate release from the presynaptic terminal is inhibited by several drugs, including lamotrigine and riluzole. Lamotrigine has recently been introduced as an antiepileptic drug; and both agents are under study as neuroprotective agents.

Glutamate Pathways

Most of the excitatory pathways in the brain are known to use glutamate as a neurotransmitter (Fig. 8.4). These include the cortical output pathways to subcortical structures, which include the basal ganglia, thalamus, pons, brainstem, and spinal cord. The long intracortical pathways are glutamatergic as are the pathways within the hippocampal formation, including the perforant pathway from the entorhinal cortex to the molecular layers of the dentate gyrus and CA1, the mossy fiber pathway from the dentate granule cells to the pyramidal cells of CA3, and the Schaeffer collateral pathway from CA3 to CA1 as well as the hippocampal commisural pathway of which the Schaeffer pathway fibers are collaterals. Subthalamic nucleus neurons use glutamate. The main inputs to the cerebellum, the climbing fiber pathway from the inferior olive and the mossy fibers from the pontine nuclei, use glutamate. The only excitatory neurons in the cerebellar cortex, the cerebellar granule cells, are glutamatergic. Many, if not all, of the primary sensory fibers use glutamate as (one of) their transmitters.

A number of the other major anatomical pathways in the brain are probably glutamatergic, although the glutamatergic nature of these pathways has not been proven. These include the projections from thalamus to cortex and the

Figure 8.4. Some glutamate pathways and the presumed distribution of the α-amino-3-hydroxy-5-methylisoxazole-4-propionic acid (AMPA) subtype of excitatory amino acid receptors.

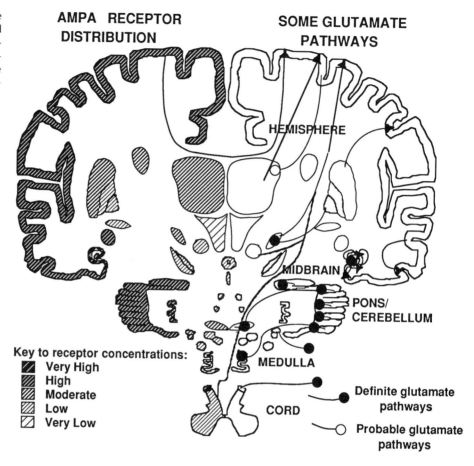

ascending sensory pathways. Some brainstem pathways such as the median longitudinal fasciculus probably also use glutamate.

Glutamate Pharmacology and Receptors

There are at least six pharmacologic types of mammalian postsynaptic excitatory amino acid receptors. Three of these receptors are linked to ion channels. Each of the ion channel-linked receptors has been named for a prototypic drug that acts specifically at that receptor.

The α-amino-3-hydroxy-5-methylisoxazole-4-propionic acid (AMPA) receptor is a monovalent cation (i.e., sodium) channel that mediates most of the fast, excitatory neurotransmission in the brain. This channel ordinarily does not allow the passage of divalent cations such as calcium. Several drugs that are antagonists of the AMPA receptor are under development as potential antiepileptics. When glutamate is released from a presynaptic terminal, the excitatory postsynaptic potential that quickly appears at the postsynaptic membrane is due to activation of AMPA receptors. AMPA receptors desensitize rapidly so that the stimulation of the postsynaptic cell by activation of an AMPA receptor is brief. This makes it likely that AMPA receptors are used to convey highly time- and location-specific information along the excitatory pathways. The other glutamate receptors are slower in onset but have

longer effects. These other receptors seem better suited to play modulatory roles at their synapses.

AMPA receptors are present throughout the brain. Their distribution is shown in Figure 8.4. They are densest in the hippocampus; dense in neocortex, on the dendrites of Purkinje cells in the cerebellum and in the dorsal horn of the spinal cord; moderate in the caudate, putamen, thalamus, and subthalamus; and of lower density in the rest of the brain.

A family of genes that carry the DNA code for the AMPA receptor have been cloned. Four genes (GluR1, GluR2, GluR3, and GluR4) are known whose sequences are about 70% identical. The functional receptor that is present on neuronal membranes probably consists of several of the proteins coded by these genes in a large complex. Each complex seems to be made up of at least one GluR2 molecule and four other molecules. The exact composition may vary from cell to cell and from region to region within a cell. In the process of DNA transcription, the noncoding "introns" that are present as inserts within the DNA coding sequence are removed from the primary RNA transcript and the "exons" that code for the amino acid sequence of the protein are "spliced" together into two patterns that differ slightly. Thus, the resultant messenger RNA, can have two different "splice variants" that have been called "flip" and "flop." In addition, the RNA sequence that codes for the second transmembrane domain of GluR2 is "edited" so that a codon that carries the instructions for a glutamine is changed into a codon that codes for an arginine. The second transmembrane domain is the region of the protein that lines the ion channel. It is this arginine that prevents calcium ions from flowing through the channel.

The second of the ion-channel linked receptors—and the most studied—is the *N*-methyl-*D*-aspartate (NMDA) receptor. It is linked to a voltage-gated calcium channel. Activation of the channel is modulated by binding sites for glycine and polyamines on the exterior of the receptor. Drugs are currently being developed that interact with the glutamate, glycine, and polyamine binding sites on the receptor. There is also a modulatory binding site for the dissociative anesthetics, such as ketamine and phencyclidine (PCP—"angel dust") within the channel itself. Under normal membrane potentials, even if glutamate binds to its receptor site on the molecule, the channel is not permeable to calcium because a magnesium ion blocks the channel. When the membrane is somewhat depolarized, however, the channel no longer binds magnesium. Thus, when glutamate binds to its receptor site under depolarized conditions, the channel opens and calcium enters the neuron. This NMDA receptor-mediated calcium entry is associated with some forms of learning. On the other hand, activation of this receptor during extremely depolarizing situations, such as ischemia and epilepsy, seems to cause neuronal death after a delay of about 24 hours.

The distribution of NMDA receptors is shown in Figure 8.5. NMDA receptors are present on practically all neurons. They are densest on the pyramidal neurons of the hippocampus. They are very dense throughout the neocortex, less dense in subcortical structures, and quite low in number in the brainstem. In the cerebellum they are located on granule cell neurons, with very few on the Purkinje cells. There are a moderate number of NMDA receptors in the dorsal horn of the spinal cord, where they may be involved in pain transmission pathways.

Recently two families of genes have been cloned that carry the DNA code for NMDA receptors. The first type of receptor gene, NMDAR1, is a single gene that is expressed in virtually all neurons. Like the AMPA receptors, the messenger RNA for this single gene is edited into a number of different splice variants before it is translated into a protein. These splice variants differ in how sensitive they are to modulation by glycine and in how many phosphorylation sites they possess. Neurons differ in which splice variant they express, thus controlling their sensitivity to glycine and phosphorylation. The NMDAR2 receptor gene family consists of at least four different genes that are highly (approximately 70%) homologous to one another but share only a 25% homology with the NMDAR1 gene. NMDAR2A is expressed throughout the brain, NMDAR2B in the forebrain, and NMDAR2C in the cerebellum. NMDAR2D is expressed in diencephalon, midbrain, and brainstem. Two more NMDAR2 genes appear to be expressed in olfactory bulb and retina, respectively. The

NMDA RECEPTOR DISTRIBUTION   **KAINATE RECEPTOR DISTRIBUTION**

Figure 8.5. Presumed distributions of the *N*-methyl-*D*-aspartate and kainate subtypes of excitatory amino acid receptors.

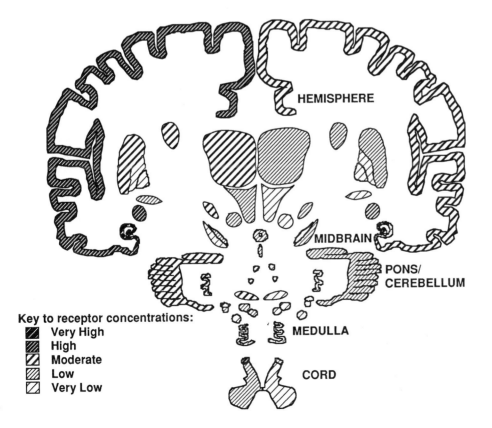

HEMISPHERE

MIDBRAIN

PONS/
CEREBELLUM

MEDULLA

CORD

Key to receptor concentrations:
- Very High
- High
- Moderate
- Low
- Very Low

Figure 8.6. Presumed distributions of two pharmacologic subtypes of metabotropic excitatory amino acid receptors.

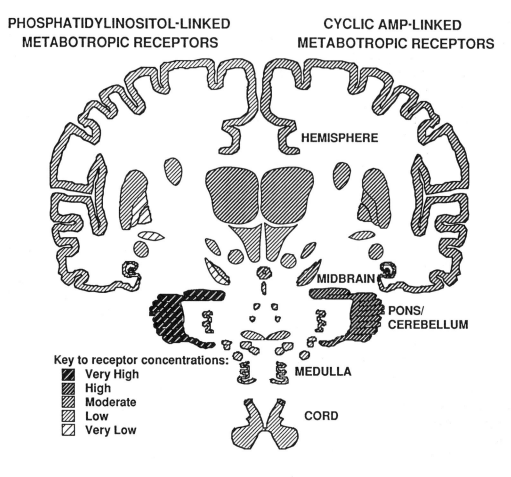

PHOSPHATIDYLINOSITOL-LINKED METABOTROPIC RECEPTORS

CYCLIC AMP-LINKED METABOTROPIC RECEPTORS

HEMISPHERE

MIDBRAIN

PONS/ CEREBELLUM

MEDULLA

CORD

Key to receptor concentrations:
- Very High
- High
- Moderate
- Low
- Very Low

proteins expressed by the different NMDAR2 genes differ in their pharmacology. The most significant difference is that the NMDAR2C receptor found in the cerebellum lacks a dissociative anesthetic binding site in its channel. It is thought that an NMDAR1 protein molecule combines with one or more NMDAR2 molecules to make the functional receptor that is present on the surface of the neuron.

The kainate receptor is linked to a monovalent cation channel that does not desensitize as rapidly as the AMPA receptor-linked channels do. Certain naturally occurring toxins that may contaminate shellfish, such as kainate itself and the more potent domoic acid, are able to stimulate this receptor so that it stays open for a long time. This allows sodium to flood into the neuron and kill it through an osmotic overload. The distribution of kainate receptors is shown in Figure 8.5. The receptors are extremely dense on postsynaptic neurons in stratum lucidum of the CA3 region of the hippocampus. This is the area where the "mossy fiber" pathway from the dentate gyrus to CA3 terminates. CA3 neurons are, by far, the most susceptible to the toxic effects of kainate and domoate. There are a moderate number of kainate receptors in the deep layers of the cortex and few to very few of them elsewhere in the brain. Five genes from two families code for kainate receptors. GluR5, GluR6, and GluR7 are in one family, while KA1 and KA2 are in the other family. How these gene products are organized to make functional receptors is not known at the time of this writing. It is speculated that members of the GluR5, 6, 7 and

KA1, 2 families must combine in a larger complex to form a functional receptor.

In addition to the three types of ion channel-linked excitatory amino acid receptors, there are also three pharmacologic types of G-protein-linked receptors that are activated by glutamate. These receptors have been labeled the "metabotropic" glutamate receptors. They have the typical seven membrane-spanning domains of the G-protein-linked receptors. At least seven genes (mGluR1 – mGluR7) are known that code for different subtypes of these receptors. The pharmacologic type 1 metabotropic receptors are coded by the genes mGluR1 and mGluR5. They are linked to phosphatidylinositol metabolism and mGluR1 is also linked to weak stimulation of cyclic AMP. The pharmacologic type 2 metabotropic receptors (coded by the genes mGluR2 and mGluR3) are linked to cyclic AMP inhibition. The distribution of the pharmacologic type 1 and 2 metabotropic receptors is shown in Figure 8.6. Type 1 receptors are extremely dense in the Purkinje cells of the cerebellum, with moderate amounts in the thalamus, and lesser amounts in basal ganglia, hippocampus and cortex. Type 2 receptors are relatively dense in cortex, hippocampus, basal ganglia, and in the cerebellum. Type 2 receptors are also present in glial cells, coded by the mGluR3 gene. The receptors coded by the mGluR4, mGluR6 and mGluR7 genes are linked to cyclic AMP stimulation. The mGluR4 and mGluR7 receptors have complementary distributions in brain with mGluR4 receptors being almost exclusively located in cerebellar granule cells with a few in thalamus, the caudate nucleus, the putamen, and the CA2 region of the hippocampus. mGluR7 receptors are located in most other neurons. mGluR6 receptors are found only in the "on" bipolar cells of the retina.

GLYCINE

Glycine, like glutamate, is an essential amino acid that is present in all cells. Because the alkaloid poison strychnine acts by blocking glycine receptors, glycine was shown to be a neurotransmitter before glutamate, even though there are many more glutamatergic than glycinergic neurons. Glycine has two major actions in the brain outside of its role in intermediary metabolism. The first is as an inhibitory neurotransmitter. There are neurons that release glycine at their synapses and remove glycine from the synaptic cleft with high-affinity glycine transporters. Glycine released at these synapses interacts with inhibitory receptors on the postsynaptic neurons. These inhibitory glycine receptors can be blocked by strychnine. The remainder of this section is devoted to this role of glycine. There is, however, another role for glycine. The glycine that is normally present in the extracellular fluid binds to a modulatory site on the NMDA type of glutamate receptors. No special neurons are known to release the glycine that interacts with this site. Glycine needs to be bound to this site in order for the NMDA receptor to be activated. The seizures that are a prominent symptom of the rare, inherited, metabolic disease nonketotic hyperglycinemia are probably caused by excess glycinergic stimulation of this modulatory site on the NMDA receptor.

This binding site is not sensitive to the actions of strychnine. Several drugs that bind to this site are under development as potential neuroprotective agents and antiepileptics.

Glycinergic Neurons

All known glycinergic neurons are inhibitory interneurons. These cells release glycine when stimulated and have high-affinity transporters for removing glycine from the synaptic cleft. The best known are the inhibitory interneurons of the ventral horn of the spinal cord. These include the Renshaw cell that mediates recurrent inhibition of the α-motor neurons and the inhibitory Ia afferent-coupled interneurons that mediate crossed inhibition of the spinal reflexes. Similar interneurons are present in the motor nuclei of the brainstem. The distribution of glycinergic neurons is shown in Figure 8.7.

Dysfunction of the synapses formed by glycinergic neurons causes a marked increase in the reflexes with spread of innervation from one spinal cord segment to another. Total failure of these synapses causes the sensory input from one contracting muscle to stimulate other muscles to contract. Shortly thereafter, all muscles are maximally contracting due to positive feedback. This leads to opisthotonus, paralysis, and respiratory failure.

Glycine Pharmacology and Receptors

The pharmacology of glycine is known because of the symptoms (just described) of failure of glycinergic synapses.

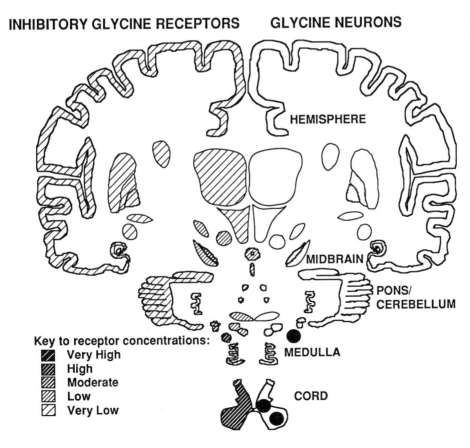

INHIBITORY GLYCINE RECEPTORS   **GLYCINE NEURONS**

HEMISPHERE

MIDBRAIN

PONS/ CEREBELLUM

MEDULLA

CORD

Key to receptor concentrations:
- Very High
- High
- Moderate
- Low
- Very Low

Figure 8.7. Location of some glycine neurons and the presumed distribution of inhibitory glycine receptors.

Tetanus toxin causes symptoms and death in this way because it blocks the release of glycine from the presynaptic terminal.

There is only one known type of inhibitory postsynaptic glycine receptor. The distribution of these receptors is shown in Figure 9.7. The receptor is a typical ligand-gated ion channel consisting of several—probably five—interacting subunits. The channel is permeable to chloride and, when open, causes the neuron to become hyperpolarized. The alkaloid poison, strychnine, interacts with a site on the receptor that prevents glycine from binding to its binding site. Strychnine thus prevents motor neurons from being inhibited and causes the same symptoms as those of tetanus.

The rare inherited syndrome hyperekplexia, characterized by excessive startle reactions, is caused by minor mutations in the α subunit of the glycine receptor.

γ-AMINOBUTYRIC ACID

γ-Aminobutyric acid (GABA) is the predominant, fast-acting, inhibitory neurotransmitter in the nervous system. GABA is synthesized from glutamate by the specific enzyme, glutamic acid decarboxylase (GAD). This enzyme occurs in two isoforms, long and short, that are under separate metabolic regulation. Some GABA neurons have only one form of the enzyme, while some have both. GAD is found only in neurons that utilize GABA as a neurotransmitter and serves as a useful immunohistochemical marker for these neurons.

GABA is ordinarily removed from the synapse by a high-affinity neuronal transport system and restored in synaptic terminals. GABA may also be transported into glia, where it is converted to succinic semialdehyde, a Krebs cycle intermediate, by the enzyme GABA transaminase.

There are several classes of drugs whose mechanism of action is to enhance GABA's actions. These drugs function as sedatives, antiepileptics, and anxiolytics. Some of these act by inhibiting the metabolism of GABA by GABA-transaminase. These include the antiepileptics gabaculin and valproate.

GABA Pathways

GABA neurons serve as the local circuit inhibitory neurons throughout the central nervous system except in the spinal and brainstem motor nuclei, where glycine serves this purpose. There are also several long projection pathways that utilize GABA. One is the Purkinje cell pathway from cerebellar cortex to the deep cerebellar nuclei. The Purkinje cell is the only output cell of the cerebellar cortex, and it functions to inhibit cells in the deep cerebellar nuclei. Similarly, the only output neurons of the caudate nucleus, putamen, and nucleus accumbens (striatum) are GABA-ergic, medium-sized neurons whose dendrites are covered with synaptic spines (medium spiny neurons). These GABA-ergic cells also contain a neuromodulatory peptide, either enkephalin or substance P. These neurons project to the globus pallidus and substantia nigra. The neurons of the globus pallidus and the pars reticulata of the substantia nigra are large, tonically firing neurons that also use GABA. These neurons project to the subthalamic nucleus and thalamus. Activation of the striatal spiny neurons thus disinhibits (inhibits the inhibitor of) the thalamus. The distribution of GABA neurons and their pathways is shown in Figure 8.8.

GABA, Benzodiazepine, and Barbiturate Pharmacology and Receptors

Many drugs—the benzodiazepines, the barbiturates, certain convulsants, and lioresal—act by modulating the activity of one of the two types of postsynaptic GABA receptors.

The first type of GABA receptor to be discovered, the $GABA_A$ receptor, is a typical ligand-gated ion channel. When open, these receptors provide a pathway for chloride ions to enter the cell and hyperpolarize it. $GABA_A$ receptors are quite dense throughout the brain, wherever there are GABA synapses. Benzodiazepines modulate the activity of these receptors through a binding site that is different from the one to which GABA binds. Benzodiazepines cannot open the channel unless GABA is present. The barbiturates bind to a site in the chloride channel and can open the channel without GABA being present. This difference in the actions of the two classes of drugs explains the greater toxicity of the barbiturates. Furthermore, not all $GABA_A$ receptors are sensitive to the benzodiazepines.

The pharmacology of the benzodiazepines is complex. There are at least two types of benzodiazepine binding sites that are associated with $GABA_A$ receptors and a third site that clearly is not. This "peripheral" benzodiazepine binding site is on a mitochondrial transporter and has nothing to do with GABA pharmacology. The "central" benzodiazepine receptors are divided into at least two types. "Type 1" benzodiazepine receptors are more associated with the anxiolytic properties of the drugs while "type 2" receptors are more associated with the benzodiazepine's sedative and antiepileptic properties. The distribution of these two types of central benzodiazepine receptors is shown in Figure 8.9.

Several large families of genes have been cloned that code for subunits of the $GABA_A$ receptor. The families of genes go by Greek alphabetical names: α, β, γ, δ, and ρ. Each of the functional receptor-ion channel complexes contains at least one α and one β subunit. A γ or δ subunit may or may not be included with the α and β subunits. The α subunit has binding sites for both GABA and benzodiazepines. However, even though a binding site for benzodiazepines is present on the α subunit, the receptor-ion channel complex will not be sensitive to benzodiazepines unless a γ or (possibly) a δ subunit is present. The β subunits contain a GABA binding site and a number of phosphorylation sites through which the receptor can be regulated by intracellular events. The α_1 subunit is associated with benzodiazepine type 1 pharmacology, while the α_2, α_3, and α_4 subunits are associated with benzodiazepine type 2 pharmacology. The α subunit is commonly co-localized with the β_2 subunit in the globus pallidus, substantia nigra and cerebellum. The α_3

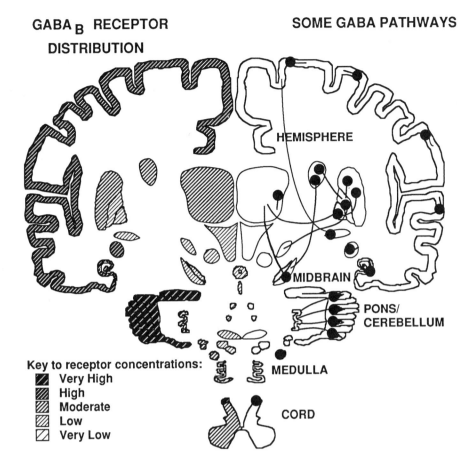

GABA$_B$ RECEPTOR DISTRIBUTION

SOME GABA PATHWAYS

HEMISPHERE

MIDBRAIN

PONS/CEREBELLUM

MEDULLA

CORD

Key to receptor concentrations:
- Very High
- High
- Moderate
- Low
- Very Low

Figure 8.8. Some γ-amino-butyric acid (GABA) pathways and the presumed distribution of GABA$_B$ receptors.

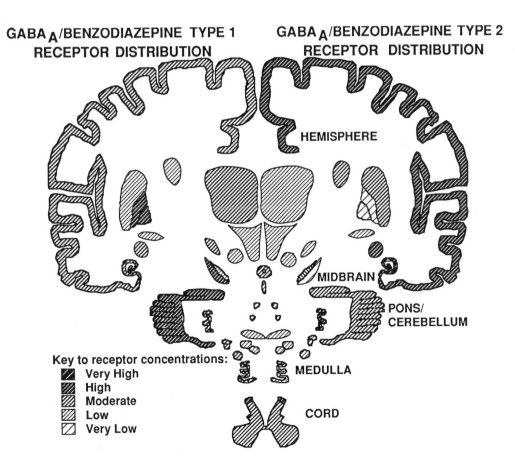

GABA$_A$/BENZODIAZEPINE TYPE 1 RECEPTOR DISTRIBUTION

GABA$_A$/BENZODIAZEPINE TYPE 2 RECEPTOR DISTRIBUTION

HEMISPHERE

MIDBRAIN

PONS/CEREBELLUM

MEDULLA

CORD

Key to receptor concentrations:
- Very High
- High
- Moderate
- Low
- Very Low

Figure 8.9. Presumed distribution of two subtypes of GABA$_A$/benzodiazepine receptors.

subunit is commonly co-localized with the β_1 subunit in the cerebral cortex. An unusual α subunit, the α_6 unit, is located on cerebellar granule cells and is not sensitive to benzodiazepines. The ρ subunit is located only in the retina. The frequent co-localization of α_1 with β_2 and α_3 with β_1 suggests that these subunits join together to make the functional receptors and that their gene expression is under a single control system.

The other major type of GABA receptor is the $GABA_B$ receptor. $GABA_B$ receptors are G-protein-linked. Activation of these receptors results in inhibition of cyclic AMP, an increase in the permeability of potassium channels, and a decrease in the permeability of sodium channels. Physiological studies have indicated that many $GABA_B$ receptors are located on presynaptic terminals of non-GABA neurons, where they function as heteroreceptors, regulating the release of other neurotransmitters. On the other hand, ligand-binding studies indicate that most $GABA_B$ receptors are located postsynaptically. Whether presynaptic or postsynaptic $GABA_B$ receptors are functionally more important remains to be resolved. The distribution of $GABA_B$ receptors as revealed by ligand-binding studies is shown in Figure 8.8. Binding is very high in the cerebellum and dorsal horn of the spinal cord. High binding is present in the cortex. The very high binding in dorsal horn or spinal cord likely represents receptors that regulate the release of neurotransmitter from primary afferents through presynaptic inhibition.

Acetylcholine

Acetylcholine was the first neurotransmitter to be clearly described. It is the major transmitter of the peripheral motor system, the presynaptic autonomic nervous system, the postsynaptic innervation of sweat glands, and the entire postsynaptic parasympathetic system. It also serves as a neurotransmitter in a number of central nervous system pathways. Acetylcholine is released from presynaptic terminals and interacts with postsynaptic receptors in a manner very similar to that of amino acids. However, its fate in the synapse differs from that of the amino acids. There is no high-affinity transport system for acetylcholine. Instead, there is an enzyme—acetylcholinesterase—present in the synapse that breaks acetylcholine down into choline and acetate. A number of drugs that are useful for treating myasthenia gravis act by blocking the activity of acetylcholinesterase. By preventing acetylcholine from being metabolized, these drugs prolong acetylcholine's actions at the synapse. Recently, centrally acting cholinesterase inhibitors such as tetrahydroaminoacridine (tacrine) have been targeted as potential treatments for Alzheimer's disease.

Acetylcholine Pathways

There are six major types of acetylcholine neurons within the central nervous system. The distribution of these neurons is shown in Figure 8.10. The most numerous are the motor neurons of the ventral horn of the spinal cord and of the motor nuclei of the brainstem. These neurons send their axons to innervate the somatic muscles. Recurrent collaterals of these neurons innervate the Renshaw cells. The second major type of neuron is the presynaptic sympathetic neurons, whose cell bodies are in the intermediolateral cell column of the spinal cord in the thoracic and lumbar regions. The first-order parasympathetic neurons in the 3rd, 7th, 9th, 10th, and 11th cranial nerves and the sacral spinal cord are also cholinergic.

Within the central nervous system there are two major cholinergic projections. One arises in the pedunculopontine nuclei of the midbrain and projects to the medulla, substantia nigra, thalamus, and globus pallidus. These neurons are part of the ascending reticular activating system. These neurons may play an important role in regulating the sleep/wake cycles. A second major central nervous system projection for acetylcholine is provided by a complex of nuclei, including the medial septal nucleus, the diagonal band of Broca, and the basal nucleus of Meynert. These neurons innervate all the cortical structures including the neocortex, the hippocampus, and the amygdala. The acetylcholine provided by these neurons seems to be vital for normal learning and memory function. The degeneration of these neurons is one of the major hallmarks for Alzheimer's disease.

There are a few acetylcholine neurons within the neocortex that function as local circuit neurons. However, the major region where acetylcholine neurons serve as local circuit neurons is within the caudate nucleus and the putamen. Here, approximately 5% of the neurons are large cholinergic neurons that have no long projections. These neurons participate in the cholinergic/dopaminergic balance that characterizes the pharmacology of the movement disorders.

Acetylcholine Receptors

There are two major classes of acetylcholine receptors. The nicotinic receptors at the neuromuscular junction are the prototypic ligand-gated ion channel receptor complex. These are the only receptors that have been purified to homogeneity and that are known to exist in a pentamer confirmation. Each receptor complex usually consists of two α and two β subunits with one γ, δ, or ϵ subunit. The ion channel opened by the receptor is a sodium channel, and activation of the receptor stimulates an excitatory postsynaptic potential.

The nicotinic receptors located on neurons in the central nervous system and sympathetic ganglia are pharmacologically different from those located at the neuromuscular junction. They are coded by a different family of genes, and different neurons may express different nicotinic receptors. All these receptors are linked to ion channels for cations, particularly channels that convey both sodium and calcium. Many of these receptors are located on presynaptic terminals, where they may govern neurotransmitter release. They are also particularly dense on the postsynaptic neurons of the interpeduncular nucleus and the superior colliculus.

MUSCARINIC RECEPTOR DISTRIBUTION

ACETYLCHOLINE PROJECTIONS

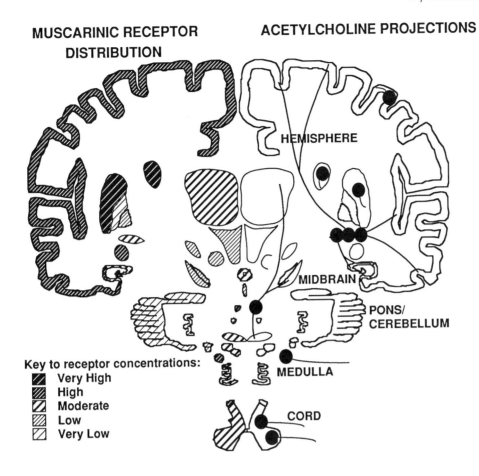

Figure 8.10. Some acetylcholine pathways and the presumed distribution of muscarinic acetylcholine receptors.

HEMISPHERE

MIDBRAIN

PONS/ CEREBELLUM

MEDULLA

CORD

Key to receptor concentrations:
- Very High
- High
- Moderate
- Low
- Very Low

The other major type of acetylcholine receptor is the muscarinic receptor. These receptors are present at the synapses where the postsynaptic parasympathetic neurons terminate, such as those in the heart, intestine, and sweat glands. Atropinic (antimuscarinic) drugs produce their tachycardia, constipation, and decreased sweating by blocking these peripheral muscarinic receptors.

Two pharmacologic subclasses of central nervous system muscarinic receptors have been described: M_1 receptors that are susceptible to pirenzepine and M_2 receptors that are not. The M_1 receptors are located postsynaptically and are G-protein-coupled receptors often linked to cyclic AMP and/or phosphatidylinositol metabolism. The M_2 receptors are located on the presynaptic terminals of acetylcholine neurons and function as autoreceptors governing acetylcholine release. The distribution of the M_1 receptors is shown in Figure 8.10.

Blockade of central muscarinic receptors can profoundly affect learning and memory. Drugs that block these receptors include not only the well-known anticholinergics but also tricyclic antidepressants, antihistamines, and many of the atypical neuroleptics.

Four genes that code for the muscarinic receptors have been isolated. The m_1 and m_3 proteins are linked to phosphatidylinositol systems. The m_2 protein corresponds to the M_2 type of receptor. Thus, m_2 proteins are mainly expressed by acetylcholine neurons, and are located on presynaptic acetylcholine terminals. They are linked to cyclic

AMP inhibition and to stimulation of potassium conductance. The m_4 protein is linked to cyclic AMP inhibition in postsynaptic neurons.

Amine neurotransmitters

DOPAMINE

Dopamine was first discovered about 40 years ago. Research soon revealed that this neurotransmitter plays major roles in governing both motor activity and behavior. Only long after the discovery of its central actions was its ability to act as a cardiac ionotropic agent discovered.

The rate-limiting step in the synthesis of dopamine, and for the other catecholamines, norepinephrine and epinephrine, is the conversion of tyrosine to L-Dopa by tyrosine hydroxylase. Tyrosine hydroxylase is a specific marker for catecholamine neurons throughout the nervous system. L-Dopa is converted to dopamine by the actions of L-aromatic acid decarboxylase. Dopamine is metabolized by a combination of monoamine oxidase and catechol-*o*-methyltransferase to homovanillic acid. However, the actions of dopamine at dopamine synapses are usually terminated by high-affinity transport back into the presynaptic dopamine terminal by a transporter that is specific for dopamine. The stimulant drugs of abuse, cocaine and the amphetamines, act by blocking the reuptake of dopamine via this transporter. In addition, amphetamines can stimulate the release of dopamine.

Dopamine Pathways

Dopamine cell bodies are located in a number of distinct nuclei in the brainstem and hypothalamus. The location of these nuclei and their pathways are shown in Figure 8.11. There are dopamine neurons in the area postrema and dorsal motor nucleus of the vagus nerve that may be involved in the generation of emesis. There is a descending dopaminergic pathway from the zona incerta that projects to the dorsal horn of the spinal cord and regulates some aspects of pain sensation. There are also dopamine neurons located in the median eminence of the hypothalamus. These neurons govern the release of pituitary hormones, particularly prolactin release, which dopamine inhibits. Thus, prolactin-secreting pituitary tumors can be treated with dopamine agonists. Therefore use of drugs that affect dopamine neurotransmission will have an effect on pituitary function. The major source of dopamine for the brain, however, is the chain of cells running from the substantia nigra pars compacta through the ventral tegmental area (VTA). The nigral neurons project to the caudate nucleus and putamen, where they govern motor activity. Dysfunction of these neurons produces the symptoms of parkinsonism. The VTA neurons project to the nucleus accumbens and the entire cortex, particularly the frontal lobe. Dysfunction (hyperactivity?) of these neurons is thought to contribute to the symptoms of Tourette's syndrome and schizophrenia.

Dopamine Receptors

All dopamine receptors are G-protein-linked receptors. There are two main pharmacologic classes of such receptors. D_1 receptors are linked to the stimulation of cyclic AMP, while D_2 receptors are linked to cyclic AMP inhibition. The distribution of these receptors is shown in Figure 8.12. Both receptor subtypes are extremely high in the caudate nucleus, putamen, and nucleus accumbens. D_1 receptors are located on postsynaptic striatal neurons. They are also located on the terminals of these neurons in the medial global pallidus and substantia nigra pars reticulata. Most striatal D_2 receptors are also on intrinsic striatal neurons, although some exist as autoreceptors on dopamine neuron terminals, where they govern dopamine release. The D_2 receptors are blocked by the classic neuroleptics, such as haloperidol, and the antiemitics, such as metoclopramide. Blockade of these receptors produces parkinsonism as a prominent side effect.

Five genes that code for dopamine receptors have been cloned. The d_1 and d_5 proteins have D_1 pharmacology and stimulate adenylate cyclase. The other three proteins, the d_2, d_3, and d_4 proteins, all have a D_2 pharmacology. The d_1 and d_5 proteins are primarily located in striatum, with a few cortical cells expressing the d_1 receptor protein. The d_2 receptor gene is expressed in the striatum, hypothalamus, and substantia nigra. These nigral d_2 receptors presumably represent autoreceptors. d_3 Receptors are expressed in nucleus accumbens, and parts of caudate and may be responsible for mediating some of the mental effects of dopamine. However, most of the mental effects of dopamine

Figure 8.11. Some dopamine pathways and the presumed distribution of the dopamine D4 receptor.

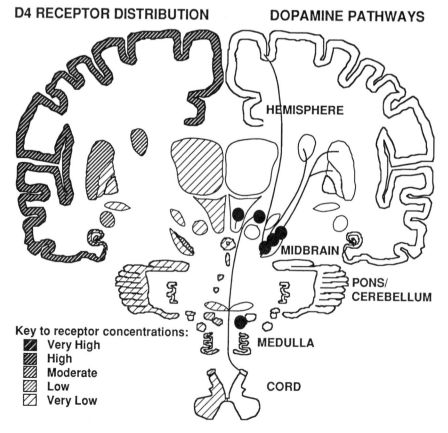

D4 RECEPTOR DISTRIBUTION

DOPAMINE PATHWAYS

HEMISPHERE

MIDBRAIN

PONS/CEREBELLUM

MEDULLA

CORD

Key to receptor concentrations:
- Very High
- High
- Moderate
- Low
- Very Low

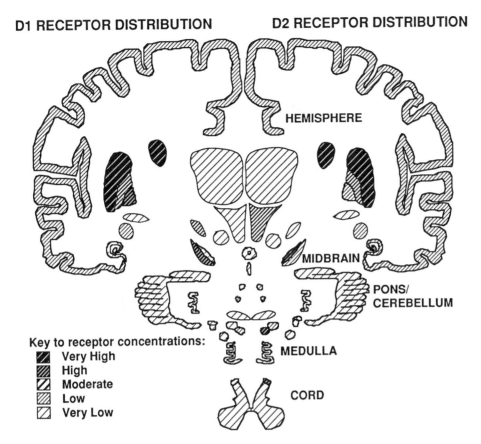

D1 RECEPTOR DISTRIBUTION

D2 RECEPTOR DISTRIBUTION

HEMISPHERE

MIDBRAIN

PONS/
CEREBELLUM

MEDULLA

CORD

Key to receptor concentrations:
- Very High
- High
- Moderate
- Low
- Very Low

Figure 8.12. Presumed distribution of the dopamine D1 and D2 receptors.

are probably mediated by the d_4 receptor protein which is expressed mainly in the cortex. The d_4 receptor protein is sensitive to the atypical neuroleptics, such as clozapine, as well as to the traditional neuroleptics. d_4 receptors are not susceptible to the antiemetics, such as metoclopramide. Thus, quite possibly, the behavioral effects of dopaminergic drugs can be separated from the motor effects by finding drugs that selectively interact with either the d_4 or d_2 type of receptor protein.

There is abundant evidence for interaction between the D_1 and D_2 receptor subtypes. Both are required for normal motor activity. However, it is not clear whether the two receptor subtypes are localized on the same cells in the caudate nucleus and putamen. Some studies have shown a complete segregation of receptors, with D_1 receptors being located on striatal output cells that project to the medial globus pallidus and substantia nigra and contain substance P. D_2 receptors are located on cells that project to the lateral globus pallidus and that contain enkephalin. Some studies have found an approximately 25% overlap of cells that express these two receptor subtypes; other studies have found complete overlap with all striatal neurons expressing both types of receptors. Further studies will be needed to measure the amount of overlap between the neurons that express the different pharmacologic subtypes.

NOREPINEPHRINE

Norepinephrine is synthesized from dopamine by the enzyme dopamine-β-hydroxylase. The presence of this enzyme in cells distinguishes norepinephrine from dopamine neurons. Like dopamine, norepinephrine is metabolized by monoamine oxidase and catechol-*o*-methyltransferase. Again, like dopamine, the major route of inactivation of norepinephrine at the synapse is via a high-affinity transport system into the presynaptic terminal. Paroxetine is a specific inhibitor of the norepinephrine transport system. Tricyclic antidepressants, particularly desipramine, also block norepinephrine reuptake. This may be part of their mechanism of action.

Norepinephrine is thought to play major roles in arousal, memory, and affect.

Norepinephrine Pathways

In the peripheral nervous system, norepinephrine is the major transmitter of the postsynaptic sympathetic nervous system. These neurons have their cell bodies in the chain of sympathetic ganglia that lie bilaterally in the paravertebral gutter from the lower cervical to the lumbar regions. The axons of these neurons are distributed to the blood vessels throughout the body, irides, salivary glands, heart, lungs, intestines, and bladder. These neurons play important roles in the regulation of blood pressure, pupilary dilatation, cardiac strength and rhythm, pulmonary airway dilatation, and intestinal and vesicle mobility.

There are several major norepinephrine-containing cell groups in the mammalian brain. The distribution of these neurons is shown in Figure 8.13. One group is distributed in the reticular formation of the lateral medulla. Descending

Figure 8.13. Some norepinephrine pathways and the presumed distribution of β-adrenergic receptors (receptors for norepinephrine and epinephrine).

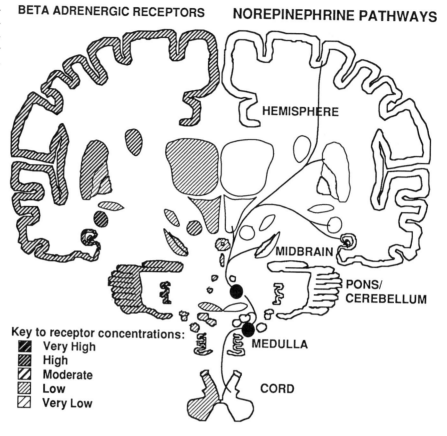

BETA ADRENERGIC RECEPTORS   **NOREPINEPHRINE PATHWAYS**

Key to receptor concentrations:
- Very High
- High
- Moderate
- Low
- Very Low

axons of these neurons project into the spinal cord, where they play an inhibitory role on muscle tone and spinal cutaneous pain reflexes. Ascending projections of these neurons go to the locus ceruleus. The locus ceruleus itself serves as the major source of norepinephrine for the forebrain. This dense cluster of pigmented neurons is located in the dorsal lateral pons. A few cells project from there to the cerebellum, but most project rostrally. The axons of the ceruleus neurons project in the median forebrain bundle, where they distribute to the hypothalamus, thalamus, basal ganglia, amygdala, hippocampus, and the entire neocortex. Norepinephrine terminals are distributed most densely in layers 2, 5, and 6. These projections from the locus ceruleus are thought to play an important role in arousal, memory (being responsible for the hippocampal theta rhythm), and affect.

Norepinephrine Receptors

Norepinephrine receptors are all of the G protein coupled type. There are two main pharmacologic subtypes of these receptors, α and β receptors. α Receptors are linked to the inositol phosphate system and to the inhibition of cyclic AMP, while β receptors are linked to stimulation of cyclic AMP. Both receptors are found not only in the brain but also in the periphery. Each major pharmacologic class has several subtypes as well.

The distribution of α receptors in the brain is shown in Figure 8.14. α_1 Receptors are located postsynaptically

throughout the brain and periphery. They are high in thalamus and hippocampus, moderate in basal ganglia, cerebral, and cerebellar cortices and some brainstem nuclei, while they are low elsewhere. α_2 Receptors, on the other hand, are located postsynaptically and as autoreceptors on the synaptic terminals of norepinephrine neurons, where they regulate norepinephrine release. They are particularly abundant in cerebral cortex and locus ceruleus. β Receptors are also distributed throughout the brain and spinal cord. Distribution of these receptors is shown in Figure 8.13. They are particularly concentrated in basal ganglia structures, caudate nucleus, globus pallidus, and subthalamic nucleus as well as in the deep nuclei of the cerebellum. β Receptors have been found to be increased in some cases of drug-free suicide. There is evidence that β receptors downregulate with antidepressant treatment. Perhaps this plays a role in the therapeutic response to tricyclics.

At least 11 distinct adrenergic genes are known to exist. There are four different genes that code for α_1 proteins. All of these proteins are linked to phosphatidylinositol metabolism. Three other genes code for slightly different pharmacologic types of α_2 receptors. All are linked to cyclic AMP inhibition. One of these, α_{2B}, is found largely in the kidney, while the other two, α_{2A} and α_{2C}, are found throughout the brain. α_{2A} is located both pre- and postsynaptically on neurons. It is also found in the pituitary, blood, lungs, spleen, and muscles, where it mediates postsynaptic α effects. Postsynaptically, these α_2 receptors modulate smooth muscle tone in the arteries and play roles in sodium excretion by the kidney in platelet aggregation and in fat and carbohydrate metabolism. There are three genes that code for β receptor proteins. All are linked to cyclic AMP stimulation.

Serotonin

While serotonin has a small role in regulating the gut, the majority of its actions are in the central nervous system. Serotonin is synthesized from tryptophan in a manner entirely analogous to that by which norepinephrine is synthesized from tyrosine. 5-hydroxytryptophan is the immediate precursor for serotonin and has had some success as a drug in the treatment of myoclonus. Serotonin is metabolized to 5-hydroxyindole acetic acid (5-HIAA). Like norepinephrine, serotonin is thought to play a major role in the arousal, sleep, and affective systems within the brain.

Serotonin is mostly inactivated at the synapse by a high-affinity transport system. The specific serotonin transport inhibitors fluoxetine and sertraline are useful antidepressants. Tricyclic antidepressants are also potent serotonin reuptake inhibitors. The usefulness of these drugs has led to the hypothesis that serotonin plays a major role in depression.

Serotonin Pathways

All serotonin pathways have their origin in a series of nuclei that are located on the midline of the brainstem, the raphe nuclei. Serotonin pathways are shown in Figure 8.15. Some serotonin axons descend to the spinal cord, where they modulate pain transmission. Within the brainstem, serotonin neurons play a role in arousal and sleep. Ascending pathways from the raphe nuclei distribute to the substantia nigra, the rest of the basal ganglia, the thalamus, hypothalamus, cortex, amygdala, and hippocampi. Within the cortex, the serotonin terminals are concentrated in the superficial layers.

Serotonin Receptors

Pharmacologic studies originally divided serotonin receptors into three main subtypes. 5HT1 receptors were defined as those having a high affinity for serotonin itself, while 5HT2 receptors were defined as those with a high affinity for lysergic acid diethylamide (LSD). The distribution of those currently defined 5HT1 and 5HT2 receptors is shown in Figure 8.16. Both of these receptors turned out to be G-protein-linked. However, the 5HT3 receptor, which is found only on peripheral sensory nerve fibers, turned out to be a classic ligand-gated ion channel that permits the passage of cations. Signal transduction, cloning, and more refined pharmacologic studies have since revealed that the original nomenclature was inappropriate. The receptor originally named 5HT1C was found to be a member of the 5HT2 gene family and has been renamed 5HT2C. The 5HT1 receptors were found to be linked to cyclic AMP inhibition, while the 5HT2 receptors were found to be linked to phosphatidylinositol metabolism. A 5HT4 receptor that was linked to cyclic AMP stimulation has been described pharmacologi-

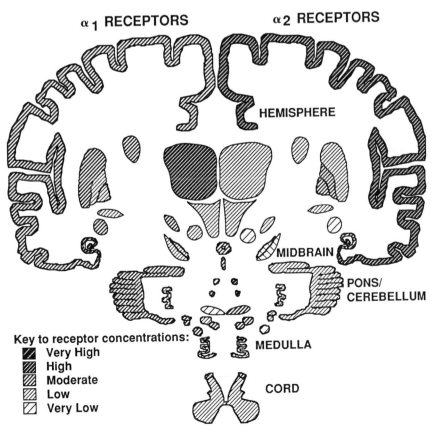

Figure 8.14. Presumed distributions of the α_1 and α_2 subtypes of adrenergic receptors.

α_1 RECEPTORS α_2 RECEPTORS

HEMISPHERE

MIDBRAIN

PONS/ CEREBELLUM

Key to receptor concentrations:
- Very High
- High
- Moderate
- Low
- Very Low

MEDULLA

CORD

Figure 8.15. Some serotonin pathways and the distribution of nitric oxide-producing neurons.

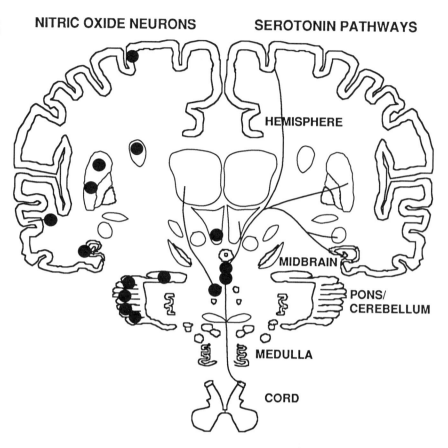

NITRIC OXIDE NEURONS

SEROTONIN PATHWAYS

HEMISPHERE

MIDBRAIN

PONS/CEREBELLUM

MEDULLA

CORD

Figure 8.16. Presumed distribution of two of the 5HT1 subtypes of serotonin receptors.

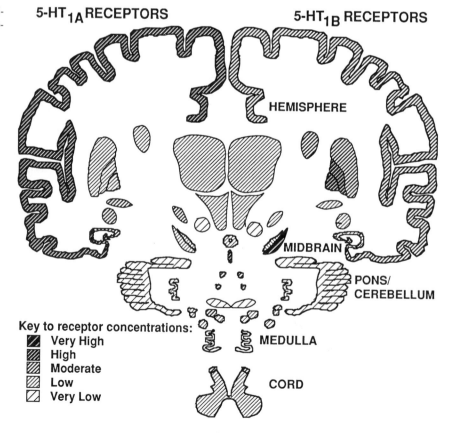

5-HT$_{1A}$ RECEPTORS

5-HT$_{1B}$ RECEPTORS

HEMISPHERE

MIDBRAIN

PONS/CEREBELLUM

Key to receptor concentrations:
- Very High
- High
- Moderate
- Low
- Very Low

MEDULLA

CORD

5-HT$_{2A}$ RECEPTORS   5-HT$_{2C}$ RECEPTORS

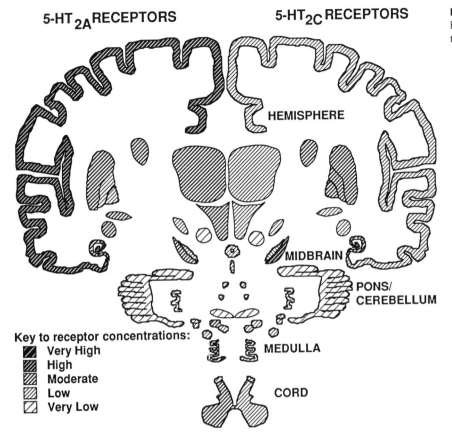

HEMISPHERE

MIDBRAIN

PONS/
CEREBELLUM

MEDULLA

CORD

Key to receptor concentrations:
- Very High
- High
- Moderate
- Low
- Very Low

Figure 8.17. Presumed distribution of two of the 5HT2 subtypes of serotonin receptors.

cally, but the gene (genes) for this receptor have not yet been cloned.

At least five true 5HT1 receptor genes have been cloned. All are linked to the inhibition of adenylate cyclase. The 5HT1A receptor is particularly prominent in the limbic system, including the hippocampus, septum, and thalamus. 5HT1A receptors also appear to be present as presynaptic autoreceptors on raphe nuclei terminals. Human 5HT1B (defined by genetic homology) receptors are located in substantia nigra and globus pallidus preferentially, where they are present on the terminals on striatal output neurons. The 5HT2B receptor has the same pharmacology (high affinity for sumatriptan) as the rat 5HT1D receptor and was originally called the human 5HT1D receptor, therefore contributing to the confusion in the nomenclature. The 5HT1E receptor has a widespread distribution of brain and spinal cord. The 5HT1F receptor (also called 5HT1Eβ and 5HT6) has a high affinity for sumatriptan and has a limited distribution in layer 5 of cerebral cortex, in pyramidal cells of CA1–CA3 regions of the hippocampus and, in the raphe nuclei to a slight extent. All the 5HT1 receptors are more closely related in their DNA sequences to the adrenergic receptors than they are to the other families of serotonin receptors.

Yet another serotonin receptor that stimulates cyclic AMP and is concentrated in the striatum has recently been cloned. Unfortunately, this receptor has also been named "5HT1F." The receptor has a high affinity for LSD and neuroleptic drugs. This receptor may therefore be involved in the pathogenesis and/or treatment of thought disorders.

The 5HT2A and the 5HT2C receptors are closely related to one another and are both linked to stimulation of the phosphatidylinositol pathway. The distribution of these receptors is shown in Figure 8.17. The 5HT2A receptor is found in high abundance only in the cerebral cortex. This provides a substrate for the actions for LSD. It is present in much lower amounts in the hypothalamus, hippocampus, spinal cord, platelets, and muscle cells. The 5HT2C receptor was originally described as a binding site in the choroid plexus. High numbers of these receptors are also present in the pyramidal cells of the hippocampus and to a lesser extent in the cerebral cortex as a whole. They are also present in sensory nuclei of the thalamus, in the dopaminergic neurons of the pars compacta of the substantia nigra, and in the raphe nuclei themselves. In addition, they are found in pain transmission areas, such as the periaqueductal gray, descending raphe serotonin neurons, and in the spinal thalamic tract, suggesting that these receptors play a role in the pain system.

Adenosine

The purine adenosine has recently been identified as a neuromodulator in the central nervous system. Adenosine has a well-established role as a precursor to both DNA and RNA. It is also a precursor to ATP, ADP, and cyclic AMP. Thus, enzymes for its synthesis and metabolism are ubiqui-

Figure 8.18. Presumed distribution of two subtypes of adenosine receptors.

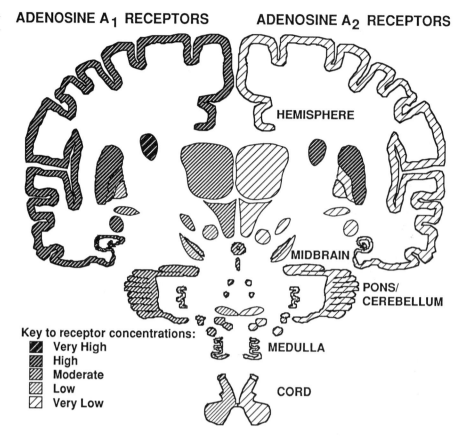

tously distributed. There is also a high-affinity transport system for adenosine. However, specific neurons that use adenosine as their neurotransmitter have not been identified.

Adenosine interacts with two types of postsynaptic receptors. The pharmacology of these receptors is important because the xanthines, such as caffeine, act as antagonists at adenosine receptors. In fact, studies have concluded that adenosine antagonism may be responsible for the major pharmacologic effects of caffeine rather than inhibition of phosphodiesterase. The distribution of these receptors is shown in Figure 8.18. Adenosine A1 receptors have a wide distribution with high binding in cortex (particularly the outer layers), basal ganglia, hippocampus, amygdala, and thalamus. Lower amounts are found in hypothalamus brainstem structures and the spinal cord. There are two subtypes of adenosine A2 receptors. The $A2_a$ receptor is found only in the striatum, while the $A2_b$ receptor is found only the periphery and is not thought to play a role in neurotransmission.

Peptide Neurotransmitters

A bewildering variety of peptides have been shown to act as neuromodulators within the central nervous system. Most of these peptides were originally isolated in another bodily system and then shown to be present in brain either by purification, demonstration of physiological action, or (most commonly) their presence has been inferred by immunohis-

tochemical staining. Localization of antigens such as peptides by immunohistochemistry presumes that the antigen in brain to which the antibody binds is identical to that which is found in the periphery.

In every case that has been studied, neuropeptides are found to be co-transmitters with some other neuroactive compound such as GABA or serotonin, being released at the same synapse. The best studied of these neuromodulators are the endogenous opiates and substance P. These compounds are reviewed in some detail here.

ENDORPHINS

The endorphins were all isolated as endogenous compounds that have activity at opiate receptors. Unsuccessful attempts have since been made to isolate endogenous ligands for other receptors such as the benzodiazepine receptor.

The endorphins are all synthesized by cleavage of much larger peptide precursor molecules. The three known precursors are proopiomelanocortin (POMC), proenkephalin, and prodynorphin. Methionine enkephalin is derived from both POMC and proenkephalin. Leucine enkephalin is derived from proenkephalin and prodynorphin. In addition, the two dynorphins, dynorphin A and dynorphin B are derived from prodynorphin. Since the dynorphins and enkephalins are distributed in different cells, the enzymes that cleave them from the precursor are probably different in the different cell types.

Endorphin Pathways

The distribution of enkephalin neurons is shown in Figure 8.19. Enkephalin neurons serve as local interneurons in the primary sensory receiving areas of the dorsal horn of the spinal cord and the spinal tract of the trigeminal nucleus. It is thought that this is a primary site where the enkephalins suppress pain sensation. There is light to moderate enkephalinergic innervation of the solitary nucleus and the other dorsal tegmental nuclei of the medulla. There is also dense enkephalinergic innervation of the central gray and periaqueductal gray from the floor of the 4th ventricle through the entire midbrain. In addition, the interpeduncular nucleus has dense enkephalinergic innervation. There are enkephalinergic neurons in the parabrachial nucleus that appear to be important for enkephalinergic innervation of the substantia nigra. Within the forebrain there are some enkephalinergic neurons in the cortex and hippocampus, although no cell contains a high concentration of this neuromodulator. There is relatively dense enkephalinergic innervation of the central nucleus of the amygdala. In the bed nucleus of the stria terminalis, there are large numbers of enkephalinergic neurons. These serve as a relay nucleus for the amygdala's projection to the hypothalamus and nucleus accumbens. However, the major source of enkephalin in the forebrain is in the striatum. Approximately half of the spiny neurons of the caudate nucleus and putamen contain enkephalin as a co-neurotransmitter. These neurons send their projections almost exclusively to the lateral segment of the globus pallidus, with recurrent collaterals innervating the striatum itself. The concentration of enkephalin in the globus pallidus is by far the highest of any place in the brain. The precise role of enkephalin in this structure remains unknown. It appears to have nothing to do with the pain system.

Dynorphin neurons are distributed very similarly to the enkephalin neurons, with concentrations in the pain-receiving areas of the spinal cord and spinal tract of the 5th nerve being particularly prominent. A major difference between enkephalin and dynorphin systems occurs, however, in the basal ganglia. Here, dynorphin is co-localized with substance P in striatal neurons that project to the medial segment of the globus pallidus and the substantia nigra rather than in the striatal cells, which project to the lateral globus pallidus. The lateral globus pallidus is the region that enkephalin densely innervates.

Opiate Receptors

A number of different binding sites for opiates have been described using ligand-binding techniques. The three that are probably most specific for opiate actions are the μ, δ, and κ receptors. μ Receptors seem to bind the morphine-like opiate pain medications most specifically. δ Receptors are most specific for the enkephalins, while the κ receptors are most specific for the dynorphins. The paradox of these binding sites and binding sites for ligands that bind to many

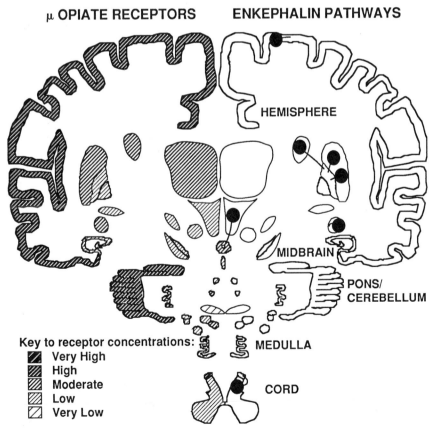

Figure 8.19. Some enkephalin pathways and the presumed distribution of μ-opiate receptors.

μ OPIATE RECEPTORS   ENKEPHALIN PATHWAYS

HEMISPHERE

MIDBRAIN

PONS/CEREBELLUM

MEDULLA

CORD

Key to receptor concentrations:
- Very High
- High
- Moderate
- Low
- Very Low

Figure 8.20. Presumed distribution of the δ and κ subtypes of opiate receptors.

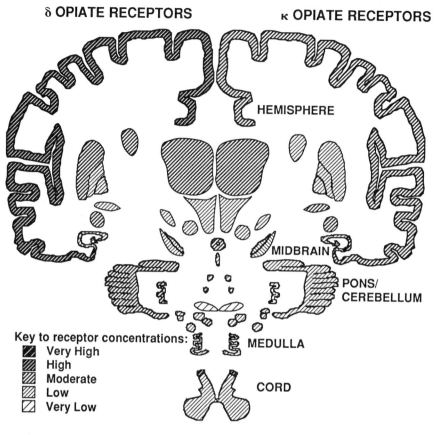

δ OPIATE RECEPTORS

κ OPIATE RECEPTORS

HEMISPHERE

MIDBRAIN

PONS/
CEREBELLUM

MEDULLA

CORD

Key to receptor concentrations:
- Very High
- High
- Moderate
- Low
- Very Low

of the other peptide transmitters is that the distribution of ligand-binding sites is radically different from the distribution of peptide-containing nerve terminals. Whether the receptors are present in places to which the peptides can diffuse over long distances, whether the peptides are somehow paradoxically present in great concentrations at places where they have no functional role, or whether the presence of high concentrations of peptide causes downregulation of receptor numbers, remains to be determined.

The distribution of μ opiate receptors is shown in Figure 8-19. These receptors are found selectively throughout the brain, with significant numbers in the dorsal horn of the spinal cord and spinal trigeminal nucleus. There are also receptors present in cerebellum, where there is no enkephalinergic innervation, or in the central gray of the brainstem. In the forebrain they are found in the cortex, particularly in association cortices, being most concentrated in layers 1, 2, and 4. There are numerous μ binding sites in the amygdala, whereas there are virtually no binding sites in the hippocampus or claustrum. The basal ganglia contain numerous sites in the caudate nucleus and putamen but practically no binding sites in the globus pallidus, particularly in the lateral segment. μ Receptors are also in high concentration in the medical dorsal nucleus of the thalamus.

The distribution of δ receptors is shown in Figure 8.20. This distribution closely resembles that of μ receptors being present in the dorsal horn or spinal cord and trigeminal nucleus, in layers 1 and 2 of the cortex, caudate nucleus, and putamen, medial dorsal nucleus of thalamus, and amygdala

with low binding in the globus pallidus. The δ sites are different from the μ sites in that there are significant numbers of δ receptors in the hippocampal formation, particularly in the dentate gyrus, while there are very few δ receptors in the cerebellum.

K-Receptor distribution is also shown in Figure 8.20. K receptors are concentrated in the deep layers of the cortex, particularly layers 5 and 6. It has been suggested that this deep layer binding is responsible for the sedative properties of K-agonist drugs. There is relatively little binding in the caudate nucleus and putamen except in the striosomes. There is slightly more binding in globus pallidus for K receptors than there is for either μ or K receptors. There is also a significant concentration of K receptors in the basal lateral nucleus of the amygdala. K-receptor sites are also found in the granule cell layer of the cerebellum, while the μ receptors seem to be more concentrated in the molecular cell layer.

TACHYKININS

Three main tacyhkinins have been described in the mammalian brain: substance P, neurokinin A, and neuromedin K. By far, the best described of these is substance P. The tachykinins all share the same carboxyterminal amino acid sequence, phenylalanine—an amino acid-glycine-leucine-amino terminal.

The preprotachykinin A gene is processed by differential splicing into either α-preprotachykinin A messenger RNA (the resultant protein is then cleaved to give substance P) or into β- and γ-preprotachykinin A messenger RNAs, which contain the coding sequences for both substance P and neurokinin A. Subsequent processing would therefore produce both compounds. These alternate transcription and RNA splicing mechanisms occur in both the periphery and in the central nervous system.

Neuromedin K is spliced from the preprotachykinin B gene, which is present in both the central nervous system and in the periphery. Preprotachykinin A—and therefore substance P and neurokinin A—are mainly expressed in the trigeminal ganglion, dorsal root ganglia and in the striatum while preprotachykinin B and thus, neuromedin K is primarily synthesized in the hypothalamus and in the intestines.

Substance P Distribution

The distribution of substance P neurons is shown in Figure 8.21. Substance P is a major neurotransmitter of primary afferent nerve terminals. Its primary roles seem to be in pain transmission via the small, unmyelineated, primary afferent nerve fibers. There is dense innervation of substantia gelatinosa of the spinal cord and spinal tract of the trigeminal nerve with substance P fibers. Stimulation of substance P fibers produces burning pain. Capsaicin, the active ingredient in chili peppers, stimulates the release of substance P both where it is applied locally to a nerve, such as the skin, or the mucous membranes of the mouth and centrally.

Capsaicin applications produce a temporary sensation of burning, followed by relative anesthesia as the substance P in the affected nerve is first released and then depleted.

Within the central nervous system (Fig. 8.21), substance P neurons are densely concentrated within the nucleus of the solitary tract, moderately around the cranial nerve nuclei, and moderately in the other medullary tegmental nuclei. There is also a dense cluster of substance P neurons in the parabrachial nucleus. These neurons innervate other pontine nuclei as well as the caudal parts of the substantia nigra.

In the forebrain there are a few substance P neurons in the cortex. These are mainly located in layer 6 and in deep parts of layer 5. They seem to project to the upper three layers. The dentate gyrus of the hippocampus contains some substance P innervation, while the central nucleus of the amygdala contains more. As with enkephalin about half of the spiny neurons of the striatum contain substance P. This is a different population from that of the enkephalin neurons. These neurons project to the medial segment of the globus pallidus and the substantia nigra pars reticulata rather than to the lateral segment of the globus pallidus.

Tachykinin Receptors

The tachykinin receptors are coupled by G proteins to the activation of the phosphatidylinositol system. There are three receptors named the NK1 (formerly called the substance P receptor). NK2 (formerly called the substance K or substance E receptor) and the NK3 (formerly the

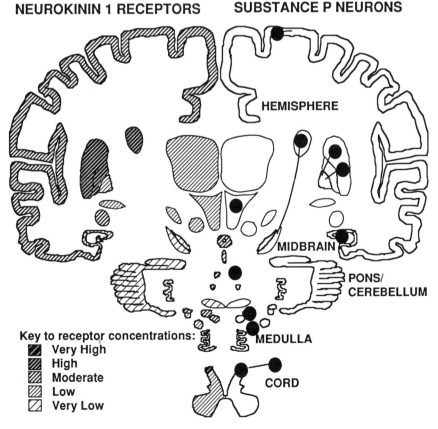

NEUROKININ 1 RECEPTORS   **SUBSTANCE P NEURONS**

HEMISPHERE

MIDBRAIN

PONS/ CEREBELLUM

MEDULLA

CORD

Key to receptor concentrations:
- Very High
- High
- Moderate
- Low
- Very Low

Figure 8.21. Some substance P pathways and the presumed distribution of NK1 receptors.

neurokinin B receptor). The three receptors share approximately 60% homology in the seven transmembrane regions, which makes them a family as closely related as the adrenergic or muscarinic receptors. The NK1 receptor is most susceptible to substance P. It is found in both nervous system and in the periphery. The NK2 is most susceptible as neurokinin A and is found only in the periphery. The NK3 receptor gene is expressed in both the central nervous system and in the periphery. However, NK3 binding sites have not been clearly demonstrated in binding studies of human brain.

The NK1 receptor is widely distributed in both the central nervous system and the periphery (Fig. 8.21). It is highly expressed in the hypothalamus, dorsal horn in the spinal cord, the olfactory bulb, and the striatum within the central nervous system. In the periphery it is expressed in the bladder, salivary glands, and the intestines. The NK2 receptor is restricted to peripheral tissues, particularly the bladder, the stomach, the large intestine, and the adrenal gland. The NK3 receptor gene, similar to the NK1 receptor gene, is more highly expressed in the central nervous system than in the periphery. The highest densities of expression are in the cerebellum, hypothalamus, and cortex.

Similar to the opiates, there is a large divergence between the location of the neuropeptides and the location of their receptors. For example, neurokinin A is present in the brain but the receptor is not located either in the brain or in the spinal cord. Thus, the actual role of these neuromodulators play in central nervous system function remains in doubt because of the lack of correlation between presence of the neuromodulator and presence of its effector.

SOMATOSTATIN

Somatostatin is a peptide that was first discovered to play a role in the control of growth hormone secretion. It was also found to be present in the intestinal system as well as in scattered interneurons throughout the brain. These interneurons are particularly prominent in layer 4 of the neocortex, in the hippocampus, and in the striatum. Four subtypes of somatostatin receptors have been described. In contrast to the opiate and neurokinin receptors, these receptors seem to be located in regions in close proximity to the location of somatostatinergic presynaptic terminals.

OTHER PEPTIDES

A large number of other peptides that were first discovered because they had a role in bodily functions outside the brain have subsequently been identified within the brain. For the most part the distribution of these neuropeptides is much more restricted than that of either the endorphins, somatostatin, or the tachykinins. Few data have been gathered about the distribution and role of receptors for these peptides in the central nervous system. The three main locations of these other neuropeptides are primary afferent neurons, the medulla, and the hypothalamus. Thus, these peptides are positioned to influence sensation through the primary afferents and vegetative functions through the medulla and hypothalamus.

Among these peptides are two that were originally discovered to play hormonal roles in intestinal functions. These are cholecystokinin and bombesin. Both are present in primary afferents. In addition, cholecystokinin is found in the dopamine neurons that project from the ventral tegmental area to the nucleus accumbens in the rat, although not in higher primates. Cholecystokinin is found in the caudate nucleus of humans, but the source of this projection is unknown. Both peptides are thought to play roles in the sensation of satiety.

Several regulators of vascular tone (angiotensin, atrial natiuretic hormone, bradykinin, and vasoactive intestinal peptide) are present in hypothalamus and medulla.

The peptides that were originally described as hormones (calcitonin gene-related peptide, melatonin, oxytocin, and vasopressin) have projecting axons within hypothalamus, outside of the pituitary stalk.

Finally, recently several of the interleukins have been shown to be used as neuromodulators by cells of the hypothalamus. Interleukins are peptides used as intercellular-signaling messengers by the cells of the immune system. They are involved in the inflammatory response to foreign antigens. Injection of interleukins into the cerebral spinal fluid produces a febrile response. Therefore, it has been speculated that the interleukin pathways within the hypothalamus are those that stimulate the febrile response occurring as a result of infection.

Gases

Recently it has been discovered that at least two diffusible gases are used as intercellular messengers within the central nervous system and the periphery. Several years ago such a role was described for nitric oxide (NO). More recently it has been proposed that carbon monoxide is also a neurotransmitter. The mechanism of action of the gases is completely different from that of the other neurotransmitters and neuromodulators because they are so diffusable. They are not stored in vesicles. There is no release mechanism at the synaptic terminal and there is no postsynaptic receptor for these gases. The gases are synthesized in presynaptic terminals. They then diffuse freely throughout the tissues including across the synaptic cleft where they interact directly with second messenger systems within the "postsynaptic" neuron.

NITRIC OXIDE

The first gas to be discovered to play a role as a neurotransmitter was nitric oxide. It had long been known that in addition to the acetylcholine and norepinephrine systems, there was at least one more transmitter involved in the autonomic nervous system. This noncholinergic/nonadrenergic neurotransmitter was responsible for relaxation of arterioles and was called endothelial-relaxing factor. It has recently been shown that nitric oxide is the endothelial relaxing factor. It is synthesized by a specific enzyme, nitric oxide synthase, in endothelial cells, and it diffuses from there into the smooth muscle cells that surround the arterioles. There it stimulates guanylate cyclase, the synthetic enzyme for the second messenger molecule, cyclic GMP. It is the cyclic GMP that produces relaxation of the arteriolar smooth muscle. This NO/cyclic GMP mediated system is vital to the arteriolar relaxation that allows blood to engorge the penis. Thus, nitric oxide is the neurotransmitter responsible for penile erections.

The distribution of nitric oxide neurons in the brain is shown in Figure 8.15. (These cells are easy to detect because NO synthase is the enzyme responsible for the histochemical NADPH diaphorase stain. Thus, cells containing nitric oxide synthase, and only those cells, are colored by the histochemical reaction.) Nitric oxide synthase is located densely in the granule cells of the cerebellum, where nitric oxide is synthesized and diffuses to other cells, where it then stimulates guanylate cyclase. Other cells containing nitric oxide synthase are scattered throughout the brain, including the cortex, striatum, and hippocampus. In these locations, the nitric oxide synthase-containing neurons are interneurons with large numbers of local axon collaterals. It has recently been shown that nitric oxide may play a very important role in the stimulation of long-term potentiation, a model of memory formation in the hippocampus. Current

evidence suggests that a message is sent retrogradely from the postsynaptic neuron to the presynaptic terminal to increase the presynaptic terminal's firing ability as part of the learning process. Nitric oxide appears to be the messenger molecule that is sent in a retrograde fashion. However, within the hippocampus nitric oxide synthase is not located in the postsynaptic pyramidal neurons. Instead, it is synthesized in local interneurons and if it is involved in actual learning process, these neurons must somehow be specifically stimulated as part of the long-term potentiation process.

Nitric oxide has been proposed as a potential neurotoxin because exposure of neurons to excess amounts of this compound causes neurons to die. Two proposed mechanisms can possibly make nitric oxide toxic. The simpler theory is that nitric oxide is a free radical and can combine with oxygen to form even more toxic free radicals. This is how neutrophils are thought to use nitric oxide to kill bacteria. The second proposed mechanism is that nitric oxide causes inhibition of glyceraldehyde-3-phosphate dehydrogenase, a vital enzyme in the metabolism of glucose. Thus, excessive stimulation of nitric oxide may make neurons unable to metabolize glucose, their primary energy source. Interestingly, the nitric oxide-containing neurons themselves are quite resistant to neurotoxic processes such as ischemia and Huntington's disease. It has been proposed that as producers of nitric oxide, these neurons may somehow have extra protective mechanisms against its neurotoxic actions.

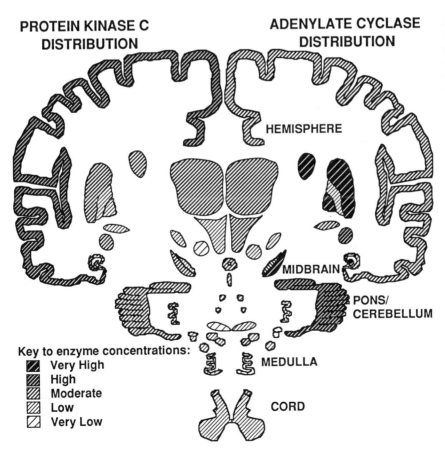

Figure 8.22. Presumed distribution of two important second messenger system enzymes, adenylate cyclase, which forms cyclic AMP, and protein kinase C, which is involved in phosphatidylinositol metabolism.

PROTEIN KINASE C DISTRIBUTION

ADENYLATE CYCLASE DISTRIBUTION

HEMISPHERE

MIDBRAIN

PONS/ CEREBELLUM

MEDULLA

CORD

Key to enzyme concentrations:
- Very High
- High
- Moderate
- Low
- Very Low

CARBON MONOXIDE

It has recently been found that carbon monoxide can also be produced in the brain by the enzyme hemeoxygenase-2. Like nitric oxide, carbon monoxide is a freely diffusible compound. Once synthesized it appears to be able to stimulate guanylate cyclase, just as nitric oxide can. Thus, carbon monoxide and nitric oxide both stimulate the same enzyme, and carbon monoxide can greatly potentiate the response to nitric oxide. Hemeoxygenase-2 is enriched in olfactory structures, pyramidal cells of the hippocampus, and Purkinje cells of the cerebellum, but it is present throughout the brain.

SECOND MESSENGERS

There are two extremely well-described second messenger systems within the brain. Both are ordinarily stimulated by G-protein-coupled receptors. One is the cyclic AMP system, which is stimulated by adenylate cyclase. The other is the phosphatidylinositol cycle in which phosphatidylinositol bis (phosphate) is cleaved by phospholipase C to inositol triphosphate and diacylglycerol. Diacylglycerol in turn stimulates protein kinase C and calcium influx. Recently ligands have been found that bind with high affinity to adenylate cyclase and to protein kinase C, thus making it possible to identify the sites in the brain where these two second messenger systems are located (Fig. 8.22).

Adenylate cyclase is extremely dense in both neurons of the striatum and in their terminals within the medial globus pallidus and substantia nigra. Very high levels are present in the cerebellar granule cell axon terminals within the cerebellar molecular layer and in the hippocampal formation. There it is found in the dendrites of dentate gyrus granule cells and in their mossy fiber terminals in the CA3 region. Lesser amounts of adenylate cyclase are found throughout the rest of the brain, including the cortex, thalamus, and hypothalamus. Adenylate cyclase is present in both dorsal and ventral horns of the spinal cord, being denser within the dorsal horn.

Protein kinase C is also located throughout the brain, but it is not nearly as dense as adenylate cyclase is in the striatum and its terminals. The densest distribution of protein kinase C is in the cell bodies, dendrites, and axons of CA3 and CA1 pyramidal cells of the hippocampus and in the Purkinje cells of the cerebellum. Moderate levels are found in cortex, sriatum, thalamus, substantia nigra, and brainstem. In the spinal cord protein kinase C is largely located in the substantia gelatinosa.

Interestingly, there is a significant negative correlation between the dense regions of cyclic AMP and the dense regions of protein kinase C localization. Thus, cyclic AMP is located in cerebellar granule cells, while protein kinase C is located in Purkinje cells. Similarly, adenylate cyclase is located in the granule cells of the dentate gyrus in the hippocampus, while protein kinase C is located in the postsynaptic CA3 and then CA1 neurons. Thus, the first cell in both the hippocampal and cerebellar chains of neurons are sensitive to cyclic AMP, while the subsequent neurons are sensitive to the inositol phosphate system.

Other signal transduction systems exist, including the guanylate cyclase system, to which nitric oxide and carbon monoxide are linked, growth factor systems, protooncogene systems, and immediate early genes. Clearly, the future will bring greater understanding of the distribution and roles of these systems in the brain, just as research in the last 25 years has enhanced our knowledge of neurotransmitters significantly.

Acknowledgments

The author thanks Rita Zollo for secretarial assistance. This work was supported by USPHS grants NS19613 and AG08671.

Suggested Readings

General

Mendelsohn FAO, Paxinos G, eds. Receptors in the human nervous system. San Diego: Academic Press, 1991.
Paxinos G, ed. The human nervous system, San Diego: Academic Press, 1990.
Watson S, Girdlestone D. TIPS receptor nomenclature supplement. Trends Pharmacol Sci 1993;14 (suppl).

Transporters

Amara SG, Kuhar MJ. Neurotransmitter transporters: recent progress. Annu Rev Neurosci 1993;16:73–93.
Kanai Y, Smith CP, Hediger MA. The elusive transporters with a high affinity for glutamate. Trends Neurol Sci 1993;16:365–370.

Glutamate Receptors

Collingridge GL, Singer W. Excitatory amino acid receptors and synaptic plasticity. Trends Pharmacol Sci 1990;11:290–296.
Meldrum B, Garthwaite J. Excitatory amino acid toxicity and neurodegenerative disease. Trends Pharmacol Sci 1990;11:379–387.
Nakanishi S. Molecular diversity of glutamate receptors and implications for brain function. Science 1992;258:597–603.
Seeburg PH. The TINS/TIPS lecture: The molecular biology of mammalian glutamate receptor channels. Trends Neurol Sci 1993;16:359–364.

GABA Receptors

Burt DR, Kamatchi GL. GABA$_A$ receptor subtypes: from pharmacology to molecular biology. FASEB J 1991;5:2916–2923.

Acetylcholine Receptors

Sargent PB. The diversity of neuronal nicotinic acetylcholine receptors. Annu Rev Neurosci 1993;16:403–443.

Dopamine Receptors

Sibley DR, Monsma FJ. Molecular biology of dopamine receptors. Trends Pharmacol Sci 1992;13:61–68.

Norepinephrine Receptors

Kobilka B. Adrenergic receptors as models for G protein-coupled receptors. Annu Rev Neurosci 1992;15:87–114.

Serotonin Receptors

Julius D. Molecular biology of serotonin receptors. Annu Rev Neurosci 1991;14:335–360.

Humphrey PPA, Hartig P, Hoyer D. A proposed new nomenclature for 5-HT receptors. Trends Pharmacol Sci 1993;14:233–236.

Adenosine Receptors

Fastbom J, Pazos A, Probst A, Palacios JM. Adenosine A1 receptors in the human brain: a quantitative autoradiographic study. Neuroscience 1987;22:827–839, 1987.

Peptide Receptors

Herkenham M. Mismatches between neurotransmitter and receptor localizations in brain: observations and implications. Neuroscience 1987;23:1–38.

Nakanishi S. Mammalian tachykinin receptors. Annu Rev Neurosci 1991;14:123–136.

Gases

Snyder SH, Bredt DS. Biological roles of nitric oxide. Sci Am 1992;266:68–77.

Verma A, Hirsch DJ, Glatt CE, Ronnett GV, Snyder SH. Carbon monoxide: a putative neural messenger. Science 1993;259:381–384.

Second Messengers

Worley PF, Baraban JM, De Souza EB, Snyder SH. Mapping second messenger systems in the brain: differential localizations of adenylate cyclase and protein kinase C. Proc Nat Acad Sci USA 1986;83:4053–4057.

9

PSYCHONEUROENDOCRINOLOGY

Beatriz M. DeMoranville and Ivor M.D. Jackson

The central nervous system (CNS) has a fundamental role in the regulation of the endocrine system. The hypothalamus, part of the diencephalon, secretes specific neuroregulatory hormones or releasing factors that can activate or inhibit anterior pituitary function. Additionally, within the CNS itself there are peptide hormone-producing neurons (neuroendocrine cells) responsible for interneuronal communication and neuromodulation, but not directly involved in pituitary regulation (1–3).

Hypothalamic peptidergic neurons are regulated by monoamine neurotransmitters: dopamine (DA), norepinephrine (NE), and serotonin (5HT). Peptidergic neurons act as "neuroendocrine transducers," converting neural information from the brain into chemical (hormonal) information (4, 5). The hypothalamic-releasing hormones are part of a family of neural peptides with a widespread distribution throughout the CNS.

Alterations in monoamine neurotransmitters play a major role in the pathophysiology of psychiatric and neurological disorders. For this reason, the hypothalamic-pituitary axis has been extensively investigated in neuropsychiatric disorders as a window on CNS pathophysiology.

PSYCHONEUROENDOCRINOLOGY: DEFINITION

Psychoneuroendocrinology is the field of experimental and clinical neurosciences in which psychiatry, neurology, and endocrinology intersect. Study of this discipline enhances knowledge about the relationships between the neurosecretory systems and behavior and leads to a better understanding of the pathogenesis and management of psychiatric disorders (Fig. 9.1).

Objectives of Psychoneuroendocrinology

The field of psychoneuroendocrinology involves the following objectives (1):

1. To define the hormonal, neurotransmitter, or neuromodulatory defect in a psychiatric or neurological disorder;

2. To utilize this information to elucidate the differential diagnosis of psychiatric disorders;
3. To predict the response to treatment and its prognosis by attempting to correct underlying neuroendocrine abnormalities; and
4. To utilize this approach to characterize the mechanisms of action of the neuroactive compounds used for therapy of psychiatric conditions.

HYPOTHALAMIC-PITUITARY SYSTEM: ANATOMICAL CONSIDERATIONS

This section reviews the anatomy of the hypothalamic-pituitary system. Familiarity with it is important for the understanding of the neuroendocrine system's role in psychiatric disorders.

Hypothalamus

The hypothalamus is part of the diencephalon (6). Anteriorly, it is limited by the optic chiasm and the lamina terminalis, and it is continuous with the preoptic area, the substantia innominata, and the septal region. Posteriorly, it is limited by an imaginary plane defined by the posterior mammillary bodies ventrally and the posterior commissure dorsally. Caudally, the hypothalamus merges with the midbrain periaqueductal gray and tegmental reticular formation. The dorsal limit of the hypothalamus is determined by the horizontal level of the hypothalamic sulcus on the medial wall of the third ventricle, at the horizontal level of the anterior commissure. Here the hypothalamus is continuous with the subthalamus and the zona incerta. Laterally, the hypothalamus is limited by the internal capsule and the basis of the cerebral peduncles (7).

The hypothalamic area involved with the regulation of the anterior pituitary has been named the hypophysiotropic area (6). Neuroendocrine cells in this area form the following nuclei: the supraoptic (SON), paraventricular (PVN), periventricular, medial preoptic, and arcuate nuclei of the hypothalamus (3, 6). These nuclei project to the median

173

Figure 9.1. Diagram representing psychoneuroendocrinology and its interactions with
endocrinology, psychiatry, and
neurology.

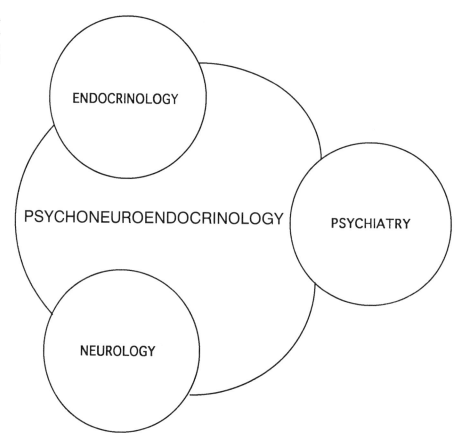

eminence (6) and secrete the hypophysiotropic factors that
regulate pituitary function.

Median Eminence

The *median eminence* or *infundibulum* gives rise to the
pituitary stalk at the base of the hypothalamus, in the floor of
the third ventricle. The median eminence is the site where:
(*a*) the hypothalamic neuroendocrine cells release their secretions to the primary plexus of the hypophysial portal system
for regulation of the adenohypophysis (i.e., the anterior
pituitary); (*b*) hypothalamic neural fibers that end in the
neurohypophysis and intermediate lobe (the hypothalamic
neurohypophysial tract) pass through; and (*c*) the portal
venous system, which provides the only significant blood
flow to the anterior pituitary, originates (6, 8).

The Pituitary Gland or Hypophysis

The *pituitary gland* or *hypophysis* lies close to the medial
basal hypothalamus, to which it is connected by the pituitary
stalk (7). In most vertebrates it is divided into three lobes:
the anterior lobe or adenohypophysis, the posterior lobe or
neurohypophysis, and the intermediate lobe (6, 8). In the
adult human, there are only rudimentary vestiges of the
intermediate lobe (6, 8). During fetal life and pregnancy,
however, an intermediate lobe is evident (8).

THE ANTERIOR PITUITARY OR ADENOHYPOPHYSIS

The *anterior pituitary* or *adenohypophysis* contains cells that
secrete the following hormones: adrenocorticotropin hormone (ACTH), thyroid-stimulating hormone (TSH),
luteinizing-hormone (LH), follicle-stimulating hormone
(FSH), growth hormone (GH) and prolactin (PRL)
(Fig. 9.2).

Five cell types have been recognized in the adenohypophysis and are responsible for the synthesis of the classic
anterior pituitary hormones: somatotropes, mammotropes,
corticotropes, thyrotropes and gonadotropes. The somatotropes are the GH-producing cells, which account for 50%
of the cells in the adenohypophysis. The mammotropes are
the prolactin-producing cells, which account for 15–25% of
the cells. They increase in number and size with pregnancy,
lactation, and with estrogen therapy. The corticotropes are
ACTH-producing cells, which constitute about 20% of the
anterior pituitary cells. Thyrotropes produce TSH and
constitute about 5% of the cells in the anterior pituitary.
Gonadotropes, the least numerous hormone-secreting cells
in the anterior pituitary, produce LH and FSH. Each of these
cell types can also be identified histologically by immuno-
staining techniques using specific antisera against the specific
hormone produced (9), or by in situ hybridization. Additionally, there are other cell types within the anterior
pituitary, including the folliculostellate cells shown to
contain interleukin-6. Furthermore, there are numerous

neural peptides produced within the anterior pituitary, including vasoactive intestinal polypeptide (VIP), which regulates prolactin and substance P (10). It is likely that these peptides modulate anterior pituitary hormone secretion, especially under conditions of stress (11, 12). VIP may have a role in regulating the pulsatile secretion of LH (13) and in determining circadian rhythms (14, 15, 16), along with substance P (17, 18).

NEUROHYPOPHYSIS

The *neurohypophysis* includes the neural stalk, the neural lobe or posterior pituitary, and the specialized neurons at the base of the hypothalamus. The major nerve tracts of the neurohypophysis arise from the accessory magnocellular, the SON, the PVN, and from cells scattered in the periformical and lateral hypothalamic areas and the bed nucleus of the stria terminalis. The supraoptic nucleus is located above the optic tract, and the PVN is located on each side of the 3rd ventricle. Most of their unmyelinated fibers descend through the infundibulum and neural stalk within the zona interna to

end in the neural lobe. The majority of these fibers contain arginine-vasopressin (AVP) (also known as antidiuretic hormone or ADH) and oxytocin. Some vasopressin or oxytocin fibers derived from the parvocellular division descend in the zona externa of the median eminence, where they are involved in the regulation of the anterior pituitary, specifically, ACTH release during stress (19). Other neuropeptides, including thyrotropin-releasing hormone (TRH), corticotropin releasing hormone (CRH), VIP, and neurotensin, have been found to be secreted from smaller cells or parvicellular neurons (8). In addition, enkephalins, dynorphins, galanin, cholecystokinin, and angiotensin II have been found in the fibers of the supraopticohypophysial tract and in neuronal terminals in the neurohypophysis (3).

HYPOTHALAMIC HYPOPHYSIOTROPIC FACTORS

It is known that the hypothalamic neurons produce neuropeptides that regulate the function of the adenohy-

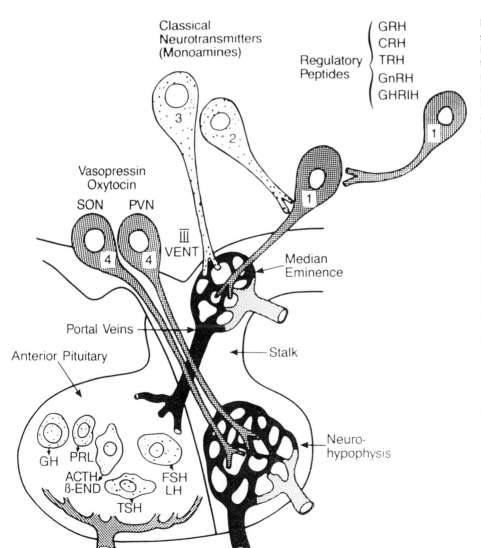

Figure 9.2. Diagram representing the hypothalamic-pituitary axis. Neuron 4 represents the magnocellular peptidergic neurons of the hypothalamo-neurohypophysial tract with cell bodies in the supraoptic (SON) and paraventricular (PVN) nuclei and terminals in the neurohypophysis. Neurons 2 and 3 are monoaminergic neurons. Neuron 2 represents a neuron contacting the cell body of a peptidergic neuron, whereas neuron 3 represents a dopaminergic neuron projecting to the median eminence, where release of dopamine occurs. The neurons 1 are the peptidergic neurons, which secrete regulatory peptides into the pituitary portal plexus. The regulatory peptides as well as dopamine are involved in the control of the secretion of different anterior pituitary hormones (β-END = β-endorphin). (Reproduced with permission from Pelletier G. Anatomy of the hypothalamic-pituitary axis. In Jasmin G, Cantin M, eds. Stress revisited. 1. Neuroendocrinology of stress. Methods Achievements in Experimental Pathology. Basel: Karger 1992;14:2.)

pophysis. Two regulators are inhibitory: dopamine, a monoamine tonic inhibitory factor for PRL, and somatostatin (also known as somatotropin inhibitory factor, or SRIF), which inhibits the production of GH. The other known factors stimulate the release of anterior pituitary hormones and are therefore referred to as releasing factors.

The hypophysiotropic factors or hormones are synthesized by neurons in the hypothalamus, transported to nerve endings in the stalk-median eminence, released into the interstitial space in contiguity with the primary portal capillary plexus, and distributed to the anterior pituitary by means of the portal circulation (Fig. 9.2)(5).

The arcuate nucleus of the hypothalamus contains growth-hormone-releasing hormone (GHRH), paraventricular nucleus contains mainly TRH and CRH, and the preoptic nucleus contains mainly gonadotropin releasing hormone (GnRH or LHRH). SRIF is found in the periventricular nucleus. These nuclei also contain many other peptides, including proopiomelanocortin (POMC) and derived peptides ACTH, β-endorphin, and α-melanocyte-stimulating hormone (MSH); neuropeptide Y, galanin, substance P, enkephalins, atrial natriuretic peptide, angiotensin II, cholecystokinin, and dynorphins (3, 20).

Although the actions of each of the hypophysiotropic factors are not limited to a single pituitary hormone, these factors have been named in accordance to the anterior pituitary hormone first recognized to be regulated. Releasing factors are synthesized in neuronal cell bodies, then migrate in dense core vesicles to the median eminence, where they are stored in axonal endings, ready for their release into the pituitary portal circulation upon stimulation. The hypophysiotropic neurons are regulated by neurotransmitters and neuropeptide modulators and by feedback effects. These are exerted both by the hormones produced by the end organs and by pituitary hormones—"short-loop" feedback (Fig. 9.3).

Hypophysiotropic factors of the hypothalamus in relationship to the corresponding pituitary-end organ axis are shown schematically in Figure 9.4.

Gonadotropin-Releasing Hormone (GnRH) or Luteinizing Hormone-Releasing Hormone (LHRH)

This decapeptide was the first hypophysiotropic factor to be localized by immunohistochemistry. In humans, the GnRH neurons are located in the highest concentrations in the medial basal hypothalamus (infundibular and mammillary nuclei) and the preoptic area (6). GnRH stimulates the release of LH and FSH by the pituitary gland. In the female, it controls the menstrual cycle. In males, it controls testosterone secretion and spermatogenesis. It has been shown to stimulate sexual activity in rats of both sexes, independently of its hypophysiotropic action, suggesting a direct influence on brain functions relevant to sexual drive. For example, LHRH enhances lordosis behavior and sexual

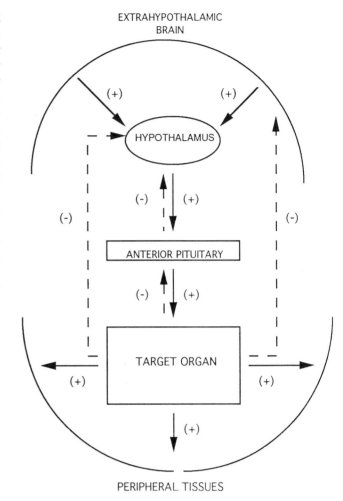

Figure 9.3. Interactions of the neuroendocrine system with the extrahypothalamic brain and peripheral tissues. Lines indicate regulatory interactions.

receptivity in ovariectomized, estradiol-benzoate treated rats (21–23).

Corticotropin releasing hormone (CRH). This 41-peptide is found in neuronal cell bodies of the PVN of the human hypothalamus (24, 25). CRH is responsible for stimulating the secretion of ACTH and other POMC-related peptides from the anterior pituitary. ACTH regulates the secretion of cortisol from the adrenal cortex. The hypothalamic-pituitary-adrenal (HPA) axis is essential to the neuroendocrine response to physical or mental stress. Additionally, cerebral CRH is involved in the stress response independently of its pituitary-adrenal effects (26, 27).

Thyrotropin-releasing hormone. In the rat brain, cell bodies containing immunoreactive TRH and its precursor, pro-TRH, have been demonstrated in the preoptic nucleus, parvocellular subdivision of the PVN, perifornical region, dorsomedial nucleus, and basolateral hypothalamus (6). The TRH-containing cells of the PVN are most important to the regulation of the pituitary-thyroid axis. TRH regulates the thyroid axis by stimulating the release of TSH from the anterior pituitary, which acts directly on receptors on the secretory cells of the thyroid gland. TRH is also a potent stimulatory factor for prolactin (PRL) secretion, but its physiological role in the regulation of PRL is uncertain at this time. TRH neurons are also present in extrahypothalamic tissues, particularly the raphe nucleus, where there is colocalization with serotonin (5HT). The relevance of this colocalization is not yet known. TRH may be a neurotransmitter or neuromodulator in view of its localization in nerve endings and the presence of TRH receptors in brain tissue.

Growth hormone-releasing hormone. In primates, neuronal bodies containing GHRH are found in high concentrations in the arcuate nucleus (6). GHRH stimulates GH secretion. GH is required for normal growth and development.

Somatostatin. Bodies of the neurons containing this tetradecapeptide are mainly found in the anterior portion of the arcuate nucleus close to the infundibular recess in humans (28). Somatostatin inhibits GH release. It is widely distributed throughout the nervous system and in extraneuronal tissues, including the gastrointestinal tract and endocrine pancreas. Somatostatin inhibits the secretion of TSH and, under certain circumstances, PRL and ACTH. In addition, it has inhibitory effects on endocrine and exocrine secretions of the pancreas, the gallbladder, and the gut.

Prolactin (PRL) regulatory factors—Dopamine. The most important is the inhibitory factor *dopamine.* Dopamine acts on the lactotrope to inhibit the biosynthesis and release of PRL.

PSYCHONEUROENDOCRINE APPROACH OF THE HYPOTHALAMIC-PITUITARY AXIS

In the following section we review the different hypothalamic-pituitary systems in the context of neuropsychiatric conditions.

The Hypothalamic-Pituitary Adrenocortical Axis

The HPA system has been the subject of much of the literature and research in the field of psychoneuroendocrinology since it was recognized that hypercortisolism is a consequence of stress, and a frequent accompaniment of depression.

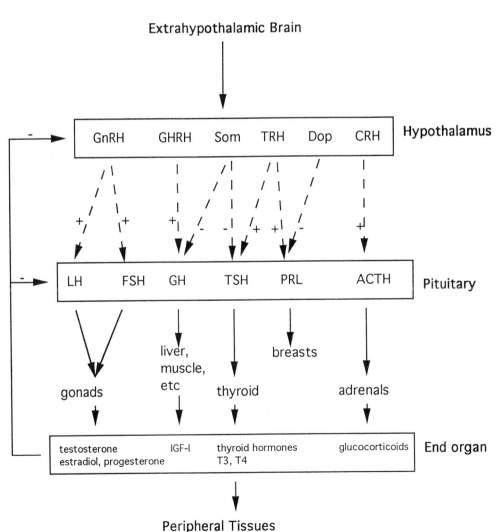

Figure 9.4. Diagram representing the interactions of the different hypothalamic-pituitary-end-organ axes.

REGULATION OF THE HPA AXIS

At the highest level, a variety of neurotransmitter pathways (including serotoninergic and cholinergic excitatory pathways and adrenergic and possibly GABAergic inhibitory pathways) influence the release of CRH and co-secretagogues, including arginine-vasopressin (AVP) and oxytocin, into the portal circulation. In response to CRH, a large precursor molecule, POMC is synthesized in the anterior pituitary and is cleaved into ACTH and other neuropeptides, including β-endorphin. ACTH is then secreted into the systemic circulation. At the adrenal cortex, ACTH stimulates the release of cortisol (19, 29, 30). The major HPA neuropeptides, CRH and ACTH, not only coordinate the neuroendocrine response to stress, but also facilitate behavioral adaptation. They play a key role as regulators of cell development, homeostatic maintenance, and adaptation to environmental challenges.

Regulation of the HPA axis is dependent upon three major mechanisms (30, 31): (*a*) pulsatile CRH release linked to the endogenous circadian rhythm of the CNS. This mechanism involves an oscillator located in the suprachiasmatic nucleus and is mediated by serotonergic pathways; (*b*) physical and psychological stresses, which affect the input from the limbic and the reticular-activating systems to CRH-secreting neurons. Vasopressin secretion, which is increased by stress, enhances the CRH-induced release of ACTH from corticotrophs; (*c*) feedback loops, by which circulating glucocorticoids feed back to the pituitary, the hypothalamus, and certain extrahypothalamic regions to inhibit HPA activity (29). The hippocampus appears to have an important role in this inhibitory action of glucocorticoids. There are numerous glucocorticoid receptors in the hippocampus. A reduction in number of these receptors, as by prenatal dexamethasone treatment of experimental monkeys (32), or by hippocampal lesions such as those of Alzheimer's disease, is associated with hypersecretion of glucocorticoids, increased hypothalamic levels of CRH and reduced suppression of ACTH by exogenous glucocorticoid administration (29, 33–35). Chronic but variable stress down-regulates glucocorticoid receptors in both the hippocampus and the paraventricular nucleus of the hypothalamus, thereby reducing the suppression of CRH by glucocorticoids and leading to tonic hypersecretion of cortisol (36).

HPA AXIS IN STRESS AND DEPRESSION

Stress can be defined as any threat—real or perceived—to homeostasis or survival (37). Stimuli in this category include injury, hemorrhage, significant illness, fear, and bereavement. In recent years, immune activation has been found to be a stimulus for HPA activation as well through the role of interleukins. Interleukin-1, for example, has been shown to directly stimulate the release of both CRH and ACTH (37–31) in experimental animals; it also down-regulates prolactin secretion (31a). Interleukin effects, recently reviewed by Rivier and Abraham (37, 41), are discussed in detail in Chapter 10 of this book.

In 1936, Hans Seyle (43) was the first to describe the stress syndrome produced by noxious agents, which included three stages: the "alarm reaction," "resistance," and "exhaustion." There is a major role for glucocorticoids during the alarm reaction. Glucocorticoids are highly catabolic and they induce lipolysis, glycogenolysis, and proteolysis, thus increasing the levels of free fatty acids, glucose and amino acids as readily available fuels for the body (29, 44). The ultimate effect is to prepare the organism for strenuous activity by increasing the availability of energy substrates. In addition, glucocorticoids suppress immunological function and decrease the inflammatory response (44), involving alterations in both T- and B-cell function and interleukin release (41). The suppression of immunity during stress may protect the animal at a time where maximal mobility may be important (29), but also may explain the increased incidence of infection after injury (41). Other physiological changes induced by prolonged stress include suppression of thyroid and GH activity, as well as of sexual and reproductive behavior (44–46). Growth and reproduction are subordinated to the need to make energy readily available to confront an immediate danger.

Psychological stressors are less potent stimuli of the HPA axis than physical stressors, but they can cause changes in ACTH and cortisol production. However, patients with uncomplicated anxiety or panic disorder do not demonstrate excess urinary free cortisol (UFC) levels, except when their anxiety is accompanied by depression (47).

In depression, there is both increased secretion of CRH and a neurally mediated hyper-responsivity of the adrenal gland to ACTH (48).

MEASURES OF BASAL HPA ACTIVITY

Several measures of HPA activity have been employed in neuroendocrine studies of depression.

1. *Basal plasma cortisol:* This increases with increased activity at any level of the HPA axis. It shows a good correlation with levels of urinary free cortisol.
2. *Urinary free cortisol:* This is an integrated measure of HPA activity over time and it directly measures the unbound portion of total plasma cortisol. It reflects the cortisol secretion rate. It is less sensitive to time of collection.
3. *Cortisol in saliva and CSF:* These correlate well with unbound plasma cortisol. The former provides a potential means for frequent noninvasive sampling of ambient circulating levels, while the latter provides a direct indication of the levels of glucocorticoids to which CNS is exposed.

DYNAMIC MEASURES OF HPA AXIS ACTIVITY

The Dexamethasone Suppression Test

The lack of inhibition of the HPA axis by exogenous glucocorticoid was first observed by Carrol et al. (49) in the presence of severe depression. It is found in children and adolescents as well as in adults (50). A "psychiatric" dexamethasone suppression test (DST) is normal if there is suppression of plasma cortisol level to less than 5 μg/dl from 8–24 hours after an oral dose of 1 mg dexamethasone given at 11 PM (51, 52). An abnormal DST is found in approximately 45% of patients with depression. The test has shown a specificity of up to 80% in some studies, but the specificity depends on the population tested. Abnormal DSTs are seen in other psychiatric disorders, including anorexia nervosa (53), obsessive-compulsive disorder (54), degenerative dementia (55), mania (56), schizophrenia (57), alcoholism (58), psychosexual dysfunction (59), and schizoaffective psychosis (60), as well as gross brain diseases, including Parkinson's disease (61) and stroke. Other variables, such as weight loss, acute hospitalization, and drug and alcohol withdrawal, can affect the test significantly, as can many commonly prescribed medications (62, 63). The DST is a more sensitive test for major depression in older persons and in children and adolescents (64). It is abnormal more frequently in patients with psychotic affective disorders and melancholia (> 50%) than in those with minor depression (23%) or with grief reactions (10%) (51, 65).

Several hypotheses have been proposed to explain the nonsuppression of the DST in major depression (66), including increased metabolism of dexamethasone, decreased sensitivity of the pituitary glucocorticoid receptors to dexamethasone, hyperresponsivity of the adrenal gland to ACTH stimulation, and increased central drive of the pituitary from hypothalamic/limbic structures that overrides the action of the dexamethasone. The latter seems to be the most coherent and is supported by the blunted ACTH response to exogenous CRH administration (67–69) and to insulin-induced hypoglycemia (70), which reflects the down-regulation of corticotrophin receptors (71) in the pituitary from prolonged hypothalamic CRH hypersecretion and the consequent feedback by the elevated cortisol levels.

The DST has not evolved into a routine diagnostic test in clinical psychiatry because of its lack of specificity. There is, however, some evidence that an abnormal DST identifies depressed patients who respond more slowly to treatment and that nonsuppression persisting after treatment may predict earlier relapse (65, 72).

The DST also has been applied to patients with neurologic diseases, with and without a concomitant major depression. In *Parkinson's disease,* one study showed 74% nonsuppression in patients with concurrent major depression, and 25% suppression in those with PD alone (73); another study showed 14% nonsuppression among depressed patients and no nonsuppression among those with PD alone (74). *Alzheimer's disease* yields nonsuppression rates comparable with those seen in primary melancholia (75). *Stroke* is associated with an abnormal DST in 25% or more of patients without clinical depression (76), but with nonsuppression in more than half of patients with concomitant major depression (76–79).

ACTH Stimulation Test

Adrenocortical hyperresponsiveness to exogenous ACTH is associated with the hypercortisolism of Cushing's syndrome. Depressed patients also may show an increased response to ACTH, which correlates with adrenal enlargement found by computerized tomography (80) and in postmortem studies of adrenals of subjects who committed suicide (81). The enhanced response to ACTH stimulation may represent a persistent and prolonged state of endogenous ACTH elevation, leading to adrenal hyperplasia.

CRH Stimulation Test

Patients with melancholia show blunted ACTH and cortisol response and to exogenous CRH administration (67–69). Corticotropes in the anterior pituitary are down-regulated by hypercortisolism and persistent CRH release. This decreased response to exogenous CRH distinguishes depressed patients from Cushing's disease patients, who have both an ACTH and a cortisol hyperresponse to exogenous CRH. In Cushing's disease, endogenous CRH secretion is decreased; in depression, it is increased.

ROLE OF CRH IN STRESS AND DEPRESSION

Since its identification and sequencing in 1981, CRH has been recognized as the principal organizer of the neuroendocrine stress response (82). In addition, CRH plays a major role in coordinating the endocrine autonomic, behavioral, and immune responses to stress through actions in the brain and peripheral tissues. In autoradiographic studies, CRH receptors are localized in highest densities in anterior and intermediate lobes of the pituitary, the olfactory bulb, cerebral cortex, amygdala and cerebellum, and the spleen (83). In addition to activation of the HPA axis, CRH causes behavioral arousal, sympathetic stimulation, and a decrease in appetite (82, 84).

Intracerebroventricular (i.c.v.) administration of CRH in rats produces behavioral activation (85). When the CRH-antagonist, α-helical CRF9-41 (αhCRF) was given to rats prior to experimental stress, it attenuated expected increases in norepinephrine in several brain regions, including the locus ceruleus region, the cerebral cortex, the hippocampus, the amygdala, and the hypothalamus. Plasma corticosterone levels were not significantly decreased. These findings suggest that CRH is necessary for stress-induced norepinephrine release in these regions (86). A study by Matzusaki et al. (85) showed that i.c.v. administration of CRH in rats increased dopamine utilization in the frontal cortex, striatum, hippocampus and amygdala.

CRH release from the hypothalamus is subject to stimulatory serotoninergic control. Owens et al. (87) showed that acute administration of serotonin agonists to rats activates the HPA axis, with increased plasma ACTH and corticosterone levels. Chronic administration of serotonin agonists does not increase CRH levels in the median eminence or CRH receptor number or receptor affinity in the anterior pituitary. It does, however, increase concentrations of CRH in the piriform cortex and hippocampus (87).

In depression, neuroendocrine and catecholamine dysfunctions may be linked to CRH effects on locus coeruleus (LC) neurons, via persistent elevated levels of LC discharge and diminished responses to phasic sensory stimuli (27, 88). Antidepressant drugs appear to decrease LC sensory evoked discharge after acute administration. Desipramine and mianserin appear to attenuate LC activation by suppressing endogenous CRH release (27, 88).

Stress leads to activation of both the HPA axis and the catecholaminergic systems (which include the sympathetic nervous systems and CNS catecholamines) (89). CRH stimulates noradrenergic neurons in the locus ceruleus (90), suggesting that brain CRH coordinates the behavioral and autonomic nervous system responses in stress with the neuroendocrine response (91). There is evidence for a reciprocal effect of norepinephrine on CRH; α_1-adrenergic agonists raise the levels of CRH within the CNS (90). How much of this cerebral CRH emanates from hypothalamic PVN neuronal outflow or arises in situ from other limbic system neuronal sources such as the amygdala is unknown, but it is likely that the most of the CRH in the brain is derived from extrahypothalamic neurons.

Some forms of depression are associated with hyperactivity of the noradrenergic system (92), which, by direct or indirect connections, leads to enhanced CRH production in the hypothalamic PVN. This causes activation of the HPA axis, as well as increased sympathetic outflow. Evidence in favor of a major role for CRH in depression is shown by studies from Nemeroff et al. (93) documenting reduced CRH binding sites in the frontal cortex of suicide victims and the increased levels of CRH in the CSF of depressed patients (93–95). However, the latter finding was not confirmed in a subsequent study (96).

SUICIDE

Postmortem studies of brains of suicide victims support an association with altered serotonin levels and HPA axis activation. Levels of both serotonin and its metabolite 5-hydroxyindoleacetic acid (5-HIAA) are lower in brains of suicide victims than in control brains (97–99). A positive DST has been reported in 80% of violent suicide attempters (100, 101); elevated plasma and urine corticosteroid levels have also been reported (102, 103). Brain CRH levels are increased (93–95), as discussed earlier. However, reports from other studies of suicide attempters (101, 104–106) and studies of depressed people with suicidal ideation showed no difference in DST response from those without suicidal ideation (107). In a recent study of 57 medication-free schizophrenics, those with a history of suicide attempts had higher levels of post-dexamethasone cortisol control than those who did not (108).

HYPOTHALAMIC-PITUITARY-THYROID AXIS

Primary thyroid disorders may present with mental and behavioral symptoms, and both physical and psychological stress can affect hypothalamic-pituitary-thyroid (HPT) axis function. Knowledge of these phenomena aids in the management of mood disorders and in the early recognition of thyroid disease.

REGULATION OF THE HPT AXIS

The synthesis and secretion of the thyroid hormones, thyroxine (T4) and triidiothyronine (T3), by the thyroid gland is regulated primarily by TSH or thyrotropin, a glycoprotein synthesized by the thyrotropic cells of the anterior pituitary. TSH is secreted from the pituitary in a circadian rhythm determined by rhythmic TRH secretion by suprachiasmatic nucleus of the hypothalamus. The highest serum TSH concentrations occur between 9 PM and 5:30 AM. The TSH nadir occurs between 4 and 7 PM. Although negative feedback of T4 and T3 on the pituitary is the most potent factor affecting TSH secretion, the hypothalamus plays an important role through releasing and inhibiting factors. TRH is a tripeptide synthesized in the "thyrotropic" area of the hypothalamus, principally the parvocellular division of the PVN (109). It is the dominant hypophysiotropic factor modulating the secretion of TSH through a tonic stimulating action. TRH interacts with high-affinity receptors on the pituitary thyrotrophs. Two other hypothalamic factors, dopamine (110) and somatostatin (111), have inhibitory effects on TSH secretion at the level of the thyrotrope and may function as physiological thyrotropin-inhibitory factors; they reduce the degree of TSH release by TRH. Antiserum to somatostatin increases basal TSH secretion and potentiates the TSH response to exogenous TRH (112). Drugs that block pituitary dopamine receptors, such as metoclopramide or neuroleptics, have a similar effect (7, 113). TSH secretion and its responsivity to TRH are also modulated by the levels of cortisol (114), sex steroids, and growth hormone in the peripheral circulation (109).

The hypothalamic neurons that secrete TRH are regulated by monoamine neurotransmitters. Serotonin, norepinephrine and histamine can all stimulate the release of TRH (115, 116).

Stress inhibits TSH release. In rats, this effect may be due to stress-induced release of somatostatin (112). In humans subjected to physical stress, such as in the euthyroid sick syndrome, TSH levels do not compensate for the low T3 and T4 levels found in these situations (117). Patients with this syndrome have decreased levels of TSH secretion, as well as a diminished circadian periodicity of TSH release (118).

EXTRAHYPOTHALAMIC TRH

TRH is widely distributed throughout the mammalian brain, and is also found in the pancreas, gastrointestinal tract, and reproductive system (90). Its widespread presence in the brain may suggest that TRH functions as a neurotransmitter or neuromodulator in addition to its hypophysiotropic actions. Despite the fact that TRH crosses the brain-blood barrier poorly, effects on the CNS occur after systematic administration. In the rat, TRH reverses the CNS depression induced by barbiturate and ethanol administration, and it causes increased motor activity in hypophysectomized mice pretreated with pargyline and then given L-dopa (119).

In normal human subjects, TRH administration produces mild euphoria. In subjects undergoing alcohol withdrawal, TRH increases subjective well-being. Antidepressant actions of TRH are controversial. Intravenous administration of TRH in normal subjects often produces a transient increase or fall in blood pressure, as well as a sensation of urinary urgency (120, 121). These responses reflect central effects of TRH on the autonomic nervous system.

THYROID AXIS AND PSYCHIATRIC DISORDERS

About one-quarter of patients with unipolar major depression have a blunted TSH response to TRH administration (121–124). Although increased cortisol levels reduce the thyrotropin response to TRH in patients with endocrine disorders and in normal individuals (114, 125), investigations have not confirmed a significant correlation between excess endogenous cortisol and the blunted TRH responses seen in depression (122). Because an abnormality in brain catecholamine metabolism may underlie some depressive disorders (124), it is conceivable that a dopamine excess, for example, may account for this blunted TSH response to TRH seen in depression, but this notion has not been confirmed (109, 123). Additionally, neurotensin and somatostatin, which may inhibit TSH secretion, also have been suggested as possible factors in the blunted TSH responses seen in depressed patients. Other hypotheses include an altered pituitary receptor sensitivity (126) and the possibility that the blunted TRH response might reflect enhanced endogenous TRH secretion with down-regulation of TRH receptors.

People who abuse amphetamines and patients with paranoid schizophrenia may develop hyperthyroxinemia (increased T4). Interestingly, amphetamine is structurally similar to phenylethylamine, an endogenous brain amine that may be elevated in some cases of paranoid schizophrenia (127, 128). Activation of the HPT axis by endogenous biogenic amines may be responsible for the hyperthyroxinemia found in many patients who are hospitalized for acute psychosis.

THYROID AXIS IN DEPRESSION

Although the majority of depressed patients appear to be euthyroid, several studies have found either high normal or borderline low thyroid hormone levels in a substantial minority of depressed samples. Reverse T3 (rT3), the inactive analogue of T3, is increased in patients with unipolar depression. In general, thyroid hormone levels are not correlated with severity of depression (123), though some measures of HPT axis function have been found to be altered in patients with major depression.

TRH Test

This test consists of the measurement of serum TSH before and after administration of exogenous TRH. A standardized dose of 200–500 μg of TRH is injected intravenously after an overnight fast, with the subject recumbent throughout the procedure. Blood samples for serum TSH are drawn at baseline and at 30-minute intervals for 3 hours. A blunted response is defined as a peak response that is less than 5 μU/ml above baseline. With this definition, about 30% of patients with primary depression will have a blunted response (122). Hyperthyroid patients will have suppressed TSH and a flat response to TRH (< 1 μU/L). Hypothyroid patients will show a high normal or elevated TSH and an exaggerated response because of lack of feedback inhibition (> 30 μU/L) (128). Several factors may influence the thyrotropin response; therefore, the clinical value of the TRH test is controversial. Age, especially in males over 60 years, acute starvation, chronic renal failure, Klinefelter's syndrome, and numerous medications also can reduce the response of TSH to TRH to as little as 2 μg/ml (109). There appears to be no association of the response with severity of depression or previous intake of antidepressant drugs (except for long-term lithium use). The test does not seem to aid in the distinction between primary or secondary depression or between unipolar and bipolar subgroups. However, blunted TSH responses are more common in patients with chronic depression. In addition, there is a negative association between the TSH peak value and a history of violent suicidal behavior. In a study by Linkowski et al. (129), 12 of 51 female patients with a history of suicidal behavior had an absent thyrotropin response to TRH, and of these, seven had a history of violent suicidal behavior. In contrast, only four of 39 patients with a TSH response greater than 1 μU/ml had a history of violent suicidal behavior. Also, during a 5-year follow-up study, there was a higher frequency of suicides in the group with absent TSH response to TRH stimulation.

Many studies have evaluated the TRH test as a "marker" of depression and as a tool of prognostic value regarding outcome of treatment, but their results have been discrepant. In some patients, a blunted TSH response to TRH stimulation is a "state" marker, abnormal during a state of depression and normal upon recovery. In others, it persists even after remission, suggesting that it is a biological "trait" that identifies the patient as at risk for depression (123, 130).

Hypotheses advanced to explain this blunted response include suppression of TSH secretion by increased levels of dopamine, somatostatin, and/or neurotensin secretion. Another suggested mechanism is down-regulation of TRH receptors in the anterior pituitary, possibly due to depression-associated hypersecretion of TRH (126). Prior studies show that TRH is elevated in the spinal fluid of depressed patients (131) and that chronic administration of TRH to healthy subjects causes blunted TSH response to TRH (132) as well as loss of the normal diurnal rhythm (133).

Other investigators have suggested a role for inhibition of the pituitary by an increased T3/T4 ratio, or by hypercortisolism (114, 134, 135).

Loss of Nocturnal TSH Surge

The loss of the nocturnal TSH surge is a more sensitive indicator of HPT axis alterations in depressive illness than the TRH test. Bartalena et al. (136) found that the normal nocturnal TSH surge was abolished in 14 of 15 depressed patients. Six of them had low morning TSH levels and a blunted response to the TRH test: all of them lacked the normal nocturnal TSH surge. The nine depressed patients with normal morning TSH values all had normal response to TRH test, but the TSH surge was lost in all but one. The suprachiasmatic nucleus, which rhythmically secretes TRH, may be suppressed by the elevated circulating glucocorticoids (128), although a direct effect on the nucleus through its neural input is also possible. Similar loss of the nocturnal TSH surge has been reported in Cushing's Syndrome (137) and during the rigors of military "boot camp" (138).

THYROID HORMONE THERAPY IN DEPRESSION

Triiodothyronine (T3) can accelerate the antidepressant effect of tricyclic antidepressants in women, and can induce a response to tricyclics in individuals previously unresponsive to it in both sexes (139, 140). In addition, administration of TRH can induce an increased sense of well-being and relaxation in healthy volunteers and in some depressed patients (141). In some schizophrenic subjects, administration of oral or intravenous TRH improved emotional rapport and diminished apathy without affecting serum prolactin or thyroid hormone levels (142). The mechanism of action of TRH in this context may be independent of its functions on the pituitary-thyroid axis. The beneficial effect of T3 in potentiating the therapeutic efficacy of tricyclic antidepressants raises the possibility that there may be a diminished conversion of T4 to T3 (the bioactive thyroid hormone) in depression, leading to functional CNS hypothyroidism despite apparently normal systemic thyroid function tests.

Should patients with psychiatric illness be treated with thyroid hormone? At least 5% of patients with depression have an elevated TSH or hyperresponse to TRH despite normal serum T4 levels, suggestive of latent or subclinical hypothyroidism. In such patients a therapeutic trial of thyroid hormone, such as levothyroxine (T4) or liothyronine (T3 – Cytomel) may be indicated, aiming to keep the serum TSH as measured by a sensitive assay within the normal range, but not suppressed (128). There are no studies to support a choice of T4 over T3 in antidepressant therapy. Although several studies have shown a positive effect of T3 (140, 143), it produces fluctuating levels of T3 and may cause clinical signs of hyperthyroidism even when usual thyroid studies fall within normal limits (128).

The role for thyroid supplementation is well established for rapid-cycling bipolar disorder, in which as many as 50% of patients have a subclinical hypothyroidism (144–147). High doses of levothyroxine or of T3, given with lithium or other mood stabilizing agents, can stop the rapid cycling, suggesting the influence of thyroid hormone in the phenotypic expression of bipolar illness (144, 146). As with depression, it is not settled whether T3 is superior to T4 for this purpose.

LITHIUM AND THYROID FUNCTION

Drugs frequently used in psychiatry can affect thyroid function. Lithium at therapeutic levels inhibits thyroid hormone release by decreasing endocytosis of T3- and T4-laden thyroglobulin on the luminal side of the thyroid follicle. At higher levels, it can inhibit iodine uptake and organification. Clinical hypothyroidism develops in approximately 7% of patients taking lithium, over and above the rate expected for patients of the same age and sex not on lithium. Women and patients with positive antithyroid antibodies are especially vulnerable. In some cases lithium unmasks a subclinical case of autoimmune thyroiditis. Lithium inhibits the conversion of T4 to T3 in the rodent brain and pituitary, suggesting that part of the therapeutic effect of lithium in patients with bipolar disorder may be achieved by reducing brain T3 levels (128) – the converse of the effect of the administration of T3 (along with tricyclic antidepressants) in unipolar depression.

Carbamazepine, a commonly-prescribed alternative or adjunct to lithium in the treatment of bipolar disorder, can lower levels of T4 and free T4 without a compensatory increase in TSH (148). While T4 may fall to 70% of the basal level within 2 weeks after starting carbamazepine, patients usually remain clinically euthyroid (149). However, cases of overt hypothyroidism have been reported (150).

REPRODUCTIVE AXIS

In this section, we discuss several issues of clinical relevance. These are stress and reproductive function, neuroendocrine accompaniments of eating disorders, and reproductive endocrine aspects of epilepsy.

Sexual Dimorphism of the CNS: Sex Hormones and CNS Function

Sexual brain organization is dependent on sex hormone and neurotransmitter levels occurring during critical developmental periods, including peri- and neonatal life (151–156) (see also Chapter 32). In males, studies have suggested that somatic components of the testes may contribute to a male type of differentiation of germ cells from the beginning of sexual differentiation (157). The testes actively produce androgens in utero, while physiologically important steroid hormone production by the ovary does not start until puberty (158). Androgens can produce a male phenotype, regardless of genotypic gender. Their action is mediated by the androgen receptor (159). Higher androgen levels during brain organization cause a characteristically male pattern of brain development.

The levels of androgen necessary at the time of differentiation in the second trimester of pregnancy are only three times greater in male fetuses than female fetuses during the 2nd trimester, as compared with 20 times higher levels of free testosterone in the adult male than in the adult female. Androgen excess in females can be caused by genetic conditions, such as the 21-hydroxylase deficiency, or by exogenous androgenic drugs. Studies in rats showed a significant sex-related difference in the hypothalamic somatostatin and GHRH mRNA levels after full sexual maturation was attained. In addition, ovariectomized rats that received dihydrotestosterone had a GH secretory pattern that was indistinguishable from that of intact male rats, with the higher somatostatin and GHRH mRNA levels typical of male rats (160). These effects on the genetic expression of GH were therefore mediated by androgen receptors. A functional androgen receptor is an absolute requirement for male sexual differentiation (159).

Estrogens are also important during brain differentiation. Estrogen exposure during fetal development is necessary for the sex-specific organization of gonadotropin secretion, including positive estrogen feedback (152) and the establishment of the cyclic LH surge mechanism. In the rat, fetal estrogen exposure is necessary for the expression of lordosis behavior in the adult (154).

Many neuroanatomical sex differences have been identified in both animals and humans that may underlie sex-specific behavior in both reproductive and nonreproductive functions. For instance, in the adult pig, the cell count and volume of the vasopressin- and oxytocin-containing nucleus is 260% larger in the male than in the female. Hoffman and Swaab (161) reviewed observations on the human hypothalamus. They observed that the suprachiasmatic nucleus (SCN)—a structure involved in the regulation of circadian rhythms and reproductive cycles—is ellipsoidal in females and more spherical in males. In addition, an extremely large SCN was observed in the brains of homosexual men who died from acquired immunodeficiency syndrome (AIDS). Both the volume of the SCN and the number of vasopressin neurons were about twice as large as in the male reference group. The volume and cell count of the so-called sexually dimorphic nucleus of the preoptic area (SDN-POA) shows a marked sexual dimorphism. The mean volume of the SDN-POA is 2.2 times larger in males than in females and contains about twice as many cells. This area might be involved in the control of male sexual behavior. Asymmetries in temporoparietal regions of the brain also differ between men and women (162). However, a correlation between these findings and gender-specific behaviors has not yet been established.

Studies performed by LeVay (163) on autopsy material from 41 subjects—19 homosexual men who died from AIDS, 16 heterosexual men, and six heterosexual women, showed that the third interstitial nuclei of the anterior hypothalamus (INAH-3) were twice as large in heterosexual men as in the women or the homosexual men. Studies by Allen and Gorski (164) on postmortem tissue, have shown that there are neuroanatomical differences in the area of both the anterior commissure and the massa intermedia, being both areas larger in females than in males.

Play behavior in children seems to be affected by the history in their mothers of exposure to progestational agents. In this case, the history of progesterone exposure in the prenatal period was associated with hypomasculinization effects (155). Progesterone exposure also reduces play-fighting in male rats (165). Perinatal androgen exposure masculinizes social play in children, but after this period of critical neuronal differentiation, androgen levels apparently have no effect on the expression of social play. This effect may involve androgen receptors in the amygdala (165).

There are also large sex differences in the incidence or age of onset of many mental disorders. For example, depression is more prevalent in women, and antisocial personality is more prevalent in men. Also, schizophrenia tends to have a later onset in women. These differences are likely to involve both social and biological factors (166, 167).

Stress and Reproductive Function

Stress-related hormones, i.e., CRH, the POMC-derivatives ACTH and β-endorphin, and adrenal corticosteroids, can influence reproductive function at three different levels of the hypothalamic-pituitary-gonadal (HPG) axis: in the brain, by inhibiting GnRH secretion, in the pituitary, by interfering with LH release, and in the gonads, by interfering with the stimulatory effect of gonadotropin on sex steroid secretion (168).

The mechanisms through which CRH suppresses GnRH and LH in stress are not fully understood. In rats, direct anatomical connections have been demonstrated between CRH axon terminals and dendrites of GnRH-secreting neurons (169). But, again, there are CRH-immunoreactive cells and fibers in many telencephalic, diencephalic and brainstem structures (170). Studies suggest that the effect of CRH on GnRH may involve the activation of several pathways, including those dependent on endogenous opiates (171) and on catecholamines (172). Infusion of CRH into both sides of the medial preoptic area significantly decreases GnRH release and plasma LH levels in ovariectomized rats (168).

Endogenous opiates (POMC derivatives) and morphine decrease GnRH concentrations (173, 174) in rats, whereas naloxone increases GnRH release from hypothalamic fragments (175). CRH stimulates the release of POMC-derived peptides, including β-endorphin. Both CRH and POMC-derived peptides may be directly released onto GnRH neurons of the POA, and act synergistically to reduce their activity (168, 176, 177).

There is substantial evidence that the stress inhibition of gonadotropin secretion is mediated mainly by the direct and indirect effects of CRH on GnRH secretion. CRH infusions inhibit LH secretion in women (178, 179). In rats, inhibition of LH secretion by experimental stress can be prevented by prior administration of a CRH antagonist (α-helical CRH9-41) (180).

Eating Disorders: Anorexia Nervosa and Bulimia

Eating disorders, especially anorexia nervosa, are associated with alterations in the reproductive endocrine system.

Other neuroendocrine systems are altered simultaneously, i.e., the HPA, the GH, and the HPT axis.

ANOREXIA NERVOSA

Anorexia nervosa (AN) is a psychiatric disorder characterized by voluntary emaciation because of an intense fear of weight gain and a disturbance in body image. The criteria include a weight below 15% of expected body weight and at least a 3-month history of amenorrhea (181). Multiple endocrine disturbances are present in this condition, which are not explained by weight loss alone. Some of them may persist despite weight recovery.

The amenorrhea of AN is a form of hypothalamic dysfunction, in which LH and FSH secretion reverts to a prepubertal pattern; that is, LH and FSH secretion are significantly decreased when compared with control women. LH shows a greater depression than FSH. The number of their secretory spikes is also reduced (182, 183). These abnormalities may be mild or severe, ranging from a luteal phase defect to the complete picture of hypogonadotropic hypogonadism, with loss of the LH and FSH response to a clomiphene challenge (183). The response of LH to GnRH is blunted, whereas the FSH response may be increased (182, 183). The characteristic immature pattern of 24-hour LH secretion has been reproduced in experimental starvation of healthy individuals. However, the onset of amenorrhea and return to menses in anorexia nervosa is poorly correlated with body weight (182). The circadian rhythm of other hormones has also been found to be altered. Growth hormone is significantly higher in many women with AN, and the elevation is inversely proportional to the deviation of body weight from the ideal. Basal GH levels are elevated in 29% of women with AN, and 22% of AN patients do not exhibit a significant GH nocturnal peak (184). An abnormal GH increase after TRH stimulation has been found in about 50% of patients (185). IGF-I is decreased. These abnormalities are most likely tied to starvation. Elevated GH levels are found in protein or caloric malnutrition states, and the levels revert to normal after refeeding (186).

Cortisol levels are also significantly elevated in AN patients, and are inversely correlated with body mass index (BMI) and directly correlated with the percent decrease from ideal body weight (IBW) and Hamilton Rating Scale (HRS) scores for depression (184). Endogenous hypothalamic CRH levels are also likely elevated, and the ACTH/cortisol response to CRH is decreased, as in depression (182). These findings indicate a significant relationship between the HPA axis abnormalities and the severity of weight loss and depressive symptoms in AN.

A delayed TSH response is found in 86% of anorectics and it may, but not always, normalize with recovery of weight. This abnormal TSH response is not correlated with depressive symptoms (185). Prolactin levels and the prolactin response to TRH stimulation usually are normal (185), but occasionally are decreased.

BULIMIA

Bulimia is an eating disorder characterized by recurrent binge eating with fear or inability to stop eating voluntarily, alternating with behavior directed toward losing weight or avoiding weight gain, such as self-induced vomiting, laxative or diuretic abuse, dieting and exercising to lose weight, accompanied by depressed mood after binge eating (187). About one-third of patients with bulimia nervosa have a history of anorexia nervosa.

Studies performed in bulimic patients by Fichter et al. (188) showed that there was a tendency toward nonsuppression of cortisol in the DSTs of patients with bulimia. This was more pronounced in patients with evidence of restricted caloric intake, but there was no association with depressive symptoms. However, plasma dexamethasone levels following a standard dose were lower in bulimics than in controls. TRH stimulation produced blunted responses in TSH levels in 80% of patients with both bulimia and AN, and in 22% of those with bulimia alone (185). Prolactin response was blunted in one study (188), but normal in another (185). LH and FSH were reduced in bulimics with evidence of reduced caloric intake (188). Increased basal GH levels were found in 33% of bulimic patients, regardless of food restriction. A paradoxical increase of GH levels upon TRH stimulation was found in 15–20% of patients with bulimia (185). All these results indicate that multiple neuroendocrine disturbances occur in bulimia, but to a lesser degree than in anorexia nervosa. This also suggests that caloric intake is an important factor, but not the only one, in the maintenance of a normal neuroendocrine function.

Gonadotropin levels to GnRH stimulation in bulimic patients were found to be abnormal in bulimic patients (157). LH response to GnRH as well as the number of LH peaks in 24 hours tend to be very heterogenous. FSH response, as in AN, is sometimes greater than that of LH.

REPRODUCTIVE ENDOCRINE ASPECTS OF EPILEPSY

Epilepsy is associated with reduced fertility in women, with impotence in men, and with hyposexuality in both men and women. Often, these changes are due to hormonal phenomena that may be affected by pharmacologic treatment.

In one recent study of 37 adult male epileptics on who were seizure-free on monotherapy, 8 were impotent, and 2 of those lacked desire. Patients with epilepsy had significantly lower levels of free testosterone and dihydrotestosterone than healthy controls, and those with impotence had higher levels of estradiol than those with normal sexual function. (189). Other authors have observed that both carbamezepine and phenytoin increase serum levels of sex hormone binding globulin (SHBG), which, without an increase in total testosterone, reduces the free fraction present (190). Measurement of free testosterone and estradiol would thus be expected to aid in understanding impotence or hyposexuality in a treated epileptic man.

The decreased fertility of women with epilepsy is due to impairment of ovulation (191). More than one-third of 17 women with temporal lobe epilepsy had anovulatory cycles, in contrast to none of 7 women with primary generalized epilepsy studied recently by Cummings and colleagues. Women with epilepsy and anovulation may have either hypothalamic amenorrhea or the polycystic ovary syndrome (192). In both cases, the pulsatile secretion of LH is altered—Drislane et al. found it to be both lower and more variable among patients with temporal lobe epilepsy than among healthy controls (193). In contrast, Meo et al. studied 11 drug free epileptic women with normal menstrual cycles, and found them to have increased pulsatility of LH secretion, with increased basal secretion during increases in interictal activity (194).

Herzog has presented impressive evidence for laterality effects of temporal lobe foci. In a study of 30 women with unilateral temporal lobe foci, complex partial seizures and reproductive endocrine abnormality, 15 of the 16 with polycystic ovary syndrome had left-sided EEG discharges, and 12 of 14 with hypothalamic hypogonadism had right-sided EEG discharges (195).

The specific choice of drug therapy for epilepsy in women apparently affects its reproductive endocrine consequences. Menstrual disturbances, polycystic ovaries by ultrasound, and elevated serum testosterone all are more common in women taking valproate than those taking carbamazepine or other medications (196). In fact, the majority of women taking valproate for epilepsy in the just-cited Finnish study had either elevated testosterone, polycystic ovaries, or both. Women who had started valproate before age 20 had the highest rate of reproductive endocrine problems—80%.

Serum prolactin is known to increase following generalized seizures and complex partial seizures with bilateral medial temporal involvement (197, 198). Prolactin peaks at 2–3 times normal in 15 to 20 minutes and returns to baseline within 3 hours. Unilateral temporal lobe activity, by contrast, does not raise prolactin levels (199). Failure of prolactin to rise after an apparent generalized seizure suggests pseudoseizures.

In summary, specific reproductive endocrine abnormalities can be demonstrated in most patients with epilepsy and altered sexual or menstrual function. While patients with such abnormalities should be offered endocrine treatment if they are troubled by their symptoms, the efficacy of endocrine interventions in fully restoring sexual function in epileptic patients is not known.

HYPOTHALAMIC-PITUITARY-SOMATOTROPIC SYSTEM

GH release is regulated by the noncompetitive antagonism of GHRH and somatostatin (126). The effects of other hormones appear to be mediated via alterations in the secretion of both GHRH and somatostatin.

It has been observed that somatostatin concentration is decreased in the CSF of patients with depression (200), and its levels are inversely related to the maximum postdexamethasone plasma cortisol concentration (201, 202).

Somatostatin-containing neuronal cell bodies, terminals, and receptors are distributed throughout the brain where it likely plays a role in neuronal function unrelated to regulation of pituitary GH secretion. There is a widespread reduction of somatostatin immunoreactivity in the cerebral cortex of patients with Alzheimer's disease caused by degeneration of intrinsic somatostatin cortical neurons (203, 204). The somatostatin reduction correlates with impaired cognitive function and brain hypometabolism on PET scanning (205). It is not known whether the somatostatin changes play an etiologic role in the dementia or are a secondary response to the neuronal degeneration.

PROLACTIN

Conflicting results on basal prolactin levels and response to TRH have been reported in depression. Basal prolactin has been found low, normal, and elevated. Similarly, the response to TRH has been variable (129). The underlying cause of the disturbances in PRL regulation in affective disorders is still not clear. Increased activity of the hypothalamic tuberoinfundibular dopaminergic neurons or deficiency of central 5-HT pathways could account for the suppressed TRH-induced PRL response. DA is the principal physiological regulator of PRL secretion; however, a number of neurotransmitters, including γ-aminobutyric acid (GABA), 5-HT, histamine and several neural peptides (VIP, β-endorphin, neurotensin, substance P) affect PRL secretion. This effect may occur either at the pituitary or hypothalamic level (125), and a disturbance in any of these peptides may account for the abnormalities found in psychiatric disorders.

ENDOCRINE DISEASES PRESENTING AS PSYCHIATRIC DISORDERS

Hypothalamic Lesions

Experiments of nature demonstrate in vivo the role of the CNS, particularly, the hypothalamus in human behavior. Anatomical lesions of the hypothalamus can present as mental or behavioral disorders, such as explosive disorder (206), polyphagia and morbid obesity (207), hypodipsia (208, 209), primary polydipsia (210), hypersomnolence (211), and dementia (212, 213).

The etiologies cited are varied and they include not only parasellar tumors, but also granulomatous disorders such as sarcoidosis (207, 210), eosinophilic granuloma (214), histiocytosis X (212, 215), congenital defects (208), pseudotumor cerebri (209), hemochromatosis (216), whole brain irradiation (Table 9.1)(213). The role of hypothalamic lesions in violent and aggressive behavior is discussed in depth in Chapter twenty-four by Saver et al.

Table 9.1.   Hypothalamic Lesions Presenting as Psychiatric Disorders

Hypothalamic Lesions	Psychiatric Manifestations
Granulomatous disorders	Explosive disorder
Sarcoidosis	Polyphagia
Eosinophilic granuloma	Hypodypsia
Histiocytosis X	Polydipsia
Congenital defects	Hypersomnolence
Hemochromatosis	Dementia
Pseudotumor cerebri	
Whole brain irradiation	

Table 9.2.   Psychiatric Manifestations of Thyroid Disease

Hyperthyroidism	Hypothyroidism
Anxiety	Depression
Dysphoria	Inattention
Irritability	Poor memory
Insomnia	Sleepiness
Difficulty concentrating	Difficulty concentrating
Restlessness	Slow motor function
Manic symptoms	Paucity of speech
Decreased energy	Hallucinations
Delusions	Bizarre behavior
Paranoia	Lethargy
Apathy	Drowsiness
Lethargy	Stupor
Depression	Coma

Hypo- and Hyperthyroidism

Disturbances of thyroid function can cause mental and behavioral symptoms. Thus, appropriate treatment directed to the thyroid gland is a necessary and often sufficient condition for their total reversal. In addition, patients with subtle defects in thyroid function may be more susceptible to mental disorders because the prevalence of thyroid autoantibodies is higher in psychiatric patients than in the general population (Table 9.2)(217).

The neuropsychiatric features of adult-onset hypothyroidism are not specific and consist of ill-defined complaints and disturbances in cognition and/or mood. There is lack of attention, concentration, and poor memory. Symptoms may resemble those of depression, with apathy, social withdrawal, paucity of speech, and slow motor function. In severe hypothyroidism, delusions and hallucinations may occur, giving rise to bizarre behavior and paranoid ideas. This may be followed by lethargy, drowsiness, and finally, stupor and coma (218). The pathophysiology of these symptoms and signs probably involves both direct effects of T3 on neurons, and indirect effects via other neurotransmitters. T3-nuclear receptors are present in neurons, with high concentrations in the amygdala and hippocampus, and with the lowest concentrations in the brainstem and cerebellum (219).

Patients with *hyperthyroidism* may present with anxiety and dysphoria, emotional liability, insomnia, difficulty concentrating, irritability, restlessness, and tremulousness. This may resemble mania because motor activity is increased,

Table 9.3.   Psychiatric Manifestations of Hypercortisolism

Emotional lability
Depression
Lack of energy
Loss of libido
Irritability
Anxiety
Panic attacks
Paranoia
Increased appetite

but unlike mania, energy is usually decreased (218). In some cases severe thyrotoxicosis may present as a psychotic illness, with delusional and paranoid thoughts. Elderly individuals, however, may present with apathy, lethargy, and depression ("apathetic thyrotoxicosis"). The clinical diagnosis of apathetic thyrotoxicosis is often delayed, with the patient developing a tachyarrhythmia or congestive heart failure before thyroid disease is appreciated. It is probable that the interactions between the thyroid hormones and the catecholaminergic system play an important role in the development of symptoms and signs of hyperthyroidism. Catecholamines and thyroid hormones share the amino acid tyrosine as a precursor and have synergistic cellular actions. In hyperthyroidism, the turnover of catecholamines is decreased, but β-adrenergic receptor numbers are increased (218). These mechanisms may explain the role of β-adrenergic antagonists in the reduction of thyrotoxic symptoms. Successful treatment of thyrotoxicosis with antithyroid agents, thyroidectomy, or radioactive iodine usually leads to the resolution of the neuropsychiatric syndrome.

Hypo- and Hypercortisolism

Patients with severe or chronic adrenal insufficiency may present with mild to moderate cognitive impairment (5–20%); apathetic depression (20–40%); or psychosis (20–40%). Symptoms may include irritability, social withdrawal, poor judgment, hallucinations, paranoid delusions, bizarre thinking, and even catatonic posturing (220).

Hypercortisolism, such as in Cushing's syndrome or exogenous glucocorticoid excess presents with mental or behavioral symptoms in up to 50% of cases (Table 9.3). Symptoms and signs include emotional lability, depression, loss of energy and poor libido, irritability, anxiety, panic attacks, and paranoia. Occasional patients present with a manic psychosis. A study performed by Martignoni et al. (221) in 24 patients with Cushing's disease (hypercortisolism induced by an ACTH-pituitary tumor) matched with same number of control subjects, showed significant difficulty with everyday tasks and impairment in verbal and nonverbal episodic memory, which did not correlate with plasma ACTH levels, urinary-free cortisol or DST response. Memory impairment was worse in older patients. The behavioral abnormalities were significantly reversed after surgical treatment of the pituitary tumor.

The brain represents one of the principal targets for steroid hormones. Steroids secreted by the adrenal cortex, such as glucocorticoids, mineralocorticoids, and stress hormones, easily cross the blood-brain barrier and exert their actions in the CNS at classic steroid receptors (221). Glucocorticoids have prominent actions on the hippocampus, which is the area of the brain with the major number of glucocorticoid receptors. Either a lack or an excess of glucocorticoids can produce significant functional impairment or structural change in CA3 cells in the hippocampus. Studies in monkeys subjected to stress showed degenerative changes at the level of the hippocampus (222). Furthermore, in humans subjected to severe stress, such as concentration camp survivors (223) and war sailors (224), cognitive and psychological disturbances have been documented. Brain CT scans of political prisoners who were subjected to physical torture showed cerebral atrophy (225).

Exogenous glucocorticoids have been shown to produce impairment of higher brain functions in humans. The term "steroid psychosis" has been used to describe a psychotic syndrome in patients who are given high doses of corticosteroids for medical illnesses that have not directly affected the CNS (226). A cognitive impairment syndrome was described by Varney et al. (227) in such patients, consisting of decreased attention, concentration, retention, and mental speed. Administration of exogenous glucocorticoids in healthy subjects has also been associated with cognitive impairment, with poor performance on memory tasks (228). It has been postulated that corticosteroids may impair selective attention (228) and may suppress the activity of the hippocampus, where the stimuli may be initially filtered (229).

Endocrine dysfunction is a common accompaniment of neuropsychiatric disorders, and neuropsychiatric symptoms frequently are part of the preservation of primary endocrine disorders. Clinical assessment of endocrine function, and, where appropriate, laboratory investigation of endocrine function, is an integral part of comprehensive neuropsychiatric evaluation. Endocrine interventions are likely to find an increasing role in neuropsychiatric therapy.

References

1. Müller EE. The neuroendocrine approach to psychiatric disorders: a critical appraisal. J Neural Transm [GenSect] 1990,81:1–15.
2. Palkovits M. Neuropeptides in the median eminence. Neurochem Int 1986;9:131–137.
3. Palkovits M. Peptidergic neurotransmitters in the endocrine hypothalamus. In: Functional anatomy of the neuroendocrine hypothalamus. Wiley, Chichester (Ciba Foundation Symposium 168) 1992:3–5.
4. Wurtman RJ, Hefti F, Melamed E. Precursor control of neurotransmitter synthesis. Pharmacological Rev 1980;32:315–335.
5. Jackson IMD. Hypothalamic releasing hormones: mechanisms underlying neuroendocrine dysfunction in affective disorders. In Brown GM et al., eds. Neuroendocrinology of psychiatric disorders. New York: Raven Press, 1984:255–266.
6. Pelletier G. Anatomy of the hypothalamic-pituitary axis. In Jasmin G, Cantin M, eds. Stress revisited. 1.Neuroendocrinology of stress. Methods Achiev Exp Pathol, Karger, Basel: 1991, 14:1–22.
7. Martin J, Reichlin S. Clinical neuroendocrinology. Philadelphia: FA Davis, 1987:11–44.
8. Reichlin S. Neuroendocrinology. In Wilson JD, Foster DW, eds. Williams textbook of endocrinology. Philadelphia: WB Saunders, 1992: 135–219.
9. Kovacs K, Horvath E, Ezrin C. Anatomy and histology of the normal and abnormal pituitary gland. In DeGroot L, ed. Endocrinology. Philadelphia: WB Saunders 1989: 264.
10. Denef C, Schramme C, Baes M. Stimulation of growth hormone release by vasoactive intestinal peptide and peptide PHI in rat anterior pituitary reaggregates. Permissive action of a glucocorticoid and inhibition by thyrotropin releasing hormone. Neuroendocrinology. 1985; 40:88–91.
11. Nowak M, Markowska A, Nussdorfer GG, Tortorella C, Malendowicz LK. Evidence that endogenous vasoactive intestinal peptide (VIP) is involved in the regulation of rat pituitary-adrenocortical function: in vivo studies with a VIP antagonist. Neuropeptides 1994;27(5):297–303.
12. Youngren OM, Silsby JL, Rozenboim I, Phillips RE, el Halawani ME. Active immunization with vasoactive intestinal peptide prevents the secretion of prolactin induced by electrical stimulation of the turkey hypothalamus. Gen Comp Endocrinol 1994;95(3):330–336.
13. Lafuente A, Marco J, Esquifino AI. Possible changes in the regulatory mechanisms of pulsatile luteinizing hormone secretion in adult pituitary-grafted female rats. Proc Soc Exp Biol Med 1995;209(2):163–169.
14. Shibata S, Ono M, Tominaga K, Hamada T, Watanabe A, Watanabe S. Involvement of vasoactive intestinal polypeptide in NMDA-induced phase delay of firing activity rhythm in the suprachiasmatic nucleus in vitro. Neurosci Biobehav Rev 1994;18(4):591–595.
15. Aguilar-Roblero R, Morin LP, Moore RY. Morphological correlates of circadian rhythm restoration induced by transplantation of the suprachiasmatic nucleus in hamsters. Exp Neurol 1994;130(2):250–260.
16. Peters RV, Zoeller RT, Hennessey AC, Stopa EG, Anderson G, Albers HE. The control of circadian rhythms and the levels of vasoactive intestinal peptide mRNA in the suprachiasmatic nucleus are altered in spontaneously hypertensive rats. Brain Res 1994;639(2):217–227.
17. Mick G, Shigemoto R, Kitahama K. Localization of substance P receptors in central neural structures controlling daily rhythms in nocturnal rodents. C R Acad Sci III 1995;318(2):209–217.
18. Mick G, Maeno H, Kiyama H, Tohyama M. Marginal topography of neurons expressing the substance P receptor in the rat suprachiasmatic nucleus. Brain Res Mol Brain Res 1994;21(1–2):157–161.
19. Makara GB. The relative importance of hypothalamic neurons containing corticotropin-releasing factor or vasopressin in the regulation of adrenocorticotropic hormone secretion. In Functional anatomy of the neuroendocrine hypothalamus. Wiley, Chichester (Ciba Foundation Symposium) 1992:43–53.
20. Hokfelt T, Meister B, Everitt B, et al. Chemical neuroanatomy of the hypothalamo-pituitary axis: focus on multimessenger systems. In McCann SM, Weiner RI, eds. Integrative neuroendocrinology: molecular, cellular and clinical aspects. Basel: Karger 1987:1–34.
21. Dudley CA, Moss RL. LHRH and mating behavior: sexual receptivity versus sexual preference. Pharmacology, Biochemistry and Behavior 1985;22:967–972.
22. Dudley CA, Moss RL. Facilitation of lordosis in female rats by CNS-site specific infusions of an LHRH fragment, Ac-LHRH-(5-10). Brain Res 1988;44:161–167.
23. Moss RL, Dudley CA. Differential effects of a luteinizing-hormone (LHRH) antagonist analogue on lordosis behavior induced by LHRH and the LHTH fragment Ac-LHRH 5-10. Neuroendocrinology 1990;52:138–142.
24. Vale W, Spiess J, Rivier C, Rivier J. Characterization of a 41 residue ovine hypothalamic peptide that stimulates secretion of corticotropin and β-endorphin. Science 1981;213:1394–1397.
25. Pelletier G, Desy L, Cote J, Vaudry H. Immunocytochemical

localization of corticotropin-releasing factor-like immunoreactivity in the human hypothalamus. Neurosci Lett 1983;41:259–263.

26. Dunn AJ, Berridge CW. Physiological and behavioral responses to corticotropin-releasing factor administration: is CRF a mediator of anxiety or stress responses? Brain Res-Brain Res Rev 1990;15: 71–100.

27. Valentino RJ, Page ME, Curtis AL. Activation of noradrenergic locus coeruleus neurons by hemodynamic stress is due to local release of corticotropin-releasing factor. Brain Res 1991;555:25–34.

28. Desy L, Pelletier G. Immunohistochemical localization of somatostatin in the human hypothalamus. Cell Tiss Res 1977;184:491–497.

HPA Axis

29. Meaney JM, Viau V, Bhatnagar S, et al. Cellular mechanisms underlying the development and expression of individual differences in the hypothalamic-pituitary-adrenal stress response. J Steroid Biochem Molec Biol 1991;39:265–274.

30. Stokes PE, Sikes CR. The hypothalamic-pituitary-adrenocortical axis in major depression. Endocrinol Metab Clin North Am 1988; 17:1–17.

31. Stokes PE, Sikes CR. Hypothalamic-pituitary-adrenal axis in psychiatric disorders. Annu Rev Med 1991;42:519–531.

32. Uno H, Eisele S, Sakai A, Shelton S, Baker E, DeJesus O, Holden J. Neurotoxicity of glucocorticoids in the primate brain. Horm Behav 1994;28(4):336–348.

33. Sapolsky RM, Krey LC, McEwen BS. Glucocorticoid sensitive hippocampal neurons are involved in terminating the adrenocortical stress response. Proc Natl Acad Sci USA 1984;81:6147–6177.

34. Herman JP, Schafter MK, Young EA, et al. Evidence for the hippocampal regulation of neuroendocrine neurons of the hypothalamo-pituitary-adrenocortical axis. J Neurosci 1989;9:3072–3082.

35. McEwen BS, De Kloet ER, Rostene WH. Adrenal steroid receptors in the nervous system. Physiol Rev 1986;66:1121–1150.

36. Herman JP, Adams D, Prewitt C. Regulatory changes in neuroendocrine stress-integrative circuitry produced by a variable stress paradigm. Neuroendocrinology 1995;61(2):180–190.

37. Rivier C. Role of interleukins in the stress response. In Jasmin G, Cantin M, eds. Stress revisited. 1. Neuroendocrinology of stress. Meth Achieve Exp Pathol, Basel: Karger, 1991;14:63–79.

38. Woloski BM, Smith EM, Meyer WI, et al. Corticotropin-releasing activities of monokines. Science 1985;230:1035–2037.

39. Ovadia H, Abramsky O, Barak V, et al. Effect of interleukin-1 on adrenocortical activity in intact and hypothalamic deafferentated rats. Exp Brain Res 1989, 76:246–249.

40. Harbuz MS, Stephanou A, Sarlis N, et al. The effects of recombinant human interleukin (IL)-1 alpha, IL-1 beta or IL-6 on hypothalamo-pituitary-adrenal axis aviation. J Endocrinology 1992;133:349–355.

41. Abraham E. Effects of stress on cytokine production. In Jasmin G, Cantin M, eds. Stress revisited. 1. Neuroendocrinology of stress. Meth Achieve Exp Pathol, Basel: Karger, 1991;14:45–62.

42. Jorgensen C, Sany J. Modulation of the immune response by the neuro-endocrine axis in rheumatoid arthritis. Clin Exp Rheumatol 1994;12(4):435–441.

43. Seyle H. General adaption syndrome and diseases adaption. J Clin Endocrinol Metab 1946;6:117–230.

44. Van der Kar LD, Richardson-Morton KD, Rittenhouse P. Stress: neuroendocrine and pharmacological mechanisms. In Jasmin G, Cantin M, eds. Stress revisited. I. Neuroendocrinology of stress. Meth Achieve Exp Pathol, Basel: Karger, 1991;14:133–173.

45. Opstad PK, Aakvaag A. Decreased serum levels of oestradiol, testosterone and prolactin during prolonged physical strain and sleep deprivation. Eur J Appl Physiol 1981;49:343–348.

46. Opstad PK. Androgenic hormones during prolonged physical stress, sleep and energy deficiency. J Clin Endocrinol Metab 1992;74:1174–1183.

47. Kathol RG, Noyes R, Lopez A. Similarities in hypothalamic adrenal axis activity between patients with panic disorder and those experi-

encing external stress. Psychiatr Clin North Am 1988;11:335–348.

48. Charlton BG, Ferrier IN. Hypothalamo-pituitary-adrenal axis abnormalities in depression: a review and a model. Psychol Med 1989;19: 331–336.

49. Carrol BJ, Martin FI, Davis BM. Resistance to suppression by dexamethasone of plasma 11(OH)CS levels in severe depressive illness. Br Med J 1968;3:285–287.

50. Weller EB, Weller RA. Neuroendocrine changes in affectively ill children and adolescents. Neurol Clin 1988;6:41–54.

51. Arana GW, Mossman D. The dexamethasone suppression test and depression. Endocrinol Metab Clin North Am 1988;17:21–39.

52. Carrol BJ. The dexamethasone suppression test for melancholia. Br J Psychiatry 1982;140:293–304.

53. Gerner R, Gwirtsman HE. Abnormalities of dexamethasone suppression and urinary MPHG in anorexia nervosa. Am J Psychiatry 1981;138:650.

54. Insel TR, Kalin HH, Guttmacher LB, et al. The dexamethasone suppression test in patients with primary obsessive-compulsive disorder. Psychiatry Res 1982;6:153.

55. Spar JE, Gerner R. Does the dexamethasone suppression test distinguish dementia from depression? Am J Psychiatry 1982;139: 238–240.

56. Graham PM, Booth H, Boranga G, et al. The dexamethasone suppression test in mania. J Affect Disord 1982;4:201–211.

57. Dewan MJ, Pandurangi AK, Boucher ML, et al. Abnormal dexamethasone suppression test results in chronic schizophrenic patients. Am J Psychiatry 1982;131:1501.

58. Kroll P, Palmer C, Greden JF. The dexamethasone suppression test in patients with alcoholism. Biol Psychiatry 1983;14:441–450.

59. Rupprecht R, Noder M, Jecht E, et al. Pre- and post dexamethasone cortisol and prolactin levels in sexual dysfunction and normal controls. Biol Psychiatry 1988;23:527–530.

60. Greden JF, Kronfol Z, Gardner R, et al. Neuroendocrine evaluation of schizoaffectives with the dexamethasone suppression test. Biol Psychiatry 1984;145:372–382.

61. Frochtengarten ML, Villares JCB, Maluf E, et al. Depressive symptoms and the dexamethasone suppression test in parkinsonian patients. Biol Psychiatry 1987;22:386–389.

62. Berger M, Pirke KM, Doerr P. The limited utility of the dexamethasone suppression test for the diagnostic process in psychiatry. Br J Psychiatry 1984;145:372–382.

63. Berger M, Krieg C, Bossert S, et al. Past and present strategies of research on the HPA-axis in psychiatry. Acta Psychiatr Scand(Suppl) 1988;341:112–125.

64. Weller E, Weller R. Neuroendocrine changes in affectively ill children and adolescents. Endocrinol Metab Clin North Am 1988;17:41–54.

65. Arana GW, Baldessarini RJ, Ornsteen M. The dexamethasone suppression test for diagnoses and prognosis in psychiatry: commentary and review. Arch Gen Psychiatry 1985;42:1193–1204.

66. Kathol RG, Jaeckle RS, Lopez JF, et al. Pathophysiology of HPA axis abnormalities in patients with major depression: an update. Am J Psychiatry 1989;146:311–317.

67. Gold PW, Chrousos GP. Clinical studies with corticotropin releasing factor: implications for the diagnosis and pathophysiology of depression, Cushing disease and adrenal insufficiency. Psychoneuroendocrinology 1985;10:401–419.

68. Gold PW, Loriaux DL, Roy A, et al. Responses to corticotropin-releasing hormone in the hypercortisolism of depression and Cushing's disease: pathophysiologic and diagnostic implications. N Engl J Med 1986;314:1329–1335.

69. Amsterdam JD, Maislin G, Winokur A, et al. Pituitary and adrenocortical responses to the ovine corticotropin releasing hormone in depressed patients and healthy volunteers. Arch Gen Psychiatry 1987;44:775–781.

70. Lopez JF, Kathol RG, Jaeckle RS, et al. The HPA axis response to insulin hypoglycemia in depression. Biol Psychiatry 1987;22: 153–166.

71. Reisine T, Hoffman AA. Desensitization of corticotropin-releasing

factor receptors. Biochem Biophys Res Commun 1983;3:919–925.

72. Brown GM. Psychoneuroendocrinology of depression. Psychiatric Journal of the University of Ottawa 1989;14:344–348.

73. Kostic VS, Sternic NC, Bumbasirevic LB, et al. Dexamethasone suppression test in patients with Parkinson's disease. Movement Disord 1990;5:23–26.

74. Frochtengarten ML, Villares JCB, Maluf E, et al. Depressive symptoms and the dexamethasone suppression test in Parkinsonian patients. Biol Psychiatry 1987;22:386–389.

75. Skare S, Pew B, Dysken M: The dexamethasone suppression test in dementia: a review of the literature. J Geriatr Psychiatry Neurol 1990;3(3):124–138.

76. Lipsey JR, Robinson RG, Pearlson GD, et al. Dexamethasone suppression test and mood following strokes. Am J Psychiatry 1985;142:318–323.

77. Finklestein S, Benowitz LI, Baldessarini. Mood, vegetative disturbance, and dexamethasone suppression test after stroke. Ann Neurol 1981;12:463–468.

78. Bauer M, Gans JS, Harley JP, et al. Dexamethasone suppression test and depression in a rehabilitation setting. Arch Phys Med Rehabil 1983;64:421–422.

79. Olsson T, Astrom M, Eriksson S, et al. Hypercorticolism revealed by the dexamethasone suppression test with acute ischemic stroke. Stroke 1989;20:1685–1690.

80. Amsterdam JD, Winokur A, Abelman E, et al. Cosyntropin stimulation test in depressed patients and healthy controls. Am J Psychiatry 1983;140:907–909.

81. Zis AP, Dorovini-Zis K. Increased adrenal weight in victims of violent suicides. Am J Psychiatry 1987;144:1214–1215.

82. Ur E, Grossman A. Corticotropin releasing hormone in health and disease: an update (Review). Acta Endocrinol 1992;127:193–199.

83. Grigoriadis DE, Heroux JA, De Souza EB. Characterization and regulation of corticotropin releasing factor receptors in the central nervous, endocrine and immune systems. Ciba Found Symp 1993;172:85–101.

84. Sawchenko PE, Imaki T, Potter E, et al. The functional neuroanatomy of corticotropin releasing factor. Ciba Found Sym 1993;172:5–29.

85. Matsuzaki I, Takamatsu Y, Moroji T. The effects of intracerebroventricularly injected corticotropin-releasing factor (CRF) on the central nervous system: behavioral and biochemical studies. Neuropeptides 1989;13:147–155.

86. Emoto H, Koga C, Ishii H, et al. The effect of CRF antagonist on immobilization stress induced increases in noradrenaline release in rat brain regions. Yakubutsu Seishin Kodo 1993;13:81–87.

87. Owens MJ, Edwards E, Nemeroff CB. Effects of 5-HT1A receptor agonists on hypothalamo-pituitary adrenal axis activity and corticotropin-releasing factor containing neurons in the rat brain. Eur J Pharmacol 1990;190:113–122.

88. Valentino RJ, Curtis AL. Pharmacology of locus coeruleus spontaneous and sensory evoked activity (Review). Prog Brain Res 1991;88:249–256.

89. Axelrod J, Reisine TD. Stress hormones: their interaction and regulation. Science 1984;224:452–459.

90. Dunn AJ, Berridge CW. Physiological and behavioral responses to corticotropin-releasing factor administration: is CRF a mediator of anxiety or stress responses? Brain Res Brain Res Rev 1990;15:71–100.

91. Koob GF, Bloom FE. Corticotropin-releasing factor and behavior. Fed Proc 1985;44:259–263.

92. Butler PD, Weiss JM, Stout JC, et al. Corticotropin releasing factor produces fear-enhancing and behavioral activating effects following infusion into the lucus coeruleus. J Neurosci 1990;10:176–183.

93. Nemeroff CB, Owens MJ, Bissette G, et al. Reduced corticotropin releasing factor binding sites in the frontal cortex of suicide victims. Arch Gen Psychiatry 1988;45:577–579.

94. Banki CM, Bissette G, Arato M, et al: CSF corticotropin-releasing factor-like immunoreactivity in depression and schizophrenia. Am J Psychiatry. 1987;144:873–877.

95. Arato M, Banki CM, Bissette G, et al. Elevated CSF CRF in suicide victims. Biol Psychiatry 1989;25:355–359.

96. Geracioti TD, Orth DN, Ekhator NN, et al. Serial cerebrospinal fluid corticotropin releasing hormone concentrations in healthy and depressed humans. J Clin Endocrinol Metab 1992;74:1325–1330.

Suicide

97. Stahl SM. Neuroendocrine markers of serotonin responsivity in depression. Prog Neuropsychopharmacol Biol Psychiatry 1992;16:655–659.

98. Beskow J, Gottfries EF, Ross BE. Determination of monoamine metabolites in the human brain: postmortem studies in a group of suicides and in a control group. Acta Psychiatr Scand 1976;53:7–20.

99. Lloyd KG, Farley IJ, Deck JHN, et al. Serotonin and 5-hydroxyindoleacetic acid in discrete areas of the brain stem of suicide victims and control patients. Adv Biochem 1974;11:387–398.

100. Banki CM, Arato M, Papp Z, et al. Biochemical markers in suicidal patients. Investigations with cerebrospinal fluid amine metabolites and neuroendocrine test. J Affect Disord 1984;6:341–350.

101. Roy A. Hypothalamic-pituitary adrenal function and suicidal behavior in depression. Biol Psychiatry 1992;32:812–816.

102. Bunney WE, Fawcett JA, Davis JM, et al. Further evaluation of urinary hydroxycorticosteroid in suicidal patients. Arch Gen Psychiatry 1969;21:138–150.

103. Krieger J. The plasma level of cortisol as a predictor of suicide. J Dis Nerv Sys 1974;35:273–240.

104. De Leo D, Pellegrini C, Serraiotto L, et al. Assessment of severity of suicide attempts. A trial with the dexamethasone suppression test and 2 rating scales. Psychopathology 1986;19:186–191.

105. Modestin J, Ruef C. Dexamethasone suppression test (DST) in relation to depressive somatic and suicidal manifestations. Acta Psychiatr Scand 1987;75:491–494.

106. Wilmotte J, Van Wettere JP, Depauw Y, et al. Dexamethasone suppression test repeated after a suicide attempt. Acta Psychiatr Belg 1986;86:242–248.

107. Maes M, Vandewoude M, Schotte C, et al. Hypothalamic-pituitary-adrenal and thyroid axis dysfunctions and decrements in the availability of L-tryptophan as biological markers of suicidal ideation in major depressed females. Acta Psychiatr Scand 1989;80:13–17.

108. Jones JS, Stein DJ, Stanley B, Guido JR, Winchel R, Stanley M. Negative and depressive symptoms in suicidal schizophrenics. Acta Psychiatr Scand 1994;89(2):81–87.

HPT Axis

109. Jackson, IMD. Thyrotropin releasing hormone. N Engl J Med 1983;306:145–155.

110. Scanlon MF, Weightman DR, Shale DJ, et al. Dopamine is a physiological regulator of thyrotropin (TSH) secretion in normal man. Clin Endocrinol 1979;10:7–15.

111. Tanjasiri P, Kozbur X, Floersheim WH. Somatostatin in the physiologic feedback control of thyrotropin secretion. Life Sci 1976;19:657–660.

112. Arimura A, Schally AV. Increases in basal and thyrotropin releasing hormone (TRH)-stimulated secretion of thyrotropin (TSH) by passive immunization with antiserum to somatostatin in rats. Endocrinology 1976;98:1069–1072.

113. Birkhaeuser MH, Staubb JC, Crani R, et al. Dopaminergic control of TSH response to TRH e = in depressive patients. Abstracts of the XIth International Congress of the International Society of Psychoneuroendocrinology, Florence, Italy, 1980: 61.

114. Nicoloff JT, Fisher DA, Appleman MD. The role of glucocorticoids in the regulation of thyroid function in man. J Clin Invest 1979;49:1922–1929.

115. Weiner RL, Ganong WF. Role of brain monoamines and histamine

in regulation of anterior pituitary secretion. Physiol Rev 1978;58: 905–976.

116. Burger HG, Patel YC. TSH and TRH: their physiological regulation and the clinical applications of TRH. In Martini L, Besser GM (eds). Clinical neuroendocrinology. New York: Academic Press, 1977: 67–131.

117. Wartofsky L, Burman KD. Alterations in thyroid function in patients with systemic illness: the "euthyroid sick syndrome." Endocr Rev 1982;3:164–217.

118. Custro N, Scafidi V, Gallo S, Notarbartolo A. Deficient pulsatile thyrotropin secretion in the low-thyroid-hormone state of severe non-thyroidal illness. Eur J Endocrinol 1994;130(2):132–136.

119. Yarbrough GG. On the neuropharmacology of thyrotropin releasing hormone (TRH). Prog Neurobiol 1979;12:291–312.

120. Hershman JM. Clinical application of thyrotropin-releasing hormone. N Engl J Med 1974;290:886–890.

121. Prange AJ, Numeroff CB, Loosen PT, et al. Behavioral effects of thyrotropin releasing hormone in animals and man: a review. In Collu R, Brabeau A, Ducharme JR, et al., eds. Central nervous system effects of the hypothalamic hormones and other peptides. New York: Raven Press, 1979:75–96.

122. Loosen PT, Prange AJ. Serum thyrotropin response to thyrotropin-releasing hormone in psychiatric patients: a review. Am J Psychiatry 1982;139:405–416.

123. Loosen PT. Thyroid function in affective disorders and alcoholism. Endocrinol Metab Clin North Am 1988;17:55–81.

124. Terry LC. Catecholamine regulation of growth hormone and thyrotropin in mood disorders. In Brown GM, ed. Neuroendocrinology and psychiatric disorders. New York: Raven Press, 1984: 237–254.

125. Re RB, Kourides IA, Ridgway EC, et al. The effect of glucocorticoid administration on human pituitary secretion of thyrotropin and prolactin. J Clin Endocrinol Metab 1976;43:338–346.

126. Lesch KP, Rupprecht R. Psychoneuroendocrine research in depression. J Neural Transm 1989;75:179–194.

127. Morley JE, Shafer RB, Elson MK, et al. Amphetamine induced hyperthyroxinemia. Ann Intern Med 1980;93:707–709.

128. Hein MD, Jackson IMD. Review: thyroid function in psychiatric illness. Gen Hosp Psychiatry 1990;12:232–244.

129. Linkowski P, VanWettere JP, Kerkhofs M, et al. Thyrotropin response to thyreostimulin in affectively ill women: relationships to suicidal behavior. Br J Psychiatry 1983;143:401–405.

130. Prange AJ, Loosen PT. Findings in affective disorders relevant to the thyroid axis, meanotropin, oxytocin and vasopressin. In Brown GM, ed. Neuroendocrinology and psychiatric disorder. New York: Raven Press, 1984:191–200.

131. Kirkegard C, Faber J, Hummer L. Increased levels of TRH in cerebrospinal fluids from patients with endogenous depression. Psychoneuroendocrinology 1979;4:227–235.

132. Snyder PJ, Utiger RD. Repetitive administration of thyrotropin-releasing hormone results in small elevations of serum thyroid hormones and marked inhibition of thyrotropin response. J Clin Invest 1973;52:2305–2312.

133. Spencer CA, Greenstadt MA, Wheeler WS, et al. The influence of long-term low dose thyrotropin-hormone infusions on serum thyrotropin and prolactin concentrations in man. J Clin Endcrinol Metab 1980;51:771–775.

134. Otsuki M, Dakoda M, Baba S. Influence of glucocorticoids in TRF induced TSH response in man. J Clin Endocrin Metab 1973;36: 95–102.

135. Wilber JF, Utiger RD. The effects of glucocorticoids on thyrotropin secretion. J Clin Invest 1969;48:2096–2103.

136. Bartalena L, Placidi GF, Martin, et al. Nocturnal serum thyrotropin (TSH) surge and TSH response to TSH-releasing hormone: dissociated behavior in untreated depressives. J Clin Endocrinol Metab 1990;71:650–655.

137. Adriaanse R, Brabant G, Endert E, Wiersinga WM. Pulsatile thyrotropin secretion in patients with Cushing's syndrome. Metabolism 1994;43(6):782–786.

138. Opstad K. Circadian rhythm of hormones is extinguished during prolonged physical stress, sleep and energy deficiency in young men. Eur J Endocrinol 1994;131(1):56–66.

139. Prange AJ, Wilson IC, Rabon AM, et al. Enhancement of imipramine antidepressant activity by thyroid hormone. Am J Psychiatry 1969; 126:457.

140. Coppen A, Whybrow PC, Noguera R, et al. The comparative antidepressant value of L-tryptophan and imipramine with and without attempted potentiation by liothyronine. Arch Gen Psychiatry 1972;26:234.

141. Loosen PT. Hormones of the hypothalamic-pituitary-thyroid axis: a psychoneuroendocrine perspective. Pharmacopsychiatry 1986;19: 401–415.

142. Kobayashi K, Nakaoka K, Tsuji N, et al. Effects of thyrotropin releasing hormones in chronic schizophrenic patients. Acta Med Okayama 1980;34:263–273.

143. Whybrow PC, Coppen A, Prange AJ, et al. Thyroid function and the response of L-thyronine in depression. Arch Gen Psychiatry 1972; 26:242.

144. Bauer MS, Whybrow PC, Winokur A. Rapid cycling bipolar affective disorder I: association with grade I hypothyroidism. Arch Gen Psychiatry 1990;47:427.

145. Cowdry RW, Wehr TA, Zis AP, et al. Thyroid abnormalities associated with rapid cycling bipolar illness. Arch Gen Psychiatry 1983;40:414.

146. Bauer MS, Whybrow PC. Rapid cycling bipolar affective disorder II; treatment of refractory rapid cycling with high dose levothyroxine: a preliminary study. Arch Gen Psychiatry 1990;4:435.

147. Whybrow PC, Prange AJ Jr. A hypothesis of thyroid catecholamine receptor interaction: its relevance to affective illness. Archives of General Psychiatry 1981;38:106–113.

148. Isojarvi JIT, Pakarinen AJ, Ylipalosaari, Myllyla VV. Serum hormones in male epileptic patients receiving anticonvulsant medication. Arch Neurol 1990;47:670–676.

149. Rootwelt K, Ganes T, Johannessen SI. Effect of carbamazepine, phenytoin and phenobarbitone on serum levels of thyroid hormone and thyrotropin in humans. Scand J Clin Lab Invest 1978;38: 731–736.

150. Aanderud S, Strandjord RE. Hypothyroidism induced by antiepileptic therapy. Acta Neurol Scand 1980;61:330–332.

Sexual Dimorphism

151. Dörner G, Poppe I, Stahl F, et al. Gene- and environment- dependent neuroendocrine etiogenesis of homosexuality and transsexualism. Exp Clin Endocrinol 1991;98:141–150.

152. Dörner G. Neuroendocrine response to estrogen and brain differentiation in heterosexuals, homosexuals and transsexuals. Arch Sex Behav 1988;17:57–75.

153. Dörner G. Hormone-dependent brain development and neuroendocrine prophylaxis. Exp Clin Endocrinol 1989;94:4–22.

154. Dohler KD. The pre- and post-natal influence of hormones and neurotransmitters on sexual differentiation of the mammalian hypothalamus. Int Rev Cytol 1991;131:1–57.

155. Meyer-Bahlburg HF, Feldman JF, Cohen P, et al. Perinatal factors in the development of gender-related play behavior: sex hormones versus pregnancy complications. Psychiatry 1988;51:260–271.

156. Vanderticele H, Eechaute W, Lacroix E, Leusen I. The effects of neonatal androgenization of male rats on testosterone metabolism by the hypothalamus-pituitary-gonadal axis. J Steroid Biochem Mol Biol 1987;26:493–497.

157. Francavilla S, Cordeschi G, Properzi G, et al. Ultraestructure of fetal human gonad before sexual differentiation and during early testicular and ovarian development. J Submicrosc Cytol Pathol 1990;22: 389–400.

158. Huhtaniemi I. Endocrine function and regulation of the fetal and neonatal testis. Int J Dev Biol 1989;33:117–123.
159. Mowszowics I, Stamatiadis D, Wright F, et al. Androgen receptor in sexual differentiation. J Steroid Biochem Mol Biol 1989;32:157–162.
160. Hasegawa O, Sugihara H, Minami S, et al. Masculinization of growth hormone (GH) secretory pattern by dihydrotestosterone is associated with augmentation of hypothalamic somatostatin and GH-releasing hormone mRNA levels in ovariectomized adult rats. Peptides 1992;13:475–481.
161. Hoffman MA, Swaab DF. Sexual dimorphism of the human brain: myth and reality. Exp Clin Endocrinol 1991;98:161–170.
162. Witelson SF. Neural sexual mosaicism: sexual differentiation of the human temporoparietal region for functional asymmetry. Psychoneuroendocrinology 1991;16:131–153.
163. LeVay SA. A difference in hypothalamic structure between heterosexual and homosexual men. Science 1991;253:1034–1037.
164. Allen LS, Gorski RA. Sexual dimorphism of the anterior commisure and massa intermedia of the human brain. J Compar Neurol 1991;312(1):97–104.
165. Meaney MJ. The sexual differentiation of social play. Psychiatric Developments 1989;7:247–261.
166. Seeman MV. Prenatal gonadal hormones and schizophrenia in men and women. Psychiatric Journal of the University of Ottawa 1989;14:473–475.
167. Sikich L, Todd RD. Are the neurodevelopmental effects of gonadal hormones related to sex differences in psychiatric illnesses? Psychiatric Developments 1988;6:277–309.

Stress and Reproductive Function

168. Rivier C, Rivest S. Review: effect of stress on the activity of the hypothalamic-pituitary-gonadal axis: peripheral and central mechanisms. Biol Reprod 1991;45:523–532.
169. MacLuskey NJ, Naftolin F, Leranth C. Immunocytochemical evidence for direct synaptic connections between corticotropin releasing factor (CRF) and gonadotropin releasing hormone (GnRH)-containing neurons in the preoptic area of the rat. Brain Res 1988;439:391–395.
170. Sawchenko PE, Swanson LW. Organization of CRF immunoreactive cells and fibers in the rat brain: immunohistochemical studies. In DeSouza EB, Numeroff CB, eds. Corticotropin-releasing factor: basic and clinical studies of a neuropeptide. Boca Raton: CRC Press; 1990:29–51.
171. Almeida OFX, Nikolarakis KE, Herz A. Evidence for the involvement of endogenous opioids in the inhibition of luteinizing hormone by corticotropin releasing factor. Endocrinology 1988;122:1034–1041.
172. Butler PD, Weiss JM, Stout JC, et al. Corticotropin-releasing factor produces fear-enhancing and behavioral activating effects following infusion into the locus coeruleus. J Neurosci 1990;10:176–183.
173. Sarkar D, Yen S. Hyperprolactinemia decreases the luteinizing hormone-releasing hormone concentration in pituitary portal plasma: a possible role for β-endorphin as a mediator. Endocrinology 1985;116:2080–2084.
174. Ching M. Morphine suppresses the proestrous surge of GnRH in pituitary portal plasma of rats. Endocrinology 1983;112:2209–2211.
175. Leadem CA, Crowley WR, Simpkins JW, et al. Effects of naloxone on catecholamine and LHRH release from the perifused hypothalamus of the steroid primed rat. Neuroendocrinology. 1985;40:497–500.
176. Sirinathsinghji DJS. Regulation of lordosis behavior in the female rat by corticotropin releasing factor, β-endorphin/corticotropin and luteinizing hormone releasing-hormone neuronal systems in the medial preoptic area. Brain Res 1986;375:49–56.
177. Gopalan C, Gilmore DP, Brown CH. Effects of different opiates on hypothalamic monoamine turnover and on plasma LH levels in pro-estrous rats. J Neurol Sci 1989;94:211–219.
178. Barbarino A, De Marinis L, Fillo G, et al. Corticotropin-releasing hormone inhibition of gonadotropin secretion during the menstrual cycle. Metabolism 1989;38:504–506.
179. Barbarino A, De Marinis L, Tofani A, et al. Corticotropin-releasing hormone inhibition of gonadotropin release and the effect of opioid blockade. J Clin Endocrinol Metab 1989;68:523–528.
180. Tazi A, Dantzer R, Le Moal M, et al. Corticotropin releasing-factor antagonist blocks stress induced fighting in rats. Regulatory peptides. 1987;18:37–42.

Anorexia and Bulimia

181. Newman MM, Halmi KA. The endocrinology of anorexia nervosa and bulimia nervosa. Endocrinol Metab Clin North Am 1988;17:195–211.
182. Devlin M, Walsh T, Katz J, et al. Hypothalamic-pituitary gonadal function in anorexia nervosa and bulimia. Psychiatry Res 1988;28:11–24.
183. Sherman BM. Hypothalamic control of the menstrual cycle: implications for the study of anorexia nervosa. In Brown GM, ed. Neuroendocrinology and psychiatric disorder. New York: Raven Press, 1984:315–324.
184. Ferrari E, Fraschini F, Brambilla F. Hormonal circadian rhythms in eating disorders. Biol Psychiatry 1990;27:1007–1020.
185. Kiriike N, Nishiwaki S, Izumiya Y, et al. Thyrotropin, prolactin, and growth hormone responses to thyrotropin-releasing hormone in anorexia nervosa and bulimia. Biol Psychiatry 1987;22:167–176.
186. Garfinkel PE. Anorexia nervosa: an overview of hypothalamic-pituitary function. In Brown GM, ed. Neuroendocrinology and psychiatric disorder. New York: Raven Press, 1984:301–314.
187. American Psychiatric Association. DSM-III-R: Diagnostic and statistical manual of mental disorders. 3rd. ed., revised. Washington, D.C.: American Psychiatric Association, 1987.
188. Fichter MM, Pirke KM, Pöllinger J, et al. Disturbances in the hypothalamo-pituitary-adrenal and other neuroendocrine axes in bulimia. Biol Psychiatry 1990;27:1021–1037.
189. Murialdo G, Galimberti CA, Fonzi S, Manni R, Costelli P, Parodi C, Solinas GP, Amoretti G, Tartara A. Sex hormones and pituitary function in male epileptic patients with altered or normal sexuality. Epilepsia 1995;36(4):360–365.
190. Isojarvi JI, Repo M, Pakarinen AJ, Lukkarinen O, Myllyla VV. Carbamazepine, phenytoin, sex hormones, and sexual function in men with epilepsy. Epilepsia 1995;36(4):366–370.
191. Cummings LN, Giudice L, Morrell MJ. Ovulatory function in epilepsy. Epilepsia 1995;36(4):355–359.
192. Nappi C, Meo R, Di Carlo C, Estraneo A, Bilo L. Reduced fertility and neuroendocrine dysfunction in women with epilepsy. Gynecol Endocrinol 1994;8(2):133–145.
193. Drislane FW, Coleman AE, Schomer DL, Ives J, Levesque LA, Seibel MM, Herzog AG. Altered pulsatile secretion of luteinizing hormone in women with epilepsy. Neurology 1994;44(2):306–310.
194. Meo R, Bilo L, Nappi C, Tommaselli AP, Valentino R, Nocerino C, Striano S, Buscaino GA. Derangement of the hypothalamic GnRH pulse generator in women with epilepsy. Seizure 1993;2(3):241–252.
195. Herzog AG. A relationship between particular reproductive endocrine disorders and the laterality of epileptiform discharges in women with epilepsy. Neurology 1993;43(10):1907–1910.
196. Isojarvi JI, Laatikainen TJ, Pakarinen AJ, Juntunen KT, Myllyla VV. Polycystic ovaries and hyperandrogenism in women taking valproate for epilepsy. N Engl J Med 1993;329(19):1383–1388.
197. Sperling MR, Pritchard PB III, Engel J Jr, et al. Prolactin in partial epilepsy: An indicator of limbic seizures. Ann Neurol 1986;20:716–722.
198. Yerby MS, vanBelle G, Friel PN, et al. Serum prolactins in the diagnosis of epilepsy. Sensitivity, specificity, and predictive value. Neurology 1987;37:1224–1226.

199. Matthew E, Woods JF. Growth hormone and prolactin in temporal lobe epilepsy. Epilepsy Res 1993;16(3):215–222.

Somatostatin

200. Rubinow DR, Gold PW, Post RM, et al. CSF somatostatin in affective illness. Arch Gen Psychiatry 1983;40:409–412.
201. Doran AR, Rubinow DR, Roy A, et al. CSF somatostatin and abnormal response to dexamethasone administration in schizophrenic and depressed patients. Arch Gen Psychiatry 1986;43:365–369.
202. Serby M, Richardson SB, Rypma B, et al. Somatostatin regulation of the CRF-ACTH-cortisol axis. Biol Psychiatry 1986;21:971–974.
203. Beal MF, Kowall NW, Mazurek MF. Neuropeptides in Alzheimer's disease. J Neural Transm Suppl 1987;24(Suppl):163–174.
204. Beal MF, Mazurek MF, Svendsen CN et al. Widespread reduction of somatostatin-like immunoreactivity in the cerebral cortex in Alzheimer's disease. Ann Neurol 1986;20:489–495.
205. Tamminga CA, Foster NL, Fedio P. Alzheimer's disease: low cerebral somatostatin levels correlate with impaired cognitive function and cortical metabolism. Neurology 1987;37:161–165.

Hypothalamic Lesions

206. Tonkonogy JM, Geller JL. Hypothalamic lesions and intermittent explosive disorder. J Neuropsychiatry Clin Neurosci 1992;4:45–50.
207. Vesely DL. Hypothalamic sarcoidosis: a new cause of morbid obesity. South Med J 1989;82:758–761.
208. Ben-Amitai D, Rachmel A, Levy Y, et al. Hypodypsic hypernatremia and hypertriglyceridemia associated with cleft lip and cleft palate: a new hypothalamic dysfunction syndrome? Am J Med Genetics 1990;36:275–278.
209. Verdin E, Smitz S, Thibaut A, et al. Adipsic hypernatremia in a patient with pseudotumor cerebri and the primary empty sella syndrome. J Endocrinol Invest 1985;8:369–372.
210. Chiang R, Marshall MC, Rosman PM, et al. Empty sella turcica in intracanial sarcoidosis. Pituitary insufficiency, primary polydipsia, and changing neuroradiologic findings. Arch Neurol 1984;41:662–665.
211. Gurewitz R, Blum I, Lavie P, et al. Recurrent hypothermia, hypersomnolence, central sleep apnea, hypodipsia, hypernatremia, hypothyroidism, hyperprolactinemia and growth hormone deficiency in a boy—treatment with clomipramine. Acta Endocrinol Suppl 1986;279:468–472.
212. Yoshikawa M, Yamamoto M, Ohba S, et al. Hypothalamic histiocytosis X with diabetes insipidous and Korsakoff's syndrome: a case report. Neurologia Medico-Chirurgica 1991;31:529–534.
213. Mechanick JI, Hochberg FH, LaRocque A. Hypothalamic dysfunction following whole-brain irradiation. J Neurosurgery 1986;65:490–494.

214. Moore JB, Kulkarni R, Crutcher DC, et al: MRI in multifocal eosinophilic granuloma: staging disease and monitoring response to therapy. Am J Pediatr Hematol Oncol 1989;11:174–177.
215. Ober KP, Alexander E, Challa VR, et al. Histiocytosis X of the hypothalamus. Neurosurgery 1989;24:93–95.
216. Williams TC, Frohman LA. Hypothalamic dysfunction associated with hemochromatosis. Ann Intern Med 1985;103:550–551.

Thyroid Disease

217. Nemeroff CB, Simon JS, Haggerty JJ, et al. Antithyroid antibodies in depressed patients. Am J Psychiatry 1983;142:840–843.
218. Whybrow PC. Behavioral and psychiatric aspects of hypothyroidism. In Braverman L, Utiger R, eds. The thyroid. Philadelphia: JB Lippincott, 1991:1078–1083.
219. Ruel J, Faure R, Dussault JH. Regional distribution of nuclear T4 receptors in rat brain and evidence for preferential localization in neurons. J Endocrinol Invest 1985;8:343.

Hypo- and Hypercortisolism

220. Orth DN, Kovacs WJ, DeBold CR. The adrenal cortex. In Wilson JD, Foster DW, eds. Williams textbook of endocrinology. Philadelphia: WB Saunders 1992:489.
221. Martignoni E, Costa A, Sinforani E, et al. The brain as a target for adrenocortical steroids: cognitive implications. Psychoneuroendocrinology 1992;17:343–354.
222. Uno H, Tarara R, Else J, et al. Hippocampal damage associated with prolonged and fatal stress in primates. J Neurosci 1988;9:1705–1711.
223. Thuggesen P, Herman K, Willanger R. Concentration camp survivors in Denmark: persecution, disease, disability, compensation. Dan Med Bull 1970;17:65–70.
224. Sjaastad O: The war sailor and KZ syndromes. Functional Neurology 1986;1:5–19.
225. Jensen T, Genefke I, Hyldebrandt N. Cerebral atrophy in young torture victims. N Engl J Med 1982;307:1341.
226. Ling M, Perry P, Tsaung M. Side effects of corticosteroid therapy. Arch Gen Psychiatry 1981;38:471–477.
227. Varney NR, Alexander B, MacIndoe JH. Reversible steroid dementia in patients without steroid psychosis. Am J Psychiatry 1984;141:369–372.
228. Wolkowitz OM, Reus VI, Weingartner H, et al. Cognitive effects of corticosteroids. Am J Psychiatry 1990;147:1297–1303.
229. McEwen BS: Glucocorticoids and hippocampus: receptors in search of a function. In Ganten D, Pfaff D, eds. Adrenal actions on brain. New York: Springer-Verlag 1982:1–22.

10

PSYCHONEUROIMMUNOLOGY: INTERACTIONS BETWEEN THE BRAIN AND THE IMMUNE SYSTEM

Robert Ader, Kelley Madden, David L. Felten, Denise L. Bellinger, and Randolph B. Schiffer

During the past 15 years, psychoneuroimmunology has developed into a bona fide field of interdisciplinary research (1). Previously unknown and unsuspected links between the nervous system, the endocrine system, and the immune system have provided a basis for the numerous observations that neuroendocrine manipulations alter immune responses and that activation of the immune system alters neural and endocrine responses. It is not surprising, then, that behavioral processes also can influence immunological reactivity and that the immune status of an organism has consequences for behavior. Research in psychoneuroimmunology addresses the functional significance of the relationship among neural, endocrine, and immune processes, not in place of, but in addition to the more traditional, disciplinary analysis of the mechanisms governing functions within a "single" system.

The research findings to date indicate that the brain and the immune system, the two most complex systems that have evolved for the maintenance of homeostasis, represent an integrated mechanism for the adaptation of the individual and the species. Within the context of neuropsychiatry, this chapter provides a brief overview of some of the evidence that behavioral factors influence immune functions and describes some of the neural and endocrine pathways that can serve as vehicles for communication between the brain and the immune system.

Although this is a relatively new field of research, the range of phenomena bearing on brain-behavior-immune system interactions is already quite broad. An old and continuing experimental and clinical literature base, for example, suggests that immune function can be altered by a variety of psychological interventions. Other data suggest that affective states and personality characteristics sometimes may be associated with differences in immunological reactivity. While provocative, these studies are difficult to replicate, and unequivocal evidence of such associations is not yet available. Our selective review will concentrate on the experimental literature dealing with the effects of behavior on immune responses and the relationships among neural, endocrine, and immune processes that could be involved in mediating such interactions.

BEHAVIOR-IMMUNE SYSTEM INTERACTIONS

Effects of "Stress"

In the context of this chapter, "stress" refers to any natural or experimentally contrived experiential, social, or environmental circumstances that intuitively, at least, pose an actual or perceived threat to the psychobiological integrity of the individual. In subhuman animals as well as in humans, psychosocial conditions that are perceived as a threat to the organism and to which the organism cannot adapt are accompanied by acute and chronic psychophysiological changes that could contribute to the development of disease, especially if the organism is coincidentally exposed to potentially pathogenic stimuli. An extensive literature testifies to the role of psychosocial factors in the susceptibility to and/or the progression of a variety of pathophysiological processes, including allergic, infectious, autoimmune, and neoplastic diseases that, to a varying extent, involve alterations in immunological defense mechanisms (2–8).

The effects of stress are not, however, uniform in nature. Experimental studies provide numerous illustrations of the fact that the outcome of stressful experiences depends upon several factors, including the nature of the stressor and the pathophysiological stimuli to which the organism is subjected. Physical restraint, for example, increases susceptibility to herpes simplex virus infection (9–11) and to the Maloney sarcoma virus (12) in rodents, but does not influence the response to an experimentally induced lymphoma (13), and decreases susceptibility to experimental allergic encephalomyelitis (14). Electric shock stimulation increases susceptibility to Coxsackie B virus and decreases susceptibility to a rodent malaria (15) and to the development of leukemia in genetically susceptible mice (16). Both electric shock and handling decrease susceptibility to a collagen-induced arthritis, whereas a different stressor, auditory stimulation, increases susceptibility. Analogous results are obtained in experiments on the development and progression of tumors in animal subjects (4, 5). Evidently, the same stressor can have different effects on different pathophysiological processes, and different stressors can exert different effects on a single disease process. Thus, the ability to predict the pathophysiological effects of stress would seem to depend upon a more complete understanding of the interaction between those responses unconditionally elicited by potentially pathogenic stimulation, and those acute and chronic psychophysiological (including immunological) changes elicited by the stressful circumstances upon which pathogenic conditions are superimposed.

Although the literature documents the influence of psychosocial factors on alterations in the susceptibility to or progression of a variety of diseases, only a few studies provide direct evidence that such effects are mediated by psychosocially induced changes in immunocompetence. Such evidence can only come from studies that examine psychosocially induced changes in immune function that are relevant to the potential mechanisms underlying the disease process under study. Feng et al. (17), for example, observed a delay in the production of virus-specific antibody in restrained mice infected with influenza virus, and Bonneau et al. (9) found that repeated and prolonged periods of restraint suppressed natural killer (NK) cell activity and the primary development of cytotoxic T lymphocytes of mice inoculated with herpes simplex virus (HSV). Also, higher titers of infectious HSV were recovered from the restrained animals.

In another study (10), it was found that restraint inhibited the activation of HSV-specific memory cells. Similar results were obtained by Kusnecov et al. (18), using electric shock stimulation. Other examples include the observations of immune responses and neoplastic disease (19, 20). Using a tumor model in which lung metastases are thought to be related to NK cell function, Ben-Eliyahu et al. (19) found that, depending upon when the stressor was imposed in relation to the effect of NK cells on the metastatic process, forced swimming decreased NK cell activity and increased lung metastases.

As an initial step in examining the link among psychosocial factors, alterations in immune function, and disease, some current research is focused on quantifying the changes in immune function induced by different stressful circumstances. The death of a family member, for example, is rated highly on scales of stressful life events and bereavement, and has been associated with depression and an increased morbidity and mortality in the case of some diseases (21, 22). Also, bereavement has been associated with changes in some components of immunological reactivity, such as reduced lymphoproliferative responses to mitogenic stimulation (23, 24) and impaired NK cell activity (25). Other reports have described similar changes in immune function associated with the affective responses to other "losses," such as marital separation and divorce (26). Although the clinical relevance of these alterations of immune function may appropriately be questioned, changes in immune function may constitute a potential link between psychosocial factors and an altered susceptibility to or progression of some diseases. This chain of psychophysiological events, however, has not yet been firmly established.

Changes in immune function in humans can be observed in response to a variety of common (stressful) situations. In 1938, Farris (27) reported immunological changes in response to football games in the players and in the spectators. In response to forthcoming examinations, medical students display increased levels of distress that are accompanied by transient impairments in several parameters of immune function (26). Relative to nonstressful baseline levels, there are decreases in mitogen responsiveness, NK cell activity, the percentage of helper T lymphocytes in the blood, and interferon production by stimulated lymphocytes during the examination periods. Medical students who are seropositive for Epstein-Barr virus (EBV) also show elevated anti-EBV antibody titers during examination periods (28). These are interpreted to reflect reduced cell-mediated control over the latent virus. There is, at the same time, an increase in the incidence of self-reported symptoms of infectious illness (29). Thus far, personality tests have failed to discriminate between students who volunteered for these studies and their classmates. In addition, other life events that could influence immunological reactivity were minor and did not correlate with the documented changes in immunological reactivity.

In experimental animals, "losses" also have immunological consequences. Periodic interruptions of mother-litter interactions and/or early weaning in rodents decreases lymphoproliferative responses to mitogenic stimulation and reduces the response to subsequent antigenic challenge (30, 31). Whether the immunological sequelae of premature weaning—or extended maternal care (32)—are the result of nutritional deficits, inadequate body temperature regulation, and/or maternally mediated influences on neural and/or endocrine development has not yet been determined.

In response to separation, infant monkeys and their mothers show a transient depression of in vitro mitogen responsiveness. Like the results of bereavement studies in humans, these effects are not correlated with plasma cortisol levels (33, 34). Separating squirrel monkeys from their mothers results in a decrease in complement protein level (an effector mechanism in humoral immunity), macrophage function, and the IgG antibody response to immunization with a benign bacteriophage. The magnitude of these effects depends upon the social environment in which the animals are caged following the separation (35, 36). Rhesus macaque monkeys show essentially the same behavioral reactions to separation from the mother as squirrel monkeys, but they display a different pattern of endocrine responses and do not show immunological changes following separation.

Various behavioral manipulations and social and environmental conditions evocative of stress responses can influence a variety of immune responses in different species. Stress is generally but not uniformly immunosuppressive. Here again, the literature indicates that the effects of stress on acquired antibody- and cell-mediated immunity as well as on natural immune reactions such as NK cell activity depend on (a) the quality as well as the quantity of the stressful stimulation (37–45) and the immunogenic stimulation (46); (b) the temporal relationship between stressful stimulation and immunogenic stimulation (47–49); (c) the immune response (or compartment) under study (38, 43, 47, 50–53); and (d) several host factors such as strain, sex, and age (54, 55). As in the case of disease susceptibility, predicting the outcome of such experiments depends upon an understanding of the interaction between the effects unconditionally elicited by immunogenic stimulation and the acute and chronic psychophysiological effects of the stressful stimulation upon which the immunological stimulation is superimposed.

The most sophisticated experimental paradigms for inducing stress responses are those that are ethologically appropriate and involve no direct physical damage to the animal. One such example is the observation that the exposure of mice to the odors emitted by stressed conspecifics (animals of the same species) is sufficient to influence immunological reactivity (56) — or those that entail noxious stimulation that is predictable or unpredictable, escapable or inescapable, or avoidable or unavoidable. Such experiments hold the physical elements of the stressor constant, while enabling some animals to adapt to or control their environment. Acute and chronic exposure to these experimental situations have yielded interesting but inconsistent results. Preliminary findings suggest that escapable footshock prevents the suppression of splenic NK cell activity observed in animals subjected to inescapable shock (41) and that inescapable but not escapable footshock results in a suppression of mitogen-induced lymphoproliferation (57). Although these latter findings have been difficult to reproduce (58), others (53) have described immune changes among animals subjected to electric shock with and without a warning signal, or among animals that could or could not avoid electric shock. The direction of the observed effects varied with the parameter of immune function being measured. The limited number of studies on the "control" of stressful conditions by human subjects (59, 60) has also yielded inconsistent effects.

Depression and Immunity

Associations between depressive clinical states and immune function are of importance to neuropsychiatry for two reasons. Depressive clinical states may be clinical manifestations of certain autoimmune diseases, and functional impairments of the immune system may be associated secondarily with depressive disease, rendering such patients more vulnerable to infectious or neoplastic disease.

A variety of clinical studies have described an association between certain diseases of the immune system and clinical depression. Multiple sclerosis (MS) is the best example of a T-cell-mediated autoimmune disease that has been associated with depressive syndromes. Systemic lupus erythematosus (SLE) is an example of a B-cell-mediated autoimmune disease in which depressive features are frequently reported. In syndromes caused by the human immunodeficiency virus I (HIV), depressive features also have been described frequently.

MS is a T-cell-mediated autoimmune disease of the central nervous system (CNS) in which there is inflammatory destruction of the myelin sheaths. Specific subsets of CD4+ and CD8+ T lymphocytes are involved in this process, along with macrophages (61–65). There are genetically determined risk factors for the disease (65–68), but also environmental determinants that are still undetermined. (69–71). Hormonal modulation of some sort is also important in MS because the disease is more common among women by a ratio on the order of 1.8:1 (72).

The association of affective disorders with MS has been the subject of a recent review (73). Point prevalence estimates for diagnosable depressive disorders in MS patients are at least 27% in better-designed epidemiological studies. Phenomenologically, these depressions tend to be moderately severe as opposed to the more psychotic or agitated states sometimes seen among psychiatric patients. Such prevalence rates of depressive illness are higher than those observed in control groups comprised of normal subjects, patients with various medical and neurological illnesses, and patients with non-brain-related neural disorders such as spinal cord injury. MS patients with primarily cerebral disease may have greater rates of depressive illness than MS patients with primarily spinal cord disease. Patients in exacerbation are more depressed than patients in remission.

From all such observations, it remains difficult to conclude that affective disturbance can be produced in some direct manner by the CNS autoimmune pathology. Psychological explanations can also apply to such mood disorders, and possibly both psychological and neurobiological processes are at work. We lack the sort of neuroanatomical or neuroimmunological data that might definitively link these mood disorders with CNS disease. Such studies will constitute the next research horizon in MS patients with mood disorders, and some early examples of such studies have appeared. One example of the application of new technologies to this problem is that of Honer and colleagues (74). These authors performed magnetic resonance imaging (MRI) studies on eight MS patients with psychiatric disorders, six of whom had bipolar or unipolar depression, and on eight matched nonpsychiatric MS controls. Although the two groups did not differ with regard to total MS plaque volume, the psychiatric group had a greater proportion of plaques within temporal lobe structures.

Very few studies to date concern therapy for the depressive episodes associated with MS. Schiffer et al. (75) have described a series of time-limited psychotherapeutic strategies, primarily to be used by nonpsychiatric clinicians. This same group has also conducted a double-blind, placebo-controlled study of the effectiveness of desipramine in 28 MS patients with major depression, finding significantly greater improvement in the desipramine-treated patients (76).

In SLE we have the opportunity to observe a primarily antibody-mediated autoimmune disease in which mood disorders also occur with some frequency. SLE is a relatively common multisystem inflammatory disease of connective tissue which, like MS, is sometimes characterized by exacerbations and remissions. The psychiatric features associated with SLE have not been as well characterized as those associated with MS, but clearly include cognitive blunting, psychosis, and affective disorder (77, 78). The prospective prevalence risk for SLE patients to develop such behavioral disturbances over 1 to several years approaches 50% in studies that have included longitudinal follow-up (79–81). Some of these mood disturbances may be related to the variety of circulating anti-self-antibodies that occur in SLE (82, 83). Increased circulating oligoclonal IgG is known to occur commonly in the cerebrospinal fluid (CSF) of these patients (84, 85). Certain antilymphocytic antibodies from SLE patients are known to cross-react with neurons in vitro (86, 87). Serum antiribosomal antibodies have also been reported in association with psychosis and severe affective disorder, and possibly, titers of these antibodies vary with behavioral fluctuation (88). There is also some evidence (89) that levels of antineuronal antibodies in CSF are elevated in those SLE patients who have "organic mental disorders."

The data available from these studies are too preliminary to allow an understanding of specific connections between circulating autoantibodies in these patients and behavioral disturbance. There is a suggestion of such a link; these patients have a variety of neurobehavioral disturbances, and many of them have circulating brain-reactive autoantibodies in sera. Exciting neuropsychiatric possibilities remain open for future investigators who might approach this question.

Depressive and other psychiatric disturbances have also been commonly reported in patients infected by the HIV (90, 91). Again, it has been difficult to develop evidence that there is a specific neurological connection between the T-cell tropic virus that causes the disease and the mood disorders. It does not appear that there is a direct relationship between the mood disorder and severity of HIV illness, as measured by clinical staging or by CD4 cell counts. Moreover, many of the persons affected by HIV have positive lifetime histories for affective disturbance. We cannot yet conclude that there is a direct mediation by HIV in the production of these mood disorders.

Because of the frequently cited relationship between bereavement and depression, investigators have begun to study the immune changes that accompany depression. Several recent reviews have described the occurrence of immunological alterations in the setting of stress, depression, and bereavement (92–96). There is substantial evidence that in vitro measures of immune function are altered during depressive states, especially in the more severe depressive states. Persuasive evidence of alteration in immunity associated with depressive states appears when studies of immune system function are performed in depressed patients. Lymphocyte proliferation in response to mitogens and antigens, for example, seems to be impaired or decreased in some patients with clinical depression. In Stein et al.'s review (93), there are 14 cited studies in which lymphocyte responses to phytohemagglutinin (PHA), concanavalin A (conA) and pokeweed mitogen were measured. Six of these studies found the mitogen-stimulated responses to be decreased among depressed patients compared with controls, and only one found an increase in the PHA response. Schleifer and his colleagues (97) suggest that this blunting of mitogen responsiveness is more specifically linked with the more severe, hospitalized depressive patients. Their studies indicate that an additional variable of importance might be age, because older depressed patients in the series showed an absence of age-related changes in T4-helper cell counts.

Immune alterations in depression are not as consistent when relatively crude measures of immune function are used, such as the enumeration of total white cells in blood, the differential count of major white cell types, or even lymphocyte subtype counts. Some investigators have observed a significant suppression of one or another parameter of immunity (98–103); others have not (99, 104–106). Stein and his coauthors (93), for example, reviewed 11 studies of cellular enumeration in depressed patients, most of which found no differences between depressed and control groups in total white blood cell (WBC) count, differential count of neutrophils, or total lymphocytes, or total T-cell or B-cell subsets. However, on the basis of their meta-analysis of the literature on depression and immune changes, Herbert and Cohen (95) came to the conclusion that clinical depression, particularly in older and hospitalized populations, is reliably associated with both functional and enumerative measures of immunity. In conducting and interpreting such data, it is necessary to consider a variety of interacting factors, such as the age and sex of the patients; the nature of the depression (endogenous vs. nonendogenous, dexamethasone suppressors or nonsuppressors); whether patients are experiencing acute depression or are in remission; the severity and/or duration of depression that may be related to whether patients are hospitalized or ambulatory; whether patients are drug-free (and for how long); and the presence or absence (and kind) of therapy. Of particular concern would be the nature of the immune response being measured and its relationship to some disease outcome.

The functional response of NK cells to malignant and virus-infected cells in vitro has also been used as a measure of immune responsiveness. Most studies that have assessed NK function in depressed patients have found it to be impaired compared with control populations (107–109).

Depression and altered B-cell function have not been correlated extensively. There are some reports of elevated circulating antibody titers to herpes virus and cytomegalovirus among depressed patients (95). Others have found no evidence of oligoclonal IgG or IgM in such patients (106). Recently, some interesting data bearing on B cell function as a potential mechanism in the causation of some mood disorders have come from Roy's laboratory (110). These investigators have been exploring levels of circulating antibodies to endogenous neuropeptides, which might be of relevance to psychiatric disorders. Such peptide systems include somatostatin and endorphins, among others, and preliminary data have suggested that some depressed subjects may have increased levels of such circulating autoantibodies.

The clinical significance of the in vitro immunological changes that accompany bereavement or clinical depression remains a primary and, as yet, unresolved concern. Because the trend in most of these studies has primarily shown decreased cellular immune function, one might expect that depressed patients would be more vulnerable to certain nonpyogenic infections or malignancies. Clearly, there is a general clinical wisdom on this point, imputing an increased risk for death and disease among bereaved spouses, or to people with cancer who develop an attitude of "giving up." Early clinical observations suggested such a connection, but large, elegant epidemiological studies of patients with various psychiatric diagnoses have generally not corroborated an increased mortality from medical disease among such patients. Excess mortality among such patients seems to be attributable either to unnatural causes (suicide, accidents) or to selection bias (111–113). On the other hand, there are suggestions of specific connections between subgroups of these patients and disease-specific mortality. Such connections derive from post hoc data analyses only, however. One large twin study has found evidence for broadly increased mortality from all medical diseases among psychiatric patients (114). Ideally, conclusions could be drawn from epidemiological studies in which associations between diseases related to immunological surveillance (infection, malignancy) and affective disorders are tested.

These data concerning immune function and depression are quite preliminary in several ways. In many studies the psychiatric diagnoses were not rigorously performed. None of the studies has been prospective, to include retesting of subjects after resolution of depression, so we do not know whether the immunological alterations are trait or state variables. We do not know the clinical relevance of the in vitro immunological alterations that have been seen in some depressed patients. There are no studies that have convincingly linked these in vitro changes with clinical changes in health or disease. We do not know the mechanism by which such functional changes in the immune system appear in certain depressed patients. Also, abnormalities of cortisol regulation are known to occur in many depressed individuals, and hypercortisolism can suppress at least some T-cell-related immune functions (115–119). Clearly, a range of laboratory and clinically based investigations is needed to help us understand the mechanisms and significance of immunological alterations associated with affective disorders.

Neuroendocrine states constitute the internal milieu within which immune responses take place. Normal and abnormal affective states, different prenatal and early life experiences and social interactions, and environmental circumstances over which the individual has no control are all associated with neuroendocrine changes that are implicated in the modulation of immune responses. Our understanding of the interactions between neuroendocrine and immune function under normal and stressful conditions, however, is incomplete. For example, glucocorticoids are usually immunosuppressive, and it is frequently assumed that an elevation in adrenal steroids, a common manifestation of the effects of different stressors, accounts for suppression of immunological reactivity associated with stressful experiences. There are many examples of stressor-induced, adrenocortically mediated changes in immunological reactivity, particularly in vitro. However, there are several other observations of stressor-induced alterations in immune function that are independent of adrenocortical activation (13, 40, 48, 50, 120–125). The immunological changes associated with stressful stimulation or different affective states involve complex interactions among neural, endocrine, and compartmentalized immune responses. Activation of the immune system will, in turn, alter levels of circulating hormones and neurotransmitters. It is likely, therefore, that complex feedback and feedforward mechanisms characterize the interactions within and between these "systems."

Conditioned Alterations of Immunity

Immune responses can be modified by classical (Pavlovian) conditioning. The conditioned modulation of natural and acquired host defense mechanisms and immune responses was first investigated by Russian scientists in the 1920s, using the principles and procedures of the day (126, 127). After multiple pairings of a neutral conditioned stimulus (CS) and an injection of antigen, the unconditioned stimulus (UCS), presentation of the CS, alone, was purported to elicit conditioned increases in nonspecific defense responses and increases in antibody titers, as well. A detailed review of these experiments, taking into account their scientific controls and statistical analysis, has been provided elsewhere (128).

Current interest in conditioned alterations of immunity began with a study by Ader and Cohen (129). Using a taste aversion learning paradigm (a passive-avoidance conditioning situation), water-deprived rats were provided with a novel, distinctively flavored drinking solution (saccharin), the CS. Consumption of the CS solution was followed by an intraperitoneal injection of cyclophosphamide (CY), an immunosuppressive unconditioned stimulus (UCS) that also causes a transient gastrointestinal malaise. Three days later, the animals were immunized with sheep red blood cells (SRBC), and the conditioned population was randomly divided into three subgroups: Group CS was reexposed to the CS previously paired with the immunosuppressive drug and injected with saline; to control for the effects of conditioning per se, Group CSo was provided with plain water and not otherwise manipulated; Group UCS was also given plain water but was injected with CY to define the unconditioned immunosuppressive effects of the drug. A nonconditioned group initially received CY without the saccharin drinking solution and, following immunization, was provided with the saccharin solution whenever any subsample of Group CS was reexposed to the CS. A placebo group was initially injected with saline following the consumption of plain water.

The pairing of saccharin consumption and an injection of CY resulted in an aversion to saccharin-flavored water when conditioned animals were reexposed to the CS, and, as hypothesized, conditioned animals reexposed to the CS also showed an attenuated antibody response to SRBC compared with nonconditioned animals and animals that were conditioned but not reexposed to the CS. These results, since verified by other investigators (130, 131), have been taken as evidence for a conditioned suppression of immunological reactivity. The acquisition and extinction of the conditioned suppression or enhancement of antibody- and cell-mediated immune responses, as well as nonimmunologically specific host defense reactions, has been documented repeatedly using different CSs, different UCSs, different antigens, and different outcome measures (131, 132). Although much of this research has involved taste aversion conditioning using an immunomodulating drug as the UCS, the phenomenon is not confined to conditioned immunopharmacological effects. The immunological effects of stress have been conditioned (133) and, most impressively, conditioning has been accomplished using antigens as unconditioned stimuli (134, 135).

The frequent use of aversive unconditioned stimuli (immunosuppressive drugs or electric shock) raises the issue of an association between conditioned avoidance and immune responses. The literature, however, reveals no consistent relationship between conditioned behavioral and immunological responses; taste aversions have been observed without parallel changes in immune function, and conditioned changes in immunological reactivity have been noted in the absence of conditioned avoidance responses (131). As is the case with conditioned behavioral and autonomic responses, current data suggest that multiple and independent processes are involved.

Extensions of this research have implicated conditioning processes in the development of tolerance to an immuno-modulating agent (136, 137) in much the same way as conditioning has been found to play a role in the development of tolerance to other pharmacological substances (138, 139). The potential biological significance of conditioned alterations of immune responses, in general, and conditioned immunosuppressive responses, in particular, have been elaborated in several studies. In the course of a 2-month regimen of pharmacotherapy in lupus-prone mice, the substitution of a saccharin solution (CS) previously associated with the immunosuppressive effects of CY for some of the scheduled treatments with active drug delayed the progression of autoimmune disease using a cumulative amount of drug that was not, by itself, sufficient to alter the course of the disease (140, 141). Conditioned immunosuppressive effects have also been found to alter the development of adjuvant-induced arthritis (142–144) and mortality to a transplanted plasmacytoma (145) in rats. The therapeutic potential of conditioning is further suggested by data obtained from rodents indicating that reexposure to a CS previously paired with an immunosuppressive drug could prolong the survival of a skin allograft (146) and extend the survival of a heterotypic heart transplant (147).

Extensions of this research have also documented conditioned alterations of immunity in human subjects. Bovbjerg et al. (148), for example, found that the anticipatory nausea that frequently accompanies immunosuppressive cancer chemotherapy was associated with anticipatory suppression of the in vitro proliferative response to T cell mitogens. In another recent study, Buske-Kirschbaum et al. (149) paired a distinctive flavor with injections of adrenalin and found an enhancement of blood NK cell activity when the subjects were subsequently reexposed to the gustatory CS alone. These studies lend credence to earlier clinical and experimental observations of what would appear to be conditioned alterations of immunity in human subjects or patients (150–154).

The physiological mechanisms underlying conditioned alterations of immunity are not known. Originally, conditioned immunosuppressive responses were considered the result of the "stressful" treatment because an increase in glucocorticoid elevations, equated with stress, could suppress immune responses. The hypothesis provided a ready explanation of an observation for which no other theory existed. The data, however, do not support the hypothesis that an elevation in circulating "stress hormones," particularly adrenocortical steroids, mediates the conditioned modulation of immune responses (131). Although there are problems in inferring causal relationships from the results of extirpation experiments, one study (155) failed to observe a conditioned immunosuppressive response in adrenalectomized mice. Most of the available data, however, directly contradict the "stress mediation" hypothesis. For example, invoking the ubiquitous elevation of adrenocortical steroids cannot account for the observations that lithium chloride, which is an effective UCS for inducing conditioned aversions and an elevation in corticosterone, is ineffective for inducing a conditioned suppression of antibody production (129, 156).

Several studies (134, 157–159) have demonstrated that the conditioned suppression and/or enhancement of antibody- and/or cell-mediated responses can be observed in the absence of or with equivalent changes in adrenocortical activity. When total fluid consumption is equated among the several conditioned groups by using a preference testing procedure in nonfluid-deprived animals (which also obviates the conflict inherent in a one-bottle or forced exposure to the CS solution), one can still observe a conditioned suppression of the antibody response to T-dependent and T-independent antigens (159, 160), a graft-vs.-host reaction (159), and the WBC response to cyclophosphamide (161). In a discriminative conditioning paradigm, both the CS paired with the UCS (CS+) and a novel gustatory stimulus not previously paired with the UCS (CS−) induce adrenocortical steroid elevations, but only the CS+ elicits a conditioned release of histamine (162). It is quite reasonable to suppose that conditioned alterations of immune function may be mediated by *conditioned* neuroendocrine responses, but the data collected thus far are inconsistent with the hypothesis that these effects are mediated simply by nonspecific (stressor-induced) changes in circulating hormones. Recently, attention has focused on opioid (42, 163–165) and catecholamine (166–169) responses as potential mediators of both conditioned and stressor-induced alterations of immunologically and nonimmunologically specific responses.

Although the mechanism(s) underlying conditioned or stressor alterations of immune function have not been elaborated, there is no scarcity of possible mediators. Most likely, multiple processes are involved. The fact that conditioned immunosuppression occurs when conditioned animals are reexposed to the CS before as well as after immunization could indicate that the mechanisms do not involve antigen-induced immune or neuroendocrine changes; it could also imply that different mechanisms are involved when conditioning is superimposed on a resting system in contrast to an antigen-activated system. Also, different immunomodulating drugs have different sites of action, and the same immunomodulating agent may have different effects on activated or nonactivated lymphocytes. As discussed later, the immune system is innervated, leukocytes and neurons share certain neuropeptide/neurotransmitter receptors, activated lymphocytes produce several neuroendocrine factors, and both cells of the immune and nervous systems produce and respond to the same cytokines. Conditioned and stressor-induced changes in the pattern of increases or decreases of neural and/or endocrine activity that can be recognized by activated lymphocytes or, conversely, the effects of conditioning on the release of immune products that can be recognized by the nervous system constitute potential pathways for the mediation of behaviorally induced alterations of immune function.

Immunological Effects on Behavior

Just as there are reciprocal relationships between neural and immune functions and endocrine and immune functions, there are immunological influences on behavior as well as behavioral influences on immune function. The behavioral effects of viral infections (particularly during early life), the cognitive and emotional sequelae of autoimmune disease, and the differences in the behavior of normal mice and those genetically susceptible to autoimmune disease are summarized elsewhere (170–175).

There is now evidence suggesting that the behavioral changes associated with immunological dysfunctions can be adaptive with respect to the maintenance or restoration of homeostasis within the immune system. Lupus-prone mice of the genetically susceptible (NZBxNZW)F1 strain fail to display conditioned taste aversions in response to doses of CY that are effective in inducing avoidance responses in healthy control (C57BL/6) mice (172). Similarly, MRL-lpr/lpr mice with lymphadenopathy and elevated autoantibody titers who manifest symptoms of autoimmune disease, do not avoid flavored solutions paired with doses of CY that evoke taste aversions in congenic (MRL+/+) control mice (176). These behavioral differences do not reflect a learning deficit in the lupus-prone mice because there are no observable differences between these substrains before the development of symptoms of disease—nor are there substrain differences when a nonimmunosuppressive agent is used as the UCS.

Also, MRL-lpr/lpr mice displaying symptoms of autoimmune disease voluntarily consume greater quantities of a CY-laced flavored drinking solution than asymptomatic controls—a quantity sufficient to attenuate lymphadenopathy and anti-DNA antibody titers (177). Such observations have not been reported with regard to the immune system, but such data are consistent with numerous studies on the behavioral regulation of other physiological states (172). It is not yet known whether such animals are responding to immunologically induced but nonspecific pathophysiological changes in one or more target organs or, consonant with the bidirectional pathways linking the CNS and immune system, the brain is capable of receiving and processing information emanating directly from the dysregulated immune system. To the extent that the brain does respond to immunological signals, behavioral processes could serve an in vivo immunoregulatory function.

Central Nervous System Lesions and Intracerebroventricular Infusions

A neuroanatomical approach has been used to evaluate the immunomodulatory capacity of specific regions of the CNS. This work complements the behavioral and psychological evidence for CNS communication with the immune system by demonstrating the presence of specific brain circuitry that can influence immune reactivity in the periphery.

Autonomic preganglionic neurons receive direct fiber projections from brainstem nuclei (nucleus solitarius, raphe nuclei, tegmental noradrenergic nuclei), hypothalamic nuclei (paraventricular nucleus, oxytocin and vasopressin neurons, lateral hypothalamus, posterior hypothalamus, dorsal hypothalamus), limbic forebrain structures (central amygdaloid nucleus), and regions of the cerebral cortex (frontal, cingulate, and insular cortical areas, mainly zones of "limbic" cortex). In addition, indirect regulation of these systems arises from regions such as the parabrachial nuclei, central gray, and reticular formation of the brainstem, numerous hypothalamic nuclei and cell groups, limbic forebrain areas such as the hippocampal formation and septum, and cortical association areas. These structures interconnect with the hypothalamus, the structure that lies at the crossroads of the limbic forebrain and brainstem nuclei.

This integrated circuitry has extensive ascending and descending connections among the regions cited. These regions also share many similarities. They are sites intimately involved in visceral, autonomic, and neuroendocrine regulation. The cortical and limbic forebrain regions mediate both affective and cognitive processes and may be involved in the response to stressors, in affective states and disorders such as depression, in aversive conditioning, and in the emotional context of sensory inputs from the outside world as well as the inside world. From an immunological perspective, these regions are the sites in which lesions result in altered responses of cells of the immune system; they are the regions that respond to immunization or cytokines by altered neuronal activity or altered monoamine metabolism; and they are the regions that possess the highest concentration of glucocorticoid receptors and link some endocrine systems with neuronal outflow to the autonomic and neuroendocrine systems. Thus, this circuitry is the major system of the CNS suspected to play a key role in responding to immune signals and regulating CNS outflow to the immune system.

Discrete lesions in the brain, particularly in specific nuclei of the hypothalamus and limbic system, resulted in structural and functional changes in the immune system (178). Cross et al. observed thymic involution and transiently decreased ConA-stimulated spleen cell proliferation after electrolytic lesioning of the anterior hypothalamus (179). Removal of adherent, macrophage-like suppressor cells abrogated this reduction in ConA responsiveness, suggesting CNS regulation of this splenic suppressor cell population (180). Forni et al. reported virtual abrogation of NK cell activity following destruction of the tuberoinfundibular region of the hypothalamus (181). Lesions in the amygdaloid complex and the hippocampus in rats led to increased numbers of thymocytes and spleen cells, and enhanced their proliferative responses to ConA (182). Nance and colleagues (183) showed that kainic acid-induced lesions of the lateral septal area resulted in decreased antibody production (IgG, IgA, IgM), while similar lesioning of the hippocampus resulted in elevated IgM and IgG antibody production in response to ovalbumin challenge. These alterations were sustained over time following subsequent reimmunization. These studies suggest that specific regions of the brain may modulate immune activity. However, the usefulness of stereotaxic ablation as an experimental approach is limited because of the inability to destroy specific nuclei without damaging passing tracts from other regions. In addition, even careful removal or destruction of a circuit is a rather drastic alteration in the CNS that often induces compensatory adjustments by remaining intact circuitry, and may not reveal a role for that same circuit in normal daily physiological fluctuations and regulation of CNS outflow.

Another approach to studying CNS-immune system links in vivo is intracerebroventricular (ICV) administration of agents that alter CNS communication with the periphery. For example, injection of gp120, the envelope protein of HIV into rat lateral ventricles induced interleukin-1 (IL-1) in the brain and elevated plasma corticosteroid levels and reduced immune responses in the periphery (184). IL-1 administered ICV, but not intravenously, induced similar peripheral effects (185, 186). These results suggest that IL-1 production in the brain can mediate signaling from the CNS to the immune system, but further substantiation of this contention awaits additional evidence besides ICV injections. Irwin et al. demonstrated that ICV corticotropin-releasing factor (CRF) reduced splenic NK cell activity via activation of the sympathetic subdivision of the autonomic nervous system (ANS) (187, 188). Thus, chemical stimulation of specific brain regions can generate a signal in the CNS that is transduced by mediators to alter immune function in the periphery.

The two main pathways by which the CNS may communicate with the periphery are: (*a*) neuroendocrine outflow via the hypothalamopituitary-target organ axes; and (*b*) the autonomic nervous system (ANS) through direct nerve fiber connections with cells of the immune system. In the next two sections of this review, evidence for endocrine hormone and ANS interactions with the immune system is presented.

Endocrine-Immune System Interactions

Early studies identified the pituitary as an essential component in the regulation of immune system development and function. Surgical removal of the pituitary gland (hypophysectomy) reduced antibody responses and impaired contact sensitization (189, 190). The Snell-Bagg and Ames strains of mice, both genetically predisposed to a hypopituitary dwarfism, exhibit severely impaired lymphoid organ development marked by reductions in T- and B-cell activity (191–193). Susceptibility to infection by *Salmonella typhimurium* was much greater in hypophysectomized rats compared with pituitary-intact rats (194). A discussion of the impact of products of the hypothalamopituitary target organ axes on immune reactivity and disease processes follows and has been reviewed in more detail (195).

HYPOTHALAMOPITUITARY-ADRENAL AXIS: GLUCOCORTICOIDS AND ADRENOCORTICOTROPIC HORMONE

Glucocorticoids (GCs) and their synthetic analogues have been used clinically at supraphysiological levels as immunsuppressive agents in inflammatory and autoimmune diseases. Endogenous GCs regulate lymphokine production, inhibit responses to self-antigens, and limit inflammatory processes (196–199). GCs act by binding to cytosolic GC receptors in T and B lymphocytes and macrophages (200, 201). Upon receptor binding, the GC-receptor complex undergoes a conformational change to allow penetration of the nuclear membrane. GC binds to specific regions of DNA, termed glucocorticoid regulatory elements (GRE), to activate or silence GRE-containing genes. This alteration in gene expression translates into multiple mechanisms of immunoregulation in vivo.

GCs limit immune responsiveness in vivo by *(a)* initiating programmed cell death (apoptosis), *(b)* altering lymphocyte distribution and trafficking, and *(c)* regulating lymphocyte cytokine production. GC-induced apoptosis is dependent on the maturational state of the lymphocyte: immature T cells in the thymic cortex and follicular B cells in secondary lymphoid organs exhibit greater susceptibility to lysis by glucocorticoids than mature (medullary) T cells and activated B cells (202). Lymphopenia induced by infusion of the synthetic analogue prednisolone or dexamethasone was associated with a redistribution of circulating cells from blood to the bone marrow and retention of circulating lymphocytes within secondary lymphoid organs (203, 204). GC-induced impairment of lymphocyte emigration may inhibit immune reactivity by limiting lymphocyte encounters with antigen. Thus, glucocorticoids cause cell death in T and B cells and induce alterations in lymphocyte circulation and trafficking, both of which lead to reduced immune reactivity.

GCs can also directly influence inflammatory processes and immune reactivity by altering cytokine production. Anti-inflammatory and immunosuppressive effects of GCs are mediated in part by inhibition of macrophage production of IL-1, tumor necrosis factor, and IL-6 (205–207). GC-induced inhibition of T-cell proliferation was correlated with reduced IL-2 production (208, 209). Daynes et al. demonstrated the potential for a more complex role for endogenous GC. In mice, GC inhibited IL-2 production and enhanced IL-4 production by activated T cells in vivo and in vitro (210). This pattern of cytokine production leads to inhibition of cell-mediated responses and to enhanced antibody production. By shifting from a cell-mediated response to an antibody response, the chances of acquiring cell-mediated reactivity to self is reduced, but the risk of infection by viral and bacterial pathogens that require cell-mediated immunity for elimination is increased. Endogenously produced GC may be important for regulating the critical balance between elimination of an infectious agent and limiting inflammatory processes and unwanted cell-mediated responses against self-antigens.

Another product of the adrenal medulla, dehydroepiandrosterone (DHEA), has recently been recognized for its lymphokine-regulating activities. DHEA increased IL-2 production in young animals, and in old animals shifted the pattern of lymphokine production from predominantly IL-4/IL-5 to predominantly IL-2 (211, 212). Impaired antibody responses in aged animals were elevated by DHEA to that of young animals (211, 212). DHEA can also counteract effects of GC; it prevented GC-induced thymic atrophy, suppression of lymphocyte proliferation, and reduction IL-2 production (211, 213, 214). Further studies are required to determine the conditions under which this steroid may interact with GCs to maintain immunological homeostasis.

Adrenocorticotropic hormone (ACTH) itself may have immunoregulatory properties; it was reported to reduce mouse spleen cell antibody responses and interferon-γ

(INF-γ) production in vitro (215, 216). High- and low-affinity ACTH receptors have been demonstrated on normal T and B lymphocytes (217). ACTH and pro-opiomelanocorticotropin (POMC), the mRNA encoding ACTH and the opioids, can be produced by endotoxin or viral-stimulated lymphocytes and macrophages, suggesting that ACTH may regulate immune reactivity locally (218–220). However, the cell type(s) capable of producing POMC mRNA is controversial, and requires further investigation before extra-pituitary ACTH can be considered a regulator of local immune responses (221, 222).

Animal models have been used to examine the role of the HPA axis in autoimmune disease (199). Studies comparing two histocompatible rat strains, Lewis/N (Lewis) and Fischer 344/N (F344), linked susceptibility to experimentally induced arthritis to defects in the HPA axis (223). Streptococcal cell wall (SCW) fragments initiate an inflammatory disease in Lewis rats that is characterized by an acute and chronic phase arthritis similar to rheumatoid arthritis in humans. Female Lewis rats are unable to produce a GC response to SCW, IL-1, and other HPA-activating agents that act at the level of hypothalamic CRF neurons. The susceptibility of Lewis rats to arthritis has been linked to the inability to generate a sufficient GC increase following SCW injection, and treatment with dexamethasone following SCW injection greatly reduced arthritis severity. On the other hand, F344 rats, which can elevate GC when exposed to SCW and other HPA stimuli, are resistant to SCW-induced arthritis. When GC access to the GC receptor was blocked by treatment with the GC blocker RU486, F344 rats developed severe SCW-induced inflammation and arthritis.

Endogenous GCs play a role in the pathology of another autoimmune disease, experimental allergic encephalomyelitis (EAE), a model for MS. Induction of EAE with myelin basic protein in complete Freund's adjuvant is accompanied by a rapid increase in serum glucocorticoid levels and mild hind limb paralysis from which the animals recover spontaneously (224). Adrenalectomized animals given cortisone replacement to mimic resting GC levels died following induction of EAE. Increasing replacement cortisone levels to concentration reached during the disease process elicited spontaneous recovery. Therefore, the presence of high levels of GCs was required for recovery of rats from an acute episode of EAE. These findings strongly implicate the HPA axis as an important component of the physiological mechanisms to prevent or limit autoimmune processes.

When the immunosuppressive and anti-inflammatory effects of the GCs were discovered, ACTH-induced release of adrenal GCs was widely considered the mechanism underlying stress-induced immunosuppression. Elevated GC levels induced by stressful stimuli have been correlated with immunosuppression, and ACTH or cortisone treatment mimicked the diminished immune reactivity (37, 189, 225). However, not all CNS-mediated changes in immune responses, even those that are immunosuppressive, are mediated by this axis. For example, conditioned immunosuppression was not correlated with increased GC levels (156). Others have shown that stress-induced alterations in immune responsiveness are not always dependent on the presence of the adrenal gland or synthesis of adrenal corticoids (40, 48, 50, 167). The CRF-ACTH-GC pathway must be viewed as an important, but by no means exclusive, intermediary of CNS-immune interactions.

OPIOID PEPTIDES

The opioid peptides consist of a series of low-molecular weight (< 4500 kD) peptides found in the pituitary, brain, and peripheral structures, such as the adrenal medulla; they include the endorphins, the enkephalins, and the dynorphins. In the brain, ligand interaction with opioid receptors induces profound analgesia and complex behavioral effects, many of which are blocked by naloxone and other opioid antagonists. With the finding that serum levels of β-endorphin increase in parallel with ACTH following some stressors, the search for peripheral opiate targets has focused on the cells of the immune system (226). Indeed, in one report, stress-induced reduction in NK activity was blocked by naloxone, suggestive of an opioid-mediated mechanism (42), but the target site of naloxone was not determined. Opioids may influence the immune system indirectly via the CNS through the sympathetics or the HPA axis, or directly through effects of opioid peptides on cells of the immune system.

Functional evidence for opioid receptors on human T lymphocytes was first reported by Wybran et al. (227), followed by numerous confirming reports; at present, a clear functional role has not yet emerged for the opioid peptides (218, 228). Although α-, γ-, and β-endorphins and met-enkephalin have identical *N*-termini, they have different immunological effects in vitro. For example, α-endorphin and met-enkephalin, but not β- or γ-endorphin, diminished antibody production by murine spleen cells (215). Furthermore, the immunological effects of opioids are not always blocked by nalaxone or other classical opioid receptor blockers, indicating a heterogeneity of receptors on cells of the immune system.

Opioid and nonopioid-mediated effects of β-endorphin in vitro include altered T-cell proliferation and enhanced production of IL-1, IL-2, IL-4, IL-6, and IFN-γ (207, 229–234.) β-Endorphin inhibited production of a T-lymphocyte-chemotactic factor by ConA-stimulated human peripheral blood mononuclear cells (235). β-Endorphin, met-enkephalin and leu-enkephalin may themselves serve as chemotactic factors; in the presence of these opioid peptides, increased migration of human T lymphocytes was demonstrated in vitro (236).

Taub et al. used alkyloid compounds with selective activity for δ-, μ-, or κ-opioid receptors to investigate which subtypes are involved in immune regulation (237). The κ agonists U50,488H and U69,593 at concentrations as low as 10^{-10} M reduced in vitro antibody production by unfractionated mouse spleen cells. The μ-selective agonists,

morphine and DAMGE, also were inhibitory, but only at high doses, 10^{-7} M and 10^{-6} M, respectively. A δ-agonist had no effect up to 10^{-5} M. The κ-induced inhibition was stereoselective, and both μ and κ effects were inhibited by naltrexone or naloxone. These results provide strong evidence for the presence of classical μ- and κ-opioid receptors on the surface of mouse spleen cells. Using highly selective radiolabeled ligands, δ- and κ-opioid receptors on normal lymphocytes and lymphoid lines have been reported (238–240). Further work is required to characterize specific opioid receptors and their functions on cells of the immune system.

The detection of POMC mRNA, the gene for ACTH and the opioids, in viral- or endotoxin-stimulated lymphocytes and macrophages, suggests that endorphins may be produced by cells of the immune system. Kavelaars et al. demonstrated β-endorphin production by human B cells that was induced by CRF and arginine-vasopressin (AVP), a regulatory mechanism similar to pituitary-derived β-endorphin (241). However, the cell type(s) capable of synthesizing POMC mRNA and the conditions under which it is produced is still under investigation (221, 222). Zurawski et al. found that ConA-stimulated, but not unstimulated, T-helper cell lines synthesized mRNA for preproenkephalin, precursor of the enkephalins; met-enkephalin was detected in the culture supernatants of these stimulated cell lines (242). Preproenkephalin A mRNA has been detected in thymocytes as well as mature T and B cells, and may be important in lymphocyte activation (243–245). This body of work points to potential local or regional regulation of the immune response by the opioid peptides, and a means by which the immune system may convey noncognitive stimuli such as viral and bacterial infection to the CNS.

GROWTH HORMONE

In several species, growth hormone (GH, somatotropin) deficiency resulted in small, hypocellular primary and secondary lymphoid organs that possessed abnormal morphology (193, 246). Reconstitution with GH restored normal morphology and restored the impaired immune reactivity observed in hypophysectomized animals (189–191) and GH-deficient animals (247–250). In aged rats, implantation of a GH- and prolactin-secreting pituitary adenoma restored thymic morphology and partially restored ConA-induced spleen cell proliferation and IL-2 production (251). Consistent with an immuno-enhancing role for GH, generation of cytotoxic T lymphocyte activity by mouse spleen cells in vitro was potentiated in the presence of GH (252). In macrophages and neutrophils, GH stimulated superoxide anion release at levels comparable to that achieved by INF-γ, a potent macrophage activator (253). Kelley and his colleagues demonstrated the relevance of these findings to susceptibility to infectious disease (194). Hypophysectomy increased susceptibility to lethal infection with *S. typhimurium* in rats, and GH administration restored disease resistance to hypophysectomized animals. In patients with GH deficiency, decreased T4/T8 ratios, increased circulating B cells, impaired responsiveness to alloantigen, and diminished NK activity have been reported (254, 255). Lymphocyte secretion of immunoreactive (ir) GH has been demonstrated, and T and B lymphocyte proliferation was inhibited by antisense oligodeoxynucleotide to GH mRNA (256, 257). These findings demonstrate that GH is an important regulator of immune function in vivo, and suggest that lymphocytes may provide an extrapituitary source of GH (258).

PROLACTIN

Prolactin binding sites have been identified on macrophages, T lymphocytes, and B lymphocytes (259–261). Similar to GH, prolactin completely restored impaired immune reactivity in hypophysectomized animal (190, 262). Treatment of mice with bromocriptine, a dopamine agonist and inhibitor of pituitary prolactin secretion, inhibited graft-vs.-host responses and mixed lymphocyte reactions (263). In another study, bromocriptine treatment induced an increase in the number of deaths following infection of mice with the bacterial pathogen, *Listeria monocytogenes* (264). This increase corresponded to markedly diminished macrophage activation, a consequence of reduced production of INF-γ, a T-lymphocyte-derived macrophage activator. Thus, like GH, prolactin may be an important factor in host resistance to infectious disease.

Prolactin may be a cell cycle progression factor, necessary but not sufficient for lymphocyte proliferation. Antiprolactin antibodies inhibited proliferation of T cell lines and normal lymphocytes in response to T- and B-cell mitogens (265–267). Clevenger et al. showed that nuclear prolactin is required for IL-2-induced T-cell proliferation (265, 268, 269). These experiments suggest that prolactin produced by lymphocytes may be an important potentiator of antigen-specific immune responses. Indeed, prolactin treatment of dwarf (DW/J) mice, and to a lesser extent, their heterozygous litter mates, increased the proliferative response of primed lymph node cells to antigen (250). Lymphocytes may be an extra-pituitary source of prolactin. Lymphocyte secretion of a prolactin-like molecule, which appears to be a structural variant of pituitary-derived prolactin, has been reported, and prolactin mRNA is expressed in activated murine lymphocytes (270, 271).

A potential link between prolactin and cyclosporine A-mediated immunosuppression has been described. Cyclosporine decreased prolactin receptors on human lymphocytes in vitro (260, 261) and blocked prolactin-induced polyamine synthesis (259). This suggests that cyclosporine may block or down-regulate prolactin receptors on lymphocytes in vivo, hindering prolactin-mediated potentiating effects on immune function. In addition, the immunosuppressive effects of cyclosporine were blocked by treatment with a prolactin-releasing agent in mice (263). These results suggest that prolactin, characterized initially as a lactogenic hormone, has important immunopotentiating effects that may be useful in clinical applications.

THYROID-STIMULATING HORMONE AND THYROID HORMONES

Thyroid-stimulating hormone (TSH) receptors have been reported on several B cell lines and LPS-stimulated B cells (272). In vitro, TSH enhanced antibody responses by mouse spleen cells to both T-dependent and T-independent antigens (273, 274). In a subsequent study, thyroid-releasing hormone (TRH) was shown to stimulate TSH mRNA and (ir) TSH production by murine lymphocytes, a regulatory mechanism similar to pituitary-derived TSH (275). TRH in picomolar concentrations also enhanced antibody production to a T-independent antigen in vitro; this enhancement was prevented by anti-TSH antibody. These results suggest that endogenous production of TSH is regulated in a fashion similar to pituitary-derived TSH and that lymphocyte-derived TSH has biological activity, that is, enhancement of murine antibody responses.

The TSH-induced thyroid hormones, triiodothyronine (T3) and thyroxin (T4), also have immunomodulating activities. Thyroidectomy in neonatal and adult rats, or thiouracil-induced hypothyroidism in chickens, led to decreased lymphoid organ weight, reduced numbers of circulating lymphocytes, diminished antibody responses, and decreased PHA or PWM-induced proliferative responses (276–278). T3 or T4 administration to thyroidectomized animals restored these deficiencies (276, 277). In euthyroid animals, T3 or T4 administration enhanced antibody and mitogen responses (276, 277). In old mice, treatment with T4 restored NK cell activity to levels observed in young mice, but did not alter NK cell activity in young mice (279). In vitro, T4 had no effect on NK cell activity, even in the presence of NK cell-activating factors, IL-2 or IFN-γ. Thus, the restoration of immune activity with T3 and T4 presumably may be achieved indirectly through interactions with nonlymphoid cells.

GONADAL STEROIDS

The sex steroids are important regulatory hormones of the immune system, and have been implicated in autoimmune processes (280, 281). Females have higher levels of serum IgG, IgG$_1$, IgM, and IgA than males in several species (282, 283). Antibody responses to T-independent and T-dependent antigens are greater in magnitude and more prolonged in females than in males (284, 285). Estrogen may enhance antibody production with specificity for foreign and self-antigens. Ansar Ahmed et al. demonstrated increased production of naturally occuring autoantibodies in normal female mice and in orchidectomized mice implanted with an estrogen-containing pellet, compared with male mice and orchidectomized testosterone-implanted mice (286). Cytokines that alter B cell antibody differentiation are altered by estrogens. In vitro, estrogen increased INF-γ mRNA production in ConA-stimulated mouse lymphocytes (287), and dihydrotestosterone (dhT, a metabolite of testosterone) inhibited IL-4, IL-5, and IFN-γ production by anti-CD3 stimulated mouse spleen cells (213). These results suggest that gonadal steroids may act through regulation of T-cell cytokine production to alter B-cell antibody production. T and B lymphocyte expression of androgen and estrogen receptors by lymphocytes have been reported (288–290).

Females experience a higher incidence of autoimmune diseases such as SLE and rheumatoid arthritis (RA) (291–293). Pharmacological manipulation of estrogen and testosterone levels can alter the course of experimental autoimmune disease in laboratory animals (293, 294). For example, treatment of NZB/W F$_1$ female mice, a mouse model for SLE, with a drug that blocks estrogen interaction with its receptor delayed the onset of several manifestations of this genetic disease (292). Administration of dihydrotestosterone to nonobese diabetic (NOD) female mice after the onset of insulitis prevented the islet cell destruction and spontaneous development of diabetes (295). Contrasting effects of estrogen treatment were reported in lupus-prone MRL-lpr/lpr mice (296). Estrogen was reported to enhance immune complex-mediated glomerulonephritis, a consequence of polyclonal B cell activation. In contrast, renal vasculitis and other T-cell-mediated pathologies in these animals were suppressed in estrogen-treated lpr/lpr mice.

The sex steroids may influence the immune system via T-cell differentiation in the thymus. Androgen and estrogen binding sites have been reported in thymic cytosol fractions and in thymic epithelium (283, 297, 298). Removal of the thymus prevented gonadectomy-induced hyperplasia of the thymus and other lymphoid organs (283, 297). Estradiol treatment in mice reduced T-cell differentiation in the thymus (decreased CD4$^+$CD8$^+$ thymocytes) and activated T cell differentiation in the liver, detected by an increase in "forbidden" T-cell clones (Vβ3$^+$) (299, 300). T-cell differentiation in the liver has been reported under conditions that can be associated with reactivity to self, including aging, infectious disease, autoimmunity, and athymia in nude mice. The mechanisms of gonadal steroid regulation of normal immunity and autoimmune processes have yet to be completely elucidated.

NEUROHORMONES OF THE POSTERIOR PITUITARY

The neuropeptides derived from the posterior pituitary (neurohypophysis), vasopressin and oxytocin, exhibit immunoregulatory properties. Vasopressin and oxytocin can induce INF-γ production by staphylococcal enterotoxin A (SEA)-stimulated mouse spleen cells (301). Receptor-ligand binding studies demonstrated that the effect was mediated through interactions with vasopressin receptors on lymphocytes (302). Immunohistochemical evidence has demonstrated colocalization of oxytocin with vasopressin and IL-1 in thymic epithelial cells (303). Oxytocin and its protein carrier neurophysin is present in human thymic extracts and is similar to the pituitary form by molecular weight, bioactivity, and the 1:1 ratio of oxytocin to neurophysin (304). Concentrations of oxytocin were much higher in the thymus than circulating levels, and they declined with age.

These results constitute evidence that oxytocin is synthesized in the thymus and plays a role in T cell differentiation.

Neural-Immune Interactions

The ANS communicates with target organs via a two-neuron chain. Preganglionic neuronal cell bodies are located in the thoracic and lumbar (T1–L2) spinal cord intermediolateral cell column (sympathetic) or in the sacral (S2–S4) intermediate gray or brainstem autonomic nuclei (parasympathetic). These preganglionic neurons send cholinergic myelinated axons to ganglia found in the sympathetic chain or in plexuses associated with the great vessels (collateral sympathetic ganglia) or found in or near the target organ (intramural parasympathetic ganglia). Postganglionic noradrenergic (NA) sympathetic nerve fibers arborize widely in target organs, in association with smooth muscle compartments as well as directly in the parenchyma, giving rise to various sites of release that may provide neurotransmitters for extensive interaction with target cells of the immune system, even from a few or a single postganglionic axon. Norepinephrine (NE) can diffuse widely, and can interact with cells immediately adjacent to, or even distant from, the sites of release. The extent to which many peptides can diffuse away from their nerve terminals of origin has not yet been determined.

AUTONOMIC INNERVATION OF LYMPHOID ORGANS

Early studies of lymphoid tissue innervation focused on the networks of NA nerve fibers in the spleen associated with smooth muscle of the vasculature, trabeculae, and splenic capsule (305–307). This work led to the notion that splenic NE serves to regulate capsular contraction, vascular resistance, and blood flow. Further analysis of sympathetic neural innervation of spleen and other lymphoid organs has revealed additional distribution of NA nerve fibers in the parenchyma, with compartmentalization in regions distinct from vascular or trabecular smooth muscle, and suggests that cells of the immune system may serve as target cells for neurally derived NE (308), particularly those cells possessing functional receptors for neurotransmitters.

Primary Lymphoid Organs

Innervation of tissues responsible for lymphocytic and monocytic stem cell development have been studied at the light and electron microscopic level. Both myelinated and nonmyelinated nerves have been demonstrated in the bone marrow (309). Fluorescence histochemistry for catecholamines and immunohistochemical localization of tyrosine hydroxylase (TH), the rate-limiting enzyme for NE synthesis, has revealed extensive networks of NA nerve fibers along the vasculature and among hemopoietic and lymphopoietic cells in the substance of the bone marrow, suggesting a functional role for NA innervation of the bone marrow. A functional role for NA innervation of the bone marrow was suggested by Maestroni et al. (310), who demonstrated that chemical sympathectomy with the neurotoxin 6-hydroxy-dopamine (6-OHDA) increased the number of peripheral blood leukocytes after syngeneic bone marrow transfer. Prazosin, an α_1-adrenergic antagonist, mimicked this effect and also increased myelopoiesis. The finding that the sympathetic nervous system (SNS) can be manipulated to increase hematopoietic output from the bone marrow has potential clinical applicability, especially in the area of bone marrow transplantation, but further studies are required to more fully understand how NA innervation influences stem cell development in the bone marrow.

In the thymus, networks of NA nerve fibers, detected by fluorescence histochemistry and TH immunocytochemistry, are found in plexuses associated with blood vessels and intralobular septa as well as directly in the cortical parenchyma (311–315). Nerve fibers that travel with intralobular septa branched deeply within the cortex, and were found adjacent to thymocytes; even in sites where very fine septa were present, no barrier to diffusion of NE existed. The densest NA innervation was found in the superficial cortical regions and along the vasculature of the corticomedullary boundary. Scattered fibers associated with the vasculature were located in the medulla.

The origin of these thymic sympathetic nerves was assessed with retrograde tracing (316). Labeling of nuclei was found in the sympathetic chain ganglia from the superior cervical ganglia caudal to the T3 ganglia. No labeling was found in the brainstem and spinal cord by these investigators, suggesting that direct or preganglionic innervation of the thymus from the CNS is unlikely; a postganglionic origin for NA innervation appears to be the major source. Neuropeptide Y (NPY) also is found in nerve fibers in the rat thymus and may be colocalized in the NA postganglionic sympathetic nerve fibers (317).

A functional role for thymic NA innervation has been investigated by surgical or chemical removal of NA fibers (317, 318). The results suggest that the presence of NA nerve fibers inhibit thymocyte proliferation and immigration. Adrenergic agonists in vitro have been reported to increase the expression of markers (Thy-1, TL) associated with thymocyte differentiation (319, 320). Further investigation of the role of the SNS in the development of T lymphocytes in the thymus may reveal an important means of regulating T-cell tolerance and development of the T-cell repertoire. Manipulation of NE in the thymus may provide a means of boosting thymocyte proliferation in physiological circumstances where such cells could be beneficial, such as aging, in which naive T cells are diminished.

Secondary Lymphoid Organs

Spleen. In the spleen tyrosine hydroxylase (TH) + (i.e., noradrenergic [NA]) nerve fibers have been localized to sites adjacent to T cells, B cells, and macrophages using fluorescence histochemistry and immunocytochemistry. NA nerve fibers enter the spleen with the splenic artery and then further distribute with the central artery, with the capsular and trabecular systems, and into the parenchyma (308, 311, 312, 321–323). Some NA fibers distribute into the parenchyma of the periarteriolar lymphatic sheath (PALS), where they arborize among T lymphocytes and along the macrophage zone at the marginal sinus, lined with ED3 + macrophages and IgM + B cells. Some fibers travel along the margin of follicles, among OX-19 + T cells and sIgM + B cells. Very fine, single TH + fibers distribute into B cell follicles, previously thought to be devoid of NA innervation by fluorescence histochemical analysis. The appearance of scattered NA fibers was noted in the red pulp, especially in zones adjacent to the trabecular and venous plexuses (306, 311). Splenic NE is primarily neurally derived, because chemical destruction of NA nerve terminals with the neurotoxic drug, 6-OHDA or with ganglionectomy resulted in loss of fluorescent nerve profiles, and more than 90% reduction in NE levels, as measured by high-performance liquid chromatography (311, 313, 321, 324). The origin of sympathetic neural innervation in rat spleen is mainly the superior mesenteric/coeliac ganglion (324, 325).

In previous studies, electron microscopy had shown close associations between neurons and reticular cells or other cell types in the spleen (326–328). However, the results were often interpreted very cautiously because of the inability to definitively distinguish between a nerve terminal and other cell types with vesicles and inclusions, such as platelets (328). Staining with specific antisera for TH has allowed visualization of direct contacts between TH + nerve terminals and lymphocytes in the PALS and marginal zone of the rat spleen by light and electron microscopy (321, 329). Controls with ganglionectomy or 6-OHDA treatment demonstrated that these TH + profiles are nerve terminals and that such staining completely disappears with these neural-depleting procedures. These associations, often distant from vascular smooth muscle cells, even at the adventitial zone along the central artery, consisted of parallel membrane appositions of 6 nm or more.

No cell processes (e.g., Schwann cell, interdigitating cell) were interposed between these neuroeffector junctions, unlike the ubiquitous intervening basement membrane, and frequent cell processes between TH + nerve terminals and smooth muscle cells. No specialized pre- or postganglionic features were noted for these neuroeffector junctions. Thus, TH + nerve terminals demonstrate very close appositions with lymphocytes and macrophages, at the adventitial zone along the central artery, throughout the PALS, and along the marginal sinus. These appositions appear to be the closest neuroeffector contacts thus far identified in the periphery.

Lymph nodes and gut-associated lymphoid tissue. Cervical, mesenteric, and popliteal lymph nodes, as well as Peyer's patch and lymphoid tissue associated with the appendix exhibit the same general pattern of innervation as that observed in the spleen (313, 321, 323, 330–334). NA nerves enter the lymph nodes at the hilus with the vasculature and distribute throughout the medullary cords among mixed populations of lymphocytes and macrophages and in the subcapsular region. Fibers from these regions then contribute to the innervation of the paracortical and cortical regions, where T lymphocytes are abundant. Fine varicosities, not associated with blood vessels, run between nodules with little distribution into the B cell-containing follicles. The gut-associated lymphoid tissue (GALT) contains NA nerve fibers that distribute through the T-dependent zones and within the lamina propria, including along the inner region of immunoglobulin-secreting plasma cells at the luminal surface.

Cholinergic innervation of lymphoid tissues has been difficult to demonstrate experimentally. Putative cholinergic innervation in the subcapsular region and at the corticomedullary boundary (335) of the thymus, was proposed on the basis of staining for acetylcholinesterase (AChE), the enzyme that rapidly degrades acetylcholine. Unfortunately, AChE stains some reticular elements, some NA nerve fibers, and other unidentified nerve fibers (336). Bellinger et al. (337) investigated choline acetyltransferase (ChAT) activity in lymphoid organs and found it absent in spleen and lymph nodes and very low (less than twice background, with a sizable proportion of noncholine carnitine acetyltransferase) in the thymus. Furthermore, NA nerve fibers overlapped with AChE+ nerve fibers, and other AChE+ profiles were distinctly nonneural, suggesting that AChE is not a good marker to definitively identify cholinergic nerves and that AChE may have some function other than metabolic degradation of acetylcholine (311). These findings have resulted in serious questioning of the existence of cholinergic innervation of thymus, spleen, and lymph nodes (336). There are reports, however, of receptors for acetylcholine (muscarinic and nicotinic) on lymphocytes (338–344). Cholinergic innervation is found in the periphery in the gut, salivary glands, and other sites supplied by parasympathetic postganglionic nerve fibers. Lymphocyte cholinergic receptors may be important during migration through, for example, the gut, suggesting that the physiological function of cholinergic receptors on lymphocytes may be selective, assuming importance in tissues with the availability of the appropriate ligand.

Peptidergic Innervation and Influences on the Inflammatory and Immune Processes

Several peptides have been described that can modulate splenic vascular resistance and capsule contraction following autonomic stimulation (345). In addition, many neuropeptides may have direct influences on immunological reactivity, and are found in nerve fibers innervating T- and B-cell-containing compartments of primary and secondary lymphoid organs (314). One such peptide, NPY, is colocalized in NA nerve terminals in the rat spleen and thymus (317, 346), while others, such as vasoactive intestinal peptide (VIP) and substance P (SP) appear to be associated with non-NA nerve fibers of the arteries, veins, trabeculae, and parenchyma of the spleen (314, 345). Analysis of the regulatory role of these neuropeptides in inflammatory and immune processes has revealed that they can influence lymphocyte and accessory cell activity (195, 314).

Substance P and somatostatin.   Substance P (SP) is an 11-amino acid peptide found in the CNS, in peripheral sensory neurons, and in nerve plexuses of the gut, spleen, lymph nodes, and thymus (347–350). SP levels are elevated in chronically inflamed tissue, implicating SP as a neural regulator of inflammatory processes (351–353). SP evokes vasodilation and vascular permeability, potentiates the activities of vasoactive amines, such as histamine, and enhances phagocytosis by neutrophils (354). Substance P can induce release of histamine by mast cells; numerous mast cells can be found in contact with SP$^+$ nerve fibers in the intestine and thymus (349, 355, 356). The proinflammatory cytokines IL-1, tumor necrosis factor-α (TNF-α), and IL-6 can be induced by SP in the absence of endotoxin or other stimulators (357). These findings suggest that SP is an early inducer of local and systemic host defense responses to inflammation and injury.

SP also can regulate cell-mediated and humoral immune responses via interactions with SP receptors on T and B lymphocytes (358, 359). Destruction of SP-containing nerves with capsaicin reduced primary antibody responses to SRBC in draining popliteal LN (360). Local administration of SP restored the response, demonstrating that SP depletion, and not capsaicin toxicity, diminished antibody responsiveness. T-cell proliferation and IL-2 production were enhanced by SP; these effects were blocked by a nonfunctional analogue, indicative of a receptor-mediated event (361, 362). Polyclonal IgA production by Peyer's patch and mesenteric LN cells in vitro was enhanced significantly by SP, whereas IgM production was less affected, and IgG production was unchanged (363).

SP has been implicated in the pathogenicity of an autoimmune/inflammatory disease, adjuvant-induced arthritis. In Lewis/N rats, denervation of SP nerve fibers in popliteal and inguinal lymph nodes by capsaicin treatment prolonged the onset and reduced severity of adjuvant-induced arthritis (350). Ablation of SP nerve fibers in the joint with capsaicin also ameliorated the inflammatory response in affected joints (364). These results demonstrate that SP innervation can influence the cells of the immune system involved in the disease process and is an inflammatory mediator at the site of inflammation.

Somatostatin has immunoregulatory effects that are generally opposite to those of SP. Somatostatin inhibited proliferation of human T lymphocytes in vivo and in vitro (361, 365). Somatostatin reduced INF-γ production stimulated by the T-cell mitogen staphylococcal enterotoxin A (SEA) (366). In vitro polyclonal IgA and IgM production by lymphocytes from murine Peyer's patch, spleen, and mesenteric lymph nodes were reduced by somatostatin (363). High- and low-affinity somatostatin receptors have been reported on human T- and B-cell lines. SP and somatostatin thus mediate isotype- and organ-specific regulation of B-cell differentiation in vitro, suggesting that in vivo, they may act as neurophysiological regulators to influence tissue-specific synthesis of particular immunoglobulin isotypes.

Vasoactive intestinal peptide. Vasoactive intestinal peptide (VIP) is a 28-amino acid neuropeptide found in central and peripheral sites. Immunohistochemical staining of the thymus has revealed immunoreactive (ir) VIP-containing nerve fibers in the cortex, subcapsular region, and septal zones, but rarely in the medulla (311, 317), suggesting a possible role for VIP in T cell maturation. In the bursa fabricii of the chicken, (ir) VIP-containing nerves were found in association with B cells and macrophages (367), suggesting a role for VIP in B-cell development as well. Specific, high-affinity binding sites for VIP have been reported on human and mouse T cells, as well as two human B-cell lines (368–370). In vitro, VIP inhibited lymphocyte proliferation to T-cell mitogens, but not B-cell mitogens (363, 369). VIP also may influence T-lymphocyte trafficking and localization through modulation of lymphocyte interactions with specialized endothelial cells lining the postcapillary venules in lymph nodes and Peyer's patch (371). Together, these studies indicate that VIP may provide a neurophysiological signal for regulating lymphocyte migration in vivo.

α- and β-Adrenoceptors on cells of the immune system. The presence of adrenoceptors on lymphocytes and monocytes is an important criterion in defining cells of the immune system as targets of sympathetic innervation in lymphoid tissues. The neurotransmitters NE and epinephrine (EPI) have affinity for both α- and β-adrenoceptors. The presence of β-adrenoceptors on T and B lymphocytes (372, 379), macrophages (380), and neutrophils (381, 382) in numerous species is well established, but the presence of α-adrenoceptors on lymphocytes has been difficult to detect by ligand binding studies. Only a few such reports exist (383–385), but there are reports of α-adrenergic effects on immunological activity in vivo and in vitro. This activity is blocked solely by α-adrenergic antagonists and suggests that α-adrenoceptors may be expressed on a minor subset of cells or on a wider range of cells transiently, perhaps depending on their activational or maturation state.

Lymphocyte β-adrenoceptors behave similarly to β-adrenoceptors expressed on other tissues innervated by the SNS. The receptors are up-regulated in the presence of β-blockers (386, 387), and down-regulated in the presence of β-agonists (388, 389). β-receptors on lymphocytes are linked intracellularly to the adenylate cyclase system to generate cyclic adenosine monophosphate (cAMP) (390). Lymphocyte activation or differentiation can alter cell surface density of β-adrenoceptors. For example, immature thymic T cells express fewer β-adrenoceptors than mature thymic T cells (315, 391, 392), but the β-adrenoceptors on immature thymocytes are linked to adenylate cyclase (393). Increased and decreased β-adrenoceptors have been reported in draining lymph node and spleen following contact sensitization and intraperitoneal injection of SRBC, respectively (391, 394), suggesting that lymphocyte sensitivity to catecholamines can be regulated at the level of the target cell, and that such regulation may occur during an immune response. However, more careful studies assessing purified cell types and correlating β-adrenoceptor density with changes in intracellular signaling mechanisms are required to gain a fuller understanding of the significance of these findings. In view of the influence of catecholamines on a wide range of immune reactivity, the intracellular control of adrenoceptor expression takes on great significance.

In vivo immune regulation by catecholamines. Peripheral administration of the catecholamines EPI and NE has been employed to demonstrate that catecholamines can modulate lymphocyte responses to antigenic challenge in vivo. This modulation of immune reactivity may occur directly via lymphocyte adrenoceptors or indirectly through interactions with other cell types, such as reticular cells, endothelial cells, or smooth muscle cells associated with the vasculature. Direct effects of β-adrenoceptor stimulation were demonstrated by incubating lymphocytes with catecholamines in vitro, followed by their transfer into syngeneic mice (395). Recipients of EPI-treated immune spleen cells had elevated antibody responses in untreated recipients compared to antibody responses of animals that received untreated immune cells. No alterations in antibody production were observed in EPI-treated recipients of untreated immune lymphocytes.

The effect of EPI on antibody production was dependent on the timing of EPI administration relative to immunization (395). EPI injected 6 hours before primary or secondary challenge with SRBC changed the kinetics of the antibody response, so the peak IgM and IgG response occurred a day earlier than in control mice. However, EPI administered 2–4 days before immunization inhibited the primary antibody response at all times examined. These results are indicative of the complexity of catecholamine effects on the immune system.

Other studies have demonstrated that perturbations in catecholamines can alter lymphocyte migration. In humans, a single EPI injection induced transient increases in the number of circulating blood lymphocytes and monocytes and decreased proliferative responsiveness to T-cell mitogens (396, 397). These functional alterations were accompanied by reduced CD4$^+$ T helper cells and increased HNK-1$^+$ natural killer cells (398). In guinea pigs, increased lymphocyte and granulocyte release from the spleen was observed after administration of NE, EPI, or the β-adrenergic receptor agonist, isoproterenol (ISO) in immune and nonimmune animals (399, 400). No change in splenic blood flow or smooth muscle contraction could be demonstrated, suggesting that a direct interaction with lymphocyte adrenoceptors was necessary for the enhanced cellular release.

Chemical sympathectomy with the neurotoxin 6-hydroxydopamine (6-OHDA) selectively destroys sympathetic nerve terminals in the periphery of adult or neonatal animals. Immune reactivity in the absence of neural NE has been assessed in mice and rats after treatment with 6-OHDA (334). Chemical sympathectomy in nonimmune adult mice enhanced cellular proliferation in spleen, bone marrow, and peripheral lymph nodes in vivo (401), but the effect of sympathectomy on lymphocyte responses in vitro differed between lymph nodes and spleen (402). Sympathectomy enhanced in vitro lymph node cell proliferation to the B-cell mitogen lipopolysaccharide (LPS), but inhibited LPS-induced proliferation by spleen cells. Sympathectomy dramatically increased IgG production and reduced IgM production by LPS-stimulated lymph node cells, but not spleen cells. The increased IgG production by lymph node cells was accompanied by increased IFN-γ production in vitro; IFN-γ production was reduced by sympathectomy in the spleen. In immunized adult animals, chemical sympathectomy reduced cell-mediated responses, including delayed type hypersensitivity, IL-2 production, and cytotoxic T-lymphocyte activity (394, 403). Primary antibody responses to T-dependent antigens were inhibited in spleen and draining lymph nodes (404–406), but antibody responses to T-independent responses were enhanced (407). When neonates were sympathectomized or when adult rats were surgically sympathectomized, a T-dependent antibody response was enhanced (313, 408). Neonatal 6-OHDA treatment results in central catecholamine depletion, which may itself influence immune responsiveness (409). Surgical cutting of the splenic nerve produces a pan-denervation of NA nerve fibers and neuropeptide-containing fibers. Results using these procedures cannot be directly compared with adult sympathectomy.

The differing responses between lymphoid organs indicate that SNS regulation of the immune system in vivo cannot be characterized as a simple enhancement or inhibition. Each cell type participating in the specific response may be affected differentially by catecholamines, based on environmental and temporal factors. A more detailed mechanistic assessment of individual lymphocyte and monocyte function by catecholamines is required, as discussed below.

In several animal models of autoimmune disease, experimental evidence is beginning to emerge that the SNS is an important regulator of immune reactivity to self. Sympathectomy with 6-OHDA enhanced the severity of autoimmune disease in two animal models, experimental allergic encephalomyelitis (EAE) and rheumatoid arthritis in Lewis/N rats (350, 410, 411). In the EAE model, sympathectomy was achieved with systemic neonatal administration of 6-OHDA. In the adjuvant-induced arthritis model, selective denervation with 6-OHDA of the reactive secondary lymphoid organs, the popliteal and inguinal lymph nodes, resulted in earlier onset and enhanced severity of inflammation and bone erosions compared with sham injected rats (411). These results suggest that the effects of ablation of NA nerves are exerted via influence on the reactive lymph nodes themselves. Levine et al. (412) showed that systemic β-adrenoceptor blockade either before or after the onset of disease symptoms attenuated clinical symptoms in the Lewis/N arthritis model, suggesting that both the lymphoid organs and target tissue of autoimmune reactivity (the joints) may be affected by catecholamines. The MRL lpr/lpr mouse, an animal model of SLE, demonstrated a

significant reduction in NA sympathetic innervation of secondary lymphoid organs in conjunction with the onset of autoimmune symptoms (413). This is consistent with findings of diminished NA innervation in other autoimmune mouse models, such as the NZB and the NZBxNZW F1 mouse (414). Together, the evidence points to a tonic inhibitory role for the SNS in certain autoimmune states, but the mechanism(s) by which the SNS may modulate autoimmune disease require further investigation.

In vitro immune regulation by catecholamines.   Early studies reported that antibody responses, proliferation, and lytic activity could be reduced by β-adrenergic stimulation and enhanced by α-adrenergic stimulation in vitro (415–421). Prostaglandins, dibutyryl cAMP, and other means of inducing intracellular cAMP have similar inhibitory effects in lymphocytes. Elevation of intracellular cAMP was viewed as a way to limit lymphocyte proliferation and effector function, and by extension, suppress immune responsiveness (422). More recent examination of the effects of adrenergic agonists on immune reactivity suggests a more intricate and complex role for catecholamines in the modulation of immune function.

Micromolar concentrations of NE and a $β_2$-adrenergic agonist, terbutaline, enhanced the antibody response to SRBC by unfractionated mouse spleen cells on the day of peak antibody production in vitro (423–425). β-blockade with propranolol blocked the stimulatory effects of NE and terbutaline, confirming that this was a β-adrenoceptor-mediated response. The $α_1$-agonist methoxamine enhanced antibody production early in the response; this effect was blocked by the α-blocker, phentolamine. The β-adrenoceptor-mediated enhancement of antibody production was further examined in a simplified in vitro system requiring only T cells for lymphokine production and B cells for antigen presentation and for antibody production (426). The β-adrenoceptor-mediated increase in the IgM antibody response was related to an increase in the number of antigen-specific B-lymphocyte precursors, indicating a direct effect on B cell differentiation. Potential β-adrenoceptor-mediated effects on T-cell lymphokine production were eliminated by the inability to show changes in major histocompatibility (MHC) class II or isotype class switching to IgG_1, functions induced by the T-helper, cell-derived IL-4.

Similar effects have been reported in T cell systems requiring cell maturation, such as the generation of alloreactive cytotoxic T lymphocytes (CTL) in vitro (321, 427). Hatfield et al. reported that stimulation of β-adrenoceptors with ISO (10^{-7} M), EPI (10^{-6} M), or NE (10^{-5} M) in a murine-mixed lymphocyte culture potentiated the generation of CTL activity (427). This increase was mimicked by 10^{-5} M terbutaline; both the ISO and terbutaline effects were blocked by propranolol. A $β_2$-antagonist, butoxamine, but not a $β_1$-antagonist, atenolol, blocked the EPI-induced enhancement. α-Blockade with phentolamine potentiated the NE-induced enhancement, suggesting opposing α-and β-adrenoceptor-mediated effects in this system.

Catecholamines also can regulate macrophage and NK

cell function either directly or through regulation of cytokine production. NE and EPI ($\geq 10^{-7}$ M) suppressed the killing of virus-infected cells and tumor cells by IFN-γ-activated macrophages (428, 429). Reduced macrophage function was associated with an increase in cAMP levels, and a similar effect was observed following incubation of macrophages with dbcAMP. The neuropeptide VIP, an inducer of cAMP, potentiated NE-induced inhibition of tumor cell killing. LPS-induced TNF production by activated murine peritoneal macrophages was enhanced in the presence of nanomolar concentration of NE and an α_2-agonist, UK-14304 (430). The α_2-adrenergic antagonist yohimbine blocked this enhancement. However, EPI or ISO added at the same time as LPS to human whole blood cells or the human monocyte line, THP-1, inhibited TNF production; the effect of EPI was blocked by the β-blocker, oxprenolol, but not by the α-blocker, phentolamine. When EPI was added to THP-1 cells 24 hours before LPS, subsequent TNF production was dramatically enhanced. The changes in TNF production in these experiments corresponded inversely to cAMP levels. Increased human monocyte production of complement components was observed in the presence of EPI, NE, or phenylephrine (an α-adrenergic agonist) (431), which was blocked by phentolamine, and by prazosin, an α_1-antagonist, but not by propranolol.

Human NK cell activity was reported in one study to be inhibited by ISO and other cAMP-inducers when added directly to target and effector cells in a ^{51}Cr-release assay (432). More complex effects were reported by Hellstrand and colleagues in which EPI at 10^{-6} M inhibited, while 10^{-8} M potentiated, lysis; propranolol prevented both of these changes (433). Pretreatment of effector cells with EPI yielded similar results, demonstrating that EPI and ISO stimulated β-adrenoceptors on the NK cells, and not the target cells. It also must be remembered that NE or EPI effects in vivo may be exerted by altering compartmentation and trafficking of NK cells between spleen, blood, and reactive target sites where NK cells reside (e.g., lung and liver).

Studies of intracellular signaling mechanisms have focused on cAMP, the second messenger generated following β-adrenoceptor stimulation. Carlson et al. reported that ISO inhibited lymphocyte proliferation in response to the T cell mitogen, PHA (390). PHA alone did not alter cAMP levels, but PHA in the presence of ISO elevated cAMP synergistically, compared to ISO alone. This same effect occurred using the T cell activator, anti-CD3 to stimulate the T-cell receptor and NE as the β-adrenergic agonist (434). These results demonstrate that β-adrenoceptor stimulation may act synergistically with the T-cell receptor to modulate lymphocyte activity. In B cells, increased cAMP did not predict the effect of β-adrenoceptor stimulation; instead, the effect was dependent on the B cell stimulus. NE and ISO enhanced lipopolysaccharide (LPS)-induced proliferation and differentiation through a β-adrenoceptor-mediated mechanism, whereas proliferation stimulated with antibodies directed toward surface IgM was inhibited by NE (435, 436). The

β-adrenoceptor-mediated enhancement correlated with increased cAMP, but the cAMP-inducers dbcAMP and forskolin inhibited proliferation. Studies of intracellular signaling and dual or synergistic influences using fractionated lymphocyte populations should lead to a more coherent understanding of interactions between the nervous and immune systems and will help predict the outcome of such encounters in vitro and in vivo.

Immune System Communication with the Nervous System

Several investigators have reported changes in hypothalamic activity following antigen challenge (437–440). Furthermore, NE concentration in the hypothalamus and brainstem was reduced after intraperitoneal injection of supernatants from ConA-stimulated spleen cells (441), demonstrating that secreted products of activated lymphocytes can stimulate specific regions of the CNS. IL-1 has become a prime candidate for an immune mediator capable of communicating with the CNS. In vivo administration of IL-1, but not IL-2, IFN-γ, or TNF elevated glucocorticoid secretion by direct stimulation of hypothalamic CRF neurons in vivo (442–445). Other investigators have reported IL-1 regulation of pituitary-derived hormones in vitro (446–448). The mechanism(s) by which IL-1 signals the CNS in vivo is under active investigation. Immunoreactive IL-1-staining nerves have been demonstrated in human hypothalamus, and IL-1 is synthesized by microglia and astrocytes in the brain (449–451). IL-1 produced peripherally also may act through secondary mediators via circumventricular organs or sensory neurons.

The observation that NE levels in spleen were inversely proportional to immunological activity suggested that the immune system can influence sympathetic activity. This relationship was observed following initiation of a primary antibody response (452, 453), and in germ-free animals compared with animals raised in the specific pathogen-free environment (452). Furthermore, high responders to SRBC exhibited greater and more prolonged reductions in splenic NE levels, whereas NE levels of low responders were reduced transiently, and to a lesser degree (454). More recently, intravenous injection of recombinant IL-1 was demonstrated to increase sympathetic nerve firing rates in the adrenal gland and in spleen in rats (455). NE turnover rate was increased following i.p. injection of IL-1 in spleen and lung, but not in heart and other tissues in the rat (456), suggesting that the decreased concentration of NE in the spleen noted in previous reports resulted from increased turnover.

Modulation of sympathetic activity by the immune system may be achieved by two routes: (a) through control of hypothalamic autonomic centers, or (b) at a local level, through reciprocal interactions between the cells of the immune system and nerve terminals within lymphoid organs. Evidence for the first mode of regulation is found in the changes in firing rates and NE levels in discrete regions of the hypothalamus following antigenic challenge (438). These central autonomic sites can influence sympathetic activity and subsequent NA outflow to lymphoid organs. Recent evidence suggests that central CRF (188, 457) and IL-1 (185) can alter immune responses via descending influences on sympathetic outflow. Only indirect evidence exists for local regulation of sympathetic activity: (*a*) IL-1 influences on NE release (456); (*b*) the close association between nerve terminal and lymphocytes, demonstrated by electron microscopy in the rat spleen (329); and (*c*) the findings that the presence of ConA-activated spleen cells altered tyrosine hydroxylase gene expression by sympathetic nerve cells in vitro and that TNF reduced NE release from polarized superior cervical ganglia neurons in vitro (458). These results suggest that secretory products of the immune system may be influential in the physiological activity of the SNS in vivo. Local regulation of sympathetic activity would allow rapid responsiveness to activation or perturbations of specific compartments and sites of the immune system, whereas communication through the CNS would permit systemic coordination of the neuroendocrine, autonomic, and immune systems.

Investigators in the field of psychoneuroimmunology have just begun to identify the numerous modes of interactions possible between the nervous and immune systems. Perhaps the operational definition or physiological constituents of the nervous and immune "systems" should be expanded to include each other. What lies ahead is the determination of how these systems interact physiologically under homeostatic and stressful conditions. Although immunologists have generally considered the immune system to be an autonomously regulated system, from the evidence presented here, it is clear that a better understanding of communication pathways between the immune system and the nervous system is required to determine the etiologies of pathological conditions, such as cancer and autoimmune disease. Furthermore, factors may be identified that contribute to a host becoming more or less susceptible to these diseases. This will be achieved only through integration of behavioral, pharmacological, neurological, and immunological methods. What is likely to emerge from this field at the cellular and molecular levels is a more unified understanding of biological signaling in general.

SUMMARY

It is a testament to the research conducted over the past 10–15 years that the subject of immunity is being incorporated within a textbook of neuropsychiatry. The observations and research described in this chapter represent a nontraditional view of the "immune system," but also a perspective, based on interactions between behavioral and physiological events, that is not foreign to a neuropsychiatric audience. Perhaps the complex mechanisms underlying these interactions and their relationship to health and illness are not well understood. Nonetheless, using "stress" effects, clinical depression, and conditioning

phenomena as illustrations, we have described recent research showing that psychological factors are, in fact, capable of influencing immune function. We have also reviewed data indicating that the immune system can receive and respond to neural and endocrine signals. Conversely, behavioral, neural, and endocrine processes are influenced by an activated immune system. It is hardly surprising, then, that a traditional view of immunity, one that is confined to the analysis of autoregulatory processes, needs to be expanded to account for those changes in immunity that are observed under conditions that prevail in the real world and, particularly, in health and disease.

Although recent research raises basic questions about the autonomy of the immune system, the immune system is, indeed, capable of considerable self regulation; immune responses can be made to take place in vitro. Ultimately, however, the adaptive significance of the "immune system" must refer to those immunological reactions that occur in vivo. There are now compelling data to justify the view that in vivo immunoregulatory processes influence and are influenced by the neuroendocrine environment in which they take place—an internal milieu that is exquisitely sensitive to the individual's perception of and capacity to adapt to the demands of the external environment. In turn, that environment generates signals that resting and/or activated leukocytes are capable of receiving. Immune responses appear to be modulated by feedback mechanisms mediated through neural and endocrine processes, as well as by feedforward mechanisms. The immunological effects of conditioning, an essential feedforward mechanism, suggest that, like neural and endocrine processes, there are circumstances under which behavior can serve an in vivo immunoregulatory function.

We do not yet understand the nature of all the pathways connecting the brain and the immune system—or the functional significance of those neural and endocrine interrelationships that have been identified thus far.

The research presented in this chapter originates from different levels of biological organization, all of which argue for an integrated approach to an analysis of the adaptive functions of the immune system. This research provides compelling evidence that, like any other system operating in the interests of homeostasis, the immune system is integrated with other psychophysiological processes and is therefore influenced by and capable of influencing the brain.

Acknowledgments

This review of the literature is an updated and expanded version of a paper published earlier. Preparation of this chapter was supported by a Research Scientist Award (KO-5 MH06318) from the National Institute of Mental Health (RA), and was completed during the senior author's tenure as a Fellow at the Center for Advanced Study in the Behavioral Sciences with support from the John D. and Catherine T. MacArthur Foundation (#8900078).

References

1. Ader R, Felten DL, Cohen N, eds. Psychoneuroimmunology. 2nd ed. New York: Academic Press, 1991.

2. Weiner H. Psychobiology and human disease. New York: Elsevier, 1977.

3. Plaut SM, Friedman SB. Psychosocial factors in infectious disease. In: Ader R, ed. Psychoneuroimmunology. New York: Academic Press, 1981:3–30.

4. Sklar LS, Anisman H. Stress and cancer. Psychol Bull 1981;89:369–406.

5. Justice A. Review of the effects of stress on cancer in laboratory animals: importance of time of stress application and type of tumor. Psychol Bull 1981;98:108–138.

6. Mor V, McHorney C, Sherwood S. Secondary morbidity among the recently bereaved. Am J Psychiatry 1986;143:158–163.

7. Cohen S, Williamson GM. Stress and infectious disease in humans. Psychol Bull 1991;109:5–24.

8. Ader R. Presidential address. Psychosomatic and psychoimmunologic research. Psychosom Med 1980;42:307–321.

9. Bonneau RH, Sheridan JF, Feng N, Glaser R. Stress-induced suppression of herpes simplex virus (HSV)-specific cytotoxic T lymphocyte and natural killer cell activity and enhancement of acutepathogenesis following local HSV infection. Brain Behav Immun 1991;5:170–192.

10. Bonneau RH, Sheridan JF, Feng N, Glaser R. Stress-induced effects on cell mediated innate and adaptive memory components of the murine immune response to herpes simplex virus infection. Brain Behav Immun 1991;5:274–295.

11. Rasmussen AF Jr, Marsh JT, Brill NQ. Increased susceptibility to herpes simplex in mice subjected to avoidance-learning stress or restraint. Proc Soc Exp Biol Med 1957;96:183–189.

12. Seifter E, Rettura G, Zisblatt M, et al. Enhancement of tumor development in physically stressed mice incubated with an oncogenic virus. Experientia 1973;29:1379–1382.

13. Greenberg AH, Dyck DG, Sandler LS, Pohajdak B, Dresel KM, Grant D. Neurohormonal modulation of natural resistance to a murine lymphoma. J Natl Cancer Inst 1984;72:653–659.

14. Levine S, Strebel R, Wenk EJ, Harman PJ. Suppression of experimental allergic encephalomyelitis by stress. Proc Soc Exp Biol Med 1962;109:294–298.

15. Friedman SB, Ader R, Glasgow LA. Effects of psychological stress in adult mice inoculated with Coxsackie B viruses. Psychosom Med 1965;27:361–368.

16. Plaut SM, Esterhay RJ, Sutherland JC, et al. Psychological effects on resistance to spontaneous AKR leukemia in mice. Psychosom Med 1981;42:72.

17. Feng N, Pagniano R, Tovar A, Bonneau RH, Glaser R, Sheridan JF. The effect of restraint stress on the kinetics, magnitude, and isotype of the humoral immune response to influenza virus infection. Brain Behav Immun 1991;5:370–382.

18. Kusnecov AV, Grota LJ, Schmidt SG, et al. Decreased herpes simplex viral immunity and enhanced pathogenesis following stressor administration in mice. J Neuroimmunol 1992;88:129–138.

19. Ben-Eliyahu S, Yirmiya R, Liebeskind JC, Taylor AN, Gale RP. Stress increases metastatic spread of a mammary tumor in rats: evidence for mediation by the immune system. Brain Behav Immun 1991;5:193–205.

20. Brenner GJ, Cohen N, Ader R, Moynihan JA. Increased pulmonary metastases and natural killer cell activity in mice following handling. Life Sci 1990;47:1813–1819.

21. Jacobs S, Ostfeld A. An epidemiological review of the mortality of bereavement. Psychosom Med 1977;39:344–357.

22. Helsing KJ, Szklo M, Comstock GW. Factors associated with mortality after widowhood. Am J Public Health 1981;71:802–809.

23. Bartrop RW, Luckhurst E, Lazarus L, Kiloh LG, Penny R. Depressed lymphocyte function after bereavement. Lancet 1977;1:834–836.

24. Schleifer SJ, Keller SE, Camerino M, Thornton JC, Stein M. Suppression of lymphocyte stimulation following bereavement. JAMA 1983;250:374–377.

25. Irwin M, Daniels M, Smith TL, Bloom E, Weiner H. Impaired natural killer cell activity during bereavement. Brain Behav Immun 1987;1:98–104.

26. Kiecolt-Glaser JK, Glaser R. Psychological influences on immunity. Psychosomatics 1986;27:621–624.

27. Farris EJ. Increase in lymphocytes in healthy persons under certain emotional states. Am J Anat 1938;63:297–323.

28. Glaser R, Thorn BE, Tarr KL, Kiecolt-Glaser JK, D'Ambrosio SM. Effects of stress on methyltransferase synthesis: an important DNA repair enzyme. Health Psychol 1985;4:403–412.

29. Glaser R, Rice J, Sheridan J, et al. Stress-related immune suppression: health implications. Brain Behav Immun 1987;1:7–20.

30. Michaut R-J, Dechambre R-P, Doumerc S, Lesourd B, Devillechabrolle A, Moulias R. Influences of early maternal deprivation on adult humoral immune response in mice. Physiol Behav 1981;26:189–191.

31. Ackerman SH, Keller SE, Schleifer SJ, et al. Premature maternal separation and lymphocyte function. Brain Behav Immun 1988;2:161–165.

32. Pierpaoli W, Fabris N, Sorkin E. Developmental hormones and immunological maturation. Ciba Found Study Group 1970;36:126–143.

33. Reite M, Harbeck R, Hoffman A. Altered cellular immune response following peer separation. Life Sci 1981;29:1133–1136.

34. Laudenslager ML, Reite M, Harbeck RJ. Suppressed immune response in infant monkeys associated with maternal separation. Behav Neural Biol 1982;36:40–48.

35. Coe CL, Weiner SG, Rosenberg LT, Levine S. Endocrine and immune responses to separation and maternal loss in nonhuman primates. In: Reite M, Field T, ed. The psychobiology of attachment and separation. New York: Academic Press, 1985;163–220.

36. Coe CL, Rosenberg LT, Levine S. Prolonged effect of psychological disturbance on macrophage chemiluminescence in the squirrel monkey. Brain Behav Immun 1988;2:151–160.

37. Monjan AA, Collector ML. Stress-induced modulation of the immune response. Science 1977; 196:307–308.

38. Keller SE, Weiss JM, Schleiffer SJ, Miller NE, Stein M. Suppression of immunity by stress: effect of a graded series of stressors on lymphocyte stimulation in the rat. Science 1981;213:1397–1400.

39. Blecha F, Barry RA, Kelley KW. Stress-induced alterations in delayed-type hypersensitivity to SRBC and contact sensitivity to DNFB in mice. Proc Soc Exp Biol Med 1982;169:239–246.

40. Blecha F, Kelley KW, Satterlee DG. Adrenal involvement in the expression of delayed-type hypersensitivity to SRBC and contact sensitivity to DNFB in stressed mice. Proc Soc Exp Biol Med 1982;169:247–252.

41. Shavit Y, Ryan SM, Lewis JW, et al. Inescapable but not escapable stress alters immune function. Physiologist 1983;26:A64.

42. Shavit Y, Lewis JW, Terman GW, Gale RP, Liebeskind JC. Opioid peptides mediate the suppressive effect of stress on natural killer cell cytotoxicity. Science 1984; 223:188–190.

43. Lysle DT, Lyte M, Fowler H, Rabin BS. Shock-induced modulation of lymphocyte reactivity: suppression, habituation, and recovery. Life Sci 1987;41:1805–1814.

44. Moynihan J, Brenner G, Koota D, Breneman S, Cohen N, Ader R. The effects of handling on antibody production, mitogen responses, spleen cell number, and lymphocyte subpopulations. Life Sci 1990;46:1937–1944.

45. Rinner I, Schauenstein K, Mangge H, Porta S. Opposite effects of mild and severe stress on in vitro activation of rat peripheral blood lymphocytes. Brain Behav Immun 1992;6:130–140.

46. Moynihan JA, Ader R, Grota LJ, Schachtman TR, Cohen N. The effects of stress on the development of immunological memory following low-dose antigen priming in mice. Brain Behav Immun 1990;4:1–12.

47. Okimura T, Nigo Y. Stress and immune responses. I. Suppression of T cell function in restraint-stressed mice. Jpn J Pharmacol 1986;40:505–511.

48. Esterling B, Rabin BS. Stress-induced alteration of T-lymphocyte

subsets and humoral immunity in mice. Behav Neurosci 1987;101: 115–119.

49. Zalcman S, Minkiewicz-Janda A, Richter M, Anisman H. Critical periods associated with stressor effects on antibody titers and on the plaque-forming cell response to sheep blood cells. Brain Behav Immun 1988;2:254–266.

50. Keller SE, Weiss JM, Schleiffer SJ, Miller NE, Stein M. Stress-induced suppression of immunity in adrenalectomized rats. Science 1983;221: 1301–1304.

51. Okimura T, Ogawa M, Yamauchi T. Stress and immune responses III. Effect of restraint stress on delayed type hypersensitivity (DTH) response, natural killer (NK) activity, and phagocytosis in mice. Jpn J Pharmacol 1986;41:229–235.

52. Cunnick JE, Lysle DT, Armfield A, Rabin BS. Shock-induced modulation of lymphocyte responsiveness and natural killer activity: differential mechanisms of induction. Brain Behav Immun 1988;2: 102–113.

53. Mormede P, Dantzer R, Michaud B, Kelley KW, Le Moal M. Influence of stressor predictability and behavioral control on lymphocyte reactivity, antibody responses and neuroendocrine activation in rats. Physiol Behav 1988;43:577–583.

54. Raymond LN, Reyes E, Tokuda S, Jones BC. Differential immune response in two handled inbred strains of mice. Physiol Behav 1986;37:295–297.

55. Rabin BS, Lyte M, Hamill E. The influence of mouse strain and housing on the immune response. J Neuroimmunol 1987b;17: 11–16.

56. Cocke R, Moynihan JA, Cohen N, Grota LJ, Ader R. Exposure to conspecific alarm chemosignals alters immune responses in BALB/c mice. Brain Behav Immun 1993;7:36–46.

57. Laudenslager ML, Ryan SM, Drugan RC, Hyson RL. Maier SF. Coping and immunosuppression—inescapable but not escapable shock suppresses lymphocyte proliferation. Science 1983;221:568–570.

58. Maier SF, Laudenslager ML. Inescapable shock, shock controllability, and mitogen stimulated lymphocyte proliferation. Brain Behav Immun 1988;2:87–91.

59. Weisse CS, Pato CN, McAllister CG, et al. Differential effects of controllable and uncontrollable acute stress on lymphocyte proliferation and leukocyte percentages in humans. Brain Behav Immun 1990;4:339-351.

60. Sieber WJ, Rodin J, Larson L, et al. Modulation of human natural killer cell activity by exposure to uncontrollable stress. Brain Behav Immun 1992;6:141–156.

61. Estes ML, Rudick RA, Barnett GH, Ransohoff RM. Stereotactic biopsy of an active multiple sclerosis lesion. Arch Neurol 1990;47: 1299–1303.

62. Traugott U. Characterization and distribution of lymphocyte subpopulations in multiple sclerosis plaques versus autoimmune demyelinating lesions. Springer Semin Immunopathol 1984;8:71–95.

63. Hauser SL, Bhan AK, Gilles F, Komp M, Kerr C, Weiner HL. Immunohistochemical analysis of the cellular infiltrate in multiple sclerosis lesions. Ann Neurol 1986;19:578–587.

64. Woodroofe MN, Bellamy AS, Feldmann M, Davison AN, Guzner ML. Immunocytochemical characterization of the immune reaction in the central nervous system in multiple sclerosis: possible role for microglia in lesion growth. J Neurol Sci 1986;74:135–152.

65. Traugott U. Multiple sclerosis: relevance of Class I and Class II MHC-expressing cells to lesion development. J Neuroimmunol 1987;16:283–302.

66. Haile RW, Hodge SE, Iselius L. Genetic susceptibility to multiple sclerosis: a review. Int J Epidemiol 1983;2:8–16.

67. Stewart GJ, Kirk RL. The genetics of multiple sclerosis: the HLA system and other genetic markers. In: Hallpike JF, Adams CWM, Tourtellotte WW, eds. Multiple sclerosis. Baltimore: Williams & Wilkins, 1983.

68. Spielman RS, Nathanson N. The genetics of susceptibility to multiple sclerosis. Epidemiol Rev 1982;4:45–65.

69. Kurtzke JF. A reassessment of the distribution of multiple sclerosis, Parts I and II. Acta Neurol Scand 1975;51:110–157.

70. Kurtzke JF. Epidemiologic contributions to multiple sclerosis. An overview. Neurology 1980;30:61–79.

71. Kurtzke JF. Search for the cause of multiple sclerosis and other chronic diseases of the central nervous system. In: A. Boese, ed. First International Symposium of Hertie Foundation in Frankfurt on Main, September 1979. Verlag Chemie, Weinheim-Deerfield Beach, FL-Basel; 1980:393–404.

72. Weitkamp LR. Multiple sclerosis susceptibility: interaction between sex and HLA. Arch Neurol 1983;40:339–401.

73. Minden SL, Schiffer RB. Affective disorders in multiple sclerosis: review and recommendations for clinical research. Arch Neurol 1990;47:98–104.

74. Honer WG, Hurtwitz T, Li DKB, Palmer M, Paty DW. Temporal lobe involvement in multiple sclerosis patients with psychiatric disorders. Arch Neurol 1987;44:187–190.

75. Schiffer RB. The spectrum of depression in multiple sclerosis: an approach for clinical management. Arch Neurol 1987;44: 596–599.

76. Schiffer RB, Wineman NM. Antidepressant pharmacotherapy of depression associated with multiple sclerosis: a double-blind placebo controlled trial. Am J Psychiatry 1990;147:1493–1497.

77. Carr RI, Shucard DW, Hoffman SA, Hoffman AA, Bardana EJ, Harbeck RJ. Neuropsychiatric involvement in systemic lupus erythematosus. In: Bergsma D, Goldstein AL, eds. Neurochemical and immunologic components in schizophrenia. New York: Alan R. Liss, 1978:209–235.

78. Hall RCW, Stickney SK, Gardner ER. Psychiatric symptoms in patients with systemic lupus erythematosus. Psychosomatics 1981; 22:15–24.

79. Abel T, Gladman DD, Urowitz MB. Neuropsychiatric lupus. J Rheumatol 1980;7:325–333.

80. Adelman DC, Saltiel E, Klinenberg JR. The neuropsychiatric manifestations of systemic lupus erythematosus: an overview. Semin Arthritis Rheum 1986;15:185–199.

81. Grigor R, Edmonds J, Lewkonia R, Bresnihan B, Hughes GRV. Systemic lupus erythematosus: a prospective analysis. Ann Rheum Dis 1978;37:121–128.

82. Calabrese LH. Diagnosis of systemic lupus erythematosus. Postgrad Med 1984;75:103–112.

83. Levine SR, Welch KMA. The spectrum of neurologic disease associated with antiphospholipid antibodies. Arch Neurol 1987;44: 876–883.

84. Ernerudh J, Olsson T, Lindstrom F, Skogh T. Cerebrospinal fluid immunoglobulin abnormalities in systemic lupus erythematosus. J Neurol Neurosurg Psychiatry 1985;48:807–813.

85. Hirohata S, Migamoto T. Increased intrathecal immunoglobulin synthesis of both kappa and lambda types in patients with systemic lupus erythematosus and central nervous system involvement. J Rheumatol 1986;13:715–721.

86. How A, Dent PB, Lia SK, Denburg SD. Antineuronal antibodies in neuropsychiatric systemic lupus erythematosus. Arthritis Rheum 1985;28:789–795.

87. Temesvari P, Denburg J, Denburg S, Carbotte R, Bensen W, Singal D. Serum lymphocytotoxic antibodies in neuropsychiatric lupus: a serial study. Clin Immunol Immunopathol 1983;18:243–251.

88. Bonfa E, Golombek SJ, Kaufman LD. Association between lupus psychosis and anti-ribosomal P protein antibodies. N Engl. J Med 1987;317:265–271.

89. Bluestein HG, Williams GW, Steinberg AD. Cerebrospinal fluid antibodies to neuronal cells: association with neuropsychiatric manifestations of systemic lupus erythematosus. Am J Med 1981;70: 240–246.

90. Rabkin JG, Williams JBW, Remien RH, Goety R, Kertzner R, Gorman JM. Depression, distress, lymphocyte subsets, and human immunodeficiency virus symptoms on two occasions in HIV-positive homosexual men. Arch Gen Psychiatry 1991;48:111–119.

91. Williams JBW, Rabkin JG, Remien RH, Gorman JM, Ehrhardt AA. Multidisciplinary baseline assessment of homosexual men with and without human immunodeficiency virus infection II. Standardized

clinical assessment of current and lifetime psychopathology. Arch Gen Psychiatry 1991;48:124–130.

92. Miller AH, ed. Depressive disorders and immunity. Washington DC: American Psychiatric Press, 1989.

93. Stein M, Miller AH, Trestman RL. Depression, the immune system and health and illness. Findings in search of a meaning. Arch Gen Psychiatry 1991;48:171–177.

94. Calabrese JR, Kling MA, Gold PW. Alterations in immunocompetence during stress, bereavement and depression: focus on the interplay between the immunologic apparatus and neuroendocrine regulation. Am J Psychiatry 1987;144:1123–1134.

95. Herbert TB, Cohen S. Depression and immunity: a meta-analytic review. Psychol Bull 1993;113:472–486.

96. Weisse CS. Depression and immunocompetence: a review of the literature. Psychol Bull 1992;111:475–489.

97. Schleifer SJ, Keller SE, Bond RN, Cohen J, Stein M. Major depressive disorder and immunity. Arch Gen Psychiatry 1989;46:81–87.

98. Schleifer SJ, Keller SE, Meyerson AT, Raskin MJ, Davis KL, Stein M. Lymphocyte function in major depressive disorder. Arch Gen Psychiatry 1984;41:484–486.

99. Schleifer SJ, Keller SE, Siris SG, Davis KL, Stein M. Depression and immunity: lymphocyte function in ambulatory depressed patients, hospitalized schizophrenic patients, and patients hospitalized for herniorrhaphy. Arch Gen Psychiatry 1985;42:129–133.

100. Jankovic BD, Jakulic S, Horvat J. Delayed skin hypersensitivity reactions to brain S-100 protein in psychiatric patients. Biol Psychiatry 1982;17:687–697.

101. Kiecolt-Glaser JK, Stephens RE, Lipetz PD, Speicher CE, Glaser R. Distress and DNA repair in human lymphocytes. J Behav Med 1985;8:311–320.

102. Irwin M, Gillin JC. Impaired natural killer cell activity among depressed patients. Psychiatry Res 1987;20:181–182.

103. Kronfol Z, Silva J Jr, Greden J, Dembrinski S, Gardner R, Carroll B. Impaired lymphocyte function in depressive illness. Life Sci 1983; 33:241–247.

104. Syvhalti E, Eskola J, Ruuskanen O, Laine T. Nonsuppression of cortisol in depression and immune function. Prog Neuropsychopharmacol Biol Psychiatry 1985;9:413–422.

105. Sengar DPS, Waters BGH, Dunne JV, Bouer IM. Lymphocyte subpopulations and mitogenic responses of lymphocytes in manic-depressive disorders. Biol Psychiatry 1982;17:1017–1022.

106. Albrecht J, Helderman JH, Schlesser MA, Rush AJ. A controlled study of cellular immune function in affective disorders before and during somatic therapy. Psychiatry Res 1985; 15:185–193.

107. Roos RP, Davis K, Meltzer HY. Immunoglobulin studies in patients with psychiatric disease. Arch Gen Psychiatry 1985;42:124–128.

108. Mohl PC, Huang L, Bowden C, Fischbach M, Vogtsberger K, Talal N. Natural killer cell activity in major depression. Am J Psychiatry 1987;144:1619.

109. Nerozzi D, Santoni A, Bersani G, et al. Reduced natural killer cell activity in major depression: neuroendocrine implications. Psychoneuroendocrinology 1989;14:295–301.

110. Roy BF, Rose JW, Sunderland T, Morihisa JM, Murphy DL. Antisomatostatin IgG in major depressive disorder. Arch Gen Psychiatry 1988;45:924–928.

111. Eastwood MR, Stiasny S, Meier HMR, Woogh CM. Mental illness and mortality. Compr Psychiatry 1982;23:377–385.

112. Martin RL, Cloninger CR, Guze SB, Clayton PJ. Mortality in a follow-up of 500 psychiatric outpatients I. Total mortality. Arch Gen Psychiatry 1985;42:47–54.

113. Tsuang MT, Woolson RF, Fleming JA. Causes of death in schizophrenia and manic-depression. Br J Psychiatry 1980;36:239–242.

114. Kendler KS. A twin study of mortality in schizophrenia and neurosis. Arch Gen Psychiatry 1986;43:643–649.

115. Dyck DG, Greenberg AH. Immunopharmacological tolerance as a conditioned response: dissecting the brain immune pathways. In: Ader R, Felten DL, Cohen N, eds. Psychoneuroimmunology. 2nd ed. New York: Academic Press, 1991:663–684.

116. Chrousos GP, Gold PW. The concepts of stress and stress disorders: overview of physical and behavioral homeostasis. JAMA 1992;267: 1244–1252.

117. Dupont E, Schandene L, Devos R, et al. Depletion of lymphocytes with membrane markers of helper phenotype: a feature of acute and chronic drug-induced immunosuppression. Clin Exp Immunol 1983; 51:345–350.

118. Glasser L, Hicks MJ, Lindberg RE, et al. The effect of in vivo dexamethasone on lymphocyte subpopulations: differential response of ea rosette-forming cells. Clin Immunol Immunopathol 1981;18: 22–31.

119. Haynes BF, Fauci AS. The differential effect of in vivo hydrocortisone on the kinetics of subpopulations of human peripheral blood T lymphocytes. J Clin Invest 1978;61:703–707.

120. Landi MS, Kreider JW, Lang CM, Bullock LP. Effects of shipping on the immune function in mice. Am J Vet Res 1982;43: 1654–1657.

121. Feldman RD, Limbird LE, Nadeau J, Fitzgerald GA, Robertson D, Wood AJJ. Dynamic regulation of leukocyte beta adrenergic receptor-agonist interactions by physiological changes in circulating catecholamines. J Clin Invest 1983;72:164–170.

122. Ito Y, Mino K, Ago Y, Nakagawa T, Fujiwara M, Ueki S. Attack stress and IgE antibody production in rats. Pharmacol Biochem Behav 1983;19:883–886.

123. Rocha B. The effects of stress in normal and adrenalectomized mice. Eur J Immunol 1985;15:1131–1135.

124. Rabin BS, Salvin SB. Effect of differential housing and time on immune reactivity to sheep erythrocytes and candida. Brain Behav Immun 1987;1:267–275.

125. Odio M, Brodish A, Ricardo MJ. Effects on immune response by chronic stress are modulated by aging. Brain Behav Immun 1987;1: 204–215.

126. Metal'nikov S, Chorine V. Role des reflexes conditionnels dans l'immunite. Annals of the Pasteur Institute, Paris 40:893–900.

127. Metal'nikov S, Chorine V. Role des reflexes conditionnels dans la formation des anticorps. Compte Rendu Seances Soc Biol 1928;99: 142–145.

128. Ader R. A historical account of conditioned immunobiologic responses. In: Ader R, ed. Psychoneuroimmunology. New York: Academic Press, 1981:3231–3254.

129. Ader R, Cohen N. Behaviorally conditioned immunosuppression. Psychosom Med 1975;37:333–340.

130. Ader R, Cohen N. CNS-immune system interactions: conditioning phenomena. Behav Brain Sci 1985;8:379–395.

131. Ader R, Cohen N. The influence of conditioning on immune responses. In: Ader R, Felten DL, Cohen N, eds. Psychoneuroimmunology. 2nd ed. New York: Academic Press 1991:611–646.

132. Ader R, Cohen N. Psychoneuroimmunology: conditioning and stress. Ann Rev Psychol 1993;44:53–85.

133. Lysle DT, Cunnick JE, Fowler H, Rabin BS. Pavlovian conditioning of shock-induced suppression of lymphocyte reactivity: acquisition, extinction, and preexposure effects. Life Sci 1988;42:2185–2194.

134. Gorczynski RM, Macrae S, Kennedy M. Conditioned immune response associated with allogeneic skin grafts in mice. J Immunol 1982;129:704–709.

135. MacQueen GM, Marshall J, Perdue M, Siegel S, Bienenstock J. Pavlovian conditioning of rat mucosal mast cells to secrete rat mast cell protease II. Science 1989;243:83–85.

136. Dyck DG, Greenberg AH, Osachuk TAG. Tolerance to drug-induced (Poly I:C) natural killer cell activation: congruence with a pavlovian conditioning model. J Exp Psychol Anim Behav Proc 1986;12: 25–31.

137. Dyck DG, Dreidger SM, Nemeth R, Osachuk TAG, Greenberg AH. Conditioned tolerance to drug-induced (Poly I:C) natural killer cell activation: effect of drug dosage and context specificity parameters. Brain Behav Immun 1987;1:251–266.

138. Siegel S. Morphine analgesia tolerance: its situation specificity supports a Pavlovian model. Science 1976;193:323–325.

139. Siegel S. Classical conditioning, drug tolerance, and drug dependence. In: Israel Y, Gaser FB, Kalant H, Popham RE, Schmidt W, Smart RG,

eds. Research advances in alcohol and drug problems. New York: Plenum, 1983:207–246.

140. Ader R, Cohen N. Behaviorally conditioned immunosuppression and murine systemic lupus erythematosus. Science 1982;215:1534–1536.

141. Ader R. Conditioned immunopharmacological effects in animals: implications for a conditioning model of pharmacotherapy. In: White L, Tursky B, Schwartz GE, eds. Placebo: theory, research, and mechanisms. New York: Guilford Press, 1985;306–323.

142. Klosterhalfen W, Klosterhalfen S. Pavlovian conditioning of immunosuppression modifies adjuvant arthritis in rats. Behav Neurosci 1983;97:663–666.

143. Klosterhalfen S, Klosterhalfen W. Conditioned immunopharmacologic effects and adjuvant arthritis: further results. In: Spector NH, ed. Neuroimmunomodulation: proceedings of the first international workshop on neuroimmunomodulation. Bethesda:IWGN, 1985:183–187.

144. Lysle DT, Luecken LJ, Maslonek KA. Suppression of the development of adjuvant arthritis by a conditioned aversive stimulus. Brain Behav Immun 1992;6:64–73.

145. Gorczynski RM, Kennedy M, Ciampi A. Cimetidine reverses tumor growth enhancement of plasmacytoma tumors in mice demonstrating conditioned immunosuppression. J Immunol 1985;134:4261–4264.

146. Gorczynski RM. Conditioned enhancement of skin allografts in mice. Brain Behav Immun 1990;4:85–92.

147. Grochowicz P, Schedlowski M, Husband AJ, King MG, Hibberd AD, Bowen KM. Behavioral conditioning prolongs heart allograft survival in rats. Brain Behav Immun 1991;5:349–356.

148. Bovbjerg DH, Redd WH, Maier LA, et al. Anticipatory immune suppression and nausea in women receiving cyclic chemotherapy for ovarian cancer. J Consult Clin Psychol 1990;5:153–157.

149. Buske-Kirschbaum A, Kirschbaum C, Stierle H, Lehnert H, Hellhammer S. Conditioned increase of natural killer cell activity (NKCA) in humans. Psychosom Med 1992;54:123–132.

150. Mackenzie JN. The production of the so-called "rose cold" by means of an artificial rose. Am J Med Sci 1896;91:45–57.

151. Smith GH, Salinger R. Hypersensitiveness and the conditioned reflex. Yale J Biol Med 1933;5:387–402.

152. Dekker E, Pelser HE, Groen J. Conditioning as a cause of asthmatic attacks. J Psychosom Res 1957;2:97–108.

153. Ottenberg P, Stein M, Lewis J, Hamilton C. Learned asthma in the guinea pig. Psychosom Med 1958;20:395–400.

154. Ikemi Y, Nakagawa S. A psychosomatic study of contagious dermatitis. Kyushu J Med Sci 1962;13:335–350.

155. Gorczynski RM, Macrae S, Kennedy M. Factors involved in the classical conditioning of antibody responses in mice. In: Ballieux R, Fielding R, L'Abbate A, eds. Breakdown in human adaptation to stress: towards a multidisciplinary approach. Boston: Martinus Nijhof, 1984:704–712.

156. Ader R, Cohen N, Grota LJ. Adrenal involvement in conditioned immunosuppression. Int J Pharmacol 1979;1:141–145.

157. Ader R, Cohen N, Bovbjerg D. Conditioned suppression of humoral immunity in the rat. J Comp Physiol Psychol 1979;96:517–521.

158. Kusnecov AW, Sivyer M, King MG, Husband AJ, Cripps AW, Clancy RL. Behaviorally conditioned suppression of the immune response by antilymphocyte serum. J Immunol 1983;130:2117–2120.

159. Bovbjerg D, Ader R, Cohen N. Acquisition and extinction of conditioned suppression of a graft-vs-host response in the rat. J Immunol 1984;132:111–113.

160. Cohen N, Ader R, Green N, Bovbjerg D. Conditioned suppression of a thymus-independent antibody response. Psychosom Med 1979;41:487–491.

161. Klosterhalfen S, Klosterhalfen W. Classically conditioned cyclophosphamide effects on white blood cell counts in rats. Ann N Y Acad Sci 1987;496:569–577.

162. Peeke HVS, Ellman G, Dark K, Salfi M, Reus VI. Cortisol and behaviorally conditioned histamine release. Ann N Y Acad Sci 1987;496:583–587.

163. Shavit Y, Terman GW, Lewis J W, Zane CJ, Gale RP, Liebeskind JC. Effects of footshock stress and morphine on natural killer lymphocytes in rats: studies of tolerance and cross-tolerance. Brain Res 1986;372:382–385.

164. Lysle DT, Luecken LJ, Maslonek KA. Modulation of immune function by a conditioned aversive stimulus: evidence for the involvement of endogenous opioids. Brain Behav Immun 1992;6:179–188.

165. Solvason HB, Hiramoto RN, Ghanta VK. Naltrexone blocks the expression of the conditioned elevation of natural killer cell activity in BALB/c mice. Brain Behav Immun 1989;3:247–262.

166. Gorczynski RM, Holmes W. Neuroleptic and anti-depressant drug treatment abolishes conditioned immunosuppression in mice. Brain Behav Immun 1989;3:312–319.

167. Cunnick JE, Lysle DT, Kucinski BJ, Rabin BS. Evidence that shock-induced immune suppression is mediated by adrenal hormones and peripheral β-adrenergic receptors. Pharmacol Biochem Behav 1990;36:645–651.

168. Zalcman S, Irwin J, Anisman H. Stressor-induced alterations of natural killer cell activity and central catecholamines in mice. Pharmacol Biochem Behav 1991;39:361–366.

169. Sonnenfeld G, Cunnick JE, Armfield AV, Wood PG, Rabin BS. Stress-induced alterations in interferon production and class II histocompatibility antigen expression. Brain Behav Immun 1992;6:170–178.

170. McFarland D, Hotchin J. Animal models in behavioral neurovirology. In: Kurstak E, Lipowski ZJ, Morozov PV, eds. Viruses, immunity, and mental disorders. New York: Plenum, 1987;189–198.

171. Ader R, Grota LJ, Cohen N. Conditioning phenomena and immune function. Ann N Y Acad Sci 1987;496:532–544.

172. Ader R, Grota LJ, Moynihan JA, Cohen N. Behavioral adaptations in autoimmune disease-susceptible mice. In: Ader R, Felten DL, Cohen N, eds. Psychoneuroimmunology. 2nd ed. New York: Academic Press, 1991;685–708.

173. Forster J, Lal HM. Brain reactive antibodies and learning. In: Ader R, Felten DL, Cohen N, eds. Psychoneuroimmunology. 2nd ed. New York: Academic Press, 1991;709–748.

174. Crnic L. Behavioral consequences of virus infection. In: Ader R, Felten DL, Cohen N, eds. Psychoneuroimmunology. 2nd ed. New York: Academic Press, 1991:749–769.

175. Schiffer RB, Hoffman SA. Behavioral sequelae of autoimmune disease. In: Ader R, Felten DL, Cohen N, eds. Psychoneuroimmunology. 2nd ed. New York: Academic Press, 1991:1037–1066.

176. Grota LJ, Ader R, Cohen N. Taste aversion learning in autoimmune Mrl-lpr/lpr and Mrl +/+ mice. Brain Behav Immun 1987;1:238–250.

177. Grota LJ, Schachtman R, Moynihan JA, Cohen N, Ader R. Voluntary consumption of cyclophosphamide by Mrl mice. Brain Behav Immun 1989;3:263–273.

178. Felten DL, Cohen N, Ader R, Felten SY, Carlson SL, Roszman TL. Central neural circuits involved in neural-immune interactions. In: Ader R, Felten DL, Cohen N, eds. Psychoneuroimmunology-II. New York: Academic Press, 1991:3–25.

179. Cross RJ, Markesbery WR, Brooks WH, Roszman TL. Hypothalamic-immune interactions. I. The acute effect of anterior hypothalamic lesions on the immune response. Brain Res 1980;196:79–87.

180. Roszman TL, Cross RJ, Brooks WH, Markesbery WR. Hypothalamic-immune interactions II. The effect of hypothalamic lesions on the ability of adherent spleen cells to limit lymphocyte blastogenesis. Immunology 1982;45:737–742.

181. Forni G, Bindoni M, Santoni A, Belluardo N, Marchese AE, Giovarelli M. Radiofrequency destruction of the tuberoinfundibular region of hypothalamus permanently abrogates NK cell activity in mice. Nature 1983;306:181–184.

182. Brooks WH, Cross RJ, Roszman TL, Markesbery WR. 1982. Neuroimmunomodulation: neural anatomical basis for impairment and facilitation. Ann Neurol 12:56–61.

183. Nance DM, Rayson D, Carr RI. The effects of lesions in the lateral septal and hippocampal areas on the humoral immune response of adult female rats. Brain Behav Immun 1987;1:292–305.

184. Sundar SK, Cierpial MA, Kamaraju LS, et al. Human immunodeficiency virus glycoprotein (gp120) infused into rat brain induces interleukin 1 to elevate pituitary-adrenal activity and decrease peripheral cellular immune responses. Proc. Natl. Acad. Sci. U. S. A. 1991;88:11246-11250.

185. Sundar SK, Becker KJ, Cierpial MA, et al. Intracerebroventricular infusion of interleukin 1 rapidly decreases peripheral cellular immune responses. Proc. Natl. Acad. Sci. (USA) 1989;86:6398–6402.

186. Brown R, Li Z, Vriend C, et al. Suppression of splenic macrophage interleukin-1 secretion following intracerebroventricular injection of interleukin-1B: Evidence for pituitary-adrenal and sympathetic control. Cell Immunol 1991;132:84–93.

187. Irwin M, Vale W, Rivier C. Central corticotropin-releasing factor mediates the suppressive effect of stress on natural killer cytotoxicity. Endocrinology 1990;126:2837–2844.

188. Irwin M, Hauger RL, Brown M, Britton KT. CRF activates autonomic nervous system and reduces natural killer cytotoxicity. Am J Physiol 1988;255:R744–R747.

189. Gisler RH, Schenkel-Hulliger, L. Hormonal regulation of the immune response. II. Influence of pituitary and adrenal activity on immune responsiveness in vitro. Cell Immunol 1971;2:646–657.

190. Nagy E, Berczi I, Friesen HG. Regulation of immunity in rats by lactogenic and growth hormones. Acta Endocrinol 1983;102: 351–357.

191. Pierpaoli W, Baroni C, Fabris N, Sorkin E. Hormones and immunological capacity. II. Reconstitution of antibody production in hormonally deficient mice by somatotropic hormone, thyrotropic hormone and thyroxin. Immunology 1969;16:217–230.

192. Duquesnoy RJ, Kalpaktsoglou PK, Good RA. Immunological studies of the Snell-Bagg pituitary dwarf mouse. Proc. Soc. Exp. Biol. Med. 1970;133:201–206.

193. Duquesnoy RJ. Immunodeficiency of the thymus-dependent system of the Ames dwarf mouse. J Immunol 1972;108:1578–1590.

194. Edwards CK III, Yunger LM, Lorence RM, Dantzer R, Kelley KW. The pituitary gland is required for protection against lethal effects of Salmonella typhimurium. Proc. Natl Acad Sci (USA) 1991;88: 2274–2277.

195. Johnson HM, Downs MO, Pontzer CH. Neuroendocrine peptide hormone regulation of immunity. In: Neuroimmunoendocrinology, chemical immunology. Blalock JE, ed. Basel: Karger, 1992: 49–83.

196. Munck A, Guyre PM. Glucocorticoids and immune function. In: Psychoneuroimmunology-II. Ader R, Felten, DL, Cohen N, eds. San Diego: Academic Press, 1991:447–474.

197. Munck A, Guyre PM, Holbrook NJ. Physiological functions of glucocorticoids in stress and their relation to pharmacological actions. Endocrinol Rev 1984;5:25–44.

198. Stam WB, Van Oosterhout AJM, Nijkamp FP. Pharmacologic modulation of TH1- and TH2-associated lymphokine production. Life Sci 1993;53:1921–1934.

199. Wick G, Hu Y, Kroemer G. Immunoendocrine communications via the hypothalamo-pituitary-adrenal axis in autoimmune diseases. Endocrinol Rev 1993;14:539–563.

200. Cupps TR, Fauci AS. Corticosteroid-mediated immunoregulation in man. Immunol Rev 1982;65:133–155.

201. Werb Z, Foley R, Munck A. Interaction of glucocorticoids with macrophages. Identification of glucocorticoid receptors in monocytes and macrophages. J Exp Med 1978;147:1684–1694.

202. Cohen J, Duke RC. Glucocorticoid activation of a calcium-dependent endonuclease in thymocyte nuclei leads to cell death. J Immunol 1984;132:38–42.

203. Cox JH, Ford WL. The migration of lymphocytes across specialized vascular endothelium. IV. Prednisolone acts at several points on the recirculation pathways of lymphocytes. Cell Immunol 1982;66: 407–422.

204. Hall JG. Sulphated polysaccharides, corticosteroids and lymphocyte recirculation. Immunology 1986;57:275–279.

205. Snyder DS, Unanue ER. Corticosteroids inhibit macrophage Ia expression and interleukin 1 production. J Immunol 1982;129: 1803–1805.

206. Barber AE, Coyle SM, Marano MA, et al. Glucocorticoid therapy alters hormonal and cytokine responses to endotoxin in man. J Immunol 1993;150:1999–2006.

207. Van Den Bergh P, Dobber R, Ramlal S, Rozing J, Nagelkerken L. Role of opioid peptides in the regulation of cytokine production by murine CD4+ T cells. Cell Immunol 1994;154:109–122.

208. Gillis S, Crabtree GR, Smith KA. Glucocorticosteroid induced inhibition of T cell growth factor production. I. The effect on mitogen-induced lymphocyte proliferation. J Immunol 1979;123: 1624–1631.

209. Pinkston P, Saltini C, Muller-Quernheim J, Crystal RG. Corticosteroid therapy suppresses spontaneous interleukin 2 release and spontaneous proliferation of lung T lymphocytes of patients with active pulmonary sarcoidosis. J Immunol 1987;139:755–760.

210. Daynes RA, Araneo BA. Contrasting effects of glucocorticoids on the capacity of T cells to produce the growth factors interleukin 2 and interleukin 4. Eur J Immunol 1989;19:2319–2325.

211. Daynes RA, Dudley DJ, Araneo BA. Regulation of murine lymphokine production in vivo II. Dehydroepiandrosterone is a natural enhancer of interleukin 2 synthesis by helper T cells. Eur J Immunol 1990;20:793–802.

212. Araneo BA, Woods ML II, Daynes RA. Reversal of the immunosenescent phenotype by dehydroepiandrosterone: hormone treatment provides an adjuvant effect on the immunization of aged mice with recombinant hepatitis B surface antigen. J Infect Dis 1993;167: 830–840.

213. Daynes RA, Araneo BA, Dowell TA, Huang K, Dudley D. Regulation of murine lymphokine production in vivo III. The lymphoid tissue microenvironment exerts regulatory influences over T helper cell function. J Exp Med 1990;171:979–996.

214. Blauer KL, Poth M, Rogers WM, Bernton EW. Dehydroepiandrosterone antagonizes the suppressive effects of dexamethasone on lymphocyte proliferation. Endocrinology 1991;129:3174–3179.

215. Johnson HM, Smith EM, Torres BA, Blalock JE. Regulation of the in vitro antibody response by neuroendocrine hormones. Proc Natl Acad Sci (USA) 1982;79:4171–4174.

216. Johnson HM, Torres BA, Smith EM, Dion LD, Blalock JE. Regulation of lymphokine (gamma-interferon) production by corticotropin. J Immunol 1984;132:246–250.

217. Clarke BL, Bost KL. Differential expression of functional adrenocorticotropic hormone receptors by subpopulations of lymphocytes. J Immunol 1989;143:464–469.

218. Heijnen CJ, Kavelaars A, Ballieux RE. β-endorphin: cytokine and neuropeptide. Immunol Rev 1991;119:41–63.

219. Blalock JE. A molecular basis for bidirectional communication between the immune and neuroendocrine systems. Physiol Rev 1989;69:1–32.

220. Carr DJJ, Blalock JE. Neuropeptide hormones and receptors common to the immune and neuroendocrine systems: bidirectional pathway of intersystem communication. In: Psychoneuroimmunology-II. Ader R, Felten DL, Cohen N, eds. San Diego: Academic Press, 1991: 573–588.

221. Woudenberg AD, Metzelaar MJ, Van Der Kleij AAM, De Wied D, Burbach JPH, Wiegant VM. Analysis of proopiomelanocortin (POMC) messenger ribonucleic acid and POMC-derived peptides in human peripheral blood mononuclear cells: No evidence for a lymphocyte-derived POMC system. Endocrinology 1993;133: 1922–1933.

222. Mechanick JI, Levin N, Roberts JL, Autelitano DJ. Proopiomelanocortin gene expression in a distinct population of rat spleen and lung leukocytes. Endocrinology 1992;131:518–525.

223. Sternberg EM, Hill JM, Chrousos GP, Kamilaris T, Listwak SJ, Gold PW, Wilder RL. Inflammatory mediator-induced hypothalamic-

pituitary-adrenal axis activation is defective in streptococcal cell wall arthritis-susceptible Lewis rats. Proc Natl Acad Sci (USA) 1989;86: 2374–2378.

224. MacPhee IAM, Antoni FA, Mason DW. Spontaneous recovery of rats from experimental allergic encephalomyelitis is dependent on regulation of the immune system by endogenous adrenal corticosteroids. J Exp Med 1989;169:431–455.

225. Folch H, Waksman BH. The splenic suppressor cell. I. Activity of thymus-dependent adherent cells: changes with age and stress. J Immunol 1974;113:127–139.

226. Guillemin R, Vargo T, Rossier J, et al. β-Endorphin and adrenocorticotropin are secreted concomitantly by the pituitary gland. Science 1977;197:1368–1369.

227. Wybran J, Appelboom T, Famaey J-P, Govaerts A. Suggestive evidence for receptors for morphine and methionine-enkephalin on normal human blood T lymphocytes. J Immunol 1979;123:1068–1070.

228. Sibinga NES, Goldstein A. Opioid peptides and opioid receptors in cells of the immune system. Annu Rev Immunol 1988;6:219–249.

229. Gilman SC, Schwartz JM, Milner RJ, Bloom FE, Feldman JD. β-Endorphin enhances lymphocyte proliferative responses. Proc Natl Acad Sci (USA) 1982;79:4226–4230.

230. Gilmore W, Weiner LP. The opioid specificity of beta-endorphin enhancement of murine lymphocyte proliferation. Immunopharmacology 1989;17:19–30.

231. Van Den Bergh P, Rozing J, Nagelkerken L. Two opposing modes of action of β-endorphin on lymphocyte function. Immunology 1991;72:537–543.

232. Apte, RN, Oppenheim JJ, Durum SK. β-Endorphin regulates interleukin 1 production and release by murine bone marrow macrophages. International Immunology 1989;1:465–470.

233. Mandler RN, Biddison WE, Mandler R, Serrate SA. β-Endorphin augments the cytolytic activity and interferon production of natural killer cells. J Immunol 1986;136:934–939.

234. Mathews PM, Froelich CJ, Sibbitt WL Jr, Bankhurst AD. Enhancement of natural cytotoxicity by β-endorphin. J Immunol 1983;130:1658–1662.

235. Brown SL, Van Epps DE. Suppression of T lymphocyte chemotactic factor production by the opioid peptides β-endorphin and metenkephalin. J Immunol 1985;134:3384–3390.

236. Heagy W, Laurance M, Cohen E, Finberg R. Neurohormones regulate T cell function. J. Exp. Med. 1990;171:1625–1633.

237. Taub DD, Eisenstein TK, Geller EB, Adler MW, Rogers TJ. Immunomodulatory activity of μ- and κ-selective opioid agonists. Proc Natl Acad Sci (USA) 1991;88:360–364.

238. Carr DJJ, DeCosta BR, Kim C-H, et al. Opioid receptors on cells of the immune system: evidence for δ- and κ- classes. J Endocrinol 1989;122:161–168.

239. Carr DJJ, Kim C-H, DeCosta B, Jacobson AE, Rice KC, Blalock JE. Evidence for a δ-class opioid receptor on cells of the immune system. Cell Immunol 1988;116:44–51.

240. Bidlack JM, Saripalli LD, Lawrence DM. κ-Opioid binding sites on a murine lymphoma cell line. Eur J Pharmacol 1992;227:257–265.

241. Kavelaars A, Ballieux RE, Heijnen CJ. The role of IL-1 in the corticotropin-releasing factor and arginine-vasopressin-induced secretion of immunoreactive β-endorphin by human peripheral blood mononuclear cells. J Immunol 1989;142:2338–2342.

242. Zurawski G, Benedik M, Kamb BJ, Abrams JS, Zurawski SM, Lee FD. Activation of mouse T-helper cells induces abundant preproenkephalin mRNA synthesis. Science 1986;232:772–775.

243. Linner KM, Beyer HS, Sharp BM. Induction of the messenger ribonucleic acid for proenkephalin A in cultured murine CD4-positive thymocytes. Endocrinology 1991;128:717–724.

244. Behar OZ, Ovadia H, Polakiewicz RD, Abramsky O, Rosen H. Regulation of proenkephalin A messenger ribonucleic acid levels in normal B lymphocytes: specific inhibition by glucocorticoid hormones and superinduction by cycloheximide. Endocrinology 1991;129:649–655.

245. Rosen H, Behar O, Abramsky O, Ovadia H. Regulated expression of proenkephalin A in normal lymphocytes. J Immunol 1989;143:3703–3707.

246. Roth JA, Kaeberle ML, Grier RL, Hopper JG, Spiegel HE, McAllister HA. Improvement in clinical condition and thymus morphologic features associated with growth hormone treatment of immunodeficient dwarf dogs. Am J Vet Res 1984;45:1151–1155.

247. Marsh JA, Gause WC, Sandhu S, Scanes CG. Enhanced growth and immune development in dwarf chickens treated with mammalian growth hormone and thyroxine. Proc Soc Exp Biol Med 1984;175:351–360.

248. Fabris N, Pierpaoli W, Sorkin E. Hormones and the immunological capacity. IV. Restorative effects of developmental hormones or of lymphocytes on the immunodeficiency syndrome of the dwarf mouse. Clin Exp Immunol 1971;9:227–240.

249. Murphy WJ, Durum SK, Longo DL. Role of neuroendocrine hormones in murine T cell development. Growth hormone exerts thymopoietic effects in vivo. J Immunol 1992;149:3851–3857.

250. Murphy WJ, Durum SK, Longo DL. Differential effects of growth hormone and prolactin on murine T cell development and function. J Exp Med 1993;178:231–236.

251. Kelley KW, Brief S, Westly HJ, et al. GH3 pituitary adenoma cells can reverse thymic ageing in rats. Proc Natl Acad Sci (USA) 1986;83:5663–5667.

252. Snow, EC, Feldbush TL, Oaks JA. The effect of growth hormone and insulin upon MLC responses and generation of cytotoxic T lymphocytes. J Immunol 1981;126:161–164.

253. Edwards CK, Ghiasuddin SM, Schepper JM, Yunger LM, Kelley KW. A newly defined property of somatotropin: priming of macrophages for production of superoxide anion. Science 1988;239:769–771.

254. Gupta S, Fikrig SM, Noval MS. Immunological studies in patients with isolated growth hormone deficiency. Clin Exp Immunol 1983;54:87–90.

255. Kiess W, Doerr H, Eisl E, Butenandt O, Belohradsky BH. Lymphocyte subsets and natural killer activity in growth hormone deficiency. N Engl J Med 1985;314:321.

256. Weigent DA, Blalock JE, LeBoeuf RD. An antisense oligodeoxynucleotide to growth hormone messenger ribonucleic acid inhibits lymphocyte proliferation. Endocrinology 1991;128:2053–2057.

257. Weigent DA, Baxter JB, Wear WE, Smith LR, Bost KL, Blalock JE. Production of immunoreactive growth hormone by mononuclear leukocytes. FASEB J 1988;2:2812–2818.

258. Kelley KW. Growth hormone in immunobiology. In: Ader R, Felten DL, Cohen N, eds. Psychoneuroimmunology-II. San Diego: Academic Press, 1991:377–402.

259. Russell DH, Larson DF. Prolactin-induced polyamine biosynthesis in spleen and thymus: specific inhibition by cyclosporine. Immunopharmacology 1985;9:165–174.

260. Russell DH, Kibler R, Matrisian L, Larson DF, Poulos B, Magun BE. Prolactin receptors on human T and B lymphocytes: antagonism of prolactin binding by cyclosporine. J Immunol 1985;134:3027–3031.

261. Russell DH, Matrisian L, Kibler R, Larson DF, Poulos B, Magun BE. Prolactin receptors on human lymphocytes and their modulation by cyclosporine. Biochem Biophys Res Commun 1984;121:899–906.

262. Berczi I, Nagy E, Kovacs K, Horvath E. Regulation of humoral immunity in rats by pituitary hormones. Acta Endocrinol 1981;98:506–513.

263. Hiestand PC, Mekler P, Nordmann R, Grieder A, Permmongkol C. Prolactin as a modulator of lymphocyte responsiveness provides a possible mechanism of action for cyclosporine. Proc Natl Acad Sci (USA) 1986;83:2599–2603.

264. Bernton EW, Meltzer MS, Holaday JW. Suppression of macrophage activation and T-lymphocyte function in hypoprolactinemic mice. Science 1988;239:401–404.

265. Clevenger CV, Russell DH, Appasamy PM, Prystowsky MB. Regulation of interleukin 2-driven T-lymphocyte proliferation by prolactin. Proc Natl Acad Sci (USA) 1990;87:6460–6464.

266. Hartmann DP, Holaday JW, Bernton EW. Inhibition of lymphocyte proliferation by antibodies to prolactin. FASEB J 1989;3:2194–2202.

267. Sabharwal P, Glaser R, Lafuse W, et al. Prolactin synthesized and secreted by human peripheral blood mononuclear cells: An autocrine growth factor for lymphoproliferation. Proc Natl Acad Sci (USA) 1992;89:7713–7716.

268. Clevenger CV, Altmann SW, Prystowsky MB. Requirement of nuclear prolactin for interleukin-2 stimulated proliferation of T lymphocytes. Science 1991;253:77–79.

269. Clevenger CV, Sillman AL, Hanley-Hyde J, Prystowsky MB. Requirement for prolactin during cell cycle regulated gene expression in clone T-lymphocytes. Endocrinology 1992;130:3216–3222.

270. Montgomery DW, LeFevre JA, Ulrich ED, Adamson CR, Zukoski CF. Identification of prolactin-like proteins synthesized by normal murine lymphocytes. Endocrinology 1990;127:2601–2603.

271. Shah GN, Laird HE II, Russell DH. Identification and characterization of a prolactin-like polypeptide synthesized by mitogen-stimulated murine lymphocytes. International Immunology 1991;3:297–304.

272. Harbour DV, Leon S, Keating C, Hughes TK. Thyrotropin modulates B-cell function through specific bioactive receptors. Progress in Neuroendocrinimmunology 1990;3:266–276.

273. Blalock JE, Johnson HM, Smith EM, Torres BA. Enhancement of the in vitro antibody response by thyrotropin. Biochem Biophys Res Commun 1984;125:30–34.

274. Kruger TE, Blalock JE. Cellular requirements for thyrotropin enhancement of in vitro antibody production. J Immunol 1986;137:197–199.

275. Kruger TE, Smith LR, Harbour DV, Blalock JE. Thyrotropin: an endogenous regulator of the in vitro immune response. J Immunol 1989;142:744–747.

276. Fabris N. Immunodepression in thyroid-deprived animals. Clin Exp Immunol 1973;15:601–611.

277. Chatterjee S, Chandel AS. Immunomodulatory role of thyroid hormones: in vivo effect of thyroid hormones on the blastogenic response of lympoid tissues. Acta Endocrinol 1983;103:95–100d.

278. Scott T, Glick B. Organ weights, T-cell proliferation, and graft vs host capabilities of hypothyroidic chickens. Gen Comp Endocrinol 1987;67:270–276.

279. Provinciali M, Muzzioli M, DiStefano G, Fabris N. Recovery of spleen cell natural killer activity by thyroid hormone treatment in old mice. Nat Immun Cell Growth Regul 1991;10:226–236.

280. Lahita RG. Sex hormones and the immune system-part 1. Human data. Baillieres Clin Rheumatol 1990;4:1–12.

281. Ansar Ahmed S, Talal N. Sex hormones and the immune system—part 2. Animal data. Baillieres Clin Rheumatol 1990;4:13–31.

282. Butterworth M, McClellan B, Allansmith M. Influence of sex on immunoglobulin levels. Nature 1967;214:1224–1225.

283. Grossman CJ. Interactions between the gonadal steroids and the immune system. Science 1985;227:257–261.

284. Terres G, Morrison SL, Habicht GS. A quantitative difference in the immune response between male and female mice. Proc Soc Exp Biol Med 1968;127:664–667.

285. Eidinger D, Garrett TJ. Studies of the regulatory effects of the sex hormones on antibody formation and stem cell differentiation. J Exp Med 1972;136:1098–1116.

286. Ansar Ahmed S, Dauphinee MJ, Montoya AI, Talal N. Estrogen induces normal murine CD5+ B cells to produce autoantibodies. J Immunol 1989;142:2647–2653.

287. Fox HS, Bond BL, Parslow TG. Estrogen regulates the IFN-γ promoter. J Immunol 1991;146:4362–4367.

288. Danel L, Souweine G, Monier JC, Saez S. Specific estrogen binding sites in human lymphoid cells and thymic cells. J Steroid Biochem Mol Biol 1983;18:559–563.

289. Luster MI, Hayes HT, Korach K, et al. Estrogen immunosupression is regulated through estrogenic responses in the thymus. J Immunol 1984;133:110–116.

290. Stimson WH. Oestrogen and human T lymphocytes: presence of specific receptors in the T-suppressor/cytotoxic subset. Scand J Immunol 1988;28:345–350.

291. Masi AT, Kaslow RA. Sex effects in systemic lupus erythematosus. A clue to pathogenesis. Arthritis Rheum 1978;21:480–483.

292. Duvic M, Steinberg AD, Klassen LW. Effect of the anti-estrogen, nafoxidine, on NZB/W autoimmune disease. Arthritis Rheum 1978;21:414–417.

293. Grossman CJ, Roselle GA, Mendenhall CL. Sex steroid regulation of autoimmunity. J Steroid Biochem Mol Biol 1991;40:649–659.

294. Ansar Ahmed S, Penhale WJ, Talal N. Sex hormones, immune responses, and autoimmune diseases. Am J Pathol 1985;121:531–551.

295. Fox HS. Androgen treatment prevents diabetes in nonobese diabetic mice. J Exp Med 1992;175:1409–1412.

296. Carlsten H, Nilsson N, Jonsson R, Backman K, Holmdahl R, Tarkowski A. Estrogen accelerates immune complex glomerulonephritis but ameliorates T cell-mediated vasculitis and sialadenitis in autoimmune MRL lpr/lpr mice. Cell Immunol 1992;144:190–202.

297. Pearce P, Khalid BAK, Funder JW. Androgens and the thymus. Endocrinology 1981;109:1073–1077.

298. Reichman ME, Villee CA. Estradiol binding by rat thymus cytosol. J Steroid Biochem Mol Biol 1978;9:637–641.

299. Screpanti I, Morrone S, Meco D, et al. Steroid sensitivity of thymocyte subpopulations during intrathymic differentiation. J Immunol 1989;142:3378–3383.

300. Okuyama R, Abo T, Seki S, et al. Estrogen administration activates extrathymic T cell differentiation in the liver. J Exp Med 1992;175:661–669.

301. Johnson HM, Torres BA. Regulation of lymphokine production by arginine vasopressin and oxytocin: modulation of lymphocyte function by neurohypophyseal hormones. J Immunol 1985;135:773s–775s.

302. Torres BA, Johnson HM. Arginine vasopressin (AVP) replacement of helper cell requirement in INF-γ production. Evidence for a novel AVP receptor on mouse lymphocytes. J Immunol 1988;140:2179–2183.

303. Robert F, Geenen V, Schoenen J, et al. Co-localization of immunoreactive oxytocin, vasopressin, and interleukin 1 in human thymic epithelial neuroendocrine cells. Brain Behav Immun 1991;5:102–115.

304. Geenen V, Legros JJ, Franchimont P, Baudrihaye M, Defresne MP, Boniver J. The neuroendocrine thymus: coexistence of oxytocin and neurophysin in the human thymus. Science 1986;232:508–510.

305. Ayers AB, Davies BN, Withrington PG. Responses of the isolated, perfused human spleen to sympathetic nerve stimulation, catecholamines and polypeptides. Br J Pharmacol 1972;44:17–30.

306. Reilly FD, McCuskey RS, Meineke HA. Studies of the hemopoietic microenvironment. VIII. Adrenergic and cholinergic innervation of the murine spleen. Anat Rec 1975;185:109–118.

307. Reilly FD. Innervation and vascular pharmacodynamics of the mammalian spleen. Experientia 1985;41:187–192.

308. Felten SY, Felten DL. The innervation of lymphoid tissue. In: Ader R, Felten DL, Cohen N, eds. Psychoneuroimmunology. 2nd ed. New York: Academic Press, 1991:27–68.

309. Calvo W. The innervation of the bone marrow in laboratory animals. Am J Anat 1968;123:315–328.

310. Maestroni GJM, Conti A, Pedrinis E. Effect of adrenergic agents on hematopoiesis after syngeneic bone marrow transplantation in mice. Blood 1992;80:1178–1182.

311. Felten DL, Felten SY, Carlson SL, Olschowka JA, Livnat S. Noradrenergic and peptidergic innervation of lymphoid tissue. J Immunol 1985;135:755s–765s.

312. Williams JM, Felten DL. Sympathetic innervation of murine thymus and spleen: A comparative histofluorescence study. Anat Rec 1981;199:531–542.

313. Williams JM, Peterson RG, Shea PA, Schmedtje JF, Bauer DC, Felten DL. Sympathetic innervation of murine thymus and spleen: Evidence

for a functional link between the nervous and immune systems. Brain Res Bull 1981;6:83–94.

314. Bellinger DL, Lorton D, Romano T, Olschowka JA, Felten SY, Felten DL. Neuropeptide innervation of lymphoid organs. Ann N Y Acad Sci 1990;594:17–33.

315. Ackerman KD, Bellinger DL, Felten SY, Felten DL. Ontogeny and senescence of noradrenergic innervation of the rodent thymus and spleen. In: Ader R, Felten DL, Cohen N, eds. Psychoneuroimmunology, 2nd ed. New York: Academic Press, 1991:71–125.

316. Nance DM, Hopkins DA, Bieger D. Re-investigation of the innervation of the thymus gland in mice and rats. Brain Behav Immun 1987;1:134–147.

317. Kendall MD, Al-Shawaf AA. Innervation of the rat thymus gland. Brain Behav Immun 1991;5:9–28.

318. Singh U. Lymphopoiesis in the nude fetal mouse thymus following sympathectomy. Cell Immunol 1985;93:222–228.

319. Singh U, Owen JJT. Studies on the maturation of thymus stem cells. The effects of catecholamines, histamine, and peptide hormones on the expression of T alloantigens. Eur J Immunol 1976;6:59–62.

320. Scheid MP, Hoffmann MK, Komuro K, et al. Differentiation of T cells induced by preparations from thymus and by nonthymic agents. J Exp Med 1973;138:1027–1032.

321. Felten DL, Felten SY, Bellinger DL, et al. Noradrenergic sympathetic neural interactions with the immune system: structure and function. Immunol Rev 1987;100:225–260.

322. Ader R, Felten DL, Cohen N. Interactions between the brain and the immune system. Ann Rev Pharmacol Toxicol 1990;30:561–602.

323. Felten SY, Felten DL, Bellinger DL, Olschowka JA. Noradrenergic and peptidergic innervation of lymphoid organs. In: Chemical immunology: neuroimmunoendocrinology. Blalock JE, ed. Basel: S Karger, 1992:25–48.

324. Bellinger DL, Felten SY, Lorton D, Felten DL. Origin of noradrenergic innervation of the spleen in rats. Brain Behav Immun 1989;3:291–311.

325. Nance DM, Burns J. Innervation of the spleen in the rat: evidence for absence of afferent innervation. Brain Behav Immun 1989;3:218–230.

326. Reilly FD, McCuskey PA, Miller ML, McCuskey RS, Meineke HA. Innervation of the periarteriolar lymphatic sheath of the spleen. Tissue Cell 1979;11:121–126.

327. Galindo B, Imaeda T. Electron microscopic study of the white pulp of the mouse spleen. Anat Rec 1962;143:399–415.

328. Heusermann U, Stutte HJ. Electron microscopic studies of the innervation of the human spleen. Cell Tissue Res 1977;184:225–236.

329. Felten SY, Olschowka JA. Noradrenergic sympathetic innervation of the spleen: II. Tyrosine hydroxylase (TH)-positive nerve terminals form synaptic-like contacts on lymphocytes in the splenic white pulp. J Neurosci Res 1987;18:37–48.

330. Felten DL, Livnat S, Felten SY, Carlson SL, Bellinger DL, Yeh P. Sympathetic innervation of lymph nodes in mice. Brain Res Bull 1984;13:693–699.

331. Giron LT, Crutcher KA, Davis JN. Lymph nodes—a possible site for sympathetic neuronal regulation of immune responses. Ann Neurol 1980;8:520–522.

332. Ackerman KD, Felten SY, Bellinger DL, Livnat S, Felten DL. Noradrenergic sympathetic innervation of spleen and lymph nodes in relation to specific cellular compartments. In: Cinader B, Miller RG, eds. Progress in immunology IV. Orlando: Academic Press, 1987:588–600.

333. Felten DL, Overhage JM, Felten SY, Schmedtje JF. Noradrenergic sympathetic innervation of lymphoid tissue in the rabbit appendix: further evidence for a link between the nervous and immune systems. Brain Res Bull 1981;7:595–612.

334. Madden KS, Livnat S. Catecholaminergic influences on immune reactivity. In: Ader R, Felten DL, Cohen, N, eds. Psychoneuroimmunology, second edition. New York: Academic Press, 1991:283–310.

335. Bulloch K, Pomerantz W. Autonomic nervous system innervation of thymic related lymphoid tissue in wild-type and nude mice. J Comp Neurol 1984;228:57–68.

336. Felten DL, Felten SY. Innervation of the thymus. In: Kendall, MD, Ritter MA, eds. Thymus Update. London: Harwood Academic Publishers, 1989:73–88.

337. Bellinger DL, Lorton D, Hamill R, Felten SY, Felten DL. Acetylcholinesterase staining and choline acetyltransferase activity in the young adult rat spleen: lack of evidence for cholinergic innervation. Brain Behav Immun 1992;7:191–204.

338. Shaskan EG, Ballow M, Lederman M, Margoles SL, Melchriet R. Spiroperidol binding sites on mouse lymphoid cells. Effects of ascorbic acid and psychotropic drugs. J Neuroimmunol 1984;6:59–66.

339. Lefur G, Phan T, Uzan A. Identification of a stereospecific 3H-spiroperidol binding sites in mammalian lymphocytes. Life Sci 1980;1139–1148.

340. Gordon MA, Cohen JJ, Wilson IG. Muscarinic cholinergic receptors in murine lymphocytes: Demonstration by direct binding. Proc Natl Acad Sci (USA) 1978;79:5097–5100.

341. Adem A, Nordberg A, Slanina P. A muscarinic receptor type in human lymphocytes: A comparison of 3H-QNB binding to intact lymphocytes and lysed lymphocyte membranes. Life Sci 1986;38:1359–1368.

342. Ovadia H, Abramsky O. Dopamine receptors on isolated membranes of rat lymphocytes. J Neurosci Res 1987;18:70–74.

343. Shapiro HM, Strom TB. Electrophysiology of T lymphocyte cholinergic receptors. Proc Natl Acad Sci (USA) 1980;77:4317–4321.

344. Maslinski W, Laskowska-Bosek H, Ryzewski J. Nicotinic receptors of rat lymphocytes during adjuvant polyarthritis. J Neurosci Res 1992;31:336–340.

345. Lundberg JM, Änggård A, Pernow J, Hökfelt T. Neuropeptide Y-, substance P- and VIP-immunoreactive nerves in cat spleen in relation to autonomic vascular and volume control. Cell Tissue Res 1985;239:9-18.

346. Romano TA, Felten SY, Felten DL, Olschowka JA. Neuropeptide-Y innervation of the rat spleen: another potential immunomodulatory neuropeptide. Brain Behav Immun 1991;5:116-131.

347. Payan DG, Goetzl EJ. Modulation of lymphocyte function by sensory neuropeptides. J Immunol 1985;135:783s.-786s.

348. Lorton, D, Bellinger DL, Felten SY, Felten DL. Substance P innervation of spleen in rats: nerve fibers associate with lymphocytes and macrophages in specific compartments of the spleen. Brain Behav Immun 1991;5:29-40.

349. Müller S, Weihe E. Interrelation of peptidergic innervation with mast cells and ED1-positive cells in rat thymus. Brain Behav Immun 1991;5:55-72.

350. Felten DL, Felten SY, Bellinger DL, Lorton D. Noradrenergic and peptidergic innervation of secondary lymphoid organs: role in experimental rheumatoid arthritis. Eur J Clin Invest 1992;22 (suppl 1):37-41.

351. Payan DG, Goetzl EJ. Substance P receptor-dependent responses of leukocytes in pulmonary inflammation. Am Rev Respir Dis 1987;36:S39-43.

352. Payan DG. Neuropeptides and inflammation: the role of substance P. Ann Rev Med 1989;40:341-352.

353. McGillis JP, Mitsuhaski M, Payan DG. Immunologic properties of substance P. In: Psychoneuroimmunology. 2nd ed. Ader R, Felten DL, Cohen N, eds. New York: Academic Press, 1991: 209–223.

354. McGillis JP, Organist ML, Payan DG. Substance P and immunoregulation. Fed Proc 1987;46:196-199.

355. Shanahan F, Denburg JA, Fox J, Bienenstock J, Befus D. Mast cell heterogeneity: effects of neuroenteric peptides on histamine release. J Immunol 1985;135:1331-1337.

356. Stead RH, Tomioka M, Quinonez G, Simon G, Felten SY, Bienenstock J. Intestinal mucosal mast cells in normal and nematode-infected rat intestines are in intimate contact with peptidergic nerves. Proc Natl Acad Sci (USA) 1987;84:2975-2979.

357. Lotz M, Vaughan JH, Carson DA. Effect of neuropeptides on production of inflammatory cytokines by human monocytes. Science 1988; 241:1218-1221.

358. Stanisz, AM, Seicohitano R, Dazin P, Bienenstock J, Payan DG. Distribution of substance preceptors on murine spleen & Peyer's patch T and B cells. J Immunol 1987;139: 749–754.

359. Payan DG, Brewster DR, Goetzl EJ. Stereospecific receptors for substance P on cultured human IM-9 lymphoblasts. J Immunol 1984;133:3260-3265.

360. Helme RD, Eglezos A, Dandie GW, Andrews PV, Boyd RL. The effect of substance P on the regional lymph node antibody response to antigenic stimulation in capsaicin-pretreated rats. J Immunol 1987;139:3470-3473.

361. Payan DG, Hess CA, Goetzl EJ. Inhibition by somatostatin of the proliferation of T-lymphocytes and Molt-4 lymphoblasts. Cell Immunol 1984;84:433-438.

362. Calvo C-F, Chavanel G, Senik A. Substance P enhances IL-2 expression in activated human T cells. J Immunol 1992;148:3498-3504.

363. Stanisz AM, Befus D, Bienenstock J. Differential effects of vasoactive intestinal peptide, substance P, and somatostatin on immunoglobulin synthesis and proliferation by lymphocytes from Peyer's patches, mesenteric lymph nodes, and spleen. J Immunol 1986;136:152–156.

364. Levine JD, Clark R, Devor M, Helms C, Moskowitz MA, Basbaum AI. Intraneuronal substance P contributes to the severity of experimental arthritis. Science 1984;226:547-549.

365. Malec P, Zeman K, Markiewicz K, Tchorzewski H, Nowak Z, Baj Z. Short-term somatostatin infusion affects T lymphocyte responsiveness in humans. Immunopharmacology 1989;17:45-49.

366. Muscettola M, Grasso G. Somatostatin and vasoactive intestinal peptide reduce interferon-gamma production by human peripheral blood mononuclear cells. Immunobiology 1990;180:419-430.

367. Zentel HJ, Weihe E. The neuro-B cell link of peptidergic innervation in the bursa Fabricii. Brain Behav Immun 1991;5:132-147.

368. Danek A, O'Dorisio MS, O'Dorisio TM, George JM. Specific binding sites for vasoactive intestinal polypeptide on nonadherent peripheral blood lymphocytes. J Immunol 1983;131: 1173–1177.

369. Ottaway CA, Greenberg GR. Interaction of vasoactive intestinal peptide with mouse lymphocytes: Specific binding and the modulation of mitogen responses. J Immunol 1984;132:417-423.

370. O'Dorisio MS, Shannon BT, Fleshman DJ, Campolito LB. Identification of high affinity receptors for vasoactive intestinal peptide on human lymphocytes of B cell lineage. J Immunol 1989; 142:3533–3536.

371. Ottaway CA. In vitro alteration of receptors for vasoactive intestinal peptide changes in the in vivo localization of mouse T cells. J Exp Med 1984;160:1054-1069.

372. Brodde OE, Engel G, Hoyer D, Block KD, Weber F. The beta-adrenergic receptor in human lymphocytes–Subclassification by the use of a new radio-ligand (±) [125 Iodo]cyanopindolol. Life Sci 1981;29:2189-2198.

373. Bishopric NH, Cohen HJ, Lefkowitz RJ. Beta adrenergic receptors in lymphocyte subpopulations. J Allergy Clin Immunol 1980;65:29-33.

374. Pochet R, Delespesse G, Gausset PW, Collet H. Distribution of beta-adrenergic receptors on human lymphocyte subpopulations. Clin Exp Immunol 1979;38:578-584.

375. Loveland BE, Jarrott B, McKenzie IFC. The detection of beta adrenoceptors on murine lymphocytes. Int J Immunopharmacol 1981;3:45-55.

376. Miles K, Atweh S, Otten G, Arnason BGW, Chelmicka-Schorr E. Beta-adrenergic receptors on splenic lymphocytes from axotomized mice. Int J Immunopharmacol 1984;6:171-177.

377. Landmann R, Burgisser E, West M, Buhler FR. Beta adrenergic receptors are different in subpopulations of human circulating lymphocytes. J Recept Res 1985;4:37-50.

378. Williams LT, Snyderman R, Lefkowitz RJ. Identification of β-adrenergic receptors in human lymphocytes by (--)[3H]-alprenolol binding. J Clin Invest 1976;57:149-155.

379. Nahorski SR, Barnett DB, Howlett DR, Rugg EL. Pharmacological characteristics of beta-adrenoceptor binding sites in intact and sympathectomized rat spleen. Naunyn Schmiedebergs Arch Pharmacol 1979;307:227-233.

380. Abrass CK, O'Connor SW, Scarpace PJ, Abrass IB. Characterization of the β-adrenergic receptor of the rat peritoneal macrophage. J Immunol 1985;135:1338-1341.

381. Galant SP, Durisetti L, Underwood S, Insel PA. Decreased beta-adrenergic receptors on polymorphonuclear leukocytes after adrenergic therapy. N Engl J Med 1978; 299:933–936.

382. Motulsky HJ, Insel PA. Adrenergic receptors in man. N Engl J Med 1982;307:18-29.

383. Spengler RN, Allen RM, Remick DG, Strieter RM, Kunkel SL. Stimulation of alpha-adrenergic receptor augments the production of macrophage-derived tumor necrosis factor. J Immunol 1990;145:1430-1434.

384. McPherson GA, Summers RJ. Characterization and localization of [3H]-clonidine binding in membranes prepared from guinea-pig spleen. Clin Exp Pharmacol Physiol 1982;9:77-87.

385. Titinchi S, Clark B. Alpha2-adrenoceptors in human lymphocytes: Direct characterisation by [3H]yohimbine binding. Biochem Biophys Res Commun 1984;121:1-7.

386. Aarons RD, Molinoff PB. Changes in the density of beta adrenergic receptors in rat lymphocytes, heart, and lung after chronic treatment with propranolol. J Pharmacol Exp Ther 1982;221:439-443.

387. Aarons RD, Nies AS, Gal J, Hegstrand LR, Molinoff PB. Elevation of β-adrenergic receptor density in human lymphocytes after propranolol administration. J Clin Invest 1980;65:949-957.

388. Aarons RD, Nies AS, Gerber JG, Molinoff PB. Decreased beta adrenergic receptor density on human lymphocytes after chronic treatment with agonists. J Pharmacol Exp Ther 1983;224:1-6.

389. Motulsky HJ, Cunningham EMS, Deblasi A, Insel PA. Desensitization and redistribution of β-adrenergic receptors on human mononuclear leukocytes. Am J Physiol 1986;250:E583-E590.

390. Carlson SL, Brooks WH, Roszman TL. Neurotransmitter-lymphocyte interactions: dual receptor modulation of lymphocyte proliferation and cAMP production. J Neuroimmunol 1989;24:155-162.

391. Fuchs BA, Campbell KS, Munson AE. Norepinephrine and serotonin content of the murine spleen: its relationship to lymphocyte β-adrenergic receptor density and the humoral immune response in vivo and in vitro. Cell Immunol 1988;117:339-351.

392. Radojcic T, Baird S, Darko D, Smith D, Bulloch K. Changes in β-adrenergic receptor distribution on immunocytes during differentiation: an analysis of T cells and macrophages. J Neurosci Res 1991;30:328–335.

393. Bach, MA. Differences in cyclic AMP changes after stimulation by prostaglandins and isoproterenol in lymphocyte subpopulations. J Clin Invest 1975;55:1074-1081.

394. Madden KS, Felten SY, Felten DL, Sundaresan PR, Livnat S. Sympathetic neural modulation of the immune system. I. Depression of T cell immunity in vivo and in vitro following chemical sympathectomy. Brain Behav Immun 1989;3:72-89.

395. Depelchin A, Letesson JJ. Adrenaline influence on the immune response. II. Its effects through action on the suppressor T-cells. Immunol Lett 1981;3:199-205.

396. Gader AMA. The effects of β adrenergic blockage on the responses of leukocyte counts to intravenous epinephrine in man. Scand J Haematol 1974;13:11-16.

397. Crary B, Borysenko M, Sutherland DC, Kutz I, Borysenko JZ, Benson H. Decreased in mitogen responsiveness of mononuclear cells from peripheral blood after epinephrine administration in humans. J Immunol 1983;130:694-697.

398. Crary B, Hauser SL, Borysenko M, et al. Epinephrine-induced

changes in the distribution of lymphocyte subsets in peripheral blood of humans. J Immunol 1983;131:1178-1181.

399. Ernström U, Sandberg G. Effects of adrenergic alpha- and beta-receptor stimulation on the release of lymphocytes and granulocytes from the spleen. Scand J Haematol 1973;11:275-286.

400. Ernström U, Söder O. Influence of adrenaline on the dissemination of antibody-producing cells from the spleen. Clin Exp Immunol 1975;21:131-140.

401. Madden KS, Felten SY, Felten DL, Hardy CA, Livnat S. Sympathetic nervous system modulation of the immune system. II. Induction of lymphocyte proliferation and migration in vivo by chemical sympathectomy. J Neuroimmunol 1994;49:67-75.

402. Madden KS, Moynihan JA, Brenner GJ, Felten SY, Felten DL, Livnat S. Sympathetic nervous system modulation of the immune system. III. Alterations in T and B cell proliferation and differentiation in vitro following chemical sympathectomy. J Neuroimmunol 1994;49: 77-87.

403. Livnat S, Madden KS, Felten DL, Felten SY. Regulation of the immune system by sympathetic neural mechanisms. Prog Neuropsychopharmacol Bio Psychiatry 1987; 11:145–152.

404. Livnat S, Felten SY, Carlson SL, Bellinger DL, Felten DL. Involvement of peripheral and central catecholamine systems in neural-immune interactions. J Neuroimmunol 1985;10:5-30.

405. Hall NR, McClure JE, Hu S-K, Tare NS, Seals CM, Goldstein AL. Effects of 6-hydroxydopamine upon primary and secondary thymus dependent immune responses. Immunopharmacology 1982;5: 39-48.

406. Kasashara K, Tanaka S, Ito R, Hamashima Y. Suppression of the primary immune response by chemical sympathectomy. Res Commun Chem Pathol Pharmacol 1977;16:687-693.

407. Miles K, Quintáns J, Chelmicka-Schorr E, Arnason BGW. The sympathetic nervous system modulates antibody response to thymus-independent antigens. J Neuroimmunol 1981;1:101-105.

408. Besedovsky HO, del Rey A, Sorkin E, Da Prada M, Keller HH. Immunoregulation mediated by the sympathetic nervous system. Cell Immunol 1979;48:346-355.

409. Cross RJ, Roszman TL. Central catecholamine depletion impairs in vivo immunity but not in vitro lymphocyte activation. J Neuroimmunol 1988;19:33-45.

410. Chelmicka-Schorr E, Checinski M, Arnason BGW. Chemical sympathectomy augments the severity of experimental allergic encephalomyelitis. J Neuroimmunol 1988;17:347-350.

411. Lorton D, Bellinger DL, Duclos M, Felten SY, Felten DL. Sympathectomy of lymph nodes exacerbates the expression of experimental arthritis. [Abstract] Soc Neurosci Abstr 1990;16:1210.

412. Levine JD, Coderre TJ, Helms C, Basbaum AI. β_2-Adrenergic mechanisms in experimental arthritis. Proc Natl Acad Sci 1988;85: 4553-4556.

413. Breneman SM, Moynihan JA, Grota LJ, Felten DL, Felten SY. Splenic norepinephrine is decreased in MRL-lpr/lpr mice. Brain Behav Immun 1993;7:135-143.

414. Bellinger DL, Felten SY, Felten DL. Noradrenergic sympathetic innervation of lymphoid organs during development, aging, and autoimmunity. Amenta F, ed. In: Aging of the autonomic nervous system. Boca Raton: CRC Press, 1993:243–284.

415. Hadden JW, Hadden EM, Middleton E Jr. Lymphocyte blast transformation. I. Demonstration of adrenergic receptors in human peripheral lymphocytes. Cell Immunol 1970; 1:583–595.

416. Watson J. The influence of intracellular levels of cyclic nucleotides on cell proliferation and the induction of antibody synthesis. J Exp Med 1975;141:97-111.

417. Goodwin JS, Messner RP, Williams RC Jr. Inhibitors of T-cell mitogenesis: effect of mitogen dose. Cell Immunol 1979;45:303-308.

418. Johnson DL, Ashmore RC, Gordon MA. Effects of beta-adrenergic agents on the murine lymphocyte response to mitogen stimulation. J Immunopharmacol 1981;3:205-219.

419. Melmon KL, Bourne HR, Weinstein Y, Shearer GM, Kram J, Bauminger S. Hemolytic plaque formation by leukocytes in vitro. Control by vasoactive hormones. J Clin Invest 1974;53:13-21.

420. Watson JR, Epstein R, Cohn M. Cyclic nucleotides as intracellular mediators of the expression of antigen-sensitive cells. Nature 1973; 246:405-409.

421. Strom TB, Carpenter CB, Garovoy MR, Austen KF, Merrill JP, Kaliner M. The modulating influence of cyclic nucleotides upon lymphocyte-mediated cytotoxicity. J Exp Med 1973;138:381-393.

422. Bourne HR, Lichtenstein LM, Melmon KL, Henney CS, Weinstein Y, Shearer GM. Modulation of inflammation and immunity by cyclic AMP. Science 1974;184:19-28.

423. Sanders VM, Munson AE. Kinetics of the enhancing effect produced by norepinephrine and terbutaline on the murine primary antibody response in vitro. J Pharmacol Exp Ther 1984;231:527-531.

424. Sanders VM, Munson AE. Beta adrenoceptor mediation of the enhancing effect of norepinephrine on the murine primary antibody response in vitro. J Pharmacol Exp Ther 1984;230:183-192.

425. Sanders VM, Munson AE. Role of alpha adrenoceptor activation in modulating the murine primary antibody response in vitro. J Pharmacol Exp Ther 1985;232:395-400.

426. Sanders VM, Powell-Oliver FE. β^2-adrenoceptor stimulation increases the number of antigen specific precursor B lymphocytes that differentiate into IgM-secreting cells without affecting burst size. J Immunol 1992;148: 1822-1828.

427. Hatfield SM, Petersen BH, DiMicco JA. Beta adrenoceptor modulation of the generation of murine cytotoxic T lymphocytes in vitro. J Pharmacol Exp Ther 1986;239:460–466.

428. Koff WC, Dunegan MA. Modulation of macrophage-mediated tumoricidal activity by neuropeptides and neurohormones. J Immunol 1985;135:350-354.

429. Koff WC, Dunegan MA. Neuroendocrine hormones suppress macrophage-mediated lysis of herpes simplex virus-infected cells. J Immunol 1986;136:705-709.

430. Severn A, Rapson NT, Hunter CA, and Liew FY. Regulation of tumor necrosis factor production by adrenaline and β-adrenergic agonists. J Immunol 1992;148:3441-3445.

431. Lappin D, Whaley K. Adrenergic receptors on monocytes modulate complement component synthesis. Clin Exp Immunol 1982;47: 606-612.

432. Katz P, Zaytoun AM, Fauci, AS. Mechanisms of human cell-mediated cytotoxicity. I. Modulation of natural killer cell activity by cyclic nucleotides. J Immunol 1982;129:287-296.

433. Hellstrand K, Hermodsson S, Strannegård Ö. Evidence for a β-adrenoceptor-mediated regulation of human natural killer cells. J Immunol 1985;134:4095-4099.

434. Roszman TL, Carlson SL. Neurotransmitters and molecular signaling in the immune response. In: Psychoneuroimmunology-II. Ader R, Felten DL, Cohen N, eds. New York: Academic Press, 1991. p. 311-335.

435. Kouassi E, Li YS, Boukhris W, Millet I. Revillard J-P. Opposite effects of the catecholamines dopamine and norepinephrine on murine polyclonal B-cell activation. Immunopharmacology 1988;16:125-137.

436. Li YS, Kouassi E, Revillard JP. Differential regulation of mouse β-cell activation of β-adrenoceptor stimulation depending on type of mitogens. Immunology 1990;69:367-372.

437. Besedovsky H, Sorkin, Felix D, Haas H. Hypothalamic changes during the immune response. Eur J Immunol 1977;7:323-325.

438. Carlson SL, Felten DL, Livnat S, Felten SY. Alterations of monoamines in specific central autonomic nuclei following immunization in mice. Brain Behav Immun 1987; 1:52–63.

439. Saphier D, Abramsky O, Mor G, Ovadia H. Multiunit electrical activity in conscious rats during an immune response. Brain Behav Immun 1987;1:40-51.

440. Dunn AJ. Systemic interleukin-1 administration stimulates hypothalamic norepinephrine metabolism parallelling the increased plasma corticosterone. Life Sci 1988;43:429-435.

441. Besedovsky HO, del Rey A, Sorkin E, Da Prada M, Burri R,

Honegger C. The immune response evokes changes in brain noradrenergic neurons. Science 1983;221:564-565.

442. Besedovsky HO, Sorkin E, Keller M, Müller J. Changes in blood hormone levels during the immune response. Proc Soc Exp Biol Med 1975;150:466-470.

443. Besedovsky HO, del Rey A, Sorkin E, Dinarello CA. Immunoregulatory feedback between interleukin-1 and glucocorticoid hormones. Science 1986;233:652-654.

444. Berkenbosch J, van Oers J, del Rey A, Tilders F, Besedovsky H. Corticotropin-releasing factor-producing neurons in the rat activated by interleukin-1. Science 1987;238:524-526.

445. Sapolsky R, Rivier C, Yamamoto G, Plotsky P, Vale W. Interleukin-1 stimulates the secretion of hypothalamic corticotropin-releasing factor. Science 1987;238:522-524.

446. Brown SL, Smith LR, Blalock JE. Interleukin 1 and interleukin 2 enhance proopiomelanocortin gene expression in pituitary cells. J Immunol 1987;139:3181-3183.

447. Woloski BMRNJ, Smith EM, Meyer WJ III, Fuller GM, Blalock JE. Corticotropin-releasing activity of monokines. Science 1985;230:1035-1037.

448. Bernton EW, Beach JE, Holaday JW, Smallridge RC, Fein HG. Release of multiple hormones by a direct action of interleukin-1 on pituitary cells. Science 1987;238:519-521.

449. Breder CD, Dinarello CA, Saper CB. Interleukin-1 immunoreactive innervation of the human hypothalamus. Science 1988;240:321-324.

450. Giulian D, Baker TJ, Shih LN, Lachman LB. Interleukin 1 of the central nervous system is produced by ameboid microglia. J Exp Med 1986;164:594–604.

451. Lieberman AP, Pitha PM, Shin HS, Shin ML. Production of tumor necrosis factor and other cytokines by astrocytes stimulated with lipopolysaccharide or a neurotropic virus. Proc Natl Acad Sci 1989;86:6348-6352.

452. del Rey A, Besedovsky HO, Sorkin E, Da Prada M, Arrenbrecht S. Immunoregulation mediated by the sympathetic nervous system. Cell Immunol 1981;63:329-334.

453. Carlson SL, Felten SY, Livnat S, Felten DL. Splenic norepinephrine turnover is increased during an immune response in mice. Soc.Neurosci.Abstr. 1987;13:380.(Abstract)

454. del Rey A, Besedovsky HO, Sorkin E, Da Prada M, Bondiolotti GP. Sympathetic immunoregulation: Difference between high- and low-responder animals. Am J Physiol 1982;242:R30-R33.

455. Niijima A, Hori T, Aou S, Oomura Y. The effects of interleukin-1β on the activity of adrenal, splenic and renal sympathetic nerves in the rat. J Autonom Nerv Syst 1991;36:183-192.

456. Akiyoshi M, Shimizu Y, Saito M. Interleukin-1 increases norepinephrine turnover in the spleen and lung in rats. Biochem Biophys Res Commun 1990;173:1266-1270.

457. Irwin M, Vale W, Britton KT. Central corticotropin-releasing factor suppresses natural killer cytotoxicity. Brain Behav Immun 1987;1:81-87.

458. Barbany G, Friedman WJ, Persson H. Lymphocyte-mediated regulation of neurotransmitter gene expression in rat sympathetic ganglia. J Neuroimmunol 1991;32:97-104.

11
DRUG THERAPY IN NEUROPSYCHIATRY

Barry S. Fogel

Although various psychotherapeutic, psychoeducational, environmental, and behavioral interventions may be useful in patients with neuropsychiatric disorders, the use of drugs acting on the central nervous system (CNS) is the cornerstone of therapy for most patients seen in practice. This chapter discusses ways in which drug therapy in neuropsychiatry is distinguished from general psychopharmacological practice. Advice is offered concerning the selection and monitoring of drug therapy for patients with neuropsychiatric disorders, including the decision to use drug treatment, the choice of target symptoms and syndromes, methods of monitoring treatment response and adverse effects, use of drug combinations, and concerns regarding side effects and drug interactions. Specific guidance is also provided for the use of antidepressants, neuroleptics, antianxiety drugs, stimulants, anti-Parkinson drugs, antiepileptic drugs, autonomic agents, and opiate antagonists. Discussion of clinical trials of drug therapy for specific conditions, however, is limited to illustration of general principles; further details are found in the chapters on each of the specific neuropsychiatric conditions.

DISTINCTIVE FEATURES OF DRUG THERAPY IN NEUROPSYCHIATRY

Limits of Diagnosis and the Need to Extrapolate from the Literature

In general psychopharmacology, the indications for drug treatment usually are (primary) mental disorders as defined in the American Psychiatric Association *Diagnostic and Statistical Manual* (1) or in the International Classification of Diseases (2). The efficacy of treatment for these conditions is established by randomized, controlled clinical trials (RCTs). For many standard psychopharmacological agents, such as the tricyclic antidepressants, literally hundreds of RCTs support efficacy for their principal indication — in this case, major depression (3). In contrast, the syndromes of mood and behavior due to gross brain diseases — though they have a special place in systems of diagnostic classification — may differ in important ways from the primary mental disorders that have been so intensively studied. Even when patients with a specific neurological disease have a syndrome that meets formal criteria for a common mental disorder such as major depression, RCTs specifically addressing drug efficacy for that disorder in that specific population are few, and the aggregate number of patients studied is small. Thus, for example, only three RCTs address the treatment of major depression following stroke (4; 4a): one studied nortriptyline, one studied trazodone, and one studied citalopram.

The limitations of the RCT literature place the clinician in the position of choosing therapy based on extrapolation from studies in which either the patients did not have exactly the same syndrome, or they did not suffer from the neurological disease that afflicts the current patient. When a clinician undertakes the treatment of a poststroke major depression using a selective serotonin reuptake inhibitor (SSRI), the empirical basis consists of studies of the efficacy of the SSRIs for major depression in patients without strokes, plus one RCT of an SSRI in poststroke depression that involves an agent, citalopram, not available in the U.S. (4a) (An additional trial of citalopram showed its utility for pathological crying after stroke [4b].)

Atypical and Subsyndromal Conditions

In general, patients with syndromes that do not meet criteria for established mental disorders do not necessarily have milder or less functionally significant problems. Criteria sets are chosen by consensus, with the aim of maximizing accuracy, not eliminating all false-negative classifications (5). The presence of brain disease adds another issue to the interpretation of syndromes that do not meet conventional criteria — the modification of the expression of psychopathology by brain dysfunction. Among the ways in which regional brain dysfunction modifies the symptomatic expression of mental disorders are: *(a)* producing indifference or shallowness of affect, as in frontal lobe or right-hemisphere dysfunction; *(b)* affecting the ability to organize a coherent account of symptoms, as with diffuse dysfunction or frontal system dysfunction; *(c)* producing apathy regarding one's condition, as with subcortical and basal ganglia dysfunction; and *(d)* affecting the expression of problems in spoken language, as when left-hemisphere dysfunction produces aphasia.

In patients with mental syndromes that do not meet consensus criteria for a major mental disorder, the clinical decision in favor of drug therapy is based on the severity, persistence, tolerability, and functional consequences of the symptoms. To this, an additional bias in favor of treatment is added if there is an obvious neurological deficit that would be expected to prevent expression of the full syndrome if it were present.

Major mental disorders in patients with neurological disease may represent either coincident diagnoses, or true secondary effects of the neurological disease itself. A history of a chronic, recurrent, or relapsing-remitting mental disorder similar to the current problem and preceding the onset of the neurological disease favors coincident diagnoses, as does a family history of a similar problem in a neurologically healthy first-degree relative. When a patient with a neurological disease has a coincident psychiatric diagnosis, a choice of therapy based on RCTs for the mental disorder in question involves less extrapolation, and can be made with greater confidence. A true secondary mental disorder, even if it comprises the same syndrome as a primary mental disorder, may have different biology and a different pattern of drug response. For example, secondary major depression in patients with significant medical illness may respond to lower doses of antidepressants than are usually necessary to treat primary major depression (6).

Behavioral Syndromes of Gross Brain Dysfunction

In addition to psychiatric syndromes and partial versions of such syndromes, neuropsychiatrists also apply drug therapy to symptoms and syndromes that are primarily found in populations with gross brain dysfunction. Such symptoms and syndromes, when they occur in connection with primary mental disorders, usually are seen as dimensions of illness, rather than as the objects of drug treatment in their own right. Such symptoms and syndromes include:

1. Affective instability or emotional lability;
2. Apathy or abulia;
3. Aggressive behavior—either spontaneous or reactive to provocation;
4. Irritability without overt aggression;
5. Impaired attention;
6. Disordered sleep;
7. Pain;
8. Involuntary movements;
9. Paroxysmal phenomena; and
10. Recurrent self-injurious behavior.

Obviously, patients may have these phenomena either in isolation or in connection with disturbances of cognition and mood. As a rule, if a symptom (e.g., apathy) is part of a major disorder (e.g., depression) the disorder will be treated. However, the symptom may become the focus of subsequent or concurrent treatment if it does not resolve with treatment of the accompanying polysymptomatic disorder. Thus, drug treatment is given for apathy that persists after successful treatment of depression, for aggressiveness that persists after successful treatment of a delusional disorder, and for sleep disturbance that persists after optimal remediation of the cognitive deficits of dementia.

Increased Sensitivity to CNS Side Effects of Drugs

Patients with gross brain disease are known to be more sensitive to CNS side effects of psychotropic drugs. Appropriate cautions are given to start with low dosages of drugs and slowly increase dosage, and if possible to avoid drugs known to have an especially high rate of CNS toxicity. When a drug is chosen, its specific CNS toxicities should be considered in relation to the patient's specific CNS vulnerabilities. Thus, when giving a benzodiazepine for anxiety, the major concern in a young epileptic would be effects on cognition; in an older person with cerebellar degeneration, the major concern would be the potential for falls. Medications given for incidental medical conditions that have high rates of CNS side effects should be eliminated or replaced whenever possible. CNS toxicity of drugs usually is greater if the patient is depressed, sedated, or otherwise underaroused. Successful treatment of depression facilitates the treatment of other neuropsychiatric conditions. Elimination of sedating drugs may improve the tolerability of other drugs. In the author's experience, the addition of a stimulant to a drug regimen can lead to a generalized improvement in CNS tolerability of the entire regimen, if the patient is underaroused or sedated prior to stimulant therapy.

Potential for Personality Change

Gross changes in brain structure or function have the potential to change a person's enduring patterns of social interaction. Such personality changes interact with the patient's premorbid personality. Premorbid traits may either disappear or become more intense. An example of the latter case is when a demanding, irritable person becomes physically agitated and violent in the early stages of a dementing illness. When premorbid traits are intensified by gross brain disease, drug therapy can be directed at the premorbid trait (7). In the given example, an SSRI might be administered to reduce the patient's constitutional irritability. If the behavioral manifestations of the trait had not been intensified by brain disease, it is unlikely that it would be treated with psychotropic drugs.

Frequency of Comorbid Medical Conditions

In addition to brain diseases and mental disorders, neuropsychiatric patients often have general medical diseases that are related to their neurological conditions as causes or consequences. Patients with cerebrovascular disease usually have hypertension; patients with debilitating conditions frequently develop infectious complications. Treatment of these general medical diseases must be compatible with the treatment of the patient's neurological and psychiatric problems. In addition to screening patients for the well-known pharmacokinetic interactions that now are summarized in electronic databases, this requires consideration of the CNS actions of the drugs given for the medical condition. For example, theophylline generally should not be used to treat bronchospasm in a person with epilepsy and an associated anxiety disorder, because of its proconvulsant and anxiogenic effects (8). CNS actions of general medical drugs can on occasion be exploited for neuropsychiatric benefit. Thus, patients with recurrent agitation who also have hypertension can be treated with agents such as propranolol that both lower blood pressure and may decrease the frequency and severity of agitation (9, 10).

Co-morbid endocrine disorders are of particular importance in neuropsychiatric patients because of the effect of hormones on central neurotransmission. When there is a relatively mild disorder of endocrine function, such as hypothalamic hypogonadism in a man with limbic epilepsy (11), or "subclinical" hypothyroidism with a normal thyroxine level and an elevated TSH (12), the neuropsychiatric bias is to offer treatment for the endocrine disorder. Experience suggests that interventions to normalize endocrine status facilitate the effectiveness of psychotropic drug treatment, even when they do not in themselves eliminate the patient's mental and behavioral symptoms.

A Broader Pharmacopeia

Neuropsychiatrists use the full range of traditional psychotropic drugs. In addition, they frequently use "neurological" drugs to modify behavior. Specific categories of neurological drugs widely used by neuropsychiatrists as psychotropics include antiepileptic drugs, anti-Parkinson drugs, agents that affect adrenergic function, and opiate agonists and antagonists. In contrast to general psychiatrists, neuropsychiatrists appear more likely to use these agents for behavioral indications before their efficacy has been established by RCTs. Thus, neuropsychiatrists widely used carbamazepine for mood stabilization for years before RCTs in bipolar disorder brought it into the general psychiatric mainstream.

Hypothesis-Driven Prescribing Versus Indication-Driven Prescribing

Indication-driven prescribing matches drugs with disorders for which RCTs have demonstrated drug efficacy. Hypothesis-driven prescribing begins with a hypothesis about the biochemical or physiological basis of the patient's symptoms or syndrome, and selects a drug with a mechanism of action relevant to the hypothesis. Because of the short-

comings of both classification systems and the literature of neuropsychiatric RCTs, neuropsychiatrists often must resort to hypothesis-driven prescribing. Prescription of drugs on this basis amounts to conducting an "N of 1" drug study (a clinical trial with a single subject). A poor response to the drug suggests, but does not prove, that the hypothesis is flawed.

As an example of hypothesis-based prescribing, consider the initial use of the opiate-receptor blocker naltrexone in the treatment of self-injurious behavior in a patient with severe mental retardation. The neuropsychiatric hypothesis is that self-inflicted pain releases endogenous opiates, which in turn reinforce the behavior (13). Initial successes with naltrexone led to RCTs (14, 15), which showed effectiveness for some autistic patients and an apparent adverse effect in patients with Rett's syndrome. The neuropsychiatrist who now prescribes naltrexone in this situation combines an indication-based approach with a hypothesis-based approach. If a particular patient does not respond, the neuropsychiatrist suspects that opiate-related mechanisms may not be the essential driver of the self-injurious behavior in the individual case.

Need for Combining Drug Therapy with Nonpharmacological Therapy

Like general psychiatric patients, neuropsychiatric patients often need a combination of drug therapy with nonpharmacological therapy to get a satisfactory outcome. In neuropsychiatry, there are important situations where appropriate drug therapy will have little benefit unless it is combined with environmental or behavioral intervention. These situations involve patients with major impairments in executive cognitive function, who are extremely responsive to immediate environmental contingencies because of their deficits in working memory and self-regulation (16). Drug therapy for such patients, beyond treating established psychiatric syndromes, aims to optimize patients' attention and arousal so that they can make use of whatever residual executive functions remain. However, if the optimal level of executive function attainable with drug therapy remains low, well-planned external contingencies will still be essential for behavioral management.

Presenting Neuropsychiatric Drug Therapy to Patients and Caregivers

Drug therapy in neuropsychiatry requires the consent and cooperation of the patient, or, if the patient is incompetent, the responsible caregiver or guardian. Obtaining consent and cooperation is based on explaining to the patient and/or caregiver the hypotheses on which the drug trial is based, the background from relevent RCTs or case series, the desired result of treatment, the expected risks, and how therapy will be monitored. When there is a reasonable choice of therapies, or several therapies to be tried in sequence until one is effective, the patient and/or caregiver should participate in the decision of which to try first.

The process of obtaining informed consent and eliciting cooperation has the same general features in neuropsychiatry as in other specialties, but the presentation tends to emphasize more of what is *not* known about the field, and the physician's reasons for recommending treatment that is not thoroughly established by RCTs. Patients or their caregivers sometimes fear that the patient will be treated as an experimental animal; an emphasis on the individualization of treatment, close monitoring, and the human situation that compels a trial of drug treatment will help to alleviate these fears.

DECISION TO USE DRUG THERAPY

The decision to use drug therapy in a neuropsychiatric patient is based on the traditional balancing of risks and benefits, taking into account the wishes of the patient and/or caregiver or guardian. With regard to expected benefits, considerations include: the results of RCTs addressing the syndrome from which the patient suffers, or those similar to it, the results described in case studies or case series in which the patients reported most closely resemble the patient being treated, the condition of the patient without drug treatment, and the likely natural history of the patient's symptoms or syndrome, drawn both from the literature and from the clinician's experience. The impact of the mental and behavioral symptoms or syndrome on the patient's everyday function is considered, and the likely functional consequences of improvement are estimated. Risk is estimated from the literature on the drug to be used, emphasizing literature in which the drug was used in a population sharing important clinical and demographic features with the patient to be treated. Risks of permanent injury are carefully distinguished from risks of temporary discomfort.

Before initiating drug therapy, the relevance and implementation of nonpharmacological therapies should be carefully reviewed, and general medical or environmental factors influencing the patient's mental or behavioral symptoms should be addressed. If the need for symptom control is urgent, drug therapy can be proposed in combination with efforts to modify environmental or general medical factors. Patients and caregivers should be aware that a holistic approach will be taken, and that drug therapy will not substitute for attention to general medical and environmental issues, or for psychotherapeutic and psychoeducational efforts.

CHOICE OF TARGET SYMPTOMS

Neuropsychiatric patients may present with well-recognized mental syndromes and disorders, such as major depression. When they do, drug therapy is directed at the disorder, rather than at a specific symptom. When a specific symptom, such as aggressiveness, is the impetus for drug therapy, it is first determined whether the aggressiveness is directly related to a mental disorder such as hypomania or a delusional disorder. If it is, the disorder is the focus of treatment. If it is not, the aggressiveness as such becomes the focus of treatment.

Even when a recognized mental disorder is the basis for selecting treatment, the symptoms should be identified that are most closely connected to the patient's distress and disability. These key symptoms may direct the choice of drug among equally reasonable alternatives, and form the basis of ancillary measures of treatment response.

MONITORING TREATMENT RESPONSE AND ADVERSE EFFECTS

Monitoring the drug therapy in neuropsychiatry is based on the principle that optimal therapy should improve the patient's function and well-being, as well as reducing or eliminating symptoms and signs that cause distress or concern to others. Thus, monitoring emphasizes a multidimensional approach that incorporates measures of function and measures of symptoms that are most distressing to the patient.

When patients are treated for recognized mental disorders, such as major depression or obsessive-compulsive disorder (OCD), a standard rating scale is used to monitor treatment response. The choice of rating scale takes into account any limitations the patient may have in self-reporting symptoms. Thus, when monitoring treatment for major depression in dementia, an observer-rated scale such as the Cornell Scale for Depression in Dementia (17) would be used, because a self-rated instrument like the Geriatric Depression Scale (18) is known to underestimate depressive symptoms in this situation (19).

Whether or not a disorder-specific scale is used, a determination is made regarding the symptom or syndrome causing the patient the greatest distress or disability. A scale is used to periodically measure the response of this symptom or syndrome to the drug treatment. For some syndromes, such as for aggression (20) and for apathy (21), well-validated multi-item scales are available. When no such scale is relevant, an alternative is to use a Visual Analogue Scale (22), or have the patient or caregivers rate the symptom on a scale of 1 to 10, with mutually agreed-upon anchor points. This latter approach has shown considerable value in monitoring the treatment of chronic pain (23) (see also Chapters 21 and 22 on chronic pain management).

In addition to measures of disorders, symptoms, and syndromes, patients should be periodically assessed for functional performance. In patients with more severe neurological impairment, this can be done with standard scales of physical activities of daily living and instrumental activities of daily living, such as those used regularly by occupational therapists (24). For less severely impaired outpatients, general-purpose self-rating questionnaires are available that measure the impact of illness on everyday physical and social activities. A popular choice is the SF-36, an instrument with 36 multiple choice questions about self-assessed health, mental health, and function (25).

Monitoring for adverse reactions is based on two lists of potential adverse effects: those that are uncommon but serious and require immediate action, and those that are common but not immediately dangerous. The patient and caregivers are informed of both kinds of potential problems, and are instructed to notify the physician immediately about problems of the first type. When specific monitoring of blood tests or other examinations are needed to evaluate the more serious type of adverse reaction, clear responsibility for these must be taken by one individual. Patients and caregivers are encouraged to tell the physician about less serious but common adverse reactions, and the more common ones are asked about systematically on each follow-up visit with the patient. When the patient is an outpatient who is seen infrequently, telephone follow-up should include a systematic review of common or potentially serious adverse reactions.

USE OF DRUG COMBINATIONS

There is a long tradition in general psychiatry of avoiding drug combinations, which has gradually yielded to scientific evidence on additive and synergistic therapeutic effects. Neurologists have come to accept the necessity of drug combinations for some cases of epilepsy (26) and for some cases of Parkinson's disease (27). Notwithstanding, "polypharmacy" continues to be viewed with suspicion by both consumers and providers, in part because of the greater complexity of monitoring multiple drug therapy, and the much greater incidence of drug interactions.

In a limited number of situations in neuropsychiatry, drug combinations are supported by well-designed RCTs of combined therapy. Studies of add-on therapy for poorly controlled epilepsy are an outstanding example (28, 29). In most cases, however, drug combinations are justified either by the presence of multiple coincident diseases, or by a hypothesis of multiple mechanisms contributing to the patient's mental or behavioral syndrome. In the former case, the justification for multiple drug therapy is clear, and the major precaution to be taken is checking a recent text or database for potential drug interactions. In the latter case, clarity regarding the hypothesis of multiple causation is the best way to prevent inappropriate prescribing. As an example, consider a patient with recent traumatic brain injury (TBI), a premorbid irritable personality, and a current syndrome of affective instability, emotional lability, and irritable outbursts. The working hypothesis is that the affective instability and emotional lability are consequences of diffuse cerebral injury, but that the irritability represents a premorbid personality trait. Initial treatment of the affective instability with a valproate reduces the patient's mood swings, but he remains irritable. A serotonin reuptake inhibitor is added, directed at the hypothesis of an underlying irritable temperament. A third type of rational polypharmacy is the application of two treatments that work on the same neurotransmitter system in different ways, as when levodopa-carbidopa and a direct dopamine agonist are combined in the treatment of advanced Parkinson's disease.

SIDE EFFECTS AND INTERACTIONS

Comprehensive treatment of drug side effects is beyond the scope of this chapter, as is a comprehensive review of all potentially relevant drug interactions. Neuropsychiatric patients often have general medical illnesses, and take multiple medications. The implications of these for choosing and monitoring psychotropic drugs are discussed in detail by Alan Stoudemire and the author in a series of analytic reviews (30–32). This chapter focuses specifically on neurological side effects of drugs, and on drug interactions that are either very common or illustrate a important principle of drug interaction.

ANTIDEPRESSANT DRUGS

Efficacy

The efficacy of antidepressant drugs is best established for the treatment of primary major depression, but a relatively small number of RCTs support their efficacy for major depression secondary to common neurological diseases. Successful trials have been reported for nortriptyline (32a), for citalopram (4a), and for trazodone (33) in the treatment of poststroke depression. Nortriptyline (33a), amitriptyline (33b), and citalopram (4a) have been shown to help pathologic crying after stroke. Reifler et al. (34) failed to find imipramine superior to placebo in the treatment of major depression associated with Alzheimer's disease, though numerous case series and uncontrolled studies suggest that usual antidepressant drug treatments are efficacious. Schiffer and Wineman (35) found desipramine superior to placebo in the treatment of major depression associated with multiple sclerosis. Four RCTs support the efficacy of tricyclic antidepressants for major depression associated with Parkinson's disease (36–39). The benefit of selegiline for depressed patients as well as for Parkinsonism per se is supported by a well-designed study by Allain et al. (39a). An open trial supported a combined antidepressant–antiparkinson effect of bupropion (39b). RCTs of antidepressants for major depression following traumatic brain injury, and of depression accompanying multi-infarct dementia, have not been carried out.

In contrast to the paucity of RCTs, there are numerous case reports, case series, and open trials suggesting that antidepressants of various classes will relieve symptoms of major depression in patients with common brain diseases. This uncontrolled literature does not support the choice of one antidepressant type over another in any specific neurological disease. Peyser and Folstein (40) observe in their review of depression in Huntington's disease that even though there is a known genetic lesion on chromosome 4 that underlies all cases, not all patients respond to the same antidepressant medication.

With regard to efficacy in primary nonmelancholic nondelusional major depression, there is reasonable consensus that all currently available antidepressants are of equivalent efficacy (41, 42). In cases of melancholia, tricyclic antidepressants and venlafaxine may be superior to the SSRIs, although the issue remains unresolved because there have been few direct comparative studies with severely ill patients (42–45). Delusional depression requires treatment with an antidepressant-neuroleptic combination or with electroconvulsive therapy (ECT).

Apart from major depression, the best established indication for antidepressants is the treatment of OCD. Here, clomipramine, fluoxetine, and fluvoxamine have proven efficacious by RCTs sufficient to satisfy the U.S. Food and Drug Administration.

Neuropsychiatric Applications Other Than Major Depression and OCD

In the past several years, a number of reports have appeared regarding the application of antidepressant drugs to neuropsychiatric problems other than major depression. These applications have included:

1. *Dysthymia in patients with mental retardation.* Jancar and Gunaratne (46) reported two cases of successful treatment with SSRIs and psychotherapy.
2. *Adult attention deficit disorders.* Wilens et al. (47) review several studies supporting the effectiveness of tricyclic antidepressants in some cases;
3. *Self-injurious behavior in developmentally disabled persons.* Case reports, summarized by Aman (48) suggest that SSRIs may inhibit this behavior. The evidence for their efficacy, however, lags behind the evidence supporting thioridazine, lithium, and naltrexone.
4. *Chronic fatigue syndrome and fibromyalgia.* Twelve double-blind studies, reviewed by Goodnick and Sandoval (49) support the efficacy of serotonergic antidepressants for pain relief in these conditions, and the efficacy of the catecholaminergic agents maprotiline and bupropion for depressive symptoms as such.
5. *Chronic nonmalignant pain.* A meta-analysis of 39 controlled studies of antidepressants suggested that the average chronic pain patient who received an antidepressant drug had less pain than 74% of comparison patients who received a placebo (50). The study suggested that antidepressants have analgesic effects. More recent articles continue to support the role of antidepressants as analgesics (51) (See chapters 21 and 22.)
6. *Miscellaneous disorders of impulse control.* Pathological gambling and certain sexual compulsions and paraphilias have been conceptualized as part of a continuum of obsessive-compulsive spectrum disorders that also include OCD itself and body dysmorphic disorder. These conditions may respond to treatment with SSRIs (52, 53).
7. *Emotional lability, including pathological laughing and crying, in patients with brain injury.* Fluoxetine and tricyclic antidepressants have both been shown effective for this symptom in case series (54, 55).
8. *Posttraumatic stress disorder (PTSD).* High-dose SSRIs were given for 8 weeks to PTSD patients by Sutherland and Davidson (56). They found improvement, especially in psychic numbing and avoidant behavior.
9. *Tourette's syndrome with attention deficits* Sweeney & Henry (57) reported efficacy of imipramine.

Neurotoxicity of Antidepressant Drugs

In choosing an antidepressant drug for a patient with gross brain disease, CNS toxicity of antidepressants will be a primary concern. Other aspects of antidepressant toxicity, such as cardiac toxicity of tricyclic antidepressants, are of course important, but are not discussed here. The reader is referred to the comprehensive reviews of Stoudemire et al. (30–32; 58) for detailed discussion of general medical issues in the choice of antidepressants.

The SSRIs, which have emerged as the antidepressants of first choice for most physicians (42, 59), rarely cause delirium or gross cognitive impairment. However, at high doses, they can produce an apathetic frontal lobe syndrome in some patients (60, 61). SSRIs also increase neuromuscular excitability, and can produce or aggravate tremor or myoclonus. Overt extrapyramidal disorders, such as akathisia and parkinsonism, occur more rarely, but have been seen in patients not exposed to neuroleptics either concurrently or in the past (62). Although the mechanism is not known for certain, SSRIs may produce extrapyramidal effects by indirect down-regulation of dopamine turnover by increased synaptic serotonin (63). Among the SSRIs fluoxetine is most likely to cause nervousness or restlessness. Although there is some question about whether this represents akathisia in all cases, it frequently requires dosage reduction or switching to a different SSRI. Finally, all of the SSRIs can cause headaches. In the author's experience, these headaches can either be of the tension type or of the vascular type. In some of the author's cases, these were relieved by adding 10–25 mg of doxepin at bedtime.

Tricyclic antidepressants, all of which have potent anticholinergic properties, can cause hallucinations or delirium, particularly in elderly patients and those with dementia. Like the SSRIs, they can cause or aggravate tremor or myoclonus, but, with the exception of the antidepressant-neuroleptic amoxapine, they are rarely associated with extrapyramidal reactions such as akathisia and acute dyskinesia (64). Tricyclic antidepressants have been associated with speech arrest, particularly at high dosages. They can have discrete effects on memory in the absence of delirium (65).

The monoamine oxidase inhibitors increase neuromuscular excitability. In usual dosages, they do not cause delirium, cognitive impairment, or extrapyramidal reactions.

Bupropion has the greatest propensity to induce seizures of all of the currently marketed antidepressants. In patients without neurological risk factors for seizures who are taking a full therapeutic dose, the risk is approximately 0.4%. Accordingly, patients with risk factors for seizures should be on a prophylactic antiepileptic drug if bupropion is to be prescribed. Bupropion is a stimulating antidepressant, and can produce agitation or a delirious psychosis in occasional vulnerable individuals (66).

Nefazodone has a relatively benign neurological side-effect profile. Sedation and ataxia are the most common limiting neurological side effects. However, nefazodone is a fairly weak antidepressant, and must be pushed to the upper end of its therapeutic range (i.e., 400–600 mg/day) to have equivalent efficacy to tricyclic antidepressants or conventional SSRIs (67). At this higher dosage, sedation and/or ataxia can pose significant problems in patients with preexisting brain disease. In one animal model, nefazodone significantly potentiates opioid analgesia (68). It is not known whether this is an applicable effect in humans at usual clinical dosage.

Venlafaxine has a neurological side-effect profile resembling that of the SSRIs. In addition, it is associated with hypertension: the rates are 3–5% on dosage less than 200 mg/day, 7% on dosage of 201–300 mg/day, and 13% on dosaes over 300 mg/day (69). Paroxysmal sweats, sometimes drenching the patient's bed or clothing, can also be seen. Cognitive side effects appear minimal.

Drug Interactions

Concern about drug interactions is greatest with the SSRIs and with nefazodone, which are potent inhibitors of the hepatic cytochrome P450 system. The inhibition of the cytochromes leads to clinically significant increases in drug levels when a drug is coadministered that is primarily metabolized by the isoenzyme that is inhibited. The SSRIs inhibit isoenzyme CYP2D6. This isoenzyme metabolizes the tricyclic antidepressants (TCAs) (70). It is well established that TCA levels are significantly higher in patients taking SSRIs concomitantly (70, 71). Levels of clozapine, the atypical neuroleptic, are raised by as much as an order of magnitude when the SSRI fluvoxamine is given concomitantly (72). Fluvoxamine inhibits several cytochrome isoenzymes; it has clinically significant effects to slow the metabolism and increase the blood level of TCAs, alprazolam, diazepam, theophylline, propranolol, warfarin, methadone, and carbamazepine (73). The size and clinical importance of pharmacokinetic interactions of other drugs with SSRIs depends in part on genetic polymorphism of CYP2D6; different alleles corresponding to different levels of metabolic activity are distributed in the general population (74). Nefazodone is a potent inhibitor of CYP3A4, the enzyme that metabolizes terfenadine and astemizole, as well as carbamazepine. Because of the risk of ventricular arrhythmia at high serum levels of terfenadine or astemizole, these drugs should not be used together with nefazodone. When given together with nefazodone, carbamazepine dosage should be reduced, and blood levels monitored frequently during dosage adjustments.

A particularly neuropsychiatric concern is the interaction of antidepressant drugs with antiepileptic drugs. The concurrent administration of an SSRI and carbamazepine may raise carbamazepine levels. The concurrent administration of carbamazepine, phenytoin, or primidone together with a TCA may lower tricyclic levels (74a, 74b). In general, when an antidepressant and an antiepileptic drug are given together, the level of the antiepileptic drug should be monitored frequently until a stable and therapeutic blood level is confirmed. TCA blood levels as well as carbamazepine levels should be monitored when combining the two drugs. The choice of desipramine or nortriptyline, which have meaningful blood levels and no significant active metabolites, facilitates this task.

Pharmacodynamic drug interactions involving antidepressant drugs usually are related to additive effects of the antidepressant and other drugs on neurotransmitter receptors, specifically α-adrenergic, serotonergic, and cholinergic receptors. Thus, hypotension can occur when tricyclic antidepressants or trazodone are combined with antihypertensive α-adrenergic blockers. The "serotonin syndrome" — a state of delirium, tremulous rigidity, and autonomic instability — can occur when an SSRI is combined with a monoamine oxidase inhibitor or with clomipramine. An anticholinergic delirium can occur when TCAs are combined with other drugs that have central anticholinergic effects, such as first-generation antihistamines.

Choice of Antidepressant in the Neuropsychiatric Patient

Table 11.1 summarizes some of the issues relevant to choosing and initiating antidepressant therapy in a neuropsychiatric patient.

The process of choosing an antidepressant begins by ruling out any that are contraindicated. In practical terms, this means rejecting tricyclic antidepressants for patients with heart block, and rejecting drugs to which the patient has shown a significant hypersensitivity reaction in the past.

The second step is to consider whether the patient has significant melancholic features, especially substantial weight loss and early morning awakening. Such patients may do better on a TCA or venlafaxine.

Next, the patient should be placed on a continuum between apathetic-retarded and agitated-anxious. Patients with significant agitation and anxiety are more likely to tolerate sertraline, paroxetine, or nefazodone than bupropion or fluoxetine, both of which are stimulating. Patients with apathy and retardation may benefit from the activating effects of bupropion or fluoxetine.

Among anxious patients, those with obsessions, compulsions, or premorbid obsessive-compulsive personality should receive SSRIs, with fluvoxamine an additional consideration. Those with predominant anxiety and insomnia might be treated with nefazodone. Patients with

Table 11.1. Issues Relevant to Choosing and Instituting an Antidepressant for Neuropsychiatric Patients

Drug	Benefits	Precautions	Relevant Controlled Trials	Initial Daily Dosage
Amitriptyline	Sedation, analgesia	Strongly anticholinergic; quinidine-like cardiac effects; orthostatic hypotension	Pathologic laughing and crying; post stroke depression; pain; headache	10-25 mg, usually given at bedtime
Nortriptyline	Meaningful blood levels; less hypotension, sedation, and anticholinergic effect than amitriptyline	Quinidine-like cardiac effects; anticholinergic effects	Pathologic laughing and crying; poststroke depression	10-25 mg, usually given at bedtime (target blood level 50-150 ng/ml)
Imipramine	Antipanic and antiphobic actions; less sedating than amitriptyline	Quinidine-like cardiac effects; orthostatic hypotension; anticholinergic effects	Depression in Parkinson's disease	10-25 mg
Desipramine	Least anticholinergic of tricyclic antidepressants; can be stimulating	Quinidine-like cardiac effects; orthostatic hypotension anticholinergic effects	Depression in multiple sclerosis; depression in Parkinson's disease	10-25 mg (target blood level >125 ng/ml).
Clomipramine	Potent antiobsessional effects	As for amitriptyline, plus myoclonus	None	12.5-25 mg
Protriptyline	Potent stimulant; alternative to direct stimulants	As for amitriptyline	None; case reports suggest utility as a stimulant in TBI patients	5 mg
Fluoxetine	Helpful for dysphoria and irritability; can be activating; effective for OCD at higher dosages	Akathisia, agitation, anxiety may appear on treatment initiation; apathy at very high doses: drug interactions due to P450 inhibition	None; numerous case series suggest efficacy for depression due to general medical diseases, including neurologic diseases	5-10 mg
Fluvoxamine	Specific for OCD	Potent enzyme inhibitor with significant drug interactions; sedation, myoclonus, GI side effects from hyperserotonergic state all possible	None	25-50 mg
Paroxetine	Less activating than fluoxetine; may cause less sedation and lower GI symptoms than sertraline; chief benefits are relief of dysphoria and irritability	Drug interactions from P450 inhibition; nausea; potential for sedation	None	5-10 mg
Sertraline	Helpful for dysphoria and irritability; may enhance executive cognitive function	Sedation, lower GI side effects; drug interactions from P450 inhibition	None	12.5-25 mg
Trazodone	Sedating and anxiolytic; may help agitation in dementia	Orthostatic hypotension, excessive sedation, priapism risk in men	Poststroke depression (improved rehabilitation outcome)	25 mg, usually at bedtime
Nefazodone	Anxiolytic, less sedating than trazodone; promotes sleep without disrupting sleep architecture	Sedation (orthostatic hypotension rare and priapism not seen); drug interactions due to inhibition of P450 3A4	None	50 mg at bedtime, or 50 b.i.d.
Bupropion	Stimulating, antiapathy, mildly antiparkinson, no cardiotoxicity	Risk of seizures, especially with single doses >150 mg or total daily dosage >450 mg; mild anticholinergic effects; insomnia; weight loss possible	Depression in Parkinson's disease (levodopa requirement reduced)	75 mg b.i.d.
Tranylcypromine	Stimulating, antiapathy, no cardiotoxicity, broad spectrum of antidepressant efficacy	Orthostatic hypotension, insomnia, risk of drug interactions or hypertensive crisis from tyramine rich foods	None; case series suggest utility in subcortical vascular dementia with apathetic depression	10 mg morning and noon
Phenelzine	Antianxiety and antiphobic effects; analgesic and antimigraine effects	As for tranylcypromine; more likely to be sedating; may cause major weight gain	Migraine	15 mg morning and noon
Selegiline	Well-tolerated; stimulating and antiparkinson effects	Risk of drug interactions or drug-food interactions with dose >10 mg/day; can cause nausea	Early Parkinson's disease—helps motor symptoms, mood, cognition	5 mg b.i.d.

compulsive behaviors such as paraphilias and compulsive gambling should be treated with SSRIs.

Monoamine oxidase inhibitors (MAOIs) generally should be regarded as second-line agents. Consideration of a MAOI as first-line therapy would be given for patients with severe phobic symptomatology, or with an active migraine problem in need of prophylaxis. Regarding the latter, phenelzine is a well-established agent for migraine prophylaxis.

Patients with a history of poor response to antidepressant drugs, with rapid cycling of mood induced by antidepressants, or with a mixture of depressive symptoms and paroxysmal symptoms typical of partial seizures, should not be initially treated with antidepressants. Instead, the first line treatment would be a mood-stabilizing antiepileptic drug such as carbamazepine (75).

Titration of Antidepressant Therapy

Starting dosages of antidepressants in patients with gross brain disease should be low enough to test the patient for unusual sensitivity to the drug. The author's recommended starting dosages are therefore below the manufacturer's recommended starting dosages. They are:

1. TCAs (excluding protriptyline): 10 mg q.h.s.;
2. Fluoxetine and paroxetine: 5 mg q.d.;
3. Sertraline: 25 mg q.d.;
4. Nefazodone: 50 mg q.h.s.;
5. Bupropion: 75 mg q.d.; and
6. MAOIs: tranylcypromine 10 mg qam and noon; phenelzine 15 mg b.i.d.
7. Protriptyline: 5 mg q.d.

If the patient tolerates the test dose of the drug, the daily dose may be increased every 2–3 days until limiting side effects develop, a conventional therapeutic dosage is reached, or, in the case of the secondary amine tricyclics, a therapeutic blood level is attained. Along the way, if the patient experiences significant improvement in symptoms, dosage is held at that level for at least a week. If the patient is continuing to improve, the dose is not increased further. If a plateau has been reached and there are persistent symptoms, dosage increases are resumed. The increment of dosage increase is approximately the same as the initial dose, with the proviso that bupropion and the MAOIs are given on a t.i.d. schedule and venlafaxine and nefazodone are given on a b.i.d. schedule.

Generally, a slow start is emphasized because of the greater vulnerability of neuropsychiatric patients to CNS side effects. But there will be some patients who, because of some combination of fast metabolism and pharmacodynamic insensitivity, will require dosages at the top of the recommended range for physically healthy patients, or even slightly beyond it. If a patient does not experience significant side effects from an SSRI, venlafaxine, nefazodone, or an MAOI, one may continue dosage increases to the following limits:

1. Fluoxetine and paroxetine: 80 mg per day;
2. Sertraline: 300 mg per day;
3. Nefazodone: 600 mg per day; and
4. MAOIs: tranylcypromine 90 mg per day; phenelzine 90 mg per day.

Bupropion is not raised beyond 450 mg per day (150 mg t.i.d.) because of an unacceptable risk of seizures at higher dosages. TCAs may on occasion be raised beyond 300 mg per day for desipramine or imipramine or 150 mg per day for nortriptyline. When this is done, a tricyclic serum level and an electrocardiogram (ECG) should be done to establish the safety of going to a higher dosage.

Duration of Therapy

When antidepressants are used to treat primary major depression, maximal treatment response takes 4–8 weeks. Therapy, if successful, is continued for at least 6 months at the dosage used to induce a remission of depression. It is not known whether these durations apply equally to major depression secondary to gross brain diseases. However, in the absence of other data, one should allow at least 4 weeks at full dosage (or maximum tolerated dosage) before determining that an antidepressant trial is unsuccessful. And, if a drug is helpful, treatment should be continued for several months at the remission-inducing dose before attempting to taper the dose of antidepressant.

ANTIPSYCHOTIC DRUGS

Efficacy

Antipsychotic drugs, or neuroleptics, have extremely well-established efficacy for the treatment of schizophrenia and of mood disorders with delusions. They have also been tested in numerous RCTs for pscyhotic symptoms and behavioral disturbances in dementia and in mental retardation. In patients with dementia, they have their most clear-cut benefit for delusions and hallucinations (76–78). When used to treat agitation without overt psychotic symptoms, they are superior to placebo, but less than half of patients treated will benefit (79). No particular antipsychotic drug has shown consistent superiority to any other in the treatment of psychotic complications of dementia. In mental retardation, RCTs have not shown consistent benefit of neuroleptics over placebo for behavioral disturbances in general, though low-dose neuroleptics have been shown to alleviate stereotypies in some small controlled studies (78, 79). Risperidone was recently shown to be superior to placebo for aberrant behavior in a group of 30 mentally retarded individuals (80).

The efficacy of haloperidol and of pimozide for reducing tics in Tourette's syndrome has been established by numerous clinical trials (81); with more than three-quarters of patients showing some benefit.

Haloperidol has been tested for efficacy in children with autism (pervasive developmental disorder), where it has been shown to reduce hyperactivity, stereotypies, and conduct problems (83, 84). However, the drug is associated with a high rate of dyskinesias—both acute dyskinesia and withdrawal dyskinesia—in this population (84).

Other Neuropsychiatric Indications

Substantial published experience, but not RCTs, support the use of neuroleptics for several common neuropsychiatric problems:

1. *The chorea of Huntington's disease.* Halpoperidol, perphenazine, and sulpiride have all been reported to be effective (85). Agitated behavior, hallucinations, and paranoia in patients with delirium. Lipowski (86), in his comprehensive synthesis of the literature on delirium, concluded that haloperidol was the drug of first choice for delirious agitation;
2. *Some cases of late-life delusional disorder.* However, there is general agreement that neuroleptics are less effective for delusional disorder than for schizophrenia (87);
3. *Psychosis in Parkinson's disease.* Clozapine is the only neuroleptic consistently reported to alleviate hallucinations and delusions in patients with treated Parkinson's disease, without aggravating the patients' movement disorder (88). Doses as low as 6.25 mg per day may provide substantial improvement. Risperidone, despite its lower rate of parkinsonian side effects in the schizophrenic population, nonetheless aggravates rigidity when given to patients with Parkinson's disease (88); and
4. *Obsessive-compulsive symptoms poorly responsive to SSRIs alone, and accompanied by tics or psychotic features* (89, 89a). In a controlled clinical trial, McDougle et al. (89b) showed that patients with obsessive-compulsive disorder and tics usually improved when haloperidol was added to fluvoxamine, but those without tics did so only occasionally.

In summary, the neuroleptics have their most consistent beneficial effects on positive symptoms of psychosis and on motor tics, chorea, and stereotypies. In addition, they appear to help a poorly defined subset of persons with agitation due to gross brain disease or cerebral metabolic dysfunction.

Neurotoxicity of Neuroleptics

Significant neurological toxicity is a feature of all of the neuroleptics, and their propensity to cause neurological side effects parallels their antipsychotic potency. The atypical neuroleptics, which include clozapine and risperidone, have fewer neurological side effects than the typical agents for an equivalent degree of antipsychotic efficacy.

Neurological toxicity of neuroleptics is divided into two kinds: *acute* toxicity, seen within days to weeks of drug administration, and *tardive* toxicity, which develops after more prolonged exposure and which may persist, even permanently, after drug discontinuation. Advanced age is a risk factor for two of the most common neuroleptic side effects—drug-induced parkinsonism and tardive dyskinesia.

Acute neurological toxicity includes parkinsonism, akathisia, dystonia (usually an axial dystonia), dyskinesia of the face or limbs, akinesia, and apathy. More rarely, patients can show extreme rigidity exceeding that typical of ordinary parkinsonism. One of the rigid conditions, neuroleptic-induced catatonia, may be prolonged but does not necessarily lead to dire systemic complications. The other, neuroleptic malignant syndrome, is a combination of tremulous rigidity, fever, delirium, autonomic instability, and rhabdomyolysis that has the potential for death due to renal failure, pneumonia, and shock.

Chronic neurological toxicity includes tardive dyskinesia, tardive dystonia, tardive akathisia, tardive dysmentia, and dopamine supersensitivity psychosis. Tardive dyskinesia characteristically involves the buccal, oral, and lingual muscles, but may also include choreoathetosis of the upper extremities or dyskinesia of the larynx and pharynx, leading to dysphagia and dysarthria. Tardive dystonia, like acute dystonia, is usually axial. Tardive akathisia resembles acute akathisia. Tardive dysmentia is a chronic disturbance of attention, concentration, and executive cognitive function that usually accompanies a tardive movement disorder. Dopamine supersensitivity psychosis is a state of agitation, confusion, and affective instability that emerges after neuroleptics are withdrawn after long-term use, and which is different from the psychosis that originally led to neuroleptic use (90).

All of the neuroleptic drugs also can cause or provoke seizures. However, neuroleptic-induced seizures are most common with the atypical agent clozapine, with which the incidence rate reaches 10% at doses of 900 mg per day or higher. Among the typical agents, chlorpromazine is the most likely to cause seizures. The agent least likely to cause seizures is not definitively established, although molindone and fluphenazine were least likely to produce seizure discharges in one *in vitro* model (91).

An extensive literature on risk factors for tardive dyskinesia, recently surveyed by Kane (91a), intermittently suggests that gross brain disease is a risk factor, but only advanced age and female sex have been established as risk factors beyond all doubt. Tardive dyskinesia in older patients is more likely to be irreversible. Regarding acute side effects, age is a risk factor for drug-induced parkinsonism.

Drug Interactions

The neuroleptics are metabolized by oxidative enzymes in the liver; specific cytochromes are responsible for the metabolism of each specific drug. There is substantial interindividual variability in drug metabolism (92–94). Most of the neuroleptic drugs have many active metabolites, complicating the interpretation of blood levels. Haloperidol is notable for not having significant active metabolites.

Pharmacokinetic interactions with neuroleptics are primarily related to effects of hepatic enzyme induction or inhibition on oxidative metabolism. Carbamazepine, a potent enzyme inducer, lowers blood levels of haloperidol. On the other hand, phenothiazine and thioxanthine neuroleptics can raise carbamazepine levels by inhibiting carbamazepine metabolism (94). As noted above, fluvoxamine raises the blood level of clozapine when the two drugs are given together; other SSRIs may have similar but weaker effects. It is not clear whether the enzyme inhibition associated with valproate reduces neuroleptic metabolism to a clinically significant degree.

However, in practice, pharmacodynamic interactions with the neuroleptics are far more common and clinically relevant. The principle is that neuroleptics, which block dopamine receptors, will have additive or synergistic effects when combined with drugs that reduce dopamine release or affect dopamine's interaction with second messengers. These additive or synergistic effects may either be therapeutic, toxic, or both. When they are toxic, one sees usual neuroleptic toxicity, or, in more severe cases, sedation or delirium. Drugs that interact in this way with neuroleptics include carbamazepine, lithium, and calcium channel blockers.

A second set of pharmacodynamic interactions, which may also be either beneficial or problematic, occurs between the neuroleptics and drugs that potentiate inhibition by the γ-aminobutyric acid (GABA) system, such as benzodiazepines and barbiturates. On the therapeutic side, tranquilizing effects may be enhanced, with less likelihood of tremor or akathisia. On the other hand, sedation, lethargy, quiet delirium, or apathy and akinesia may be more common.

Choice of Neuroleptic

Considerations relevant to the choice and initiation of neuroleptic therapy are presented in Table 11.2.

Prior to the availability of atypical agents, choosing a neuroleptic was primarily an issue of deciding among a high-potency, mid-potency, or low-potency agent, taking into account past experiences that a patient encountered with any specific drug. The high-potency agents, of which haloperidol is the prototype, have less sedating, anticholinergic, and hypotensive effects, but frequently cause extrapyramidal reactions, while the low-potency agents, of which thioridazine is the prototype, are associated with a lower incidence of extrapyramidal side effects (i.e., acute neurotoxicity). The mid-potency agents represent a compromise. Among mid-potency agents, molindone has the distinguishing characteristic of being the only neuroleptic that does not cause weight gain and actually causes a modest weight loss; it is also the neuroleptic with the least effect on nondopaminergic systems. Perphenazine may have an anxiolytic effect disproportionate to its antipsychotic effect.

Marked patient preferences for particular antipsychotic drugs may reflect patients' subjective experience of pharmacokinetic differences among drugs, or the relevance for them of a particular drug's effects on nondopamine systems. Such preferences are associated with better therapeutic outcomes and better adherence to treatment (95). Drugs of equal potency should not be presumed therapeutically equivalent for all patients.

The atypical agent risperidone is a high-potency D_2 receptor blocker that also has potent $5HT_2$ antagonist effects. Risperidone, particularly at doses of 6 mg per day or less, causes substantially less extrapyramidal side effects than haloperidol. Also, it probably causes less extrapyramidal side effects than therapeutically equivalent doses of thioridazine, although a head-to-head comparison has not been done. The most commonly encountered side effects are weight gain, sedation, orthostatic hypotension, and hyperprolactinemia.

The role of risperidone in the treatment of schizophrenia is evolving. Compared with typical agents, risperidone appears to have more effect on so-called "negative symptoms" (e.g., apathy, anhedonia, social disengagement) (96), and it also may relieve symptoms in patients unresponsive to typical agents. Because of its cost and the lack of availability of a parenteral preparation, it is not considered a first-line drug for schizophrenia.

Risperidone's relative lack of extrapyramidal side effects at lower dosages, combined with its high potency, make it an appealing antipsychotic drug for neuropsychiatric patients. Early, uncontrolled reports of its use in patients with dementia and psychotic features suggest it may be better tolerated than haloperidol, with at least equal efficacy.

Clozapine, the first atypical neuroleptic available in the United States, is a low-potency agent that is a relatively weak blocker of D_2 receptors, a significant blocker of D_3 and D_4 receptors, and a potent blocker of $5HT_2$ receptors. It has an extremely low rate of extrapyramidal side effects. When a movement disorder occurs, it usually consists of bradykinesia or mild akathisia, rather than rigidity or tremor (97). Clozapine can be given to patients with severe Parkinson's disease without aggravating their movement disorder, and may actually ameliorate tardive dyskinesia and tardive dystonia—not merely mask them (98, 99). Clozapine always alters the EEG, and it causes seizures at a rate that increases with dosage: the annual incidence is 1% at dosages below 300 mg/day, 2.7% at dosages from 300–599 mg/day, and 4.4% at dosages between 600–900 mg/day. It has many systemic side effects, including fever, hypotension, anticholinergic effects, weight gain, hypersalivation, and suppression of the bone marrow. Agranulocytosis occurs in approximately 1% of patients, requiring weekly monitoring of blood counts and immediate discontinuation of the drug if the white blood count falls below 3000/mm^3.

In the treatment of schizophrenia, clozapine is effective in more than one-third of patients who are unresponsive to typical neuroleptics. Also, clozapine is more effective than typical agents for relieving negative symptoms, and may alleviate some of the cognitive impairments associated with chronic schizophrenia. At present, a trial of clozapine is indicated for all patients with schizophrenia who fail to respond to a typical neuroleptic and to risperidone. It has not

Table 11.2. Issues Relevant to Choosing and Initiating a Neuroleptic in Neuropsychiatric Patients

Drug	Initial Dose (in mg)	Usual Max.	Motor	Anticholinergic	Hypotensive	Sedative	Special Benefits	Special Concerns
Haloperidol	0.5-1.0	5-10	+++	+	±	+	Can give IV; depot form; cardiac safety	Frequent extrapyramidal effects, some malignant
Fluphenazine	0.5-1.0	5-10	+++	+	±	+	Depot form; least effect on seizures	Same as haloperidol
Thiothixene	1.0-2.0	10	++	+	±	+	Somewhat less motor effect than haloperidol	
Perphenazine	2-4	16-24	++	++	±	++	Anti-anxiety effect; combines well with TCA for psychotic depression	Drug interaction: Raises TCA blood levels
Molindone	5-10	50-100	++	0	0	+	Lack of systemic side effects; does not cause weight gain	No IM preparation available; not sedative; poor choice for behavioral crises
Chlorpromazine	10-25	100	+	+++	+++	+++	Marked sedation may be useful in crises; good antiemetic	Systemic side effects risky in frail elders; causes seizures
Thioridazine	10-25	100-150	+	+++	++	++	Lowest motor effect of "typical" anti-psychotics	Strong quinidine like effects on heart; lack of IM preparation
Mesoridazine	10-25	100	+	+++	++	++	Like thioridazine, but available IM	Like thioridazine
Risperidone	0.25-0.5	4-6	±	±	+	++	Rare motor side effects at low doses	High cost; hypotension, especially if dose raised quickly; no IM prep.
Clozapine	12.5-25	200	0	+++	+	+++	Virtually no motor side effects; drug of choice in patients with Parkinson's and psychosis	Weekly blood counts required; many systemic side effects; may cause seizures

been established whether it is beneficial to routinely attempt to switch clozapine responders to risperidone because of the latter's lesser systemic toxicity. A related issue of specifically neuropsychiatric interest is whether a person with schizophrenia who has good control of positive symptoms on a typical agent, but who has negative symptoms and cognitive impairment, should have a trial of an atypical neuroleptic in the hope of improving motivation and cognition (100). Neuropsychiatrists, with a tradition of attending to cognitive and motivational deficits in patients with brain diseases, may favor an aggressive position toward trials of atypical neuroleptics in this situation, particularly if the cognitive and motivational symptoms are causing distress to the patient, or are producing functional disability.

When choosing a neuroleptic for neuropsychiatric indications, the following guidelines may be useful:

1. In acute behavioral emergencies where a neuroleptic is to be used for short-term stabilization or "chemical restraint," haloperidol is the best established agent. When it cannot be given orally, it may be given by either the intramuscular or intravenous route; the intravenous route, while not FDA-approved, offers the advantage of not causing muscle damage that might later obscure the interpretation of a creatine phosphokinase (CPK) level. Dosage is titrated in increments every hour, with increments of 0.5–2 mg for fragile patients, and 5–10 mg for patients who are physically robust. A combination of haloperidol with lorazepam (0.5–1 mg for fragile patients; 2 mg for robust patients) gives a more rapid behavioral response and may prevent some acute extrapyramidal symptoms.

2. When the patient's primary problem appears to be overwhelming anxiety with some psychotic features such as mild paranoia or disorganization, the patient may be treated with a sedative neuroleptic such as thioridazine or perphenazine. Typical starting dosages of thioridazine would be 10 mg t.i.d. for fragile patients and 25 mg t.i.d. for more robust patients; dosage is increased as tolerated, with sedation, hypotension, and anticholinergic effects usually the limiting factors. Perphenazine can be used similarly; this midrange agent presents fewer problems with sedation, hypotension, and anticholinergic effects but is more likely to cause acute extrapyramidal effects. Starting dosage would be 2 mg b.i.d. at the lower end and 4 mg t.i.d. at the higher end.

3. For psychotic phenomena such as delusions and hallucinations in persons with gross brain disease—who do not present a behavioral emergency—risperidone is an appealing first choice because of its low rate of motor side effects. However, it can cause substantial sedation at first, so the dose should be built up slowly. Starting doses range from 0.5 mg at bedtime to 1.0 mg b.i.d. in a more severely disturbed yet physically robust person. Dosage is increased if necessary and as tolerated to 3 mg, b.i.d. Above this level, risperidone's distinctive lack of extrapyramidal side effects is less evident, and the use of a high-potency or mid-potency typical agent should be considered, because of the lower cost and lesser sedation.

As mentioned earlier, clozapine is the drug of choice for psychosis in Parkinson's disease. Risperidone has not proved to be a good alternative, because it aggravates the movement disorder even at low dosage. Clozapine is probably the best currently-available drug for treating psychosis in patients with system degenerations with parkinsonian features (101).

Titration of Antipsychotic Drug Therapy

Titration of neuroleptic treatment in neuropsychiatric patients comprises several issues: dosage increase in emergent and nonemergent situations; dosage reduction when behavior or symptoms have stabilized; the use of adjuncts to minimize neuroleptic dose; and the use of anti-Parkinson drugs. Particularly in the neuropsychiatric population, there are essentially no comparative studies of dosage titration strategies, so what follows must be regarded only as informed opinion. However, dosage strategy should take into account that neuroleptics alter behavior first, affect second, and thought and perception last, and that the full effect of a given dose on thought and perception may take several weeks.

In the emergency situation, a neuroleptic (typically haloperidol) is given every hour until the patient's behavior is manageable. Then, the total dose used to stabilize the patient is repeated every 24 hours, usually in divided doses. Doses are reduced or withheld if the patient appears excessively sedated. Once the neurological, medical, or psychiatric condition underlying the behavioral emergency is diagnosed and treatment is under way, neuroleptics should be tapered. If the patient has a psychotic disorder and will need longer-term neuroleptic therapy, the taper should aim for a typical long-term maintenance dose within 2 weeks. If the patient has a transient psychosis due to an underlying medical condition that is resolved, the neuroleptic should be tapered and discontinued over 1 week. If problematic behavioral symptoms recur, the dosage should be raised to the lowest dosage that controlled the symptoms, and withdrawal should be reattempted in another week.

When a neuroleptic is to be used for a nonemergent indication, the therapeutic dosage is approached from below rather than from above. Dosage is increased weekly until behavioral symptoms are clearly improved; the dosage is then kept at that level for another month to assess its effect on thought disorder before considering further dosage increases.

Frequently, neuroleptics will suppress specifically psychotic symptoms such as hallucinations and delusions, while leaving the patient with residual symptoms such as affective instability, irritability, anxiety, or intermittent explosive behavior. Because neuroleptics are the most neurotoxic of the psychotropic classes, it is generally preferable to use adjunctive drugs to treat these symptoms rather than to raise neuroleptic dosage in an effort to control them. Preferred options include mood-stabilizing antiepileptic drugs or lithium for affective instability; SSRIs or buspirone for irritability; SSRIs, buspirone, or benzodiazepines for anxiety, and mood-stabilizing antiepileptic drugs, propranolol, or clonidine for intermittent explosive behavior.

Neuropsychiatric patients may be more likely than general psychiatric patients to develop extrapyramidal reactions to neuroleptics, and may be more likely to suffer significant functional impairment as a consequence of those reactions. For example, an aged stroke patient is at increased risk for parkinsonism and tardive dyskinesia because of age, and the effects of a movement disorder on mobility and activities of daily living (ADL) performance will add to the effects of the stroke itself. For this reason, special efforts are warranted to identify extrapyramidal reactions early, and to treat them effectively.

When extrapyramidal reactions occur, the first consideration is whether dosage reduction or a switch to risperidone is reasonable in the given patient. If these measures are not feasible, or have been done, drug treatment of the reaction comes next (102). First-line drugs for treatment of extrapyramidal reactions are benztropine or trihexyphenidyl for tremor, acute dystonia, or acute dyskinesia, amantadine or bromocriptine for rigidity and akinesia, and propranolol for akathisia. There is substantial interindividual variability in response to the anti-Parkinson drugs for pharmacokinetic reasons alone. Typical starting dosages are: benztropine 2 mg bid-qid; trihexyphenidyl 5 mg b.i.d.-q.i.d., amantadine 100 mg b.i.d.-t.i.d.; bromocriptine 2.5 mg q.d.-b.i.d., and propranolol 20 mg t.i.d. Fragile patients should begin at approximately half of the usual dose. Rapid upward dosage titration should be carried out until symptoms are relieved. Usual maximum doses are benztropine 10 mg per day, trihexyphenidyl 20 mg per day, amantadine 300 mg per day, bromocriptine 30 mg per day, and propranolol 360 mg per day. If maximal dosage is reached with persistent extrapyramidal symptoms, either the neuroleptic or its dosage should be changed, or a different anti-Parkinson agent should be used.

Duration of Therapy

The duration of neuroleptic therapy depends on the indication for which the drug is used. Strategy for dosage reduction in schizophrenia is beyond the scope of this chapter. When neuroleptics are used for psychotic symptoms or for severe agitation in patients with dementia or with gross brain disease, periodic efforts at drug discontinuation are warranted because changes in the brain and in the patient's situation over time may have removed the necessity for neuroleptic use. A reasonable approach is to attempt a taper after the patient has had stable behavior or well-controlled psychotic symptoms for 3 months. The drug should then be tapered over the next 3 months, with an interruption of the taper if clinically significant symptoms recur.

Patients with chronic neuropsychiatric disorders may present for neuropsychiatric attention on neuroleptic therapy of uncertain duration, for which the original indications are unclear. In this situation, vigorous detective work is warranted to determine preneuroleptic mental status and whether the indications for the drug were sound. If it cannot be determined that the patient is receiving neuroleptics for an appropriate indication, a gradual taper should be attempted over no less than 3 months. The value of withdrawing unnecessary neuroleptics is illustrated by a recent study of Thapa et al. in elderly nursing home residents (103), in which withdrawal of neuroleptics prescribed for questionable indications did not increase behavior problems, but led to a highly significant improvement in patients' affect. Excessively rapid tapering of neuroleptics can cause somatic withdrawal symptoms, especially anorexia and weight loss. Also, patients may show a mental disorder characterized by confusion, agitation, and affective instability without the thought disorder typical of schizophrenia. This "dopamine supersensitivity psychosis" can be treated with mood-stabilizing antiepileptic drugs. The rate of tapering of the neuroleptic should be slowed, but the effort to discontinue the neuroleptic should not be abandoned unless a convincing indication for its use can be established.

ANTIANXIETY DRUGS

The category of antianxiety drugs reviewed in this section comprises the benzodiazepines and the $5HT_{1A}$ partial agonist drug buspirone. However, many other classes of drugs have been used to treat specific anxiety disorders. The SSRIs are the drugs of choice of OCD, and numerous antidepressants have been effective for treating recurrent panic attacks. The more sedating neuroleptics may be the drugs of choice for anxiety associated with paranoid phenomena and disorganized thinking. Anxiety due to hypomania is appropriately treated with lithium or a mood-stabilizing antiepileptic drug. The unique role of "antianxiety drugs" is in the acute, short-term treatment of anxiety, panic, and insomnia. Antianxiety drugs are also used for the treatment of generalized anxiety disorder and chronic anxious traits. Antidepressants are an acceptable alternative therapy for many of these patients.

Efficacy

The efficacy of benzodiazepines for symptoms of anxiety, and for insomnia, has been established by hundreds of RCTs conducted in patients without significant neurological disease (104, 105). The benzodiazepines are especially effective for autonomic symptoms of anxiety, and for hypervigilance. Buspirone is more effective than placebo for symptoms of generalized anxiety, but is less consistently effective than the benzodiazepines (106). It may be more effective than benzodiazepines for cognitive symptoms and less for hypervigilance and autonomic arousal. It does not block panic attacks, and it does not have a direct hypnotic effect, although it can sometimes improve sleep through relieving anxiety.

Although there are no RCTs specifically confirming the antianxiety effects of benzodiazepines or buspirone in neurologically ill populations, there is general consensus among clinicians that benzodiazepines are therapeutically effective for anxiety in patients with gross brain disease. Concerns about the use of benzodiazepines in neuropsychiatric populations center around side effects rather than efficacy.

Other Neuropsychiatric Indications

Clonazepam is an established antiepileptic drug. It is discussed in more detail in the section on antiepileptic drugs. Benzodiazepines have been used effectively for the following additional indications:

1. *Myoclonus, including nocturnal myoclonus.* Clonazepam is the benzodiazepine of choice (107, 107a, 107b). It also can be used to suppress myoclonus associated with antidepressants;
2. *Parasomnia associated with slow-wave sleep.* These can be alleviated by any of the benzodiazepines, which suppress stage 4 sleep;
3. *Rapid behavioral stabilization of acutely agitated patients.* The combination of a short-acting benzodiazepine such as lorazepam, with a neuroleptic such as haloperidol, is more effective and safer than single-drug neuroleptic therapy. The combination of midazolam and droperidol has been used at some institutions; and
4. *Catatonia.* Both lorazepam and diazepam have been reported to reverse the motor manifestations of catatonia without affecting the underlying disorder of thinking or mood.

Benzodiazepines generally are not used in the treatment of aggressive or self-injurious behavior, because they may disinhibit behavior, and such disinhibition may occur unpredictably. Buspirone has been efficacious for such problems. Neuropsychiatric indications for buspirone supported by recent uncontrolled experience include:

1. *Self-injurious behavior in some adults with mental retardation.* A modest reduction was seen with an average of 30 mg per day of buspirone (108);
2. *Agitated and impulsive behavior in patients with "organic" mental syndromes.* Partial response of this behavior has been reported (109, 110);
3. *Tardive dyskinesia.* Relatively high doses, up to 180 mg per day, partially relieved dyskinesia in five of seven patients in an open study (111); and
4. *Hostility and irritable "type A" behavior.* Buspirone treatment was associated with decreased hostility, impatience, and anxiety in an 8-week open trial of therapy in 10 men with coronary artery disease and no psychiatric diagnosis (112).

Neurological Toxicity

The neurological side effects of the benzodiazepines are directly related to their effect on the benzodiazepine receptor to facilitate GABA-related inhibitory neurotransmission. They include cognitive impairment, memory impairment, decreased alertness, and impaired coordination. The more severe forms of these side effects include confusion, amnesia, lethargy, apathy, or somnolence, ataxia, and falls. These neurological side effects are more likely to occur in elderly patients (113).

The neurological side effects of buspirone are less predictable. Both insomnia and sedation can occur, but most patients do not have measurable cognitive impairment at usual doses. Akathisia and dyskinesia have been reported as rare occurrences; the mechanism of these movement disorders is not known.

Drug Interactions

The benzodiazepines subdivide into two groups according to their metabolism: some are metabolized by hepatic oxidation; others are conjugated with glucuronide and are eliminated by the kidney. The benzodiazepines that are oxidized are more often involved in pharmacokinetic interactions, because any drug that inhibits the relevant hepatic oxidative enzymes can raise benzodiazepine levels and prolong the drug's half-life. Likewise, agents that induce hepatic oxidative enzymes can reduce blood levels of these benzodiazepines and shorten their effective duration of action. Diazepam, chloridazepoxide, alprazolam, and clonazepam all undergo oxidative metabolism; oxazepam and lorazepam do not. Common drugs that induce benzodiazepine metabolism include theophylline and carbamazepine, with clinically significant effects of the latter drug on the metabolism of alprazolam (114a, 115) and clonazepam (114b). Common drugs that inhibit benzodiazepine metabolism include valproate, SSRIs, nefazodone, erythromycin, and cimetidine.

Choice of Antianxiety Drug

After determining that a patient should be treated with an antianxiety drug, rather than a drug of another class, the first decision is whether to use buspirone or a benzodiazepine. Buspirone is most likely to be helpful when the indication is either generalized anxiety disorder, chronic anxiety traits and symptoms falling short of diagnostic criteria for generalized anxiety disorder, or chronic tension-irritability. It tends to work best in patients who either never have used benzodiazepines or who do not like benzodiazepines. Patients rarely experience buspirone as a satisfactory substitute for chronic benzodiazepine therapy if they found such therapy helpful and well tolerated.

Benzodiazepines are the drugs of first choice in situations of acute anxiety or panic and in situations where a specific benzodiazepine effect such as an antiepileptic action is desired. For some indications, e.g., myoclonic epilepsy, only one benzodiazepine is known to be efficacious. For others, such as panic attacks or generalized anxiety, there is a choice of many agents. Choice of drug in the latter case can be guided by these principles:

1. Patients on a complex, multiple-drug regimen usually should be given a benzodiazepine that is eliminated by the kidney, does not require extensive oxidative metabolism, and does not have active metabolites. Oxazepam is the paradigm for such a drug.

2. Patients who have panic attacks are more likely to respond to alprazolam or clonazepam than to other benzodiazepines. Alprazolam, with a relatively short duration of action, is more likely to cause problems with rebound anxiety or interdose anxiety than clonazepam. Therefore, clonazepam usually is preferable. However, clonazepam does cause more sedation and ataxia, so alprazolam would be preferable for patients with unsteady gait or apathy at baseline.

3. When benzodiazepines are to be used for treating insomnia, the important distinction is between use for a day or two and use for a week or more. For very short-term use, long-acting drugs such as flurazepam or quazepam offer the advantage of minimal rebound insomnia after the drug is stopped, and their propensity to accumulate is not relevant. When a drug is to be used for a week or more, accumulation is a problem for the longer-acting drugs, and a drug with a medium half-life, such as temazepam, would be a better choice. The ultrashort-acting drug triazolam is not advisable in the neuropsychiatric population. Although the issue remains controversial, it may have slightly more behavioral toxicity than the other hypnotic agents.

Dosage Titration

Dosage titration for buspirone must deal with the wide interindividual variability in first-pass metabolism for this drug. For some patients, 5 mg t.i.d. is an adequate dose; for others, 20 t.i.d. will have little effect. Excessively high blood levels of buspirone give patients unpleasant side effects such as nausea, dizziness, and tinnitus. Accordingly, patients should be started on 2.5 mg b.i.d. to t.i.d. if they are fragile and 5 mg t.i.d. if they are not, and then, if there are neither therapeutic effects nor side effects, the dose should be raised every 2–3 days until the patient gets relief, develops a limiting side effect, or a dose of 20 mg t.i.d. is reached. Increments are 2.5–5 mg at a time in fragile patients and 5–10 mg at a time in healthier patients. Once limiting side effects have been reached, dosage should be reduced to the highest level that does not cause unpleasant side effects, and kept there for 3–4 weeks. If a patient reaches 20 mg t.i.d. without side effects but without benefit, the dose should be maintained for 2 weeks. If there is still no effect, the dosage may be raised to 30 mg t.i.d. for an additional 2 weeks.

When short-acting benzodiazepines are used, patients are started on one-half of the manufacturer's recommended dosage, given as divided doses according to the manufacturer's recommendation. Every other day, the dose can be raised until the patient gets relief or limiting side effects develop. When long-acting agents are used, 2 weeks should be allowed between dosage increases. If necessary, as-needed doses of a shorter-acting agent can be used to alleviate severe symptoms during the titration period.

During upward dosage titration of benzodiazepines, the patient should be checked periodically for effects of the drug on gait and coordination, alertness, and memory. Patients without insight, or with a history of drug misuse, should be tested directly for side effects; the clinician should not rely only on the patient's self-reports.

When patients on long-term benzodiazepine therapy develop brain diseases, they may become intolerant to their usual benzodiazepine dosage, and show side effects, most often decreased alertness, memory disturbance, or impaired gait or coordination. Under such circumstances, a slow withdrawal of benzodiazepines is indicated. Dosage should be reduced by no more than 10% per week, unless the clinical situation is urgent. If the patient is known to have an underlying anxiety disorder, alternative therapy for that anxiety disorder should be initiated during the benzodiazepine taper, before severe symptoms break through.

Duration of Therapy

Anxiety disorders can have either a relapsing-remitting or a chronic course. Once it is established that a patient has a chronic course, he or she can be kept on antianxiety drugs indefinitely, as long as there are few or no side effects. If the patient's course is unknown, or the patient has never had a trial off medication since it was started, gradual withdrawal of medication may be attempted 3–6 months after the patient is free of major symptoms of the anxiety disorder. Buspirone should be tapered over about 1 month; benzodiazepines over 2–3 months. Benzodiazepine tapering usually is easier with longer-acting agents, and crossover from short- to long-acting benzodiazepines should be considered if the patient is on a short-acting agent. If anxiety symptoms emerge during the taper, nonpharmacological treatment should be provided. Ideally, such treatment would precede an effort to taper a patient off benzodiazepine therapy. If an unacceptable level of symptoms recur, dosage should be restored to the minimum that controls the symptoms, and a taper should be reattempted in another 3–6 months. Nonpharmacological therapy should be offered in the interim. A patient who fails three well-implemented attempts to taper antianxiety drugs probably has a chronic condition. Alternate drug therapy, such as antidepressants, should be considered if there is a problem with the use of benzodiazepines in the individual patient.

LITHIUM

Lithium, a simple monovalent cation, has an impressive range of effects on neurochemical processes in the brain.

Among these are: enhancement of serotonergic neurotransmission, at least at some subtypes of serotonergic synapses; prevention of dopamine receptor supersensitivity induced by receptor blockade; facilitation of norepinephrine release; reduction of the adenylate cyclase response to β-adrenergic stimulation; stimulation of acetylcholine synthesis and release; and prevention of up-regulation of muscarinic receptors in response to chronic blockade. Lithium also affects neurochemical signal transduction through effects on phosphoinositide turnover, adenylate cyclase activity, G proteins, and protein kinase C (116). This broad range of pharmacodynamic actions is the basis of lithium's applicability to several different neuropsychiatric disorders, and may be the basis of pharmacodynamic interactions between lithium and other CNS drugs.

Efficacy

Lithium has been shown by RCTs to be an effective agent for acute mania in 70–80% of manic patients. Well-designed, double-blind studies have shown it to prevent relapses in about two-thirds of bipolar patients (116). RCTs have not been extended to the population of patients with mania secondary to gross brain diseases, e.g., right-hemisphere stroke.

Substantial literature, albeit with fewer RCTs, supports the use of lithium for augmentation of antidepressants in major depression, and combined use with neuroleptics in the treatment of schizoaffective disorder (118).

Other Neuropsychiatric Indications

TREATMENT OF IMPULSIVE AGGRESSION

For over 20 years, reports with varying levels of rigor have supported an antiaggressive effect of lithium at blood levels similar to those used to treat bipolar disorder (118, 119). Studies and case reports have been conducted mainly with institutionalized populations, including people with mental retardation (119, 120), hospitalized children with conduct disorder (121), prison inmates (122), and a patient recovering from a severe traumatic brain injury (123).

SELF-INJURIOUS BEHAVIOR

Self-injurious behavior (SIB) in people with mental retardation has been treated successfully with lithium (124). A chart review study examining 3 months of care before and after institution of lithium therapy in 11 mentally retarded patients showed a significant reduction in episodes of SIB in the treated period.

HUNTINGTON'S DISEASE

Irritability and aggression in patients with Huntington's disease have also been reduced by lithium. Reports suggest that lithium may improve these behavioral features, without affecting the movement disorder (125, 126).

PREVENTION OF CLUSTER HEADACHE

This application has been established by RCTs (127).

Neurological Toxicity of Lithium

Lithium is associated with numerous neurological side effects, all of which are dose related. The occurrence of neurological side effects rises very rapidly with lithium levels greater than 1.5 mEq/ml (128). At lithium levels in the therapeutic range, some patients have virtually no neurological side effects apart from a barely detectable action tremor. For others, including many patients with gross brain disease or dementia, neurological side effects at levels within the usual therapeutic range are limiting factors in the use of lithium.

Neurological side effects of lithium seen within the usual therapeutic range include impaired concentration or memory, apathy, restlessness, myoclonus, and tremor. The tremor typically seen at therapeutic doses is a fine action tremor. With lithium levels in the toxic range, the tremor is more coarse and proximal, and may be accompanied by asterixis. Other side effects seen with toxic levels of lithium are confusion, hallucinations, and rigidity resembling that produced by neuroleptics. At extreme levels of lithium (e.g., over 2.5 mEq/L) patients can develop seizures and may develop muscular weakness due to anterior horn cell damage and/or interference with the function of the neuromuscular junction. Elderly patients and patients with Parkinson's disease and related disorders can show rigidity and coarse tremor with lithium levels within the usual therapeutic range.

Neurological side effects of lithium can also be produced indirectly through lithium's effect on the endocrine system (129). Lithium-induced diabetes insipidus can lead to hypernatremia, and thereby cause a typical metabolic encephalopathy. Lithium-induced hyperparathyroidism can cause the typical neurological syndromes of hypercalcemia. The most common lithium-induced endocrinopathy, hypothyroidism, causes depression, ataxia, and slowed cognition; it also increases the patient's sensitivity to adverse effects of other drugs on alertness, cognition, or gait and coordination. Accordingly, when a patient on lithium therapy develops new neurological side effects, the diagnostic assessment should include not only a lithium level, but also measures of electrolytes, calcium, renal function, and thyroid function.

Lithium Versus Alternatives

When lithium is considered as a mood-stabilizing agent, the major alternatives are the mood-stabilizing antiepileptic drugs (AEDs), of which carbamazepine and valproate are best established. Both of the latter drugs have been shown to be as efficacious as lithium in the treatment of mania appear to work for the prophylaxis of bipolar disorder. Although individual patients may respond to lithium and not to AEDs, to AEDs but not to lithium, or to either one, there is no well-established way to know in advance which drug will be best for a given individual. However, the relatively poor response of patients with dysphoric mania or rapid cycling to lithium has led some authors to recommend that valproate or carbamazepine be the first choice for such patients (130). Also, the presence of "organic" features in patients with bipolar disorder has been shown to favor a good response to valproate therapy (131). In my practice, lithium is the first-line mood stabilizer in patients with typical bipolar disorder, and AEDs are the first-line mood stabilizers in all other situations, including rapid cycling, mixed manic and depressive symptoms, dysphoric mania, and mood instability accompanying gross brain disease or epilepsy. When mania results from a specific brain lesion, such as a right-hemisphere stroke, AEDs are preferred, because the embolic strokes that usually cause secondary mania are potential seizure foci. The use of an AED both addresses the mania and minimizes the risk of seizures. If AEDs are the mood stabilizers of choice except for classic primary bipolar disorder, electroencephalography (EEG) is not needed as an aid to choosing treatment. It may, however, be useful for diagnostic purposes.

When lithium is considered as an antiaggressive agent, its competition includes the AEDs, adrenergic agents such as propranolol and clonidine, and serotonergic agents such as the SSRI antidepressants and buspirone. Various authors have suggested sequences of drug trials in this situation, with different rationales for the order in which drugs are tried (130–133). Unless there is a contraindication, lithium should be tried in any seriously aggressive but nonpsychotic patient before accepting long-term neuroleptic therapy. Lithium is tried first, or early on, in patients with either: (*a*) a family history of bipolar disorder or another lithium-responsive mental disorder; (*b*) long periods of elevated mood, energy, or rate alternating with periods of normal or decreased function; (*c*) grandiosity or expansiveness; or (*d*) recurrent depression with clearcut discrete episodes.

Drug Interactions

Like all electrolytes, lithium is eliminated by the kidney. It is processed by the proximal tubule in parallel with sodium; drugs and clinical situations that increase sodium retention also increase lithium retention. Most significant pharmacokinetic interactions involving lithium arise in situations where a drug increases proximal tubular reabsorption of sodium, thereby raising lithium levels for a given oral dose. Drugs that can raise lithium levels in this way include thiazide diuretics and nonsteroidal anti-inflammatory drugs (NSAIDs). When starting lithium in a patient taking a diuretic or an NSAID, the dose should be decreased by about half. When adding a diuretic or NSAID to the regimen of a patient already taking lithium, a similar adjustment should be made, and lithium levels should be checked frequently (e.g., every other day) until they are stabilized in the desired therapeutic range.

Pharmacodynamic interactions with lithium are many, and most can be understood by considering lithium's manifold effects on neurotransmitters and second messengers. Coadministration of lithium with a neuroleptic increases the risk of an acute extrapyramidal reaction over the risk associated with the neuroleptic alone. Coadministration of lithium with an antidepressant increases the risk of tremor, myoclonus, or cognitive side effects. Coadministration of lithium with an AED increases the risk of confusion, ataxia, sedation, or tremor. However, all of these combinations have greater therapeutic effectiveness for mania, depression, and bipolar disorder, respectively, than either drug given alone.

Titration of Lithium Dosage

In patients not deemed to be at increased risk for lithium neurotoxicity, the target blood level for dosage titration is 1.2–1.4 mEq/L. In elderly, demented, or parkinsonian patients, where the risk is higher, the target blood level is 0.8–1.0 mEq/L. The oral dose needed to attain the target blood level will depend on renal function and the size of the patient (i.e., the volume of distribution). A small, fragile patient with normal or perhaps slightly decreased renal function might be started on 300 mg b.i.d. A large, robust patient with known normal renal function might be started on 600 mg t.i.d.

During aggressive dosage titration, as would be carried out for acute mania, blood levels are determined every other day. The patient is also examined for neurological symptoms, which are correlated with the blood level obtained at the time of the examination. Dosage is adjusted as needed to rapidly attain the desired blood level; if unacceptable neurological symptoms occur at a level lower than the original target, the target is lowered.

Gradual dosage titration, as might be carried out for an outpatient with intermittent explosiveness and no behavioral emergency, would be based on a weekly blood level determinations. Incremental changes in dosage would be conservative, to minimize the risk of overshooting the target blood level.

Duration of Therapy

The usual psychiatric indication for lithium, prophylaxis of bipolar disorder, implies very long-term treatment. When lithium is used for mood disorders or aggressiveness associated with gross brain diseases, there are no rigorous studies of continuation therapy to supplant clinical judgment as the criterion for continued therapy. My recommendation is to determine first whether the patient has bipolar disorder that is simply altered in its presentation because of brain disease (e.g., mental retardation or dementia). If so, prolonged treatment would be carried out, in keeping with the hypothesis of an underlying case of primary bipolar disorder. If the current syndrome is the consequence of an acute brain insult, such as stroke or TBI, it would be reasonable to attempt a taper of lithium after the patient had more time to recover from the insult. For example, if the patient's mental and behavioral symptoms were well-controlled for 3 months, and neurological recovery is proceeding well, an attempt would be made to taper the lithium. Dosage would be reduced and the drug discontinued over about 2 weeks. If symptoms recurred, the drug would be reinstated for another 3 months, and another attempt might be made at that time.

If the patient's behavioral syndrome is related to a progressive or degenerative brain disease, a reasonable time to attempt tapering of lithium is when clinically significant progression of the disease has been noted. Under those circumstances, it is possible that the lithium is no longer necessary, or that the relative risk:benefit ratio has changed.

If a patient has a stable, lifelong neurological basis for mood instability or aggressiveness, long-term therapy with lithium may be justified if the lithium has substantially improved safety, enhanced function, relieved distress, or permitted greater freedom in the patient's life. Under these circumstances, an annual reassessment of the patient's symptoms and drug treatment is a valuable precaution.

ANTIEPILEPTIC (AND MOOD-STABILIZING) DRUGS

The use of AEDs for mood and behavior, as well as for seizure disorders, is one of the distinguishing features of the neuropsychiatric practitioner. Neuropsychiatrists used antiepileptic drugs for a wide range of indications long before they entered the mainstream of general psychiatry. As of the mid-1990s, clonazepam has been broadly accepted by general psychiatrists as a treatment for anxiety and panic, and both carbamazepine and valproate have been accepted as efficacious treatments for mania and the prophylaxis of bipolar disorder. Issues relevant to choosing and initiating lithium or a mood-stabilizing antiepileptic drug are presented in Table 11.3.

Efficacy

The efficacy of the AEDs for seizures has been established by multiple RCTs. Among AEDs approved in the United States in the past 30 years, valproate, carbamazepine, clonazepam, and felbamate have been shown to be effective as monotherapy, while lamotrigine and gabapentin have been shown to be effective as add-on therapy. However, lamotrigine in particular has been used effectively as monotherapy in Europe.

The efficacy of carbamazepine for the treatment of acute mania, and its comparability to lithium for this purpose, has been demonstrated by 11 RCTs (134). Five studies, only one placebo-controlled, demonstrate the efficacy of carbamazepine in the prophylaxis of mania in patients with bipolar disorder. The efficacy of valproate for acute mania is supported by six RCTs. Its efficacy for prophylaxis of mania is supported by open studies only (134). None of the controlled studies of carbamazepine or valproate addressed the use of those agents in patients with mood disorders secondary to gross brain disease, epilepsy, or dementia.

The newer AEDs, felbamate, lamotrigine, and gabapentin, have not yet been evaluated for psychiatric indications. Anecdotally, both lamotrigine and gabapentin are in use by mood disorder specialists as alternatives or adjuncts to carbamazepine and valproate for the treatment of bipolar disorder, particularly atypical or treatment-refractory cases.

Other Neuropsychiatric Indications

The AEDs have been used empirically in neuropsychiatric conditions in which paroxysmal brain activity is part of a hypothesized mechanism of symptom production. Numerous case reports, case series, and open studies have been reported. Some of the potential indications for AEDs include:

1. *Posttraumatic stress disorder (PTSD).* Both carbamazepine and valproate (135–137) have been found to reduce symptoms in PTSD patients, especially the symptom of episodic hyperarousal.
2. *Neuropathic pain.* While carbamazepine for trigeminal neuralgia is recognized as indicated by the Food and Drug Administration (FDA), clinical experience and numerous reports, some based on controlled studies, suggest that carbamazepine, valproate, and clonazepam are effective for a wide range of neuropathic pain syndromes (138, 139) (See also Chapter 21).
3. *Aggressive behavior.* Carbamazepine has been used to suppress aggressive outbursts in patients with and without epilepsy, in clinical populations with dementia (140, 141), as well as in other "organic" populations (142–144). Similar positive reports of clinical experience and open trials have appeared for valproate in the treatment of aggressive behavior (145–148).
4. *Treatment-resistant depression with partial seizure-like symptoms.* Carbamazepine led to improvement in 11 of 13 tricyclic-unresponsive patients in a recent open trial (149).
5. *Self-injurious behavior in mentally retarded persons.* Open trials have supported the efficacy of carbamazepine for some patients with this condition, although it has not been shown to be generally useful (150).
6. *Withdrawal from long-term benzodiazepine therapy.* Carbamazepine during benzodiazepine withdrawal increased the success of the withdrawal attempt in a sample of 40 patients with a history of difficulty withdrawing from benzodiazepines. The trial was conducted under placebo-controlled, double–blind conditions, with a 25% per week reduction in benzodiazepine dosage (151).
7. *Affective symptoms in people with mental retardation.* Kastner et al. (152) gave valproate to a cohort of 18 mentally retarded patients with three of four of the following symptoms: behavioral cycling, aggressive or self-injurious behavior, sleep disturbance, and irritability. Fourteen of the 18 improved and continued to be improved on valproate over 2 years of follow-up.

Table 11.3. Issues in Choosing and Initiating Lithium or AEDs.

Drug	Benefits	Precautions	Controlled Trials	Initial Dose
Lithium	Low cost; very well-known side effects and established monitoring schedule	Low therapeutic index; may induce hypothyroidism; causes tremor and may aggravate parkinsonism; synergistic toxicity with neuroleptics	None; case series support efficacy for mania due to gross brain disease, impulsive aggression, and self-injurious behavior	300 mg b.i.d.; usual target blood level approximately 1.0 mEq/ml
Carbamazepine	Efficacy for rapid cycling; antiepileptic effects	Quinidine-like cardiac effects; anticholinergic effects; drug interactions due to enzyme induction; rare hematologic side effects require patient warning but not routine monitoring of CBC	None; case series support efficacy for mania due to gross brain disease and impulsive aggression	100 mg b.i.d.; slow titration to target blood level of 8 to 12 µg/dl when the drug is used as sole therapy
Valproate	Efficacy for rapid cycling, antianxiety effects; antiepileptic effects	Rare hepatic toxicity requires warning but not routine monitoring of enzymes; can cause pancreatitis or hyperammonemia; weight gain common; may cause tremor	None; case series support efficacy for mania due to gross brain disease, and for mood instability and aggression in mentally retarded persons and dementia patients	250 mg b.i.d. (125 mg if unusually sensitive to side effects); gradual titration to blood level of 50-100 µg/ml; may load rapidly in case of behavioral emergency due to mania
Clonazepam	Strong antianxiety and antipanic effects; sedative; treats myoclonus	Long half-life predisposes to accumulation and risk of falling; ataxia and sedation the main side effects that limit therapy; some risk of disinhibition	None; case series support efficacy for anxiety, panic, and agitation due to gross brain disease	0.25-0.5 mg, usually at bedtime
Gabapentin	Antianxiety and mood-stabilizing actions suggested by patients' experiences in epilepsy trials; no significant drug interactions	Additive sedation and ataxia with other drugs	No systematic trials of psychotropic activity	100 mg t.i.d.; may raise gradually to maximum of 900 t.i.d., but mechanism of action implies diminishing effect of increases
Lamotrigine	Subjective well-being improved in patients enrolled in epilepsy clinical trials	Interactions with valproate; can cause severe skin rashes, especially if dose raised rapidly	None; anecdotes support efficacy for rapid-cycling mood disorders	50 mg at bedtime or b.i.d.; 25 mg every other day if patient is on valproate because of increased risk of rash

Neurological Toxicity

The AEDs, with the exception of felbamate, all share the tendency to cause sedation, ataxia, nystagmus, and other signs of CNS depression. These signs can be seen if the serum drug concentration is too high, if dosage is raised too rapidly, or if the patient is unusually sensitive to the depressant effects of the drug. In addition, several of the AEDs have characteristic neurological side effects.

Carbamazepine toxicity frequently manifests with diplopia. Carbamazepine also is anticholinergic, and can cause typical signs of anticholinergic toxicity in susceptible patients, usually elderly persons or those with Alzheimer's disease.

Valproate often causes an action tremor; at times this is severe enough to be a limiting side effect. Valproate raises serum ammonia; signs of hepatic encephalopathy can develop in patients with occult liver disease treated with this drug. Phenytoin usually produces nystagmus and ataxia at toxic levels. Prolonged exposure to phenytoin at excessive levels can cause permanent cerebellar damage.

Clonazepam toxicity typically presents with sedation and ataxia. An apathetic confusional state can also occur. Lamotrigine and gabapentin tend to have "generic" AED side effects of sedation, dizziness, ataxia, or impaired coordination. Remarkably, patients on lamotrigine frequently describe a sense of increased well-being (153). Felbamate can cause headache, insomnia, or agitation; more severe toxicity can include an agitated confusional state. Felbamate is the only AED that commonly produces side effects related to CNS stimulation.

Phenobarbital, primidone, phenytoin, and ethosuximide are prescribed as AEDs, but are very rarely used as psychotropics. Phenobarbital and primidone, in particular, are generally regarded as psychotoxic, with a propensity to cause either depression, cognitive impairment, or behavioral disturbances. Common neuropsychiatric practice is to replace these medications by other AEDs if patients develop significant cognitive, behavioral, or emotional problems while being treated for epilepsy with one of them.

Drug Interactions

Pharmacokinetic interactions involving AEDs usually result from the induction or inhibition of oxidative enzymes. In these interactions, the AED may either be the cause of altered metabolism or the drug affected by it. Some typical and clinically relevant interactions are summarized here.

Carbamazepine levels are increased by drugs that inhibit the enzymes that metabolize it, or compete with carbamazepine at the active sites of those enzymes. Calcium channel blockers (verapamil and diltiazem), macrolide antibiotics (erythromycin and clarithromycin), and cimetidine all can raise carbamazepine levels to a clinically significant degree. Carbamazepine itself can induce enzymes that metabolize other drugs, as well as carbamazepine itself. Four

important examples are warfarin, oral contraceptives, opiate analgesics, and tricyclic antidepressants. In each of these cases, the other drug may lack expected efficacy if given at its usual dosage.

Valproate inhibits both oxidative metabolism and glucuronide conjugation of a number of drugs. Its effect on glucuronide conjugation is relevant to the combination of valproate with lorazepam; with coadministration, lorazepam has a higher level and a longer elimination half-life. Its impairment of oxidation affects the metabolism of carbamazepine 10-11% epoxide (CBZ-E). When valproate and carbamazepine are given together, CBZ-E can accumulate, leading to typical symptoms of carbamazepine toxicity at an apparently therapeutic level of the parent compound, carbamazepine. Valproate also prolongs the metabolism of lamotrigine, raising its half-life by 15–25% (154). This interaction necessitates slower dosage titration of lamotrigine when it is added on to valproate therapy. Valproate is highly bound to serum albumin. Aspirin displaces valproate from serum albumin, raising the free drug level, sometimes to the toxic range.

Felbamate is an inhibitor of oxidative enzymes, particularly CYP2C19. This isoenzyme metabolizes omeprazole, imipramine, and diazepam, any of which can have increased levels for a given dose if given concurrently with felbamate. It raises levels of valproate by a mechanism not fully elucidated. On the other hand, concurrent felbamate lowers carbamazepine levels by 20–25% while raising levels of carbamazepine epoxide 10–11% (155). Lamotrigine does not induce or inhibit oxidative enzymes, so it does not influence the metabolism of other drugs. Gabapentin, which is excreted by the kidney unchanged, is essentially free from pharmacokinetic drug interactions (156).

Pharmacodynamic interactions involving the AEDs generally consist of additive CNS depression. However, carbamazepine also decreases dopamine turnover, and can intensify extrapyramidal side effects when coadministered with neuroleptics. This interaction may be offset by a pharmacokinetic interaction that lowers the blood level of the neuroleptic drug.

A common and clinically important interaction occurs between theophylline and AEDs. Theophylline, a drug still prescribed for bronchospasm, despite its being superseded as a drug of choice by inhaled bronchodilators and inhaled corticosteroids, is a proconvulsant agent. It antagonizes the antiepileptic effect of a number of AEDs, including carbamazepine and diazepam.

Choice of Antiepileptic Drug

Neuropsychiatrists are called upon to choose AEDs either for epilepsy, for mood stabilization, or for one of the other neuropsychiatric indications mentioned previously. In the treatment of epilepsy, guidance is provided by standard references on AED therapy (157, 158). At this point, because of their behavioral toxicity, barbiturates and primidone are no longer first-line agents for the treatment of epilepsy.

When choosing an AED for treatment of bipolar disorder, the fact the valproate has a U.S. FDA indication for the treatment of mania is a point in its favor, though the evidence for the therapeutic efficacy of carbamazepine is just as good. When choosing an AED for mood stabilization in a patient with gross brain disease, the FDA indication is not relevant, and the drugs can be viewed as equivalent. In some cases, however, safety favors one drug over the other. For example, carbamazepine would be preferred to valproate in a patient with a history of pancreatitis or the possibility of occult liver cirrhosis, because of the tendency of valproate to raise amylase and to cause hyperammonemia. Valproate would be preferred to carbamazepine in a patient with heart block that might be aggravated by carbamazepine's quinidine-like effects.

When an AED is used as an antidepressant, a case can be made for preferring carbamazepine to valproate, because there is slightly more uncontrolled evidence of its antidepressant efficacy.

When carbamazepine and valproate are ineffective or not tolerated, the neuropsychiatric picture might still suggest that an AED might be helpful. For example, a patient with a right-hemisphere lesion might have a very rapidly cycling mood disorder, or a patient with a history of TBI might have sudden rages associated with a paroxysmal EEG. In these situations, the author's preference is to employ lamotrigine. Other neuropsychiatrists use gabapentin in this situation. Both drugs are considered as promising neuropsychiatric drugs because of reports of positive effects on mood when the drugs underwent clinical testing as antiepileptic agents (159, 159a).

An extensive earlier literature described psychotropic actions of phenytoin. Because these were not confirmed by subsequent controlled clinical trials, and the robust psychotropic actions of valproate and carbamazepine became evident, phenytoin fell out of use as a psychotropic. It is actually unknown whether phenytoin might be useful as a psychotropic drug for carefully selected patients and indications.

Dosage Titration

In the absence of data suggesting that an alternative would be better, the dosages and blood levels appropriate for the treatment of epilepsy are followed when using AEDs as psychotropics. Therapeutic dosages and levels usually are approached gradually. When AEDs are discontinued for reasons other than serious adverse reactions, discontinuation is by gradual taper. A typical, conservative dosage strategy might be as follows:

1. *Carbamazepine.* Start with 100 mg q.h.s. If tolerated, increase every 2–3 days by 100 mg, building up to an evenly divided t.i.d. schedule (thus, 100 mg b.i.d., 100 mg t.i.d., 100–100–200 on a t.i.d. schedule, etc.) A pre-dose blood (trough) level would be checked after reaching 200 mg t.i.d. The target level would be 8–12

μg/ml. Dosage increases would continue until the target range is reached; the dosage would then be held constant for another 2 weeks. The blood level would be checked again and further dosage adjustment made if necessary.
2. *Valproate.* Start with 250 mg q.h.s. If tolerated, increase every 2–3 days by 250 mg, building up to a t.i.d. schedule (thus, 250 b.i.d., 250 t.i.d., 250–250–500, etc.) A trough blood level would be checked on 1000 mg per day, and weekly thereafter. Dosage increases would continue until the target range of 75–100 μg/ml was reached.
3. *Lamotrigine.* Start with 50 mg q.h.s. If tolerated, increase by 50 mg every week on a b.i.d. schedule, eventually reaching 200 mg b.i.d.
4. *Gabapentin.* Start with 100 mg q.h.s. Build up in 100 mg increments every 2–3 days, on a t.i.d. schedule, eventually reaching 600 mg t.i.d. after reaching 300 mg t.i.d., increments may be 300 mg.

In all cases, dosage increases are stopped if the desired therapeutic effect is attained, or if limiting side effects develop.

An exception to gradual dosage is in the treatment of acute mania, where the need to rapidly attain a therapeutic blood level outweighs the greater incidence of side effects with high initial dosage. When treating acute mania, the drug dose likely to produce a therapeutic level in steady state (e.g., valproate 500 mg t.i.d.; carbamazepine 200 t.i.d.) is estimated and dosage is initiated at that dose.

Duration of Therapy

Considerations regarding the duration of therapy with AEDs as mood stabilizers are identical with those presented earlier for lithium therapy. When AEDs are used for epilepsy, contemporary guidelines for AED discontinuation are followed if the patient has been seizure-free for more than 1 year.

STIMULANTS

Stimulants—dextroamphetamine, methylphenidate, and pemoline—are the well-established drug treatment for attention-deficit/hyperactivity disorder (ADHD). In sleep medicine, they are the treatment of choice for narcolepsy. In consultation psychiatry, they are used to rapidly mobilize hospitalized medically ill patients with apathy and depressed mood (160). In neuropsychiatric practice, additional applications draw upon the stimulants' capacity to enhance arousal, motivation, and the ability to sustain attention.

Efficacy

The efficacy of the stimulants for ADHD has been established by over 100 RCTs (161). However, up to 30% of ADHD patients treated with any given stimulant will not improve. Some will respond to a different stimulant, others to an alternate therapy, such as a TCA.

The efficacy of stimulants for patients with narcolepsy has been established by sleep laboratory studies using the Multiple Sleep Latency Test or the Maintenance of Wakefulness Tests as measures. These studies have shown that pemoline is inferior to methylphenidate and dextroamphetamine. Also, they suggest that patients with narcolepsy are still sleepier than control subjects, even after therapy with relatively high doses of stimulants (162).

Methylphenidate has been shown to produce significant improvement in depressive symptoms within 1 week, in a double-blind randomized placebo-controlled crossover trial in 16 older medically ill patients (163). This recent RCT is in accord with a large anecdotal literature on the effectiveness of stimulants for depression in the medically ill.

Other Neuropsychiatric Indications

POSTSTROKE DEPRESSION

Methylphenidate may be able to produce a remission of depressive symptoms following stroke in about half of patients treated. Lazarus et al. (164) retrospectively reviewed the treatment of 58 elderly stroke patients for poststroke major depression, 28 of whom received methylphenidate, and 30 of whom received nortriptyline. Fifteen (53%) of the methylphenidate group had a complete remission of depression, while 13 (43%) of the nortriptyline group had a complete remission. The difference was not statistically significant. However, the average response time was 2.4 days in the methylphenidate group, and 27 days in the nortriptyline group (p < .001).

ATTENTION DEFICIT HYPERACTIVITY DISORDER AMONG PATIENTS WITH DEVELOPMENTAL DISABILITIES

ADHD symptomatology in patients with mental retardation and other developmental disabilities has improved with the use of stimulants. The improvement rate of ADHD in blind methylphenidate trials does not differ significantly between children with ADHD alone and those with ADHD plus other neurodevelopmental disorders (165). However, the comparison did not include severely and profoundly retarded children.

APATHY

Methylphenidate or dextroamphetamine can reduce apathy in patients with a variety of causes for apathy, including depression, TBI, and side effects of AEDs, antidepressants, or neuroleptics (166–168). The use of stimulants for the treatment of apathy has not been subjected to RCTs.

Neurological Toxicity

In usual therapeutic doses, neurological side effects of the stimulants include insomnia, irritability, nervousness, headache, and tremor. Acute overdose can produce an agitated confusional state with hyperreflexia and seizures; a manic-like psychosis is also possible. Prolonged use at unusually high doses can produce a paranoid psychosis with features of acute schizophrenia. Withdrawal from long-term use can be associated with headache, apathy, fatigue, and hypersomnia.

Between 5–10% of children with ADHD treated with stimulant medications will develop tics or dyskinesias (169). Most are transient, with less than 1% of treated children developing Tourette's syndrome. Although risk factors have not been fully evaluated, a personal or family history of tics may increase the risk of developing persistent tics on stimulant therapy (169).

Drug Interactions

Methylphenidate inhibits oxidative enzymes that metabolize tricyclic antidepressants, warfarin, and AEDs, including phenobarbital, phenytoin, and primidone. All of these drugs may require downward dosage adjustments to avoid toxicity.

All of the stimulants have pharmacodynamic interactions with psychotropic drugs. They enhance antidepressant effects. Their stimulating and anorexiant effects are antagonized by neuroleptics and by lithium.

Stimulants Versus Other Therapies

For the treatment of ADHD, stimulants are first-line therapy, and other therapies would be used only if the patient objected to stimulants, did not tolerate them, did not respond to them, had a personal or family history of tics or Tourette's syndrome, or was deemed to be at an unacceptably high risk for abusing or diverting stimulant drugs. For these patients, therapeutic alternatives include most of the nonsedating antidepressants (desipramine, nortriptyline, imipramine, phenelzine, tranylcypromine, bupropion, sertraline, and fluoxetine), and the adrenergic agents clonidine and propranolol (170).

For depression, stimulants are preferred to antidepressants when apathy is a prominent feature of the depression, and when a prompt response to treatment is of great importance to the patient. For example, a patient with a recent stroke who is depressed and too apathetic to participate in physical therapy would be an ideal candidate for stimulant therapy. Patients with anxious or delusional depressions should not be treated with stimulants, nor should stimulants be primary treatment for a physically healthy person with a primary unipolar depression.

Dopamine agonist drugs are the present alternative therapy for apathy. Stimulants are preferred when an apathetic patient is sleepy or lethargic and maximal efforts had already been made to remove sedating drugs from the patient's regimen. Dopamine agonists are preferred when the patient has rigidity, bradykinesia, or other motor signs of parkinsonism. For apathy with neither sleepiness nor parkinsonian features, either a stimulant or a dopamine agonist is a reasonable first choice.

Choice of Stimulant

Issues related to the choice of stimulant and to initiating therapy are mentioned in Table 11.4, along with similar details for the dopamine agonist drugs.

Patients may respond to dextroamphetamine or methylphenidate but not to pemoline; the reverse situation can occur, but it is uncommon. Therefore, one of the former two drugs usually should be tried first. During dose titration, the drug is given two or three times a day. Once a dose has been established, the use of long-acting preparations may allow q.d. or b.i.d. dosing. Pemoline can be given on a q.d. schedule at the outset, as it is long-acting.

Dosage Titration

Initial dosage of dextroamphetamine or methylphenidate is 2.5 mg AM and noon in a fragile or small person; 5 mg AM and noon in a more robust and larger person. Therapeutic effects, if any, are immediate. If there are neither side effects nor an apparent therapeutic response, the dose is increased the next day to 5 mg AM and noon or 10 mg AM and noon, respectively. Dosage may be increased further if needed, in units of 2.5 mg for the small or fragile patient, and 5 mg for the larger and healthier patient. When the patient feels some change for the better in attention, mood, or motivation, or the clinician sees an apparent change, the dose is maintained at the same level for a week, after which the response is reevaluated and dosage adjusted if necessary to maximize response or to minimize side effects.

Pemoline is started at 18.75 mg once a day. The dose is raised by 18.75 mg once a week until the patient improves, limiting side effects develop, or a dose of 112.5 mg per day is reached.

Duration of Therapy

Treatment for ADHD and other attentional disorders is continual and long term. However, in children, drug-free intervals are given when feasible to allow for growth unimpeded by stimulants' anorexic and potential growth-suppressing effects. Weekends and school vacations are natural opportunities in children whose behavior at home without medication is tolerable. For adults with attentional disorders, growth is not an issue, but tolerance or tachyphylaxis to stimulants may be. If an adult on stimulant therapy for ADHD finds that the benefits of stimulants are wearing off, a drug holiday should be considered. Vacations or periods of relatively lower work demand may be suitable times.

When stimulants are used to treat illness-associated depressions, the drug should be withdrawn once the acute illness has resolved or stabilized. If the patient's depression persists after withdrawal of the stimulant, a standard antidepressant should be initiated. For the patient's comfort, the stimulant could be restarted until there was time for the antidepressant to take effect. If stimulants are given for a week or more, they should be withdrawn gradually, ideally by no more than 25% every 2–3 days.

When stimulants are used to treat apathy, therapy, if effective, may continue until the underlying cause of the apathy has resolved. If the cause of the apathy is permanent, stimulant therapy may continue, unless tachyphylaxis or tolerance develops. In that case, a planned drug holiday might restore sensitivity to the stimulant. Alternatively, the specific stimulant might be rotated to a different member of the class.

DOPAMINE AGONISTS

The dopamine agonist anti-Parkinson drugs selegiline, amantadine, bromocriptine, and pergolide have recently been used for neuropsychiatric indications other than Parkinson's disease, drug-induced parkinsonism, and other movement disorders. The best established neuropsychiatric indication is bromocriptine for treatment-resistant depression.

Efficacy

Bromocriptine has been tested as an antidepressant in three RCTs with a total N of 125 (171). An open trial of pergolide as an adjunct to standard antidepressants in 20 patients with treatment-resistant depression converted 11 cases to remissions (172).

Other Neuropsychiatric Indications

Dopamine agonists have other neuropsychiatric indications. These include:

1. *Neuroleptic-induced apathy and abulia.* Amantadine has a stimulating effect on patients with neuroleptic-treated schizophrenia (173).
2. *Agitation and assaultiveness during recovery from traumatic coma.* Amantadine was reported to suppress agitation in two patients with traumatic frontotemporal lesions (174), and was then tested by Gualtieri et al. (174a) in a group of patients recovering from coma who were agitated and emotionally labile. Over 50% responded in this open trial; doses of 100–400 mg/day were given in this study. The response was all-or-nothing—either dramatic improvement or no benefit.
3. *Akinetic mutism.* Ross and Stewart (175) reported a case in which bromocriptine relieved stimulated spontaneous speech and movement in a man with akinetic mutism from hypothalamic damage.
4. *Hemineglect.* Fleet et al. (176) reported alleviation of neglect when bromocriptine was administered to two patients with right-hemisphere strokes.
5. *Amnesia due to mediobasal forebrain injury.* In a single surgical case of damage to the area of the septum and nucleus accumbens, bromocriptine partially alleviated anterograde amnesia (177).

Table 11.4. Issues Relevant to Choosing and Initiating a Dopamine Agonist or Stimulant

Drug	Benefits	Precautions	Controlled Trials	Initial Daily Dose
Bromocriptine	Antidepressant, antiparkinson, anti-apathetic effects	Orthostatic hypotension; nausea; confusion; depression or mania; ergot hypersensitivity (pulmonary or retroperitoneal fibrosis)	Many for Parkinson's disease and several for primary major depression; case series support for apathy and abulia from gross brain disease, and for drug-induced parkinsonism	2.5-5 mg; drug is usually given on a b.i.d. schedule
Pergolide	Can be given once a day because of long half-life; may be less expensive because of its high potency; otherwise like bromocriptine	As for bromocriptine; however, some patients do better on one than another	Many for Parkinson's disease; case series support for depression; case reports for apathy and abulia	0.05-0.10 mg q.d.
Amantadine	Antiparkinson, anti-apathetic; rapid onset of action	Orthostatic hypotension, confusion, anticholinergic effects	In drug-induced parkinsonism has fewer cognitive side effects than benztropine	50-100 mg b.i.d.
Dextroamphetamine	Improves alertness, attention, motivation	May increase anxiety or induce mania; subject to abuse because of euphoriant effects	For narcolepsy; case series support benefit for apathy and for depression in the medically ill	2.5-5 mg morning and noon
Methylphenidate	Improves alertness, attention, motivation	May increase anxiety or induce mania; subject to abuse because of euphoriant effects	Many for ADHD; one for depression in the medically ill; case series support benefit for apathy	2.5-5 mg morning and noon
Pemoline	Improves alertness, attention, motivation; less subject to abuse than dextroamphetamine and less tightly controlled; longer duration of action permits once a day dosing	Onset of action may take weeks; dysphoric reactions more common than with dextroamphetamine; overall efficacy probably lower; may induce mania or anxiety	Many for ADHD; no studies in other neuropsychiatric conditions	18.75 mg q.d.

6. *Transcortical motor aphasia*. Albert et al. (178) reported recovery of spontaneous speech when bromocriptine was given, which relapsed when bromocriptine was discontinued.

In summary, there is evidence for an antidepressant, psychomotor activating effect of dopamine agonist drugs, but insufficient empirical study to determine the appropriate indications for dopamine agonist therapy.

Neurological Toxicity

The most serious neurological side effects of the dopamine agonist drugs are changes in mental status. The dopamine agonists can cause confusion, agitation, insomnia, hallucinations, paranoid ideation, disorganized thinking, incoherent speech, emotional lability, hypersexuality, hypomanic and manic phenomena, depression, or anxiety. They also can cause involuntary movements, including choreoathetosis, dyskinesia, and tremor. Although the list of potential side effects is long, many patients take those drugs with no side effects at all.

Drug Interactions

Drug interactions with selegiline may become problematic if the dose of selegiline is raised above 10 mg per day. At higher doses, selegiline, a selective MAO-B inhibitor, loses its selectivity. When MAO is nonselectively inhibited, patients can develop serious hypertension from indirect adrenergic agents, or manifest a serotonin syndrome if they take an SSRI.

Combination therapy, using multiple dopamine agonists, typically the case in the treatment of Parkinson's disease, increases both therapeutic effect and the risk of side effects, particularly the adverse effects on mental status discussed previously.

Choice of Dopamine Agonist

The choice of dopamine agonist drugs for Parkinson's disease is beyond the scope of this chapter. When a dopamine agonist drug is to be used for neuroleptic-induced parkinsonism, amantadine usually is selected first because of ease of administration and extensive experience with its use for this indication. If amantadine at a full dose does not relieve the patient's symptoms, bromocriptine is used next, because the combination of bromocriptine and neuroleptics in schizophrenia treatment is documented, and bromocriptine rarely appears to cause aggravation of psychosis during neuroleptic treatment.

When a dopamine agonist drug is to be used as a primary or adjunctive treatment for depression resistant to usual treatments, bromocriptine should be considered as a first choice, in view of support for its use from RCTs. If bromocriptine were not tolerated, pergolide would be substituted.

When a dopamine agonist is to be used to treat apathy or to attempt pharmacological remediation of a focal cortical deficit (as in the reported cases of hemineglect and transcor-

tical motor aphasia), there is no strong reason to prefer bromocriptine over pergolide. Because successful cases have been reported using bromocriptine, some clinicians might prefer to begin with that agent.

Dosage Titration

The starting dose of amantadine is 50 mg b.i.d. in a small or fragile person; 100 mg b.i.d. in a larger and more robust person. Dosage increases should be in 50-mg increments in the former case; 100-mg increments in the latter case. Dosage usually should not exceed 100 mg t.i.d. Dosage must be reduced in renal insufficiency.

The starting dose of selegiline is 5 mg q.d. This can be increased to 5 mg b.i.d. after 2 days, if the initial dose is tolerated.

The starting dose of bromocriptine is 1.25 mg b.i.d. in a smaller or more fragile patient, and 2.5 mg b.i.d. in a larger and more robust person. Dosage increases are in steps of 1.25 mg in the former type of patient; 2.5 mg in the latter type. There is no absolute maximum dosage for neuropsychiatric indications if the drug is well tolerated; however, the dose should not be raised beyond 10 mg t.i.d., unless there is clear evidence of benefit.

The starting dose of pergolide is 0.05 mg q.d. in a small or fragile person; 0.1 mg q.d. in a larger and more robust person. Dosage increments begin at 0.05–0.1 mg, and gradually rise to 0.1–0.25 mg per day. Dosage would not ordinarily be raised beyond 5 mg per day, unless partial benefit is observed.

Duration of Therapy

Duration of therapy for major depression is 6–12 months, followed by an attempt to taper the medication. When dopamine agonists are used for drug-induced parkinsonism, efforts should be made periodically (e.g., at 2 and at 4 months) to see if they are still needed, because some patients become more tolerant of neuroleptics. If extrapyramidal effects recur promptly on two or three attempts to taper dopamine agonists, they probably will be needed long term, unless the patient is switched to an atypical neuroleptic.

When dopamine agonists are used to partially reverse cognitive deficits caused by acquired lesions such as strokes and contusions, the clinical hope is that further recovery of function in the brain will make pharmacological palliation of deficits unnecessary, or that the drug-induced improvement will be relevant to everyday functioning. Attempts to taper the drugs should be made every 3 months or so during the recovery process. Deficits persisting at 3 years following acquisition of the lesion are likely to be permanent. At that point, if the drug makes a meaningful difference to the patient's function and well-being, it may be continued indefinitely.

ADRENERGIC AGENTS

The adrenergic agents most often used in neuropsychiatry are the β-adrenergic blockers, especially propranolol, and clonidine, a mixed α_1-α_2 agonist. In addition to their original indication of hypertension, these agents have well-established efficacy for several neuropsychiatric indications, and have been tried for numerous other ones. The appeal of these agents, which either block adrenergic receptors or indirectly decrease adrenergic activity, is their ability to diminish the autonomic component of emotional response. Through feedback to the limbic system, decreased autonomic response can lead to decreased cognitive and affective responses.

Efficacy

The efficacy of propranolol has been established by RCTs for migraine prophylaxis (179), and for treatment or essential tremor (180). The efficacy of clonidine has been established by RCTs for reducing tics in Tourette's syndrome (181), and decreasing the intensity of withdrawal symptoms after discontinuation of opiates (182).

Other Neuropsychiatric Indications

Both propranolol and clonidine have been used in a number of conditions in which anxiety or symptoms of anxiety are present or inferred. These include:

1. *ADHD.* Clonidine (183, 184) has shown efficacy and is a primary therapy for ADHD. The dose, reached by gradual titration, is 3–10 μg/kg/day. Propranolol has been used as an adjunct to stimulants, to reduce impulsive behavior, at a dose of 2–8 mg/kg/day (185). Recently, guanfacine, a more selective α_2 agonist than clonidine, was shown in an open study of 13 outpatients with ADHD to substantially improve hyperactivity, inattention, and immaturity, with less sedation than would be expected with an equivalent dosage of clonidine (186).
2. *Agitation in dementia.* There have been several double-blind studies showing propranolol to be superior to placebo for assaultiveness and agitation; dosages have varied greatly, from 10 mg per day to 600 mg per day (187, 188).
3. *Rage attacks in children, adolescents, and adults with "organic" brain dysfunction.* Williams et al. (188), and Yudofsky and his colleagues (189) have summarized a number of early studies supporting an antiaggressive action of propranolol.
4. *Akathisia due to neuroleptics.* Propranolol has been found to be superior to benztropine and to placebo in the treatment of akathisia, at doses up to 120 mg per day (190, 191).

Neurological Toxicity

The most common neurological side effects of propranolol and clonidine are fatigue, sedation, and decreased libido. The fatigue and sedation occasionally combine with other symptoms to form a depressive syndrome, although it is unclear whether the drugs actually can cause a major depression in a person with no psychiatric vulnerability.

Rarely, and especially in patients with preexisting cognitive impairment, either drug can cause a delirious or agitated state, with visual or auditory hallucinations.

Drug Interactions

Pharmacokinetic interactions with propranolol are related to its oxidative metabolism. Propranolol levels are raised by coadministration of chlorpromazine or cimetidine; they are lowered by coadministration of phenytoin or phenobarbital. Propranolol inhibits the metabolism of theophylline, leading to increased serum drug concentrations at a fixed dose.

The major reported interaction of clonidine is with TCAs; coadministration decreases the hypotensive effect of clonidine. Pharmacodynamic interactions are mainly with other antihypertensive drugs (additive or synergistic antihypertensive effect) and with other drugs with sedative or CNS depressant effects (increased lethargy, fatigue, and depressive symptoms).

Decision to Use an Adrenergic Agent

Issues related to the choice and initiation of an adrenergic agent are summarized in Table 11.5.

Propranolol is a first-choice agent for migraine and for essential tremor; clonidine is a second-line agent for Tourette's syndrome. For akathisia, propranolol is preferred, and is almost always more effective than either benzodiazepines or anticholinergics. For aggressive behavior and rage attacks, there is no general way to choose between a mood-stabilizing drug, an antidepressant, and propranolol as a first treatment. In a specific patient, affective instability or cycling of behavior suggests trying a mood stabilizer first, chronic irritability suggests trying an SSRI, and marked autonomic arousal at the time of behavioral display suggests propranolol. If more than one picture fits, such considerations as vulnerability to side effects and past experiences of the patient or the physician will affect the decision. At present, no laboratory test, including the EEG, supersedes clinical considerations in drug choice.

Clonidine should be regarded as a potential adjunct in the treatment of ADHD, Tourette's syndrome, or the combination of the two, to address attentional impairment, impulsivity, and autonomic arousal, if these persist after first-line treatments are instituted. It is possible that guanfacine, with its lesser sedation and possibly greater benefit than clonidine, may become more of a routine agent in the treatment of ADHD and related conditions.

OPIATE RECEPTOR BLOCKERS

Oral opiate receptor blockers, of which naltrexone is the only one currently available in the United States, were introduced as an aid in the treatment of opiate abuse, and subsequently in the treatment of alcoholism (203). However, neuropsychiatrists have perennially speculated on the role of endogenous opiate mechanisms in sustaining other

Table 11.5. Issues Relevant to Choosing and Initiating an Adrenergic Agent

Drug	Benefits	Precautions	Controlled Trials	Initial Daily Dose
Propranolol	Antianxiety, helpful for migraine, tremor, irritability, impulsive aggression	Sedation; hypotension; can aggravate asthma or heart failure; various drug interactions related to its oxidative metabolism	Migraine, essential tremor; case series support utility for agitation and aggression, and for neuroleptic induced akathisia	20-40 mg t.i.d.
Nadolol	Less fat-soluble and more β_1 selective; therefore less sedation and aggravation of asthma; may help impulsive aggression; long half-life so may be taken once a day	Same as propranolol	None; open trials support benefit for aggression in mental retardation	40 mg
Clonidine	Major anxiolytic effects, including blocking of anxiety from drug withdrawal—decreases firing of locus ceruleus	Sedation, hypotension, confusion	ADHD, Tourette syndrome, opiate or nicotine withdrawal; case series support use for impulsive aggression and memory loss in Korsakoff syndrome	0.1 mg q.d. to t.i.d., depending on indication
Guanfacine	Decreases firing of locus ceruleus; stimulates frontal lobe α_2 receptors to improve executive function; long duration of action permits once daily dosing	As with clonidine, but less sedation; can cause dyspepsia or nausea	ADHD; anecdotal support for use in impulsive aggression	1 mg q.d.

forms of habitual behaviors, particularly those that involve some self-inflicted pain or discomfort. Theoretically, patients with self-inflicted injuries may be releasing substantial amounts of endogenous opiates when they perform self-injurious acts.

The evidence for the efficacy of naltrexone in addiction treatment is provided in Chapter 30. Other neuropsychiatric indications for naltrexone include:

1. *Self-injurious behavior in mentally retarded adults.* Sandman (192), reviewing studies of naloxone and naltrexone in SIB, concluded that sometimes they worked, and sometimes they did not. Gillberg (193) reached similar conclusions. Herman et al. (194) reported that patients with the severe SIB of head and face hitting improved with naltrexone. Possibly, more severe forms of SIB are related to opiate mechanisms, and less severe forms represent a form of stereotypic behavior with a different pattern of pharmacological response (195). In a study of SIB in eight mentally retarded adults, naltrexone decreased the number of days with frequent SIB, and increased the number of days with infrequent SIB (196).
2. *Autism.* Because of the role of opiates in systems mediating attachment, there has been speculation that opiate antagonists might restore more normal social behavior. In a RCT of naltrexone in autistic children, Campbell et al. (197) found that the naltrexone-treated patients communicated more and withdrew less. Kolman (198) found improved social behavior in eight of 13 autistic children treated with naltrexone. Lensing et al. (199) reported a case of a 5-year-old boy in whom treatment with naltrexone increased smiling, crying, and playing. However, Zingarelli et al. (200) failed to find benefit in a trial of naltrexone in eight autistic young adults. Apparently, naltrexone affects social behavior, but the response may be dependent on the measures used, the individuals' level of function before treatment, and the social environment.
3. *Bulimia.* A study comparing low-dose and high-dose naltrexone in the treatment of bulimia found a lower rate of binge eating and purging in the high-dose group (201). Subsequently, a single case appeared reporting that naltrexone reduced a bulimic patient's subjective urge to binge-eat (202).
4. *Tourette's syndrome.* Kurlan et al. (203) found that naltrexone reduced tics, and also improved patients' concentration.

Neurological Toxicity

As might be expected from a drug used exclusively in populations with mental illness or substance abuse, patients on naltrexone have reported a wide range of mental symptoms, including restlessness, insomnia, nightmares, confusion, hallucinations, paranoia, and fatigue. The relation of these symptoms to drug effects is not clear.

Drug Interactions

There is only one drug interaction of consequence—the precipitation of an acute and severe withdrawal state if the drug is given to a person still taking narcotics on a regular basis.

When to Consider Using Naltrexone

In the neuropsychiatric context, naltrexone should be considered as an option for the treatment of recurrent SIB. It might be expended for other repetitive behaviors that are hypothesized to be drawn by opiate-related mechanisms. The use of naltrexone in the treatment of alcohol and drug abuse is discussed fully by Ling et al. in Chapter 30.

Dosage Titration

No titration is needed. A fixed dose of 50 mg per day, 100 mg every other day, or 150 mg every third day should provide adequate opiate receptor blockade.

Duration of Therapy

After blocking opiate receptors, there theoretically can be a brief rebound of the behavior that was previously reinforced by endogenous opiate release. Such a rebound was actually observed in a case reported by Benjamin et al. (204). An adequate therapeutic trial should permit this rebound period to pass. After that, behavioral and environmental therapies to extinguish the unwanted behavior should be instituted, taking advantage of the change in internal reinforcement. An attempt to taper and discontinue naltrexone could be made once the patient had a stable period without significant self-injury. If the self-injury recurred, therapy with naltrexone would be reinstated.

CONCLUSION

RCTs focusing specifically on neuropsychiatric populations are limited. Still, the combination of RCTs in general psychiatric populations and a rich literature of case series and open trials should provide the neuropsychiatrist with an empirical basis for planning drug therapy in a neuropsychiatric practice. Neuropsychiatrists working with well-defined and homogenous populations would greatly advance the field by conducting methodologically rigorous tests of the drug therapies they find clinically useful in their populations of interest.

References

1. American Psychiatric Association. *Diagnostic and statistical manual of mental disorders.* 4th ed. Washington, DC: American Psychiatric Association, 1994.
2. World Health Organization. *International classification of diseases.* 10th ed. Geneva: World Health Organization, 1994.
3. Burke MJ, Preskorn SH. Short-term treatment of mood disorders with standard antidepressants. In: Bloom FE, Kupfer DJ, eds.

Psychopharmacology: the fourth generation of progress. New York: Raven Press, 1995:1053–1066.

4. Starkstein SE, Robinson RG. Depression in cerebrovascular disease. In: Starkstein SE, Robinson RG. Depression in neurologic disease. Baltimore: Johns Hopkins University Press, 1993:28–49.

4a. Andersen G, Vestergaard K, Lauritzen L. Effective treatment of post-stroke depression with the selective serotonin reuptake inhibitor citalopram. Stroke 1994;25:1099–1104.

4b. Andersen G, Vestergaard K, Riis JO. Citalopram for post-stroke pathological crying. Lancet 1993;342:837–839.

5. Berrios GE. History of descriptive psychopathology. In: Mezzich JE, Jorge MR, Salloum IM, eds. Psychiatric epidemiology: assessment concepts and methods. Baltimore: Johns Hopkins University Press, 1994:47–68.

6. Lakshamanan M, Mion LC, Frengley JD. Effective low dose tricyclic antidepressant treatment for depressed geriatric rehabilitation patients. A double-blind study. J Am Geriatr Soc 1986;34: 421–426.

7. Fogel BS, Ratey JJ. A neuropsychiatric approach to personality and behavior. In: Ratey JJ. Neuropsychiatry of personality disorders. Cambridge: Blackwell Science, 1995:1–16.

8. Wlaz P, Rolinski Z, Kleinrok Z, Czuczwar SJ: Influence of chronic aminophylline on antielectroshock activity of diazepam and aminophylline induced convulsions in mice. Pharmacol Biochem Behav 49(3):609-13, 1994.

9. Yudofsky S, Williams D, Gorman J. Propranolol in the treatment of rage and violent behavior in patients with chronic brain syndromes. Am J Psychiatry 1981;138:218–220.

10. Silver JM, Yudofsky SC. Aggressive behavior in patients with neuropsychiatric disorders. Psychiatric Annals 1987;17:367–370.

11. Herzog AG. Reproductive endocrine considerations and hormonal therapy for men with epilepsy. Epilepsia 1991;32(6)(Suppl): S34–S37.

12. Haggerty JJ, Prange AJ. Borderline hyperthyroidism and depression. In: Coggins CH, Hancock EW, Levitt LJ, eds. Annual review of medicine: selected topics in the clinical sciences. Palo Alto: Annual Reviews, Inc., 1995:37–46.

13. Sandman CA, Datta PC, Barrum J, et al. Noloxone attenuates self abusive behavior in developmentally disabled clients. Applied Research in Mental Retardation 1983;4:5–11.

14. Campbell M, Anderson LT, Small AM, Adams P, Gonzales NM, Ernst M. Naltrexone in autistic children: behavioral symptoms and attentional learning. J Am Acad Child Adolesc Psychiatry 1993;32: 1283–1291.

15. Percy AK, Glaze DG, Schultz RJ, et al. Rett syndrome: controlled study of an oral opiate antagonist, naltrexone. Ann Neurol 1994;35: 464–470.

16. Royall DR, Mahurin RK, True JE, et al. Executive impairment among the functionally dependent: comparisons between schizophrenic and elderly subjects. Am J Psychiatry 1993;150:1813.

17. Alexopoulous GS, Abrams RC, Young RC, et al. Cornell scale for depression in dementia. Biol Psychiatry 1988;23:271–284.

18. Yesavage JA, Brink TL, Rose TL, et al. Development and validation of a geriatric depression screening scale: a preliminary report. Psychiatry Research 1983;17:37–39.

19. Ott B, Fogel BS. Measurement of depression in dementia: self vs. clinician rating. International Journal of Geriatric Psychiatry 1993;7: 899–904.

20. Yudofsky SC, Silver JM, Jackson W, et al. The overt aggression scale for the objective rating of verbal and physical aggression. Am J Psychiatry 1986;143:35–39.

21. Marin RS, Biedrzyck RC, Firinciogullari. Reliability and validity of the apathy evaluation scale. Psychiatry Res 1991;38:143–162.

22. Huskisson EC. Visual analogue scales. In: Melzack R, ed. Pain measurement and assessment. New York: Raven Press, 1983:33–37.

23. Melzack R, ed. Pain measurement and assessment. New York: Raven Press, 1983.

24. Siu AL, Reuben DB, Hays RD. Hierarchical reaction of physical function in ambulatory geriatrics. J Am Geriatr Soc 1990;38: 1113–1119.

25. Stewart AL, Hays RD, Ware JE. The MOS short form health survey. Med Care 1988;26:724–732.

26. Jenner P. The rationale for the use of dopamine agonists in Parkinson's disease. Neurology 1995;45:6.

27. Koller WC, Silver DE, Lieberman A. An algorithm for the management of Parkinson's disease. Neurology 1994;44(Suppl 10): S1–S52.

28. Leach JP, Brodie MJ. Lamotrigine—clinical use. In: Levy RH, Mattson RH, Meldrum BS, eds. Antiepileptic drugs. 4th ed. New York: Raven Press, 1995:889–896.

29. Chadwick D. Gabapentin—Clinical use. In: Levy RH, Mattson RH, Meldrum BS, eds. Antiepileptic drugs. 4th ed. New York: Raven Press, 1995:851–856.

30. Stoudemire A, Fogel BS. Psychopharmacology update. In: Stoudemire A, Fogel BS, eds. Medical psychiatric practice, vol 1. Washington, DC: American Psychiatric Press, 1991:29–98.

31. Stoudemire A, Fogel BS. New psychotropics in medically ill patients. In: Stoudemire A, Fogel BS, eds. Medical psychiatric practice, vol 2. Washington, DC: American Psychiatric Press, 1993:69–112.

32. Stoudermire A, Fogel BS. Psychopharmacology in medical patients: an update. In: Stoudemire A, Fogel BS, eds. Medical psychiatric practice, vol 3. Washington, DC: American Psychiatric Press, 1995:79–150.

32a. Lipsey JR, Robinson, RG, Pearlson FD, et al. Nortriptyline treatment of post-stroke depression: a double-blind treatment trial. Lancet 1:297–323, 1985.

33. Reding MJ, Orto LA, Winter SW, et al. Antidepressant therapy after stroke: a double-blind trial. Arch Neurol 47:785–789, 1986.

33a. Robinson RG, Parikh RM, Lipsey JR, et al. Pathologic laughing and crying following stroke: validation of a measurement scale and a double-blind treatment study. Am J Psychiatry 193;150:286–293.

33b. Schiffer RB, Herndon RM, Rudick RA. Treatment of pathological laughing and weeping with amitriptyline. NEJM 1985;312:1480–1482.

34. Reifler BV, Teri L, Rasking M, et al. Double blind trial of imipramine in Alzheimer's disease patients with and without depression. Am J Psychiatry 1989;146:45–49.

35. Schiffer RB, Wineman NM. Antidepressant pharmacotherapy of depression associated with multiple sclerosis. Am J Psychiatry 1990; 147:1493–1497.

36. Denmark JC, Powell JD, McComb SG. Imipramine hydrochloride in parkinsonism. Br J Clin Pract 1961;15:523–524.

37. Laitinena L. Desipramine in treatment of Parkinson's disease. Acta Neurol Scand 1969;45:109–113.

38. Strang RR. Imipramine in the treatment of parkinsonism: a double blind placebo study. Br Med J 1965;2:33–34.

39. Andersen J, Aabro E, Gulmann N, et al. Antidepressive treatment in Parkinson's disease. Acta Neurol Scand 1980;62:210–219.

39a. Allain H, Cougnard, Neukirch HC, et al. Selegiline in de novo parkinsonian patients: The French Multicenter Trial (FSMT). Acta Neurol Schand 1991;84(Suppl 136):73–78.

39b. Goetz CG, Tanner CM, Klawans HL. Bupropion in Parkinson's disease. Neurology 1984; 34:1092–1094.

40. Peyser CE, Folstein SE. Huntington's disease as a model for mood disorders: clues from neurpathology and neurochemistry. Mol Chem Neuropathol 1990;12:99–119.

41. Moller HJ, Fuger J, Kasper S. Efficacy of new generation antidepressants: meta-analysis of imipramine-controlled studies. Pharmacopsychiatry 1994;27:215–23.

42. Montgomery SA, Henry J, McDonald G, et al. Selective serotonin reuptake inhibitors: meta analysis of discontinuation rates. Int Clin Psychopharmacol 1994;9:47–53.

43. Andrews JM, Nemeroff CB. Contemporary management of depression. Am J Med 1994;97:24S–32S.

44. Clerc GE, Ruimy P, Verdeau Palles J. A double-blind comparison of venlafaxine and fluoxetine in patients hospitalized for major depres-

sion and melancholia. The Venlafaxine French Inpatient Study Group. Int Clin Psychopharmacol 1994;9:139–143.

45. Nierenberg AA, Feighner JP, Rudolph R, Cole JO, Sullivan J. Venlafaxine for treatment resistant unipolar depression. J Clin Psychopharmacol 1944;14:419–423.

46. Jancar J, Gunaratne JJ. Dysthymia and mental handicap. Br J Psychiatry 1994;164:691–693.

47. Wilens TE, Biederman J, Mick E, Spencer TJ. A systematic assessment of tricyclic antidepressants in the treatment of adult attention-deficit hyperactivity disorder. J Nerv Ment Dis 1995;183:48–50.

48. Aman MG. Efficacy of psychotropic drugs for reducing self-injurious behavior in the developmental disabilities. Ann Clin Psychiatry 1993; 5:171–188.

49. Goodnick PJ, Sandoval R. Psychotropic treatment of chronic fatigue syndrome and related disorders. J Clin Psychiatry 1993; 54:13–20.

50. Onghena P, Van Houdenhove B. Antidepressant induced analgesia in chronic non-malignant pain: a meta-analysis of 39 placebo controlled studies. Pain 1992;49:205–219.

51. Philipp M, Fickinger M. Psychotropic drugs in the management of chronic pain syndromes. Pharmacopsychiatry 1993;26:221–234.

52. Hollander E, Wong CM. Body dysmorphic disorder, pathological gambling, and sexual compulsions. J Clin Psychiatry 1995;56(Suppl 4) 7–12.

53. Kafka MP. Sertraline pharmacotherapy for paraphilias and paraphilia-related disorders: an open trial. Ann Clin Psychiatry 1994;6: 189–195.

54. Sloan RL, Brown KW, Pentland B. Fluoxetine as a treatment of emotional lability after brain injury. Brain Inj 1992;6:315–319.

55. Panzer MJ, Mellow AM. Antidepressant treatment of pathologic laughing or crying in elderly stroke patients. J Geriatr Psychiatry Neurol 1992;5:195–199.

56. Sutherland SM, Davidson JR. Phamacotherapy for post-traumatic stress disorder. Psychiatr Clin North Am 1994;17:409–423.

57. Sweeney S, Henry A. The use of imipramine in Tourette's syndrome and attention deficit disorder. J Clin Psychiatry 1994;46:348.

58. Stoudemire A, Fogel BS, Gulley L, Moran MG. Psychopharmacology in the medical patient. In: Stoudemire A, Fogel S, eds. Psychiatric care of the medical patient. New York: Oxford University Press, 1993: 155–206.

59. Cassano GB, Musetti L, Soriani A, Savino M. The pharmacologic treatment of depression: drug selection criteria. Pharmacopsychiatry 1995;26(Suppl 1):17–23.

60. George MS, Trimble MR. A fluvoxamine-induced frontal lobe syndrome in a patient with comorbid Gilles de la Tourette's syndrome and obsessive compulsive disorder. J Clin Psychiatry 1992;53:379.

61. Hoehn SR, Harris GJ, Pearlson GD, et al. A fluoxetine induced frontal lobe syndrome in an obsessive compulsive patient. J Clin Psychiatry 1991;52:131–133.

62. Coulter DM, Pillans PI. Fluoxetine and extrapyramidal side effects. Am J Psychiatry 1995;152:122–125.

63. Kahn RS, David KL. New developments in dopamine and schizophrenia. In: Floom FE, Kupfer DJ, eds. Psychopharmacology: the fourth generation of progress. New York: Raven Press, 1995: 1193–1204.

64. Lejoyeux M, Rouillon F, Ades J, Gorwood P. Neural symptoms induced by tricyclic antidepressants: phenomenology and pathophysiology. Acta Psychiatr Scand 85(4):1992;249–256.

65. Knegtering H, Eijck M, Huijsman A. Effects of antidepressants on cognitive functioning of elderly patients. A review. Drugs and Aging. 1994;5:192–199.

66. Ames D, Wirshing WC, Szuba MP. Organic mental disorders associated with bupropion in three patients. J Clin Psychiatry 1992;53,53–55.

67. Ansseau M, Darimont P, Lecoq A, et al. Controlled comparison of nefazodone and amitriptyline in major depressive inpatients. Psychopharmacology Berl 1994;115:254–260.

68. Pick CG, Paul D, Eison MS, Pasternak GW. Potentiation of opioid analgesia by the antidepressant nefazodone. Eur J Pharmacol 1992; 211:375–381.

69. Feighner JP. The role of venlafaxine in rational antidepressant therapy. J Clin Psychiatry 1994;55(Suppl A):62–68.

70. Jerling M, Bertilsson L, Sjoqvist F. The issue of therapeutic drug monitoring data to document kinetic drug interactions: an example with amitriptyline and nortriptyline. Ther Drug Monit 1994;16: 1–12.

71. Von Moltke LL, Greenblatt DJ, Cotreau Bibbo MM, Duan SX, Harmatz JS, Shader RI. Inhibition of desipramine hydroxylation in vitro by serotonin reuptake inhibitor antidepressants and by quinidine and ketoconazole: a model system to predict drug interactions in vivo. J Pharmcol Exp Ther 1994;268:1278–1283.

72. Jerling M, Lindstrom L, Bondesson U, Bertilsson L. Fluvoxamine inhibition and carbamazepine induction of the metabolism of clozapine: evidence from a therapeutic drug monitoring service. Ther Drug Monit 1994;16:368–374.

73. Perucca E, Gatti G, Spina E. Clinical pharmacokinetics of fluvoxamine. Clin Pharmcokinet 1994;27:175–190.

74. DeVane CL, Ware MR, Lydiard RB. Pharmacokinetics, pharmacodynamics, and treatment issues of benzodiazepines: alprazolam, adinazolam, and clonazepam. Psychopharmacol Bull 1991;27: 463–473.

74a. Brathwaite RA, Flanagan RA, Richens A. Steady state plasma nortriptyline concentrations in epileptic patients. Br J Clin Pharmacol 1975;2:469–471.

74b. Brøsen K, Kragh Sørensen P. Concomitant intake of nortriptyline and carbamazepine. Ther Drug Monit 1993;15:258–260.

75. Akiskal HS. Dysthymic and cyclothymic depressions: therapeutic considerations. J Clin Psychiatry 1994;55(Suppl)46–52.

76. Wragg RE, Jeste DV. Neuroleptics and alternative treatments: management of behavioral symptoms and psychosis in Alzheimer's disease and related conditions. Psychiatr Clin North Am 1988;11: 195–213.

77. Schneider LS, Pollock VE, Lyness SA. A metaanalysis of controlled trials of neuroleptic treatment in dementia. J Am Geriatric Soc 1990; 38:553–563.

78. Feinstein C, Leroy D. Pharmacotherapy of severe psychiatric disorders in mentally retarded individuals. In: Stoudemire A. Fogel BS, eds. Medical Psychiatric Practice, vol. 1. Washington, DC: American Psychiatric Press, 1991:501–537.

79. Aman MG, Singh NN. A critical appraisal of recent drug research in mental retardation: the coldwater studies. J Ment Defic Res 1988;30: 203–216.

80. Vanden Borre R, Vermote R, Buttiens M, et al. Risperidone as add-on therapy in behavioral disturbances in mental retardation: a double-blind placebo controlled cross over study. Acta Psychiatr Scand 1993; 87(3):167–171.

81. Shapiro AK, Shapiro E. Neuroleptic drugs. In Kurlan R, ed. Handbook of Tourette's syndrome and related tic and behavioral disorders. New York: Marcel Dekker, 1993:347–377.

82. Cohen DJ. The pathology of the self in primary childhood autism and Gilles de la Tourette syndrome. Psychiatr Clin North Am 1980;3: 383–402.

83. Locascio JJ, Malone RP, Small AM, et al. Factors related to haloperidol response and dyskinesias in autistic children. Psychopharmacol Bull 1991;27:119–126.

84. Campbell M, Adams P, Perry R, et al. Tardive and withdrawal dyskinesia in autistic children: a prospective study. Psychopharmacol Bull 1988a;24:251–255.

85. Morris M, Tyler A. Management and therapy. In: Harper PS, ed. Huntington's disease. Philadelphia: WB Saunders, 1991:205–250.

86. Lipowski ZJ. Delirium: acute confusional states. New York: Oxford University Press, 1990.

87. Mori E, Yamadori A. Acute confusional state and acute agitated delirium. Occurrence after infection in the right middle cerebral artery. Arch Neurol 1987;44:1139–1143.

88. Rich SS, Friedman JH. Treatment of Psychosis in Parkinson's disease.

In Stoudemire A, Fogel BS, eds. Medical psychiatric practice Washington, DC: American Psychiatric Press, 1995:151–182.

89. McDougle CJ, Price LH, Goodman WK. Fluvoxamine treatment of coincident autistic disorder and obsessive-compulsive disorder: a case report. J Autism Dev Disord 1990;20:537–543.

89a. McDougle CJ, Goodman WK, Price LH, et al. Neuroleptic addition in fluvoxamine-refractory obsessive-compulsive disorder. Am J Psychiatry 1990;147:652–654.

89b. McDougle CJ, Goodman WK, Leckman JF, et al. Haloperidol addition to fluvoxamine-refractory obsessive-compulsive disorder: a double-blind, placebo-controlled study in patients with and without tics. Arch Gen Psychiatry 1994;51:302–308.

90. Chouinard G, Sultan S. Treatment of supersensitivity psychosis with antiepileptic drugs: report of a series of 43 cases. Psychopharmacol Bull 1990;26:337–341.

91. Luchins DJ, Oliver AP, Wyatt RJ. Seizures with antidepressants: an in vitro technique to assess relative risk. Epilepsia 1984;25:25–32.

91a. Kane JM. Tardive dyskinesia: epidemiological and clinical presentation. In: Bloom FE, Kupfer DJ, eds. Psychopharmacology: The Fourth Generation of Progress. New York: Raven Press, 1995:1485–1495.

92. Balant-Gorgia AE, Balant LP, Andreoli A. Pharmacokinetic optimisation of the treatment of psychosis. Clin Pharmacokinet 1993;25:217–236.

93. Javaid JI. Clinical pharmacokinetics of antipsychotics. J Clin Pharmacol 1994;34:286–295.

94. Daniel W, Janczar L, Danek L, Legrum W, Netter KJ. Pharmacokinetic interaction between carbamazepine and neuroleptics after combined prolonged treatment in rats. Naunyn-Schmiedebergs Arch Pharmacol 1992;345:598–605.

95. Awad AG. Subjective response to neuroleptics in schizophrenia. Schizophr Bull 1993;19:609–618.

96. Schooler NR. Negative symptoms in schizophrenia: assessment of the effect of risperidone. J Clin Psychiatry 1994;55(Suppl):22–28.

97. Gerlach J, Peacock L. Motor and mental side effects of clozapine. J Clin Psychiatry 1994;55(Suppl B):107–109.

98. Chengappa KN, Shelton MD, Baker RW, Schooler NR, Baird J, Delaney J. The prevalence of akathisia in patients receiving stable doses of clozapine. J Clin Psychiatry 1994;55:142–145.

99. Friedman JH. Clozapine treatment of psychosis in patients with tardive dystonia: report of three cases. Mov Disord 1994;9:321–324.

100. Lindstrom LH. Long-term clinical and social outcome studies in schizophrenia in relation to the cognitive and emotional side effects of antipsychotic drugs. Acta Psychiatr Scand 1994;380:74–76.

101. Safferman AZ, Kane JM, Aronowitz JS, Gordon MF, Pollack S, Lieberman JA. The use of clozpine in neurologic disorders. J Clin Psychiatry 1994;55(Suppl B):98–101.

102. Bezchlibnyk-Butler, KZ, Remington GJ. Antiparkinsonian drugs in the treatment of neuroleptic-induced extrapyramidal symptoms. Can J Psychiatry 1994;39:74–84.

103. Thapa PB, Meador KG, Dieon P, Fought RL, Ray WA. Effects of antipsychotic withdrawal in elderly nursing home residents. J Am Geriatr Soc 1994;42:280–286.

104. Shader RI, Greenblatt DJ. Use of benzodiazepines in anxiety disorders. N Engl J Med 1993;328:1398–1405.

105. Woods JH, Katz JL, Winger G: Benzodiazepine use, abuse, and consequences. Pharmacol Rev 1992;44:151–347.

106. Jann MW, Kurtz NM. Treatment of panic and phobic disorders. Clin Pharmacol 1987;6:947–962.

107. Tarsy D. Restless legs syndrome. In: Joseph AB, Young RR, eds. Movement disorders in neurology and neuropsychiatry. Boston: Blackwell Scientific Publications, 1992:397–400.

107a. Ronthal M. Myoclonus and asterixis. In: Joseph AB, Young RR, eds. Movement disorders in neurology and neuropsychiatry. Boston: Blackwell Scientific Publications, 1992:479–486.

107b. Joseph AB. Catatonia. In: Joseph AB, Young RR, eds. Movement

disorders in neurology and neuropsychiatry. Boston: Blackwell Scientific Publications, 1992:335–342.

108. Ricketts RW, Goza AB, Ellis CR, et al. Clinical effects of buspirone on intractable self-injury in adults with mental retardation. J Am Acad Child Adolesc Psychiatry 1994;33:270–276.

109. Stanislav SW, Fabre T, Crismon ML, Childs A. Buspirone's efficacy in organic induced aggression. J Clin Psychopharmcol 1994;14:126–130.

110. Ratey J, Sovner R, Parks A, Rogentine K. Buspirone treatment of aggression and anxiety in mentally retarded patients: a multiple-baseline, placebo lead in study. J Clin Psychiatry 1991;52:159–162.

111. Moss LE, Neppe M, Drevets WC. Buspirone in the treatment of tardive dyskinesia. J Clin Psychopharmacol 1993;13:204–209.

112. Littman AB, Fava M, McKool K, Lamon-Fava S, Pegg E. Buspirone therapy for type A behavior, hostility, and perceived stress in cardiac patients. Psychother Psychosom 1993;59:107–110.

113. Salzman C. Treatment of anxiety. In Salzman C, ed. Clinical geriatric psychopharmacology, 2nd ed. Baltimore: Williams and Wilkins, 1992, pp. 189–212.

114. Regestein R. Effects of lithium on behavioral reactivity: relation to increases in brain cholinergic activity. Psychopharmacology 1981;73:120–125.

114a. Arana GW, Epstein S, Molloy M, et al. Carbamazepine-induced reduction of plasma alprazolam concentrations: a clinical case report. J Clin Psychiatry 1988;49:448–449.

114b. Lai AA, Levy RH, Cutler RE. Time course of interaction between carbamazepine and clonazepam in normal man. Clin Pharmacol Ther 1978:24:316–323.

115. Tuncok Y, Akpina R, Guven H, Akkoclu A. The effects of theophylline on serum alprazolam levels. Int J Clin Pharmacol Ther 1994;32:642–645.

116. Lenox RH, Manji HK. Lithium. In: Schatzberg AF, Nemeroff CB, eds. Textbook of psychopharmacology. Washington, DC: American Psychiatric Press, 1995:303–358.

117. Goodwin FK, Jamison KR. Manic depressive illness. New York: Oxford University Press, 1990.

118. Schou M. Use in other psychiatric conditions. In: Johnson FN, ed. Depression and mania: modern lithium therapy. Oxford: IRL Press, 1987:44–50.

119. Dale PG. Lithium therapy in aggressive mentally subnormal patients. Br J Psychiatry 1980;137:469–474.

120. Smith DA, Perry PJ. Nonneuroleptic treatment of disruptive behavior in organic mental syndromes. Ann Pharmacother 1992;26:1400–1408.

121. Campbell M, Small AM, Green WH, et al. Behavioral efficacy of haloperidol and lithium carbonate—a comparison in hospitalized aggressive children with conduct disorder. Arch Gen Psychiatry 1984;41:650–656.

122. Sheard MH, Marini JL, Bridges C, et al. The effects of lithium in impulsive aggressive behavior in man. Am J Psychiatry 1976;133:1409–1413.

123. Haas JF, Cope N. Neuropharmacologic management of behavior sequelae in head injury: a case report. Arch Phys Med Rehabil 1985;66:472–474.

124. Luchins DF, Dojka D. Lithium and propranolol in aggression and self-injurious behavior in the mentally retarded. Psychopharmacol Bull 1989;25:372–375.

125. Leonard DP, Kidson MA, Shannon PJ, et al. Double-blind trial of lithium carbonate and haloperidol in Huntington's chorea. Lancet 1974;2:1208–1209.

126. Morris M, Tyler A. Management and therapy. In: Harper PS, ed. Huntington's disease. Philadelphia: WB Saunders, 1991:205–250.

127. Bussone G, Leone M, Peccarisi C, et al. Double-blind comparison of lithium and verapamil in cluster headache prophylaxis. Headache 1990;30:411–417.

128. Delgado PL, Gelenberg AJ. Antidepressant and antimanic medication. In Gabbard GO (ed). Treatments of psychiatric disorders.

Washington DC; American Psychiatric Press, 1995, pp. 1132–1168.

129. Lazarus JH. Endocrine and metabolic effects of lithium. New York, Plenum, 1986.

130. McElroy SL, Keck PE. Antiepileptic drugs. In: Schatzberg AF, Nemeroff CB, eds. Textbook of psychopharmacology. Washington DC: American Psychiatric Press, 1995:351–376.

131. Stoll AL, Banov M, Kolbrener M, et al. Neurologic factors predict a favorable valproate response in bipolar and schizoaffective disorders. J Clin Psychopharmacol 1994;14:311–313.

132. Fogel BS, Duffy J. Elderly patients. In: Silver JM, Yudofsky SC, Hales RE, eds. Neuropsychiatry of traumatic brain injury. Washington, DC: American Psychiatric Press, 1994:413–442.

133. Silver JM. Yudofsky SC. Aggressive disorders. In: Silver JM, Yudofsky SC, Hales RE, eds. Neuropsychiatry of traumatic brain injury. Washington DC. American Psychiatric Press, 1994: 313–356.

134. Gualtieri CT. Neuropsychiatry and Behavioral Pharmacology. New York: Springer-Verlag, 1991.

135. Keck PE, McElroy SL, Friedman LM. Valproate and carbamazepine in the treatment of panic and posttraumatic stress disorders, withdrawal states, and behavioral dyscontrol syndromes. J Clin Psychopharmacol 1992;12:36S–41S.

136. Fesler FA. Valproate in combat-related posttraumatic stress disorder. J Clin Psychiatry 1991 Sep;52(9):361–364.

137. Silver JM, Sandberg DP, Hales RE. New approaches in the pharmacotherapy of posttraumatic stress disorder. J Clin Psychiatry 1990 Oct. 51(Suppl):33–38.

138. McQuay H, Carroll D, Jadad AR, et al. Anticonvulsant drugs for management of pain: a systematic review. BMJ 1995 Oct 21; 311(7012):1047–1052.

139. Guiec R, Mesdjian E, Rochat H, et al. Central analgesic effect of valproate in patients with epilepsy. Seizure 1993 Jun;2(2):147–150.

140. Lemke MR. Effect of carbamazepine on agitation in Alzheimer's in patients refractory to neuroleptics. J Clin Psychiatry 1995 Aug;56(8):354–357.

141. Tariot PN, Erb R, Leibovici A, et al. Carbamazepine treatment of agitation in nursing home patients with dementia: a preliminary study. J Am Geriatr Soc. 1994 Nov;42(11):1160–1166.

142. Young JL, Hillbrand M. Carbamazepine lowers aggression: a review. Bull Am Acad Psychiatry Law 1994;22:53–61.

143. Barratt ES. The use of anticonvulsants in aggression and violence. Psychopharmacol Bull 1993;29(1):75–81.

144. Lewin J, Sumners D. Successful treatment of episodic dyscontrol with carbamazepine. Br J Psychiatry 1992 Aug;161(8):261–262.

145. Lott AD, McElroy SL, Keys MA. Valproate in the treatment of behavioral agitation in elderly patients with dementia. J Neuropsychiatry Clin Neurosci 1995 Summer;7(3):314–319.

146. Geracioti TD. Valproic acid treatment of episodic explosiveness related to brain injury. J Clin Psychiatry 1994;55:416–417.

147. Mazure CM, Druss BG, Cellar JS. Valproate treatment of older psychotic patients with organic mental syndromes and behavioral dyscontrol. J Am Geriatr Soc 1992;40:914–916.

148. Mellow AM, Solano Lopez C, Davis S. Sodium valproate in the treatment of behavioral disturbance in dementia. J Geriatr Psychiatry Neurol 1993;6:205–209.

149. Varney NR, Garvey MJ, Cook BL, Campbell DA, Roberts RJ. Identification of treatment resistant depressives who respond favorably to carbamazepine. Ann Clin Psychiatry 1993;5:117–122.

150. Winchel RM, Stanley M. Self-injurious behavior: a review of the behavior and biology of self-mutilation. Am J Psychiatry 1991;148:306–317.

151. Schweizer E, Rickels K, Case WG, Greenblatt DJ. Carbamazepine treatment in patients discontinuing long-term benzodiazepine therapy. Effects on withdrawal severity and outcome. Arch Gen Psychiatry 1991;48:448–452.

152. Kastner T, Finesmith R, Walsh K. Long-term administration of valproic acid in the treatment of affective symptoms in people with mental retardation. J Clin Psychopharmacol 1993;13(6):448–451.

153. Pellock JM. The clinical efficacy of lamotrigine as an antiepileptic drug. Neurology 1994;44:S29–35.

154. Yau MK, Wargin WA, Wolf KB, et al. Effect of valproate on the pharmacokinetics of lamotrigine at steady state. Epilepsia 1992; 33(Suppl 3):82.

155. Howard JR, Dix RK, Shumaker RC, et al. Effect of felbamate on carbamazepine pharmacokinetics. Epilepsia 1992;33(Suppl 3); 84–85.

156. McLean MJ. Gabapentin: Chemistry, absorption, distribution, and excretion. In: Levy RH, Mattson RH, Meldrum BS, eds. Antiepileptic Drugs, 4th ed. New York: Raven Press, 1995:843–849.

157. Levy RH, Mattson RH, Meldrum BS, eds. Antiepileptic Drugs, 4th ed. New York: Raven Press, 1995.

158. Laidlaw J, Richens A, Chadwick D, eds: A Textbook of Epilepsy, 4th ed. Edinburgh: Churchill Livingstone, 1993.

159. Saletu B, Grunberger J, Linzmayer L. Evaluation of encephalotropic and psychotropic properties of gabapentin in man by pharmaco-EEG and psychometry. Int J Clin Pharmacol Ther Toxicol 1986;24:364–373.

159a. Smith D, Baker G, Davies G, et al. Outcomes of add-on treatment with lamotrigine in partial epilepsy. Epilepsia 1993;34:312–322.

160. Kaplitz SE. Withdrawn, apathetic geriatric patients responsive to methylphenidate. J Am Geriatric Soc 1975;23:271–276.

161. Wilens TE, Biederman J. The stimulants. Psychiatric Clin North Am 1992;15:191–222.

162. Mitler MM. Evaluation of treatment with stimulants in narcolepsy. Sleep 1993;17(8 Suppl):S103–S106.

163. Wallace AE, Kofoed LL, West AN. Double blind, placebo controlled trial of methylphenidate in older, depressed, medically ill patients. Am J Psychiatry 1995;152:929–931.

164. Lazarus LW, Moberg PJ, Langsley PR, Lingam VR. Methylphenidate and nortriptyline in the treatment of poststroke depression: a retrospective comparison. Arch Phys Med Rehabil 1994;75:403–406.

165. Mayes SD, Crites DL, Bixler EO, Humphrey FJ 2nd, Mattison RE. Methylphenidate and ADHD: influence of age, IQ and neurodevelopmental status. Dev Med Child Neurol 1994;36:1099–1107.

166. Marin R, Fogel BS, Hawkins J, et al. Apathy: a treatable disorder. J Neuropsychiatr Clin Neurosci 1995;7:23–30.

167. Pritchard JG, Mykyta LJ. Use of a combination of methylphenidate and oxyprenolol in the management of physically disabled, apathetic, elderly patients: a pilot study. Curr Med Res Opinion 3:26–29, 1975.

168. Chiarello RJ, Cole JO: The use of psychostimulants in general psychiatry. Arch Gen Psychiatry 44:286–295, 1987.

169. Lipkin PH, Goldstein IJ, Adesman AR. Tics and dyskinesias associated with stimulant treatment in attention deficit hyperactivity disorder. Arch Pediatr Adolesc Med 1994;148:859–861.

170. Biederman J, Spencer T, Wilens TE, Spirch-Buckminster S. Attention deficit hyperactivity disorder: pharmacotherapy. In: Gabbard G, ed. Treatment of psychiatric disorders. Washington, DC: American Psychiatric Press, 1995.

171. Wells BG, Marken PA. Bromocriptin in the treatment of depression DICP: Annals of Pharmacotherapy 1989;23:600–601.

172. Bouckoms A, Manigini L. Pergolide: an antidepressant adjuvant for mood disorders? Psychopharmacol Bull 1993;29:207–211.

173. Borison RI. Amantadine in the management of extrapyramidal side effects. Clin Neuropharmacol 1983;6:557–563.

174. Chandler MC, Barnhill JB, Gualtiere CT. Amantadine for the agitated head injury patient. Brain Inj 1988;2:309–311.

174a. Gualtieri CT, Chandler M, Coons T, Brown L. Amantadine: a new clinical profile for traumatic brain injury. Clin Neuropharmacol 1989; 12:258–270.

175. Ross ED, Stewart RM. Akinetic mutism from hypothalamic damage: successful treatment with dopamine agonists. Neurology 1981; 31:1435–1439.

176. Fleet WS, Valenstein E, Watson RT, Heilman KM. Dopamine agonist therapy for neglect in humans. Neurology 1987;37:1765–1770.

177. Dobkin BH, Hanlon R. Dopamine agonist treatment of anterograde amnesia from a mediobasal forebrain injury. Ann Neurol 1993; 33:313–316.

178. Albert ML, Bachman DL, Morgan A, et al. Pharmacotherapy for aphasia. Neurology 1988;38(6):877–879.

179. Ziegler DK, Hurwitz A, Hassanein RS, et al. Migraine prophylaxis: a comparison of propranolol and amitriptyline. Arch Neurol 1987; 44:486–489.

180. Larsen TA, Teravainen H. Beta I versus nonselective blockade in therapy of essential tremor. Adv Neurol 1983;37:247–251.

181. Leckman JF, Knorr AM, Rasmusson AM, Cohen DJ. Basal ganglia research and Tourette's syndrome. Trends Neurosci 1991;14:94.

182. Jasinski DR, Johnson RE, Kocher TR. Clonidine in morphine withdrawal: differential effects on signs and symptoms. Arch Gen Psychiatry 1985;42:1063–1065.

183. Hunt RD. Treatment effects of oral and transdermal clonidine in relation to methylphenidate: an open pilot study in ADD-H. Psychopharmacol Bull 1987;23:111–114.

184. Steingard RJ, Biederman J, Spencer T, et al. Comparison of clonidine response in the treatment of attention deficit hyperactivity disorder with and without comorbid tic disorders. J Am Acad Child Adolesc Psychiatry 1993;32:350–353.

185. Ratey JJ, Greenberg MS, Lindem DJ. Combination of treatments for attention deficit hyperactivity disorder in adults. J Nerv Ment Dis 1991;179:699–701.

186. Hunt RD, Arnsten AF, Asbell MD. An open trial of guanfacine in the treatment of attention deficit hyperactivity disorder. J Am Acad Child Adolesc Psychiatry 1995;34:50–54.

187. Schneider LS, Sobin PB. Non-neuroleptic treatment of behavioral symptoms and agitation in Alzheimer's disease and other dementias. Psychopharmacol Bull 1992;28:71–79.

188. Williams DT, Mehl R. Yudofsky S, Adams D, Roseman D. The effect of propranolol on uncontrolled rage outbursts in children and adolescents with organic brain dysfunction. J Am Acad Child Psychiatry 1982;21:129–135.

189. Yudofsky SC, Silver JM, Schneider SE. Pharmacologic treatment of aggression. Psychiatric Annals 1987;17:397–407.

190. Adler LA, Angrist B, Reiter S, et al. Neuroleptic induced akathisia: a review. Psychopharmacology 1989;97:1–11.

191. Fleischhacker W, Roth SD, Kane JM. The pharmacologic treatment of neuroleptic-induced akathisia. J Clin Psychopharmacol 1990; 10:12–21.

192. Sandman CA. The opiate hypothesis in autism and self injury. J Child Adolesc Psychopharmacol 1991;1:237–248.

193. Gillberg C. Endogenous opioids and opiate antagonists in autism: Brief review of empirical findings and implications for clinicians. Dev Med Child Neurol 37(3):239–245, 1995.

194. Herman BH, Hammock MK, Egan J, Arthur-Smith A, Chatoor R, Werner A. Role for opioid peptides in self-injurious behavior: dissociation from autonomic nervous system functioning. Dev Pharmacol Ther 1989;12:81–89.

195. Gillberg C. Endogenous opioids and opiate antagonists in autism: brief review of empirical findings and implications for clinicians. Dev Med Child Neurol 1995;37:239–245.

196. Thompson T, Hackenberg T, Cerutti D, Baker D, Axtell S. Opioid antagonist effects on self-injury in adults with mental retardation: response form and location as determinants of medication effects. Am J Ment Retard 1994;99:85–102.

197. Campbell M, Anderson LT, Small AM, et al. Naltrexone in autistic children: a double-blind and placebo-controlled study. Psychopharmacol Bull 1990;26:130–135.

198. Kolman D. The use of opiate antagonists in treatment of bulimia: a study of low-dose versus high-dose naltrexone. Psychiatry Res 1988; 24:195–199.

199. Lensing P, Klingler D, Lampl C, et al. Naltrexone open trial with a 5 year old boy. A social rebound reaction. Acta Paedopsychiatr 1992; 55:169–173.

200. Zingarelli G, Ellman G, Hom A, Wymore M, Heidorn S, Chicz DA. Clinical effects of naltrexone on autistic behavior. Am J Ment Retard 1992;97:57–63.

201. Jonas JM, Gold MS. The use of opiate antagonists in treating bulimia: a study of low-dose versus high-dose naltrexone. Psychiatry Res 1988;24:195–199.

202. Chatoor I, Herman BH, Hartzler J. Effects of the opiate antagonist, naltrexone, on binging antecedents and plasma beta-endorphin concentrations. J Am Acad Child Adolesc Psychiatry 1994;33: 748–752.

203. Kurlan R, Majumdar L, Deeley C, Mudholkar GS, Plumb S, Como PG. A controlled trial of propoxyphene and naltrexone in patients with Tourette's syndrome. Ann Neurol 1991;30:19–23.

204. Benjamin E, Buot Smith T. Naltrexone and fluoxetine in Prader-Willi syndrome. J Am Acad Child Adolesc Psychiatry 1993;32:870–873.

12

NEUROBIOLOGICAL MECHANISMS OF HUMAN ANXIETY

Dennis S. Charney, Linda M. Nagy, J. Douglas Bremner, Andrew W. Goddard, Rachel Yehuda, and Steven M. Southwick

The anxiety disorders discussed in this chapter are those included in the *Diagnostic and Statistical Manual of Mental Disorders,* 4th Edition (DSM-IV: panic disorder and agoraphobia, social phobia, specific phobia, posttraumatic stress disorder [PTSD], acute stress disorder, and generalized anxiety disorder). Obsessive Compulsive Disorder (OCD) is not included because of the evidence that the etiology and treatment of OCD substantially differs from other anxiety disorders. (OCD is discussed in Chapter 35.) Initially, the neurobiological foundation needed to understand the etiology of the major anxiety disorders is described. Subsequently, for each disorder, epidemiologic data, a basic description of the syndrome, comparisons to other psychiatric and nonpsychiatric disorders, and current etiologic theories are reviewed.

FUNCTIONAL NEUROANATOMICAL CORRELATES OF ANXIETY AND FEAR

Evidence accumulated from a large body of preclinical studies provides a basis for proposing a functional neuroanatomy of anxiety and fear. The brain structures constituting a neural circuit of anxiety or fear should have several features:

1. There must be sufficient afferent sensory input to permit assessment of the fear- or anxiety-producing nature of external or internal stimuli;
2. The neuronal interactions among the brain structures must be capable of incorporating an individual's prior experience (memory) into the cognitive appraisal of stimuli. These interactions are important in the attachment of affective significance to specific stimuli and the mobilization of adaptive behavioral responses; and
3. The efferent projections from the brain structures should be able to mediate an individual's neuroendocrine, autonomic, and skeletal motor responses to threat in order to facilitate survival, as well as account for the pathological reactions that result in anxiety-related signs and symptoms.

The major afferent arms of the neural circuitry of anxiety include the exteroceptive sensory systems of the brain (auditory, visual, somatosensory), consisting of serially organized relay channels that convey directly or through multisynaptic pathways information relevant to the experience of fear or anxiety. The sensory information contained in a fear- or anxiety-inducing stimulus is transmitted from peripheral receptor cells to the dorsal thalamus (1). An exception is the olfactory system, which does not relay information through the thalamus, and whose principal targets in the brain are the amygdala and entorhinal cortex (2). Visceral afferent pathways alter the function of the locus ceruleus and the amygdala, either through direct connections or via the nucleus paragigantocellularis (PGI) and the nucleus tractus solitarius (3–5).

The thalamus relays sensory information to the primary sensory receptive areas of the cortex. In turn, these primary sensory regions project to adjacent unimodal and polymodal cortical association areas (6–8). The cortical association areas of visual, auditory, and somatosensory systems send projections to other brain structures, including the amygdala, entorhinal cortex, orbitofrontal cortex, and cingulate gyrus (9–11). The hippocampus receives convergent, integrated inputs from all sensory systems by way of projections from entorhinal cortex (12). (See Chapter 7 for further details.)

Thus, much of the sensory information of fear- and anxiety-inducing stimuli are first processed in the sensory cortex prior to transfer to subcortical structures, which are more involved in affective, behavioral, and somatic responses. It is noteworthy that the amygdala also receives sensory information directly from the thalamus. The medial geniculate nuclei of the thalamus (acoustic thalamus) sends projections to the amygdala and hypothalamus. The thalamic areas associated with the visual system also innervate the amygdala. These data support a pivotal role for the amygdala in the transmission and interpretation of fear- and anxiety-inducing sensory information because it receives afferents from thalamic and cortical exteroceptive systems, as

258 *Neuropsychiatry*

well as subcortical visceral afferent pathways (13). The neuronal interactions between the amygdala and cortical regions, such as the orbitofrontal cortex, enable the individual to initiate adaptive behaviors to threat based upon the nature of the threat and prior experience.

The efferent pathways of the anxiety-fear circuit mediate autonomic, neuroendocrine, and skeletal-motor responses. The structures involved in these responses include the amygdala, locus ceruleus, hypothalamus, periaqueductal gray (PAG), and striatum.

Many of the autonomic changes produced by anxiety- and fear-inducing stimuli are produced by the sympathetic and parasympathetic neural systems. Stimulation of the lateral hypothalamus results in sympathetic system activation—increases in blood pressure and heart rate, sweating, piloerection, and pupil dilatation. Activation of the paraventricular nucleus of the hypothalamus promotes the release of a variety of hormones and peptides. The hypothalamus integrates information it receives from a variety of brain structures into a coordinated pattern of sympathetic responses. The sympathetic activation and hormonal release associated with anxiety and fear are probably mediated, in part by stimulation of the hypothalamus via projections from the amygdala and locus ceruleus (14–16). In addition, the PGI also plays an important role in regulating sympathetic function and may account for the parallel activation of the peripheral sympathetic system and the locus ceruleus.

The vagus and splanchnic nerves are major projections of the parasympathetic nervous system. Afferents to the vagus include the lateral hypothalamus, paraventricular nucleus, locus ceruleus, and the amygdala. There are afferent connections to the splanchnic nerves from the locus ceruleus (17, 18). This innervation of the parasympathetic nervous system may relate to visceral symptoms associated with anxiety, such as gastrointestinal and genitourinary disturbances.

The regulatory control of skeletal muscle by the brain in response to emotions is complex. Both subtle movements involving a few muscle groups (facial muscles) as well as fully integrated responses requiring the entire musculoskeletal system for fight or flight may be required. Adaptive mobilization of the skeletal motor system to respond to threat probably involves pathways between the cortical association areas and motor cortex, cortical association areas and the striatum, and the amygdala and striatum.

The amygdala has strong projections to most areas of the striatum, including the nucleus accumbens, olfactory tubercle, and parts of the caudate and putamen. The portion of the striatum that is innervated by the amygdala also receives efferents from the orbitofrontal cortex and the ventral tegmental area. The amygdalocortical and amygdalostriatal projections are topographically organized and occur in register. Individual areas of the amygdala, and in some cases individual amygdaloid neurons, can integrate information from the cortico-striato-pallidal systems. The dense innervation of the striatum and prefrontal cortex by the amygdala indicates that the amygdala can powerfully regu-

late both of these systems (19, 20). These interactions between the amygdala and the extrapyramidal motor system may be very important for generating motor responses to threatening stimuli, especially those related to prior adverse experiences.

Effects of Prior Experience

Memories and previously learned behaviors influence the responses to anxiety- and fear-inducing stimuli via such neural mechanisms as fear conditioning, extinction, and sensitization (see discussion that follows). Although within the medial temporal lobe memory system, emotional responsiveness (amygdala) and memory (hippocampus) may be separately organized, there is considerable interaction between storage and recall of memory and affect. This is exemplified by the critical role of the amygdala in conditioned fear acquisition, sensitization, extinction, and the attachment of affective significance to neutral stimuli (21, 22).

The hippocampus and amygdala are sites of convergent reciprocal projections from widespread unimodal and polymodal cortical association areas. It is probably through these interactions, as well as cortical-cortical connections, that memories stored in the cortex—which are continually being reinforced by ongoing experience—are intensified, and develop greater coherence (23).

The hippocampal memory system is essential to short-term memory. However, long-term memory storage may be organized such that, as time passes, with subsequent additional retrieval opportunities and the acquisition of related material, the role of the hippocampus diminishes until it may no longer be necessary for memory. The repository of long-term memory may be in the same areas of cortex where the initial sensory impressions take place (24). The shift in memory storage to the cortex may represent a shift from conscious representational memory to unconscious memory processes that indirectly affect behavior.

Therefore, once a fear- or anxiety-inducing sensory stimulus is relayed through the thalamus into neural circuits involving the cortex, hippocampus, and amygdala, relevant memory traces of posttraumatic experiences are stimulated. Most likely, the potency of the cognitive and somatic responses to the stimulus will be strongly correlated with prior experiences, due to the strengthening of neural connections within the circuit. These functional neuroanatomical relationships can explain how a single sensory stimulus such as a sight or sound can elicit a specific memory. Moreover, if the sight or sound was associated with a particular traumatic event, a cascade of anxiety- and fear-related symptoms will ensue, probably mediated by the efferent arm of the proposed circuit.

NEURAL MECHANISMS OF ANXIETY AND FEAR

Fear Conditioning

In many patients with anxiety disorders such as panic disorder with agoraphobia, simple phobias, and posttraumatic stress disorder (PTSD), vivid memories of a traumatic event, autonomic arousal, and even flashbacks can be elicited by diverse sensory and cognitive stimuli that have been associated with the original trauma (25, 26). Consequently, patients begin to avoid these stimuli in their everyday life, or a numbing of general emotional responsiveness occurs. Modality-specific and contextual fear conditioning, which are easily demonstrated in the laboratory, may explain some of these observations. Animals exposed to emotionally neutral, visual, or auditory conditioned stimuli (CS) in conjunction with an aversive unconditioned stimulus (UCS), will subsequently exhibit a conditioned emotional response (CER) to the CS in the absence of the UCS. CERs are also produced when an animal is placed in an environment in which an aversive UCS has previously been experienced. In this circumstance the CER are not elicited by a modality-specific stimulus that was paired with a UCS, but instead by complex, polymodal contextual stimuli that were present in the environment when the UCS originally occurred and are present upon reexposure to the environment (27). CERs can last for years in laboratory animals (28) and are used to establish that a state of fear has been produced (29). Therefore, a neural analysis of fear conditioning in animals may be useful in identifying the neurochemicals and brain structures involved in learning and remembering associations of stimuli with traumatic events, which may form the basis of many of the symptoms associated with human anxiety disorders.

Contextual fear conditioning, which involves more complex stimuli from multiple sensory modalities, may require projections to the amygdala from higher-order cortical areas that integrate inputs from many sources and the hippocampus. It is noteworthy that lesions of the hippocampus 1 day after fear conditioning abolish contextual fear. Lesions 7 days or longer after fear conditioning have no effect. These findings suggest the hippocampus may have a time-limited role in associative fear memories evoked by contextual sensory (polymodal), but not unimodal sensory stimuli (27, 30). Contextual fear conditioning appears to require exposure to more aversive UCS than modality-specific fear conditioning. Apparently, as the intensity of the UCS increases, the organism becomes more sensitive to a wider range of stimulus factors in the environment. This is consistent with clinical observations that severely traumatized individuals can develop anxiogenic responses to a much broader spectrum of environmental stimuli than those initially related to the trauma. Such patients frequently suffer from chronic and severe emotional distress.

Several behavioral paradigms indicate an important role for noradrenergic neuronal systems in the processes involved in fear conditioning. Neutral stimuli paired with shock produce increases in brain norepinephrine metabolism and behavioral deficits similar to those elicited by the shock (31, 32). In the freely moving cat, the firing rate of cells in the locus ceruleus can be increased by presenting a neutral acoustic stimulus previously paired with an air puff to the whiskers, which also increases firing and is aversive to the cat

(33). There is also a body of evidence indicating that an intact noradrenergic system may be necessary for the acquisition of fear-conditioned responses. (34, 35).

Extinction

It is possible that the continued ability of conditioned stimuli to elicit a spectrum of anxiety and fear behaviors results from a deficit in the neural mechanisms involved in response reduction or extinction. Experimental extinction is defined as a loss of a previously learned conditioned emotional response following repeated presentations of a conditioned fear stimulus in the absence of a contiguous traumatic event. Extinction has been explained in terms of either an 'erasure' of the original associations that led to the production of the conditioned response (36) or the acquisition of new associations that compete with or "mask" the expression of the still intact, response-producing associations (37). The "erasure" hypothesis predicts that following nonreinforcement, the response-producing associations no longer exist and, therefore, the conditioned response can no longer be performed. The "masking" hypothesis predicts that the response-producing associations remain after nonreinforcement and, therefore, if it were possible to temporarily remove the masking associations, the conditioned response could be performed.

Results in several studies suggest that the original associations are intact following extinction. Expression of extinction may be specific to the stimulus context in which nonreinforcement occurred (38–40). Re-presentation of the unconditioned stimulus, even up to 1 year after extinction, is sufficient for reinstating extinguished response to a preextinction level (41–44). These data indicate the essentially permanent nature of conditioned fear and the apparent fragility of extinction. This phenomenon may help to explain the common clinical observation that traumatic memories may remain dormant for many years, only to be elicited by a subsequent stressor or unexpectedly by a stimulus long ago associated with the original trauma (45, 46).

Clearly, these studies indicate that extinction does not erase the original aversive memory, but instead involves the learning of a new memory that masks or inhibits the original one. It is important to emphasize, however, that although extinction can be overcome, in normal animals extinction does result in a reduction of the conditioned fear response. Using traditional measures of conditioned fear, such as freezing, potentiated startle, or autonomic indices, nonreinforcement leads to a reduction in all these measures. In healthy humans, many childhood fears become extinguished and do not intrude daily in adulthood. In contrast, patients with a variety of phobias, and PTSD patients, describe persistent traumatic memories that do not disappear. Thus, it is conceivable that some anxiety disorder patients have deficits in brain systems involved in extinction.

The amygdala is not only involved in the acquisition and expression of conditioned fear responses, but may also be necessary for extinction. NMDA antagonists infused into the amygdala prevent the extinction of fear-potentiated startle (47). Thus, activity in the amygdala during nonreinforced stimuli presentations may be essential for extinction of conditioned fear stimuli. This may result from processes within the amygdala itself or via structures that project to the amygdala (e.g., hippocampus, prefrontal cortex, septal area) and have been implicated in extinction in several experimental paradigms. Extinction of conditioned fear responses may represent an active suppression by the cortex of subcortical neural circuits (thalamus, amygdala) that maintain learned associations over long time periods (48).

Behavioral Sensitization

Sensitization generally refers to the increase in behavioral or physiological responsiveness that occurs following repeated exposure to a stimulus. Behavioral sensitization can be generally context-dependent or conditioned, such that animals will not demonstrate sensitization if the stimulus is presented in a different environment (49). However, if the intensity of the stimulus or drug dose is high enough, behavioral sensitization will occur even if the environments change. It has been suggested that different mechanisms are called into play with environment-independent sensitization (50).

In addition to stimulus intensity and drug dose, the number and temporal sequencing of exposures are important determinants of the degree of sensitization produced. Repeated intermittent exposures produce more robust sensitization (51). Another critical variable involves the time interval between the initial stimulus and subsequent exposure. Thus, a single stimulus can elicit behavioral sensitization, provided that sufficient time has elapsed between the initial presentation and subsequent reexposure (52). Moreover, cross-sensitization (augmented response to a different stimulus than the original evoking stimulus) may occur (53).

The neurochemical and neuroanatomical systems mediating environment-dependent and environment-independent behavioral sensitization have begun to be investigated. The mechanisms of the development and maintenance of stress-induced sensitization in mammals have been most extensively studied in catecholaminergic systems.

Single or repeated exposure to a stressor potentiates the capacity of a subsequent stressor to increase dopamine function in the forebrain (54, 55) without apparently altering basal dopamine turnover (56–58). Recently it has been shown that the conditioned components of sensitization is related to increased dopamine release in the nucleus accumbens (59). Behavioral sensitization to stress may also involve alterations in noradrenergic function. Animals previously exposed to a stressor exhibit increased norepinephrine release in the hippocampus (60), hypothalamus (60), and prefrontal cortex (61), upon stressor reexposure.

Dopamine D_2 receptor antagonists block the development but not the maintenance of sensitization. Conversely, α_2-receptor agonists and benzodiazepine agonists block the

maintenance but not the development of sensitization (50). In addition, lesions of the amygdala or the nucleus accumbens block the development of cocaine-induced behavioral sensitization. In contrast, lesions of the hippocampus and frontal cortex have no effect (Pert A, Weiss SRB, unpublished observations).

NEUROTRANSMITTERS IMPLICATED IN ANXIETY AND FEAR

Numerous preclinical studies have been conducted to identify the neurotransmitters and neuropeptides that mediate the behavioral responses associated with anxiety and fear. This work has generally taken the form of determining the neurotransmitters and neuropeptides altered by stress. The next section briefly describes the evidence implicating specific neurotransmitter and neuropeptide systems in anxiety and fear.

Noradrenergic System

EFFECTS OF STRESSFUL AND FEAR-INDUCING STIMULI ON BIOCHEMICAL INDICES OF NORADRENERGIC FUNCTION

Stressful stimuli of many types produce marked increases in brain noradrenergic function. Stress produces regional selective increases in NE turnover in brain regions identified as part of the neural circuitry of anxiety, including the locus ceruleus (LC), hypothalamus, hippocampus, amygdala, and cerebral cortex. It has recently been demonstrated that immobilization stress, footshock stress, tail-pinch stress, and conditioned fear increase noradrenergic metabolism in the hypothalamus and amygdala (62–64). Stress also increases tyrosine hydroxylase levels in the LC (65). Anxiolytic agents reverse the effects of stress on noradrenergic metabolism (62, 66, 67). Consistent with these findings, acute cold-restraint stress results in decreased density of α_2-adrenergic receptors in the hippocampus and amygdala (68). The stress-induced decrease in NE turnover is also associated with a decrease in postsynaptic β-receptor density (69). The heightened responsiveness of the noradrenergic system to stress is consistent with the notion that the elevated sense of fear or anxiety connected to stress may be a critical factor in the neurochemical effects observed.

LOCUS CERULEUS ACTIVITY AND BEHAVIORAL STATES ASSOCIATED WITH STRESS AND FEAR

In laboratory rats, chronic stress results in an increased firing of the LC (70, 71). Animals exposed to chronic inescapable shock, which is associated with learned helplessness, have an increase in responsiveness of the LC to an excitatory stimulus compared with animals exposed to escapable shock (71).

The effect of stressful and fear-inducing stimuli on LC activity has been assessed in freely moving cats (72, 73). Conditions that are behaviorally activating but not stressful, such as visual exposure to other rats or to food that is physically inaccessible, do not increase LC firing. In contrast, stressful and fear-inducing stimuli, such as loud white noise, air puff, restraint, and confrontation with a dog, produce a rapid, robust, and sustained increase in LC activity (72). Interestingly, these increases in LC function are accompanied by sympathetic activation. Generally, the greater the sympathetic activation in response to the stressor, as indicated by heart rate, the greater the correlation observed. Thus, a stimulus intensity threshold for coactivation of central and peripheral NE systems may exist.

A parallel activation of LC neurons and splanchnic sympathetic nerves is produced by noxious stimuli. The LC-like sympathetic splanchnic activity is highly responsive to various peripheral cardiovascular events, such as alterations in blood volume or blood pressure. Internal events that must be responded to for survival, such as thermoregulatory disturbance, hypoglycemia, blood loss, an increase in pCO_2, or a marked reduction in blood pressure, cause robust and long-lasting increases in LC activity (67).

There are also peripheral visceral influences on LC activity. In rats, distention of the urinary bladder, distal colon, or rectum activate LC neurons. These findings suggest that changes in autonomic or visceral function may result in specific behavioral responses via the brain LC-norepinephrine system. The LC-norepinephrine network may help determine whether, under threat, an individual turns attention toward external, sensory stimuli or to internal vegetative events. The system, when functioning normally, may be important in facilitating the planning and execution of behaviors important for survival (67).

BEHAVIORAL EFFECTS OF LOCUS CERULEUS STIMULATION

Electrical stimulation of the LC produces a series of behavioral responses similar to those observed in naturally occurring or experimentally induced fear (74). These behaviors are also elicited by administration of drugs, such as yohimbine and piperoxone, which activate the LC by blocking α_2-adrenergic autoreceptors. Drugs that decrease the function of the LC by interacting with inhibitory opiate (morphine), benzodiazepine (diazepam), and α_2- (clonidine) receptors on the LC decrease fearful behavior and partially antagonize the effects of electrical stimulation of the LC in the monkey (75). These studies suggest that abnormally high levels of LC activity, producing increased release of NE at postsynaptic projection sites throughout the brain, may augment some forms of fear or pathological anxiety, depending on the environmental conditions (76).

Dopaminergic System

Acute stress increases dopamine release and metabolism in a number of specific brain areas. However, the dopamine innervation of the medial prefrontal cortex (mPFC) appears to be particularly vulnerable to stress; sufficiently low-intensity stress (such as that associated with conditioned fear) or brief exposure to stress increases dopamine release and metabolism in the prefrontal cortex in the absence of overt changes in other mesotelencephalic dopamine regions (77, 78). Low-intensity electric footshock increases in-vivo tyrosine hydroxylase and dopamine turnover in the mPFC, but not the nucleus accumbens or striatum (79–81). Benzodiazepine anxiolytics prevent selective increases in dopamine utilization in mPFC following mild stress (81). Anxiogenic benzodiazepine inverse agonists exert an opposite effect (81, 82). Selective activation of mPFC dopamine neurons can also be induced by intracerebroventricular injection of corticotropin-releasing factor (CRF), which has anxiogenic properties (80).

Stress can enhance dopamine release and metabolism in other areas receiving dopamine innervation, provided greater-intensity or longer-duration stress is used (77, 83). Thus the mPFC dopamine innervation is preferentially activated by stress compared to mesolimbic and nigrostriatal systems, and the mesolimbic dopamine innervation appears to be more sensitive to stress than the striatal dopamine innervation (77, 84, 85).

Serotonergic Function

The effects of stress on serotonin systems have been studied less thoroughly than noradrenergic and dopamine systems, and the data are somewhat contradictory. Animals exposed to a variety of stressors including footshock, tail shock, tail pinch, and restraint stress have all been shown to produce an increase in serotonin turnover in the mPFC (80, 86–91).

On the other hand, inescapable stress paradigms producing "learned helplessness" behavioral deficits have been associated with reduced in-vivo release of serotonin in cerebral cortex (92, 93). Serotonin antagonists produce behavioral deficits resembling those seen following inescapable shock (94). Drugs that enhance serotonin neurotransmission (SSRIs) are effective in reversing "learned helplessness" (95).

The effect of stress to active serotonin turnover may stimulate a system that has both anxiogenic and anxiolytic pathways within the forebrain (96, 97). A primary distinction in the qualitative effects of serotonin may be between the dorsal and median raphe nuclei—the two midbrain nuclei that produce most of the forebrain serotonin. The serotonergic innervation of the amygdala and the hippocampus by the dorsal raphe are believed to mediate anxiogenic effects via 5-HT2 receptors. In contrast, the median raphe innervation of hippocampal 5-HT1A receptors has been hypothesized to facilitate the disconnection of previously learned associations with aversive events, or to suppress the formation of new associations, thus providing a resilience to aversive events (96, 98). Chronic stress increase cortical 5-HT2 receptors (99–101) and reduce hippocampal 5-HT1A receptors (101–106).

Establishing the precise role of serotonin in the behavioral effects of uncontrollable stress is complicated because different animal models reflect different types of anxiety and fear, and serotonin neurons are involved in some but not all forms of anxiety—adding to the confusion. Also, important functional interactions between noradrenergic and serotonin may be important in the modulation of anxiety and fear behaviors. The stress-induced increases in brain tryptophan and serotonin metabolism depend on sympathetic nervous system activity (107). The elevation of cortical 5-HT2 receptors by stress depend on the integrity of brain noradrenergic neurons (108). In addition, there is considerable preclinical evidence that serotonin has inhibitory effects on noradrenergic function in the LC and the cortex (109).

Benzodiazepine Receptor Systems

Benzodiazepine receptors are present throughout the brain (110), with the highest concentration in cortical grey matter (111). Benzodiazepines potentiate and prolong the synaptic actions of the inhibitory neurotransmitter γ-aminobutyric acid (GABA) (112). Central benzodiazepine receptors and GABA receptors are part of the same macromolecular complex. These receptors have distinct binding sites, although they are functionally coupled and regulate each other in an allosteric manner. A correlation has also been found between the efficacy of the benzodiazepines and their potency at displacing [3H]diazepam binding, which suggests that these compounds are physiologically relevant (113, 114). The hypothesis that alterations in benzodiazepine receptor function play a role in the pathophysiology of the anxiety disorders is supported by several lines of preclinical evidence (115).

Administration of inverse agonists of benzodiazepine receptors, such as B-carboline-3-carboxylic acid ethyl ester (B-CCE) (116), result in behavioral and biological effects similar to those seen in anxiety, including increases in heart rate, blood pressure, plasma cortisol, and catecholamines. Administration of the β-carboline FG7142 results in an increase in local cerebral glucose utilization in brain structures involved in memory, including lateral septal nucleus, mammillary bodies, and anterior thalamic nuclei (117). The effects of the β-carbolines are blocked by administration of benzodiazepines (118).

Studies using the animal model of uncontrollable stress, a putative animal model for the anxiety disorders, suggest alterations in benzodiazepine receptor function associated with uncontrollable stress (119, 120). Most studies have found that animals exposed to acute inescapable stress develop a decrease in benzodiazepine-receptor binding in cerebral cortex, frontal cortex, and hippocampus, with conflicting results for hypothalamus, and no change in striatum, midbrain, thalamus, cerebellum, and pons. Chronic stress has been associated in most studies with decreases in benzodiazepine-receptor binding in cerebral cortex, frontal cortex, hippocampus, and hypothalamus, with mixed results for cerebellum, midbrain, and striatum, and no changes in pons.

Decreases in benzodiazepine-receptor binding are associated with alterations in memory manifested by deficits in maze escape behaviors (121, 122). Changes in benzodiazepine-receptor function appear to be specific to uncontrollable stress, as opposed to controllable stress, and are prevented by preadministration of benzodiazepines (123). A decrease in benzodiazepine-receptor binding has been demonstrated in the Maudsley genetically fearful strain of rat in comparison with nonfearful rats in several brain structures, including the hippocampus (124).

Neuropeptides Implicated in Anxiety and Fear

CORTICOTROPIN-RELEASING FACTOR

Considerable data now indicate that corticotropin-releasing factor (CRF), the hypothalamic hypophysiotropic hormone that activates the pituitary-adrenal axis, is also a neurotransmitter at extra-hypothalamic brain sites (125). In laboratory animals, CRF has anxiogenic-like properties when injected centrally (126). Furthermore, CRF appears to play an important role in the neuroendocrine, autonomic, and behavioral responses to stress (127, 128). Severe stressors produce increases in CRF concentrations in the amygdala, hippocampus, and the LC (129). Recently, it has been demonstrated that early-life trauma can produce persistent changes in CRF receptors.

The brain sites mediating the CRF responses to stress have not been established. However, there is increasing evidence that these effects of CRF may be produced by interactions with LC noradrenergic neurons: intraventricular infusion of CRF increases norepinephrine turnover in several forebrain areas (130). CRF in a dose-dependent fashion increases the firing rate of LC-norepinephrine neurons (131), and a stressor that activates norepinephrine neurons markedly increases CRF concentrations in the LC (129). Moreover, it has recently been demonstrated that infusion of CRF into the LC has anxiogenic activity and produces significant increases in the norepinephrine metabolite 3,4-dihydroxyphenylglycol (MPHG) in forebrain areas such as the amygdala and hypothalamus (132). Bilateral lesions of the amygdala selectively decrease CRF concentrations in the LC (133). The anxiolytic benzodiazepine, alprazolam, selectively decreases CRF concentrations in the LC (134). These data suggest that under stressful conditions CRF and norepinephrine regions, like the LC, may participate in a mutually reinforcing feedback loop.

CRF may also have important effects on dopamine neuronal function. Intraventricular administration of the peptide increases dopamine metabolism in the prefrontal cortex in a manner similar to stress (135). It is not clear, however, if the mechanism through which the prefrontal cortex dopamine system is activated is the same as that subserving the stress-induced effect (136).

OPIOID PEPTIDES

A primary behavioral effect of uncontrollable stress is analgesia, which results from the release of endogenous opiates (137). Significant analgesia is observed following only uncontrollable (137–140) and is also seen following presentation of neutral stimuli previously paired with aversive stimuli (141). There is also evidence that sensitization occurs because reexposure to less intense shock in rats previously exposed to uncontrollable shock also results in analgesia (142).

These effects are likely to be mediated, in part, by a stress-induced release of endogenous opiates in the brainstem because the analgesia is blocked by naltrexone (137, 140, 142) and shows cross-tolerance to morphine analgesia (139). Moreover, opiate peptides are elevated after acute uncontrollable shock (143, 144) and uncontrollable, but not controllable, shock decreases the density of μ-opiate receptors (145).

CHOLECYSTOKININ

Recently, preclinical investigations support the involvement of the peptide cholecystokinin (CCK) in anxiety and fear. CCK, an octopeptide originally discovered in the gastrointestinal tract, has been found to be present in high concentrations in the cerebral cortex, amygdala, and hippocampus in mammalian brain (146). CCK has anxiogenic effects in laboratory animals and appears to act as a neurotransmitter or neuromodulator in the brain. Interactions with benzodiazepine receptors are of particular interest. Benzodiazepine anxiolytics antagonize the excitatory neuronal and anxiogenic effects of CCK and CCK_B antagonists have anxiolytic actions in animal models (147). Studies in healthy human subjects have demonstrated that CCK-4 induces severe anxiety or short-lived panic attacks. This effect is reduced by lorazepam (148).

NEUROPEPTIDE Y

Low doses of neuropeptide Y administered intraventricularly have anxiolytic effects in several animal models of anxiety (149, 150). These actions may be mediated by neuropeptide Y in the amygdala. Administration of an antisense oligonucleotide targeted at the neuropeptide Y_1-receptor message, which led to a 60% decrease in the B_{max} of Y_1 receptors, was accompanied by marked "anxiogenic-like" effects in the elevated plus-maze, a test in which neuropeptide Y itself is markedly "anxiolytic" (151). This suggests that endogenous neuropeptide Y could be anxiolytic by activating Y_1 receptors and that disturbed neuropeptide Y transmission might have a role in symptoms of anxiety (152).

ANXIETY DISORDERS: DESCRIPTION AND PATHOPHYSIOLOGY

The large body of preclinical studies designed to identify the brain structures' neural mechanisms, neurotransmitters, and neuropeptides involved in the development and expression of anxiety and fear has provided a foundation from which to improve the understanding of the pathophysiology of human anxiety disorders. The section that follows, after an initial description of each disorder, reviews the current knowledge of the pathophysiology of the major anxiety disorders.

Panic Disorder and Agoraphobia

Panic disorder is characterized by recurrent discrete attacks of anxiety accompanied by several somatic symptoms, such as palpitations, paresthesias, hyperventilation, diaphoresis, chest pain, dizziness, trembling, and dyspnea. Usually the condition is accompanied by agoraphobia, which consists of excessive fear (and often avoidance) of situations, such as driving, crowded places, stores, or being alone, in which escape or obtaining help would be difficult. Current DSM-IV classifications include "panic disorder without agoraphobia," "panic disorder with agoraphobia," and "agoraphobia without history of panic disorder."

EPIDEMIOLOGY

The Epidemiologic Catchment Area Study (ECA) reports prevalence estimates based on DSM-III diagnoses, which were separated into agoraphobia (analogous to DSM-IV diagnoses of "agoraphobia without history of panic attacks" and "panic disorder with agoraphobia") and panic disorder (analogous to DSM-IV, diagnosis of "panic disorder without agoraphobia"). Lifetime prevalence rates at the three sites varied between 7.8 and 23.3% for all phobias (including social and simple) and between 1.4 and 1.5% for panic disorder. Six-month prevalence rates were 2.7 to 5.8% for agoraphobia and 0.6 to 1.0% for panic disorder. The lifetime rate for females was 2.4 to 4.3 times greater than that for males diagnosed with agoraphobia and 1.3 to 3.5 times greater for panic disorder; however, 6-month prevalence rates for panic disorder were either similar between sexes or increased in males (153, 154). Most researchers agree that there may be underreporting of these disorders by men either because of reluctance to admit to having these symptoms or through disguise by alcoholism. Alternatively, there may be higher rates than reported in females because of hormonal, social, or other gender differences.

Age of onset is typically in the late teens to early 30s and is unusual after the age of 40 years. The majority (78%) of patients describe the initial attack as spontaneous (occurring without an environmental trigger). In the remainder the first attack is precipitated by confrontation with a phobic stimulus or use of a psychoactive drug. Onset of the disorder often follows within 6 months of a major stressful life event, such as marital separation, occupational change, or pregnancy (155).

These disorders appear to be less prevalent in the elderly. Both 6-month and lifetime rates are lower in the over-65 age group, suggesting possible underreporting, decreased survival of those with the disorder, or a cohort effect, such that the frequency of the disorder is increased in the middle-age groups. Rates are generally similar for blacks and whites, and higher for noncollege graduates and unmarried individuals. It is not yet established whether these differences reflect predisposing factors, noncausal associations, or consequences of the disorder. Panic disorder is increased among family members of those with the disorder. A history of childhood separation anxiety disorder is reported by 20 to 50% of patients. Preliminary findings of high rates of behavioral inhibition in the offspring of patients with panic disorder are consistent with the hypothesis that the disorder may have developmental antecedents.

DESCRIPTION AND DIFFERENTIAL DIAGNOSIS

Panic disorder usually begins with a spontaneous panic attack that often leads the individual to seek medical treatment, such as presenting to an emergency room believing that he or she is having a heart attack, stroke, losing his or her mind, or experiencing some other serious medical event. Some time may pass before subsequent attacks, or the patient may continue to have frequent attacks. Patients may feel constantly fearful and anxious after the first attack, wondering what is wrong and fearing it will happen again. Some patients experience nocturnal attacks that awaken them from sleep. Usually patients gradually become fearful of situations (*a*) that they associate with the attacks; (*b*) in which they would be unable to flee if the attack occurred; (*c*) in which help would not be readily available; or (*d*) in which they would be embarrassed if others should notice they are experiencing an attack (although attacks are not usually evident to others). Less frequently, a history of phobia may precede the first panic attack. Before patients are educated about the symptoms of the disorder, they believe they are suffering from a serious medical condition. They are often embarrassed about their symptoms and will try to hide them from others, often making excuses not to attend functions or enter phobic situations.

The differential diagnosis of panic disorder and agoraphobia includes secondary anxiety disorder due to medical conditions; substances such as caffeine, cocaine, or amphetamines; withdrawal from alcohol, sedative-hyponotics or benzodiazepines; as well as other phobic conditions, generalized anxiety disorder, and psychosis. Medical illness that can produce symptoms similar to panic attacks must be excluded. Endocrine disturbances, such as pheochromocytoma, hyperthyroidism, or hypoglycemia, can produce similar symptoms and can be excluded with appropriate clinical history and laboratory evaluations.

When gastrointestinal symptoms of attacks are prominent, the diagnosis of colitis may need to be excluded. Symptoms of tachycardia, palpitations, chest pain or pressure, and dyspnea may be confused with cardiac or respiratory conditions. Lightheadedness, faintness, dizziness, derealization, shaking numbness, and tingling may suggest a neurological condition. The association between mitral valve prolapse and panic disorder is controversial. The presence of mitral valve prolapse in panic disorder patients does not appear to alter treatment response or course, so the diagnosis of panic disorder should be made independently of mitral valve prolapse.

Panic disorder differs from generalized anxiety disorder in that the former is distinguished by recurrent discrete, intense episodes of panic symptoms, although in both disorders anticipatory anxiety and generalized feelings of anxiety may be present. Although some of the same situations may be feared, agoraphobia differs from social and simple phobias in that the fear is related to feeling trapped or being unable to escape and that the fears often become generalized. Agoraphobics may additionally have a history of other phobias.

Panic disorder is frequently associated with major depression, other anxiety disorders, and alcohol and substance abuse. In clinical samples, as many as two-thirds of panic patients report experiencing a major depressive episode at some time in their lives. Similarly, studies of patients seeking treatment for major depression report high rates of panic in these patients and their relatives. Once symptoms begin, patients often describe becoming demoralized as a result of fear related to the symptoms and their imagined causes, and because of impairment when their activities are restricted by their agoraphobia. Unlike depressed patients, panic disorder patients usually lack vegetative symptoms and have a normal desire to engage in activities but avoid them because of their phobias.

The disorder may cause personality changes. Patients' premorbid personalities may be highly independent, outgoing, and active, but while symptoms are active, they can become very dependent, passive, and overly agreeable, with an extreme need to please others, and may resist making appointments or social engagements.

Attempts to self-medicate the intolerable anxiety may increase the risk of alcoholism and substance abuse. Patients may require a drink before entering phobic situations. Approximately 20% of patients report a history of alcohol abuse, but the onset of alcoholism precedes the first attack in almost all patients (155). Alcoholism may also alter the course of the disorder. Preliminary data suggest panic disorder precipitated by cocaine use may be less likely to respond well to the usual pharmacologic treatments and may have less association with a family history of panic disorder.

GENETIC EPIDEMIOLOGY

Genetic epidemiologic studies have consistently demonstrated increased rates of panic disorder among first- and second-degree relatives of panic disorder probands. This observation could result from genetic, nongenetic biological, and/or cultural factors shared by family members. The reported recurrence risk of illness in first-degree relatives of panic disorder probands is 15 to 18% by patient report vs. 0 to 5% in controls, and is 20 to 50% by direct interview of relatives of panic probands compared to 2 to 8% in relatives of controls (156). Segregation analysis indicates the pattern of familial transmission is consistent with single-locus, autosomal-dominant transmission with incomplete penetrance, although a multifactorial mode of inheritance (additive effects of more than one gene) or genetic heterogeneity (different gene defects producing similar clinical syndromes) have not been excluded as possibilities (157). Comparison of concordance rates in monozygotic vs. dizygotic twins is used to differentiate between genetic and environmental factors in families, since monozygotic twins share 100% of their genetic material and dizygotic twins on average share half. Torgersen (158) found concordance for anxiety disorder with panic attacks in four of 13 monozygotic and 0 of 16 dizygotic twin pairs. Other preliminary reports suggest identical HLA genotypes in sibling pairs concordant for panic disorder, but genetic linkage studies thus far have been negative (159).

Pathophysiology

STUDIES OF NORADRENERGIC FUNCTION IN PANIC DISORDER

Among all of the anxiety disorders, the evidence for an abnormality in noradrenergic function is most compelling for panic disorder and posttraumatic stress disorder (PTSD). Panic disorder and PTSD patients frequently report cardiovascular, gastrointestinal, and respiratory symptoms. Because the LC is responsive to peripheral alterations in the function of these systems, minor physiological changes in these patients may result in abnormal activation of LC neurons and, consequently, panic attacks and flashbacks. These functional interactions may explain the association of anxiety symptoms with tachycardia, tachypnea, hypoglycemia and visceral and organ distention, as well as the marked sensitivity of panic disorder and PTSD patients to interoceptive stimuli. The important role of the noradrenergic system in fear conditioning may account for the development of phobic symptoms in these patients. Finally, the involvement of noradrenergic neurons in learning and memory may relate to the persistence of traumatic memories in both disorders.

Peripheral Catecholamine Levels

Generally, measurement of peripheral norepinephrine and its metabolites have revealed concentrations in panic disorder patients similar to controls. Several studies have not found elevated plasma catecholamines following spontaneous or situationally-provoked panic attacks (160, 161). Moreover, plasma and urinary catecholamines (162, 163), and plasma and CSF 3methoxy-4hydroxyphenylethylene glycol (MHPG) levels in panic disorder patients are generally not different from healthy controls (164, 165).

A wide variety of investigations have been conducted to evaluate sympathetic nervous system (SNS) function in panic disorder. These studies have produced markedly divergent findings, yielding no firm consensus on whether a SNS dysfunction exists in panic disorder (166).

REGULATION OF NORADRENERGIC FUNCTION IN PANIC DISORDER

The regulation of noradrenergic neuronal function has been examined by determining the behavioral, biochemical, and cardiovascular effects of oral and intravenous yohimbine, an α_2-adrenergic receptor antagonist, in a spectrum of psychiatric disorders, including schizophrenia, major depression, obsessive-compulsive disorder, generalized anxiety disorder, panic disorder, and PTSD (167). Specific abnormalities have been identified in panic disorder and PTSD. Approximately 60 to 70% of panic disorder patients experience yohimbine-induced panic attacks. These patients have larger yohimbine-induced increases in plasma MHPG, blood pressure, and heart rate, compared with healthy subjects and other psychiatric disorders (168–170). The effects of yohimbine on regional cerebral blood flow (rCBF) and metabolism have been evaluated in panic-disorder and PTSD patients. In panic-disorder patients, yohimbine significantly reduced frontal rCBF rates in patients compared with healthy subjects (171).

A consistent finding in the literature is that the growth hormone rise induced by clonidine is blunted in panic disorder patients (172). In a recent investigation, a blunted growth hormone response was found primarily in the patients who experienced yohimbine-induced panic attacks (170). This suggests that the diminished postsynaptic α_2-adrenergic receptor function reflected by the blunted clonidine-growth hormone response may relate to presynaptic noradrenergic neuronal hyperactivity.

Several previous investigations observed that clonidine produced greater decreases in plasma MHPG and blood pressure in panic disorder patients compared to healthy subjects (170, 173, JD Coplan and colleagues, personal communication, December, 1993). The clonidine-induced decreases in plasma MHPG may be greatest in the panic disorder patients who experienced yohimbine-induced panic attacks (170), suggesting that there is a distinct subgroup of panic disorder patients who manifest noradrenergic neuronal dysfunction.

β-Adrenergic Receptor Function

Infusion of isoproterenol, a peripherally acting compound that is selective for the β-adrenoceptor, has been reported to trigger anxiety responses in panic patients compared with controls (174). Successful treatment of panic patients with tricyclic antidepressants blunted isoproterenol-induced anxiety and systolic blood pressure responses (175). These studies are consistent with the hypothesis of increased β_1-adrenoceptor sensitivity in panic disorder, which is normalized by effective pharmacotherapy (175).

Noradrenergic Function and Treatment for Panic Disorder

Evidence is emerging that the efficacy of some tricyclic and monoamine oxidase inhibitor drugs against panic may be related to their regulatory effects on noradrenergic activity (176). The effects of chronic treatment with these agents on the regulation of noradrenergic activity are complex. Some of these effects, such as reduced tyrosine hydroxylase activity, LC firing rate, NE turnover, and postsynaptic β-adrenergic receptor sensitivity, diminish noradrenergic function. It is interesting that antidepressant drugs that do not exhibit antipanic efficacy—bupropion and trazodone—have effects on noradrenergic function that are different from those of the tricyclic and monoamine inhibitors (177). In the rat brain, bupropion does not down-regulate β-adrenergic receptors or decrease NE turnover. While trazodone does down-regulate the β-adrenergic receptors, it does not decrease the LC firing rate or the spontaneous activity of cortical neurons receiving noradrenergic innervation.

Benzodiazepines are highly effective treatments for panic disorder, generally at higher doses than those needed for generalized anxiety disorder. Clearly, the anxiolytic effects of benzodiazepines are related to their agonist actions on benzodiazepine receptors at a variety of brain sites. However, it has been hypothesized that the antipanic properties of benzodiazepines may also relate to inhibitory effects on noradrenergic function because these drugs reduce LC neuronal activity (178).

The antipanic efficacy of the potent serotonin reuptake inhibitors (SRIs) like clomipramine, fluvoxamine, zimelidine, and fluoxetine is well documented. The mechanism of action of SRIs in panic disorder has not been established. However, 5-HT$_2$, 5-HT$_{1C}$, and 5-HT$_{1A}$ receptors are unlikely to be directly involved because ritanserin, a 5-HT$_2$ and 5-HT$_{1C}$ antagonist, and buspirone, a 5-HT$_{1A}$ agonist, lack antipanic efficacy (179).

It is possible that interactions between the serotonin (5-HT) and noradrenergic systems may be related to the antipanic properties of SRIs. Preclinical studies suggest that 5-HT-NE interactions occur between the LC and the dorsal raphe. Direct application of 5-HT to LC neurons results in a tonic inhibition of electrical activity (180). Phasic 5-HT inhibition of LC function may be mediated by an excitatory amino acid (EAA) pathway from the nucleus paragigantocellularis, possibly via a 5-HT$_{1A}$ receptor (181). In this context it is notable that fluvoxamine has been found to alter EAA receptor mRNA expression throughout the brain. Interactions between the noradrenergic and serotonin systems have been documented because fluvoxamine, but not placebo treatment, reduced yohimbine-induced anxiety in panic disorder patients (182).

If the noradrenergic system is dysregulated in panic disorder, the mechanism of action of anti-panic therapy may be its ability to decrease the wide and unpredictable fluctuations in noradrenergic activity. Likewise, it can improve efficiency by reducing basal activity (decreasing noise) while effecting a more specific responsiveness to specific stimuli (increasing signal-to-noise ratio).

SEROTONIN FUNCTION AND PANIC DISORDER

Peripheral Serotonin Function

Platelet imipramine binding (a marker of the serotonin reuptake site), which is generally reduced in depression, has been found to be normal in panic disorder (183, 184), while platelet 5-HT uptake in panic disorder has been reported to

be elevated (185), normal (186), or reduced (187). One study found that panic disorder patients had lower levels of circulating 5-HT in comparison to controls (188). Thus, no clear pattern of abnormality in 5-HT function in panic disorder has emerged from analysis of peripheral blood elements.

REGULATION OF SEROTONIN FUNCTION

To date, pharmacologic challenge studies of 5-HT in panic disorder have also been unable to establish a definite role for 5-HT in the pathophysiology of panic. Challenges with the 5-HT precursors, L-tryptophan (189) and 5-hydroxytryptophan (5-HTP) (190) did not discriminate between panic disorder and controls on neuroendocrine measures. Conversely, tryptophan depletion was not anxiogenic in unmedicated panic-disorder patients (191). However, challenge with the 5-HT releasing agent, fenfluramine, has been reported to be anxiogenic and to produce greater increases in plasma prolactin and cortisol in panic disorder compared with controls (192). Studies with the 5-HT agonist m-chloromethylpiperazine (mCPP), a probe of postsynaptic 5-HT$_{1C}$ and 5-HT$_2$ receptor function, have produced equivocal findings. Increases in anxiety and plasma cortisol in panic disorder patients as compared with controls has been reported with oral (193) but not IV administration of mCPP (194, 195).

Recent advances in 5-HT receptor pharmacology have identified at least seven distinct families of 5-HT receptor and multiple subtypes within those families. The challenge studies just reviewed have manipulated "global" 5-HT functioning in "panic disorder" or have used probes that lack selectivity (e.g., mCPP) without taking into account the full complexity of the 5-HT system and subsystems. In an attempt to address this problem, a more recent study used the selective 5-HT$_{1A}$ partial agonist ipsapirone (IPS) as a challenge agent (196). Corticotropin (ACTH), cortisol, and hypothermic responses to IPS were blunted in panic disorder patients, but their anxiety responses did not differ from controls. These data, if replicated, would implicate 5-HT$_{1A}$ receptor subsensitivity in the pathophysiology of panic disorder. In conclusion, the 5-HT system or one of its subsystems may have a role in the pathophysiology of panic disorder, the precise nature of which needs to be delineated by further investigation.

BENZODIAZEPINE-RECEPTOR FUNCTION IN PANIC DISORDER

Despite the preclinical support for the involvement of benzodiazepine systems in anxiety, clinical investigations of the function of this system in anxiety disorder patients have been difficult to design. The inability to identify measurable variables that are reflective of central benzodiazepine system function in living human subjects has contributed to the paucity of research in this area. However, evidence from clinical studies performed to date suggests a possible role for alterations in benzodiazepine receptor function in the anxiety disorders (197).

Administration of the benzodiazepine-receptor antagonist flumazenil to patients with panic disorder results in an increase in panic attacks and subjective anxiety in comparison with controls (198, 199). Both oral (199) and intravenous flumazenil (198) have been shown to produce panic in a subgroup of panic disorder patients, but not in healthy subjects. The benzodiazepine-receptor inverse agonist, FG7142, induces severe anxiety resembling panic attacks and biological characteristics of anxiety in healthy subjects (200). This observation raises a question regarding the existence of endogenous equivalents to FG7142 that might be released to provoke panic attacks. One candidate for such an endogenous ligand is tribulin, a substance with benzodiazepine-receptor binding and monoamine oxidase (MAO)-inhibiting properties, found in human urine (201). Increased levels of tribulin have been found in patients with anxiety and after lactate-induced panic attacks (202). Other candidates described include diazepam-binding inhibitor (DBI): this too is an inverse agonist (203). However, CSF levels of DBI are normal in panic disorder patients (204–206).

Benzodiazepine-induced sedation and changes in cortisol levels, as well as saccadic eye movement velocity, have been suggested as indicators of benzodiazepine-receptor-mediated actions. A preliminary clinical investigation revealed that panic disorder patients are less sensitive than controls to diazepam using saccadic eye movement velocity as a dependent measure. This finding suggests that panic disorder is associated with a functional subsensitivity of the GABA-benzodiazepine complex in brainstem regions controlling saccadic eye movements (207). Other evidence suggests lesser suppression of plasma norepinephrine, epinephrine, and pulse following administration of diazepam in panic disorder patients compared to controls (208).

The benzodiazepine receptors are highly concentrated in gray matter structures, including cortical areas such as temporal, parietal, and frontal cortex, and subcortical areas such as the hippocampus. Patients with panic disorder may have abnormalities of the right temporal lobe, with some studies suggesting atrophy and areas of increased signal activity detectable by MRI (209, 210).

Despite the modest findings of the currently available investigations regarding abnormalities in benzodiazepine receptor function in panic disorder patients, clearly, more direct assessments of benzodiazepine-receptor systems in anxiety disorders are indicated. These include measuring the density of benzodiazepine receptors and the behavioral and cerebral metabolic effects of benzodiazepine-agonist and inverse-agonist drugs, using PET and SPECT imaging techniques.

HYPOTHALAMIC-PITUITARY-ADRENAL (HPA) AXIS FUNCTION IN PANIC DISORDER

In contrast to HPA axis hyperactivity frequently found in depressive disorders, HPA axis function, in studies conducted to date, does not appear to be markedly disturbed in panic disorder (211–213). The majority of dexamethasone suppression test studies in panic disorder have shown normal suppression (214–219). Twenty-four-hour urinary-free cortisol levels are normal in panic disorder patients (220). The cortisol response to clonidine is also normal in panic disorder (220).

As reviewed previously, numerous studies indicate that CRH plays an important role in mediating the activation of endocrine, autonomic, and behavioral systems associated with the stress response. CRH has anxiogenic effects in laboratory animals. These actions of CRH involve important interactions with other brain neurochemical systems. Of particular relevance to the pathophysiology of anxiety syndromes are the findings that CRH stimulates central sympathetic outflow and the firing of the LC. Therefore, it is possible that the etiology of panic disorder is related to dysfunction in the functional linkages between brain CRH and noradrenergic systems. There is preliminary evidence that the ACTH and cortisol responses to CRH are blunted in panic disorder. However, CSF levels of CRH have been reported to be elevated in depressed patients but normal in panic disorder patients (204–206).

CHOLECYSTOKININ HYPOTHESIS OF PANIC DISORDER

Preclinical studies have shown that CCK agonists are anxiogenic in laboratory animals. DeMontigny (148) has demonstrated that in healthy volunteers intravenous administration of CCK4 (a tetrapeptide that crosses the blood-brain barrier more readily than CCK8) can induce severe anxiety or short-lived panic attacks. The anxiogenic effect of CCK was blocked by the benzodiazepine lorazepam, although this may merely be pharmacologic opposition and not true antagonism.

Recently, several investigations have shown that panic disorder patients are more sensitive to the anxiogenic effects of CCK4 and a closely related peptide, pentagastrin, and that these effects are blocked by CCK antagonists. The mechanism responsible for the enhanced sensitivity to CCK4 has not been elucidated. Patients may have an elevated production or turnover of CCK or increased sensitivity of CCK receptors. Since CCK has important functional interactions with other systems implicated in anxiety and fear (noradrenergic, dopaminergic, benzodiazepine), these interactions need to be evaluated in panic disorder patients. CCK$_B$ antagonists are now being tested as antipanic drugs (147, 221, 222).

RESPIRATORY SYSTEM DYSFUNCTION IN PANIC DISORDER

Pitts and McClure (223) made the first observation that an intravenous infusion of lactate produces panic anxiety in susceptible individuals but not in normal subjects. Subsequently, the reliability of panic provocation by sodium lactate has been well established. Lactate response appears to be specific for panic disorder compared with other anxiety disorders and psychiatric conditions (224, 225). Moreover, treatment of panic with imipramine will block the effects of lactate (226, 227).

The panicogenic mechanism of lactate has not been established. One theory is based upon the fact that systemic alkalosis causes vasoconstriction of cerebral vessels, which in turn induces cerebral ischemia, with a rise in the intracellular lactate: pyruvate ratio. Further, infused lactate results in a rapid passive elevation in the lactate: pyruvate ratio in localized brain regions outside the blood-brain barrier, such as the chemoreceptor zones. These two mechanisms lower the intracellular pH in medullary chemoreceptors. This theory suggests that in panic patients there is dysregulation (greater sensitivity to alterations in pH) in this region; thus, a panic response is triggered. Accordingly, this theory predicts that panic could be triggered in any subject if medullary pH was changed sufficiently (228).

The limitations of the model include that it is not yet known whether the pH changes in the local circulation are mirrored intracellularly. Recent evidence on the physiological effects of sodium bicarbonate have revealed a paradoxical intracellular acidosis, so the same may be true of lactate. Still, there is no clear evidence that intracellular acidosis will initiate neural activity, as the theory requires. Secondly, the model predicts that hypoxia is a profound stimulus for chemoreceptor stimulation, contradicting experiments in which removal of CO_2 from inspired air leads to loss of consciousness without anxiety or air hunger (229).

Another major hypothesis of lactate's panicogenic effect is via the induction of a metabolic alkalosis. Infused lactate is metabolized to bicarbonate. Bicarbonate is further metabolized to CO_2, which quickly permeates the central nervous system. This central buildup of CO_2 increases the ventilatory rate, via a direct stimulation of ventral medullary chemoreceptors. Increasing brain pCO_2 concentration has been shown to be a profound stimulus for locus ceruleus activation, which could cause panic via central noradrenergic activation (230).

Although the lactate-CO_2 theory has considerable appeal, initial studies with the isomer d-lactate suggest that this may not be the whole explanation. There is a preliminary report that this isomer also is panicogenic (231) but is not metabolized to CO_2. Comparisons of the behavioral effects of lactate and bicarbonate infusion have recently been made (232). Both substances provoke panic in susceptible patients; however, bicarbonate is somewhat less anxiogenic than lactate. This finding argues against alkalosis alone being the panicogenic stimulus. The researchers conclude that stimulation of respiratory centers to produce increased ventilation, hypocapnia, and respiratory alkalosis was the common factor in producing panic by both infusions, with lactate doing this very early in the infusion.

Panic can also be provoked in increases in pCO_2 (hypercapnia). This can be done slowly, such as by rebreathing air or by breathing 5–7% CO_2 in air (231, 232). Alternatively, panic attacks can be provoked by breathing only one of two deep breaths of 35% CO_2 (233, 234).

Recently, Klein has hypothesized that panic disorder patients suffer from a physiological misinterpretation of a suffocation monitor, which evokes a suffocation alarm system. This produces sudden respiratory distress quickly followed by hyperventilation, panic, and an urge to flee. This model posits that hypersensitivity to CO_2 is due to the deranged suffocation alarm systems (235).

BRAIN IMAGING STUDIES IN PANIC DISORDER PATIENTS

SPECT Studies of Cerebral Blood Flow in Panic Disorder

Patients with panic disorder, compared with healthy controls, have been shown to have a relative decrease from baseline in the ratio of frontal cortex to cerebellar blood flow measured with SPECT and ^{99m}Tc-labeled hexamethylpropylenamine oxime (HMPAO) following administration of yohimbine (236). Patients with panic disorder who had a panic attack during lactate infusion have also been shown to have no change after lactate infusion in cerebral blood flow as measured with SPECT and inhaled xenon-133; normal controls and nonpanicking patients had an increase in global blood flow with lactate. In addition, panicking patients had a slightly lower lactate-induced occipital cortex increase in blood flow compared with nonpanicking patients (237).

PET Studies in Panic Disorder

Using $H_2^{15}O$ to measure cerebral blood flow, lactate-sensitive panic disorder patients have been shown to have a decreased left-to-right parahippocampal ratio of blood flow, in comparison to controls (238, 239). Studies initially interpreted as showing an increase in temporal lobe blood flow during lactate-induced panic in panic disorder patients (240) and in healthy subjects during the anticipatory anxiety of receiving an electric shock (241) have subsequently been suggested to represent increased blood flow in the temporalis muscle due to teeth clenching (242).

Investigations of cerebral metabolism using ^{18}F-deoxyglucose have found decreases in left inferior parietal lobule metabolism and decreased left hippocampal/right hippocampal ratio of metabolism in panic disorder patients in comparison with controls (243).

POSTTRAUMATIC STRESS DISORDER

Posttraumatic stress disorder (PTSD) can be an immediate or delayed response to a catastrophic event. This disorder has become the focus of intensive research, which will lead to a rapid growth of information. One difficulty in establishing PTSD has been the frequent complication of compensation and legal issues. Therefore, because this disorder clearly occurs in the absence of secondary gain, research on populations where these issues are not present minimizes a potential source of inaccuracy or bias.

Epidemiology

Posttraumatic stress disorder was not recognized as an independent diagnosis until the publication of DSM-III in 1980, although descriptions of the syndrome date at least to the Crimean and American Civil Wars. In a remarkable epidemiologic survey, the National Vietnam Veterans Readjustment Study (244) examined PTSD in Vietnam theater veterans and matched civilian controls. The lifetime rate of PTSD in male theater veterans was 31%, and 15% had current PTSD. Rates in females were 26.9% and 8.5%, respectively. There was a direct relationship between level of combat and risk for PTSD, even when premilitary factors were taken into account; Hispanic race also increased risk. Future analyses will evaluate pretrauma and posttrauma risk factors and aspects of the trauma. Rates of most other psychiatric disorders were elevated among those with PTSD. An epidemiologic survey of adult women (245) revealed alarmingly high rates of traumatic events, particularly being the victim of a crime; lifetime and current prevalence estimates of PTSD were 13% and 3%, respectively. Victims of sexual assault were at especially high risk for subsequent mental health problems and suicide. One site of the ECA Study estimated a population prevalence of 1 to 2%, which may be an underestimate. A survey of 20- to 30-year-olds in a large HMO (246) found that 39.1% had been exposed to a traumatic event, and the lifetime rate of PTSD in those exposed was 23.6% (i.e., lifetime population prevalence 9.2%). Risk factors for exposure to traumatic events included family history of any psychiatric disorder, history of conduct disorder symptoms, male sex, extroversion, and neuroticism. Risk factors for PTSD following exposure to trauma included separation from parents during childhood, family history of anxiety, preexisting anxiety or depression, family history of antisocial behavior, female sex, and neuroticism.

A latent period of months or years may intervene between the trauma and the onset of symptoms, or an exacerbation or relapse can occur after a period of remission. The disorder can occur in childhood. Individuals with posttraumatic stress disorder may be at increased risk for impulsive behavior or suicide.

Description and Differential Diagnosis

The mental status examination should routinely include questions about exposure to trauma or abuse. The symptoms are clustered into three categories: reexperiencing the trauma, psychic numbing or avoidance of stimuli associated with the trauma, and increased arousal. Reexperiencing phenomena include intrusive memories, flashbacks, nightmares, and psychological or physiological distress in response to trauma reminders. Intrusive memories are spontaneous, unwanted, distressing recollections of the traumatic event. Repeated nightmares contain themes of the trauma or a highly accurate and detailed re-creation of the actual event(s). Flashbacks are dissociative states in which compo-

nents of the event are relived, and the person feels as if he or she is experiencing the event for a few seconds to as long as days. Reactivity to trauma-related stimuli can involve intense emotional distress or physical symptoms similar to those of a panic attack when exposed to sights, sounds, smells, or events that were present during the traumatic event. Avoidance may include thoughts, feelings, situations, or activities that are reminders of the trauma. Numbing may occur through amnesia, emotional detachment, restricted affect, or loss of interest in activities. Increased arousal may include insomnia, irritability, hypervigilance, increased startle response, or impaired concentration. This disorder can have pervasive effects on an individual's interpersonal behavior and all spheres of her or his life. Because events of this magnitude would be markedly distressing to anyone and are commonly followed by transient PTSD symptoms, distinguishing between a normal reaction and clinically relevant symptoms can be difficult. The level of distress, impairment, and duration of the symptoms can be difficult but are important measures. Recent research suggests that a 3-month duration may be a threshold between "acute" and "chronic" PTSD. However, a 1-month duration is the threshold for diagnostic criteria at the time of this writing.

In adjustment disorder, the stressor is usually less severe, and the characteristic symptoms of posttraumatic stress disorder, such as reexperiencing and avoiding, are not present. Avoidance of trauma-associated stimuli may resemble a phobia; however, in posttraumatic stress disorder the avoidance is limited to reminders of the trauma. The physiological response to events symbolizing the trauma may resemble panic attacks, but in pure posttraumatic stress disorder no spontaneous attacks occur, nor do attacks occur apart from trauma-related stimuli. Many of the symptoms of posttraumatic stress disorder resemble those of major depression. If a full depressive syndrome also exists, both diagnoses should be made. The same is true of coexisting anxiety disorders. Amnesia and impaired concentration may resemble an organic mental disorder; if the trauma involved head injury, organic brain impairment should be considered. Reexperiencing phenomena, such as flashbacks, can be mistaken for psychosis. Very commonly, patients are referred for medication to help with sleep. It is important to inquire about nightmares and other trauma-related symptoms in order to recognize the underlying disorder and not mistake it for other causes of insomnia.

Pathophysiology

NORADRENERGIC FUNCTION IN PTSD

Effects of Stress on Noradrenergic Function in Healthy Subjects

Accumulated evidence suggests that brain noradrenergic systems play a role in mediating normal-state anxiety and the response to stress in healthy human subjects. Increases in heart rate, blood pressure, and alerting behaviors, essential for the response to life-threatening situations, may be mediated by brain noradrenergic systems, although the evidence of this activation is largely peripheral.

States of anxiety or fear appear to be associated with an increase in norepinephrine release in healthy subjects (247). Inexperienced privates in the Air Force have an increase in urinary epinephrine during flight in transport planes in comparison to ground activity. Pilots of the airplane have an increase in both urinary norepinephrine and epinephrine during flight in comparison to ground activity (248). During public speaking epinephrine levels increase twofold, while during physical exercise, norepinephrine levels increase threefold (249). Among young physicians making a presentation at grand rounds, epinephrine levels rose sharply before and at the onset of the talk, while norepinephrine levels increased gradually and remained elevated throughout the duration of the talk. These increases in catecholamines were associated with increases in heart rate and electrocardiographic abnormalities and were blocked by administration of a β-adrenergic receptor antagonist (250). Plasma epinephrine and norepinephrine levels increase over baseline in healthy subjects during cognitive stressors (mental arithmetic), physical stressors (knee bends), and pain stressors (cold pressor and venipuncture). Epinephrine levels were greatest during cognitive stressors in this study, while painful stressors evoked the greatest norepinephrine response (251). In race car drivers assessed during race car driving, there was a gross elevation of catecholamines, which was highest near the start of the race, and which was largely due to norepinephrine (252). All of these findings were attributed to emotional stress and anxiety. Studies have not consistently found, however, a relationship between the severity of subjective anxiety and plasma norepinephrines and epinephrine (253).

Levels of the norepinephrine metabolite, MHPG, have also been found to increase in healthy subjects during emotional stress (254). Urinary MHPG increased in naval aviators after landings of aircraft on aircraft carriers, an extremely dangerous and potentially stressful undertaking, in comparison to a nonflying control day. Plasma MHPG was correlated with state anxiety in healthy subjects exposed to the anticipatory stress of receiving an electric shock, while there was no such correlation in the absence of the electric shock threat (255, 256). Significant within-individual correlations between changes in urinary MHPG and changes in state anxiety have been found in healthy human subjects (257).

STUDIES OF NORADRENERGIC FUNCTION IN PTSD PATIENTS

Considering the broad functions of the noradrenergic system, abnormal regulation of this system could account for many of the clinical features of PTSD.

Peripheral Catecholamine Levels

Two studies have found significantly elevated 24-hour urine norepinephrine excretion in combat veterans with PTSD compared to healthy subjects or patients with schizophrenia or major depression (258, 259).

Peripheral Noradrenergic Receptor Function

The density of platelet α_2-adrenergic receptors is reduced in PTSD, perhaps reflecting adaptive "down-regulation" in response to chronically elevated levels of circulating endogenous catecholamines (260). The relevance of these studies to brain α receptor function is questionable because of the lack of evidence demonstrating that platelet α-adrenergic receptors reflect brain α-receptor function (261).

Plasma lymphocyte β-adrenergic receptors are downregulated in PTSD (262, 263). The functional significance of these findings is unclear because the β receptors located on lymphocytes are of the β_2 subtype, whereas the β_1 receptor is predominant in the brain.

Peripheral Sympathetic System Function

Most of the early clinical investigations of the pathophysiology of PTSD identified a relationship between severe stress exposure, increased peripheral sympathetic nervous system activity, and conditioned physiological and emotional responses (264–266). Since the early 1980s there have been a series of well designed psychophysiological studies that have further documented heightened autonomic or sympathetic nervous system arousal in combat veterans with PTSD. Combat veterans with PTSD have been shown to have higher resting mean heart rate and systolic blood pressure, as well as greater increases in heart rate, when exposed to visual and auditory combat-related stimuli compared to combat veterans without PTSD, patients with generalized anxiety disorder, or healthy subjects (267–273). Further, several psychophysiological studies have found hyperreactive responses to combat-associated stimuli but not to other stressful noncombat-related stimuli. These data are consistent with the hypothesis that noradrenergic hyperreactivity in patients with PTSD may relate to the conditioned or sensitized responses to specific traumatic stimuli. Studies evaluating the efficacy of psychotherapeutic techniques emphasizing desensitization to reduce hyperarousal responses to stimuli associated with the psychological trauma represent a current focus of investigation (274, 275).

Regulation of Noradrenergic Function in PTSD

Similar to the panic disorder patients, approximately two-thirds of PTSD patients experience yohimbine-induced panic attacks. In addition, 40% of PTSD patients report flashbacks after yohimbine. As a group, PTSD patients also have greater yohimbine-induced increases in plasma MHPG, sitting systolic blood pressure, and heart rate than healthy subjects. In the PTSD patients, yohimbine induced significant increases in core PTSD symptoms such as intrusive traumatic thoughts, emotional numbing, and grief (276).

POSSIBLE SITES OF NORADRENERGIC DYSFUNCTION IN PANIC DISORDER AND PTSD

The data just reviewed suggest that some panic disorder and PTSD patients may share a common abnormality in noradrenergic system function. The etiology of the disturbance in noradrenergic function may differ in the two disorders. Panic disorder is generally believed to be familial, suggesting that the noradrenergic dysfunction may represent an inherited trait. On the other hand, the frequency of panic disorder in the family members of PTSD patients is no more frequent than in the general population (277). Thus, the abnormalities in noradrenergic function in PTSD may be more related to the effects of extreme and repeated trauma than to genetic factors.

The abnormal noradrenergic function observed in panic disorder and PTSD may reflect abnormalities in the LC-NE system at the level of the LC, the LC projection areas, and the interaction of the peripheral sympathetic with the central noradrenergic system. Dysfunction at the LC, producing noradrenergic hyperactivity, could be due to decreased functional sensitivity of the α_2-adrenergic autoreceptor or at one or more of the neuronal systems that have regulatory actions on LC activity. Unfortunately, methods have not been developed to directly evaluate brain α_2-adrenergic autoreceptor function in humans.

Another explanation for the noradrenergic hyperactivity in panic disorder and PTSD might be that excitatory inputs from the nucleus paragigantocellularis to the LC are increased in function (278). An increase in CRF secretion is also a prime candidate for an abnormal excitatory input to the LC because of the considerable evidence that CRF has anxiogenic properties (279). Preclinical data suggest that CRF produces its behavioral activating and anxiogenic effects, in part, by increasing LC activity. Consequently, it is important to develop clinical paradigms capable of evaluating central CRF activity and the interaction of CRF and noradrenergic function in panic disorder and PTSD patients.

There is abundant evidence implicating the opiate, endogenous benzodiazepine, and serotonin neuronal systems in the development of anxiety and fear. Because each of these systems has inhibitory effects on LC activity, it is possible that decreased activity of any one of these systems could account for the increased response to drugs, such as yohimbine, which activate noradrenergic neurons.

Projection areas of the LC are likely to be involved in the enhanced anxiogenic effects of yohimbine in panic disorder and PTSD. The LC projects to many brain regions implicated in the pathophysiology of anxiety and fear, including the amygdala, hypothalamus, thalamus, hippocampus, and cerebral cortex. An enhancement of norepinephrine metabolism occurs in these brain areas following a variety of stressful stimuli. It is possible that the behavioral responses to yohimbine in panic disorder and PTSD are due to abnormal regulation of noradrenergic neurotransmission by terminal α_2-adrenergic autoreceptors in brain structures such as the amygdala or increased sensitivity of β-adrenergic receptors, which are widely distributed in the cortex, limbic brain structures, and the spinal cord.

TRAUMATIC MEMORIES AND NORADRENERGIC FUNCTION

A striking effect of yohimbine is its ability to increase the severity of the core symptoms associated with PTSD, such as intrusive traumatic thoughts, emotional numbing, and grief. This may be due to the involvement of noradrenergic systems in the mechanisms by which memories of traumatic experiences remain indelible for decades and are easily reawakened by a variety of stimuli and stressors.

Indeed, the strength of traumatic memories may relate to the degree to which certain neuromodulatory systems are activated by the traumatic experience. Experimental and clinical investigations have demonstrated that memory processes are susceptible to modulating influences after the information has been acquired. Stimulation of noradrenergic receptors on the amygdala after a learning experience has memory-enhancing effects (280, 281). Activating the LC-norepinephrine system that projects to the amygdala by frightening and traumatic experiences may facilitate the encoding of memories associated with the experiences. Moreover, it is possible that reproducing a neurobiological state (noradrenergic hyperactivity in specific brain regions), similar to the one that existed at the time of the memory encoding, can elicit the traumatic memory.

HYPOTHALAMIC-PITUITARY-ADRENAL AXIS FUNCTION IN PTSD

Baseline Studies

The finding of low urinary cortisol excretion in PTSD compared with other psychiatric groups and normal controls has now been replicated in several studies. In an initial investigation, lower mean 24-hour urinary cortisol excretion was observed in nine PTSD patients compared with patients in four other diagnostic groups (282). A second study similarly found low urinary cortisol in PTSD patients compared to the amounts found in patients with major depression, panic disorder, bipolar mania, and schizophrenia (283). This finding has been replicated in inpatient and outpatient combat veterans with PTSD as compared with nonpsychiatric, healthy controls (284), and more recently in nontreatment-seeking Holocaust survivors with chronic PTSD compared to Holocaust survivors without PTSD and to demographically matched controls (285). The only other study examining 24-hour urinary cortisol excretion reported an increased urinary cortisol level in PTSD (286). However, this study was different in the method of urine collection and radioimmunoassay. A recent attempt to replicate the original findings using improved methodologies for urine collection was not successful (Pitman R., personal communication).

Lymphocyte Glucocorticoid Receptors

Because hormones cannot exert their genomic effects unless they are bound to steroid receptors, it has been suggested that steroid-receptor binding parameters are important in interpreting studies examining basal hormone secretion. Further, lymphocytes and brain glucocorticoid receptors share similar regulatory and binding characteristics, suggesting that lymphocyte glucocorticoid receptor function reflects aspects of both peripheral and central cortisol regulation (287). Results from three studies have now demonstrated an increased lymphocyte glucocorticoid receptor number in combat veterans with PTSD compared to nonpsychiatric and psychiatric comparison groups (288–290). These findings are consistent with observations of low cortisol levels in chronic PTSD. In general, low circulating levels of a hormone or neurotransmitter are associated with an up-regulation or increased number of receptors.

Dexamethasone Suppression Test

Dexamethasone is a synthetic glucocorticoid that mimics the effect of cortisol and directly inhibits the release of CRF and ACTH. The dexamethasone suppression test (DST) involves the administration of 1 mg dexamethasone at 11:00 PM, when normal cortisol secretion is at its nadir in the diurnal cycle. The inhibition of CRF and ACTH results in a decrease in the amount of cortisol released from the adrenal gland. Within hours after the administration of dexamethasone, cortisol secretion is substantially lowered in normal individuals. In normals, a dose of 1 mg usually suppresses plasma cortisol to a level below 5 µg/dl at 8:00 AM; it remains below that level at 4:00 PM. Studies examining the cortisol response to dexamethasone in psychiatric disorders, most notably in major depressive disorder, have repeatedly shown a "nonsuppression" of cortisol in about 40 to 60% of depressed patients (291–293), that likely results from either a reduced ability of glucocorticoids to suppress the release of CRF and ACTH or adrenal cortisol hypersecretion.

The cortisol response to 1 mg of dexamethasone has been investigated in five studies of PTSD. These studies have all reported that PTSD patients without major depression show a "normal" suppression to dexamethasone (294–298). However, closer examination reveals that PTSD patients as a group show an exaggerated response to dexamethasone. A recent meta-analysis of the psychiatric DST literature (299), averaging the mean cortisol data across all published studies, revealed a cortisol value in nondepressed PTSD subjects of 1.74 µg/dl, a value well below the established cutoff 5.0 µg/dl.

Most of the DST studies in PTSD were conducted before it was appreciated that cortisol levels in PTSD patients tended to be low and the number of glucocorticoid receptors high. Therefore, these earlier studies were designed to test for "nonsuppression" in PTSD, and did not focus on the possibility of an exaggerated cortisol response, or hypersuppression to dexamethasone. Failure to find the classic nonsuppression response to cortisol, coupled with reported

HPA axis alterations that appeared distinct from those in depression, led to studies designed to detect a potential enhanced suppression of the cortisol response to dexamethasone.

Recently, the question of enhanced cortisol suppression to dexamethasone was explored using 0.50 (283) and 0.25 (290) mg of dexamethasone. A hyperresponsiveness to low doses of dexamethasone, as reflected by significantly lower postdexamethasone cortisol levels, was observed in PTSD patients as compared with normals. The enhanced suppression of cortisol was accompanied by a decreased number, or down-regulation, of cystolic lymphocyte glucocorticoid receptors (290). Interestingly, the hyperresponsiveness to dexamethasone was also present in combat veterans with PTSD who met the diagnostic criteria for major depressive disorder (293), and importantly, was not present in combat veterans without PTSD (290). The hypersuppression of cortisol observed following dexamethasone is compatible with the notion that patients with PTSD do not exhibit a "classic" stress response as defined by Selye. Furthermore, this hypersuppression has not been described in other psychiatric disorders and may serve as a relatively specific marker for PTSD.

Corticotropin-Releasing Factor

The corticotropin-releasing factor (CRF) challenge test measures the pituitary adrenocorticotropin hormone (ACTH) and adrenal cortisol response to exogenous infusion of the neuropeptide CRF. Investigators have demonstrated an attenuation of the normal ACTH response to CRF in patients with major depressive disorder (300–303). The blunted ACTH response typically occurs in hypercortisolemic patients and is thought to reflect a decreased number of pituitary CRF receptors caused by hypothalamic CRF hypersecretion (301–303), and/or an increased negative feedback inhibition of the pituitary secondary to abnormally high circulating cortisol levels.

A single study of eight PTSD subjects suggests that the ACTH response to CRF is also blunted (304). However, the attenuated ACTH response in PTSD patients occurred in the presence of normal, not elevated, evening plasma cortisol levels. Thus, the response to CRF in PTSD may be due to a decreased pituitary sensitivity to CRF or to an enhanced effect of glucocorticoid negative feedback on the pituitary, rather than because of a decrease in the number of pituitary CRF receptors as is thought to occur in major depression.

SEROTONIN FUNCTION AND PTSD

Although only two studies have directly examined the 5-HT system in PTSD, there is a large body of indirect evidence suggesting that this neurotransmitter may be important in the pathophysiology of trauma-related symptomatology. In humans, low 5-HT functioning has been associated with aggression (305), impulsivity, and suicidal behavior (306). Patients with PTSD are frequently described as aggressive or impulsive and often suffer from depression, suicidal tendencies, and intrusive thoughts that have been likened to obsessions.

More direct evidence of serotonergic dysregulation in PTSD comes from the results of electrophysiological studies by Paige et al. (307). Paige et al. demonstrated a predominance of "reducing" patterns to auditory evoked potential paradigms in combat veterans with PTSD compared to normal controls. Meanwhile, Hegerl et al. (308) suggested that the slope of the stimulus-response curve to auditory tones is positively associated with serotonergic activity. Based on their findings, it is possible that Paige et al.'s discoveries are, at least in part, related to low serotonergic activity in PTSD. This hypothesis gains further support from the observation that serotonin reuptake inhibitors have been found to be partially effective in treating PTSD symptoms such as intrusive memories and avoidance symptoms (309, 310).

The first report of serotonergic function in PTSD is a study examining paroxetine binding in blood platelets of 20 combat veterans with PTSD under baseline conditions (311). In this study, platelet 5-HT uptake was significantly decreased in PTSD patients compared with normals, and with PTSD patients meeting criteria for co-morbid major depressive disorder. Because decreased platelet 5-HT uptake has also been reported in patients with depression and alcoholism, the specificity of these findings has yet to be determined.

More recently, the behavioral effects of *m*-chloro-phenyl-piperazine (M-CPP) have been examined in a preliminary study of 14 combat veterans with PTSD (312). Five of the 14 patients with PTSD had a panic attack, and four had a flashback following M-CPP administration. In contrast, no patient had a panic attack, and one patient experienced a flashback following the infusion of placebo saline. Thus, a subgroup of patients with PTSD exhibited a marked behavioral sensitivity to serotonergic provocation, raising the possibility of pathophysiological subtypes among traumatized combat veterans. Clearly, further studies are needed to delineate possible serotonergic alterations in PTSD.

OPIOID PEPTIDE FUNCTION AND PTSD

Stress causes a release of endogenous opiates, increased opiate peptide levels, and diminished pain sensitivity (313–315). Stress-induced analgesia can be blocked by the administration of an opiate antagonist, naltrexone hydrochloride. This finding supports the notion that stress, endogenous opiates, and analgesia may be related (316–318). Additionally, there is evidence to suggest that analgesia can accompany neutral stimuli previously paired with aversive stimuli (319). Further, it appears that the endogenous opiate system can become sensitized so that reexposure to lower levels of uncontrollable shock results in the same degree of analgesia previously induced by significantly greater degrees of shock (320). Given these facts, it is reasonable to study opiate systems in individuals who have been severely traumatized.

There have been only two laboratory reports describing baseline opioid peptide metabolism in traumatized humans. Hoffman et al. (321) reported significantly lower AM and PM plasma β-endorphin levels in 21 PTSD patients compared with 20 controls. The results were viewed as support for van der Kolk's hypothesis (322) that patients with PTSD have a chronic depletion of endogenous opioids and that hyperresponsiveness is related to endogenous opiate withdrawal. According to this hypothesis, patients with PTSD seek out or provoke recurrent stressors and trauma in order to increase opiate release and hence decrease endogenous opiate withdrawal.

The second study (323) measured circulating levels of methionine-enkephalin and its in vitro plasma degradation half-life in 13 Vietnam combat veterans with PTSD compared to controls. While plasma methionine-enkephalin levels were similar in PTSD patients and controls, degradation half-life was significantly higher in the PTSD group. The author suggests the possible existence of a circulating endogenous inhibitor of methionine-enkephalin degradation; however, such a substance has never been isolated. The authors further speculate that decreased degradation in the face of normal plasma methionine-enkephalin levels suggest a decreased production and release of this peptide.

To date, there is only one pharmacologic challenge study focused on the opiate system in PTSD. Eight combat veterans with PTSD and eight combat controls were exposed to the stress of a combat film (324). Following the film, subjects were exposed to a pain sensitivity test. Veterans with PTSD showed reduced pain sensitivity compared to veterans without PTSD. This effect was reversible by the opiate antagonist naloxone. These findings suggest that stress-induced analgesia, is, at least in part, mediated by endogenous opiates and that patients with PTSD show an enhanced release of endogenous opiates following exposure to stress.

Whether alterations in endogenous opiates contribute to the core symptoms seen in PTSD is not clear. However, based on the studies, it has been hypothesized that symptoms of avoidance and numbing are related to a dysregulation of opioid systems in PTSD (325). Further, it has been suggested that the use of opiates in chronic PTSD may represent a form of self-medication. Animal studies have shown that opiates are powerful suppressants of central and peripheral noradrenergic activity. If, as suggested earlier in this chapter, some PTSD symptomatology is mediated by noradrenergic hyperactivity (326), then opiates may serve to "treat" or weaken that hypersensitivity and accompanying symptoms. On the other hand, during opiate withdrawal, when opiates are decreased and noradrenergic activity increased, PTSD symptoms may become acutely exacerbated. In fact, many symptoms of PTSD have been compared to symptoms experienced during opiate withdrawal (327).

PHOBIAS

Social Phobia

Social fears are commonly experienced by healthy subjects, especially in initial public-speaking experiences. For some people, this fear becomes persistent and overwhelming, limiting their social or occupational functioning because of intense anxiety and, often, avoidance. Social phobia is an area of active research; therefore, our knowledge base will be expanding rapidly in the next several years.

EPIDEMIOLOGY

Preliminary estimates of 6-month prevalence rates of social phobia ascertained by screening questionnaires in the Epidemiologic Catchment Area (ECA) Study are 1.2 to 2.2%; 0.9 to 1.7% in men; and 1.5 to 2.6% in women. The distribution is fairly even across the age span, although rates may be lower in the over-65 age group. Onset is usually between 15 and 20 years of age, and the course tends to be chronic and unremitting. Complications include interference with work or school, social isolation, and abuse of alcohol or drugs. In inpatient alcoholism treatment programs, 20 to 25% report social phobia beginning before the onset of alcoholism or persisting after 1 year of abstinence. Significant depressive symptoms may also occur in social phobia; in one study, one-third of social phobia patients reported a history of major depression.

DESCRIPTION AND DIFFERENTIAL DIAGNOSIS

Social phobia is characterized by a persistent and exaggerated fear of humiliation or embarrassment in social situations, leading to high levels of distress and possibly avoidance of those situations. Patients may become fearful that their anxiety will be evident to others, which may intensify their symptoms or even produce a situational panic attack. The fear may be of speaking, meeting people, eating, or writing in public, and relates to the fear of appearing nervous or foolish, making mistakes, being criticized, or being laughed at. Often physical symptoms of anxiety such as blushing, trembling, sweating, and tachycardia are triggered when the patient feels he or she is being evaluated or scrutinized.

Probably the most difficult diagnostic distinctions are between social phobia and normal performance anxiety, or social phobia and panic disorder. Normal fear of public speaking usually diminishes as the individual is speaking or with additional experience, whereas in social phobia the anxiety may worsen or fail to attenuate with rehearsal. Social phobics may experience situational panic attacks resulting from anticipation or exposure to the feared social situation. Some panic disorder/agoraphobia patients avoid social situations due to fear of embarrassment if a panic attack should occur, but usually their initial panic attack is unexpected (occurs in a situation they previously did not fear), and the subsequent development of phobias is generalized beyond social phobia situations. Sometimes social phobia and panic disorder coexist. Social phobia can be differentiated from simple phobias in that the latter do not involve social situations involving scrutiny, humiliation, or embarrassment. In major depression, social avoidance may develop from apathy rather than fear and resolves with remission of the depressive episode. In schizoid personality disorder, social isolation results from a lack of interest rather than from fear. In avoidant personality disorder, the avoidance is of personal relationships; however, if the patient develops a marked anxiety about and avoidance of most social situations, the additional diagnosis of social phobia should be made.

GENETIC EPIDEMIOLOGY

Animal studies demonstrate heritability of various fear, anxiety, and exploratory, escape, or avoidant behaviors, often mediated by combinations of genes. These are reviewed by Marks (328) and may be relevant to social phobia and other anxiety disorders. Human studies of general population samples have suggested some genetic heritability for traits such as fear of strangers, shyness, social introversion, and fear of social criticism. There is greater monozygotic than dizygotic twin concordance for social phobic features such as discomfort when eating with strangers, or when being watched eating, writing, working, or trembling. The strong heritability of blood-injury phobia has led to the hypothesis that blushing, for example, may be an autonomic response under genetic influence that is tied to social cues and might lead to social phobia. A family history study found familial aggregation of social phobia, and a direct-interview family study found that relatives of social phobics without other anxiety disorders had a threefold increased risk for social phobia but not for other anxiety disorders (329). A study of female twins found higher concordance for social phobia among monozygotic as compared with dizygotic twins. This same study supported the role of both genetic and random environmental factors (330).

Specific Phobia

Specific phobia shares many of the basic features of the general phobias, but the fear is limited to a specific object or situation, such as dogs or heights, so the extent of interference in a patient's life tends to be mild.

EPIDEMIOLOGY

Six-month prevalence rates of specific phobia reported in the ECA Study are between 4.5 and 11.8%; rates are higher for females than for males. The onset of animal phobia is usually in childhood. Blood-injury phobia usually begins in adolescence or early adulthood and may be associated with vasovagal fainting on exposure to the phobic stimulus. Age of onset may be more variable for other simple phobias. Many childhood-onset phobias may remit spontaneously. Impairment depends on the extent to which the phobic object or situation is routinely encountered in the individual's life. Simple phobias may coexist with social phobia and panic disorder, but are believed to be unrelated.

DESCRIPTION AND DIFFERENTIAL DIAGNOSIS

Specific phobia is usually a circumscribed fear of a specific object or situation. As with the other phobias, the fear is excessive and unrealistic; exposure to the phobic stimulus produces an anxiety response; expectation of exposure may produce anticipatory anxiety; and the object or situation is either avoided or endured with considerable discomfort. However, unlike social phobia, the fear does not involve scrutiny or embarrassment, and, unlike agoraphobia, the fear is not of being trapped or of having a panic attack. The nature of the fear is specific to the phobia, such as a fear of falling or loss of visual support in height phobia, or fear of crashing in a flying phobia. Isolated fears are common in the general population; a diagnosis of simple phobia is reserved for situations in which the phobia results in marked distress or some degree of impairment in activities or relationships.

Pathophysiological Studies of Social and Specific Phobias

NORADRENERGIC FUNCTION

Few studies have examined noradrenergic function in patients with phobic disorders. In patients with specific phobias, increases in subjective anxiety and increased heart rate, blood pressure, plasma norepinephrine, and epinephrine have been associated with exposure to the phobic stimulus (331). This finding may be of interest from the standpoint of the model of conditioned fear, reviewed earlier, in which a potentiated release of norepinephrine occurs in response to a reexposure to the original stressful stimulus.

Patients with social phobia have been found to have greater increases in plasma norepinephrine on orthostatic challenge, compared to healthy controls and patients with panic disorder (332). In contrast to panic disorder patients, the density of lymphocyte β-adrenoceptors is normal in social phobic patients (333).

NEUROENDOCRINE STUDIES

Neuroendocrine studies in phobic patients are extremely limited. Patients with social phobia have been shown to have greater blood pressure and heart rate responses to thyrotropin-releasing hormone than panic disorder patients and healthy control subjects (334). The growth hormone response to intravenous clonidine is blunted in both panic disorder and social phobia patients (335).

GENERALIZED ANXIETY DISORDER

Generalized anxiety disorder (GAD) is characterized by excessive and uncontrollable worry about multiple life circumstances. It is accompanied by symptoms of muscle tension, restlessness, fatigue, concentration problems, diffi-

culty falling or staying asleep, and irritability. The anxiety is unrelated to panic attacks, phobic, stimuli, obsessions, having an illness, or traumatic events (in PTSD). The validity of GAD as a diagnosis distinct from other anxiety disorders or depression, or whether it is a homogenous category, is still being examined.

EPIDEMIOLOGY

An epidemiologic study in New Haven, Connecticut, estimated a 2.5% 1-month prevalence rate for GAD using research diagnostic criteria. Of the patients with GAD, 80% had at least one other anxiety disorder in their lifetime, and 7% had major depression. In this study GAD was slightly more common in young to middle-aged females, nonwhites, those not currently married, and those of lower socioeconomic status. Rates for GAD were not reported in the ECA Study. Age at onset is variable but is usually in the 20s to 30s. GAD may begin as childhood overanxious disorder. In clinical samples the prevalence in males and females appears to be equal and the course tends to be chronic (336).

DESCRIPTION AND DIFFERENTIAL DIAGNOSIS

The most common diagnostic error made by novices is to misdiagnose GAD when another anxiety disorder is present, which leads to inappropriate and ineffective treatment decisions. The symptom of anxiety is prominent in a number of conditions, including depressive, psychotic, substance use, and somatoform disorders as well as some medical conditions (particularly those associated with dyspnea) and medication side-effects (e.g., sympatomimetic), so careful questioning is necessary to differentiate among the multiple causes of anxiety.

GAD is characterized by chronic excessive anxiety about life circumstances accompanied by symptoms of motor tension, autonomic hyperactivity, vigilance, and scanning. The individual often "awakens with" apprehension and unrealistic concern about future misfortune. One patient described experiencing the anxiety of a final exam with every task he was assigned at work. The current diagnostic criteria require 6-month duration of symptoms to differentiate the disorder from more transient forms of anxiety, such as adjustment disorder with anxious mood. GAD is no longer a residual diagnosis covering a heterogeneous group of anxiety conditions that do not fit other diagnoses. Recently, an attempt has been made to refine the definition of this syndrome and determine if it is truly distinct from other diagnoses.

DSM-IV revamped this diagnosis considerably. The criteria emphasize that the worry is out of proportion to the likelihood or impact of the feared events, is pervasive (focused on many life circumstances), is difficult to control, is not related to hypochondriacal concerns or part of PTSD, and that anxiety secondary to substance-induced or non-psychiatric medical etiologies will be excluded. This is accompanied by tension or nervousness as manifested by at least three of the following symptoms: restlessness, quick fatigue, feeling keyed up or on edge, difficulty concentrating/mind going blank, and irritability. In addition, significant functional impairment or marked distress is required for the diagnosis.

Generalized persistent anxiety may develop between attacks in panic disorder. GAD symptoms are often present in episodes of depression. In patients with somatization disorder, the thrust of concern regards health and physical symptoms rather than apprehensive worry about life circumstances. As with panic disorder, medical conditions that may produce anxiety symptoms, such as hyperthyroidism or caffeinism, must be excluded. If an anxiety disorder is present that does not fit the criteria of any of the anxiety disorders, somatization, psychoactive substance-related, or medical conditions, then the diagnosis of anxiety disorder, not otherwise specified, may be considered. However, careful assessment will usually reveal the presence of a more specific diagnosis. If in doubt, obtain consultation from an anxiety disorders specialist.

GENETIC EPIDEMIOLOGY

Torgersen's twin study (158) found no evidence for genetic transmission of GAD. Diagnostic heterogeneity of GAD is suggested by the high frequency of nonanxiety psychiatric disorders in co-twins. However, a family study of GAD probands reports an increased rate of GAD but not other anxiety disorders in first-degree relatives, suggesting some degree of familial transmission and separation of GAD from panic disorder and agoraphobia (337).

Pathophysiology

NORADRENERGIC FUNCTION

There is little clinical evidence supporting a primary role for the noradrenergic system in the pathophysiology of GAD. Plasma MHPG levels have been shown to be both increased (338, 339) and not different (340) compared to normal controls. Similarly, increases in resting plasma norepinephrine in GAD patients have been reported in some studies (339, 341, 342) but not others (338, 341).

Alpha-$_2$adrenergic receptor number as measured by specific binding of tritiated yohimbine on platelet membranes has been found to be reduced (339) or unchanged (343) in GAD patients. Growth hormone response to clonidine has been found to be blunted in GAD patients (344). Patients with GAD have been found to have normal responses to the α_2-antagonist, yohimbine (340).

BENZODIAZEPINE FUNCTION

Patients with generalized anxiety disorder have been found to have decreases in peripheral-type benzodiazepine receptor binding as assessed by [3$_H$]PK11195 binding to lymphocyte membranes, although the relationship to central benzodiazepine receptor function is unclear (345). In addition, reduced binding to [3$_H$]PK11195 has been

reversed with benzodiazepine therapy in patients with anxiety disorders (346).

BRAIN IMAGING STUDIES IN GENERALIZED ANXIETY DISORDER

Patients with generalized anxiety disorder (GAD) have been found to have a decrease in metabolism at baseline measured with positron emission tomography in basal ganglia and white matter, and an increase in normalized left occipital cortex, right posterior temporal lobe, and right precentral frontal gyrus metabolism in comparison to healthy controls (347). Administration of benzodiazepine therapy in patients with GAD results in a decrease in glucose metabolism in the occipital cortex, a brain region high in benzodiazepine receptors (348).

CONCLUDING COMMENTS

Pathophysiology and Treatment of Anxiety Disorders

The proposed brain structures, neural mechanisms, and neural circuit related to anxiety and fear provide a basis to increase the understanding of the pathophysiology of anxiety disorders, such as panic disorder, PTSD, phobic disorders, and generalized anxiety disorder (GAD). To date, the primary focus of neurobiological research of these conditions has focussed more on single neurotransmitter or neuropeptide theories, such as the role of noradrenergic, benzodiazepine, serotonergic, and CCK systems, than on interactions among neurotransmitter and neuropeptides and specific brain structures, or of the neural mechanisms involved in the genesis of the symptoms of anxiety and fear.

Brain imaging techniques, such as positron emission tomography (PET), single photon emission computerized tomography (SPECT), and functional magnetic resonance imaging, provide a means to further the pathophysiological investigations of anxiety along these lines of inquiry. Despite the potential of these techniques, relatively few functional imaging studies have been completed in patients with anxiety disorders. Although definitive patterns have not yet emerged, alterations in cerebral blood flow or metabolism have been identified in cortical association areas, orbitofrontal cortex, cingulate cortex, and the hippocampus, during anxiety states.

There are several levels within the neural circuitry of anxiety and fear that may be dysfunctional in anxiety disorders. There may be abnormalities in peripheral sensory receptor systems, the relay of sensory information through the thalamus, the processing of sensory data in cortical and subcortical structures, the attachment of affect based upon prior experience by the amygdala, and the autonomic, neuroendocrine, neurochemical, and neuromotor efferent responses.

Panic disorder, which is characterized initially by spontaneous panic attacks, may be due to dysfunction in the efferent arm of the circuit. For example, increased responsiveness of the locus ceruleus-norepinephrine system have been proposed. Alternatively, Klein suggests that spontaneous panic attacks may be due to a basic defect in the suffocation alarm system (235). The neuroanatomical site for such a dysfunction in respiratory control could reside in a number of structures, including the parabrachial nucleus and nucleus of the solitary tract (349). Based upon the neural circuit outlined earlier in this chapter, additional functional neuroanatomic hypothesis can be developed to account for spontaneous panic attacks. Situational panic attacks and agoraphobia more likely result from modality-specific and contextual fear conditioning and the associated brain structures and neurotransmitters.

Posttraumatic stress disorder (PSTD) is characterized by intrusive traumatic memories manifested by recurring dreams, flashbacks, and psychological distress following exposure to events that symbolize or resemble the original trauma, persistent avoidance of stimuli associated with the trauma or a numbing of general responsiveness, and persistent symptoms of increased arousal. The neurobiological basis of some of the symptoms of PTSD can be understood in the context of neural circuits and neural mechanisms of anxiety and fear. Persistent intrusive memories may be due to the strength of neuronal interactions between cortical regions, where many such memories are stored, and subcortical regions, such as the amygdala, which serve to attach affect to the memories. The psychological distress and physiological responses to trauma reminders involve the mechanisms of fear conditioning and extinction. Contextual fear conditioning may be particularly relevant to severe cases of PTSD, in which stimulus generalization is a cardinal feature. The autonomic hyperarousal may be symptoms that are mediated by brain structures of the efferent arm of the anxiety circuit.

Simple phobias are a persistent fear of a circumscribed object or stimulus. Exposure to the phobic stimulus invariably provokes an anxiety response that includes somatic symptoms, such as sweating, tachycardia, and dyspnea. This disorder is likely to be mediated, in part, through the neural mechanisms underlying fear conditioning.

The essential feature of GAD is unrealistic or exaggerated anxiety about several life circumstances. The anxiety is frequently accompanied by symptoms of motor tension, autonomic hyperactivity, and excessive vigilance. It is frequently questioned whether GAD represents a homogeneous anxiety disorder. Some GAD symptoms overlap considerably with the hyperarousal category in the PTSD criteria. Further, many GAD patients suffer from limited symptom panic attacks or infrequent full criteria panic attacks. In this context, the etiology of GAD is likely to be heterogeneous. The symptoms of many GAD patients may relate to early childhood or adult traumatic experiences. Thus, the etiology of GAD in these patients may be similar to patients with PTSD. On the other hand, GAD patients with panic symptomatology may have an etiology related to panic disorder.

Many anxiety disorders, especially panic disorder and PTSD, are chronic illnesses. It has been suggested that the pathophysiology of these disorders should be viewed as a continuously evolving neural process. Panic disorder and PTSD are characterized by recurrent panic attacks, flashbacks, conditioned phobic behavior, and illness exacerbation by stressful life events. Through the process of sensitization, these experiences may lead to the formation of neural substrates and new vulnerability factors, resulting in autonomous anxiety symptoms that were previously elicited only by environmental triggers (350, 351).

The neural circuits and neural mechanisms of anxiety and fear described in this chapter may have implications for the psychotherapy and pharmacotherapy of anxiety disorders. As noted, fear conditioning may contribute to the symptoms of panic disorder, PTSD, and a variety of phobias. Cognitive-behavior therapies have been designed to reverse the impact of fear conditioning. Panic control treatment, which focuses on reversing the effects of fear conditioning on somatic symptoms associated with the efferent arm of the circuit, has been shown to be particularly effective (352, 353). Brain imaging studies can now be conducted before and after the therapy to determine which brain regions are involved in its therapeutic effects. Some patients may not respond to such therapies because of an inability to extinguish intrusive memories and maladaptive behaviors. For such patients, therapies need to be developed that are specifically designed to facilitate extinction through the use of conditioned inhibitors and the learning of "new memories."

Some authors have emphasized that psychotherapy is essentially a learning process (354, 355, 356). This concept binds together traditional notions of mind and brain and provides a context by which psychotherapy can reverse the neurobiological dysfunctions associated with anxiety disorders. In simple animals, learning has been shown to produce structural and functional alterations in specific neurons (357–361). Furthermore, there is evidence that learning can alter the functional interactions between sensory and motor systems. Cortical sensory maps can be changed by learning and are subject to constant modification on the basis of use or activity of the peripheral sensory pathways (362–366). It is possible that the learning associated with psychotherapy will result in changes in the neuronal systems that mediate anxiety and fear responses.

It is even conceivable that psychotherapy may work by affecting the function of genes associated with anxiety and fear behaviors. Stress and learning alter gene expression by modifying the binding of transcriptional activator proteins to each other and to the regulatory regions of genes (367–372). The most heritable of the anxiety disorders is panic disorder, perhaps reflecting alterations in the nucleotide sequence of DNA, leading to abnormal messenger RNA and protein (373). In contrast, other anxiety disorders, exemplified by PTSD, are environmentally caused, possibly resulting in stress-induced altered binding of specific proteins to regulatory regions that control the expression of certain genes. In either case, psychotherapy may bring about therapeutic changes in behavior by altering gene expression.

The concepts discussed in this chapter also suggest potentially fruitful approaches toward development of new therapeutic drugs for anxiety disorders. Given the central role of the amygdala in the neural mechanisms of fear conditioning, extinction, and sensitization, drugs that act on receptors located on amygdaloid neurons and reduce amygdala activity may be effective in reducing the symptoms associated with these mechanisms. Drugs that act selectively on the sensory pathways afferent to the anxiety-fear circuitry (by presynaptically decreasing the release of neurotransmitters or neuropeptides connecting cortical or subcortical afferents) could be effective in blocking conditioned fear. Alternatively, drugs that selectively decrease the function of brain regions in the efferent arm of the circuit may be effective in reducing the signs and symptoms of anxiety.

There has been too great an emphasis on norepinephrine, serotonin, and benzodiazepine systems in the development of new anxiolytic drugs. Identification of the relevant brain structures mediating anxiety and fear symptoms, and knowledge of the functions of neurotransmitters and neuropeptides located within these structures may permit the discovery and testing of drugs that act on neurochemicals heretofore not associated with anxiety or fear. Thus, the proposed relationships among dysfunction of specific brain structures, neural mechanisms, neurochemical systems, and clinical symptoms raise the possibility of discovering new pharmacotherapies for anxiety disorders.

References

1. LeDeux JE. Nervous System V. Emotion. In Blum F, ed. Handbook of physiology. Washington: American Physiological Society, 1987; 419–459.
2. Turner B, Gupta KC, Mishkin M. The locus and cytoarchitecture of the projection areas of the olfactory bulb in Macaca mulatta. J Comp Neurol 1978;177:381–396.
3. Whitlock DG, Nauta WJH. Subcortical projections from the temporal neocortex in Macaca mulatta. J Comp Neurol 1956;106:183–212.
4. Saper CB. Convergence of autonomic and limbic connections in the insular cortex of the rat. J Comp Neurol 1982;210:163–173.
5. Elam M, Svensson THE, Thoren P. Locus coeruleus neurons in sympathetic nerves: activation by visceral afferents. Brain Res 1986;375:117–125.
6. Jones EG. The thalamus. In: Emson P, ed. Chemical neuroanatomy. New York: Raven Press, 1983;257–293.
7. Jones EG, Powell TPSS. An experimental study of converging sensory pathways within the cerebral cortex of the monkey. Brain 1970;93: 793–820.
8. Mesulam MM, Van Hoesen G, Pandya DN, Geschwind N. Limbic and sensory connections of the IPL in the rhesus monkey. Brain Res 1977;136:393–414.
9. Turner BH, Mishkin M, Knapp M. Organization of the amygdalopetal projections from modality-specific cortical association areas in the monkey. J Comp Neurol 1980;191:515–543.
10. VanHoesen GW, Pandya DN, Butters N. Cortical afferents to the entorhinal cortex of the rhesus monkey. Science 1972;175:1471–1473.
11. Vogt BA, Miller MW. Cortical connections between rat cingulate cortex and visual, motor, and postsubicular cortices. J Comp Neurol 1983;216:192–210.
12. Swanson LW. The hippocampus and the concept of the limbic system. In: Seifert W, ed. Neurobiology of the hippocampus. London: Academic Press, 1983;3–19.
13. Amaral DG, Price JL, Pitanken A, Carmichael ST. Anatomical organization of the primate amygdala complex. In: Aggleton JP, ed. The amygdala: neurobiological aspects of emotion, memory and mental dysfunction. New York: Wiley-Liss, 1992;1–66.
14. LeDoux JE, Iwata J, Cicchetti P, Reis DJ. Different projections of the central amygdaloid nucleus mediate autonomic and behavioral correlates of conditioned fear. J Neurosci 1988;8:2517–2529.
15. Sawchenko PE, Swanson LW. The organization of forebrain afferents to the paraventricular and supraoptic nucleus of the rat. J Comp Neurol 1983;218:121–144.
16. Sawchenko PE, Swanson LWW. Central noradrenergic pathways for the integration of hypothalamic neuroendocrine and autonomic responses. Science 1982;214:685–687.
17. Westlund KN, Coulter JDD. Descending projections of the locus coeruleus and subcoeruleus/medial brachial nuclei in monkey: axonal transport studies and dopamine beat hydroxylase immunocytochemistry. Brain Res Rev 1980;2:235–264.
18. Clark FM, Proudfit HK. The projection of locus coeruleus neurons to the spinal cord in the rat determined by anterograde tracing combined with immunocytochemistry. Brain Res 1991;538:231–245.
19. McDonald AJ. Organization of amygdaloid projections to prefrontal cortex and associated striatum in the rat. Neuroscience 1991;44: 1–14.
20. McDonald AJ. Topographical organization of amygdaloid projections to the caudatoputamen, nucleus accumbens, and related striatal-like areas of the rat brain. Neuroscience 1991;44:15–33.
21. Veening JG, Swanson LW, Sawchenko PE. The organization of projections from the central nucleus of the amygdala to brain stem sites involved in central autonomic regulation: a retrograde transport-immunohistochemical study. Brain Res 1984;303:337–357.
22. Charney DS, Deutch AY, Krystal JH, Southwick SM, Davis M. Psychobiologic mechanisms of posttraumatic stress disorder. Arch Gen Psychiatry 1993;50:294–305.
23. Squire LR. Memory and the hippocampus: a synthesis from findings with rats, monkeys, and humans. Psychol Rev 1992;99:195–231.
24. Squire LR, Zola-Morgan S. The medial temporal lobe memory system. Science 1991;253:2380–2386.
25. Litz BT, Keane TM. Information processing in anxiety disorders: application to the understanding of post-traumatic stress disorder. Clin Psychol Rev 1989;9:243–257.
26. McNally RJ, Luedke DL, Besyner JK, Peterson RA, Bohm K, Lips OJ. Sensitivity to stress relevant stimuli in post traumatic stress disorder. Journal of Anxiety Disorders 1987;1:105–116.
27. Phillips RG, LeDoux JE. Differential contribution of amygdala and hippocampus to cued and contextual fear conditioning. Behav Neurosci 1992;106:274–285.
28. Hoffman HS, Selekman W, Fleishler M. Stimulus aspects of aversive controls: long term effects of suppression procedures. J Exp Anal Behav 1966;9:659–662.
29. Davis M. Animal models of anxiety based upon classical conditioning: the conditioned emotional response and fear potentiated startle effect. Pharmacol Ther 1990;47:147–165.
30. Kim JJ, Fanselow MS. Modality-specific retrograde amnesia of fear. Science 1992;256:675–677.
31. Cassens G, Kuruc A, Roffman M, Orsulak P, Schildkraut JJ. Alterations in brain norepinephrine metabolism and behavior induced by environmental stimuli previously paired with inescapable shock. Behav Brain Res 1981;2:387–407.
32. Tanaka M, Ida Y, Tsuda A, Nagasaki N. Involvement of brain noradrenaline and opioid peptides in emotional changes induced by stress in rats. In: Oomura Y, ed. Emotions: neural and chemical control. Tokyo, Japan: Scientific Societies Press, 1986;417–427.
33. Rasmussen K, Marilak DA, Jacobs BL. Single unit activity of the locus

coeruleus in the freely moving cat. I: during naturalistic behaviors and in response to simple and complex stimuli. Brain Res 1986;371:324–334.

34. Tsaltas E, Gray JA, Fillenz M. Alleviation of response suppression to conditioned aversive stimuli by lesions of the dorsal noradrenergic bundle. Behav Brain Res 1987;13:115–127.

35. Cole BJ, Robbins TW. Dissociable effects of lesions to dorsal and ventral noradrenergic bundle on the acquisition performance, and extinction of aversive conditioning. Behav Neurosci 1987;101:476–488.

36. Estes WK. Statistical theory of spontaneous recovery and regression. Psychol Rev 1955;62:145–154.

37. Konorski J. Conditioned reflexes and neuronal organization. London: Cambridge University Press, 1948.

38. Bouton ME, Bulles RC. Contexts, event memories, and extinction. In: Balsam PDD, Tomic KA, eds. Context and learning. Hillsdale, NJ: Lawrence Erlbaum Associates, 1985;133–166.

39. Bouton ME, King DA. Contextual control of conditioned fear: tests for the associative value of the context. J Exp Psychol [Anim Behav] 1983;9:248–256.

40. Bouton ME, King DA. Effect of context with mixed histories of reinforcement and nonreinforcement. J Exp Psychol [Anim Behav] 1986;12:4–15.

41. Bouton ME, Bolles RC. Role of contextual stimuli in reinstatement of extinguished fear. J Exp Psychol [Anim Behav] 1979;5:368–378.

42. Pavlov JP. Conditioned reflexes. Oxford, England: Oxford University Press, 1927.

43. Rescola RA, Heth CD. Reinstatement of fear to extinguished conditioned stimulis. J Exp Psychol [Anim Behav] 1975;104:88–96.

44. McAllister WR, McAllister DE. Reconditioning of extinguished fear after a one-year delay. Bulletin of Psychonomic Society 1988;26:463–466.

45. VanDyke C, Zilberg NJ, MacKinnon JA. Post traumatic stress disorder: a thirty year delay in a World War II veteran. Am J Psychiatry 1985;142:1070–1073.

46. Solomen Z, Garb K, Bleich A, Grupper D. Reactivation of combat related post traumatic stress disorder. Am J Psychiatry 1987;144:51–55.

47. Falls WA, Miserendino MJD, Davis M. Excitatory amino acid antagonists infused into the amygdala block extinction of fear-potentiated startle. Society of Neuroscience Abstracts 1990;16:767.

48. Teich AH, McCabe PM, Gentile CC, et al. Auditory cortex lesions prevent extinction of pavlovian differential heart rate conditioning to tonal stimuli in rabbits. Brain Res 1989;480:210–218.

49. Post RM. Transduction of psychosocial stress into the neurobiology of recurrent affective disorders. Am J Psychiatry 1992;149:999–1010.

50. Weiss SRB, Post RM, Pert A, Woodward R, Murman D. Context-dependent cocaine sensitization: differential effect of haloperidol on development versus expression. Pharmacol Biochem Behav 1989;34:655–661.

51. King GR, Joyner C, Lee T, Kuhn C, Ellinwood EH Jr. Intermittent and continuous cocaine administration: residual behavioral states during withdrawal. Pharmacol Biochem Behav 1992;43:243–248.

52. Antelman SM. Time dependent sensitization as the cornerstone for a new approach to pharmacotherapy: drugs as foreign or stressful stimuli. Drug Development and Research 1988;14:1–30.

53. Sorg B, Kalivas PW. Behavioral and neurochemical cross-sensitization between footshock stress and cocaine. Brain Res 1991;559:29–36.

54. Caggiula AR, Antelman SM, Aul E, Knopf S, Edwards DJ. Prior stress attenuates the analgesic response but sensitizes the corticosterone and cortical dopamine responses to stress 10 days later. Psychopharmacology 1989;99:233–237.

55. Kalivas PW, Duffy P. Similar effects of daily cocaine and stress on mesocorticolimbic dopamine neurotransmission in the rat. Biol Psychiatry 1989;25:913–928.

56. Kalivas PW, Duffy P, Abhold R, Dilts RP. Sensitization of mesolimbic dopamine neurons by neuropeptides and stress. In: Kalivas PW,

57. Kalivas PW, Striplin CD, Steketee JD, Klitenick MA, Duffy P. Cellular mechanisms of behavioral sensitization to drugs of abuse. Ann NY Acad Sci 1992;654:128–135.

58. Criswell HE, Mueller RA, Breese GR. Long-term D1-dopamine receptor sensitization in neonatal 6-OHD-lesioned rats is blocked by an NMDA antagonist. Brain Res 1990;512:284–290.

59. Fontana DJ, Post RM, Pert A. Conditioned increase in mesolimbic dopamine overflow by stimuli associated with cocaine. Brain Res, in press.

60. Nisenbaum LK, Zigmand MJ, Sved AF, Abercrombie ED. Prior exposure to chronic stress results in enhanced synthesis and release of hippocampal norepinephrine in response to a novel stressor. J Neurosci 1991;11:1478–1484.

61. Finlay JM, Abercrombie ED. Stress induced sensitization of norepinephrine release in the medial prefrontal cortex. Society for Neuroscience Abstracts 1991;17:151.

62. Ida Y, Tanaka M, Tsuda A, Tsujimaru S, Nagasaki N. Attenuating effect of diazepam on stress-induced increases in noradrenaline turnover in specific brain regions of rats: Antagonism by Ro 15-1788. Life Sci 1985;37:2491–2498.

63. Tanaka T, Yokoo H, Mizoguchi K, Yoshida M, Tsuda A, Tanaka M. Noradrenaline release in rat amygdala is increased by stress: Studies with intracerebral microdialysis. Brain Res 1991;544:174–181.

64. Tanaka T, Yokoo H. Tsuda A, Tanaka M. Stress increased hypothalamic noradrenaline release studied by intracerebral dialysis method. Neuroscience 1990;16:293–300.

65. Melia KR, Nestler EJ, Duman RS. Chronic imipramine treatment normalized levels of tyrosine hydroxylase in the locus coeruleus of chronically stressed rats. Psychopharmacology 1992;108:23–26.

66. Shirao I, Tsuda A, Yoshisshige I, et al. Effect of acute ethanol administration on noradrenaline metabolism in brain regions of stressed and nonstressed rats. Pharmacol Biochem Behav 1988;30:769–773.

67. Svensson TH. Peripheral, autonomic regulation of locus coeruleus noradrenergic neurons in brain. Putative implications for psychiatry and psychopharmacology. Psychopharmacology 1987;92:1–10.

68. Torda T, Kvetnansky R, Petrikova M. Effect of repeated immobilization stress on rat central and peripheral adrenoceptors. In: Usdin E, Kvetnansky R, Axelrod J, eds. Stress: the role of catecholamines and other neurotransmitters. New York: Gordon & Breach, 1984;691–701.

69. U'Prichard DC, Kvethansky R. Central and peripheral adrenergic receptors in acute and repeated immobilization stress. In: Usdin E, Kvetnansky R, Kopin IJ, eds. Catecholamines and stress: recent advances. Amsterdam: Elsevier, 1980;299–308.

70. Pavcovich LA, Cancela LM, Volosin M, Molina VA, Ramirez OA. Chronic stress-induced changes in locus coeruleus neuronal activity. Brain Res Bull 1990;24:293–296.

71. Simson PE, Weiss JM. Altered activity of the locus coeruleus in an animal model of depression. Neuropsychopharmacology 1988;1:287-295.

72. Levine ES, Litto WJ, Jacobs BL. Activity of cat locus coeruleus noradrenergic neurons during the defense reaction. Brain Res 1990;531:189–195.

73. Rasmussen K, Morilak DA, Jacobs BL. Single unit activity of locus coeruleus neurons in the freely moving cat. I. During naturalistic behaviors and in response to simple and complex stimuli. Brain Res 1986;371:324–334.

74. Redmond DE Jr, Huang YH, Snyder DR, Maas JW. Behavioral effects of stimulation of the locos coeruleus in the stumptail monkey (Macaca arctoides). Brain Res 1976;116:502–507.

75. Redmond DE Jr. Studies of the nucleus locus coeruleus in monkeys and hypotheses for neuropsychopharmacology. In: Meltzer HY, ed. Psychopharmacology: the third generation of progress. New York: Raven Press, 1987;467–974.

76. Charney DS, Woods SW, Price LH, Goodman WK, Glazer WM, Heninger, GR. Noradrenergic dysregulation in panic disorder. In: Ballenger JC, ed. Neurobiology of panic disorders. New York: Alan R. Liss, 1990;91–105.

77. Deutch AY, Roth RH. The determinants of stress induced activation of the prefrontal cortical dopamine system. Prog Brain Res 1990; 85:367–403.

78. Herman J-P, Guilloneau PP, Dantzer R, Scatton B, Semerdjian-Roquier S, LeMoal M. Differential effects of inescapable footshocks and of stimuli previously paired with inescapable footshocks on DA turnover in cortical and limbic areas of the rat. Science 1982;23: 1549–1556.

79. Fadda F, Argiolas A, Melis MR, Tissari A, Onali P, Gessa GL. Stress-induced increase in 3,4-dihydroxyphenylacetic acid (DOPAC) levels in the cerebral cortex and in *n. accumbens:* reversal by diazepam. Life Sci 1978;23:2219–2224.

80. Dunn AJ. Stress-related activation of cerebral dopaminergic systems. Ann NY Acad Sci 1988;537:188–205.

81. Roth RH, Tam S-Y, Ida Y, Yang J-X, Deutch AY. Stress and the mesocorticolimbic dopamine systems. Ann NY Acad Sci 1988;537: 138–147.

82. Bradberry CW, Lory JS, Roth RH. The anxiogenic beta-carboline FG 7142 selectively increases dopamine release in rat prefrontal cortex as measured by microdialysis. J Neurochem 1991;56:748–752.

83. Roth RH, Tam S-Y, Ida Y, Yang J-XX, Deutch AY. Stress and the mesocorticolimbic dopamine systems. Ann NY Acad Sci 1988;537: 138–147.

84. Abercrombie ED, Keefe KA, DiFrischia DS, Zigmund MJ. Differential effect of stress on in vivo dopamine release in striatum, nucleus accumbens, and medial frontal cortex. J Neurochem 1989;52:1655–1658.

85. Mantz J, Thierry AM, Glowinski J. Effect of noxious tail pinch on the discharge rate of mesocortical and mesolimbic dopamine neurons: selective activation of the mesocortical system. Brain Res 1989;476: 377–381.

86. Adell A, Trullas R, Gelpi E. Time course of changes in serotonin and noradrenaline in rat brain after predictable or unpredictable shock. Brain Res 1988;459:54–59.

87. Pei Q, Zetterstrom T, Fillenz M. Tail pinch-induced changes in the turnover and release of dopamine and 5-hydroxytryptamine in different brain regions of the rat. Neuroscience 1990;35: 133–138.

88. Dunn AJ. Stress-related activation of cerebral dopaminergic systems. Ann NY Acad Sci 1988;537:188–205.

89. Heinsbroek RPW, Van Haaven F, Fecustra MGP, Boon P, Van de Poll NE. Controllable and uncontrollable footshock and monoaminergic activity in the frontal cortex of male and female rats. Brain Res 1991;551:247–255.

90. Kramer GL, Petty F. Inhibition of stress-induced increase in dopamine and serotonin metabolism in frontal neocortex by diazepam in vivo using brain micordialysis perfusion. J Neurochem 1989;52: S155.

91. Rasmussen AM, Goldstein LE, Bunney BS, Roth RH. Non-sedative dose lorazepam dissociates the neurochemical and behavioral correlates of fear conditioning in the rat. Society for Neuroscience Abstracts 1992;18:813.

92. Petty F, Sherman AD. Learned helplessness induction decreases in vivo cortical serotonin release. Pharmacol Biochem Behav 1983;18: 649–650.

93. Hellhammer DH, Rea MA, Bell L, Belkien L, Ludwig M. Learned helplessness effects on brain monoamines and the pituitary gonadal axis. Pharmac Biochem Behav 1984;21:481–485.

94. Petty F, Sherman AD. Reversal of learned helplessness by imipramine. Communications in Psychopharmacology 1980;3:371–375.

95. Martin P, Soubrie P, Pueech AJ. Reversal of helpless behavior by serotonin uptake blocker. Psychopharmacology 1990;101:403–407.

96. Graeff F. Role of 5-HT in defensive behavior and anxiety. Rev Neurosci 1993;4:181–211.

97. Watanabe Y, Gould E, Daniels D, Cameron H, McEwen BS. Tianeptine attenuates stress-induced morphological changes in the hippocampus. Eur J Pharmacol 1992;222:157–162.

98. Deakin W, Graeff F. 5-HT and mechanisms of defense. Journal of Psychopharmacology 1991;5:305–315.

99. Kuroda Y, Mikuni M, Ogawa T, Takahashi K. Effect of ACTH, adrenalectomy and the combination treatment on the density of 5-HT$_2$ receptor binding sites in neocortex of rat forebrain and 5-HT$_2$ receptor-mediated wet-dog shake behaviors. Psychopharmacology 1992;108:27–32.

100. Kuroda Y, Mikuni M, Nomura N, Takahashi K. Differential effect of subchronic dexamethasone treatment on serotonin-$_2$ and β-adrenergic receptors in the rat cerebral cortex and hippocampus. Neurosci Lett 1993;155:195–198.

101. McKittrick CR, Blanchard D, Blanchard R, McEwen BS, Sakai R. Effects of chronic social stress on serotonin receptor binding. Society for Neuroscience Abstracts 1993;593.

102. Martire M, Navarra P, Pistritto G, Preziosi P. Adrenal steroid-induced chances in serotonin receptors in rat hippocampus and hypothalamus. Pharmacol Res 1988;20:415–416.

103. Mendelson S, McEwen BS. Autoradiographic analyses of the effects of restraint-induced stress on 5-HT$_{1A}$, 5-HT$_{1C}$ and 5-HT$_2$ receptors in the dorsal hippocampus of male and female rats. Neuroendocrinology 1991;54:454–461.

104. Mendelson S, McEwen BS. Autoradiographic analyses of the effects of adrenalectomy and corticosterone on 5-HT$_{1A}$ and 5-HT$_{1B}$ receptors in the dorsal hippocampus and cortex of the rat. Neuroendocrinology 1992;55:444–450.

105. Chalmers D, Kwak S, Mansour A, Akil H, Watson S. Corticosteroids regulate brain hippocampal 5-HT$_{1A}$ receptor mRNA expression. J Neurosci 1993;13:914–923.

106. Burnet P, Mefford I, Smith C, Gold P, Sternberg E. Hippocampal 8-[3H]hydroxy-2-(di-n-propylamino) tetralin binding site densities, serotonin receptor (5-HT$_{1A}$) messenger ribonucleic acid abundance and serotonin levels parallel the activity of the hypothalamopituitary-adrenal axis in rat. J Neurochem 1992;59: 1062–1070.

107. Dunn AJ, Welch J. Stress- and endotoxin-induced increases in brain tryptophan and serotonin metabolism: Depend on sympathetic nervous system activity. J Neurochem 1991;57:1615–1622.

108. Torda T, Murgas K, Cechova E, et al. Adrenergic regulation of 3H-ketanserin binding sites during immobilization stress in the rat frontal cortex. Brain Res 1990;527:198–203.

109. Segal M. Serotonergic innervation of the locus coeruleus from the dorsal raphe and its action on responses to noxious stimuli. J Physiol 1979;286:401–415.

110. Mohler H, Okada T. Benzodiazepine receptor demonstration in the central nervous system. Science 1977;198:849–851.

111. Hirsch JD, Garrett KM, Beer B. Heterogeneity of benzodiazepine binding sites. A review of recent research. Pharmacol Biochem Behav 1985;23:681–685.

112. Costa E, Greengard P. Mechanism of action of benzodiazepines. New York: Raven Press, 1975.

113. Tallman JF, Gallagher DW. The GABA-ergic system: a locus of benzodiazepine action. Annu Rev Neurosci 1985;8:21–44.

114. Squires RF, Braestrup C. Benzodiazepine receptors in rat brain. Nature 1977;266:732–734.

115. Guidotti A, Baraldi M, Leon A, Costa E. Benzodiazepines: a tool to explore the biochemical and neurophysiological basis of anxiety. Federation Proceedings 1990;39:1039–1042.

116. Braestrup C, Schmiechen R, Neef G, Nielsen M, Petersen EN. Interaction of convulsive ligands with benzodiazepine receptors. Science 1982;216:1241–1243.

117. Ableitner A, Herz A. Changes in local cerebral glucose utilization induced by the β-carbolines FG 7142 and DMCM reveal brain structures involved in the control of anxiety and seizure activity. J Neurosci 1987;7:1047–1055.

118. Ninan PT, Insel TM, Cohen RM, Cook JM, Skolnick P, Paul SM.

Benzodiazepine receptor-mediated experimental "anxiety" in primates. Science 1982;218:1332–1334.

119. Bremner JD, Charney DS. Anxiety disorders. In Rakel RE, ed. Conn's current therapy. Philadelphia: WB Saunders, 1994;1103–1108.

120. Charney DS, Deutch AY, Krystal JH, Southwick SM, Davis M. Psychobiologic mechanisms of posttraumatic stress disorder. Arch Gen Psychiatry 1993;50:294–299.

121. Weizman R, Weizman A, Kook KA, Vocci F, Deutsch SI, Paul SM. Repeated swim stress alters brain benzodiazepine receptors measured in vivo. J Pharmacol Exp Ther 1989;249:701-707.

122. Drugan RC, Morrow AL, Weizman R, et al. Stress-induced behavioral depression in the rat is associated with a decrease in GABA receptor-mediated chloride ion flux and brain benzodiazepine receptor occupancy. Brain Res 1989;487:45–51.

123. Drugan RC, Ryan SM, Minor TR, Maier SF. Librium prevents the analgesia and shuttlebox escape deficit typically observed following inescapable shock. Pharmacol Biochem Behav 1984;21:749–754.

124. Robertson HA, Martin IL, Candy JM. Differences in benzodiazepine receptor binding in Maudsley-reactive and nonreactive rats. Eur J Pharmacol 1978;50:455–457.

125. Wynn PC, Hauger RL, Holmes MC, Millon MA, Catt KJ, Aguilera G. Brain and pituitary receptors for corticotropin releasing factor: localization and differential regulation after adrenalectomy. Peptides 1984;5:1077–1084.

126. Koob GF, Bloom FE. Corticotropin-releasing factor and behavior. Federation Proceedings 1985;44:259–263.

127. Gold PW, Goodwin FK, Chrousos GP. Clinical and biochemical manifestations of depression. N Engl J Med 1988;319:413–420.

128. Dunn AJ, Berridge CW. Physiological and behavioral responses to corticotropin-releasing factor administration: is CRF a mediator of anxiety or stress responses. Brain Res Rev 1990;15:71–100.

129. Chappell PB, Smith MA, Kitts CD, et al. Alterations in corticotropin-releasing factor-like immunoreactivity in discrete rat brain regions after acute and chronic stress. J Neurosci 1986;6:2908–2914.

130. Dunn AJ, Berridge CW. Corticotropin-releasing factor administration elicits a stress like activation of cerebral catecholaminergic systems. Pharmacol Biochem Behav 1987;27:685–691.

131. Valentino RJ, Foote SL. Corticotropin-releasing hormone increases tonic but not sensory-evoked activity of noradrenergic locus coeruleus neurons in unanesthetized rats. J Neurosci 1988;8:1016–1025.

132. Butler PD, Weiss JM, Stout JC, Nemeroff CB. Corticotropin-releasing factor produces fear-enhancing and behavioral activating effects following infusion into the locus coeruleus. J Neurosci 1990;10:176–183.

133. Koegler SM, Kilts CD, Owens MJ, Ervin GN, Bissette G, Nemeroff CB. The effect of bilateral electrolytic lesions of the central amygdaloid nucleus on the concentration of corticotropin-releasing factor (CRF) in microdissected brain regions. Society of Neuroscience Abstracts 1991;17:663.

134. Owens MJ, Vargas MA, Knight DL, Nemeroff CB. The effects of alprazolam on corticotropin releasing factors neurons in rat brain: acute time course, chronic treatment, and abrupt withdrawal. J Pharmacol Exp Ther 1991;258:349–356.

135. Dunn AJ, Berridge CW. Corticotropin-releasing factor administration results in a stress-like activation of cerebral catecholaminergic systems. Pharmacol Biochem Behav 1987;27:685–691.

136. Kalivas PW, Duffy P, Latimer LG. Neurochemical and behavioral effects of corticotropin-releasing factor in the ventral tegmental area of the rat. J Pharmacol Exp Ther 1987;252:757–763.

137. Jackson RL, Maier SF, Coon DJ. Long term analgesic effects of inescapable shock and learned helplessness. Science 1979;206:91–93.

138. Hyson RL, Ashcraft LJ, Drugan RC, Grau JW, Maier SF. Extent and control of shock affects naltrexone sensitivity of stress-induced analgesia and reactivity to morphine. Pharmacol Biochem Behav 1982;17:1019–1025.

139. Williams JL, Drugan RC, Maier SF. Exposure to uncontrollable stress alters withdrawal from morphine. Behav Neurosci 1984;98:836–846.

140. Hemingway RB, Reigle TG. The involvement of endogenous opiate systems in learned helplessness and stress-induced analgesia. Psychopharmacology 1987;93:353–357.

141. Fanselow MS. Conditioned fear-induced opiate analgesia: a competing motivational state theory of stress analgesia. Ann NY Acad Sci 1986;467:40–54.

142. Maier SF. Stressor controllability and stress induced analgesia. Ann NY Acad Sci 1986;467:55–72.

143. Madden J, Akil H, Patrick RL, Barchas JD. Stress induced parallel changes in central opioid levels and pain responsiveness in the rat. Nature 1977;265:358–360.

144. Amir S, Brown ZW, Amit Z. The role of endorphins in stress: evidence and speculations. Neurosci Biobehav Rev 1986;4:77–86.

145. Stuckey J, Marra S, Minor T, Insel TR. Changes in μ opiate receptors following inescapable shock. Brain Res 1989;476:167–169.

146. Woodruff GN, Hill DR, Boden P, Pinnock R, Singh L, Hughes J. Functional role of brain CCK receptors. Neuropeptides 1991;19(suppl):45–56.

147. Bradwejn J, Koszyck D, Couetoux du Terte A, Bourin M, Palmour R, Ervin F. The cholecystokinin hypothesis of panic and anxiety disorders. J Psychopharmacol 1992;6:345–351.

148. deMontigny C. Cholecystokinin tetrapeptide induces panic like attacks in healthy volunteers. Arch Gen Psychiatry 1989;46:511–517.

149. Heilig M, Soderpalm B, Engel JA, Widerlov E. Centrally administered neuropeptide Y (NPY) produces anxiolytic-like effects in animal anxiety models. Psychopharmacology 1989;98:524–529.

150. Heilig M, McLeod S, Koob GF, Britton KT. Anxiolytic-like effect of neuropeptide Y (NPY), but not other peptides in an operant conflict test. Regul Pept 1992;41:61–69.

151. Wahlestedt C, Pich EM, Koob GF, Yee F, Heilig M. Modulation of anxiety and neuropeptide Y-Y$_1$ receptors by antisense oligodeoxynucleotides. Science 1993;259:528–531.

152. Heilig M, Koob GF, Ekman R, Britton KT. Corticotropin releasing factor and neuropeptide Y: role in emotional integration. Trends in Neuroscience 1994;17:80–85.

153. Robins LN, Helzer JE, Weissman MM, et al. Lifetime prevalence of specific psychiatric disorders in three sites. Arch Gen Psychiatry 1984;41:949–958.

154. Myers JK, Weissman MM, Tischler GL, et al. Six-month prevalence of psychiatric disorders in three communities. Arch Gen Psychiatry 1984;41:959–967.

155. Breier A, Charney DS, Heninger GR. Agoraphobia with panic attacks: development, diagnostic stability, and course of illness. Arch Gen Psychiatry 1986;43:1029–1036.

156. Crowe RR. The genetics of panic disorder and agoraphobia. Psychiatric Developments 1985;2:171–186.

157. Pauls DL, Bucher KD, Crowe RR, Bucher D, Crowe RR, Noyes R Jr. A genetic study of panic disorder pedigrees. Am J Hum Genet 1980;32:639–644.

158. Torgersen S. Genetic factors in anxiety disorders. Arch Gen Psychiatry 1983;40:1085–1089.

159. Crowe RR. Panic disorder: genetic considerations. J Psychiatr Res 1990;24(suppl 2):129–134.

160. Cameron OG, Lee MA, Curtis GC, McCann DS. Endocrine and physiological changes during spontaneous panic attacks. Psychoneuroendocrinology 1987;12:321–331.

161. Woods SW, Charney DS, McPherson CA, Gradman AH, Heninger GR. Situational panic attacks: behavioral, physiological, and biochemical characterization. Arch Gen Psychiatry 1987;44:365–375.

162. Nesse RM, Cameron OG, Buda AJ, McCann DS, Curtis CG, Huber-Smith MJ. Urinary catecholamines and mitral valve prolapse in panic anxiety patients. Psychiatry Research 1985;14:67–75.

163. Nesse RM, Cameron OG, Curtis GC, McCann DS, Huber-Smith MJ. Adrenergic function in patients with panic anxiety. Arch Gen Psychiatry 1984;41:771.

164. Edlund MJ, Swann AC, Davis CM. Plasma MHPG in untreated panic disorder. Biol Psychiatry 1987;22:1491–1495.

165. Finaly JM, Abercrombie ED. Stress induced sensitization of norepinephrine release in the medial prefrontal cortex. Soc Neurosci Abstr 1991;17:151.

166. Roth WT, Margraf J, Ehlers A, et al. Stress reactivity in panic disorder. Arch Gen Psychiatry 1992;49:301–310.

167. Charney DS, Woods SW, Price LH, Goodman WK, Glazer WM, Heninger, GR. Noradrenergic dysregulation in panic disorder. In: Ballenger JC, ed. Neurobiology of panic disorders. New York: Alan R. Liss, 1990;91–105.

168. Charney DS, Heninger GR, Breier A. Noradrenergic function in panic anxiety: effects of yohimbine in healthy subjects and patients with agoraphobia and panic disorder. Arch Gen Psychiatry 1984;41:751–763.

169. Charney DS, Woods SW, Goodman WK, Heninger GR. Neurobiological mechanisms of panic anxiety: biochemical and behavioral correlates of yohimbine-induced panic attacks. Am J Psychiatry 1987;144:1030–1036.

170. Charney DS, Woods SW, Krystal JH, Nagy LM, Heninger GR. Noradrenergic neuronal dysregulation in panic disorder: the effects of intravenous yohimbine and clonidine in panic disorder patients. Acta Psychiatr Scand 1992;86:273–282.

171. Woods SW, Hoffer PB, McDougle CJ, et al. Cerebral noradrenergic function in panic disorder. Biol Psychiatry, in press.

172. Uhde TW, Murray MB, Vittone BJ, et al. Behavioral and physiological effects of short-term and long-term administration of clonidine in panic disorder. Arch Gen Psychiatry 1989;46:170–177.

173. Nutt DJ. Altered alpha₂-adrenoceptor sensitivity in panic disorder. Arch Gen Psychiatry 1989;46:165–169.

174. Pohl R, Yeragani VK, Balon R, et al. Isoproterenol induced panic attacks. Biol Psychiatry 1988;24:891–902.

175. Pohl R, Yeragani VK, Balon R. Effects of isoproterenol in panic disorder patients after antidepressant treatment. Biol Psychiatry 1990;28:203–214.

176. Charney DS, Heninger GR. Noradrenergic function and the mechanism of action of antianxiety treatment. II: The effect of long-term imipramine treatment. Arch Gen Psychiatry 1985;41:473–481.

177. Sheehan DV, Davidson J, Manschrek T. Lack of efficacy of a new antidepressant (bupropion) in the treatment of panic disorder with phobias. J Clin Psychopharmacol 1983;3:28–31.

178. Charney DS, Heninger GR. Noradrenergic function and the mechanism of action of antianxiety treatment. I. The effect of long-term alprazolam treatment. Arch Gen Psychiatry 1985;42:458–467.

179. DenBoer JA, Westenberg HGM. Serotonin function in panic disorder: a double blind placebo controlled study with fluvoxamine and ritanserin. Psychopharmacology 1990;102:85–94.

180. Segal M. Serotonergic innervation of the locus coeruleus from the dorsal raphe and its action on responses to noxious stimuli. J Physiol 1979;286:401–415.

181. Aston-Jones G, Akaoka H, Charlety P, Chouvet G. Serotonin selectively attenuates glutamate-evoked activation of noradrenergic locus coeruleus neurons. J Neurosci 1991;11:760–769.

182. Goddard AW, Woods SW, Sholomska DE, Goodman WK, Charney DS, Heninger GR. Effects of the serotonin reuptake inhibitor fluvoxamine on noradrenergic function in panic disorder. Psychiatry Res 1993;48:119–133.

183. Uhde TW, Berrettini WH, Roy-Byrne PP, Boulenger J-P, Post RM. Platelet ₃H-imipramine binding in patients with panic disorder. Biol Psychiatry 1987;22:52–58.

184. Innis RB, Charney DS, Heninger GR. Differential ₃H-imipramine platelet binding in patients with panic disorder and depression. Psychiatry Res 1987;21:33–41.

185. Norman TR, Judd FK, Gregory M, et al. Platelet serotonin uptake in panic disorder. J Affect Disord 1986;11:69–72.

186. Balon R, Poh R, Yeragani V, Rainey J, Oxenkrug GF. Platelet serotonin levels in panic disorder. Acta Psychiatr Scand 1987;75:315.

187. Pecknold JC, Suranyi-Cadotte B, Chang H, Nair NPV. Serotonin uptake in panic disorder and agoraphobia. Neuropsychopharmacology 1988;1:173–176.

188. Schneider LS, Munjack D, Severson JA, Palmer R. Platelet ₃H-imipramine binding in generalized anxiety disorder, panic disorder, and agoraphobia with panic attacks. Biol Psychiatry 1987;21:33–41.

189. Charney DS, Heninger GR. Serotonin function in panic disorders. The effects of intravenous tryptophan in healthy subjects and panic disorder patients before and during alprazolam treatment. Arch Gen Psychiatry 1986;43:1059–1065.

190. DenBoer JA, Westenberg HGM. Behavioral, neuroendocrine, and biochemical effects of 5-hydroxytryptophan administration in panic disorder. Psychiatry Res 1990;31:367–378.

191. Goddard AW, Goodman WK, Woods SW, Charney DS, Heninger GR, Price LH. Effects of tryptophan depletion on panic anxiety. Soc Neurosci Abstr 1993;19:244.

192. Targum SD, Marshall LE. Fenfluramine provocation of anxiety in patients with panic disorder. Psychiatry Res 1989;28:295–306.

193. Kahn RS, Asnis GM, Wetzler S, Asnis GM, Barr G. Serotonin and anxiety revisited. Biol Psychiatry 1988;23:189–208.

194. Charney DS, Woods SW, Goodman WK, Heninger GR. Serotonin function in anxiety: II. Effects of the serotonin agonist MCPP in panic disorder patients and healthy subjects. Psychopharmacology 1987;92:14–24.

195. Germine M, Goddard AW, Sholomskas DE, Woods SW, Charney DS, Heninger GR. Response to m-chlorophenylpiperazine (MCPP) in panic disorder patients and healthy subjects. Influence of reduction in intravenous dosage. Psychiatry Res, in press.

196. Lesch KP, Wiesmann M, Hoh A, et al. 5-HT1A receptor-effector system responsivity in panic disorder. Psychopharmacology 1992;106:111–117.

197. Hommer DW, Skolnick P, Paul SM. The BZ/GABA receptor complex and anxiety. In: Meltzer HY, ed. Psychopharmacology: the third generation of progress. New York: Raven Press, 1987.

198. Nutt DJ, Glue P, Lawson C, Wilson S. Flumazenil provocation of panic attacks: evidence for altered benzodiazepine receptor sensitivity in panic disorder. Arch Gen Psychiatry 1990;47:917–925.

199. Woods SW, Charney DS, Silver JM, Krystal JH, Heninger GR. Behavioral, biochemical and cardiovascular responses to benzodiazepine receptor antagonist flumazenil in panic disorder. Psych Res 1991;36:115–124.

200. Dorow R, Horowski R, Paschelke G, Amin M, Braestrup C. Severe anxiety induced by FG 7142, a β-carboline ligand for benzodiazepine receptors. Lancet 1983;7:98–99.

201. Clow A, Glover V, Armando I, Sandler M. New endogenous benzodiazepine receptor ligand in human urine. Identity with endogenous monoamine oxidase inhibitor? Life Sci 1983;33:735–741.

202. Clow A, Glover V, Sandler M, Tiller J. Increased urinary tribulin output in generalized anxiety disorder. Psychopharmacology 1988;95:378–380.

203. Clow A, Glover V, Weg WM, et al. Urinary catecholamine metabolism and tribulin output during lactate infusion. Brit J Psychiatry 1989;152:122–126.

204. George D, Adinoff B, Ravitz B. A cerebrospinal fluid study of the pathophysiology of panic disorder associated with alcoholism. Acta Psychiatr Scand 1990;82:1–7.

205. Roy A, Pickar D, Gold P. Diazepam binding inhibitor and corticotropin releasing hormone in cerebrospinal fluid. Acta Psychiatr Scand 1989;80:287–291.

206. Payeur R, Lydiard RB, Ballenger JC, Laraia MT, Fossey MD, Zealberg J. CSF diazepam-binding inhibitor concentrations in panic disorder. Biol Psych 1992;32:712–716.

207. Roy-Byrne PP, Cowley DS, Greenblatt DJ, Shader RL, Hommer D. Reduced benzodiazepine sensitivity in panic disorder. Arch Gen Psychiatry 1990;47:534–538.

208. Roy-Byrne PP, Lewis N, Villacres E, et al. Preliminary evidence of benzodiazepine subsensitivity in panic disorder. Biol Psychiatry 1989;26:744–748.

209. Ontiveros A, Fontaine R, Breton G, Elie G, Fontaine S, Dery R. Correlation of severity of panic disorder and neuroanatomical changes

on magnetic resonance imaging. J Neuropsychiatr Clin Neurosci 1989;1:404–408.

210. Fontaine R, Breton G, Dery R, Fontaine S, Elie R. Temporal lobe abnormalities in panic disorder. An MRI study. Biol Psychiatry 1990;27:304–310.

211. Avery DH, Osgood TB, Ishiki DM, Wilson LG, Kenny M, Dunner DL. The DST in psychiatric outpatients with generalized anxiety disorder, panic disorder, or primary affective disorder. Am J Psychiatry 1985;142:844–848.

212. Coryell W, Noyes R Jr, Clancy J, Crowe R, Chaudhry D. Abnormal escape from dexamethasone suppression in agoraphobia with panic attacks. Psychiatry Res 1985;15:301–311.

213. Faludi G, Kasko M, Perenyi A, Arato M, Frecska E. The dexamethasone suppression test in panic disorder and major depressive episodes. Biol Psychiatry 1986;21:1008–1014.

214. Curtis GC, Cameron OG, Nesse RM. The dexamethasone suppression test in panic disorder and agoraphobia. Am J Psychiatry 1982;139:1043–1046.

215. Lieberman JA, Brenner R, Lesser M, Coccaro E, Borenstein M, Kane JM. Dexamethasone suppression tests in patients with panic disorder. Am J Psychiatry 1983;140:917–919.

216. Sheehan DV, Claycomb JS, Surman OS, Baer L, Coleman J, Gelles L. Panic attacks and the dexamethasone suppression test. Am J Psychiatry 1983;140:1063–1064.

217. Roy-Byrne PP, Bierer LM, Uhde TW. The dexamethasone suppression test in panic disorder: comparison with normal controls. Biol Psychiatry 1985;20:1237–1240.

218. Peterson GA, Ballenger JC, Cox DP, et al. The dexamethasone suppression test in agoraphobia. J Clin Psychopharmacol 1985;5:100–102.

219. Bridges M, Yeragani VK, Rainey JM, Pohl R. Dexamethasone suppression test in patients with panic attacks. Biol Psychiatry 1986;21:853–855.

220. Stein MB, Uhde TW. Cortisol response to clonidine in panic disorder: comparison with depressed patients and normal controls. Biol Psychiatry 1988;24:322–330.

221. Bradwejn J, Koszycki D, Annable L, Couetoux du Tertre A, Reines S, Karkanias C. A dose-ranging study of the behavioral and cardiovascular effects of CCK-tetrapeptide in panic disorder. Biol Psychiatry 1992;32:903–912.

222. Bradwejn J, Koszycki MA. Imipramine antagonism of the panicogenic effects of the cholecystokinin tetrapeptide in panic disorder. Arch Gen Psychiatry 1994;151:261–263.

223. Pitts FM, McClure JN. Lactate metabolism in anxiety neurosis. N Engl J Med 1967;277:1329–1336.

224. Liebowitz MR, Fyer AJ, Gorman JM, et al. Specificity of lactate infusions in social phobia versus panic disorders. Am J Psychiatry 1985;142:947–950.

225. Cowley DS, Arana GW. The diagnostic utility of lactate sensitivity in panic disorder. Arch Gen Psychiatry 1990;47:277–284.

226. Rifkin A, Klein DF, Dillon DF, Dillon D, Levit M. Blockade by imipramine or desipramine of panic induced by sodium lactate. Am J Psychiatry, 1981;138;676–677.

227. Liebowitz MR, Fyer AJ, Gorman JM, et al. Lactate provocation of panic attacks. Arch Gen Psychiatry 1984;41:764–770.

228. Carr DB, Sheehan DV. Panic anxiety: a new biological model. J Clin Psychiatry 1984;45:323–330.

229. Nutt D, Lawson C. Panic attacks: a neurochemical overview of models and mechanisms. Br J Psychiatry 1992;160:165–178.

230. Gorman JM, Battista D, Goetz RR, et al. A comparison of sodium bicarbonate and sodium lactate infusion in the induction of panic attacks. Arch Gen Psychiatry 1989;46:145–150.

231. Gorman JM, Goetz RR, Dillon D, et al. Sodium d-lactate infusion in panic disorder patients. Neuropsychopharmacology 1990;3:181–189.

232. Gorman JM, Fyer MR, Goetz R, et al. Ventilatory physiology of patients with panic disorder. Arch Gen Psychiatry 1988;45:31–39.

233. Van Den Hout MA, Griez E. Panic symptoms after inhalation of carbon dioxide. Br J Psychiatry 1984;144:503–507.

234. Griez E, Lousberg H, Van Den Hout, MA, van der Molen GM. Carbon dioxide vulnerability in panic disorder. Psychiatry Res 1987;20:87–95.

235. Klein DF. False suffocation alarms, spontaneous panics, and related conditions. Arch Gen Psychiatry 1993;50:306–317.

236. Woods SW, Koster K, Krystal JH, et al. Yohimbine alters regional cerebral blood flow in panic disorder [Letter]. Lancet 1988;2:678.

237. Stewart RS, Devous MD, Rush AJ, Lane L, Bonte FJ. Cerebral blood flow changes during sodium-lactate-induced panic attacks. Am J Psychiatry 1988;145:442–449.

238. Reiman EM, Raichle ME, Butler FK, Herscovitch P, Robins E. A focal brain abnormality in panic disorder: a severe form of anxiety. Nature 1984;310:683–685.

239. Reiman E, Raichle ME, Robins E, et al. The application of positron emission tomography to the study of panic disorder. Am J Psychiatry 1986;143:469–477.

240. Reiman EM, Raichle ME, Robins E, et al. Neuroanatomical correlates of a lactate-induced anxiety attack. Arch Gen Psychiatry 1989;46:493–500.

241. Reiman EM, Fusselman MJ, Fox PT, Raichle ME. Neuroanatomical correlates of anticipatory anxiety. Science 1989;243:1071–1074.

242. Drevets WC, Videen TO, MacLeod AK, Haller JW, Raichle ME. PET images of blood flow changes during anxiety. Correction. Science 1992;256:1696.

243. Nordahl TE, Semple WE, Gross M, et al. Cerebral glucose metabolic differences in patients with panic disorder. Neuropsychopharmacology 1990;3:261–271.

244. Kulka RA, Schlenger WE, Fairbank JA, et al. Trauma and the Vietnam war generation. New York: Brunner/Mazel, 1990.

245. Kilpatrick DG, Best CL, Veronen LJ, Amick AE, Villeponteaux LA, Ruff GA. Mental health correlates of criminal victimization: a random community survey. J Consult Clin Psychol 1985;53:866–873.

246. Breslau N, Davis GC, Andreshi P, Peterson E. Traumatic events and posttraumatic stress disorder in an urban population of young adults. Arch Gen Psychiatry 1991;48:216–222.

247. Weiner H. The psychobiology of anxiety and fear. In: Gorman JA, ed. Diagnosis and treatment of anxiety disorders. Washington, DC: American Psychiatric Press, 1984;33–62.

248. Von Euler US, Lundberg U. Effect of flying on epinephrine excretion in Air Force personnel. J Appl Physiol 1954;6:551–558.

249. Dimsdale J, Moss J. Plasma catecholamines in stress and exercise. JAMA 1980;243:340–342.

250. Taggart P, Carruthers M, Sommerville W. Electrocardiogram, plasma catecholamines, and lipids, and their modification by oxprenolol when speaking before an audience. Lancet 1973;2:341–346.

251. Ward MM, Mefford IN, Parker DS, et al. Epinephrine and norepinephrine responses in continuously collected plasma to a series of stressors. Psychosom Med 1983;45:471–486.

252. Taggart P, Carruthers M. Endogenous hyperlipidemia induced by emotional stress of racing driving. Lancet 1971;1:363–366.

253. Morrow GR, Labrum AH. The relationship between psychological and physiological measures of anxiety. Psychol Med 1978;8:95–101.

254. Lader M. The peripheral and central role of the catecholamines in the mechanisms of anxiety. International Pharmacopsychiatry 1974;9:125–137.

255. Uhde TW, Boulenger J-P, Post RM, et al. Fear and anxiety: relationship to noradrenergic function. Psychopathology 1984;17(suppl 3):8–23.

256. Uhde TW, Siever IJ, Post RM, Jimerson DC, Boulenger J-P, Buchsbaum MS. The relationship of plasma-free MHPG to anxiety and psychophysical pain in normal volunteers. Psychopharmacol Bull 1982;18:129–132.

257. Sweeney DR, Maas JW, Heninger GR. State anxiety, physical activity, and urinary 3-methoxy-4-hydroxyphenethylene glycol excretion. Arch Gen Psychiatry 1978;35:1418–1423.

258. Kosten TR, Mason JW, Giller EL, Ostroff RB, Harkness L. Sustained urinary norepinephrine and epinephrine elevation in posttraumatic stress disorder. Psychoneuroendocrinology 1987;12:13–20.

259. Yehuda R, Southwick SM, Giller EL. Urinary catecholamine excretion and severity of post-traumatic stress disorder in Vietnam combat veterans. J Nerv Ment Dis 1992;180:321–325.

260. Perry BD, Giller EL, Southwick SM. Altered platelet alpha2-adrenergic binding sites in posttraumatic stress disorder. Am J Psychiatry 1987;144:1511–1512.

261. Nutt DJ. Increased central alpha-2 adrenoceptor sensitivity in panic disorder. Psychopharmacology 1986;90:268–269.

262. Brown SL, Charney DS, Woods SW, Heninger GR, Tallman J. Lymphocyte beta-adrenergic receptor binding in panic disorder. Psychopharmacology 1988;94:2428–2434.

263. Krystal JH, Kosten TR, Perry BD, Southwick S, Mason JW, Giller EL Jr. Neurobiological aspects of PTSD: review of clinical and preclinical studies. Behav Ther 1989;20:177–198.

264. Grinker RR, Spiegle JJ. Men under stress. New York: McGraw-Hill, 1945:219.

265. Meakes JC, Wilson RM. The effect of certain sensory stimulations on respiratory and heart rate in case of "so-called" irritable heart. Heart 1918;7:17–22.

266. Peabody FW, Clough HD, Sturgis LC, Wearn JJ, Thompkins EH. Effects of injection of norepinephrine in soldiers with "irritable heart." JAMA 1918;21:1912–1917.

267. Blanchard EB, Kolb LC, Pallmeyer TP, Gerardi RJ. A psychophysiological study of post-traumatic stress disorder in Vietnam veterans. Psychiatr Q 1982;54:220–229.

268. Kolb LC. The post traumatic stress disorders of combat: a subgroup with a conditioned emotional response. Mil Med 1984;149:237–243.

269. Malloy PF, Fairbank JA, Keane TM. Validation of a multimethod assessment of post-traumatic stress disorders in Vietnam veterans. J Consult Clin Psych 1983;51:488–494.

270. McFall MF, Murburg MM, Ko GM, Veith RC. Autonomic responses to stress in Vietnam veterans with post traumatic stress disorder. Biol Psych 1990;27:1165–1175.

271. Orr SP. Psychophysiologic studies of post traumatic stress disorder. In: Giller EL, ed. Biological assessment and treatment of post traumatic stress disorder. Washington, DC: American Psychiatric Press, 1990:114–120.

272. Pallmeyer TP, Blanchard EB, Kolb LC. The psychophysiology of combat-induced post-traumatic stress disorder in Vietnam veterans. Behav Res Ther 1986;24:645–652.

273. Pitman RK, Orr SP, Forgue DF, deJong JB, Claiborn JM. Psychophysiologic assessment of post-traumatic stress disorder in Vietnam combat veterans. Arch Gen Psychiatry 1987;44:970–975.

274. Boudewyns PA, Hyer L. Psychophysiological response to combat memories and preliminary treatment outcome in Vietnam veteran PTSD patients treated with direct therapeutic exposure. Behav Ther 1990;21:63–87.

275. Keane T, J Fairbank, Caddell JM, Zimering RT. Implosive therapy reduces symptoms of PTSD in Vietnam combat veterans. Behav Ther 1989;20:245–260.

276. Southwick SM, Krystal JH, Morgan CA, et al. Abnormal noradrenergic function in post-traumatic stress disorder. Arch Gen Psychiatry 1993;181:31–37.

277. Nagy L, Merikangas K, Southwick S, et al. Family relationship between panic disorder and PTSD. Program and Abstracts of the 144th Annual Meeting of the American Psychiatric Association, New Orleans, LA, May, 1991:NR182.

278. Aston-Jones G, Valentino RJ, Van Bockstaele EJ, Meyerson AT. Locus coeruleus, stress and post traumatic stress disorder: neurobiological and clinical parallels. In: Murburg M, ed., Catecholamine function in post traumatic stress disorder: emerging concepts. Washington, DC: American Psychiatric Press, in press.

279. Butler PD, Weiss JM, Stout JC, Nemeroff CB. Corticotropin-releasing factor produces fear-enhancing and behavioral activating effects following infusion into the locus coeruleus. J Neurosci 1990;10:176–183.

280. McGaugh JL. Involvement of hormonal and neuromodulatory systems in the regulation of memory storage: endogenous modulation of memory storage. Annu Rev Neurosci 1989;12:255–287.

281. McGaugh JL. Significance and remembrance: the role of neuromodulatory systems. Psychol Sci 1990;1:15–25.

282. Mason JW, Giller EL, Kosten TR, Ostroff RB, Podd L. Urinary free-cortisol levels in post-traumatic stress disorder patients. J Nerv Ment Dis 1986;174:145–159.

283. Yehuda R, Antelman S. Criteria for rationally evaluating animal models of posttraumatic stress disorder. Biol Psychiatry 1993;33:479–486.

284. Yehuda R, Southwick SM, Nussbaum G, Wahby V, Mason JW, Giller EL. Low urinary cortisol excretion in patients with PTSD. J Nerv Ment Dis 1990;178:366–309.

285. Yehuda R, Boisoneau D, Mason JW, Giller EL. Dose-response changes in plasma cortisol and lymphobyte glucocorticoid receptors following dexamethasone administration in combat veterans with and without posttraumatic stress disorder. Am J Psychiatry, in press.

286. Pitman RK, Orr SP, Forgue DF, Altman B, deLong JB, Herz LR. Psychophysiologic responses to combat imagery of Vietnam veterans with posttraumatic stress disorder versus other anxiety disorders. J Abnorm Psychol 1990;99:49–54.

287. Lowy MT, Reder AT, Antel J, Meltzer HY: Glucortocoid resistance in depression: the dexamethasone suppression test and lymphocyte sensitivity to dexamethasone. Am J Psychiatry 1985;141:1365–1370.

288. Yehuda R, Giller EL, Southwick SM, Lowy MT, Mason JW. Hypothalamic-pituitary-adrenal dysfunction in post-traumatic stress disorder. Biol Psychiatry 1991;30:1031–1048.

289. Yehuda R, Boisoneau D, Mason JW, Giller EL. Relationship between lymphocyte glucocorticoid receptor number and urinary-free cortisol excretion in mood, anxiety, and psychotic disorder. Biol Psychiatry 1993;34:18–25.

290. Yehuda R, Boisoneau D, Mason JW, Giller EL. Dose-response changes in plasma cortisol and lymphocyte glucocorticoid receptors following dexamethasone administration in combat veterans with and without posttraumatic stress disorder. Arch Gen Psychiatry, in press.

291. Carroll BJ, Feinberg M, Gredan JF, et al. A specific laboratory test for the diagnosis of melancholia. Arch Gen Psychiatry 1981;38:15–22.

292. Carroll BJ. The dexamethasone suppression test for melancholia. Br J Psychiatry 1982;140:292–304.

293. APA Task Force on Laboratory Tests in Psychiatry. The dexamethasone suppression test: an overview of its current status in psychiatry. Am J Psychiatry 1987;144:1253–1262.

294. Kudler H, Davidson J, Meador K, Lipper S, Ely T. The DST and post-traumatic stress disorder. Am J Psychiatry 1987;144:1068–1071.

295. Kosten TR, Wahby V, Giller E Jr, Mason J. The dexamethasone test and TRH stimulation test in post-traumatic stress disorder. Biol Psychiatry 1990;28:657–664.

296. Olivera AA, Fero D. Affective disorders, DST, and treatment in PTSD patients: clinical observations. Journal of Traumatic Stress 1990;3:407–414.

297. Halbreich U, Olympia J, Carson S, et al. Hypothalamo-pituitary-adrenal activity in endogenously depressed posttraumatic disorder patients. Psychoneuroendocrinology 1989;14:365–370.

298. Dinan TG, Barry S, Yatham LN, Mobayed M, Brown I. A pilot study of neuroendocrine test battery in post traumatic stress. Biol Psychiatry 1990;28:665–672.

299. Yehuda R, Lowy MT, Southwick SM, Shaffer D, Giller EL Jr. Lymphocyte glucocorticoid receptor number in post traumatic stress disorder. Am J Psychiatry 1991;144:499–504.

300. Gold PW, Chrousos GP. Clinical studies with corticotropin releasing factor implications for the diagnosis and pathophysiology of depression, Cushing's disease and adrenal insufficiency. Psychoneuroendocrinology 1985;10:401–420.

301. Gold PW, Loriaux DL, Roy A. Responses to corticotropen-releasing hormone in the hypercortisolism of depression and Cushing's disease. N Engl J Med 1986;314:1329–1335.

302. Holsboer F, Gerken A, Stalla GK, Muller OA. ACTH cortisol and corticosterone output after ovine corticotropin-releasing factor challenge during depression and after recovery. Biol Psychiatry 1985;20:276–286.

303. Holsboeer F, Geerken A, von Bardelenben U. Human corticotropin-releasing hormone in depression: correlation with thyrotopin secretion following thyrotropin releasing hormone. Biol Psychiatry 1986;21:601–611.

304. Smith MA, Davidson J, Ritchie JC, et al. The corticotropin releasing hormone test in patients with posttraumatic stress disorder. Biol Psychiatry 1989;26:349–355.

305. Brown GL, Linnoila MI. CSF serotonin metabolite (5-HIAA) studies in depression, impulsivity, and violence. J Clin Psychiatry 1990;51:31–41.

306. Stanley M, Stanley B. Postmortem evidence for serotonin's role in suicide. J Clin Psychiatry 1990;51:22–28.

307. Paige S, Reid G, Allen M. Psychophysiological correlates of post traumatic stress disorder. Biol Psychiatry 1990;27:419–430.

308. Hegerl U, Ulrich G, Muller-Oerlinghausen B. Auditory evoked potentials and response to lithium prophylaxis. Pharmacopsychiatry 1987;20:213–216.

309. McDougle C, Southwick SM, Charney DS, St. James RL. An open trial of fluoxetine in the treatment of post traumatic stress disorder. J Clin Psychopharmacol 1992;1:325–327.

310. Nagy LM, Morgan CA, Southwick SM, Charney DS. Open prospective trial of fluoxetine for posttraumatic stress disorder. J Clin Psychopharmacol 1993;13:107–113.

311. Arora RC, Fitchuer CT, O'Connor F. Paroxetine binding in the blood platelets of posttraumatic stress disordered patients. Life Sci 1993;53:919–928.

312. Southwick SM, Krystal JH, Morgan CA, et al. Yohimbine and m-chloro-phenylpiperazine in PTSD. New Research Abstracts of the American Psychiatric Association 144th Annual Meeting, 1991: NR3481.

313. Amir S, Brown ZA, Arnit A. The role of endorphins in stress: evidence and speculations. Neurosci Biobehav Rev 1986;4:77–86.

314. Hemingway RB, Reigle TG. The involvement of endogenous opiate systems in learned helplessness and stress-induced analgesia. Psychopharmacology 1987;3:353–357.

315. Pitman RK, Orr S. Twenty-four hour urinary cortisol and catecholamine excretion in combat-related posttraumatic stress disorder. Biol Psychiatry 1990;27:245–247.

316. Jackson RL, Maier SF, Coon DL. Long term analgesic effects of inescapable shock and learned helplessness. Science 1979;206:91–93.

317. Maier SF. Stressor controllability and stress induced analgesia. Ann NY Acad Sci 1986;467:55–72.

318. Pitman RK, Orr S. Twenty-four hour urinary cortisol and catecholamine excretion in combat-related posttraumatic stress disorder. Biol Psychiatry 1990;27:245–247.

319. Fanselow MS. Conditioned fear-induced opiate analgesia: a competing motivational state theory of stress analgesia. Ann NY Acad Sci 1986;467:40–54.

320. Maier SF. Stressor controllability and stress induced analgesia. Ann NY Acad Sci 1986;467:55–72.

321. Hoffman L, Watgson PD, Wilson G, et al. Low plasma beta-endorphin in post-traumatic stress disorder. Aust N Z J Psychiatry 1989;23:268–273.

322. Van der Kolk BA, Greenberg MS, Orr SP, et al. Endogenous opioids, stress induced analgesia and posttraumatic stress disorder. Psychopharmacol Bull 1981;25:417–421.

323. Wolf M. Plasma methionine enkephalin in PTSD. Biol Psychiatr 1991;29:295–308.

324. Pitman RK, van der Kolk BA, Orr SP, Greenberg MS. Naloxone-reversible analgesic response to combat-related stimuli in post traumatic stress disorder. Arch Gen Psychiatry 1990;47:541–544.

325. Charney DS, Keutch A, Krystal J, Southwick SM, Davis M. Psychobiologic mechanisms of post traumatic stress disorder. Arch Gen Psychiatry 1993;50:294-305.

326. Kosten TR, Mason JW, Giller EL, Ostroff RB, Harkness L. Sustained urinary norepinephrine and epinephrine elevation in post-traumatic stress disorder. Psychoneuroendocrinology 1987;12:13–20.

327. Salloway S, Southwick S, Sadowsky M. Opiate withdrawal presenting as posttraumatic stress disorder. Hosp Community Psychiatry 1990;41:666–667.

328. Marks IM. Genetics of fear and anxiety disorders. Br J Psychiatry 1986;149:406–418.

329. Fyer AJ, Mannuzza S, Gallops MS, et al. Familial transmission of simple phobias and fears. A preliminary report. Arch Gen Psychiatry 1990;47:252–256.

330. Kendler KS, Neale MC, Kessler RC, Heath AC, Eaves LJ. The genetic epidemiology of phobias in women. Arch Gen Psychiatry 1992;49:273–282.

331. Nesse RM, Curtis GC, Thyer BA, McCann DS, Huber-Smith MJ, Knopf RF. Endocrine and cardiovascular responses during phobic anxiety. Psychosom Med 1985;47:320–332.

332. Stein MB, Tancer ME, Uhde TW. Heart rate and plasma norepinephrine responsivity to orthostatic challenge in anxiety disorders. Comparison of patients with panic disorder and social phobia and normal control subjects. Arch Gen Psychiatry 1992;49:311–317.

333. Stein MB, Huzel LL, Delaney SM. Lymphocyte β-adrenoceptors in social phobia. Biol Psychiatry 1993;34:45–50.

334. Tancer ME, Stein MB, Uhde TW. Effects of thyrotropin-releasing hormone on blood pressure and heart rate in phobic and panic patients: a pilot study. Biol Psychiatry 1990;27:781–783.

335. Tancer ME, Stein MB, Unde TW. Growth hormone response to intravenous clonidine in social phabia: comparison to patients with panic disorder and healthy volunteers. Biol Psychiatry 1993;34:591–595.

336. Merikangas KM, Weissman MM. Epidemiology of anxiety disorders in adulthood. In: Cavenar JO, ed. Psychiatry, vol. 3, Philadelphia: JB Lippincott, 1986:86–102.

337. Noyes R, Clarkson C, Crowe RR, Yates WR, McChesney CM. A family study of generalized anxiety disorder. Am J Psychiatry 1987;144:1019–1024.

338. Cedarbaum JM, Aghajanian GK. Afferent projections to the rat locus coeruleus as determined by a retrograde tracing technique. J Comp Neurol 1978;178:1–16.

339. Sevy S, Papadimitriou GN, Surmont DW, Goldman S, Mendlewicz J. Noradrenergic function in generalized anxiety disorder, major depressive disorder, and healthy subjects. Biol Psychiatry 1989;25:141–152.

340. Charney DS, Woods SW, Heninger GR. Noradrenergic function in generalized anxiety disorder. Effects of yohimbine in healthy subjects and patients with generalized anxiety disorder. Psychiatry Res 1987;27:173–182.

341. Mathew RJ, Ho BT, Francis DJ, Taylor DL, Weinman ML. Catecholamines and anxiety. Acta Psychiatrica Scand 1982;65:142–147.

342. Mathew RJ, Ho BT, Kralik P, Taylor DL, Claghorn JL. Catecholamines and monoamine oxidase activity in anxiety. Acta Psychiatr Scand 1981;63:245–252.

343. Cameron OG, Smith CB, Lee MA, Hollingsworth PJ, Hill EM, Curtis GC. Adrenergic status in anxiety disorders. Platelet alpha-2-adrenergic receptor binding, blood pressure, pulse, and plasma catecholamines in panic and generalized anxiety disorder patients and in normal subjects. Biol Psychiatry 1990;28:3–20.

344. Curtis G, Lee MA, Glitz DA, Cameron OG, Abelson J, Bronzo M. Growth hormone response to clonidine in anxiety disorders. Biol Psychiatry 1989;25:6A.

345. Rocca P, Ferrero P, Gualerzi A, et al. Peripheral type benzodiazepine receptors in anxiety disorders. Acta Psychiatr Scand 1992;84:537–544.

346. Weizman R, Tanne Z, Granek M, et al. Peripheral benzodiazepine

binding sites on platelet membranes are increased during diazepam treatment of anxious patients. Eur J Pharmacol 1987;138:289–292.

347. Wu JC, Buchsbaum MS, Hershey TG, Hazlett E, Sicotte N, Johnson JC. PET in generalized anxiety disorder. Biol Psychiatry 1991;29: 1181–1199.

348. Buchsbaum MS, Wu J, Haier R, et al. Positron emission tomography assessment of the effect of benzodiazepines on regional glucose metabolic rate in patients with anxiety disorder. Life Sci 1987;40: 2392–2400.

349. Mitchell RA, Berger AJ. Neural regulation of respiration. In: Hornbein TF, ed. Regulation of breathing. New York: Marcel Dekker, 1981:541–621.

350. Post RM, Weiss SRB, Smith MD. Sensitization and kindling: implications for the evolving neural substrate of PTSD. In: Friedman MJ, Charney DS, Deutch AY, eds. Neurobiological and clinical consequences of stress: from normal adaptation to PTSD. New York: Raven Press, in press.

351. Post RM, Weiss SRB, Uhde TW, Clark M, Rosen JB. Preclinical neuroscience advances pertinent to panic disorder: implications of cocaine kindling, induction of the proto-oncogene c-fos, and contingent tolerance. In: Hoehn-Saric R, ed. Biology of anxiety disorders: recent developments. Washington, DC: American Psychiatric Press, 1993;129–187.

352. Craske MG, Cerny JA, Barlow DH. Behavioral treatment of panic disorder. Behav Res Ther 1989;20:261–282.

353. Klosko JS, Barlow DH. A comparison of alprazolam and behavioral therapy. J Consult Clin Psychotherapy 1990;58:77–84.

354. Reiser MF. Memory in mind and brain. New York: Basic Books, 1990;218.

355. Reiser MF. The relationship of psychoanalysis to neuroscience. In: Kopf J, Nersessian H, eds. Textbook psychoanalysis. Washington, DC: American Psychiatric Press, in press.

356. Kandel ER. Genes, nerve cells and the remembrance of things past. J Neuropsychiatry 1989;1:103–125.

357. Kandel ER. Cellular mechanisms of learning and the biological basis of individuality. In: Kandel ER, Schwartz JM, Jessell TM, eds. Principles of neural science. East Norwalk, CT: Appleton-Century-Crofts, 1991;1009–1031.

358. Frost WN, Castellucci VF, Hawkins RD, Kandel ER. Monosynaptic connections from the sensory neurons participate in the storage of long term memory for sensitization of the gill-and siphon-withdrawal reflex in aplysia. Proc Natl Acad Sci, U S A 1985;82: 8266–8269.

359. Bailey CH, Chen M. Morphological basis of long term habituation and sensitization in aplysia. Science 1983;220:91–93.

360. Bailey CH, Chen M, Keller F, Kandel ER. Serotonin mediated endocytosis of apCAM: an early step of learning related synaptic growth in aplysia. Science 1992;256:645–649.

361. Rose SP. How chicks make memories: the cellular casacade from c-fos to dendritic remodeling. Trends Neurosci 1991;14:390–397.

362. Merzenich MM, Nelson RJ, Stryker MP, Cynander MS, Schoppmann A, Zook JM. Somatosensory, cortical map changes following digit amputation in adult monkeys. J Comp Neurol 1984;224:591–605.

363. Pons TD, Garraghty PE, Mishkin M. Lesion induced plasticity in the second somatosensory cortex of adult macaques. Proc Natl Acad Sci U S A 1988;85:5279–5281.

364. Ramachandran VS, Stewart M, Rogers-Ramachandran. Perceptual correlates of massive cortical reorganization. Neuroreport 1993;3: 583–586.

365. Halligan PW, Harshall JC, Wade DT, Davey J, Morrison D. Thumb in-cheek? Sensory reorganization and perceptual plausticity after limb amputation. Neuroreport 1993;4:233-236.

366. Mogilner A, Grossman JA, Ribary V, et al. Somatosensory cortical plasticity in adult humans revealed by magnetoencephalography. Proc Natl Acad Sci 1993;90:3593–3597.

367. Campean S, Hayward MD, Hope BT, Rosen JB, Nestler EJ, Davis M. Induction of the c-fos proto-oncogene in rat amygdala during unconditioned and conditioned fear. Brain Res 1991;565:349–352.

368. Smith MA, Banerjee S, Gold PW, Glowa J. Induction of c-fos in mRNA in rat brain by conditioned and unconditioned stressors. Brain Res 1992;578:135–141.

369. Kandel ER. Genes, nerve cells and the remembrance of things past. J Neuropsychiatry 1989;1:103–125.

370. Kandel ER. Cellular mechanisms of learning and the biological basis of individuality. In: Kandel ER, Schwartz JM, Jessell TM, eds. Principles of neural science. East Norwalk, CT: Appleton-Century-Crofts, 1991;1009–1031.

371. Deutch AY, Lee MC, Gillham MH, Cameron DA, Goldstein M, Ladarola MJ. Stress selectively increases fos protein in dopamine neurons innervating the prefrontal cortex. Cerebral Cortex 1991;1: 273–292.

372. Pezzone MA, Lee WS, Hoffman GE, Rabin BS. Induction of c-fos immunoreactivity in the rat forebrain by conditioned and unconditioned aversive stimuli. Brain Res 1992;597:41–50.

373. Skre I, Onstad S, Torgersen S, Lygren S, Kinglen E. A twin study of DSM-III-R anxiety disorders. Acta Psychiatr Scand 1993;88:85–92.

13

NEUROPSYCHIATRY OF MOOD DISORDERS

Robert G. Robinson and Javier I. Travella

The neuropsychiatry of mood disorders is based primarily on the study of patients with structural brain lesions such as stroke, traumatic brain injury, and Parkinson's disease. The clinical manifestations of affective disorder include a wide range of emotional and cognitive disturbances and can be divided based on type of mood disorder and the underlying neuropsychiatric disorder. Although studies providing empirical data about individual neuropsychiatric disorders have only begun to emerge within the last few years, these kinds of investigations are essential to build a firm empirical database for our understanding of the clinical manifestations, treatments, and mechanisms of these disorders.

A confounding factor in our understanding of affective disorders associated with brain disease is the tendency of investigators to intermix different types of brain disorders when studying emotional problems in patients with brain injury. For example, the early work of Babinski (1) or Denny-Brown et al. (2), as well as the systematic study of emotional disorders in patients with brain injury by Gainotti (3), included patients with various types of brain injuries such as traumatic closed head injury, penetrating head injury, thromboembolic stroke, surgical incision, and intracerebral hemorrhage (ICH). Although it is generally assumed that neuronal death produced by a variety of mechanisms will result in similar clinical symptoms, depending on the size and location of the lesion, that is not necessarily the case. Moreover, rarely will two conditions producing brain injury result in identical types of lesions. For example, closed head injury generally produces widespread brain injury with multiple small areas of shear or torsion injury, whereas cerebral embolism produces a focal lesion with an area of transient peripheral ischemia. This much of the early information about emotional disorders associated with brain disease has drawn on data obtained from a heterogeneous group of patients, some with clearly defined and localized brain disease and others without it.

In this chapter we briefly review the historical development of neuropsychiatric aspects of affective disorder and then present the disturbances (depressive, mania, and bipolar disorders) associated with the specific neuropsychiatric disorders of stroke, traumatic brain injury, and Parkinson's disease (PD).

HISTORICAL BACKGROUND

The first reports of mood disorders following brain damage (usually caused by cerebrovascular disease) were made by neurologists and psychiatrists in case descriptions. Meyer (4) proposed that in some cases there may be a relationship between traumatic insanities and specific locations and causes of brain injury. Babinski (1) noted that patients with right-hemisphere disease frequently displayed the symptoms of anosognosia, euphoria, and indifference. Bleuler (5) wrote that after stroke, "melancholic moods lasting for months and sometimes longer appear frequently." Kraepelin (6) recognized an association between manic depressive insanity and cerebrovascular disease when he wrote:

> The diagnosis of states of depression may, apart from the distinctions discussed, offer difficulties especially when the possibility of arteriosclerosis has to be taken into consideration. It may, at a time, be an accompanying phenomenon of manic depressive disease, but at another time may itself engender states of depression.

The affective disorders associated with brain injury have frequently been attributed to the existence of aphasia (7). In the middle of the 19th century, Broca (8) localized the process of speech to the inferior left frontal lobe and deduced that the left brain was endowed with different functions from the right brain. Hughlings Jackson (9) regarded language as an extension of brain function existing in two basic forms: the intellectual (conveying content) and the emotional (expressing feeling). He suggested that these components may be separated by disease.

Goldstein (10) was the first to describe an emotional mood disorder thought to be uniquely associated with brain disease: the catastrophic reaction. The catastrophic reaction

(CR) is an emotional outburst involving various degrees of anger, frustration, depression, tearfulness, refusal, shouting, swearing, and sometimes aggressive behavior. Goldstein ascribed this reaction to the inability of the organism to cope when faced with a serious defect in its physical or cognitive functions. In his extensive studies of brain injury in war, Goldstein (11) described two symptom clusters: those related directly to physical damage of a circumscribed area of the brain and those related secondarily to the organism's psychological response to the injury. Emotional symptoms, therefore, represented the latter category (i.e., the psychological response of an organism struggling with physical or cognitive impairments).

A second abnormality unique to brain injury, also involving a disturbance of (this time an absence of) mood, was the indifference reaction described by Hecaen et al. (12) and Denny-Brown et al. (2). The indifference reaction associated with right-hemisphere lesions, consists of symptoms of indifference toward failures, lack of interest in family and friends, enjoyment of foolish jokes, and minimization of physical difficulties. It is associated with neglect of the opposite half of the body and space.

A third "mood" disorder associated with brain injury, such as cerebral infarction, is pathological laughter or crying. Ironside (13) described the clinical manifestations of this disorder. Such patients' emotional displays are characteristically unrelated to their inner emotional state. Crying, for example, may occur spontaneously or after some seemingly minor provocation. This phenomenon has been given various names such as emotional incontinence, emotional lability, pseudobulbar affect, or pathological emotionalism.

The first systematic study to contrast the mood disorders of patients with right- and left-hemisphere brain damage was done by Gainotti (3). He reported that depressive catastrophic reactions were more frequent among patients with left-hemisphere brain damage, particularly those with aphasia, when compared to patients with right-hemisphere lesions. Gainotti agreed with Goldstein's explanation (11) that it is a desperate reaction of the organism when confronted with a severe physical disability. The indifference reaction, on the other hand, was not easy to understand. Gainotti suggested that denial of illness and organization of the nonverbal type of synthesis may play an important role in this emotional disorder.

Despite the assertions by Kraepelin (6) and others (14) that mood disorder may be produced directly by focal brain injury, many investigators have adopted "psychological" explanations for the affective disorders associated with brain injury. Studies examining the emotional symptoms associated specifically with cerebrovascular disease (CVD) began to appear in the early 1960s. Ullman and Gruen (15) reported that stroke was a particularly severe stress to the organism, as Goldstein (11) had suggested, because the organ governing the emotional response to injury had itself been damaged. Fisher (16) described depression associated with cerebrovascular disease as reactive and understandable because "the brain is the most cherished organ of humanity."

Thus, depression was viewed as a natural emotional response to a decrease in self-esteem from a life-threatening injury and the resulting disability and dependence.

Systematic studies, however, led other investigators, who were impressed by the frequency of association between brain injury and mood disorders, to hypothesize more direct causal links. In a study of 100 elderly patients with affective disorders, Post (14) stated that the high frequency of brain ischemia associated with first episodes of depressive disorder suggested that the causes for atherosclerotic disease and depression may be linked. Folstein et al. (17) compared 20 stroke patients with 10 orthopedic patients. Although the functional disability in both groups was comparable, more of the stroke patients were depressed. The authors concluded that "mood disorder is a more specific complication of stroke than simply a response to motor disability."

In summary, there have been two primary lines of thought in the study of affective disorders that are associated with structural brain disease. One attributes mood disorders to an understandable psychological reaction to the associated impairment; the other, based on a lack of association between severity of impairment and severity of emotional disorder, suggests a direct causal connection between mood disorders and structural brain damage.

DEPRESSIVE DISORDERS

Depression Associated with Stroke

Cerebrovascular disease is one of the most common life-threatening problems among the elderly in the U.S., and it ranks only behind heart disease and cancer as the third leading cause of death in patients over age 50. The incidence of stroke increases steadily with age, rising from 10/100,000 under age 35 to 5970/100,000 over age 75 (18). The American Heart Association estimates there will be 400,000 new victims of stroke each year. During the past 10 years, however, there has been a steady decline in the incidence of stroke, which most investigators have attributed to the improved control of hypertension (18,19). Nevertheless, 75% of stroke survivors are left with physical or intellectual impairments of sufficient severity to limit their vocational capacity (19).

PREVALENCE

Depression is the most common emotional disorder associated with CVD. Investigators who have utilized structured psychiatric interviews, and established diagnostic criteria have usually identified two forms of depressive disorder associated with brain disease. One type is major depression, which has been defined by DSM-III or DSM-III-R criteria (excluding the criteria which precludes an organic factor). The second type of depression is dysthymic depression as defined by DSM-III or DSM-III-R criteria (excluding the 2-year duration criterion and the exclusionary organic factor).

The prevalence of these depressions varies, depending upon the duration of the underlying illness as well as the nature and location of the brain disorder. In a study of 103 consecutive patients admitted to hospital with acute cerebrovascular lesions, Robinson et al. (20) reported that 27% met symptom criteria for major depression, while 20% met symptom criteria for dysthymic (minor) depression (termed minor depression because the 2-year duration criteria was not met). Most other studies of patients with cerebrovascular lesions have reported similar frequencies of depression ranging from 25–50% of the population studied (21–23).

PHENOMENOLOGY

The phenomenology of poststroke depression (PSD) appears to be virtually identical to that found in patients with functional or primary mood disorders.

Lipsey et al. (24) compared the frequency and type of depressive symptoms in a group of 43 patients with poststroke major depression and a group of 43 age-comparable patients with primary major depression. Both groups showed the same frequency and types of depressive symptoms, even those symptoms that were not part of the diagnosis criteria. The only exception was that major PSD patients had a greater frequency of "slowness" than the functional depressives, and the primary depression patients had a greater frequency of loss of interest and concentration than the patients with PSD. This study demonstrated that major PSD is not an atypical form of depression and that these patients present with symptoms that appear identical to those of elderly patients with primary major depression.

LONGITUDINAL COURSE OF DEPRESSION

The longitudinal course of PSD was investigated by Robinson et al. (26), Morris et al. (27), and Astrom et al. (28). In the first study, Robinson and Price (25) found that about one-third of 103 patients examined were depressed. By 8–9 months after the initial evaluation, 67% of the patients who were depressed initially remained depressed. By the 1-year follow-up, however, none of the patients seen was depressed. In a second study (26), a consecutive series of 103 acute stroke patients were prospectively studied over a 2-year period. At the time of the initial evaluation, 26% of the patients had major depression, while 20% had symptoms of minor (dysthymic) depression. Although patients with major depression fully recovered between 1–2 years poststroke, minor depression had a less favorable prognosis, with only 30% having recovered by 2 years poststroke. In addition, about 30% of patients who were not depressed in the hospital, became depressed after discharge.

Morris et al., (27) found that among a group of 99 patients in a stroke rehabilitation hospital, those with major depression had a duration of illness of 40 weeks, whereas those with adjustment disorders (minor depression) had a duration of depression of only 12 weeks.

Astrom et al., (28) showed that the majority of patients with early-onset major depression recover by 1 year (eight of

14), but among those who were still depressed, only one of six had recovered by 3 years follow-up.

In summary, the available data suggest that PSD is not a transient but a long-standing disorder with a natural course of somewhat less than 1 year for major depression and, perhaps a more variable course for minor depression. Some major depressions, however, last more than 3 years, and some minor depressions evolve into major depression and may last for several years.

BIOLOGICAL MARKERS

The dexamethasone suppression test (DST; 29) has been investigated as a possible biological marker for functional melancholic depression. Although several studies have demonstrated that there is a statistical association between major depression and failure to suppress serum cortisol, in response to administration of dexamethasone, the specificity of the test is insufficient to allow it to be diagnostically useful (30–32).

In a study of 65 patients whose acute strokes had occurred within the preceding year, Lipsey et al., (33) found that 67% of the patients with major depression failed to suppress serum cortisol, compared to 25% of patients with minor depression, and 32% of nondepressed patients. The sensitivity of the DST for major depression was 67%, but the specificity was only 70%. False-positive tests, found in 30% of patients, seemed to be related to large lesion volumes. Similarly, Reding et al. (32) reported a sensitivity of 47% and specificity of 87%, with more extensive strokes having a greater likelihood of producing an abnormal DST response.

A recent study by Barry and Dinan (34) examined growth-hormone response to desipramine as a biological marker of PSD. They found that growth hormone responses were significantly blunted in patients with PSD, suggesting that diminished α_2-adrenergic receptor function may be an important marker for PSD. The sensitivity of the test was 100%, and the specificity was 75%. Future studies may further examine the validity of this biological marker.

RELATIONSHIP TO IMPAIRMENT IN ACTIVITIES OF DAILY LIVING

Although many clinicians have assumed that the most powerful determinant of depression after stroke was the severity of associated physical impairment, empirical studies have consistently failed to find a strong relationship between severity of depression and severity of physical impairment (20, 22, 27). This is not to say, however, that there is no relationship. Numerous studies have demonstrated that severity of physical impairment is one of several factors that contributes to depression and, in some subpopulations, may be an important contributing factor to depression (20, 22, 28, 35).

Although the effect of impairment on depression appears to be fairly weak, there is a significant influence of PSD on recovery in activities of daily living (ADL). In a recent study,

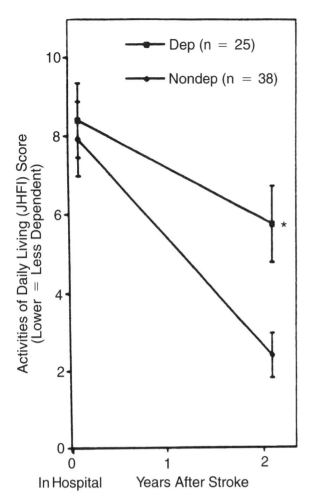

Figure 13.1. Change in ADL scores for depressed (major or minor) patients and nondepressed patients at the time of the in-hospital evaluation and 2 years later. Depressed patients show less recovery than nondepressed patients. (Reprinted with permission from Parikh RM, Robinson RG, Lipsey JR. The impact of poststroke depression on recovery in activities of daily living over a 2 year follow-up. Arch Neurol 1990; 47:787.)

Parikh et al. (36) compared 25 patients with PSD (either major or minor depression) and 38 stroke patients with no mood disorders who were matched for severity of ADL impairments in hospital. After controlling for all the variables that have been shown to influence stroke outcome such as acute treatment on a stroke unit, size, nature and location of brain injury, age, education, and duration of rehabilitation services, patients with in-hospital PSD were found to have a significantly poorer recovery than nondepressed stroke patients, even after their depression had subsided (Fig. 13.1).

RELATIONSHIP TO COGNITIVE IMPAIRMENT

A study comparing the presence of cognitive impairments in depressed and nondepressed stroke patients found that patients with major PSD after left-hemisphere lesions had significantly more cognitive deficits than nondepressed patients with a similar size and location of brain lesion (37).

These cognitive deficits were observed in a wide range of neuropsychological tasks, including orientation, language, visuoconstructional ability, executive motor functions, and frontal lobe tasks (38). In contrast, among patients with right-hemisphere lesions, patients with major depression did not differ from nondepressed patients on any of the measures of cognitive impairment.

In a recent follow-up study, Downhill and Robinson (39) found that patients with major depression had more severe intellectual impairment than nondepressed patients after 3, 6, and 12 months following stroke but only among patients with left-hemisphere lesions. The effect of depression on cognitive function was greatest during the acute poststroke period, but no effect could be demonstrated even among patients with left-hemisphere lesions and major depression at 2 years poststroke.

These findings suggest that left-hemisphere lesions (particularly left frontal and left basal ganglia) that lead to major depression may produce a different kind of depression from depression caused by comparable right-hemisphere lesions. Left-hemisphere lesions can produce a dementia of depression; this does not occur or may be less severe with major depression following right-hemisphere lesions. Although there are several reports of improved intellectual function in stroke patients treated with antidepressants, these studies are inconclusive. Double-blind controls are needed to determine whether these dementias of depression will improve with the treatment of depression (40).

RELATIONSHIP TO APHASIA

The diagnoses of depression among patients with severe comprehension deficits are very difficult, and most investigators have excluded these patients from studies of PSD. Some investigators (41) made the suggestion that a diagnosis of depression should be based upon behavioral observations (i.e., diminished sleep, food intake, restlessness and agitation, retarded or tearful behavior). However, the sensitivity and specificity of those methods for detecting depression have not yet been demonstrated.

Robinson and Benson (42), in a study of depression in patients with fluent or nonfluent aphasias, found that 53% were depressed and that those findings were similar to the frequencies of major and minor depression seen in nonaphasic patients with comparable-sized left-hemisphere lesions (43). This study also found that patients with nonfluent aphasia had a significantly higher frequency of depression than patients with fluent aphasia (42).

Perhaps the higher frequency of depression among nonfluent aphasic patients is attributable to the greater awareness related to the language impairment. But in a recent study, Starkstein and Robinson (44) concluded that the most important variable in the association between PSD and nonfluent aphasia was lesion location, suggesting that nonfluent language impairment and depression may not be casually related but may be independent outcomes of the same lesion.

RELATIONSHIP TO LESION LOCATION

Robinson et al. (43) and Starkstein et al. (45) have systematically examined the association between lesion location and PSD. They found in different series of patients with acute stroke that major or minor PSD showed a significantly higher frequency of lesions in anterior areas of the left hemisphere (i.e., 14 of 22 patients with left-anterior hemisphere injury), namely the left frontal dorsolateral cortex. They also found a relationship between PSD and specific subcortical lesions (46). Basal ganglia lesions (caudate and/or putamen) produced major depression in seven of eight patients with left-sided lesions, while only one of seven patients with right-sided lesions became depressed. None of the patients with left or right thalamic lesions showed PSD. Similar findings have also recently been reported by Astrom et al. (28). In summary, the frequency of depression appears to be higher among patients with lesions of the left anterior hemisphere (left frontal dorsolateral cortex) and left basal ganglia, than among those patients with any other lesion locations.

Among patients with right-hemisphere stroke lesions, those with frontal or parietal damage showed the highest frequency of depression (47). Similar results were reported by Finset (48), who found that patients with lesions in the right parietal white matter had a higher frequency of depression than patients with lesions involving other locations in the right hemisphere.

Perhaps the most consistent finding in PSD has been the association of depressive symptoms with intrahemispheric lesion location. In 1981 Robinson and Szetela (49) first reported that, in a group of 29 patients with left-hemisphere lesions produced by trauma or stroke, there was an inverse correlation between severity of depression and distance of the anterior border of the lesion from the frontal pole

($r = .76$, p < .001)(Fig. 13.2). Since then, using CT scan imaging, Robinson et al. (43) reported the same phenomenon in another group of 10 patients with single stroke lesions of the left-anterior hemisphere ($r = -.92$, p < .001). When patients with left-posterior lesions were added (n = 18), the correlation decreased to $r = -.54$, p < .05. This phenomenon was also found in other groups of patients with purely cortical lesions of the left hemisphere (n = 16) ($r = -.52$, p < 0.5) (45), purely left subcortical lesions (n = 13) ($r = -.68$, p < .01) (45), single left-hemisphere lesions among left-handed patients (n = 13) ($r = -.78$, p < .01) (50). This phenomenon has now been replicated by four different groups of investigators using patients from Canada (21, 22), England (51) and Australia (52). Some of these investigators found a correlation between severity of depression and proximity of the lesion to the frontal pole in combined right- and left-hemisphere lesion groups (21, 51), while others found it only with left-sided lesions (22, 52). Longitudinal studies have found that proximity of the lesion to the frontal pole is significantly associated with severity of depression most strongly during the first 6 months poststroke, suggesting that this phenomenon is a dynamic one that changes over time (28, 53).

Although there is some difference in the strength of this correlation (and therefore the amount of variance in severity of depression explained by lesion location), this phenomenon has emerged as one of the most consistent and robust clinical-pathological correlations ever described in neuropsychiatry.

In summary, several studies conducted by different investigators support the hypothesis that depressive disorders after stroke are more severe if the lesion is closer to the frontal pole and that left-anterior hemisphere lesions are the most likely lesions to show this relationship.

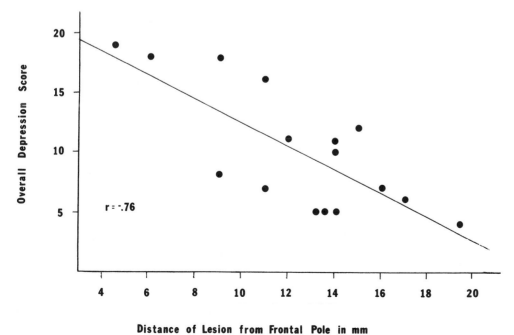

Figure 13.2. Relationship between severity of depression and proximity of the CT scan visualized lesion to the frontal pole for patients with stroke or TBI involving the left hemisphere. Lesions whose anterior border was closer to the frontal pole were associated with more depressive symptoms. (Reprinted with permission from Robinson RG, Szetela B. Mood change following left hemisphere brain injury. Ann Neurol 1981; 9:450.)

Figure 13.3. The area of the lateral and third ventricle on C.T. scans of 13 pairs of patients with or without depression who were paired for having the same size and location of stroke lesion. Patients with major depression had significantly larger ventricles, indicating mild subcortical atrophy.

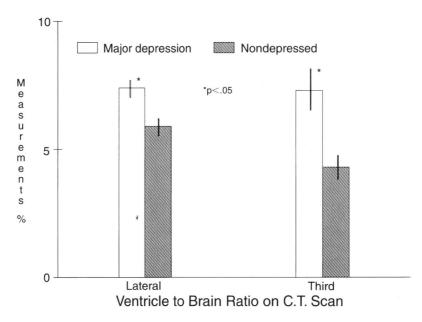

RELATIONSHIP TO VASCULAR TERRITORY OF STROKE

Starkstein et al. (54) reported that patients with middle cerebral artery (MCA) lesions showed a higher incidence and longer course of PSD when compared to those with posterior circulation (PC) lesions (i.e. temporo-occipital and cerebellar/brainstem region). Major or minor depression occurred in 48% of the patients in the MCA and in 35% of patients in the PC group. At 6-month follow-up, frequencies of depression among the patients with in-hospital depression were 82% and 20% respectively. At follow-up 1 to 2 years poststroke, frequencies of depression were 68% and 0% respectively.

This finding suggests that the mechanism of depression after MCA infarcts may differ from posterior lesions. It has been suggested that the shorter duration may be related to the smaller size and to the possibility that cerebellar/brainstem lesions produce less injury to the biogenic amine pathways than middle cerebral artery distribution lesions.

RISK FACTORS FOR DEPRESSION FOLLOWING STROKE

Although a significant number of patients with left-anterior hemisphere or right-posterior hemisphere lesions develop PSD, not every patient with a lesion in these locations develops a depressive mood. That raises the question of why clinical variability occurs and why some but not all patients with lesions in these locations develop depression. Starkstein et al. (55) examined these questions by comparing 13 patients with major PSD to 13 stroke patients without depression, who had lesions of the same size and location. The groups did not differ on important demographic variables, such as age, sex, socioeconomic status, or education. They also did not differ on family or personal history of psychiatric disorders or neurological

deficits. Patients with major PSD, however, had significantly more subcortical atrophy as measured by the ratio of third ventricle to brain (i.e., the area of the third ventricle divided by the area of the brain at the same level), and the ratio of lateral ventricle to brain (i.e., the area of the lateral ventricle contralateral to brain lesion divided by the brain area at the same level) (p < .05) (Fig. 13.3). Because most patients' CT scans were obtained immediately after the stroke, it is likely that the subcortical atrophy preceded the stroke. Thus, a mild degree of subcortical atrophy may be a premorbid risk factor that increases the risk of developing major depression following stroke.

Starkstein et al. (47) also found that patients who develop PSD after a right-hemisphere lesion had a significantly higher frequency of family history of psychiatric disorders than nondepressed patients with right-hemisphere or left-hemisphere lesions. This suggests that a genetic predisposition for depression may play a role in the development of major depression after right-hemisphere lesions.

In summary, lesion location is not the only factor that influences the development of PSD. Subcortical atrophy that probably precedes the stroke and a family or personal history of affective disorders also seem to play an important role in determining whether patients develop depression after stroke.

MECHANISM OF DEPRESSION FOLLOWING STROKE

Although the cause of PSD is not known, it has been hypothesized that disruption of the amine pathways by the stroke lesion may play an etiological role (43). The noradrenergic and serotonergic cell bodies are located in the brainstem and send ascending projections through the median forebrain bundle to the frontal cortex. The ascending axonsi then arc posteriorly and run longitudinally through the deep layers of the cortex, arborizing and sending terminal projections into the superficial cortical layers (56). Lesions that disrupt these pathways in the frontal cortex or the basal ganglia may affect many downstream fibers. Based on these neuroanatomical facts and the clinical findings that the severity of depression correlates with the proximity of the lesion to the frontal pole, Robinson et al., (43) suggested that PSD may be the consequence of severe depletion of norepinephrine and/or serotonin produced by frontal or basal ganglia lesions.

Supporting this hypothesis, some investigations have shown (in rats) that biogenic amines are depleted in response to ischemic lesions. This biochemical response to ischemia is also lateralized. Right-hemisphere lesions produce depletions of norepinephrine and an accompanying behavior change of locomotor hyperactivity, while lesions of the left hemisphere do not (57). Mayberg et al. (58), also reported that patients with stroke lesions in the right hemisphere had significantly higher ratios of ipsilateral-to-contralateral spiperone binding (predominantly 5-HT$_2$ [serotonin] receptor binding) in noninjured temporal and parietal cortex than patients with comparable left-hemisphere strokes (p < .05). Patients with left-hemisphere lesions showed a significant inverse correlation between the amount of spiperone binding in the left temporal cortex and depression scores (i.e., higher depression scores were associated with lower serotonin receptor binding—p < .05).

Thus, a greater depletion of biogenic amines in patients with right-hemisphere lesions as compared to those with left-hemisphere lesions could lead to a compensatory up-regulation of receptors that might protect against depression. On the other hand, patients with left-hemisphere lesions may have moderate depletions of biogenic amines but without a compensatory up-regulation of 5-HT receptors and, therefore, a dysfunction of biogenic amine systems in the left hemisphere. This dysfunction ultimately may lead to the clinical manifestations of depression.

Another possibility is that both the frontal dorsal lateral cortex and the dorsal caudate play an important role in mediating motor, intellectual, and instinctive behavior through their connection with the supplementary motor area, temporoparietal association cortex, and limbic system. A lesion of these anterior brain areas may result in low activation of motor, sensory, or limbic areas, and produce the autonomic and affective symptoms of depression.

TREATMENT OF DEPRESSION FOLLOWING STROKE

Although there have been relatively few studies that have examined the effectiveness of the treatment of depression among patients with brain disease, two randomized double-blind studies of the efficacy of antidepressant treatment have been published. Lipsey et al., (24) examined 14 patients treated with nortriptyline and 20 patients given placebo. Patients received 25 mg for 1 week, 50 mg for 2 weeks, 75 mg for 1 week, and 100 mg for 2 weeks. The group on the active drug (11 completed the study) showed a significant decrease in depression scores compared to the placebo group (15 completed) (Fig. 13.4). Side effects were observed in six of 17 patients: three developed delirium, one had syncope, one complained of oversedation, and one complained of dizziness. Patients receiving nortriptyline showed a significantly greater improvement in depression, as measured by the Hamilton Depression Rating Scale and the Zung Self-Rating Depression Scale. Active and placebo groups, however, did not differ significantly in their mean Hamilton Depression Scores until weeks 4 and 6 of treatment.

The other controlled study, that which demonstrated the usefulness of another antidepressant drug (trazodone) for PSD, was carried out by Reding et al. (59). In this study 27 patients participating in a stroke rehabilitation program

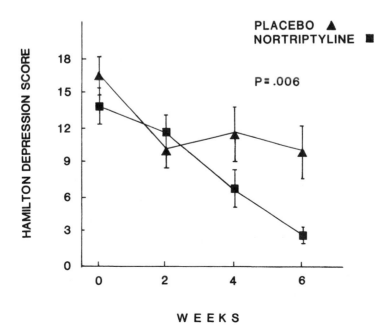

Figure 13.4. Hamilton depression scores during a 6-week double-blind treatment trial of nortriptyline vs. placebo for patients with depression (major or minor) following stroke. Patients receiving active treatment showed significantly greater improvement than those receiving placebo. (Reprinted with permission from Lipsey JR, Robinson RG, Pearlson GD. Nortriptyline treatment for poststroke depression: a double blind trial. Lancet 1984; 1:299.)

were randomly assigned to treatment. Depressed patients taking trazodone were found to have greater improvements in ADL scores than patients treated with placebo. This trend became statistically significant when the treatment groups were restricted to patients with abnormal dexamethasone tests. Although antidepressants are effective in the treatment of PSD, the high rate of complications—such as delirium—dictate that tricyclic drugs should be used cautiously in elderly patients. (See Chapter 11 for more information on drug therapy.)

In summary, although additional controlled treatment trials using a variety of antidepressant medications need to be conducted, current data support the efficacy of antidepressant medication in the treatment of PSD. In the future, the development of clinical techniques or laboratory markers highly specific to major depression may add to our ability to recognize and treat affective disorders among stroke patients whose mental status is difficult to determine.

Depression Associated with Parkinson's Disease

As with stroke, depression is a frequent finding in patients with PD. Although the frequent association of emotional disorders with PD was recognized more than 50 years ago (60), it has only been within the past several years that investigators have begun to empirically examine the nature of the relationship. Some investigators have suggested that the high frequency of depression in PD is the understandable consequence of progressive physical impairment (61). Other investigators, however, have not found a significant correlation between the severity of depression and the severity of the physical impairment, and have suggested that depression may be a consequence of neurochemical changes in specific brain areas (62, 63).

PREVALENCE

In several studies, the frequency of depression was reported to be around 40% (62, 64, 65). In a recent prospective study of a consecutive series of 105 patients, Starkstein et al. (66) found that 21% met DSM-III criteria for major depression, while 20% met DSM-III criteria for dysthymic (minor) depression. The highest frequency of depression was found in the early and the late stages of PD (Fig. 13.5).

RELATIONSHIP TO COGNITIVE IMPAIRMENT

In PD, cognitive impairments may range from subtle deficits in frontal lobe-related tasks to an overt dementia (67). Mayeux et al. (68), using a modified Mini-Mental State Examination (MMSE) reported a significant correlation between cognitive deficits and severity of depression (i.e., severe depression was associated with severe cognitive impairments). This relationship was also reported by Starkstein et al. in three studies. In the first study, the association between depression, cognitive impairments, and stage of PD was examined (69). Patients in the late stages showed significantly greater overall cognitive impairments than patients in the early stages; and those impairments were restricted to tasks involving motor-related functions (Fig. 13.6). Depressed patients in the late stages of the disease showed the most significant impairment (70). Taken together, these findings suggest that cognitive deficits may primarily be a result of motor impairments; but when depression also occurs, the cognitive deficits are greater and increase in severity as the PD progresses (69). In the second study, the association between cognitive impairments and type or severity of depression (major or minor) among patients with PD was examined. No differences were found

Figure 13.5. The percentage of patients (total of 105 patients) at each stage of Parkinson's disease (PD) who were depressed. All patients were attending an outpatient care clinic and ranged in duration of disease from a few months to more than 15 years. The relative frequency of depression was higher in both the early and late stages of the illness compared with the middle stages.

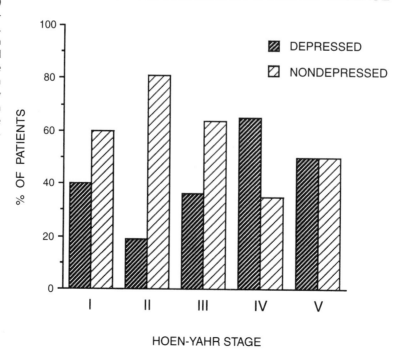

FREQUENCY OF DEPRESSION BY STAGE OF DISEASE

DEPRESSED
NONDEPRESSED

% OF PATIENTS

HOEN-YAHR STAGE

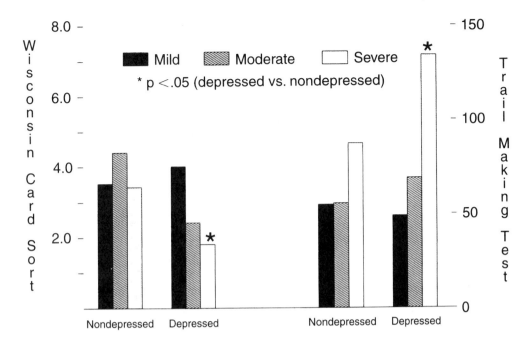

Figure 13.6. Cognitive performance as measured by the number of correctly selected categories in the Wisconsin Card Sorting Task and seconds to complete the Trail Making Test in Parkinson's disease patients with and without depression. Depressed patients were significantly (p < .05) more impaired than nondepressed patients during the moderate and severe stages of PD. Among the depressed patients, performance on these "frontal lobe" tasks, declined with advancing stages of PD.

on cognitive tasks between minor and nondepressed patients, but patients with major depression showed the worst cognitive performance. This impairment was greatest on frontal lobe-related tasks, such as the Wisconsin Card Sorting test (70). In the third study, the influence of depression upon the longitudinal evolution of cognitive deficits was examined in a 3-4-year follow-up. Both groups—depressed and nondepressed patients—showed significant declines in MMSE scores over time, but depressed patients had significantly greater cognitive decline than nondepressed subjects (66).

These findings demonstrate that depression may not only be associated with cognitive impairments at the time depression is present, but may also be associated with more rapid cognitive deterioration. These findings support Sano et al.'s (71) speculation that depression may be an early finding in patients with PD who later show dementia (Chapter 34).

MECHANISM

Several studies have demonstrated that patients with PD and dementia may show senile plaques and neurofibrillary tangles compatible with the diagnosis of Alzheimer's disease (AD) as well as severe depletion of cholinergic neurons in the nucleus basalis of Meynert or Lewy bodies in cortical regions (72). Few neuropathological studies, however, have been carried out in patients with PD and depression. Torack and Morris (73) have recently reported a marked loss of pigmented neurons in the ventral tegmental area (VTA) in a small group of patients with PD, dementia, and depression. The VTA contains cell bodies of dopaminergic neurons that provide most of the dopaminergic innervation to the prefrontal cortex, nucleus accumbens, and amygdala. Thus, dysfunction of the mesocorticolimbic dopaminergic system may play an important role in the production of deficits in

"frontal-lobe" tasks among patients with PD and major depression.

Depression in PD may also be related to changes in other biogenic amines. Mayeux et al.(62) showed that patients with PD and depression had significantly lower 5-HIAA (a metabolite of serotonin) levels in the CSF than patients with PD without depression. However, patients with PD and both dementia and depression had the lowest 5-HIAA CFS values (71).

In a recent study, the metabolic abnormalities associated with depression in PD were examined using neuroimaging techniques (74). Regional cerebral glucose metabolism was determined in depressed (n = 5) and nondepressed (n = 4) patients with PD using [^{18}F]-fluoro-1-deoxy-D-glucose (FDG) positron emission tomography (PET). Patients with PD and major depression had significantly lower metabolic activity in the head of the caudate and the inferior frontal cortex than nondepressed PD patients of comparable age, duration, and stage of illness. Moreover, there was a significant correlation between Hamilton Depression Scale scores and the relative regional metabolism in the inferior frontal cortex ($r = 0.73, p < .05$ (i.e., the lower the relative regional metabolic activity in the inferior frontal cortex, the more severe the depression).

How can these findings be reconciled with the finding of cortical serotonergic and dopaminergic dysfunction in depressed patients with PD? In a recent article, Mayberg et al.(74) proposed a tentative hypothesis. While dopaminergic projections from the ventral tegmental area show regional specificity for the orbitofrontal cortex (75), the serotonergic projections are more diffusely distributed (76). On the other hand, the major cortical outflow back to the mesencephalon originates in the orbitofrontal cortex (77). Thus, degeneration of the mesocorticolimbic dopaminergic systems in patients with PD may lead to dysfunction of the orbitofrontal cortex, which may secondarily affect cell bodies in the dorsal raphe. This combination of dopamine (DA) and serotonergic deficits may account for the presence of cognitive impairments and depression in patients with PD.

TREATMENT

A question that remains unanswered is whether the treatment of depression may influence the progression of intellectual impairments in patients with PD. In the longitudinal 3–4-year follow-up study (66), six patients in the depressed group who had received treatment for depression had only an 11% decrease in cognitive scores compared to a 23% decrement in cognitive scores among nontreated depressed patients. Moreover, the two patients who were receiving the highest doses of tricyclics did not show decline in their MMSE scores. These preliminary findings are very encouraging, and further prospective double-blind treatment studies are needed to determine whether the use of antidepressants may delay the progression of cognitive impairment in patients with PD.

Depression Associated with Traumatic Brain Injury

Traumatic brain injury (TBI) has an annual incidence of 2 million cases and represents the most common cause of brain injury and the most common cause of death in people under age 45 in the U.S. (78). Although there is an extensive literature on the neurobehavioral consequences of head injury, very few studies have examined the frequency or course of mood disorders that occur following TBI.

PREVALENCE

Most of the studies of emotional or depressive symptoms among patients with TBI have relied on rating scales or relatives' reports rather than on structured interviews and established diagnostic criteria (e.g., DSM-III-R). Perhaps as a result the frequency of depression has varied from one study to the next. For example, Rutherford and colleagues (79) found that 6% of 145 patients with minor head injury had a significant number of depressive symptoms within 6 weeks after injury. On the other hand, McKinlay and others (80) reported indirect evidence of a depressed mood in about 50% of their patients at 3, 6, or 12 months following severe head injury. Kinsella and others (81), reported that in a series of 39 patients, 33% were classified as depressed and 26% as suffering from anxiety within 2 years of severe head injury.

In recent studies by Fedoroff et al. (82) and Jorge et al. (83), 28 of 66 patients (42%) admitted to a head trauma unit developed major depression at some point during a 1-year follow-up. Of 66 patients admitted to the hospital with acute closed head injury without significant spinal cord or other organ system injury, 17 (26%) met diagnostic criteria for major depression at the time of the initial in-hospital evaluation. In addition, 3% met criteria for minor (dysthymic) depressive disorder. This frequency is consistent with

the finding of several other investigators (84, 85). These data suggest that major depression constitutes a significant psychiatric complication in this population.

LONGITUDINAL COURSE OF DEPRESSION

Mood disorders following TBI may be transient syndromes lasting for a few weeks, or they may be persistent disorders lasting for many months (86). Other authors have suggested that transient disorders may be the result of neurochemical changes provoked by brain injury while prolonged depressive disorders, on the other hand, may be of a more complex nature and may be reactive to physical or

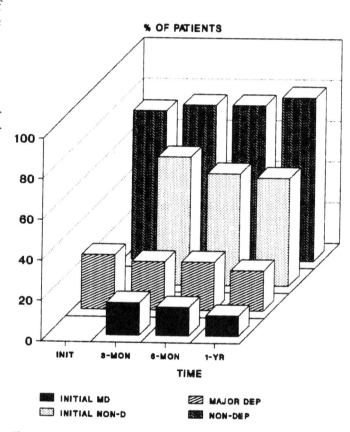

Figure 13.7. The percentage of patients who had major depression or were nondepressed during the 1-year longitudinal study are shown by columns. The column indicating initial in-hospital evaluation shows the percent of depressed and nondepressed patients. The columns for 3-month, 6-month, and 1-year follow-up indicate in Row 1 the percent of patients who remained depressed from the group of patients (n = 17) with major depression during the acute hospitalization. Row 2 indicates the total number of patients with major depression at that exact point (i.e., unresolved cases plus new-onset cases). Row 3 indicates the percent of patients who were never depressed, and Row 4 indicates the total nondepressed patients at that point. Note that the number of persistent initial major depressions declines over time, with a more gradual decline in the total major depressions, indicating fewer overall depressions but a significant number of delayed-onset cases. (Reprinted with permission from Jorge RE, Robinson RG, Arndt SV, Forrester AW, Geisler F, Starkstein SE. Depression and traumatic brain injury: a longitudinal study. J Affect Disord 1993a; 27:236.)

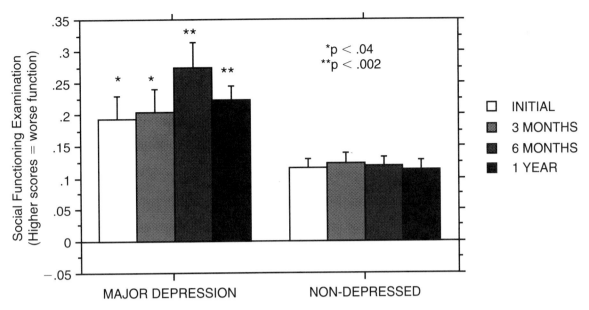

Figure 13.8. Social functioning exam (SFE) scores for patients with major depression or nondepressed during 1 year following traumatic brain injury (TBI). The SFE scores reflect function during the month prior to evaluation. Therefore, the initial score indicates social functioning prior to TBI. Both before and after head injury, patients with depression had significantly more impaired social functioning than nondepressed patients. This probably reflects both the effect of depression on social functioning and vice versa.

cognitive impairment (87–89). Empirical data supporting these suggestions have recently been reported by Jorge et al. (83). Diagnoses of depression were based on a semistructured psychiatric interview (90) and DSM-III-R criteria for major or minor (dysthymic) depression (91). Of the original 66 patients evaluated with acute TBI, 54 were reevaluated at 3 months, 43 at 6 months, and 43 at 1 year. The prevalence of depression was 30% at 3 months, 26% at 6 months, and 26% at 1 year (92) (Fig. 13.7). The mean duration of major depression was 4.7 months. There were, however, a group of seven patients (41% of the depressed group) who had transient depressions lasting 1.5 months, while the nine remaining depressed patients had a mean duration of 7 months. The patients with transient depressions showed a strong association with left-anterior lesion location (Fischer exact p = .006). Prolonged depressions, on the other hand, were associated with impaired social functioning, suggesting that biological factors may lead to transient depression, while prolonged depressions may result from psychological factors.

Risk Factors for Depression Following Traumatic Brain Injury

Several premorbid factors may influence patients' emotional responses to acute traumatic brain injury and may therefore be relevant to the etiology of depressive disorders following TBI (93). In the study of 66 patients with acute TBI, there was significantly greater frequency of previous personal history of psychiatric disorder in the major depressed group compared with the nondepressed patients (82). In addition, this group had significantly more impaired social functioning as measured by the Social Functioning

Examination (SFE) (94) (Fig. 13.8). The SFE, during the initial evaluation, measured the quality and personal satisfaction with social functioning during the period prior to brain injury. This suggests, as other investigators have reported, that patients with poor social adjustment and social dissatisfaction prior to the brain injury were more prone to develop depression.

RELATIONSHIP TO LESION LOCATION

There is some empirical evidence supporting an association between post-TBI depression and specific lesion locations. Lishman (95) reported that several years after penetrating brain injury, depressive symptoms were more common among patients with right-hemisphere lesions. Depressive symptoms were also more frequent among patients with frontal and parietal lesions compared with other lesion locations. Grafman et al. (96) also reported that several years following head injury, depressive symptoms were more frequently associated with penetrating injuries involving the right-hemisphere (right-orbitofrontal) lesions than any other lesion location.

TBI is characterized by the presence of diffuse and focal lesions that may be the direct result of traumatic shear injury or secondary to ischemic complications (97).

Of the 66 patients previously described, 42 (64%) had a diffuse pattern of brain injury on their CT scans, and 24 (36%) presented with focal lesions. There were no significant differences between major depressed and nondepressed groups in the frequency of diffuse or focal patterns of injury. In addition, no significant differences were found in the frequency of extraparenchymal hemorrhages, contusions, intracerebral or intraventricular hemorrhages, hydrocephalus, or CT findings suggestive of brain atrophy. There was, however, a significant association between lesion location and the development of major depression. The presence of left-anterior hemisphere lesions (i.e., left dorsolateral frontal cortex or left basal ganglia) was the strongest correlate of major depression (Fig. 13.9). On the other hand, other frontal lesions (i.e., left, right or bilateral frontal lesions (i.e., left, right or bilateral frontal lesions, including orbitofrontal cortex) were associated with a lesser probability of developing major depression (82).

These results are consistent with previous findings in stroke patients of an increased frequency of depression among patients with left dorsolateral cortical and left basal ganglia lesions (45). These findings are also consistent with a previous study in which patients with anterior left-hemisphere lesions were found to have more severe depressive symptoms than patients with left-posterior-hemisphere lesions in both stroke and TBI (42). However, the analysis of the data revealed that this relationship is not intact after the initial in-hospital evaluation. This finding contrasts with stroke patients, where the association between lesion location and major depression is not lost until after 6 months follow-up (53). This difference between stroke and TBI

depressions may be the result of differences in the nature of the brain injury with TBI, leading to reorganization (e.g., pruning, reactive synaptogenesis, regenerative sprouting) (98, 99) and perhaps clinical recovery from depression.

In conclusion, some acute-onset depressions appear to be related to lesion characteristics and may have their etiology in biological responses such as neurochemical changes. Left dorsolateral frontal and left basal ganglia lesions are strongly associated with major depression during the initial in-hospital evaluation and may represent a strategic lesion location that elicits biochemical responses that finally lead to depression. In addition, however, other major correlates of depression were previous history of psychiatric disorder and impaired social functioning, suggesting psychosocial factors in the mechanism of some post-TBI depressions.

RELATIONSHIP TO IMPAIRMENT VARIABLES

Empirical studies have reported conflicting findings with regard to the relationship between impairment and depressive symptoms following TBI (100, 101). In the previously described study of 66 patients with TBI, there was no significant association between depression and severity of intellectual impairment (i.e., MMSE exam score) or ADL (82). Social functioning, however, was the clinical variable that had the most consistent relationship with depression throughout the whole follow-up period (83). Although it is likely that lack of social support contributed to the development of depression, the existence of depression may have negatively influenced social functioning. This suggestion is supported by the finding that depression scores correlated with SFE only at the onset of depression and not with the initial SFE scores (92). One might infer from these findings that social intervention as well as the treatment of depression may be necessary to alleviate these severe and long-lasting mood disorders.

TREATMENT OF TRAUMATIC BRAIN INJURY DEPRESSION

There have been no double-blind, placebo-controlled studies of the efficacy of pharmacological treatments of depression in TBI patients.

The selection of antidepressant drugs for the treatment of post-TBI depression is usually guided by their side effect profiles. Mild anticholinergic activity, minimal lowering of seizure threshold, and low sedative effect are the most important factors to be considered in the choice of an antidepressant drug in this population (102) (See Chapter 11).

Tricyclic antidepressants have important anticholinergic effects that may interfere with cognitive and memory functions. In addition, they may lower the seizure threshold. Fluoxetine, a serotonin reuptake inhibitor, is an antidepressant that appears to have a less adverse side-effect profile (103). Initial dosing should be 20 mg/day given as a single morning dose. The dose may be increased up to 80 mg/day given on a twice-a-day schedule. The most common side effects include headache, gastrointestinal complaints, and insomnia.

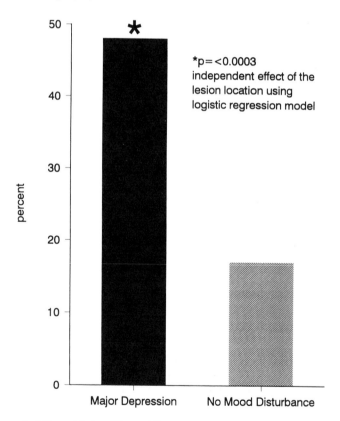

*p= <0.0003 independent effect of the lesion location using logistic regression model

Left Dorsal Lateral Frontal Cortex or Basal Ganglia Lesions

Figure 13.9. The proportion of patients with major depression or no mood disturbance at 1 month following traumatic brain injury (TBI) who had evidence on CT scan of injury involving the left dorsal lateral frontal cortex and/or left basal ganglia. Because patients with TBI frequently have multiple areas of injury, a logistic regression analysis was used to examine the independent effects of each area of injury. The strongest independent effect of lesions on depression was found in this left anterior brain region.

Trazodone is an alternative antidepressant that also inhibits serotonin reuptake. Treatment is started at low doses (50–100 mg) at bedtime following a snack. The dose may be gradually increased every 3–4 days up to 400 mg. The most troublesome side effects are sedation and orthostatic hypotension (104).

There are case reports of successful treatments of post-TBI depression with psychostimulants (105). These include dextroamphetamine (8–60 mg/day), methylphenidate (10–60 mg/day), and pemoline (56–75 mg/day). They are given twice a day with the last dose at least 6 hours before sleep, to prevent initial insomnia. Treatment is begun at lower doses, which are then gradually increased. Patients taking stimulants need close medical monitoring to prevent abuse or toxic effects. The most common side effects are anxiety, dysphoria, headaches, irritability, anorexia, insomnia, cardiovascular symptoms, dyskinesias, or even psychotic symptoms (104).

Buspirone, a drug that has an agonist effect on $5HT_{1a}$ receptors and an antagonist effect on D_2-dopaminergic receptors, has proved to be a safe and efficacious anxiolytic. Initial dosing is 15 mg/day given in three divided doses, and it may gradually be increased (5 mg every 4 days) up to 60 mg/day. The most common side effects are dizziness and headaches (104, 106).

Electroconvulsive therapy (ECT) is not contraindicated in TBI patients and may be considered if other methods of treatment prove to be unsuccessful.

Finally, the role of social interventions and adequate psychotherapeutic support may be included in the treatment of depression. Psychological and pharmacological treatments, however, need to be examined in controlled treatment trials.

MANIA

Mania Associated with Stroke

Mania is a relatively rare consequence of acute stroke lesions. Although prevalence studies have not yet been conducted, Robinson et al. (107) reported that less than 1% of patients with acute stroke have mania. Most of the patients included in studies of mania following stroke present with manic symptoms and are only secondarily found to have brain injury. These patients, however, have typical manic syndromes and their symptoms are not significantly different from patients with mania who do not have brain injury (108).

RELATIONSHIP TO LESION LOCATION

In a series of 17 patients with post-brain-injury mania, Robinson et al. (107) reported a significantly increased frequency of right-hemisphere lesions compared with 31 depressed patients and 28 nonmood-disordered controls. These lesions involved the basal and polar areas of the right temporal lobe as well as subcortical areas of the right hemisphere, such as the head of the caudate and right

thalamus. In another recent study using PET with 18-fluorodeoxyglucose, metabolic abnormalities were examined in three patients with mania following right basal ganglia strokes (109). These patients were found to have focal hypometabolic deficits in the right basotemporal cortex. This finding suggests that lesions that lead to secondary mania may do so through their distant effects on the right basotemporal cortex. This phenomenon, called diaschisis (i.e., lesions producing distant effects), is a well-recognized consequence of some brain lesions.

RISK FACTORS FOR MANIA FOLLOWING STROKE

Because not every patient with a right orbitofrontal or basotemporal lesions develops a manic syndrome, the question arises as to whether there are potential predisposing factors for secondary mania (107, 108). Patients with secondary mania were found to have a significantly higher frequency of familial history of psychiatric disorders, as well as significantly more subcortical brain atrophy (as determined by increased ventricular to brain ratios) than patients with similar brain lesions but without mania. Interestingly, patients without a genetic predisposition had significantly more subcortical atrophy than secondary manics with a genetic burden, suggesting that subcortical atrophy and genetic predisposition may be independent risk factors for mania following brain injury (108).

MECHANISM

To postulate a mechanism for secondary mania, two clinical-pathological correlations need to be explained with regard to the studies. First, most lesions associated with secondary mania involved—directly or indirectly—limbic or limbic-related area of the brain. Second, virtually all of these lesions were localized to the right hemisphere.

Several studies have demonstrated that the amygdala (located in the limbic portion of the temporal lobe) plays an important role in the production of instinctive reactions and the association between stimulus and emotional response (110). The amygdala receives its main afferents from the basal diencephalon (which in turn receives psychosensory and psychomotor information from the reticular formation), and the temporopolar and basolateral cortices (which receives main afferents from heteromodal association areas) (111, 112). The basotemporal cortex receives afferents from association cortical areas and the orbitofrontal cortex, and it sends efferent projections to the entorhinal cortex, hippocampus, and amygdala. By virtue of these connections, the basotemporal cortex may represent a cortical link between sensory afferents and instinctive reactions (113).

The orbitofrontal cortex may be subdivided into two regions: a posterior one, which is restricted to the limbic functions and should be considered part of the limbic system; and an anterior one, which exerts a tonic inhibitory control over the amygdala by means of its connection through the uncinate fasciculus with the basotemporal cortex (77). Lesions or dysfunction of these areas may result in motor disinhibition (e.g., hyperactivity, pressured speech), intellectual disinhibition (e.g., flight of ideas, grandiose delusions), and instinctive disinhibition (e.g., hyperphagia and hypersexuality).

The second finding that needs to be incorporated into an explanation of mania following stroke is that it almost always occurs following right-hemisphere lesions. Laboratory studies of the neurochemical and behavioral effects of brain lesions in rats found that small suction lesions in the right (but not the left) frontal cortex of rats produced a significant increase in locomotor activity (57). Similar abnormal behavior was also found after electrolytic lesions of the right (but not left) nucleus accumbens (which is considered part of the ventral striatum) (114). Moreover, right frontocortical suction lesions also produced a significant increment in dopaminergic turnover in the nucleus accumbens that was not seen with left-hemisphere lesions (37). Thus, it is possible that in the presence of predisposing factors such as a genetic burden or subcortical atrophy, significant increments in biogenic amine turnover in the nucleus accumbens produced by specific right-hemisphere lesions may be part of the mechanism that results in manic syndrome.

A case report (115) suggested that the mechanism of secondary mania is not related to the release of transcallosal inhibitory fibers (i.e., the release of left limbic areas from tonic inhibition due to a right-hemisphere lesion). A patient who developed secondary mania after bleeding from a right basotemporal arteriovenous malformation underwent a Wada test before the therapeutic embolization of the malformation. Amytal injection in the left carotid artery did not abolish the manic symptoms (which would be the expected finding if the "release" theory were correct).

In conclusion, secondary mania is a rare complication of stroke lesions. Three risk factors for mania following stroke have been identified: *(a)* a genetic burden for psychiatric disorders (107), *(b)* increased subcortical atrophy (108), and *(c)* seizure disorder (116). Most patients with secondary mania have right-hemisphere lesions, which involve the orbitofrontal and/or basotemporal cortex, or subcortical structures such as the thalamus or head of the caudate. Secondary mania may result from disinhibition of dorsal cortical and limbic areas and/or dysfunction of asymmetric biogenic amine pathways.

TREATMENT

Although no systematic treatment studies of secondary mania have been conducted, one recent report suggests several potentially useful treatment modalities. Bakchine et al. (117) carried out a double-blind, placebo-controlled treatment study in a single patient with secondary mania. Clonidine (600 mg/day) rapidly reversed the manic symptoms, whereas carbamazepine (1200 mg/day) was associated with no mood changes, and levodopa (375 mg/day) was associated with an increase in manic symptoms. Other treatment modalities, such as antiepileptic drugs (valproate

and carbamazepine), neuroleptics, and lithium, have been reported to be useful in treating secondary mania (107). None of these treatments has been evaluated in double-blind, placebo-controlled studies (Chapter 11).

Mania Associated with Traumatic Brain Injury

PREVALENCE

Mania is more frequent among patients with TBI than among patients with stroke lesions (107, 116, 118). In the previously described study of 66 patients with acute TBI, six cases (9%) with secondary mania were found (118). One of these patients (17%) presented a bipolar course. The manic episodes, however, were short-lived, with a mean duration of 2 months. The mean duration of the elevated mood (without meeting other diagnostic criteria for mania), however, was 5.7 months. In addition, three of the six secondary manic patients developed brief episodes of violent behavior at some point during the 1-year follow-up. Aggressive behavior was significantly more frequent in the secondary mania group than among those who did not experience an affective disorder. Although at the time of the diagnosis, three patients were receiving drug treatment (two patients received lorazepam and 1 patient haloperidol), the duration of mania did not appear to be significantly different from those who were not treated.

RELATIONSHIP TO IMPAIRMENT VARIABLES

In the previously described study of 66 patients with mania following TBI, the severity of mania was not associated with severity of brain injury, degree of physical or cognitive impairment, personal or family history of psychiatric disorder, or the availability of social support or quality of social functioning (118). Thus, although further studies of the relationships between impairment or risk factors and the development of mania need to be conducted, the present data suggest that mania is not a response to the associated impairments.

RELATIONSHIP TO LESION LOCATION

The cortical areas most frequently affected by closed head injury are the ventral aspects of frontal and temporal lobes. There is also evidence that damage to subcortical, diencephalic, and brainstem structures are involved (119).

The Jorge et al. (118) study of secondary manic syndromes found that the major correlate of mania was the presence of anterior temporal lesions. This finding is consistent with the finding in patients with stroke that mania is associated with right basotemporal lesions. The trauma study did not have sufficient numbers of patients with unilateral lesions to examine the right- vs. left-hemisphere effect. Factors such as personal history of mood disorders or posttraumatic epilepsy did not appear to significantly influence the frequency of secondary mania in this group of patients.

MECHANISM

It has been suggested that the development of abnormal electrical activation patterns in limbic networks, functional changes in aminergic inhibitory systems, and the presence of aberrant regeneration pathways, may play an important role in the genesis of these syndromes (120, 121).

BIPOLAR DISORDER

Bipolar Disorder Associated with Stroke or Trauma

Starkstein et al. (122), studied 19 patients with the diagnosis of secondary mania, in an effort to determine which factors played a role in the development of bipolar or unipolar affective disorder.

The bipolar (manic-depressive) group consisted of seven patients who, after the brain lesion, met the DSM-III-R criteria for organic mood syndrome, mania, followed or preceded by organic mood syndrome, depression. The unipolar mania (mania only) consisted of 12 patients who met the criteria for mania just described not followed or preceded by depression. All the patients had CT scan evidence of vascular, neoplastic, or traumatic brain lesion and no history of other neurological, toxic, or metabolic conditions.

There were no significant between group differences in age, sex, race, education, handedness, or personal history of psychiatric disease. Also, no significant differences were found on neurological examination. On psychiatric examination, which was carried out during the index manic episode, no significant differences were observed in the type or frequency of manic symptoms. The bipolar group, however, showed significantly greater intellectual impairment as measured by MMSE scores (p < .05).

Patients with bipolar disorder had lesions restricted to the right hemisphere, which involved the head of the caudate or thalamus. One patient developed a bipolar illness after surgical removal of a pituitary adenoma. In contrast to these subcortical lesions, the unipolar mania group had lesions involving the right basotemporal and orbitofrontal cortex.

This suggests that patients with bipolar disorder tend to have subcortical lesions (mainly involving the right head of the caudate or right thalamus), while patients with pure mania tend to show a higher frequency of cortical lesions, particularly in the right orbitofrontal and right basotemporal cortex.

The question that now arises is why subcortical lesions might produce a bipolar disease? The causes of both bipolar and unipolar mood disorder remain unknown and are a major goal of future investigation. Numerous hypotheses have been proposed to explain these disorders. Pappata et al. (123) reported that subcortical lesions induce hypometabolic effects in many regions, including contralateral brain areas (i.e., crossed-hemisphere and crossed-cerebellar diaschisis). It is therefore possible that subcortical lesions may induce metabolic changes in left frontocortical regions, which are associated with depression. Mania may develop at a later stage, when these changes become restricted to the orbitofrontal and basotemporal cortices of the right hemisphere.

SUMMARY AND CONCLUSIONS

The neuropsychiatry of mood disorders involves the investigation of similarities and differences in mood disorders associated with several neurological disorders. This chapter has focused on mood disorders associated with stroke, PD, and TBI.

Depression occurs in about 40% of patients with acute stroke lesions, and its natural evolution is from 1–2 years, although patients with subcortical or brainstem lesions may show depressions of shorter duration. Both intrahemispheric and interhemispheric lesion location appear to contribute to the development of depression. Major depression is significantly more frequent among patients with left-hemisphere lesions involving anterior cortical (frontal) or subcortical (basal ganglia) regions than any other lesion location. On the other hand, depressions following right-hemisphere lesions are sometimes associated with a genetic vulnerability and frontal or parietal lobe damage. Finally, an important risk factor for the development of PSD is the presence of subcortical atrophy before the stroke lesion.

Mania that develops after stroke has a phenomenology similar to that of mania without known neuropathology. Secondary mania, a rare complication in stroke patients, is almost always the consequence of lesions involving right cortical (orbitofrontal or basotemporal) or right subcortical (head of the caudate or thalamus) limbic-related regions. Among these areas, dysfunction of the basotemporal cortex seems to be particularly important to the development of secondary mania, and basotemporal dysfunction may be produced by direct or indirect (diaschisis) damage. Risk factors for secondary mania include a familial history of psychiatric disorders or prior subcortical atrophy.

Among patients with TBI, the frequency of major depression is about 26%. Although some patients remain depressed for more than a year, the average duration of depression is 4–5 months. Risk factors for depression include previous history of psychiatric disorder and poor social functioning. Intellectual or physical impairment is not associated with the degree of depression. In addition, transiently depressed patients are more likely to have sustained injury to left dorsal lateral frontal or left basal ganglia structures than patients with more prolonged depressions. Similarly, manic patients are significantly more likely to have temporal basopolar lesions than depressed or nondepressed patients.

There are many areas that are ripe for future research. The most important elements of social functioning that contribute to depression need to be explored as well as the effect of social intervention. The role of antidepressants in treating these depressive disorders has not been systematically explored and deserves study.

Finally, the mechanism of these depressions, both those associated with psychosocial factors and those associated with neurobiological variables (e.g., strategic lesion locations), need to be investigated. It is only through the discovery of their mechanism that specific and rational treatment strategies for these disorders will be developed.

Acknowledgments

The authors are indebted to Drs. Sergio E. Starkstein, Thomas R. Price, John R. Lipsey, Rajesh M. Parikh, J. Paul Fedoroff, Helen S. Mayberg, and Karen Bolla, who participated in many of these studies. This work was supported by the following NIMH grants: Research Scientist Award MH00163 and MH40355.

References

1. Babinski J. Contribution a l'etude des troubles mentaux dans l'hemiplegie organique cerebrale (anosognosie). Rev Neurol (Paris) 1914;27:845–848.
2. Denny-Brown D, Meyer JS, Horenstein S. The significance of perpetual rivalry resulting from parietal lesions. Brain 1952;75:434–471.
3. Gainotti G. Emotional behavior and hemispheric side of the brain. Cortex 1972;8, 41–45.
4. Meyer A. The neuroanatomical facts and clinical varieties of traumatic insanity. American Journal of Insanity 1904;60:373.
5. Bleuler EP. Textbook of psychiatry. New York: Dover Publications, 1951.
6. Kraepelin E. Manic depressive insanity and paranoia. Edinburg: Churchill Livingstone, 1921.
7. Benson DF. Psychiatric aspects of aphasia. Br J Psychiatry 1976;123:555–556.
8. Broca P. Sur la faculte du langage articule, suivi d'une observation d'aphemie. Bulletin of the Anatomical Society (Paris) 1861;2-230-357.
9. Hughlings Jackson J. On affections of speech from disease of the brain. Brain 1915;138:106–174.
10. Goldstein K. The organism: a holistic approach to biology derived from pathological data in man. New York: American Books, 1939:35.
11. Goldstein K. After-effects of brain injuries in war. New York: Grune & Stratton, 1942.
12. Hecaen H, Ajuriaguerra J de, Massonet J. les troubles visoconstructifs par lesion parieto occipitale droit. Encephale 1951;40:122–179.
13. Ironside R. Disorders of laughter due to brain lesions. Brain 1956;79:589–609.
14. Post F. The significance of affective symptoms in old age (Maudsley Monograph No. 10). London: Oxford University Press, 1962.
15. Ullman M, Gruen A. Behavioral changes in patients with strokes. Am J Psychiatry 1960;117:1004–1009.
16. Fisher S. Psychiatric considerations of cerebral vascular disease. Am J Cardiol 1961;7:379.
17. Folstein MF, Folstein SE, Mc Hugh PR. Mood disorder as a specific complication of stroke. J Neurosurg Psychiatry 1977;40:1018–1020.
18. Wolfe PA, Kannel WB, Verter J. Cerebrovascular disease in the elderly; epidemiology. In: Albert ML, ed. Clinical neurology of aging. New York: Oxford University Press, 1984:458–477.
19. Hachinsk V, and Norris JW. The Acute Stroke, Philadelphia: FA Davis, 1985.
20. Robinson RG, Starr LB, Kubos KL. A 2 year longitudinal study of post-stroke mood disorders: findings during the initial evaluation. Stroke 1983;14:736–741.
21. Sinyor D, Jacques P, Kaloupek DG, Becker R, Goldemberg M, Coopersmith HM. Post-stroke depression and lesion location: an attempted replication. Brain 1986;109:537–546.
22. Eastwood MR, Rifat SL, Nobbs H, Ruderman J. Mood disorder following cerebro vascular accident. Br J Psychiatry 1989;154:195–200.
23. Adams GF, Hurwitz LJ. Mental barriers to recovery from strokes. Lancet 1963;2:533–537.
24. Lipsey JR, Robinson RG, Pearlson GD. Nortryptiline treatment for post stroke depression: a double blind trial. Lancet 1984;1:297–300.
25. Robinson RG, Price TR. Post stroke depressive disorders: a follow-up study of 103 patients. Stroke 1982;13:635–641.
26. Robinson RG, Bolduc PL, Price TR. Two-year longitudinal study of post-stroke mood disorders: diagnosis and outcome at one and two years. Stroke 1987;18:837–843.
27. Morris PLP, Robinson RG, Raphael B. Prevalence and course of post stroke depression in hospitalized patients. Int J Psychiatry Med 1990;20:349–364.
28. Astrom M, Adolfsson R, Kjell A. Major depression in stroke patients. A 3 year longitudinal study. Stroke 1993;24 - No.7 (976–982).
29. Carrol BJ, Feinberg M, Gredent JF. A specific laboratory test for the diagnosis of melancholia: standardization, validation and clinical utility. Arch Gen Psychiatry 1981;38:15–22.
30. Finklestein S, Benowitz LI, Baldessarini RJ. Mood, vegetative disturbance, and dexamethasone suppression test after stroke. Ann Neurol 1981;12:463–468.
31. Olsson T, Astrom M, Erikson S. Hypercortisolism revealed by dexamethasone suppression test with acute ischemic stroke. Stroke 1989;20:1685–1690.
32. Reding MJ, Orto LA, Willenski P. The dexamethasone depression test: an indicator of depression in stroke but not a predictor of rehabilitation outcome. Arch Neurol 1985;42:209–212.
33. Lipsey JR, Robinson RG, Pearlson GD. Dexamethasone suppression test and mood following strokes. Am J Psychiatry 1985;14:318–323.
34. Barry S, Dinan TG. Alpha-2 adrenergic receptor function in post stroke depression. Psychol Med 1990;20:305–309.
35. Morris PLP, Robinson RG, Raphael B, Samuels J, Molloy P. The relationship between risk factors for affective disorder and post-stroke depression in hospitalized stroke patients. Aust N Z J Psychiatry 1992;26:208–217.
36. Parikh RM, Robinson RG, Lipsey JR: The impact of post stroke depression on recovery in activities of daily living over a 2 year follow-up. Arch Neurol 1990;47:785–789.
37. Starkstein SE, Moran TH, Bowersox JA, Robinson RG. Behavioral abnormalities induced by frontal cortical and nucleus accumben lesions. Brain Res 1988;473:74–80.
38. Bolla-Wilson K, Robinson RG, Starkstein SE, Boston J, Price TR. Lateralization of dementia of depression in stroke patients. Am J Psychiatry 1989;146:627–634.
39. Downhill J, Robinson RG. Longitudinal assessment of depression and cognitive impairment following stroke. J Nerv Ment Dis 1994;182:425–431.
40. Fogal BS, Sparadeo FR. Focal cognitive deficits accentuated by depression. J Nerv Ment Dis 1985;173:119–124.
41. Ross ED, Rush AJ. Diagnosis and neuroanatomical correlates of depression in brain damage patients. Arch Gen Psychiatry 1981;38:1344–1354.
42. Robinson RG, Benson DF. Depression in aphasic patients: frequency, severity and clinical pathological correlations. Brain Lang 1981;14:282–291.
43. Robinson RG, Kubos KL, Starr LB, Rao K, Price TR. Mood changes in stroke patients: relationship to lesion location. Brain 1984;107:81–93.
44. Starkstein SE, Robinson RG. Aphasia and depression. Aphasiology 1988;2:1–20.
45. Starkstein SE, Robinson RG, Price TR. Comparison of cortical and subcortical lesions in the production of post-stroke mood disorders. Brain 1987;110:1045–1059.
46. Starkstein SE, Robinson RG, Berthier ML. Differential mood changes following basal ganglia vs. thalamic lesions. Arch Neurol 1988;45:725–730.

47. Starkstein SE, Robinson RG, Honig MA, Parikh RM, Joselyn R, Price TR. Mood changes after right hemisphere lesion. Brit J Psychiatry 1989;155:79–85.
48. Finset A. Depressed mood and reduced emotionality after right hemisphere brain damage. In: Kinsbourne M, ed. Cerebral hemisphere function in depression. Washington, DC: American Psychiatric Press, 1988:49–64.
49. Robinson RG, Szetela B. Mood change following left hemisphere brain injury. Ann Neurol 1981;9:447–453.
50. Robinson RG, Lipsey JR, Bolla-Wilson K, et al. Mood disorders in left handed stroke patients. Am J Psychiatry 1985;142:1424–1429.
51. House A, Dennis M, Warlow C, Molyneux K. Mood disorders after stroke and their relation to lesion location. A CT scan study. Brain 1990;113:1113–1130.
52. Morris PLP, Robinson RG, Raphael B. Lesion location and depression in hospitalized stroke patients: evidence supporting a specific relationship with left hemisphere. Neuropsychiatry Neuropsychology and Behavioral Neurology 1992;3:75–82.
53. Parikh RM, Lipsey JR, Robinson RG, Price TR. A two year longitudinal study of post-stroke mood disorders: Prognostic factors related to one and two year outcome. Int J Psychiatr Med 1988; 18:45–56.
54. Starkstein SE, Robinson RG, Berthier ML, Price TR. Depressive disorders following posterior circulation as compared with middle cerebral artery infarcts. Brain 1988;11:375–387.
55. Starkstein SE, Robinson RG, Price TR. Comparison of patients with and without post-stroke major depression matched for size and location of lesion. Arch Gen Psychiatry 1988;45:247–252.
56. Morrison JH, Molliver ME, Grzanna R. Noradrenergic inervation of the cerebral cortex: widespread effects of local cortical lesions. Science 1979;205:313–316.
57. Robinson RG. Differential behavioral and biochemical effects of right and left hemispheric cerebral infarction in the rat. Science 1979; 205:707–710.
58. Mayberg HS, Robinson R, Wong D, et al. PET imaging of cortical S2 serotonin receptors following stroke: lateralized changes and relationship to depression. Am J Psychiatry 1988;143:527–529.
59. Reding MJ, Orto LA, Winter SW. Antidepressant therapy after stroke: a double blind trial. Arch Neurol 1986;43:763–765.
60. Lewy FH. Die Lehre von Tonus und der Bewegung. Berlin: Springer, 1923.
61. Mindham RHS. Psychiatric symptoms in parkinsonism. J Neurol Neurosurg Psychiatry 1970;33:188–191.
62. Mayeux R, Williams JBW, Stern Y: Depression in Parkinson disease. Adv Neurol 1984;40:242–250.
63. Mayeux R, Stern Y, Williams JBW. Clinical and biochemical features of depression in Parkinson's disease. Am J Psychiatry 1986; 143:756–759.
64. Celesia GG, Wanamaker WM. Psychiatric disturbances in Parkinson's disease. Diseases of the Nervous System 1972;33:577–583.
65. Gotham AM, Brown RG, Marsden CD. Depression in Parkinson's disease: a quantitative and qualitative analysis. J Neurol Neurosurg Psychiatry 1986;49:381–389.
66. Starkstein SE, Bolduc PL, Mayberg HS, Preziosi TJ, Robinson RG. Cognitive impairment and depression in Parkinson's disease; a follow up study. J Neurol Neurosurg Psychiatry 1990;53:597–602.
67. El-Awar M, Bekcer JT, Hammond KM. Learning deficits in Parkinson's disease: comparison with Alzheimer's disease and normal aging. Arch Neurol 1987;44:180–184.
68. Mayeux R, Stern Y, Rosen J. Depression, intellectual impairment and Parkinson disease. Neurology 1981;32:645–650.
69. Starkstein SE, Bolduc PL, Preziosi TJ. Cognitive impairments in different states of Parkinson disease. Journal of Neuropsychiatry and Clinical Neuroscience 1989;1:243–248.
70. Starkstein SE, Preziosi TJ, Berthier ML. Depression and cognitive impairment in Parkinson's disease. Brain 1989;112:1141–1153.
71. Sano M, Stern Y, William J. Coexisting dementia and depression in Parkinson's disease. Arch Neurol 1989;46:1284–1286.

72. Perry EK, Curtis M, Dick DJ. Cholinergic correlates of cognitive impairment in Parkinson disease: comparisons with Alzheimer's disease. J Neurol Neurosurg Psychiatry 1985;48:413–421.
73. Torack RM, Morris JC. The association of ventral tegmental area histopathology with adult dementia. Arch Neurol 1988;45: 211–218.
74. Mayberg HS, Starkstein SE, Sadzot T, et al. Selective hypometabolism in the inferior frontal lobe in depressed patients with Parkinson's disease. Ann Neurology 1990;28:57–64.
75. Simon H, LeMoal M, Calas A. Efferents and afferents of the ventral tegmental A-10 region studied after local injection of [3H]-leucine and horseradish peroxidase. Brain Res 1979;178:17–40.
76. Azmitia EC, Gannon PJ. Primate serotonergic system: a review of human and animal studies and a report on Macacca fascicularis. Adv Neurol 1986;43:407–468.
77. Nauta WJH. The problem of the frontal lobe: a reinterpretation. J Psychol Res 1971;8:167–187.
78. Silver JM, Hales RE, Yudofsky SC. Depression in traumatic brain injury. Neuropsychiatry, Neuropsychology and Behavioral Neurology 1991;4:12–23.
79. Rutherford WH, Merret JD, Mc Donald JR. Sequelae of concussion caused by minor head injuries. Lancet 1977;1:1–4.
80. McKinlay WW, Brooks DN, Bond MR, Martinage DP, Marshall MM. The short term outcome of severe blunt head injury as reported by the relatives of the head injury person. J Neurol Neurosurg Psychiatry; 1981;44:527–533.
81. Kinsella G, Moran C, Ford B. Emotional disorders and its assessment within the severe head injured population. Psychol Med 1988; 18:57–63.
82. Fedoroff JP, Starkstein SE, Forrester AW, Geisler F, Jorge RE, Robinson RG. Depression in patients with acute brain injury. Am J Psychiatry 1992;149:7.
83. Jorge RE, Robinson RG, Arndt SV, Forrester AW, Geisler F, Starkstein SE. Depression and traumatic brain injury: a longitudinal study. J Affect Disord 1993;27:233–243.
84. Gualtieri CT, Cox DR. The delayed neurobehavioral sequelae of traumatic brain injury. Brain Inj 1991;5:219–232.
85. Brooks N, Campsie L, Symington C. The five year outcome of severe blunt head injury: a relative's view. J Neurosurg Psychiatry 1986; 49:764–770.
86. Grant I, Alves W. Psychiatric and psychological disturbances in head injury. In: Levin HS, Grafman J, Eisemberg HM, eds. Neurobehavioral recovery from head injury. Oxford: Oxford University Press, 1987;232–261.
87. Prigatano GP. Psychiatric aspects of head injury: problem areas and suggested guidelines for research. In: Levin HS, Grafman J, Eisemberg HM, eds. Neurobehavioral recovery from head injury. Oxford: Oxford University Press, 1987:215–232.
88. Lishman WA. Physiogenesis and Psychogenesis in the post concussional syndrome. Br J Psychiatry 1988;153:460–469.
89. Van Zomeren AH, Saan RJ. Psychological and social sequelae of severe head injury. In: Braakman R, ed. Handbook of clinical neurology, vol 13 (57). Elsevier, 1990:397–420.
90. Wing JK, Cooper E, Sartorius N. Measurement and classification of psychiatric symptoms. Cambridge: Cambridge University Press.
91. American Psychiatric Association, Diagnostic and statistical manual III-revised. Washington, DC: American Psychiatric Press, 1987.
92. Jorge RE, Robinson RG, Arndt SV, Forrester AW, Geisler F, Starkstein SE. Comparison between acute and delayed onset depression following traumatic brain injury. J Neuropsychiatry 1993; 5:43–49.
93. Lishman WA. The psychiatric sequelae of head injury: a review. Psychol Med 1973;3:304–318.
94. Starr LB, Robinson RG, Price TR. Reliability, validity and clinical utility of the social functioning exam in the assessment of stroke patients. Exp Aging Res 1983;9:101.
95. Lishman WA. Brain damage in relation to psychiatric disability after head injury. Br J Psychiatry 1968;114:373–410.

96. Grafman J, Vance SC, Swingartner H. The effects of lateralized frontal lesions on mood regulation. Brain 1986;109:1127–1148.

97. Katz DI. Neuropathology and neurobehavioral recovery from closed head injury. J Head Trauma Rehabil 1992;7:1–15.

98. Chollet F, DiPiero V, Wise RJS, Brooks DJ, Dolan RJ, Frackowiak RSJ. The functional anatomy of motor recovery after stroke in humans: a study with positron emission tomography. Ann Neurol 1991;29:63–71.

99. Steward O. Reorganization of neuronal connections following CNS trauma: principles and experimental paradigms. J Neurotrauma 1989; 6:99–152.

100. Prigatano GP. Neuropsychological rehabilitation after brain injury. Baltimore: Johns Hopkins University Press, 1986.

101. Bornstein RA, Miller HB, Van Schoor JT. Neuropsychological deficit and emotional disturbance in head injured patients. J Neurosurg 1989;70:509–513.

102. Silver JM, Hales RE, Yudofsky SC. Psychopharmacology of depression in neurologic disorders. J Clin Psychiatry; 1990;51:33–39.

103. Cassidy JW. Fluoxetine: a new serotonergically active antidepressant. J Head Trauma Rehabil 1989;4:67–69.

104. Zasler ND. Advances in neuropharmacological rehabilitation for brain dysfunction. Brain Inj 1992;6:1–14.

105. Gualtieri CT. Pharmacotherapy and the neurobehavioral sequelae of traumatic brain injury. Brain Inj 1988;2:101–129.

106. Gualtieri CT. Buspirone: neuropsychiatric effects. Journal of Head Trauma and Rehabilitation 1991;6:90–92.

107. Robinson RG, Boston JD, Starkstein SE, Price TR. Comparison of mania with depression following brain injury. Am J Psychiatry 1988; 145:172–178.

108. Starkstein SE, Pearlson GD, Robinson RG: Mania after brain injury: a controlled study of etiological factors. Arch Neurol 1987;44:1069–1073.

109. Starkstein SE, Bolduc PE, Preziosi TJ. Depression in Parkinson's disease. J Nerv Ment Dis 1990;178:27–31.

110. Gloor P. Role of the human limbic system in perception, memory and affect: lessons for temporal lobe epilepsy. In: Doane BK, Livingstone KE, eds. The limbic system: functional organization and clinical disorders. New York: Raven Press, 1986.

111. Beck E. A cytoarchitectural investigation into the boundaries of cortical areas 13 and 14 in the human brain. J Anat 1949; 83:145–157.

112. Crosby E, Humphrey T, Lauer E. Correlative anatomy of the nervous system. New York: Macmillan, 1962.

113. Goldar JC, Outes DL. Fisiopatologia de la desinhibicion instintiva. Acta Psiquiatrica y Psicologica de America Latina 1972;18:177–185.

114. Kubos KL, Moran TH, Robinson RG. Mania after brain injury: a controlled study of etiological factors. Arch Neurol 1987;44:1069–1073.

115. Berthier ML, Starkstein SE, Robinson RG, Leiguarda R. Limbic lesions in a patient with recurrent mania. Journal of Neuropsychiatry and Clinical Neuroscience 1990;2:235–236.

116. Shukla S, Cook BL, Mukherjee S. Mania following head trauma. Am J Psychiatry 1987;144:93–96.

117. Bakchine S, Lacomblez L, Benoit N. Manic-like state after orbito-frontal and right temporoparietal injury: Efficacy of clonidine. Neurology 1989;39:777–781.

118. Jorge RE, Robinson RG, Starkstein SE, Arndt SV. Manic syndromes following traumatic brain injury. Am J Psychiatry, 1993; 150:916–921.

119. Teasdale G, Mendelow D. Pathophysiology of head injuries. In: Brooks N, ed. Closed head injury. Psychological, social and family consequences. New York: Oxford University Press, 1984;4–36.

120. Stevens JR. Psychiatric consequences of temporal lobectomy for intractable seizures. Psychol Med 1990;20:529–545.

121. Csernansky JG, Mellentin J, Beauclair L, Lombrozo L. Mesolimbic dopaminergic supersensitivity following electrical kindling of the amygdala. Biol Psychiatry, 1988;23:285–294.

122. Starkstein SE, Federoff JP, Berthier ML, Robinson RG. Manic depressive and pure manic states after brain lesions. Biol Psychiatry 1991;29:149–158.

123. Pappata, Dinh ST, Baron JC, Cambon H, Syrota A. Remote metabolic effects of cerebrovascular lesions: magnetic resonance and positron tomography imaging. Neuroradiology 1987;29:1–6.

Suggested Readings

Bamrah JS, Johnson J. Bipolar affective disorder following head injury. Br J Psychiatry 1991;158:117–119.

Blackwell MJ: Rapid-cycling manic depressive illness following subarachnoid hemorrhage. Br J Psychiatry 1991;159:279–280.

Bryer JB, Starkstein SE, Votypka V, Parikh RM, Price TR, Robinson RG: Reduction of CSF monoamine metabolites in post-stroke depression. Journal of Neuropsychiatry Clinical Neuroscience 1992;4:440–442.

Corn TH, Checkley SA: A case of recurrent mania with recurrent hyperthyroidism. Br J Psychiatry 1983;143:74–76.

Cummings JL, Mendez MF: Secondary mania with focal cerebrovascular lesions. Am J Psychiatry 1984;141:1084–1087.

Davison C, Kelman H. Pathological laughing and crying. Arch Neurol Psychiatry 1939;42:595–643.

Fawcett RG: Cerebral infarct presenting as mania. J Clin Psychiatry 1991; 52:352–353.

Fedoroff UP, Starkstein SE, Parikh RM: Are depressive symptoms non-specific in patients with acute stroke? Am J Psychiatry 1991; 148:1172–1176.

Folstein MF, Folstein SE, Mc Hugh PR: Mini-Mental State: a practical method for grading the cognitive state of patients for the clinician. J Psychiatr Res 1975;12:189–198.

Goggans FC: A case of mania secondary to vitamin B12 deficiency. Am J Psychiatry 1984;141:300–301.

Goldemberg G, Oder W, Spatt J, Podreka I: Cerebral correlates of disturbed executive function and memory of survivors of closed head injury: a SPECT study. J Neurol Neurosurg Psychiatry 1992;55:362–368.

Isles LJ, Orrell MW: Secondary mania after open-heart surgery. Br J Psychiatry 1991;159:280–282.

Jamielson RC, Wells CE: Manic psychosis in a patient with multiple metastatic brain tumors. J Clin Psychiatry 1979;40:280–283.

Khanna R, Nizamie SH, Das A: Electrical trauma, non-ictal EEG changes and mania: a case report. J Clin Psychiatry 1991;52:280.

Lees AJ, Smith E: Cognitive deficits in the early stages of Parkinson's disease. Brain 1983;106:257–270.

Mayberg HS, Moran TH, Robinson RG: Remote lateralized changes in cortical 3H-spiperone binding following focal frontal cortex lesions in the rat. Brain Res 1990;516:127–131.

Morris PLP, Raphael B, Robinson R: Clinical depression impairs recovery from stroke. Med J Aust 1992;157:239–242.

Oder W, Goldemberg G, Spatt J: Behavioral and psychosocial sequelae of severe closed head injury and regional cerebral blood flow: a SPECT study. J Neurol Neurosurg Psychiatry 1992;55:475–480.

Robinson RG, Bolla-Wilson K, Kaplan E: Depression influences intellectual impairment in stroke patients. Br J Psychiatry 1986;148:541–547.

Robinson RG, Parikh RM, Lipsey JR, Starkstein SE, Price TR: Pathological laughing and crying following stroke: validation of a measurement scale and a double blind treatment study. Am J Psychiatry 1993; 150:286–293.

Robinson RG, Starr LB, Kubos KL: Mood disorders in stroke patients: importance of lesions location. Brain 1984;107:81–93.

Stoudermire A, Miller J, Schmitt F, Logue P, Shelton D: Development of an organic affective syndrome during a hyperbaric diving experiment. Am J Psychiatry 1984;141:1251–1254.

Thienhaus OJ, Khosla N: Meningeal cryptococosis misdiagnosed as a manic episode. Am J Psychiatry 1984;141:1459–1460.

Thomas CS, Neale TJ: Organic manic syndrome associated with advanced uremia due to polycystic kidney disease. Br J Psychiatry 1991; 158:119–121.

Wade DT, Legh-Smith JE, Hewer RA: Depressed mood after stroke: a community study of its frequency. Br J Psychiatry 1987;141:200–205.

Wells CE: Pseudodementia. Am J Psychiatry 1979;136:895–900.

Wilson JTL, Wyper D: Neuroimaging and neuropsychological functioning following closed head injury. Journal of Head Trauma and Rehabilitation 1992;7:29–39.

Wolf PA, Dawber TR, Thomas HE: Epidemiology of stroke. In: Thompson RA, Green JR, eds. Advances in neurology, vol 16. New York: Raven Press, 1977:5–19.

Zolese G, Henryk-Gutt R. Mania induced by biochemical imbalance resulting from low energy diet in patient with undiagnosed myxoedema. Br Med J 1987;295:1026–1027.

14

HALLUCINATIONS AND DELUSIONAL THINKING

D. Frank Benson and D. Gregory Gorman

Premier among the clinical findings indicative of psychiatric disorder, delusions and hallucinations are not only the most dramatic but also the most visible. For most psychiatrists, a delusion establishes the presence of psychosis (1) and for almost all physicians, the presence of either delusions or hallucinations implies psychiatric disorder. These dramatic clinical aberrations have been observed and described since antiquity, albeit under a variety of names; both entities are significant in medical lore (2, 3). Interpretations of hallucinatory experiences and delusional beliefs have varied with the wide shifts in accepted psychiatric reasoning over the years, but have almost always been accepted as prime examples of "functional" (nonorganic) mental disorder. Current changes in viewing psychiatric symptomatology prompt reevaluation of both hallucinations and delusions.

DEFINITIONS

Delusions and hallucinations are dynamic entities, resistant to rigid definition. *In both disorders the fundamental component concerns incorrect interpretation.* Both can vary in the tenacity with which the incorrect impression is held. Variations in content and degree have led to numerous categorizations and subclassifications.

An *hallucination* can be defined rather simply as "a sensory perception without external stimulation of the relevant sensory organ" (4). Unfortunately, this definition—and most others—fails to exclude many nonstimulated experiences, such as daydreaming; the key difference is the ability to gauge the reality of the image. A sensory experience without external stimulation and firmly accepted as real is considered pathological; a similar mental experience recognized as unreal is normal. An hallucinatory experience may appear real at the time and only in retrospect be recognized as unreal. Determining if the experience is actually hallucinatory can be difficult, at times almost impossible.

Attempts to define hallucinatory experience produce some clinically useful distinctions. First, hallucinations are distinguished from *illusions,* which are actual external

stimuli, perceived but misinterpreted. In contrast, the hallucinatory experience occurs in the absence of relevant external stimulus. *Pseudohallucinations* are partial hallucinatory states in which clear, vivid images are perceived and misinterpreted but are recognized as unreal. The distinction, however, is so subtle that most psychiatrists have abandoned the term. *Hallucinosis,* an ongoing series of hallucinatory experiences, is most often linked to toxic brain disorders, has an acute onset, and tends to persist or recur. While often considered distinct, hallucinations and hallucinosis differ mostly in degree. Although distinct by definition, hallucinatory experiences and delusional thinking are often intertwined, as we will discuss later in this chapter.

Almost all definitions of *delusion* emphasize two points: the presence of a false belief and the persistent, unshakable acceptance of the false belief. Both points, however, must have qualifiers if they are to encompass the range of elegantly complex but confusing symptoms occurring in different delusional states. Thus, existential and phenomenological explanations, psychoanalytic and dynamic theories, and biological or molecular approaches to psychiatric disorders all define a delusion as an unshakable false belief but feature significant qualifying variations. One basic definition of delusion is as follows:

... a false personal belief based on incorrect inference about external reality and firmly sustained in spite of what almost everyone else believes and in spite of what constitutes incontrovertible and obvious proof or evidence to the contrary. The belief is not one ordinarily accepted by other members of the person's culture or subculture (i.e., it is not an article of religious faith) (4).

A more dynamically oriented definition of delusion is:

... an unshakable personal belief that is obviously mistaken or unreal, which directs a significant aspect of the individual's behavior; an attempt to explain events or interpersonal relations of importance to the individual, but incorrect on both logical and realistic grounds. The explanation fits an already held distorted view of self and others; it excludes group, professional or religious beliefs that persist in the face of logic or contrary evidence; it must have some consequence for the individual's behavior (5).

A basic distinction between hallucinations and delusions concerns content. With hallucinatory experiences sensory input is improperly processed; a delusion is an idea or belief—a complex thought content—that is abnormal. Although rarely emphasized in formal definitions, this distinction provides the base for most classifications of the two phenomena. Delusions are almost universally categorized in terms of thought content, while the most consistently used classifications of hallucinations are based on the sensory modality involved. This chapter breaks down this definition accordingly—sensory modality for hallucinations, thought contents for delusions—but, as will be obvious, the distinction is not absolute, so that one entity can fade into the other.

HALLUCINATIONS

Classification of hallucinatory experiences varies considerably. One categorization suggested by neurologists (6) features *release hallucinations* and *ictal hallucinations*. In release hallucinations a normal sensory processing channel is blocked and, as a replacement, stored images are experienced. Ictal hallucinations, in contrast, are produced by abnormal neuronal discharges. Release hallucinations consist of formed images that persist for minutes or hours, may be modified by altering the sensory input, and more often follow right hemisphere damage. Ictal hallucinations tend to be brief, stereotyped, and, when formed, often represent recollections of past experience.

A second way to categorize hallucinations is based on etiology. Five varieties have been suggested (7): *(a)* brain damage/disorder (e.g., tumor, epilepsy, metabolic alteration), *(b)* sensory deprivation, *(c)* suggestibility, *(d)* emotion, and *(e)* psychiatric disease. Although this etiologic classification is consistent and complete, it has not proved particularly helpful.

The most commonly used means to classify hallucinations is based on the misperceived sensory element. Division into visual, auditory, olfactory/gustatory, somesthetic (haptic), and vestibular categories has proved most practical for identifying types of hallucinatory experiences. In this chapter, discussion of hallucinatory experiences is based on the sensory modality and, where possible, the described entities start from external and move to central involvement.

Visual Hallucinations

The most readily demarcated and, therefore, most clearly categorized hallucinatory experiences are those involving the visual system. Disorder may occur at the end organ (retina) during sensory transmission or be based on abnormal cortical reception, perception, and/or interpretation.

Several purely ophthalmalogic entities meet the definition of hallucination. Thus, *Moore's lightning streaks,* vertical bands of light that occur in the temporal visual fields during eye movement, represent true hallucinations; most often they indicate vitreous detachment (8). *Ocular phosphenes,* the phenomenon produced by vigorously rubbing the eyes, are similar to Moore's lightning streaks; they can occur spontaneously in the aging eye or in cases of optic neuritis (9). *Auditory-visual synesthesias* are photisms induced by sound and can occur in some patients with ocular pathology (10, 11). Many unusual visual phenomena (e.g., particles floating in the vitreous, nerve bundles swollen with macular edema, or blood cells circulating in the paramacular region) represent actual entities and do not fit the definition of hallucination.

Following enucleation of one eye, hallucinations that are analogous to the phantom limb syndrome and appropriately called *phantom vision* can occur (12). Phantom vision is common; over one-half of 104 patients with acute bilateral visual loss reported spontaneous visual phenomena (13). A related phenomenon, *palinopsia* (the persistence of a visual image in a disordered or blind visual field) is well known (14, 15). A single image (e.g., flower, face) can appear wherever the patient fixes a gaze and may persist from minutes to days. Palinopsia has been described in such diverse entities as nonketotic hyperglycemia (16), cocaine abuse (17), and occipital lobe seizures (18–20). When persistent, and if the etiology is not obvious, palinopsia is easily misinterpreted as a psychiatric symptom (21).

The Charles Bonnet syndrome has been used to describe certain hallucinations that are not frightening and occur without delusions in the elderly (22). Charles Bonnet was a Swiss naturalist who reported (in 1760) that his 89-year-old grandfather, blind because of cataracts, was entertained by complex visions but was fully cogent of their unreality and could still lecture in a clear, coherent fashion, an indication that he was not demented. While the phenomenon is always related to ocular pathology (23–26), its occurrence in old age suggests that brain alterations plus ocular disorder may be essential to the phenomenon (27–29).

A better known variety of visual hallucination, *hypnagogic hallucinations,* are vivid, often terrifying hallucinatory experiences that accompany or precede sleep paralysis and usually occur in individuals with narcolepsy. The hallucination may be auditory, vestibular, or somesthetic but most often features a strong visual component (30).

Peduncular hallucinations are dream-like states in which small (Lilliputian) people, animals, or objects carry out activities. They occur in individuals who have both vision and insight preserved. The patient's relationship with the hallucination is characteristic, almost diagnostic. At first the hallucination may be troubling but then becomes interesting and pleasantly entertaining. Eventually, however, the patient becomes irritated by the persistence of the hallucinatory experience (31). Lhermitte (32) originally described the syndrome and suggested that a structural change in the midbrain peduncular region was the source. Subsequent reports indicate that a variety of disorders affecting the upper midbrain can be associated with these characteristic hallucinatory experiences (33). McKee and colleagues (34) reported a single case of peduncular hallucinosis with evidence of infarction in the substantia nigra-pars reticulata, a portion of the serotonergic neurotransmitter system. Others (35–37) suggest that decreased blood flow in the vessels feeding the occipital and medial temporal regions is the true source of these hallucinations. None of the localization theories has been substantiated.

Visual release hallucinations have traditionally been associated with visual field defect. Weinberger and Grant (38) found that the phenomenon could occur with pathology involving any portion of the visual system from the retina through the occipital cortex and into the temporal cortex. Visual release hallucinations tend to last minutes or hours, are variable in content, and can be modified by altering visual input (e.g., opening or closing the eye). In a broad sense, all of the visual hallucinatory phenomena described thus far can be considered examples of release hallucinations.

Visual ictal hallucinations tend to be stereotyped in content, are often geometric in design, or produce a recollection of previously experienced visual images. They are not confined to any single portion of the visual field. They may be experienced as auras or distortions (e.g., micropsia, macropsia, or metamorphopsia) and can be artificially produced by direct brain stimulation (39). While these experiences are most commonly related to epilepsy, similar hallucinatory experiences have been described with ecstasy (40) and migraine (41).

ETIOLOGY OF VISUAL HALLUCINATIONS

Disorders that decrease or alter the level of conscious awareness have been associated with visual hallucinations. About a third of the patients who suffer acute confusion (delirium) report hallucinatory experiences; most of the hallucinations seen in acute confusion are visual and increase with diminished visual stimulation (sundowning) (42). Sleep deprivation and narcolepsy are often associated with visual hallucinations, and a vast array of drugs can produce visual hallucinatory experiences. Three groups of drugs are particularly likely to produce visual hallucinations (43): *(a)* hallucinogens, *(b)* sedative/hypnotic drugs, and *(c)* toxic quantities of certain other drugs.

Hallucinogenic drugs such as lysergic acid diethylamide (LSD), mescaline, or psilocybin are defined by their ability to produce hallucinations. Drug-induced hallucinations, particularly from LSD, mescaline, and the like, can recur at a later, drug-free time; these experiences, called "flashbacks," may occur up to several years after LSD use (44). Flashbacks rarely cause diagnostic misinterpretation because the subject is well aware of both the experience and the source. Many other substances can produce hallucinations, including drugs such as the bromides, most of the narcotic substances, levodopa, bromides, barbiturates, benzodiazapines, sedative/hypnotic drugs, and substance of abuse such as alcohol. Most of these tend to produce hallucinations during periods of withdrawal. Any type of hallucination may be produced, but visual experiences predominate.

Visual hallucinations occur in many traditional psychiatric disorders but, in general, these tend to be different phenomena. The visual hallucinations associated with psychiatric disorders are often complex, may be enhanced by auditory misperceptions, and often lead to delusional belief. Although auditory hallucinations are far more common in schizophrenic subjects (45), visual hallucinations are reported in a sizable number, particularly by those most severely afflicted.

It should be recognized that hallucinatory-like experiences also occur in normal individuals. Thus, dreams, the transient mental (mostly visual) experiences that occur in the sleep state are, by any definition, perceptions without immediate external stimulus. Daydreams and fantasies are similar hallucinatory experiences occurring during the waking state. In some societies, "visions" of this type are valued as a source of guidance and inspiration. Eidetic imagery, daydreams, the imaginary friends of childhood, sleep deprivation, narcolepsy, hypnosis, sensory deprivation, and intense emotional experiences (such as hostage situations) are all capable of producing visual hallucinations in the absence of either primary brain disorder or significant psychiatric disease.

Auditory Hallucinations

Standard medical teaching suggests that auditory hallucinations most often indicate primary psychiatric problems, whereas visual hallucinations occur in organic disorder. In general this concept is correct (45) but many causes of auditory hallucinations other than traditional psychiatric disorders exist and deserve consideration.

Tinnitus, the perception of ringing, whistling, buzzing, or even a drumbeat, represents an auditory experience without external stimulus. In some instances, tinnitus can be experienced as a complex series of sounds, a state resembling release hallucinations. When auditory input is decreased (total or partial deafness), this form of auditory hallucination becomes more notable and may resemble articulate speech; hallucinations of threatening or disparaging voices may be an important factor leading to the paranoid state of acquired deafness (46).

Palinacousis, the continued recurrence (echo) of a prior auditory perception, resembles palinopsia (47) but is less common. Some cases have been related to temporal lobe seizures (48).

Musical hallucinations, a variation of release hallucinations featuring the perception of music without an external source, are seen in many disorders ranging from simple deafness (49, 50) to focal temporal lobe pathology. When based on brain pathology, musical hallucinations are more often correlated with right hemisphere disorder (51).

Auditory hallucinations are commonly reported as *auras of epilepsy.* Thus, Currie (52) found 17% of a group of over 500 epileptic patients noted auditory hallucinations as their aura. At times, focal pathology in the temporal lobe may be associated with sounds or voices that are independent of reality but occur without overt seizure activity (53), a situation easily confused with primary psychiatric disorder.

Withdrawal states, particularly from alcohol, are well recognized as causes of auditory hallucinations (54) and have been called *alcoholic hallucinosis* (55). The hallucinations most often feature voices that are self-deprecating and/or threatening (56). They tend to affect older individuals with a long record of heavy alcohol consumption. A past history of trauma or long-standing dietary inadequacy may produce compromised function in an aging brain. A combination of these problems plus alcohol withdrawal may produce alcoholic hallucinosis.

A variety of psychiatric disorders are known to cause auditory hallucinations. Auditory hallucinations due to primary mental illness are often difficult for the patient to localize in space (often sensed as occurring inside the head), and the gender and age of the voice are often vague. The voice most often comments on the patient's behavior and/or echoes the patient's thoughts. In attempts to rid themselves of these voices, psychotic patients will sometimes play loud music or stuff material such as cotton into their ears. Monotonous sounds (white noise) such as traffic noise may be troublesome, leading to increased auditory hallucinations in schizophrenic patients. While auditory hallucinations are often considered an indication of primary mental illness, the possibility of a secondary psychosis always deserves consideration. Perez and Trimble (57) noted that a significant number of patients with ictal psychosis will present Schneiderian first-rank symptoms, suggesting schizophrenia. Psychiatric conditions other than schizophrenia may also produce auditory hallucinations. Psychotically depressed or manic patients often have periods in which voices speak to them. Patients with multiple personality disorder report auditory hallucinations at times, leading to misinterpretation of the disorder as schizophrenia (58).

Olfactory/Gustatory Hallucinations

Disorders of smell and taste are difficult to distinguish from hallucinatory experiences. Thus, apparent hallucinations of smell or taste can be the result of damage to the olfactory bulb, and at times the symptom can be "cured" by surgical resection of the olfactory bulb (59). Tumors at the base of the brain that extend into the olfactory apparatus can produce apparent olfactory hallucinations. Migraine patients occasionally describe auras of olfactory or gustatory type; if present, these tend to occur in patients who are depressed or present some other suggestion of limbic dysfunction (60).

Patients with complex partial seizures commonly report indescribable odors or tastes, traditionally called *uncinate fits.* A seizure focus, if present, is most often localized in the insula or opercular area, but olfactory hallucinations have been reported in patients with parietal and temporal area lesions (61) and even with a colloid cyst of the third ventricle (62). Olfactory hallucinations have been described by some demented patients, particularly those with Alzheimer's disease; one study contends that the olfactory hallucinations of Alzheimer's disease are based on a greatly increased number of neurofibrillary tangles in the limbic areas (63). Olfactory hallucinations may occur in drug abuse situations (64). Among patients with primary mental illness, olfactory/gustatory hallucinations are most commonly seen in those who present a delusion of being poisoned.

The complaint that one's body is malodorous and socially offensive, the *olfactory reference syndrome,* can be seen in severe depressive states; while this represents a symptom based on involvement of a single sensory system, it is usually accompanied by other incorrect perceptions, often systematized, and is thus classed as a delusion. The olfactory reference syndrome has also been reported in a patient with seizure disorder (65).

Haptic/Pain Hallucinations

Somesthetic (haptic) hallucinations include both unusual body experiences and pain. Following limb amputation, an hallucination of *phantom limb* is almost universal and pain in the nonexisting limb is present in as many as 85% of postamputation patients (66, 67). Similar phantom hallucinatory experiences are seen following amputation of breasts, genitals, or other body parts and are commonly reported to affect the body in areas below spinal cord transection. Over time, the phantom hallucination changes, most often perceived as a shrinking in size of the affected body area. Other hallucinatory experiences include a cutting type of pain (most often reported following surgery) or cramping pain, which may be helped by interventions that reduce muscle spasm. Even children born without limbs have phantom experiences, and Melzack (68, 69) has suggested that the brain contains a genetically inherited template of the body image that is the source of these haptic hallucinations.

Hallucinatory duplication of a limb or other body segment or a sensation of distorted body shape may occur with migraine, as an epileptic aura, with toxic encephalopathy, or following use of hallucinogenic drugs. Reports of abnormal body segments tend to be sufficiently fantastic that the observer may accept the phenomenon as a delusion and relate it to schizophrenia. Experiences of complete bodily transformation, such as becoming an animal or a person of the opposite sex or the impression that a segment or all of the body are absent, are usually categorized as delusions, rather than hallucinations.

Formication hallucinations, the feeling that bugs are crawling on the skin, occur in a variety of neurological and psychiatric conditions (23). They are common in alcohol and drug withdrawal states and occur in a number of toxic/metabolic conditions. They are also common in schizophrenia and affective disorder (45). If the sensation is unilateral, formication hallucinations may indicate thalamic or parietal lesions (70, 71).

Vestibular Hallucinations

Vestibular hallucinations, producing a feeling of giddiness or vertigo, are almost impossible to distinguish from primary vestibular disease. Better-defined experiences, such as sinking into a hard object, the sense of flying off through the air, of walking on waves or cork, or perceiving the ground as rising, lowering, or turning, suggest that the experience is hallucinatory. Nonetheless, a careful search for primary vestibular pathology as the source of these experiences is indicated.

Haptic/vestibular hallucinations, in which the patient describes abnormal heaviness, lightness to the point of levitation, and similar feelings, have been reported in schizophrenia, drug withdrawal, and seizure disorders. Combined visual/vestibular hallucinations and the sense of flying, are said to be characteristic of intoxication with the *Datura* plant and can occur in atropine or scopolamine intoxication. Closely related mixed vestibular hallucinatory experiences have been described in the context of Tantric and Yogic practices.

Synesthesia

Synesthesia is a term used to represent crossed modality hallucinations, e.g., the experience of hearing a vision or seeing a sound. Taste may be geometrically structured, and smells may provoke a color identification (72). *Auditory-visual synesthesia* (sound-induced photisms) may occur as release hallucinations, particularly if there is a defect in the visual field (10). A similar situation has been described in a patient with a medial temporal mass (73). Synesthesia may occur in the presence of impaired primary sensory pathways, with brainstem impingement, or with multimodal association area involvement. LSD is a well-known cause of synesthesia. Crossed modality hallucinatory experiences are only rarely reported by schizophrenics.

DELUSIONAL THINKING

Delusions involve thought contents and, as such, tend to be idiosyncratic and richly varied. They are formed from and colored by the individual's background, including personal, family, social and group experiences, educational background, and cultural (including religious) influences. Delusions are sufficiently idiosyncratic that sharp distinctions and inclusive classifications have remained elusive. In his discussion of delusions, Nash (74) lists 44 varieties and admits that the list is not complete. Vast differences can be seen in the content of any single variety of delusion. An individual with totally psychotic delusions in one line of thought may be perfectly rational and competent in other respects.

Numerous attempts have been made to demonstrate an underlying psychological basis for delusions. Early in his career, Freud (75) attempted to explain selected types of delusion as the product of latent homosexuality; the subject's attempts to deny (repress) the problem gave rise to delusions of persecution, erotomania, jealousy, and grandeur. Non-Freudian psychiatrists have not accepted latent homosexuality as the sole basis for these four types of delusion, and most subsequent attempts to demonstrate a psychological cause have produced unsatisfactory explanations (76). While no single classification of the varieties of delusion is satisfactory, most emphasize alterations of thought content. Nine of the most common and dramatically distinct types of delusion are presented here.

Delusions of Persecution

Commonly referred to as paranoid delusions, delusions of persecution are common, occur in a wide variety of neuropsychiatric disorders, and can take many different forms.

DELUSIONS OF REFERENCE

One common presentation of the delusion of persecution features belief by patients that people are talking about, slandering, or spying on them. When associated with depression, this belief can become a delusion of guilt in which the patients insist that they are being persecuted, justifiably, on the basis of some previous or ongoing action. Delusions of reference are frequent in individuals with paranoid schizophrenia, and similar symptomatology also occurs in a variety of organic conditions. In these situations the persecutors may be specified individuals such as members of the family, business or employment contacts, or neighbors; they may be organized groups such as Communists, Catholics, or Jews, or police organizations such as the FBI or CIA; often, however, the persecutors are identified only as "they," and close questioning as to the identity of "they" produces only vague responses from the patient. Everyday occurrences may be interpreted as clear evidence of the ongoing persecution; often a vast delusional network is built.

DELUSIONS OF LOSS OF PROPERTY

Some individuals are convinced that "they" are attempting to rob them, deprive them of an inheritance, or cheat them out of earnings from an invention, written material, or a business arrangement. In many instances "they" will be identified as family members, business or professional associates, or other known figures; just as frequently the persecutors remain vague.

DELUSIONS OF POISON OR INFECTION

Some patients, particularly those suffering morbid jealousy, develop a firm belief that they are being poisoned.

These individuals tend to blame their current mental or physical problems on sinister alterations to their environment. Delusions of poisoning are often accompanied by hallucinations of smell and/or taste. In some instances the individual attempting the poisoning is named but more often remains unknown, and the patient expresses wonder at why "they" should be doing this to him/her.

DELUSIONS OF INFLUENCE

Delusions of influence include feelings of passivity under the influence of hypnotism or control of the individual's movements or thoughts through radio waves, atomic rays, radar, or other mysterious manipulations. Delusions of influence are most commonly seen in schizophrenics and have long been considered a significant diagnostic criterion for this diagnosis (77, 78). Delusions of influence are related to and, in fact, are often an aspect of a delusion of persecution (7).

DELUSIONS OF INNOCENCE

Opposite in nature but apparently related to the delusion of influence is the delusion of innocence, the firmly held belief in self-justification or acquittal noted in some individuals accused—or who believe themselves accused—of crime, cowardice, or other unacceptable behavior (74). A complex justification, usually based on a matrix of loosely related circumstances, is offered as evidence of innocence or justification for the act. The delusion of innocence appears to exist only in combination with a more primary delusion, almost always that of persecution.

Delusions of persecution occur in a wide and disparate variety of disorders. They make up the major, almost the defining, manifestation of most paranoid states, including paranoid schizophrenia (79), and are often present in individuals suffering severe depression or other overwhelming breakdown of personal integrity. In addition, delusions of persecution occur in both acute and chronic organic mental states (80). Of these, the best known are the psychotic states produced by certain intoxications; amphetamine (81) and cocaine (82), both of which tend to produce bizarre, complex delusions of persecution and fear, are the prime examples.

Treatment for delusions of persecution depends on the underlying etiology. Those produced by chemical intoxicants sometimes respond to simple withdrawal, but intractable persecutory delusions often remain after successful withdrawal from cocaine addiction. The long-lasting fixed delusions seen with structural brain disorder (e.g., frontal brain tumor, traumatic brain injury) and those associated with major psychiatric disorders, such as schizophrenia or depression, demand disease-specific treatment. High-potency neuroleptic medication or electroshock therapy (ECT) may be indicated. Skillful management, including a secure environment (often in the hospital), carefully molded behavioral modification measures, and supportive psycho-

therapy are often necessary. While intense treatment tends to be successful, the results are often transient.

Nihilistic Delusions

For some psychotic patients, parts of themselves (e.g., heart, brain), routinely used objects (e.g., home, telephone), or standard external phenomena (e.g., daylight, time) cease to exist. Originally described in France as a syndrome of negation, nihilistic delusions are also known as *Cotard's syndrome* (83, 84). Many phenomenological variations exist, all based on sharply focused negation. These patients may assert that they have no mind, no intelligence, no existence, or that selected parts of the entire body do not exist. They may deny their own existence or state that the world has stopped and that everyone around them is actually dead. Typically, patients with a nihilistic delusion feel apathetic, hopeless, and internally impoverished; everything is bleak.

Nihilistic delusions can complicate a number of clinical states. The most frequent association is with depression, either agitated depression or melancholia, but severe negation has been reported in schizophrenia, in patients with mixed psychiatric diagnoses, and in states of delirium.

Treatment of nihilistic delusions must be centered on the underlying cause, not the symptom. The disorder is often difficult to treat.

Delusions of Ill Health

Worrying about one's personal health, particularly with advancing age, is extremely common—almost ubiquitous—and excessive concern about the presence of ill health is a frequent psychiatric problem. Delusions of ill health are probably the most common of all delusions (74). Many variations are recognized, with severity ranging from mild anxiety to disabling psychosis. The basic disturbance is a fixed belief that some serious or potentially serious problem of personal health is present. Delusions of ill health are often accompanied by a distrust of the medical profession and family members who ignore the "obvious" predicament described by the patient.

A broad variety of etiologies can produce delusions of ill health. There appears to be little or no correlation between the etiology and the symptom picture described by the patient. Delusions of ill health are common among depressed patients, who may insist that they have an incurable disease such as cancer or a brain tumor or, patients may have the delusional belief that they are incurably insane.

HYPOCHONDRIASIS

Different degrees of hypochondriacal delusion, while traditionally given separate names, have considerable overlap. The described types are differentiated more by degree of complaint than as specific or definable symptom complexes. Although usually ranked as a milder disorder (neurosis), concern about bodily health can become sufficiently severe to be considered delusional. *Briquet's syndrome* (85–87), is a true *hypochondriasis fantastica;* by definition, the patient with this syndrome presents, over a period of years, a series of physical complaints that involve at several different physical systems (e.g., reproductive, nervous, cardiac, pulmonary). The fourth edition of the *Diagnostic and Statistical Manual of Mental Disorders* (4) simplified the clinical description and renamed the problem *somatization disorder.* To fulfill this definition, the patient, predominantly (but not exclusively) female, must have presented at least 8 complaints before age 30, for which no medical justification could be found. In both instances multiple treatments, including extensive use of pharmaceuticals and multiple surgical procedures, cloud the clinical picture. Whether either of these disorders deserves recognition as a delusional system is debatable, but a relationship between a severe degree of hypochondriasis and a delusion of ill health is obvious. (See Chapter 28 for a more extensive discussion of somatization.)

MONOSYMPTOMATIC HYPOCHONDRIASIS

In some patients only a single symptom, organ system, or body part becomes the source of a fixed delusion. The patient may complain that the stomach is being eaten away, that the brain is dissolving, that the body is infested by insects or worms, or that a blemish represents a severe, disfiguring anatomical defect (dysmorphophobia or body dysmorphic disorder). One of the most common variations concerns infestations with bugs, parasites, or other unseeable objects. Parasitosis, also called Ekbom's syndrome, is common in dermatological practice. Published reports (71, 88–90) suggest that many cases of parasitosis have an organic basis (e.g., vascular insufficiency, metabolic disorders). Musalek and colleagues (91) reported good outcome for psychopharmacologic treatment (antidepressants) when parasitosis was based on psychiatric problems, such as depression, but poor results when it was based on organic brain disorders. Monosymptomatic hypochondriacal delusions are relatively common and can be extremely difficult to treat. Body dysmorphic disorder, however, may respond to SSRIs.

SOMATIC DELUSIONS

The most severe and bizarre examples of delusions of ill health, termed somatic delusions, are usually linked with serious mental disorders. The health problem is often fantastic, bizarre, and unbelievable and is tenaciously maintained against all efforts to reassure or disprove. The most dramatic somatic delusions tend to be incongruous (e.g., that a rat is eating away the subject's brain) and tenaciously held despite insistence that the situation is impossible. Treatment of the delusion (rather than the somatic complaint) is actively resisted. Antipsychotic medications can be helpful in some cases, and if depression is the cause, electroshock therapy (ECT) may be of considerable help. If the patient does not respond to more conventional therapy, ECT may also be tried for other suspected causes of the delusion. If there is an organic etiology, the prognosis for the fixed somatic delusion is even worse; while specific therapy (e.g., correction of a thyroid deficiency) may be successful, the delusion often remains unchanged. If the cause is not correctable (e.g., vascular lacunes, progressive dementia), response to empiric approaches, such as psychotropic medications, is usually unsuccessful.

Delusions of Grandeur

Also known as grandiose delusions, expansive delusions, or happiness psychosis, delusions of grandeur are known to occur in a variety of disorders. Some individuals will believe themselves to be God, Jesus, the Virgin Mary, the King of England, or some other exalted person. More often the delusion takes the form of business success, athletic prowess, an ingenious invention, or great wealth. The delusion is often supported by fantastic confabulations, detailed accounts of business or political accomplishments, great athletic feats, international honors, and so forth. At times the degree of confabulation may be sufficient to warrant the term fantastic hallucinosis.

In the 19th century, delusions of grandeur were often described in the general paresis variant of tertiary neurosyphilis. Lues is rarely seen in current practice but until the past few decades, grandiose delusions associated with neurosyphilis remained common in some countries such as India (92) and China (93). Dewhurst (94) suggested that the grandiose delusions associated with syphilis were particularly common in patients from the higher echelons of society, a group that has had little involvement with the disease for many years. Delusions of grandeur have been reported in primitive groups (e.g., cargo cults) (95), but currently mania is by far the most common underlying cause of delusions of grandeur.

Typically, the grandiose patient tends to be bombastic and expansive, expressing delusions of power, wealth, or social position. Manic patients may spend large amounts of money, based on belief of their great wealth. Ecstatic delusions, frequently with strong religious coloring, and megalomania, the belief in one's own supreme importance, are well-known manifestations of manic psychosis. While the patient may boast of fantastic riches, exploits in battle, or superior athletic or sexual prowess, a shallowness and naive quality to the delusion is apparent.

If treated, the delusion of grandeur is usually short-lived and without residuals. In some instances, however, the involved individual may influence others and develop a following, with the potential of producing a political or cult organization; this scenario is especially likely to occur among primitive or oppressed people.

Treatment for delusions of grandeur is closely tied to the etiology. Penicillin and related antispirochetal agents are the treatment of choice for neurosyphilis; adequate treatment of the luetic infection is usually effective in controlling the delusions. Many treatments are currently suggested for mania; the basic therapy consists of lithium, carbamazepine, or valproate, often in conjunction with a neuroleptic. In most instances the delusional quality of the manic episode is either self-limited or comes under control with appropriate treatment.

Delusions of Poverty

The opposite of the grandiose delusion is an unreal belief of extreme poverty. The involved individual feels depleted, impoverished, and, despite adequate finances or even considerable wealth, expresses a feeling of being destitute or in immediate danger of becoming so. Delusions of poverty tend to be associated with a broader, more pervasive nihilistic delusion, a general belief by the patient that he/she is of no value.

Delusions of poverty are most often seen in psychotic depression, and the course usually mirrors the response to the treatment of depression. Both medications and electroshock treatments have been successful. While the delusion may disappear with appropriate therapy, an underlying feeling of monetary concern often persists as part of an ongoing depressive personality.

Delusions of Possession

The belief that one's body is possessed by God, by a mystic power figure, by the Devil, by a lesser demon, or by an animal dates to antiquity (96). Supernatural possession ranks among the earliest explanations of illness and is still employed to explain incompletely understood phenomena, particularly by the poorly educated. Serious mental illnesses, such as schizophrenia, severe depression, delirium, or dementia can produce possession states. Of 1,029 psychotic patients surveyed in Japanese mental hospitals (97), possession states were reported by 20.7%; females were involved more often, but no relationship was demonstrated between the possession state and any specific psychiatric diagnosis. Organic factors are seldom suggested as the source of possession states. Mesulam (98), however, reported four individuals from an epilepsy clinic who told of demonic possession, and he suggested a correlation between temporal lobe epilepsy and possession state.

Typically, possession is embedded in a rich, cohesive supernaturalistic belief system that pervades some or all of an individual's actions. Belief in demonic possession is limited, however, even in primitive cultures, and tends to be associated with a particular sociocultural milieu. Possession states have been linked with an individual's inability to cope with the evils of society (99–101). As Pattison (102) explains, "Demonic possession is highly correlated with social oppression and stagnation; it expresses both individual and social unrest." Another factor—the suspension of critical self-analysis—must be present. Possession states, particularly if maintained for any significant duration, demand a strong supernaturalistic belief system, an inability to cope effectively with problems inherent in the individual's society, and a problem in reality testing.

Delusions of possession are difficult to treat. Understanding an individual case of demonic possession requires comprehension of the underlying cultural construct as well as the individual's personal problems. Successful management involves culturally-sensitive treatment of the patient's mental illness.

Delusions of Love

Although often considered a variant of the common paranoid syndromes (74, 84) and providing dramatic, difficult-to-overlook, presentations, erotic delusions are relatively uncommon. Pertinent literature is sparse, and categorization within the disorder remains difficult. Two documented variations—the phantom lover syndrome, and erotomania (belief that one is loved by a powerful and/or prominent person)—have been detailed (7, 103). Whether the object of the delusion is imagined (phantom lover) or a real person (as in de Clerambault's syndrome) is the distinguishing feature. In both, the predominant finding is a *feeling* by the patient, most often female, that she is loved, admired, and adored by another person, often of a high social rank (e.g., royalty, movie star). The patient is firmly convinced that the person is madly in love with her, although the two may never have spoken or met. The object of the delusion usually remains stable, often for many years. In some instances, however, the "lover" changes with circumstances; thus, a female, convinced that her psychiatrist was madly in love with her, changed the lover's identity when she came under the care of a new psychiatrist.

Best known of the delusions of love is *de Clerambault's syndrome "psychose passionelle,"* erotomania) (103–105). Many thoughts and actions of the individual are devoted to the delusional relationship with many everyday occurrences misinterpreted as proof of the man's love. The object of the passion may be pestered with letters, and the patient's attentions may become so forward as to be dangerous to the love object or his family. Based on the delusional level of misinterpretation, erotomania is often considered a variant of paranoid schizophrenia, but other schizophrenic symptoms are not present. More recent investigations suggest a heterogeneous group of diagnoses, including delusional disorder, schizophrenia, and schizo-affective disorder (106). With the exception of the delusion of love, thinking tends to be well-organized in the involved individuals.

All of the originally reported cases of de Clerambault's syndrome were described as free of organic disorder, but several later reports (107, 108) have presented examples of the syndrome in individuals with brain damage or epilepsy. The relationship of erotomania to any recognized neurological or psychiatric entity remains uncertain.

Management of an erotic delusion, either the phantom lover syndrome or de Clerambault's syndrome, is difficult and may actually be dangerous. Psychotropic medications or ECT can reduce the power of the delusion, occasionally bringing about a total cure but more often producing a state of loss. The patient may act out against the loss, threatening self-harm or an attack on the object of the delusion. Careful, skillful psychotherapy is essential. A delusion of love is powerful, and attempts to remove the delusion demand extreme caution on the part of the treating physician.

Delusions of Jealousy

Delusions of jealousy, also known as morbid jealousy or delusions of infidelity, are fairly common and occur in a variety of organic and "functional" states. The patient is often said to have had a sensitive, suspicious, and mildly jealous nature before onset of the psychosis. Metabolic intoxications, particularly alcohol addiction, are common in individuals who describe morbid jealousy (109). During the course of the illness, a suspicious, insecure person becomes convinced of infidelity by his/her spouse or significant other. The severity of the delusion fluctuates; during psychotic episodes the patient may question his/her spouse incessantly, keep him/her awake for hours at night, search his/her clothes for stains or body hairs, and proffer physical stigmata on the part of the spouse (e.g., insomnia, poor appetite, tired look, bags under the eyes) as "evidence" of infidelity. The spouse may be beaten or tortured by the patient in attempts to extract a confession; even murder can occur. Except for the morbid jealousy, the patient often displays no symptoms suggestive of serious mental disorder. In general the delusion tends to run a more benign course than other types of delusions (110). Rarely does the patient develop other evidence of psychosis.

Delusions of Reduplication

While not common in either psychiatric or neurological practice, delusions of reduplication, including the delusion that a person has been replaced by an imposter or that a building or possession has been duplicated elsewhere, deserve consideration among the recognized delusions. The findings are consistently dramatic and tend to be sufficiently bizarre that psychiatric consultation is requested. Reduplication of place has traditionally been associated with organic brain disease, whereas reduplication of person was, until recent years, classed as an unusual variation of psychiatric disorder. Phenomenologically, reduplication syndromes are related, differing only in the object being duplicated. Four variations are described here.

REDUPLICATIVE PARAMNESIA

Reduplication of place has been recognized for many years. Originally described in brain-injured subjects (111, 112), reduplicative paramnesia has always been considered a brain abnormality. The patient involved almost invariably recognizes and remembers the name of the hospital or institution but insists that it is located in a different community or area, usually closer to his or her own home. The patient may be normally competent in other cognitive functions (e.g., memory or visuospatial skills) but adamantly maintains, against constantly reiterated proof, that the institution is located elsewhere. The disorder is most commonly described as a stage of recovery from severe brain trauma. The cases reported since the availability of brain imaging have almost always had demonstrable frontal pathology (113, 114); some suggest that the syndrome represents frontal pathology plus right parietal damage (115). While often occurring in individuals who have suffered and are recovering from serious memory disorder, reduplicative paramnesia demands, by definition, some ability to learn new information (e.g., the name of the hospital). In the best described cases, only the geographical repositioning of place is held in a fixed delusional manner and the disorder tends to be transient.

REDUPLICATION OF PERSON

First described by French psychiatrists (116), reduplication of person has come to be known as the *Capgras syndrome* and is usually discussed as an unusual psychiatric problem (84, 117). The patient with this disorder holds a strong, fixed belief that a person or persons (usually a family member or someone closely associated with the patient) has been replaced by an imposter of nearly identical physical appearance and possessing similar identifying features (e.g., same name, age, number of children, location of home). Despite constant assurances by the individual who is the object of the delusion and by multiple friends, acquaintances, and therapists, the patient remains convinced that the individual is an imposter.

The bizarre nature and strongly fixed quality of the delusion has suggested schizophrenia, and most cases of Capgras syndrome are seen and reported by psychiatrists. More recently, the Capgras syndrome has been described in patients with obvious organic brain disease (118, 119). Most contemporary descriptions now suggest that organic brain disorder is significant in the genesis of the syndrome (120–122). Merrin and Silberfarb (119) noted that the age of onset of the Capgras syndrome averaged 61, far later than the usual age of onset of schizophrenia. In 1986, Hay (123) reported two individuals who developed the Capgras phenomenon following a course of ECT; the reduplication syndrome remitted as the ECT-induced organic brain syndrome cleared.

A related but phenomenologically distinct disorder, the *delusion of de Fregoli* (124, 125) identifies a situation in which a specific person, usually a suspected tormentor, is believed by the patient to change into different people encountered by the patient. Many dissimilar individuals are misidentified by the patient as the specified person (the opposite of the Capgras phenomenon). Even though the physical differences of the misidentified individuals can be adequately described by the patient, he or she remains firmly convinced that they all represent the same individual, either in disguise or magically transformed.

MISIDENTIFICATION OF SELF

A rare variation of delusional reduplication concerns the self. The patient has a fixed, delusional belief that his/her persona is actually occupied by some other person or by an identical person (self-double; *doppelgänger*) (126). The delusion of self-misidentification is often related to delusions of persecution, including delusions of guilt.

MISIDENTIFICATION OF OBJECTS

Some individuals, particularly those suffering persecutory feelings, will insist that an object (e.g., their coat, their car, an object on their dressing table) has been moved or has been replaced with a similar item. While relatively common as a symptom, particularly in paranoid populations, only rarely does this phenomenon reach sufficient severity to disable the patient and warrant classification as an individual delusion.

Reduplicative phenomena have been considered evidence of schizophrenia or have been given psychodynamic or psychoanalytic explanations (124, 127, 128). Signer (129) found that 46% of the cases of reduplication of person in the literature had been considered depressed; Foerstl (121) proposed that a combination of psychiatric disorder plus organic brain damage was present in reduplicative syndromes. Benson and Studd (130), based on brain trauma cases, noted that reduplicative phenomena occur when frontal damage/dysfunction is present. They also suggested that, although frontal disorder alone was not sufficient to produce the phenomenon, it is an essential element for psychotically held reduplications and the presence of frontal dysfunction in other psychotic syndromes is a currently popular concept (131, 132).

Along with the altered ideas concerning etiology, treatment for the delusions of reduplication has changed over the years. Psychodynamically directed behavioral conditioning therapy was attempted, particularly in cases with the Capgras syndrome (127, 133), but reduplicative phenomena have not, in general, been aided by psychotherapy (134). If an acute organic psychosyndrome is the cause (e.g., post-ECT or recent brain trauma), the prognosis for eventual recovery is relatively good (113). If, however, a stable, noncorrectable organic problem (such as an old stroke or chronic residua of brain trauma) is the source of the reduplicative syndrome, the prognosis for recovery must be considered guarded. Indirect therapy aimed at symptom control, such as behavioral conditioning or psychotropic medication, becomes necessary.

DISCUSSION

As the previous sections have illustrated, multiple variations of hallucinations and delusions are documented and recognized. Phenomenologically, hallucinations and delusions are discrete entities, easily distinguished from each other by definition. There are many similarities, however, and the boundaries are insecure. The defining difficulty underlying hallucinatory experiences is an *abnormality of percept,* whereas the difficulty underlying delusions is an *abnormality of thought.* In both disorders, the basic problem can be considered misinterpretation. The boundary between hallucinations and delusions, while distinct, is also artificial, as they share the essential feature of disordered interpretation.

To evaluate distinctions between hallucinations and delusions, we provide three approaches. Each is significant for the neuropsychiatrist. One stresses an anatomical distinction, the second concerns disordered mechanisms, and the third focuses on the psychological state in which the problem develops.

Anatomical Basis of Hallucinations and Delusions

From an anatomical viewpoint, a significant differentiation can be suggested. Hallucinations, involving only a single perceptual modality, are truly unimodal neural activities. In contrast, delusions involve a more complex system, utilizing experiential data from multiple modalities, a polymodal brain activity. The separation is not trivial; totally different cortical regions are the sites of unimodal and multimodal associations.

For purposes of discussion, refer to the simple hierarchy of cortical function shown in Table 14.1. Each of the four cortical areas is, to a large degree, anatomically discrete. In addition, many clinical observations and mountains of experimental data indicate that the functions subserved by these four areas are entirely different. Thus, an obvious difference between hallucinatory experiences and delusional thinking concerns the area of cortex involved.

Each major sensory modality (vision, audition, somesthesis) has an area of primary or isotypical cortex dedicated to the reception of signals from that sensory system. Each primary sensory (and motor) cortex is anatomically distinct, both histologically and in location (Fig. 14.1). Each region has a contiguous, sizable territory of cortex dedicated to processing stimuli from that modality (unimodal association cortex).

Although the primary cortex is relatively limited in size, the surrounding unimodal association cortex is extensive (Fig. 14.2). Within the unimodal sensory cortex, sensory stimuli are processed through stages of quantitative and qualitative discriminations, differentiated from simultaneously received stimuli and compared to previous experiences of a similar nature. These processing functions increase in complexity to form a unimodal percept, a composite realization of the perceived stimulus as related to previously

Table 14.1.   Cortical Areas

Primary (isotypical) cortex
Unimodal association cortex
Heteromodal association cortex
Supramodal association cortex

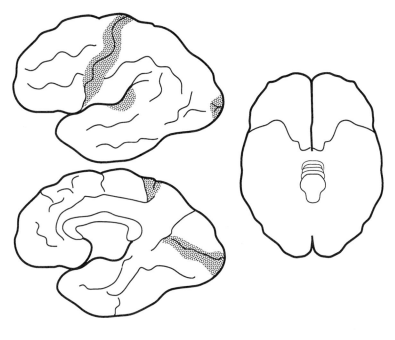

Figure 14.1 Outlines of lateral, sagittal, and inferior views of human brain with areas of primary (isotypical) sensory and motor cortex indicated with stippling.

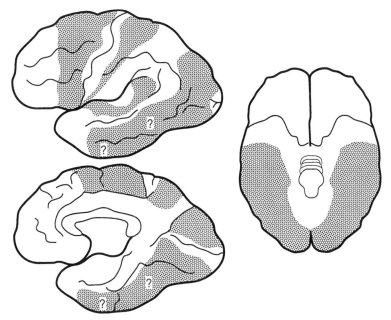

Figure 14.2 Outlines of human brain with unimodal association cortex indicated with stippling. The question marks indicate areas of advanced unimodal association that may involve some cross-modal activity.

experienced stimuli. The comparison process demands a massive memory bank to maintain previously experienced stimuli. Processing is performed through multiple synaptic connections in tightly interrelated loops to form reverberating circuits within the unimodal territory. Malfunction at any step within the single modality neural matrix (from the source of stimulation to the unimodal association cortex) can lead to an hallucinatory experience.

In the next step, unimodal percepts are combined (associated) with other unimodal percepts, with memories of prior events and, eventually, with emotional and limbic influences to form the complex concepts of a cognitive process (thought). Much of this process occurs in heteromodal association cortex (135). The original associations made in this region, simple cross-modality associations that

link unimodal percepts with memories of prior multimodality experiences, occur, to a large degree, in the parietotemporal heteromodal association cortex. In all but the most elementary instances, however, cognition demands additional processing, including serial management over time. The phenomenon of maintaining and processing serial data has been called working memory (136, 137), temporal gradient (138), or sequencing (115). Both clinical observations and animal experimental data indicate that serial information is processed in the anterior heteromodal association cortex, primarily the lateral prefrontal area. Heteromodal association cortex, therefore, consists of two sizable areas of association cortex (anterior and posterior) containing the neural circuits that carry out cognitive processing. Figure 14.3 illustrates these areas. Polymodal circuits in-

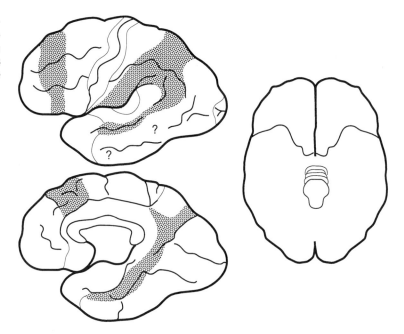

Figure 14.3 Outlines of human brain with heteromodal association cortex indicated with stippling. The question marks indicate areas that may have some cross-modal function.

clude neural structures located at a distance from each other and often involve both hemispheres. They are large, complex networks capable of processing multimodality cognitive experiences. Delusions can be said to arise from abnormal function within the heteromodal association system.

An anatomical basis for the disturbed competency in reality testing of both hallucinations and delusions can be suggested as another factor common to both.

Clinical experience indicates that a separate and relatively distinct cortical area is critical for reality testing. It has long been recognized that individuals who suffer anterior frontal pathology, particularly trauma or tumor, tend to lose the ability to anticipate, inhibit verbal or motor activities, maintain concentration, and test reality. Anterior prefrontal cortex (supramodal association cortex) appears to monitor the multiple, simultaneously active cognitive neural networks, make judgments (based in part on limbic input), inhibit most cognitive activities, and thereby select the cognitive activities to receive prime awareness. When the monitoring function is deficient, reality testing becomes incompetent, and both hallucinatory experiences and delusions can be interpreted as real. Dysfunction of supramodal association cortex (Fig. 14.4) appears to be a key factor in the formation of both hallucinatory experiences and delusional thinking.

Mechanisms of Hallucinations and Delusions

Table 14.2 presents five mechanisms that have been suggested as a genesis for hallucinatory experiences. Each is discussed separately in the sections that follow.

DISORDERS OF ATTENTION/AROUSAL

The most common mechanism for hallucination production is a disturbance of *attention and/or arousal* (139). Sleep deprivation, narcolepsy, dream states, drug intoxications,

and the hallucinations of acute confusion all feature disturbed attention/arousal. Impaired information processing is combined with a failure of cerebral gating and decreased ability to inhibit extraneous thoughts, allowing hallucinatory experiences to arise.

SENSORY INPUT DISORDERS

Sensory input disorders, such as the sudden onset of blindness, can lead to hallucinatory experiences. Apparently, associations formed in the unimodal association cortex continue functioning as though receiving input, producing an hallucinatory experience, a so-called release hallucination.

STIMULATION DISORDERS

Stimulation disorders, such as seizures, can produce hallucinatory experiences in the absence of an external stimulation. Epileptic auras represent a prime example of a hallucinatory stimulation disorder. The electrical studies of Penfield and Jasper (140) and many others (141–143) demonstrate genesis of hallucinations by electrical stimulation.

LIMBIC OVERLOAD DISORDERS

Excessive stimulation of the limbic circuits responsible for the affective tone of life experiences can produce overvaluation of certain stimuli. When limbic input is thus manipulated (e.g., hostage situations), the resulting hallucinations often lead to delusional thinking. It is reasonable to hypothesize that many classic psychiatric disorders are based on limbic malfunction; as yet, however, there is no firm experimental validation.

EXECUTIVE CONTROL DISORDERS

The final suggested mechanism, *executive control disorder,* refers to a disturbance of self-criticism, with decreased ability

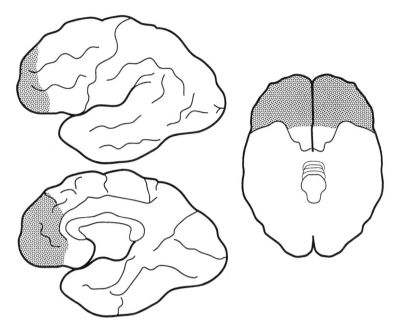

Figure 14.4 Outlines of human brain with supramodal association cortex indicated with stippling.

Table 14.2. Mechanisms of Hallucination Production[a]

Arousal/attention disorders
Sensory input disorders
Stimulation disorders
Limbic overload disorders
Executive control disorders

[a]Adapted from Benson DF, Gorman DG. The neural basis of hallucinations. In: Appel SH, ed. Current neurology, vol. 13. Chicago: Mosby-Year Book (in press).

to separate the experiences being processed into categories of reality or fantasy. Firmly held hallucinatory experiences occurring in individuals with other evidence of judgment disorder would fall into this category.

While most hallucinatory experiences can be subsumed within the mechanistic categorization suggested above, no similar classification of the mechanisms of delusions has been satisfactory. Freud's attempted explanation of delusions based on latent homosexuality has not survived. One later attempt, that of the Heidelberg School (Jaspers, Schneider, Gruhle, Meyer-Gross), divided delusions into primary and secondary variations. Primary delusional experiences represented formation of new meaning for psychological events. Three variations were suggested—delusional mood, delusional perception, and sudden delusional ideation. Primary delusions were considered evidence of schizophrenia. Secondary delusions were thought to arise from a morbid experience. Delusions associated with depressive mood or with ill health, and many of the projective (paranoid) delusions would fit into this categorization. Unfortunately, this categorization fails to explain the mechanisms leading to the delusions.

Other schools of psychiatric thought have produced theoretical mechanisms for delusions. Existentialists attempt to explain delusions as altered interpretations of world design or inner attitudes. Pathological affect is suggested as the basic cause of delusions. Advocates of behavior therapy have explained delusions as a pathological learning process in which the delusion represents a learned method of avoiding unpleasant emotions. The increasing recognition that delusions can occur in organic mental states provides an additional potential for explaining delusions but, to date, organic explanations remain mysterious; why some individuals develop delusions with amphetamine or other drug abuse while others do not remains enigmatic.

Psychological Basis of Hallucinations and Delusions

Attempts to explain hallucinations and/or delusions on a psychological basis have also encountered considerable difficulty. The ubiquitous occurrence and on/off status make many hallucinatory experiences difficult to explain on a psychological basis. On the other hand, it has been noted that the content of hallucinatory experiences may reflect the psychological background (144). Table 14.3 presents a number of proposed psychological explanations of hallucinatory mechanisms.

The *conditioning theory* of hallucination formation is derived from classic conditioning experimentation—production of an hallucinated image (unconditioned stimulus) from a conditioning stimulus. The *seepage theory* suggests that a decrease in cortical scanning ability (an arousal/attention disorder) can alter image strength sufficiently to produce an hallucination. The opposite, the *imagery theory*, holds that exceptionally vivid imagery (plus a defect in reality testing) can lead to hallucinations. The *subvocalization theory* is more limited—auditory hallucinations may be due to either inappropriately monitored inner speech or incursion of right hemisphere speech into left hemisphere language comprehension (or vice versa). Finally, *integration theory* recognizes that the problem may lie in differentiating real from imagined stimuli.

Table 14.3. Theories of Psychological Mechanisms Producing Hallucinations

Conditioning theory
Seepage theory
Imagery theory
Subvocalization theory
a. Disordered inner speech
b. Incursion by right hemisphere speech
Integration theory

[a]Adapted from Bentall RP. The illusion of reality: a review and integration of psychological research on hallucinations. Psychol Bull 1990; 107:82–95.

Delusional thinking may have proved difficult to explain by consistent psychological mechanisms (76) but the nature of the disorder has led to many suggested psychological explanations (145). Anomalous perceptual experiences that lead to thought disorder are often suggested (146) and the relationship between psychotic delusions and less deviant but still aberrant beliefs has been explored (147). Disturbing social experiences establishing delusional defense mechanisms has been a suggested explanation (148), and reasons for an individual's vulnerability to delusional belief have been explored (149). Personality disorder, situational stresses (particularly recurrent), and cultural background have been proposed as significant in the formation of delusional beliefs (150). There is a growing tendency for investigators to study such factors in a longitudinal manner and to suggest that delusional thinking is a product of repeated stress, not a disorder based on a single, acute situational problem (151). Variations in the content of delusional beliefs, both with and without pharmaceutical intervention, have been studied. Also, response to psychological manipulation as a means of treatment of delusion has been reported, with inferences drawn concerning the basis of the delusion (152).

Despite the many psychological approaches proposed over the years, a consistent psychological explanation for delusional beliefs remains elusive. Psychological factors are, nonetheless, obviously significant in the content and quite possibly govern the formation and longitudinal consistency of a delusion. Psychological factors clearly affect both the genesis and course of delusional thinking.

SUMMARY

The information presented in this chapter proposes that hallucinatory experiences and delusional thinking are products of disturbed neural function and that the primary difference between the two phenomena reflects the cortical regions involved. One common thread, the abnormality of reality testing, is prominent in both disorders and indicates malfunction in yet another cortical area. The simple, anatomical view of hallucinations and delusions suggested here, although parsimonious, is inadequate. Many mechanisms have been demonstrated that help explain hallucinations; similar explanations of the mechanisms that can lead to delusions have been less successful. To some degree for hallucinations, and to a considerable degree for delusions, a psychological basis can be established for the contents of the experience. Whether the specific contents are important in the genesis or merely represent the subject of a delusion remains uncertain. Three factors—anatomical basis, mechanical operations, and psychological composition—appear significant.

For purposes of treatment, the most approachable of the multiple factors active in the production of hallucinations and/or delusions must be selected. In some instances an anatomical basis can be demonstrated and appropriate treatment instituted. Far more often the cause of abnormality is explicable only as a disorder affecting one of the functional mechanisms; treatment can be based on this knowledge. Finally, in some instances the composition of the abnormal experience is of prime significance, and appropriately directed manipulation will be the therapy of choice.

While remaining exotic and mysterious, a sizable number of hallucinations and delusions become explicable within the framework just outlined. Continued investigations within this multifaceted structure will lead to better understanding of these dramatic neuropsychiatric disturbances.

References

1. Maltbie AA. Psychosis. In: Cavenar JO, Brodie HKH, eds. Signs and symptoms in psychiatry. Philadelphia: JB Lippincott, 1983:413–432.
2. Ellenberger HF. The discovery of the unconscious. New York: Basic Books, 1970.
3. Veith I. Hysteria, the history of a disease. Chicago: University of Chicago Press, 1965.
4. American Psychiatric Association. Diagnostic and statistical manual of mental disorders. 4th ed.—revised. Washington: American Psychiatric Association, 1994.
5. Buss AH. Psychopathology. New York: John Wiley & Sons, 1966.
6. Cummings JL, Syndulko K, Goldberg Z. Palinopsia reconsidered. Neurology 1982;32:444–447.
7. Hamilton M, ed. Fish's clinical psychopathology. 2nd ed. Bristol: Wright, 1985.
8. Zaret BS. Lightning streaks of Moore: a cause of recurrent stereotypic visual disturbance. Neurology 1985;35:1078–1081.
9. Davis FA, Bergen D, Schauf C, McDonald I, Deutsch W. Movement phosphenes in optic neuritis: a new clinical sign. Neurology 1976;26:1100–1104.
10. Jacobs L, Karpik A, Bozian D, Gothgen S. Auditory-visual synesthesia. Arch Neurol 1981;38:211–216.
11. Lessell C, Cohen MM. Phosphenes induced by sound. Neurology 1979;29:1524–1527.
12. Cohn R. Phantom vision. Arch Neurol 1971;25:468–471.
13. Lepore FE. Spontaneous visual phenomena with visual loss: 104 patients with lesions of retinal and neural afferent pathways. Neurology 1990;40:444–447.
14. Bender MD, Feldman M, Sobin AJ. Palinopsia. Brain 1968;91:321–338.
15. Critchley M. The parietal lobes. London: Edward Arnold and Co., 1953.
16. Johnson SF, Loge RV. Palinopsia due to nonketotic hyperglycemia. West J Med 1988;148:331–332.
17. Hughes MS, Lessell S. Trazodone induced palinopsia. Arch Ophthalmol 1990;108:339–400.
18. Lefebre C, Kolmel HW. Palinopsia as an epileptic phenomenon. Eur Neurol 1989;29:323–327.
19. Michel EM, Troost BT. Palinopsia: cerebral localization with computed tomography. Neurology 1980;30:887–889.

20. Young WB, Heros DO, Ehrenberg BL, Hedges TR. Metamorphopsia and palinopsia. Arch Neurol 1989;46:820–822.

21. Gates TJ, Stagno SJ, Gulledge AD. Palinopsia posing as a psychiatric depression. Br J Psychiatry 1988;153:391–393.

22. Morsier G. Les hallucinations. Rev Oto-neuro-ophthalmol 1938;16:244–352.

23. Berrios GE, Brook P. The Charles Bonnet syndrome and the problem of visual perceptual disorders in the elderly. Age Ageing 1982;11:17–23.

24. Berrios GE, Brook P. Visual hallucinations and sensory delusions in the elderly. Br J Psychiatry 1984;144:662–664.

25. Damas-Mora J, Skelton-Robinson M, Jenner FA. The Charles Bonnet syndrome in perspective. Psychol Med 1982;12:251–261.

26. Saitkowski M, Zimmer B, Rosenberg PR. The Charles Bonnet syndrome. J Clin Neurol Ophthalmol 1990;10:215–218.

27. Cogan DG. Neurology of the visual system. Springfield, IL: Charles C Thomas, 1966.

28. Gold K, Rabins PV. Isolated visual hallucinations and the Charles Bonnet syndrome: a review of the literature and presentation of six cases. Compr Psychiatry 1989;30:90–98.

29. Podoll K, Osterheider M, Noth J. [The Charles Bonnet syndrome] Neurologische Klinik mit Klinischer Neurophysiologie Essen. Fortschr Neurol Psychiatr 1989;57:43–60.

30. Adams RD, Victor M. Principles of neurology. 4th ed. New York: McGraw-Hill, 1989.

31. Kolmel HW. Peduncular hallucinations. J Neurol 1991;238:457–459.

32. Lhermitte J. Syndrome de la calotte pédoncle cérébral. Les troubles psychosensorielles dans les lesions du mesencéphale. Rev Neurol (Paris) 1922;38:1359–1365.

33. Dunn DW, Weisberg LA, Nadell J. Peduncular hallucinations caused by brainstem compression. Neurology 1983;33:1360–1361.

34. McKee AC, Levine DN, Kowall NW, et al. Peduncular hallucinosis associated with isolated infarction of the substantia nigra pars reticulata. Ann Neurol 1990;27:500–504.

35. Brust JC, Behrens MM. "Release hallucinations" as the major symptom of posterior cerebral artery occlusion. Ann Neurol 1977;2:432–436.

36. Rozanski J. Peduncular hallucinosis following vertebral angiography. Neurology 1952;2:341–349.

37. Smith RA, Gelles DB, Vanderhaegen JJ. Subcortical visual hallucinations. Cortex 1971;7:162–168.

38. Weinberger LM, Grant FC. Visual hallucinations and their neurooptical correlates. Arch Ophthalmol 1940;23:166–199.

39. Penfield W. Engrams in the human brain. Proc R Soc Med 1968;61:831–840.

40. Naito H, Matsui N. Temporal lobe epilepsy with ictal ecstatic state and interictal behavior of hypergraphia. J Nerv Ment Dis 1988;176:123–124.

41. Ardila A, Sanchez E. Neuropsychological symptoms in the migraine syndrome. Cephalalgia 1988;8:67–70.

42. Mendez M. Acute confutional state. In: Bradley WG, Daroff RB, Fenichel GM, Marsden CD, eds. Neurology in clinical practice. Boston: Butterworth-Heinemann 1991:31–42.

43. Cummings JL. Clinical neuropsychiatry. Orlando, FL: Grune & Stratton, 1985.

44. Abraham K. Selected papers on psychoanalysis. New York: Basic Books, 1953.

45. Mueser KT, Bellack AS, Brady EU. Hallucinations in schizophrenia. Acta Psychiatr Scand 1990;82:26–29.

46. Houston F, Royse AB. Relationship between deafness and psychotic illness. J Ment Sci 1954;100:990–993.

47. Jacobs L, Feldman M, Diamond SP, et al. Palinacousis: persistent or recurring auditory sensations. Cortex 1973;9:275–287.

48. Patterson MC, Tomlinson FH, Stuart GG. Palinacousis: a case report. Neurosurgery 1988;22:1088–1090.

49. Miller TC, Crosby TW. Musical hallucinations in a deaf elderly patient. Ann Neurol 1979;5:301–302.

50. Ross ED, Jossman PB, Bell B. Musical hallucinations in deafness. JAMA 1975;231:620–622.

51. Berrios GE. Hallucinosis. In: Frederiks JAM, ed. Handbook of clinical neurology, vol 2(46): neurobehavioral disorders. New York: Elsevier, 1985:561–572.

52. Currie S, Heathfield KWG, Henson RA, Scott DF. Clinical course and prognosis of temporal lobe epilepsy. Brain 1971;94:173–190.

53. Sherwin I, Peron-Magnan P, Bancaud J, Bonis A, Talairach J. Prevalence of psychosis in epilepsy as a function of the laterality of the epileptogenic lesion. Arch Neurol 1982;39:621–625.

54. Victor M. Neurologic disorders due to alcoholism and malnutrition. In Joynt RJ, ed. Clinical neurology, vol 4. Philadelphia: JB Lippincott, 1986:1–94.

55. Victor M, Hope JM. The phenomenon of auditory hallucinations in chronic alcoholism. J Nerv Ment Dis 1958;126:451–481.

56. Glass IB. Alcoholic hallucinosis. A psychiatric enigma. Br J Addict 1989;84:29–41.

57. Perez MM, Trimble MR, Murray NMF, Reider I. Epileptic psychosis—an evaluation of PSE profiles. Br J Psychiatry 1985;146:155–163.

58. Kluft RP. First-rank symptoms as a diagnostic clue to multiple personality disorder. Am J Psychiatry 1987;144:393–398.

59. Kaufman MD, Lassiter KR, Shenoy BV. Paroxysmal unilateral dysosmia: a cured patient. Ann Neurol 1988;24:450–451.

60. Morrison DP. Abnormal perceptual experiences in migraine. Cephalalgia 1990;10:273–277.

61. Hausser-Hauw C, Bancaud J. Gustatory hallucinations in epileptic syndromes. Electrophysiological, clinical and anatomical correlates. Brain 1987;110:339–359.

62. Faris AA, Terrence CF. Limbic system symptomatology associated with a colloid cyst of the third ventricle. J Neurol 1989;236:60–61.

63. Takahashi H, Takeda S, Ikuta F, Homma Y. Progressive supranuclear palsy with limbic system involvement: report of a case with ultrastructural investigation of neurofibrillary tangles in various locations. Clin Neuropathol 1987;6:271–276.

64. Siegel RK. Cocaine hallucinations. Am J Psychiatry 1978;135:309–314.

65. Toone BK. Psychomotor seizures, arterio-venous malformation and the olfactory reference syndrome. A case report. Acta Psychiatr Scand 1978;58:61–66.

66. Jensen TS, Krebs B, Nielsen J, Rasmussen P. Phantom limb, phantom pain and stump pain in amputees during the first 6 months following limb amputation. Pain 1983;17:243–256.

67. Sherman RA, Sherman CJ. Prevalence and characteristics of chronic phantom limb pain among American veterans. Results of a trial survey. Am J Phys Med 1983;62:227–238.

68. Melzack R. Labat lecture. Phantom limbs. Reg Anaesth 1989;14:208–211.

69. Melzack R. Phantom limbs and the concept of a neuromatrix. Trends Neurosci 1990;13:88–92.

70. Awada A. Isolated cheiro-facial formication caused by a thalamic hematoma. Rev Neurol (Paris) 1989;145:861–862.

71. Flynn FG, Cummings JL, Scheibel J, Wirshing W. Monosymptomatic delusions of parasitosis associated with ischemic cerebrovascular disease. J Geriatr Psychiatry Neurol 1989;2:134–139.

72. Cytowic RE, Wood FB. Synesthesia. I. A review of major theories and their brain basis. Brain Cogn 1982;1:23–25.

73. Vike J, Jabbari B, Maitland CG. Auditory-visual synesthesia. Arch Neurol 1984;41:680–681.

74. Nash JL. Delusions. In: Cavenar JO Jr, Brodie HK, eds. Signs and symptoms in psychiatry. Philadelphia: JB Lippincott, 1983:455–481.

75. Freud S. Psychoanalytische Bemerkungen über einen autobiographische beschreibenen Fall von Paranoia (Dementia Paranoides). Jahrbuch für psychoanalytische und psychopathologische Forschungen 1911. The works of Sigmund Freud, collected papers (Strachey J, transl). London: Hogarth, 1955:387–470.

76. Oltmanns TF, Maher BA. Delusional beliefs. New York: John Wiley & Sons, 1988.

77. Mellor CS. First rank symptoms of schizophrenia. Br J Psychiatry 1970;117:15–23.
78. Schneider C. Die Schizophrenen Symptomverbande. Berlin: Springer, 1942.
79. Lucas CJ, Sainsbury P, Collins JG. A social and clinical study of delusions in schizophrenia. J Ment Sci 1962;108:747–758.
80. Lishman WA. Organic psychiatry. 2nd ed. Oxford: Blackwell Scientific Publications, 1987.
81. Connell PH. Amphetamine psychosis (Maudsley monograph no. 5). London: Chapman and Hall, 1958.
82. Siegel RK. Cocaine hallucinations. Am J Psychiatry 1978;135:309–314.
83. Arieti S, Bemporad JR. Rare, unclassifiable and collective psychiatric syndromes. In: Arieti S, ed. American handbook of psychiatry, vol 3. 2nd ed. New York: Basic Books 1974:710–722.
84. Rudnick FD. The paranoid-erotic syndromes. In: Friedmann CTH, Faguet RA, eds. Extraordinary disorders of human behavior. New York: Plenum Press, 1982:99–120.
85. Bibb RC, Guze SB. Hysteria (Briquet's syndrome) in a psychiatric hospital. Am J Psychiatry 1972;129:224–228.
86. Briquet P. Traite Clinique et Therapeutique a l'Hysterie. Paris: Bailliere et Eils, 1859.
87. Guze SB, Perley MJ. Observations on the natural history of hysteria. Am J Psychiatry 1963;119:960–965.
88. de Leon J, Antelo RE, Simpson G. Delusions of parasitosis, or chronic tactile hallucinosis. Comparative Psychiatry 1992;33:25-33.
89. de Leon OA, Schlager H, Kravcio JT. Pathogenesis of the delusional formation in Ekbom's syndrome. Rev Med Panama 1990;15:42–49.
90. Liebowitz R, Nuetzel EJ, Bowser AE, Klein DF. Phenelzine and delusions of parasitosis. Am J Psychiatry 1978;135:1565–1566.
91. Musalek M, Bach M, Gerstberger K, Lesch OM. Drug therapy of delusional parasitosis. Wien Medicine Wochenschrift 1989;139:297–302.
92. Varma P. The incidence and clinical features of general paresis. Indian Journal of Neurology and Psychiatry 1952;3:141–163.
93. Liu MC. General paresis of the insane in Peking between 1933 and 1943. J Ment Sci 1960;106:1082–1092.
94. Dewhurst K. The neurosyphilitic psychoses today: a survey of 91 cases. Br J Psychiatry 1969;115:31–38.
95. Burton-Bradley BG. Cargo cult syndromes. In: Friedmann CTH, Faguet RA, eds. Extraordinary disorders of human behavior. New York: Plenum Press, 1982:191–202.
96. Oesterreich TK. Possessions: demonical and other among primitive races in antiquity, the middle ages and modern times. New York: NYU Press, 1966.
97. Iida J. The current situation in regard to the delusion of possession in Japan. Japn J Psychiatry Neurol 1989;43:19–27.
98. Mesulam M-M. Dissociative states with abnormal temporal lobe EEG. Arch Neurol 1981;38:176–181.
99. Bourguignon E. Possessions. San Francisco: Chandler and Sharp, 1976.
100. Carstairs GM, Kapur RL. The Great universe of Kota. Stress, change and mental disorder in an Indian village. Berkeley: University of California Press, 1976.
101. Wijesinghe CP, Dissanayake SAW, Mendis N. Possession in a semi-urban community in Sri Lanka. Aust N Z J Psychiatry 1976;10:135–139.
102. Pattison EM. Possession states and exorcism. In: Friedmann CTH, Faguet RA, eds. Extraordinary disorders of human behavior. New York: Plenum Press, 1982:203–213.
103. Seeman MV. Delusional loving. Arch Gen Psychiatry 1978;35:1265–1267.
104. de Clerambault GG. Oeuvre Psychiatrique. Paris: Presses Universitaires, 1942.
105. Raskin DE, Sullivan KE. Erotomania. Am J Psychiatry 1974;131:1033–1035.
106. Rudden M, Sweeney J, Frances A. Diagnosis and clinical course of erotomanic and other delusional patients. Am J Psychiatry 1990;147:625–628.
107. Gaddal Y. De Clerambault's syndrome (erotomania) in organic delusional syndrome. Br J Psychiatry 1989;154:714–716.
108. Signer SF, Cummings JL. De Clerambault's syndrome with organic and affective components: two cases. Br J Psychiatry 1987;151:853–855.
109. Soyka M, Sass H, Volcker A. Alcoholic delusion of jealousy—psychopathologic characteristics. Psychiatr Prax 1989;16:189–193.
110. Crowe RR, Clarkson C, Tsai M, Wilson R. Delusional disorder: jealous and non-jealous types. Europena Archives of Neurological Science 1988;237:179–183.
111. Paterson A, Zangwill OL. Recovery of spatial orientation in the post-traumatic confusional state. Brain 1944;67:54–68.
112. Pick A. On reduplicative paramnesia. Brain 1903;26:242–267.
113. Benson DF, Gardner H, Meadows JC. Reduplicative paramnesia. Neurology 1976;26:147–151.
114. Ruff RL, Wolpe BT. Environmental reduplication associated with right frontal and parietal lobe injury. J Neurol Neurosurg Psychiatry 1981;44:382–386.
115. Stuss DT, Benson DF. The frontal lobes. New York: Raven Press, 1986.
116. Capgras J, Reboul-Lachaux J. L'illusion des sosies dans un de'lire systématisé clinique. Bulletin de la Societe Clinique de Medicine Mentale 1923;11:6–16.
117. Enoch MD, Trethowan WH. Uncommon psychiatric syndromes. Bristol: Wright, 1979.
118. Alexander MP, Stuss DT, Benson DF. Capgras syndrome: a reduplicative phenomenon. Neurology 1979;29:334–339.
119. Merrin EL, Silberfarb PM. The Capgras phenomenon. Arch Gen Psychiatry 1976;33:965–968.
120. Fishbain DA. The frequency of Capgras delusions in a psychiatry emergency service. Psychopathology 1987;20:42–47.
121. Foerstl H. Capgras delusion: an example of coalescent psychodynamic and organic factors. Compr Psychiatry 1990;31:447–449.
122. Neitch SM, Zaggara A. A misidentification delusion in two Alzheimer's patients. J Am Geriatr Soc 1991;39:513–515.
123. Hay GG. Electroconvulsive therapy as a contributor to the production of delusional misidentification. Br J Psychiatry 1986;148:667–669.
124. Christodoulou GN. The syndrome of Capgras. Br J Psychiatry 1977;130:555–564.
125. Courbon P, Fail G. Syndrome d'illusion de Fregoli et schizophrenie. Bull Soc Clin Med 1927;15:121–128.
126. Kalmanitz JR, e-Mallakh RS, Tosman A. Delusional misidentification involving the self. J Nerv Mental Dis 1989;177:658–659.
127. Enoch MD. The Capgras syndrome. Acta Psychiatr Scand 1963;39:437–462.
128. Weinstein EA, Kahn RL. Denial of illness: symbolic and physiologic aspects. Springfield, IL.: Charles C Thomas, 1955.
129. Signer SF. Capgras syndrome: the delusion of substitution. J Clin Psychiatry 1987;48:147–150.
130. Benson DF, Stuss DT. Frontal lobe influences on delusions: a clinical perspective. Schiz Bull 1990;16:403–411.
131. Buchsbaum MS. The Frontal lobes, basal ganglia and temporal lobes as sites for schizophrenia. Schiz Bull 1990;16:379–390.
132. Hyde TM, Ziegler JC, Weinberger DR. Psychiatric disturbances in metachromatic leukodystrophy: insights into the neurobiology of psychosis. Arch Neurol 1992;49:401–406.
133. Moskowitz J. Communicative meaning in Capgras syndrome [Letter]. Am J Psychiatry 1973;130:1297.
134. Coleman SM. Misidentification and non-recognition. J Ment Sci 1933;79:42–49.
135. Mesulam M-M. Patterns in behavioral neuroanatomy: association areas, the limbic system and hemispheric specialization. In: Mesulam M-M, ed. Principles of behavioral neurology. Philadelphia: FA Davis, 1985:1–70.
136. Baddeley A. Working memory. Science 1992;255:556–559.

137. Goldman-Rakic PS. Cellular and circuit basis of working memory in prefrontal cortex of nonhuman primates. In: Uylings HBM, Van Eden CG, De Bruin JPC, Corner MA, Feenstra MGP, eds., Progress in brain research, vol 85. Amsterdam: Elsevier, 1990:325–336.

138. Fuster JM. The prefrontal cortex. 2nd ed. New York: Raven Press, 1989.

139. West LJ. A clinical and theoretical overview of hallucinatory phenomena. In: Siegel RK, West LJ, eds. Hallucinations: behavior, experience, and theory. New York: John Wiley & Sons, 1975:287–311.

140. Penfield W, Jasper H. Epilepsy and the functional anatomy of the human brain. Boston: Little, Brown & Co. 1954.

141. Gloor P, Olivier A, Quesney LF, Andermann F, Horowitz S. The role of the limbic system in experimental phenomena of temporal lobe epilepsy. Ann Neurol 1982;12:129–144.

142. Halgren E, Walter RD, Cherlow DG, Crandall PH. Mental phenomena evoked by electrical stimulation of human hippocampal formation and amygdala. Brain 1978;101:83–117.

143. Ojemann GA, Engel J Jr. Acute and chronic intracranial recording and stimulation. In: Engel J Jr, ed. Surgical treatment of the epilepsies. New York: Raven Press, 1987:263–288.

144. Bentall RP. The illusion of reality: a review and integration of psychological research on hallucinations. Psychol Bull 1990;107:82–95.

145. Strauss ME. On the experimental psychopathology of delusion. In: Oltmanns TF, Maher BA, eds. Delusional beliefs. New York: John Wiley & Sons, 1988:157–164.

146. Maher BA, Ross JS. Delusions. In: Adams HE, Sutker PB, eds. Comprehensive handbook of psychopathology. New York: Plenum Press, 1984.

147. Chapman LJ, Chapman JP, Miller EN. Reliabilities and intercorrelations of eight measures of proneness to psychosis. J Consult Clin Psychol 1982;50:187–195.

148. Higgins ET. Self-discrepancy: a theory of relating self and affect. Psychol Rev 1987;9:319–340.

149. Neale JM, Oltmanns TF, Harvey PD. The need to relate cognitive deficits to specific behavioral referents of schizophrenia. Schiz Bull 1985;2:286–291.

150. Westermeyer J. Psychiatric diagnosis across cultural boundaries. Am J Psychiatry 1985;142:798–805.

151. Harrow M, Marengo JT, McDonald C. The early course of schizophrenic thought disorder. Schiz Bull 1986;12:208–224.

152. Goldstein AP, Heller K, Sechrest LB. Psychotherapy and the psychology of behavior. New York: John Wiley & Sons, 1966.

153. Benson DF, Gorman DG. The neural basis of hallucinations. In: Appel SH, ed. Current neurology, vol. 13. Chicago: Mosby-Year Book (in press).

15

NEUROPSYCHIATRIC ASPECTS OF THE SCHIZOPHRENIAS

Dilip V. Jeste, Douglas Galasko, Jody Corey-Bloom, Stanley Walens, and Eric Granholm

Schizophrenia is a serious psychiatric illness that can involve massive disruptions of thinking, perception, emotions and behavior. With a worldwide lifetime prevalence rate of 1%, schizophrenia is a major cause of long-term psychiatric disability.

At the turn of the century, Kraepelin (1) distinguished dementia praecox from manic-depressive psychoses, and noted that the two conditions differed in both course and outcome. Dementia praecox had an earlier onset and a progressively deteriorating course with no return to the premorbid level of functioning, whereas the mood disorders had episodic periods of severe psychopathology followed by periods of normal functioning. Kraepelin also noted that no single pathognomonic symptom or cluster of symptoms served to characterize schizophrenia.

The startling cognitive, affective, and conative dysfunctions in schizophrenia present clinicians and theoreticians with a conundrum whose understanding is essential to the understanding of many other psychopathological disorders. Yet despite the amount of research that has been devoted to schizophrenia, it remains an enigmatic condition, and its etiology and pathophysiology remain obscure. Although schizophrenia has often been conceptualized as a monadic entity, current theories have moved toward viewing schizophrenia as a collection of etiologically disparate disorders with similar clinical presentations — as a syndrome with heterogeneous symptoms.

Current approaches to schizophrenia acknowledge it to be essentially a neurobiological disorder and have focused on neurophysiological approaches to its pathogenesis (2,3). However, schizophrenia presents no consistent or gross neuropathology, unlike Alzheimer's disease, and the localization and nature of the lesion(s) that "produce" schizophrenia remain unknown. It is likely schizophrenia is not a single disease but a syndrome with heterogeneous manifestations, implicating a diffuse and diverse neuropathology. Recent technological innovations in brain imaging have improved our ability to map and examine the structure and functioning of the brain, and have given new impetus to neuropathological studies of schizophrenia.

This chapter considers the following aspects of schizophrenia: neuropsychology, brain imaging, neuropathology, neurochemistry, late-onset schizophrenia, secondary psychoses, neuroleptic-induced tardive dyskinesia, and management.

NEUROPSYCHOLOGY

The neuropsychological approach assumes that the cognitive functions measured by specific tests are associated with specific brain regions/systems and, thus, impairment on a specific test may be taken as evidence of dysfunction in the specific brain region/system associated with the test (See Chapter 3). Several extensive reviews (4–10) have described numerous neuropsychological deficits in patients with schizophrenia. The most consistently replicated deficits in schizophrenia patients have been observed on tasks measuring attention/information-processing, learning/memory, and executive (i.e. frontal systems) functions. Impairment of schizophrenia patients on motor tasks is often attributable to medication effects on performance, which include both motor and cognitive side effects (8,11). Findings of impairment in basic language and visuospatial functions have been inconsistent, and deficits are typically reported on complex tasks that make significant demands on attention (e.g., distraction) or executive (e.g., planning) functions (8). With regard to language functions, some patients with schizophrenia produce abnormal utterances (e.g., neologisms); however, an area of debate is whether these utterances are the result of disordered language or disordered thought (12).

The brief selective review focuses on the more robust findings of deficits in attention/information-processing, learning/memory, and executive functions. This pattern of neuropsychological impairments in patients with schizophrenia has led to the hypothesis that specific frontal-subcortical brain systems are involved in the pathophysiology of schizophrenia.

Attention and Information Processing

Tasks in this domain are designed to measure the ability to select one stimulus or channel (e.g., ear) over another for processing, to divide processing between two stimuli or channels, or to sustain processing over time (vigilance). The extensive literature on the performance of schizophrenia patients on these tasks has shown deficits, which are most apparent when the processing demands (workload) of the tasks are increased by increasing the number or complexity of cognitive operations that must be completed at a given moment (9,13,14). For example, on the span of apprehension (SOA) task, which is designed to assess the number of items that can be apprehended or attended to at one time, subjects must report whether a "T" or "F" target letter is among a group of distractor letters flashed briefly in a visual display. In numerous SOA task studies reviewed (15), schizophrenia patients accurately reported significantly fewer target letters than healthy controls with 8-, 10- or 12-letter arrays (higher processing demands), but the schizophrenia patients' detection accuracy did not differ significantly from the controls' with smaller array sizes (lower processing demands).

One of the most consistently replicated impairments in this domain in schizophrenia patients has been found on reaction time (RT) tasks (16). Schizophrenia patients show slower RT relative to normal individuals on RT tasks that require a rapid response to a single imperative stimulus (IS), e.g., a tone. Also, schizophrenia subjects, unlike normal controls, do not benefit (i.e., show faster RT to the IS) when a warning stimulus is presented at regular preparatory intervals before the IS, if the intervals are relatively long (16). (The loss of benefit with a longer interval is called the Shakow crossover effect.) This finding may suggest a failure to establish a preparatory set or a failure to sustain attention over longer, more attention-demanding intervals (16).

On the Continuous Performance Test (CPT), which measures sustained (from 8–30 minutes) attention, subjects are typically required to press a response key every time a critical target stimulus (e.g., an "X" or a "7") appears in a random sequence of individually presented letter or digit distractors, which are shown at 40–100 msec exposure durations in a visual display. Schizophrenia patients obtain significantly lower target hit rates than normal control subjects on this version of the CPT (17). Deficits are not always observed on the CPT in schizophrenic subjects, however, unless distraction or other factors that increase processing burden are present. For example, the CPT deficits in schizophrenia patients are more evident when subjects are required to actively ignore distracting digits presented aurally, when a sequential target version of the CPT is used (e.g., one which incorporates a memory component by requiring that subjects respond only when a "5" occurs on

one trial *and* a "9" occurs on the next trial), or when stimulus encoding operations are debilitated by degrading (e.g., blurring) stimuli (9).

Studies utilizing dichotic listening tasks have also shown that schizophrenia patients are abnormally susceptible to the effects of distraction. On these tasks, subjects are asked to listen to a message and repeat (shadow) it out loud, while ignoring an irrelevant message played simultaneously either in a different ear or in a different voice. When shadowing word lists, schizophrenia patients commonly make more shadowing omission errors than normal controls on random, irrelevant word lists (18,19). These impairments are, however, reduced or eliminated when shadowing semantically and syntactically structured textual information (20,21), which has inherent syntactical organization that can be more automatically deciphered and decoded than random messages (reduced processing demand) (21). Deficient shadowing during distraction in schizophrenia patients has also been shown with faster (50 items per minute), but not with slower (25 items per minute) presentation rates (19), which again suggests that greater processing demand (increased pressure for rapid processing) leads to information-processing overload and cognitive impairment in schizophrenia.

Impairments on some of these attentional and information-processing tasks (e.g., SOA, CPT) have been observed in schizophrenic subjects in a remitted state, in nonpsychotic biological mothers of schizophrenia patients, in foster children whose biological mothers have schizophrenia, and in individuals in the general population with schizotypal or "psychosis-prone" characteristics (9,15). These findings of impairment in individuals across the schizophrenia spectrum suggest that some of these tasks are sensitive, not only to the psychotic state, but also to more subtle "core" deficits of schizophrenia that may mark a genetic vulnerability and possibly a genetically transmitted pathophysiology of schizophrenia (22).

In summary, patients with schizophrenia show deficits on attention and information-processing tasks when the intensity or complexity of task-processing demands is higher, but not when the task-processing demands are lower. This finding that schizophrenia patients are relatively easily overloaded by the information-processing demands of cognitive tasks has led some researchers to conceptualize the cognitive impairments of schizophrenia patients within the framework of processing "resource" (or "capacity") theories from contemporary cognitive psychology (9,13,14). Processing "resources" are broadly defined here as the limited pool(s) of fuel(s), processes, and structures that are available at a given moment for performance of cognitive tasks. "Resources" are a hypothetical commodity to be utilized and consumed for the purpose of information processing. The use of this concept simply provides a means of describing the human brain as a resource-dependent system—that is, there are clear limits to its capacity to perform. Resource models of schizophrenia stress that patients with schizophrenia perform poorly only when processing loads (i.e., resource demands) are higher. This finding that schizophrenia patients are probably more adversely affected by higher processing resource demands than are normal controls is consistent with the hypothesis that these patients deplete their available resources at lower processing loads than do normal individuals (9,13,14).

The brain systems that govern the availability of processing resources are thought to involve frontal-basal ganglia-thalamic-reticular circuits (23). Kinsbourne and Hicks (24) have suggested that different functional regions of the cerebral cortex constitute different processing resource pools. The frontal lobes modulate sensory input to cortical resource pools through connections with the nucleus reticularis thalami and modulate activation of cortical resource pools in accordance with task demands through connections (directly or through the basal ganglia) with the midbrain reticular formation (25). Reduced cortical resource availability in patients with schizophrenia may result from a failure to mobilize appropriate cortical resources by midbrain reticular centers, or from a failure to gate information flow through the thalamus to the cortex. These abnormalities would lead to information overload of cortical resources either due to insufficient arousal of cortical resources, or due to wasteful processing of information normally gated at lower brain centers, which would result in reduced availability of cortical resources for processing task-relevant information. Several schizophrenia researchers (26) have hypothesized that information-processing impairment in schizophrenia may involve dysfunction in these frontal-basal ganglia-thalamic-reticular circuits involved in the control of information flow to cortical resource pools.

Learning and Memory

A common finding is that recall, but not recognition, performance is deficient in patients with schizophrenia (13,27). Intact recognition is, however, not universally found in schizophrenia patients. Several studies (28-30) provide evidence of a similar level of impairment on recall and recognition tasks in patients with schizophrenia, when tasks require subjects to use semantic or other strategic encoding operations to improve performance. Unlike normal controls, schizophrenia patients do not make normal use of semantic categorical clustering of word lists. They also do not benefit from affective clustering of word lists based on "pleasantness," show normal levels of idiosyncratic, subjective organization of random word lists, or show normal release from proactive interference (i.e., the interference of previously learned material on the learning of new material) (27,28). These findings have led to the conclusion that schizophrenia patients fail to spontaneously carry out semantic or other organizational mnemonic processes necessary for effective memory encoding and retrieval (27). Memory for visual stimuli has received less attention in neuropsychological studies of schizophrenia, but these patients typically show comparable levels of impairment on verbal and nonverbal memory tasks (8,31).

Several studies have examined the learning (or automation) of perceptual and motor skills with practice (i.e., procedural learning) in schizophrenia patients. Intact motor procedural learning in schizophrenic subjects has been reported in two studies on the pursuit rotor task, which requires that subjects keep a hand-held stylus on a target stimulus rotating on a turntable (32,33), on a motor sequencing RT task, which requires subjects to learn a repeating pattern of key presses (34), and on the Tower of Hanoi task, which requires subjects to learn a problem-solving "rule" involved in moving stacks of disks from one of three pegs to another (35). Finally, schizophrenia patients demonstrate the ability to automate attentional skills on the multiple-frame visual search task, which is a task similar to the SOA task described above and requires subjects to automate target detection operations (36). This consistent pattern of results across studies of procedural learning suggests that, despite impairments in the ability to learn verbal and nonverbal factual (declarative) information (29,35), schizophrenia patients do learn procedural skills involving motor, problem-solving, and attentional functions.

In summary, the learning and memory deficits in schizophrenia appear to be related to a failure to spontaneously use contextual cues (e.g., semantic categories) and strategic processes to organize their encoding and retrieval of information (27). Because patients with frontal lobe dysfunction show similar impairments in the spontaneous use of strategic mnemonic processes, and patients with temporal-hippocampal dysfunction show similar impairment in the encoding of semantic information, the memory impairments in schizophrenia have been interpreted as being consistent with frontal and/or temporal-limbic abnormalities (28,31,33). In addition, because superior recognition over recall memory is commonly observed in patients with primarily subcortical (e.g., Huntington's disease) rather than cortical (e.g., Alzheimer's disease) neuropathology (37), the general finding of superior recognition over recall performance in schizophrenia may suggest subcortical (e.g, basal ganglia) pathology (38). On the other hand, basal ganglia dysfunction has been shown to lead to impaired procedural learning (37), but schizophrenia patients generally show intact procedural learning, which may be indicative of greater dysfunction in frontal and/or temporal-limbic, rather than basal ganglia, structures.

Executive Functions

Numerous studies have reported impairments in schizophrenia subjects on tasks measuring executive functions that are mediated by frontal lobe systems (i.e., neural circuitry involving the frontal cortex and its basal-ganglia, limbic, and reticular connections). Executive functions are those neuropsychological processes important for adapting to the environment, such as preparation, initiation, and modulation of action, maintenance of arousal, cognitive set maintenance and set shifting, abstract reasoning, hypothesis testing, and monitoring of ongoing purposeful behavior. The executive function deficits shown by schizophrenia patients include sorting fewer categories and making more perseverative errors than normal controls on the Wisconsin Card Sorting Task (WCST) (39–41); increased errors on the Halstead Category Task (40), reduced verbal fluency on Benton's Controlled Oral Word Association Task (42), psychomotor slowing on the Trail Making Test – Part B (40), and impaired memory for the temporal ordering of information (35).

These executive impairments are consistent with frontal system dysfunction in schizophrenia patients. Even stronger evidence for such dysfunction in schizophrenia is found in functional brain imaging studies, as discussed in the next section.

Conclusions and Caveats

Since the time of Kraepelin and Bleuler, many researchers have viewed schizophrenia as resulting from frontal lobe pathophysiology. The modern version of this hypothesis considers the frontal cortex in the context of its subcortical connections with basal ganglia, thalamus, and reticular structures. Robbins (43) suggested that dysfunction in the flow of information through frontostriatal cognitive and motor "loops" is involved in schizophrenia. Several investigators (e.g., 44) have proposed a diffuse lesion in schizophrenia subjects involving the periventricular limbic and diencephalic nuclei and connections between these structures and the dorsolateral prefrontal cortex, which occurs early in development, but results in symptoms later when the brain areas involved reach maturity. Carlsson and Carlsson (43) described a negative feedback loop, involving frontal, striatal, thalamic and reticular structures, which together modulate cortical sensory input (through thalamic nucleus reticularis sensory gating) and cortical tone (through arousal centers in the midbrain reticular formation). They further postulated that disruption in the balance of glutamate and dopamine in this system leads to inability to modulate the influx and processing of information, which may lead to psychosis. Andreasen and colleagues (26) also hypothesized that deficient gating of sensory input due to an abnormality in the thalamus and related circuitry could explain the symptoms of schizophrenia. Again, the neuropsychological deficits in schizophrenia patients are consistent with these hypotheses that the pathophysiology of schizophrenia involves dysfunction in the complex interactions between frontal cortex and the limbic structures, basal ganglia, thalamus, and reticular structures connected with the frontal lobes.

Several important caveats, however, require mention. The localization of brain pathophysiology on the basis of neuropsychological test results is complicated because impairment on a specific neuropsychological test does not *necessarily* implicate pathophysiology in a specific region of the brain. The validity of this association between impaired test performance and localized brain pathophysiology is

based on the assumption that diffuse brain damage, poor motivation or arousal, variations in task difficulty and other nonspecific factors do not explain the impairment. In addition, psychotropic medications taken by schizophrenia patients may also affect neuropsychological test performance. Long-term treatment with antipsychotic medications tends to normalize schizophrenia patients' performance on several neuropsychological measures (especially attention/information-processing tasks), while anticholinergic medications tend to impair performance on many memory tasks (7,45,46). Finally, although the neuropsychological deficits in schizophrenia in this brief review were interpreted as being consistent with frontal-subcortical circuit system dysfunction, alternative interpretations of the neuropsychological findings exist. Some researchers (6) have described a more "generalized deficit" syndrome in schizophrenia patients, involving significantly lower performance and verbal IQ, more diffuse impairments, and possibly a deteriorating course. Other researchers (4,42) have suggested that left-hemisphere deficits are more common than right-hemisphere deficits in schizophrenia patients.

The possibility of different profiles of neuropsychological deficits (e.g., more frontal, lateralized, or diffuse deficits) in schizophrenia patients, as well as findings that a considerable number (up to 60%) of schizophrenic subjects may demonstrate intact performance on neuropsychological tasks (15,40,42), has led to the notion of various subgroups of schizophrenia patients. One subgrouping hypothesis with a fair amount of support is that neuropsychological impairment is more common in patients with predominantly negative, rather than positive, symptoms (11,47). Identifying different subgroups of schizophrenia patients on the basis of different neuropsychological test profiles has important implications for treatment and outcome prediction. Neuropsychological test performance has been shown to predict medication response (15,48), success in social and community functioning (18,49), and effectiveness of social skills training (50). Future neuropsychological research will have obvious etiological and treatment implications if subgrouping issues are examined more closely.

BRAIN IMAGING

Abundant neuroimaging evidence suggests that structural and functional cerebral pathology exists in schizophrenia. The localization of the site(s) responsible for the pathophysiology of schizophrenia has remained elusive, however. The following discussion presents a selective review of structural and functional neuroimaging studies of schizophrenia.

Structural Neuroimaging

One of the most consistent findings in the myriad of computed tomographic (CT) and magnetic resonance imaging (MRI) studies of schizophrenia has been that of enlarged ventricular spaces. It remains unclear, however, what the significance of the enlarged ventricles is to the pathophysiology of the disease and whether the ventricular enlargement reflects tissue loss. If it does, the nature and locus of this tissue loss remains uncertain. Most CT and many early MRI studies of schizophrenia subjects have relied on clinical ratings, essentially visual inspection, or linear and area measurements of selected sections. A new generation of MRI techniques has recently made it possible to quantify the volume of both whole brain and specific small brain structures. The advantages of quantitative volumetric measurements for evaluating and comparing this or any population of subjects are many. Even so, methodology for the semiautomated computerized approaches varies greatly across investigative groups and it is often difficult to compare results from different laboratories. Sagittal, axial, and coronal sections of the brain have been utilized by various investigators to compare volumes of different cerebral structures. In addition, differences in MRI scanners, scanning sequences, section thickness, and image analysis algorithms have likely contributed to variations in results.

Enlargement of the lateral ventricles of the brain was first demonstrated on CT in 1976 by Johnstone et al. in a group of chronic schizophrenia patients (51). This was confirmed by Weinberger et al. (52) and by others (53). Both lateral and third ventricular enlargement has also been noted by a number of investigators. More recently, decreases in brain area and volume have been described in schizophrenia patients (54,55). Additionally, there appears to be CT evidence of a relationship between brain asymmetry and the schizophrenia disease process (56,57), especially when handedness is taken into account. When unilateral abnormalities have been reported, they have typically involved the left hemisphere (56).

MRI, with its ability to detect relatively small structural brain abnormalities, has not only confirmed the ventricular findings of CT (26,58–61), but also has revealed evidence of significantly reduced volumes of important cerebral structures. The advantages of MRI also include better soft tissue contrast, lack of bone artifact, and no ionizing radiation exposure. In MRI studies of schizophrenia, the most frequently described morphologic abnormalities have involved the temporal lobes, frontal lobes, and basal ganglia; however, the pattern and magnitude of findings varies from one study to another. A number of recent MRI studies have reported reductions in temporal lobe volumes (59,60,62–68) in chronic schizophrenia subjects as compared with controls, especially on the left (63,65,67,69–71). Others, however, have not been able to replicate these findings (58,72,73). Shenton et al. (73) described decreased gray matter volume in the left hippocampus, left parahippocampal gyrus, and left superior temporal gyrus without a decrease in overall left temporal lobe volume. It is unclear to what extent these discrepancies are secondary to differences between subjects or between measurement techniques.

Morphologic abnormalities of the frontal lobe have also been described in schizophrenia. Several studies using MRI have reported decreased prefrontal volumes in schizophrenia subjects (26,66,72,74,75). Others, however, have failed to find any differences in the frontal lobes between schizophrenia patients and normal healthy controls (58,59,71,76,77). Most of the negative studies included more posterior regions in their computations, however, instead of restricting their measurements to the prefrontal area.

The basal ganglia also have been implicated in the pathophysiology of schizophrenia. Larger left caudate volumes have been observed by a number of investigators in chronic schizophrenia subjects (65,66). Although Jernigan et al. (64) were unable to corroborate this finding, enlargement of another basal ganglionic structure, the lenticular nucleus, was noted.

Abnormalities of the corpus callosum (78,79) plus adjacent septum pellucidum (76,80,81) and decreased thalamic volumes (58,82) have also been described in MRI studies of schizophrenia patients. The variability in the MRI findings from different studies probably relates to both differences in patient populations studied and in the MRI methods used.

Functional Neuroimaging

Available techniques for imaging brain function or activity include measurement of cerebral perfusion, referred to as regional cerebral blood flow (rCBF), and measurement of cerebral energy metabolism as provided by blood glucose or local cerebral metabolic rate of glucose (LCMRGlu). Both rCBF and LCMRGlu are believed to reflect neuronal activity and thus serve as markers of brain function. rCBF is commonly quantified by the nontomographic ^{133}Xe inhalation method; single photon emission computed tomography (SPECT) using ^{133}Xe or IV radiopharmaceuticals; or positron emission tomography (PET) using ^{15}O labeled water. At present, the best method for measuring LCMRGlu appears to be PET with ^{18}F-FDG (^{18}Fluorodeoxyglucose).

Two-dimensional ^{133}Xe inhalation rCBF is a nontomographic strategy that allows measurement of blood flow of individual cortical regions. It is relatively inexpensive, and technically easy to carry out. The test evaluates the cortical surface and is unable to "see" deeper structures. Also, its poor spatial resolution (2 cm) makes precise localization of the areas of functional activity difficult. Unfortunately, most of the studies to date that have used the xenon inhalation method to measure cerebral blood flow have used the two-dimensional method rather than SPECT.

SPECT utilizes radioxenon ^{133}Xe or radionuclides such as ^{99m}Te and ^{123}I, which are commercially available and widely used in nuclear medicine departments of most hospitals. Spatial resolution is of the order of 1 cm and there is no requirement for an on-site cyclotron for radionuclide production. It is less invasive, less expensive, and even more flexible than PET, because scans can be performed many hours after administering the radiotracer. An important disadvantage includes lower spatial and temporal resolution, and partial volume effects that have greater relevance because of the relatively large voxel size. PET has better resolution and is more quantitative than SPECT, but is also significantly more expensive and less widely available. It utilizes radiotracers such as ^{15}O and ^{18}F which are positron-emitting isotopes that must be generated in an on-site cyclotron. In addition, PET is more invasive, requiring not only venous access for administration of the radiotracer, but also insertion of an arterial line to continuously monitor the amount of isotope delivered to the brain.

Numerous studies have demonstrated abnormalities of cerebral perfusion and glucose metabolism in patients with schizophrenia. Initial efforts focused on the measurement of either perfusion or glucose utilization during the "resting state." There is, however, substantial variance in the resting state among individuals. Therefore, more recent studies have emphasized the use of paired examinations of control conditions and cognitive challenges in the same individual.

Thus far, the data that have emerged from functional brain imaging studies have generated a number of important hypotheses about the neural basis of schizophrenia. Frontal, temporal, and basal ganglia dysfunction have all been demonstrated.

Beginning with the seminal studies of Ingvar and Franzen (83) using intracarotid ^{133}Xe rCBF, numerous functional imaging studies have reported diminished cerebral activity in the frontal lobes of schizophrenia patients. A substantial literature now exists that has addressed the "hypofrontality issue." Many studies have confirmed this effect, but not all, perhaps because of marked heterogeneity of patient samples. A variety of potential confounders, including use of neuroleptics, chronicity of illness, clinical presentation, and nature of the cognitive task during functional imaging, appear to be important factors. The effects of neuroleptics and other medications on frontal lobe metabolism, for example, are not yet clear. Treatment with neuroleptic medication most likely increases metabolism in the basal ganglia in keeping with its known effect of increasing dopamine turnover. Many investigators try to get around this by assessing patients following 2–4 week drug-free intervals, but it is doubtful that even a 4-week washout completely avoids effects of persistent medication or medication withdrawal effects. Clearly, evaluation of metabolic activity in the frontal lobes and other brain structures is best ascertained in patients who have never previously been treated with neuroleptics. Large sample studies of neuroleptic-naive patients are rare, however. A recent study by Potkin et al. (84) indicated that clozapine tended to normalize asymmetry, but exaggerated hypofrontality.

In addition to medication effects, many investigators have expressed concern about the chronicity of illness in the patient samples studied. Of the numerous studies reporting hypofrontality, most have included primarily chronic schizophrenia patients. With few notable exceptions, studies failing to find hypofrontality have included patients with more acute schizophrenia (85). At present, it remains unclear whether hypofrontality is a primary problem in schizophrenia or, as some propose, secondary to either long-term neuroleptic treatment or duration of illness. A third possibility is that hypofrontality is a variable feature, whose presence increases chronicity and disability, and worsens the response to neuroleptics.

The nature of the clinical presentation of schizophrenia patients may help explain some of the variations in results across studies. Some schizophrenia patients have prominent positive symptoms while others have primarily negative symptoms; still others present with a mixture of the two. Whether there is a relationship between frontal lobe hypometabolism and negative symptoms, as reported by some investigators, remains unsettled, although one recent study (86) strongly supports such an association.

Concerns have also been raised about the nature of the patient samples. Differences in rCBF and glucose utilization between men and women have been observed. Women may have higher metabolic rates than men (87). In addition, differences have been described with aging (88) and between right- and left-handed individuals. Therefore, any careful study of brain metabolism will require that groups be matched for gender, age, and handedness. Controlling for education may be necessary but difficult because many schizophrenia patients are educationally limited as a consequence of their illness. Obviously, a full exploration of the confounding variables of gender, age, handedness, and education will require much larger samples than are presently available.

Another area of disparity across studies is in the methods used to define hypofrontality. Some studies have used ratio methods in which the activity of the frontal lobes is expressed relative to that of the occipital cortex, for example, to generate a "frontal index" that is compared across groups during the resting condition. Others have attempted to normalize data to correct for overall brain blood flow. With the introduction of cognitive tasks in the evaluation paradigm, each subject is used as his or her own control. With this approach, the inability of the subject to increase frontal blood flow when stimulated with a frontal cognitive task as compared to his own baseline, is defined as hypofrontality. Unfortunately, significant variability exists in the nature of the cognitive challenges that have been used to assess prefrontal cortical function, which may depend on different frontal subsystems or be of unequal difficulty. For example, some studies have utilized the WCST, while others have used the Continuous Performance Task (CPT) or number matching tasks. Whether these cognitive tests are stimulating the same or different areas of cortex and their specificity for cortical regions remains undetermined.

Despite all of the uncertainties and variability among studies, results of many functional evaluations to date suggest that there may be a disturbance in frontal lobe function in schizophrenia. A number of 2D-rCBF studies have reported hypofrontality in both medicated (89–92) and drug-free schizophrenia patients (44,93). Most were evaluated in the resting condition only; however, some (44,92) also included "prefrontal" and control tasks. Hypofrontality was not demonstrated in two studies of schizophrenic subjects evaluated during the acute stages of their illness (94,95).

Results from numerous controlled studies with ^{18}F-FDG PET, both during the resting state and performance of frontal tasks, have likewise been inconsistent. Hypofrontality has been reported in schizophrenic subjects by a number of authors (96–102). In all cases, however, except for one study (102), patients were on neuroleptic medications as recently as 2 weeks prior to scanning. Studies utilizing ^{11}C glucose (100) and ^{11}C deoxyglucose (103), have reported similar decreases in frontal lobe metabolism. Using ^{15}O (103–105), ^{11}C deoxyglucose (89), and ^{18}FCG (85,106), several investigators failed to find evidence of hypofrontality, however. About half of the patients in the studies by Sheppard et al. (104) and Early et al. (105) were drug-naive; as were all of the patients in the Sedvall et al. study (107), who, unfortunately, were not matched for gender. One study (108) consisted of acute unmedicated patients only and therefore differed radically from most other cohorts. The authors (108) not only failed to find evidence of hypofrontality, but actually observed increased frontal metabolism in their eight drug-naive acutely psychotic patients. Similarly, hyperfrontality was reported by Szechtman et al. (106) in both neuroleptic-free and neuroleptic-treated patients, while Warkentin et al. (109) found relative hypofrontality in patients with schizophrenia in remission.

Thus, while the literature is not entirely consistent, hypofrontality remains a frequently observed functional abnormality in schizophrenia. This finding is representative of a subgroup of patients but the clinical characterization of that subgroup has not been consistent. In addition, the possible role of the neuroleptic treatment in producing this finding remains ambiguous.

The basal ganglia have also been implicated in the pathophysiology of schizophrenia. Using ^{11}C deoxyglucose and PET, Sedvall et al. (107) found decreased left lenticular nucleus activity in a study of 13 medication-free schizophrenia patients. Sheppard et al. (104), using ^{15}O, also noted decreased basal ganglia metabolism in twelve schizophrenia patients, half of whom were drug-naive. Decreased absolute (85,99,102) and relative (96,102) basal ganglia activity has been reported by a number of investigators, primarily in patients who were never medicated or had been off medications for some time. On the other hand, increased absolute basal ganglia activity has been described in 18 chronic schizophrenia patients on medication (103).

Finally, several investigators have reported an increase in relative basal ganglia metabolism in schizophrenia (85,99,103,110). Except for one study (110), most patients were either on medication at the time of scanning or had been on neuroleptics for various intervals prior to examination. Quite possibly, then, striatal metabolism in schizophrenia better correlates with neuroleptic treatment than with disease-related pathophysiology.

It is now possible to examine neuroreceptors in vivo in schizophrenia, using radioligands for the dopamine receptor with PET and SPECT technology. This is an exciting and important application of functional brain imaging because alterations in dopamine receptors have been suggested in this illness. Ideally, these studies should be carried out in medication-naive patients since neuroleptics themselves produce striatal dopamine receptor increases.

Using SPECT and ^{77}Br-bromospiperone, Crawley et al. (111) found elevated values of dopamine receptors in a small group of schizophrenia subjects off medication for 6 months. Whether a 6-month washout period is enough to nullify the effects of long-term use of neuroleptics on striatal receptors is uncertain. Using PET and ^{11}C-N-methyl-spiperone, Wong et al. (112) found highly elevated dopamine receptor densities in the caudates of both treated and nontreated schizophrenia patients before and after administration of 7.5 mg of haloperidol. These findings were not confirmed by other PET receptor ligand studies, however. Farde et al. (113), for example, found no increase in dopamine receptor binding in 18 neuroleptic-naive schizophrenia patients as compared to controls using ^{11}C raclopride.

Conclusions

Neuroimaging techniques have provided unique opportunities for exploring brain anatomy and function in schizophrenia. The precise morphologic and physiological substrates of this disabling disorder remain ambiguous, however. Evidence suggests that the frontal lobes, temporal lobe structures, the basal ganglia, and thalamus, either alone or in concert, may be involved in the pathophysiology of schizophrenia. As the technology improves and measurements are standardized and refined, these techniques will likely become an even more powerful aid in understanding the primary brain lesions responsible for producing the symptoms and signs of schizophrenia. Future studies should involve combined structural and functional modalities in large cohorts of well-characterized and carefully selected subjects and appropriate controls.

NEUROPATHOLOGY AND NEUROCHEMISTRY

In parallel with neuroimaging studies, neuropathological examination of the brains of schizophrenia patients has provided evidence of a high prevalence of structural abnormalities. However, findings are variable and have not led as yet to conclusions regarding any "core" neuropathology of the disorder. Studies have addressed two important questions: where are the lesions in the brains of schizophrenia patients, and what type of pathological process is likely to result in the changes that are found?

Older studies of brain weight, gross brain structure, and histological appearance in schizophrenia were inconclusive—a consequence of flaws in methodology and sampling (114). Efforts were hampered by a lack of quantitative methods, confounding factors such as postmortem shrinkage of tissue and brain changes due to neurological diseases such as stroke or agonal coma, and failure to match with controls for potential confounding factors such as age and gender. Recent studies have established the existence of structural brain abnormalities in schizophrenia, suggesting an "organic" basis for the psychosis. Three sets of studies that controlled for variables such as age, gender, weight, and height, found that the overall brain weight was decreased in schizophrenia patients (115–117). The extent of the decrease was modest but consistent, about 5 to 8%. In one of these studies, the decrease in volume of the hemispheres in schizophrenia patients compared to controls was accounted for more strongly by a loss of cortical gray matter (12%) rather than by a loss of central gray matter (6%), while white matter volume did not differ (116).

In agreement with neuroimaging studies on living patients, autopsy studies on the brains of schizophrenia patients have generally shown ventricular enlargement. Ventriculomegaly exceeds that attributable to normal aging alone (56,115). The increase mainly affects the lateral ventricles, especially the temporal horn, and the left temporal horn may be more severely affected than the right (118). In contrast to Alzheimer's disease, where enlargement of the lateral ventricles is generalized, in schizophrenia the temporal horns are enlarged to a much greater extent than the rest of the ventricles (118). This selective enlargement suggests that structures adjacent to the temporal horn bear the brunt of the pathology, including the temporal cortex, hippocampus, and amygdala.

Planimetric studies (115,119–122) have shown decreased volumes or areas on cross-section of temporal lobe structures, notably the hippocampus, parahippocampal gyrus, amygdala and inner pallidal segment. The parahippocampal cortex was thinner in the brains of schizophrenia patients, and correlated with the extent of ventricular enlargement (115). Studies have found no differences in the volumes of basal ganglia structures, or the cingulate or insular cortex (115,119,123). In patients chronically treated with neuroleptics, striatal volumes may be slightly increased (124). A quantitative study of the major subnuclei of the thalamus showed no significant difference between schizophrenia patients and controls, apart from volume loss in gray matter adjacent to the third ventricle (125), although other studies have noted neuron loss in some thalamic nuclei (126). A report of an altered gyral pattern of the temporal lobe in some schizophrenia patients (127) was not confirmed in a larger study (117).

Histological studies carried out over the past decade have used quantitative microscopic methods and a variety of staining and immunohistochemical techniques to study the number and arrangement of neurons in various brain areas in schizophrenia. Apart from being technically demanding, these studies have a number of potential clinical difficulties. Cases and controls need to be carefully matched for age and gender. Many schizophrenia patients die at a relatively advanced age, when the effects of aging, chronic medications, co-morbidity, and factors such as alcohol abuse may need to be considered. Indeed, studies have found an increased frequency of neuropathological lesions caused by Alzheimer's disease, Parkinson's disease, or infarcts in schizophrenia patients compared to elderly controls (117,128). This factor needs to be considered before drawing conclusions about schizophrenia.

Recent studies have paid special attention to matching cases with controls, studying brains "blind" to clinical diagnoses, and using computer-assisted cell-counting methods of serial thin sections. Several investigators have reported decreased numbers and disordered arrangement of neurons in temporal lobe structures (121,127,129–131)—especially the parahippocampal gyrus, where neuron loss as high as 20% has been reported (121). Other studies have found a more modest degree of neuron loss in several layers of the prefrontal and cingulate cortex (132,133) and to a lesser extent in other brain areas. Only rarely do recent studies disagree with these findings (134). Although the nature and extent of neuron loss described in these studies are not entirely consistent across studies, this is likely to be the result of different methods of histologic analysis. The balance of evidence from these controlled studies supports the presence of nonspecific pathology in temporolimbic areas in the brains of schizophrenia patients.

The reported changes are relatively subtle, and unlike neurodegenerative diseases such as Alzheimer's disease or Parkinson's disease, there are no characteristic neuronal ultrastructural changes or inclusion bodies. Instead, a variety of alterations of neuronal size and/or arrangement has been noted. This includes loss of small interneurons (133) or large pyramidal cells (129), neuronal disarray (135–138), and decreased neuronal size in some areas (131). The disorganized orientation of neurons described is subtle and not unique to the brains of schizophrenia patients, but is more common in schizophrenia than in controls. The severity of neuron loss or other changes does not seem to increase in proportion to the duration of illness. This implies that the pathology is established at the time of initial clinical presentation, and does not necessarily progress. The concept of schizophrenia as a neurodevelopmental lesion that manifests clinically in adolescence is thus supported.

A recent study shed further light on the timing and nature of neuronal changes. In it, the brains of schizophrenia patients and controls were stained with an antibody against NADPH-diaphorase, which labels a class of neurons resistant to the neurodegeneration of Alzheimer's disease and other conditions. In the schizophrenia patients, diaphorase-positive neurons were decreased in the cortical gray matter, and increased in the white matter deep to the cortex in the frontal lobes (139), temporal lobes, and hippocampus (140). This suggests failure of migration toward the cortical plate, which normally occurs between 6 and 14 weeks of gestation. How these out-of-position cells affect cerebral dysfunction and later brain development, and their relationship to the etiology of schizophrenia, remain to be determined, but the findings further support frontal and temporolimbic sites of pathology.

Many studies have consistently reported that inflammation or gliosis does not accompany neuronal abnormalities or atrophy in the brains of schizophrenia patients (56,121,126,141,142). Studies that excluded cases with acquired pathology, such as infarcts, supported this conclusion most clearly. This further supports the notion that the pathology likely reflects a developmental event, occurring in utero, because acquired lesions generally elicit a glial response. Gliosis occurs from the 3rd trimester onward, again narrowing the window during which abnormalities may arise. Obstetrical injuries and perinatal infections should leave a trail identified by gliosis, and are, therefore, less strongly favored than genetic or developmental factors.

Although the events that incite the pathology of schizophrenia remain elusive, clues — and theories — abound. Infectious agents have been sought with great effort, including molecular biological techniques of testing for viral DNA, without avail. More recent theories attribute neuronal misarrangements to abnormal migration of developing neurons in cortical columns. This migration is genetically controlled, and it is conceivable that a disturbance in the genetic regulation of brain development may result in the types of abnormalities just described. Twin studies have demonstrated that although heredity does increase the risk of schizophrenia, the concordance rate in monozygotic twins is substantially less than 100%. This suggests that environmental factors are probably important in many cases.

The neurochemical basis of schizophrenic symptoms has been a separate focus of inquiry. Until recently, the most accepted explanation was the dopamine hypothesis, which attributed the illness to an excess of dopaminergic neurotransmission. The dopamine hypothesis derived from two major findings. First, neuroleptics, which block D_2 receptors, improve the positive symptoms of schizophrenia. Their clinical efficacy is roughly proportional to their affinity for D_2 receptors (143,144). Second, amphetamine and other aminergic agents, which increase the activity of transmission of dopamine and other catecholamines, can provoke a psychotic state or worsen the symptoms of some schizophrenia patients, especially those who are more treatment-resistant (145,146). These observations indicate that manipulating the dopaminergic system can regulate psychotic symptoms. Nevertheless, they do not directly implicate a central excess of dopamine as the cardinal cause of schizophrenic symptoms.

More direct evidence to support the dopamine hypothesis has been sought from studies of brain tissue-, serum- and cerebrospinal fluid (CSF)-monoamine neurotransmitters, and neuroimaging techniques such as PET. The least ambiguous evidence should come from brains of patients not exposed to neuroleptics, with tissue frozen within a few hours of death. In the absence of large numbers of such patients, it is not surprising that neurochemical studies of catecholamine concentrations in schizophrenia patients' brains have been difficult to interpret. Modest increases in dopamine and its metabolites were reported in several early studies in the caudate, putamen, nucleus accumbens (147-149), and amygdala (150). There were also trends toward increased dopamine levels in the temporal and frontal cortex. Later studies did not, however, confirm these findings (151,152). In general, increased levels of dopamine and its metabolites were more apparent in younger patients and in patients who had received neuroleptics (153). In

neuroleptic-free patients, there was no consistent finding of an overall hyperdopaminergic state.

The technique of radioligand receptor-binding studies was used to examine the distribution and levels of dopamine receptors in schizophrenia. Findings of increased D_2 receptors in the caudate and nucleus accumbens, targets of mesolimbic catecholaminergic projections, have been attributed to the effect of treatment with neuroleptics, rather than to the disease itself (149,154,155). Nonetheless, neuroleptic-treated patients with Alzheimer's or Huntington's disease treated with neuroleptics show lesser degrees of increased D_2 receptor binding, implying indirectly that medications do not fully account for the increased receptor binding found in schizophrenia.

Studies of dopamine and its metabolites in the CSF, especially HVA, have yielded inconsistent findings. Reported results have included an increase, no difference, and a decrease in dopamine levels in schizophrenia subjects compared with normal controls (156). Inconsistencies may be related to variables such as neuroleptic treatment, diet and activity that affect CSF neurotransmitters, as well as to assay variability, but even those studies with "positive" results have shown considerable overlap between concentrations in schizophrenia patients and in controls. Plasma amines, especially HVA, have been extensively studied in schizophrenia subjects before and after neuroleptic treatment (153,156). Although no clear and consistent difference at baseline distinguishes schizophrenia patients from controls, higher pretreatment levels of HVA may predict patients who are more likely to respond to neuroleptics.

In light of these inconclusive findings, and because important negative or deficit symptoms of apathy and withdrawal are not readily explained by augmented dopamine transmission, the original theory has undergone several revisions (153,157). These have tried to explain both the positive and negative symptoms associated with schizophrenia by alterations in limbic dopaminergic circuits, particularly the projections of the ventral tegmental area (VTA) or mesolimbic projections. These neurons have extensive connections to the frontal lobes, as well as the nucleus accumbens and amygdala. Damage to the VTA system may potentially explain hypofrontality, thought to be an important basis of the deficit syndrome of schizophrenia. In animals, prefrontal neurons inhibit subcortical dopaminergic pathways which may possibly trigger positive phenomena such as delusions and hallucinations. Thus, frontal hypodopaminergic function accompanied by episodic hyperdopaminergic function in temporolimbic areas may account more closely for the clinical features of schizophrenia (153). The atypical antipsychotics such as risperidone and clozapine may shed light on other important neurochemical pathways in schizophrenia. These drugs block serotonin *and* dopamine receptors, control both positive and negative symptoms of schizophrenia, and are less likely to induce extrapyramidal side effects. The cloning of several subtypes of dopamine receptors indicates that the regulation and effects of aminergic neurotransmission are more complicated than previously thought. Clozapine binds strongly to D_4 receptors, but poorly to other subtypes (158), while typical neuroleptics show relatively greater binding to D_2 than to D_4 receptors.

Several neuropeptide and amino acid transmitters have also been studied in schizophrenia. Normal levels of GABA, the major inhibitory neurotransmitter in the brain, have been found in cortical and subcortical areas, making it unlikely that positive symptoms result from inadequate inhibition of neuronal circuits. Decreased density of GABA uptake sites was found in the hippocampus, possibly reflecting neuron loss (159). Several neuropeptides have been measured in the brains of schizophrenia patients, the rationale being that these either co-localized with dopamine or interacted with aminergic pathways. Although levels of neurotensin are normal (160), slight reductions of the neuropeptides somatostatin and cholecystokinin (CCK) have been found in the hippocampus and amygdala and in the frontal cortex (161) of schizophrenia subjects (162,163). The implications of these findings are unclear, but they could reflect loss of neurons, or specific neurotransmitter deficits. Several studies of glutamate receptor binding have been carried out, and are likely to continue as newer ligands for these excitatory transmitters are developed. Binding to the kainate subtype of glutamate receptor has been reported as decreased in the left hemisphere (164) and increased in the frontal lobe (165). Numerous studies of neuropeptides and neurotransmitters in CSF and plasma have been carried out without yielding consistent markers favoring specific circuits or pathways.

Substantial progress has been made in neuropathological and neuroanatomical studies of the schizophrenic brain. Insights from physiological imaging studies in living patients, studies of brain development and its genetic control, and pharmacological studies using newer agents such as clozapine and risperidone, are promising stepping stones that may lead to a better understanding of the pathogenesis of schizophrenia.

LATE-ONSET SCHIZOPHRENIA

The possible development of schizophrenia in mid- or late life has been a topic of continuing controversy with important implications for the understanding of schizophrenia. Historically, schizophrenia has been defined as a condition for which early onset is an intrinsic criterion (166–168). Until recently, the etiology of late-onset psychoses has been attributed almost exclusively to "organic" illnesses or brain lesions, substance abuse, mood disorders, and sensory deficits. The DSM-III (168) restricted the diagnosis of schizophrenia to patients with an age of onset of the illness less than 45 years. Although the criterion for age of onset under 45 was eliminated in the DSM-III-R (169), and late-onset schizophrenia (LOS) was acknowledged as a recognizable clinical form, the validity of LOS as a discriminate nosological entity (or group of entities) and the relationship between LOS and other subtypes of

schizophrenia are still not well understood. The DSM-IV (170) does not include any age-cutoff for the diagnosis of schizophrenia nor does it specify LOS as a distinct subcategory of schizophrenia.

Despite problems in methodology, inconsistent or incompatible terminology and nosological criteria, and difficulties in accurately diagnosing schizophrenia and determining a date of onset in any clinical instance, clearly, a fair number of patients demonstrate their first recognizable symptoms of schizophrenia only after age 40 or 45 (171). LOS is characterized by many of the typical symptoms of schizophrenia, especially of paranoid type: persecutory delusions, auditory hallucinations, schizoid or paranoid traits in premorbid personality, a tendency toward chronicity, and improvement in positive symptoms with neuroleptics. In contrast to early-onset schizophrenia (EOS), there is a preponderance of women among LOS patients (166,172–174). Several researchers have noted that hearing and/or vision impairment may be an important factor for LOS (175–177), although this causality has been questioned by others (178).

A literature review by Harris and Jeste (171) estimated that approximately 13% of hospitalized schizophrenia patients had onset in the 5th decade, 7% in the 6th decade, and 3% thereafter. Although these estimates must be taken as preliminary, they do provide evidence that schizophrenia with onset after age 40 is not rare.

An analysis of family histories shows that both EOS and LOS patients have greater numbers of first-degree relatives with schizophrenia than normal controls. Some studies suggest that a "positive" family history may be more common in EOS than in LOS. The premorbid personality of LOS patients sometimes includes schizoid or paranoid traits. The proportion of LOS patients who are, or were married is higher than that in the EOS group. A diagnosis of schizophrenia in the LOS patients is also supported by the numerous similarities between the EOS and LOS groups on neuropsychological and psychopathological measures (179,180). The degree of neuropsychological impairment in LOS is, however, somewhat milder than that in EOS (180).

There has been a modest number of CT and MRI studies of LOS (181–184). Although the relationship of this entity to EOS remains uncertain, in general, these investigations have demonstrated similar increases in ventricular size in LOS and EOS patients compared with age-matched normal controls. A higher prevalence of white matter abnormalities has been described by Breitner et al. (185) and Miller et al. (177) in the late-onset group. A recent preliminary study (186) reported that LOS patients had larger thalami on MRI than age- and education-comparable patients with EOS. In view of other reports of smaller thalami in EOS (82), one wonders if the larger thalamus could be a protective factor contributing to the delayed onset of symptoms in patients with LOS.

Investigations of the course and prognosis of LOS have concluded that the course tends to be chronic but the prognosis may not be as unfavorable as in EOS

(171,173,187–190). There have been only a few studies on the use of neuroleptics in treating LOS patients. These (191) suggest that treatment with neuroleptics is as effective in counteracting the symptoms of schizophrenia in LOS as in EOS, and that the risk of relapse after neuroleptic withdrawal is similar in both groups. There is a fairly high risk of side effects associated with neuroleptic treatment in older patients, including tardive dyskinesia (180,192). Pharmacokinetic and pharmacodynamic changes associated with aging require that any clinical treatment of LOS patients always weigh the significant risk/benefit issues involved. It is also important to gauge the extent to which the sedative or anticholinergic properties of different neuroleptics may adversely affect patients suffering from other medical problems.

Many research questions about LOS remain unanswered: What are the factors that protect patients from schizophrenia until later, or perhaps which prolong the preclinical and/or prodromal phases of the disease? How do LOS patients compare with EOS patients as well as with normal cohorts in neuropsychological performance, brain imaging measures, psychosocial stressors, and other biological and sociocultural factors associated with schizophrenia? Why is there such a gender difference in the incidence of LOS? What do treatment response patterns of older patients tell us about the characteristics of and the neurobiological mechanisms involved in schizophrenia in general? Research on these and other questions must be based on a consistent set of diagnostic criteria and on carefully planned and clinically sophisticated experiments.

SECONDARY PSYCHOSES — (PSYCHOSES SECONDARY TO GENERAL MEDICAL CONDITIONS OR FOCAL BRAIN LESIONS) AND GROSS BRAIN DISEASES ASSOCIATED WITH SCHIZOPHRENIC SYMPTOMS

"Secondary psychosis" is diagnosed in patients with brain lesions who have prominent delusions or hallucinations. Typically in secondary psychoses, fragments of the schizophrenic syndrome, especially delusions, occur rather than the full repertoire of positive and negative symptoms. Many reports of secondary psychosis have been incompletely documented and lack details of the precise symptoms and their time course, or the presence of previous psychopathology, affective symptoms, or a family history of schizophrenia. Most reports take the form of case reports or small series, and it is difficult to assess how frequently psychotic symptoms occur in various neurological conditions. With these reservations in mind, the relationship between psychotic symptoms and brain lesions is discussed below, with conditions being grouped as neurodegenerative diseases, infections, focal lesions, and metabolic or toxic encephalopathies. For more complete lists of disorders reported in combination with delusions or hallucinations, the reader is referred to other reviews (193,194).

Neurodegenerative Diseases

In dementing conditions, delusions and hallucinations may be prominent. In Alzheimer's disease (AD), the prototypical cortical dementia, about 30–40% of patients have delusions at some point during the illness (195). These are most common during intermediate stages, and less so in advanced dementia, presumably because functioning cortical areas are necessary to generate delusions or because severely demented patients cannot verbalize their delusions. Usually the delusions in AD are simpler than those in schizophrenia, and are not systematized. They often have a paranoid quality and may be related to memory impairment, for example, blaming people for stealing items that the subject misplaces. Spousal infidelity, Capgras's syndrome—the belief that a significant person (most commonly the spouse) has been replaced by an identical impostor, beliefs that strangers are entering the house, and paranoid delusions that people are plotting to hurt the patient or are spying are also common in AD. Psychotic symptoms occur less often in Pick's disease and Creutzfeldt—Jakob disease.

Idiopathic Parkinson's disease is associated with psychotic symptoms in two situations: in patients who develop dementia, usually late in the course of the illness, and as a result of overstimulation with L-dopa. The latter occurs more commonly in patients with severe parkinsonism that is less responsive to L-dopa, and tends to produce hallucinations rather than delusions. Postencephalitic parkinsonism, now rare, was linked to a variety of psychotic symptoms, especially delusions. Clozapine has been reported as being beneficial for psychosis in Parkinson's disease, a situation where "typical" neuroleptic agents (especially the high potency ones such as haloperidol) are disfavored because they worsen extrapyramidal function (196).

Approximately 50% of Huntington's disease patients develop psychosis, sometimes as the presenting feature. Rarer conditions involving the basal ganglia, such as Wilson's disease and idiopathic calcification of the basal ganglia, and cerebellar or multisystem degenerations may also produce psychosis (197).

Delusions are somewhat less common in demyelinating diseases. They have been reported in multiple sclerosis (MS), and in inherited dysmyelinating conditions such as metachromatic leukodystrophy and adrenoleukodystrophy.

Infections and Focal Lesions

Although the result of an infectious agent, HIV encephalopathy is convenient to group along with neurodegenerative conditions because of its association with dementia. Psychotic symptoms occur in a small proportion of subjects with HIV encephalopathy (198,199) and respond symptomatically to relatively low doses of neuroleptics.

Many focal brain lesions have been reported as potential causes of psychotic symptoms, which are often transient.

The highest risk occurs with temporolimbic lesions. Left-sided lesions are reportedly more likely to produce persecutory delusions, while right-sided lesions may be more likely to cause visual hallucinations and sometimes delusions. Infarcts, arteriovenous malformations, tumors, trauma, Herpes simplex encephalitis (and other infections), hydrocephalus and anoxic encephalopathy are among the list of culprits, although more common than any of these is the psychosis associated with epilepsy. The relationship between epilepsy and psychosis has been extensively studied and comprehensively reviewed (198,200) and is dealt with by Trimble.

In brief, complex partial seizures are more likely than other types of seizures to manifest with psychosis, which may be ictal, interictal, or postictal and may bear a poor relationship to the adequacy of seizure control (201,202). Interictal psychosis can be a major management problem in patients with complex partial seizures. The content of delusions and hallucinations may closely resemble that of schizophrenia (203). Rarely, marked improvement in seizure control by medications (forced normalization) may precipitate psychotic symptoms (204). Left-sided seizure foci and structural lesions of the temporal lobe are risk factors for interictal psychosis (205–207).

Metabolic (and Toxic) Encephalopathies

Most systemic illnesses and metabolic derangements have the potential to produce psychotic symptoms, although delirium is far more common. Psychosis may appear in the setting of delirium or fluctuation of consciousness. Renal, hepatic, or pulmonary failure, hypoxemia, disorders of the thyroid, parathyroid, or adrenal glands, collagen-vascular diseases such as SLE and temporal arteritis, vitamin deficiencies (B_{12}, folate, thiamine) are examples of such conditions. The psychoses seen in intensive care units or postoperatively are usually multifactorial.

Toxic or medication-induced encephalopathies may present with prominent delusions or hallucinations. An extensive list of medications reported as being potentially associated with delusions or hallucinations has been compiled by Cummings (208). Therapeutic drugs affecting neurotransmitter function, such as anticholinergics, dopaminergic agents, antidepressants, anticonvulsants, antihistamines, and antihypertensive agents, may provoke psychotic symptoms, as may many other drugs such as cimetidine, benzodiazepines, corticosteroids, and digoxin. Many drugs of abuse may produce psychiatric symptoms that include hallucinations or delusions. LSD, phencyclidine (PCP), psilocybin and cocaine may cause acute excited states with hallucinations. More sustained psychotic symptoms that sometimes persist after withdrawal of the drug occur with amphetamines, LSD, PCP, and mescaline, and with inhalation of glue or other organic solvents. Withdrawal from alcohol, barbiturates, and opioids, and, more rarely, other drugs may precipitate psychosis.

In the face of such a large array of lesions and disorders

that can result in psychotic symptoms, it is difficult to extract general principles regarding secondary psychoses. Clinically there are several important distinctions between these secondary psychoses and schizophrenia. The secondary psychoses usually have a later age of onset, and a family history of schizophrenia is usually absent. The delusions are often less chronic and indolent than those in schizophrenia and often respond well to low doses of neuroleptics. First-rank Schneiderian delusions can, however, occur in many of the conditions just listed. In patients whose overall level of cognition is impaired, the content of delusions is less complex than that in schizophrenia.

From the plethora of conditions associated with secondary psychotic symptoms, some patterns emerge linking brain sites of lesions and specific symptoms. Delusions associated with disease processes affecting the cortex tend to be less elaborate than those related to subcortical or limbic lesions. Left-hemisphere lesions are overrepresented in case series and case reports, as are temporal lobe lesions. This is especially evident in conditions that can arise in various areas of the brain, such as seizures or tumors, where delusions are far more common if the temporal lobe is affected.

Investigation and Treatment of Secondary Psychotic Symptoms

Most of the aforementioned neurological conditions display prominent neurological and cognitive deficits and usually do not pose diagnostic problems in the setting of psychosis. Apart from the physical examination findings, patients with secondary psychosis are generally distinguished from those with schizophrenia by a later age of onset. Many toxic or metabolic disturbances produce psychotic symptoms in association with delirium. These patients may need a period of observation and relevant blood and urine tests to establish the diagnosis. Neuroimaging studies are needed in patients in whom the underlying disease process is not evident on clinical examination and laboratory tests.

TARDIVE DYSKINESIA

Neuroleptic-induced tardive dyskinesia (TD) is a serious problem in the psychopharmacology of schizophrenia. The TD syndrome, whose defining characteristics and mechanisms are still being delimited, consists of abnormal, involuntary movements, usually of choreoathetoid type, sometimes stereotyped (209). Many different hyperkinetic movements, excluding tremor, have been reported as manifestations of TD. Typically, however, orofacial and upper extremity musculature is involved, with orofacial dyskinesias occurring in about 80% of patients. In some patients the trunk, lower extremities, pharynx, and diaphragm are also affected (210). Other tardive syndromes, such as tardive dystonia and tardive akathisia, may be dominated by single particular forms of hyperkinesis (211-214), but TD usually presents multiple and disparate hyperkinesias simultaneously. Whether these tardive manifestations imply disparate syndromes or are variants within a unitary TD syndrome remains unclear.

Neuroleptic treatment is a primary and necessary factor in the etiology of and development of TD. Although various drugs have been implicated in producing choreoathetoid movements and possibly TD (210), persistent TD has been associated only with the use of neuroleptics. Usually the syndrome appears after at least 3 months of neuroleptic treatment (except in older patients in whom 1 month of treatment may be sufficient), and other than withdrawal from neuroleptics, treatments for TD are still experimental. These include noradrenergic agents such as clonidine and propranolol, GABAergic agents such as benzodiazepines, and antioxidants such as vitamin E (192).

Differential diagnosis of TD from other disorders with hyperkinetic and hypokinetic manifestations is critical (210). TD has also been found to coexist with many other disorders that present with movement-related symptoms (210,215–219). It can be difficult to separate stereotypies seen in schizophrenia, autism, catatonia, and mental retardation from those of TD, or from illnesses such as Huntington's disease and Wilson's disease, where psychiatric symptoms manifested in the early stage of the disease may be treated with neuroleptics. Separating TD from akathisia is important, and Munetz and Cornes (220) have proposed a set of clinical guidelines. A number of studies have reported that TD and neuroleptic-induced parkinsonism can coexist (221–223).

Prevalence and Incidence

Given the problems in recognition and diagnosis, it is not surprising that reported TD prevalence in various subgroups of neuroleptic-treated patients has ranged from less than 10% to greater than 60%. True prevalence and incidence rates may be significantly higher than casual clinical observation might suggest, because neuroleptics suppress or mask some of the symptoms of TD that may emerge only upon reduction or withdrawal from neuroleptic treatment. Accurate assessment may require newer instrumental procedures for objectively measuring and quantifying normal and abnormal movements, and for differentiating the features of TD from other disorders (192).

Yassa and Jeste (224) evaluated data from 76 published studies of TD, involving a total of nearly 40,000 patients. They noted that the mean reported prevalence of TD varied from 13.5% during the 1960s, to 28.6% in the 1970s, to 25.1% in the 1980s.

In a study of patients with a mean age of 29 years and a median length of lifetime exposure to neuroleptics at baseline of 12 months, Kane et al. (225) found that at least for the first several years the rate was linear at about 4-5% per year. Saltz et al. (226) reported a 31% incidence of TD after 43 weeks of neuroleptic treatment in an elderly patient population (mean age = 77 years; 72% female).

A recent study of 266 psychiatric outpatients (227)

determined the incidence of TD to be approximately 26% after one year of treatment, in patients over the age of 45 (mean age = 66 years, 83% male), being treated with relatively low doses of neuroleptics. The incidence was 52% after 2 years and 60% after 3 years.

Risk Factors

Older age is the most important patient-related risk factor for TD. Patients over the age of 45 are several times more likely to develop TD than younger subjects, and the prevalence, severity of dyskinetic symptoms, and intractability of the course of the disease increase with advancing age (228,229).

Gender may be another risk factor for TD. Many researchers have reported a significantly greater incidence of TD in women. In their review of the published literature, Yassa and Jeste (224) calculated a global mean value of 26.6% for women and 21.6% in men. Moreover, women tended to have more severe TD and a higher prevalence of spontaneous dyskinesia than men.

Psychiatric diagnosis has some relevance as a risk factor for TD. Schizophrenia patients may be at lower risk than patients with affective and schizoaffective disorders treated with antipsychotics (230,231). Unipolar and bipolar affective disorders (232-235) and phenylketonuria (236) have been identified as risk factors.

Ganzini et al. (237) found a higher prevalence of TD in diabetic than in nondiabetic patients, and Sewell and Jeste (238) suggested diabetes mellitus as a risk factor for metoclopramide-induced TD. The evidence for organic mental syndromes as risk factors for TD so far has been inconclusive (239–243). Patients who react to antipsychotic drugs with acute or subacute extrapyramidal symptoms may be at greater risk for developing TD with continued treatment (229). Our recent study (227) of older patients found that greater cumulative amounts of neuroleptics, especially the high-potency ones, were a significant risk factor for TD. Metoclopramide, a D_2-receptor blocker used commonly for gastroparesis, can also produce persistent TD (244), as can amoxapine, an antidepressant with neuroleptic metabolites.

Neurochemistry

TD has frequently been thought to result from supersensitivity of striatal dopamine receptors. But although all neuroleptic-treated patients probably develop some degree of supersensitivity to dopamine, only a minority develop the movements associated with TD. Jeste and Wyatt (209) summarized the evidence against the supersensitivity hypothesis of TD.

There is some evidence that noradrenergic hyperfunction may be a factor in the pathogenesis of TD. γ-Aminobutyric acid (GABA) is also thought to be involved in the regulation of the activity of norepinephrine, dopamine, and acetylcholine, all of which have been implicated in the etiology of TD (245,246).

MANAGEMENT

There is no cure for schizophrenia, and the goal of any treatment program must be to alleviate the suffering of the patient and those around him or her and to help the patient to function better in the world cognitively, affectively and socially. Medication alone is insufficient: management of schizophrenia patients requires psychosocial care conjoined with pharmacotherapy.

Any management of schizophrenia must be based on an accurate diagnosis. Before diagnosing schizophrenia, a clinician must perform an appropriate diagnostic workup both to rule out conditions in the differential diagnosis and to identify any coexisting medical conditions that may affect treatment. There is no standard schizophrenia work-up; it varies with each individual case. Given the lack of insight that characterizes schizophrenia patients, it is important that a complete psychiatric and other medical history be gathered from the patient's relatives, friends, significant others, colleagues, physicians, and medical records to the greatest feasible extent. Thorough neurological and other medical examinations are also critical.

It is especially important that the diagnostician rule out mood disorders, delusional disorder, and secondary psychoses. This may involve the use of brain imaging CT, MRI, blood chemistry, neuropsychological testing, and other related tests.

Neuroleptic medications have been shown to be the most effective treatment modality for schizophrenia in general (191,247,248). In a significant proportion of schizophrenia patients, many of the positive symptoms and some negative symptoms of the disorder can be brought under control by the use of neuroleptic drugs, although functioning may not improve to the premorbid level of social adjustment. In approximately two-thirds of acute schizophrenia patients, neuroleptic medication can reduce the psychotic symptoms, sometimes within a matter of weeks. In addition, a maintenance program of continuous neuroleptic medication can aid in preventing psychotic relapses in remitted patients (249). Some patients are treatment-resistant; there is little evidence that intensive treatment with massive prolonged doses of neuroleptics has any beneficial effect in these cases. Atypical antipsychotics such as clozapine should be considered in these patients.

Neuroleptic drugs carry a significant risk of side effects, including but not limited to sedation, hypotension, dryness of the mouth, blurred vision, tachycardia, cardiac effects, amenorrhea, galactorrhea, hyperpyrexia, pigmentary retinopathy, allergic reactions, and seizures (250). Some patients experience extrapyramidal side effects, including dystonia, akathisia, and parkinsonism that may respond to anticholinergic medication. Prolonged use of neuroleptics can produce TD, and a small number of patients may develop neuroleptic malignant syndrome, a potentially fatal condition (251,252). Pharmacokinetic and pharmacodynamic changes attributable to aging may significantly intensify response to neuroleptic medications. Accordingly, consider-

able caution should be exercised in the prolonged use of neuroleptics in patients over age 45. The relationship between serum neuroleptic levels and neuroleptic bioavailability is not yet well understood.

Given the potential side effects of neuroleptic drugs, the current conventional clinical strategy is to minimize the total lifetime amount of neuroleptic medication administered to a patient by prescribing the lowest effective dosage and avoiding unnecessary use of neuroleptics. Because commonly prescribed typical or conventional neuroleptic medications seem to be equally efficacious in equivalent dosages in controlling the active symptoms of schizophrenia, selection of a specific neuroleptic drug in a given instance is often dictated by careful consideration of the drug's side effects and the patient's particular medical condition. Atypical antipsychotics, such as clozapine and risperidone, are useful in controlling the symptoms of schizophrenia and may carry a reduced risk of TD, although they do have their own side effects. A unique feature of these drugs, which block serotonin and dopamine receptors, is their efficacy against negative symptoms of schizophrenia (253). The ultimate decision on suitability of a given neuroleptic medication must be determined in each case after evaluating the risk/benefit ratios of each drug. A trial of an atypical neuroleptic is indicated in patients who are unresponsive to treatment with typical neuroleptics.

Acute or subacute extrapyramidal symptoms that occur commonly with typical neuroleptics include dystonia, akathisia, and parkinsonism. Acute dystonia responds rapidly to antihistaminic or anticholinergic medications. Akathisia and parkinsonism respond less well to anticholinergic or dopaminergic medications, and these agents have their own side effects. It is best to use neuroleptics in doses that are effective, yet low enough not to produce extrapyramidal reactions. Alternatively, the atypical neuroleptics risperidone or clozapine may be used in view of their generally excellent efficacy and a low potential to cause extrapyramidal side effects. Clozapine is, however, officially indicated only for treatment-resistant schizophrenia.

In the treatment of schizophrenia, neuroleptic medications usually must be administered for long periods. Such long term treatment exposes the patient to increased risks of deleterious side effects. Ostensibly, the goal would be to remove the patient from neuroleptic medication except when needed, but intermittent neuroleptic treatment schedules may actually increase the risk of psychotic relapse and even of persistent TD (254,255) and increase the rate of episodes of both psychotic and dysphoric-neurotic symptoms (256). It is imperative that any neuroleptic taper be very gradual, and accompanied by careful monitoring and follow-up (249).

Schizophrenia has an organic, neurophysiological basis, and pharmacotherapy is an essential part of its treatment, but pharmacotherapy must be supplemented by psychosocial support. Successful treatment requires that each patient be engaged in a therapeutic process fashioned to his or her personal situation and directed toward providing the patient with an expanded repertoire of interpersonal skills. The therapy should involve behavior modification designed to help the patient to develop necessary social or other skills. A trusting therapist-patient relationship can facilitate the success of other modes of treatment, providing a secure environment in which the patient can learn and practice strategies of interpersonal relationship and communication. The risk of psychotic exacerbation or relapse increases with greater stress, which in turn could result from excessive stimulus load or from too high expectations about performance. The goals of supportive psychosocial therapy should, therefore, include keeping the stress level low, and avoiding unnecessary distractions and pressure to perform quickly.

Acknowledgments

This work was supported, in part by: Scottish Rite Benevolent Foundation's Schizophrenia Research Program, N.M.J., U.S.A.; NIMH grants MH 43693, MH 45132, MH 49671-01; and by the Department of Veterans Affairs.

REFERENCES

1. Jellinger K: Neuropathological findings after neuroleptic long-term therapy. In: Roizen L, Sharki H, Grevil N (eds): Neurotoxicology, New York, Raven Press, 1977, pp 25–42.
2. Gottesman II, Shields J: Schizophrenia: The Epigenetic Puzzle. Cambridge, Cambridge University, 1982.
3. Nasrallah HA, Weinberger DR:. Handbook of Schizophrenia. The Neurology of Schizophrenia. Amsterdam, Elsevier, 1986.
4. Flor-Henry P: Influence of gender in schizophrenia as related to other psychopathological syndromes. Schizophr Bull 16:211–227, 1990.
5. Isaacman DJ, Verdile VP, Kohen FP, Verdile LA: Pediatric telephone advice in the emergency department: Results of a mock scenario. Pediatrics 89:35–39, 1992.
6. Goldstein G: The Neuropsychology of Schizophrenia. In: Grant I, Adams KM (eds): Neuropsychological Assessment of Neuropsychiatric Disorders, New York, NY, Oxford University Press, 1986.
7. Heaton RK, Crowley TJ: Effects of Psychiatric Disorders and Their Somatic Treatments on Neuropsychological Test Results. In: Filskov SB, Ball TJ (eds): Handbook of Clinical Neuropsychology. New York, Wiley-Interscience, 1981, pp 481–525.
8. Levin S, Yurgelun-Todd D, Craft S: Contributions of clinical neuropsychology to the study of schizophrenia. J Abnorm Psychol 98:341–356, 1989.
9. Nuechterlein KH, Dawson ME: Information processing and attentional functioning in the course of schizophrenic disorder. Schizophr Bull 10:160–203, 1984.
10. Seidman L: Schizophrenia and brain dysfunction: An integration of recent neurodiagnostic findings. Psychol Bull 94:195–238, 1983.
11. Nuechterlein KH, Edell WS, Norris M, Dawson ME: Attentional vulnerability indicators, though disorder, and negative symptoms. Schizophr Bull 12:408–426, 1986.
12. Maher BA: Language and Schizophrenia. In Steinhauer S, Gruzelier JH, Zubin J (eds). In: Handbook of Schizophrenia, Volume 4, Neuropsychology, Psychophysiology, and Information Processing, Amsterdam, Elsevier, 1991, pp 437–464.
13. Gjerde PF: Attentional capacity dysfunction and arousal in schizophrenia. Psychol Bull 93:57–72, 1983.
14. Granholm E: Processing resource limitations in schizophrenia: Implications for predicting medication response and planning attentional training. In Margolin DI (ed): In: Cognitive Neuropsychology in Clinical Practice, New York, Oxford University Press, 1992, pp 43–69.
15. Asarnow RF, Granholm E, Sherman T: Span of Apprehension in Schizophrenia. In: Steinhauer S, Gruzelier JH, Zubin J (eds). Handbook of Schizophrenia, Vol. 4, Neuropsychology, Psychophysi-

ology, and Information Processing, Amsterdam, Elsevier, 1991, pp 335–370.
16. Nuechterlein KH: Reaction time and attention in schizophrenia: A critical evaluation of the data and the theories. Schizophr Bull 3:373–428, 1977.
17. Orzak MH, Kornetsky C: Attention dysfunction in chronic schizophrenia. Arch Gen Psychiatry 14:323–326, 1966.
18. Perlick D, Mattis S, Stastny P, Teresi J: Neuropsychological discriminators of long-term inpatient or outpatient status in chronic schizophrenia. J Neuropsychiat Clin Neurosci 4:428–434, 1992.
19. Wishner J, Wahl O: Dichotic listening in schizophrenia. J Consult Clin Psychol 42:538–546, 1974.
20. Wielgus MS, Harvey PD: Dichotic listening and recall in schizophrenia and mania. Schizophr Bull 14:689–700, 1988.
21. Pogue-Geile MF, Oltmanns TF: Sentence perception and distractibility in schizophrenic, manic and depressed patients. J Abnorm Psychol 89:115–124, 1980.
22. Asarnow RF, Granholm E: The Contributions of Cognitive Psychology to Vulnerability Models. In: Hafner H, Gattaz WF (eds): Search for the Causes of Schizophrenia, Vol. II, Heidelberg, Springer-Verlag, 1991, pp 205–220.
23. Goldberg TE, Ragland JD, Torrey EF, Gold JM, Bigelow LB, Weinberger DR: Neuropsychological assessment of monozygotic twins discordant for schizophrenia. Arch Gen Psychiatry 47:1066–1072, 1990.
24. Kinsbourne M, Hicks RE: Functional Cerebral Space: A Model for Overflow, Transfer and Interference Effects in Human Performance. In: Requin J (ed): Attention and Performance, VII, Hillsdale, Erlbaum, 1978, pp 345–362.
25. Luria RR: The Working Brain. New York, Basic Books, 1973.
26. Andreasen NC, Flashman L, Flaum M, Arndt S, Swayze V, O'Leary DS, Ehrhardt JC, Yuh WTC: Regional brain abnormalities in schizophrenia measured with magnetic resonance imaging. JAMA 272:1763–1769, 1994.
27. Koh SD: Remembering of verbal materials by schizophrenic young adults. In: Schwartz S (ed): Language and Cognition in Schizophrenia, Hillsdale, NJ, Lawrence Erlbaum, 1978, pp 55–99.
28. Gold JM, Randolph C, Carpenter CJ, Goldberg TE, Weinberger DR: Forms of memory failure in schizophrenia. J Abnorm Psychol 101(3):487–494, 1992.
29. Russell PN, Bannatyne PA, Smith JF: Associative strength as a mode of organization in recall and recognition: A comparison of schizophrenics and normals. J Abnorm Psychol 84:122–128, 1975.
30. Bauman E: Schizophrenic short-term memory: The role of organization at input. J Consult Clin Psychol 36:4–19, 1971.
31. Saykin AJ, Gur RC, Gur RE, Mozley PD, Mozley LH, Resnick SM, Kester B, Stafiniak P: Neuropsychological function in schizophrenia: Selective impairment in memory and learning. Arch Gen Psychiatry 48:618–624, 1991.
32. Granholm E, Bartzokis G, Asarnow RF, Marder SR: Preliminary associations between motor procedural learning, basal ganglia T2 relaxation times, and tardive dyskinesia in schizophrenia. Psychiatry Research: Neuroimaging 50:33–44, 1993.
33. Goldberg TE, Saint-Cyr JA, Weinberger DR: Assessment of procedural learning and problem solving in schizophrenia patients by Tower of Hanoi type tasks. Journal of Neuropsychiatry 2:165–173, 1990.
34. Schmand B, Brand N, Kuipers T: Procedural learning of cognitive and motor skills in psychotic patients. Schizophr Res 8:157–170, 1992.
35. Schwartz BL, Rosse RB, Deutsch SI: Toward a neuropsychology of memory in schizophrenia. Psychopharmacol Bull 28:341–351, 1992.
36. Granholm E, Asarnow RF, Marder SR: Controlled information processing resources and the development of automatic detection responses in schizophrenia. J Abnorm Psychol 100:22–30, 1991.
37. Butters N, Salmon DP, Granholm E, Heindel W, Lyon L: Neuropsychological Differentiation of Amnesiac and Dementing States. In: Stahl S, Iversen S, Goodman E (eds): Cognitive Neurochemistry, Oxford, Oxford University Press, 1987, pp 3–20.

38. Pantelis C, Barnes RRE, Nelson HE: Is the concept of frontal-subcortical dementia relevant to schizophrenia. Br J Psychiatry 76:185–193, 1970.

39. Daniel DG, Weinberger DR, Jones DW, Zigun JR, Coppola R, Handel S, Bigelow LB, Goldberg TE, Berman KF, Kleinman JE: The effect of amphetamine on regional cerebral blood flow during cognitive activation in schizophrenia. J Neurosci 11(7):1907–1917, 1991.

40. Braff DL, Heaton R, Kuck J, Cullum M, Moranville J, Grant I, Zisook S: The generalized pattern of neuropsychological deficits in outpatients with chronic schizophrenia with heterogeneous Wisconsin Card Sorting Test results. Arch Gen Psychiatry 48:891–898, 1991.

41. Weinberger D: The pathogenesis of schizophrenia: A neurodevelopment theory. In: Nasrallah HA, Weinberger DR (eds): Handbook of Schizophrenia, Vol. I: The Neurology of Schizophrenia, New York, Elsevier Science, 1986, pp 397–406.

42. Gruzelier J, Seymour K, Wilson L, Jolley A, Hirsch S: Impairments on neuropsychologic tests of temporohippocampal and frontohippocampal functions and word fluency in remitting schizophrenia and affective disorders. Arch Gen Psychiatry 45:623–629, 1988.

43. Carlsson M, Carlsson A: Schizophrenia: A subcortical neurotransmitter imbalance syndrome? Schizophr Bull 16:425–432, 1990.

44. Weinberger DR, Berman KF, Zec RF: Physiological dysfunction of dorsolateral prefrontal cortex in schizophrenia, I: Regional cerebral blood flow evidence. Arch Gen Psychiatry 43:114–124, 1986.

45. Bilder RM, Turkel E, Lipschutz-Broch L, Lieberman JA: Antipsychotic medication effects on neuropsychological functions. Psychopharmacol Bull 28:353–366, 1992.

46. Spohn HE, Strauss ME: Relation of neuroleptic and anticholinergic medication to cognitive functions in schizophrenia. J Abnorm Psychol 98:367–380, 1989.

47. Cornblatt BA, Lenzenweger MF, Dworkin RH, Erlenmeyer-Kimling L: Positive and negative schizophrenia symptoms, attention, and information processing. Schizophr Bull 11:397–408, 1985.

48. Smith RC, Largen J, Vroulis G, Ravichandran GK: Neuropsychological test scores and clinical response to neuroleptic drugs in schizophrenic patients. Compr Psychiatry 33:139–145, 1992.

49. Breier A, Schreiber JL, Dyer J, Pickar D: National Institute of Mental Health longitudinal study of chronic schizophrenia-Prognosis and predictors of outcome. Arch Gen Psychiatry 48:239–246, 1991.

50. Kern RS, Green MF, Satz P: Neuropsychological predictors of skills training for chronic psychiatric patients. Psychiatry Res 43:223–230, 1992.

51. Johnstone EV, Crow TJ, Frith CD, Husband J, Kreel L: Cerebral ventricular size and cognitive impairment in chronic schizophrenia. Lancet ii:924–926, 1976.

52. Weinberger D, Torrey E, Neophytides A, Wyatt R: Lateral cerebral ventricular enlargement in chronic schizophrenia. Arch Gen Psychiatry 36:735–739, 1979.

53. Owens D, Johnstone E, Crow T, Frith C, Jagoe J, Kreel L: Cerebral ventricular enlargement in schizophrenia: relationship to the disease process and its clinical correlates. Psychol Med 15:27–41, 1985.

54. Pearlson G, Kim W, Kubos K, et al: Ventricle-brain ratio, computed tomographic density, and brain area in 50 schizophrenics. Arch Gen Psychiatry 46:690–697, 1989.

55. Nasrallah H, Coffman J, Schwarzkopf S, Olson S: Reduced cerebral volume in schizophrenia. Schizophr Res 3:17, 1990.

56. Crow T, Ball J, Bloom S, Brown R, Bruton C, Colter N, Frith C, Johnstone E, Owens D, Roberts G: Schizophrenia as an anomaly of development of cerebral asymmetry: A post mortem study and a proposal concerning the genetic basis of the disease. Arch Gen Psychiatry 46:1145–1150, 1989.

57. Daniel D, Myslobodsky M, Ingraham L, Coppola R, Weinberger D: The relationship of occipital skull asymmetry to brain parenchymal measures in schizophrenia. Schizophr Res 2:465–472, 1989.

58. Andreasen NC, Ehrhardt JC, Swayze VW, Alliger RJ, Yuh WTC, Cohen G, Ziebell S: Magnetic resonance imaging of the brain in schizophrenia. Arch Gen Psychiatry 47:35–44, 1990.

59. Suddath RL, Casanova MF, Goldberg TE, Daniel DG, Kelsoe JR, Weinberger DR: Temporal lobe pathology in schizophrenia: a quantitative magnetic resonance imaging study. Am J Psychiatry 146:464–472, 1989.

60. Suddath RL, Christison GW, Torrey EF, Casanova MF, Weinberger DR: Anatomical abnormalities in the brains of monozygotic twins discordant for schizophrenia. N Engl J Med 322:789–794, 1990.

61. Gur R, Mozley P, Resnick S: Magnetic resonance imaging in schizophrenia: I. Volumetric analysis of brain and cerebrospinal fluid. Arch Gen Psychiatry 48:407–412, 1991.

62. DeLisi LE, Dauphinais ID, Gershon E: Perinatal complications and reduced size of brain limbic structures in familial schizophrenia. Schizophr Bull 14:21–32, 1988.

63. Bogerts B, Ashtari M, Degreeef G, Alvir J, Bilder RM, Lieberman JA: Reduced temporal limbic structure volumes on magnetic resonance images in first episode schizophrenia. Psychiatry Res: Neuroimaging 35:1–13, 1990.

64. Jernigan TL, Zisook S, Heaton RK, Moranville JT, Hesselink JR, Braff DL: Magnetic resonance imaging abnormalities in lenticular nuclei and cerebral cortex in schizophrenia. Arch Gen Psychiatry 48:881–890, 1991.

65. DeLisi L, Hoff A, Schwartz J, Shields GW, Halthore SN, Simhadri MG, Henn FA, Anand AK: Brain morphology in first-episode schizophrenic like psychotic patients: A quantitative magnetic resonance imaging study. Biol Psychiatry 29:159–175, 1991.

66. Breier A, Buchanan RW, Elkashef A, Munson RC, Kirkpatrick B, Gellad F: Brain morphology and schizophrenia: A magnetic resonance imaging study of the limbic, prefrontal cortex, and caudate structures. Arch Gen Psychiatry 49:921–926, 1992.

67. Rossi A, Stratta P, Mancini F, Gallucci M, Mattei P, Core L, Di Michele V, Casacchia M: Magnetic resonance imaging findings of amygdala-anterior hippocampus shrinkage in male patients with schizophrenia. Psychiatry Res 52:43–53, 1994.

68. Flaum M, Swayze VW, O'Leary DS, Yuh WTC, Ehrhardt JC, Arndt SV, Andreasen NC: Effects of Diagnosis, Laterality, and Gender on Brain Morphology in Schizophrenia. Am J Psychiatry 152:704–714, 1995.

69. Johnstone E, Owens D, Crow T: Temporal lobe structure as determined by nuclear magnetic resonance in schizophrenia and bipolar affective disorder. J Neurol Neurosurg Psychiatry 52:736–741, 1989.

70. Rossi A, Stratta P, D'Albenzio L: Reduced temporal lobe areas in schizophrenia: Preliminary evidences from a controlled multiplanar magnetic resonance imaging study. Biol Psychiatry 27:61–68, 1990.

71. Young A, Blackwood D, Roxborough H, McQueen J, Martin M, Kean D: A magnetic resonance imaging study of schizophrenia: Brain structure and clinical symptoms. Br J Psychiatry 158:158–164, 1991.

72. DeMyer M, Gilmor R, Hendrie H, DeMyer W, Augustyn G, Jackson R: Magnetic resonance brain images in schizophrenic and normal subjects: Influence of diagnosis and education. Schizophr Bull 14:21–37, 1988.

73. Shenton ME, Kikinis R, Jolesz FA, Pollak SD, LeMay M, Wible C, Hokama H, Martin J, Metcalf D, Coleman M, McCarley RW: Abnormalities of the left temporal lobe and thought disorder in schizophrenia: A quantitative magnetic resonance imaging study. N Engl J Med 327:604–612, 1992.

74. Raine A, Lencz T, Reynolds GP, Harrison GP, Sheard C, Medley I, Reynolds LM, Cooper JE: An evaluation of structural and functional prefrontal deficits in schizophrenia: MRI and neuropsychological measures. Psychiatry Res: Neuroimaging 45:123–137, 1992.

75. Schlaepfer TE, Harris GJ, Tien AY, Peng LW, Lee S, Federman EB, Chase GA, Barta PE, Pearlson GD: Decreased regional cortical gray matter volume in schizophrenia. Am J Psychiatry 151:842–848, 1994.

76. Uematsu M, Kalya H: Midsagittal cortical pathomorphometry of schizophrenia: A magnetic resonance imaging study. Psychiatry Res 30:11–20, 1989.

77. Wible CG, Shenton ME, Hokama H, Kikinis R, Jolesz FA, Metcalf

D, McCarley RW: Prefrontal cortex and schizophrenia. A quantitative magnetic resonance imaging study. Arch Gen Psychiatry 52:279–288, 1995.

78. Casanova M, Sanders R, Goldbert T: Morphometry of the corpus callosum in monozygotic twins discordant for schizophrenia: A magnetic resonance imaging study. J Neurol Neurosurg Psychiatry 53:416–421, 1990.

79. Raine A, Harrison G, Reynolds G, Sheard C, Cooper J, Medley I: Structural and functional characteristics of the corpus callosum in schizophrenics, psychiatric controls, and normal controls. A magnetic resonance imaging and neuropsychological evaluation. Arch Gen Psychiatry 47:1060–1064, 1990.

80. Mathew R, Partain C, Prakash R, Kulkami M, Logan T, Wilson W: A study of the septum pellucidum and corpus callosum in schizophrenia with MR Imaging. Acta Psychiatr Scand 72:414–421, 1985.

81. Nasrallah HA, Olson SC, McCalley-Whitters M, Chapman S, Jacoby CG: Cerebral ventricular enlargement in schizophrenia: A preliminary follow-up study. Arch Gen Psychiatry 43:157–159, 1986.

82. Andreasen NC, Arndt S, Swayze VI, Cizadlo T, Flaum M, O'Leary D, Ehrhardt JC, Yuh WTC: Thalamic abnormalities in schizophrenia visualized through magnetic resonance image averaging. Science 266:294–298, 1994.

83. Ingvar D, Franze G: Abnormalities of cerebral blood flow distribution in patients with chronic schizophrenia. Acta Psychiatr Scand 50:425–462, 1974.

84. Potkin SG, Buchsbaum MS, Jin Y, Tang C: Clozapine effects of glucose metabolic rate in striatum and frontal cortex. Long Island Jewish Medical Center and Case Western Reserve University School of Medicine: Symposium on clozapine. J Clin Psychiatry 55:63–66, 1994.

85. Gur RE, Resnick SM, Alavi A, Gur RC, Caroff S, Dann R, Silver F, Saykin AJ, Chawluk JB, Kushner M, Reivich M: Regional brain function in schizophrenia, I: A positron emission tomography study. Arch Gen Psychiatry 44:119–125, 1987.

86. Schroder J, Buchsbaum MS, Siegel BV, Geider FJ, Niethammer R: Structural and functional correlates of subsyndromes in chronic schizophrenia. Psychopathology 28:38–45, 1995.

87. Baxter L, Mazziotta J, Phelps M, Selin C, Guze B, Fairbanks L: Cerebral glucose metabolic rates in normal human females versus normal males. Psychiatry Res 21:237–245, 1987.

88. Jernigan T, Sargent T, Pfefferbaum A, Kusubov N, Stahl S: 18-Fluorodeoxyglucose PET in schizophrenia. Psychiatry Res 16:317–330, 1985.

89. Mubrin Z, Knezevic S, Koretic D, et al. Regional cerebral blood flow patterns in schizophrenic patients. Cerebral Blood Flow Bull 3:43–46, 1982.

90. Ariel RN, Golden CJ, Quaife MA, Dirksen JW, Forsell T, Wilson J, Graber B: Regional cerebral blood flow in schizophrenics. Arch Gen Psychiatry 40:258–263, 1983.

91. Kurachi M, Kobayashi K, Malsubara R: Regional cerebral blood flow in schizophrenic disorders. Eur Neurol 24:176–181, 1985.

92. Berman KF, Zec RF, Weinberger DR: Physiologic dysfunction of dorsolateral prefrontal cortex in schizophrenia: II. Role of neuroleptic treatment. Arch Gen Psychiatry 43:126–135, 1986.

93. Chabrol H, Guell A, Bes A, Moron P: Cerebral blood flow in schizophrenic adolescents. Am J Psychiatry 143:130, 1986.

94. Gur RE, Skolnick BE, Gur RC, Carol S, Rieger W, Obrist WD, Younkin D, Reivich M: Brain function in psychiatric disorder, I: Regional cerebral blood flow in medicated schizophrenics. Arch Gen Psychiatry 40:1250–1254, 1983.

95. Gur RE, Gur RC, Skolnick BE, Caroff S, Obrist WD, Resnick S, Reivich M: Brain function in psychiatric disorders: III Regional cerebral blood flow in unmedicated schizophrenics. Arch Gen Psychiatry 42:329–334, 1985.

96. Buchsbaum M, Ingvar D, Kessler R: Cerebral glucography with positron emission tomography. Arch Gen Psychiatry 39:251–259, 1982.

97. Buchsbaum M, DeLisi L, Holcomb H: Anterior gradients in cerebral glucose use in schizophrenia and affective disorders. Arch Gen Psychiatry 41:1159–1166, 1984.

98. Farkas T, Wolf A, Jaeger J, Brodie J, Christman D, Fowler J: Regional brain glucose metabolism in chronic schizophrenia: A positron emission transaxial tomographic study. Arch Gen Psychiatry 41:293–300, 1984.

99. Wolkin A, Jaeger J, Brodie J: Persistence of cerebral metabolic abnormalities in chronic schizophrenia as determined by positron emission tomography. Am J Psychiatry 142:564–571, 1985.

100. Kishimoto H, Kuwahara H, Ohno S: Three subtypes of chronic schizophrenia identified using 11C-glucose positron emission tomography. Psychiatry Res 21:285–292, 1987.

101. Buchsbaum MS: The frontal lobes, basal ganglia, and temporal lobes as sites for schizophrenia. Schizophr Bull 16 (3):379–389, 1990.

102. Buchsbaum MS, Haier RJ, Potkin SG, Nuechterlein K, Bracha HS, Katz M, Lohr J, Wu J, Lottenberg S, Jerabek PA, Trenary M, Tafalla R, Reynolds C, Bunney WE: Frontostriatal disorder in cerebral metabolism in never-medicated schizophrenics. Arch Gen Psychiatry 49:935–942, 1992.

103. Volkow N, Wolf A, Van Gelder P: Phenomenological correlates of metabolic activity in 18 patients with chronic schizophrenia. Am J Psychiatry 144:151–158, 1987.

104. Sheppard G, Gruzelier J, Manchanda R, Hirsch SR, Wise R, Frackowiak R, Jones T: O-15 Positron emission tomographic scanning in predominantly never-treated acute schizophrenic patients. Lancet 2:1448–1452, 1983.

105. Early TS, Reiman EM, Raichle ME, Spitznagel EL: Left globus pallidus abnormality in never-medicated patients with schizophrenia. Proc Natl Acad Sci U S A 84:561–563, 1987.

106. Szechtman H, Nahmias C, Garnett E: Effects of neuroleptics on altered cerebral glucose metabolism in schizophrenia. Arch Gen Psychiatry 45:523–532, 1988.

107. Sedvall G, Blomquist G, DePaulis T, et al: PET Studies on Brain Energy Metabolism and Dopamine Receptors in Schizophrenia Patients and Monkeys, in Psychiatry. In Pichot P, Berner P, Wolf R, et al (eds): The State of the Art. Biological Psychiatry, Higher Nervous Activity, New York, Pleniun, 1985.

108. Cleghorn J, Garnett E, Nahmias C: Increased frontal and reduced parietal glucose metabolism in acute untreated schizophrenia. Psychiatry Res 28:119–133, 1989.

109. Warkentin S, Nilsson A, Risberg J: Regional cerebral blood flow in schizophrenia: Repeated studies during a psychotic episode. Psychiatry Res 35:27–38, 1990.

110. Cleghorn J, Szechtman H, Garnett E: Apomorphine effects on brain metabolism in neuroleptic naive schizophrenic patients. Psychiatry Res 40:135–153, 1991.

111. Crawley J, Crow T, Johnstone E: Dopamine D2 receptors in schizophrenia studied in vivo. Lancet 2:224–225, 1986.

112. Wong D, Wagner H, Tune L: Positron emission tomography reveals elevated D2 dopamine receptors in drug-naive schizophrenic patients. Science 234:1558–1563, 1986.

113. Farde L, Wiesel F, Stone-Elander S: D2 dopamine receptors in neuroleptic-naive schizophrenic patients: A positron emission tomography study with (11C0 raclopride. Arch Gen Psychiatry 47:213–219, 1990.

114. Corsellis J: Psychoses of Obscure Pathology. In Blackwood W, Corsellis J (eds): Greenfield's Neuropathology, London, E. Arnold, 1976, pp 903–915.

115. Brown R, Colter N, Corsellis J, Crow FJ, Frith CD, Jagoe R, Johnstone EC, Marsh L: Postmortem evidence of structural brain changes in schizophrenia: Differences in brain weight, temporal horn area, and parahippocampal gyms compared with affective disorder. Arch Gen Psychiatry 43:36–42, 1986.

116. Pakkenberg B: Post-mortem study of chronic schizophrenic brains. Br J Psychiatry 151:744–752, 1987.

117. Bruton C, Crow T, Frith C, et al: Schizophrenia and the brain: a prospective clinico-neuropathological study. Psychol Med 20:285–304, 1990.

118. Crow T, Colter N, Brown R, Bruton C, Johnstone E: Lateralized asymmetry of temporal horn enlargement in schizophrenia. Schizophr Res 1:155–156, 1988.

119. Bogerts B, Meertz E, Schonfeldt-Bausch R: Basal ganglia and limbic system pathology in schizophrenia: A morphometric study of brain volume and shrinkage. Arch Gen Psychiatry 42:784–791, 1985.

120. Bogerts B, Falkai P, Haupts M, et al: Post-mortem volume measurements of limbic systems and basal ganglia structures in chronic schizophrenics. Schizophr Res 3:295–301, 1990.

121. Falkai P, Bogerts B, Rozumek M: Limbic pathology in schizophrenia: the entorhinal region: a morphometric study. Biol Psychiatry 24:515–521, 1988.

122. Atlshuler L, Casanova M, Goldberg T, Kleinman J: The hippocampus and parahippocampus in schizophrenic, suicide and control brains. Arch Gen Psychiatry 47:1029–1034, 1990.

123. Stevens J: Clinicopathological correlations in schizophrenia. Arch Gen Psychiatry 43:715–716, 1986.

124. Heckers S, Heinsen H, Heinsen Y, Beckmann H: Cortex white matter, and basal ganglia in schizophrenia: a volumetric postmortem study. Biol Psychiatry 29:556–566, 1991.

125. Lesch A, Bogerts B: The Diencephalon in Schizophrenia: Evidence for reduced thickness of the periventricular grey matter. Eur Arch Psychiatry Neurol Sci 234:212–219, 1984.

126. Pakkenberg B: Pronounced reduction of total neuron number in mediodorsal thalamic nucleus and nucleus accumbens in schizophrenia. Arch Gen Psychiatry 47:1023–1028, 1990.

127. Jakob H, Beckmann H: Gross and histological criteria for developmental disorders in brains of schizophrenics. J R Soc Med 39:1131–1139, 1989.

128. Stevens JR: Neuropathology of schizophrenia. Arch Gen Psychiatry 39:1131–1139, 1982.

129. Falkai P, Bogerts B: Cell loss in the hippocampus of schizophrenics. Eur Arch Psychiatry Neurol Sci 236:154–161, 1986.

130. Lawson WB, Jeste DV, Kopp V, Wyatt RJ, Hanin I: RBC and plasma choline in neuroleptic-treated schizophrenic patients. Psychiatry Res 29:45–53, 1989.

131. Benes F, Sorensen I, Bird E: Reduced neuronal size in posterior hippocampus of schizophrenic patients. Schizophr Bull 17:597–608, 1991.

132. Benes F, Majocha R, Bird E, Marotta C: Increased vertical axon numbers in the cingulate cortex of schizophrenics. Arch Gen Psychiatry 4417:1017–1021, 1987.

133. Benes F, McSparren J, Bird E, SanGiovanni J, Vincent S: Deficits in small interneurons in prefrontal and cingulate cortices of schizophrenic and schizoaffective patients. Arch Gen Psychiatry, 1993.

134. Heckers S, Heinsen H, Geiger B, Beckman H: Hippocampal neuron number in schizophrenia-a stereological study. Arch Gen Psychiatry 48:1002–1008, 1993.

135. Kovelman J, Scheibel A: A neurohistological correlate of schizophrenia. Biol Psychiatry 19:1601–1621, 1984.

136. Benes F, Bird E: An analysis of the arrangement of neurons in the cingulate cortex of schizophrenic patients. Arch Gen Psychiatry 44:608–616, 1987.

137. Conrad A, Abebe T, Austin R, Forsythe S, Scheibel A: Hippocampal pyramidal cell disarray in schizophrenia. Arch Gen Psychiatry, 1993.

138. Christian G, Casanova M, Weinberger D, et al. A quantitative investigation of parahippocampal pyramidal cell size, shape and variability of orientation in schizophrenia. Arch Gen Psychiatry 46:1027–1032, 1989.

139. Akbarian S, Bunney JW, Potkin S, et al.: Altered distribution of nicotinamide-adenine dinucleotide phosphate-diaphorase cells in frontal lobe of schizophrenics implies disturbances of cortical development. Arch Gen Psychiatry 50:169–177, 1993.

140. Akbarian S, Vinuela A, Kim J, Potkin S, Bunney JW, Jones E: Distorted distribution of nicotinamide-adenine dinucleotide phosphate-diaphorase neurons in temporal lobe of schizophrenics implies anomalous cortical development. Arch Gen Psychiatry 40:178–187, 1993.

141. Roberts G, Colter N, Lofthouse R, et al. Is there gliosis in schizophrenia? Investigation of the temporal lobe. Biol Psychiatry 22:1459–1486, 1987.

142. Casanova M, Saunders R, Stevens J, Kleinman J: Quantitation of astrocytes in the molecular layer of the dentate gyms in schizophrenic patients. Biol Psychiatry 1993.

143. Creese I, Burt D, Snyder S: Dopamine receptor binding predicts clinical and pharmacological potencies of antischizophrenic drugs. Science 192:481–483, 1976.

144. Seeman P, Lee T, Chau Wong K: Antipsychotic drug doses and neuroleptic/dopamine receptors. Nature 261:717–719, 1976.

145. Lieberman J, Kane J, Gadaleta D, Brenner R, Lesser M, Kinon B: Methylphenidate challenge as a predictor of relapse in schizophrenia. Am J Psychiatry 141:633–638, 1984.

146. Davidson M, Keefe R, Mohs R, et al. L-Dopa challenge and relapse in schizophrenia. Am J Psychiatry 144:934–938, 1987.

147. Bird E, Barnes J, Iversen L, Spokes E, Mackay A, Shepherd M: Increased brain dopamine and reduced glutamic acid decarboxylase and choline acetyltransferase activity in schizophrenia and related psychoses. Lancet ii:1157–1159, 1977.

148. Owen F, Crow T, Poulter M, et al. Increased dopamine-receptor sensitivity in schizophrenia. Lancet ii:223–225, 1978.

149. Mackay AVP, Iversen LL, Rosser M, Spokes E, Bird E, Arregui A, Creese I, Synder SH: Increased brain dopamine and dopamine receptors in schizophrenia. Arch Gen Psychiatry 39:991–997, 1982.

150. Reynolds G: Increased concentrations and lateral asymmetry of amygdala dopamine in schizophrenia. Nature 305:527–529, 1983.

151. Crow T, Baker H, Cross A, et al. Monamine mechanisms in chronic schizophrenia: Post-mortem neurochemical findings. Br J Psychiatry 134:249–256, 1979.

152. Reynolds G, Czudek C, Bzowej N, et al. Dopamine receptor asymmetry in schizophrenia. Lancet i:979, 1987.

153. Davis KL, Kahn RS, Ko G, Davidson M: Dopamine in schizophrenia: A review and reconceptualization. Am J Psychiatry 148:1474–1486, 1991.

154. Mackay A, Bird E, Spokes E, et al. Dopamine receptors and schizophrenia: Drug effect or illness? Lancet ii:925–926, 1980.

155. Lee T, Seeman P, Tourtellotte W, Farley I, Hornykeiwicz O: Binding of 3H-neuroleptics and 3H-apomorphine in schizophrenic brains. Nature 274:897–900, 1978.

156. Widerlov E: A critical appraisal of CSF monoamine metabolite studies in schizophrenia. Ann N Y Acad Sci 537:309–323, 1988.

157. Bartokis G, Garber HJ, Marder SR, Olendorf WH: MRI in tardive dyskinesia: Shortened left caudate T2. Biol Psychiatry 28:1027–1036, 1990.

158. Van Tol H, Bunjow J, Guan H, et al. Cloning of the gene for a human dopamine D4 receptor with high affinity for the antipsychotic clozapine. Nature 350:610–614, 1991.

159. Benes F, Davidson J, Bird E: Quantitative cytoarchitectural studies of the cerebral cortex of schizophrenics. Arch Gen Psychiatry 43:31–35, 1986.

160. Bissette G, Nemeroff C, Mackay A: Peptides in Schizophrenia. In: Enson P, Rosser M, Tohyama M (eds): In: Progress in Brain Research, 66th ed. Amsterdam, Elsevier, 1986.

161. Farmery S, Owen F, Poulter M, et al. Reduced high affinity cholecystokinin binding in hippocampus and frontal cortex of schizophrenic patients. Life Sci 36:473–477, 1985.

162. Ferrier I, Roberts G, Crow T, et al. Reduced cholecystokinin-like and somatostatin-like immunoreactivity in limbic lobe is associated with negative symptoms in schizophrenia. Life Sci 33:475–482, 1983.

163. Roberts G, Ferrier I, Lee Y, et al. Peptides, the limbic lobe and schizophrenia. Brain Res 288:199–211, 1983.

164. Kerwin R, Patel S, Maldrum B, et al. Asymmetrical loss of glutamate receptor subtype in left hippocampus in schizophrenia. Lancet i:583–584, 1988.

165. Nishikawa T, Takashima M, Toru M: Increased (3H) kainic acid binding in the prefrontal cortex in schizophrenia. Neurosci Lett 40:245–250, 1983.

166. Bleuler M: The Schizophrenic Disorders: Long-term Patient and Family Studies. Translated by S.M. Clemens. New Haven and London, Yale University Press, 1978.

167. Feighner JP, Robins E, Guze SB, Woodruff RA, Winokur G, Munoz R: Diagnostic criteria for use in psychiatric research. Arch Gen Psychiatry 26:57–63, 1972.

168. American Psychiatric Association: Diagnostic and Statistical Manual of Mental Disorders. Washington, DC, American Psychiatric Press, 1980.

169. American Psychiatric Association: Diagnostic and Statistical Manual of Mental Disorders, Third Edition-Revised. Washington, DC, American Psychiatric Press, 1987.

170. American Psychiatric Association: Diagnostic and Statistical Manual of Mental Disorders, Fourth Edition-Revised. Washington, DC, American Psychiatric Press, 1994.

171. Harris MJ, Jeste DV: Late-onset schizophrenia: An overview. Schizophr Bull 14:39–55, 1988.

172. Kay DWK, Beamish P, Roth M: Old age mental disorders in Newcastle-Upon-Tyne. Br J Psychiatry 110:146–158, 1964.

173. Castle DJ, Murray RM: The neurodevelopmental basis of sex differences in schizophrenia. Psychol Med 21:565–575, 1991.

174. Pearlson GD, Kreger L, Rabins RV, Chase GA, Cohen B, Wirth JB, Schlaepfer TB, Tune LE: A chart review study of late-onset and early-onset schizophrenia. Am J Psychiatry 146:1568–1574, 1989.

175. Cooper JK, Mungas D, Weiler PG: Relations of cognitive status and abnormal behaviors in Alzheimer's Disease. J Am Geriatr Soc 38:867–870, 1990.

176. Cooper AF, Porter R: Visual acuity and ocular pathology in the paranoid and affective psychoses of later life. J Psychosom Res 20:107–114, 1976.

177. Miller BL, Lesser IM, Boone KB, Hill E, Mehringer CM, Wong K: Brain lesions and cognitive function in late-life psychosis. Br J Psychiatry 158:76–82, 1991.

178. Prager S, Jeste DV: Sensory impairment in late-life schizophrenia. Schizophr Bull 19(4):755–772, 1993.

179. Jeste DV, Harris MJ, Zweifach M: Late-onset Schizophrenia. In: Michels R, Cavenar JO, Jr., Brodie NKH, et al (eds): Psychiatry, Revised Edition., Philadelphia, J.B. Lippincott Co., 1988, pp 1–8.

180. Jeste DV, Harris MJ, Krull A, Kuck J, McAdams LA, Heaton R: Clinical and neuropsychological characteristics of patients with late-onset schizophrenia. Am J Psychiatry 152:722–730, 1995.

181. Naguib M, Levy R: Neuropsychological impairment and structural brain abnormalities on computed tomography. International Journal of Geriatric Psychiatry 2:83–90, 1987.

182. Rabins P, Pearlson G, Jayaram G, Steele C, Tune L: Elevated VBR in late-onset schizophrenia. Am J Psychiatry 144:1216–1218, 1987.

183. Burns A, Carrick J, Ames D, Naguib M, Levy R: The cerebral cortical appearance in late paraphrenia. International Journal of Geriatric Psychiatry 4:31–34, 1989.

184. Krull AJ, Press G, Dupont R, Harris MJ, Jeste DV: Brain imaging in late-onset schizophrenia and related psychoses. International Journal of Geriatric Psychiatry 6:651–658, 1991.

185. Breitner J, Husain M, Figiel G, Krishnan K, Boyko O: Cerebral white matter disease in late-onset psychosis. Biol Psychiatry 28:266–274, 1990.

186. Corey-Bloom J, Jernigan T, Archibald S, Harris MJ, Jeste DV: Quantitative magnetic resonance imaging in late-life schizophrenia. Am J Psychiatry 152:447–449, 1995.

187. Kay DWK, Roth M: Environmental and hereditary factors in the schizophrenias of old age ("late paraphrenia") and their bearing on the general problem of causation in schizophrenia. Journal of Mental Science 107:649–686, 1961.

188. Post F: Persistent Persecutory States of the Elderly. London, Pergamon Press, 1966.

189. Herbert ME, Jacobson S: Late paraphrenia. Br J Psychiatry 113:461–469, 1967.

190. Rabins P, Pauker S, Thomas J: Can schizophrenia begin after age 44? Compr Psychiatry 25:290–293, 1984.

191. Jeste DV, Lacro JP, Gilbert PL, Kline J, Kline N: Treatment of late-life schizophrenia with neuroleptics. Schizophr Bull 19(4):817–830, 1993.

192. Jeste DV, Caligiuri MP: Tardive dyskinesia. Schizophr Bull 19:303–315, 1993.

193. Davison K, Bagley C: Schizophrenia-like Psychoses Associated with Organic Disorders of the Central Nervous System-A Review of the Literature. In Hetherington R (ed): Current Problem in Neuropsychiatry, Kent, Hetherington R. 1969, pp 113–184.

194. Cummings JL: Organic Delusions: Phenomenology, Anatomical Correlations, and Review. Br J Psychiatry 146:184–197, 1985.

195. Jeste DV, Wragg RE, Salmon DP, Harris MJ, Thal LJ: Cognitive deficits of patients with Alzheimer's disease with and without delusions. Am J Psychiatry 149:184–189, 1992.

196. Friedman J, Lannon M: Clozapine in the treatment of psychosis in Parkinson's disease. Neurology 39:1219–1221, 1989.

197. Jeste DV, Wyatt RJ: Neuropsychiatric Movement Disorders. Washington, D.C. American Psychiatric Press, 1984.

198. Harris MJ, Jeste DV, Gleghorn A, Sewell DD: New-onset psychosis in HIV-infected patients. J Clin Psychiatry 52:369–376, 1991.

199. Sewell DD, Jeste DV, Atkinson JH, Heaton RK, Hesselink JR, Wiley C, Thal L, Chandler JL, Grant I, HNRC Group: HIV-associated psychosis: A longitudinal study of 20 cases. Am J Psychiatry 151(2):237–242, 1994.

200. Trimble M: Interictal Psychosis. In Trimble M (ed): The Psychoses of Epilepsy, New York, Raven Press, 1991, pp 109–149.

201. Gibbs A: Ictal and non-ictal psychiatric disorders in temporal lobe epilepsy. Journal of Nervous and Mental Disease 113:522–528, 1951.

202. Bear D, Levin K, Blumer D, Chetham D, Ryder J: Interictal behavior in hospitalized temporal lobe epileptics: Relationship to idiopathic psychiatric syndromes. J Neurol Neurosurg Psychiatry, 1993.

203. Perez M, Trimble M: Epileptic psychosis: Diagnostic comparison with process schizophrenia. Br J Psychiatry, 1993.

204. Pakalnis A, Drake M, John K, Kellum J: Forced normalization: acute psychosis after seizure control in seven patients. Arch Neurol, 1993.

205. Sherwin I, Peron-Magnan P, Bancaud J, Bonis A, Talairach J: Prevalence of psychosis in epilepsy as a function of the laterality of the epileptogenic lesion. Arch Neurol 39:621–625, 1982.

206. Roberts GW, Done DJ, Bruton C, Crow TJ: A "mock up" of schizophrenia: Temporal lobe epilepsy and schizophrenia-like psychosis. Biol Psychiatry 28:127–143, 1990.

207. Mendez M, Grau R, Doss R, Taylor J: Schizophrenia in epilepsy: seizure and psychosis variables. Neurology 43:1073–1077, 1993.

208. Cox DR: A note on the graphical analysis of survival data. Biometrika 66(1):188–190, 1979.

209. Jeste DV, Wyatt RJ: Understanding and Treating Tardive Dyskinesia. New York, Guilford Press, Inc. 1982.

210. Lohr J, Wisniewski A, Jeste DV: Neurological Aspects of Tardive Dyskinesia. In Nasrallah HA, Weinberger DR (eds): The Neurology of Schizophrenia. Amsterdam, Elsevier Science Publishers, 1986, pp 97–119.

211. Burke RF, Fahn S, Jankovic J, Marsden CD, Lang AE, Gollomp S, Ilson J: Tardive dystonia: Late-onset and persistent dystonia caused by antipsychotic drugs. Neurology 32:1335, 1982.

212. Gimenez-Roldan S, Mateo D, Bartolome P: Tardive dystonia and severe tardive dyskinesia: a comparison of risk factors and prognosis. Acta Psychiatr Scand 44:417, 1985.

213. Weiner WJ, Luby ED: Tardive akathisia. J Clin Psychiatry 44:417, 1983.

214. Stahl SM: Tardive Tourette syndrome in an autistic patient after long-term neuroleptic administration. Am J Psychiatry 137:1267, 1980.

215. Nasrallah HA, Pappas NJ, Crowe RR: Oculogyric dystonia in tardive dyskinesia. Am J Psychiatry 137:850–851, 1980.

216. Weiner WJ, Nausieda PA, Glantz RH: Meige syndrome (blepharospasmoromandibular dystonia) after long-term neuroleptic therapy. Neurology 31:1555, 1981.

217. Weiss KJ, Ciraulo DA, Shader RI: Physostigmine test in the rabbit syndrome and tardive dyskinesia. Am J Psychiatry, 1993.
218. Klawans HL, Barr A: Prevalence of spontaneous lingual-facial-buccal dyskinesias in the elderly. Neurology 32:558–559, 1982.
219. Koller WC: Eduntulous orodyskinesia. Ann Neurol 13:97, 1983.
220. Munetz MR, Cornes CL: Distinguishing akathisia and tardive dyskinesia: A review of the literature. J Clin Psychopharmacol 3:343, 1983.
221. Crane GE: Pseudoparkinsonism and tardive dyskinesia. Arch Neurol 27:426–430, 1972.
222. Richardson MA, Craig TJ: The coexistence of parkinsonism-like symptoms and tardive dyskinesia. Am J Psychiatry 139:341, 1982.
223. Britton V, Melamed E: Coexistence of severe parkinsonism and tardive dyskinesia as side effects of neuroleptic therapy. J Clin Psychiatry 45:28, 1984.
224. Yassa R, Jeste DV: Gender differences in tardive dyskinesia: A critical review of the literature. Schizophr Bull 18 (4):701–715, 1992.
225. Kane JM, Woerner M, Lieberman J: Tardive dyskinesia: prevalence, incidence, and risk factors. J Clin Psychopharmacol 8(4):52S–56S, 1988.
226. Saltz BL, Woerner MG, Kane JM, Lieberman JA, Alvir JM, Bergmann KJ, Blank K, Koblenzer J, Kahaner K: Prospective study of tardive dyskinesia incidence in the elderly. JAMA 266:2402–2406, 1991.
227. Jeste DV, Caligiuri MP, Paulsen JS, Heaton RK, Lacro JP, Harris MJ, Bailey A, Fell RL, McAdams LA: Risk of tardive dyskinesia in older patients: A prospective longitudinal study of 266 patients. Arch Gen Psychiatry 52:756–765, 1995.
228. Dworkin RH, Bernstein G, Kaplansky LM, Lipsitz JD, Rinaldi A, Slater SL, Cornblatt BA, Erlenmeyer-Kimling L: Social competence and positive and negative symptoms: A longitudinal study of children and adolescents at risk for schizophrenia and affective disorder. Am J Psychiatry 148:1182–1188, 1991.
229. Kane JM, Jeste DV, Barnes TRE, Casey DE, Cole JO, Davis JM, Gualtieri CT, Schooler NR, Sprague RL, Wettstein RM: Tardive Dyskinesia: A Task Force Report of the American Psychiatric Association. Washington, D.C. American Psychiatric Association, 1992.
230. Lang AE, Marsden CD: Alphamethylparatyrosine and tetrabenazine in movement disorders. Clin Neuropharmacol 5:375–387, 1982.
231. Casey DE, Keepers GA: Neuroleptic Side Effects: Acute Extrapyramidal Syndromes and Tardive Dyskinesia. In Casey DE, Christensen AV (eds): Psychopharmacology: Current Trends. Berlin, Springer-Verlag, 1988, pp 74–93.
232. Davis KL, Berger PA, Hollister LE: Tardive dyskinesia and depressive illness. Psychopharmacology Communications 2:125–130, 1976.
233. Rosenbaum AH, Niven RG, Hanson NP, Swanson DW: Tardive dyskinesia: Relationship with a primary affective disorder. Diseases of the Nervous System 38:423–427, 1977.
234. Mukherjee S, Rosen AM, Caracci G, Shukla S: Persistent tardive dyskinesia in bipolar patients. Arch Gen Psychiatry 43:342–346, 1986.
235. Casey DE: Affective disorders and tardive dyskinesia. L'Encephale 14:221–226, 1988.
236. Richardson MA, Pass R, Craig TJ, Fickers E: Factors influencing the prevalence and severity of tardive dyskinesia. Psychopharmacol Bull 20/1:33, 1984.
237. Ganzini L, Heintz RT, Hoffman WF, Casey DE: The prevalence of tardive dyskinesia in neuroleptic-treated diabetics: A controlled study. Arch Gen Psychiatry 48:259–263, 1991.
238. Sewell DD, Yoshinobu BH, Caligiuri MP, Jeste DV: Metoclopramide-associated tardive dyskinesia in hemodialysis patients with diabetes mellitus: Two case reports. Gen Hosp Psychiatry 14:416–419, 1992.
239. Yassa R, Nair V, Schwartz G: Tardive dyskinesia: a two-year follow-up study. Psychosomatics 25:852–855, 1984.
240. Manschreck TC, Keuthen NJ, Schneyer ML, Celada MT, Laughery J, Collins P: Abnormal involuntary movements and chronic schizophrenic disorders. Biol Psychiatry 27:150–158, 1990.
241. Mion CC, Andreasen NC, Arndt S, Swayze VW, Cohen GA: MRI abnormalities in tardive dyskinesia. Psychiatry Research: Neuroimaging 40:157–166, 1991.
242. Gold JM, Egan MF, Kirch DG, Goldberg TE, Daniel DG, Bigelow LB, Wyatt RJ: Tardive dyskinesia: Neuropsychological, computerized tomographic, and psychiatric symptom findings. Biol Psychiatry 30:587–599, 1991.
243. Brown KW, White T: The influence of topography on the cognitive and psychopathological effects of tardive dyskinesia. Am J Psychiatry 149:1385–1389, 1992.
244. Sewell DD, Jeste DV: Metoclopramide-associated tardive dyskinesia: An analysis of 67 cases. Archives of Family Medicine 1:271–278, 1992.
245. Scatton B, Bartholini G: Gamma-aminobutyric acid (GABA) receptor stimulation. IV. Effect of progabide (SL 76002) and other GABAergic agents on acetylcholine turnover in rat brain areas. J Pharmacol Exp Ther 220:689, 1982.
246. Scatton B, Zivkovic B, Dedek J, Lloyd KG: Gamma-aminobutyric acid (GABA) receptor stimulation. III. Effect of progabide (SL 76002) on norepinephrine, dopamine and 5-hydroxytryptamine turnover in rat brain areas. J Pharmacol Exp Ther 220:678, 1982.
247. Kane JM: Drug Maintenance Strategies in Schizophrenia. Washington DC, American Psychiatric Press, 1984.
248. Davis JM, Barter JT, Kane JM: Antipsychotic Drugs. In Kaplan HI, Sadock BJ (eds): Comprehensive Textbook of Psychiatry, volume 2, 5th ed. Baltimore, Williams and Wilkins, 1989, pp 1591–1626.
249. Gilbert PL, Harris MJ, McAdams LA, Jeste DV: Neuroleptic withdrawal in schizophrenic patients. Arch Gen Psychiatry 52:173–188, 1995.
250. Kane JM, Marder SR: Psychopharmacologic treatment of schizophrenia. Schizophr Bull 19:287–302, 1993.
251. Levensen JL: Neuroleptic malignant syndrome. Am J Psychiatry 142:1137–1145, 1985.
252. Sewell DD, Jeste DV: Neuroleptic Malignant Syndrome: Clinical Presentation, Pathophysiology, and Treatment. In Stoudemire A, Fogel BS (eds): Medical Psychiatric Practice, Washington, D.C. American Psychiatric Press, 1991, pp 425–452.
253. Meltzer HY: Atypical Antipsychotic Drugs. In Bloom FE, Kupfer DJ (eds): Psychopharmacology: The Fourth Generation of Progress, New York, Raven Press, Ltd. 1995, pp 1277–1286.
254. Jeste DV, Potkin SG, Sinha S, Feder SL, Wyatt RJ: Tardive dyskinesia - reversible and persistent. Arch Gen Psychiatry 36:585–590, 1979.
255. Goldman MB, Luchins DJ: Intermittent neuroleptic therapy and tardive dyskinesia: A literature review. Hosp Community Psychiatry 35:1215–1219, 1984.
256. Jolley AG, Hirsch SR, McRink A, Manchanda R: Trial of brief intermittent neuroleptic prophylaxis for selected schizophrenic outpatients: Clinical outcome at one year. British Medical Journal 298:985–990, 1989.

16

PERCEPTUAL DISTURBANCES IN FOCAL NEUROLOGICAL DISEASES

Lynn C. Robertson

Knowledge of how damage to different neural systems affects perception in humans has grown substantially over the past decade. This can be attributed in no small part to the advent of new imaging techniques such as magnetic resonance imaging (MRI) and positron emission tomography (PET). However, without behavioral methods to measure functioning at various levels of complexity, these new technologies would be of little value in addressing brain-behavior relationships. Measurement of both sides of the brain-behavior scale must evolve if advances in understanding these relationships are to occur.

Historically, neuropsychology focused on large chunks of behavior. Clinically, deficits were categorized as "memory," "attention," "thought disorder," "language," as if there were only about four or five categories of cognition that could be affected. When further parsing was attempted, the deficits often reflected little more than a description of the behavioral manifestation. For instance, "visual-spatial" deficits could be divided into difficulties with parts versus wholes or Gestalts. Or they could be described as unilateral neglect, meaning that patients would not respond to unilaterally presented stimuli in the contralesional field. A diagnosis of Balint's syndrome meant that patients would respond to only one object, had difficulty with visually guided reaching (optic ataxia) and visual tracking deficits. A diagnosis of Gerstman syndrome meant that patients had difficulty with left-right discrimination, calculation (acalculia), naming digits of the hand (finger agnosia), and writing (agraphia). These are but a few examples that demonstrate that neuropsychological classifications do not specify the underlying cognitive processes that are affected in any given syndrome. Rather, they are examples of descriptions that refer to the type of behavior one is likely to observe in a particular patient; descriptions that are not very useful in elucidating the cognitive mechanisms that are involved.

The broadly thrown cloth of traditional clinical neuropsychology was developed for the purposes of assessing patient's neurological status, and it is too large to relate biological systems to cognitive function in meaningful ways. This limitation has been altered substantially by the application to neurological populations of cognitive theory and chronometric measures derived from the study of cognition in healthy young college students.

This chapter presents some of the important advances in understanding components of visual-spatial functioning and how they relate to neural systems. The focus is on anatomical correlates of visual-perceptual function, but this does not imply that psychopharmacological or electrophysiological correlates are not equally important. Some evidence using the latter methods are mentioned in passing, but the emphasis in this chapter is on deficits that are caused by structural damage in the human brain and their application in understanding both normal brain function and dysfunction.

LESION METHOD—CAVEATS AND CREDENCE

Neuropsychology's history is couched in the lesion method. In clinical neuropsychology there was a pragmatic reason for knowing how behavior related to the affected region. Before the advent of techniques to image the human brain, clinicians were forced to rely on behavioral data to determine the probable neural regions of damage. Despite well-known variability in functional damage between individuals, accuracy in determining the neural regions involved was rather impressive, given the limited technological tools of the time. Clearly, localization of deficit occurs in the sense that performance on certain tasks is likely to be affected by a lesion to a given location, while performance on other tasks is not. Given the superiority of radiological measures in localizing neurological damage, the use of psychometric measures for this purpose in neuropsychology has become increasingly less important. In clinical neuropsychology, concerns have shifted from an emphasis on locating the lesion to an emphasis on articulating the specific cognitive deficits and intact cognitive capacities that patients possess.

Despite its historical record, the lesion method has been challenged, both in animal and human research. One problem in relating damaged regions directly to a behavioral deficit is that the region of injury may be in the pathway of other regions that are integrally involved in the behavior. To take a simple example, a left or right field cut or homonymous hemianopia can be due to subcortical disconnection of the optical fibers, to an infarct that directly affects primary visual centers in striate cortex, or to damage in areas that directly receive information from primary centers. This type of relationship between regions has led some investigators to question the idea of specialization of function and argue for a systems approach (1–4). In this case, the system that supports vision in the contralateral visual field is one that begins after the optic chiasm and includes tectal, thalamic, striate, and extrastriate regions and all the connecting pathways and structures in between.

However, proposed systems or networks continue to include specialization *within* a network. For instance, Mesulam (3) has proposed an attentional network in which association cortices are involved in sensory representation of the stimulus, the frontal lobe in motor representation, the cingulate in motivation, and the reticular structures in arousal. All interact with parietal function. This approach is clearly superior to older approaches that made claims such as "attention is a parietal lobe function," but there is still localization of function within the network. One of the most important benefits of the network approach is that it demonstrates the necessity to consider the underlying operations associated with different regions that then interact with other (perhaps quite distant) sites. When the attentional network is intact, it results in behavior that we call "attending," and damage to different parts of it will disrupt attending in different ways. One traditional way to determine the function of each region within the network is studying the effects of damage to each region, and in fact, network theorists like Mesulam have relied heavily on this method.

Another difficulty with the lesion method is that compensatory strategies often occur after neural damage. This possibility is extremely difficult to test using the lesion method alone. Due to complications such as diaschisis after acute insult, investigators who wish to specify the neural structures that correspond to a cognitive process must test subjects well after lesions occur, whether in humans or in animals. If subjects are tested too soon, it is unclear if the observed performance deficit is caused by dysfunction of the dead tissue or by secondary dysfunction in other sites due to effects such as those caused by edema. Depending on a number of factors, stability can take up to 6 months (5). This leaves plenty of time for compensatory strategies to emerge.

A third concern in interpreting data from studies using the lesion method is that neural plasticity can allow remaining structures to take over the function of a damaged region. For instance, Merzenich and Kaas (6) showed that in primates, neural reorganization occurs rapidly, even in primary somatic sensory cortex. When monkeys lose the use of one of their digits, somatic cortex associated with that digit is reorganized to produce a similar function for adjacent digits. A similar reorganization has been observed after the introduction of small retinal scotomas (7).

The problem of neural plasticity is less of a concern in older than younger subjects, although it still must be considered. On the other hand, there is no reason to believe that the probability of developing compensatory strategies is decreased in aged subjects.

One way to address problems associated with the lesion method is to collect converging evidence in different populations of subjects and to use various techniques to address the questions of interest. For instance, if the posterior parietal lobe is associated with a particular attentional deficit in stroke patients, and the parietal lobe shows abnormal activity during similar procedures in PET studies in normals, then confidence in the parietal lobe's role in attention is increased. Or, if hemisphere laterality effects found in groups of patients with focal lesions are supported by converging evidence in normals using lateralized visual field presentation or evoked potentials, then theories derived from patients with unilateral lesions is given substantial support. Additionally, if the distinct component operations that are affected with different lesions can be disassociated in measures of normal performance, then there is far more confidence that the deficits observed in patient groups are not due to compensatory strategies.

So why perform studies using the lesion method at all if it is fraught with such difficulties? Perhaps the most important and obvious reason is to determine what deficits are caused by strokes and trauma, events that afflict thousands of people every day. For purposes of basic research into normal behavior, the lesion method continues to be important because there is no foolproof method to replace it. All techniques have their strengths and weaknesses, but only the lesion method can reveal whether or not a certain region is both sufficient and *necessary* to perform a given task.

Another reason to use the lesion method in basic research is to study the division of labor between neural subregions. If a certain lesion affects one aspect of cognition while leaving others intact, we can be reasonably sure that there are areas of the brain that perform distinct operations, and we can study what those operations may be. The best evidence for separate systems is the double dissociation. If damage to one region affects process x without affecting process y, while damage to another affects process y without affecting process x, evidence for functional separation receives strong support. For instance, damage to the left angular gyrus can affect language comprehension without affecting semantic comprehension of pictures, while damage to right parietal regions can affect spatial orientation without disrupting language comprehension. This observation demonstrates that one process associated with the left hemisphere functions in a way that disrupts language when damaged, while another involving the right hemisphere functions in a different way that disrupts spatial orientation when damaged. Notice that this interpretation is not the same as saying that the left hemisphere is specialized for language and the right for space. Rather, it poses the question of what different computations occur in the right and left hemispheres that will disrupt language on the one hand and spatial orientation on the other. This is an important conceptual change in neuropsychological investigation that should be kept in mind throughout this chapter.

Finally, the lesion method can be as valuable in studying deficits associated with damage in different areas as in studying the functions that remain intact. If a lesion does not disrupt a cognitive operation of interest, it suggests that the structures that support the process are probably intact. For instance, Grabowecky et al. (8) found that certain preattentive processes involved in the perception of stimulus mass were intact in subjects with unilateral visual neglect tested in acute states. Although these subjects showed similar deficits on neuropsychological measures, damaged areas and lesion size varied tremendously across subjects. Nevertheless, the magnitude of neglect in each subject was affected by stimulus mass on their neglected side. These data are discussed more fully in a subsequent section. For now, keep in mind that preattentive visual responses that compute the spatial extent of a stimulus were intact in each subject even in acute stages, despite lesions that varied from frontal to basal ganglia to posterior regions.

VISUAL PATHWAYS TO CORTEX

Two visual pathways that transmit visual information from the retina to the cortex have been studied extensively. The retinotectal pathway sends information from the retina through the superior colliculus (SC). The geniculostriate pathway sends information through the lateral geniculate nucleus (LGN) of the thalamus to striate visual cortex (V1) or Brodmann's area 17 in the occipital lobe. There are also massive backprojections to the reciprocal subcortical areas as well.

These two systems contribute to vision in different ways. The retinotectal pathway is considered more primitive. Cells within this system respond most vigorously to light occurring within the peripheral visual field. As a result, the system appears very good at detecting and localizing luminance changes. Functionally, it seems well suited to act as a monitor for potentially relevant changes in the visual field, to attract attention, and then to align the eyes with the attended location for further identification. Consistently, the retinotectal system is directly involved in the initiation of saccadic eye movements.

The geniculostriate pathway responds to features that are critical for pattern perception such as shape, color, and orientation. Nearly 90% of the projections from the retina are within this pathway, and this system is considered the major source of information for higher-level visual analysis.

Although SC, FEF, and visual striate cortex or V1 all contain a topographic map of the contralateral visual field, cells in V1 have not been found that respond when saccades occur, and V1 is not considered an area involved in eye movements. Conversely, cells in the deep layers of SC increase their response just prior to saccade initiation, and cortical cells in the frontal eye field (FEF) act in concert with SC responses (see 9, 10, for reviews). Consistently, bilateral ablation of SC and FEF in primates causes severe and permanent impairment of saccadic activity (11). Interestingly, ablation of SC or FEF alone causes only temporary impairment in initiating saccades. Damage to both areas is necessary to observe permanent deficits. Damage to SC or FEF in one hemisphere will cause eye deviations in the ipsilesional direction, and electrical stimulation of FEF produces saccades in the contralateral direction to the stimulated hemisphere.

Cells in monkey parietal cortex (area 7a) also respond before saccades are made, but primarily when the animal is motivated to attend to a particular location. Lynch et al. (12) found that these cells increase the frequency of their response before a saccade is made to a peripheral light when it predicts food. When the light is unpredictive or when saccades occur during visual scanning in a dark room, increased firing rate does not occur in these cells. Unlike FEF and SC responses, parietal responses associated with saccades also respond when manual responses are made to a target in a location.

Retinotectal System and Progressive Supranuclear Palsy

Acute insults to the tectal area generally causes severe morbidity or death. However, there are several investigations of patients with a degenerative disease that affects tectal areas, known as progressive supranuclear palsy (PSP). Patients with PSP present with similar symptoms to patients with Parkinson's disease but with a distinctive saccade deficit. This deficit is more pronounced along the vertical axis than the horizontal axis. As the disease progresses, the ability to initiate a saccade in any direction is lost. Autopsies show massive bilateral damage in the midbrain (superior colliculus and peritectal region).

In tests of covert orienting, these patients are slow to orient attention to a bright light. Perhaps more interestingly, they also lose a normal inhibitory response to the light after long delays. This abnormality occurs along the same axis as their saccade deficit, namely vertical. Rafal et al. (13) asked eight PSP patients to press a switch the moment they detected a target (an asterisk), and measured their response time to do so. The target was preceded by a bright box that acted as a cue to the subject that the target was likely to occur in the location of the box. On 80% of the trials, the target did appear in that cued location (valid trials), but on the remaining trials the target appeared in the homologous location on the other side of fixation (invalid trials). The interval between cue and target was varied. Under such conditions normal subjects exhibit facilitation of target detection for the validly cued location at early cue-target intervals (under 300 msec) compared to target detection at invalidly cued locations. However, at longer cue-target intervals, this relationships switches. Target detection at invalidly cued locations is faster than at cued locations. This slowing at longer cue-target intervals is called "inhibition of return" and is reminiscent of the inhibition in saccades back to a location where the eyes have just been focused (14, 15).

Inhibition of return, whether in covert attentional orienting or overt saccades, is believed to facilitate visual search in normals by keeping track of where attention has been (16). Inhibiting those locations that have been attended would encourage search of other, perhaps more relevant, locations.

PSP patients show virtually no inhibition of return in covert attention, but only along the same axis as their saccadic deficits. These findings demonstrate that at least one elementary operation of normal spatial orienting, the inhibition of return, is eliminated in patients who also have a saccade deficit due to damage in a primary structure of the retinotectal pathway. Somewhat puzzling, but nevertheless interesting to the psychiatric community, unmedicated patients with paranoid schizophrenia lose inhibition of return, while schizophrenics without paranoid symptoms show normal inhibition (17).

It is also important to note that inhibition of return in normals occurs only with exogenous cuing (e.g., a bright light) and not with symbolic or endogenous cuing, such as an arrow at fixation pointing in the direction of a target's likely location (15). In addition, facilitation at short cue-target intervals happens with exogenous cues, even when the probability of the target being at the cued location is 0.5 (i.e, the cue is uninformative). Attentional orienting is automatic when a bright flash of light appears in the peripheral field, even when the eyes themselves do not move. Endogenous cues do not produce facilitation unless there is a clear advantage in moving attention to a cued location. When endogenous cues predict a target location with a high probability, targets preceded by valid cues are responded to more rapidly than targets preceded by invalid cues. Thus, endogenous cuing does not *automatically* orient visual attention. More importantly, for the present purposes, inhibition of return does not appear with endogenous cues, even under cuing conditions that include unequal probability.

In sum, inhibition of return is linked to automatic covert attentional orienting but not to controlled or intentional covert attentional orienting. Patients with PSP lose inhibition of return in visual attentional orienting as well as saccade initiation. This finding strongly suggests that inhibition of return in covert attention is associated with the same system that is involved in initiating saccades.

Retinotectal System and Blindsight

Total ablation of primary visual cortex in one hemisphere will cause blindness in the contralateral field. Blindsight refers to residual visual capacity in a hemifield "blind" due to damage to primary visual cortex. The most intense and thorough study of blindsight was performed in one case (DB) by Weiskrantz and his colleagues (18). Basically, they found that DB could detect and locate light sources

and motion well above chance within his blind field. In addition, he denied any conscious awareness of stimulation when it occurred within this field.

Evidence for blindsight is rather important because it suggests that the retinotectal system is capable of transmitting sufficient visual information to affect performance (although not sufficient to culminate in full awareness of the stimulation). The major question among investigators of blindsight has been whether residual visual capacity can be attributed solely to the intact tectal system in hemianopic cases or to undetected visual capacities that remain functional in the geniculostriate system. Recently, Fendrich et al. (19) showed that residual pockets of intact visual functioning could be found in the "blind" field of a hemianopic subject. Standard perimetry tests showed the patient to be blind in peripheral locations in the hemianopic field. By using a special perimetry device with finer resolution than standard devices and with more precise measures of eye fixation, they found that detection of light in several parts of the hemianopic field was above chance. They argued that without such testing, no conclusions can be made concerning the role of the tectal system in blindsight phenomena. Subjects may simply respond on the basis of information projected to intact pockets of striate cortex.

Clearly, more fine-grained visual field testing is needed to determine whether or not patients who are considered blind in one field can detect and locate light sources because they have residual geniculostriate function. However, a different way to test the role of the retinotectal system in hemianopic patients is to use tasks that can distinguish between retinotectal and geniculostriate responses. Rafal et al. (20) approached the problem of blindsight in a different way by exploiting anatomical differences in the two systems. As in primary visual cortex, each SC responds to stimulation in the contralateral visual field. However, unlike the geniculostriate system, information from the temporal field from each eye is more strongly represented in the contralateral SC than information from the nasal side. Rather than asking subjects to detect information in their blind field, Rafal et al. (20) measured saccade latency to lights presented monocularly in the *good* field. Subjects were simply asked to move their eyes to wherever they saw a light. Under conditions where one eye is covered, the light in the blind field is presented in the nasal field, and when the other eye is covered, the light in the blind field is presented in the temporal field. The important question was whether or not a second light presented in the blind field would affect saccade latency, and, if so, would it affect latency more when the "blind" light was presented temporally than when it was presented nasally. Three patients with dense hemonomous hemianopia were tested. In all three cases, latencies were slowed to lights within their good field when lights also occurred in their blind field. More importantly, this slowing was found only when the light in the blind field was projected to the temporal side of the eye, which is more strongly represented in SC.

These data are difficult to explain by reference to residual pockets of functioning in the geniculostriate system. Nevertheless, the findings of Fendrich et al. demonstrate that caution must be taken in interpreting above-chance detection in hemianopic patients. Patients with deep inferior lesions that affect the visual radiation from thalamus to primary visual cortex or lesions that directly ablate primary cortex may respond to visual stimulation in their "blind" field because their retinotectal system is intact, because they have pockets of intact striate cortex, or both.

Effects of Frontal and Parietal Lesions

In acute stages after insult, patients with frontal and/or parietal damage often deviate their eyes in an ipsilesional direction. Saccades in the contralesional direction are difficult and sometimes impossible to make. Studies of patients with frontal or parietal damage have begun to shed light on the cortical visual centers involved in different aspects of this deficit.

Although saccade latency to the onset of light is typically normal in patients with dorsolateral frontal damage who do not show clinical signs of ocular-motor deficits, inhibiting a saccade to the light is very poor in such cases. When subjects are told to look in the opposite direction of light onset (i.e., make an antisaccade), patients with frontal lobe damage have extreme difficulty (21). More recently, Braun et al. (22) found that the number of express saccades (i.e., latencies roughly between 100–150 msec) to a target in the peripheral visual field were more frequent in patients with frontal lobe damage that included FEF than normals or patients with frontal lobe damage without FEF involvement. The difference was observed when a fixation point disappeared 200 msec before a target but not when the fixation point remained on the screen. The authors concluded that volitional inhibition of reflexive saccades is affected in patients with lesions extending into FEF. The relationship between these deficits and higher-order visual cognition is not yet known.

Conversely, there is rather good correspondence between eye movement deficits associated with parietal lesions and attentional mechanisms associated with unilateral visual neglect. Patients with moderate to severe unilateral visual neglect (typically associated with inferior parietal lobe in humans) often have eye deviations in the ipsilesional direction, especially during initial stages after insult. In most of these patients, eye deviations resolve over time. Clinical observation suggests that patients who have recently suffered insult cannot overcome this problem. If told to "look left," they may move their eyes to the center and then move their heads toward the left, but often cannot follow the instructions at all. It is as if the endogenous command cannot overcome involuntary eye movements into the ipsilesional field. With time these patients will be able to look left upon instruction, but their eyes will drift back toward the right side. As with the syndrome of unilateral neglect, these deficits are more pronounced in patients with right-hemisphere damage than in patients with left-hemisphere damage. De Renzi (23) found that saccadic deficits into the contralateral field in patients with right- or left-hemisphere damage (not necessarily having unilateral neglect) were more frequent with posterior than anterior lesions. Although gaze paresis toward the ipsilesional side was observed in about 5% of patients with anterior damage, it was equally frequent for patients with right or left involvement. For the posterior group, 61% with right hemisphere damage and 13% with left hemisphere damage exhibited such deficits. The asymmetry in the frequency of gaze paresis in patients with posterior damage is an intriguing and potentially critical step in understanding the relationship between FEF, SC, and parietal lobe in guiding eye movements in humans.

One question raised by these findings is whether eye movements and the covert orienting of visual spatial attention to locations in space are related to the same neural function. This question is addressed more fully in a later section, but it is intriguing to note that patients with right-parietal lobe damage are more likely to deviate *covert* attention to ipsilesional locations than contralesional locations, even when they do not exhibit overt eye movement deficits (24,25).

VISUAL PATHWAYS THROUGH THE CORTEX

Studies in primates have revealed two main processing streams in cortical vision. One stream is associated with inferior occipital-temporal pathways and is involved in object identification, or determining "what" is there. The other is associated with occipital-parietal pathways and is involved in analyzing spatial relationships, or "where" objects are (26). The separation of these streams appears to begin in the retina, continues divided in geniculate and primary visual cortex, and is relatively separate (although by no means completely) as information flows anteriorly. The two major streams correspond roughly to the parvocellular and magnocellular systems respectively (Fig. 16.1). The receptive field size of both the magnocellular and parvocellular systems increases as information is processed through progressively higher levels, but this increase in size is more pronounced in the magnocellular system that projects to the parietal lobe (27,28). Cells in parietal lobe often have receptive fields that include the ipsilateral and contralateral visual fields (28). Large receptive fields are well suited for large-scale analysis, such as for motion, low spatial frequency, figure/ground, and relative location of objects. The parvocellular system has smaller receptive fields that respond to features such as color, brightness, shape, and higher spatial frequencies. These features likely provide some of the building blocks of object perception (29).

Primate studies have also revealed several functionally separate areas within each of the cortical visual pathways that act together to analyze objects and their spatial relationships. The number of visual areas increases in invertebrates as the ratio of brain to body weight increases across species. In 1989, Kaas reported that there were somewhere between 15

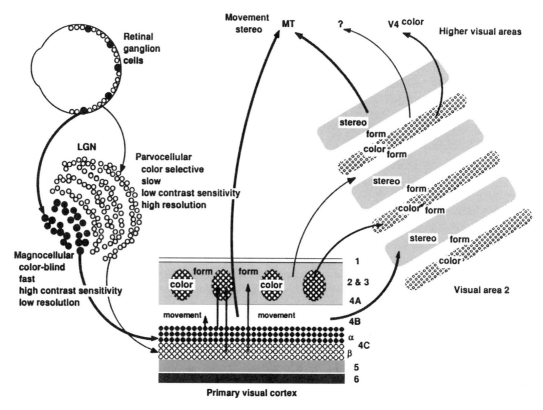

Figure 16.1. Schematic of visual pathways. (Reprinted from Livingstone M, Hubel D. Segregation of form, color, movement, and depth: anatomy, physiology and perception. Science 1988;240:740–749.

and 30 visual areas in new and old world monkeys, and additional areas have been identified since then (30). A vast majority of posterior cortex in monkeys contains neurons that respond to visual stimuli. It is likely that more areas exist within the human brain. Although the animal work has been critical in mapping visual areas, the existence of the two pathways that correspond to identification of an object (knowing what) versus the spatial location of objects (knowing where) was first reported in humans. Upon extensive neuropsychological testing of English war veterans with gunshot wounds to the head, Newcombe and Russell (31) showed that penetrating wounds in parietal lobe produced difficulty locating objects but not in identifying them, while occipital-temporal damage produced difficulty identifying objects but not in locating them. Consistently, posterior ventral lesions produce object agnosias, while dorsal lesions produce spatial deficits, as seen in unilateral visual neglect, visual extinction or Balint's syndrome.

Despite the evidence that two processing streams are differentially involved in determining "what" and "where," this can be but a first approximation. Studies of patients with Balint's syndrome associated with bilateral parietal lobe damage have shown that the perception of spatial relationships between objects can be altered without affecting spatial relationships within objects. That is, these patients may know where a part of an object is in relation to other parts but not know where the object is in relation to other objects. In a simple task of reporting whether there were one or two colors in a display with many circles, Humphreys and

Riddoch (32) found that a patient with Balint's syndrome reported that there were two colors 75% of the time when the circles were unconnected (Fig. 16.2*A*). However, when lines were placed so that the circles on one end of the lines were one color and circles on the other end were another color (Fig. 16.2*B*), his accuracy increased to 90%. Patients with Balint's syndrome are often mistaken as blind. They typically report their vision as "hazy" or "blurred." However, in-depth testing reveals that these patients are able to recognize individual objects, but have great difficulty recognizing two objects placed next to each other, either side by side or behind one another along the same line of sight.

In addition to deficits in perceiving spatial relations between objects, eye movements in patients with Balint's syndrome appear fixed, and there is great difficulty tracking an object through space. These patients also suffer from a severe spatial reaching problem with no accompanying motor deficits.

We recently had the opportunity to test a patient diagnosed with Balint's syndrome and found a similar profile (33, 34). RM suffered embolic infarcts separated by about 7 months to each parietal-occipital region (Fig. 16.3). Testing began approximately 5 months after the second infarct. As with all Balint's patients, RM could easily identify single objects in a visual scene, but could not accurately reach for the object or track it. He could not accurately reach for an object where reaching was visually guided, nor could he point to the location of an object if he moved his hand and arm to do so.

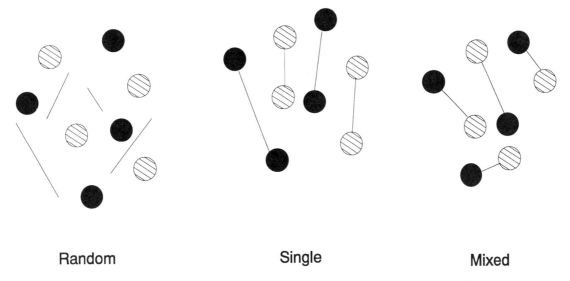

Random   Single   Mixed

Figure 16.2. Example of stimuli. (Adapted from Humphreys GW, Riddoch MJ. Interactions between object and space systems revealed through neuropsychology. In: Meyer DE, Kornblum S, eds. Attention and performance, XIV. Hillsdale, NJ. Lawrence Erlbaum & Associates, 1993. with permission.

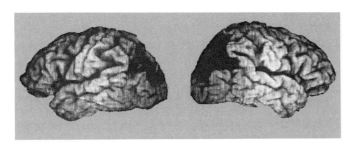

Figure 16.3. Reconstruction of CT scans of a patient with Balint's syndrome.

Further experimental testing showed that when a single object was tilted away or toward RM, he was able to determine which side of the object was nearer to him, but when two objects were presented closer or farther from him, he would guess which one was nearer to him. He could readily report the color of an object presented briefly in his peripheral vision, but could not do so when a second object was presented foveally. He could name single pictures of everyday objects without difficulty and could do so even when critical features were covered over (e.g., the trunk of an elephant). When two pictures were presented, he named the two only in frequency, and then only with a great deal of effort.

We also tested RM's ability to respond to part/whole relationships by presenting hierarchically structured patterns that have local objects nested within a more global object. These patterns represent a different type of spatial relationship between objects, with one object being a part of the other. For instance, the pattern in Figure 16.4 contains a global H created from the repetition of local S's. The local S's are parts of the global H. We presented a series of hierarchical patterns and asked RM to report what letters he saw. He invariably reported the identity of the local letter (H out of S), and did so whether the local patterns were large (25 cm) or small (2.5 cm). When prodded to identify the

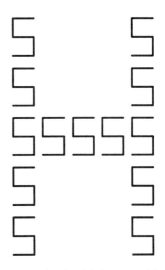

Figure 16.4. Example of a global H created from local S's.

global letter, he was able to do so less than 1% of the time, and when forced to choose what the global level might be, he could only guess. Yet when shown patterns with "neutral" forms taking the place of the local letters (Fig. 16.5) RM could identify the global pattern. In other words, RM perceived the level with the smallest-sized pattern that seemed to contain meaningful, frequent, or overlearned forms. Once such an object captured his attention, he could not move it to the global form.

An MRI scan revealed bilateral parietal-occipital involvement of nearly equal location and volume (Fig. 16.3). There were also cerebellar infarcts that were unlikely to contribute to his perceptual deficits. Standard tests of his primary vision, including the perception of random dot stereograms, contrast sensitivity, color perception, acuity, shape from shading, and shape from motion (by V. Ramachandran), showed that his vision was intact.

Intact parietal lobes appear necessary for normal spatial vision between objects, whether presented side by side or

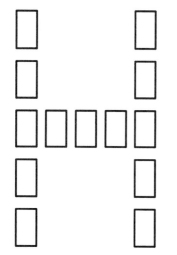

Figure 16.5. Example of a global H created from local rectangles.

one within the other. Data from patients with Balint's syndrome suggest that the what and where distinction for the respective ventral and dorsal systems is a good heuristic that captures some of the functional distinctions between the two systems but not all. It is not space per se that is disrupted, but rather some interaction between overall spatial processing and objects seems affected. Yet determining what features predict when spatial relationships between items will be perceived as part of an object and when they will be perceived as separate objects is not a trivial matter. In fact, one of the more perplexing problems in the study of pattern perception concerns what constitutes an object. Abrupt changes in color and contrast can distinguish one object from another, but not always. A pattern carved in a table is not a separate object from the table. A contour change in a swatch of fabric does not divide the cloth in two perceptually. The screen of a monitor is not perceived as a completely independent object from the casing that houses it. It is part of the object we perceive as a computer monitor. To understand the dorsal and ventral processing streams fully, we need to understand the cognitive mechanisms involved in how the visual system determines when luminance flux in the visual field is perceived as part of an object and when it is perceived as space between or within objects. These questions have just begun to be addressed in neuropsychology, partly because the questions have only recently been posed in this manner. Whatever the answers may ultimately be, they must explain both normal vision and the way in which visual perception breaks down.

DEFICITS IN PERCEIVING OBJECTS

The perception of objects can break down in highly specific ways. The investigation of deficits in recognizing objects (visual agnosias) has had an important influence on recent theories of normal and abnormal object perception (see 35). Studies of visual agnosia have also focused attention on certain brain regions as more important in

object perception than others. Generally, visual agnosia occurs with ventral damage along occipital and temporal lobes. "Pure" agnosias are seldom as specific as one would like for scientific investigations, and pure cases are difficult to find. Nevertheless, the purest cases demonstrate some interesting problems that limit the way in which investigators should conceptualize normal object perception.

Associative Agnosia

Normal individuals cannot look at a picture of a dog without perceiving a dog. Perceiving objects seems to happen effortlessly, and the concept of an object appears impossible to inhibit. When looking at or attending to a dog, one recognizes a dog. It appears that part of seeing a dog is knowing that what one sees is a dog (i.e., having a "form concept").

Neuropsychological evidence does not support this simple-minded view. There are patients who can see patterns that normals perceive as a dog, draw what they see, discriminate one dog from another, match pictures of dogs, yet may not be able to report that the object is a dog or even that it is generally kept as a pet. In other words, these patients lose both the name and the meaning of the object upon visual presentation.

This problem has been historically called "associative agnosia." One striking aspect of this syndrome is that the meaning and name of an object is readily available to the patient through other modalities. They will easily identify a dog by touch or when it barks.

Shallice (36) reports that in a review of the literature he found only two patients with "pure" associative agnosia. That is, there were no other visual deficits that could account for the phenomenon. These two patients had posterior left-hemisphere lesions with lesion extension into white matter areas that disrupted posterior callosal transfer. Commissurtomized subjects do not exhibit associative agnosia. It appears that a left occipital-temporal lesion combined with disrupted interhemispheric communication between posterior regions is necessary to produce a disassociation between an intact visual representation of the object and its meaning.

Notice that these patients are able to perceptually isolate objects. They "see" objects and they "see" the spatial relationship between objects. They have no reported spatial deficits. This is a case where damage to the ventral processing stream that presumably identifies objects does not disrupt the percept of the object. Rather, it disrupts the connection between the object's function and its meaning.

Integrative Agnosia and Simultanagnosia

Some patients have trouble perceiving an object as a whole but little difficulty seeing its parts. They may perceive the parts such as the four feet, the body, and the trunk of an elephant, but they either cannot integrate the parts to form the internal representation of the elephant or are very slow to do so. If these patients do perceive a part that uniquely defines the object, such as the trunk, they are likely to guess correctly that the object is an elephant, but objects with few distinctive features are very difficult for such patients to recognize. Thus, unlike patients with associative agnosia, patients with integrative agnosia do have form concept access, but they do not have the ability to perceive the integration of parts in the same way as normals. Riddoch and Humphreys (37) were the first to use the term integrative agnosia as opposed to simultanagnosia to refer to this type of deficit. Wolpert (38) introduced the term "simultaneous agnosia" and referred to it as an "integration apperception." His patient could not comprehend the meaning of a scene, but probably had a different underlying deficit. Although he could identify objects in a scene, he could not report the meaning of the scene. Yet individual objects were readily apprehended.

Humphreys and Riddoch (39) reported an in-depth study of their patient HJA, who was previously categorized as having associative agnosia on neuropsychological examination. They found that the patient's deficit was an extreme slowness in integrating the pieces of objects. HJA would laboriously trace a picture of an object and construct objects piece by piece. Once the object was perceptually integrated, the identity and function could be reported without difficulty. A CT scan revealed bilateral deep lesions in the inferior, posterior occipital temporal region (39).

A different way to think about HJA's deficit is that they reflect a problem in "perceptual organization" (in HJA's case, a specific organizational deficit that required the strategy of piecemeal processing). Once organization was achieved, he could readily access the meaning of the object. This patient showed abnormally slow perceptual organization for visually presented patterns but could recognize simple patterns if given enough time. He could report only one piece of the whole at a time. This occurred despite the fact that in-depth tests showed that his vision was intact.

Several lesion locations produce a deficit in seeing two objects simultaneously, or more accurately, in seeing two objects in the same amount of time that it takes normals to see two objects. Reaction time measures demonstrate that neurologically normal subjects recognize objects serially, but in a much shorter time window than patients (29, 40). Although the description of this timing deficit is captured in the terms "simultanagnosia" or "integrative agnosia," it does not mean that patients who show a timing deficit do so for the same reason, nor should they necessarily have the same or similar lesions. For instance, unilateral extinction could be classified as simultanagnosia, yet it is associated with parietal or frontal lesions (24). Extinction is a deficit in recognizing or detecting contralesional stimuli in the presence of ipsilesional stimuli. Recognition is normal when the contralesional stimulus is presented in isolation. Global/local deficits also qualify, as these deficits are defined as an abnormal ability to see either the local or the global form

within normal time limits. Yet deficits of this sort have been associated with asymmetries in temporal-parietal junction in the right or left hemispheres (41, 42). Difficulties in perceiving two objects in patients with Balint's syndrome could also be and have been described as simultanagnosia. Yet this deficit is found in patients with bilateral parietal-occipital damage.

Piecemeal or serial processing is often a consequence of brain insult. For instance, patients with pure alexia (an inability to read with intact ability to write) are known as letter-by-letter readers, a deficit associated with left occipital-temporal damage. One way to circumvent a reading deficit is to spell words letter by letter, just as one way to circumvent a perceptual organization problem is to construct objects part by part. This serial process in pure alexics is not a normal way in which reading occurs. Letter-by-letter reading may mean that all pure alexics have the same underlying deficit or it may mean that there are various visual and/or language deficits that produce the loss of whole word reading (see 43). When this occurs, one option is to spell out the word. Similarly, visual agnosias may lead to feature-by-feature or line-by-line processing in order to overcome deficits in perceiving a pattern as a whole.

It is not clear what constitutes perceiving a whole, and this question poses one of the challenges for investigators of object perception. One thread that does appear throughout the history of psychology is the observation that wholes are often perceived before the parts that constitute them (46-48). Until there is better understanding about how objects are perceived as objects and how an object can be perceived before seeing its parts, the underlying cause of integrative agnosia or simultanagnosia as it occurs in vision will remain unresolved.

Prosopagnosia

Prosopagnosia refers to a recognition deficit limited to faces, although thorough testing has revealed that other categories can also be affected, such as automobiles, breeds of dogs, and species of birds. Many investigators have argued that the deficit is one of accessing the meaning of the face as with pure associative agnosia for objects. However, unlike patients with associative agnosia for objects, patients with prosopagnosia can identify a face as a face; they simply cannot classify it as a particular person nor accurately report whether or not they have seen the face before. Lesions that produce this deficit are most commonly linked to inferior right temporal-occipital damage. However, there is much debate about whether a right-hemisphere lesion alone is sufficient to cause prosopagnosia, or if bilateral lesions are required (see discussion in ref. 35). Damasio (49) rather convincingly argues that the fussiform gyrus of the mesial occipital-temporal region bilaterally must be affected.

Prosopagnosia has been considered a deficit in accessing the memory trace or structural description of a particular face (49, 50). However, Farah (51) notes that visual discrimination of *unfamiliar* faces has accompanied prosopagnosia in every case in which it has been tested consistent with a primary deficit in facial discrimination. She argues that there are higher-order perceptual deficits that may disproportionately affect face recognition. Identification of any one individual requires expertise in making subtle visual distinctions along a number of dimensions. Farah's argument can also account for cases like the prosopagnosic farmer who lost the ability to discriminate his cows (52) or another prosopagnosic patient who lost the ability to discriminate racehorses (53). Although Farah's conclusion makes a great deal of sense, it cannot account for all the data. Other evidence collected in prosopagnosic patients demonstrates that there is intact visual analysis of faces at a preconscious level. Tranel and Damasio (54) demonstrated an increased galvanic skin response (GSR) to familiar faces in two prosopagnosics. Although these patients could not accurately report which faces were familiar, physical responses demonstrated below-threshold knowledge of which faces had been seen and which had not. GSR was greater to familiar faces than to unfamiliar faces. Visual discrimination must be intact at some level for such responses to occur. Thus, the issue of whether or not there are visual areas that respond uniquely to faces in the human brain is far from resolved.

Animal studies are often cited as support for the idea that face perception is special, consistent with the idea that specific regions exist that uniquely support the perception of faces. Although the biological significance of facial discrimination is difficult to deny, there is little evidence in the animal literature that is helpful in settling debates about critical sites that produce prosopagnosia in humans. Electrophysiological responses to faces have been found in the temporal lobe and along the superior temporal sulcus in the monkey (55, 56). Between 5–10% of the visually sensitive cells in facially sensitive areas respond uniquely to faces. Cells in the mesial occipital-temporal area have not been found that respond uniquely to faces. Yet this is the primary area that causes prosopagnosia in humans. Anterior temporal damage in humans does not produce pure or even relatively pure prosopagnosia.

Agnosia for Features

Some individuals with neurological damage in posterior regions involved in extrastriate occipital, temporal, and parietal lobes have difficulty with more fundamental visual analysis, including the perception of color (achromatopsia), orientation, or motion. These types of agnosias are considered primary deficits, or bottom-up deficits, and are generally classified as "apperceptive agnosias." These agnosias represent basic visual deficits produced by cortical lesions. Each has been observed in isolation in patients with lesions and can be evident when visual sensory function is normal (57). These dissociations are consistent with PET studies showing that identifying shape, color, and velocity have different profiles in extrastriate cortex (see ref. 58 for discussion).

Color agnosia over the full visual field is associated with lesions similar to those that produce prosopagnosia. In fact, prosopagnosia typically occurs simultaneously with achromatopsia. However, achromatopsia can exist in isolation and can affect only one quadrant or one hemifield. Damasio (49) reports that patients with such deficits may describe what they see as "dirty" or "dulled," a "washing out" of colors. Some patients do not lose the ability to discriminate between monochromatic colors but cannot accurately report the color that is presented (see ref. 59).

Achromatopsia has been associated with inferior occipital-temporal damage. Single-unit recordings from animal studies are consistent with the human literature. Although color per se (i.e., the spectrum of the visual systems response to monochromatic colors) is first extracted in the lateral geniculate nucleus of the thalamus (60), the color that is perceived in more complex settings appears to be associated with higher visual analysis in temporal-occipital association areas. The absolute color (or more accurately the wavelength projected to the retina) may change as a function of lighting, but the relationship between wavelengths at contiguous locations remains perceptually constant as lighting changes. There is "color constancy" across various lighting conditions. Single-unit recordings in V4 in monkeys have revealed responses to *relative* color, which is consistent with color constancy (61). Thus, when damage occurs to areas that may include V4 in humans, discrimination of one monochromatic color from another need not suffer, but the experience of color may change to disrupt color constancy.

As noted before, identification of shape can also suffer with damage in similar regions. Again, the animal literature is consistent with these clinical observations. Single-unit responses in inferior occipital-temporal regions show sensitivity to color, brightness, orientation, and shape.

A rare case of motion agnosia has been reported. Zihl et al. (62) studied a woman who had difficulty detecting motion and reported that objects in motion looked as if they jumped from place to place. Continuous motion, as in running water, looked frozen. There is some controversy whether or not motion perception deficits can occur in isolation (see ref. 49). Animal work in areas MT and MTS in the posterior superior temporal sulcus of monkey has shown convincingly that cells in this region are sensitive to direction and velocity of movement (63). However, cells in parietal regions are also sensitive to movement, which may explain why movement deficits in isolation are extremely rare in humans.

In sum, the animal and human literature demonstrate that inferior posterior association cortices are extensively involved in higher-order vision. Given the number of visual centers that lie in close proximity to one another and often abut one another, it is not surprising that only rare cases of isolated feature agnosias occur. Clearly, patients with posterior temporal-parietal and extrastriate occipital lesions should show some form of visual deficit, even if visual acuity is intact. The exact nature of the deficit will depend on what visual areas have been affected.

DEFICITS ASSOCIATED WITH VISUAL SPACE

A great deal of evidence has shown that parietal lobes are extensively involved in spatial analysis. Animal data have demonstrated that cells in parietal lobe are involved in the computation of abstract space. Parietal regions appear to be critical for maintaining stable spatial structure to allow accurate movement through the world (64). Cells in this area attend to locations in space independent of eye movements. They appear to be involved in the covert movement of attention over the visual field, but only in particular ways as described at length below.

It is well established that parietal lobes are involved in location analysis and the analysis of spatial relationships. However, parietal lobes in humans are involved in covert attentional processes that selectively attend to spatial locations but also to object features as well. The evidence for this claim is the subject of this section.

Unilateral Visual Neglect

To many neuropsychologists, unilateral neglect is considered the quintessential example of a spatial deficit. Patients with left neglect often act as if they are attempting to escape from their left side, sometimes to the point that they will deny left paresis or other problems on the left side of their body. Upon neuropsychological examination, patients with unilateral visual neglect will respond to the right side of drawings and will bisect a horizontal line well to the right side of the line, as if the length of the line toward the left side was misperceived (65).

The magnitude of neglect varies tremendously between subjects, and more so in acute stages. Eye deviations to the right with left neglect are often observed, but need not be present for neglect to occur. Patients may interact normally with a person standing on their right side and be completely unaware of a person standing on their left side.

The bulk of the evidence from studies of unilateral visual neglect suggests that right inferior parietal lobe produces neglect more often than other areas of the brain (66). However, neglect has been found in patients with thalamic, basal ganglia, frontal, and cingulate damage (3). Left or right parietal lesions can also produce an extinction-like deficit that is equal in frequency and severity, but the full-blown neglect syndrome is clearly more severe and more frequent with right-hemisphere damage (67). This asymmetry suggests that left neglect due to right hemisphere damage is a combination of an attentional deficit (that produces an extinction-like phenomenon) plus some other cognitive deficit that is more associated with right-hemisphere function (see 68).

Unilateral neglect typically resolves into extinction. Patients with extinction will respond to an object in their contralesional visual field if it is presented alone, but will not respond to the object if presented at the same time with another object in their ipsilesional visual field. Current neuropsychological theories of neglect disagree over whether neglect is a reflection of a direct deficit in spatial attention or a deficit in the visual representation of one side of space with secondary effects on attention (4, 24, 66, 69–73). The resolution of this debate is important in understanding the neuropsychological syndrome itself, but it is also important in determining what cognitive functions involve the parietal lobe. For this reason, evidence related to this matter is discussed at length here.

Both human and animal research have shown that parietal lobes contribute to the covert movement of attention across the visual field (74, 75). Morrow and Ratcliffe (73) reported that right-parietal damage produced more severe effects on covert attention (moving attention without accompanying eye movements) than left. In accordance with Posner et al. (24), they argued that the deficit was in one particular elementary operation that contributes to attentional orienting, namely the ability to "disengage" attention from an attended location. In other words, the patient's attention gets "stuck" on the "good" side because they have difficulty disengaging attention from their ipsilateral side. Theoretically, the intact hemisphere orients attention into the good field, but the signal to disengage to move attention in the contralesional direction is disrupted by the damaged hemisphere, and attention remains fixed at a location on the ipsilesional side.

Posner et al. (24) used a simple detection task where subjects had to press a button when they detected a target. The targets could appear ipsilesionally or contralesionally and were preceded by a cue. The cue told the subject whether the target would more likely appear on the left or the right of the screen. Thus, the cue set up an expected location where the target would appear. On 80% of the trials, the target appeared in the cued location (valid targets), and on 20% it appeared in the opposite location (invalid targets). Groups of patients with right- or left-parietal damage responded to valid targets about equally well in the ipsilesional and contralesional fields. Both patient groups also had difficulty in responding to invalid targets when they occurred in the contralesional field. That is, for both groups, attention got "stuck" in the ipsilesional field. The right-parietal group took longer to detect an invalidly cued target than the left-parietal group in their contralesional field.

Posner et al. (24) concluded that the parietal lobe is involved in the "disengagement" of attention from one location to move it to a new location. Covert attentional orienting can be broken down into its component parts, and right parietal damage disrupts one part disproportionately. Posner et al. argued that successful covert orienting within the visual field required (a) moving attention in the direction of an expected location, (b) engaging attention at that location, and (c) disengaging attention from that location to move it elsewhere. Patients with parietal lobe damage are especially deficient at the latter, or "disengaging" process. Both hemispheres appear to be involved in disengaging attention from its current location to move it in the contralateral direction (24). However, the strength of the disengagement process is asymmetrically represented (76). This conclusion was also supported using a similar paradigm in patients with clear signs of unilateral visual neglect (24, 73). Posner et al.'s (1984) cuing paradigm has been used in a variety of patient populations, including subjects with psychosis, to examine left/right differences in disengagement deficits (17, 77). The evidence is consistent with a spatial attentional deficit associated with left-parietal function.

Although these studies represent very good support for the idea that neglect is an attentional disorder, this is not necessarily the conclusion that is demanded by the evidence from the cuing paradigm. Bisiach and his colleagues (69, 78) argued that attention is indirectly affected in unilateral neglect; that the primary deficit is one in which information on one side is absent or distorted in the internal representation. Bisiach and Luzzatti (69) found that patients with visual neglect generalized the deficit to internally generated images. When subjects were asked to imagine themselves at one end of a plaza and report the places along the plaza, they reported those on the right side of their image. When they were then asked to imagine themselves at the other end of the plaza, facing back to where they had originally imagined themselves standing, they again reported those places on the right side of their image. Notice that places on the left that were neglected in the first image would be on the right in the second image, where they were reported.

Bisiach and Luzzatti argued that attention was not summoned to the left in the internally generated image because the left side of the image was not visually represented by the patients. The internal representation of the plaza was deficient on the left side for right-hemisphere-damaged subjects. Obviously, if the representation of an object on the

left is weak, whether in a visual image or not, then attention will not be summoned. People do not generally attend to something they have no evidence for which it exists. Thus, attentional mechanisms could be intact in patients with unilateral visual neglect but appear disrupted only because such patients see no reason to move attention into an area of the field that is weakly represented or is subjectively lacking in stimulation.

Several studies have attempted to untangle this problem with only partial success. For instance, Eglin et al. (79) showed that the speed subjects searched for a target, although elevated overall, was similar on both sides of a display once attention was directed to the target side. However, starting to search for a target on the neglected side took up to 30 seconds or more in relatively uncomplicated displays like that shown in Figure 16.6.

Extensive research in neurologically healthy subjects demonstrates that such arrays produce a serial attentional search, and that the time taken to find the target increases linearly with the number of distractors in the display (28, 80). This is also the case for patients with visual neglect, but they are much slower. The elevated search rates in these patients could indicate difficulty in utilizing space over the entire field, while the "contralateral delay" is consistent with a problem in disengaging attention from one side of space to move it in the contralesional direction. This delay could be due to a lag in time in representing contralesional space with unilateral lesions, or it could be due to a lag in cuing attention to move into contralesional space.

A subsequent study (81) showed that the contralateral delay was present but greatly reduced in stable patients with unilateral parietal lobe lesions and no clinical signs of neglect. However, unlike patients in acute stages after stroke, search rates for a target were completely normal. The

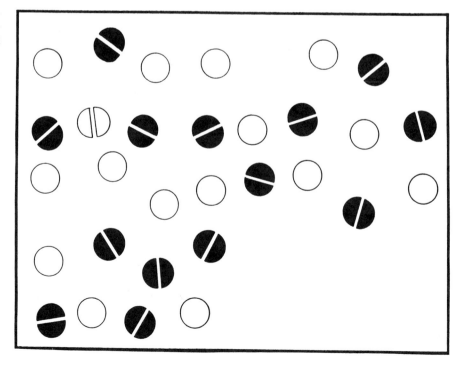

Figure 16.6. Stimulus requiring a serial search to find the target (a white split circle) among distractors of white circles and black split circles. The target is on the left with 19 same side distractors and 10 opposite side distractors. Time to locate a contralateral target increased as the number of opposite side distractors increased in patients with unilateral visual neglect.

directional bias in space remained, while the rate of search was normal in stable patients well past the acute stages of insult. These data suggest that some component operations of spatial attention can be permanently affected after unilateral damage, while others recover completely. They are also consistent with contributions of both spatial and attentional deficits to unilateral visual neglect.

More recent visual search studies showed that the magnitude of neglect was affected by information in the contralesional field in a manner consistent with intact preattentive perception of the spatial extent of the display as a whole. Yet awareness of this space appears to remain below conscious awareness in patients with neglect. Grabowecky et al. (8) used a visual search task similar to Eglin et al. (79) but presented the target in a small area in the center of the display and told subjects that the target would always appear in this area. In some conditions irrelevant distractors were placed around the central area either on the left side, the right side, or both sides. Subjects were informed and understood that the distractors were irrelevant. When irrelevant distractors were placed only on the ipsilesional side of the display (Fig 16.7), the contralateral delay in visual search was profound, as would be expected. However, when the irrelevant distractors on the ipsilesional side were "balanced" by irrelevant distractors on the contralesional side, the contralateral delay returned to baseline (i.e., baseline was defined as a condition with no irrelevant distractors). The addition of irrelevant distractors or "mass" in the contralateral field pulled initiation of visual search back toward the center, and the magnitude of neglect returned to baseline. This occurred even though the irrelevant information on the ipsilesional side was the same whether the contralesional distractors were present or not. One of the challenges in this area for future research will be to explain how spatial information that a patient with unilateral visual neglect cannot access continues to affect performance. It is possible that a more complete understanding of how spatial representations and attention interact will hold the key.

Attention, Objects, and the Parietal Lobes

One question about attentional orienting is whether attention is directed to a spatial location per se or to objects, which obviously cannot exist without a spatial location. These two possibilities are difficult to separate experimentally, but the answer appears to be that both locations in space and objects are attended. Hemispheric differences for attention to space and attention to objects have been observed in groups of patients with inferior parietal damage. Egly et al. (82) used Posner's cuing paradigm, as described earlier, in patients with parietal lesions but on invalid trials presented cues and targets either within or between objects (Fig. 16.8). They found that a right parietal group was affected equally by movements over space whether within or between objects, while a left inferior parietal group was also affected by whether the movement was within objects.

Inferior parietal lobe lesions also disrupts the ability to

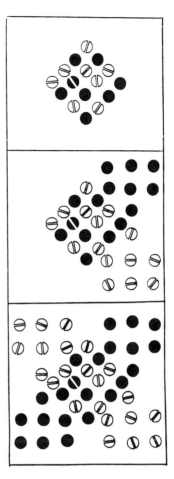

Figure 16.7. Examples of stimuli that require serial search of the central 4 × 4 matrix with no irrelevant flankers *(top)*, right-sided flankers, *(middle)* or bilateral flankers *(bottom)*. The example contains a target (black split-circle) among distractors of white split-circles and black circles. Neglect was more severe for the middle stimulus than the bottom or top stimulus.

redistribute attention across different levels of an object in a hierarchical pattern, such as that shown in Figure 16.4. This has been observed in groups of patients with left-inferior parietal damage (42), but not in patients with right-parietal damage. When a target is expected at the global level of the pattern, performance is better when identifying global forms, and when a target is expected at the local level, performance is better when identifying local forms. This occurs in groups of younger and older normals as well as in patient groups with posterior temporal lobe lesions or dorsolateral frontal lobe lesions (42, 83). However, groups with left-inferior parietal lesions do not show these tradeoffs in performance. When attentional shifts are required within an object, such as between levels of the pattern in Figure 16.4, damage to the left-inferior parietal lobe reduces the shifts.

The type of attention involved in this effect is more categorical in nature. That is, it divides attention between features of the global pattern and features of the local pattern, independent of their spatial location or overall size. In addition, it shows facilitation for specific levels that carry

INVALID CONDITION

Figure 16.8. Examples of two invalid conditions in a study by Egly et al. (111) that tested for within-object versus between-object shifts of attention. Only left-parietal patients had abnormal difficulty with within object shifts. Nothing in common with the target or distractors (off-colored triangles) produced a similar pattern of performance.

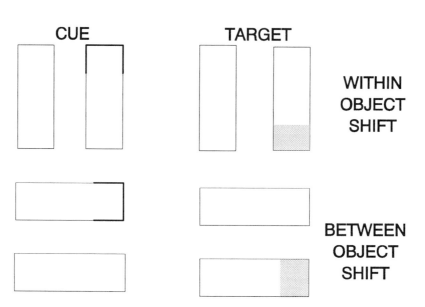

over from one trial to the next. Analysis of trial-by-trial sequential effects show that attending to a global level on trial N facilitates response time to a global letter on trial $N + 1$, and attending to a local level on trial N facilitates response time to a local letter on trial $N + 1$. This level-specific facilitation is the same, whether the consecutive patterns appear in the same location in the visual field or in different locations (84). It appears that the inferior parietal lobe on the left responds to object features. This attentional mechanism is deficient in patient groups with left inferior parietal lesions but not in other groups, including those with right inferior parietal lesions (85, 86). Interestingly, Filoteo et al. (87) reported a similar analysis in a group of patients with Alzheimer's disease. This group also showed an abnormal disengaging deficit in switching attention between levels that was due to level-specific facilitation or inhibition between trials.

The right hemisphere is involved in a different type of attentional process when responding to such patterns; one more associated with space. Studies in normals have revealed that both spatial attention and object attention are involved in responding to a hierarchical pattern (86). The spatial extent of an attentional "spotlight" can be either small or large (88–90). If the extent is large, both global and local information will be within the spotlight, and response to both is facilitated. If it is small, the global level would be outside the spotlight, and facilitation accrues only for local information. Control conditions showed that the process that occurs when a small cue is presented is best explained by an active inhibition of the space surrounding the cue. Studies in patients with parietal damage demonstrated that superior, but not inferior, parietal lesions eliminated the ability to inhibit the surround (85).

It would be wrong to conclude that the left inferior parietal lobe is *specialized* to attend to objects, while superior

parietal lobes are *specialized* to attend to space. Other areas surely contribute to such complex attentional analyses. For instance, spatial inhibition of a surround has been linked to pulvinar function in PET studies with normals (91). Given that the pulvinar connects to a large area of the posterior cortex, it is quite likely that pulvinar–superior parietal connections are part of a network that determines the size of the spatial area that will be attended at any given moment. It is clear that distributed networks within the brain support higher-order visual processes, and spatial and object attention should be no exceptions.

FUNCTIONAL HEMISPHERIC ASYMMETRIES

Although few contemporary scientists would accept the oversimplification of hemispheric specialization that proposes that the left hemisphere is dedicated to language and the right hemisphere to spatial analysis, it is obvious from clinical observation that in humans the hemispheres differ in the pattern of deficits that occur when lesioned. Generally, it is assumed that theories of hemispheric specialization refer to differences in function between homologous structures of the two hemispheres and not to the hemispheres as a whole (although there seems to be some confusion about this point in the lay press and unfortunately even in the neuropsychological literature). When studying patients with focal lesions, keep in mind that functional hemispheric differences would probably not be implicated if patients with left frontal damage perform differently on a task from patients with right parietal damage. Care must be taken that damage is in homologous regions.

This is no small matter. Although the example using left anterior and right posterior areas obviously makes this point, the caveat holds as well for regions that are closer in proximity. This problem is magnified by the fact that there are large anatomical differences between right and left hemispheres. For instance, the Sylvian fissure of the right hemisphere is typically shorter and steeper than the left, and the posterior regions of the left hemisphere are larger than the right, while the frontal regions of the right are larger than the left (92). One way to test the generality of asymmetric deficits found in patients with right or left damage is to use converging evidence from different procedures and different populations, including visual field presentation in normals, PET and evoked potential procedures. It is also desirable to test groups of patients with overlapping lesions in neighboring regions in right- or left-hemisphere damaged groups. For instance, if right temporal-parietal damage produces the same performance as left inferior parietal damage, it may mean that homologous functional areas are simply in slightly different places in the two hemispheres. But if subjects with right- or left-temporal-parietal damage exhibit an asymmetry and subjects with damage in neighboring areas show normal performance, then confidence in asymmetric responses in the two hemispheres is increased.

Studies using primates do not regularly test for functional hemispheric differences (although see ref. 93), and this lack of interest is especially prevalent in electrophysiological investigations. The fact that there are two hemispheres is often omitted from discussions entirely, as if the two halves of the brain were functionally mirror images of each other. Conversely, the human literature has often offered all or no dichotomies. The truth probably lies somewhere between the two extremes; that is, although right hemisphere damage produces more severe and long-lasting spatial deficits in humans, left hemisphere damage also produces spatial deficits.

Evidence from human subjects has increasingly supported hemispheric laterality in visual processing in relatively early stages of analysis (51, 76, 94–100). The amount of data on visual spatial processing and hemispheric function is simply too large to review here, and hemispheric differences have been mentioned along the way in earlier sections.

Rather than review all the different types of visual and spatial deficits that have been associated with one hemisphere or another, I will discuss the historically accepted notion that the right hemisphere analyzes Gestalts or wholes, while the left hemisphere analyzes details or parts. This has been one of the guiding principles of hemispheric specialization for decades, but the answers have often been circular because of the difficult task of determining a priori what constitutes a part and what constitutes a whole or Gestalt. This question has been one of the driving forces behind much of my own work over the past decade. Undoubtedly with a large bias, I believe this work has helped a great deal in understanding the underlying mechanisms that result in the phenomenology of Gestalt versus part processing deficits associated with the two hemispheres.

First, it is important to recognize that describing the functions of the two hemispheres as processing Gestalts or parts is nothing more than a description of the way we, as human beings with normal vision, describe how we perceive

our world. When we describe a deficit as one of missing parts, we are describing it in a way that has face validity for us. We perceive what the subject has missed as a part. This is not entirely wrong. Our own phenomenology does suggest that the visual system transforms sensory input into something that allows the experience of different aspects of a stimulus array as parts and wholes. So perhaps it is not surprising that damage to one area of the brain can disrupt the comprehension of the whole, while damage to another area disrupts the comprehension of parts in a way that fits our own experience of the world.

We have shown repeatedly that damage extending into regions of the left superior temporal lobe with adjacent parietal involvement (T-P) disrupts identification of the local form in hierarchical patterns (Fig. 16.4), while right hemisphere damage in similar regions disrupts identification of the global form. But to understand what has been disrupted, the more important question is how the visual system gets from raw sensory information to comprehension of different forms as parts of other forms. What are the computations that occur between input and output that can explain our own phenomenology as well as the phenomena we observe in patients?

The role of attention and parietal lobes in responding to global and local levels has already been discussed, but there is much more to relate. Patients with T-P lesions (patients who show evidence for hemispheric laterality) show normal performance related to attention, at least for some types of manipulations that are used to study attention. Patients with right T-P damage are generally faster to respond to local than global patterns, and patients with left T-P damage are generally faster to respond to global than local patterns, all else being equal. But attentional manipulations that have been used to study perception of hierarchical objects alter performance in normal ways relative to baseline measures (42). These findings are consistent with two different types of mechanisms—one that is associated with T-P junction responding to features that differentiate global and local levels, and another attentional system associated with parietal areas that can modulate the signal in the T-P region.

As discussed in a previous section, attentional mechanisms associated with left inferior parietal function appear to modulate global and local identification in a categorical manner, while attentional mechanisms associated with superior parietal function modulate it by adjusting the spatial dimensions of the attended region in the visual field. These attentional mechanisms should operate over a variety of stimulus conditions. Conversely, features of the stimulus that define what forms are global and what forms are local rely on selected relevant dimensions from the sensory array. One dimension that differentiates global and local levels is the spatial frequencies at the two levels. Several studies in normals have shown that global/local processing changes are a function of the spatial frequencies in the stimulus (101–104). Simply put, spatial frequency refers to the periodicity of light and dark over the stimulus array at a given resolution. This periodicity is coded at different spatial scales, hence the nomenclature of higher and lower spatial frequencies. If one blurs vision and looks at the stimulus in Figure 16.4, the local elements become more difficult to see, while the global element remains very clearly an H. Blurring reduces the high spatial frequencies, which affects the perception of local more than global elements. However, the global H contains lower spatial frequencies, and is still visible. Global forms invariably contain lower frequencies than local forms. This relationship is true whether the pattern as a whole is expanded to become larger or reduced to become smaller.

One question we addressed recently was whether T-P mechanisms were responding to the absolute size of the global and local levels or to their relative size. We addressed this question by testing left and right T-P groups with different-sized hierarchical patterns. The right T-P group showed a global deficit over the different sizes, while the left T-P group showed a local deficit over the different sizes relative to baseline measures established by healthy controls (41). In other words, the asymmetry, in terms of spatial frequency would have to be linked to the *relative* frequencies in the stimulus. Absolute size or frequency was not the critical dimension.

The most direct evidence for hemispheric differences for spatial frequency analysis has been reported in normals using visual half-field presentation. Kitterle et al. (98) showed that higher frequencies in a stimulus set were identified more rapidly when presented in the right visual field (projected directly to the left hemisphere, while lower frequencies were identified more rapidly when presented in the left visual field — projected directly to the right hemisphere).

Animal work has revealed single cells in striate visual cortex that respond to higher or lower spatial frequencies (105). However, there is no evidence of an asymmetry in this area. Consistently, there is no visual field asymmetry in humans when subjects are simply asked to detect the presence or absence of a frequency grating (whether high or low (106)). Subjects must identify which grating is present for asymmetric performance to appear. Also important is that the asymmetry in young healthy subjects has been found when relative frequency was varied (94).

Work in monkeys has shown that unlike striate cortex, cells in V4 respond to spatial frequency gratings in a way more consistent with an analysis of relative frequencies in a stimulus display (Schein et al.) (106a), reminiscent of cells in MT that respond to relative motion (107). These cells respond more frequently when the differences between frequencies is greater. V4 is a part of the inferior processing stream that is involved in object identification and would be a prime target for relating hemisphere differences found in patients to the animal literature.

When the evidence from various populations and various methods are considered as a whole, there are very good reasons to conclude that T-P lesions in people produce global/local deficits that probably originate in an analysis of the relatively higher and lower spatial frequencies in a stimulus pattern or stimulus set. It could also be argued that

relative frequency analysis is one of the early building blocks in perceiving a multileveled object as a hierarchical form with global patterns that contain local parts.

Certainly, relative frequency information would be more valuable for the way in which we see the world than absolute frequency. A hierarchical figure does not become a different figure when it is reduced or expanded, nor does it become a different figure when it is varied in depth, producing looming and shrinking in a different way. For a hierarchical pattern to be perceived as the same two-leveled form over these spatial transformations (referred to in the perceptual literature as size or object constancy), there must be some mechanism that can respond to the relative feature values at the different levels. For reasons that are not yet clear, it appears to be at this point that hemispheric asymmetries arise in early vision.

This is not to say that every time a patient misses a global form, or is slow to respond to it, temporal-parietal damage should be suspected. RM, the patient with Balint's syndrome discussed in a previous section, had a severe deficit in identifying global forms (much more even than the right T-P groups we tested). However, the data on the role of attentional processes in modulating the speed of response to global and local forms in normals suggest that RM did not, and perhaps could not, allocate attention to a broad region of space once attention was locked onto an object. He did not disengage attention from objects to move to other objects in other spatial locations. Under such circumstances global information could not be reported because it was never attended. In this context, it is interesting to note that interference from global forms was found to be normal in RM (34). When he reported the local form (which he nearly always did), inconsistent global information (a global S made of local H's) slowed his response over consistent global information (a global H made of local H's). The nature of the global form affected his performance, even though he could not identify what the global form was. This is consistent with intact preattentive processing of global spatial information. We conclude that for RM, who had bilateral parietal lesions, the global information was processed, but he could not attend to it and therefore could not report it.

One can see that simple descriptions of hemisphere laterality and visual spatial processing are not very informative. Although nothing I have said is inconsistent with the idea that the right hemisphere is more involved in the perception of wholes and the left hemisphere in the perception of parts, studies of the underlying mechanisms and the neural regions involved have advanced understanding of these asymmetries substantially. It is also obvious that classifications like "simultanagnosia" that have been used to refer to deficits of dual-object or dual-level processing, can capture the essence of the observed behavior but are not explanations of the underlying mechanisms. Simultanagnosia is not a diagnostic for where neural damage has occurred and, for that matter, neither is the absence or slowness to respond to global forms. We need to know what the observed deficit represents in terms of the underlying cognitive mechanisms involved, and this often requires long and careful evaluation.

LIMITATIONS IMPOSED BY DISCIPLINARY CLASSIFICATIONS

The advent of cognitive neuroscience has begun to merge the interests of investigators from diverse backgrounds who have roots in interconnected but different fundamental interests. For investigators interested in the relationship between cognition and the brain, it is important to emphasize the need to break through institutional and professional barriers that often limit scientific thinking. Merging disciplines not only requires interdisciplinary cooperation, but also requires interdisciplinary understanding.

The questions that initially motivate individuals to study brain-behavior relationships are often very different. Neurologists or psychiatrists typically emphasize questions concerning behavioral deficits that are associated with damage to some neural system or disease process. They may ask what behavioral deficits are associated with Alzheimer's disease or what cognitive deficits appear with basal ganglia damage, if any? These questions do not require an answer to how abnormal cognition is mapped onto normal cognition. Rather, an understanding of normal functioning is important to the extent that it establishes normal baselines on which definitions of abnormal can be based. The interest is not initiated by a question specifically about the elementary operations and underlying cognitive processes but in the neural systems that underly disruption of measures of these processes. Obviously, this necessitates the study of normal brain-cognition relationships, even though the original goal was to understand abnormal cognition.

Similarly, clinical neuropsychologists are generally concerned with what cognitive deficits underly observed behavioral deficits. The main goal is to outline those processes that are intact and those that are deficient to perform everyday activities. Although there is increasing concern about subtle deficits in many different diseases that may go undetected with traditional measures (see ref. 108, for example), the emphasis is on the patient's cognitive profile and how well that profile fits a particular syndrome or disease. Again, defining normal cognition is important to the extent that it establishes a baseline for the definition of abnormal. This does not mean that clinical researchers are not interested in evidence for elementary operations and the cognitive and neural architecture of healthy normals. It is simply a reminder that the issues that initiated research interests for individuals from different disciplines are different, and therefore the data and methods that are emphasized in theory construction and everyday practice will be different, even if they are motivated by data from the same studies.

These different fundamental interests also lead to a different classification scheme by scientists from different disciplines. If asked what their interests are, psychiatrists may say schizophrenia or depression. Neurologists may say Alzheimer's disease or hippocampal damage. Clinical neuropsychologists may say unilateral neglect or dementia.

Neuropsychologists trained in experimental psychology programs have long been interested in individuals with damaged brains, but the emphasis has been on normal rather than abnormal function. One way to answer questions about normal functioning is to study abnormal function, so the distinction often becomes somewhat blurred. However, the fundamental questions that drive these investigators concern normal brains. What cognitive mechanisms are associated with the parietal lobe in normals? How does the hippocampus support normal memory? What processing differences best describe differences in normal hemisphere functioning? Obviously, the answers to these questions will influence how one proceeds in interpreting deficits by clinically trained scientists.

In contrast to all of these issues, cognitive psychologists need not take notice of the brain at all. Although this often strikes scientists in the medical community as ludicrous, it is clear that a great deal of behavior can be understood without reference to biological evidence. In fact, the information processing approach within psychology that formed the basis for the "cognitive revolution" was based on the premise that cognition could be studied without knowing anything about the brain. The metaphor was and is the computer, where one can theoretically understand how the software of a system works without knowing how the machine is put together nor even whether the machine is made from chips or neurons. This conceptualization means that the questions that motivate cognitive psychologists are quite different from those discussed so far. They may ask how many types of attentional mechanisms exist? How do attentional mechanisms contribute to object perception? What cognitive processes are automatic and what processes are controlled? What mechanisms determine what information will be selected for further processing? Whether one agrees or disagrees with ignoring the brain, it is becoming clear that the answers to these questions will guide interpretations of cognitive dysfunction.

Cognitive neuropsychology is the integration of cognitive psychology and neuropsychology, as the name implies. It therefore must include the study of brain-cognition relationships. The driving questions are derived from the cognitive part of the equation, but the assumption is that the brain is a special type of hardware, and knowledge of the way it works can guide theoretical development. There are at least two camps who do not agree on the definition of the term. One camp argues for a science based entirely on single case studies with the brain side of the equation having to await a full understanding of how cognitive mechanisms can break down in individual cases (see ref. 109). Members of this camp claim that patients are too heterogeneous to form meaningful groups. Only single cases can provide meaningful data for issues concerning normal cognition and only if tested in hypothesis driven designs.

The other camp argues for the use of converging evidence from a variety of sources, including groups of patients and single cases. Members of this camp suggest that meaningful links between developments in normal cognition, abnormal cognition, and neurobiology are the most optimal way to meet the goal of understanding abnormal cognition and its relationship to normal cognition. It is argued that this goal will be attained only through the use of a variety of methods and subject populations, including the single case design (see ref. 110). In this view, one side of the brain-cognition scale need not await a full understanding of the other. Whatever the resolution of this debate may be, the goal of relating abnormal cognition to normal cognition is a driving pursuit in the field of cognitive neuropsychology.

CONCLUSION

The merging of interests from different disciplines has begun to produce a new wave of investigation under the umbrella of "cognitive neuroscience." In addition to the disciplinary classifications I have discussed, this field includes anatomists, physiologists, computer scientists, linguists, philosophers, psychopharmacologists, and others. This merging of disciplines has created an explosion of new information concerning functional neural systems and the different elementary cognitive operations and specific behaviors they support. I have had space in this chapter to discuss only a subset of these advances in relating visual spatial deficits to lesions in humans. This chapter is not exhaustive on this point. The topics were selected to emphasize the integrative nature of the enterprise and to give examples of what can be accomplished by interdisciplinary communication. A great deal remains to be done. We have only scratched the surface, but clearly the exchange of ideas in tandem with advances in technology have offered an exciting and promising new adventure for everyone interested in the human mind and its relationship to the physical material from which it emerges.

Acknowledgments

The preparation of this chapter was supported by the Medical Review Council of the Veterans Administration and by NIH grant award AA06637 to the author. I wish to thank Robert Rafal for his many helpful comments on an earlier draft.

References

1. Efron R. The decline and fall of hemispheric specialization. Hillsdale NJ:Lawrence Erlbaum & Associates, 1990.
2. Goldman-Rakic PS. Circuitry of primate prefrontal cortex and regulation of behavior by representational memory. In Mountcastle VB, Plum F, Geiger SR, eds. Handbook of Physiology I. Bethesda, MD: American Physiological Society, 1987.
3. Mesulam M-M. Attention, confusional states and neglect. In Mesulam M-M, ed. Principles of behavioral neurology. Philadelphia: F.A. Davis, 1985.
4. Rizzolatti G, Camarda R. Neural circuits for spatial attention and unilateral neglect. In Jeannerod M, ed. Neurophysiological and neuropsychological aspects of spatial neglect. Amsterdam: Elsevier Science Publishers, 1987.
5. Baron JD, D'Antoni R, Pantano P, Serdau M, Samson Y, Boussu MC. Brain 1986;109:1243–1259.
6. Merzenich MM, Kaas JH. Reorganization of mammalian somatosensory cortex following peripheral nerve injury. Trends Neurosci 1982;5:434–436.
7. Kaas JH, Krubitzer LA, Chino YM, Langston AL, Polley EH, Blair M. Reorganization of retinotopic cortical maps in adult mammals after lesion of the retina. Science 1990;248:229–231.
8. Grabowecky M, Robertson LC, Treisman A. Preattentive processes guide visual search: Evidence from patients with unilateral visual neglect. J Cogn Neurosci 1993;5:288–302.
9. Wurtz RH, Albano JE. Visual-motor function of the primate superior colliculus. Annu Rev Neurosci 1980;3:189–226.
10. Sparks DL, Mays LE. Signal transformations required for the generation of saccadic eye movements. Annu Rev Neurosci 1990; 13:309–336.
11. Schiller PH, True SD, Conway JL. Deficits in eye movements following frontal eye field and superior colliculus ablations. J Neurophysiol 1980;44:1175–1189.
12. Lynch JC, Mountcastle VB, Talbot WH, Yin TCT. Directed visual attention. J Neurophysiol 1977;40:362–389.
13. Rafal RD, Posner MI, Friedman JH, Inhoff AW, Bernstein E. Orienting of visual attention in progressive supranuclear palsy. Brain 1988;111:267–280.
14. Posner MI, Rafal RD, Choate L, Vaughn J. Inhibition of return: Neural basis and function. Cogn Neuropsychol 1985;2:211–228.
15. Rafal RD, Calabresi PA, Brennan CW, Sciolto TK. Saccade preparation inhibits reorienting to recently attended locations. J Exp Psychol [Hum Percept], 1989;15:673–685.
16. Posner MI, Cohen Y. Components of performance. In Bouma H, Bowhuis D, eds. Attention & Performance X. Hillsdale, NJ: Lawrence Erlbaum & Associates, 1984.
17. Carter CS, Robertson LC, Chaderjian MR, O'Sora-Celaya L, Nordahl RE. Attentional asymmetries in schizophrenia: the role of illness subtype and symptomatology. Prog Neuropsychopharmacol Biol Psychiatry 1994;18:661–683.
18. Weiskrantz L. Blindsight: a case study and implications. New York:Oxford University Press, 1986.
19. Fendrich R, Wessinger CM, Gazzaniga MS. Residual vision in a scotoma: implications for blindsight. Science 1992;258:1489–1491.
20. Rafal R, Smith J, Krantz J, Cohen A, Brennan C. Extrageniculate vision in hemianopic humans: Saccade inhibition by signals in the blind field. Science 1990;250:118–121.
21. Guitton D, Buchtel HA, Douglas RM. Frontal lobe lesions in man cause difficulties in suppressing reflexive glances and in generating goal-directed saccades. Exp Brain Res 1985;58:455–472.
22. Braun D, Weber H, Mergner TH, Schulte-Monting J. Saccadic reaction times in patients with frontal and parietal lesions. Brain 1992;115:1359–1386.
23. De Renzi E. Oculomotor disturbances in hemispheric disease. In Johnston CW, Pirozzolo FJ, eds. Neuropsychology of eye movements. Hillsdale, NJ: Lawrence Erlbaum & Associates, 1988.
24. Posner MI, Walker JA, Friedrich FJ, Rafal RD. Effects of parietal injury on covert orienting of attention. J Neurosci 1984;4:1863–1874.
25. Morrow L, Ratcliff G. The disengagement of covert attention and the neglect syndrome. Psychobiology 1988;16:261–269.
26. Ungerleider LG, Mishkin M. Two cortical visual systems. In Ingle DJ, Goodale MA, Mansfield RJW, eds. Analysis of visual behavior. Cambridge:MIT Press, 1982.
27. Gattass R, Sousa APB, Covery E. Cortical visual areas of the macaque: possible substrates for pattern recognition mechanisms. In Chagas C, Gattass R, Gross C, eds. Pattern recognition mechanisms. Berlin: Springer-Verlag, 1985.
28. Livingstone M, Hubel D. Segregation of form, color, movement, and depth: anatomy, physiology and perception. Science 1988;240: 740–749.

29. Treisman A, Gelade G. A feature-integration theory of attention. Cognitive Psychology 1980;12:97–136.

30. Kaas JH. Why does the brain have so many visual areas? J Cognitive Neurosci 1989;1:121–135.

31. Newcombe F, Russell WR. Dissociated visual perceptual and spatial deficits in focal lesions of the right hemisphere. J Neurol, Neurosurg Psychiatry 1969;32:73–81.

32. Humphreys GW, Riddoch MJ. Interactions between object and space systems revealed through neuropsychology. In Meyer DE, Kornblum S, eds. Attention and Performance, XIV. Hillsdale, NJ: Lawrence Erlbaum, 1992.

33. Grabowecky M, Egly R, Robertson LC, Rafal, RD. Attentional control in a patient with bilateral parietal lesions. Annual meeting of the Society for Neuroscience. Washington, DC, November, 1993.

34. Egly R, Grabowecky M, Rafal RD, Robertson LC (submitted). Visual stimuli that cannot be reported affect performance in a patient with Balint's syndrome.

35. Farah MJ, Brunn JL, Wong AB, Wallace MA, Carpenter PA. Frames of reference for allocating attention in space: Evidence from the neglect syndrome. Neuropsychologia 1990;28:335–347.

36. Shallice T. From neuropsychology to mental structure. Melbourne: Cambridge University Press, 1988.

37. Riddoch MJ, Humphreys GW. A case of integrative agnosia. Brain 1987;110:1431–1462.

38. Wolpert I. Die Simultanagnosie: Storung der Gesamtauffassung. Z. f. d. gesamte Neurol. u. Psychiatr., 93, 397–425 (as referenced by A. Benton, [1985]). Visuoperceptual, visuospatial and visuoconstructive disorders. In Heilman KM, Valenstein E, eds. Clin Neuropsychol. NY: Oxford University Press, 1924.

39. Humphreys GW, Riddoch MJ. To see but not to see: a case study of visual agnosia. Hillsdale, NJ: Lawrence Erlbaum & Associates, 1987.

40. Kinsbourne M, Warrington EK. The localizing significance of limited simultaneous form perception. Brain 1962;85:461–486.

41. Lamb MR, Robertson LC, Knight RT. Component mechanisms underlying the processing of hierarchically organized patterns: inferences from patients with unilateral cortical lesions. J Exp Psychol [Learn Mem Cogn] 1990;16:471–483.

42. Robertson LC, Lamb MR, Knight RT. Effects of lesions of temporal-parietal junction on perceptual and attentional processing in humans. J Neurosci 1988;8:3757–3769.

43. Farah MJ, Wallace MA. Pure alexia as a visual impairment: a reconsideration. Cognitive Neuropsychology 1991;8:313–334.

44. Broadbent DA. The hidden preattentive process. Am Psychologist 1977;32:109–118.

45. Koffka KA. Principles of Gestalt psychology. NY: Harcourt, Brace & World, 1935.

46. Krech D, Calvin A. Levels of perceptual organization and cognition. J Abnorm Soc Psychol 1953;48:394–400.

47. Krechevsky I. An experimental investigation of the principle of proximity in the visual perception of the rat. J Exp Psychol 1938;22:497–523.

48. Navon D. Forest before trees: the precedence of global features in visual perception. Cognitive Psychology 1977;9:353–383.

49. Damasio AR. Disorders of complex visual processing: agnosias, achromatopsia, Balint's syndrome, and related difficulties of orientation and construction. In Mesulum M-M, ed. Principles of behavioral neurology. Philadelphia: FA Davis, 1985:259–288.

50. Bruce V, Young A. Understanding face recognition. Br J Psychol 1986;77:305–327.

51. Farah MJ. Visual agnosia: disorders of object recognition and what they tell us about normal vision. NY: Academic Press, 1990.

52. Bornstein B, Stroka H, Munitz H. Prosopagnosia with animal face agnosia. Cortex 1969;5:164–169.

53. Newcombe F. The processing of visual information in prosopagnosia and acquired dyslexia: functional versus physiological interpretation. In Oborne DJ, Gruneberg MM, Eiser JR, eds. Research in Psychology and Medicine. London: Academic Press, 1979.

54. Tranel D, Damasio AR. Knowledge without awareness: an autonomic index of facial recognition by prosopagnosics. Science 1985; 228:1453–1454.

55. Perrett DI, Rolls ET, Caen W. Visual neurones responsive to faces in the monkey temporal cortex. Exp Brain Res 1982;47:329–342.

56. Rolls ET. The processing of face information in the primate temporal lobe. In Bruce V, Burton M, eds. Processing images of faces. Norwood, NJ: Ablex Publishing, 1992.

57. Warrington EK. Visual deficits associated with occipital lobe lesions in man. Exp Brain Res 1986;11 (Suppl):247–261.

58. LaBerge D. Thalamic and cortical mechanisms of attention suggested by recent positron emission tomographic experiments. J Cogn Neurosci 1990;4:358–372.

59. Davidoff J. Cognition through color. Cambridge: Bradford Book/ MIT Press, 1991.

60. DeValois RL. Analysis and coding of color vision in the primate visual system. Cold Spring Harbor Symposium on Quantitative Biology 1965;30:567–579.

61. Desimone R, Schein SJ, Albright TD. Form, color and motion analysis in prestriate cortex of the Macaque. In Chagas C, Gattass R, Gross C, eds. Pattern recognition mechanisms. NY: Springer-Verlag, 1985.

62. Zihl J, Von Cramon D, Mai N. Selective disturbance of movement vision after bilateral brain damage. Brain 1983;106:313–340.

63. Maunsell JHR, Newsome WT. Visual processing in monkey extrastriate cortex. Annu Rev Neurosci 1987;10:363–401.

64. Andersen R.A. Inferior parietal lobule function in spatial perception and visuomotor integration. In Mountcastle VB, Plum F, Geiger SR, eds. Handbook of physiology I. Bethesda, MD: American Physiological Society, 1987:483–518.

65. Marshall JC, Halligan PW. When right goes left: an investigation of line bisection in a case of visual neglect. Cortex 1989;25:503–515.

66. Heilman KM, Watson RT and Valenstein E. Neglect and related disorders. In Heilman KM, Valenstein E, eds. Clinical neuropsychology, 2nd ed. NY: Oxford U Press, 1985.

67. Ogden JA. The "neglected" left hemisphere and its contribution to visuospatial neglect. In Jeannerod M, ed. Neurophysiological and neuropsychological aspects of spatial neglect. Amsterdam: Elsevier Science Publishers, 1987.

68. Robertson LC, Eglin M. Attentional search in unilateral neglect. In Robertson I, Marshall J, eds. Unilateral neglect: Clinical and experimental studies. London: Taylor & Francis, 1993:169–191.

69. Bisiach E, Luzzatti C. Unilateral neglect of representational space. Cortex, 1978;14:129–133.

70. Bisiach E, Luzzatti C, Perani D. Unilateral neglect, representational schema and consciousness. Brain 1979;102:609–618.

71. Kinsbourne M. Mechanisms of unilateral neglect. In Jeannerod M, ed. Neurophysiological and neuropsychological aspects of spatial neglect. Amsterdam: Elsevier Science Publishers, 1987.

72. Kinsbourne M. Orientational bias model of unilateral neglect: evidence from attentional gradients within hemispace. In Robertson I, Marshall J, eds. Unilateral neglect: Clinical and experimental studies. Hillsdale: Lawrence Erlbaum & Associates, 1993.

73. Morrow LA, Ratcliff G. Attentional mechanisms in clinical neglect. J Clin Exp Neuropsychol 1987;9:74–75.

74. Lynch JC. The functional organization of posterior parietal association cortex. Behav Brain Sci 1980;3:485–534.

75. Posner MI, Petersen SE. The attention system of the human brain. Annu Rev Neurosci 1990;13:25–42.

76. Corbetta M, Miezin FM, Shulman GL, Petersen AE. Shifts of visuo-spatial attention: a PET study. J Neurosci, 1993;13:1202–1226.

77. Posner MI, Early RS, Reiman E, Pardo PJ, Dhawan M. Asymmetries of attentional control in schizophrenia. Arch Gen Psychiatry 1988; 45:814–821.

78. Bisiach E, Berti A. Dyschiria: an attempt at its systemic explanation. In Jeannerod M, ed. Neurophysiological and neuropsychological

aspects of spatial neglect. Amsterdam: Elsevier Science Publishers, 1987.

79. Eglin M, Robertson LC, Knight RT. Visual search performance in the neglect syndrome. J Cogn Neurosci 1989;1:372–385.

80. Eglin M, Robertson LC, Knight RT. Cortical substrates supporting visual search in humans. Cerebral Cortex 1991;1:262–272.

81. Treisman A, Souther J. Search asymmetry: A diagnostic for preattentive processing of separable features. J Exp Psychol. [Gen] 1985;114:285–210.

82. Egly R, Driver J, Rafal RD. Deficits following parietal damage: space based or object based? Paper presented at the annual meeting of Psychonomic Society, St. Louis, November, 1992.

83. Robertson LC, Lamb MR, Knight RT. Dorsolateral frontal lobe lesions and global-local analysis. Neuropsychologia 1991;29:959–967.

84. Robertson LC. Attention and the parietal lobes. Paper presented at the annual meeting of the Winter Conference for Brain Research, Whistler, BC, January, 1993.

85. Robertson LC. The role of perceptual organization and search in attentional disorders. In Margolin DI, ed. Cognitive neuropsychology in clinical practice. New York: Oxford University Press, 1992.

86. Robertson LC, Egly R, Lamb MR, Kerth L. Spatial attention and cuing to global and local levels of hierarchical structure. J Exp Psychol [Hum Percept] 1993;19:471–487.

87. Filoteo JV, Delis DC, Massman PJ, Demadura T, Butters N, Salmon DP. Directed and divided attention in Alzheimer's disease: impairment in shifting of attention to global and local stimuli. J Clin Exp Neuropsychol 1992;14:871–883.

88. Eriksen CW, St James JD. Visual attention within and around the field of focal attention: a zoom lens model. Perception and Psychophysics 1986;40:225, 240.

89. Eriksen CW, Yeh Y. Allocation of attention in the visual field. Journal of Experimental Psychology: Human Perception and Performance 1985;11:583, 597.

90. LaBerge D, Brown V. Variations in size of the visual field in which targets are presented: An attentional range effect. Perception & Psychophysics 1986;40:188–200.

91. LaBerge D, Buchsbaum MS. Positron emission tomographic measurements of pulvinar activity during an attention task. J Neurosci 1990;10:613–619.

92. Geschwind M, Galaburda AM. Cerebral lateralization. Cambridge: Bradford Books, MIT Press, 1987.

93. Bradshaw J, Rogers L. The evolution of lateral asymmetries, language, tool use, and intellect. San Diego: Academic Press, 1993.

94. Christman S, Kitterle FL, Hellige J. Hemispheric asymmetry in the processing of absolute versus relative spatial frequency. Brain Cogn 1991;16:62–73.

95. Ivry RB, Lebby PC. Hemispheric differences in auditory perception are similar to those found in visual perception. Psychological Science 1993;4:41–45.

96. Ivry RB, Robertson, (in press). Hemispheric processing of frequency information: A general model. Cambridge: MIT Press.

97. Jonsson JE, Hellige JB. Lateralized effects of blurring: a test of visual spatial frequency model of cerebral hemisphere asymmetry. Neuropsychologia 1986;24:351–362.

98. Kitterle F, Christman S, Hellige J. Hemispheric differences are found in the identification, but not detection of low versus high spatial frequencies. Perception & Psychophysics 1990;48:297–306.

99. Sergent J. The cerebral balance of power: Confrontation or cooperation? J Exp Psychol [Hum Percept] 1982;8:253–272.

100. Sergent J. Failures to confirm the spatial-frequency hypothesis: Fatal blow or healthy complication? Can J Psychol 1987;41:412–428.

101. Hughes HC, Fendrich R, Reuter-Lorenz PA. Global versus local processing in the absence of low spatial frequencies. J Cogn Neurosc 1990;2:272–282.

102. LaGasse LL. Effects of good form and spatial frequency on global precedence. Perception & Psychophysiology 1993;53:89–105.

103. Shulman GL, Sullivan MA, Gish K, Sadoda WJ. The role of spatial-frequency channels in the perception of local and global structure. Perception 1986;15:259–273.

104. Shulman GL, Wilson J. Spatial frequency and selective attention to local and global information. Perception 1987;16:89–101.

105. DeValois RL, Albrecht DG, Thorell LG. Spatial frequency selectivity of cells in macaque visual cortex. Vision Res 1982;22:545–559.

106. Kitterle FL, Kaye RS. Hemispheric symmetry in contrast and orientation sensitivity. Perception & Psychophysics 1985;37:391–396.

106a. Schein SJ, Desimone R, de Monasterio FM. Spectral properties of area V4 cells of Macaque monkey. Invest Ophthalmol Vis Sci 1983;24:107.

107. Allman J, Miezin F, McGuinness E. Stimulus specific responses from beyond the classical receptive field: neurophysiological mechanisms for local-global comparisons in visual neurons. Annu Rev Neurosci 1985;8:407–430.

108. Martin EM, Sorensen DJ, Edelstein HE, Robertson LC. Decision-making speed in early HIV-1 infection. AIDS 1992;6:109–113.

109. McCloskey, M. Theory and Evidence in Cognitive Neuropsychology: A "Radical" Response to Robertson, Knight, Rafal & Shimamura. J Exp Psychol [Mem Learn Cogn] 1993;19:718–734.

110. Robertson LC, Rafal RD, Knight RT, Shimamura A. Cognitive neuropsychology is more than single case studies. J Exp Psychol [Learn Mem Cogn] 1993;19:710–717.

111. Egly R, Driver J, Rafal RD. Shifting visual attention between objects and locations: Evidence from normal and neurological populations. J Exp Psychol Gen 1994;123:161–177.

17

MEMORY

Dean C. Delis and John A. Lucas

This chapter describes several aspects of learning and memory. We begin by reviewing the neuronal bases of learning and memory, followed by a discussion of some of the more common definitions of memory constructs and the neuroanatomical substrates underlying memory functioning. We then review a number of clinical neuropsychological techniques used to assess learning and memory, and conclude with a discussion of memory disorders typically seen in clinical populations and normal aging.

NEURONAL BASES OF MEMORY

Most organisms have the ability to change their behavior in response to events that occur during the course of their lifetimes. This is due to the capacity of the animal's nervous system to be modified by experience—a capacity that gives the animal the ability to learn and remember. Learning and memory exhibit different phenomenological aspects, depending upon the level of organization observed. They may be seen as changes in complex behaviors and interactions between the organism and its environment, in neuronal communication and the functional relationships of brain structures, or in signal processing and transduction at the molecular level (1).

Most neurobiologists view memory as a special case of the general phenomenon known as neuronal plasticity, that is, the ability of neurons to change their structure or function in a lasting way. Early investigators hypothesized that memory reflected modification of the existing structure of the nervous system either through growth or change (2). This basic premise formed the foundation of numerous theories of memory functioning that have appeared over the last half century (3–5). Today, there is a consensus that the neuronal changes associated with learning and memory occur at the level of the synapse; however, this was not always the accepted theory. With advances in the study of molecular biology during the 1960s and 1970s, investigators began to question whether learned information could be coded in the brain in terms of specific molecules or unique proteins, such as RNA or DNA. It was hypothesized that each neuron in the brain could have its own individual

molecular label, and that when learning occurred, new molecules were created, reflecting the combination of neurons involved in the learned experience. The structure of the "learned" molecule itself would then contain a code representing the learned experience.

Based on this assumption, it was believed that the molecular code for a learned experience could be extracted from one individual and transferred into the brain of another individual. In fact, the first investigations of this hypothesis reported that learned behaviors, such as initiation of food-seeking behavior in response to a neutral signal, could indeed be transferred from trained rats to untrained rats via the injection of brain homogenates (6). A large number of subsequent investigations, however, failed to replicate these findings. By 1971, over 250 studies had been published on the subject. A review of these studies failed to find cumulative experimental evidence for molecular hypothesis (7), and it was abandoned by the end of the 1970s. Today, investigations of the biochemical aspects of memory focus not on the search for unique molecules associated with learned experiences, but with identification of those biochemical processes that may underlie synaptic modification and/or changes in neuronal connectivity (8).

Memory as Change of Synaptic Efficacy

Studies of neuronal interaction and organization have shown that each neuron in the brain is interconnected with many other neurons in a network of feedback loops. Hebb (4) proposed that psychologically important events such as memory were manifestations of the flow of activity within a given neuronal loop or set of loops. When neurons in a given loop were excited together, the synapses in that pathway were believed to become functionally connected and form what Hebb called a "cell assembly." This functional connection could be maintained over time by repeated or persistent activity flow within the loop. This would eventually lead to a growth process or metabolic change that would make the connection more efficient. Hebb (4) believed that this was accomplished via the development of additional synaptic terminals, which served to increase the area of contact between the axon of the afferent neuron and the cell body of the efferent neuron.

Hebb's theory of functional connections and synaptic growth provided a useful heuristic for understanding memory functioning and continues to be incorporated into models of neural networks of memory. Some of his originally proposed mechanisms of memory development, however, were not supported by subsequent research. For example, Hebb (4) assumed that changes at the level of the synapse were dependent upon continued activity in the cell assembly after the initial stimulation ceased; he referred to this activity as a "reverberatory trace." Specifically, he wrote that the "reverberatory trace might cooperate with the structural change, and carry the memory until the growth change is made" (4, p. 62). According to Squire (2), however, sustained electrical activity of the sort proposed by Hebb has never been observed. Instead, recent evidence suggests that the neurons themselves can hold information temporarily, and thus do not require mechanisms such as reverberatory circuits to sustain information over brief time intervals (2).

Hebb's basic hypothesis that memory is reflected in structural changes of the neuronal synapses, however, is well supported by the literature. Studies have shown that animals trained to perform specific tasks or exposed to enriched environments not only develop new synapses, but also demonstrate changes in existing synapses. These changes include postsynaptic thickening and increases in the number of presynaptic vesicles, dendritic branching, and density of dendritic spines (9, 10). Such changes have been observed in both young and adult animals, and they can occur subsequent to a single learning experience. Patel and Stewart (11), for example, presented a 1-day-old chick with a small, shiny bead coated with a distasteful, bitter substance. Following a single peck, the chick avoided similar beads when presented thereafter. Twenty-five hours later, the density of dendritic spines on a neuron from a region of the brain known to be important to memory function was found to be 60% greater than that of a control chick presented with a bead coated with water. This type of training has also been associated with increases in the area of the active regions between pre- and postsynaptic sites and in the number of synaptic vesicles (2).

The findings of synaptic changes associated with learning and memory raise the question of where in the brain these changes occur. It is not likely that every neuronal synapse is modified by every experience, nor does it seem likely that each experience is represented by a change to only one corresponding neuron. Research has shown that damage to any of a number of distinct brain regions can affect memory functioning; however, because memory is not a unitary construct, the type of difficulties experienced subsequent to such damage can vary, depending upon the site of involvement. Consequently, before we address the question of which neuroanatomical structures underlie memory, we must first define the various constructs that comprise memory functioning.

CONCEPTUAL DIVISIONS OF MEMORY

Perhaps more than any other cognitive domain, memory has inspired researchers to hypothesize numerous conceptual divisions. Questions about the validity of these divisions and their interrelationships, however, often prompt lively debate. Such responses are partly the result of the lack of a universally accepted terminology, which can lead to confusion in the literature (12,13). For example, different investigators may use the same terminology to reflect different constructs, or different terminology to reflect the same construct. This section describes several of the more widely accepted conceptual divisions of memory; however, the reader is referred elsewhere for more comprehensive reviews (2, 12–14).

Short-term Versus Long-term Memory

In 1890, William James distinguished between memory that endured for a very brief time and memory that lasted after the experience had been "dropped from consciousness" (15, p. 648). The former, known as short-term memory (or primary memory), generally refers to recall of material immediately after it is presented or during uninterrupted rehearsal. The latter, known as long-term memory (or secondary memory), refers to the ability to remember information after a delay interval, during which the individual's attention is focused away from the target information (16). Short-term memory is thought to be of limited capacity, holding an average of seven "bits" of information at any one time. This information may be retained for up to several minutes, but will be lost or replaced by new information if it is not sustained by rehearsal. In contrast, long-term memory is believed to have an extraordinarily large capacity, with the potential for holding information indefinitely without the need for continued rehearsal (17).

Hebb (18) conducted an experiment that illustrates the dichotomy of short-term and long-term memory. Subjects were read sets of nine digits and asked to recall them immediately following each presentation. As just noted, short-term memory has a capacity of approximately seven pieces of information; thus, the average person has a short-term memory span of approximately seven digits. Nine digits are beyond the span of most normal individuals; thus, relatively few of Hebb's subjects could recall all nine digits correctly. Without the subjects' knowledge, however, one set of digits was repeated on every third trial. Results of the study revealed that the repeated set of digits was recalled correctly by an increasingly greater percentage of subjects as the number of presentations increased. In contrast, recall of the novel sets of digits remained at baseline levels (Fig. 17.1). This demonstrates that a type of memory distinct from immediate memory span develops as information is learned.

The clinical significance of the distinction between short- and long-term memory is best exemplified in cases of amnesia (19–23). In perhaps the most famous case study in

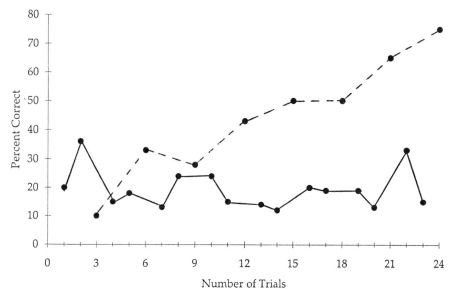

Figure 17.1 Results of Hebb's Recurring Digits Test. Subjects were asked to recall sets of nine digits, not knowing that the same set of digits was repeated on every third trial. Over time, a greater percentage of subjects recalled the repeated set correctly while continuing to do poorly in recalling novel sets of digits. This illustrates the dichotomy between short-term, or immediate, memory and long-term memory. (From Hebb DO. Distinctive features of learning in the higher animal. In: Delafresnay JF, ed. Brain mechanisms and learning. Oxford: Blackwell, 1961.)

the neuropsychological literature, a patient, H.M., underwent surgical resection of the medial temporal lobes for treatment of intractable epilepsy. The surgery successfully treated the seizure disorder; however, H.M. was left with profound deficits in new learning and memory. One striking finding was that H.M. could repeat information immediately following presentation and hold new information via active rehearsal, but he would rapidly forget that information over time or with distraction. In other words, he demonstrated intact short-term memory in the presence of severely impaired long-term memory. This phenomenon has also been demonstrated in other cases of amnesic patients, such as N.A. (22) and P.Z. (19).

Despite the rather eloquent demonstrations of how short- and long-term memory can be dissociated, there is some controversy in the experimental literature surrounding this dichotomy. First, there is disagreement regarding the temporal definitions of short- and long-term memory. For example, the criterion used by one investigator to define short-term memory may overlap with that which another investigator uses to define long-term memory (24, 25). Second, there is disagreement over whether it is appropriate to dichotomize memory processes. Some investigators have argued that a two-stage model of memory is inadequate, preferring instead to conceptualize memory into three or more separate stages (e.g., immediate, short-term, long-term). Others believe that the division of memory into discrete stages is altogether spurious and that levels of successful encoding of information into memory exist on a continuum (26, 27). Squire (2) contends, however, that the abrupt decline in memory seen in amnesic patients when they are distracted from target material provides strong clinical justification for the distinction between a short-term and long-term memory store, and that there is little compelling evidence in the literature to warrant further subdivision of this dichotomy (2).

Encoding Versus Retrieval

Encoding refers to the process by which information is transformed into a stored, mental representation, while retrieval is the process of bringing the stored memory back into consciousness. Patients with brain damage can vary considerably in terms of whether their memory problems are at the level of encoding or retrieval. One common way to illustrate this distinction is to present new information, such as a story or word list, and to compare the patient's memory for that information using both a free recall and recognition paradigm. If information has been encoded successfully but cannot be retrieved, performance will be poor on free recall, which places maximal demands on retrieval. In contrast, patients whose deficits lie in the encoding of information will perform equally poorly on free recall and recognition testing.

Retroactive Versus Proactive Interference

Events or information encountered before or after the presentation of information to be remembered can interfere with recall of the target information. The two mechanisms fundamental to such memory failure are retroactive and proactive interference. Retroactive interference refers to the disrupting effect that later learning has on the ability to recall previously learned information. This is illustrated by a study of verbal learning by Slamecka (28). Subjects were given eight trials to learn a long, complex sentence. After the eighth trial, some subjects were given a rest period, while others were asked to learn a second sentence. As seen in Figure 17.2, the presentation of new information (i.e., the second sentence) is related to poorer recall of the target sentence. Moreover, the amount of target information forgotten is a function of the number of interference trials administered.

The effect of retroactive interference is also a function of the similarity between the target and interference informa-

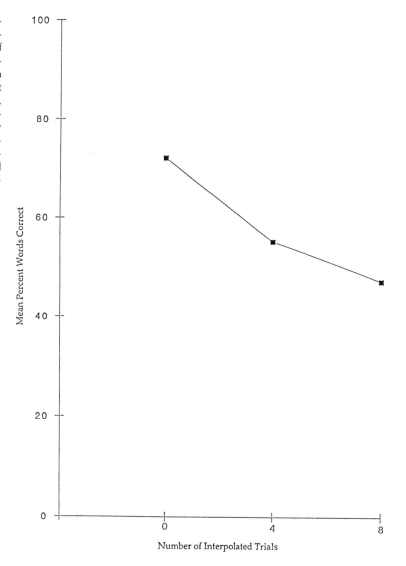

Figure 17.2. The effect of retroactive interference on sentence retention. Accuracy of sentence recall is negatively affected by the presentation of a new sentence after the target sentence is learned. Moreover, poorer recall of the target sentence is a function of the number of interference trials administered. (From Slamecka NJ. Retroactive inhibition of connected discourse as a function of practice level. J Exp Psychol 1960; 59:104–108.)

tion. The more similar the interference information is to the target information, the greater the degree of interference and the poorer the recall of the target stimuli.

Proactive interference refers to the situation in which earlier learning interferes with the subject's ability to learn new information at a later time. In one of a series of studies on memory for nonsense syllables, Underwood (29) noticed that some subjects demonstrated substantial forgetting rates from one day to the next. It seemed unlikely that this was due to retroactive interference, because subjects would not likely encounter nonsense syllables in their activities between the day they were presented the information and the next day, when recall was assessed. Underwood noted, however, that many of the subjects in his experiment had also served as subjects in several of his previous experiments on learning and memory of nonsense syllables. He suspected that the subjects' *previous* exposure to similar material may have interfered with their ability to recall new lists learned later.

Underwood plotted the percentage of correct recall of the new list of nonsense syllables as a function of the number of past nonsense syllable experiments in which each subject had participated. He found that as the number of previous

experiments in which subjects took part increased, the percentage of correct 24-hour recall of information from the new list decreased, thus providing evidence for a proactive form of interference.

As with retroactive interference, studies show that the degree of proactive interference in recall is dependent upon the degree of similarity between the target items and the interfering information. The more similar the interference items are to the target items and the more times these items are presented, the greater the interference and the poorer the recall of the target items (25, 30). Conversely, recall can be *facilitated* by making target items dissimilar to the interference information. In a study by Randolph et al. (31), subjects were shown different series of word triplets (e.g., cat-dog-rabbit) over five trials. After each trial, subjects engaged in an interference task (i.e., color naming) for 15 seconds and were then asked to recall the previously seen words. Half of the subjects were presented words from the same semantic category (e.g., animals) on all five trials. The other half were presented words from the same category on the first four trials only; on the fifth trial, the words shifted to an unrelated semantic category (e.g., articles of clothing).

Data from normal subjects are presented in Figure 17.3. The effect of proactive interference on recall can be seen quite clearly on trials in which similar words were to be recalled. Note, however, the improved recall on trial 5 of the shift condition. This phenomenon is known as release from proactive interference.

Anterograde Versus Retrograde Amnesia

Patients with memory disorders have been studied extensively, and two dissociable disturbances of memory have been observed. Anterograde amnesia refers to the inability to recall or recognize new information or events that have been encountered since the onset of the amnesic condition. In contrast, retrograde amnesia refers to the inability to recall or recognize information or events that were encountered prior to the onset of amnesia. Evidence of both anterograde and retrograde deficits are typically seen in all amnesic patients; however, the relative severity of each type of deficit may differ from patient to patient (2, 14, 32–35).

Anterograde amnesia typically affects a wide variety of new learning. Observing H.M., the patient who became amnesic following surgical intervention for intractable epilepsy, Milner (36) wrote: "He could no longer recognise the hospital staff, apart from Dr. Scoville himself, whom he had known for many years; he did not remember and could not relearn the way to the bathroom, and he seemed to retain nothing of the day-to-day happenings in the hospital. . . ." (p. 113). On formal testing, H.M. demonstrated severely impaired memory for new verbal and nonverbal information, such as stories, faces, figures, or sequences beyond his immediate memory span (20, 21, 37). His intellectual functioning, however, remained within normal limits for his age.

Patients with retrograde amnesia are unable to remember events that occurred prior to the onset of the amnesic syndrome. In most cases, however, the ability to recall factual information not related to specific contexts or experiences remains fairly intact (see discussion of episodic vs. semantic memory later in this chapter). For example, patients with true retrograde amnesia will typically retain previously acquired factual knowledge such as the name of the first U.S. President or state capitals, as well as salient personal facts, such as their name. They may also retain basic, albeit vague, recollections of their career, marital status, and family (38). Patients who suffer complete loss of personal history and identity are rare and typically reflect psychological, rather than neurological, etiologies (39).

Recent Versus Remote Memory

The distinction between recent and remote memory is typically applied to the temporal dimension of retrograde amnesia. Recent memory most often refers to the information acquired just prior to the onset of an amnesic syndrome, while remote memory refers to information regarding events or experiences acquired years or decades before the amnesia began. Patients with retrograde amnesia often demonstrate a temporal gradient in which memory for more recent events is disrupted to a greater extent than memory for remote events. This gradient is illustrated clearly by the case study of patient P.Z., a distinguished scientist who became amnesic secondary to alcoholic Korsakoff syndrome (40). Several

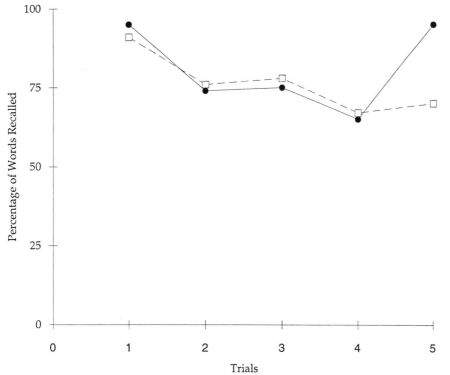

Figure 17.3. An illustration of proactive interference (PI). On each of the first four trials, subjects were asked to recall sets of words from the same semantic category (e.g., animals). The effect of PI can be seen in the decline in performance over these trials. On the fifth trial, subjects who were asked to recall another set of words from the same category continued to demonstrate PI, while subjects asked to recall words from a new semantic category (e.g., clothing) demonstrated improved recall. This illustrates the phenomenon known as release from PI. (From Randolph C, Gold JM, Carpenter CJ, Goldberg TE, Weinberger DR. Release from proactive interference: determinants of performance and neuropyschological correlates. J Clin Exp Neuropsychol 1992;14:785–800.)

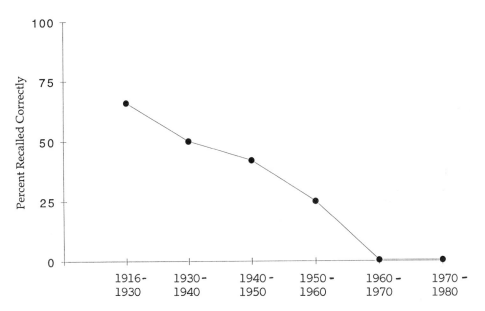

Figure 17.4. Temporal gradient of retrograde amnesia for autobiographical information in a patient with alcoholic Korsakoff syndrome (P.Z.). Information from earlier decades are recalled better than that from more recent decades. (From Butters N, Cermak LS. A case study of the forgetting of autobiographical knowledge: implications for the study of retrograde amnesia. In: Rubin D, ed. Autobiographical memory. New York: Cambridge University Press, 1986:253–272.)

years prior to the onset of his amnesic syndrome, P.Z. completed an autobiography. This allowed the investigators to assess the patient's ability to recall past events that he had been able to recall premorbidly. The percentage of correct recall of autobiographical questions as a function of the decades during which the events occurred is presented in Figure 17.4. These data illustrate a clear temporal gradient, with memory for recent experiences and events substantially worse than memory for events from his early life.

Declarative Versus Nondeclarative Memory

One of the most important insights to emerge from modern neuropsychological research is the distinction between declarative and nondeclarative memory, also known as explicit and implicit memory. Declarative memory refers to the acquisition of facts, experiences, and information about events. It is memory that is directly accessible to conscious awareness and can be declared. In contrast, nondeclarative memory refers to various forms of memory that are not directly accessible to consciousness. These include skill and habit learning, classical conditioning, the phenomenon of priming, and other situations in which memory is expressed through performance rather than recollection (2, 41).

According to Squire and colleagues (41), declarative memory is relatively fast and flexible. Fact-based information, for example, can usually be expressed quickly via a number of different response systems. Declarative memory, however, is not always reliable, as is evident in everyday problems with retrieval of information and forgetting. In contrast, nondeclarative memory is considered quite reliable, but is often slow and inflexible. The information present in a learned skill, for example, can often be expressed most readily only by the response systems that were involved in the original learning of that skill.

EPISODIC VERSUS SEMANTIC MEMORY

Declarative knowledge can be divided into episodic and semantic memory (42). Episodic memory refers to infor-

mation learned at a particular place and time in one's life. Asking an individual to recall what he or she ate for breakfast that morning, what they were doing when they first heard of the Space Shuttle *Challenger* disaster, or what words were presented on list they heard earlier all tap into episodic memory. To recall the target information correctly, the individual must be able to access information regarding the time and place of the original event. Semantic memory, on the other hand, refers to general knowledge of the world that is not linked to a particular temporal or spatial context. This might include asking an individual to define the word "breakfast," to state what a space shuttle is, or to recall the alphabet. None of these tasks requires recall of where or when the information was learned. Both episodic and semantic memory are declarative, however, in that retrieval of information is carried out explicitly, on a conscious level.

TYPES OF NONDECLARATIVE MEMORY

The study of nondeclarative memory is relatively new, and a complete classification scheme for all nondeclarative forms of memory has yet to be developed. At present, nondeclarative memory includes several different forms of learning and memory abilities, including procedural memory, some forms of classical conditioning, and the phenomena of priming. Although these constructs are reviewed here briefly, the interested reader is referred elsewhere for a more comprehensive discussion of the types of nondeclarative memory (2, 41).

Procedural Memory

Procedures are motor, perceptual, or cognitive skills that are learned and used by an individual to operate effectively in the world. They include such behaviors as tying a shoe, riding a bicycle, or driving a car. Procedural memory refers to the process of retrieving information that underlies these skilled performances. Although some aspects of skills can be declared, the skill itself is most often performed automatically, without conscious retrieval of information regarding the procedure. For example, an individual skilled at riding a bicycle does not consciously retrieve information about bicycle riding in order to get on a bicycle and ride. The procedure is automatic and is performed without conscious attention to the mechanics involved. In fact, conscious attention to procedural information can often disrupt performance of the skill.

Habits are another form of procedural memory similar to that of skill learning and performance; they are dispositions and tendencies that are specific to particular sets of stimuli and help guide behavior (41). Consider, for example, the situation in which an individual drives to a familiar destination (e.g., home from work) along a familiar route. He or she will make turns at various points and slow down when approaching a dip in the road without conscious processing of the specific details of that particular trip. Although the procedure of driving the car is a skilled performance, the knowledge of driving the route could be considered a habit. This information is often accessible to conscious retrieval if needed (e.g., if a colleague asks for directions from work to your home); however, habits, like skills, are most often revealed in their performance and can be carried out automatically without conscious awareness.

Conditioning

Classical conditioning is one of the most basic forms of learning and illustrates another type of nondeclarative memory. In such a learning paradigm, a stimulus that naturally produces a desired response is identified and paired with a neutral stimulus. After repeated pairings, the neutral stimulus alone will elicit the desired response. For example, a dog will naturally begin to salivate when presented food, but not when presented with the sound of a bell ringing. If, however, a bell is rung immediately prior to the presentation of food, and this pairing is repeated over several trials, presentation of the bell alone will produce salivation. The food in this situation is called an unconditioned stimulus (UCS) because it is a behavior that required no training. Likewise, salivation in response to food is called an unconditioned response (UCR). The sound of the bell ringing is called a conditioned stimulus (CS) because the dog becomes conditioned to salivate to the once neutral stimulus. Once this occurs, the salivation in response to the bell is called a conditioned response (CR).

Some researchers have argued that conditioning in humans requires conscious awareness of the CS-UCS contingency (43); however, studies of patients with amnesic disorders strongly suggest that associations can be conditioned without declarative knowledge (44). In one such study, Weiskrantz and Warrington (45) paired the presentation of a puff of air to the eye with a sound and flash of light. The puff of air is an UCS that reflexively elicits an eye-blink (UCR). Amnesic patients were able to acquire a conditioned eye-blink response to the sound and light flash despite their inability to recall any relevant details about the

training session. Conditioning in amnesic patients has not, however, been compared with that of normal control subjects. Therefore, although conscious awareness may not always be necessary for conditioning to occur, it has not been established that amnesics acquire the conditioned response at a normal rate. If differences in acquisition exist between amnesic subjects and normal controls, it would suggest that some aspects of conditioning may indeed be reliant upon declarative knowledge.

Priming

Priming is a phenomenon in which prior experience with perceptual stimuli temporarily and unconsciously facilitates the subject's ability to later detect or identify those stimuli. At present, priming is the most extensively studied aspect of nondeclarative memory. Although discussion here is limited to key features of priming, the interested reader may refer to several sources in the literature for a more exhaustive review (46–48).

In the typical priming experiment, sets of verbal or nonverbal stimuli, such as lists of words, pictures of common or novel objects, or line drawings, are presented to subjects who, at a later time, are tested using both old and new stimuli. Test procedures may involve asking subjects to identify items from fragments or to make rapid decisions concerning items. Priming is said to have occurred when task performance for previously presented stimuli is superior to that for new stimuli. For example, Salmon and his colleagues (49) showed subjects 10 words (e.g., motel, abstain) one at a time, asking them to judge the pleasantness of each word as a means to ensure attention to the stimuli. Subjects were later given 20 three-letter word stems (e.g., mot-, abs-) and asked to complete each stem with the first word that came to mind. Half of the word stems could be completed by using words presented previously, while the other half could not. Subjects in this study displayed a significantly greater tendency (relative to baseline guessing rates) to complete the word stems with words that had been presented previously, thus demonstrating what is known as a lexical priming effect.

Warrington and Weiskrantz (50) demonstrated that priming is independent of the subject's ability to consciously recall or recognize stimuli. Amnesic subjects and normal controls were presented printed lists of words and later tested by one of three techniques: free recall, recognition, or the aforementioned stem-completion task. As expected, amnesic subjects performed significantly worse than normal controls on recall and recognition measures; however, they performed as well as normal controls on the stem-completion task. That is, amnesics and controls demonstrated equivalent increases in the number of stems completed with previously presented words. Normal priming effects in the presence of impaired declarative memory have also been reported in patients with alcoholic Korsakoff syndrome (49, 51, 52) and in nondemented patients with subcortical disease processes such as Huntington's disease and Parkinson's disease (49, 52–55).

NEUROANATOMY OF MEMORY

The majority of information known about the neuroanatomy and organization of memory comes from two primary sources. The first is the study of acquired human memory dysfunction. These studies typically attempt to correlate the types of memory difficulties that accompany various brain traumas or diseases, such as head injury, cerebrovascular accidents, or degenerative disorders, with the structures damaged by those disease processes. The advantage to such a paradigm is that behavioral data can be obtained fairly easily and the affected memory processes can be evaluated in detail. Unfortunately, brain damage in human populations rarely respects known anatomical boundaries, and in many cases a patient's disorder will involve more than a single lesion. Consequently, the location and extent of cerebral involvement often varies from one patient to the next. Brain imaging techniques, such as magnetic resonance imaging (MRI), have improved our ability to correlate neuropsychological data with estimated loci of pathology. These techniques, however, do not always provide conclusive anatomical evidence, and postmortem verification studies are often lacking. This combination of patient variability and imprecise lesion localization limits the usefulness of this line of inquiry in the identification of individual structures responsible for the various aspects of memory functioning.

The disadvantages of using human studies as a basis for our understanding of the neuroanatomy of memory led many investigators to study nonhuman primates and other animal species. The advantages of animal studies include the ability to control the site of the anatomical lesion and the ability to compare pre- and postlesion behavior in the same individual. Although these studies often provide useful heuristics for our understanding of human memory, they are limited because many aspects of complex behaviors such as memory are often difficult to generalize across species. In addition, there are several aspects of human memory functioning that are difficult or impossible to assess in nonhuman species (e.g., semantic memory).

Together, the cumulative literature of studies of memory functioning in humans and nonhuman animals provides a broad outline of the major neuroanatomical structures and connections believed to be important for memory. In light of the preceding review of the constructs of memory functioning, we can divide our discussion into two sections. Most of the discussion focuses on the neuroanatomical substrates of declarative memory because this has been most extensively researched. We then review what is known about the brain structures and systems believed to underlie nondeclarative memory.

Neuroanatomical Correlates of Declarative Memory

Several regions of the brain have been implicated in declarative memory functioning. These include the temporal lobes, the medial diencephalon, and the basal forebrain. The location of these brain regions and their relationship to each other are illustrated in Figure 17.5.

TEMPORAL LOBES

As in the case of H.M., described earlier, bilateral surgical removal of the medial portion of the temporal lobe results in profound deficits in declarative memory functioning. In a series of abstracts published in 1981, Corkin and her colleagues described H.M.'s memory deficits 28 years after his original surgery (56–58). In these studies, H.M. continued to demonstrate profound anterograde amnesia; he could not recall new episodic or semantic memories, such as his age, the current year, or what he had eaten during his most recent meal. Like most amnesics, however, H.M. demonstrated evidence of some occasional new learning. He could, for example, tell the examiner what an astronaut was (a term not in use at the time of his surgery), and he was able to recall that a public person named Kennedy had been assassinated.

Although the case of H.M. and of other patients with bilateral medial temporal lobe lesions established the importance of this region in memory functioning, the investigation of patients with unilateral temporal lobe lesions and resections has provided evidence for differential, lateralized contributions of each temporal lobe to memory. Patients who have had surgical resection of the left temporal lobe have more difficulty learning and remembering verbal material, such as stories, paired verbal associations, word lists, and sequences of digits beyond their immediate memory span than do patients with right temporal lobectomy (59, 60).

In contrast, patients with right temporal lobe resection are typically more impaired on tasks that require memory for nonverbal material, such as tonal patterns, visually presented, abstract geometric patterns, and faces (60–62). Their ability to learn verbal associations between relatively abstract nouns (e.g., liberty – judgment) is also fairly intact; however, they demonstrate significant impairment when instructed to use visual imagery to form associations between concrete nouns (e.g., tree – chair; 63).

The right temporal lobe is believed to play an important role in spatial memory. Smith and Milner (64) presented patients who had undergone either right or left temporal lobectomy a display board on which 16 toys had been arranged randomly. Subjects were asked to estimate the cost of each toy (a procedure employed to ensure that subjects attended to each stimulus), after which the board was removed. Subjects were then asked to recall as many of the previously seen objects as possible, and to indicate where on the board each object was located. Recall was again assessed 24 hours later. Subjects did not differ in the amount of difficulty they experienced recalling the various objects; however, the patients with right temporal lobe resection evidenced significantly greater impairment in spatial recall than left temporal lobectomy patients.

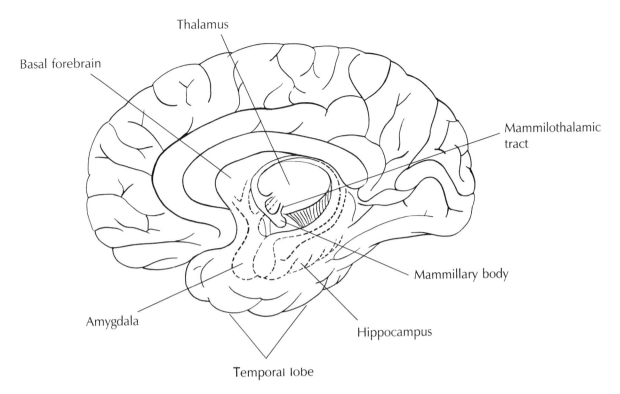

Figure 17.5. Brain regions implicated in declarative memory functioning. (Modified from Kolb B, Whitshaw I. Fundamentals of human neuropsychology. New York: WH Freeman and Co.)

Despite the severity of declarative memory deficits in patients with medial temporal lobe damage or resection, the capacity for skill learning, priming, and certain kinds of conditioning remains relatively intact. In a study by Cohen and Corkin (56), H.M. was trained to solve the Tower of Hanoi puzzle, a challenging, rule-based problem involving three pegs and a number of blocks of different sizes. The subject is presented all the blocks on one "source" peg, stacked from largest to smallest in ascending order. The subject is then instructed to move the blocks one at a time in such a way as to reconstruct the tower onto a "goal" peg. At no time is the subject allowed to place a larger block on top of a smaller block. H.M. engaged in this task four times a day over 4 consecutive days, followed by a 7-day rest interval and then 4 more days of testing. Despite his inability to recall the task or recognize the apparatus at each testing session, H.M., like normal control subjects, demonstrated systematic improvement in his ability to solve the puzzle. This and similar studies suggest that the temporal lobes may not be necessary for aspects of nondeclarative memory such as learning and retention of skills and procedures.

The temporal lobe is a fairly large brain region with several anatomically distinct areas. The majority of the temporal lobectomy studies just described involved resections that included a number of neuroanatomical structures, many of which have been implicated in various aspects of memory functioning. Most investigators agree, however, that the hippocampus with its anatomically related cortex (i.e., entorhinal cortex, perirhinal cortex, and parahippo-

campal gyrus) and the amygdala hold primary importance for declarative memory functioning.

Hippocampus and Related Structures

One major observation of temporal lobectomy patients was that memory impairment developed only when the resection extended far enough posteriorly to include the hippocampal formation and associated cortical areas (65). Studies of hippocampal functioning in animals further supported the role of these structures in memory. Kesner and Conner (66) showed that disruption of hippocampal functioning in rats via electrical stimulation immediately following training impaired memory for bar-pressing behavior 24 hours later. A number of studies by Olton and his colleagues on the effects of hippocampal lesions on maze-learning in rats yielded similar results (67–69).

The human hippocampal formation is located bilaterally in the cerebral hemispheres, forming a ridge that extends along the temporal horn of each lateral ventricle. The ventricular surface of the hippocampal formation is covered by a layer of myelinated axons, called the alveus, which arise primarily from the cells of the hippocampus. These fibers converge on the medial surface of the hippocampus to form the fimbria, which is continuous with the fornix (Fig. 17.6).

As illustrated in Figure 17.7, the hippocampal formation and its associated cortices are convoluted in structure. Proceeding from the collateral sulcus, the parahippocampal gyrus curves dorsally, transitioning into the regions of the

Figure 17.6. Illustration of a brain dissection showing the gross anatomy of the temporal lobe memory system, including the hippocampal formation and fornix. (Modified from Carpenter MB. Core text of neuroanatomy. 3rd ed. Baltimore: Williams & Wilkins, 1985:226–264.)

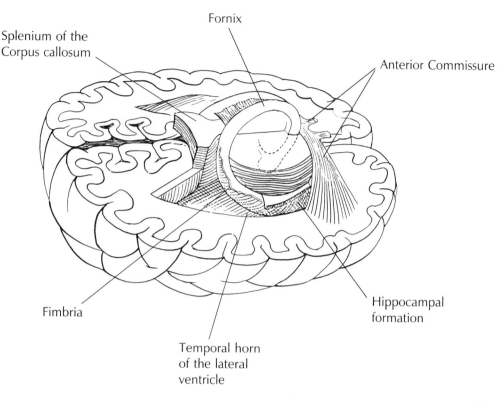

Figure 17.7. Illustration of a transverse section through the human hippocampal formation and parahippocampal gyrus. (Modified from Carpenter MB. Core text of neuroanatomy. 3rd ed. Baltimore: Williams & Wilkins, 1985:226–264.)

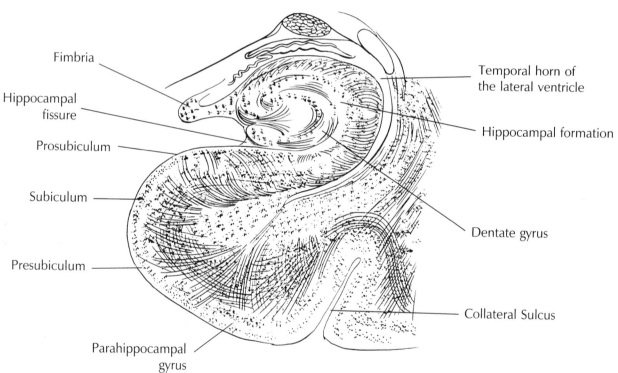

presubiculum and subiculum. At that point, the subiculum curves medially and transitions into the prosubiculum and hippocampus, which then curves inward again, forming the hippocampal fissure. When the hippocampal fissure is opened, a narrow layer of cortex can be observed between the hippocampal fissure and the fimbria; this is known as the dentate gyrus. The hippocampus proper is composed of three substructures, which can be distinguished based on their cytoarchitecture and functional connections; these are known as areas CA1, CA2, and CA3. These areas, together with the dentate gyrus, comprise the hippocampal formation.

In 1978, two proposals were advanced that challenged the theory that the hippocampal formation was critical to memory. The first suggested that the memory dysfunction exhibited by temporal lobe amnesic patients like H.M. reflected damage not to the hippocampus, but to the temporal stem white matter (70). The temporal stem lies above the lateral ventricle near the hippocampus and connects the lateral temporal neocortex to subcortical structures and diencephalic nuclei (e.g., thalamus). Given the nature of the surgical resection, the temporal stem would always be damaged by the procedure, and thus could have accounted for the observed memory deficits. To test this hypothesis, Zola-Morgan and his colleagues (71) examined the effects of hippocampal and temporal stem lesions on delayed nonmatching to sample in monkeys. This is a test of recognition memory, in which a monkey is first presented a sample object. After a delay, the monkey is presented the original object and a novel object together, and the monkey must displace the novel object in order to obtain a food reward. Results showed that monkeys with bilateral medial temporal lobe lesions comparable to those sustained by H.M. demonstrated significantly greater impairment on this task than monkeys with lesions only to the white matter tracts that form the temporal stem. Thus, it seems unlikely that damage to the temporal stem white matter is responsible for the temporal lobe amnesic syndrome in humans.

Amygdala

The second hypothesis to challenge the role of the hippocampus in memory suggested that hippocampal damage alone was not sufficient to cause severe amnesia, but that damage to the amygdala must also be present (72). The amygdala is a complex of nuclei and specialized cortical areas situated in the dorsomedial portion of the temporal lobe rostral and dorsal to the tip of the temporal horn of the lateral ventricle (Fig. 18.5). Although the earliest investigations suggested that the amygdala was primarily an olfactory structure, later studies revealed substantial inputs from other sensory systems as well. Reciprocal fibers connect the amygdala to the visual areas in the inferior temporal gyrus, the auditory areas in the superior temporal gyrus, and the somatosensory areas of the insula; autonomic connections to and from the brainstem are also present (73). In addition, the nuclei of the amygdala have axonal projections to many other parts of the brain, including the hypothalamus, thalamus, hippocampal formation, prefrontal cortex, basal forebrain, and corpus striatum.

The amygdala has long been believed to play a role in the control of emotional, autonomic, reproductive, and feeding behaviors. Electrical stimulation of the amygdala in animals typically results in a constellation of aggressive and fear-related responses. Bilateral lesions to the amygdala result in a condition known as Klüver-Bucy syndrome, a disorder characterized by excessive docility, lack of fear response,

hypersexuality, and changes in dietary habits. In addition, almost all objects within reach are examined, smelled, and placed in the mouth; if the object is inedible, it is subsequently discarded. Our understanding of the role of the amygdala in memory functioning, however, has developed only recently.

Relative Contributions of the Hippocampus and Amygdala to Memory

Examination of the role of the hippocampus alone in human amnesia was made possible in a case study of the patient R.B. (33). R.B. was a 52-year-old male who developed a striking anterograde memory impairment following an episode of global brain ischemia (i.e., obstruction of blood flow). He lived for 5 years following his ischemic attack, during which time he continued to demonstrate marked memory deficits in the absence of other significant cognitive dysfunction. Following his death, histological examination of R.B.'s brain revealed bilateral, well-circumscribed lesions restricted to area CA1 of the hippocampus. This finding suggested that damage to the hippocampus alone was sufficient to disrupt new learning and memory. R.B. did not, however, demonstrate as severe an amnesic syndrome as H.M. For example, R.B.'s performance on a standard neuropsychological test of memory was 1–2 standard deviations below his general intellectual ability, while the average difference between memory and intellectual functioning for H.M. across five evaluations from 1955–1983 was approximately 3 standard deviations.

Because R.B. was not as severely amnesic as H.M., it is logical to assume that temporal lobe structures other than area CA1 of the hippocampus are also important for memory (33). In fact, studies of amnesic patients using high-resolution MRI of the hippocampal region demonstrate that atrophic changes restricted to the region of the hippocampus proper, fimbria, dentate gyrus, and subiculum are associated with less severe levels of memory impairment than lesions caused by more radical loss of tissue in the medial temporal lobe (74,75).

These findings have been supported by studies of nonhuman primates. In the discussion of these studies that follows, we utilize the short-hand terminology employed by Squire and Zola-Morgan (65), in which a lesion to the hippocampal formation is denoted "H" and a lesion to the amygdala is denoted "A;" lesions involving cortical regions adjacent to the hippocampal formation and amygdala are denoted " + ."

Consistent with the evidence found in human amnesics, when lesions in monkeys are limited to the hippocampal formation and the adjacent cortical region of parahippocampal cortex (H +), a memory impairment results that is less severe than when lesions extend beyond this area and involve the amygdala and its adjacent cortices (H + A + ; 65, 76, 77). There are three possible explanations for this. As the lesion to the hippocampal formation and adjacent cortex extends anteriorly to include the amygdala and its adjacent cortical regions, the exacerbation of the memory impairment could be accounted for by damage sustained to the amygdala (A), its adjacent cortex (+), including the perirhinal and entorhinal cortex, or the combination of damage to both the amygdala and the adjacent cortex (A+). To date, the experimental evidence appears to favor the second of these possibilities—that the additional memory impairment noted in the H+A+ lesions results from damage sustained by the cortex adjacent to the amygdala.

This conclusion was drawn from several sources, including studies that compared memory performances among monkeys with controlled lesion combinations. Figure 17.8 illustrates the results of such comparisons on a delayed nonmatching to sample test. As expected, monkeys with the H+ lesions were impaired on this and similar memory tasks, but to a lesser degree than the monkeys with the H+A+ lesions. In contrast, monkeys with an A lesion alone performed no differently from normal, nonlesioned monkeys. Moreover, monkeys with H+A lesions had no greater impairment than monkeys with H+ lesions. When the H+ lesion was extended forward to include the entorhinal and perirhinal cortex, but not the amygdala (the H++ lesion), the memory deficit was exacerbated to a level comparable to the H+A+ lesion.

Although lesions to the amygdala do not appear to contribute to deficits in new learning and memory such as those assessed by the delayed nonmatching to sample test, studies of rats and monkeys suggest that the amygdala is important to other types of memory. One example, is the

learning of conditioned fear and other types of affective memory in which the valence of a neutral stimulus is altered by experience. Such instances appear to be strongly reliant upon the integrity of the amygdala, as described later in this chapter and by other researchers (78, 79).

MEDIAL DIENCEPHALON

Damage to the medial diencephalic region has been linked to human amnesic disorders since the turn of the century (80); however, our understanding of the specific structures involved in memory functioning and the nature of the amnesia that occurs following damage to this system has come to light only recently. The diencephalon is a region of several important nuclei located at the most rostral part of the brainstem (Figs. 17.9 and 17.10). It is bounded superiorly by the lateral ventricles, corpus callosum, and fornix, and laterally by the fibers of the posterior limb of the internal capsule, the stria terminalis, and the body and tail of the caudate nucleus. The diencephalon extends caudally to the posterior commissure, and is separated into two symmetrical parts by the third ventricle. Note, however, that it is common to see an interthalamic adhesion, called the massa intermedia, where the medial surfaces of the thalami of the diencephalon are continuous.

The diencephalon can be divided into four major parts: the epithalamus, thalamus, hypothalamus, and subthalamus (also known as ventral thalamus). The epithalamus makes up the superior surface of the diencephalon and consists of the

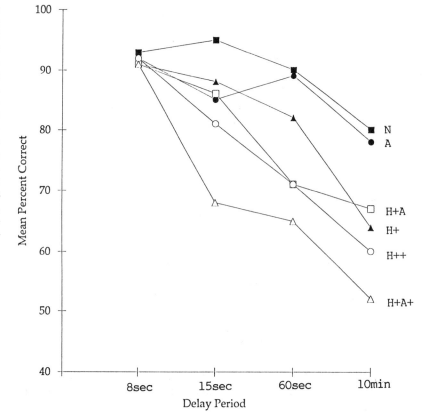

Figure 17.8. Performance on a delayed nonmatching to sample test in normal monkeys (N) and monkeys with controlled lesions in the amygdala (A), hippocampus (H), hippocampus and its associated cortical regions (H+), hippocampus, its associated cortical regions, and the amygdala (H+A), hippocampus, its associated cortical regions, and cortical regions associated with the amygdala (H++), and hippocampus, amygdala, and both associated cortical regions (H+A+). (From Squire LR, Zola-Morgan S. The medial temporal lobe memory system. Science 1991;253:1380–1386.)

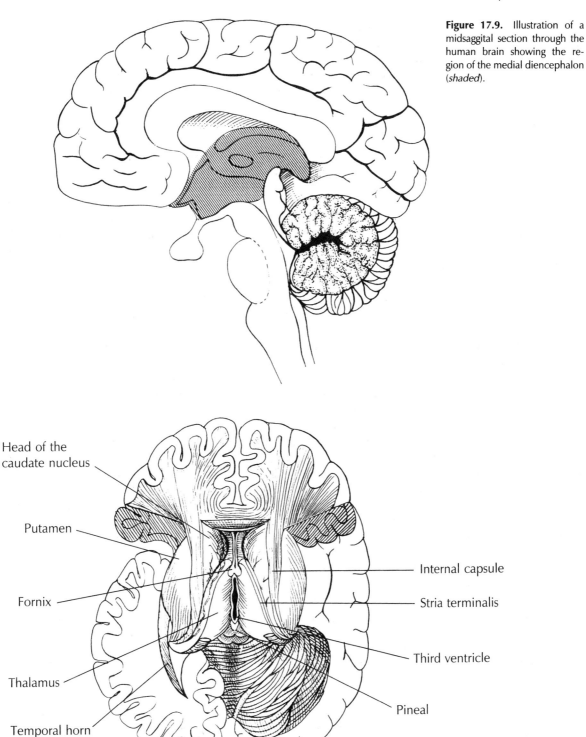

Figure 17.9. Illustration of a midsaggital section through the human brain showing the region of the medial diencephalon (*shaded*).

Head of the caudate nucleus

Putamen

Fornix

Thalamus

Temporal horn of the lateral ventricle

Internal capsule

Stria terminalis

Third ventricle

Pineal

Figure 17.10. Illustration of a brain dissection showing the gross relationship of the thalamus and related structures. (From Carpenter MB. Core text of neuroanatomy. 3rd ed. Baltimore: Williams & Wilkins, 1985:226–264.)

pineal body, stria terminalis, and stria medullaris. The thalamus is the largest subdivision of the diencephalon and is comprised of the pulvinar, lateral, and medial geniculate bodies, and numerous histopathologically distinct nuclei (81). The hypothalamus, as the name suggests, lies below the thalamus and extends from the optic chiasm caudally to the mammillary bodies. Finally, the subthalamus is a transition zone lying ventral to the thalamus between the hypothalamus and internal capsule. It consists primarily of the subthalamic nucleus and is traversed by many important fibers projecting to the thalamus.

With few exceptions, the phenomenon of diencephalic

amnesia involves damage to regions along the midline of the thalamus and hypothalamus. There has been considerable controversy, however, concerning which of the many neuroanatomical structures and connections in this region must be damaged to cause memory dysfunction. Compared to the study of the medial temporal lobe system, identification of the neuroanatomical substrates of diencephalic amnesia has been relatively slow. This is primarily because of technological limitations and a lack of patients with well-circumscribed lesions in this area. Although animal models have increased our understanding of this system, much remains to be explored.

To date, the structures that have been most often implicated in diencephalic amnesia are the dorsomedial nucleus of the thalamus, the mammillary bodies of the hypothalamus, and the mammillothalamic white matter tract (Fig. 17.5). The basis for this originated from the study of patients with alcoholic Korsakoff syndrome. The etiology of this syndrome is believed to be a severe thiamine deficiency related to the malnutrition associated with chronic alcoholism (82). The patient who enters the first stage of the disorder presents with an acute, global confusional state, occulomotor abnormalities, ataxia, and peripheral polyneuropathy; this is known as Wernicke's encephalopathy. Without immediate treatment (i.e., administration of massive doses of thiamine), the patient is in danger of suffering potentially fatal hemorrhages to the midbrain. With appropriate treatment, however, most patients experience a rapid recovery from the confusion and from the aforementioned neurological signs. Approximately 25% of patients who reach this point in the disorder regain the majority of their premorbid cognitive abilities. The remaining 75% demonstrate enduring deficits in declarative memory, including a severe anterograde and retrograde amnesia, despite maintaining relatively intact intellectual functioning (83).

The mammillary bodies and dorsomedial nucleus of the thalamus are both frequently damaged in patients with alcoholic Korsakoff syndrome. In two thorough postmortem studies of four patients with Korsakoff syndrome, marked neuronal loss was noted in the medial mammillary bodies together with evidence of damage to the dorsomedial nucleus along the wall of the third ventricle (84, 85). The findings of damage to both structures in Korsakoff syndrome has led to continued debate as to which site of damage is of greater importance to the observed amnesic symptoms. Is it possible that damage to one structure or the other is sufficient to produce memory impairment, or is damage to both structures necessary?

Cases of medial diencephalic damage of nonalcoholic origin suggest that damage to the dorsomedial nucleus of the thalamus may be the critical focus of memory impairment. Severe memory disturbances have been reported in patients with tumors of the third ventricle in the area of the dorsomedial nucleus that did not involve the mammillary bodies or the mammillothalamic tract (86). Similar findings have been reported by studies of patients with diencephalic amnesia of various other origins as well (87).

Equally strong evidence, however, has been found for mammillary involvement in memory functioning. In one study, computerized tomography (CT) scans of six amnesic patients with hemorrhagic lesions to the medial diencephalon suggested that the mammillothalamic tract and the ventral portion of the internal medullary lamina (i.e., the connections to and from the medial thalamus) were the structures critical to the patient's memory dysfunction and not the dorsomedial nucleus (88). A second neuroimaging study of two amnesic patients with bilateral thalamic infarctions found that damage was sustained primarily to the mammillothalamic tract and the inferior thalamic peduncle at the level of the anterior nucleus of the thalamus (89).

Lesion localization within the medial diencephalon, however, is quite difficult to establish based solely on neuroimaging results, especially CT scans. An example of the need for caution can be seen in the case of the patient N.A., who suffered a severe anterograde and mild retrograde amnesia following a penetrating stab wound to the base of the brain (22). Analyses of N.A.'s head CT scan initially indicated a focal lesion in the left dorsomedial nucleus of the thalamus. A reanalysis of the site of damage 10 years later using MRI, however, revealed that the damage was in fact more extensive within the left thalamus, and likely involved the mammillothalamic tract and mammillary bodies as well (90).

In monkeys, bilateral lesions restricted to the mammillary bodies result in a mild but measurable anterograde memory deficit. The severity of this impairment is substantially less than that caused by lesions to the hippocampal formation and its associated cortices (91); however, impairment increases when the anterior, dorsomedial, and midline thalamic nuclei are included in the lesion (92). When lesions are limited to either the dorsomedial or the anterior thalamic nucleus, mild to moderate memory impairment is seen, while lesions to both regions produce severe deficits (93).

In contrast, a series of studies using an animal model of alcoholic Korsakoff syndrome in rats has suggested that the internal medullary lamina is the critical structure in diencephalic amnesia. In these studies, diencephalic damage was induced in rats via an experimentally controlled thiamine deficiency (94). The rats subsequently developed lesions bilaterally in the mammillary bodies, dorsomedial nucleus of the thalamus, and internal medullary lamina of the thalamus. The thiamine-deficient rats were later compared to rats with radio frequency-induced lesions to either the mammillary bodies, midline thalamus, or the internal medullary lamina on a test of spatial memory. Results showed that the animals with damage to the internal medullary lamina performed as poorly as the rats with thiamine deficiency, while rats with lesions to the mammillary bodies or midline nuclei performed normally (95, 96).

In summary, although it is clear that the structures of the medial diencephalon are important to memory functioning, the relative contributions of these structures remain under investigation. The dorsomedial nucleus of the thalamus and the mammillary bodies of the hypothalamus are frequently identified as the critical neuroanatomical substrates of diencephalic amnesia; however, other structures and/or pathways may also be involved in memory. Indeed, some of these (e.g., the internal medullary lamina) may be of primary importance.

BASAL FOREBRAIN

Significant memory dysfunction has also been associated with damage to the basal forebrain (35, 97, 98). The basal forebrain is a somewhat loose term used to describe the area of the brain superior to the optic chiasm. It includes the medial septal nuclei, nucleus accumbens, anterior hypothalamus, diagonal band of Broca, nucleus basalis of Meynert, and part of the prefrontal cortex (i.e., Brodmann's area 13). The structures within the basal forebrain project widely throughout the brain. For example, the septal nuclei and nucleus basalis of Meynert are known to have extensive connections to and from the hippocampal formation, amygdala, and the frontal, parietal, and temporal cortices (99). The majority of evidence suggests that these two basal forebrain structures, as well as the diagonal band of Broca may be fundamental to memory functioning (80).

Basal forebrain involvement in memory functioning is implicated primarily from the study of two patient groups: patients with ruptured aneurysm of the anterior communicating artery and patients with Alzheimer's disease. The region of the basal forebrain is perfused primarily by branches of the anterior communicating artery; thus, disturbances within this flow of circulation result in infarction and necrosis of basal forebrain tissue. A number of amnesic patients have suffered damage to this region secondary to stroke or surgical repair of anterior communicating artery aneurysms (98); however, the damage to the basal forebrain following such events is typically too variable and extensive to identify specific structures that may be responsible for the amnesic syndrome in these patients.

The basal forebrain has also been implicated in the development of Alzheimer's disease, a disorder in which anterograde memory deficits are a prominent early symptom. Postmortem studies of patients with Alzheimer's disease reveal degenerative lesions within the basal forebrain, specifically involving the cholinergic neurons of the nucleus basalis of Meynert (100). These neurons produce the neurotransmitter acetylcholine, and represent the major source of cholinergic input to the neocortex. This finding initially led investigators to propose that cholinergic depletion was of etiological significance to the memory disorder seen in Alzheimer's disease. Subsequent studies, however, revealed that other neurotransmitter systems are equally depleted in Alzheimer's disease and that treatment with cholinergic agonists is ineffective in improving memory functioning in patients with dementia of the Alzheimer type (101).

These and similar findings prompted many investigators to question the specific role of the nucleus basalis of Meynert in memory functioning. In a series of studies on basal forebrain lesions and memory, Aigner and colleagues (102, 103) evaluated the performance of monkeys on a delayed nonmatching to sample task. Results revealed that combined lesions to the nucleus basalis of Meynert, medial septal nuclei, and diagonal band of Broca resulted in significant memory impairment; however, no significant impairment was noted when each structure was lesioned separately or when lesions were produced in combinations of two of the three structures. Apparently, extensive damage to the basal forebrain, rather than specific damage to any given structure, is necessary to produce memory impairment. Given these findings and the presence of strong anatomical connections between the basal forebrain and medial temporal lobe structures, some have suggested that the primary role of the basal forebrain in memory may be to modulate medial temporal lobe processing (2, 98).

PREFRONTAL CORTEX

Although often not considered a memory center, *per se,* damage to the association area of the frontal lobes, commonly called the prefrontal cortex, can nevertheless result in memory disturbance. It has long been recognized that the frontal lobes play an important role in the attentional and organizational processes necessary for the registration and retrieval of information (104); however, recent studies provide evidence that the prefrontal cortex may be of primary importance for specific memory functions.

Patients with damage to the prefrontal cortex can typically retrieve factual information with little difficulty; however, information regarding when and where the information was obtained is frequently forgotten (105). This phenomenon is known as a source memory deficit; that is, the inability to recall the origin of learned information. A recent study by Glisky and her colleagues (106) examined source memory in a sample of elderly patients who were grouped according to their scores on a composite measure of frontal lobe functioning. Subjects were asked to listen to a series of sentences expressing common everyday events (e.g., "The boy went to the store to buy some apples and oranges."). Half the sentences were recorded in a female voice, the other half in a male voice. After all sentences were presented, subjects were given recognition and source memory tests. In the recognition memory test, subjects were asked to identify which sentences they had heard previously, while in the source memory test, they were asked to determine whether the sentence they were hearing was originally presented in a male or female voice. Results showed that subjects with high frontal lobe functioning had significantly better recall for the original voice (i.e., source memory) than subjects with low frontal lobe functioning. Groups did not, however, differ in their ability to recognize which sentences had been presented previously (i.e., recognition memory). The reverse pattern was seen when these subjects were regrouped according to their scores on a composite measure of medial temporal lobe functioning. That is, subjects with high temporal lobe functioning performed better than subjects with low temporal lobe functioning on the recognition memory test, but were no different from each other on the source memory measure.

Another memory function believed to be mediated by the prefrontal cortex is temporal ordering. Corsi (cited in 107) studied this phenomenon by presenting unilateral frontal lobectomy patients series of cards, each containing pairs of either concrete words (e.g., cowboy, railroad), representational drawings, or abstract paintings. Subjects viewed each card, one at a time, for several seconds before going on to the next card. At several points throughout the deck, a response card would appear containing either two previously viewed items, or one old and one new item. Each time a response card appeared, the subject was asked to identify which of the two stimuli was presented most recently. Choosing between two previously viewed items assessed temporal ordering, while choosing between an old item and a novel item assessed recognition memory. Results showed that temporal ordering was impaired in these patients while recognition memory remained intact. Moreover, an interaction between stimulus type and lesion site was identified. Patients with left frontal lobe lesions showed temporal ordering deficits only on verbal stimuli, while patients with right frontal lobe lesions demonstrated greater deficits on the pictorial stimuli than on verbal stimuli. Verbal temporal ordering deficits are believed to be related specifically to damage or dysfunction of the middorsolateral region of the left frontal lobe; however, studies have failed to identify a corresponding critical area for impaired pictorial temporal ordering in the right frontal lobe (108).

Brain Systems as Memory Systems

The available data strongly suggest that medial temporal lobe and medial diencephalic structures are components of a single memory system essential to the formation of long-term declarative memory. According to Zola-Morgan and Squire (80), sensory information is processed by the neocortex and sent to the parahippocampal and perirhinal cortices. From there, the information is sent to the entorhinal cortex, hippocampal formation, and medial diencephalon, where associations are created between events and/or stimulus features. These associations bind together the cortical sites, where different aspects of the given information were originally processed and serve as an index of memory (65).

This indexing system is believed to be relatively temporary in nature. Although memory for newly acquired information is initially dependent upon the integrity of the hippocampal formation, the memory gradually becomes reorganized over time and becomes less and less dependent upon these structures (41, 65, 80). Patients with medial temporal lobe or diencephalic damage, for example, frequently demonstrate spared remote memories despite marked deficits in anterograde memory functioning. This suggests that the medial temporal lobes and medial diencephalon are not the storage sites for long-term memories.

Rather, as time passes after learning, a more permanent memory store develops elsewhere, presumably in the neocortex (109).

Neuroanatomical Correlates of Nondeclarative Memory

As discussed earlier, nondeclarative memory is a performance-based behavior comprised of phenomena such as skill learning, conditioning, and priming. Unlike declarative memory, nondeclarative memory is not believed to be reliant upon the medial temporal lobe/medial diencephalic system. Instead, memories underlying acquired skills or conditioned or primed responses are believed to be a function of the sensory and motor systems inherent in the involved behaviors. Consequently, no one brain system can likely account for all types of nondeclarative memory.

PROCEDURAL MEMORY AND SKILL LEARNING

Recent work suggests that the brain structures important for skill and procedure learning are those of the corticostriatal system. This system is comprised of the corpus striatum and its projections from the neocortex. The corpus striatum represents the largest component of the basal ganglia—the subcortical nuclei located deep in the cerebral hemispheres at the upper brainstem. The basal ganglia consist of two distinct parts: the neostriatum, which includes the putamen and the caudate nucleus, and the paleostriatum, which includes the globus pallidus. The putamen and caudate nucleus receive a wide range of inputs, including projections from the thalamus, amygdala, mesencephalic structures such as the raphe nuclei and substantia nigra, and broad regions of the neocortex. The primary outputs are to the globus pallidus and back to the substantia nigra. The globus pallidus receives input from the caudate nucleus, the putamen, the nucleus accumbens, and the subthalamic nucleus, and projects primarily to the thalamus, habenula, substantia nigra, and subthalamic nucleus.

The corpus striatum is important for motor planning and for performing motor programs. Patients with Parkinson's disease and Huntington's disease (disorders caused by damage or deterioration of the substantia nigra and basal ganglia, respectively) typically demonstrate impaired performance on a wide variety of skill learning tasks, including prism adaptation (110), sequence-specific procedural learning (111), cognitive skill learning (112,113), and motor skill learning (54, 114, 115). In contrast, patients with disorders of medial temporal lobe memory systems (e.g., Alzheimer's disease, amnesic patients) demonstrate normal performances on many of these same measures (54, 110, 115, 116).

Heindel, Salmon, and Butters (117) propose that learning a skill depends upon the development and modification of increasingly accurate motor programs that allow the performer to combine appropriate motor movements into both the correct serial order and the correct temporal pattern within that order. A feedback system detects errors made as the skill is learned, and generates new, more accurate motor commands as a result. As these programs are acquired and modified, the performer can begin to organize sequences of motor movements prior to performance, thus leading to more facile and coordinated movement. In patients with Huntington's and Parkinson's disease, deficits in skill learning are believed to result from the lack of integrity of the neostriatum (54, 110, 118). The ensuing interruption of complex motor and sensory circuits between the neostriatum, and the supplementary motor cortex, prefrontal cortex, and the pyramidal and extrapyramidal motor systems interferes with the ability to generate and/or modify motor programs, thus preventing the acquisition of skill based knowledge.

CONDITIONING

Within the past few years, considerable progress has been made in identifying the brain structures and systems that underlie the processes of conditioned learning and memory. This is especially true with regard to aversive conditioning (119). Stimuli that are normally neutral in emotional valence, such as lights or tones, can rapidly become conditioned to elicit fear-responses when associated with aversive unconditioned stimuli, such as electric shock.

A number of studies have shown that experimental manipulation of the amygdala and/or its connections can affect fear conditioning. Ablation of the amygdala in a variety of mammalian species results in disrupted acquisition and retention of innate and experimentally induced fear responses, such as increased blood pressure (120), startle response (121), and defensive behavioral inhibition (122). Electrophysiological recordings from the central nucleus of the amygdala reveal that neuronal activity in this region changes during fear conditioning (123). In one study, a fear response was elicited in rabbits via the pairing of an electrical shock with a neutral tone (124). Recordings from cells in the central nucleus of the amygdala in these animals revealed increased activity when the conditioned tone was presented; however, presentation of a different tone unrelated to shock elicited little to no change in recorded activity.

Although the amygdala appears to be crucial to the learning of conditioned fear, it does not appear to be the site of storage for long-term fear-related memory. Retention of fear responses is disrupted by lesions to the amygdala shortly after conditioning, but no such disruption is noted if the amygdala is lesioned several days later (125). To date, the brain areas that have been implicated as possible storage sites for fear memories include the insular cortex and the vermis of the cerebellum (119).

PRIMING

The study of the neuroanatomical bases of priming effects is a relatively recent pursuit, and hypotheses about which brain structures and systems underlie this phenomenon continue to be formulated. In divided visual field studies of word-stem completion priming in normal subjects, Mar-

solek and others (126) found that priming was greater when word stems were presented to the right hemisphere than to the left, but only when the words were presented in the same sensory modality and the same structural format (i.e., upper vs. lower case) during both initial presentation and later testing. In a similar study, Squire and his colleagues used positron emission tomography (PET) to determine the locus of cerebral activity during a word-stem completion task (41). Each item was presented visually, in uppercase letters. Results revealed a significant reduction of cerebral blood flow in the right posterior cortex in the region of the lingual gyrus during priming. This locus of reduced activity corresponds to the area of the brain that is known to respond to the physical features of words (127), suggesting that once those features have been analyzed, it requires less neuronal activity to process the same word at a subsequent time.

Because of the numerous components that make up the physical aspects of presented words, it has been suggested that perceptual priming may occur in any of more than 30 different cortical areas known to be involved in visual information processing (128). Thus, the importance of a particular brain region to a specific case of priming is most likely dependent upon the stimulus qualities and external demands inherent to the individual priming task.

In a groundbreaking study of neuroanatomical correlates to word priming and recognition memory, Jernigan and Ostergaard (129) examined MRI scans of 30 subjects, including normal subjects and patients with memory disorders of various etiologies, including Alzheimer's disease, Huntington's disease, alcoholic Korsakoff syndrome, and amnesic disorders secondary to hypoxic episodes. Volumetric measures were calculated in each of three brain regions: the caudate nuclei, the gray matter of the medial temporal lobe (including amygdala, hippocampus, parahippocampal gyrus, and uncus), and the posterior nonlimbic cortex of the temporal, parietal, and occipital lobes. Using a tachistoscope, identification thresholds for words were established for each subject. Subjects were then asked to read a list of 68 words presented one at a time on a computer screen. After a delay, identification thresholds for new words and words from the previously presented word list were measured, after which subjects were asked to state whether or not each word had been presented on the earlier list. The mean difference in identification threshold between old words (i.e., those presented on the original word list) and novel words was used to indicate the degree of priming, while the number of correct classifications of words as new or old was used to measure recognition memory. A third measure of "lexical processing efficiency" was also calculated. This was defined as the identification threshold of new words presented during the priming procedure.

As expected, a significant specific association was found between recognition memory (i.e., the declarative memory task) and medial temporal lobe volume, with decreased volume associated with poorer memory. In contrast, priming was significantly correlated to volume measurements of two of the brain regions studied: the caudate nuclei and the medial temporal lobe gray matter. These effects were in opposite directions; medial temporal lobe volume loss was associated with decreased priming, while caudate volume loss was associated with increased priming. Finally, an impressive association was found between all three brain regions and efficiency of lexical processing, with volume loss to the caudate most strongly related to inefficient lexical processing (i.e., increased identification threshold).

This study raises several questions regarding the nature of the brain systems responsible for priming. First, why would volume loss to the medial temporal lobe, a region responsible for declarative memory, interfere with a nondeclarative memory process such as priming? Also, why would damage to the caudate nuclei, as indicated by volume loss to this region, serve to facilitate priming? Based on the results of their studies, Ostergaard and Jernigan (129, 130) suggest that priming may be influenced by at least two factors: one related to memory and the other related to efficiency of information processing. They suggest that the memory component of priming is related to recognition memory, and thus is reliant upon the integrity of medial temporal lobe structures. The processing efficiency component of priming, on the other hand, is related to the integrity of the caudate. Studies of lexical processing and priming in normal subjects show that when stimuli are manipulated in such a way as to make lexical processing more difficult (e.g., by use of very low-frequency words or degraded stimuli), priming for those items increases (131). Jernigan and Ostergaard (129) showed that caudate volume loss was strongly associated with impaired lexical processing. Consequently, the increased difficulty in lexical processing caused by caudate dysfunction (i.e., decreased caudate volume) may serve to increase priming effects in much the same way as presentation of degraded stimuli.

CLINICAL ASSESSMENT OF MEMORY

The last two decades have witnessed a proliferation of memory tests, particularly in the experimental literature. Because of space limitations, however, only a sampling of commonly used clinical memory tests and recently developed instruments are described here. For a more detailed discussion, the interested reader is referred to several excellent reviews by Butters and Cermak (19), Lezak (17), Loring and Papanicolaou (132), and Spreen and Strauss (133).

Memory Scales

Spreen and Strauss (133) note that the clinical assessment of memory should cover a number of different abilities, including immediate retention of information, rate and pattern of learning, efficiency of retrieval of recent and remote information, and susceptibility to proactive and retroactive interference. Moreover, each of these components should be evaluated for both verbal and nonverbal information. Several batteries of tests have been developed over the years in an attempt to provide a thorough assessment of memory; the success of this endeavor, however, has been somewhat limited.

WECHSLER MEMORY SCALE-REVISED

Perhaps more than any other clinical test of memory, the revised version of the Wechsler Memory Scale (WMS-R) (134) reflects the strength of the impact that neuropsychological research can have on clinical practice. The original WMS (135) consisted of seven subtests assessing different aspects of memory, including span of attention, immediate recall of stories, learning and recall of verbal paired associates, and immediate memory for novel geometric figures. The scores for these subtests were summed and added to an age-correction factor to obtain a summary score known as a Memory Quotient (MQ). Over the years, the WMS was criticized extensively for a number of weaknesses involving its validity, standardization, and psychometric properties (132, 136, 137). These weaknesses included inadequate normative data, reliance on immediate recall to the exclusion of evaluation of retention over time, vague scoring criteria, and unequal treatment of verbal and nonverbal memory. In addition, the entire concept of the MQ was assailed for confounding several cognitive and memory constructs.

The WMS-R represents a significant improvement over the original WMS. It contains 13 subtests, including updated versions of the original seven subtests, plus six additional measures. Delayed recall procedures are included, as are more tests of visuospatial memory. The scoring rules have been improved considerably, more extensive normative studies have been conducted, and the singular MQ index has been eliminated.

Based empirically on factor analytic results from a sample of 316 normal subjects and 346 clinical patients, five composite standardized scores have been derived for the WMS-R. These include: General Memory, Attention/Concentration, Verbal Memory, Visual Memory, and Delayed Recall. In addition, percentile scores have been computed for several of the more widely used subtests (e.g., Digit Span, Logical Memory, Visual Reproduction; these subtests are discussed in later sections), and normative studies are available for patients up to 94 years of age (138). Recent investigations indicate that the WMS-R has considerable utility in characterizing the memory disorders of patients with Alzheimer's disease, Huntington's disease, multiple sclerosis, alcoholic Korsakoff syndrome, long-term alcoholism, closed head injury, exposure to neurotoxins, schizophrenia and depression (129, 139, 140–143).

Despite its improvement over the original WMS, the WMS-R met with almost immediate criticism upon publication (144). Some of the criticisms represent limitations of any relatively brief battery that attempts to measure a broad spectrum of memory functions, but others reflect more serious limitations. For example, although delayed recall procedures are included in the revised WMS, there are no cued recall or recognition procedures to help dissociate problems of encoding, retrieval, and retention. In addition, subtests designed to measure visual memory are subject to varying degrees of verbal encoding and are confounded by perceptual and visuomotor factors. Finally, although the WMS-R normative sample included representative proportions of the population with regard to numerous demographic variables (e.g., sex, education), normative data are not stratified by these variables.

RANDT MEMORY TEST

The Randt Memory Test (145) is comprised of seven subtests, including tests of general information, immediate span of auditory-verbal attention, verbal learning and recall, picture recognition, and an incidental learning test of the names of the previous tasks. On some of the subtests, a Brown-Peterson distraction task is used in which the examinee must count backwards by threes between presentation and recall. Twenty-four-hour delayed recall is also solicited. As the authors state, the test attempts to provide a "global survey" of patients' memory complaints; it is *not* intended to help localize brain lesions or functions, nor is it intended to tap every type of normal human memory.

An advantage of the test is that five alternative forms are available, thus allowing for multiple testing over short intervals of time. There are, however, several disadvantages. First, test instructions are at times complex and difficult to understand, especially if the examinee suffers from a moderate memory disturbance. In addition, the manual instructs the examiner to change the nature of the distraction task (i.e., count backwards by twos or ones) if the patient is too impaired to count backwards by threes. Such unsystematic variation in administration may lessen the test's psychometric rigor. Another problem is that examinees are told before tasks of new learning that they will have to remember the material "again tomorrow." This instruction may be a confound because highly motivated examinees have the opportunity to write down and study target items after leaving the examination. Finally, visuospatial memory is not adequately assessed by this battery. This is because the stimuli presented for picture recognition are common objects (e.g., telephone) and can be encoded verbally with little or no difficulty.

LURIA-NEBRASKA NEUROPSYCHOLOGICAL BATTERY MEMORY SCALE

The Luria-Nebraska Neuropsychological Battery (LLNB) (146) contains 14 scales, one of which is a memory scale. This scale has drawn extensive criticism, primarily because of low content validity, heterogeneity of items (e.g., confounding memory and nonmemory questions and verbal and visuospatial items), and failure to assess delayed recall (147–149). Although the LLNB itself has been found to be useful in identifying cerebral dysfunction, the psychometric weaknesses of the Memory Scale makes it impossible to use this measure to determine the integrity of specific memory functioning.

Rather than rely on standardized memory scales, a large number of neuropsychologists prefer to create their own battery of memory tests and procedures from various sources, including the scientific literature. Lezak (17) recommends choosing tests that provide a general review of memory systems, and following up on any detected memory deficits with more detailed assessment measures. Some common individual memory tests are reviewed in the following sections.

Verbal Tests

IMMEDIATE RECALL SPAN

The repetition of information immediately after its initial presentation requires attentional abilities and what many researchers call short-term memory capacity (see discussion earlier in this chapter). Patients with classic amnesic syndromes often perform within, or close to, the normal range on such tests, while individuals with impaired attentional skills, such as patients with severe depression, often perform poorly (150, 151).

Digit Span

The most commonly used attention span tests are those found on Wechsler's scales (134, 152). The examiner presents increasingly long sequences of digits, and the examinee is asked to repeat each sequence in the same order presented. Once a maximum digit span is achieved in the forward direction, a second series of increasingly long digits is presented, and the examinee is asked to repeat them backwards.

One major criticism of using this particular method to determine immediate recall span is that digits forward and backward have traditionally been collapsed into one score. It is widely recognized, however, that each taps different cognitive processes (i.e., digits backwards places more demand on mental control and symbol transformation than digits forward). Thus, a single score can obscure findings in which only one or the other process is impaired. Amnesic patients, for example, will typically show a normal forward digit span and an impaired backward span. Strictly speaking, only the number of digits an examinee is able to repeat in the forward direction should be used as an indication of immediate recall span. Clinical analysis of this has been facilitated in the WMS-R (134) by the provision of separate percentile scores for both digits forward and backwards.

Some researchers have argued that repeating digits exactly as presented in the forward direction may not be the best measure of an examinee's immediate verbal recall span either. Most tests of verbal memory do not require that the target items be recalled in the exact order in which they were presented. Consequently, the length of a digit sequence accurately repeated, regardless of the order of the digits, may be the better measure of immediate recall span. A method of evaluating this has been incorporated into a new scoring system for Wechsler's Digit Span subtest developed by Kaplan and her colleagues (153).

Word and Sentence Span

Tests have been developed that require the examinee to repeat increasingly long sequences of words or sentences (154-156). As Lezak (17) points out, however, a number of variables can confound interpretation of such tests, including the number of syllables per word and the frequency, abstractness, imageability and meaningfulness of words, phrases, or sentences used.

MEMORY FOR WORD LISTS

Verbal Paired Associates

This subtest of the WMS-R (129) assesses differential learning of high-frequency and low-frequency associations. A large number of different paired-associate learning tasks can be found in the experimental literature; however, most follow procedures similar to that of the WMS-R. The examinee is first read eight word pairs, one at a time. Four of the word pairs are difficult associates (e.g., "House-Majesty") and four are relatively easy (e.g., "Boy-Girl"). The examiner then states the first word of each pair and asks the examinee to provide its associate. Errors are corrected and the procedure is repeated for up to six learning trials in order to provide ample opportunity for the examinee to learn the associations. Examiners then have the option of assessing recall for the word pairs after an intervening delay period.

In her revision of this subtest, Kaplan includes an additional recall trial after the first three learning trials are completed. In this procedure, the examiner reads the *second* word of each pair and the examinee must report the first word. Patients who encode word pairs on a more superficial, phonetic level, rather than a "deeper" semantic level, will often perform worse on this trial compared to the third trial because the phonemic sequence of the word pairs is altered.

Selective Reminding

In this procedure, a word list is presented once, after which subjects are asked to recall as many words as possible. On the next trial, only those words the examinee failed to recall on the preceding trial are presented, after which recall for the entire list is again elicited. This procedure is repeated for several trials until the examinee recalls all the target words or until a predetermined number of trials has been administered. A number of different versions of this procedure have been developed (145, 157–160).

The selective reminding procedure represents one of the first attempts to bridge the gap between clinical assessment and cognitive science. Several memory constructs are operationally defined and quantified by the procedure, including "short-term retrieval" (STR; i.e., the number of words recalled that were presented on a given trial), "long-term retrieval" (LTR; i.e., the number of words recalled that were *not* presented on the immediately preced-

ing trial), "long-term storage" (LTS; i.e., the total number of words that were recalled on two consecutive trials at least once), and "consistent long-term retrieval" (CLTR; i.e., the subset of long-term retrieval items that are recalled on all successive trials following their initial recall). The validity of some of these constructs has, however, been challenged. For example, Loring and Papanicolaou (132) argue that the distinction made between long-term storage and retrieval appears arbitrary. They note that:

> According to Buschke's definition, a word has entered [long-term storage] if it has been successfully recalled on two consecutive trials. Therefore, by definition, and definition only, failure to recall is due to retrieval failure. Just as plausible and conceptually appealing, however, is that these 'memory traces' have been stored in a weak or degraded form [i.e., an ecoding/storage deficit].... Therefore, operationally defined retrieval may have in fact little to do with retrieval itself (p. 349).

As discussed earlier in this chapter, inferences about the relative integrity of encoding and retrieval processes can often be made by contrasting free-recall and recognition performance. Therefore, the addition of a recognition procedure to the selective reminding task may help clarify such questions for individual patients (159).

It has also been suggested that the selective reminding procedure's definition of LTS may be invalid for certain patient populations. Ober and her colleagues (160) found that patients with moderate to severe dementia of the Alzheimer's type actually showed better LTS than mild Alzheimer patients on a selective reminding test. Review of the test data revealed that the moderate-to-severe patients tended to perseverate one or two words across the majority of trials, thus artificially inflating their LTS score. Consequently, labeling these perseverations as responses from LTS would be an incorrect characterization of a pathological performance.

Auditory Verbal Learning Test

On this test, a list of 15 unrelated words is presented over five trials, with immediate recall assessed following each presentation (17). Next, a second list of unrelated words is presented for one trial (i.e., an interference task), followed by recall and then recognition testing of the original 15 words. Many examiners also test for recall of the first list again after a delay interval. Normative data are available for many of the indices that can be derived from the Auditory Verbal Learning Test (AVLT) (17, 133), including subjects in the oldest age groups (161). In addition, the examiner can make qualitative interpretations about various learning parameters, such as primacy-recency effects and vulnerability to interference.

California Verbal Learning Test

The general format of the California Verbal Learning Test (CVLT) (162) was modeled after the AVLT. One major difference between the two tests is that the 16-item word lists of the CVLT contain four words from each of four different semantic categories (e.g., fruits, tools). Words from the same category are never presented consecutively, which affords an assessment of the degree to which an examinee uses an active semantic clustering strategy in recalling the words. Another difference between the tests is that the CVLT scoring system quantifies and provides normative data for numerous learning and memory variables in addition to total levels of recall and recognition. Normative data from 273 normal subjects and 145 carefully diagnosed neurological patients are provided for 26 memory variables up to age 79. An alternate form is available, and a children's version of the CVLT has also been developed.

Hopkins Verbal Learning Test

The Hopkins Verbal Learning Test (HVLT) (163) is similar in structure to the CVLT; however, the HVLT is shorter, takes only 10 minutes to administer, and has six equivalent forms. The 12-item word lists contain four words each from three semantic categories. The list is presented over three learning trials (compared with five learning trials of the AVLT and CVLT), after which recognition memory is tested. Normative data are provided based on 129 healthy subjects from ages 19–77. Only seven subjects, however, comprise the oldest age group of subjects over age 70. The HVLT has been shown to be useful in differentiating patients with Alzheimer's disease from normal elderly subjects (163) and with further research may prove to be a suitable alternative to the CVLT or AVLT when patients are too impaired for these tests or when frequent, repeated testing is necessary. The HVLT does not, however, provide many of the more comprehensive measures of verbal learning and memory obtained by the CVLT.

MEMORY FOR STORIES

The most commonly used story memory test is the Logical Memory subtest of the WMS-R (134). In its standardized format, a brief paragraph is read to the examinee, who then recalls immediately as much of the story as possible. This procedure is repeated with a second, different story. Recall is assessed again following a 30-minute delay period. Other clinical tests of story memory have been developed by Babcock (164), Lezak (17), Randt and Brown (145), and Heaton and his colleagues (165). Most of these, like Logical Memory, test memory following a single presentation of the story. Heaton et al. (165), however, present one story repeatedly until a learning criterion is reached or up to a maximum of five learning trials. This affords an assessment of learning as well as free recall, which is measured following a 4-hour delay. Normative data for close to 200 normal subjects are available for this test (165).

It is not uncommon for a patient to perform considerably better in recalling stories than word lists. These examinees often have difficulty adopting an active learning strategy

such as semantic clustering in recalling word lists, but they are able to benefit from the thematic organization inherent in stories.

Visuospatial Tests

Visuospatial memory is often more difficult to assess than verbal memory. Finding procedures that do not confound deficits in visuospatial analysis and construction with memory, as well as stimuli that are difficult to encode verbally has proven challenging. Often, confounds can be sorted out at least in part by assessing visuoperceptual abilities, asking patients to copy stimuli, and by employing recognition techniques. The confound of verbal encoding, however, is typically more difficult to control.

IMMEDIATE RECALL SPAN

Corsi Blocks

On this test, nine, 1-inch cubes are fastened in a random but standardized pattern on a board (17). The examiner touches increasingly long sequences of blocks and the examinee is asked to re-create each sequence in the same order. In the backwards condition, the examinee touches each sequence in the reverse order from the examiner. The Corsi Block Test assesses an examinee's attentional skills and span capacity for visuospatial stimuli. It represents a spatial analog of the Digit Span subtest (discussed earlier), and the same cautions apply. A similar, 10-block test is included as a supplemental neuropsychological subtest of the Wechsler Adult Intelligence Scale - Revised neuropsychological instrument (WAIS-R NI) (153), while a two-dimensional, pictorial version of this task is included in the WMS-R (134).

MEMORY FOR VISUALLY PRESENTED STIMULI

Benton Visual Retention Test

The Benton Visual Retention Test (BVRT) (166) is a test of memory for geometric designs. The examinee is presented 10 stimulus cards, one at a time. The first two stimuli consist of one geometric shape each, and the remaining eight contain three figures each: two large "main" figures and one small "peripheral" figure (Fig. 17.11). The examiner can choose between three alternate forms and four different administration conditions (e.g., immediate versus delayed recall). The BVRT is one of the first clinical instruments to use a scoring system that quantifies and provides normative data for multiple variables, including accuracy and error types.

The BVRT has been used extensively in neuropsychological investigations (166–168) and has been found to be sensitive to hemispatial processing deficits in unilateral brain-damaged patients (169). Most designs on the BVRT, however, can be verbalized easily (e.g., "large bisected triangle"), and it is often difficult to ascertain the degree to which an examinee uses a spatial and/or verbal learning

Figure 17.11. An example of a stimulus similar to that used in the Benton Visual Retention Test. (From Benton AL. The Revised Visual Retention Test. 4th ed. New York: The Psychological Corporation, 1974.)

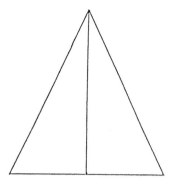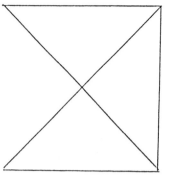

strategy on this test. In addition, the constructional (i.e., drawing) component on this and similar visual memory tests can present another confounding factor.

As mentioned earlier, impaired performance on a visuospatial memory test such as this may be caused by perceptual, constructional or memory difficulties. Asking the examinee to copy the same designs he or she previously drew from memory will often clarify the nature of the impairment. If the patient's copied drawings are deficient, then a matching task in which the examinee selects the target design displayed with several similar designs will help determine whether the patient has a perceptual or constructional problem. Benton and his colleagues have developed tests of copying, visual discrimination, and visual recognition memory for greater diagnostic specificity (133, 166).

Visual Reproduction

On this subtest of the WMS-R (134), the examinee studies each of four stimulus cards for 10 seconds, and attempts to recall each one immediately after its presentation. Memory for these figures is assessed again following a 30-minute delay. The first three stimulus cards display one design each, and the last one displays two designs side by side. Like the BVRT, the figures are relatively simple, can be easily verbalized, and can be confounded by perceptual and/or constructional deficits.

Prior to its revision in 1987, the Visual Reproduction subtest consisted of only three stimulus cards (two single-figure cards and one with two figures) and assessed immediate recall only. Heaton and his associates (165) employ these original stimuli in a Figure Memory Test that assesses both learning and recall. The designs are displayed one at a time for 10 seconds each; however, the examinee is not allowed to draw them until after all three cards (i.e., four designs) have been presented. This procedure is repeated for up to five trials or until the examinee reaches a criterion score; recall for the drawings is assessed following a 4-hour delay. Normative data for over 150 normal subjects are available for this test (165).

Recognition Memory Test for Faces

This test assesses recognition memory for 50 photographs of unfamiliar faces (170). Examinees are presented each

photograph one at a time and rate each one as "pleasant" or "unpleasant" (in order to ensure attention to each stimulus). After all 50 stimuli have been viewed, pairs of photographs are presented side by side. One photograph is new; the other was presented among the original 50. Subjects are asked to identify which of the two faces they have seen before. Normative data for this and a verbal analog (recognition of 50 printed words following the same procedure just described) are provided for over 300 subjects. This test affords a rigorous assessment of modality-specific recognition memory and has been found to be sensitive to unilateral brain damage (170).

Rey-Osterrieth Complex Figure Test

In this test, the examinee is shown a complex figure (Fig. 17.12), and asked to copy it. When the copy is completed, both the stimulus and the copy are removed, and the examinee is asked to draw the figure a second time from memory. Recall following a delay interval is also commonly assessed (see 133). Taylor (171) developed a second complex figure that serves as an alternative form of the original test.

One advantage of this test is that the examiner can assess the relationship between the examinee's organizational strategy and subsequent recall performance. To analyze constructional strategy, Kaplan recommends that the examiner record exactly what a patient draws, numbering the lines to indicate the order in which they are generated and placing arrows on the lines to indicate directionality of construction (172). Another frequently used method of determining organizational strategy is to give the examinee different colored pencils at specified time intervals (e.g., every 15 seconds) during their copy of the design or when each section of the drawing is completed (17).

A second advantage of the Rey-Osterrieth Test is that the drawing contains both larger, configural features (e.g., the large rectangle) and smaller internal details (e.g., the dots and circle). This configural/detail stimulus parameter can help dissociate the differential processing strategies of patients with unilateral brain damage. As detailed later in this chapter, patients with left-hemisphere dysfunction often have difficulty remembering the internal details, whereas patients with right-hemisphere dysfunction are often impaired in their recall of the general configuration (17, 173, 174).

Different scoring systems for the Rey-Osterrieth Test are available (174–176). The system developed by Taylor (176) yields a single achievement score that reflects final accuracy only, while the scoring systems developed by Binder (174) and Shorr et al. (175) quantify an examinee's constructional strategy in addition to providing an achievement index of the final product.

California Global-Local Learning Test

Unilateral brain pathology tends to disrupt analysis of wholes and parts selectively (177), and the California Global-Local Learning Test (CGLT; see 178) was developed specifically to quantify this phenomenon more rigorously. The test involves the presentation of visual hierarchical stimuli consisting of a larger letter or shape constructed from numerous smaller letters or shapes (Fig. 17.13). These stimuli provide precise demarcation between features perceived as larger wholes (i.e., the "global" letter or shape) and smaller details (i.e., the "local" letter or shape). To control for the ease of verbalizing the stimuli, three types of stimuli are used: linguistic forms (i.e., letters), high-frequency nonlinguistic forms (i.e., shapes with established names, such as a square or trapezoid), and low-frequency nonlinguistic forms (i.e., shapes without established names). Stimuli are presented in pairs, with one stimulus in each hemispace. Each of three paired stimuli are presented for 5 seconds, followed by recall drawing of each pair immediately after its presentation. The pairs are presented for three trials to assess learning; free recall, recognition, and copy are assessed following a 20-minute delay.

The CGLT provides indices and normative data for learning rate and retention of forms that are global or local, linguistic or nonlinguistic, and presented in the left or right hemispace. Studies have found that left-hemisphere-damaged patients are selectively impaired in learning local forms, especially when they are presented in the right hemispace, whereas right-hemisphere-damaged patients are selectively impaired in learning global forms, especially when they are presented in the left hemispace (178, 179).

Tactile Memory Tests

TACTUAL PERFORMANCE TEST

Although primarily a measure of psychomotor problem solving, the Tactual Performance Test (TPT) (180) is also used to measure memory for tactually presented information. The examinee sits blindfolded in front of a formboard and is asked to place cut-out shapes of high-frequency geometric figures (e.g., square, star) into their appropriate spaces as quickly as possible. This procedure is performed first with the preferred hand, then with the nonpreferred hand, and finally with both hands. Once the test is completed, the equipment is removed, the blindfold is taken off, and the examinee is asked to draw the shapes and their respective locations. Normative data for close to 500 normal subjects have been gathered for this test (165). This test is also useful in evaluating nonverbal memory in blind persons.

Retrograde Memory Tests

The assessment of memory for events that occurred prior to the onset of brain dysfunction can often be done

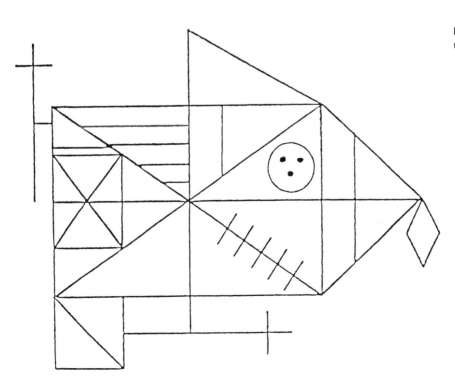

Figure 17.12. The Rey-Osterrieth complex figure.

Figure 17.13. An example of a pair of hierarchical visual stimuli from the California Global-Local Learning Test. (From Delis DC, Kiefner M, Fridlund AJ. Visuospatial dysfunction following unilateral brain damage: dissociations in hierarchical and hemispatial analysis. J Clin Exp Neuropsychol 1988;10:421–431.)

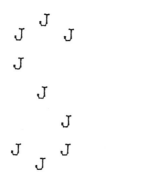
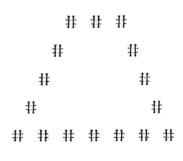

informally by eliciting autobiographical recall. When using this technique, however, it is important to obtain verification of memories from relatives or ask the same questions a second time after a delay interval, because patients with retrograde amnesia are occasionally prone to confabulation (i.e., fabricating answers) (181). If the responses are valid, a time-line can be constructed reflecting the presence, nature, and extent of a patient's retrograde amnesia (182).

BOSTON RETROGRADE AMNESIA BATTERY

A second method of testing retrograde amnesia is to ask patients about past general information, such as past public figures and events. The Boston Retrograde Amnesia Battery (BRAB) (183) is one such test battery, assessing familiarity with events, politicians, celebrities, and other individuals who were in the public spotlight from the 1930s to the 1970s. There are three components to the battery: a famous faces test, a verbal recall questionnaire, and a multiple-choice recognition questionnaire, all of which have been updated to include stimuli from the 1980s and 1990s (N. Butters, personal communication). Memory for information from each decade is graphed, revealing whether an existing retrograde amnesia is equally severe across all decades (i.e., flat retrograde amnesia) or less severe for more remote decades (i.e., temporally graded). A creative feature of the famous faces portion of this test is that some of the pictures presented were taken during different decades of an individual's popularity (e.g., Jimmy Stewart during the 1930s and 1970s); patients whose retrograde amnesia adheres to a temporal gradient will often recognize the earlier but not the later picture.

TELEVISION TEST

A methodological problem inherent in testing retrograde memory is possible differences in item difficulty across decades. Amnesics, for example, may show better memory for celebrities from the remote past than from the recent past because celebrities from the remote past have had a longer period of exposure and fame, thereby making them easier to recall. To circumvent this problem, Squire and Slater (184) developed a test to maximize the potential for equivalent public exposure across years. They used as test items television programs that were broadcast for only one season, and they employed both recall and recognition techniques.

This test has been useful in documenting the nature of retrograde amnesia in depressed patients who have undergone electroconvulsive (ECT) treatment (185) and in amnesic patients (186), and has been validated by repeated administrations of updated versions to subjects over a 7-year period (187).

INFORMATION

Many clinicians use this subtest of the WAIS-R (152) as a rough indication of retrograde amnesia. The test consists of 29 questions that require the examinee to recall famous people and information of the sort normally learned in school (e.g., scientific facts, geography). For middle-aged and older individuals, this subtest can serve as a gross measure of memory for remote semantic information. The items of this subtest, however, are neither selected systematically from different decades nor equated for ease of recall. Consequently, important qualitative features of a patient's retrograde memory cannot be evaluated. Moreover, because most of the items tap knowledge acquired during school years, older patients with retrograde amnesia extending only a few years or decades prior to their disease onset often perform well on this test.

MEMORY PROFILES OF SELECTED CLINICAL POPULATIONS

A brief overview of the memory profiles of selected patient populations reveals how different components of learning and memory can be selectively disrupted or spared.

Unilateral Brain Damage

For years it was believed that patients with left-hemisphere damage (LHD) demonstrated impaired memory only for verbal material, whereas right-hemisphere damage (RHD) disrupted only memory for visuospatial material (188, 189). Subsequent findings, however, have indicated that patients with RHD suffer subtle deficits in verbal memory functioning, while patients with LHD are impaired in remembering certain types of visual stimuli.

On tests of story memory, for example, patients with RHD may remember an equivalent number of idea units as normal controls; however, they are more prone to lose the gist of the story (190). They tend to recall the exact wording of idea units rather than using the more efficient strategy of paraphrasing the words of stories that do not fit into their everyday vocabulary. These patients also tend to introject personal information into their recall, which can further obscure the original gist of the story (190). On tests of word-list learning and recall such as the CVLT, patients with RHD do not adopt an active semantic clustering strategy; consequently, the number of words they recall is lower than that of normal controls (191).

As a group, however, patients with LHD show significantly greater impairment than patients with RHD and normal controls on tests of story recall and memory for word lists (188–190). This is sometimes confounded by the presence of an aphasic disorder, and the examiner may conclude that language impairment, if present, precludes a valid assessment of verbal memory function. Recognition testing, however, can often be used to circumvent difficulties with expressive language and dissociate some aspects of memory from language dysfunction in patients with aphasia.

With regard to visuospatial memory following unilateral brain damage, Kaplan (177) observed that patients with LHD displayed more impairment in memory for internal details relative to the outer configural features of complex stimuli such as the Rey-Osterrieth figure. In contrast, patients with RHD showed the opposite pattern (Fig. 17.14). As discussed earlier, Delis et al. (178) found that patients with LHD were selectively deficient in remembering local forms of visual hierarchical stimuli, especially when they were presented in right hemispace. In contrast, patients with RHD were selectively impaired in remembering global forms, especially when the stimuli were presented in left hemispace. These findings occurred regardless of whether or not the patients displayed visual field cuts, hemi-inattention, or aphasic deficits (Fig. 17.15). (178, 179, 192).

Alcoholic Korsakoff Syndrome

Alcoholic Korsakoff syndrome results from damage to medial diencephalic structures, including the dorsomedial nucleus of the thalamus, the mammillary bodies (see discussion earlier in this chapter). For these patients, intelligence and immediate recall span ranges from the average to low average range, but the ability to encode new information into more permanent storage is very severely impaired (19). This severe anterograde amnesia is restricted to declarative knowledge; nondeclarative memory, including procedural learning and semantic priming, are preserved (52, 186). The declarative amnesia encompasses all stimulus categories (e.g., verbal and visuospatial material) and stimulus features (e.g., global and local forms). On delayed recall tasks, these patients frequently have no recollection of the target items, or of having been presented any information at all. At times, however, they will confabulate memories and present them in a matter-of-fact fashion.

Confabulation and the tendency to make intrusion errors on memory testing may reflect the combination of

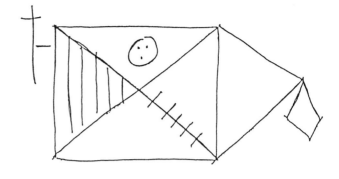

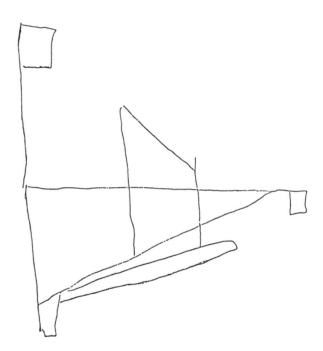

Figure 17.14. Examples of 30-minute delayed recall of the Rey-Osterrieth complex figure by a patient with left-hemisphere damage (LHD; *top*) and a patient with right-hemisphere damage (RHD; *bottom*). Note that the patient with LHD demonstrates better recall of the outer configuration but recalls few details. The patient with RHD has greater difficulty than the LHD patient in recalling the outer configuration.

severely impaired declarative memory in conjunction with intact linguistic skills (19, 193). For example, when asked, "Tell me all the shopping items I read to you earlier," patients with Korsakoff's syndrome often respond as if they are free-associating to the cue "shopping items." In cases such as this, the patient appears to rely heavily upon his or her cognitive strength in language functioning. Confabulation can also be seen in visuospatial memory in these patients. When asked to recall the Rey-Osterrieth figure, for example, a Korsakoff patient may instead draw a house. This and similar case studies suggest that severely impaired memory in the presence of the preserved ability to draw

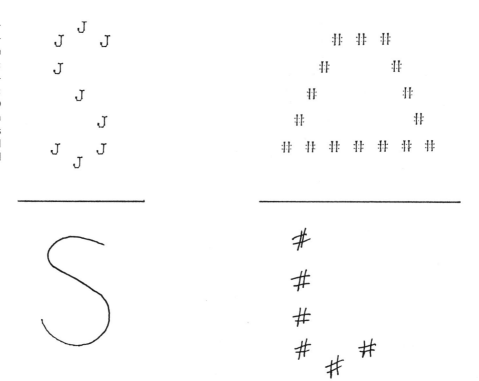

Figure 17.15. Examples of immediate free recall of global-local stimuli by a patient with left-hemisphere damage (LDH; *left*) and a patient with right-hemisphere damage (RHD; *right*). The patient with LHD recalls only the global form. In contrast, the RHD patient recalls the local form but not the global configuration of the presented stimulus.

common objects may contribute to these patients' tendency to confabulate memories on delayed recall testing of visuospatial material.

On yes/no recognition testing, Korsakoff patients typically adopt a liberal response bias, saying that they recognize all stimuli, including both target items and distractors (139). Consequently, their overall recognition discriminability is often as severely impaired as their free-recall performance.

When recall of past autobiographical events and public information is assessed, Korsakoff patients typically demonstrate a severe retrograde amnesia characterized by a temporal gradient. Generally, memory for events from the 20–30 year period immediately preceding onset of the disorder is much worse than memory for remote events from childhood and early adulthood (83). Some researchers have suggested that the temporal gradient of retrograde amnesia in Korsakoff patients is an artifact of a primary progressive deficit in anterograde memory over the period of their alcohol abuse (183, 194). That is, chronic alcoholics with Korsakoff syndrome may recall less information from more recent times because they were able to acquire fewer and fewer new memories over that period of time.

Perhaps the most convincing evidence against this hypothesis comes from the case study of P.Z., discussed earlier in this chapter (40). P.Z. developed Korsakoff syndrome at age 65, 3 years after completing an extensive autobiography. Like most alcoholic Korsakoff patients, P.Z. demonstrated a temporally graded retrograde amnesia, with no memory for personal episodes or facts from the immediately preceding 20-year period (refer to Fig. 17.4). By all accounts and documentation, however, he possessed complete autobiographical knowledge just 3 years prior to his development of the disorder. Thus, in the case of P.Z., the

temporally graded amnesia cannot be attributed to not having acquired past information in the first place.

An alternative explanation for the temporal gradient in Korsakoff syndrome is proposed by Cermak (12), who suggests that there may be a dichotomy of remote memories. Autobiographical knowledge and relatively recently acquired information may be more episodic in nature; that is, they are more reliant upon temporal and spatial contexts. With time, however, these memories may become less dependent upon temporal and spatial contexts and become part of semantic memory. The temporally graded retrograde amnesia seen in Korsakoff syndrome may therefore represent a specific vulnerability of episodic memory to the damage incurred in the disorder (i.e., medial diencephalic damage).

CHRONIC ALCOHOLISM

Detoxified chronic alcoholics often display mild to moderate deficits on more challenging tests of new learning and memory (143, 195–197). Memory for visuospatial stimuli is often worse than for verbal material (196), which parallels the findings that these patients tend to show greater dysfunction in visuospatial skills relative to verbal abilities (198–200). Some researchers have interpreted these findings in accordance with the traditional verbal/visuospatial theory of hemispheric specialization, concluding that the right hemisphere is more vulnerable than the left to the toxic effects of alcohol (196, 201). However, neuropathological changes have not been found to be greater in the right hemisphere compared with the left (202–204), and studies indicate that chronic alcoholics do not show the same type of visuospatial memory dysfunction as found in patients with RHD (205).

In testing chronic alcoholics, a period of 3–6 weeks of sobriety prior to conducting the evaluation is typically recommended. This is because acute intoxication and/or the detoxification process will often exacerbate the patient's cognitive dysfunction (206). Relatively young alcoholics (in their 30s) may show little neuropsychological impairment due to alcohol (206); however, alcoholics frequently incur head injuries from falls, altercations, and/or driving accidents. This may result in additional focal and/or diffuse damage and a varied assortment of memory and cognitive deficits on neuropsychological testing.

Older alcoholics may show continued improvement in cognitive functioning for at least 5 years of sobriety (195). Some chronic alcoholics, however, develop a global dementia that persists despite abstinence from alcohol. This alcoholic dementia is typically characterized by severe impairment of memory, conceptualization, problem-solving, and visuospatial abilities (207). The memory disturbance is characterized by rapid forgetting of information over time, rather than retrieval or encoding difficulties. In addition, patients with alcoholic dementia are more sensitive to proactive interference. Priming abilities, however, remain relatively preserved (49, 52).

DRUG-INDUCED MEMORY DEFICITS

Alcohol is not the only substance known to affect memory functioning. Other drugs with sedating effects, such as barbiturates, are known to negatively affect memory functioning, while stimulants and euphoriants may augment memory, at least temporarily (208). Likewise, several of the most commonly used prescription medications may also affect memory functioning. The elderly are particularly susceptible to this because of drug interactions secondary to polypharmacy and alterations in drug metabolism, distribution, binding, and excretion associated with aging. Katzman, Lasker, and Bernstein (209) reported that medication-induced cognitive dysfunction was the most common reversible form of dementia in the elderly, accounting for 2.7% of all cases. Moreover, studies show that the incidence of medication-related cognitive difficulties increases substantially with the number of medications the patient is taking, from 2.7% for those taking two or three prescription drugs, to 9.3% for those taking four to five, and to 13.7% for those taking six or more medications (210). The medications most commonly associated with cognitive impairment include the sedative-hypnotics, especially long-acting benzodiazepines, and the anticholinergic agents.

Benzodiazepines

It has been known for over a quarter century that even a single dose of benzodiazepine can impair cognitive functioning (211, 212). One of the most pronounced cognitive effects is impaired ability to learn new information. The ability to recall information that has been previously learned, however, is not disrupted by benzodiazepine use. In fact, administration of benzodiazepine immediately after learning new information has been known to enhance recall of that information (211). This phenomenon is known as "retrograde facilitation" and is believed to be due to the reduction of retroactive interference caused by the supressed ability to learn new information following drug administration.

The learning deficit associated with benzodiazepine use can differ depending on which medication is used. With diazepam use, the most pronounced deficits occur within the first hour or two after taking the medication; however, learning deficits are not seen with lorazepam use until the third to fourth hour after ingestion (211). The time that is required to recover from these cognitive effects depends on the specific agent used, the dose given, and the sensitivity of the memory measures used, but can often last up to 6 hours. The mechanism by which benzodiazepines affect memory functioning remains unclear. Part of the effect is believed to be due to the general central nervous system (CNS) depressant effect of the medication; however, many believe that benzodiazepine action extends beyond the sedating effects of the medication.

Interestingly, the cognitive effects of benzodiapines may diminish with repeated administration (211). Studies of long-term benzodiazepine use, however, have shown that patients taking higher dosages for long periods of time perform poorly on tasks requiring sustained attention, and report improved concentration and increased sensory perception following discontinuation of the medication (213, 214). In the elderly, substantial impairment in arousal, attention, memory, and psychomotor abilities are often seen even with brief benzodiazepine use (215). Moreover, the duration of cognitive impairment following a single dose is prolonged in the elderly compared with younger patients (216).

Anticholinergics

Anticholinergic agents such as atropine and scopolamine are also known to cause significant memory impairment. In addition, a wide variety of commonly used medications can disrupt memory because of significant anticholinergic side effects. These include most heterocyclic antidepressants (e.g., imipramine, amitriptyline), over-the-counter sleep and cold preparations containing antihistamines, several antiparkinsoninan medications (e.g., benztropine), and some neuroleptics (e.g., phenothiazines). It is believed that anticholinergic agents produce an imbalance in the cholinergic and adrenergic pathways of the reticular activating system and thalamocortical projections, thereby disrupting arousal and attentional capabilities (210). At higher doses, anticholinergics can cause memory impairment and acute confusional episodes. The presence of any preexisting neurodegenerative process, combined with the pharamacokinetic changes associated with aging noted earlier make the elderly brain most susceptible to the cognitive side effects of these medications. Fortunately, alternative medications with minimal anticholinergic effects are typically available for many of the indications just described. For example, monoamine oxidase inhibitors (e.g., phenelzine) and many of the newer selective serotonin-reuptake inhibitors (e.g., paroxetine, sertraline) have strong antidepressant effects with little to no cognitive sequelae. Similarly, neuroleptics such as clozapine and thiothixene have significantly less effect on memory functioning than the phenothiazines and butyrophenones.

Other Medications

In addition to benzodiazepines and drugs with anticholinergic effects, a number of other prescription medications can cause memory disturbance. Anticonvulsant medications such as phenobarbital, phenytoin, and primidone have been found to cause significant memory impairment, while carbamazepine (i.e., Tegretol) has been found to have minimal cognitive sequelae (210, 217). Other drugs reported to cause cognitive impairment include lithium, corticosteroids, antineoplastic agents such as interferon and azothioprine, and antihypertensive medications, including β-blockers (e.g., propranolol), anti-adrenergic agents (e.g., clonidine, reserpine, methyldopa), hydralazine, and hydrochorothiazide.

ALZHEIMER'S DISEASE

Anterograde amnesia for declarative knowledge is often one of the first neuropsychological findings in Alzheimer's disease (AD) (218). Memory difficulties begin insidiously, progress gradually over time, and are typically characterized by poor learning and rapid forgetting of information (160, 219, 220). Patients with AD tend to recall most items from the recency region of word lists, reflecting a highly passive learning style (162, 220). They also make numerous intrusion errors (221). On delayed recall, AD patients recall few target items (160, 219, 220) and tend to adopt a liberal response bias on recognition testing, endorsing high numbers of both target hits and false-positive errors (221).

On tests of retrograde memory, patients with moderate to severe AD demonstrate impaired memory for past events from all periods of their lives equally (i.e., flat retrograde amnesia) (222, 223). The retrograde amnesia of patients in earlier stages of AD, however, may be characterized by a temporal gradient (224).

Several studies have shown a dissociation of subtypes of nondeclarative memory abilities in AD. These patients demonstrate deficits in priming (49, 52), as well as in the classical conditioning of an eye-blink response (225). Procedural learning, however, remains intact in AD (115, 116).

As with any progressive disease, there is considerable variability in the spared and impaired cognitive functions of AD patients. One source of variability is individual difference in emotional reaction to the disease. Some patients develop a reactive depression in the earlier stages that exacerbates their memory impairment (226). There is also variability in the cerebral regions most affected by the neuropathological process. PET indicates that AD patients show significantly more lateral asymmetry of brain glucose metabolism than age-matched normal subjects (227, 228).

Especially in the early stages of the disease, patients with greater metabolic dysfunction in one or the other cerebral hemisphere tend to demonstrate asymmetry of memory deficits consistent with the hemisphere most affected (see earlier discussion of left- and right-hemisphere damage; see also 229).

A recent study by Massman and his colleagues (230) demonstrated asymmetric visuospatial memory profiles in some patients with AD. Patients were divided into three subgroups based on their performance on clinical tests of verbal and visuospatial ability. One subgroup consisted of patients who performed significantly better on verbal measures than on visuospatial measures (high-verbal); the second was comprised of patients who performed significantly better on visuospatial than verbal measures (high-spatial). Patients who obtained similar normative scores on tests of both verbal and visuospatial functioning comprised the third subgroup (equal). All patients were administered a modified version of the California Global-Local Learning Test (CGLT). The investigators found pronounced dissociations among the AD subgroups on this test. Patients in the high spatial subgroup had particular difficulty processing details (i.e., "local" forms), whereas patients in the high verbal subgroup exhibited marked deficits in processing the configural aspects (i.e., "global" forms). No significant dissociation in global or local processing was seen in the equal subgroup.

HUNTINGTON'S DISEASE

Patients with Huntington's disease (HD), a subcortical degenerative disorder, display equally impaired immediate free recall of information when compared to AD patients with equivalent overall severity of cognitive dysfunction. HD patients, however, show better retention of information over delay intervals (112). When presented with multiple trials of different verbal stimuli, HD patients reveal normal sensitivity to proactive interference (231), and they make significantly fewer intrusion and perseveration errors than AD patients and amnesics (221).

Recognition performance, though impaired, tends to be disproportionately better in HD patients than in AD or amnesic patients (112, 221). This has led some researchers to propose that the mechanism of memory failure in HD patients may be deficient retrieval search (232). A recent study, however, reported that HD patients in the most advanced stages of illness are as impaired as Alzheimer patients in recognition discriminability (221). This suggests that although retrieval failure may account for memory deficits throughout much of the disease process, encoding abilities may become progressively more affected as the disease advances.

HD patients have impaired retrograde memory, but their performance differs qualitatively from that of Korsakoff patients. HD patients show a flat retrograde amnesia, with equally deficient recall of events from all decades (224, 233).

The performance of recently diagnosed HD patients improves on recognition testing of remote events, which further implicates a retrieval search deficit in this group of patients (224).

Martone et al. (114) reported a crossover effect between declarative and procedure learning in HD and Korsakoff patients. HD patients showed better recognition memory for declarative knowledge than amnesics, whereas amnesics displayed superior procedural learning (in this case, mirror reading) than HD patients. Although oculomotor defects associated with HD may have contributed to these patients' difficulty on this particular skill-learning task, other studies have reported similar degrees of impairment on perceptual-motor tasks which place much less demand on eye movements (112, 115). Interestingly, HD patients have been found to show normal semantic priming (52), suggesting that the subcortical structures affected in HD (i.e., corpus striatum) may be important for skill learning but not for the processes central to semantic priming (115).

FRONTAL LOBE DEMENTIA

The frontal lobes account for approximately one-half of the cerebrum. Given their size, the chances that the frontal lobes will be involved in any diffuse pathological process are high. Some dementing disorders, however, preferentially affect the frontal lobes. These include one variant of Pick's disease and Jakob-Creutzfeldt disease, both of which are rare conditions. Recent evidence suggests that another more common degenerative dementia specific to the frontal lobes may exist that is histopathologically distinct from these and other known dementing illnesses (see 234–236).

Although it may be too early to establish frontal lobe dementia as a distinct diagnostic entity, there are several features that appear to be indicative of dementia associated with frontal lobe dysfunction. The patient with frontal lobe features typically presents with reports of a change in personality or adaptive behaviors that precede the onset of cognitive symptoms. When cognitive deficits appear, they typically involve disorders of planning, organization, mental flexibility, and memory (237). The memory deficits associated with frontal lobe dementia typically reflect poor organization, use of inefficient learning strategies, and increased susceptibility to interference (85). Ability to sustain attention is disturbed; however, there is no evidence of rapid forgetting of information, such as is seen in AD (238). Errors in recall are quite common, and include perseverations, intrusions, and source memory problems (see earlier discussion of the prefrontal cortex). There is some evidence that release from proactive interference may also be disturbed in frontal lobe dementia; however, this is not a consistent finding (238).

AFFECTIVE DISORDERS

Patients suffering from depression represent a heterogeneous group in terms of their cognitive profiles (239).

Depressed patients whose vegetative symptoms are not too severe but who are highly self-critical often show considerable variability in their ability to do well on tests of memory and other cognitive functioning. Effort, motivation, and subsequent performance typically wax and wane with the intensity of the depressed state. In many cases, perception of a poor performance will feed upon itself and cause the patient to feel more self-critical and anxious. This, in turn, can lead to additional poor performances.

Depressed patients frequently show impaired immediate recall of span and supra-span material, presumably because their attention capacity is consumed with dysphoric preoccupation and obsessive thinking (150). They are deficient in adopting active encoding strategies (240) and tend to give minimal responses, reporting only few target items and making few errors (i.e., intrusions and perseverations). The information they do report on immediate recall trials is typically retained to a normal degree after a delay interval. Their memory performance often improves with recognition testing, which probably compensates for retrieval difficulties that arise from being minimal responders (241). Errors on recognition testing are more likely to be missed targets than false positives, reflecting a negative response bias (242). Note, however, that at least one study found that depressed patients also make an elevated number of false-positive errors (243).

Patients with severe vegetative symptoms of psychomotor retardation, weight loss, and insomnia appear to be a more homogeneous group cognitively. This is because they often perform close to or at the lowest levels on neuropsychological tests. A "floor effect" such as this is especially common on tests assessing high-order functions such as memory and novel problem solving.

In general, patients with depression present with difficult diagnostic dilemmas. Depression can coexist with CNS damage and mask the impaired and spared cognitive functions related to the structural damage. Patients in the early stages of Alzheimer's disease, for example, can develop a depression that obscures the initial pattern of cognitive strengths and weaknesses, thus making the disorder difficult to detect (226). A clinical rule of thumb when seeing patients with clinically significant depressive symptomatology is to treat the depression and repeat the assessment. Memory and other test results then become diagnostically important for documenting improvement in mental functioning corresponding with alleviated mood disturbance, and/or declines in cognition associated with progressive neuropathology.

A common referral question for clinical neuropsychologists is to determine whether the memory and cognitive dysfunction in a depressed patient is "organic" versus "functional" (with elderly patients, this is typically phrased as "dementia" versus "pseudodementia"). There is increasing evidence that the cognitive abnormalities of depressed patients may occur secondary to genuine neuropathology, often related to changes in neurotransmitter systems such as serotonin and norepinephrine (241). A more sophisticated clinical examination would thus inquire whether cognitive dysfunction in a depressed patient is consistent with reversible neurochemical changes associated with the psychiatric disorder, irreversible structural changes, or some combination of the two.

Sensitive neuroimaging techniques such as MRI will play an increasing role in this difficult differential diagnosis. In a preliminary study by Dupont and her colleagues (244) eight of 14 patients with bipolar mood disorder showed focal areas of signal hyperintensity within the deep white matter and periventricular regions. Those patients with positive MRI findings had significantly greater memory dysfunction and higher numbers of psychiatric hospitalizations for mood disturbance than patients with normal MRI scans. For subgroups of psychiatric patients with chronic affective disorders, small subcortical lesions and subsequent neurochemical changes may affect both cognitive and emotional functioning.

NORMAL AGING

Decrements in memory functioning are apparent with advancing age in normal populations. The elderly commonly report that their memory is not as good as it once was, and they perform more poorly than younger subjects on standard tests of learning and recall (see 245 for review). In general, the decrements in memory functioning associated with normal aging are more apparent in some aspects of memory than in others, and appear to reflect decreased efficiency of processing rather than a true breakdown or loss of component structures (246).

Studies show that elderly subjects do not differ significantly from younger controls on tests of immediate recall span *unless* the task requires the subject to manipulate and/or transform the information (such as recalling digits backward; see 246). With regard to long-term memory, several investigators have demonstrated that the normal elderly can usually manage to perform tasks that are driven directly by the stimulus or that are strongly influenced or supported by the environment (247). Conversely, memory impairment is greatest when the situation requires self-initiation and/or the establishment of new routines or patterns. For example, substantial declines in free recall of stories and word lists are evident by age 50 (248). These declines do not appear to reflect differences in forgetting rates between younger and older subjects; instead, the elderly appear less efficient than younger subjects in their encoding and retrieval of information. When structure is provided via the use of recognition testing or cuing during encoding and free recall, the magnitude of age-related memory decrements is reduced significantly (249, 250).

Changes in nondeclarative memory with advanced age appears dependent upon the measure used. There does not appear to be a significant decline with age on measures of priming; however, skill learning, procedural memory, and the rate of developing classically conditioned responses appear to be affected negatively by age (251).

CONCLUSION

The past 25 years have witnessed substantial changes in our understanding of the neurological and cognitive processes that comprise memory. This has produced a generation of improved assessment measures incorporating constructs from the cognitive psychological literature, such as encoding strategies, recall measures, recognition discriminability, sensitivity to interference, and forgetting rates. As the investigation of cognitive processes comprising memory functioning progresses, so will our ability to measure and characterize memory disorders at both the structural and functional level. The recognition of the existence of two dissociable memory systems, for example, has led to an explosion of interest in the neurology of memory and the search for brain structures that mediate nondeclarative memory systems.

Because publishers of psychological tests must often assume a conservative stance regarding experimental "breakthroughs" in cognitive science, there is often a lag of several years between the development of experimental procedures and the incorporation of these techniques in clinical assessment measures. Thus, the revolution study of nondeclarative types of memory in the laboratory has thus far had little impact on how memory is assessed in clinical settings. The next few years, however, should witness the introduction of standardized measures of nondeclarative memory into clinical practice. This will provide a means of better defining the extent and nature of memory impairment in patient populations and will aid in differential diagnosis. Whether patients with declarative memory disorders can be trained to use intact nondeclarative memory systems to ameliorate or circumvent these deficits has yet to be determined.

References

1. Matthies H. Neurobiological aspects of learning and memory. Annu Rev Psychol 1989;40:381–404.
2. Squire LR. Memory and brain. Oxford: Oxford University Press, 1987.
3. Konorski J. Conditioned reflexes and neuron organization. Cambridge, England: Cambridge University Press, 1948.
4. Hebb DO. The organization of behavior. New York: John Wiley & Sons, 1949.
5. Eccles JC. The neurophysiological basis of mind: the principles of neurophysiology. Oxford: Clarendon Press, 1953.
6. Babich FR, Jacobsen AL, Bubash S, Jacobson A. Transfer of a response to naive rats by injection of ribonucleic acid extracted from trained rats. Science 1965;149:656–657.
7. Dyal JA. Transfer of behavioral bias: reality and specificity. In: Fjerdingstad EJ, ed. Chemical transfer of learned information. New York: Elsevier Science Publishers, 1971.
8. Rose SPR. The biochemistry of memory. Essays in biochemistry 1991;26:1–12.
9. Rosenzweig MR, Bennett EL. Experiential influences on brain anatomy and brain chemistry in rodents. In: Gottlieb G, ed. Studies on the development of behavior and the nervous system. New York: Academic Press, 1978:289–327.
10. Turner AM, Greenough WT. Differential rearing effects on rat visual cortex synapses. I. Synaptic and neuronal density and synapses per neuron. Brain Res 1985;329:195–203.

11. Patel SN, Stewart MG. Changes in the number and structure of dendritic spines 25hr after passive avoidance training in the domestic chick, *Gallus domesticus*. Brain Res 1988;449:34–46.
12. Cermak LS. The episodic-semantic distinction in amnesia. In: Squire LR, Butters N, eds. Neuropsychology of memory. New York: Guilford Press, 1984:55–62.
13. Warrington EK, Weiskrantz L. An analysis of short-term and long-term memory defects in man. In: Deutsch JA, ed. The physiological basis of memory, 1973:365–395.
14. Butters N, Miliotis P. Amnesic disorders. In: Heilman KM, Valenstein E, eds. Clinical neuropsychology. 2nd ed. Oxford: Oxford University Press, 1985:403–452.
15. James W. Principles of psychology. New York: Holt, Rinehart & Winston, 1890.
16. Miller GA. The magical number seven: plus or minus two. Some limits on our capacity for processing information. Psychol Rev 1956;9;81–97.
17. Lezak MD. Neuropsychological assessment. 2nd ed. Oxford: Oxford University Press, 1983.
18. Hebb DO. Distinctive features of learning in the higher animal. In: Delafresnay JF, ed. Brain mechanisms and learning. Oxford: Blackwell, 1961:37–51.
19. Butters N, Cermak LS. Alcoholic Korsakoff's syndrome. New York: Academic Press, 1980.
20. Milner B, Corkin S, Teuber HL. Further analysis of the hippocampal amnesic syndrome: a 14-year follow-up study of H.M. Neuropsychologia 1968;6:215–234.
21. Scoville WB, Milner B. Loss of recent memory after bilateral hippocampal lesions. J Neurol Neurosurg Psychiatry 1957;20:11–21.
22. Squire LR, Moore RY. Dorsal thalamic lesions in a noted case of chronic memory dysfunction. Ann Neurol 1979;6:503–506.
23. Teuber HL, Milner B, Baughan HG. Persistent anterograde amnesia after stab wound of the basal brain. Neuropsychologia 1968;6:267–282.
24. Cermak LS. Human memory: research and theory. New York: Ronald Press, 1972.
25. Klatzky, RL. Human memory: structures and processes. 2nd ed. San Francisco: Freeman, 1980.
26. Crowder, RG. The demise of short-term memory. Acta Psychol 1982;50:291–323.
27. Wickelgren WA. The long and short of memory. Psychol Bull 1973;80:425–438.
28. Slamecka, NJ. Retroactive inhibition of connected discourse as a function of practice level. J Exp Psychol 1960;59:104–108.
29. Underwood BJ. Interference and forgetting. Psychol Rev 1957;64:49–60.
30. Reitman JS. Mechanisms of forgetting in short-term memory. Cogn Psychol 1971;2:185–195.
31. Randolph C, Gold JM, Carpenter CJ, Goldberg TE, Weinberger DR. Release from proactive interference: determinants of performance and neuropsychological correlates. J Clin Exp Neuropsychol 1992;14:785–800.
32. Corkin S. Lasting consequences of bilateral medial temporal lobectomy: clinical course and experimental findings in H.M. Semin Neurol 1984;4:249–259.
33. Zola-Morgan S, Squire LR, Amaral DG. Human amnesia and the medial temporal lobe region: enduring memory impairment following a bilateral lesion limited to field CA1 of the hippocampus. J Neurosci 1986;6:2950–2967.
34. Goldberg E, Antin SP, Bilder RM, Hughes JEO, Mattis S. Retrograde amnesia: possible role of mesencephalic reticular activation in long-term memory. Science 1981;213:1392–1394.
35. Damasio AR, Eslinger PJ, Damasio H, Van Hoesen GW, Cornell S. Multimodal amnesic syndrome following bilateral temporal and basal forebrain damage. Arch Neurol 1985;42:252–259.
36. Milner B. Amnesia following operation on the temporal lobes. In: Whitty CWM, Zangwill OL, eds. Amnesia. London: Butterworths, 1966:113.
37. Drachman DA, Arbit J. memory and the hippocampal complex. II. Is memory a multiple process? Arch Neurol 1966;15:52–61.
38. McCarthy, RA, Warrington EK. Cognitive neuropsychology: a clinical introduction. San Diego: Academic Press, 1990.
39. Kopelman MD. Amnesia: organic and psychogenic. Br J Psychiatry 1987;150:428–442.
40. Butters N, Cermak LS. A case study of the forgetting of autobiographical knowledge: implications for the study of retrograde amnesia. In: Rubin D, ed. Autobiographical memory. New York: Cambridge University Press, 1986:253–272.
41. Squire LR, Knowlton B, Musen G. The structure and organization of memory. Annu Rev Psychol 1993;44:453–495.
42. Tulving E. Elements of episodic memory. Oxford: Clarendon Press, 1983.
43. Marinkovic K, Schell AM, Dawson ME. Awareness of the CS-UCS contingency and classical conditioning of skin conductance responses with olfactory CSs. Biolo Psychol 1989;29:39–60.
44. Daum I, Channon S, Canavar A. Classical conditioning in patients with severe memory problems. J Neurol Neurosurg Psychiatry 1989;52:47–51.
45. Weiskrantz L, Warrington EK. Conditioning in amnesic patients. Neuropsychologia 1979;17:187–194.
46. Simamura AP. Priming effects in amnesia: evidence for a dissociable memory function. Q J Exp Psychol 1986;38a:619–644.
47. Schacter DL, Chiu C-YP, Ochsner KN. Implicit memory: a selective review. Annu Rev Neurosci 1993;16:159–182.
48. Tulving E, Schacter DL. Priming and human memory systems. Science 1990;247:301–306.
49. Salmon DP, Shimamura AP, Butters N, Smith S. Lexical and semantic priming deficits in patients with Alzheimer's disease. J Clin Exp Neuropsychol 1988;10:477–494.
50. Warrington EK, Weiskrantz L. Amnesic syndrome: consolidation or retrieval? Nature 1970;228:628–230.
51. Cermak LS, Talbot N, Chandler K, Wolbarst LR. The perceptual priming phenomenon in amnesia. Neuropsychologia 1985;23:615–622.
52. Shimamura AP, Salmon DP, Squire LR, Butters N. Memory dysfunction and word priming in dementia and amnesia. Behav Neurosci 1987;101:347–351.
53. Bondi MW, Kaszniak AW. Implicit and explicit memory in Alzheimer's disease and Parkinson's disease. J Clin Exp Neuropsychol 1991;13:339–358.
54. Heindel WC, Salmon DP, Shults CW, Walicke PA, Butters N. Neuropsychological evidence for multiple implicit memory systems: a comparison of Alzheimer's, Parkinson's and Huntington's disease patients. J Neurosci 1989;9:582–587.
55. Heindel WC, Salmon DP, Butters N. Pictorial priming and cued recall in Alzheimer's and Huntington's disease. Brain Cogn 1990;13:282–295.
56. Cohen NJ, Corkin S. The amnesic patient H.M.: learning and retention of a cognitive skill. Abstracts of the Society of Neuroscience 1981;80:235.
57. Corkin S, Sullivan E, Twitchell T, Grove E. The amnesic patient H.M.: clinical observations and test performance 28 years after operation. Abstracts of the Society of Neuroscience 1981;80:235.
58. Nissen M, Cohen N, Corkin S. The amnesic patient H.M.: learning and retention of perceptual skills. Abstracts of the Society of Neuroscience 1981;80:235.
59. Hermann BP, Wyler AR, Bush AJ, Tabatabai FR. Differential effects of left and right anterior temporal lobectomy on verbal learning and memory performance. Epilepsia 1992;33:289–297.
60. Gerner P, Ommaya A, Fedio P. A study of visual memory: verbal and nonverbal mechanisms in patients with unilateral lobectomy. Int J Neurosci 1972;4:231–238.
61. Kimura D. Right temporal lobe damage: perception of unfamiliar stimuli after damage. Arch Neurol 1963;8:264–267.
62. Milner B. Visual recognition and recall after right temporal-lobe excision in man. Neuropsychologia 1968;6:191–210.

63. Jones-Gotman M, Milner B. Right temporal-lobe contribution to image-mediated verbal learning. Neuropsychologia 1978;16:61–71.

64. Smith ML, Milner B. The role of the right hippocampus in the recall of spatial location. Neuropsychologia 1981;19:781–793.

65. Squire LR, Zola-Morgan S. The medial temporal lobe memory system. Science 1991;253:1380–1386.

66. Kesner RP, Conner HS. Independence of short- and long-term memory: a neural system analysis. Science 1972;176:432–434.

67. Olton DS. Memory functions and the hippocampus. In: Siefert W, ed. Neurobiology of the hippocampus. New York: Academic Press, 1983:335–373.

68. Olton DS, Becker JT, Handlemann GE. A re-examination of the role of hippocampus in working memory. Behav Brain Sci 1979;2:353–359.

69. Olton DS, Collison C, Werz MA. Spatial memory and radial-arm maze performance in rats. Learning and Motivation 1977;8:289–314.

70. Horel JA. The neuroanatomy of amnesia: a critique of the hippocampal memory hypothesis. Brain 1978;101:403–445.

71. Zola-Morgan S, Squire LR, Mishkin M. The neuroanatomy of amnesia: amygdala-hippocampus versus temporal stem. Science 1982;218:1337–1139.

72. Mishkin M. Memory in monkeys severely impaired by combined but not by separate removal of amygdala and hippocampus. Nature 1978;273:297–298.

73. Price, JL. Amygdaloid complex. In: Adelman G, ed. Encyclopedia of neuroscience. Boston: Birkhauser, 1987:40–42.

74. Press GA, Amaral DG, Squire LR. Hippocampal abnormalities in amnesic patients revealed by high resolution magnetic resonance imaging. Nature 1989;341:54–57.

75. Squire LR, Amaral DG, Press GA. Magnetic resonance measurements of hippocampal formation and mammillary nuclei distinguish medial temporal lobe and diencephalic amnesia. J Neurosci 1990;10:3106–3117.

76. Mahut HS, Zola-Morgan S, Moss M. Hippocampal resections impair associative learning and recognition in the monkey. J Neurosci 1982;2:1214–1229.

77. Zola-Morgan S, Squire LR. Memory impairment in monkeys following lesions of the hippocampus. Behav Neurosci 1986;100:155–160.

78. Davis M. Pharmacological and anatomical analysis of fear conditioning using the fear-potentiated startle paradigm. Behav Neurosci 1986;100:814–824.

79. Kesner RP. Learning and memory in rats with an emphasis on the role of the amygdala. In: Aggleton J, ed. The amygdala. New York: John Wiley & Sons, 1992:379–400.

80. Zola-Morgan S, Squire LR. Neuroanatomy of memory. Annu Rev Neurosci 1993;16:547–563.

81. Carpenter MB. Core text of neuroanatomy. 3rd ed. Baltimore: Williams & Wilkins, 1985:226–264.

82. Victor M, Adams RD, Collins GH. The Wernicke-Korsakoff syndrome. Philadelphia: FA Davis, 1971.

83. Butters N, Stuss DT. Diencephalic amnesia. In: Boller F, Grafman J, eds. Handbook of neuropsychology, vol. 3. Amsterdam: Elsevier Science Publishers, 1989:107–148.

84. Mair RG, Warrington EK, Weiskrantz L. Memory disorder in Korsakoff's psychosis: a neuropathological and neuropsychological investigation of two cases. Brain 1979;102:749–783.

85. Mayes A, Meudell P, Mann D, Pickering A. Location of lesions in Korsakoff's syndrome: neuropsychological and neuropathological data on two patients. Cortex 1988;24:367–388.

86. McEntee WJ, Biber MP, Perl DP, Benson DF. Diencephalic amnesia: a reappraisal. J Neurol Neurosurg Psychiatry 1976;39:436–441.

87. Guberman A, Stuss D. The syndrome of bilateral paramedian thalamic infarction. Neurology 1983;33:540–546.

88. Cramon DV, Hebel N, Schuri U. A contribution to the anatomical basis of thalamic amnesia. Brain 1985;108:993–1008.

89. Graff-Radford NR, Tranel D, Van Hoesen GW, Brandt J. Diencephalic amnesia. Brain 1990;113:1–25.

90. Squire LR, Amaral DG, Zola-Morgan S, Kritchevsky M, Press DG. Description of brain injury in amnesic patient N.A. based on magnetic resonance imaging. Exp Neurol 1989;105:23–35.

91. Zola-Morgan S, Squire LR, Amaral DG. Lesions of the hippocampal formation but not lesions of the fornix or the emammillary nuclei produce long-lasting memory impairment in monkeys. J Neurosci 1989;9:897–912.

92. Aggleton JP, Mishkin M. Visual recognition impairment following medial thalamic lesions in monkeys. Neuropsychologia 1983;21:189–197.

93. Aggleton JP, Mishkin M. Memory impairments following restricted medial thalamic lesions. Exp Brain Res 1983;52:199–209.

94. Mair RG, Anderson CD, Langlais PJ, McEntee WJ. Behavioral impairments, brain lesions, and monoaminergic activity in the rat following a bout of thiamine deficiency. Behav Brain Res 1988;27:223–239.

95. Mair RG, Lancourse DM. Radio-frequency lesions of thalamus produce delayed non-matching to sample impairments comprable to pyrithiamine-induced encephalopathy in rats. Behav Neurosci 1992;106:634–645.

96. Mair RG, Robinson JK, Koger SM, Fox DG, Zhang YP. Delayed non-matching to sample is impaired by extensive, but not by limited lesions of the thalamus in the rat. Behav Neurosci 1992;106:646–656.

97. Alexander MP, Freedman M. Amnesia after anterior communicating artery aneurysm rupture. Neurology 1984;34:752–757.

98. Damasio AR, Graff-Radford NR, Eslinger PJ, Damasio H, Kassell N. Amnesia following basal forebrain lesions. Arch Neurol 1985;42:263–271.

99. Mesulam MM, Mufson EJ, Levey AI, Wainer BH. Cholinergic innervation of cortex by the basal forebrain: cytochemistry and cortical connections of the septal area, diagonal band nuclei, nucleus basalis (substantia innominata), and hypothalamus in the rhesus monkey. J Com Neurol 1983;214:170–197.

100. Whitehouse PJ, Price DL, Struble RG, Clark AW, Coyle JL, DeLong MR. Alzheimer's disease and senile dementia: loss of neurons in the basal forebrain. Science 1982;215:1237–1239.

101. Bartus RT, Dean RL, Beer B, Lippa AS. The cholinergic hypothesis of geriatric memory dysfunction. Science 1982;217:408–417.

102. Aigner T, Mitchell S, Aggleton J, et al. Recognition deficit in monkeys following neurotoxic lesions of the basal forebrain. Society for Neuroscience Abstracts 1984;10:386.

103. Aigner TG, Mitchell SJ, Aggleton JP, et al. Transient impairment of recognition memory following ibotenic acid lesions of the basal forebrain in macaques. Exp Brain Res 1991;86:18–26.

104. Mayes AR, Meudell PR. Problems and prospects for research on amnesia. In: Squire LR, Butters N, eds. Neuropsychology of memory. New York: Guilford, 1984:134–144.

105. Knight RT, Grabowecky MF, Scabini D. Role of human prefrontal cortex in attention control. In: Jasper HH, Riggio S, Goldman-Rakic PS, eds. Advances in neurology. Vol. 66: Epilepsy and the functional anaotmy of the frontal lobe. New York: Raven Press, 1995:21–36.

106. Glisky EL, Polster MR, Routhieaux BC. Double dissociation between item and source memory. Neuropsychology 1995;9:229–235.

107. Milner B. Aspects of human frontal lobe function. In: Jasper HH, Riggio S, Goldman-Rakic PS, eds. Advances in neurology. Vol. 66: Epilepsy and the functional anatomy of the frontal lobe. New York: Raven Press, 1995:67–84.

108. Milner B, Corsi P, Leonard G. Frontal-lobe contribution to recency judgments. Neuropsychologia 1991;28:803–813.

109. Squire LR. Memory and the hippocampus: a synthesis from findings with rats, monkeys, and humans. Psychol Rev 1992;99:195–231.

110. Paulsen JS, Butters N, Salmon DP, Heindel WC, Swenson MR. Prism adaptation in Alzheimer's and Huntington's disease. Neuropsychology 1993;7:73–81.

111. Knopman D, Nissen MJ. Procedural learning is impaired in Huntington's disease: evidence from the serial reaction time task. Neuropsychologia 1991;29:245–254.

112. Butters N, Wolfe J, Martone M, Granholm E, Cermak LS. Memory disorders associated with Huntington's disease: verbal recall, verbal recognition, and procedural memory. Neuropsychologia 1985;23:729–743.

113. Saint-Cyr JA, Taylor AE, Lang AE. Procedural learning and neostriatal dysfunction in man. Brain 1988;111:941–959.

114. Martone M, Butters N, Payne M, Becker J, Sax D. Dissociations between skill learning and verbal recognition between amnesia and dementia. Arch Neurol 1984;41:965–970.

115. Heindel WC, Butters N, Salmon DP. Impaired learning of a motor skill in patients with Huntington's disease. Behav Neurosci 1988;102:141–147.

116. Eslinger PJ, Damasio AR. Preserved motor learning in Alzheimer's disease: implications for anatomy and behavior. J Neurosci 1986;6:3006–3009.

117. Heindel WC, Salmon DP, Butters N. Cognitive approaches to memory disorders of demented patients. In: Sutker PB, Adams HE, eds. Comprehensive handbook of psychopathology. 2nd ed. New York: Plenum Press, 1993.

118. Heindel WC, Salmon DP, Butters N. The biasing of weight judgments in Alzheimer's and Huntington's disease: a priming or programming phenomenon? J Clin Exp Neuropsychol 1991;13:189–203.

119. Lavond DG, Kim JJ, Thompson RF. Mammalian brain substrates of aversive classical conditioning. Annu Rev Psychol 1993;44:317–342.

120. Iwata J, LeDoux JE, Meely MP, Arneric S, Reis DJ. Intrinsic neurons in the amygdaloid field projected to by the medial geniculate body mediate emotional responses conditioned to acoustic stimuli. Brain Res 1986;383:161–166.

121. Hitchcock JM, Davis M. Lesions of the amygdala, but not of the cerebellum or red nucleus, block conditioned fear as measured with the potentiated startle paradigm. Behav Neurosci 1986;100:11–22.

122. Blanchard DC, Blanchard RJ. Innate and conditioned reactions to threat in rats with amygdaloid lesions. J Comp Physiol Psychol 1972;81:281–290.

123. Applegate CD, Frysinger RC, Kapp BS, Gallagher M. Multiple unit activity recorded from the amygdala central nucleus during pavlovian heart rate conditioning in the rabbit. Brain Res 1982;238:457–462.

124. Pascoe JP, Kapp BS. Electrophysiological characteristics of amygdaloid central nucleus neurons during pavlovian fear conditioning in the rabbit. Behav Brain Res 1985;16:117–133.

125. Liang KC, McGaugh JL, Martinez JL, Jensen RA Jr., Vasquez BJ, Messing RB. Post-training amygdaloid lesions impair retention of an inhibitory avoidance response. Behav Brain Res 1982;4:237–249.

126. Marsolek CJ, Kosslyn S, Squire LR. Form-specific visual priming in the right cerebral hemisphere. J Exp Psychol [Learn Mem Cogn] 1992;18:492–508.

127. Petersen SE, Fox PT, Snyder AZ, Raichle ME. Activation of extrastriate and frontal cortical areas by visual words and word-like stimuli. Science 1990;249:1041–1044.

128. Felleman D, Van Essen D. Distributed hierarchical processing in primate cerebral cortex. Cerebral Cortex 1991;1:1–47.

129. Jernigan TI, Ostergaard AL. Word priming and recognition memory are both affected by mesial temporal lobe damage. Neuropsychology 1993;7:14–26.

130. Ostergaard AL, Jernigan TL. Are word priming and explicit memory mediated by different brain structures? In: Graf P, Masson MEJ, eds. Implicit memory: new directions in cognition, development, and neuropsychology. Hillsdale, NJ: Erlbaum & Associates, 1994.

131. Norris D. The effects of frequency, repetition, and stimulus quality in visual word recognition. Q J Exp Psychol [A] 1984;36:507–518.

132. Loring DW, Papanicolaou AC. Memory assessment in neuropsychology: theoretical considerations and practical utility. J Clin Exp Neuropsychol 1987;9:340–358.

133. Spreen O, Strauss E. A compendium of neuropsychological tests: administration, norms, and commentary. New York: Oxford University Press, 1991.

134. Wechsler D. Wechsler Memory Scale-Revised. New York: The Psychological Corporation, 1987.

135. Wechsler D. A standardized memory scale for clinical use. J Psychol 1945;19:87–95.

136. Erickson RC, Scott ML, Clinical memory testing: a review. Psychol Bull 1977;84:1130–1149.

137. Prigatano GP. Wechsler Memory Scale: a selective review of the literature. J Clin Psychol 1978;34:816–832.

138. Ivnik RJ, Malec JF, Tangalos EG, Petersen RC, Kokmen E, Kurland LT. Mayo's older Americans normative studies: WMS-R norms for ages 56 to 94. The Clinical Neuropsychologist 1992;6 (Suppl):83–104.

139. Butters N, Salmon DP, Cullum CM, et al. Differentiation of amnesic and demented patients with the Wechsler Memory Scale-Revised. The Clinical Neuropsychologist 1988;2:133–148.

140. Chelune GJ, Bornstein RA. Wechsler Memory Scale-Revised patterns among patients with unilateral brain lesions. Clin Neuropsychol 1988;2:121–132.

141. Fischer JF. Using the Wechsler Memory Scale-Revised to detect and characterize memory deficits in multiple sclerosis. Clin Neuropsychol 1988;2:149–172.

142. Reference deleted.

143. Ryan JJ, Lewis CU. Comparison of normal controls and recently detoxified alcoholics on the Wechsler Memory Scale-Revised. Clin Neuropsychol 1988;2:173–180.

144. Loring DW, Lee GP, Meador KJ. Issues in memory assessment of the elderly. Clin Geriatr Med 1989;5:565–581.

145. Randt CT, Brown ER. Randt Memory Test. Bayport: Life Science Associates, 1983.

146. Golden CJ, Hammeke TA, Purisch AD. The Luria Nebraska Neuropsychological Battery. Los Angeles: Western Psychological Services, 1983.

147. Adams KM. In search of Luria's battery: a false start. J Consul Clin Psychol 1980;48:511–516.

148. Spiers P. Have they come to praise Luria or to bury him? The Luria-Nebraska Battery controversy. J Consult Clin Psychol 1981;49:331–341.

149. Russell EW. The psychometric foundation of clinical neuropsychology. In: Filskov SB, Boll TJ, eds. Handbook of neuropsychology, vol. 2. New York: John Wiley & Sons, 1986:45–80.

150. Breslow R, Kocsis J, Belkin B. Memory deficits in depression: evidence utilizing the Wechsler Memory Scale. Percept Mot Skills 1980;51:541–542.

151. Stromgren LS. The influence of depression on memory. Acta Psychiatr Scand 1977;56:109–128.

152. Wechsler D. Manual for the Wechsler Adult Intelligence Scale-Revised. New York: The Psychological Corporation, 1981.

153. Kaplan E, Fein D, Morris R, Delis DC. WAIS-R as a Neuropsychological Instrument. New York: The Psychological Corporation, 1991.

154. Miller E. Short- and long-term memory in patients with presenile dementia. Psychol Med 1973;3:221–224.

155. Benton AL, Hamsher K deS. Multilingual Aphasia Examination. Iowa City: University of Iowa, 1976.

156. Goodglass H, Kaplan E. The assessment of aphasia and related disorders. 2nd ed. Philadelphia: Lea & Febiger, 1983.

157. Buschke H. Selective reminding for analysis of memory and behavior. Journal of Verbal Learning and Verbal Behavior 1973;12:543–550.

158. Buschke H, Fuld PA. Evaluating storage, retention, and retrieval in disordered memory and learning. Neurology 1974;24:1019–1025.

159. Hannay HJ, Levin HS. Selective reminding test: an examination of the equivalence of four forms. J Clin Exp Neuropsychol 1985;7:251–263.

160. Ober BA, Koss E, Friedland RP, Delis DC. Processes of verbal

memory failure in Alzheimer-type dementia. Brain Cogn 1985;4: 90–103.

161. Ivnik RJ, Malec JF, Tangalos EG, Petersen RC, Kokmen E, Kurland LT. Mayo's older Americans normative studies: updated AVLT norms for ages 56 to 97. The Clinical Neuropsychologist 1992;6 (Suppl):83–104.

162. Delis DC, Kramer JH, Kaplan E, Ober BA. The California Verbal Learning Test. New York: The Psychological Corporation, 1987.

163. Brandt J. The Hopkins Verbal Learning Test: development of a new memory test with six equivalent forms. The Clinical Neuropsychologist 1991;5:125–142.

164. Babcock H. An experiment in the measurement of mental deterioration. Arch Psychol 1930;117:105.

165. Heaton RK, Grant I, Matthews CG. Comprehensive norms for an expanded Halstead-Reitan Battery. Odessa, FL: Psychological Assessment Resources, 1991.

166. Benton AL. The Revised Visual Retention Test. 4th ed. New York: The Psychological Corporation, 1974.

167. Marsh GG, Hirsch SH. Effectiveness of two tests of visual retention. J Clin Psychol 1982;38:115–118.

168. Sterne DM. The Benton, Porteus, and WAIS Digit Span tests with normal and brain injured subjects. J Clin Psychol 1969;25:173–175.

169. Heilbrun AB. Psychological test performance as a function of lateral localization of cerebral lesion. J Comp Physiol Psychol 1956;49: 10–14.

170. Warrington EK. Recognition Memory Test. Windsor: Nfer-Nelson, 1984.

171. Taylor LB. Psychological assessment of neurosurgical patients. In: Rasmussen T, Marino R, eds. Functional neurosurgery. New York: Raven Press, 1979.

172. Milberg WP, Hebben N, Kaplan E. The Boston process approach to neuropsychological assessment. In: Grant I, Adams KM, eds. Neuropsychological assessment of neuropsychiatric disorders. New York: Oxford University Press, 1986:65–86.

173. Goodglass H, Kaplan E. Assessment of cognitive deficit in the brain injured patient. In: Gazzaniga MS, ed., Handbook of behavioral neurobiology, vol. 2. New York: Plenum Press, 1979.

174. Binder LM. Constructional strategies of complex figure drawing after unilateral brain damage. J Clin Neuropsychol 1982;4:51–58.

175. Shorr JS, Delis DC, Massman PJ. Memory for the Rey-Osterrieth figure: perceptual clustering, encoding, and storage. Neuropsychology 1992;6:43–50.

176. Taylor EM. The appraisal of children with cerebral deficits. Cambridge, MA: Harvard University Press, 1959.

177. Kaplan E. Process and achievement revisited. In: Wapner S, Kaplan B, eds. Toward a holistic developmental psychology. Hillsdale, NJ: Erlbaum & Associates, 1983.

178. Delis DC, Kiefner M, Fridlund AJ. Visuospatial dysfunction following unilateral brain damage: dissociations in hierarchical and hemispatial analysis. J Clin Exp Neuropsychol 1988;10:421–431.

179. Delis DC, Robertson LC, Efron R. Hemispheric specialization of memory for visual hierarchical stimuli. Neuropsychologia 1986;24: 205–214.

180. Reitan RM, Wolfson D. The Halstead-Reitan neuropsychological test battery. Tucson: Neuropsychology Press, 1985.

181. Schacter D, Wang PL, Tulving E, Freedman PC. Functional retrograde amnesia: a quantitative case study. Neuropsychologia 1982;20:523–532.

182. Squire LR, Slater PC. Electroconvulsive therapy and complaints of memory dysfunction: a prospective three-year follow-up study. Br J Psychiatry 1983;142:1–8.

183. Albert MS, Butters N, Levin J. Temporal gradients in the retrograde amnesia of patients with alcoholic Korsakoff disease. Arch Neurol 1979;36:211–216.

184. Squire LR, Slater PC. Forgetting in very long-term memory as assessed by an improved questionnaire technique. J Exp Psychol [Learn Mem Cogn] 1975;104:50–54.

185. Squire LR, Slater PC, Chase PM. Retrograde amnesia: temporal gradient in very long term memory following electroconvulsive therapy. Science 1975;187:77–79.

186. Cohen NJ, Squire LR. Preserved learning and retention of pattern analyzing skill in amnesia: dissociation of knowing how and knowing that. Science 1980;210:207–209.

187. Squire LR, Fox MM. Assessment of remote memory: validation of the television test by repeated testing during a seven-year period. Behavioral Research Methods and Instruments 1980;12:583–586.

188. Gerner P, Ommaya A, Fedio P. A study of visual memory: verbal and nonverbal mechanisms in patients with unilateral lobectomy. Int J Neurosci 1972;4:231–238.

189. Milner B. Interhemispheric differences in the localization of psychological processes in man. Br Med Bull 1971;27:272–277.

190. Wapner W, Hamby S, Gardner H. The role of the right hemisphere in the apprehension of complex linguistic material. Brain Lang 1981;14:15–32.

191. Villardita C. Verbal memory and semantic clustering in right hemisphere damaged patients. Neuropsychologia 1987;25:277–280.

192. Delis DC, Kramer JH, Kiefner MG. Visuospatial functioning before and after commissurotomy: disconnection in hierarchical processing. Arch Neurol 1988;45:462–465.

193. Zangwill OL. The amnesic syndrome. In: Whitty CWM, Zangwill OL, eds. Amnesia. London: Butterworths, 1966.

194. Squire LR, Cohen NJ. Remote memory, retrograde amnesia, and the neuropsychology of memory. In: Cermak LS, ed. Human memory and amnesia. Hillsdale, NJ: Erlbaum & Associates, 1982:275–303.

195. Brandt J, Butters N, Ryan C, Bayog R. Cognitive loss and recovery in long-term alcohol abusers. Arch Gen Psychiatry 1983;40: 435–442.

196. Miglioli M, Buchtel HA, Campanin T, DeRisio C. Cerebral hemispheric lateralization of cognitive deficits due to alcoholism. J Nerv Men Disord 1979;167:212–217.

197. Ryan C, Butters N. Learning and memory impairments in young and old alcoholics: evidence for the premature aging hypothesis. Alcoholism 1980;4:288–293.

198. Glosser G, Butters N, Kaplan E. Visuoperceptual processes in brain damaged patients on the Digit Symbol Substitution test. Int J Neurosci 1977;7:59–66.

199. Kapur N, Butters N. An analysis of visuoperceptive deficits in alcoholic Korsakoffs and long term alcoholics. J Stud Alcohol 1977;38:2025–2035.

200. Wilson B, Kolb B, Odland L, Whishaw IQ. Alcohol, sex, age, and the hippocampus. Psychobiology 1987; 15:300–307.

201. Jones BM, Parsons OA. Specific versus generalized deficits in abstracting ability in chronic alcoholics. Arch Gen Psychiatry 1972; 26:380–384.

202. Hudolin V. Impairments of the nervous system in alcoholics. In: Richter D, ed. Addiction and brain damage. Baltimore: University Park Press, 1980:168–200.

203. Ron MA. The alcoholic brain: CT scan and psychological findings. Psychol Med 1983;3:1–33.

204. Parsons OA. Neuropsychological consequences of alcohol abuse: many questions–some answers. In: Parsons OA, Butters N, Nathan PE, eds. Neuropsychology of alcoholism: implications for diagnosis and treatment. New York: Guilford, 1987:256–272.

205. Kiefner MG, Delis DC. Effects of chronic alcohol abuse on visual hierarchical processing. Paper presented at the 15th annual meeting of the International Neuropsychological Society, Washington, DC, 1987.

206. Grant I, Adams K, Reed R. Aging, abstinence, and medical risk factors in the prediction of neuropsychologic deficit among long-term alcoholics. Arch Gen Psychiatry 1984;41:710–718.

207. Salmon DP, Butters N, Heindel WC. Alcoholic dementia and related disorders. In: Parks RW, Zec RF, Wilson RS, eds. Neuropsychology of Alzheimer's disease and other dementias. New York: Oxford University Press, 1993:186–209.

208. Tartar RE, Edwards KL, Van Thiel DH. Perspective and rationale for neuropsychological assessment of medical disease. In: Tartar RE, Van

Thiel DH, Edwards KL, eds. Medical neuropsychology: the impact of disease on behavior. New York: Plenum, 1988;1–10.

209. Katzman R, Lasker B, Bernstein N. Advances in the diagnosis of dementia, accuracy of diagnosis, and consequences of misdiagnosis of disorders causing dementia. Aging and the Brain 1988;32:17–62.

210. McConnell H, Duffy J. Neuropsychiatric aspects of medical therapies. In: Coffey CE, Cummings JL, eds. Textbook of geriatric neuropsychiatry. Washington, D.C.: American Psychiatric Association Press, 1994;549–574.

211. Taylor JL, Tinklenberg JR. Cognitive impairment and benzodiazepines. In: Meltzer HY, ed. Psychopharmacology: the third generation of progress. New York: Raven Press, 1987;1449–1454.

212. Bixler EO, Kales A, Manfredi RL, et al. Next-day memory impairment with triazolam use. Lancet 1991;337:827–831.

213. Golombok S, Moodley P, Lader M. Cognitive impairment in long-term benzodiazepine users. Psychol Med 1988;18:365–374.

214. Petursson H, Gudjonsson GH, Lader MH. Psychosomatic performance during withdrawal from long-term benzodiazepine treatment. Psychopharmacology 1983;81:345–349.

215. Pomara N, Deptula D, Singh R, et al. Cognitive toxicity of benzodiazepines in the elderly. In: Salzman C, Lebowitz BD, eds. Anxiety in the elderly: treatment and research. New York: Springer-Verlag, 1991;175–196.

216. Nikaido AM, Ellinwood EH Jr, Heatherly DG, et al. Age-related increase in CNS sensitivity to benzodiazepines as assessed by task difficulty. Psychopharmacology 1990;100:90–97.

217. Smith DB, Mattson RH, Cramer JA, et al. Results of a nationwide VA cooperative study comparing the efficacy and toxicity of carbamazepine, phenobarbitol, phenytoin, and primidone. Epilepsia 1987;28 (Suppl 3):S50–S58.

218. Zec RF. Neuropsychological functioning in Alzheimer's disease. In: Parks RW, Zec RF, Wilson RS, eds. Neuropsychology of Alzheimer's disease and other dementias. New York: Oxford University Press, 1993:3–80.

219. Moss MB, Albert MS, Butters N, Payne M. Differential patterns of memory loss among patients with Alzheimer's disease, Huntington's disease, and alcoholic Korsakoff's syndrome. Arch Neurol 1986;43: 239–246.

220. Wilson RS, Bacan LD, Fox JH, Kazniak AW. Primary memory and secondary memory in dementia of the Alzheimer type. J Clin Neuropsychol 1983;5:337–344.

221. Kramer JH, Delis DC, Blusewicz MJ, Brandt J, Ober BA, Strauss M. Verbal memory errors in Alzheimer's and Huntington's dementias. Developmental Neuropsychology 1988;4:1–5.

222. Albert MS, Butters N, Brandt J. Patterns of remote memory in amnesic and demented patients. Arch Neurol 1981;38:495–500.

223. Wilson RS, Kazniak AW, Fox JH. Remote memory in senile dementia. Cortex 1981;17:41–48.

224. Beatty WW, Salmon DP, Butters N, Heindel WC, Granholm EP. Retrograde amnesia in patients with Alzheimer's disease or Huntington's disease. Neurobiol Aging 1987;9:181–186.

225. Solomon PR, Levine E, Bein T, Pendlebury WW. Disruption of classical conditioning in patients with Alzheimer's disease. Neurobiol Aging 1991;12:283–287.

226. Miller NE. The measurement of mood in senile brain disease: examiner ratings and self-ratings. In: Cole J, Barret J, eds. Psychopathology in the aged. New York: Raven Press, 1980:97–118.

227. Haxby JV, Duara R, Grady CL, Cutler NR, Rapoport SI. Relations between neuropsychological and cerebral metabolic asymmetries in early Alzheimer's disease. J Cereb Blood Flow Metab 1985;5: 193–200.

228. Friedland RP, Budinger TF, Koss E, Ober BA. Alzheimer's disease: anterior-posterior and lateral hemispheric alterations in cortical glucose utilization. Neurosci Lett 1985;53:235–240.

229. Parks RW, Haxby JV, Grady CL. Positron emission tomography in Alzheimer's disease. In: Parks RW, Zec RF, Wilson RS, eds. Neuropsychology of Alzheimer's disease and other dementias. New York: Oxford University Press, 1993:459–488.

230. Massman PJ, Delis DC, Filoteo JV, Butters N, Salmon DP, Demadura TL. Mechanisms of spatial impairment in Alzheimer's disease subgroups: differential breakdown of directed attention to global-local stimuli. Neuropsychology 1993;7:172–181.

231. Butters N, Tarlow S. Cermak LS, Sax D. A comparison of the information processing deficits in patients with Huntington's chorea and Korsakoff's syndrome. Cortex 1976;12:134–144.

232. Butters N, Wolfe J, Granholm E, Martone M. An assessment of verbal recall, recognition and fluency abilities in patients with Huntington's disease. Cortex 1986;22:11–32.

233. Albert MS, Butters N, Brandt J. Development of remote memory loss in patients with Huntington's disease. J Clin Neuropsychol 1981;3:1–12.

234. Gustafson L, Brun A, Risberg J. Frontal lobe dementia of the non-Alzheimer type. In Wurtman RJ, ed. Advances in Neurology. Vol. 51: Alzheimer's disease. New York: Raven Press, 1990.

235. Knopman DS, Mastri AR, Frey WH, Sung JH, Rustan T. Dementia lacking distinctive histologic features: a common non-Alzheimer degenerative dementia. Neurology 1990;40:251–256.

236. Neary D, Snowden JS. Dementia of the frontal lobe type. J Neurol Neurosurg Psychiatry 1991;51:353–356.

237. Sungaila P, Crockett DJ. Dementia and the frontal lobes. In: Parks RW, Zec RF, Wilson RS, eds. Neuropsychology of Alzheimer's disease and other dementias. Oxford: Oxford University Press, 1993:235–264.

238. Shimamura AP, Janowski JS, Squire LR. What is the role of frontal damage in memory disorders? In: Levin HS, Eisenberg HM, Benton AL, eds. Frontal lobe function and dysfunction. Oxford: Oxford University Press, 1991:173–195.

239. Niederehe G. Depression and memory impairment in the aged. In: Poon LW, ed. Clinical memory assessment of older adults. Washington, DC: American Psychological Association, 1987.

240. Weingartner, H, Grafman J, Boutelle W, Kaye W, Martin P. Forms of memory failure. Science 1981;221:380–382.

241. Caine ED. The neuropsychology of depression: the pseudodementia syndrome. In: Grant I, Adams KM, eds. Neuropsychological assessment of neuropsychiatric disorders. New York: Oxford University Press, 1986:221–243.

242. Niederehe G, Camp CJ. Signal detection analysis of recognition memory in depressed elderly. Exp Aging Res 1985;11:207–213.

243. Frith CD, Stevens M, Johnstone EC, et al. Effects of ECT and depression on various aspects of memory. Br J Psychiatry 1983;142: 610–617.

244. DuPont RM, Jernigan TL, Gillin JC, Butters N, Delis DC, Hesselink JR. Presence of subcortical signal hyperintensities in bipolar patients detected by magnetic resonance imaging. Psychiatr Res 1987;21: 357–358.

245. Craik FIM, Rabinowitz JC. Age differences in the acquisition and use of verbal information. In: Bouma H, Bouwhuis DG, eds. Attention and performance X. Hillsdale, NJ: Erlbaum & Associates, 1984.

246. Craik FIM. Age differences in remembering. In: Squire LR, Butters N, eds. Neuropsychology of memory. New York: Guilford, 1984:3–12.

247. Cerella J, Poon LW, Williams DM. Aging and the complexity hypothesis. In: Poon LW, ed. Aging in the 1980's. Washington, DC: American Psychological Association, 1980.

248. Albert MS, Duffy FH, Naeser MA. Nonlinear changes in cognition and their neurophysiologic correlates. Can J Psychol 1987;41: 141–157.

249. Craik FIM, Byrd M, Swanson JM. Patterns of memory loss in three elderly patients. Psychol Aging 1987;2:79–86.

250. Albert MS. Cognitive function. In: Albert MS, Moss MB, eds. Geriatric neuropsychology. New York: Guilford, 1988:33–53.

251. Albert MS. Age-related changes in cognition. Presentation at the 3rd Annual West Coast Neuropsychology Conference, San Diego, April 9–11, 1994.

18

EMOTIONAL DISORDERS ASSOCIATED WITH HEMISPHERIC DYSFUNCTION

Kenneth M. Heilman and Dawn Bowers

Because the brain mediates emotion, diseases that affect the brain can induce emotional changes. In this chapter we discuss the effects of focal brain lesions on emotions. Although disorders that affect the neurotransmitter systems may also profoundly influence emotions, these are not covered in this chapter. In addition, seizures and degenerative disorders, including disorders of the basal ganglia, can also affect emotions. The behavioral effects of these disorders are described in more detail in other chapters.

There are two major aspects to emotions: cognitive/communicative and experiential. Although we discuss both of these aspects of emotion, we begin this chapter with a discussion of cognitive and communicative disorders.

EMOTIONAL COGNITION AND COMMUNICATION

Comprehension

Although patients with psychiatric disorders and seizures may experience emotions even in the absence of an exciting event, for most normal people, emotions are induced by environmental events or memories of these. The environmental events include: (*a*) seeing emotional displays and gestures of others, such as emotional facial displays and scenes; (*b*) hearing emotional prosody; and (*c*) hearing words.

Many other sensory and perceptual disorders in the visual and auditory system (e.g., blindness) may lead to impaired comprehension of the emotional significance of environmental events, but these are not specific for emotion and are not discussed here.

Disorders of Emotional Facial Recognition

Several investigators studied patients who had right-hemisphere stroke and found that, when compared with controls with left-hemisphere damage, patients with right-hemisphere damage were impaired at recognizing emotional facial displays (1–3).

The right hemisphere plays a dominant role in many visual-spatial and visual-perceptual activities. For example, patients with right-hemisphere disease are impaired in the ability to tell if two faces, previously unknown to the patient, are the same or different people (4). Therefore, the inability of patients to recognize emotional faces may be related to a visual-perceptual defect. Bowers and co-workers (5) studied subjects with right- and left-hemisphere brain damage and equated their patient groups for visual-perceptual abilities. These investigators found that when compared with controls, subjects with right-hemisphere brain damage were still impaired at naming, selecting, and discriminating facial emotions. The critical factor appeared to be impairment of "categorizing" facial emotional expressions.

Studies using patients with callosal section (6) and selective hemispheric anesthesia (7) support the ablative studies. In addition, tachistoscopic studies of normal subjects have also supported the special role of the right hemisphere in processing facial emotional gestures (8, 9). Although the mechanism underlying this hemispheric asymmetry is unknown, we (10) have proposed that the right hemisphere contains stores of prototypic facial emotional icons or facial emotional representations.

Blonder et al. (11) had patients with right- and left-hemisphere damage listen to computer-generated sentences describing emotional gestures, including facial expressions. These investigators found that, when compared with controls who had left-hemisphere- and nonhemisphere brain damage, patients with right-hemisphere brain damage were impaired at deriving the target emotions from the verbal descriptions. Because the emotional displays were described verbally, the impaired performance of the group with right-hemisphere brain damage could not be accounted for by visuospatial perceptual deficits. Blonder et al. (11) also presented subjects with sentences where the emotion had to be inferred from a verbal description (e.g., "after you drink the water, you see the sign"). In this emotionally semantic inferential task there were no significant differences between the right- and left-hemisphere-damaged subjects, suggesting that emotional knowledge or emotional semantics was not lateralized.

Bowers et al. (12) provided further evidence that the right hemisphere contains representations of facial expressions. We studied right- and left-hemisphere-damaged subjects' ability to perform facial emotion and object imagery tasks. If such patients are unable to access a hypothetical store of facial emotional representations, then they should not only be unable to recognize and discriminate emotional facial expressions, but also should be unable to answer questions about facial and emotional expressions that require subjects to image these emotional faces. Although the right hemisphere was more impaired at facial emotion imagery than object imagery, the group with left-hemisphere brain damage was more impaired in object imagery than in facial emotional imagery.

Ekman and Friesen (13) and Izard (14) have suggested there are a finite number of emotional facial expressions and that these emotional faces are universally comprehended. Their results suggest that knowledge of emotional facial expressions are not learned but rather are innate. For example, infants can recognize their mother's emotional faces, suggesting that knowledge of emotional faces is inborn. Moreover, these studies of patients with brain damage and normal subjects suggest that in the human brain the right hemisphere contains inborn representations of species' typical emotional facial expressions. Although the exact cerebral location of these representations remain unknown, most patients with impaired comprehension and discrimination of facial emotional expressions have temporal parietal lesions. Single-cell recordings of the monkey's temporal cortex reveal cells that respond selectively to emotional faces (15, 16). Intraoperative stimulation of patients undergoing epilepsy surgery has also implicated the right temporal lobe in the storage of these facial emotional representations (17).

In an earlier study (10), we described a patient who was unable to name emotional faces or point to an emotional face named by the examiner. However, this patient could tell if two faces displayed the same or different emotions. This patient had a deep lesion interfering with the white matter tracts leading to the corpus callosum. We proposed that this lesion caused a disconnection, functionally disassociating the speech and language areas of the left hemisphere from the facial and emotional representations stored in the right hemisphere. Rapcsak et al. (18) have reported a similar case. However, the case studied by Rapcsak et al. had a temporal lobe lesion.

Disorders of Emotional Scene Recognition

Unfortunately, not much research has been performed on emotional scene/recognition in patients with brain impairments. Gardner et al. (19) studied patients with right- and left-hemisphere disease by showing them cartoons. The groups were equally impaired in selecting the most humorous of a group of cartoons; however, patients with left-hemisphere disease in general performed better in the

cartoons without captions. DeKosky et al. (1) also presented right- and left-hemisphere-damaged subjects cartoons. These cartoons were of scenes that typically were associated with one of four emotions (happy, angry, sad, indifferent). For example, there was a cartoon of children playing tic tac toe on a painted wall as the mother comes home.

Although patients with right-hemisphere brain damage were more impaired than those with left-hemisphere damage, when the groups were equated for visual perceptual disorders, there was no significant difference between the groups. As mentioned earlier, when Blonder et al. (11) described emotional scenes, there was no difference between patients with left- and right-hemisphere brain damage. Therefore, patients with right-hemisphere damage may be impaired in interpreting emotional scenes; however, the defect is more likely to be related to a visual-perceptive disorder rather than to a disorder in a specific emotional system.

Disorders of Emotional Prosody

Speech prosody is conveyed by changes of pitch, amplitude, tempo, and rhythm. English speakers may use prosody as a syntactic marker. For example, in declarative sentences the pitch drops at the end of a sentence and in interrogative sentences it rises. However, English speakers use prosody most commonly to convey emotional content (20, 21). Heilman et al. (22) and Tucker et al. (23) had subjects with brain damage listen to sentences whose literal meaning was emotionally neutral. However, these sentences were intoned with four different emotional prosodies (happy, sad, angry, and indifferent). Patients with right- or left-hemisphere damage were asked to identify the emotional tone of the speaker. They were asked to base their selection not on the words the actor said but rather on the emotional tone of the actor's voice. Patients with right-hemisphere disease who had predominantly temporoparietal lesions performed worse on this task than those with left-hemisphere lesions, suggesting that the right hemisphere has a special role in decoding emotional prosody. Although Ross (24) reported similar findings, Schlanger and colleagues (25) could not find differences in the comprehension of emotional prosody between their groups with right- and left-hemisphere brain damage. Unfortunately, only a small minority of the patients of Schlanger et al. had cortical lesions that affected the temporoparietal region.

Weintraub et al. (26) studied right-hemisphere-damaged patients' ability to comprehend the prosody that is used for syntax. The researchers found that right-hemisphere-damaged patients were more impaired than normal controls. The results of this study suggest that the right hemisphere may not have a specific role in the comprehension of emotional prosody. Rather, right-hemisphere damage probably causes a global perceptual disturbance that may interfere with the comprehension of all types of prosody. Unfortunately, Weintraub et al. did not study patients with left hemisphere brain damage. Heilman and his co-workers (27), however, studied right- and left-hemisphere-damaged patients' ability to comprehend both emotional and syntactic prosody. In the syntactic prosody task, both right- and left-hemisphere damaged groups were equally impaired. However, on the emotional prosody task, the patients with right-hemisphere brain damage performed significantly worse than those with left-hemisphere brain damage, suggesting that whereas both hemispheres may be important in comprehending propositional prosody, the right hemisphere is dominant in comprehending emotional prosody.

Further support for a special role of the right hemisphere in comprehending emotional prosody comes from studies of normal subjects using dichotic listening. When subjects were asked for the words they heard, the subjects reported more words that were broadcast to the right ear (left hemisphere) than they heard words that were broadcast to the left ear (right hemisphere). However, when the subjects were asked to detect the mood of the speaker, as determined by prosody, left ear (right hemisphere) recall was superior to the right ear (left hemisphere) recall (28).

In our discussion of naming emotional faces, we noted that the inability to do so can be caused by at least two mechanisms, a disconnection of the facial emotional representations from the left-hemisphere speech systems and destruction of the facial emotional representations. The inability to name an emotion while listening to emotionally intoned speech may be induced by a similar mechanism. Tucker et al. (23) studied patients with right-hemisphere temporoparietal lesions and found that even when they did not have to verbally name or classify the prosody, they were still unable to discriminate between the same and different emotional intonations. Based on these studies, we believe that the right hemisphere also contains representations or a lexicon of emotional prosodic expressions.

Disorders of Verbal Comprehension

Several studies have attempted to learn if the right hemisphere plays a special role in deriving emotional meaning from verbal language. Morris and co-workers (29) studied subjects with right- and left-hemisphere brain damage and their ability to comprehend both the denotative and the connotative meaning of emotional and unemotional words. They found no significant differences. Etcoff (3) also studied these two groups by presenting pairs of emotional words and requiring her subjects to judge the similarity of the emotional states indicated by these words. She also found that patients with right-hemisphere brain damage did not differ from controls. Several investigators have also given patients with right-hemisphere brain damage short propositional sentences and found they were not impaired compared to controls (2, 27). As we discussed previously, Blonder et al. (11) presented patients with right- and left-hemisphere brain damage tape-recorded sentences where the nature of the emotion had to be inferred from the situational context. Both groups performed comparably. Blonder et al. (11) also did not find any difference between the two groups. However, Borod et al. (30) gave three measures of lexical emotion perception to subjects with right- and left-hemisphere brain

damage. In one task, they presented clusters of three words and asked the participants to name or point to an emotion that was best represented by each cluster. They also gave sentences and word pairs, and the subjects had to state whether the word pairs represented the same or different emotions. Borod et al. demonstrated that patients with right-hemisphere brain damage had deficits in processing emotion on these lexically based tasks. It is not clear why the results of Borod et al. are different from those of other investigators who did not find hemispheric differences. Borod et al. screened out all patients with impaired reading; perhaps this procedure created a sampling bias.

Several studies have found that the auditory and reading comprehension of patients with left-hemisphere brain damage may be improved by the use of emotional words (31, 32). Although these findings seem to support the postulate that the right hemisphere contains a special lexicon for emotional words, emotional words may also increase arousal and interest. Increased arousal and interest may be the critical factor in the improved comprehension.

Emotional Semantics

Certain environmental events can predictably lead to one or two specific emotions. For example, loss leads to sadness (or anger), gain to happiness, and potential physical harm to fear (or anger). The knowledge of the type of circumstance that may be associated with an emotion we term emotional semantics.

Although patients with right-hemisphere brain damage may have problems understanding environmental stimuli that may lead to emotion (because they have an impairment of facial emotional representations, emotional prosodic representations, or even an emotional verbal lexicon), it appears that their emotional semantics may nevertheless be intact (11). Because unilateral hemispheric disease does not impair emotional semantics, emotional knowledge may be widely distributed and bi-hemispheric. Diseases that impair widely distributed networks such as Alzheimer's disease may impair emotional semantics. Bortz et al. (33) presented patients with Alzheimer's disease and controls with complex emotional scenes. The Alzheimer's patients appeared to be impaired in being able to label scenes and match facial expressions to scenes, suggesting a defect in emotional semantics.

EMOTIONAL EXPRESSION

Emotions may be expressed through speech (e.g., words and prosody) and gesture (e.g., emotional faces).

Disorders of Facial Expression

Buck and Duffy (34) reported that compared to controls with left-hemisphere brain damage, patients with right-hemisphere brain damage appeared to display less emotional facial expressions when viewing emotion-inducing slides than did controls. Buck and Duffy's study has been replicated by Borod et al. (35) and Kent et al. (36). In a more naturalistic setting, Blonder et al. (37) videotaped patients in their homes and found patients with right-hemisphere damage were less facially expressive than those with left-hemisphere damage. In a study of deaf signers, Bellugi et al. (38) noted that right-hemisphere lesions are associated with dramatic impairments in the spontaneous use of facial affective expressions, but the facial expressions used with language remain unchanged. Bellugi et al. reported the opposite pattern in deaf signers who had left-hemisphere lesions. However, using a more formal facial muscle scoring system several investigators have found no right/left hemispheric asymmetries (39, 40). The reasons for these discrepancies are unknown. Richardson and colleagues (in preparation) suggest and provide evidence for the hypothesis that hemispheric asymmetries of emotional facial expressions may be related to the means in which the facial affect is initiated, such that when facial emotions are produced in response to verbal commands, there may be no differences. However, when facial expressions are induced by viewing emotional scenes, other emotional faces, or emotional prosody, there are right/left asymmetries, with patients who have right-hemisphere brain impairments being less expressive.

Studies of normal subjects revealed that the left half of the face, controlled by the right hemisphere, is more expressive than the right half of the face (41, 42).

Prosody

Tucker et al. (23) asked patients to emotionally intone linguistically neutral sentences and noted that patients with right-hemisphere brain damage were severely impaired. Instead of intoning a sentence, they often denoted a target emotion by changing the words in the sentence. Whereas most of the cases of Tucker et al. (23) also had emotional prosodic comprehension disturbances, Ross and Mesulam (43) described two patients who could not express emotional prosody in speech but could comprehend emotional prosody. Ross (24) also described patients who had impaired comprehension but spared repetition. Ross posited that the affective prosodic speech disturbances seen with right-hemisphere lesions could mirror the aphasic syndromes seen with left-hemisphere lesions.

Further support for the important role the right hemisphere plays in mediating prosodic expression comes from the observation of patients with left-hemisphere brain damage who, in spite of being verbally nonfluent, are able to prosodically intone stereotypic verbal expressions with a variety of appropriate emotional intonations.

Verbal Expression

In addition to being able to intone verbal expressions with emotional prosody, Hughlings Jackson (44) observed that nonfluent aphasics may become very fluent when using explicatives. Hughlings Jackson posited that the right hemisphere may be mediating this activity. Bloom et al. (45) noted that right-hemisphere-damaged patients use fewer emotional words in their spontaneous speech. Landis

et al. (32) and Roeltgen (46) showed that aphasic patients were able to write emotional words better than nonemotional words. However, the role of the right hemisphere in producing emotional words remains to be fully investigated.

Whereas the right hemisphere may contain a limited lexicon (store) for emotional words, overwhelming research clearly demonstrates left-hemisphere superiority for mediating speech output. If, as discussed, the right hemisphere is important for controlling the emotional prosodic aspects of speech, and the left is responsible for producing the phonology and the order in which they are produced (lexical syntactic aspects of speech), how are these two systems integrated? Ross (24) proposed that the propositional and prosodic elements are integrated at the brainstem level. However, it would appear that the integration of these two systems is a highly skilled activity that may require integration at the cortical level. Speedie et al (47) demonstrate that integration of the propositional and emotional messages probably occurs intrahemispherically.

Emotional Moods

Several investigators noted that patients with hemispheric lesions appeared to have a change in their emotional mood. For example, Goldstein (48) noted that patients with left-hemisphere lesions who were aphasic often appeared depressed, anxious, and agitated. Goldstein called this constellation of mood changes the "catastrophic reaction." In contrast, Babinski (49) as well as Hécaen et al. (50) and Denny-Brown et al. (51) noted that patients with right-hemisphere disease often appear to be indifferent or even mildly euphoric despite their disability, including hemiparesis. Gainotti (52) studied 160 patients with lateralized brain damage. He also noted that right-hemisphere damage was often associated with indifference and left-hemisphere damage was associated with depression and anxious agitation. Right-hemisphere lesions are often associated with anosognosia (denial of an illness), and Gainotti thought that the right-hemisphere-damaged patient's anosognosia may have been related to their indifference and that the catastrophic reaction was a normal response to the serious defects associated with left-hemisphere strokes. Terzian (53) and Rossi and Rodadini (54) studied patients undergoing barbiturate-induced hemispheric anesthesia (Wada test). They noted that injection into the left carotid, which anesthetizes the left hemisphere, was also associated with a catastrophic reaction, whereas injections into the right carotid (which induces right-hemisphere anesthesia) were associated with a euphoric response. Gilmore et al. (55) demonstrated that whereas right-hemisphere anesthesia is often associated with anosognosia, left-hemisphere anesthesia is not, thereby providing some support for Gainotti's hypothesis.

As we have discussed, patients with right-hemisphere disease have disorders of emotional expression. Those with left-hemisphere disease, however, rely more heavily on emotional expression. Therefore, patients with right-hemisphere disease who have disorders of emotional expression may appear to be indifferent and those with left hemisphere disease who rely more heavily on emotional expression may appear to have heightened emotions. Gasparrini et al. (56) administered a Minnesota Multi-Phasic Inventory (MMPI) to patients with right- and left-hemisphere dysfunction. The MMPI does not require a patient to express affectively intoned speech or to make emotional faces. It has been widely used as an index of affective experience and mood. Gasparrini et al. found that patients with left-hemisphere lesions had a marked elevation of the depression scale and patients with right-hemisphere disease did not. These findings suggest that the emotional moods of patients with hemispheric disease cannot be solely attributed to difficulties in perceiving or expressing affective stimuli.

Benson (57) and Robinson and Szetela (58) noticed that most patients with left-hemisphere brain damage who have a depressive response had left anterior perisylvian lesions with nonfluent aphasia. Starkstein et al. (59) studied the relationship between strokes and depression and found that about one-third of stroke patients had a major and long-lasting depression. He found that not only were these depressions associated with cortical lesions but also with subcortical lesions, especially in the region of the left caudate. The cortical lesions that cause the most severe depressions were located in the frontal pole. Many of his patients also had anxiety associated with depression. In addition, he found that right-hemisphere lesions, especially in the frontal lobes, were associated with indifference or even euphoria.

In contrast to these studies, House et al. (60) reported that depression could be seen with right-hemisphere disease and may be underdiagnosed because patients with right-hemisphere brain damage, as we discussed, have emotional communicative disorders. Ross (personal communication) believes that when vegetative signs of depression such as loss of appetite and sleep are assessed, there are no hemispheric asymmetries of depression. Bowers et al. (in preparation) studied patients with right- and left-hemisphere brain damage and assessed them for depression with a Zung Depression Inventory and the Self-Assessment Mannequin. They found no differences in the rate or severity of depression between the patients with left- and right-hemisphere lesions.

PSEUDOBULBAR AFFECT

Patients with hemispheric lesions may laugh or cry or both without feeling sad, happy, or being exposed to something funny. Unlike normal emotional expressions, these outbursts are stereotypic and do not have different degrees of intensity. Pseudobulbar laughing and crying are usually associated with lesions that interrupt the cortical bulbar motor pathways bilaterally and thereby release reflex mechanisms for facial expression. Wilson (61) thought that there was an area in the pons that was responsible for emotional facial expression, and when this area became disinhibited from cortical control, one saw the pseudobulbar affect. In contrast, Poeck (62) thought that the center for the

control of emotional expressions was located higher in the diencephalon.

It is not known why some patients predominantly cry and others laugh. However, Sackheim et al. (63) reported that, although most patients have bilateral lesions, when the lesion is larger in the right hemisphere, there is a greater chance for laughter to ensue. When the lesion is larger in the left hemisphere, however, crying is more likely to occur.

TREATMENT

The first goal of treatment should always be to learn the etiology that caused the focal dysfunction and then to treat the underlying disease to prevent further damage or to reverse the damage. The second important part of treatment is education of the patient and family. Although patients typically understand that weakness and language disorders may be related to focal neurological disease, emotional disorders often are attributed to psychodynamic factors. The patient and family need to focus on the appropriate problem. Patients with emotional communicative disorders can use alternative strategies. Therefore, when communicating an emotion to a patient with a right-hemisphere dysfunction, primarily propositional speech should be used. When communicating emotions to patients with left-hemisphere lesions, emotional faces and prosody should be used. In cases of mood changes (e.g., depression) drug therapy (e.g., antidepressants) may be helpful. Patients who have left-hemisphere brain damage and depression may be helped with antidepressants. In addition, pseudobulbar affect may also be helped with antidepressants (see Chapter 11).

References

1. DeKosky S, Heilman KM, Bowers D, Valenstein E. Recognition and discrimination of emotional faces and pictures. Brain Lang 1980;9: 206–214.
2. Cicone M, Waper W, Gardner H. Sensitivity to emotional expressions and situation in organic patients. Cortex 1980;16:145–158.
3. Etcoff N. Perceptual and conceptual organization of facial emotions. Brain Cogn 1984;3:385–412.
4. Benton AL, Van Allen MW. Impairment in facial recognition in patients with cerebral disease. Cortex 1968;4:344–358.
5. Bowers D, Bauer RM, Coslett HB, Heilman KM. Processing of faces by patients with unilateral hemispheric lesions. I. Dissociation between judgments of facial affect and facial identity. Brain Cogn 1985;4: 258–272.
6. Benowitz L, Bear D, Mesulam M, Rosenthal R, Zaidel E, Sperry W. Non-verbal sensitivity following lateralized cerebral injury. Cortex 1983;19:5–12.
7. Ahern G, Schumer D, Kleefield J, et al. Right hemisphere advantage in evaluating emotional facial expressions. Cortex 1991;27:193–202.
8. Suberi M, McKeever W. Differential right hemisphere memory storage of emotional and nonemotional faces. Neuropsychologia 1977;15: 737–768.
9. Ley R, Bryden M. Hemispheric differences in recognizing faces and emotions. Brain Lang 1979;1:127–138.
10. Bowers D, Heilman KM. Dissociation of affective and nonaffective faces: a case study. J Clin Neuropsychol 1984;6:367–379.
11. Blonder LX, Bowers D, Heilman KM. The role of the right hemisphere on emotional communication. Brain 1991;114:1115–1127.

12. Bowers D, Blonder DX, Feinberg T, Heilman KM. Differential impact of right and left hemisphere lesions on facial emotion and object imagery. Brain 1991;114:2593–2609.
13. Ekman P, Friesen WV. Facial action coding system. Palo Alto, CA: Consulting Psychologists Press, 1978.
14. Izard CE. Human emotions. New York: Plenum Press, 1977.
15. Baylis G, Rolls E, Leonard C. Selectivity between faces in the responses of a population of neurons in the superior temporal sulcus of the monkey. Brain Res 1985;342:91–102.
16. Leonard C, Rolls E, Wilson A. Neurons in the amygdala of the monkey with responses selective for faces. Behav Brain Res 1985;15:159–176.
17. Fried I, Mateer C, Ojemann G, Wohns R, Fedio P. Organization of visuospatial functions in human cortex. Brain 1982;105:349–371.
18. Rapcsak S, Kasniak A, Rubins A. Anomia for facial expressions: evidence for a category specific visual verbal disconnection. Neuropsychologia 1989;27:1031–1041.
19. Gardner H, Ling PK, Flam I, Silverman J. Comprehension and appreciation of humorous material following brain damage. Brain 1975;98:399–412.
20. Paul H. Principien der Sprachgeschichte. 4th ed. Germany: Niemeyer, 1909.
21. Monrad-Krohn G. The prosodic quality of speech and its disorders. Acta Psychol Scand 1947;22:225–265.
22. Heilman KM, Scholes R, Watson RT. Auditory affective agnosia: disturbed comprehension of affective speech. J Neurol Neurosurg Psychiatry 1975;38:69–72.
23. Tucker DM, Watson RT, Heilman KM. Affective discrimination and evocation in patients with right parietal disease. Neurology 1977;17:947–950.
24. Ross ED. The aprosodias: functional-anatomic organization of the affective components of language in the right hemisphere. Ann Neurol 1981;38:561–589.
25. Schlanger BB, Schlanger P, Gerstmann LJ. The perception of emotionally toned sentences by right-hemisphere damaged and aphasic subjects. Brain Lang 1976;3:396–403.
26. Weintraub S, Mesulam MM, Kramer L. Disturbances in prosody. Arch Neurol 1981;38:742–744.
27. Heilman KM, Bowers D, Speedie L, Coslett B. Comprehension of affective and nonaffective speech. Neurology 1984;34:917–921.
28. Haggard MP, Parkinson AM. Stimulus and task factors as determinants of ear advantages. QJ Exp Psychol 1971;23:168–177.
29. Morris M, Bowers D, Verfaellie M, et al. Lexical denotation and connotation in right and left hemisphere damaged patients [Abstract]. J Clin Exp Neuropsychol 1992;14:105.
30. Borod J, Andelman F, Obler L, Tweedy JR, Welkowitz J. Right hemispheric specialization for the identification of emotional words and sentences: evidence from stroke patients. Neuropsychologia 1992;30:827–844.
31. Boller F, Cole M, Vtunski P, Patterson M, Kim Y. Paralinguistic aspects of auditory comprehension in aphasia. Brain Lang 1979;7:164–174.
32. Landis T, Graves R, Goodglass H. Aphasic reading and writing: possible evidence for right hemisphere participation. Cortex 1982;18:105–122.
33. Bortz JJ, Rapcsak SZ, Kaszniak AW, Butters MA. Perception and interpretation of affect in Alzheimer's disease. J Clin Exp Neuropsychol 1993;15:28.
34. Buck R, Duffy RJ. Nonverbal communication of affect in brain damaged patients. Cortex 1980;16:351–362.
35. Borod J, Koff E, Perlman-Lorch J, Nicholas M. The expression and perception of facial emotions in brain damaged patients. Neuropsychologia 1986;24:169–180.
36. Kent J, Borod JC, Koff E, Welkowitz J, Alpert M. Posed facial and emotional expression in brain-damaged patients. Int J Neurosci 1988;43:81–87.
37. Blonder L, Burns A, Bowers D, Moore R, Heilman K. Right hemisphere expressivity during natural conversation [Abstract]. J Clin Exp Neuropsychol 1991;13:85.
38. Bellugi U, Corina D, Normal F, Klima E, Reilly J. Differential specialization for linguistic facial expressions in left and right lesioned deaf signers. Paper presented at the 27th Annual Meeting of the Academy of Aphasia, 1988.
39. Mammucari A, Caltagirone C, Ekman P, et al. Spontaneous facial expression of emotions in brain damaged patients. Cortex 1988;24:521–533.
40. Caltagirone C, Ekman P, Friesen W, et al. Posed emotional facial expressions in brain damaged patients. Cortex 1988;25:653–663.
41. Sackheim H, Gur R, Saucy M. Emotions are expressed more intensely on the left side of the face. Science 1978;202:434–436.
42. Campbell R. Asymmetries in interpreting and expressing a posed facial expression. Cortex 1978;14:327–342.
43. Ross ED, Mesulam MM. Dominant language functions of the right hemisphere? Prosody and emotional gesturing. Arch Neurol 1979;36:144–148.
44. Taylor J, ed. Selected writings of John Hughlings Jackson. London: Hodder and Stoughton, 1932.
45. Bloom R, Borod JC, Ober L, Gerstman L. Impact of emotional content on discourse production in patients with unilateral brain damage. Brain Lang 1992;42:153–164.
46. Roeltgen DP, Sevush S, Heilman KM. Phonological agraphia: writing by the lexical semantic route. Neurology 1983;33:755–765.
47. Speedie LJ, Coslett HB, Heilman KM. Repetition of affective prosody in mixed transcortical aphasia. Arch Neurol 1984;41:268–270.
48. Goldstein K. Language and language disturbances. New York: Grune & Stratton, 1948.
49. Babinski J. Contribution l'etude des troubles mentaux dans l'hemisplegie organique cerebrale (anosognosie). Rev Neurol (Paris) 1914;27:845–848.
50. Hécaen H, Ajuriagurra J, de Massonet J. Les troubles visuoconstuctifs par lesion parieto-occipitale droit. Encephale 1951;40:122–179.
51. Denny-Brown D, Meyer JS, Horenstein S. The significance of perceptual rivalry resulting from parietal lesions. Brain 1952;75:434–471.
52. Gainotti G. Emotional behavior and hemispheric side of lesion. Cortex 1972;8:41–55.
53. Terzian H. Behavioral and EEG effects of intracarotid sodium amytal injections. Acta Neurochirur (Vienna) 1964;12:230–240.
54. Rossi GS, Rodadini G. Experimental analysis of cerebral dominance in man. In: Millikan C, Darley FL, eds. Brain mechanisms underlying speech and language. New York: Grune & Stratton, 1967.
55. Gilmore RL, Heilman KM, Schmidt RP, Fennell EB. Anosognosia during WADA testing. Neurology 1992;42:925–927.
56. Gasparrini WG, Spatz P, Heilman KM, Coolidge FL. Hemispheric asymmetries of affective processing as determined by the Minnesota multiphasic personality inventory. J Neurol Neurosurg Psychiatry 1978;41:470–473.
57. Benson DF. Psychiatric aspects of aphasia. In: Benson DF, ed. Aphasia, alexia, and agraphia. New York: Churchill Livingstone, 1979.
58. Robinson RG, Szetela B. Mood change following left hemisphere brain injury. Ann Neurol 1981;9:447–453.
59. Starkstein SE, Robinson RG, Price TR. Comparison of cortical and subcortical lesions in the production of poststroke mood disorders. Brain 1987;110:1045–1059.
60. House A, Dennis M, Warlow C, Hawton K, Molyneux A. Mood disorders after stroke and their relation to lesion location. Brain 1990;113:1113–1129.
61. Wilson SAK. Some problems in neurology. II: Pathological laughing and crying. J Neurol Psychopathol 1924;16:299–333.
62. Poeck K. Pathophysiology of emotional disorders associated with brain damage. In: Vinken PJ, Bruyn GW, eds. Handbook of neurology, vol. 3. New York: Elsevier Science Publishers, 1969.
63. Sackheim HA, Greenberg MS, Weiman AL, Gur RC, Hungerbuhler JP, Geschwind N. Hemispheric asymmetry in the expression of positive and negative emotion: neurologic evidence. Arch Neurol 1982;39:210–218.

19

FRONTAL LOBE SYNDROMES

Joaquín M. Fuster

In the human, the cortex of the frontal lobe comprises over one-third of the totality of the cerebral cortex. It has three major anatomical aspects: (*a*) dorsolateral, (*b*) medial, and (*c*) inferior or orbital. All three extend to the frontal pole and are limited in the back by, respectively, the rolandic fissure, the genu of the corpus callosum, and the temporal lobe. Functionally, only the dorsolateral aspect is well demarcated, by the border between the primary motor cortex (Brodmann's area 4) and the somatosensory cortex in the depth of the rolandic fissure (Fig. 19.1). The inferior and medial faces of the frontal lobe are delimited by the limbic cortex of the cingulate and orbitotemporal regions, which is involved in emotional and autonomic functions, among others.

The disorders of motor and premotor areas of the frontal lobe, of whatever etiology, lead to well-recognized pyramidal or extrapyramidal syndromes. They are not within the purview of this chapter. Instead, in this chapter we deal with the pathological conditions of all those areas in front of motor and premotor cortex that constitute the associative cortex of the frontal lobe—in other words, the so-called *prefrontal cortex.*

The prefrontal cortex is that part of the neocortex conventionally defined as the territory of cortical projection of the nucleus medialis dorsalis of the thalamus. It is one of the last regions of the cerebral cortex to develop, phylogenetically (Fig. 19.2) as well as ontogenetically (Fig. 19.3). It reaches maximum development in the human brain, where it constitutes almost 30% of the cerebral mantle. Among its areas, those that develop most and last are the areas of the dorsolateral convexity of the lobe, notably areas 9, 10, 45, and 46 of Brodmann (Fig. 19.1). Their functions are primarily cognitive, in counterdistinction to medial and orbital areas, which have primarily attentional, affective, and emotional functions. Because the orbital and medial prefrontal regions cannot yet be clearly distinguished from each other, either physiologically or neuropsychologically, they will be discussed together here.

Although the functions of the prefrontal cortex are still largely unknown, it is becoming increasingly evident that this cortex is functionally heterogeneous. Each dorsolateral or orbitomedial area may actually play a different cognitive

or emotional role. It is rare that a traumatic or nosological agent affects only one discrete prefrontal area, however defined, cytoarchitectonically or physiologically—hence the variety of prefrontal syndromes. Indeed, no two clinical cases from prefrontal pathology are exactly alike. Nonetheless, two major syndromes stand out, each characterized by a major constellation of prevailing symptoms. Each is treated separately in the sections that follow.

NEUROLOGICAL EXAMINATION

The results of the clinical neurological examination of patients with prefrontal lobe syndrome may be entirely unremarkable, regardless of the site of the lesion. Usually, such patients show neurological signs of malfunction under two sets of circumstances:

1. If the nosological agent not only affects prefrontal cortex but extends to other regions of the frontal lobe, such as the primary motor cortex or the premotor cortex, possibly encroaching on the supplementary motor area (SMA); in such cases, the patient will commonly show signs of pyramidal involvement or motor apraxia; or
2. If the nosological agent (e.g., tumor, cerebrovascular accident [CVA], or trauma) causes, in addition to prefrontal pathology, a more generalized encephalopathy; then the patient will show signs consistent with lesion in nonfrontal (cortical or subcortical) locations or with general cerebral disorder (e.g., edema with intracranial hypertension).

In any case, magnetic resonance imaging (MRI) and other imaging methods are most helpful in revealing noninvasively the nature and extent of the prefrontal lesion.

DORSOLATERAL PREFRONTAL SYNDROME

To a large extent the clinical consequences of dorsolateral prefrontal dysfunction can be predicted from what we know about the cognitive functions of dorsolateral prefrontal cortex in the primate. Thus, it is appropriate to preface our clinical considerations with a summary of that knowledge.

Figure 19.1. Brodmann's cytoarchitectonic map of the human brain in lateral view. The designated four regions are of critical functional importance for language.

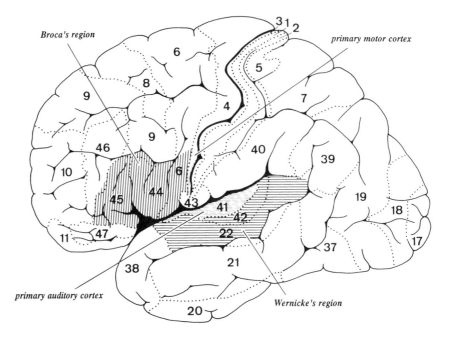

It has now been well established that, as a whole, the dorsolateral prefrontal cortex plays a critical role in the *temporal organization of behavior* (1). This role extends to all domains of voluntary *action*: to skeletal movement, to ocular motility, to speech, and even to the internal domain of logical reasoning. Wherever and whenever the organism is required to form temporally extended sequences of deliberate action, the functional integrity of the dorsolateral prefrontal cortex is needed. This is especially the case if the action is new and there are uncertainties or ambiguities in the information that determines it.

The reason why the dorsolateral prefrontal cortex is essential for temporal integration is because it—in cooperation with other cortical and subcortical structures—supports two basic and temporally complementary cognitive functions: (*a*) a temporally retrospective function of *short-term memory,* and (*b*) a temporally prospective function of *preparatory set* for action. With these two functions, the prefrontal cortex can continuously reconcile the past with the future in the course of behavior and keep the actions of the organism in logical order and on target.

Though these two temporally integrative functions are widely distributed over the dorsolateral prefrontal cortex, the behavioral domains to which they apply appear to have a somewhat discrete distribution, at least with regard to overt action. Ocular motility is probably based in area 8, the "frontal eye fields" (Fig. 19.1). Speech appears to be based mainly in Broca's area (Brodmann's areas 44 and 45) in the inferior frontal gyrus of the left or dominant hemisphere, with some extended representation also in more rostral prefrontal cortex. The cognitive substrate for skeletal motility is less clearly defined but presumed to include areas 9, 10, and 46, in the anterior cortical convexity of the frontal lobe. For reviews of the empirical evidence supporting the two temporally integrative functions of dorsolateral prefrontal cortex just mentioned, the reader is referred to previous publications by the author (1–4).

Table 19.1 presents a schematic outline of the most common clinical manifestations from prefrontal dysfunction in the human. In the table, those manifestations are subdivided by prefrontal region affected (dorsolateral versus orbitomedial), cognitive or behavioral domain affected, resulting symptoms, and deficits on formal psychological testing. The numbers in superscript refer to the prefrontal function(s) primarily impaired.

Disorders of Attention

The *disorders of attention* from dorsolateral damage can best be characterized as deficits in the intensive and selective aspects of attention. Aside from general disinterest in the world (5, 6), the patient commonly shows difficulty in attending to particularly relevant information in the external environment, or in the thinking sphere, for either prospective behavior or mental operations. This difficulty most typically manifests itself in a shortened attention span, that is, trouble concentrating and maintaining attention on any given item of information. In other words, what most often fails in the dorsolateral prefrontal syndrome is the temporal continuity of the focus of attention. This failed temporal continuity results from, and feeds into, the troubles that the patient has in short-term memory and preparatory set. Interestingly, the triad of poor concentration, poor recent memory, and poor planning may be the only symptomatology of an incipient dementia from dorsolateral prefrontal degeneration, as in some cases of Pick's or Alzheimer's disease.

The patient with dorsolateral prefrontal damage usually has no trouble retrieving items from long-term memory. Recall and recognition are intact. In fact, established memories and routines may be a refuge from a deteriorating ability to form, retain, and utilize new memories. Unlike the hippocampal or Korsakoff patient, the prefrontal patient is not totally incapacitated for those mental operations. Rather,

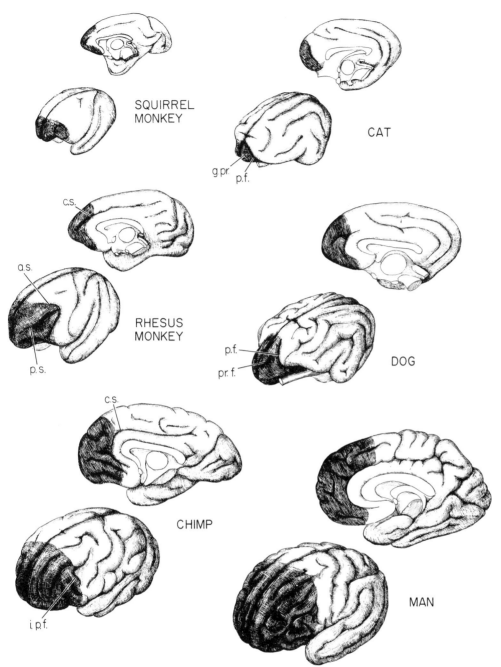

Figure 19.2. The association cortex of the frontal lobe, or prefrontal cortex *(shaded)*, in six animal species.

SQUIRREL MONKEY

CAT

g. pr. p.f.

c.s.

a.s.

RHESUS MONKEY

p. s.

p.f.

pr. f.

DOG

c.s.

CHIMP

i. p.f.

MAN

the prefrontal patient is beset with a weakened capacity to attend to new information and to retain it for prospective use. It is a weakening rather than failure of the ability to form new memory. Consequently, the memory for recent events is spotty, fragmentary, seemingly the result of lack of interest and attention. It has been said that the patient "forgets to remember."

Faced with the necessity to perform a task that requires the short-term retention of items for prospective action, the patient often fails. This can usually be made clear by testing the patient on the broad category of so-called "delayed performance tasks." (Monkeys with dorsolateral damage also perform poorly on such delayed response and delayed matching-to-sample tasks.) The patient usually also has

difficulty with the Wisconsin Card Sorting Task (WCST), a test requiring from the subject the short-term memorization of a changing principle of classification of visual items—by color, shape, or number (7). However, because some patients with nonfrontal (e.g., caudate, hippocampal) pathology may also fail delayed performance tests or the WCST, these tests in themselves cannot be considered specific for prefrontal dysfunction. Nonetheless, these tests, or simplified versions of them, should be part of the standard neuropsychological test battery whenever prefrontal pathology is suspected.

In conclusion, the patient with dorsolateral prefrontal pathology commonly manifests a deficit in active short-term memory. It is a deficit in a form of memory which, in the

Figure 19.3. Myelogenetic map of the human cortex. (After Flechsig, modified by Von Bonin G, Mehler WR. On columnar arrangement of nerve cells in cerebral cortex. Brain Res 1970; 27:1–9.) The numeration of cortical areas refers to the order of myelination of their intrinsic and extrinsic fibers.

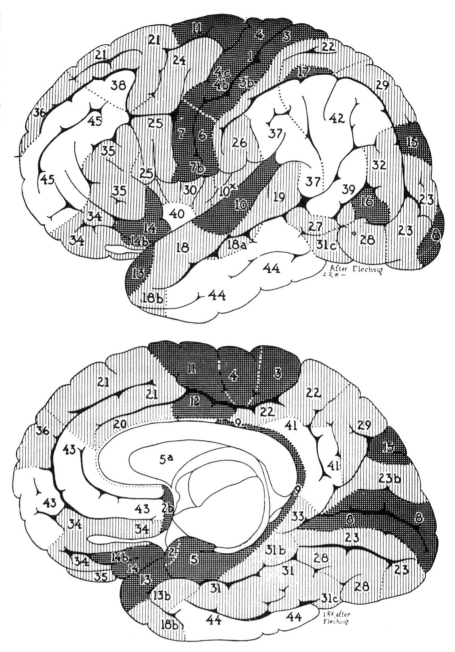

operant terms of cognitive psychology, has been called "working memory" (8). That deficit is partly but not completely attributable to the attentional deficit.

Difficulty in Planning

Perhaps the most consistent and specific symptom of dorsolateral prefrontal disorder is the patient's difficulty in planning his or her own actions. Many observers agree that this is the most characteristic manifestation of frontal lobe pathology (9, 10). The patient is unable to plan in organized fashion any novel structures of action, to keep them in mind, and to lead them to execution. This difficulty permeates all action domains, but is most apparent at the most complex levels of speech, behavior, and rational thinking. The patient cannot plan new discourse, let alone execute it; he or she

cannot plan substantial moves or departures from daily routine; cannot elaborate novel trends of thought and lead them to their logical conclusion.

Clearly, this problem in planning is temporally the mirror image—the flip side—of the patient's problem in memory. It is also a memory deficit of sorts: a faulty "memory of the future" (11). Whereas the recent-memory deficit of the frontal patient chiefly pertains to the retention of sensory material or its internal representations, the planning deficit is a deficit in representation of, and preparation for, future action. The first reflects a problem with active perceptual memory, broadly conceived; the second, a problem with active "motor memory," also broadly conceived.

The deficient "motor memory" of the dorsolateral prefrontal syndrome is most likely a derivative of an impairment of that second basic cognitive function of dorsolateral pre-

Table 19.1. Prefrontal Disorders in the Human

Affected Region	Functional Domain[a]	Symptom	Test Deficits
Dorsolateral	Attention[1,2]	Short attention span	Order and delay tasks, Wisconsin Card Sorting Test
	Memory[1]	Recent memory deficit	
	Planning[2]	Defective planning	
	Speech[1,2]	Central dynamic aphasia	
	Behavior[1,2]	Temporal concreteness, creative and executive deficit	
Orbitomedial	Attention[3]	Distractibility	Go-no go
	Behavior[3]	Disinhibition	

[a]Prefrontal function affected: [1]Active memory; [2]Set; [3]Inhibitory control

frontal cortex for which clear physiological correlates are demonstrable in the monkey: the motor set. In the patient, the preparation for action is as disturbed as the retention of recent sensory or episodic information. Both are also disturbed in the monkey with dorsolateral prefrontal lesion; both functions are accompanied by characteristic electrophysiological phenomena in dorsolateral prefrontal cortex (12, 13).

Disorders of Speech

All disorders of speech from dorsolateral prefrontal damage are attributable to malfunction of temporal integration, and thus the result of memory deficit, set deficit, or both. Of course, the best known of these disorders in the spoken language is Broca's aphasia, caused by pathology in Broca's area, in the third or inferior frontal gyrus (Brodmann's areas 44, 45) of the left side. Broca's area is part of the prefrontal cortex by definition, for it is directly connected with the nucleus medialis dorsalis of the thalamus. Broca's aphasia is the most drastic deficit observable in the articulation of speech, the most elementary form of motor aphasia. The patient's speech is characterized by a peculiar telegraphic style, with a general dearth of articles and liaison words, prepositions, and conjunctions. It has been designated *agrammatism.*

Lesions in more anterior prefrontal areas also produce speech deficits, but these are more subtle than Broca's aphasia. The anterior prefrontal speech defect is characterized by a general impoverishment of verbal expression. Spontaneous speech is diminished. So is verbal fluency. Sentences are short and mostly trite or commonplace. There is a general diminution in the number and quality of dependent clauses, reflecting what Jackson (14) called an impaired ability to "propositionise." This disorder of verbal expression from anterior dorsolateral prefrontal injury has been called "central motor aphasia" by Goldstein (15) and "frontal dynamic aphasia" by Luria (16). Like Broca's aphasia, anterior prefrontal aphasia is lateralized. It is more prevalent after lesions in the left or dominant hemisphere than in the right or nondominant one (17, 18).

In summary, all speech disorders from dorsolateral prefrontal lesion can be ascribed to an impairment of what some (19) have designated the *syntagmatic* property of language,

that is, the capability of synthesizing verbal expression in the temporal dimension. As in any other action domain, that property of the spoken language depends on the interplay of the two functions, memory and set, that we postulate are supported by dorsolateral prefrontal cortex. The speech disorders are paradigmatic of temporal integration disorders in all forms of sequential action. For this reason, I have argued (1) that the dorsolateral prefrontal cortex plays a central role in what Lashley (20) called the "syntax of action."

The problems resulting from failure of the temporal integrative functions of dorsolateral prefrontal cortex affect not only speech but behavior in general. The behavior of the patient with dorsolateral damage suffers from what can be characterized as *temporal concreteness:* his or her behavior is anchored to the "here and now," deprived of perspective either back or forward in time, driven by routine, and devoid of creativity. In cases of large lesions of dorsolateral cortex, that temporal concreteness is accompanied by apathy, lack of drive and spontaneity in all aspects of behavioral action. As a consequence, there is a global impairment of executive function in all action domains.

Schizophrenia

Because the executive and temporal-integration functions of the dorsolateral prefrontal cortex extend to the *internal action domain,* that is, to the domain of logical thinking, this cortex has been implicated in schizophrenia. Indeed, one of the cardinal symptoms of the illness is the failure in proper temporal integration of the thought process. As manifested in speech production, the thinking of the schizophrenic is commonly characterized by blocking and looseness of associations. Is schizophrenia a disease of the dorsolateral prefrontal cortex? Clearly, the etiology of the illness cannot be reduced to such simple terms. No prefrontal lesion of any cause, locus, or extent, is known to induce a schizophrenic syndrome. Quite the contrary; decades ago, frontal lobe resection was used for the *treatment* of the psychosis, a treatment that was effective presumably insofar as it alleviated anxiety. However, lobotomy did not abolish primary symptoms of thought disorder. Nonetheless, there is increasing evidence that a dorsolateral prefrontal disorder plays a role in the pathogenesis of schizophrenia. First, there is the indirect evidence that the dorsolateral prefrontal cortex is exceptionally rich in dopaminergic receptors, and that some of the most effective antipsychotic neuroleptics are dopamine antagonists. There are morphological and functional abnormalities in the prefrontal cortex of schizophrenics. Some of the morphological abnormalities are revealed by neuropathological study at the cellular level (21–23). Others are revealed by imaging techniques in the form of frontal atrophy (24, 25). The most telling evidence, however, comes from functional imaging studies. Several such studies have indicated an abnormally low level of frontal metabolism ("hypofrontality") in the schizophrenic (26–28). A striking manifestation of prefrontal dysfunction is the schizophrenic's failure to show the normal metabolic activation of dorsolateral prefrontal cortex when challenged by performance of the WCST (29). In summary, it is a plausible hypothesis that schizophrenia results from a disorder of certain neurotransmitter systems, notably but not exclusively dopaminergic, and that such a disorder impairs the normal function of the dorsolateral prefrontal cortex. (Other interpretations of the hypofrontality literature are discussed in Chapter 15.)

ORBITOMEDIAL PREFRONTAL SYNDROME

The functions of the orbital and medial aspects of the prefrontal cortex are still largely unknown. In very general terms, orbital and medial areas, in addition to engaging in certain cognitive operations related to attention, play a more important role in emotional and instinctive behavior than do the areas of the dorsolateral prefrontal convexity. This may be related to the limbic nature and connectivity of orbitomedial cortex.

A most characteristic function of orbitomedial prefrontal cortex is the *inhibitory control of interference,* that is, the suppression of extraneous sensory or internal influences on current behavior. This kind of control, which has been well documented in animal (30) and human (31) neuropsychological studies, normally facilitates the attention of the organism to relevant inputs and to the pursuit of goals. When the control of interference fails, as it does in orbitomedial lesions, the subject becomes excessively *distractible,* incapable of suppressing the interference from trivial, irrelevant, or inappropriate influences from the internal or external milieu that will tend to divert behavior away from its goal. Because not uncommonly this distractibility is accompanied by motor disinhibition (see below), the resulting syndrome in the adult human resembles that of the hyperkinetic child. For this reason, the childhood disorder has been hypothetically attributed to delayed maturation of orbitomedial prefrontal cortex (1).

Obsessive-Compulsive Disorder

Conversely, there are certain conditions in which the inhibitory control of cognition and behavior can be excessive, and this may be caused by hyperfunction of orbitomedial cortex. Attention in such cases is abnormally riveted to a given content of thought or form of behavior, which

becomes overpowering and ends up by implacably controlling the patient's mind and behavior. This may be accompanied by extreme anxiety. We are referring, of course, to obsessive-compulsive disorder (OCD). Brain-imaging studies (32, 33) have indicated hypermetabolism of orbitofrontal cortex in OCD patients. It is therefore an attractive conjecture that the OCD is a consequence of that hypermetabolic condition and the related abnormal hyperfunction of inhibitory control.

The converse disorder, that is, the failure of interference control from orbitomedial lesion can be demonstrated by formal psychological testing. Particularly sensitive to that failure is a category of behavioral tasks, named "go-no go" tasks, that require the inhibition of motor responses to certain stimuli in the course of sensory discriminations (34).

The deficit in the inhibitory control of interference is not the only kind of disinhibitory deficit observable in the orbitomedial syndrome. Indeed, quite commonly the disinhibition will affect motor activity in general, the thought process, and a variety of instinctual impulses. Orbitofrontal hypermotility gives the appearance that the patient has *excessive drive,* that he or she cannot stop and concentrate on anything, and is driven by an incessant necessity to act, albeit in haphazard and purposeless fashion. This apparently boundless energy and impulsivity may interfere with sleep and with the orderly thought process. Also disinhibited may be the basic drives: the patient may display hyperphagia and hypersexuality in utter disregard of common good judgment and mores (35). Aggressivity may also be uninhibited.

The mood of orbitomedial prefrontal patients varies greatly, depending on the case and for unknown reasons. Some patients manifest a tendency to apparent depression, which may not reflect so much a sad mood as it does the apathy ("pseudodepression") that also characterizes some cases with extensive dorsolateral lesions. More commonly, however, the orbitomedial syndrome is characterized by labile mood with a general tendency to euphoria. The latter may be accompanied by a form of silly, compulsive, and childish humor that has been called *moria* (or *Witzelsucht*).

Not surprisingly, then, because of the euphoria, the uncontrolled thinking and behavior, and the insomnia that the orbitomedial prefrontal patient often exhibits, his or her syndrome may be mistaken for mania. Only the careful history and a thorough neurological examination can exclude a primary psychiatric syndrome and confirm the "pseudomania" of a patient with orbitomedial prefrontal lesion.

The previous description can serve only as a general guideline, because cases with lesions strictly circumscribed to orbitomedial region, whether unilateral or bilateral, are uncommon. More common are cases with orbitomedial pathology plus pathology elsewhere in the frontal lobe. In such cases the syndrome may be mixed, with cognitive and affective manifestations associated with both dorsolateral and orbitomedial lesions. The picture is even more complicated when the pathology extends beyond the frontal lobe(s).

TREATMENT

The two previous sections describe in schematic form the main features of the two principal regional syndromes from prefrontal trauma or disease. Issues of etiology have been purposefully omitted in the previous discussion because they are largely irrelevant to the particular clinical picture of any given case of frontal lobe involvement. What matters for this picture, in terms of our discussion, is the extent and location of prefrontal tissue affected. However, the etiology is extremely relevant, indeed critical, for the treatment and management of the prefrontal patient. The pathological process may be acute or chronic, traumatic, infectious, neoplastic, vascular, or degenerative. The treatment, as in the case of any other brain lesion, has to be directly addressed to the cause when this is known.

Nevertheless, the judicious use of pharmacological agents can be extremely useful to treat, albeit only symptomatically, "frontal lobe behaviors." When the cognitive syndrome from a dorsolateral lesion is accompanied by severe anxiety, a benzodiazepine may be useful. Depression may be successfully treated with an antidepressant. Neuroleptics may be useful in cases (usually orbitomedial) where psychotic or manic manifestations are present. Medication has to be used with awareness of the patient's cognitive status and its functional relevance, because some drugs — especially benzodiazepines and neuroleptics — can worsen the prefrontal cognitive deficit. The application of cognitive enhancers (cholinergics, nootropics, etc.) to prefrontal syndromes is an appealing idea, but the efficacy of such drugs for this purpose has not been demonstrated. As an adjunct, psychotherapeutic grief work is important for patients accustomed to creative and executive achievements that are no longer possible as a result of frontal damage. Supportive relationships and structured environments are needed by virtually all patients with significant frontal deficits.

References

1. Fuster JM. The prefrontal cortex: anatomy, physiology, and neuropsychology of the frontal lobe. 2nd ed. New York: Raven Press, 1989.
2. Fuster JM. Prefrontal cortex in motor control. In: Brooks VB, ed. Handbook of physiology; nervous system. Vol. II: Motor control, Bethesda: American Physiological Society, 1981:1149–1178.
3. Fuster JM. The prefrontal cortex and temporal integration. In: Jones EG, Peters A, eds. Cerebral cortex, Vol. 4. New York: Plenum, 1985a:151–177.
4. Fuster JM. The prefrontal cortex, mediator of cross-temporal contingencies. Human Neurobiology 1985;4:169–179.
5. Luria AR. Higher cortical functions in man. New York: Basis Books, 1966.
6. Luria AR. Traumatic aphasia. The Hague: Mouton, 1970.
7. Milner B. Some effects of frontal lobectomy in man. In: Warren JM, Akert K, eds. The frontal granular cortex and behavior. New York: McGraw-Hill, 1964:313–334.
8. Baddeley A. Working memory. Philos Trans R Soc Lond. [Biol] 1983;302:311–324.
9. Walsh KW. Neuropsychology. Edinburgh: Churchill Livingstone, 1978.
10. Shallice T. Specific impairments of planning. Philos Trans R Soc Lond [Biol] 1982;298:199–209.
11. Ingvar DH. Memory of the future: an essay on the temporal organization of conscious awareness. Human Neurobiology 1985;4: 127–136.
12. Quintana J, Fuster JM. Mnemonic and predictive functions of cortical neurons in a memory task. Neuroreport 1992;3:721–724.
13. Fuster JM. Frontal lobes. Current Opinion in Neurobiology 1993;3: 160–165.
14. Jackson JH. On affections of speech from disease of the brain. Brain 1915;38:107–174.
15. Goldstein K. Language and language disturbances. New York: Grune & Stratton, 1948.
16. Luria AR. Traumatic aphasia. The Hague: Mouton, 1970.
17. Barbizet J, Duizabo P, Flavigny R. Rôle des lobes frontaux dans le langage. Rev Neurol 1975;131:525–544.
18. Miller, E. Verbal fluency as a function of a measure of verbal intelligence and in relation to different types of cerebral pathology. Brit J Clin Psychol 1984;23:53–57.
19. Pei MA, Gaynor F. A dictionary of linguistics. New York: Philosophical Library, 1954.
20. Lashley KS. The problem of serial order in behavior. In: Jeffress LA, ed. Cerebral mechanisms in behavior. New York: John Wiley & Sons, 1951:112–146.
21. Miyakawa T, Sumiyoshi S, Deshimaru M., et al. Electron microscopic study on schizophrenia. Acta Neuropathol 1972;20:67–77.
22. Benes FM, Davidson J, Bird ED. Quantitative cytoarchitectural studies of the cerebral cortex of schizophrenics. Arch Gen Psychiatry 1986; 43:31–35.
23. Benes FM, McSparren J, Bird ED, SanGiovanni JP, Vincent SL. Deficits in small interneurons in prefrontal and cingulate cortices of schizophrenic and schizoaffective patients. Arch Gen Psychiatry 1991;48:996–1001.
24. Weinberger DR, Torrey EF, Neophytides AN, Wyatt RJ. Lateral cerebral ventricular enlargement in chronic schizophrenia. Arch Gen Psychiatry 1979;36:735–739.
25. Andreasen N, Nasrallah HA, Dunn V et al. Structural abnormalities in the frontal system in schizophrenia. Arch Gen Psychiatry 1986;43: 136–144.
26. Ingvar DH, Franzén G. Abnormalities of cerebral blood flow distribution in patients with chronic schizophrenia. Acta Psychiatr Scand 1974;50:425–462.
27. Buchsbaum MS, Cappelletti J, Ball R, et al. Positron emission tomographic image measurement in schizophrenia and affective disorders. Ann Neurol 1984;15 (Suppl.):S157–S165.
28. Wolkin A, Jaeger J, Brodie JD, et al. Persistence of cerebral metabolic abnormalities in chronic schizophrenia as determined by positron emission tomography. Am J Psychiatry 1985;142:564–571.
29. Weinberger DR, Berman KF, Suddath R, Torrey EF. Evidence of dysfunction of a prefrontal-limbic network in schizophrenia: a magnetic resonance imaging and regional cerebral blood flow study of discordant monozygotic twins. Am J Psychiatry 1992;149:890–897.
30. Mishkin M. Perseration of central sets after frontal lesions in monkeys. In: Warren JM, Akert K, eds. The frontal granular cortex and behavior. New York: McGraw-Hill, 1964:219–241.
31. Stuss DT, Kaplan EF, Benson DF, Weir WS, Chiulli S, Sarazin FF. Evidence for the involvement of orbitofrontal cortex in memory functions: an interference effect. J Comp Physiol 1982;96:913–925.
32. Baxter LR, Phelps ME, Mazziotta JC, Guze BH, Schwartz JM, Selin CE. Local cerebral glucose metabolic rates in obsessive-compulsive disorder. Arch Gen Psychiatry 1987;44:211–218.
33. Rauch SL, Jenike MA, Alpert NM, et al. Regional cerebral blood flow measured during symptom provocation in obsessive-compulsive disorder using oxygen 15-labeled carbon dioxide and positron emission tomography. Arch Gen Psychiatry 1994;51:62–70.
34. Drewe EA. Go-no go learning after frontal lobe lesions in humans. Cortex 1975;11:8–16.
35. Erb JS, Gwirtsman HE, Fuster JM, Richeimer SH. Bulimia associated with frontal lobe lesions. International Journal of Eating Disorders 1989;8:117–121.

20

PAIN TRANSMISSION AND MODULATION

Henry J. Ralston III

Pain is a fundamental, complex sensory perception that is the product of neural processing by multiple levels of the nervous system and finally by the cerebral cortex. Usually, the experience or report of pain is readily associated with stimuli that are potentially or actively damaging to tissue. Often, however, there is no demonstrable cause of the pain, but the individual nonetheless reports that pain is present, and it is incumbent upon the therapist to attempt to diagnose and treat this pain just as arising from a more obvious cause. There are objective aspects of pain, such as its location on or in the body, and its intensity. There are also more subjective aspects, such as the memories and emotional responses with which pain is often associated.

Given these attributes of pain, it is not surprising that research on the neural networks, functional classes of neurons, neurotransmitters and their receptors, and changes in neuronal circuitry and gene expression associated with pain constitutes a complex and rapidly expanding series of topics. This chapter summarizes some of our current knowledge of pain transmission and modulation, emphasizing studies in the primate (the macaque and the human) wherever possible. To date, much of the information about neurotransmitters and their receptors and gene expression has been derived from studies in the rat, and findings resulting from these investigations are also presented. These descriptions of the neuroanatomical organization and physiology of neurons that respond to noxious stimuli are used to suggest mechanisms by which disease or injury that damages these neurons can perturb the perception of pain, leading to anesthetic or hyperpathic states. Throughout this chapter the basic biology of pain is related to discussions of the design of rational therapies for its amelioration.

TRANSMISSION AND MODULATION OF PAIN

As stated in the opening paragraph, the sensation of pain is a product of the neural networks of the brain. Therefore, there are no "pain pathways" as such, but rather neurons and the pathways arising from them that convey information arising as a result of noxious (tissue-damaging) stimuli, which may or may not result in the conscious sensory experience of pain. Noxious mechanical, thermal, or chemi-

cal stimuli activate specific peripheral nerve endings of sensory neurons (nociceptors), resulting in trains of action potentials that travel to the spinal cord or brainstem, where they are synaptically transmitted to neurons that convey the information to higher centers of the neuraxis, and ultimately to the cerebral cortex. At every level of the nervous system, from peripheral tissue to the cerebral cortex, there is the potential for modulation of the signals evoked by noxious stimuli. It is at these sites of modulation that much of the therapy designed to treat pain is targeted, either by enhancing naturally occurring suppression of noxious stimuli, such as biofeedback techniques, or by therapies designed to decrease the activation of neurons that carry nociceptive information. The following sections summarize each of these neural levels with regard to their anatomy, physiology, and neurochemistry.

Primary Afferent Neurons

SENSORY GANGLION CELLS

The cell bodies of these sensory neurons are located in the dorsal root ganglia of the spinal cord or in the trigeminal ganglia. Sensory ganglion cells are unipolar, in that they have a single process, an axon, that arises from the cell body and then bifurcates into a peripheral branch that runs in peripheral nerve to innervate cutaneous, deep, or visceral tissue, and a central branch (primary afferent axon) that carries information via dorsal or trigeminal roots into the central nervous system (CNS), either to the spinal cord or the brainstem, respectively (Fig. 20.1). As in all neurons, the cell body of sensory neurons is the metabolic center of the cell: all peptides and proteins, such as receptors (including opiate receptors), cytoskeletal precursors, enzymes, and peptide neurotransmitters, are synthesized in the cell body and then move by axonal transport within the central and peripheral axonal branches to their appropriate places within the neuron or neuronal membrane. Sensory neurons are specialized cells, in which the region of the axon where action potentials are initiated is immediately adjacent to the sensory endings in the tissue innervated (Fig. 20.1), rather than at the origin of the axon from the cell body, as in most neurons. Sensory neurons that are activated by noxious stimuli are called primary afferent nociceptors (PANs); some respond exclusively to noxious stimuli, others in a graded fashion as a stimulus becomes more intense (mechanical stimuli) or changes from innocuous to noxious (e.g., warm to hot). PANs usually have smaller-diameter cell bodies (10–15 μm) than those cells activated exclusively by nonnoxious stimuli, and these cell bodies contain one or more neuropeptides, often coexisting with excitatory amino acid neurotransmitters, such as glutamate. The best characterized neuropeptide in sensory ganglion cells (dorsal root ganglion cells: DRGs) is the undecapeptide, substance P (SP), found in about 20% of DRGs. SP is one of the class of neuropeptides called neurokinins (NK) or tachykinins. Although SP is present in some PANs, it is also found in other functional classes of DRGs. In addition, other peptides often coexist with SP in DRGs; for instance, calcitonin gene-related peptide (CGRP) is present in about 80% of SP-containing DRGs. To date, no one peptide neurotransmitter has been shown to be uniquely associated with a specific functional class of sensory neurons (1). The content of SP in DRGs can be depleted by exposure to capsaicin, a nonpeptide substance found in chili peppers that has an excitatory effect predominalty upon PANs. When neonatal rats are exposed to capsaicin, small-diameter DRGs, many of which contain SP (and CGRP), are destroyed. This finding has provided a useful model for studying animals in which a major element of the afferent somatosensory system is absent.

Noxious stimuli can induce changes in PANs. The amount of the excitatory neurotransmitter glutamate is increased in the macaque's peripheral axons, which innervate arthritic joints (2). The concentrations of peptides in DRGs change after peripheral nerve or tissue injury (1). Experimentally induced arthritis results in a significant increase in DRGs exhibiting preprotachkinin (PPT) mRNA, as well as increased concentrations of SP and CGRP. On the other hand, peripheral nerve transection results in decreases in the mRNAs of the same substances.

The axons of PANs are small in diameter: those having a myelin sheath are usually 1–3 μm in size and are functionally classified as Aδ fibers; nonmyelinated axons are usually < 1 μm diameter and are classified as C fibers (Fig. 20.2). Aδ fibers may respond to innocuous, to noxious, or to both classes of stimuli. The vast majority of C fibers in primates are activated by a variety of noxious mechanical, thermal and chemical stimuli, and have thus been termed C polymodal nociceptors.

PERIPHERAL SENSORY ENDINGS

The peripheral endings in tissue of PANs have been shown to arborize in the tissue innervated by them, leading to their being classified as free nerve endings. The peripheral terminals of PANs respond to appropriate mechanical, thermal, or chemical stimuli that evoke trains of action potentials that travel into the CNS. It is now recognized that these sensory endings are not merely the passive recipients of noxious stimuli, but that they can release neuropeptides (such as substance P) into peripheral tissues that may contribute to the inflammatory response following injury. PANs exhibit increased excitability following repeated noxious stimulation (1); this excitability change is termed sensitization, and is characterized by an increase in spontaneous activity accompanied by a lowered threshold for activation and increased firing to suprathreshold stimuli. Sensitization of PANs can be the direct result of peptides, such as interleukin-1 (IL-1) or neutrophil chemotactic peptides, arising from damaged tissue. Sensitized PANs can contribute to hyperalgesia, such as experienced with tissue inflammation, in which a normally innocuous stimulus is perceived as painful, or noxious stimuli evoke heightened sensations of pain.

The factors that affect the peripheral terminals of PANs have been the subject of intense investigation, owing to their fundamental role in pain. As mentioned earlier, they may be directly sensitized by a variety of substances released by

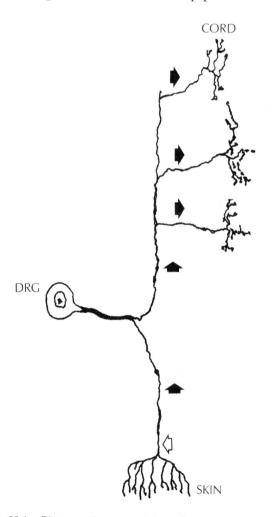

Figure 20.1. Diagrammatic representation of a sensory neuron. The unipolar cell body is located in the dorsal root ganglion (DRG) or trigeminal ganglion. The peripheral axonal branch innervates tissue (e.g., skin) and responds to various mechanical, thermal and/or chemical stimuli. The action potential is generated *(open arrow)* just proximal to the peripheral ending and travels in the direction of the *closed arrows* to enter the central nervous system (cord). (Modified from several drawings of Cajal SR. Histologie du systeme nerveux de l'homme et de vertebres, vol. 1. Paris: C.S.I.C., 1955.)

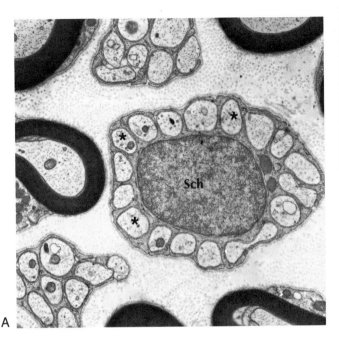
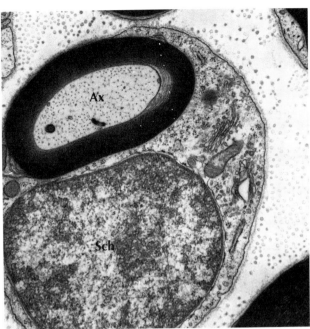

Figure 20.2. Electron micrographs of macaque peripheral nerve. **A,** Multiple nonmyelinated axons, some indicated by*, are enveloped by the cytoplasm of a Schwann cell (Sch). The nonmyelinated axons are about 0.2 μm in diameter. **B,** A myelinated axon (Ax) is invested by the Schwann cell (Sch) that forms the myelin wrapping. This axon is about 1.0 μm diameter, and is probably an Aδ fiber. In contrast to the nonmyelinated axons, Schwann cells invest only a single myelinated fiber.

damaged tissue. Also, they may be indirectly sensitized by bradykinin, or by mechanisms involving prostaglandin synthesis and/or postganglionic sympathetic axon terminals, or by the cytokine IL-1, produced by leukocytes following exposure to bacterial toxins or inflammatory mediators.

In summary, unipolar sensory ganglion cells, located in the dorsal root or trigeminal ganglia, have peripheral axonal branches, the endings of which arborize in the tissue innervated by them and respond to noxious stimuli (potentially or actually tissue damaging), these primary afferent nociceptors being termed PANs. The noxious stimuli initiate trains of action potentials that carry the information to the CNS via the central axonal branch of the sensory neuron. Repeated noxious stimuli can result in release of SP and other peptides from peripheral nerve endings that can evoke an inflammatory response in tissue. In turn, the nerve endings of PANs can be directly or indirectly sensitized by a variety of substances released by damaged tissue, by sympathetic nerve endings, and by white blood cells. Sensitized PANs have a lowered threshold and respond abnormally to innocuous or to noxious stimuli. DRGs of PANs may exhibit changes in neurotransmitter mRNA or transmitter content following inflammation or nerve injury. Therefore, the primary afferent neuron plays a dynamic role in the development and maintenance of a variety of pain states.

Dorsal Horn of the Spinal Cord

The spinal cord retains many of the organizational properties of the neural tube from which it developed. Surrounding the central canal (usually not patent in humans) is the aggregate of neurons that constitute the gray matter of

the cord, and external to these neurons are the various pathways that make up the spinal cord white matter, owing to the myelin sheaths surrounding most CNS axons (Fig. 20.3). The gray matter is subdivided into bilateral symmetrical dorsal and ventral horns, generally related to somatosensory and motor functions of the cord, respectively. The thoracic and sacral segments also contain preganglionic sympathetic and parasympathetic neurons. In 1952, Rexed (3) used cytoarchitectural characteristics to divide the dorsal horn of the cord into six laminae organized into a horizontal array, parallel to the dorsal surface of the cord (Fig. 20.4), assigning them Roman numerals I to VI. Lamina I (the marginal layer) and lamina II (the substantia gelatinosa) are often referred to as the superficial dorsal horn, laminae III and IV as the neck, and V and VI as the base of the dorsal horn. These anatomical designations have been shown to have important functional correlations, particularly with regard to pain (see later). Dorsal horn cells can be divided into three broad classes: those that send axons to rostral targets in the brainstem or diencephalon (projection neurons); those that project to other segments of the spinal cord (propriospinal neurons); and those that serve the intrinsic excitatory and inhibitory circuitry of a given spinal segment (local circuit neurons—LCNs or interneurons). Many of the lamina I neurons are larger than those of the subjacent laminae II and III, and these larger cells project to brainstem and diencephalon. Numerous LCNs in laminae II and III contain enkephalin or γ-aminobutyric acid (GABA) and are believed to participate in pain modulatory mechanisms of the superficial dorsal horn. The dendritic arbors of the neurons of laminae I–III tend to branch primarily in the rostrocaudal plane. Laminae IV, V, and VI contain a mixture

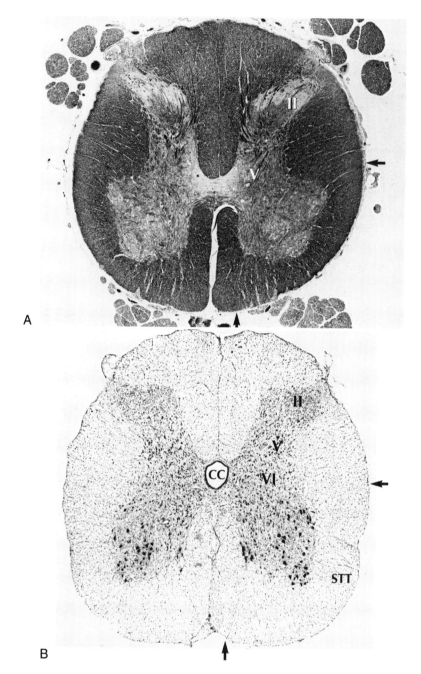

Figure 20.3. **A,** Cross section of human lumbar spinal cord, stained for myelin. The substantia gelatinosa (II) is relatively unstained. Lamina V (V) contains many spinothalamic tract cells. The *(arrows)* demarcate the approximate boundaries of the spinothalamic tract. **B,** Cross-section of macaque lumbar spinal cord, stained for neurons and glial cells (Nissl stain). Three of the dorsal horn laminae are indicated (II, III, and V). *Arrows* indicate the approximate boundaries of the spinothalamic tract (STT). *cc*-central canal.

of larger and smaller neurons: their dendritic arbors tend to be more spherical than those of the superficial laminae; and dendrites of many of the larger neurons extend dorsally into the superficial laminae, where they can be contacted by primary afferent or intrinsic axons arborizing in laminae I, II, and III (Fig. 20.5).

Ventral horn neurons have also been assigned to laminae, although they are actually grouped into clusters, such as those of lamina IX, which contains spinal motoneurons. Lamina X contains the small neurons surrounding the central canal.

PRIMARY AFFERENT AXONS

Primary afferent axons of PANs and their synaptic interactions with CNS neurons have been most extensively studied in the spinal dorsal horn, and the following description incorporates these investigations. Selected aspects of studies of trigeminal circuitry are also be presented.

Primary afferent axons are the central branches of sensory neurons located in the dorsal root ganglia (or the trigeminal ganglia) and enter the spinal cord via the dorsal roots (or the brainstem via the trigeminal roots). As in peripheral nerves, PAN axons entering the CNS are either small-diameter myelinated fibers (Aδ) or nonmyelinated (C-fibers), reaching the dorsal horn via Lissauer's tract (Figs. 20.4 and 20.5). The C-fibers in dorsal roots terminate primarily in the superficial laminae I and II (4), and form a variety of axodendritic synaptic complexes (Fig. 20.6*A*) with dorsal horn neurons (5); many C-fiber terminals in lamina II are postsynaptic to axon terminals (Fig. 20.7) or to presynaptic dendrites of intrinsic dorsal horn neurons (4). The terminals of Aδ axons are more widely distributed, being found in laminae I–V, although the majority are found in I–III (4). The larger diameter Aβ-fibers, carrying nonnoxious information, terminate in the deeper laminae (Fig. 20.6*B*) of the

dorsal horn (6) as well as in the ventral horn. As would be expected from the distribution of the afferent terminals of PANs, the neurons of the dorsal horn that receive these afferents exhibit various response properties following peripheral noxious and nonnoxious stimuli. Lamina I neurons in monkey are primarily nociceptive (nociceptive specific-NS) and signal noxious mechanical stimuli to higher centers (7). Most lamina II cells respond to noxious stimuli but are interneurons (local circuit neurons) in that they do not project to higher centers. Most laminae III and IV neurons are activated exclusively by nonnoxious stimuli. Lamina V cells exhibit convergent, or wide-dynamic-range

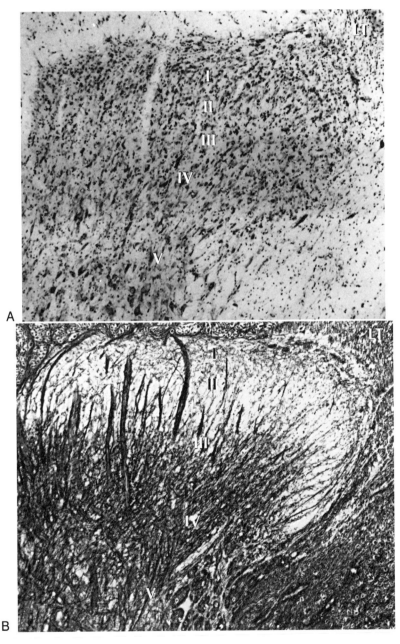

Figure 20.4. Cross-sections of the dorsal horn of the macaque spinal cord. Dorsal is up, medial is to the left. **A,** Nissl stain, to show the neuronal constituents of the horn. **B,** Axonal (neurofibrillar) stain. Five laminae of Rexed (I–V) are indicated, as is Lissauer's tract (LT), by which fine-diameter Aδ and C-fibers enter the spinal cord. The majority of spinothalamic tract neurons are in laminae I and V. The depth of lamina II, the substantia gelatinosa, is about 200 μm.

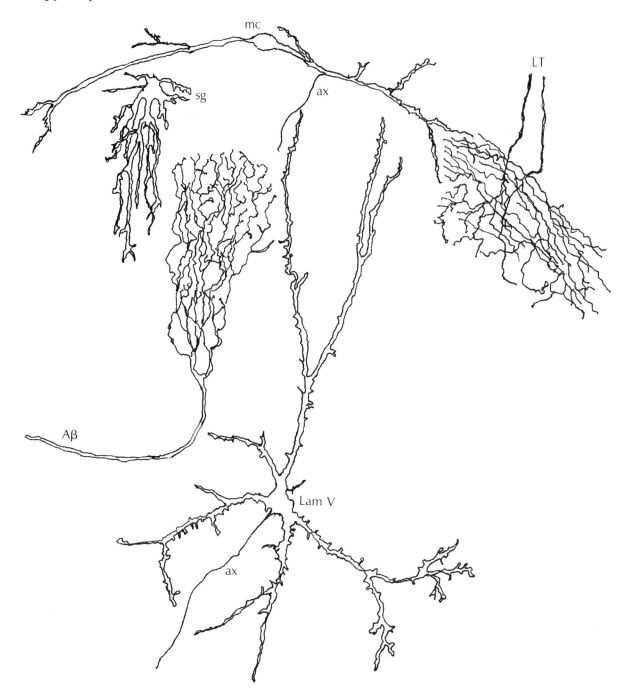

Figure 20.5.   Some of the cellular and axonal elements of the dorsal horn, drawn from Golgi-stained tissue. Dorsal is up, medial is to the left. Marginal cells (mc) of lamina I, and lamina V cells (Lam V) are the principal types of spinothalamic tract cells. Neurons of lamina II, the substantia gelatinosa (sg), are local circuit interneurons, and may contain enkephalin or other neurotransmitters. Large-diameter dorsal root axons (Aβ) arborize throughout the deeper layers of the dorsal horn, but do not reach the superficial layers, laminae I and II. Fine-diameter Aδ- and C-fibers enter the dorsal horn via Lissauer's tract (LT), and arborize primarily in laminae I and II. Aδ-fibers also extend ventrally to lamina V. Note that marginal cells would be activated primarily by fine-diameter afferents, while lamina V cells could be driven by Aβ-, Aδ-, and C-afferents. *ax*-axons of marginal and lamina V neurons. (Modified from several drawings of Cajal SR. Histologie du systeme nerveux de l'homme et de vertebres, vol. 1. Paris: C.S.I.C., 1955.)

(WDR) properties, responding to activation of Aβ-, Aδ- and C-fibers (8), following innocuous and noxious mechanical and thermal cutaneous stimuli. Many cells of laminae V and VI are also activated by a variety of stimuli arising from the viscera or from joints (see below).

Neurons that project to higher centers, such as the midbrain (spinomesencephalic tract—SMT cells) or the thalamus (spinothalamic tract—STT cells) may be iden-

tified physiologically following antidromic activation by stimulation of the target of the axons, or anatomically by injecting the target region with a retrograde tracer that is transported back to the parent cell bodies (Fig. 20.8). Using such techniques, it has been possible to identify SMT and STT projection neurons, their functional properties, and the classes of synaptic terminals that contact them.

Primary Afferent Neurotransmitters

Excitatory amino acids (EAAs), particularly glutamate (Glu), numerous peptides, and adenosine triphosphate (ATP) have been identified in dorsal root axon terminals and play a role in the transmission of afferent stimuli to dorsal horn neurons. Most DRGs, and presumably most of their terminals in the dorsal horn, exhibit coexistent neurotransmitters, most often one or more neuropeptides and an EAA. Glutamate-containing terminals have been identified synapsing on primate STT cells (9); Glu evokes a fast, short-duration depolarization of STT neurons, and both Glu and aspartate are released in the cord following activation of primary afferent axons conveying nonnoxious and noxious stimuli (10). Of the peptides, the neurokinins, particularly

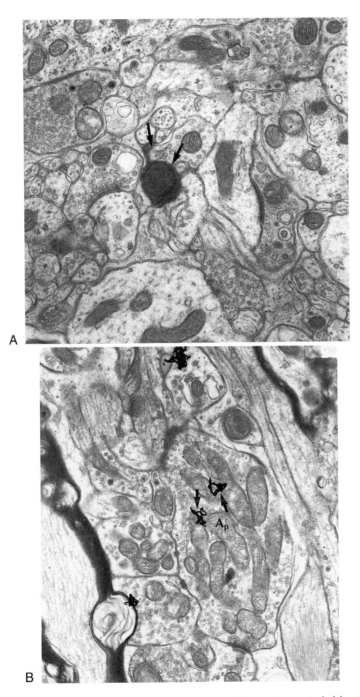

Figure 20.6.   Electron micrographs of the superficial dorsal horn of the monkey, to show the synaptic terminal of dorsal root afferent axons. **A,** A degenerating C-fiber terminal *(dark arrow)* arising from a nonmyelinated axon *(open arrow)* 1 week after dorsal rhizotomy. The degenerating terminal and an adjacent normal synaptic profile are about 0.5 μm in diameter. **B,** An Aβ terminal in lamina III, identified by silver grains *(arrows)* as a result of being made radioactive following the injection of a radioisotope into the parent dorsal root ganglion. The Aβ profile is about 2.0 μm in diameter.

SP, have been the most studied (1). SP has been identified in the terminals of PANs (11), and is found mainly in laminae I and II. SP release is evoked specifically by peripheral noxious stimulation, and iontophoretic application of SP to noxious-responding neurons results in a slow,

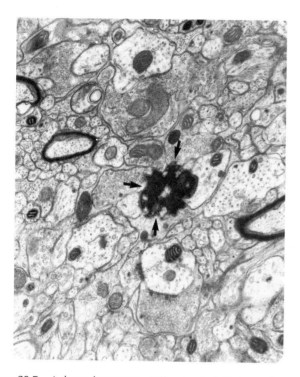

Figure 20.7. A dense degenerating C-fiber terminal *(dark arrow)* 1 week after dorsal rhizotomy. The degenerating terminal is postsynaptic *(open arrows)* to two small axon terminals arising from interneurons of the dorsal horn. It is believed that these axoaxonal synapses mediate presynaptic inhibition of dorsal root synaptic input.

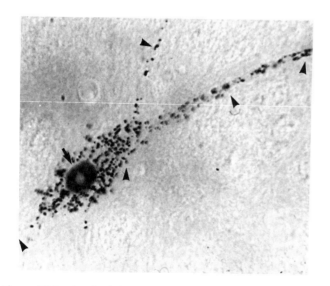

Figure 20.8. A spinothalamic tract neuron of the rat dorsal horn is identified by its content of horseradish peroxidase reaction product *(arrowheads)* that has been retrogradely transported to the spinal cord following its injection into the contralateral thalamus. The nucleus of the cell *(open arrow)* exhibits immunoreactivity for the fos protein product of the proto-oncogene, c-fos, following up-regulation of the gene by a noxious stimulus applied to the paw. (Courtesy of Dr. Allan I. Basbaum.)

long-lasting depolarization of these dorsal horn cells. Initially, SP was considered to be the specific neurotransmitter associated with signaling noxious stimuli. But neurons in the dorsal horn can be activated by peripheral noxious stimuli even when SP is depleted, so it is now suggested that SP and other neuropeptides may serve some sort of neuromodulatory role, such as by potentiating the spinal cord nociceptive neuronal responses to Glu. SP may also interact with calcitonin generated peptide (CGRP), which is found exclusively in small-diameter primary afferent axons and which is located almost entirely in laminae I and II. CGRP produces slow-onset, long-lasting depolarization of nociceptive dorsal horn neurons, and potentiates both the actions of SP and of Glu.

Several studies have demonstrated the behavioral roles of SP and other neurotransmitters associated with PANs. The intrathecal application of SP in the rat evokes the pain-related behaviors of biting and scratching, and has been shown to lower the threshold for pain avoidance behaviors, the behavior being reversed by the administration of SP receptor antagonists. As mentioned earlier, the chili pepper derivative capsaicin depletes SP from primary afferent neurons, and topical application to the skin of creams containing capsaicin have been used with some success to treat the chronic pain associated with postherpetic neuralgia. Experimentally induced arthritis in the monkey results in short-term (approximately 6 hours) decreases in dorsal horn SP and CGRP following stimulation of the affected joint, and an increase in dorsal horn Glu, regardless of joint stimulation. These findings suggest that the pain associated with Glu release may be that of the aching joint at rest, and the pain evoked by movement being associated with SP and CGRP may be activation of dorsal horn nociceptive neurons (12).

OPIATE MECHANISMS IN THE DORSAL HORN

The endogenous opiate enkephalin is present in neurons of the superficial dorsal horn, and is liberated from axons and from dendrites (presynaptic dendrites) of these cells. The terminals of Aδ- and C-fibers exhibit the three known classes of opioid binding receptors, μ, κ, and δ. Enkephalin can reduce the amount of SP released from primary afferent terminals. Morphine, acting on the μ-opioid binding site, can also reduce SP release from PANs, and this action of morphine can be reversed by the opiate antagonist naloxone. Other opiate ligands, acting at μ- and δ-binding sites can similarly reduce the release of neuropeptides and of excitatory amino acids (10) from primary afferent axons. There are also opioid binding sites on nociceptive dorsal horn neurons, including STT cells. The application of μ- and δ-opiate ligands can inhibit the responses of dorsal horn neurons to noxious stimulation. Thus, it is likely that the antinociceptive actions of opiates applied directly to the spinal cord are a result of the reduction of the release of neurotransmitters from PANs, as well as the direct inhibition of the activation of dorsal horn neurons, following peripheral noxious stimulation. Both of those types of analgesia are naloxone reversible.

Opioid binding sites can exhibit plastic changes. Following lesions of primary afferent axons produced by dorsal rhizotomy, there is a substantial decrease in μ- and δ-opioid binding sites, presumably resulting from degeneration of the axon terminals on which the binding sites are located. Within a few weeks, however, there is a gradual recovery of the binding sites, believed to be associated with sprouting of adjacent, noninjured primary afferent axons into the deafferented zone (13). There are also plastic changes in dorsal horn gene expression. For instance, the mRNAs derived from the preprotachykinin (PPT) gene that encode for the family of tachykinin peptides that includes SP are substantially increased in projection neurons of the rat dorsal horn following experimentally induced inflammation (14). These changes in neurotransmitters or their associated receptors may underlie the appearance of chronic pain states seen in many cases of peripheral nerve or dorsal root injuries.

IMMEDIATE EARLY GENES IN THE DORSAL HORN

There are a group of immediate early genes (IEGs) whose expression and protein products have served as useful markers for dorsal horn neurons that are activated by noxious—and by other—stimuli. For instance, the protein product of the c-fos proto-oncogene can be used to identify populations of dorsal horn neurons activated by peripheral noxious stimuli, and establish the relationship of the appearance of the fos protein to pain-related behavior. The changes in fos protein synthesis as a result of the administration of various opiate agonists (15), and whether the effects of opiates on IEG protein synthesis are naloxone-reversible have also been studied (Figs. 20.8 and 20.9). C-fos protein product appears in dorsal horn neurons following visceral (16) as well as somatic stimulation. There is a differential time course and varying expression of a variety of IEGs as a result of subacute or chronic somatic inflammation (17). Although it is not known why these particular genes in certain regions of the CNS have altered expression as a result of peripheral stimuli, they have formed the basis of numerous investigations correlating structural, functional, and behavioral aspects of pain mechanisms.

SPINOTHALAMIC TRACT NEURONS

The dorsal horn projection neurons of the primate that have been the most extensively studied are those that project to the thalamus, termed keep STT neurons. As described previously, STT cells can be physiologically and anatomically characterized. Most lie in lamina I or V, although they may also be found in other regions of the spinal gray, including the ventral horn (18). Those in lamina I receive Aδ- or C-fiber afferents and primarily signal noxious cutaneous stimuli (7); STT neurons in lamina V exhibit WDR convergent properties in that they receive input from Aβ-, Aδ- and C-afferents, (the latter probably terminating on distal dendrites of lamina V neurons that reach the superficial dorsal horn), and respond to a variety of innocuous and noxious peripheral stimuli. Many lamina V STT neurons are

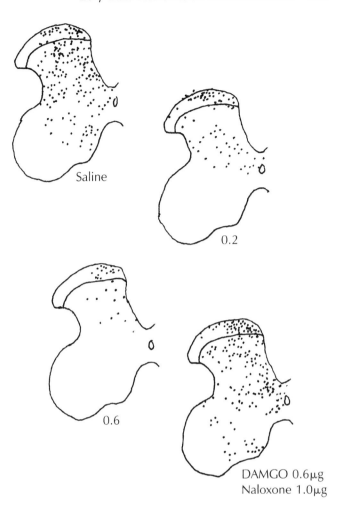

Figure 20.9. Diagrams of the distribution of neurons of the rat spinal cord that exhibit c-fos-like immunoreactivity as a result of a noxious stimulus to the paw. Saline control, in which saline was injected into the cerebral ventricles (i.c.v.), 0.2 and 0.6: show the dose-dependent distribution of c-fos cells following i.c.v. injection of μg amounts of the μ-opiate agonist D-ala, N Me-Phe, Gly-d enkephalin (DAMGO). The final drawing demonstrates the reversibility of the DAMGO effect by the i.c.v. injection of naloxone. (Modified from Gogas KR, Presley RW, Levine JD, Busbaum AI. The antinociceptive action of supraspinal opioids results in descending inhibitory control: correlation of nociceptive behavior and c-fos expression. Neuroscience 1991;42:617–628.

activated in a graded fashion by peripheral mechanical or thermal stimuli, in that the size of the evoked excitatory postsynaptic potentials (EPSPs) and the frequency of firing of the STT cells increase as the intensity of the stimuli increases, moving from the nonnoxious to the noxious range (8).

VISCERAL AND SOMATIC CONVERGENT NEURONS AND REFERRED PAIN

Numerous neurons in the deeper spinal gray matter (laminae V–VII) and in lamina X exhibit visceral and somatic convergent properties in that they respond to stimuli applied to both types of tissue. These cells are believed to play an essential role in referred pain. Referred pain of visceral origin is often perceived as arising from somatic tissues that are innervated by the same levels of the cord as is the visceral structure. Visceral pain is usually referred to the torso or to proximal regions of the limbs, but not often to the distal regions of the extremities. It is usually perceived as being of deep, rather than of cutaneous, origin. Primate STT neurons that are activated by both somatic and visceral (including bladder, gut, lung, and heart) manipulation have been shown to be driven principally by stimuli applied to deep, rather than cutaneous somatic structures, and by proximal rather than distal tissues (19). The phenomenon of counterirritation, in which noxious stimuli applied to one region of the body can reduce the sensation of pain arising from another somatic structure, has also been described for pain referred from visceral structures, in that noxious cutaneous stimuli can inhibit neuronal and reflex responses to noxious visceral stimuli (20).

MODULATION OF PAIN TRANSMISSION IN THE SPINAL CORD

It has long been known that one form of stimulus can modify the perceived quality and intensity of another. In the case of noxious stimulation, the sense of pain can be ameliorated by activation of large-diameter primary afferent fibers of the cord, a finding that led to the "gate control" theory of pain modulation (21), which states that inhibition of nociceptive STT cells by impulses in large diameter afferent axons in dorsal roots or their collaterals in the dorsal column white matter "closes the gate" via inhibitory interneurons, and the impulses carried by fine-diameter afferent leads to excitation of STT cells, thus "opening the gate" of pain transmission. Indeed, transcutaneous electrical nerve stimulation (TENS) and dorsal column stimulation modulates pain transmission similarly, following the stimulation of large-diameter afferent axons. In addition, the intensity of cold-induced painful stimuli conveyed by C-fibers can be suppressed by myelinated primary afferent fiber input (22). The gate control hypothesis has been invaluable in generating investigations of a wide variety of modulatory phenomena in the CNS, several of them demonstrating substantial roles for descending pain modulatory systems that arise in the brainstem and that are activated by noxious stimuli and follow a specific pathway in the spinal cord to terminate in the dorsal horn (23, 24). Analgesia produced by microstimulation of the periaqueductal gray (PAG) matter of the midbrain, or microinjection of morphine into PAG, has been shown to involve a descending system from PAG to medulla to the dorsolateral funiculus of the spinal cord and thence to the dorsal horn. Medullary neurons containing serotonin or pontine/midbrain cells that contain norepinephrine (25) release their neurotransmitter in the cord to either directly or indirectly (via enkephalin-containing dorsal horn LCNs) inhibit the activity of nociceptive STT neurons (23). Serotonin-containing neurons of the medullary raphe nuclei send their axons to the nucleus caudalis of the spinal cord and to the spinal dorsal horn via the dorsolateral funiculus of the cord (26). These axons then form synaptic contacts with neurons

of the superficial dorsal horn to activate modulatory mechanisms of the cord (27, 28).

Two classes of neurons in the rostral ventromedial medulla (RVM) of the rat have been identified that receive inputs from PAG and project to the dorsal horn. Stimulation of the RVM produces behavioral analgesia and has been shown to inhibit the activity of nociceptive STT cells. One of the RVM neuronal cell types, the on-cell, exhibits a burst of activity following a noxious stimulus, and this activity immediately precedes an avoidance (nocifensive) reflex, the tail-flick induced by noxious heat applied to the tail. Iontophoretic application of morphine to on-cells suppresses their activity, and is associated with behavioral hypoalgesia, in that the tail-flick response to noxious heat is also suppressed (29).

Alterations of primate STT cell activity have also been shown following stimulation of cerebral cortical projections to the spinal cord dorsal horn. PAG and cortical stimulation both evoke inhibitory postsynaptic potentials (IPSPs) in STT cells, and selectively inhibit the responses of lamina V-STT neurons activated by small-diameter afferent (noxious) input, but not those responding to large-diameter afferent (nonnoxious) fibers. These findings suggest that PAG and cortical projections to STT neurons may selectively control STT cell activation by afferent inputs, permitting switching of the coding properties of the cells according to varying behavioral states (30).

The appearance of the IEG protein product, fos, has been used to assess the neuronal populations of the cord that are affected by the administrations of opiates to produce behavioral analgesia. For instance, acute inflammation is associated with the appearance of fos protein in neurons of the superficial and deeper layers of the dorsal horn, and analgesia produced by the administration of systemic morphine reverses the expression of the fos protein in a dose-dependent, naloxone-reversible manner. The intracerebroventricular (i.c.v.) administration of a μ-opioid ligand sufficient to produce behavioral analgesia reduces fos protein expression to a greater degree in the deeper layers of the dorsal horn (the WDR cells) than in the superficial layers, chiefly populated by noxious specific neurons (Fig. 20.9), suggesting different roles for WDR and NS neurons in behavioral manifestations of pain (15). Furthermore, bilateral lesions of the spinal dorsolateral funiculus (DLF) abolish the antinociceptive effects of the opiate as well as the suppression of fos protein, providing additional evidence for the supraspinal origins of descending pain-control systems and the spinal pathway taken by the control system.

Finally, there is evidence for the modulatory effects of vagal afferent stimulation on nociception in several species, including the monkey, in that vagal stimulation can either facilitate or inhibit pain-related behavior following noxious cutaneous stimulation. A recent study in the rat (31) has shown that vagal stimulation produces inhibition of nociceptive reflexes (tail-flick) in the intact animal but facilitates this reflex if the neurotransmitters SP and CGRP, found in C-fiber afferents, had been depleted by neonatal exposure of the rats to capsaicin, suggesting that the inhibitory effects of vagal stimulation on nociception depends on C-fiber primary afferents in spinal nerves and/or the vagus.

Much of what has been described also pertains to noxious mechanisms that involve the trigeminal system, in that fine-diameter trigeminal afferents convey noxious information to the trigeminal nuclear complex of the brainstem, and these messages are synaptically transmitted to particular sets of neurons within the trigeminal nuclei using the same types of neurotransmitters as do dorsal root afferents (32). The activities of trigeminal nociceptive neurons can be modulated by similar processes as those that modulate spinal nociceptive cells. The distribution of fine-diameter nociceptive primary trigeminal afferents appears to be more complex than previously believed, in that noxious information activates neurons in almost all trigeminal subnuclei, rather than being restricted to those cells of the subnucleus caudalis. For instance, afferents from tooth pulp in the monkey, most of which carry nociceptive information, project to the principal trigeminal nucleus, and subnuclei oralis and interpolaris, with only a modest termination in the most rostral portion of subnucleus caudalis (33), explaining why trigeminal tractotomy at the level of the obex has little effect on dental pain in humans.

There is thus abundant evidence that particular populations of neurons convey noxious information from the periphery to the CNS and that specialized neurons within the CNS that receive this information send it to higher centers. At every stage of this system, excitation of neuronal networks by noxious stimuli can set in motion a variety of modulatory mechanisms to facilitate or inhibit the activities of cells that transmit the information that the brain may interpret as being painful.

Ascending Pathways Conveying Noxious Stimuli

Although ascending pathways that carry noxious information are traditionally called "pain pathways," the point once again is that the sensory experience of pain is a product of neural networks of the forebrain. Trains of stimuli ascending from the cord or trigeminal nuclei may or may not be interpreted as painful, as evident from the previous discussion of modulation of sensory processes.

This section describes four ascending systems that are concerned with pain mechanisms. The spinothalamic tract (STT) conveys information that will ultimately be transmitted to the somatosensory cerebral cortex. Regions of the cerebral cortex other than the somatosensory cortex receive the information carried by the other three ascending systems, the spinomesencephalic (SMT), the spinoparabrachial (SPB) and the spinohypothalamic (SHT) tracts. It is believed that these latter pathways are concerned with the emotional, memory, and autonomic mechanisms associated with pain.

SPINOTHALAMIC TRACT

The best-known ascending pathway, the STT (and its homologue, the trigeminothalamic pathway) conveys soma-

totopically organized information arising from peripheral noxious stimuli to several thalamic nuclei. It is believed that the STT, particularly that component that terminates in the lateral thalamus (the ventrobasal—VB, and posterior—Po nuclear complexes) is associated with the sensory-discriminative aspects of pain: the peripheral location and the intensity of the noxious stimuli.

The cells of origin of the STT are found at all levels of the spinal cord. In primates they are particularly numerous at high cervical segments of the cord. Although several laminae of the spinal gray matter contain STT neurons, they are principally found in laminae I and V (18). Lamina I cells chiefly transmit information about noxious mechanical stimuli (noxious specific—NS), and the lamina V cells transmit information about a wide variety of nonnoxious and noxious mechanical, thermal, and chemical stimuli (wide dynamic range—WDR), usually responding with a graded increase in firing rate in response to increasing stimulus intensity (34). Much of the information about noxious stimuli is carried to the spinal cord by nonmyelinated primary afferents (C-fibers). The axons of STT cells that carry this information in the CNS are myelinated as indicated by electron microscopic (35) and electrophysiological (7) studies, the latter indicating that the axons of WDR cells conduct at a faster rate (mean, 33 m/s) than do the axons of NS neurons (mean, 14 m/s).

In the primate, including the human, the axons of most (> 90%) STT neurons cross the midline to travel in the anterolateral quadrant (ALQ), a zone demarcated by the denticulate ligament laterally and the anterior median fissure medially (Fig. 20.3). The STT is intermixed with several other ascending and descending pathways of the spinal cord white matter that also lie in the ALQ of the cord. The axons of STT cells that carry noxious information are widely dispersed throughout the ALQ, but there is a segregation determined by laminar origin of the STT axons. Most of the axons of the WDR neurons of lamina V are located in the more ventral and medial regions of the ALQ; those from the NS cells of lamina I are located more dorsally and laterally, just ventral to the descending fibers of the corticospinal tract (36, 37).

The terminations of the primate STT (Fig. 20.10) are found in several nuclei of the lateral and medial thalamus (38). The STT axons ending laterally in the ventroposterolateral (VPL) nucleus arborize as "parcellated bursts" (39), which terminate on subpopulations of VPL neurons in a topographically organized manner, in that axons from caudal spinal segments (lower extremity) are located more laterally than those from cervical segments (upper extremity). Trigeminothalamic axons terminate more medially in the ventroposteromedial nucleus (VPM). VPL and VPM together constitute the major components of the ventrobasal nuclear complex (VB), which projects to the appropriate topographic regions (e.g., leg, arm, face) of the primary somatosensory cortex and which is concerned with information about the location and intensity of noxious stimuli. The VB is also the recipient of the afferent fibers from the dorsal column nuclei and from the trigeminal nuclei that

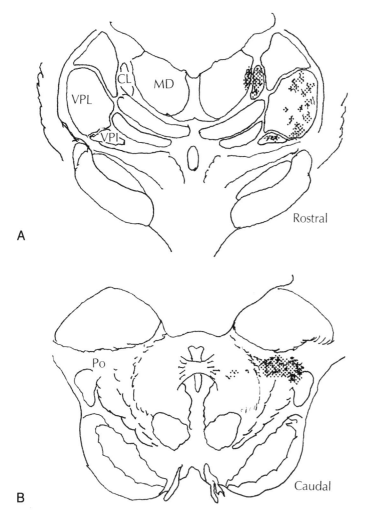

A

B

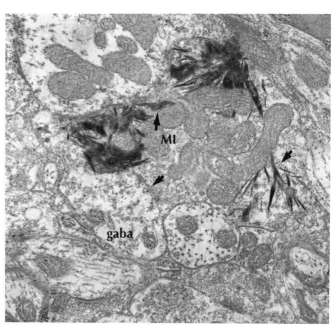

Figure 20.11. Electron micrograph of the macaque thalamus, showing a medial lemniscal terminal (ML) labeled with horseradish peroxidase reaction product *(dark arrows)* following injection of the tracer into the contralateral dorsal column nuclei. ML is presynaptic *(open arrow)* to a GABA profile, identified by the 10-nm gold particles used to label the GABA antibody. ML terminals commonly interact with GABA-ergic interneurons of the thalamus. STT afferents seldom do. (From Ralston HJ III, Ralston DD. Medial lemniscal and spinal projections to the macaque thalamus: an electron microscopic study of differing GABAergic circuitry serving thalamic somatosensory mechanisms. J Neurosci 1994;14:2485–2502.)

Figure 20.10. Projections (shown by stippling) of the spinothalamic tract (STT) to caudal **(A)** and rostral **(B)** levels of the macaque thalamus. The densest projection is to the posterior nuclear complex (Po). Electrical stimulation of Po in humans evokes reports of contralateral burning pain. Other nuclei that receive significant STT afferents are the ventral postero-lateral nucleus (VPL), in which the STT projections form "bursts," the central lateral nucleus (CL), the lateral portion of the mediodorsal nucleus (MD), and the ventral posterior inferior nucleus (VPI). Electrical stimulation of VPL does not usually elicit reports of pain. (Modified from Mehler WR, Feferman ME, Nauta WJH. Ascending axon degeneration following anterolateral cordotomy. An experimental study in the monkey. Brain 1960;83:718–750.)

convey information from nonnoxious stimuli. The other major lateral nuclear region of the thalamus that receives STT input is the posterior nuclear complex (Po/SG), which receives a major projection of STT axons (Fig. 20.10). These axons arborize just caudal to VPL and extend ventral to VPL in the ventroposterior inferior nucleus (VPI). A recent study has shown that the axons of lamina I STT neurons (NS) terminate primarily in Po/SG and in VPI, and those of lamina V STT cells end primarily in VPL (40).

STT axons also terminate more medially in the thalamus in the intralaminar nuclei (chiefly the central lateral nucleus – CL), the adjacent mediodorsal nucleus (MD), and the ventromedially placed nucleus submedius (Sm). MD and Sm project to the orbitofrontal cortex, and may thus participate in the emotional, affective aspects of pain

mechanisms (41). The cortical projections of CL are more widely distributed and may participate in generalized cortical arousal mechanisms following noxious stimuli.

Electron microscopic studies have demonstrated that medial lemniscal (ML) and STT axon terminals are large (> 2 μm diameter) profiles that form multiple synaptic contacts on dendritic segments of thalamic projection (thalamocortical relay – TCR) neurons (42). Like most other sensory afferent projections to the thalamus, ML terminals synapse upon the dendrites of thalamic projection neurons and upon GABA-ergic local circuit neurons (LCNs–interneurons) of the thalamus (Fig. 20.11). However, there appears to be little interaction between STT afferents and GABA-ergic thalamic LCNs, and this relative lack of GABA-ergic modulation of noxious input to thalamic neurons appears to be characteristic of the primate STT system (43).

The physiological responses of neurons in primate VPL are in keeping with the anatomical distribution of STT axons, which are distributed to subsets of VPL neurons, while those from the dorsal column nuclei are found throughout VPL (35). Many VPL cells respond in a graded fashion to increasing intensities of peripheral stimuli, thus exhibiting the WDR properties of lamina V neurons (44), or perhaps receiving convergent input from both the dorsal column nuclei and the spinal cord. Other VPL neurons respond only to innocuous peripheral stimuli and are driven exclusively by stimuli conveyed by large-diameter primary afferent axons, relayed in the dorsal column nuclei. Relatively small numbers of VPL cells are activated exclusively by noxious stimuli, but there are more NS neurons in Po/SG and in VPI, nuclei that receive projections from the NS cells of lamina I. STT terminations in the lateral thalamus of the cat are fundamentally different from those of the primate, in that they do not terminate in VPL but rather in a zone ventral to VPL (45), which may be analogous to primate Po/SG. Neurons in this ventral zone in the cat respond to peripheral noxious stimuli; those in VPL do not (46).

Recordings and microstimulation studies of thalamus in awake humans undergoing stereotaxic neurosurgical procedures, usually for the treatment of movement disorders, have revealed neuronal responses similar to those described in monkeys (47). In both cases, most neurons that respond to noxious stimuli, such as noxious heat, are found more ventrally and caudally in the thalamus, rather than in the central "cutaneous core" zone of the somatosensory thalamus (48). Interestingly, electrical stimulation of the human VPL does not usually elicit reports of pain, but stimulation ventral to VPL in a region analogous to the monkey Po/SG and VPI (a zone that Hassler designated Vc.Pc in the human) leads the subject to complain of burning pain in a region of the body or face contralateral to the side of the thalamus being stimulated (49). Recordings from patients having pain of central origin, usually as a result of a stroke involving the diencephalon, have revealed abnormal burst-firing of VPL neurons following both innocuous and noxious peripheral stimuli (50).

Changes in VPL neurons have also been described in animals following central injuries. In cats that have had a spinal tractotomy involving the ALQ, similar to the procedure used for treating certain forms of pain in humans, increased activity of VB neurons, both spontaneous and evoked, has been described, and this heightened activity can be reversed by the systemic administration of N-methyl-D-aspartate (NMDA) receptor antagonists, suggesting that certain central pain states following cord lesions may result from the upregulation of NMDA receptor synthesis (51). In monkeys surviving for 12 years after extensive cervical dorsal rhizotomy, transneuronal degeneration of the dorsal column nuclei and a marked reduction in GABA receptors in VPL has been reported (52). Accordingly, reduction in normally occurring GABA modulation of nonnoxious signals from the dorsal column nuclei to the thalamus may lead to the misinterpretation by the brain that the impulses arise from noxious stimuli, which usually lack GABA modulation (43).

Following injury to the CNS, some patients have burning pain referred to a particular body part, a condition called central poststroke pain, a term replacing the previous, less accurate appellation, thalamic pain syndrome. A recent study (53) of such patients found that the central lesion could involve the brainstem or spinal cord, the diencephalon (including the thalamus), or the cerebral hemispheres. All patients showed a diminished perception of pinprick or thermal stimuli, sensory modalities carried by the spinothalamic tract which are then relayed by the thalamus to the cortex. Other sensory modalities were usually normal or only somewhat altered by the central lesions. The study concluded that these central pain states were a result of deafferentation as a result of the interruption of the central pain pathways at any level of the neuraxis. The mechanisms underlying central poststroke pain are unknown, but presumably involve some sort of reorganization of central somatosensory circuits and/or changes in the expression of neurotransmitters and their receptors that participate in the central pain pathways.

A surgical procedure to treat chronic, intractable pain, usually in patients with intra-abdominal or pelvic cancer, is the transection of the ALQ of the spinal cord white matter, which contains the axons of the STT that arise from dorsal horn neurons on the contralateral side of the cord (see previous discussion). The ALQ contains many other ascending and descending pathways, so the surgically induced lesion is not only of STT axons. This procedure, spinal tractotomy, usually results in relief of pain caudal to the spinal segment of the lesion, and on the side contralateral to the lesion, because the STT axons cross the midline before they ascend in the contralateral ALQ. Most patients receiving tractotomies survive only for a few months following the lesion, because of the nature of their disease leading to the procedure. In those surviving for longer periods, the pain often returns, perhaps because of the presence of other ascending systems that are not interrupted by the lesion. Tractotomy may actually cause new pain in these patients, as a result of central deafferentation that is seen in central, poststroke pain. Surgical lesions intended to treat pain must be used with care, because damage to nerves or to central pathways that convey noxious information may actually lead to pain that is even more difficult to manage than the original pain that was being treated by the surgical procedure.

SPINOMESENCEPHALIC TRACT

In addition to their projections to the thalamus, spinal cord neurons that receive convergent input from cutaneous, muscle, joint, and visceral sources and that respond to noxious stimuli have been found to project to the midbrain, some sending collateral branches to both thalamic and mesencephalic targets (54, 55). Studies of rat, cat, and monkey (56) reveal that the major terminal fields in the midbrain of spinal afferents include the PAG, the nucleus cuneiformis (an important cholinergic nucleus of the brainstem), deeper layers of the superior colliculus that participate in visuomotor integrative mechanisms, and the intercollicular nuclei. Electrical stimulation of the region of PAG that receives SMT input results in inhibition of the responses of spinal nociceptive neurons, and microinjection of similar regions of the PAG with morphine results in analgesia (34). Thus, the SMT may contribute the ascending, afferent limb to this descending pain modulation system. The other midbrain targets of the SMT are known to participate in a variety of motor and autonomic mechanism associated with nocifensive behaviors, such as fear, flight, rage, and cardiovascular changes. Several of these same midbrain regions that receive SMT afferent projections have connections with diencephalic and telencephalic structures (57, 58). Thus, the SMT contributes ascending, primarily noxious information from all types of peripheral tissues to midbrain systems involved in pain modulation, and somatic motor and visceromotor responses.

SPINOPARABRACHIAL TRACT

The parabrachial nucleus (PB) is found bilaterally, surrounding the superior cerebellar peduncles as they exit from the cerebellum at the dorsal junction of the pons and midbrain. The PB can be cytoarchitectonically divided into several subnuclei that participate in a variety of functions, including gustation and cardiorespiratory regulation. Many PB neurons in the rat receive afferent projections from the spinal cord (59) and, in turn, these neurons project to the hypothalamus and to the amygdaloid nuclear complex of the limbic forebrain. A recent physiological study has shown that about two-thirds of these PB projection cells respond exclusively to peripheral noxious stimuli and serve to relay nociceptive information from the spinal cord and trigeminal nuclear complex to the amygdaloid nuclei (60). The possible role of this spino-ponto-amygdaloid pathway in pain mechanism is not known. However, the fact that the PB is involved in several autonomic and visceral functions suggests that this system could be concerned with autonomic and behavioral reactions to noxious stimuli. These motivational functions may be complex, as suggested by a report that bilateral PB lesions in the rat abolish the aversive motivational effects of morphine, but not the positive responses to the drug (61).

Projections from spinal cord and trigeminal lamina I neurons of cat and monkey, presumably nociceptive in function, have also been shown to terminate in the locus ceruleus (62), a pigmented cell group that lies just medial to PB. The locus ceruleus (LC) is the principal source of norepinephrine for the brain and spinal cord. The noradrenergic projections from LC to thalamus are believed to participate in arousal mechanisms, and LC fibers to the spinal cord serve descending control functions that modulate the activities of spinal neurons responding to noxious stimuli (23). Thus, the nociceptive afferent fibers from cord to LC may activate arousal as well as the descending pain modulatory circuitry of the spinal cord.

SPINOHYPOTHALAMIC TRACT

This system has been most studied in rats, although there is evidence that it also exists as a minor pathway in cats (63). There is not yet agreement concerning the existence of this system in primates. In rats, the SHT arises from neurons in both the superficial and deep regions of the dorsal horn of the cord and the medulla, the medullary dorsal horn of the subnucleus caudalis of the trigeminal nuclear complex being

comparable in structure and function to the cord dorsal horn (64). Nearly 90% of SHT neurons respond preferentially or specifically to noxious stimuli applied to cutaneous or deep structures (65), and it is assumed that this spinohypothalamic system may serve autonomic, endocrine and emotional aspects of pain mechanisms (66).

Cerebral Cortex and Pain

The somatosensory cortex receives topographically organized projections from those thalamic regions, principally the ventrobasal complex (described earlier), that receive ascending pathways conveying noxious and nonnoxious information from superficial and deep structures. Nonetheless, investigators have had great difficulty in demonstrating a particular role of the cerebral cortex in pain mechanisms in experimental animals and in humans (67). Indeed, earlier clinical studies suggested that the cerebral cortex was not essential for the perception of pain, although the cortex might participate in the localization of noxious stimuli. In their famous book reporting on the results of electrical stimulation of the exposed cerebral cortex of conscious humans, Penfield and Rasmussen (68) did not even include "pain" in the index, for their patients rarely reported painful sensations following stimulation of their cortices. Some clinical reports state that large cortical ablations did not alter pain perception, while others report that cortical lesions reduced or abolished pain and/or thermal sensitivity.

During the past decade, studies in animals and humans have demonstrated conclusively that cortical neurons can be activated by peripheral noxious stimuli, and that these neuronal responses can be correlated with the localization and intensity of the stimuli. Recordings made in the primary somatosensory cortex (SI) of barbiturate-anesthetized monkeys revealed neurons that exhibited graded responses to increasing intensities of noxious mechanical or thermal cutaneous stimuli (67), and that these neurons exhibited small peripheral receptive fields, so that they could encode the place as well as the intensity of noxious stimuli. Recordings made from SI cortical neurons in awake, behaving monkeys demonstrated that the activities of the cortical neurons could be correlated with the speed of the animals' behavioral response to noxious thermal stimuli (69).

Another somatosensory cortical area, SII (the second somatosensory cortex), lies in the upper bank of the frontoparietal operculum, adjacent to the sylvian fissure. SII is much smaller than SI and receives afferent projections from several of the same thalamic nuclei that project to SI (70). Recordings from SII and the adjacent area 7b in monkeys reveal neuronal responses that encode the duration, but not the intensity of noxious stimuli (71), and the receptive fields of the cells did not reflect the precise location of the stimuli. Therefore, this study suggested that the functional role of SII may be related to more generalized aspects of pain mechanisms, such as the initiation of avoidance behaviors following noxious stimulation.

The somatosensory cortex of the rat and cat cerebral

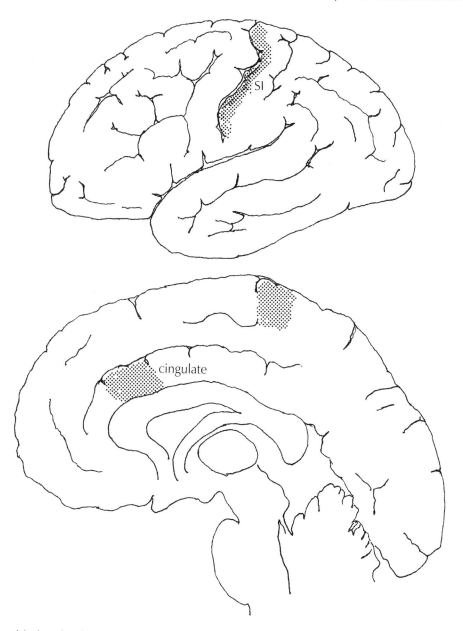

Figure 20.12. Diagrams of the lateral and medial views of the human cerebral cortex showing regions that are activated *(stipples)* by peripheral noxious stimuli. Primary somatosensory cortex — SI; cingulate cortex. The second somatosensory cortex, SII, is located in the retroinsular area, within the sylvian fissure.

cortex also contains neurons that respond to peripheral noxious stimuli (72, 73). Furthermore, in rats that have an experimentally induced inflammatory arthritis, cortical neurons significantly increase their responses to painful stimuli. Similar response changes observed in the spinal cord and thalamus can be correlated with "pain behavior" in these animals, such as guarding of the limb and heightened withdrawal from innocuous stimuli (74). Neurons that respond to noxious cold stimuli have also been reported in the orbitofrontal cortex of rats (75).

Humans are able to localize the precise location of focal pinprick stimuli, which is almost as accurate as the ability to localize the position of innocuous tactile stimuli (76), indicating the presence of a highly ordered topographic representation for the neurons responding to noxious

stimuli. One assumes that this region must be the cerebral cortex. Two recent studies in humans using positron emission tomography (PET) have found particular cortical areas that exhibit heightened cortical metabolic activity (Fig. 20.12), indicated by increased regional blood flow, that can be directly correlated with the graded intensity of noxious thermal stimuli and the reports of the degree of pain by the subjects (77, 78). Interestingly, both studies found increased activity in the anterior cingulate cortex. In addition, one (77) found elevated regional blood flow in the primary somatosensory cortex, SI, but not in the thalamus; the other (78) found thalamic activity but not SI activation.

These divergent findings illustrate the continuing problems in understanding the role of the cerebral cortex in pain perception and the substantial emotional and behavioral responses to painful stimuli. Based on these studies and on a recent review (79), patients with large lesions of the cerebral cortex can still perceive painful stimuli to the contralateral body, in contrast to individuals with thalamic lesions, who have a marked decrement in pain sensation. Such clinical findings have led to the view that the sensation of pain is a function of the thalamus, not the cortex. However, a cortical lesion leads to profound retrograde degeneration of thalamic neurons that project to the cortex; thus, a cortical lesion is also a thalamic lesion. The cingulate cortex, shown to be activated in humans receiving noxious stimuli, is on the medial surface of the hemisphere. It receives its thalamic input from several of the intralaminar thalamic nuclei, the cells of which tend to have widespread cortical projections. It could be argued that the cingulate cortex, part of the "limbic lobe," might be spared in hemispheric lesions that destroy the laterally placed SI, and thus continue to serve the perception of pain and the emotional responses to it, while the ability to distinguish the precise intensity and localization of noxious stimuli following lesions of SI would be abolished. Pain is a complex sensory and emotional experience. We have much more to learn before we can understand the forebrain mechanisms that serve it.

SUMMARY

This chapter has described the neuronal processes and pathways that transmit information arising from noxious stimuli that ultimately are interpreted by the brain as being painful. This information can be modulated at several steps of the pathway, beginning with the peripheral sensory endings of primary afferent nociceptors (PANs). Nonsteroidal anti-inflammatory drugs (NSAIDs), such as aspirin, inhibit the enzymatic action of cyclooxygenase, which participates in the breakdown of arachidonic acid to prostaglandins which, in turn, lead to the inflammatory response and the sensitization of PANs. Opiates, acting principally at μ-opiate receptor sites on the sensory endings of PANs, can inhibit the hyperalgesia resulting from tissue damage and the consequent production of prostoglandin $E_2(1)$.

In the spinal cord, the central synaptic terminations of PANs release substance P, other neuropeptides, and excitatory amino acids. Opioids applied directly to the spinal cord (intrathecally) block the behavioral responses to noxious stimuli in experimental animals and have a powerful analgesic effect in humans, probably by inhibiting the release of substance P from primary afferent terminals (1). Similarly, the application of GABA$_A$-receptor agonists to the cord can have similar analgesic effects through the inhibitory effects of these drugs on spinal cord neurons. The activity of spinothalamic tract neurons that convey noxious information to the thalamus can be modulated by descending projections (23) from the brainstem that utilize serotonin or norepinephrine as neurotransmitters to activate intrinsic neurons of the dorsal horn that contain endogenous opiate-like substances, e.g., enkephalin. The descending projections have been shown to reduce the firing of dorsal horn neurons responding to noxious input, and this system is believed to be activated normally by noxious stimuli, so that animals and humans have endogenous pain control systems. This descending control system can be accessed artificially by placing stimulating microelectrodes near the neuronal origins of the descending system, such as in the PAG of the midbrain. Such stimulus-induced analgesia was first examined in rats, and has now been used therapeutically in several thousand humans, usually relatively young individuals suffering from chronic intractable pain that has not responded to other forms of treatment.

Most analgesic drugs, whether opioids or NSAIDs, act primarily in the periphery, cord, or brainstem. Other drugs that have a role in pain therapy are not usually considered as analgesic agents, and act on the forebrain when used for their primary purpose. Tricyclic antidepressants are examples of such agents, and have been shown to be useful in a variety of painful conditions, including postherpetic neuralgia, diabetic neuropathy, and migraine headache. Animal models have shown analgesic responses to the administration of tricyclic antidepressants, and their mechanisms of action appears to be the prolongation of the actions of biogenic amine transmitters by inhibiting their reuptake into nerve terminals. The descending modulatory systems from brainstem to cord utilize serotonin or norepinephrine as neurotransmitters to inhibit pain-transmitting neurons of the dorsal horn. Prolonging the activity of these amines would be expected to enhance the analgesic effects of these descending systems. Thus, the presumed sites of action in the spinal cord of tricyclic antidepressants in producing analgesia appear to be distinct from their sites of action in the forebrain associated with their use in treating depression. The precise role of the forebrain in the perception of pain remains to be determined. Presently, drugs used to treat pain all appear to have their primary sites of action at levels caudal to the forebrain itself. One can expect that as the new functional imaging techniques of MRI continue to improve, we will gain further insights into the forebrain regions active during pain sensation, which might then yield new approaches to pain treatment targeted on forebrain activity associated with pain.

Acknowledgments

I am indebted to Diane Daly Ralston, who carried out several of our experimental studies cited in the references and shown in the accompanying figures. I thank Antonia Milroy for her skillful electron microscopic preparations, and Sandra Canchola for her photographic and laboratory assistance. The work from our laboratory is supported by NIH grants NS 23347 and NS 21445 from the National Institutes of Health.

References

1. Levine JD, Fields HL, Basbaum AI. Peptides and the primary afferent nociceptor. J Neurosci 1993;13:2273–2286.
2. Westlund KN, Sun YC, Sluka KA, Dougherty PM, Sorkin LS, Willis WD. Neural changes in acute arthritis in monkeys. II. Increased

glutamate immunoreactivity in the medial articular nerve. Brain Res Rev 1992;17:15–27.

3. Rexed B. The cytoarchitectonic organization of the spinal cord in the cat. J Comp Neurol 1952;96:415–495.

4. Ralston HJ III, Ralston DD. The distribution of dorsal root axons in laminae I, II and III of the macaque spinal cord: a quantitative electron microscope study. J Comp Neurol 1979;184:643–684.

5. Alvarez FJ, Kavookjian AM, Light AR. Ultrastructural morphology, synaptic relationships, and CGRP immunoreactivity of physiologically identified C-fiber terminals in the monkey spinal cord. J Comp Neurol 1993;329:472–490.

6. Ralston HJ III, Ralston DD. The distribution of dorsal root axons to laminae IV, V, and VI of the macaque spinal cord: a quantitative electron microscopic study. J Comp Neurol 1982;212:435–448.

7. Ferrington DG, Sorkin LS, Willis WD. Responses of spinothalamic tract cells in the superficial dorsal horn of the primate lumber spinal cord. J Physiol (Lond) 1987;388:681–703.

8. Zhang D, Owens CM, Willis WD. Intracellular study of electrophysiological features of primate spinothalamic tract neurons and their responses to afferent inputs. J Neurophysiol 1991;65:1554–1566.

9. Westlund KN, Carlton SM, Zhang D, Willis WD. Glutamate-immunoreactive terminals synapse on primate spinothalamic tract cells. J Comp Neurol 1992;322:519–527.

10. Kangrga I, Randic M. Outflow of endogenous aspartate and glutamate from the rat spinal dorsal horn in vitro by activation of low- and high-threshold primary afferent fibers. Modulation by μ-opioids. Brain Res 1991;553:347–352.

11. Knyihar-Csillik E, Torok A, Csillik B. Primary afferent origin of substance P-containing axons in the superficial dorsal horn of the rat spinal cord: depletion, regeneration and replenishment of presumed nociceptive central terminals. J Comp Neurol 1990;297:594–612.

12. Sluka KA, Dougherty PM, Sorkin LS, Willis WD, Westlund KN. Neural changes in acute arthritis in monkeys. III. Changes in substance P, calcitonin gene-related peptide and glutamate in the dorsal horn of the spinal cord. Brain Res Rev 1992;17:29–38.

13. Besse D, Lombard MC, Besson JM. Plasticity of μ and δ opioid receptors in the superficial dorsal horn of the adult rat spinal cord following dorsal rhizotomies: a quantitative autoradiographic study. Eur J Neurosci 1992;4:954–965.

14. Noguchi K, Ruda MA. Gene regulation in an ascending nociceptive pathway: inflammation-induced increase in preprotachykinin mRNA in rat lamina I spinal projection neurons. J Neurosci 1992;12:2563–2572.

15. Gogas KR, Presley RW, Levine JD, Basbaum AI. The antinociceptive action of supraspinal opioids results from an increase in descending inhibitory control: correlation of nociceptive behavior and c-fos expression. Neuroscience 1991;42:617–628.

16. Traub RJ, Pechman P, Iadarola MJ, Gebhart GF. Fos-like proteins in the lumbosacral spinal cord following noxious and non-noxious colorectal distention in the rat. Pain 1992;49:393–403.

17. Lanteri-Minet M, De Pommery J, Herdegen T, Weil-Fugazza J, Bravo R, Menetrey D. Differential time course and spatial expression of Fos, Jun, and Krox-24 proteins in spinal cord of rats undergoing subacute or chronic somatic inflammation. J Comp Neurol 1993;333:223–235.

18. Apkarian AV, Hodge CJ. Primate spinothalamic pathways: I. A quantitative study of the cells of origin of the spinothalamic pathway. J Comp Neurol 1989;288:447–473.

19. Hobbs SF, Chandler MJ, Bolser DC, Foreman RD. Segmental organization of visceral and somatic input onto C_3–T_6 spinothalamic tract cells of the monkey. J Neurophysiol 1992;68:1575–1588.

20. Ness TJ, Gebhart GF. Interactions between visceral and cutaneous nociception in the rat. I. Noxious cutaneous stimuli inhibit visceral nociceptive neurons and reflexes. J Neurophysiol 1991;66:20–28.

21. Wall PD. The gate control theory of pain mechanisms. A reexamination and re-statement. Brain 1978;101:1–18.

22. Wahren LK, Torebjork E, Jorum E. Central suppression of cold-induced C fibre pain by myelinated fibre input. Pain 1989;38:313–319.

23. Basbaum AI, Fields HL. Endogenous pain control systems: brainstem spinal pathways and endorphin circuitry. Annu Rev Neurosci. 1984; 7:309–338.

24. Zhang RX, Wang R, Chen J-Y, Qiao J-T. Effects of descending inhibitory systems on the c-Fos expression in the rat spinal cord during formalin-induced noxious stimulation. Neuroscience 1994;58:299–304.

25. Giradot M-N, Brennen TJ, Martindale ME, Foreman RD. Effects of stimulating the subcoeruleus-parabrachial region on the non-noxious and noxious responses of T1–T5 spinothalamic tract neurons in the primate. Brain Res 1987;409:19–30.

26. Westlund KN, Lu Y, Coggeshall RE, Willis WD. Serotonin is found in myelinated axons of the dorsolateral funiculus in monkeys. Neurosci Lett 1992;141:35–38.

27. Basbaum AI, Ralston DD, Ralston HJIII. Bulbospinal projections in the primate: a light and electron microscopic study of a pain modulating system. J Comp Neurol 1986;250:311–323.

28. Gerhart KD, Yezierski RP, Fang ZR, Willis WD. Inhibition of primate spinothalamic tract neurons by stimulation in periaqueductal gray or adjacent midbrain reticular formation. J Neurophysiol 1984;53:450–466.

29. Heinricher MM, Morgan MM, Fields HL. Direct and indirect actions of morphine on medullary neurons that modulate nociception. Neuroscience 1992;48:533–543.

30. Zhang D, Owens CM, Willis WD. Two forms of inhibition of spinothalamic tract neurons produced by stimulation of the periaqueductal gray and the cerebral cortex. J Neurophysiol 1991;65:1567–1579.

31. Ren K, Zhuo M, Randich A, Gebhart GF. Vagal afferent stimulation-produced effects on nociception in capsaicin-treated rats. J Neurophysiol 1993;69:1530–1540.

32. Clements JR, Magnusson KR, Hautman J, Beitz AJ. Rat tooth pulp projections to spinal trigeminal subnucleus caudalis are glutamate-like immunoreactive. J Comp Neurol 1991;309:281–288.

33. Takemura M, Nagase Y, Yoshida A, et al. The central projections of the monkey tooth pulp afferent neurons. Somatosens Mot Res 1993;10:217–227.

34. Willis WD, Coggeshall RE. Sensory mechanisms of the spinal cord. 2nd ed. New York: Plenum, 1991.

35. Ralston HJIII, Peschanski M, Ralston DD. Fine structure of spinothalamic tract axons and terminals in rat, cat, and monkey demonstrated by the orthograde transport of lectin conjugated to horseradish peroxidase. In: Fields HL, Dubner R, Cervero F, eds. Advances in pain research and therapy, vol. 9. New York: Raven Press, 1985:269–275.

36. Apkarian AV, Hodge CJ. Primate spinothalamic pathways: II. The cells of origin of the dorsolateral and ventral spinothalamic pathways. J Comp Neurol 1989;288:474–492.

37. Craig AD. Spinal distribution of ascending lamina I axons anterogradely labeled with Phaseolus vulgaris leucoagglutinin (PHA-L) in the cat. J Comp Neurol 1991;313:377–393.

38. Boivie J. An anatomical reinvestigation of the termination of the spinothalamic tract in the monkey. J Comp Neurol 1979;186:343–370.

39. Mehler WR, Feferman ME, Nauta WJH. Ascending axon degeneration following anterolateral cordotomy. An experimental study in the monkey. Brain 1960;83:718–750.

40. Ralston HJIII, Ralston DD. The primate dorsal spinothalamic tract: evidence for a specific termination in the posterior nuclei (Po/SG) of the thalamus. Pain 1992;48:107–118.

41. Craig AD, Jr., Burton H. Spinal and medullary lamina I projection to nucleus submedius in medial thalamus: a possible pain center. J Neurophysiol 1981;45:443–446.

42. Ralston HJ III. Local circuitry of the somatosensory thalamus in the processing of sensory information. Prog Brain Res 1991;87:13–28.

43. Ralston HJ III, Ralston DD. Medial lemniscal and spinal projections to the macaque thalamus: an electron microscopic study of differing GABAergic circuitry serving thalamic somatosensory mechanisms. J Neurosci 1994;14:2485–2502.

44. Chung JM, Lee KH, Surmeier DJ, Sorkin LS, Kim J, Willis WD. Response characteristics of neurons in the ventral posterior lateral nucleus of the monkey thalamus. J Neurophysiol 1986;56:370–390.

45. Boivie J. The termination of the spinothalamic tract in the cat. An experimental study with silver impregnation methods. Exp Brain Res 1971;12:331–353.

46. Kniffki K-D, Mizumura K. Responses of neurons in VPL and VPL-VL region of the cat to algesic stimulation of muscle and tendon. J Neurophysiol 1983;49:649–661.

47. Murphy JT. Single-unit analysis of the human ventral thalamic nuclear group: somatosensory responses. J Neurophysiol 1988;59:299–316.

48. Lenz FA, Seike M, Lin YC, et al. Neurons in the area of human thalamic nucleus ventralis caudalis respond to painful heat stimuli. Brain Res 1993;623:235–240.

49. Hassler R, Riechert T. Klinische und anatomische Befunde bei stereotaktischen Schmerzoperationen im Thalamus. Arch Psychiatr Zeitscrift Neurol 1959;200:93–122.

50. Lenz FA, Kwan HC, Dostrovsky JO, Tasker RR. Characteristics of the bursting pattern of action potentials that occurs in the thalamus of patients with central pain. Brain Res 1989;496:357–360.

51. Koyama S, Katayama Y, Maejima S, Hirayama T, Fujii M, Tsubokawa T. Thalamic neuronal hyperactivity following transection of the spinothalamic tract in the cat: Involvement of N-methyl-D-aspartate receptor. Brain Res 1993;612:345–350.

52. Rausell E, Cusick CG, Taub E, Jones EG. Chronic deafferentation in monkeys differentially affects nociceptive and nonnociceptive pathways distinguished by specific calcium-binding proteins and down-regulates gamma-aminobutyric acid type A receptors at thalamic levels. Proc Natl Acad Sci USA 1992;89:2571–2575.

53. Boivie J, Leijon G, Johansson I. Central post-stroke pain – a study of the mechanisms through analyses of the sensory abnormalities. Pain 1989;37:173–185.

54. Hylden JLK, Hayashi H, Dubner R, Bennett GJ. Physiology and morphology of the lamina I spinomesencephalic projection. J Comp Neurol 1986;247:505–515.

55. Yezierski RP, Broton JG. Functional properties of spinomesencephalic tract (SMT) cells in the upper cervical spinal cord of the cat. Pain 1991;45:187–196.

56. Yezierski RP. Spinomesencephalic tract: projections from the lumbosacral spinal cord of the rat, cat, and monkey. J Comp Neurol 1988;267:131–146.

57. Zemlan FP, Behbehani MM. Nucleus cuneiformis and pain modulation: anatomy and behavioral pharmacology. Brain Res 1988;453:89–102.

58. Mantyh PW. Connections of midbrain periaqueductal gray in the monkey. I. Ascending efferent projections. J Neurophysiol 1983;49:567.

59. Slugg RM, Light AR. Spinal cord and trigeminal projections to the pontine parabrachial region in the rat as demonstrated with *Phaseolus vulgaris* leucoagglutinin. J Comp Neurol. 1994;339:49–61.

60. Bernard JF, Besson JM. The spino(trigemino)pontoamygdaloid pathway: electrophysiological evidence for an involvement in pain processes. J Neurophysiol 1990;63:473–490.

61. Bechara A, Martin GM, Pridgar A, Van Der Kooy D. The parabrachial nucleus: a brain stem substrate critical for mediating the aversive motivational effects of morphine. Behav Neurosci 1993;107:147–160.

62. Craig AD. Spinal and trigeminal lamina I input to the locus coeruleus anterogradely labeled with *Phaseolus vulgaris* leucoagglutinin (PHA-L) in the cat and the monkey. Brain Res 1992;584:325–328.

63. Katter JT, Burstein R, Giesler GJ. The cells of origin of the spinohypothalamic tract in cats. J Comp Neurol 1991;303:101–112.

64. Iwata K, Kenshalo DR, Dubner R, Nahin RL. Diencephalic projections from the superficial and deep laminae of the medullary dorsal horn in the rat. J Comp Neurol 1992;321:404–420.

65. Burstein R, Dado RJ, Cliffer KD, Giesler GJ. Physiological characterization of spinohypothalamic tract neurons in the lumbar enlargement of rats. J Neurophysiol 1991;66:261–284.

66. Giesler GJ, Katter JT, Dado RJ. Direct spinal pathways to the limbic system for nociceptive information. Trends Neurosci 1994;17:244–250.

67. Kenshalo DR, Isensee O. Responses of primate SI cortical neurons to noxious stimuli. J Neurophysiol 1983;50:1479–1496.

68. Penfield W, Rasmussen T. The cerebral cortex of man. New York: Macmillan, 1950.

69. Kenshalo DR, Chudler EH, Anton F, Dubner R. SI nociceptive neurons participate in the encoding process by which monkeys perceive the intensity of noxious thermal stimulation. Brain Res 1988;454:378–382.

70. Stevens RT, London SM, Apkarian AV. Spinothalamocortical projections to the secondary somatosensory cortex (SII) in squirrel monkey. Brain Res 1993;631:241–246.

71. Dong W, Salonen LD, Kawakami Y, Shiwaku T, Kaukoranta M, Martin RF. Nociceptive responses of trigeminal neurons in SII-7b cortex of awake monkeys. Brain Res 1989;484:314–324.

72. Lamour Y, Willer J-C, Guilbaud G. Rat somatosensory (SmI) cortex: I: Characteristics of neuronal responses to noxious stimulation and comparison with responses to non-noxious stimulation. Exp Brain Res 1983;49:35–45.

73. Matsumoto N. Functional difference of tooth pulp-driven neurons in oral and facial areas of the somatosensory cortex (SI) of the cat. Exp Neurol 1984;857:437–451.

74. Vin-Christian K, Benoist JM, Gautron M, Levante A, Guilbaud G. Further evidence for the involvement of SmI cortical neurons in nociception: modifications of their responsiveness over the early stage of a carrageenin-induced inflammation in the rat. Somatosens Mot Res 1992;9:245–261.

75. Backonja M, Wang B, Miletic V. Responses of neurons in the ventrolateral orbital cortex to noxious cutaneous stimulation in a rat model of peripheral mononeuropathy. Brain Res 1994;639:337–340.

76. Koltzenburg M, Handwerker HO, Torebjork HE. The ability of humans to localise noxious stimuli. Neurosci Lett 1993;150:219–222.

77. Talbot JD, Marrett S, Evans AC, Meyer E, Bushnell MC, Duncan GH. Multiple representations of pain in human cerebral cortex. Science 1991;251:1355–1360.

78. Jones AKP, Brown WD, Friston KJ, Qi LY, Frackowiak RSJ. Cortical and subcortical localization of response to pain in man using positron emission tomography. Proc R Soc Lond 1991;244:39–44.

79. Roland P. Cortical representation of pain. Trends Neurosci 1992;15:3–5.

21

EVALUATION AND TREATMENT OF NEUROPATHIC PAIN

Howard L. Fields

Clinically, persistent pain presents a major challenge. This is because pain is subjective, and the knowledge required for optimal evaluation and treatment crosses traditional disciplinary lines. Of particular relevance to the readers of this book, severe persistent pain can have a strikingly destructive impact on the psychological state of the patient. Furthermore, psychological problems that either predate or are induced by persistent pain can add to the intractability of the problem (see Chapter 22). Ultimately, the challenge for the clinician becomes to distinguish somatic from psychological contributions to the suffering of each patient. Thus, patients with chronic pain are ideal candidates for neuropsychiatric referrals.

Evaluation of the patient with neuropathic pain represents a potentially rewarding opportunity for the diagnostically oriented neuropsychiatrist. Indeed, several therapies can significantly reduce the somatically generated components of this type of pain. Accurate diagnosis, however, is essential. Among the useful skills required for optimal evaluation and treatment of patients with persistent pain is the ability to elicit symptoms and signs consistent with the diagnosis of neuropathic pain. Most important among the findings are the location and quality of the pain and the presence of specific types of sensory abnormalities. This chapter reviews the clinical features of patients with neuropathic pain, the current thinking about the pathophysiology of different syndromes, and a strategy for the treatment of patients with this condition.

CLINICAL FINDINGS IN PATIENTS WITH PAIN DUE TO NEURAL INJURY OR DYSFUNCTION

At the outset, it is important to note that the clinical features in themselves are not sufficient for diagnosis, and rarely are all the features present in an individual. Another complication is that pain itself, regardless of the precipitating cause, can produce secondary changes such as reflex muscle contraction, guarding with immobilization of the painful area, and increased sympathetic outflow. Each of these

secondary processes can generate new (and potentially independent) sources of pain with their own characteristic features. It is not unusual for a patient to complain of several distinct pains with different anatomical locations and sensory qualities. It is essential to detail the time course and relative severity of each separate component.

The following is a list of the common features of neuropathic pain (1):

1. Association of the pain with evidence of neural damage, particularly sensory deficits. Although not conclusive, this feature is by far the most reliable indicator of neuropathic pain. Except in specific, easily identifiable syndromes such as trigeminal neuralgia or pain due to epilepsy, the absence of this feature should raise doubt about the diagnosis. Commonly, the reported location of the neuropathic pain is at least partially coextensive with a sensory disturbance. Usually this is a sensory loss, but sometimes hyperresponsiveness to sensory stimuli (see below) is present without a deficit.

2. The sensory quality of the pain is unique to the patient's experience. Burning and tingling are frequently used descriptors. Shooting, shocking, and/or electrical feelings are also common words that such patients use. Crawling, tightness, cramping, and tearing are also used. The point is that the pain is unusual and difficult to ignore. Neurologists use words like *dysethesias* (unpleasant sensation) or *paresthesias* (abnormal sensations) to describe these phenomena.

3. There is often a significant delay between the causative insult and the onset of pain. For example, in patients with pain due to central nervous system (CNS) lesions, the pain often begins after a delay of months, usually after the patient has achieved partial recovery of motor and/or sensory function.

4. Hypersensitivity phenomena are present. It is not unusual for patients with painful injuries of any type to complain of tenderness of the affected part and to avoid threatened contact with it. With neuropathic pain, such

hypersensitivity phenomena are exaggerated, often to the point of contributing in a major way to the patient's disability. For example, many patients with posttraumatic neuralgias complain that any movements involving the affected nerve trigger severe pain. Many neuropathic pain patients report that light, moving stimuli such as a gust of wind or the brushing of their skin by clothing induces rapid bursts of pain. This phenomenon, where severe pain is evoked by very light, moving tactile stimuli is termed *allodynia* and is suggestive of neuropathic pain.

Other hypersensitivity phenomena include reduced threshold for heat pain, a striking build-up of reported pain with repeated stimuli that are near threshold (summation), the spatial spread of perceived pain from the site of the noxious stimulus, and a prolonged paroxysm of pain following a brief stimulus (after discharge). These hypersensitivity phenomena are often thought of as defining the hyperpathic state.

A PATHOPHYSIOLOGY-BASED TREATMENT APPROACH TO NEUROPATHIC PAIN

Various mechanisms have been proposed to account for the paradoxical appearance of pain following injury or dysfunction of the peripheral or central nervous system. Unfortunately, little is known about the origin of any painful neuropathic condition. On the other hand, for each mechanism described here, there is a reasonable body of evidence that it contributes to some clinical condition. Where there is such evidence, it will be pointed out.

There is a major practical reason for describing a broad range of possible mechanisms in neuropathic pain; namely, that each potential mechanism suggests a particular treatment approach. In a given patient, several mechanisms may be contributing to the generation of pain (e.g., sympathetic activity, muscle spasm). Importantly, ascertaining the etiology of the neural damage (e.g., trauma, herpes zoster) does not necessarily specify the underlying mechanism of the pain. Until better diagnostic tools are developed to determine the proximate cause of the pain, the optimal strategy for treatment of an individual patient will remain a sequence of therapeutic trials targetted on specific pain-generating mechanisms. In this way, knowledge of multiple potential pain mechanisms, their expected clinical manifestations, and their sensitivity to treatments leads to a general algorithm for finding the optimal therapy in the shortest period of time for the largest number of patients.

It is essential to point out that this approach is only as good as the information upon which it is based. Currently, the relevant information is fraught with uncertainty, and many patients are not helped. On the other hand, the use of this approach gives patients the benefit of current knowledge about mechanism and available therapies. Furthermore, it is an approach that has evolved directly from clinical experience and a careful reading of the recent pertinent literature. At a minimum, this framework can help physicians organize their own clinical experience and evaluate the published work of others.

Deafferentation hyperactivity. Undoubtedly, deafferentation is associated with pain. It seems paradoxical that interruption of the pathways involved in pain transmission should result in pain. Usually, this does not occur. Loss of small-diameter primary afferents, such as occurs in some polyneuropathies, usually leads to loss of pain sensation. Furthermore, in the great majority of cases, interruption of central pain transmission pathways results in impaired pain sensation without spontaneous pain. This is the basis for the use of cordotomy for the treatment of certain pain patients. On the other hand, CNS lesions can cause pain in some patients. Such central pain syndromes are almost always accompanied by impaired pain and temperature sensation (2, 3).

The most persuasive clinical example of deafferentation pain results from avulsion of the brachial plexus. In this condition, backward hyperextension of the arm places severe traction on the brachial plexus, and some dorsal roots are anatomically separated from the spinal cord. Most of these patients have spontaneous pain referred to the anesthetic extremity (4). In animal studies, cutting the dorsal roots results in the development of high-frequency spontaneous activity in dorsal horn neurons, some of which may be pain transmission neurons (5). In support of the concept that spontaneous activity in dorsal horn neurons contributes to the pain of brachial plexus avulsion, Nashold and his colleagues (6) have shown that destructive lesions of the dorsal horn can give significant relief to patients with pain due to avulsion of the brachial plexus.

It is possible that some pain syndromes associated with lesions of the CNS are due to deafferentation hyperactivity of central pain transmission neurons. For example, thalamic pain could be caused by deafferentation of the cortical neurons to which they project. Unfortunately, there is no direct evidence that supports this proposed mechanism, nor is there any known therapy that works as well as dorsal horn lesions do for the pain of brachial plexus avulsion.

Loss of the inhibition produced by myelinated primary afferents. Primary afferents are classified by their response to peripheral stimuli, their axonal diameter, and their conduction velocity. As discussed by Ralston (Chapter 20), primary afferent nociceptors have axons that are of small diameter, mostly unmyelinated, and therefore conduct at slow velocities. Early psychophysical work had shown that when large-diameter axons in a peripheral nerve are selectively blocked by pressure/ischemia, pain threshold is unaffected, whereas discriminative aspects of sensation (joint position sense, two-point discrimination, vibration sense) are lost. More importantly, experimental blocking of myelinated axons produces an exaggerated response to noxious stimuli (7). In fact, stimuli that are usually not painful can produce significant pain when only unmyelinated primary afferents (C-fibers) are functioning in a peripheral nerve. In parallel animal studies, dorsal horn neurons that respond to noxious stimuli show an exaggerated response to nociceptor activation when their predominantly inhibitory input from myelinated axons is blocked (8).

These observations, lead to the conclusion that some central pain transmission neurons have inhibitory input from myelinated primary afferents (9). It is thus possible that pain can result from damage to peripheral nerves when it is relatively selective for myelinated fibers. Traumatic mono-neuropathies due to compression would be most likely to produce damage of this type because larger-diameter, myelinated axons are more susceptible to compression/ischemic damage. Consistent with this idea is the clinical evidence that selective electrical stimulation of large diameter axons in a peripheral nerve can be dramatically effective in relieving pain caused by traumatic nerve injury (10).

It is important to point out that even if the primary afferents are undamaged, their inhibitory effect would be reduced if the function of the dorsal horn interneurons that mediate their inhibitory effect were impaired. In fact, Bennett and his colleagues have presented evidence that certain types of peripheral nerve injury are associated with atrophy of dorsal horn neurons, some of which could be inhibitory interneurons (11).

Ectopic impulse generation.   Although it is likely that deafferentation hyperactivity of central pain transmission neurons and selective damage to large-diameter primary afferents are major contributing factors in some patients with neuropathic pain, such patients are undoubtedly a minority. Other mechanisms must be postulated for most patients. For example, patients with such common painful conditions as postherpetic neuralgia and painful diabetic neuropathy often have minimal deafferentation, and small-diameter axons may show relatively greater damage than large-diameter axons. In fact, Thomas (12) has pointed out that some painful neuropathies are associated with specific damage to small-diameter fibers.

A major breakthrough in our understanding of neuropathic pain was the discovery that many primary afferents become spontaneously active when they are damaged. In rats, when the sciatic nerve is cut, axons sprout from the proximal cut end and form a neuroma. Many of the primary afferents that grow into the neuroma, including some that are unmyelinated, develop spontaneous activity (13–15). Similarly, the small-diameter nociceptive primary afferents innervating the cornea become spontaneously active within hours following damage (16). It is important to note that when primary afferents are damaged, ectopic impulses can be generated at a site near the dorsal root ganglion as well as at the damaged and regenerating distal axon tip (17). Such spontaneous activity in primary afferent nociceptors is a likely source of pain in patients with nerve injury.

In addition to providing a possible explanation for the association of pain with damage to small-diameter primary afferents, the discovery of ectopic impulse generation may help us understand why certain patients with neuropathic pain obtain relief with membrane-stabilizing drugs. For example, the antiepileptic drugs (e.g., carbamazepine) and the antiarrhythmics (e.g., lidocaine) are not known to have general analgesic efficacy, but they can be dramatically helpful for some patients with neuropathic pain (see discussion that follows). In fact, such membrane-stabilizing drugs block the ectopic impulse generation in damaged primary afferents at concentrations that spare normal axonal conduction (16, 18).

Peripheral release of proinflammatory neuropeptides from primary afferent neurons.   Many unmyelinated primary afferent axons contain neuropeptides that are released from their peripheral terminals. There are a number of such peptides, but the most extensively studied is the 11-amino acid peptide substance P (SP). Activity of certain primary afferents causes the release of SP from their peripheral terminals. Substance P is a potent vasodilator and a chemo-attractant for white blood cells, and can also elicit the release of histamine from mast cells and serotonin from platelets (19). Clearly, by releasing biologically active peptides like SP, activity in primary afferent nociceptors can contribute to a local inflammatory process. This effector function of neurons that have traditionally been thought of as purely afferent is undoubtedly part of their normal tissue protective function. It is mentioned here to give the reader a more complete picture of the peripheral mechanisms that are capable of contributing to a clinical pain problem. One could imagine, for example, that a damaged, spontaneously firing primary afferent is capable of continual peripheral release of proinflammatory neuropeptides that perpetuate and/or amplify a patient's pain.

This scenario has clinical significance, and is supported by the observations of Ochoa and his colleagues (20). They recorded spontaneous activity in single unmyelinated axons innervating painful, vasodilated skin. They proposed that in these patients pain is produced by the peripheral release of vasoactive neuropeptides from damaged ectopically discharging primary afferent nociceptors. There is evidence that such a mechanism may contribute to the pain of some patients with postherpetic neuralgia (21).

Capsaicin, the active ingredient of the hot chili pepper, is a compound that has been shown to specifically activate unmyelinated primary afferents, primarily nociceptors. At increasing concentrations, capsaicin can activate, reversibly inactivate, peptide-deplete, or destroy primary afferent nociceptors (22, 23). In human subjects, 0.1% formulations of capsaicin produce reversible cutaneous analgesia (24). Capsaicin has been used topically as a folk remedy for pain for many years, and there is evidence that a 0.075% preparation can provide relief for patients with postherpetic neuralgia (25, 26), postmastectomy syndrome (27), and diabetic neuropathy (28, 29). Such an approach would be of obvious benefit for patients in whom antidromic release of SP from primary afferent nociceptors played a significant role in pain generation.

Sympathetic nervous system outflow.   That activity in the sympathetic nervous system can produce pain is a well-established clinical fact (30). Importantly, this does not occur in normal individuals. Thus, although electrical stimulation of the sympathetic chain is normally painless, a small percentage of patients with peripheral nerve injury develop a severe pain syndrome that is exacerbated by sympathetic activity and reversed by blockade of the sympathetic nervous system.

Mitchell (31) was the first to describe what is probably the most dramatic example of sympathetically maintained pain—causalgia. Causalgia is the syndrome of burning pain that occasionally follows peripheral nerve injury. In addition to the pain, which is the most prominent and disabling feature of the syndrome, patients with causalgia are often observed to have a cold, sweaty and swollen extremity, especially distally in the limb. In addition, there may be focal arthritis and exquisite hypersensitivity to light, moving touch. In many patients the pain is exacerbated by loud noises, movements, and cold.

A major breakthrough in understanding causalgia was Leriche's discovery (32) that early sympathectomy could cure it. Subsequently, experimental models of neuropathic pain have provided a basis for understanding how the sympathetic nervous system can elicit and/or maintain pain. For example, following partial injury to their spinal nerves, rats develop hypersensitivity to mechanical stimuli which is abolished by sympathectomy (33). Sympathetic efferent activity sensitizes primary afferent nociceptors, but only in damaged peripheral nerve (34). Furthermore, damaged nociceptive afferents that have regenerated into a neuroma can be excited by activating sympathetic efferents that have grown into the same neuroma (35). This ability of sympathetic outflow to evoke afferent activity can persist for months in rats (36).

The knowledge that sympathetic outflow can cause pain, particularly in patients with partial nerve injury, has important practical implications. First, the use of sympathetic blockade becomes a major tool in the evaluation of patients with neuropathic pain. If a patient responds to sympathetic blockade, most likely there is a major sympathetic component. Such patients should be treated with repeated sympathetic blocks, physical therapy, and anti-inflammatory drugs (37).

There are a variety of ways to carry out a sympathetic block. The traditional method is by regional blockade of the sympathetic chain with local anesthetic (38). Recently, the use of intravenous phentolamine has become popular because it is less invasive and produces little discomfort. Furthermore, it does not produce a false-positive response due to local anesthetic block of nearby somatic sensory axons (39, 40). Regional infusions with adrenergic antagonists, such as bretylium and guanethidine have also been used (41) however, the latter drug is not available in the U.S. There is anecdotal evidence that oral sympatholytic agents such as phenoxybenzamine (dibenzyline), guanethidine, or prazosin are helpful (42). On the other hand, dramatic responses are unusual, and there are no controlled clinical trials demonstrating their efficacy.

Prolonged changes in central neurons generated by synaptic activity. There is evidence from experimental studies in animals that tissue-damaging stimuli can elicit prolonged changes in the excitability of central pain-transmission neurons (43). Even brief stimuli, especially if they are intense and involve deep somatic and visceral structures, are capable of eliciting a prolonged hyperexcitable state in spinal cord pain transmission neurons (44). Depending on the stimulus intensity, duration, and the particular nerve stimulated, this hyperexcitable state may last for hours. There is evidence that a sensory barrage occurring at the time of injury can contribute to the hyperpathic syndrome that develops later (45).

These long-term changes in the CNS following intense nociceptor activation make a convincing case for the theory that there is a persistent memory trace for pain. The clinical evidence supporting this idea is controversial (46); however, there are reports that patients having preoperative or intraoperative local anesthetic block to prevent the massive sensory input from surgical trauma have less severe postoperative pain. Similarly, preoperative anesthetic block seems to lower the incidence of postamputation phantom limb pain (47).

The presence of a prolonged central hyperexcitable state, while not unique to neuropathic pain, may help to explain the hyperpathia often observed in these patients. For example, in patients with causalgia or postherpetic neuralgia, severe pain can usually be elicited with light, moving mechanical stimuli. This phenomenon, termed allodynia, is mediated by activity in large-diameter myelinated fibers, whose activity normally elicits light tactile sensations (48). Perhaps spinal pain transmission neurons can be sufficiently excited by large-diameter myelinated afferents to elicit pain sensations only when they are sensitized by prior noxious input.

Animal studies indicate that this state of hyperexcitability can be partially and selectively blocked by antagonists to the NMDA-type glutamate receptor. For example, ketamine and dextrorphan have NMDA-receptor blocking action and have been shown to reduce hyperalgesia in a rat model of neuropathic pain (49, 50). There is also evidence that the neuromodulator nitric oxide contributes to this long-term change (51). This knowledge has provided encouraging leads. For example, a recent clinical trial suggests that NMDA antagonists can relieve neuropathic pain (67).

Nociceptive nerve pain. It is important to discuss the possibility that pain may arise from activation of nociceptive primary afferents that innervate the connective tissue sheath of nerve trunks. Although such an innervation of the nerve sheath by nociceptive primary afferents is unproven, the concept is supported by the clinical observation that inflammation of nerve trunks is painful (52). Peripheral nerve sheaths are known to be innervated by nervi nervorum (53). Furthermore, there is clear evidence that the vasa nervorum are innervated by axons containing peptides, including SP (54). Because SP is a marker for unmyelinated primary afferents, mostly nociceptors, it is likely that these axons render the nerve sensitive to noxious stimuli and inflammation. Zochodnc (55) validated this concept by showing that injury of the nerve trunk produces a SP-mediated local neurogenic inflammation.

Thus, there are two mechanistically different types of pain arising from injured nerves: one due to cutting axons or otherwise interfering with normal nerve conduction, and the other due to "physiological" activation of the nociceptors that innervate the nerve sheath. We refer to this latter type of pain as nociceptive nerve pain. It may account for the deep aching pain of nerve root irritation or brachial neuritis. One would expect nociceptive nerve pain to respond well to opioids and anti-inflammatory agents.

TREATMENT APPROACHES TO PATIENTS WITH NEUROPATHIC PAIN

Carbamazepine and tricyclic antidepressants have been the mainstays for neurologists in the treatment of neuropathic pain. Carbamazepine's popularity among neurologists is no doubt based on its efficacy in trigeminal neuralgia and its relative safety. Tricyclics are popular because they have broad efficacy, which includes several types of neuropathic pain as well as both tension and migraine headache. Although useful for some patients, antiepileptic drugs and antidepressants are often either ineffective or have unacceptable side effects. Fortunately, recent research has both increased the number of therapeutic options and refined the use of previously available modalities. These alternative treatments for neuropathic pain are described in the sections that follow, along with an algorithm to optimize therapy quickly in an individual patient.

Tricyclic antidepressants. Tricyclics have a long history in the treatment of chronic pain. Tolerance and physical dependence are negligible, and they are effective for a broad range of problems including migraine and muscle contraction headache, low back pain, cancer pain, and, of course, any problem accompanied by significant depression (1). Importantly, these tricyclics are effective for a different range of conditions from those of the nonsteroidals, which is the other major category of drug that has achieved wide acceptance for chronically painful conditions.

Amitriptyline (Elavil) is the most commonly prescribed tricyclic for the treatment of pain patients. It is unclear which of its manifold pharmacological actions is responsible for its analgesic action. It not only blocks the reuptake of serotonin and norepinephrine, it blocks α-adrenergic, muscarinic, cholinergic, and histamine receptors (56). This broad range of actions produces a significant number of dose-related side effects from the harmless but annoying dry-mouth to the more serious orthostatic hypotension, urinary retention, cardiac conduction abnormalities, and memory disturbance. It also produces sedation, which is desirable in some patients and unwanted in others. So pervasive and unpleasant are the side effects that patient compliance requires starting amitriptyline at a very low dose (10 mg/qhs) and building slowly to therapeutic effect or to limiting side effects.

Other tricyclics are effective for the treatment of neuropathic pain. For example, desipramine is effective for postherpetic neuralgia (57) and is as effective as amitriptyline for diabetic neuropathy (58). Desipramine is less potent as a histamine and acetylcholine antagonist and is thus less sedating and less likely to cause memory disturbance. As with amitriptyline, it is best to initiate therapy with a very low dose of this drug (10–25 mg/day) and raise it about every third day. In nondepressed patients, relatively low doses of a tricyclic may be sufficient for optimal pain control (e.g., 75 mg amitriptyline or desipramine/day).

The newer generation, nontricyclic antidepressant agents have not been shown to affect neuropathic pain (59). Fluoxetine is a good example; it is almost a pure 5-HT uptake inhibitor and is an excellent antidepressant. Furthermore, because it has no cholinergic, adrenergic, or histamine blocking action, it is remarkably free of the troubling side effects that are common with the tricyclics. Unfortunately, it has little or no effect in patients with neuropathic pain who are not depressed (58). These clinical observations suggest that 5-HT uptake blockade is insufficient to produce pain relief. They also confirm that the pain relief produced by tricyclics is not a result of their antidepressant action (25).

It should be kept in mind that the complaint of pain is a common symptom in depressive disorders (1), and it is not unusual for pain symptoms to either clear or become less bothersome when depression is controlled. For this reason, if the patient's pain does not respond to lower doses of a tricyclic, the dose should be increased into the antidepressant range. Obtaining blood tricyclic levels is mandatory if the dose of a tricyclic is to be raised above the maximum recommended level. If the patient is depressed, fluoxetine may be a valuable drug to use because of its relative lack of serious or uncomfortable side effects.

Phenothiazines. There are some reports suggesting that drugs of the phenothiazine class are useful for neuropathic pain, especially when used as adjuncts to tricyclics (60). However, controlled studies have failed to demonstrate phenothiazine efficacy for pain management (61). Furthermore, the side-effect profile of these drugs should discourage their use. On the other hand, when more selective dopamine-receptor subtype-specific ligands become available, their use should be evaluated in patients with chronic pain.

Membrane-stabilizing agents. This group includes the anticonvulsants and the local anesthetic-antiarrhythmic drugs. Compared with the tricyclics, this group of drugs is helpful for a more restricted patient population. Carbamazepine and phenytoin have been used for a long time for the treatment of neuralgic pains. They are effective for trigeminal neuralgia, and carbamazepine has been reported to be helpful for some patients with painful diabetic neuropathy (1). Beyond these specific conditions, antiepileptic drugs are most likely to be helpful when there is a shooting, shock-like, lancinating pain. If carbamazepine and phenytoin are ineffective or are helpful but not well tolerated, alternative choices include baclofen (a second line drug for trigeminal neuralgia), clonazepam, and valproic acid.

As discussed previously, *in vitro* studies have shown that relatively low concentrations of local anesthetics can block the ectopic impulses that arise in damaged small-diameter primary afferents (16, 18). In clinical Studies, lidocaine, given by intravenous infusion, has been shown to provide immediate and often dramatic pain relief. A variety of neuropathic pains respond (62), including postherpetic neuralgia (63).

Because of the effectiveness of lidocaine-like drugs in the treatment of cardiac arrhythmias, several oral drugs of this class are available; tocainide and mexiletine are two examples. Tocainide has considerable toxicity, making mexiletine the preferred first line drug of this class. Mexiletine has been shown to be effective for diabetic neuropathy (64) and other neuropathic pains (65).

Although mexiletine helps some patients and is occasionally dramatically effective, many patients are not helped even at the maximal allowable doses, or they tolerate the drug poorly because of gastrointestinal symptoms. A promising approach for some of these patients, particularly those with cutaneous hyperpathia, is the use of topical lidocaine preparations (21, 66).

Opioids. The use of opioids in patients with neuropathic pain of nonmalignant origin is a subject of significant controversy (69, 70). Although there are open-label, uncontrolled studies indicating long-term benefit of opioids in such patients (60, 69), there are also studies that have shown no benefit (70, 71). To my knowledge, there is no prospective controlled trial of long-term opioids in any neuropathic condition. On the other hand, we have demonstrated that morphine, given acutely and in high dose, provides significant relief in patients with postherpetic neuralgia (63).

My impression is that although many patients obtain significant relief with opioids, for many the relief is incomplete and, for some, the benefit is minimal to nonexistent. Unfortunately, in the absence of a therapeutic trial, it is difficult to predict the degree of relief that will be obtained by a given patient.

Despite the controversial nature of long-term opioid use and the lack of solid longitudinal data on clinical efficacy, no patient should be denied this option. The major argument that has been raised against a trial of opioids is the possibility that the patient will become an addict. However, available evidence indicates that the risk of addiction is extremely small for patients on short-term opioid therapy (72). On the other hand, if the drug is effective, the patient may need opioids on a long-term basis, which probably increases the likelihood of addiction, especially in patients with a history of drug abuse (69). This risk should be explained to the patient. Once an effective dose is established, the patient should not be permitted to increase it on his or her own initiative.

Once the decision is made and the patient agrees to chronic opioid therapy, our preference is to use long-acting opioids. The pharmacokinetics of such compounds (methadone, levorphanol, sustained release morphine), avoids the plasma level peaks (associated with increased side effects)

and valleys (associated with breakthrough pain and mild abstinence).

Some patients treated with opioids experience a fading of their efficacy over time. This could represent a change in the underlying pain problem or the development of tolerance. Dose escalation in these patients should be undertaken cautiously and only after the patient is re-evaluated both neurologically and psychologically and adjuvant drugs have been added (e.g., tricyclic antidepressants, membrane stabilizing drugs or α_2-adrenergic agonists such as clonidine) (71).

A General Algorithm for the Management of Patients with Neuropathic Pain

This algorithm is useful as a rough guideline to evaluate and treat patients with peripheral neuropathic pain. It is unnecessary to use this approach if the diagnosis is obvious and there is an accepted treatment of choice. Examples of the latter situation include (*a*) patients with trigeminal neuralgia, who should be started immediately on carbamazepine; or (*b*) patients with a progressive compression-induced mononeuropathy, such as carpal tunnel syndrome, who should be considered for early surgical decompression. On the other hand, if the location, time-course, or quality of the pain do not suggest a diagnosis for which there is a generally accepted and effective treatment, this algorithm can provide an organized approach to a diverse patient population.

Phase I—initial evaluation, local treatments. Figure 21.1 illustrates the initial treatment process. The initial step is a diagnostic sympathetic block by phentolamine infusion, particularly in cases with pain in a single extremity that has a burning quality, is made worse by cold and is associated with swelling. If phentolamine infusion is negative but there is a high index of suspicion for sympathetically maintained pain, local anesthetic block of the paraspinal sympathetic chain should be carried out.

If the patient has pain associated with a traumatic or compressive mononeuropathy and the pain is made worse by movement, it is possible that the pain is due to traction on a mechanically sensitive neuroma at the site of injury. Such patients can often be helped by either decompression or neurotomy and/or moving the nerve to reduce the traction on it (73).

Topical agents should be considered in those patients who experience cutaneous discomfort. Such an approach seems to be especially effective if the patients have allodynia or hyperalgesia to cutaneous stimulation. Capsaicin preparations are commercially available. Topical NSAIDs and local anesthetic preparations are not currently available; however, aspirin tablets can be crushed in chloroform (74, 75), and topical lidocaine formulations can be made by a hospital pharmacist.

Phase II—oral medications. If local approaches leave the patient with significant pain, we initiate therapy with a tricyclic antidepressant (as just outlined). If further relief is needed, we proceed to a trial of a membrane-stabilizing

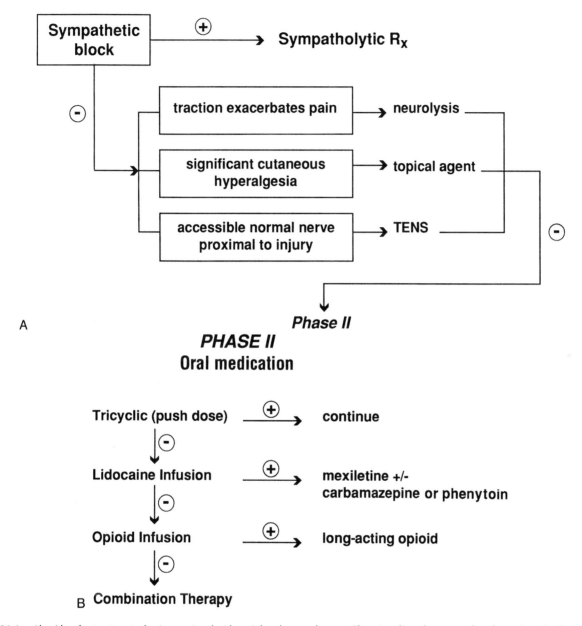

Figure 21.1. Algorithm for treatment of pain associated with peripheral nerve damage. Phase I outlines the steps to be taken prior to instituting long-term medical management. Phase II illustrates one systematic approach to long-term pharmacological treatment. (Adapted from Fields HL, Rowbotham MC. Multiple mechanisms of neuropathic pain: a clinical perspective. In: Gebhart GF, Hammond DL, Jensen TS. Progress in pain research and management, vol. 2. Seattle: IASP Press, 1994:437–454.) Transcutaneous electronic nerve stimulation (TENS): The way TENS is generally used, only local cutaneous stimulation is achieved. There is a question about whether the analgesic potency of TENS is any more than a placebo effect (77). Obviously, because the sensation produced by TENS cannot be avoided, there will always be a cue that a treatment is being given. In my experience, TENS is effective in patients with traumatic mononeuropathies when the stimulating electrodes can be placed on the trunk of the nerve proximal to the site of injury (10). Lidocaine infusion: We give 5 mg/kg body weight via continuous i.v. infusion over 90 minutes. Electrocardioram (ECG) and blood pressure monitoring are recommended (76).

drug. We use a lidocaine infusion to evaluate the usefulness of this approach. If there is no relief with lidocaine, we have found that oral membrane-stabilizing drugs will not work, and we can save the patient the time it would take to build up to the dose required for a full evaluation of related oral medications. If there is immediate and dramatic relief with the lidocaine infusion, we are willing to push oral mexiletine to high levels (up to 1200 mg per day, provided plasma levels are within the acceptable therapeutic range). Sometimes a combination of these drugs (e.g., phenytoin and mexiletine) is needed to achieve a therapeutic effect and avoid unacceptable side effects.

For many patients, tricyclics, membrane-stabilizing drugs, and oral sympatholytics either alone or in combination are inadequate. For these patients, opioids can be useful. We either begin the patient on an oral opioid or use a fentanyl infusion as a predictive test. Finally, we assess the efficacy of various combinations of the aforementioned drugs.

One can question the need for the prognostic infusions in this algorithm. Why not just proceed with the oral medications? The main argument for the prognostic infusions is to save the time required for dose-titrations of drugs that may prove to be worthless for an individual. These patients are suffering and often disabled by their pain. Thus, we try to assess as many options as quickly as possible to reduce their pain to a bearable level. The infusions also can help us to be more aggressive and patients to be more tolerant with a particular approach in the face of initial failure or bothersome side effects.

SUMMARY

This chapter has outlined a rational mechanism-based approach to the evaluation and treatment of patients with neuropathic pain. It is important to point out that this approach is still evolving and that as we learn more about the mechanisms of neuropathic pain and new treatment options become available, the algorithm will change. Furthermore, the therapeutic outcome for a given patient will be suboptimal unless the assessment and treatment of the psychosocial aspects of their problem are carried out concurrently with the somatically based algorithm outlined in this chapter.

References

1. Fields HL. Pain. New York: McGraw-Hill, 1987:133–170.
2. Leijon G, Boivie J, Johansson I. Central post-stroke pain—neurological symptoms and pain characteristics. Pain 1989; 36:13–25.
3. Cassinari V, Pagni CA. Central pain, a neurosurgical survey, Cambridge, MA: Harvard University Press, 1969.
4. Wynn-Parry CB. Pain in avulsion lesions of the brachial plexus. Pain 1980; 9:41–53.
5. Lombard MC, Larabi Y. Electrophysiological study of cervical dorsal horn cells in partially deafferented rats. In: Bonica JJ, et al, eds. Advances in pain research and therapy. New York: Raven Press, 1983.
6. Nashold BS Jr., Ostdahl RH. Dorsal root entry zone lesions for pain relief. J Neurosurg 1979; 51:59–69.
7. Landau W, Bishop GG. Pain from dermal, periosteal and fascial endings and from inflammation. Arch Neurol Psychiatry 1953; 69:490–504.
8. Price DD, Hayes RL, Ruda MA, Dubner R. Spatial and temporal transformations of input to spinothalamic tract neurons and their relation to somatic sensations. J. Neurophysiol. 1978; 41:933–947.
9. Melzack R, Wall PD. Pain mechanisms: a new theory. Science 1965; 150:971–978.
10. Meyer GA, Fields HL. Causalgia treated by selective large fibre stimulation of peripheral nerve. Brain 1972; 95:163–168.
11. Bennett GJ, Laird JM. Central changes contributing to neuropathic hyperalgesia. In: Hyperalgesia and allodynia. Willis W, Ed. New York: Raven Press, 1992:305–310.
12. Thomas PK. The anatomical substratum of pain. Can J Neurol Sci 1974; May 1974:92–97.
13. Wall PD, Gutnick M. Ongoing activity in peripheral nerves: The physiology and pharmacology of impulses originating from a neuroma. Exp Neurol 1974; 43:580–593.
14. Scadding JW. Development of ongoing activity, mechanosensitivity, and adrenaline sensitivity in severed peripheral nerve axons. Exp Neurol 1981; 73:345–364.
15. Welk E, Leah JD, Zimmerman M. Characteristics of A- and C-fibers ending in a sensory nerve neuroma in the rat. J Neurophysiol 1990; 63:759–766.
16. Tanelian DL, MacIver MB. Analgesic concentrations of lidocaine suppress tonic A-delta and C-fiber discharges produced by acute injury. Anesthesiology 1991; 74:934–936.
17. Devor M, Rappaport ZH. Pain and the pathophysiology of damaged nerve. In: Fields HL, ed. Pain syndromes in neurology. London: Butterworths, 1990:47–84.
18. Chabal C, Russell LC, Burchiel KJ. The effect of intravenous lidocaine, tocainide, and mexiletine on spontaneously active fibers originating in rat sciatic neuromas. Pain 1989; 38:333–338.
19. Levine JD, Fields HL, Basbaum AI. Peptides and primary afferent nociceptors. J Neurosci 1993; 13:2273–86.
20. Cline MA, Ochoa J, Torebjork HE. Chronic hyperalgesia and skin warming caused by sensitized C nociceptors. Brain 1989; 112:621–647.
21. Rowbotham MC, Davies PS, Fields HL. Topical lidocaine gel relieves post-herpetic neuralgia. Ann Neurol 1995; 37:246–253.
22. Lynn B. Capsaicin: actions on nociceptive C-fibres and therapeutic potential. Pain 1990; 41:61–69.
23. Holzer P. Capsaicin: cellular targets, mechanisms of action, and selectivity for thin sensory neurons. Pharmacol Rev 1991; 43:143–201.
24. Bjerring P, Arendt-Nielsen L. Use of a new argon laser technique to evaluate changes in sensory and pain thresholds in human skin following topical capsaicin treatment. Skin Pharmacol (2 (3), 1989: 161–167.
25. Watson CPN, Evans RJ, Watt VR. Post-herpetic neuralgia and topical capsaicin. Pain 1988; 33:333–340.
26. Bernstein JE, Korman NJ, Bickers DR, et al. Topical capsaicin treatment of chronic postherpetic neuralgia. J Am Acad Dermatol 1989; 21:265–270.
27. Watson CP, Evans RJ. The postmastectomy pain syndrome and topical capsaicin: a randomized trial. Pain 1992; 51:375–9.
28. Scheffler NM, Sheitel PL, Lipton MN. Treatment of painful diabetic neuropathy with capsaicin 0.075%. J Amer Podiatr Med Assoc 1991; 81:288–293.
29. Tandan R, Lewis GA, Krusinski PB, Badger GB, Freis TJ. Topical capsaicin in painful diabetic neuropathy. Controlled study with long-term follow-up. Diabetes Care 1992; 15:8–14.
30. Loh L, Nathan PW. Painful peripheral states and sympathetic blocks. J Neurol Neurosurg Psychiatry 1978; 41:664–671.
31. Mitchell SW. Injuries of nerves and their consequences. New York: Dover Publications, 1965.
32. Leriche R, ed. The surgery of pain. London: Bailliere, Tindall & Cox, 1939.
33. Kim SH, Chung JM. Sympathectomy alleviates mechanical allodynia in an experimental animal model for neuropathy in the rat. Neurosci Lett 1991; 134:131–134.
34. Sato J, Perl ER. Adrenergic excitation of cutaneous pain receptors induced by peripheral nerve injury. Science 1991; 251:1608–1610.
35. Devor M, Janig W. Activation of myelinated afferents ending in neuroma by stimulation of the sympathetic supply in the rat. Neurosci Lett 1981; 24:43–47.
36. Janig W. Activation of afferent fibers ending in an old neuroama by sympathetic stimulation in the rat. Neurosci Lett 1990; 111:309–314.
37. Kozin F, McCarty DJ, Sims J, Genant H. The reflex sympathetic dystrophy syndrome. 1. Clinical and histological studies: Evidence for

bilaterality, response to corticosteroids and articular involvement. Am J of Med 1976; 60:321–331.

38. Bonica JJ. Causalgia and other reflex sympathetic dystrophies. Adv Pain Res Ther 1979; 3:141–161.

39. Campbell JN, Meyer RA, Raja SN. Is nociceptor activation by alpha-1 adrenoreceptors the culprit in sympathetically maintained pain? APS Journal 1992; 1:3–11.

40. Arner S. Intravenous phentolamine test: diagnostic and prognostic use in reflex sympathetic dystrophy. Pain 1991; 46:17–22.

41. Hannington-Kiff JG. Intravenous regional sympathetic block with guanethidine. Lancet 1974:1019–1020.

42. Ghostine SY, Comair YG, Turner DM, Kassell NF, Azar CG. Phenoxybenzamine in the treatment of causalgia: report of 40 cases. J Neurosurg 1984; 60:1263–1268.

43. Willis WD. Central plastic responses to pain. In: Gebhart GF, Hammond DL, Jensen TS, eds. Progress in pain research and management, vol. 2. Seattle: IASP Press, 1994:301–324.

44. Woolf CJ. Excitability changes in central neurons following peripheral damage: role of central sensitization in the pathogenesis of pain. In: Willis W, ed. Hyperalgesia and allodynia. New York: Raven Press, 1992:221–243.

45. Dougherty PM, Garrison CJ, Carlton SM. Differential influence of local anesthetic upon two models of experimentally induced peripheral mononeuropathy in the rat. Brain Res 1992; 570:109–115.

46. Dahl JB, Kehlet H. The value of pre-emptive analgesia in the treatment of postoperative pain. Br J Anaesth 1993; 70:434–439.

47. Bach S, Noreng MF, Tjellden NV. Phantom limb pain in amputees during the first 12 months following limb amputation, after reoperative epidural blockade. Pain 1988; 33:297–301.

48. Ochoa JL, Yarnitsky D. Mechanical hyperalgesias in neuropathic pain patients: dynamic and static subtypes. Ann Neurol 1993; 33:465–472.

49. Mao J, Price DD, Hayes RL, Lu J, Mayer DJ, Frenk H. Intrathecal treatment with dextrorphan or ketamine potently reduces pain-related behaviors in a rat model of peripheral mononeuropathy. Brain Res 1993; 605:164–168.

50. Tal M, Bennett GJ. Dextrorphan relieves neuropathic heat-evoked hyperalgesia in the rat. Neurosci Lett 1993; 151:107–110.

51. Meller ST, Gebhart GF. Nitric oxide (NO) and nociceptive processing in the spinal cord. Pain 1993; 52:127–136.

52. Asbury AK, Fields HL. Pain due to peripheral nerve damage: an hypothesis. Neurology 1984; 34:1587–1590.

53. Hromada J. On the nerve supply of the connective tissue of some peripheral nervous system components. Acta Anat 1963; 55:343–351.

54. Appenzeller O, Dhital KK, Cowen T, Burnstock G. The nerves to blood vessels supplying blood to nerves: the innervation of vasa nervorum. Brain Res 1984; 304:383–386.

55. Zochodne DW. Epineurial peptides: a role in neuropathic pain? Can J Neurol Sci 1993; 20:69–72.

56. Richelson E. Antidepressats and brain neurochemistry. Mayo Clin Proc 1990; 65:1227–1236.

57. Kishore-Kumar R, Max MB, Schafer SC, et al. Desipramine relieves post-herpetic neuralgia. Clin Pharmacol Ther 1990; 47:305–312.

58. Max MB, Lynch SA, Muir J, Shoaf SE, Smoller B, Dubner R. Effects of desipramine, amitriptyline, and fluoxetine on pain in diabetic neuropathy. N Engl J Med 1992; 326:1250–6.

59. Sindrup SH, Gram LF, Brosen K, Eshoj O, Mogensen EF. The selective serotonin reuptake inhibitor paroxetine is effective in the treatment of diabetic neuropathy symptoms. Pain 1990; 42:135–144.

60. Taub A. Relief of postherpetic neuralgia with psychotrophic drugs. J Neurosurg 1973; 39:235–239.

61. McGee JL, Alexander MR. Phenothiazine analgesia – fact or fantasy? Am J Hosp Pharm 1979; 1:39–49.

62. Glazer S, Portenoy RK. Systemic local anesthetics in pain control. Journal of Pain Symptom Management 1991; 6:30–39.

63. Rowbotham MC, Reisner LM, Fields HL. Both intravenous lidocaine and morphine reduce the pain of post-herpetic neuralgia. Neurology 1991;41:1024–1028.

64. Dejgard A, Petersen P, Kastrup J. Mexiletine for the treatment of chronic painful diabetic neuropathy. Lancet 1988; 1:9–11.

65. Chabal C, Jacobson L, Mariano A, Chaney E, Britell CW. The use of oral mexiletine for the treatment of pain after peripheral nerve injury. Anesthesiology 1992; 76:513–717.

66. Stow PJ, Glynn CJ, Minor B. EMLA cream in the treatment of post-herpetic neuralgia. Efficacy and pharmacokinetic profile. Pain 1989; 39:301–305.

67. Eide PK, Jorum E, Stubhaug A, Bremnes J, Breivik H. Relief of postherpetic neuralgia with the N-methyl-D-aspartic acid receptor antagonist ketamine: a double-blind, cross-over comparison with morphine and placebo. Pain 1994; 58:347–354.

68. Jadad AR, Carroll D, Glynn CJ, Moore RA, McQuay HJ. Morphine responsiveness of chronic pain: double-blind randomised crossover study with patient-controlled analgesia. Lancet 1992; 339:1367–1371.

69. Portenoy R, Foley K. Chronic use of opioid analgesics in non-malignant pain: report of 38 cases. Pain 1986; 25:171–186.

70. Arner S, Meyerson B. Lack of analgesic effect of opioids on neuropathic and idiopathic forms of pain. Pain 1988; 33:11–23.

71. Max MB, Schafer SC, Culnane M, et al. Association of pain relief with drug side effects in postherpetic neuralgia: a single dose study of clonidine, codeine, ibuprofen and placebo. Clin Pharmacol Ther 1988; 43:363–371.

72. Porter J, Jick H. Addiction rare in patients treated with narcotics. N Engl J Med 1980; 302:123.

73. Dawson DM, Hallett M, Millender LH. Entrapment neuropathies. Boston: Little Brown & Co., 1983.

74. King RB. Concerning the management of pain associated with herpes zoster and of postherpetic neuralgia. Pain 1988; 33:73–78.

75. De Benedittis G, Besana F, Lorenzetti A. A new topical treatment for acute herpetic neuralgia and post-herpetic neuralgia: the aspirin/diethyl ether mixture. An open-label study plus a double-blind controlled clinical trial. Pain 1992; 48:383–390.

76. Galer BS, Miller KV, Rowbotham MC. Response to intravenous lidocaine infusion differs based on clinical diagnosis and site of nervous system injury. Neurology 1993; 43:1233–1235.

77. Marchand S, Charest J, Li J, Chenard J-R, Lavignolle B, Laurencelle L. Is TENS purely a placebo effect? A controlled study on chronic low back pain. Pain 1993; 54:99–106.

22

PAIN AND PSYCHOPATHOLOGY

David A. Fishbain

MEASUREMENT OF PAIN

Introduction

Pain is measured in two situations: experimental and clinical (1). Experimental pain is easier to study because one can measure the intensity of the pain-inducing stimulus. In clinical pain, the nature of the stimulus is often unknown and its intensity can only be measured *indirectly* (2). In addition, because pain is a complex multidimensional *subjective* experience (3), a single dimension such as intensity fails to capture the variations in pain associated with a pinprick, a toothache, or a burn. Additionally, in any given dimension, such as intensity, the reported severity of the pain is related to numerous variables such as cultural background, past experience, the meaning of the situation, personality variables, attention, arousal level, the prevailing contingencies of reinforcement, individual pain threshold and pain tolerance differences, pain responsivity differences, inability to habituate differences, suggestion, and environmental cues (1, 3, 4, 5). Because of these factors, the clinical measurement of pain has been a difficult problem, infrequently evaluated as an end point of treatment (2). Currently, the following *indirect* methods are available for the measurement of clinical pain (2, 6, 7):

1. *Rating scale* methods in which patients rate pain experiences on structured scales with clearly defined limits;
2. Psychophysical methods that attempt to define pain threshold and pain tolerance in terms of experimentally-induced pain and then ask the patient to *match* the perceived experimentally induced pain to his or her current clinical pain;
3. Measurement of *drug dosage* required to relieve the pain;
4. Measurement of observed pain *behaviors,* such as moving in bed, bracing, rubbing an affected part;
5. Magnitude estimation procedures in which judgments of perceived pain are translated into *cross-modality matching* techniques such as handgrip force;
6. Measurement of *performance ability* on laboratory tasks; and
7. Human *physiological correlates,* such as direct recording from peripheral nerves and evoked potentials.

Each of these general methods has inherent limitations (2). Thus, it is almost mandatory to use a combination of methods in most pain measurement studies. Currently, methods 5, 6, and 7 are investigational only, while 1, 2, and 3 are the most widely researched methods. Some specific approaches to the utilization of methods 1, 2, and 4 are described in the sections that follow.

Rating Scale Methods

VISUAL ANALOG SCALE

Of the rating scale methods, the Visual Analog Scale (VAS) is the most researched and accepted method, and it is the most widely utilized in measuring clinical pain (1, 2, 8–10). The VAS consists of a 10-cm line anchored by two extremes of pain, "no pain" and "pain as bad as it could be." Patients are asked to make a mark on the line that represents their level of perceived pain intensity, and the scale is scored by measuring the distance from the "no pain" to the patient's mark. There are various types of VAS scales, e.g., scaled from 0–10, but the most practical index utilizes a 101-point numerical scale (9). An example of this scale is shown in Fig. 22.1.

A common problem with the VAS is that it assumes pain to be a one-dimensional experience that varies only in intensity (2). Although the VAS is subject to response biases (2), it has been shown to be internally consistent both in experimentally induced pain and chronic clinical pain, thereby demonstrating validity (2). The VAS has been shown to be more sensitive than verbal rating scales (9), and may be more reliable (2). Also, VAS scores appear to predict chronic pain patient status at 6 months (11). Of the rating scale methods, the VAS is preferable for clinical application. However, even the VAS may have poor sensitivity to treatment effects (2). Therefore, it has been recommended that, when measuring treatment effects, two types of VAS be employed: (*a*) the absolute VAS just described and (*b*) a comparative VAS (8). The comparative VAS is 20 cm in length and has three points: less severe, unchanged (at the midline), and more severe (Fig. 22.2).

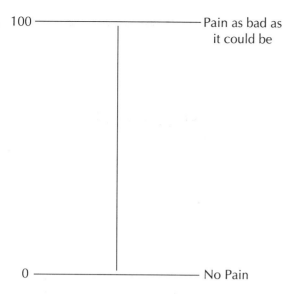

Please indicate on the line above the number between zero (0) and one hundred (100) that best describes your pain. A zero (0) would mean "no pain" and a one hundred (100) would mean "pain as bad as it could be."

Figure 22.1.   The VAS Pain Scale (10 cm).

The VAS scale can also be utilized in other ways. Depending on the *directions* given to the patient completing the VAS, a different aspects of pain can be measured. Thus, the patient can be asked to rate his/her pain at "this point in time" or as "average pain level over the last 24 hours" or "average pain over the last week." By combining visual analog scales based on different directions, the intensity, frequency, and duration of clinical pain can be indirectly assessed (2). For example, if one wanted to measure the relationship between occurrence of pain symptoms and drug use, one could construct four VAS scales with the different directions below and, of course, give them to the same patient at the same time:

1. "Rate your average pain over the last 24 hours";
2. "What level of pain do you consider intolerable?";
3. "For what level of pain would you consider taking medication?" and;
4. "What level of pain do you consider disabling?"

DESCRIPTION DIFFERENTIAL SCALE

The Description Differential Scale (DDS) consists of a list of adjectives describing different levels of pain intensity (Table 22.1) (12). Chronic pain patients (CPPs) are asked to rate the intensity of their pain as more or less than the word on the list by placing a checkmark either to the left (less) or right (more) of the word being rated. If the word describes their pain level, they place a checkmark under the word. There are 10 points to the right and left of each word, giving a 21-point rating scale. Pain intensity is defined as the mean of each rating and ranges from 0–20. The DDS scale has high internal consistency (12). The major advantage of this

Please tell us how your pain has changed in the last month by making a line on the scale. Zero (0) represents no change, +100 represents most severe increase while −100 represents the greatest possible decrease.

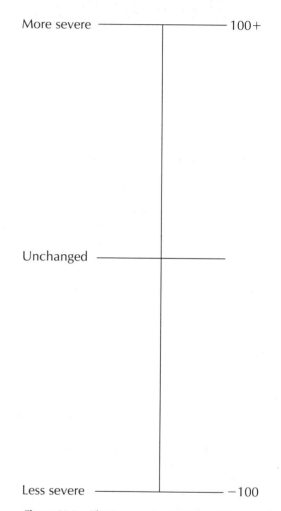

Figure 22.2.   The Comparative VAS Scale (20 cm, total).

scale is the fact that chronic pain patients (CPPs) can be checked to see how consistently they are using the scale by examining the relationship among different items. As displayed in Fig. 22.3, terms describing the intensity of pain are presented in random order. If pain is "fair" it cannot also be "very intense". Responses are checked to assure that they are consistent in this sense (Fig. 22.3).

"Pain affect" can be defined as the emotional arousal and disruption engendered by the pain experience. The pain affect component may be conceptually and empirically distinct from pain intensity (12). Multiple-item measures may be more reliable in measuring pain affect than single-item measures. Therefore, the DDS scale was modified to measure pain affect and can be used in this fashion. This scale is demonstrated in Fig. 22.4.

Pain Measurement Inventories

McGILL PAIN QUESTIONNAIRE

The McGill Pain Questionnaire (MPQ) (13) is an inventory rather than a rating scale. It is designed to quantify three dimensions of pain: sensory, affective, and valuative. The MPQ is made up of 20 sets of pain word descriptions, each set containing up to six words (2). Pain patients are asked to circle words in each set that are relevant. The investigator scores the number of words chosen on the total number of word sets that apply to the pain. Because the words within each set have been ranked, one can compute a total score. Although the MPQ is the most widely used instrument for pain measurement (14), there is little consensus over the scaling of the words (2). In addition, patients often have difficulty with the complexity of the vocabulary used (2), and the MPQ weights sensory aspects of pain more heavily than the affective and valuative aspects. This last issue may bias MPQ scores (2), but most important because of this bias, it does not focus on the most important aspect of pain treatment: the response to treatment in the valuative and affective dimension (2). In the past, caution has been urged in utilizing the MPQ for the measurement of pain intensity (15), and recently, doubt has been cast on the discriminant validity of the MPQ pain rating index (16). However, a short form of the MPQ has been developed and found to be reliable and valid (14), but has not yet been utilized widely.

MILLION SCALE

There is now convincing evidence that chronic pain intensity levels and measures of functional impairment and disability are correlated (17–26). From these data one may conclude that pain itself results in functional impairment and/or disability, or that the pain is perceived by the pain patient as a disability or both. This evidence has been utilized in developing rating scales and inventories that tap both the perceived pain and perceived functional impairment aspects of the pain experience. The Million Scale is an example of this concept. This is a 15-item inventory scored on visual analog scales concerning the association of pain with several activities, and self-perceived functional impairment (27). It appears to be valid and reliable with chronic low back pain (CLBP) patients. Low scores on this scale appear to predict return to work (28). VonKorff (26) has also developed a scale utilizing the pain/disability concept. However, the reliability and validity of this scale have not yet been determined.

PAIN BEHAVIOR METHODS

Pain behavior has been defined as "any and all outputs of the patient that a reasonable observer would characterize as suggesting pain, such as (but not limited to) posture, facial expression, verbalizing, lying down, taking medications, seeking medical assistance and receiving compensation" (29). A list of identified pain behaviors is presented in Table 22.1. Pain behaviors can often be elicited during physical examination (30) and correlate with physical examination findings, number of operations, and longer pain histories (30). In addition, pain behaviors correlate with perceived severity of pain (31, 32), extent of functional impairments (31), and scores on the Illness Behavior Questionnaire (33). As pain improves, pain behavior diminishes (2, 32, 34). Recent evidence, using pain stimulation experiments, indicates that pain behavior may be either a consequence of CLBP or an important risk factor for the development of CLBP (35). These studies highlight the importance of pain behavior measurements and the possible interrelationship of pain behavior to functional status.

To measure pain behavior in a systematic fashion, the University of Alabama (UAB) Pain Behavior Scale was developed (34). The UAB scale quantifies the observed pain behavior and has been shown to be reliable (34). In addition, ratings of pain behavior utilizing the UAB appear to be *significantly* related to both VAS sensory and VAS affective ratings (36). The concept of pain behavior has been criticized from a number of standpoints (37). However, the aforementioned studies indicate that the pain behavior concept can be operationalized as a powerful pain observational clinical tool that is particularly useful in more severely affected patients.

PAIN-MATCHING METHODS

Although the VAS scale is efficient and simple to use in pain measurement (2), it suffers from one major problem: pain threshold (level of stimulation at which the subject begins to perceive pain in a pain stimulation experiment) and pain tolerance (level of stimulation at which the subject can no longer tolerate the induced pain in a pain stimulation

Table 22.1. Behaviors Utilized in Pain Behavior Rating Scales

1. Stiffness on sitting
2. Slow movement
3. Limping
4. Frequent shifts in position
5. Stands bent forward
6. Walks bent forward
7. Distorted gait
8. Facial grimacing
9. Holds painful part
10. Rubs painful part
11. Moans
12. Groans
13. Writhes
14. Uses cane
15. Takes medications for pain
16. Moves in a guarded fashion
17. Uses heat or ice
18. Uses prosthetic devices
19. Frequent rests (lying down)
20. Avoids physical activity

Instructions: Each word represents an amount of sensation. Rate your sensation in relation to each word with a checkmark.

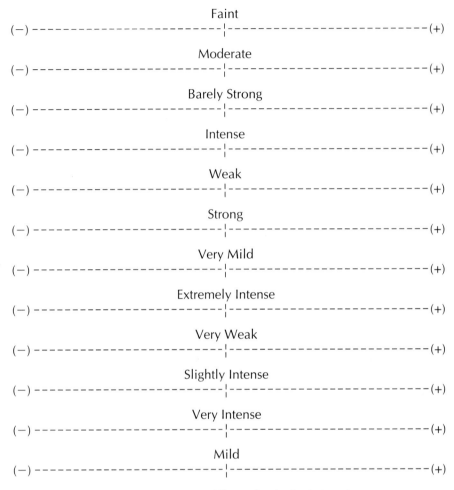

Figure 22.3. Descriptor differential scale of pain intensity.

experiment) vary among individuals (1) although a pain stimulus may approach pain tolerance or "pain as bad as it could be" for one individual, another may perceive it as mild. Pain threshold and pain tolerance mediate a patient's rating of pain intensity. As an example, CLBP patients seem to have a *higher* pain threshold and lower pain tolerance than pain-free controls, and they may not be able to habituate pain threshold like pain-free controls (38). Therefore, the VAS is most effective in measuring pain intensity and pain change in the same individual, but is less reliable when it is utilized for between subject pain comparisons. In an attempt to solve this dilemma, the pain-matching method was developed. This method allows a more *direct* measurement of the actual clinical pain a patient experiences and comes closest to the true experimental situation. Various methods can be used in humans to induce clinical experimental pain, including heat, electric shock, noise, and pressure (2). Of these, pressure has been noted to most closely approximate chronic, gnawing pain (10). A pressure algometer was developed for this type of

pain induction (39) and improved (40) to give greater reliability while producing sensations more closely related to clinical pain. This stimulator has been modified by the addition of a motor to increase the pressure in a *linear* manner over a short period of time, thereby improving reliability (41).

Before utilizing this pain stimulation method, the CLBP patient is given these instructions: "Tell us when you *first* feel the pain (pain threshold), then tell us when the pain that you feel in your finger is equal to the pain in your lower back (matching pain) and finally tell us when you can no longer tolerate the pain (pain tolerance)." In this way the pain patient's present pain can be matched to his/her pain threshold and tolerance, and thereby matched across other pain patients. Although the use of a pain-matching technique raises some ethical questions, this procedure is necessary to adequately assess pain threshold/tolerance. Again, this is the only method currently available by which pain comparisons can be made across patients.

DILEMMA OF THE SEVERITY OF PAIN AND ITS RELATIONSHIP TO FUNCTION AND DISABILITY

The major problem in the evaluation and treatment of chronic pain is the frequent discrepancy between the patient's reported level of pain and the resultant functional status versus the physician's perception of what the patient should be able to do functionally. This discrepancy in perceptions is attributable to the following complex problems:

1. Chronic pain patients perceive their pain as a disability that limits their functional status (25). The perception of pain as a disability has been investigated by Riley (25). To address this problem, he developed the Pain and Impairment Relationship Scale (PAIRS). The PAIRS was shown to covary in CLBP patients with four standardized measures of physical and overall impairment that were not intercorrelated (25). The authors interpreted this finding as indicating that patients who are more impaired are, indeed, more impaired as a function of their pain (25). The great number of patients who claim disability

based on pain alone, has forced the United States Social Security Administration Commission on the Evaluation of Pain to recommend the development of a listing based on "impairment due primarily to pain" (42a).

2. The pathology model does not predict back pain (43), making the reliability and validity of this model questionable. As a result, objective medical impairment may vary markedly from subjective disability (44). Also, chronic pain patients often lack documentation of clear structural organic pathology (45), thereby having minimum "medical impairment" as currently rated by the American Medical Association (AMA) Guides to Permanent Impairment (46). At the same time many chronic pain patients will demonstrate higher disability than medical impairment ratings (47).

3. Medical impairment ratings vary widely from one physician to another (48, 49) and so do measures of disability (50). These differences in impairment ratings have been blamed on evaluation schedules that are not scientifically based and that do not take functional status into consideration (49).

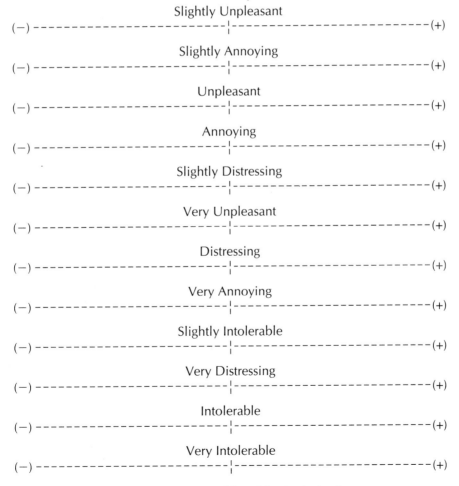

Figure 22.4. Descriptor differential scale of pain affect.

4. In cases where patients report severe pain, physicians have great difficulty in estimating patients' functional status (51). In addition, physicians have great difficulty in estimating anxiety, pain, and activity limitation from patients' self-report and the physical examination. These three dimensions are underestimated 35% of the time, and the activity limitation dimension is the one most often underestimated (52). This is because the inter-observer reliability decreases as functional status decreases (53).

5. In CLBPs, physical findings have low reliability and reproducability (54), creating a problem in the determination of medical impairment. In addition, in CLBPs, physical findings are not predictive of disability status, treatment outcome, and return to work (55, 56).

6. Patient-generated statements about severity of pain and functional impairment from pain have been shown to correlate (57, 58). However, the measures show few relationships to other measures of severity of pain: medication consumption, health care utilization, activity level, and frequency counts of engaging in a set of commonplace activities (57).

7. Chronic pain patients display a reduced activity level attributable to pain resulting in a consistent negative relationship between exercise and pain behavior, i.e., the more exercise performance, the fewer the pain behaviors (59).

8. It appears that pain behavior and movement ratings are strongly influenced by self-efficacy for movement, which in turn is determined by response expectancies for pain. Thus, the patients' movement is determined by how much pain they believe that movement will produce, how much pain they wish to avoid, and whether patients can accurately predict the pain involved in each movement (60). It has been postulated that the prediction of pain in movement promotes pain avoidance behavior, and that inaccurate prediction could promote excessive avoidance (61).

The previously reviewed studies indicate that there is little relationship between the physician's prediction of functional status based on the physical examination and the chronic pain patient's demonstrated functional status. This discrepancy relates to the inability of the physician to gauge the patient's pain and the chronic pain patient's perception of pain as a disability and differences in the chronic pain patient's willingness to risk increases in pain by increasing activities.

DILEMMA OF THE DISCREPANCY BETWEEN CHRONIC PAIN PATIENTS' SELF-REPORT OF PAIN AND OBSERVED PAIN BEHAVIOR

Pain researchers and clinicians have in the past been troubled by a concern that pain self-report and observed pain behavior might be inconsistent (62, 63). However, there is little evidence that this is a problem. Indeed, pain behavior ratings have been noted to correlate significantly with reported perceived pain (31, 32, 36, 62). As perceived pain improves, pain behavior diminishes (2, 32, 34). The question remains then: Why do some clinicians believe that in chronic pain patients (CPP) there is little correlation between reported perceived pain and observed pain behavior? The probable reasons for this perception are as follows:

1. As pointed out previously, there are discrepancies between what the CPP should be able to do according to the clinician, and what he/she actually is willing to do. Such a situation leads to this perception.

2. For a proportion of patients presenting with chronic pain, nonverbal expression may be discordant with self-reports (63). Reports of acute and severe distress may be contradicted by a calm and dispassionate manner, or displays of agony may be accompanied by denials of discomfort (63). Verbal behavior is more likely to be discounted than nonverbal behavior when the two are discordant (63). Thus, a calm CPP who demonstrates little pain behavior but reported having severe pain would lead to the "discrepancy" observation.

Conclusion

At present, there is no reliable direct method for measuring clinical pain. The VAS scale appears to be the most simple and reliable tool for that purpose. In addition, pain behavior appears to be an extremely important concept in chronic pain. The UAB scale is recommended for the measurement of pain behavior. For measurement of change in pain over time the comparative VAS is recommended along with the UAB scale.

ASSOCIATION OF PAIN WITH PSYCHIATRIC SYNDROMES

What is Chronic Pain?

There is no consensus definition of chronic pain (64). The current definitions can be summarized as follows:

1. The Institute of Medicine Committee Report on Pain and Disability (65) recognized chronic pain as a syndrome and has defined it as follows: "pain lasting for long periods of time. . .more than 6 months. . .may be associated with a residual structural defect. . .may be pain persisting past healing time without objective physical findings of residual structural defect. . .may be pain that recurs regularly and frequently over long periods." In addition, the committee pointed out that there was no agreed-upon operational definition of chronic pain in the studies reviewed.

2. The most recent issue of the American Medical Association (AMA) Guides to the Evaluation of Permanent Impairment (66) recognized chronic pain as a syndrome and pointed out that the medical profession had been slow to identify chronic pain as a specific medical disorder. The AMA defined acute pain, acute recurrent pain, and chronic pain. Acute recurrent pain

was defined as "episodic noxious sensations resulting from tissue damage in chronic disorders, e.g. arthritis, tic douloureux." Chronic pain was defined as "not a symptom of an underlying acute somatic injury. . .a pathological disorder in its own right. . .chronic. . .long-lived. . .progressive. . .tissue damage has healed and does not serve as a generator of pain. . .although applied to pain of greater than 6 months duration a chronic pain syndrome can be diagnosed two to four weeks after onset." In addition, the AMA awarded a 5% impairment (lumbar) for discal herniation or other soft-tissue lesions with a minimum of 6 months medically documented pain associated with muscle spasm and rigidity.

3. In the classification of chronic pain (67) by the International Association for the Study of Pain Subcommittee on Taxonomy, chronic pain was supposed to be coded on Axis IV as 1 month, 1–6 months, or > 6 months. In their definitions, the subcommittee advised that "many people report pain in the absence of tissue damage. . .if they regard their experience as pain, it should be accepted as pain. . .this definition would avoid tying pain to the stimulus."

Based on the previous statements, a number of conclusions can be drawn: (*a*) chronic pain is now recognized as a distinct syndrome; (*b*) the quoted authorities appear to consider pain chronic if it has lasted for more than 6 months, but they point out that chronic pain may begin earlier; (*c*) there is disagreement about the importance of presence/absence of continued tissue damage and presence/absence of objective physical findings in the definition; (*d*) overall, there appears to be no universally accepted operational definition of chronic pain.

In a recent article, this author (64) defined chronic pain as "continuous noxious output, like that of acute pain, but modulated and compounded by the prolonged or recurrent nature of the chronic state and complicated by a multitude of economic and psychosocial factors." However, the problem with the chronic pain concept is not so much the lack of a definition of chronic pain, but the lack of an operational diagnosis for chronic pain. An operational diagnosis for chronic pain would be useful for both clinical practice and research. This author made the following recommendations for the operational criteria for the diagnosis of chronic pain:

1. That the suggestion of the International Association for the Study of Pain Subcommittee on Taxonomy not to tie the definition of chronic pain to the presence or absence of noxious stimulus (67) be accepted for the operational diagnosis of chronic pain;
2. That the operational diagnosis of chronic pain should not be based on any psychiatric or psychological criteria. (Psychopathology, if present, should be investigated and diagnosed separately.)
3. That the temporal criteria of the diagnosis be flexible and defined in each individual patient either by the physician making the diagnosis of chronic pain or the patient

identifying himself/herself as having chronic pain. The last point is based on the approach to case identification as put forward in the Diagnostic Interview Schedule (DIS) for psychopathology (68). Individuals were identified as cases if they viewed their symptoms as interfering with their lives or if the symptoms led to a consultation. In other words, presumably a patient disturbed enough by his/her symptom, will seek treatment for that symptom.

4. That the category of acute recurrent pain as put forward by the AMA be eliminated and placed under acute pain (66). Those patients whose acute recurrent pain was frequent enough and severe enough as to be identified by either the physician or the patient as developing into chronic pain would be diagnosed as a chronic pain patient.

5. That the operational diagnosis of chronic pain contain some patient-perceived functional impairment (69) and patient-perceived disability criteria (70). These two criteria are suggested because many chronic pain patients link perceived pain, perceived functional impairment, and perceived disability, believing that they cannot live normal lives as long as they have pain, as their level of functioning is inversely proportional to their perceived pain (69). These two criteria (perceived functional impairment, perceived disability) become necessary in order to adequately distinguish between patient groups (using the aforementioned criteria). As an example, the patient who has chronic pain but is able to manage the pain and remain functional—perhaps because he/she has control over the pace of work at his/her job—may not seek treatment and, therefore, may not be identified as a CPP. The perceived functional impairment and perceived disability criteria are, therefore, necessary.

In summary, patients demonstrate having chronic pain through pain behavior, impaired function, and disability perception. Patients define themselves as suffering from chronic pain if the periods of what they perceive as intolerable pain are frequent enough to interfere with normal function. However, as noted earlier, there is neither a totally satisfactory definition for chronic pain nor an operational diagnosis for chronic pain. This major problem has interfered with delineating the frequency of chronic pain within the general population and within the psychiatric population.

Epidemiology of Pain and Chronic Pain in the General Population

Epidemiological data on pain are incomplete (71) but indicate that the problem is enormous. The prevalence of persistent pain in Canada is 11%, and age-specific morbidity rate for persistent pain increases with age (72). In Sweden, 40% of the general population reported "obvious pain" lasting more than 6 months (73). A statistical model applied to this population found that 25% had moderate pain and that 12% required pain treatment (73). The U.S. Nuprin Pain Report found that 5–10% of those studied report various types of pain lasting more than 3 months (74), with a reduction with age and the prevalence of chronic pain in all sites other than joints (74). The percentage of prevalent cases of low back pain with persistent pain is thought to be 16–29% (74, 75).

A recent New Zealand study indicates that 81.7% of the general population has had a pain experience severe enough to have led to a consultation with a doctor or other health professional, or led to the use of medications for the pain or interfered with life or activities "a lot" (76). In general, the prevalence of pain increased with age, except for headache and abdominal pain (76). In a suburban Australian community, 4.3% of the population were in constant pain (77). Twenty percent of hospitalized patients reported pain lasting for more than 6 months (78). Finally, it has been reported that 14.4% of the U.S. population between the ages of 25–74 may suffer from chronic pain related to the joints and musculoskeletal system (79). Based on these reports, the following observations can be drawn:

1. Pain is extremely common in the general population and is reported in 4.3–40% of the patients;
2. The lifetime prevalence of persistent pain may be as high as 80%;
3. The percentage of the reported patients who had chronic pain remains unclear. This is because of the definition variations described before. However, probably 4.3–12% of the general population has chronic pain; and
4. It is claimed that 12% of the general population required pain treatment (73). However, even if one requires pain treatment, one may not be a CPP of the type that chronic pain treatment centers treat. These patients have been shown to be distinctly different from other pain patients on many pain behavior and emotional variables (80–82). This makes them more difficult to treat, necessitating specialized treatments such as psychiatric care.

These observations lead to two major conclusions:

1. The prevalence of chronic pain patients with severe disability in the general population is unknown; and
2. The prevalence of pain complaints within the general population is uncertain. This makes comparisons with specialized populations, like the population with overt psychiatric disorders, extremely difficult.

Pain in Psychiatric Disorders

Pain is a common documented symptom in psychiatric patients (83), but there are few studies of pain complaints in these patients (84). France (84) has described a number of characteristics of the pain in psychiatric disorders. To delineate the differences between psychiatric patients with pain and chronic pain patients seen in pain centers, this author has placed France's pain characteristics into table form (Table 22.2). It is clear from this table that the pain seen in psychiatric patients differs from chronic pain seen within pain centers. In addition, although information is

Table 22.2.   Similarities and Differences in Pain Characteristics Between Psychiatric Patients and Chronic Pain Patients

	Psychiatric Patients	Chronic Pain Patients
Pain as a presenting complaint	Rarely	Always
Consistency of pain	Transient	Chronic
Location	Cephalic Trunkal	Low back Neck
Onset of pain with injury	Insidious	Usually associated
Pain sites	Multiple	Generally low back and/or neck
Neuroanatomical correlation	Poor	Poor to good
Exacerbating factors	Nonspecific	For low back pain, usually lifting, bending, sitting, or standing
Alleviating factors	Nonspecific	For low back pain, usually walking, lying down, changing positions, ice, or heat

lacking on this point, France (84) claims that chronic pain is rarely seen within the psychiatric patient group. This has also been my own clinical experience.

France (84), from his extrapolation of the literature also claims that pain complaints are common within the following psychiatric diagnostic groups: major depression, dysthymia, generalized anxiety disorder, somatoform disorder, atypical somatoform disorder, alcohol dependence, opiate dependence, conversion disorder, somatoform pain disorder, factitious disorder with physical symptoms, hypochondriasis, and personality disorders.

However, few incidence and prevalence data for pain are available within these diagnostic groups. Available incidence data indicate that 75% of nonpsychotic psychiatric inpatients had been bothered with pain within the last 3 months (85). In this study (85) pain was most frequent in patients with neurosis and personality disorders and was associated with unskilled work. The prevalence rate for chronic pain in a psychiatric outpatient clinic has been reported to be 14.37% (86, 87). These patients were usually urban, middle-aged married female housewives and were more likely to have a DSM-III diagnosis of anxiety disorder, dysthymic disorder, or no diagnosis than a pain-free psychiatric control group (86, 87). Interestingly, psychiatric patients without pain were as likely to have a DSM-III diagnosis of major depression or conversion disorder (86, 87).

Mood disorders as a group appear to have been most intensively studied for the association of a specific psychiatric disorder with pain. Here the prevalence of pain complaints is reported to vary from 30–84% (84). Data on the occurrence of pain complaints in different well-defined subtypes of depression are not available (84). It is interesting to note that pain thresholds are *increased* in depressed patients both with and without pain complaints (88). Finally, the vast majority of psychiatric patients with pain complaints report that pain developed either *before* or at the *same time* as the depression (89, 90).

Relationship Between Perceived Disability and Depression

People with physical disabilities have elevated rates of both depressive symptomatology and major depression (91–93). In older adults (60+) there is a significant relationship between disability and most mental health measures (94). Older adults with severe disabilities experience higher levels of anxiety, suicidal ideation, and overall distress than those with moderate disabilities (94). Severity of perceived disability correlates with severity of psychiatric symptoms (95).

Also, disability is a frequent accompaniment of late-onset geriatric depression (96). Conversely, psychiatric disorders (affective and anxiety) are independently associated with both acute and chronic limitations in physical functioning (97). A recent longitudinal study has demonstrated a synchronous relationship between depression and disability (93). In rheumatoid arthritis patients, depression predicts functional status ratings (98). Finally, in CPPs with headache, depression and perceived disability are significantly associated (99). Thus, there is an association between disability perception and depression.

Relationship Between Chronic Pain and Depression

Within pain treatment facilities, the vast majority of CPPs are depressed (79, 100, 101). The reported point prevalence of major depression in the chronic pain population has varied between 1.5–54.5%; the reported lifetime prevalence of major depression among CPPs varies between 20–71% (79, 102). The reported prevalence of dysthymic has ranged from 0.0–43.3% prevalence (79). Utilizing the Million Clinical Multiaxial Inventory (MCMI), more than 50% of the CPPs had clinically elevated scores for depression (103). Adjustment Disorder with Depressed Mood has been reported in 28.3% of chronic pain patients (100). We have reported (97) that 56.2% of chronic pain patients had some form of Mood Disorder (depression) as delineated by DSM-III criteria. Conversely, psychiatric outpatients who report chronic pain (14.8%), more frequently suffer from dysthymia and anxiety disorders (104), and individuals with two or more pain conditions are at elevated risk for a diagnosis of major depression (105). The differences in the reported prevalence of major depression within CPPs may be related to differences in pain center CPP selection criteria (100) and the lack of operationally-specific procedures for determining whether depressive symptoms are "due to" an organic factor, an exclusion criterion for DSM-III-R depressive disorders (106).

In addition to the reported association between pain and depression, there is strong evidence that pain affects mood (107) and the severity of depression. Pain severity has been found to be associated with negative mood (108). It also appears that negative mood increases and becomes fixed as pain continues and becomes persistent (109, 110). A number of studies (111–114) have reported a significant relationship between the level or degrees of perceived pain and the degrees of depression and the relationship between depression, pain, and pain behavior (115). Commonly used measurements of depression such as the Beck Depression Inventory are compounded by pain symptomatology (114). Finally, level of pain appears to be more important in predicting level of depression than physical dependency (116).

Major differences between authors in the reported prevalence of depression in chronic pain patients are likely to arise from problems in attributing symptoms to depression versus physical illness per se. For example, a high percentage of chronic pain patients have a sleep disorder (117–119), and many gain weight because of inactivity (100). Such a situation has confounded the utilization of the DSM criteria for major depression in this group (100). Furthermore, CPPs may demonstrate a distinctive depressive syndrome (119). This is compatible with the observation that dysthymia and atypical depression are associated with greater severity of pain than major depression or Adjustment Disorder with Depressed Mood (120).

Does the Depression Seen in Chronic Pain Patients Precede or Follow the Development of Chronic Pain?

Although depression can precede pain as an independent phenomenon, there is empirical evidence that persistent pain causes depression. A recent longitudinal study (121) of rheumatoid arthritis patients, for example, found that pain severity predicted subsequent depression. The causal relationship between pain severity and depression occurred only after the first 12 months of the study. Zarkowska and Philips (109) have also determined that as pain persists, pain intensity becomes more closely related to a number of subjective and behavioral dimensions. In two recently published studies, Gamsa (122, 123) concluded that emotional disturbance in CPPs is more likely to be a consequence than a cause of chronic pain (122), though psychological events are risk factors in the development of chronic pain (123). Finally, a recent study (124) has demonstrated that CLBP patients had significantly higher lifetime rates of major depression, alcohol use disorders, and major anxiety disorder. However, the first episode of major depression generally followed pain onset. This current evidence indicates that psychological events may be risk factors for the development of chronic pain, but that emotional disturbance is likely the result of chronic pain.

Prevalence of Other Psychiatric Diagnoses

Only a limited number of studies have addressed the issue of the prevalence of DSM-III diagnoses other than affective disorders in CPPs. These studies and the results of these studies are presented in Table 22.3. The studies support the following conclusions:

Table 22.3.   Prevalence of DSM-III Diagnoses Other Than Affective Disorder and Drug Abuse/Dependence in Chronic Pain Patients

Category and Diagnosis	Fishbain (100) Males (M) (N = 156) (%)	Fishbain (100) Females (F) (N = 127) (%)	Fishbain (100) Total (T) (N = 283) (%)	Reich (127)	Katon (251)	Large (252)	Muse (253)	Fishbain (254)
Somatoform disorders								
Somatization disorder	0.6[a]	7.9[a]	3.9	12% (F) 0% (M) 5% (T)	16.2% (T)	8% (T)		
Conversion disorder	42.3	32.3	37.8	2% (T)				
Psychogenic pain	0.6	0.0	0.3	32% (T)		8% (T)		
Hypochondriasis	0.6	0.8	0.7					
No diagnosis	5.7%	4.7%						
Anxiety disorders								
Panic disorder					11.0% (T)			
Agoraphobia with panic attacks and simple phobia	1.2	3.2	2.1					
Generalized anxiety disorder	15.4	15.0	15.2					
Obsessive-compulsive disorder	0.6	1.6	1.1					
Posttraumatic stress disorder acute and chronic	1.2	0.8	1.1				10% (T)	
Adjustment disorder with anxious mood	40.4	45.7	42.8					
Total number of patients suffering from anxiety (anxiety disorders and adjustment disorder with anxious mood)	58.8[a]	66.3[a]	62.5	7% (T)		8% (T)		
Organic mental disorders								
Delirium	0.6	0.0	0.4					
Dementia	5.1	11.0	7.8					
Substance abuse disorders								
Current alcohol abuse/dependence	5.7	2.4	4.3	2% (T)	5.4% (T)			
Alcohol abuse/dependence in remission	0.3	3.9	7.4		35.1% (T)			
Current drug dependence (opioids, barbiturates, sedatives and cannabinoid)	14.7[b]	5.5[b]	10.6	25.5% (T)	24.3% (T)			
Opioid dependence in remission	0.6	0.0	0.4					

Total current alcohol and other drug dependence	20.4[a]	7.9[a]	14.9			
Illicit drug abuse current			0%	0% (T)		
Schizophrenia	16.7	1.6	9.9			
Intermittent explosive disorder						0.14 (T)
Factitious disorder			13.0	2% (T)		
Adjustment disorder with work inhibition	17.9[a]	7.1[a]		5% (T)		
Psychological factors affecting physical condition			0%	19% (T)	0% (T)	34%
Uncomplicated bereavement	2.6	4.7	3.5			
Marital problem	7.7	8.7	8.2	7% (T)		
Personality disorders	62.3	55.1	59.0	37% (T)		
Paranoid	5.1[b]	0.0[b]	2.8			
Schizoid	3.2	0.0	1.7			
Compulsive	7.7	5.5	6.7			
Histrionic	4.5	20.5	11.7			
Dependent	21.2	12.6	17.4			
Narcissistic	4.5[b]	0.0[b]	2.4			
Borderline	0.0	2.4	1.0			
Passive-aggressive	15.4	14.2	14.9			

[a]$P < 0.01$; [b]$P < 0.05$.

1. A wide range of psychiatric disorders *besides* affective disorders are present in CPPs;
2. There are wide discrepancies between research reports on the prevalence of some DSM-III disorders;
3. The discrepancy on the prevalence of some DSM-III diagnoses within CPPs is greatest for disorders that have questionable reliability;
4. The vast majority of CPPs will have an axis I diagnosis;
5. Much work is needed in this area to resolve the conflicting data.

Is There Evidence for Preexisting Psychiatric Pathology in Chronic Pain Patients?

This issue has not been extensively explored. To the author's knowledge, there have been only three studies addressing this concern. An excellent study utilizing the DIS found that in 81% of the CPPs, alcohol use disorders preceded pain onset. CPPs, when matched against age-matched controls, had significantly higher pre-pain rates of alcohol use disorders, but not of depression (124). The second study utilized a self-designed questionnaire. In this study, 46% of the CPPs had pre-pain stress-related illness, 34% had a history of psychiatric illness, and 17% had been previously disabled (125). In the third study, the SCID-I was administered to 98 CLBP patients with a diagnosis of somatoform pain disorder. Thirty-nine percent of the CPPs admitted to a preexisting substance abuse disorder (41% males; 33% of the females). Twenty-nine percent had at least one episode of major depression prior to the onset of chronic pain (36% of the females; 25% of the males). Twenty-one percent had had preexisting symptoms consistent with an anxiety disorder (126). Finally, two studies (100, 127) have addressed this issue indirectly. Both of these studies found a high prevalence of personality disorders in CPPs: 59% (100) and 37% (127). These findings on personality disorders could be significant because apparently, axis II disorders may be less influenced by state phenomena than axis I disorders (128).

Conclusion

The general conclusions that can be drawn from this section are:

1. Chronic pain is a common complaint in the general population;
2. Psychiatric patients are unlikely to have a greater prevalence of chronic pain than the general population;
3. A wide range of psychiatric disorders are present in the chronic pain population, the most frequent being mood disorders;
4. Psychiatric disorders usually follow the development of chronic pain; and
5. There is some evidence that CPPs may have preexistent psychiatric pathology, particularly alcohol-related problems, episodes of major depression, and personality disorders.

MULTIDISCIPLINARY PAIN CENTER TREATMENT OF CHRONIC PAIN

Introduction

A multidisciplinary pain center (MPC) has been defined by Aronoff (129) as "a facility that offers multidisciplinary evaluation and treatment, a cohesive team approach directed towards the modification of pain and drug seeking behavior and towards the interruption of the disability process." MPC goals in the treatment of the CPP have been stated as follows (130–132): reduce pain; reduce medication intake; reduce psychiatric/psychological impairment; correct posture, gait, and range of motion abnormalities; educate patients in the roles that emotions, behaviors and attitudes play in chronic pain; remove rewards for pain behavior while encouraging healthy behavior; improve "up time" and thereby improve activities of daily living; improve level of function in social, familial, and household roles; improve strength and functional status; and restore occupational role function. Initially there were many questions about the efficacy of MPCS in treating chronic pain (133). However, recent evidence from well-designed outcome studies indicates that MPCs do indeed fulfill some of their goals of treatment. In his review, Aronoff concluded that MPCs do indeed return CPPs to the workplace (133). Our group has recently completed two review studies of this outcome literature, including a meta-analysis for return to work (134, 135). Both of these studies concluded that MPCs do return CPPs to work, that the increased rates of return to work are the result of treatment, and that the benefits of treatment are not temporary. At issue then is not so much whether MPC treatment is efficacious in the treatment of chronic pain, but by what mechanism it works.

Operant Conditioning

The operant conditioning model states that behavior is controlled by its consequences. Thus, when pain behavior is reinforced in a positive fashion, it is likely that pain behavior will increase (136). Fordyce was the first to propose that the behavior of CPPs fits an operant conditioning model. In a landmark study (137), he demonstrated that operant conditioning treatment could modify pain behavior. In this study, nurses withheld social reinforcement when CPPs displayed pain behaviors and provided attention when CPPs displayed "well behaviors," such as exercise. In addition, the reinforcing effects of pain medications were removed, utilizing instead, "pain cocktail" detoxification. The results demonstrated a dramatic increase in exercise tolerance and activity and a decrease in pain ratings and medication intake (137).

Since that study, Fordyce's assertion that operant conditioning is the cause of pain behavior has been severely criticized on three fronts: (*a*) there are questions as to what degree pain behavior is affected by social contingencies; (*b*) there are assertions that operant methods do not treat pain but instead teach CPPs to be more stoic about pain they experience; and (c) positive treatment outcome for operant treatment programs *is not evidence* of the importance of operant factors to the etiology and maintenance of chronic pain, i.e., pain behavior is not necessarily learned or acquired just because it can be subsequently modified (138). In addition, it has been pointed out that empirical data for this theory is lacking (138, 139) and cannot be supported experimentally (140). There are now difficulties in determining the unique contribution of contingency management techniques to modify chronic pain behavior because these techniques are usually integrated into MTPs (138). Fordyce was accused of jumping to conclusions when he stated that pain behavior is influenced by factors other than pain (138).

Fordyce has now deemphasized the role of social contingencies and now believes that CPPs are characterized by avoidance behavior (141). CPPs display pain behaviors because they anticipate that rapid movement will increase pain and thus pain behaviors are avoidance behaviors (141). The avoidance behaviors he believes are self-reinforcing, i.e., the avoidance of anticipated pain is self-reinforced (141). Fordyce then adds that the pain behaviors may lead directly to reinforcing consequences e.g., special attention, etc. (141). The avoidance learning concept for pain behaviors has some experimental support (142). These data, however, indicate that behavior treatments such as exercise quota systems are effective not because of reinforcement but because of a deconditioning process (142). At this juncture one can conclude that pain behaviors are probably not a consequence of operant conditioning but can be modified by operant conditioning. But it is unclear what the operant conditioning is acting on; that is, we may have targeted pain behavior for the operant conditioning but what is changed are the patient's beliefs about the pain, which may in turn lead to a change in pain behavior. Thus, it has been proposed that all forms of behavioral interventions, including operant conditioning, may exert an influence on chronic pain by changing the way in which the CPP thinks about his/her pain (143).

Cognitive-Behavioral Chronic Pain Treatment: Methods

Table 22.4 summarizes the pain management techniques that are currently being used within MPCs. Cognitive-behavioral methods are made up of a variety of these techniques and generally encompass A–E on Table 22.4 (144). Recent reviewers have concluded that cognitive-behavioral methods *do* indeed show that various cognitive strategies can increase pain tolerance levels (136, 144). In addition, cognitive coping strategies, a subcategory of cognitive-behavioral methods, have been shown to be more effective at alleviating pain as compared with either no treatment or expectancy controls (145).

Perhaps there is no difference in the efficacy of treatment results between the various pain management techniques. For example, one study showed operant conditioning pain treatment to be equal in efficacy to cognitive-behavioral

Table 22.4. Pain Management Techniques (260, 261)

A. Suggestion
  Information
  Direct verbal suggestion
  Programmed suggestion
  Hypnosis
  Self-hypnosis
B. Distraction
  Internal (imagination)
  External (ceiling TV)
C. Cognitive awareness
  Detailed information
  Mental preparation
  Rehearsal of strain to reduce pain
  Stimulus control (identification of stimulus and rearrangement to minimize exposure)
D. Anxiety-reduction techniques
  Relaxation
  Desensitization
E. Behavior skills training
  Social skills
  Stress management
  Self-management
  Self-improvement training
  Self-control
  Self-efficacy
  Anxiety management
  Decision making
  Social intervention
  Psychoeducation
F. Self-control
  Biofeedback
  Autogenic training
  Progressive muscle relaxation
  Imagery relaxation
  Breathing exercises
  Tension control
G. Cognitive therapy
  Transactional analysis
  Specific therapy to reevaluate meaning of pain, i.e., subjective ideas about possible aversive consequences of pain
H. Operant techniques
  Decrease attention in environment to pain behavior
I. Conditioning
J. Total push programs
  All of the above techniques

group treatment (146). In addition, individual cognitive-behavioral therapy was equal in efficacy to cognitive-behavioral group therapy (147). Cognitive-behavioral treatment effects may be additive to the effects of physical therapy. The combined condition of cognitive-behavioral group treatment with physical therapy has been shown to be superior to physical therapy alone (148). This study offers empirical support for combining various treatment disciplines in an MPC.

Indications for MPC Referral

A number of approaches are available for the treatment of chronic pain. These approaches can be categorized as follows: A—surgical, B—nerve blocks, C—psychopharmacological, D—drug detoxification, E—physical therapy, F—occupational therapy, and G—behavioral pain management techniques, as outlined in Table 22.4. MPCs utilize any combination of these approaches, depending on philosophy, the medical specialty providing leadership, and the size of the center. In addition, most MPCs utilize the "total push program" for the behavioral pain management techniques utilized. This author believes that the effectiveness of the treatment provided by MPCs rests in their ability to integrate these various treatment approaches in one setting. The larger MPCs will generally combine most of these approaches, usually in the following combinations: B–G, A and C–G, or C–G.

Indications for CPP referral to an MPC are provided in Table 22.5. Keep in mind that this table represents this author's opinions. Indications for MPC treatment have not yet been delineated in the literature. The author believes that a CPP should be referred to an MPC if he/she fulfills criterion A and *any one* of the criteria in list B (Table 22.5). However, if the CPP fulfills any of the criteria in list C, he/she should be *excluded* from MPC treatment because it is likely that the CPP will not be a treatment success. The referring doctor may be able to overcome these exclusion criteria by proper education and/or counseling of the CPP. Often the CPP is fearful or anxious about MPC treatment because he/she believes that the increased activity may increase the pain. This should be addressed directly as a risk, with the possibility that the chronic pain will eventually decrease with MPC treatment. The referring physician should also encourage realistic expectations, as many CPP wish to enter treatments that will guarantee the removal of all their pain. Care should be taken to refer the CPP to an MPC that provides the full range of disciplines and treatments.

Conclusions

A number of conclusions can be drawn from the previous discussion:

Table 22.5. Indications for Multidisciplinary Pain Center Treatment

Inclusion criterion A
  Chronic pain or chronic benign pain greater than 6 months in duration
Inclusion criteria B
  Surgical failure (failed back surgery syndrome)
  Few physical findings
  High-level pain behavior
  High-level functional disability
  Extended vocational disability (greater than 6 months)
  Drug dependence
  Severe suffering
  Significant psychopathology as a result of the chronic pain
  Failure of other modes of treatment, e.g., physical therapy alone
Exclusion criteria C
  CPP's unwillingness to participate in a pain management program
  Unrealistic expectation of what can be accomplished (e.g., that pain will be completely alleviated)

1. It is likely that operant factors are not the reason for pain behaviors;
2. Operant conditioning can, however, aid in the treatment of the CPP;
3. The most effective CPP treatment includes behavioral or other treatments that provide reduction in pain intensity. This gives the CPP an increased perception of being in personal control of the chronic pain (149);
4. The most effective CPP treatments are combinations of techniques that give the CPP this perception.

PSYCHOTROPIC DRUGS FOR THE TREATMENT OF NONNEUROPATHIC CHRONIC PAIN

Introduction

This part of the chapter deals with the use of psychotropic drugs in the treatment of chronic pain. Only the treatment of nonneuropathic chronic pain will be discussed, i.e., nociceptive pain (150). As such, this review does not present data on disease entities that appear to have a clear neuropathic component: central pain, postherpetic neuralgia, avulsion of plexus, neuroma formation, phantom limb, lancinating neuralgias, nerve compression, painful polyneuropathy, and reflex sympathetic dystrophy/causalgia (151). The treatment of neuropathic pain is addressed in Chapter 21. The utility of the following psychotropic drug groups (the World Health Organizations classification) (152) in the treatment of nonneuropathic chronic pain is discussed: Antidepressants (tricyclics, heterocyclics, serotonin reuptake inhibitors monoamine oxidase inhibitors); neuroleptics; antihistaminics; psychostimulants, and antiepileptic drugs.

Antidepressants (Tricyclic, Heterocyclics, and Serotonin Reuptake Inhibitors)—Evidence for Analgesic Efficacy in Chronic Pain

Outside of the neuropathic pain conditions, for which there is excellent evidence for the efficacy (153, 154) of antidepressants, these drugs have been utilized for numerous other syndromes for which chronic pain is believed to be either nociceptive or due to a psychological condition, or both (155). These include: headache, facial pain, arthritis/rheumatic pain, ulcer pain, fibrositis, low back pain, neck pain, pelvic pain, cancer-associated pain, depression-associated pain, and idiopathic pain. Antidepressants have also been utilized in studies where the pain conditions were *mixed* as to etiology (156). The results of the treatment studies for these various etiologies are presented in Tables 22.6–22.17. The tables attempt to list all treatment studies and/or case reports available in the literature and are organized according to number of CPPs in the study, antidepressant utilized, dosage utilized in mg per day, whether the study was controlled, percentage of CPPs reporting pain relief, and/or whether the drug was statistically better than placebo.

Table 22.6. Antidepressants for Back Pain

Author of Study/Year	N	Type of Drug	Dose (mg/day)	Controlled Study	Percentage of Patients Reporting Pain Relief
Alcoff et al., 1982 (262)	41	Imipramine	150	Yes	47% significant improvement
Goodkin et al., 1990 (263)	42	Trazodone	201 (average)	Yes	0
Hameroff et al., 1982 (264)	30	Doxepin	50–300	Yes	[a]
Hameroff et al., 1984 (265)	51	Doxepin	300	Yes	[a]
Hameroff et al., 1982 (266)	27	Doxepin	2.5 mg/kg	Yes	[a]
Jenkins et al., 1976 (267)	44	Imipramine	75	Yes	0
Pheasant et al., 1983 (268)	9	Amitriptyline	150	Yes	[a]
Ward 1986 (270)	35	Doxepin Desipramine compared	? ?	Yes (Placebo responders dropped from study)	No significant difference in pain response noted between drugs, so patient groups were collapsed. Retests indicated a statistically significant drop in pain by week 1 [a]
Ward et al., 1984 (271)	26	Doxepin Desipramine compared	188 173	Yes (Placebo responders dropped from study)	50% overall; Doxepin reduced pain severity significantly more than desipramine
Workman et al., 1991 (272)	20	Doxepin Trazodone compared	150 300	No	No change in pain for either drug but depression change scores significant for both drugs

[a]Drug significantly more effective than placebo or other comparison drug.

LOW BACK PAIN

Of 12 placebo controlled studies, six studies have demonstrated an analgesic effect significantly greater than placebo (Table 22.6). The most consistent responses are seen with doxepin and desipramine in doses above 150 mg daily (157). Although the subject requires further study, some authors (157) believe that antidepressants have been demonstrated to be effective for the treatment of low back pain.

NECK AND PELVIC PAIN

At this point, not enough studies have been completed in these two areas to make any definitive observations (Tables 22.7 and 22.8).

CANCER PAIN

Currently, there is a lack of controlled studies for antidepressant treatment of chronic pain associated with cancer (Table 22.9). However, it appears that antidepressants may be opiate-sparing in chronic pain associated with cancer (158). In the reviewed reports, the onset of analgesic action occurs in most cases in less than 6 days. Withdrawal of the antidepressant is associated with breakthrough pain in 24–48 hours (158). Thus, it is likely that the antidepressants are not acting through effects on mood. However, at present, too little information is available from which to draw conclusions regarding the utility of antidepressants for cancer pain (157, 158). Nevertheless, Magni et al. (159), using the responses to a questionnaire given to a large number of Italian oncological centers, concluded that the vast percentage of centers utilize antidepressants for pain control—with positive results. These drugs are utilized without depression being present. If antidepressants are efficacious in cancer-associated pain, the mechanism is unclear, and may vary among cases. In a large percentage of cancer patients there is a neuropathic component. For example, in a sample of 20 cancer patients closely analyzed as to whether they had nociceptive superficial somatic, nociceptive deep somatic, nociceptive visual, or neuropathic pains, 10 had a neuropathic component to their pain (160). It is therefore clear that future controlled antidepressant trials for the treatment of pain associated with cancer will

Table 22.7.   Antidepressants for Neck Pain

Author of Study/Year	N	Type of Drug	Dose (mg/day)	Controlled Study	Percentage of Patients Reporting Pain Relief
Abott et al., 1990 (273)	18	Amitriptyline	Variable	No	14 patients had decreased pain

Table 22.8.   Antidepressants for Pelvic Pain

Author of Study/Year	N	Type of Drug	Dose (mg/day)	Controlled Study	Percentage of Patients Reporting Pain Relief
Beresin, 1986 (274)	1	Imipramine	150	No	Complete resolution pelvic pain
Walker et al., 1991 (275)	7	Nortriptyline	Variable	No	6 of 7 women had complete or partial pain relief

have to control for the presence of neuropathic components to the pain (161).

ARTHRITIC/RHEUMATIC PAIN

Although a large number of controlled studies have been completed for the treatment of this syndrome with antidepressants, only a few studies have demonstrated the antidepressant utilized to be more effective than placebo (Table 22.10). It appears that the older antidepressants with some serotonergic activity (amitriptyline, imipramine) are overrepresented in the studies that have demonstrated an effect significantly better than placebo. Whether antidepressants boost the efficacy of analgesics in the management of arthritic/rheumatic pain has not been settled (157).

FIBROSITIS/FIBROMYALGIA

Here, the preponderance of studies have indicated an analgesic effect greater than that of placebo (Table 22.11). Amitriptyline appears to be superior to naproxen, while clomipramine is superior to maprotiline.

FACIAL PAIN

There are only a few controlled studies (Table 22.12). These indicate a favorable pain response (162–164). One controlled study demonstrated a reduction in pain *without* a decrease in the level of depression (164). Researchers in this area have concluded that antidepressants are a useful therapeutic modality in the treatment of chronic facial pain (165).

ULCER PAIN

Although a number of controlled studies have been done on this problem, no study has demonstrated an analgesic effect greater than placebo (Table 22.13). Doxepin, however, has been demonstrated to have equal efficacy to cimetidine for ulcer healing (166).

HEADACHE

Antidepressants have been used for various categories of headaches: migraine, tension, mixed vascular and tension, and idiopathic (167). There have been more controlled studies of antidepressants in the treatment of chronic headache than any other pain syndrome. Most of these controlled studies have found the antidepressant utilized to be significantly better than placebo (Table 22.14). In the controlled studies, the following antidepressants were shown to be efficacious: doxepin, amitriptyline, femoxetine, maprotiline, and clomipramine. The response to headache treatment often was demonstrated at a dosage lower than that used to treat major depression, e.g., dosage less than 150 mg amitriptyline. Unfortunately, posttraumatic headache has not been shown to be responsive to antidepressants (168, 169). The effect of amitriptyline for the relief for headaches was shown to be independent of its antidepressant effect (170). In fact, one study demonstrated that nondepressed patients with severe migraine were more responsive to the antidepressant than depressed patients (171). A history prior to headache treatment was shown not to predict headache response to antidepressants (170).

PAIN OF MIXED ETIOLOGY

Of seven placebo-controlled studies, four demonstrated a statistically significant effect (Table 22.15). Amitriptyline was the drug most frequently effective. A large number of nonplacebo-controlled studies have also demonstrated a positive effect on the pain of mixed etiology. However, the reduction in pain is modest (172). Many of these studies (173, 174) combined CPPs with neuropathic pain and those with nociceptive pain. This practice confounds the interpretation of study results.

PAIN AS A SYMPTOM OF DEPRESSION

It appears that antidepressants, both heterocyclics and MAOIs, are effective in alleviating depression-associated

Table 22.9. Antidepressants for Pain Associated with Cancer

Author of Study/Year	N	Type of Drug	Dose (mg/day)	Controlled Study	Percentage of Patients Reporting Pain Relief
Adjan, 1970 (276)	50	Clomipramine	50–150 i.m./p.o.	No	74% opiate sparing
Bernard & Scheuer, 1978 (277)	119	Clomipramine	400 i.v.	No	101 positive result 18 no effect
Bortz, 1967 (278)	23	Imipramine	50–150 i.m.	No	80% opiate sparing
Bourkus et al., 1978 (279)	100	Trimipramine	Up to 300	No	77 improved
Bresson, 1971 (280)	30	Clomipramine	75–150	No	75%
Brevik & Rememo, 1982 (281)	56	Amitriptyline	25–100	No	Some positive response
Buttaro et al., 1970 (282)	?	Imipramine	150	No	77%
Cohn et al., 1988 (283)	30	Piroxicam Doxepin	60–120 25–225	No	80% opiate sparing
Deutschmann, 1971 (284)	63	Imipramine	50–100 i.m.	No	79% opiate sparing
Fiorentino, 1967 (285)	40	Imipramine	150	Yes	0 (nearly significant $p < 0.06$)
Gebhardt et al., 1969 (286)	60	Clomipramine	150 i.v.	No	22 improved 12 partially improved 36 intolerant or little improvement
Hughes et al., 1963 (192)	118	Imipramine	75	No	60%
Laine et al., 1962 (287)	30	Imipramine	50–75 i.m.	No	60%
Mascles, 1976 (288)	35	Clomipramine	75–150 p.o./i.v.	No	90% opiate sparing
Monkemeier & Steffen, 1970 (289)	20	Imipramine	75–150	No	75% opiate sparing
Parolin, 1966 (290)	38	Imipramine	50–150 i.m.	No	52% opiate sparing
Paschetta, 1963 (291)	94	Imipramine	?	No	66% opiate sparing
Richlin et al., 1987 (292)	12	Methadone/amitriptyline/nonnarcotic analgesic combination	10–75	No	Good to excellent pain control in previously uncontrolled patients.
Serin, 1974 (293)	20	Clomipramine	30	No	60% opiate sparing
Stendardo, 1964 (294)	51	Imipramine	50–150 i.m.	No	82% opiate sparing
Tateno, 1969 (295)	10	Imipramine	25–150	No	80%
Ventafridda et al., 1979 (296)	?	Amitriptyline	Up to 100	No	High positive effect
Ventafridda et al., 1987 (297)	23 22	Trazodone Amitriptyline compared	225 75	No	Statistically significant drop in pain scores for both drugs—drugs equal in pain efficacy—cancer patients with neuropathic component[a]

[a]Drug significantly more effective than placebo or other comparison drug.

pain (Table 22.16). In both Raft et al.'s (175) and Ward et al.'s (176) studies, the primary diagnosis was depression. The positive response was therefore not surprising. Phenelzine was more effective than amitriptyline in one study (175).

PSYCHOGENIC (IDIOPATHIC) PAIN

There have been a surprising number of placebo-controlled studies (eight) performed for the treatment with

antidepressants for alleged psychogenic (idiopathic) pain (Table 22.17). Of these eight studies, seven demonstrated a significant improvement versus placebo. The one study that did not demonstrate a statistically significant improvement (177) demonstrated that amitriptyline reduced pain and psychotherapy alone *increased* pain. Of the other two uncontrolled studies (178, 179), both demonstrated a significant decrease in pain. It can be concluded that antidepressants are effective in the treatment of idiopathic

Table 22.10. Antidepressants for Arthritis/Rheumatic Pain

Author of Study/Year	N	Type of Drug	Dose (mg/day)	Controlled Study	Percentage of Patients Reporting Pain Relief
Caruso & Pietro Grande, 1987 (298)	734	Ademethionine (tension headaches)	200 i.m.	Yes	[a]
Frank et al., 1988 (299)		Trazodone	3.0/kg	Yes	0
Frank et al., 1988 (300)	47	Amitriptyline Desipramine Trazodone	1.5/mg/kg/d 1.5/mg/kg/d 3/mg/kg/d	Yes	Only amitriptyline greater than placebo
Frank et al., 1988 (299)		Desipramine	1.5/kg	Yes	0
Frank et al., 1988 (299)	47	Amitriptyline	1.5/kg	Yes	[a]
Ganvir et al., 1980 (301)	49	Clomipramine	25	Yes	0
Ganvir et al., 1980 (302)	49	Clomipramine	25	Yes	0
Glick & Fowler, 1979 (303)	11	Imipramine	75	Yes	[a]
Grace et al., 1985 (304)	36	Amitriptyline	75	Yes	0
Gringas, 1976 (305)	55	Imipramine	75	Yes	52
Jacobs, 1972 (306)	14	Opipramol	150	Yes	49% decrease in attacks in treated patients vs. increase in controls.
Kuipers, 1962 (307)	28	Imipramine	20–40	No	60–70
McFarland et al., 1986 (308)	27	Trimipramine	75	Yes	[a]
McDonald-Scott, 1969 (309)	22	Imipramine	75	Yes	69
Petitto et al., 1992 (171)	1	Fluoxetine	40	No	Case report: improvement of arthritic pain Arthritic symptoms without improvement of mood
Regalado, 1977 (311)	41	Clomipramine	10–25	No	57
Sarzi-Puttini et al., 1988 (312)	60	Dothiepin	75	Yes	For daytime pain only[a]
Thorpe & Marchant-Williams, 1974 (313)	19	Dibenzepine	240	Yes	[a]
Tyber, 1974 (314)	56	Amitriptyline; lithium	75	No	79
Wheatly, 1986 (315)	65	Mianserin	Various	Yes	0
Wheatly, 1986 (315)	68	Nomifensine	Various	Yes	0

[a]Drug significantly more effective than placebo or other comparison drug.

Table 22.11. Antidepressants for Fibrositis

Author of Study/Year	N	Type of Drug	Dose (mg/day)	Controlled Study	Percentage of Patients Reporting Pain Relief
Bibolotti et al., 1986 (316)	37	Maprotiline Clomipramine	75 75	Yes	Clomipramine superior to maprotiline
Carette et al., 1986 (317)	59	Amitriptyline	50	Yes	0
Caruso et al., 1987 (318)	60	Dothiepin	75	Yes	
Connolly, 1981 (319)	1	Amitriptyline	50	No	Complete pain relief
Goldenberg et al., 1986 (320)	58	Naproxen Amitriptyline	1000 25	Yes	Amitriptyline greater than placebo. Naproxen not greater.
Scudds et al., 1989 (321)	36	Amitriptyline	50	Yes	
Tavoni et al., 1987 (322)	25	Ademethionine	200 i.m.	Yes	Ademethionine significantly number of decreased tender points
Wysenbeek et al., 1985 (323)	20	Imipramine	50–75	No	2 patients responded

Table 22.12. Antidepressants for Facial Pain

Author of Study/Year	N	Type of Drug	Dose (mg/day)	Controlled Study	Percentage of Patients Reporting Pain Relief
Carasso & Yehuda, 1979 (324)	9 9	Clomipramine Amitriptyline	20–75 30–110	No	44 38
Feinmann & Harris, 1984 (164)	93	Dothiepin	150	Yes	[a]
Fishbain et al., 1993 (325)	3	Clomipramine	150	No	CPP no longer obsessing about chronic pain
Gessel, 1975 (326)	8	Amitriptyline	100	No	50
Keyser, 1992 (327)	1	Clomipramine	?	No	Total pain relief in an obsessive-type syndrome post-facial plastic surgery
Lascelles, 1966 (162)	40	Phenelzine	45	Yes	[a]
Moore & Nally, 1975 (328)	100	Amitriptyline Chlordiazepoxide	? ?	No	71
Rees & Harris, 1978-79 (329)	44	Dothiepin (28) Amitriptyline (1) Clomipramine (1) Phenelzine (4)	? ? ? ?	No	75% complete pain relief or brief mild attacks
Sharav et al., 1987 (163)	28	Amitriptyline	129 (mean)	Yes	[a]

[a]Drug significantly better than placebo or other comparison drug.

pain. Antidepressants can relieve pain even if they have no significant effect on depressed mood (164). Though overt mental symptoms, when present, resolved when pain was relieved and relapsed with drug withdrawal, pain relief was independent of CPPs' pre-treatment mental state (164). Pilowsky and Barrow recently demonstrated that level of pain predicts the response to amitriptyline in idiopathic pain (180). Onghena and Van Houdenhore (181), from a meta-analysis of 39 antidepressant placebo-controlled studies for the treatment of chronic pain, concluded that the size of the analgesic effect from antidepressants is not much different for pain having an "organic" vs. a "psychogenic"

Table 22.13. Antidepressants for Ulcer Pain

Author of Study/Year	N	Type of Drug	Dose (mg/day)	Controlled Study	Percentage of Patients Reporting Pain Relief
Berstad et al., 1980 (330)	95	Trimipramine	25	Yes	0
Guldhal, 1977 (331)	8	Trimipramine	25–75	Yes	75%
Hoff et al., 1982 (166)	25	Doxepin	50	No	78%
	25	Cimetidine comparison	1000		84% healing of ulcers with no statistical difference between drugs
Magla & Pereira, 1982 (332)	12	Doxepin	50–150	No	11 patients had complete ulcer healing
Niller et al., 1977 (333)	19	Trimipramine	50	Yes	100%
Wetterhus et al., 1977 (334)	14	Trimipramine	50	Yes	80%

basis. If idiopathic pain were truly psychogenic, one would expect the following outcomes to occur with antidepressant treatment: (*a*) no response at all; (*b*) a response equal to a placebo response; or (*c*) a response dependent on the antidepressant properties of the drug, i.e., the masked depression hypothesis (182). Neither *a, b,* or *c* has been shown in studies of antidepressant treatment of idiopathic pain. Thus, the analgesic response to antidepressants in idiopathic pain disorder questions the "psychogenic" concept. As pointed out by Davis (183), these studies suggest that these CPPs have an organically-based pain disorder.

From the reviewed studies in Tables 22.6–22.17 and from previous reviews, the following points can be made:

1. Antidepressants appear to be effective for the analgesic treatment of a wide range of nonneuropathic pain conditions. The great majority of studies show antidepressants to be superior to placebo (184). This observation has recently been supported by a meta-analysis of these data (181);
2. The beneficial effect from antidepressants for most pain conditions is not related to mood (181);
3. The beneficial effect appears to be mild to moderate (172, 184);
4. There is strong evidence for the pain effect of amitriptyline, doxepin, and clomipramine and to a lesser extent for imipramine and dothiepin (184). The antidepressants, with more selective neurochemical effects, e.g., the serotonin reuptake inhibitors, may be less effective for pain in some specific pain syndromes;
5. CPPs may have an analgesic response to lower dosages of antidepressant than usual for treating depression (184); and
6. The delay in the onset of action of the pain effect varies from a few days to several weeks (184).

In general, published antidepressant studies suffer from one or more methodological problems. Goodkin and Gullion (185), in a selective critical review of 46 antidepressant pain treatment trials, noted that only 14 trials met his minimal design and protocol criteria, while no trials met all four validity requirements: statistically significant conclusions, internal validity, construct validity, and external validity. Other frequent methodological problems are: anecdotal data; small numbers of subjects; poorly defined end-points; poor measurement of pain; lack of double-blind conditions; depression not controlled for; other drugs besides antidepressants utilized; depression poorly measured; high dropout rates; lack of true randomization, coexistent depression not specifically included or excluded, and pain duration less than 1 month. (151, 181, 186). Chronic pain, especially when related to the back and when not subject to invasive procedures, usually is a self-limiting condition.

More recently, it has been pointed out that in self-limiting conditions, it is important to compare the test drug not to placebo but to no treatment at all! (158). To my knowledge, there is not one antidepressant pain treatment study that has attempted to do this. Finally, this author believes that the largest problem with the study of antidepressants in chronic pain is difficulty in deciding if the pain has a neuropathic component. This is a major problem in cancer-associated pain (187) and may be a major problem in conditions such as low back pain and neck pain, which can involve radiculopathy. It has been suggested that researchers in this area study specific pain syndromes (188). However, researchers often mix diagnostic groups (Tables 22.6–22.8; 22.15; 22.16) and in some studies have allegedly utilized a mixed group of CPPs but chose CPPs with burning pain (189). Burning pain often is associated with a neuropathic pain component (187). Thus, future antidepressant pain studies will have to make a basic distinction in the pain that the study is trying to treat: neuropathic versus nociceptive versus both.

Table 22.14.   Antidepressants for Headaches

Author of Study/Year	N	Type of Drug	Dose (mg/day)	Controlled Study	Percentage of Patients Reporting Pain Relief
Anthony & Lance, 1969 (335)	25	Phenelzine	45	No	80
Carasso & Yehuda, 1979 (324)	?	Clomipramine Amitriptyline	20–75	No	Moderate to marked relief in 60% of tension head-ache patients
Couch & Hassanein, 1979 (336)	100	Amitriptyline	100	Yes	55.3[a]
Couch, 1976 (182)	110	Amitriptyline	75	No	72
Dalessio, 1967 (338)	100	Amitriptyline	75–100	No	64
Diamond & Baltes, 1971 (339)	56	Amitriptyline	10–25	Yes	[a]
Fogelholm & Murros, 1985 (340)	30	Maprotiline	75	Yes	[a]
Gomersall & Short, 1973 (341)	16	Amitriptyline	10–60	Yes	80
Indaco & Carriesc, 1988 (193)	15	Amitriptyline	50	Yes	[a]
Lance & Anthony, 1972 (342)	17	Cyclobenzaprine	30 60	Yes	5 headache free; 5 were 50% improved
Lance & Curran, 1964 (170)	280	Amitriptyline Imipramine	30–75 30–75	Yes	Amitriptyline >imipramine
Langemark et al., 1990 (343)	82	Clomipramine Mianserin	Variable Variable	Yes	[a]
Langohr et al., 1985 (344)	63	Clomipramine Metoprolol	100 100	Yes	0
Mahloudji, 1969 (345)	12	Amitriptyline	30–40	No	100
Martucci et al., 1985 (346)	20	Mianserin (tension headaches)	30	Yes	0
Monro et al., 1985 (347)	60	Mianserin	60	Yes	0
Morland et al., 1979 (348)	14	Doxepin	100	Yes	[a]
Noone, 1980 (349)	10	Clomipramine	30	Yes	0
Noone, 1977 (350)	8	Clomipramine	30	No	100
Okasha et al., 1973 (191)	80	Doxepin Amitriptyline	30–50 30–150	Yes	[a] (Doxepin > amitriptyline or diazepam)
Paulson, 1962 (168)	14	Imipramine	75	No	0
Saran, 1988 (169)	10	Amitriptyline	200–300	No	0
Sherwin, 1979 (351)	14	Amitriptyline Perphenazine	100–200 8–64	No	70
Sjaastad, 1983 (352)	16	Femoxetine	400	Yes	[a]
Sjaastad, 1982 (352)	60	Doxepin	175	Yes	[a]
Tyler et al., 1980 (353)	23	Amitriptyline	75–250	No	21 patients excellent or good recovery
Ziegler et al., 1987 (354)	30	Amitriptyline Propranolol	50–150 80–240	Yes	[a] [a]

[a]Drug significantly better than placebo or other comparison drug.

Table 22.15. Antidepressants for Pain of Mixed Etiologies

Author of Study/Year	N	Type of Drug	Dose (mg/day)	Controlled Study	Percentage of Patients Reporting Pain Relief
Blumer & Heilbronn, 1984 (212)	349	Various TCAs		No	89
Blumer et al., 1980 (211)	129	Amitriptyline Imipramine Doxepin	Variable Variable Variable	No	At 9 months 8% pain free, at 16 months 17% pain free
Carasso & Yehuda, 1979 (324)	15 13	Clomipramine Amitriptyline	20–75 30–110	No	66 54
Clarke, 1981 (355)	110	Amitriptyline Perphenazine	75 2	No	34
Duthie, 1977 (356)	12	Amitriptyline Trifluoperazine	75	No	67
Evans et al., 1973 (357)	22	Doxepin	150	Yes	[a]
Gourlay et al., 1986 (358)	19	Zimelidine	300	Yes	0
Hampf et al., 1989 (359)	48	Amitriptyline Amitriptyline plus Distigmine	75 75 10	No	Amitriptyline alone no significant decrease in pain. Amitriptyline plus distigmine 43% decrease in pain.
Johansson & Von Knorring, 1979 (360)	32	Zimelidine	200	Yes	[a]
Kocher, 1976 (173)	130	Desipramine Various TCAs Phenothiazine		No	82
Lindsay & Olsen, 1985 (361)	25	Maprotiline	150	No	72% responded with greater than 50% decrease in pain
McQuay et al., 1992 (189)	33	Amitriptyline	25	Yes	[a]
Merskey & Hester, 1972 (362)	30	Various TCAs + Phenothiazines		No	93
Montrastruc et al., 1985 (174)	30	Clomipramine	150	No	67
Pilowsky et al., 1982 (363)	32	Amitriptyline	150	Yes	0
Singh & Verma, 1971 (364)	60	Imipramine Amitriptyline Chlordiazepoxide		No	[a] [a]
Zitman et al., 1990 (366)	49	Amitriptyline	75	Yes	[a] (gain was modest)

[a]Drug is significantly more effective than placebo or other comparison drug.

Table 22.16. Antidepressants for Pain as a Symptom of Depression

Author of Study/Year	N	Type of Drug	Dose (mg/day)	Controlled Study	Percentage of Patients Reporting Pain Relief
Dahl et al., 1981 (367)	40	Dothiepin Amitriptyline	?	Yes	[a]
Lindsay & Wydroff, 1981 (368)	116	Various TCAs	150–300	No	83% of patients had significant relief (>50%)
Raft et al., 1981 (175)	23	Phenelzine Amitriptyline	1.5 mg/kg 3.5 mg/kg	Yes	Phenelzine more effective than amitriptyline; both superior to placebo
Ward et al., 1979 (176)	16	Doxepin	150	Yes	[a]

[a]Drug more effective than placebo or other comparison drug.

Table 22.17.   Antidepressants for Alleged Psychogenic Pain

Author of Study/Year	N	Type of Drug	Dose (mg/day)	Controlled Study	Percentage of Patients Reporting Pain Relief
Diamond & Baltes, 1971 (339)	90	Amitriptyline	10–60	Yes	[a]
Eberhard et al., 1988 (178)	40	Clomipramine	100 (mean)	No	Both drugs significantly reduced pain, with clomipramine being significantly more effective
	30	Maprotiline compared	97.2 (mean)		
Eisendrath & Kodama, 1992 (369)	1	Fluoxetine	40	No	Improvement in chronic abdominal pain; single case
Feinmann & Harris, 1983 (164, 370)	93	Dothiepin	150	Yes	[a]
Fogelholm & Murros, 1985 (340)	30	Maprotiline	75	Yes	[a] Psychogenic tension headache
Johansson & Von Knorring, 1979 (360)	32	Zimelidine	100	Yes	[a]
Lance & Anthony, 1964 (170)	27	Amitriptyline	30–75	Yes	[a]
Lascelles, 1966 (162)	40	Phenelzine	45	Yes	[a]
Loldrup et al., 1989 (371)	127	Clomipramine	150	Yes	Helpful for some specific pain locations only [a]
	124	Mianserin	60		
Okasha et al., 1973 (191)	80	Amitriptyline	50	Yes	[a]
		Doxepin	40		
Pilowsky & Barrow, 1990 (177)	102	Amitriptyline	Variable	Yes	0
		Psychotherapy			Amitriptyline reduces pain, psychotherapy increases pain
Sjaastad, 1983 (352)	16	Femoxetine	400	Yes	[a] Psychogenic tension headache
Valdes et al., 1989 (179)	31	Imipramine	100–175	No	All patients significantly improved in pain from pretreatment[a]
Zitman et al., 1991 (372)	34	Amitriptyline compared to flupenthixol	75	Yes	[a]
			3		Flupenthixol did not add
		plus amitriptyline	75		
Zitman et al., 1990 (172)	49	Amitriptyline	75	Yes	Modest gain from drug[a]

[a]Drug more effective than placebo or other comparison drug.

Mechanism of Action for the Antinociceptive Effect of Antidepressants

Based on the data given in Tables 22.6–22.17, it appears that there is a wide body of evidence indicating that antidepressants *do* have an antinociceptive effect. A number of hypotheses have been advanced as a potential explanation for the mode of action of antidepressants' antinociceptive effect. These hypotheses are summarized in Table 22.18. The accuracy of these hypotheses in light of the current evidence is discussed in the pages that follow.

It has long been observed that the analgesic effect of antidepressants appears to be independent of their antidepressant effect. Clifford (154) and Sindrup et al. (190) have summarized the evidence for the independence of analgesic and antidepressant actions of the antidepressants. This evidence includes the following observations: 1) the response of pain is more rapid than the antidepressant effect (189); 2) the dosage required for analgesia appears to be lower than that required for the treatment of depression (181, 189, 191–193); 3) when serum levels of antidepressant are measured on CPP who have an analgesic effect, these levels are lower than those required for an antidepressant effect (174, 194, 195); also, antidepressant serum levels do not correlate with a decrease in pain and/or change in depression scores in those CPPs responding to antidepressants with decreased pain (196, 197); and 4) the presence of depression is not required for an analgesic response (151, 170, 193).

Table 22.18. Hypotheses for the Mode of Action of the Antidepressant Antinociceptive Effect[a]

Antidepressant effect (manifest or masked depression)

Stabilizing aberrantly-conducting neurons or inhibiting their afferent transmission at the spinal cord (migraine headaches, neuropathic pain)

Antiepileptic (suppressing epileptiform activity in deafferented neurons)

Selective serotonin inhibition

Facilitating analgesia by facilitating central monoamine transmission (inhibiting serotonin and norepinephrine reuptake at the synapse)

Facilitating the descending pain modulation system (resultant decrease in afferent input through the spinothalamic tract)

Interaction with opioid receptors (altering binding characteristics of the receptor to morphine and enkephalins)

Affecting a "core disorder" (common psychobiological abnormalities but multiple clinical and diagnostic presentations, e.g., chronic pain and depression)

Peripheral anti-inflammatory action (inflammatory disorders)

Central skeletal muscle relaxant action (depressing polysynaptic reflexes causing muscle spasm or tension)

Sedative effect

Placebo effect

[a]From references 153, 181, 211, 367, 373, and 374.

In addition to this evidence for the independence of the antidepressant and analgesic properties of antidepressants, antidepressants have powerful analgesic effects in animal models (198). Analgesic effects of antidepressants have been demonstrated in animal models of adjuvant-induced arthritis (199). In animals, clomipramine has a powerful antinociceptive effect *in itself,* and it enhances the antinociceptive effect of morphine (200). This effect may be central rather than peripheral (201). In some animal models, antidepressants were found to be up to 70 times more potent than aspirin (202). However, the antinociceptive effects of different antidepressants may depend on the specific nociceptive test used. The relatively selective norepinephrine reuptake blockers (like desipramine and protriptyline) appear to be active in all three standard nociceptive tests in rats, while the selective serotonin reuptake inhibitors, such as fluoxetine, are only partially active in two tests and are not active in the third test (203).

Antidepressants have also been demonstrated to have an experimental antinociceptive effect against laboratory-induced pain (204, 205) and clinical acute pain (206, 207) in humans. In one human study, desipramine but not amitriptyline has been found to increase and prolong morphine analgesia (208). In another, amitriptyline and clomipramine were found to induce analgesia, as measured by pain thresholds, and to potentiate morphine analgesia. Trazodone and notriptyline did not demonstrate either property (209). A recent meta-analysis (181) of 39 placebo-controlled studies of antidepressants in chronic pain adds to the evidence that the antidepressant effect of antidepressants is independent of their analgesic effect. The meta-analysis determined that the size of the analgesic effect was not significantly different in the presence or absence of a marked or manifest depression, in the presence or absence of change in depression ratings, with drug doses smaller than versus equal to those usually effective in depression, or with sedating as opposed to nonsedating drugs.

From meta-analysis results and data from human and animal studies, Onghena and Van Houdenhove (181) concluded that the manifest depression, "masked depression," and sedation hypotheses for the analgesic mode of action of antidepressants were not correct (refer to Table 22.18). Thus, there is no support for the commonly held opinion that the response of a patient's pain to an antidepressant implies that the pain is a manifestation of some form of depression (210–212). Also, there is now enough evidence to conclude that the manifest depression, masked depression, and sedation hypotheses should be eliminated as explanations of analgesic action of antidepressants. In addition, the data do not support the theory that chronic pain is a variant of depressive disease, as Blumer has asserted (211, 212).

Onghena and Van Houdenhove (181) now believe that a biochemical hypothesis is correct: that antidepressants have hitherto unsuspected intrinsic analgesic properties. This meta-analysis did not establish the superiority of smaller antidepressant doses for analgesia, nor did they support the superiority of one antidepressant over another. Thus, one must question the hypothesis that the analgesic properties of antidepressants are related to inhibition of serotonin reuptake. Onghena and Van Houdenhove (181) found that drugs inhibiting monoamines reuptake less selectively appear to have greater analgesic efficacy than the selective antidepressants. This finding is in line with the evidence that both serotonin and norepinephrine may be involved in the analgesic effect of antidepressants (213). Finally, most studies have found that there is a significant difference between the analgesic effect of the active drug and placebo, which would rule out the placebo hypothesis.

In summary, manifest depression, masked depression, placebo, sedation, and selective serotonin inhibition are no longer viable hypotheses for the antinociceptive effect of antidepressants. The other hypotheses presented in Table 22.18 are still viable alternatives.

Practical Guidelines for the Utilization of Antidepressants in Chronic Pain

As discussed earlier, it is now clear that antidepressants have a significant antinociceptive effect independent of their antidepressant effect. In addition, although it was initially suspected that there may be a therapeutic blood level for the antinociceptive effect i.e., a therapeutic window (214), recent methodologically-sound studies (197) indicate that there is no relationship between serum antidepressant levels and their antinociceptive effect. Thus, this author believes that any practical guidelines for the treatment of the CPP with antidepressants should depend on the following variables determined during the psychiatric examination: the level and severity of depression; the level and severity of the sleep disturbance and whether it is related to the chronic pain; the degree of pain perceived by the CPP; the level of pain behavior; and the tolerance of the CPP of his/her painful condition. The treatment approach taken by the clinician for the antidepressant treatment of the CPP should utilize the clinician's knowledge of these variables in terms of how they affect the individual CPP and the clinician's knowledge that the antidepressant dosage utilized to treat pain can vary but in general will be less than the dosage usually required to treat depression. Based on these concepts, the author has developed two algorithms for the antidepressant treatment of chronic pain (Figs. 22.5 and 22.6).

When using the algorithm in Fig. 22.5, the following factors should be taken into account:

1. The presence of depression, which if severe should be treated with antidepressants at usual therapeutic doses for depression;
2. Sleep: If sleep is disturbed, insomnia should be treated by antidepressants at whatever dose facilitates sleep;
3. Pain: Here antidepressants should be utilized at a dosage tolerated by the patient but adequate to reduce pain behavior.

A final issue is which antidepressants should be utilized in the treatment of the CPP (Fig. 22.6). Here the evidence appears to favor the tricyclic antidepressants: amitriptyline, doxepin, clomipramine, and desipramine. Based on the previous discussion and the evidence for the efficacy of the tricyclic antidepressants, this author advocates the algorithm presented in Figure 22.6. In this algorithm the factors are the same as in Figure 22.5, but the drugs are chosen for their specific properties or side effects that address the problems identified in the psychiatric evaluation.

MAO Inhibitors

Table 22.19 reveals that only a few studies have evaluated MAO inhibitors for the treatment of pain. Of these, two were controlled and demonstrated a significant analgesic effect (162, 175). One study demonstrated an analgesic effect superior to that of amitriptyline (175). However, one study utilized facial pain patients (162) while the other uti-

lized patients with various pains (175). Thus, at this juncture it is not yet established that MAO inhibitors have an analgesic effect, although it is likely. In addition, while empirical data do not imply that MAO inhibitors should be prescribed first, CPPs with facial pain unresponsive to a tricyclic antidepressant have a trial of an MAO inhibitor.

Neuroleptics

Although neuroleptics such as fluphenazine and perphenazine appear to be effective in neuropathic pain (215), the situation is less clear for nonneuropathic pain. Table 22.20 delineates the available studies for the treatment of nonneuropathic chronic pain and some forms of intermittent pain, e.g., headache. This table indicates that there is strong evidence that some neuroleptics may have a significant analgesic effect. Methotrimeprazine in a number of well-designed studies (216–219) has been shown to have as strong or stronger analgesic effect than morphine. In addition, neuroleptics have been demonstrated to have a strong analgesic effect on various types of headaches; acute migraine (220–222); tension (223) and; cluster (224).

However, there continues to be controversy (225) over whether neuroleptics do indeed have a true analgesic effect, because experimentally-induced pain data do not indicate an analgesic or analgesia-potentiating effect for neuroleptics. This controversy is not yet settled. At this point, methotrimeprazine is the only neuroleptic with well-established analgesic properties. Haloperidol, however, does have a molecular structure resembling that of morphine and meperidine (226). This molecular similarity could be the basis of the analgesic effect for some neuroleptics. The risk of tardive dyskinesia associated with neuroleptics is a major deterrent to the use of neuroleptics for the treatment of chronic pain. This author recommends that neuroleptics should not be used as first-line drugs in the treatment of nonneuropathic chronic pain. These drugs should be utilized only when other drugs have failed and only with the informed consent of the patient, the latter including specific mention of the risk of tardive dyskinesia.

Antihistamines

A number of studies have attempted to utilize antihistamines for the treatment of nonneuropathic pain. These studies and their results are presented in Table 22.21. A review of this table shows that in general, antihistamines could have an analgesic effect in nonneuropathic pain and that this effect can be additive to that of other analgesics. This was also the conclusion of Runmore and Schlichting (227), who in a recent review of 27 controlled clinical trials of antihistamines, concluded that there is evidence for a direct analgesic effect of these drugs. Diphenhydramine, hydroxyzine, orphenadrine, and pyrilamine were shown to produce analgesia (227). This, however, was not the case for chlorpheniramine and phenyltoloxamine (227). One

Text continued on p. 475.

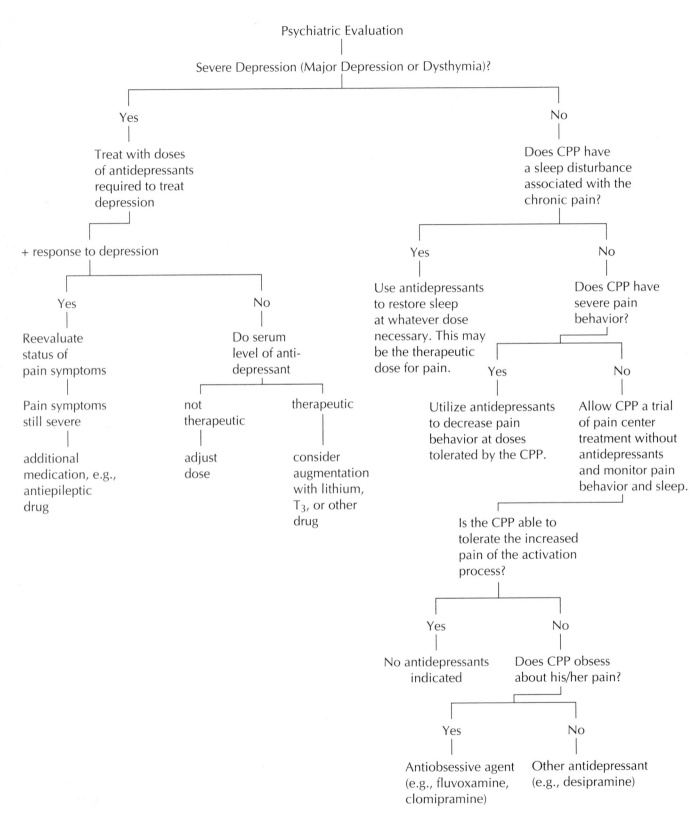

Figure 22.5. Algorithm for the use or nonuse of antidepressants with CPP.

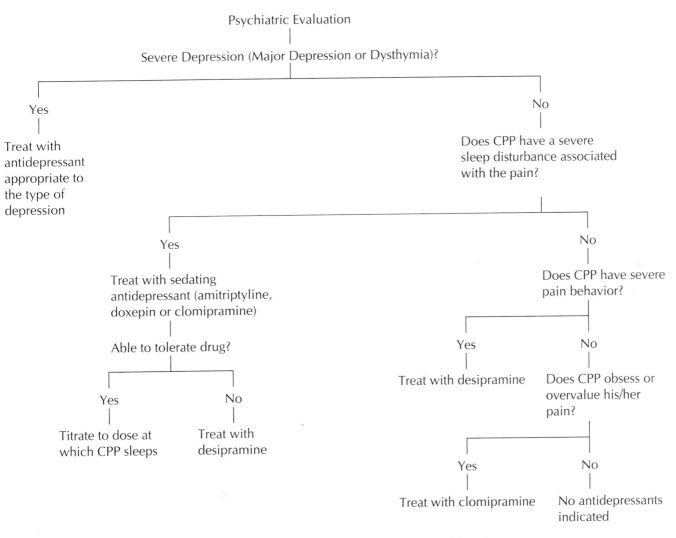

Figure 22.6. Algorithm for type of antidepressant to be used for CPPs.

Table 22.19. MAO Inhibitors in Nonneuropathic Pain

Author of Study/Year	N	Type of Pain	Type of Drug	Dose (mg/d)	Controlled Study	Percentage of Patients Reporting Pain Relief
Anthony & Lance, 1969 (335)	25	Headache	Phenelzine	45	No	80
Lascelles, 1966 (162)	40	Facial pain	Phenelzine	45	Yes	[a]
Raft et al., 1981 (175)	23	Various	Phenelzine vs. amitriptyline vs. placebo	1.5 mg/kg 3.5 mg/kg	Yes	[a] Phenelzine superior to amitriptyline and placebo for pain relief
Raskin, 1982 (375)	1	Chest pain	Tranylcypromine	30	No	Marked decrease in chest pain
Rees & Harris, 1978-79(329)	4	Facial pain	Phenelzine	?	No	100% complete pain relief or mild brief attacks

[a]Drug more effective than placebo or other comparison drug.

Table 22.20. Neuroleptics in Nonneuropathic Pain

Author of Study/Year	N	Type of Pain	Type of Drug	Dose (mg/d)	Controlled Study	Percentage of Patients Reporting Pain Relief
Beaver et al., 1966 (218)	40	Cancer pain	Morphine vs. methotrimeprazine	8 7.5, 15	No	Methotrimeprazine gave 15% more pain relief than morphine
Bell et al., 1990 (222)	24 26 26	Migraine	Chlorpromazine vs. dihydroergotamine vs. lidocaine	12.5–37.5 i.v.	No	Chlorpromazine more effective than the other two drugs
Bloomfield et al., 1964 (217)	19	Various types Chronic pain	Placebo vs. morphine vs. methotrimeprazine	15	Ye[a]	Morphine and methotrimeprazine superior to placebo and indistinguishable from each other
Caviness et al., 1970 (224)	13	Cluster headache	Chlorpromazine	75–700	No	93% headache-free
Clarke, 1981 (376)	120	Various Many with neuropathic pain	Amitriptyline Perphenazine combined	25 2	No	33.68% pain free, best results with neuropathic pain
Duthie, 1977 (377)	12	Various	Amitriptyline Trifluoperazine combined	75 3	No	67% complete relief
Hakkarainen, 1977 (223)	50	Tension headache	Fluphenazine	1	Yes	Duration and severity of headache & analgesic use decreases by drug[a]
Kast, 1966 (216)	51	Various types Chronic pain	Morphine vs. methotrimeprazine	15	Yes	No difference between drugs for pain relief
Lane et al., 1989 (220)	24 22	Acute Migraine	Comparison i.v. Chlorpromazine and i.v. Meperidine with dimenhydrinate	Variable by body weight (0.1 mg/kg chlorpromazine and 0.4 mg/kg meperidine)	Yes	Only 2 of chlorpromazine group vs. 11 in the meperidine group received inadequate pain relief[a]
Moertel et al., 1974 (378)	100	Cancer pain	Placebo vs. aspirin vs. aspirin plus promazine	25	Yes	No significant difference between groups for pain relief
Montilla et al., 1963 (219)	95	Various types	Morphine vs. methotrimeprazine		No	Similar pain relief
Peters & Friedman, 1983 (379)	4	Severe burn pain	Methotrimeprazine	37.5	No	Control of pain
Raft et al., 1979 (380)	16	Atypical facial pain	Haloperidol	2–6	No	15 patients had 85% improvement over baseline pain
Sherwin, 1979 (381)	14	Headache	Amitriptyline Perphenazine combined	100–200 8–64	No	71% stopped complaining of headache
Stiell et al., 1991 (221)	37 37	Migraine	Methotrimeprazine vs. meperidine	37.5 i.m. 75 i.m.	Yes	Methotrimeprazine as effective as meperidine at controlling pain (no statistical difference)
Zitman et al., 1991 (372)	34	Psychogenic pain	Flupenthixol	3	Yes	Flupenthixol did not add to the analgesic activity of amitriptyline but had a statistically significant effect on pain[a]

Table 22.21. Antihistaminics in Nonneuropathic Pain

Author of Study/Year	N	Type of Pain	Type of Drug	Dose (mg/d)	Controlled Study	Percentage of Patients Reporting Pain Relief
Bakris et al., 1982 (382)	38	Muscle contraction headache	Orphenadrine vs. diazepam	200 15	No	After 6 months, 79% of the diazepam and 74% of the orphenadrine group reported decreased symptoms
Batterman, 1965 (383)	78	Arthritic patients, musculoskeletal disorders	Orphenadrine vs. APC (aspirin, phenacetin, caffeine) vs. orphenadrine plus APC	25 225 + 160 + 30	Yes	In a 2–4 week trial, orphenadrine not more effective than placebo
Birkeland & Clawson, 1968 (384)	325	Muscle spasm, gunshot wounds, fractures, low back syndromes	Orphenadrine + APC vs. orphenadrine vs. APC	25 25	Yes	Orphenadrine plus APC superior to single drugs and all significantly greater than placebo in pain effect
Cass & Brederick, 1964 (385)	40	Chronic arthritis Phlebitis	Orphenadrine vs. APC vs. orphenadrine plus APC	25 25	No	Combination superior to two others while orphenadrine was superior to APC
Gilbert, 1976 (386)	160	Musculoskeletal, nonrheumatic	Phenyltoloxamine vs. acetaminophen vs. both drugs	60 325 60 + 325	Yes	Phenyltoloxamine had no significant effect on pain but added to acetaminophen
Gilbert, 1976 (387)	208	Headache	Acetaminophen vs. phenyltoloxamine vs. both drugs	650 60 650 + 60	Yes	Phenyltoloxamine effective analgesic and additive to acetaminophen[a]
Gold, 1978 (388)	60	Low back pain	Orphenadrine vs. aspirin	200 2600	Yes	Orphenadrine superior to aspirin and to placebo[a]
Hingorani, 1971 (389)	99	Low back pain	Orphenadrine plus acetaminophen vs. aspirin	210 270 1800	No	Equal pain relief for both treatments
Krabbe & Olesen, 1980 (390)	35	Muscle contraction headache, migraine	Mepyramine	.5 mg/kg i.v.	No	Headache completely abolished
McGuinness, 1983 (391)	28	Sprains, low back pain, sports injuries	Orphenadrine plus acetaminophen vs. acetaminophen	35 450 450	No	Combination superior to acetaminophen alone
Nanda, 1980 (392)	34	Migraine	Cimetidine vs. chlorpheniramine plus cimetidine	200 2 200	No	No response in either medication group
Stambaugh & Lane, 1983 (393)	30	Cancer	Meperidine vs. hydroxyzine vs. meperidine plus hydroxyzine	50 i.m. 100 i.m. 50 i.m. 100 i.m.	No	Hydroxyzine alone provided pain relief; 70% had excellent or very good response
Tek & Mellon, 1987 (228)	94	Headache	Nalbuphine i.m. vs. nalbuphine plus hydroxyzine i.m.	10 10 50	Yes	Combination not superior to nalbuphine alone
Tervo et al., 1976 (394)	50	Acute lumbago	Orphenadrine plus acetaminophen vs. acetaminophen	210 270 270	No	Combination significantly superior

[a]Drug more effective than placebo.

Table 22.22.   Psychostimulants in Nonneuropathic Pain

Author of Study/Year	N	Type of Pain	Type of Drug	Dose (mg/d)	Controlled Study	Percentage of Patients Reporting Pain Relief
Bruera et al., 1987 (395)	32	Cancer	Methylphenidate	15	Yes	[a]
Kaiko et al., 1987 (396)	19	Chronic nonmalignant pain	Cocaine	10	Yes	Not significantly better than placebo
Portenoy, 1989 (397)	48	Cancer	Methylphenidate	15	No	In most cases a significant improvement in pain was observed

[a]Drug more effective than placebo.

Table 22.23. Antiepileptic Drugs (AEDs) in the Treatment of "Nonneuropathic" Pain

Author of Study/Year	N	Type of Pain	Type of Drug	Dose (mg/d)	Controlled Study	Percentage of Patients Reporting Pain Relief
Ashley, 1984 (398)	43	Discogenic chronic pain	Clonazepam plus trifluoperazine	1 2	No	42 patients had a positive response
Bowsher, 1987 (399)	1	Tabes dorsalis with lightning pains	Valproate	?	No	Total relief
Caccia, 1975 (400)	2	Cluster headache	Clonazepam	4–8	Yes	Negligible effect
Dunsker, 1976 (243)	5	Postsurgical (laminectomy etc.) "flashing" pain	Carbamazepine	Variable	No	100% responded
Emhjellen & Skjelbred, 1990 (401)	20	Chronic orofacial pain	Clonazepam vs. amitriptyline	1 25	No	Clonazepam produced significantly more pain relief
Fishbain et al., 1991 (402)	40	Chronic myofascial pain	Clonazepam	.5–4	No	85% had partial pain relief
Hering & Kuritzky, 1989 (403)	15	Chronic cluster headache (2 patients) and episodic cluster headache (13 patients)	Valproate	600–2000	No	73.3% had positive response, 9 no pain, 2 marked improvement
Martin, 1980 (244)	14	Postlaminectomy persistent sciatic pain characterized by lightning or lancinating pains	Carbamazepine (8 pts) Clonazepam (2 pts)	Variable	No	50% of the patients responded in each drug group
Matthew & Ali, 1991 (404)	30	Chronic headache	Divalproex (valproate)	100–200	No	2/3 improved significantly
Stensrud & Sjaastad, 1979 (240)	38	Migraine	Clonazepam	2	Yes	Headache days and headache index differed significantly from pretest status, however, no difference from placebo. Eight patients continued with beneficial effects
Swerdlow, 1980 (246)	70	Various types of conditions, including neuropathic, characterized by lancinating, stabbing, or shooting pains with a burning background	Phenytoin or valproate	150 plus 600 plus	No	67% of patients improved on one or the other drug
Swerdlow & Cundill, 1981 (245)	170	Various types of conditions including neuropathic patients characterized by lancinating, stabbing, or shooting pains with a burning background	Carbamazepine (37 pts) Clonazepam (35 pts) Phenytoin (47 pts) Valproate (51 pts)	Variable	No	Proportion of patients relieved by each drug as follows: carbamazepine 30%; clonazepam 66%; phenytoin 47%; valproate 39%
Yajnik et al., 1992 (405)	75	Cancer Various etiologies	Phenytoin vs. buprenorphine vs. both combined	200 .4 SL	No	Proportion of patients relieved at least 50%: 72% for phenytoin alone; 84% for buprenorphine alone; 88% for combined treatment

Editor's note: Many of the pains treated had qualitative features of neuropathic pain, even though the investigators did not label the pains as neuropathic. See Chapter 21.

Table 22.24.   Lithium in Nonneuropathic Pain

Author of Study/Year	N	Type of Pain	Type of Drug	Dose (mg/d)	Controlled Study	Percentage of Patients Reporting Pain Relief
Bussone et al., 1990 (406)	50	Cluster headache	Lithium vs. verapamil	300–1800	Yes	Both drugs were effective in preventing chronic cluster headache attacks
Chazot et al., 1979 (407)	25	Migraine	Lithium	300–1800	No	50% had decreased number of attacks
Ekbom, 1977 (408)	5	Cluster headache	Lithium	300–1800	No	3 patients with chronic cluster had 70% improvement
Ekbom, 1981 (249)	19	Cluster headache	Lithium	300–1800	No	8 patients with chronic cluster improved
Kudrow, 1978 (409)	15	Cluster headache	Lithium vs. prednisone vs. methylsergide	300–1800	No	87% of patients had 75% or greater improvement with lithium; 41% improved with methylsergide; 50% improved with prednisone
Mathew, 1978 (410)	31	Cluster headache	Lithium	300–1800	No	Chronic cluster—80% improved; episodic cluster—84% improved
Medina et al., 1978 (411)	12	Cluster headache	Lithium	300–1800	No	All improved
Medina, 1982 (412)	22	Migraine	Lithium	300–1800	No	19 patients with cyclic form responded
Nieper, 1978 (413)	44	Migraine	Lithium	300–1800	No	39 patients had decreased severity and frequency of attacks
Peatfield & Rose, 1981 (414)	5	Migraine	Lithium	300–1800	No	All worse
Peatfield & Rose, 1981 (415)	31	Cluster headache	Lithium	300–1800	No	14 patients markedly improved; 10 showed some improvement
Tyber, 1990 (250)	3	Fibromyalgia	Lithium	300–1800	No	All 3 had sustained pain relief

hundred milligrams of hydroxyzine i.m. has been claimed to demonstrate the analgesic efficacy of 5–8 mg morphine (227). Based on these reports, it has become a common practice to combine an opioid with an antihistamine such as hydroxyzine. However, like the neuroleptics, the use of antihistamines for their analgesic properties is mired in controversy. Recent evidence indicates that antihistamines may not potentiate opiate analgesia. For example, the combination of hydroxizine plus nalbuphine was not more effective than nalbuphine alone for the treatment of acute headache (228). A recent reviewer has therefore concluded that the data do not confirm the purported clinical benefits of hydroxyzine-opioid combinations in comparison with appropriate regimens of opioids alone (229). Further research is needed to clarify this matter.

Psychostimulants

A limited number of studies have been conducted on the treatment of nonneuropathic pain with psychostimulants (Table 22.22). The studies to date indicate that, at least in cancer pain, methylphenidate may have an analgesic effect. However, in a postoperative pain study, methylphenidate did not demonstrate an analgesic effect (230). Methylphenidate does, however, appear to improve cognitive functions in cancer patients on opioids (231), thus permitting an increase in the daily opioid dose (232). Other psychostimulants may also have an analgesic effect. Dextroamphetamine has been found to potentiate the analgesic effect of morphine in acute clinical pain (233). Fenfluramine was also demonstrated to significantly increase the analgesic potency of morphine, and had a mild analgesic effect alone (234).

As a psychostimulant, cocaine presents a special case. Cocaine has been included within the Brompton cocktail for the treatment of cancer pain (235). However, there has been much controversy over the inclusion of cocaine in the mixture. Recent evidence indicates that cocaine has an analgesic effect on experimental pain (236) and potentiates opiate analgesia (237).

The reviewed studies indicate that there may be a place for the use of psychostimulants as adjuncts the treatment of cancer-associated chronic pain, especially when sedation limits opiate dosage.

Antiepileptic Drugs

It is now generally accepted that antiepileptic drugs (AEDs) do have some efficacy in neuropathic pain syndromes (238, 239). However, the issue is less clear for nonneuropathic pain as there have only been a limited number of studies for the treatment of nonneuropathic pain with AEDs. These studies are presented in Table 22.23. Note that only two of these studies were controlled (240, 241). In addition, few of the studies utilized comparable diagnoses; thus, it is difficult to compare them. However, overall, these studies indicate that AEDs could have an analgesic effect in some pain conditions. Experi-

mentally, phenytoin has been demonstrated to have an analgesic effect against suma- methonium-induced myalgia (242). However, its mechanism of action is still unclear. In addition, phenytoin, carbamazepine, valproate, and clonazepam have different modes of action (242). Therefore, it is difficult to postulate one mechanism of action for the analgesic effect of these drugs in nonneuropathic pain.

Finally, as pointed out previously, it is difficult to make a distinction between neuropathic pain and nonneuropathic pain based on diagnosis. It is unclear whether all lancinating, shooting, stabbing, and burning pains have a neuropathic component. Some authors consider these pains neuropathic in nature (238, 239, 243–246), but diagnostically these pains may not fit the diagnostic nomenclature for neuropathic pain, e.g., as diabetic neuropathy and/or herpes zoster do. In my experience, the preponderance of CPPs have these kinds of pains and yet do not have a neuropathic diagnosis. These patients are usually diagnosed as suffering from failed back surgery syndrome, or myofascial pain syndrome, among others. It is therefore possible that some or many CPPs have more than one type of pain, i.e., both neuropathic and nonneuropathic. The pain clinician needs to keep this in mind in treating CPPs. Drug choice should not only be made based on pain diagnostic category, e.g., peripheral neuropathy, but also on the pain description. This approach has recently been advocated by Jensen (247).

Lithium

Lithium has been used extensively for the treatment of migraine and cluster headache, as demonstrated in Table 22.24. An earlier reviewer concluded that lithium aggravates or exacerbates the symptoms of migraine except in cyclic migraine, where it possibly has a positive prophylactic effect (248). As far as cluster headaches are concerned, the reviewer concluded that lithium is effective for the prophylaxis of chronic cluster headache (248). Patients with chronic cluster headache may respond to lithium in the first 2 weeks of therapy. They usually respond to typical mood-stabilizing serum levels (e.g., 0.8–1.5 mE/L) (249).

This author could find only one report of lithium use in nonneuropathic pain other than headache. In this case report (250), lithium appeared to be effective for the chronic pain of fibromyalgia.

Conclusion

There is strong evidence for the analgesic effect of tricyclic antidepressants on nonneuropathic pain. The evidence for the analgesic effect of neuroleptics, MAO inhibitors, antihistamines, psychostimulants, and AEDs for nonneuropathic pain is not as strong. More extensive, well-designed research is needed to determine the appropriate role of these psychotropic drugs in pain treatment.

References

1. Price DDR, McGrath PA, Rafii A, Buckingham B. The validity of visual analogue scales as ration scale measures for chronic and experimental pain. Pain 1983; 17:45–56.
2. Chapman CR, Casey KL, Dubner R, et al. Pain measurement: an overview. Pain 1985; 22:1–31.
3. Frederiksen LW, Lynce RS, Ros J. Methodology in the measurement of pain. Behavior Therapy 1978; 9:486–488.
4. Bayer TL, Baer PE, Early C. Situational and psychophysiological factors in psychologically induced pain. Pain 1991; 44:45–50.
5. Chen ACN, Dworkin SF, Haug J, Gehrig J. Human pain responsivity in a tonic pain model: psychological determinants. Pain 1989; 37:143–160.
6. Bromm B. Modern techniques to measure pain in healthy man. Methods Find Exp Clin Pharmacol 1985; 7:161–169.
7. Chen ACN, Dworkin SF, Haug J, Gehrig J. Topographic brain measures of human pain and pain responsivity. Pain 1989; 37:129–141.
8. Huskisson EC: Measurement of pain. Lancet 1974; 1127–1132.
9. Jensen MP, Karoly P, Braver S. Measurement of clinical pain intensity: A comparison of six methods. Pain 1986; 27:117–126.
10. Malow RM, Olson RE. Changes in pain perception after treatment for chronic pain. Pain 1981; 11:65–72.
11. Yang JC, Clark WC, Janal MN. Sensory decision theory and visual analogue scale indices predict status of chronic pain patients six months later. Journal of Pain and Symptom Management. 1991; 6(2):58–64.
12. Gracely RH, Kwilosz DM: The descriptor differential scale: applying psychophysical principles to clinical pain assessment. Pain 1988; 35:279–288.
13. Melzac R. The McGill Pain Questionnaire: major properties and scoring methods. Pain 1975; 7:275–299.
14. Melzac R. The short form McGill Pain Questionnaire. Pain 1987; 30:191–197.
15. Skevington SM. Activities as indices of illness behaviour in chronic pain. Pain 1983; 15:295–307.
16. Holroyd KA, Holm JE, Keefe FJ, et al. A multi-center evaluation of the McGill Pain Questionnaire: results from more than 1700 chronic pain patients. Pain 1992; 48:301–311.
17. Gronbold M. Lukinmaa A, Konttinen YT. Chronic Low back pain: intercorrelation of repeated measures for pain and disability. Scand J Rehab Med 1990; 22:73–77.
18. Tooney TC, Mann JD, Abashian S, et al. Description of a brief scale to measure functional impairment in chronic pain patients. Pain 1990; S5:A578.
19. Millard RW, Palt RB. A comparison of measures for low back pain disability. Pain 1990; S5:A573.
20. Waddell G, Newton M, Henderson WI. Pain and disability. Pain 1990; S5:S966.
21. Sonty N, Tart RC, Chibnall JT: Use of the psychosomatic symptom checklist (PSC) as a screening instrument in patients with chronic pain. 10th Annual Meeting of the American Pain Society, New Orleans, 1991; A91404, 124.
22. Put CL, Witkower A. Pain and impairment, beliefs in patients treated in an interdisciplinary inpatient pain program. 10th Annual Meeting of the American Pain Society, New Orleans, 1991; A91408, 126.
23. Turk DC. Associations among impairment, pain perception, and disability: Results of a national survey. 10th Annual Meeting of the American Pain Society, New Orleans, 1991; A91230, 51.
24. VonKorff M, LeResche L, Whitney CW, et al. Prediction of tempomandibular disorder (TMD) pain disability. Pain 1990; S5:A631, S329.
25. Riley JF, Ahern DK, Follick MJ. Chronic low back pain and functional improvement: assessing beliefs about their relationship. Arch Phys Med Rehab 1988; 69:579–582.
26. VonKorff M, Ormel J, Keefe FJ, Dworkin SF. Grading the severity of chronic pain: Pain 1992; 50:133–149.
27. Deyo RA. Measuring the functional status of patients with low back pain. Arch Phys Med Rehab 1988; 69:1044–1053.
28. Barnes D, Smith, D. Gatchel RJ, Mayer TG. Psychosocioeconomic predictors of treatment success/failure in chronic low back pain patients. Spine 1989; 14:427–430.
29. Turk DC, Matyas TA. Pain-related behaviors–communication of pain. American Pain Society J 1992; 1(2):109–111.
30. Keefe FJ, Wilkins RH, Cook WA. Direct observation of pain behavior in low back pain patients during physical examination. Pain 1984; 20:59–68.
31. Fordyce WE, Lansky D, Calsyn DA, et al. Pain measurement and pain behavior. Pain 1984; 18:53–69.
32. Romano JM, Syrjala KL, Levy RL, Turner JA, Evans P, Keefe FJ. Overt pain behaviors: relationship to patient functioning and treatment outcome. Behav Ther 1988; 19:191–201.
33. Keefe FJ, Crisson JE, Maltbie A, et al. Illness behavior as a predictor of pain and overt behavior patterns in chronic low back pain patients. J Psychosom Res 1986; 30:543–551.
34. Richards JS, Nepomuceno C, Riles R, Suer Z. Assessing pain behavior: The UAB Pain Behavior Scale. Pain 1982; 14:393–398.
35. Brands Anne-Mieke EF, Schmidt JM. Learning processes in the persistence behavior of CLBP patients with repeated acute pain stimulation. Pain 1987; 30:329–337.
36. Gramling SE, Elliott TR. Efficient pain assessment in clinical settings. Behav Res Ther 1992; 30:71–73.
37. Keefe FJ, Dunsmore J. Pain behavior–concepts and controversies. American Pain Society J 1992; 1(2):92–100.
38. Peters ML, Schmidt AJM, VandenHout MA. Chronic low back pain and the reaction to repeated acute pain stimulation. Pain 1989; 39:69–76.
39. Merskey H, Spear FG. The reliability of the pressure algometer. Brit J Soc Clin Psychol 1964; 3:130–136.
40. Forgione AG, Barber TX. A strain gauge pain stimulator. Psychophysiology 1971; 8:102–106.
41. Asfour SS, Khalil TM, Sipes AJ, Fishbain DA, Bon E, Rosomoff HL. Quantitative measurement of pain: a new design of a pressure algometer. 6th Annual Meeting of the American Pain Society, Washington, DC, Nov. 24, 1986.
42. Atkinson JH, Slater MA, Grant I, et al. Depressed mood in chronic low back pain: relationship with stressful life events. Pain 1988; 35:47–55.
42a. Turk DC, Rudy TE, Stieg RL. The disability determination dilemma: towards a multi-axial solution. Pain 1988; 34:217–229.
43. Haldeman S. Failure of the pathology model to predict back pain. Spine 1990; 15:718–724.
44. Waddell G, Main CJ. Assessment of severity in low back pain. Spine 1984; 9:204–208.
45. Spektor S. Chronic pain and pain related disabilities. Journal of Disability 1990; 1:98–102.
46. American Medical Association. Guides to the evaluation of permanent impairment. 3rd ed (rev), Chicago: American Medical Association, 1990.
47. Brena SF, Chapman SL, Stegal PG, Chyatte SB. Chronic pain states: their relationship to impairment and disability. Arch Phys Med Rehabil 1979; 60:387–389.
48. Brand RA, Lehmann TR. Low back impairment rating practices of orthopaedic surgeons. Spine 1983; 8:75–78.
49. Clark WC, Haldeman S, Johnson P, et al. Back impairment and disability determination another attempt at objective, reliable rating. Spine 1988; 13:332–341.
50. Carey TS, Haltler NM, Gillings D, et al. Medical disability assessment of the back pain patient for the Social Security Administration: the weighing of presenting clinical features. J Clin Epidemiol 1988; 41:691–697.
51. Pettingill BF. Physicians' estimates of disability vs. patients' reports of pain. Psychosomatics 1979; 20:827–830.
52. Wartman SA, Morlock LL, Malitz FE, Palm E. Impact of divergent

evaluations by physicians and patients of patients' complaints. Public Health Rep 1983; 98:141–145.

53. Jette AM, Deniston OL: Inter-observer reliability of a functional status assessment instrument. J Chron Dis 1978; 31:573–580.

54. Waddell G, Main CJ, Morris EW, et al. Normality and reliability in the clinical assessment of backache. Br Med J 1982; 284:1519–1523.

55. Milhous RL, Hough LD, Frymoyer JW, et al. Determinants of vocational disability in patients with low back pain. Arch Phys Med Rehab 1989; 70:589–593.

56. Deyo RA, Diehe AK. Psychosocial predictors of disability in patients with low back pain. J Rheumatol 1988; 15:1557–1564.

57. Fordyce WE, Lansky D, Calsyn DA, et al. Pain measurement and pain behavior. Pain 1984; 18:53–69.

58. Linton SJ. The relationship between activity and chronic back pain. Pain 1985; 21:289–294.

59. Fordyce W, McMahon R, Rainwater G, et al. Pain complaint−exercise performance relationship in chronic pain. Pain 1981; 10: 311–321.

60. Council JR, Ahern DK, Follick CL, et al. Expectancies and function improvement in chronic low back pain. Pain 1988; 33:323–331.

61. Rachman S, Lopatka C. Accurate and inaccurate predictions of pain. Behav Res Ther 1988; 26:291–296.

62. Teske K, Daut RL, Cleeland CS. Relationships between nurses' observations and patients' self-reports on pain. Pain 1983; 16:289–296.

63. Craig KD. The facial expression of pain. American Pain Society Journal 1992; 1:153–162.

64. Fishbain DA, Rosomoff HL. What is chronic pain? Clinical Journal of Pain 1990; 6(2):164–166.

65. Osterweiss M, Kleinman A, Mechanic D, eds. Pain and disability. Clinical, behavioral, and public policy perspectives. Washington, DC: National Academy Press, Institute of Medicine Committee on Pain, Disability and Chronic Illness Behavior, 1987.

66. American Medical Association. Guides for the evaluation of medical impairment. 3rd ed. (revised), Chicago: American Medical Association, 1990.

67. International Association for the Study of Pain Subcommittee on Taxonomy. Classification of chronic pain. Pain 1986; Supplement S3.

68. Robins L, Helze J, Croughan J, et al. The National Institute of Mental Health Division Diagnostic Interview Schedule: its history and characteristics and validity. Arch Gen Psychiatry 1981; 38:381–9.

69. Riley JF, Adhera DIT, Follick MJ. Chronic low back pain and functional improvement: assessing beliefs about their relationship. Arch Phys Med Rehab 1988; 69:579–84.

70. Tait RC, Pallard CA, Margolis RB. The pain disability index: psychometric and validity data. Archives Psychometric Medicine and Rehabilitation 1987; 68:430–41.

71. Melding PS. Is there such a thing as geriatric pain? Pain 1991; 46:119–121.

72. Crook J, Rideout EL, Brown G. The prevalence of pain complaints in a general population. Pain 1984; 18:299–314.

73. Brattberg G, Thorslunce M, Wilman A. The prevalence of pain in a general population. The results of a postal survey in a country of Sweden. Pain 1989; 37:215–222.

74. Sternbach RA. Pain and "hassles" in the United States. Findings of the Nuprin pain report. Pain 1986; 27:69–80.

75. VonKorff M, Dworkin SF, LeResche L, Kruger A. An epidemiologic comparison of pain complaints. Pain 1988; 32:173–183.

76. James FR, Large RG, Bushnell JA, Wells JE. Epidemiology of pain in New Zealand. Pain 1991; 44:279–283.

77. Baum FE, Cooke RD, Kaluncy E. The prevalence of pain in a suburban Australian community. Pain 1990; S5:S335 (A642).

78. Abbott FV, Gray-Donald K, Sewitch MJ, et al. The prevalence of pain in hospitalized patients and resolution over six months. Pain 1992; 50:15–28.

79. Magni G, Caldieron C, Regatti-Luchini S, et al. Chronic musculoskeletal pain and depressive symptoms in the general population. An analysis of the First National Health and Nutrition Examination Survey Data. Pain 1990; 43:299–307.

80. Crook J, Weir R, Tunks E. An epidemiological follow-up survey of persistent pain sufferers in a group family practice and specialty pain clinic. Pain 1989; 36:49–61.

81. Merskey H, Lau CL, Russell ES, et al. Screening for psychiatric morbidity. The pattern of psychological illness and premorbid characteristics in four chronic pain populations. Pain 1987; 30: 141–157.

82. Crook J, Tinks E, Kalaher S, Roberts J. Coping with persistent pain: a comparison of persistent pain sufferers in a speciality clinic and in a family practice clinic. Pain 1988; 34:175–184.

83. Devine R, Merskey H. The desrciption of pain in psychaitric and general medical patients. J Psychosom Res 1965; 9:311–316.

84. France RD, Rama Krishnan KR, eds., Chronic pain. Washington DC. American Psychiatric Press, 1988.

85. Jensen J. Pain in non-psychotic psychiatric patients: life events, symptomatology and personality traits. Acta Psychiatr Scand 1988; 78:201–7.

86. Chaturvedi SK, Michael A. Chronic pain in a psychiatric clinic. J Psychosom Res 1986; 30:347–354.

87. Chaturvedi SK. Prevalence of chronic pain in psychiatric patients. Pain 1987; 29:231–237.

88. Davis GC, Buchsbaum MS, Bunney WE. Analgesia to painful stimuli in affective illness. Am J Psychiatry 1979; 136:1148–1151.

89. Linsey PG, Wyckoff M. The depression-pain syndrome and its response to antidepressants. Psychosomatics 1981; 22:571–577.

90. Bradley JJ. Severe localized pain associated with the depressive syndrome. Br J Psychiatry 1963; 109:741–745.

91. Turner R, Beiser M. Major depression and depressive symptomatology among the physically disabled. Assessing the role of chronic stress. J Nerv Ment Dis 1990; 178(6):343–50.

92. Turner RJ, Noh S. Physical disability and depression: a longitudinal analysis. J Health Soc Behav 1988; 29:23–27.

93. VonKorff M, Ormel J, Katon W, Lin EHB. Disability and depression among high utilizers of health care. A longitudinal analysis. Arch Gen Psychiatry 1992; 49:91–99.

94. Zautra AJ, Maxwell BM, Reich JW. Relationship among physical impairment, distress, and well being in older adults. J Behav Med 1989; 12:543–57.

95. Viney LL, Westbrook MT. Psychological reactions to chronic illness-related disability as a function of its severity and type. J Psychosom Res 1981; 25:513–23.

96. Alexopaulos GS, Meyers BS, Young RC, et al. Disability and environment in late-onset depression. 144th Annual Meeting of the American Psychiatric Association, New Orleans, May 1991; NR643.

97. Wells KB, Golding JM, Burnam MA. Psychiatric disorder and limitations in physical functioning of a Los Angeles general population. Am J Psychiatry 1988; 145:712–716.

98. Anderson KO, Keefe FJ, Bradley LA, et al. Prediction of pain behavior and functional status of rheumatoid arthritis patients using medical status and psychological variables. Pain 1988; 33:25–32.

99. Tschannen TA, Duckro PN, Margolis RB, Tomazi TJ. The relationship of anger, depression, and perceived disability among headache patients. Headache 1992; 32:501–503.

100. Fishbain DA, Goldberg M, Meagher BR, et al. Male and female chronic pain patients categorized by DSM-III Psychiatric Diagnostic Criteria. Pain 1986; 26:181–197.

101. Romano JM, Turner JA. Chronic pain and depression: does the evidence support a relationship? Psychol Bull 1985; 97:18–34.

102. Dworkin RH, Gitlin MJ. Clinical aspects of depression in chronic pain patients. Clinical Journal of Pain 1991; 7:79–94.

103. Marshall M, Helmes E, Deathe AB. A comparison of psychosocial functioning and personality in amputee and chronic pain populations. Clinical Journal of Pain 1992; 8:351–357.

104. Chaturvedi SK, Michael A. Chronic pain in a psychiatric clinic. J Psychosom Res 1986; 30(3):347–354.

105. Dworkin-Samuel F, Von-Korff Michael, LeResche LindaL. Multiple pains and psychiatric disturbance: an epidemiologic investigation. Arch Gen Psychiatry 1990; 47(3):239–244.

106. Fogel BS. Major depression versus organic mood disorder: a questionable distinction. J Clin Psychiatry 1990; 51:2:53–56.

107. Devins GM, Armstrong SJ, Mandin H, et al. Recurrent pain, illness intrusiveness, and quality of life in end-stage renal disease. Pain 1990; 42:279–285.

108. Shacham S, Dar R, Cleeland CS. The relationship of mood state to the severity of clinical pain. Pain 1984; 18:187–197.

109. Zarkowska E, Philips HC. Recent onset vs. persistent pain: Evidence for a distinction. Pain 1986; 25:365–372.

110. Dworkin RH, Hartstein G, Rosner HL, et al. Distiguishing psychological antecedents from psychological consequences of chronic pain: the prospective investigation of herpes zoster. 9th Annual Meeting of the American Pain Society, St. Louis, A278, 57, 1990.

111. Haythornthwaite JA, Sieber WJ, Kerns RD. Depression and the chronic pain experience. Pain 1991; 46:177–184.

112. Parmelee PA, Katz IR, Lawton MP. The relation of pain to depression among institutionalized aged. J Gerontology 1991; 46:15–21.

113. Doan BD, Wadden NP. Relationships between depressive symptoms and descriptions of chronic pain. Pain 1989; 36:75–84.

114. Wesley AL, Gatchel RJ, Polatin PB, et al. Differentiation between Somatic and cognitive/affective components in commonly used measurements of depression in patients with chronic low-back pain. Let's not mix apples and oranges. Spine 1991; 16:S213–S215.

115. Keefe FJ, Wilkins RH, Cook WA, et al. Depression, pain, and pain behavior. J Consult Clin Psychol 1986; 54:665–669.

116. Williams AK, Schulz R. Association of pain and physical dependency with depression in physically ill middle-aged and elderly persons. Phys Ther 1988; 68(8):1226–30.

117. Pilwosky I, Creltenden I, Townley M. Sleep disturbance in pain clinic patients. Pain 1985; 23:27–33.

118. Wittig RM, Zorick FJ, Blumer D, et al. Disturbed sleep in patients complaining of chronic pain. J Nerv Ment Dis 1982; 170(7): 429–435.

119. Bacon SF, Klapow JC, Slater MA. Characterizing subsyndromal depression in chronic low back pain. 10th Annual Meeting of the American Pain Society, New Orleans, A91251, 61, 1991.

120. Magni-Guido, SR Schifano-Fabrizio, de-Leo-Diego. Pain as a symptom in elderly depressed patients: relationship to diagnostic subgroups. Eur Arch Psychiatry Clin Neurol Sci 1985; 235(3)143–145.

121. Brown GK. A causal analysis of chronic pain and depression. J Abnorm Psychol 1990; 99:127–137.

122. Gamsa A. Is emotional disturbance a precipitator or a consequence of chronic pain? Pain 1990; 42:183–195.

123. Gamsa A, Vikis-Freibergs V. Psychological events are both risk factors in, and consequences of, chronic pain. Pain 1991; 44:271–277.

124. Atkinson JH, Slater MA, Patterson TL, et al. Prevalence, onset, and risk of psychiatric disorders in men with chronic low back pain: a controlled study. Pain 1991; 45:111–121.

125. Ciccone DS, Grzesiak RC, Psychological vulnerability to chronic back and neck pain, 9th Annual Meeting American Pain Society, St. Louis, A248, 60, 1990.

126. Polatin PB, Kinney RK, Gatchel RJ. Premorbid psychopathology in somatoform pain syndrome. American Psychiatric Association 144th Annual Meeting, New Orleans, NR553, 181, 1991.

127. Reich J, Rosenblatt RM, Tupen J. DSM-III: a new nomenclature for classifying patients with chronic pain. Pain 1983; 16:201–206.

128. Loranger AW, Lenzenweger MF, Gartner AF, et al. Trait-state artifacts and the diagnosis of personality disorders. Arch Gen Psychiatry 1991; 48:720–728.

129. Aronoff GM. Role of the pain center in the treatment of intractable suffering and disability resulting from chronic pain. Semin Neurol 1982; 3:377.

130. Aronoff GM, Evans WO, Enders PL. A review of follow-up studies of multidisciplinary pain units. Pain 1982; 16:1–11.

131. Chapman SL, Brena SF, Bradford LA. Treatment outcome in a chronic pain rehabilitation program. Pain 1981; 11:255–268.

132. Roy R. Pain clinics: reassessment of objectives and outcomes. Arch Phys Med Rehabil 1984; 65:448–451.

133. Aronoff GM, McAlary PW, Witkower A, Berdell MS. Pain treatment programs: do they return workers to the workplace? Occup Med 1988; 3:123–136.

134. Fishbain DA, Rosomoff HL, Goldberg M, et al. The prediction of return to work after pain center treatment. A review. Clinical J Pain 1993; 9:3–15.

135. Cutler RB, Fishbain DA, Rosomoff HL, et al. Does non-surgical pain center treatment of chronic pain return patients to work? A review and meta-analysis of the literature. Spine 1994; 19:643–652.

136. Keefe FJ, Bradley LA. Behavioral and psychological approaches to the assessment and treatment of chronic pain. Gen Hosp Psychiatry 1984; 6:49–54.

137. Fordyce WE, Fowler RS, Lehmann JF, DeLateur BJ, Sand PL, Trieschmann RB. Operant conditioning in the treatment of chronic pain. Arch Phys Med Rehab 1973; 54:399–408.

138. Schmidt AJM. The behavioral management of pain: a criticism of a response. Pain 1987; 30:285–291.

139. Latimer PR. External contingency management for chronic pain: critical review of the evidence. Am J Psychiatry 1982; 139:1308–12.

140. Schmidt AJM, Gierlings REH, Peters ML. Environmental and interoceptive influences on chronic low back pain behavior. Pain 1989; 38:137–143.

141. Fordyce WE. The cognitive/behavioral perspective on clinical pain. Managing the chronic pain patient, 51–64, Eds: Loeser JD, Egan KJ, New York: Raven Press, 1989.

142. Dolce JJ, Crocker MF, Moletteire C, Doleys DM. Exercise quotas, anticipatory concern and self-efficacy expectancies in chronic pain: a preliminary report. Pain 1986; 24:365–372.

143. Ciccone DS, Grzesjak RC. Cognitive dimensions of chronic pain. Soc Sci Med 1984; 19(12):1339–45.

144. Pearce S. A review of cognitive-behavioral methods for the treatment of chronic pain. J Psychosom Res 1983; 27:431–40.

145. Fernandez E, Turk DC. The utility of cognitive coping strategies for altering pain perception: a meta-analysis. Pain 1989; 38:123–135.

146. Turner JA, Clancy S. Comparison of operant behavioral and cognitive-behavioral group treatment for chronic low back pain. Clin Psychol 1988; 56:261–266.

147. Spence SH. Cognitive-behavior therapy in the management of chronic, occupational pain of the upper limbs. Behav Res Ther 1989; 27:435–446.

148. Nicholas MK, Wilson PH, Goyen J. Comparison of cognitive-behavioral group treatment an an alternative non-psychological treatment for chronic low back pain. Pain 1992; 48:339–347.

149. Toomey TC, Mann JD, Abashian S, Pope ST. Relationship between perceived self-control of pain, pain description and functioning. Pain 1991; 45:129–133.

150. Ward SJ, Portenoy RK, Yaksh TL. Nociceptive models: relevance to clinical pain states. In: Basbaum AI, Besson JM, eds. Towards a new pharmacotherapy of pain. New York, John Wiley Sons 1991; 381–392.

151. Feinmann C. Pain relief by antidepressants: possible modes of action. Pain 1985; 23:1–8.

152. Krishnan KRR, France RD. Antidepressants in chronic pain syndromes. American Family Practice 1989; 39:233–237.

153. Satterthwaite JR, Tollison CD, Kriegel ML. The use of tricyclic antidepressants for the treatment of intractable pain. Compr Ther 1990; 16:10–15.

154. Clifford DB. Treatment of pain with antidepressants. American Family Practice 1985; 31:181–185.

155. France RD, Houpt JL, Ellinwood EH. Therapeutic effects of antidepressants in chronic pain. Gen Hosp Psychiatry 1984; 6:55–63.

156. France RD. The future for antidepressants: treatment of pain. Psychopathology 1987; 20(Suppl 1):99–113.

157. Egbunike IG, Chaffee BJ. Antidepressants in the management of chronic pain syndromes. Pharmacotherapy 1990; 10(4):262–270.

158. Walsh TD. Antidepressants in chronic pain. Clinical Neuropharmacology 1983; 6(4):271–295.
159. Magni G, Arsie D, DeLeo D. Antidepressants in the treatment of cancer pain. A survey in Italy. Pain 1987; 29:347–353.
160. Ashby MA, Fleming BG, Brooksbank M, Rounsefell B, Runciman WB, Jackson K, Muirden N, Smith M. Description of a mechanistic approach to pain management in advanced cancer. Preliminary report. Pain 1992; 51:153–161.
161. Tasker RR. The problem of deafferentation pain in the management of the patient with cancer. J Palliat Care 1987; 2:8–12.
162. Lascelles RG. Atypical facial pain and depression. Br J Psychiatry 1966; 112:651–659.
163. Sharav Y, Singer E, Schmidt E, Dionne RA, Dubner R. The analgesic effect of amitripytline on chronic facial pain. Pain 1987; 31:199–209.
164. Feinmann C, Harris M. Psychogenic facial pain. Part 1: management and prognosis. Br Dent J 1984; 156(6):205–8.
165. Brown RS, Bottomley WK. The utilization and mechanism of ation of tricyclic antidepressants in the treatment of chronic facial pain: a review of the literature. Anesth Prog 1990; 37:223–229.
166. Hoff GS, Ruud RE, Tonder M, et al. Doxepin in the treatment of duodenal ulcer. An open clinical and endoscopic study comparing doxepin and cimetidine. J Clin Psychiatry 1982; 43:56–60.
167. France RD, Krishnan KRR. Assessment of chronic pain. In: France RD, Krishnan KRR, eds. Chronic pain. Washington, DC: Psychiatric Press, 1988: 265–297.
168. Paulson G: Treatment of post-traumatic headache with imipramine. Am J Psychiatry 1962; 119:368.
169. Saran A. Antidepressants not effective in headache associated with minor closed head injury. Int J Psychiatry in Medicine 1988; 18(1):74–83.
170. Lance JW, Curran DA. Treatment of chronic tension headache. Lancet 1964; 1:1236–1239.
171. Petitto JM, Mundle LB, Nagy BR, Evans DL, Golden RN. Improvement of arthritis with fluoxetine. Psychosomatics 1992; 33:338–343.
172. Zitman FG, Linssen ACG, Edelbroek PM, Stijnen T. Low dose amitriptyline in chronic pain: the gait is modest. Pain 1990; 42:35–42.
173. Kocher R. The use of psychotropic drugs in the treatment of chronic severe pains. Eur Neurol 1976; 14:458–464.
174. Montrastruc JL, Tran MA, Blanc M, et al. Measurement of plasma level of clomipramine in the treatment of chronic pain. Clin Neuropharmacol 1985; 8:78–82.
175. Raft D, Davidson J, Wasik J, et al. Relationship between response to phenelzine and MAO inhibition in a clinical trial of phenelzine, amitriptyline and placebo. Neuropsychobiology 1981; 7:122–126.
176. Ward GN, Bloom VL, Friedel RO. The effectiveness of tricyclic antidepressants in the treatment of coexisting pain and depression. Pain 1979; 7:331–341.
177. Pilowsky I, Barrow CG. A controlled study of psychotherapy and amitriptyline used individually and in combination in the treatment of chronic intractable, "psychogenic" pain. Pain 1990; 40:3–19.
178. Eberhard G, VonKnorring L, Nilsson HL, Sundequist U, Bjorling G, Linder H, Svard KO, Tysk L. A double-blind randomized study of clomipramine versus maprotiline in patients with idiopathic pain syndromes. Neuropsychobiology 1988; 19:25–34.
179. Valdes M, Garcia L, Treserra J, DePablo J, DeFlores T. Psychogenic pain in depressive disorders: an empirical study. J Affect Disord 1989; 16:21–5.
180. Pilowsky I, Barrow G. Predictors of outcome in the treatment of chronic "psychogenic" pain with amitriptyline and brief psychotherapy. Clinical Journal of Pain 1992; 8:358–362.
181. Onghena P, Van Houdenhove B. Antidepressant-Induced analgesia in chronic non-malignant pain: a meta-analysis of 39 placebo-controlled studies. Pain 1992; 49:205–219.
182. Couch JR, Ziegler DK, Hassanein R. Amitriptyline in the prophylaxis of migraine. Neurology 1976; 26:121–127.
183. Davis RW. Comments on "a controlled study of psychotherapy and amitriptyline used individually and in combination in the treatment of chronic intractable, "psychogenic" pain. I Pilowsky and CG Barrow, Pain 1990; 40:3–19.
184. Magni G. The use of antidepressants in the treatment of chronic pain. A review of the current evidence. Drugs 1991; 42:730–748.
185. Goodkin K, Gullion CM. Antidepressants for the relief of chronic pain: do they work? Annals of Behavioral Medicine 1989; 11: 83–101.
186. Rosenblatt RM, Reich J, Dehring D. Tricyclic antidepressants in treatment of depression and chronic pain. Anesth Analg 1984; 63:1025–32.
187. Lance JW, Curran DA, Anthony M. Investigations into the mechanism and treatment of chronic headache. Med J Aust 1965; 2(22):909–914.
188. Loldrup D, Langemark M, Hansen HJ, Olesen J, Bech P. Clomipramine and mianserin in chronic idiopathic pain syndrome: a placebo controlled study. Psychopharmacology 1989; 99:1–7.
189. McQuay HJ, Carroll D, Glynn CJ. Low dose amitriptyline in the treatment of chronic pain. Anaesthesia 1992; 47:646–652.
190. Sindrup SH, Brosen K, Gram LF. Antidepressants in pain treatment: antidepressant or analgesic effect? Clin Neuropharmacol 1992; 15(Suppl. 1):636A–637A.
191. Okasha A, Ghaleb HA, Sadek A. A double-blind trial for the clinical management of psychogenic headache. Br J Psychiatry 1973; 122:181–182.
192. Hughes A, Chauvergre J, Lisslour J, et Lafgarde C. L'imipramine utilisee comme antalgique majeur en carcinoligie: etude de 118 cas. Presse Med 1963; 71:1073–1074.
193. Indaco A, Carrieri PB. Amitriptyline in the treatment of headache in patients with Parkinson's disease: a double-blind placebo-controlled study. Neurology 1988; 28:1720–1722.
194. Watson CP, Evans RJ, Reed K, et al. Amitriptyline versus placebo in postherpetic neuralgia. Neurology 1982; 32:671–673.
195. Kvinesdal B, Molin J, Froland A, et al. Imipramine treatment of painful diabetic neuropathy. JAMA 1984; 251:1727–1730.
196. Rascol O, Tran MA, Bonnevialle P, et al. Lack of correlation between plasma levels of amitriptyline (and nortriptyline) and clinical improvement of chronic pain of peripheral neurologic origin. Clin Neuropharmacol 1987; 10:560–4.
197. Edelbroek PM, Linssen CG, Frans MA, Zitman G, Rooymans HGM, DeWolff FA. Analgesic and antidepressive effects of low-dose amitriptyline in relation to its metabolism in patients with chronic pain. Clin Pharmacol Ther 1986; 39:156–162.
198. Spiegel K, Klab R, Pasternak GW. Analgesic activity of tricyclic antidepressants. Ann Neurol 1983; 13:462–465.
199. Butler SH, Weil-Fugazza J, Godefroy F, Besson JM. Reduction of arthritis and pain behaviour following chronic administration of amitriptyline or imipramine in rats with adjuvant-induced arthritis. Pain 1985; 23:159–175.
200. Rosland JH, Hunskaar S, Hole K. Modification of the antinociceptive effect of morphine by acute and chronic administration of clomipramine in mice. Pain 1988; 33:349–355.
201. Ardid D, Eschalier A, Lavarenne J. Evidence for a central but not a peripheral analgesic effect of clomipramine in rats. Pain 1991; 45:95–100.
202. Spiegel K, Kalb R, Pasternak GW. Analgesic activity of tricyclic antidepressants. Ann Neurol 1983; 13:462–465.
203. Hwang AS, Wilcox GL. Analgesic properties of intrathecally administered heterocyclic antidepressants. Pain 1987; 28:343–355.
204. Bromm B, Meier W, Scharein E. Imipramine reduces experimental pain. Pain 1986; 25:245–257.
205. Deleted.
206. Nobili R, Corli O, Roma G, Morandi C, Bracco S, Panerai AE. Clomipramine and baclofen in voluntary abortion anlgesia: a placebo controlled study. Pain 31 (Suppl). 1987; 48.
207. Tiengo M, Pagnoni B, Calmi A, et al. Clomipramine compared with pentazocine as a unique treatment in post-operative pain. Int J Clin Pharmacol Res 1987; 7:141–3.

208. Levine JD, Gordon NC, Smith R, McBryde R. Desipramine enhances opiate postoperative analgesia. Pain 1986; 27:45–49.

209. Ventafridda V, Bianchi M, Ripamonti C, et al. Studies on the effects of antidepressant drugs on the antinociceptive action of morphine and on plasma morphine in rat and man. Pain 1990; 43:155–162.

210. Gupta MA. Is chronic pain a variant of depressive illness? A critical review. Can J Psychiatry 1986; 31:241–248.

211. Blumer D, Helbrom M, Pedraza E. Systematic treatment of chronic pain with antidepressants. Henry Ford Hosp Med J 1980; 28:15–21.

212. Blumer D, Heilbronn M. Antidepressant treatment for chronic pain: treatment outcome of 1,000 patients with the pain-prone disorder. Psychiatric Annals 1984; 14:796–800.

213. Taiwo YO, Fabian A, Pazoles CJ, Fields HL. Potentiation of morphine antinociception by monoamine reuptake inhibitors in the rat spinal cord. Pain 1985; 21:329–337.

214. Watson CPN. Therapeutic window for amitriptyline analgesia. Can Med Assoc J 1984; 130:105–106.

215. Getto CJ, Sorkness CA, Howell T. Antidepressants and chronic nonmalignant pain. A review. Journal of Pain and Symptom Management 1987; 2(1):9–18.

216. Kast EC. An understanding of pain and its measurement. Medical Times 1966; 94:1501–1513.

217. Bloomfield S, Simard-Savoie S, Bernier J, et al. Comparative analgesic activity of levomepromazine and morphine in patients with chronic pain. Can Med Assoc J 1964; 90:1156–1159.

218. Beaver WT, Wallenstein SL, Houde RS, et al. A comparison of the analgesic effect of methotrimeprazine and morphine in patients with cancer. Clin Pharmacol Ther 1966; 7:436–446.

219. Montilla E, Frederik WS, Cass IJ. Analgesic effects of methotrimeprazine and morphine. Arch Intern Med 1963; 111:725–728.

220. Lane PL, McLellan BA, Baggoley CJ. Comparative efficacy of chlorpromazine and meperidine with dimenhydrinate in migraine headache. Ann Emerg Med 1989; 18:53–58.

221. Stiell IG, Dufour DG, Moher D, Yen M, Beilby WJ, Smith NA. Methotrimeprazine versus meperidine and dimenhydrate in the treatment of severe migraine: a randomized, controlled trial. Ann Emerg Med 1991; 20:1201–1205.

222. Bell R, Montoya D, Shuaib A, Lee MA. A comparative trial of three agents in the treatment of acute migraine headache. Ann Emerg Med 1990; 19:1079–1082.

223. Hakkarainen H. Fluphenazine for tension headache; double-blind study. Headache 1977; 5:216–218.

224. Caviness VS, Phil D, O'Brien P. cluster headache: response to chlorpromazine. Headache 1980; 8:128–131.

225. McGee JL, Alexander MR. Phenothiazine analgesia—fact or fantasy? Am J Hosp Pharm 1979; 36:633–638.

226. Maltbie AA, Cavenar JO, Sullivan JL, Hammett EB, Zung WWK. Analgesia and haloperidol: a hypothesis. Clin J Psychiatry 1979; 57–63.

227. Rumore MM, Schlichting DA. Clinical efficacy of antihistaminics as analgesics. Pain 1986; 25:7–22.

228. Tek D, Mellon M. The effectiveness of nalbuphine and hydroxyzine for the emergency treatment of severe headache. Ann Emerg Med 1987; 16:308–13.

229. Glazier HS. Potentiation of pain relief with hydroxyzine: a therapeutic myth? DICP 1990; 24:484–8.

230. Dodson ME, Fryer JM. Postoperative effects of methylphenidate. Br J Anaesth 1980; 52:1265–70.

231. Bruera E, Miller MJ, Macmillan K, Kuehn N. Neuropsychological effects of methylphenidate in patients receiving a continuous infusion of narcotics for cancer pain. Pain 1992; 48:163–166.

232. Bruera E, Fainsinger R, MacEachern T, Janson J. The use of methylphenidate in patients with incident cancer pain receiving regular opiates. A preliminary report. Pain 1992; 50:75–77.

233. Forrest WH, Brown BW, Brown CR, et al. Dextroamphaetamine with morphine for the treatment of postoperative pain. N Engl J Med 1977; 296:712–715.

234. Coda BA, Hill HF, Schaffer RL, Luger TL, Jacobson RC, Chapman CR. Enhancement of morphine analgesia by fenfluramine in subjects receiving tailored opioid infusions. Pain 1993; 52:85–91.

235. Twycross R. Value of cocaine in opiate-containing elixirs. Br Med J 1977; 2:1348.

236. Yang JC, Clark WC, Dooley JC, Mignogna FV. Effect of intranasal cocaine on experimental pain in man. Anest Analg 1982; 61:358–61.

237. Misra AL, Pontani RB, Vadlamani NL. Stereospecific potentiation of opiate analgesia by cocaine: predominant role of noradrenaline. Pain 1987; 28:129–138.

238. Swerdlow M. Anticonvulsant drugs and chronic pain. Clin Neuropharmacol 1984; 7:51–82.

239. McQuay HJ. Pharmacological treatment of neuralgic and neuropathic pain. Cancer Surv 1988; 7:141–159.

240. Stensrud P, Sjaastad O. Clonazepam (Rivotril) in migraine prophylaxis. Headache 1979; 19:333–334.

241. Deleted.

242. Hatta V, Saxena A, Kaul HL. Phenytoin reduces suxamethonium-induced myalgia. Anaesthesia 1992; 47:664–7.

243. Dunsker SB, Mayfield FH. Carbamazepine in the treatment of the flashing pain syndrome. J Neurosurg 1976; 45:49–51.

244. Martin B. Recurrent pain of a pseudotabetit variety after laminectomy for lumbar disc lesion. J Neurol Neurosurg Psychiatry 1980; 43:283–4.

245. Swerdlow M, Cundill JG. Anticonvulsant drugs used in the treatment of lancinating pain. A comparison. Anaesthesia 1981; 36:1129–1132.

246. Swerdlow M. The treatment of "shooting" pain. Postgrad Med J 1980; 56:159–161.

247. Jensen NH. Accurate diagnosis and drug selection in chronic pain patients. Postgrad Med J 1991; 67(Suppl):S2–S8.

248. Yung CY. A review of clinical trials of lithium in neurology. Pharmacol Biochem Behav 1984; 21(Suppl 1):57–64.

249. Ekbom K. Lithium for cluster headache: review of the literature and preliminary results of long-term treatment. Headache 1981; 21:132–139.

250. Tyber MA. Lithium for persistent fibromyalgia. Can Med Assoc J 1990; 143:902–904.

251. Katon W, Egan K, Millder D. Chronic pain: lifetime psychiatric diagnoses and family history. Am J Psychiatry 1985; 142:1156–1160.

252. Large RG. DSM-III diagnoses in chronic pain - confusion or clarity? J Nerv Men Dis 1986; 174:295–302.

253. Muse M. Stress-related, posttraumatic chronic pain syndrome: criteria for diagnosis, and preliminary report on prevalence. Pain 1985; 24:295–300.

254. Fishbain DA, Goldberg M, Steele-Rosomoff R, Rosomoff HL. More Munchausen with chronic pain. Clin J Pain 1991; 7:237–244.

255. Portenoy RK, Foley KM. Chronic use of opioid analgesics in non-malignant pain: report of 38 cases. Pain 1986; 25:171–186.

256. Steele-Rosomoff R, Fishbain DA, Goldber M, Rosomoff HL. Chronic pain patients who lie in this psychiatric examination about current drug/alcohol use. Pain 1990; 5(Suppl):S299.

257. Rafii A, Haller DL, Poklis A. Incidence of recreational drug use among chronic pain clinic patients. American Pain Society Ninth Annual Meeting 1990; A33.

258. Evans PJD. Narcotic addiction in patients with chronic pain. Anaesthesia 1981; 36:597–602.

259. Medina JL, Diamond S. Drug dependency in patients with chronic headache. Headache 1977; 17:12–14.

260. Haward LRC. The stress and strain of pain. Stress Medicine 1985; 1:41–46.

261. McKegney FP, Schwartz CE. Behavioral medicine: treatment and organization issues. Gen Hosp Psychiatry 1986; 8:330–339.

262. Alcoff J, Jones E, Rust P, et al. A trial of imipramine for chronic low back pain. J Fam Pract 1982; 14:841–846.

263. Goodkin K, Gullion CM, Agras WS. A randomized, double-blind, placebo-controlled trial of trazodone hydrochloride in chronic

low back pain syndrome. J Clin Psychopharmaco 1990; 10: 269–278.

264. Hameroff SR, Cork RC, Scherer K, Crago RB, Neuman C, Womble JR, Davis RP. Doxepin effects on chronic pain, depression and plasma opioids. J Clin Psychiatry 1982; 43(8)(Sec. 2):22–26.

265. Hameroff SR, Weiss JL, Lerman JC, et al. Doxepin's effects on chronic pain and depression: a controlled study. J Clin Psychiatry 1984; 45:47–62.

266. Hameroff SR, Cork RC, Scherer K, et al. Doxepin effects on chronic pain, depression and plasma opioids. J Clin Psychiatry 1982; 43:22–26.

267. Jenkins DG, Ebbutt AF, Evans CD. Tofranil in the treatment of low back pain. J Intern Med Res 1976; 4:28–40.

268. Pheasant H, Bursk A, Goldfarb J, Azen SP, Weiss JN, Borelli L. Amitriptyline and chronic low back pain: a randomized double-blind crossover study. Spine 1983; 8:552–557.

269. Sternbach RA, Janowsky DS, Huey LY, et al. Effects of altering brain serotonin activity on human chronic pain. In: Advances in pain research and therapy, vol. 1. New York; Raven Press, 1976.

270. Ward NG. Tricyclic antidepressants for chronic low-back pain. Mechanisms of action and predictors of response. Spine 1986; 11(7):661–665.

271. Ward N, Bokan JA, Phillips M, Benedetti C, Butler S, Spengler D. Antidepressants in concomitant chronic back pain and depression: doxepin and desipramine compared. J Clin Psychiatry 1984; 45: 3(Sec.2):54–57.

272. Workman EA, Short DD, Tellian FF. A comparison of doxepin, trazodone and biofeedback therapy in the adjunctive treatment of chronic back pain. American Pain Society 10th Annual Meeting, New Orleans NR91, Pg. 70, 1991.

273. Abbott P, Rounsefell B, Fraser R, Goss A. Intractable neck pain. Clinical Journal of Pain 1990; 6:26–31.

274. Beresin EV. Imipramine in the treatment of chronic pelvic pain. Psychosomatics 1986; 27(4):294–296.

275. Walker EA, Roy-Byrne PP, Katon WJ, Jemelka R. An open trial of nortriptyline in women with chronic pelvic pain. Int J Psychiatry Med 1991; 21(3):245–52.

276. Adjan M. The treatment of pain in terminal cancer. Ther Ggw 1970; 109:1620–7.

277. Bernard A, Scheuer H. Action de la clomipramine (Anafranil) sur la douleur des cancers en pathologie cervico-faciale. J Fr de ORL 1972; 21:723–728.

278. Bortz W. The treatment of severe pain of carcinoma patients. Med Welt 1967; 18:2126–7.

279. Bourkus A, Boudouresque G, Pellet W, Fondarai J, Ponzio J, Spitalier JM. Pain infirmity and psychotropic drugs in oncology. Pain 1978; 5:263–274.

280. Bresson P. Contribution to the study of the analgesic action of a major antidepressant. Clermont Medicine 1971; 19:89–91.

281. Breivik H, Rennemo F. Clinical evaluation of combined treatment with methadone and psychotropic drugs in cancer patients. Acta Anaesth Scand 1932; (Suppl. 74):135–140.

282. Buttaro CA, Silvestri D, Turchetti A. Analgesic effects of imipramine in oncology. Minerva Med 1970; 61:485–8.

283. Cohn ML, Machado AF, Bier R, Cohn M. Piroxicam and doxepin — an alternative to narcotic analgesics in managing advanced cancer pain. West J Med 1988; 148:303–305.

284. Deutschmann W. Tofranil in the treatment of pain in cancer cases. Med Welt 1971; 22:1346–50.

285. Fiorentino M. Sperimentazione controllata dell'imipramina come analgesico maggiore in oncologia. Rivista Medica Trentina 1967; 4:387–397.

286. Gebhardt KH, Beller J, Nischk R: Treatment of carcinomatous pain using chlorimipramine (aratranie). Medizinische Klinik 1969; 64:751–756.

287. Laine E, Linquette M, Fossati P. The action of injectable imipramine in pain syndromes. Lille Med 1962; 7:711–6.

288. Mascles JC. Clinical trial of anafranil in the treatment of 35 patients with cancer. Prog Med 1976; 104:163–4.

289. Monkemeier K, Steffen U. Imipramine in the treatment of pain in malignant disease. Med Klin 1970; 65:213–5.

290. Parolin AR. The treatment of pain and anxiety in advanced carcinoma. Medical Practice (Buenos Aires) 1966; 21:3–5.

291. Paschetta V. Comparative results with drugs for pain in cancer. Nice Medicine 1963; 1:26–9.

292. Richlin DM, Jamron LM, Novick NL. Cancer pain control with a combination of methadone, amitriptyline, and non-narcotic analgesic therapy: a case series analysis. Journal of Pain Symptom Management 1987; 2:89–94.

293. Serin D. Contribution to the study of the analgesic effect of an antidepressant in the treatment of cancer. Lyon Medicine 1974; 232:483–7.

294. Stendardo B. The analgesic properties of imipramine in oncology. Riforma Medicine 1964; 44:3–12.

295. Tateno I. The therapeutic effect of tofranil in the treatment of pain in malignant disease. New Drugs Clin 1969; 18:1723–7.

296. Ventafridda V, Sganzerla EP, Fochi C. Considerazioni sull'uso di sostanze psicotrope ad azione antidepressiva in terapia antalgica. Min Med 1979; 70:667–674.

297. Ventafridda V, Bonezzsi C, Caraceni A, et al. Antidepressants for cancer pain and other painful syndromes with deafferentation component: comparison of amitriptyline and trazodone. Ital J Neurol Sci 1987; 8:579–587.

298. Caruso I, Pietro Grande V. Italian double blind multicenter study comparing S-adenosyl-methionine, naproxen and placebo in the treatment of degenerative joint disease. Am J Med 1987; 83(Suppl. 5A):66–71.

299. Frank RG, Kashani JH, Parker JC, et al. Antidepressant anaglesia in rheumatoid arthritis. J Rheumatol 1988; 15(11):1632–1638.

300. Frank RG, Kashani JH, Parker JC, Beck NC, Brownlee-Duffeck M, Elliott TR, Haut AE, Atwood C, Smith E, Kay DR: Antidepressant analgesia in rheumatoid arthritis. J Rheumatol 1988; 15(11): 1632–1638.

301. Ganvir P, Beaumont G, Seldrug J. A comparative trial of clomipramine and placebo as adjunctive therapy in arthralgia. J Intern Med Res 1980; 8(Suppl 3):60–66.

302. Ganvir P, Beaumont G, Seldrup J. A comparative trial of clomipramine and placebo: an adjunctive therapy in arthralgia. Intern Med Res 1980; 8:60–66.

303. Glick EN, Fowler PD. Imipramine in chronic arthritis. Pharmacol Med 1979; 1:94–96.

304. Grace EM, Bellamy N, Kassam Y, Buchanan WW. Controlled double blind, randomized trial of amitriptyline in relieving articular pain and tenderness in patients with rheumatoid arthritis. Curr Med Res Opin 1985; 9:426–429.

305. Gringas M. A clinical trial of tofranil in rheumatic pain in general practice. J Intern Med Res 1976; 4:41–49.

306. Jacobs H. A trial of opipramol in the treatment of migraine. J Neurol Neurosur Psychiatry 1972; 35:500–504.

307. Kuipers RK. Imipramine in the treatment of rheumatic patients. Acta Rheumatoid Scandinavica 1962; 8:45.

308. McFarland JG, Jalali S, Grace EM. Trimipramine in rheumatoid arthritis: a double-blind trial in relieving pain and joint tenderness. Curr Med Res Opin 1986; 10:89–93.

309. McDonald-Scott WA. The relief of pain with an antidepressant in arthritis. Practitioner 1969; 202:802–807.

310. Deleted

311. Regalado RG. Clomipramine (Anafranil) and musculoskeletal pain in general practice. J Intern Med Res 1977; 5:72–77.

312. Sarzi-Puttini P, Cazzola M, Bocassini L, et al. A comparison of dothiepin versus placebo in the treatment of pain in rheumatoid arthritis and the association of pain with depression. J Int Med Res 1988; 16:331–337.

313. Thorpe P, Marchant-Williams R. The role of an antidepressant,

dibenzepin (Noveril), in the relief of pain in chronic arthritic states. Med J Aust 1974; 1:264–266.

314. Tyber MA. Treatment of the painful shoulder syndrome with amitriptyline and lithium carbonate. Can Med Assoc J 1974; 111:137–140.

315. Wheatly D. Antidepressants in elderly arthritis. Practitioner 1986; 230:477–481.

316. Bibolotti E, Borghi C, Pasculli E, Regoli F, Tavoni A, et al. The management of fibrositis: a double blind comparison of maprotiline (Ludiomil), chlorimipramine and placebo. Clinical Trials Journal 1986; 23:269–280.

317. Carette S, McCain GA, Bell DA, Fam AG. Evaluation of amitriptyline in primary fibrositis: a double blind, placebo controlled study. Arthritis Rheum 1986; 29:655–659.

318. Caruso I, Sarzi Puttini PC, Boccassini L, Santandrea S, Locati M, et al. Double blind study of dothiepin versus placebo in the treatment of primary fibromyalgia syndrome. J Int Med Res 1987; 15: 154–159.

319. Connolly RG. Treatment of fibromyositis. Del Med J 1981; 53:189–91.

320. Goldenberg DL, Felson DT, Dinerman H. A randomized controlled trial of amitriptyline and naproxen in the treatment of patients with fibromyalgia. Arthritis Rheum 1986; 29:1371–1377.

321. Scudds RA, McCain GA, Rollman GB, Harth M. Improvements in pain responsiveness in patients with fibrositis after successful treatment with amitriptyline. J Rheumatol 1989; 16:98–105.

322. Tavoni A, Vitali C, Bombardieri S, Pasero G. Evaluation of S-adenasy-methionine in primary fibromyalgia: a double blind crossover study. Am J Med 1987; 83(Suppl. 5A):107–110.

323. Wysenbeek AJ, Mor F, Lurie Y, Weinberger A. Imipramine for the treatment of fibrositis: a therapeutic trial. Ann Rheum Dis 1985; 44:752–753.

324. Carasso RL, Yehuda S. Clomipramine and amitriptyline in the treatment of severe pain. Int J Neurosci 1979; 9:191–194.

325. Fishbain DA, Trescott J, Cutler B, et al. Do some chronic pain patients with atypical facial pain, overvalue and obsess about their pain. Psychosomatics 1993; 34:355–359.

326. Gessel AH. Electromyographic biofeedback and tricyclic antidepressants in myofascial pain-dysfunction syndrome: psychological predictors of outcome. J Am Dent Assoc 1975; 91:1048–1052.

327. Keyser JJ. Clomipramine for obsessive pain-type syndromes. Plast Reconstr Surg 1992; 89(1):166.

328. Moore DS, Nally FF. Atypical facial pain: an analysis of 100 patients with discussion. J Can Dent Assoc 1975; 7:396–401.

329. Rees RT, Harris M. Atypical odontalgia. Br J Oral Maxillofac Surg 1978-79; 16:212–218.

330. Berstad A, Bjerke K, Carlsen E, et al. Treatment of duodenal ulcer with antacids in combination with trimipramine or cimetidine. Scand J Gastroenterol 1980; 15(Suppl):46–51.

331. Guldhal M. The effect of trimipramine on masked depression in patients with duodenal ulcer. Scand J Gastroenterol 1977; 12(Suppl): 27–31.

332. Mangla JC, Pereira M. Tricyclic antidepressants in the treatment of peptic ulcer disease. Arch Intern Med 1982; 142:273–275.

333. Niller L, Haraoldsson A, Holck P, et al. The effect of trimipramine on the healing of peptic ulcer. Scand J Gastroenterol 1977; 12(Suppl): 39–45.

334. Wetterhus S, Aubert E, Berg CE, et al. The effect of trimipramine on symptoms and healing of peptic ulcer. Scand J Gastroenterol 1977; 12(Suppl): 33–8.

335. Anthony M, Lance JW. Monoamine oxidase inhibition in the treatment of migraine. Arch Neurol 1969; 21:263–268.

336. Deleted

337. Couch JR, Hassanein RS. Amitriptyline in migraine prophylaxis. Arch Neurol 1979; 36:695–699.

338. Dalessio DJ. Chronic pain syndrome and disordered corticol inhibition effects of tricyclic compounds. Diseases of the Nervous System 1967; 28:325–328.

339. Diamond S, Baltes BJ. Chronic tension headaches: treated with amitriptyline—a double-blind study. Headache 1971; 11:110–116.

340. Fogelholm R, Murros K. Maprotiline in chronic tension headache: a double-blind cross-over study. Headache 1985; 25:273–275.

341. Gomersall JD, Stuart A. Amitriptyline in migraine prophylaxis. J Neurol Neurosurg Psychiatry 1973; 36:684–690.

342. Lance JW, Anthony M. Cyclobenzaprine in the treatment of chronic tension headache. Med J Aust 1972; 2:1409–1411.

343. Langemark M, Loldrup D, Bech P, Olesen J. Clomipramine and mianserin in the treatment of chronic tension headache. A double-blind, controlled study. Headache 1990; 30:118–21.

344. Langohr HD, Gerber WD, Koletzki E, Mayer K, Schroth G. Clomipramine and metoprolol in migraine prophylaxis: a double blind crossover study. Headache 1985; 25:107–113.

345. Mahloudji M. Prevention of migraine. Br. Med. J. 1969; 1:182–183.

346. Martucci N, Manna V, Porto C, Agnoli A. Migraine and the noradrenergic control of vasomotricity: a study with alpha-2 stimulant and alpha-2 blocker drugs. Headache 1985; 25:95–100.

347. Monro P, Swade C, Coppen A. Mianserin in the prophylaxis of migraine: a double-blind study. Acta Psychiatr Scand 1985; 72(Suppl):98–103.

348. Morland TJ, Storli OV, Mogstad TE. Doxepin in the treatment of mixed vascular and tension headaches. Headache 1979; 19:382–383.

349. Noone JF. Clomipramine in the prevention of migraine. J Intern Med Res 1980; 8(Suppl):49–52.

350. Noone JF. Psychotropic drugs and migraine. J Intern Med Res 1977; 5:66–71.

351. Sherwin D. New method for treating "headaches". Am J Psychiatry 1979; 136:1181–1183.

352. Sjaastad O. So-called "tension headache" — the response to a 5-HT uptake inhibitor: femoxetine. Cephalalgia 1983; 3:53–60.

353. Tyler GS, McNeely HE, Dick ML. Treatment of post-traumatic headache with amitriptyline. Headache 1980; 20:213–216.

354. Ziegler DK, Hurwitz A, Hassanein RS, et al. Migraine prophylaxis: a comparison of propranolol and amitriptyline. Arch Neurol 1987; 44:486–489.

355. Clarke IMC. Amitriptyline and perphenazine in chronic pain. Anaesthesia 1981; 36:210–212.

356. Duthie AM. The use of phenothiazines and tricyclic antidepressants in the treatment of intractable pain. S Afr Med J 1977; 51:246–247.

357. Evans W, Gensler F, Blackwell B, et al. The effects of antidepressant drugs on pain relief and mood in the chronically ill. Psychosomatics 1973; 14:214–219.

358. Gourlay GK, Cherry DA, Cousins MJ, Love BL, Graham JR, McLachlan MO. A controlled study of a serotonin reuptake blocker, zimelidine in the treatment of chronic pain. Pain 1986; 25:35–52.

359. Hampf G, Bowsher D, Nurmikko T. Distigmine and amitriptyline in the treatment of chronic pain. Anesth. Prog. 1989; 36:58–62.

360. Johansson F, Von Knorring L. A double-blind controlled study of a serotonin uptake inhibitor (Zimelidine) versus placebo in chronic pain patients. Pain 1979; 7:69–78.

361. Lindsay PG, Olsen RB. Maprotiline in pain-depression. J Clin Psychiatry 1985; 46:226–8.

362. Merskey H, Hester RA. The treatment of chronic pain with psychotropic drugs. Postgrad Med J 1972; 48:594–598.

363. Pilowsky I, Hallett EC, Bassett DL, et al. A controlled study of amitriptyline in the treatment of chronic pain. Pain 1982; 14:169–179.

364. Singh G, Verma HC. Drug treatment of chronic intractable pain in patients referred to psychiatry clinic. J Indian Med Assoc 1971; 56:341–345.

365. Deleted

366. Zitman FG, Linssen ACG, Edelbroek PM, Stijnen T. Low dose amitriptyline in chronic pain: the gain is modest. Pain 1990; 42:35–42.

367. Dahl LE, Decker SJ, Lundin N. A double blind study of dothiepin (Prothiaden) and amitriptyline in outpatients with masked depression. J Int Med Res 1981; 9:103–107.

368. Lindsay PG, Wyckoff M. The depression-pain syndrome and its response to antidepressants. Psychosomatics 1981; 22:571–577.

369. Eisendrath SJ, Kodama KT. Fluoxetine management of chronic abdominal pain. Psychosomatics 1992; 33:227–229.

370. Feinmann C, Harris M. Psychogenic facial pain: the clinical presentation. Br Dent J 1984; 156:165–168.

371. Loldrup D, Langemark M, Hansen HJ, Olesen J, Bech P. Clomipramine and mianserin in chronic idiopathic pain syndrome. A placebo controlled study. Psychopharmacology 1989; (Berlin) 99:1–7.

372. Zitman FG, Linssen ACG, Edelbroek PM, Van Kempen GMJ. Does addition of low-dose flupentixol enhance the analgetic effects of low-dose amitriptyline in somatoform pain disorder? Pain 1991; 47:25–40.

373. Murphy DL, Siever LJ, Insel TR. Therapeutic responses to tricyclic antidepressants and related drugs in non-affective disorder patient populations. Prog Neuropsychopharmacol Biol Psychiatry 1985; 9:3–13.

374. Bigeon A, Samuel D. Interaction of tricyclic antidepressants with opiate receptors. Biochem Pharmacol 1980; 29:460–462.

375. Raskin DE. MAO inhibitors in chronic pain and depression. J Clin Psychiatry 1982; 43:3.

376. Clarke IMC. Amitriptyline and perphenazine (Triptafen DA) in chronic pain. Anaesthesia 1981; 36:210–212.

377. Duthie AM. The use of phenothiazines and tricyclic antidepressants in the treatment of intractable pain. S Afr Med J 1977; 51:246–7.

378. Moertel CG, Ahamann DL, Taylor WF, et al. Relief of pain by oral medications. JAMA 1974; 229:55–59.

379. Peters WJ, Friedman J. Methotrimeprazine for burn patients. Can Med Assoc J 1983; 128:894–897.

380. Raft D, Toomey T, Gregg JM. Behavior modification and haloperidol in chronic facial pain. South Med J 1979; 72:155–159.

381. Sherwin D. A new method for treating headaches. Am J Psychiatry 1979; 136:1181–3.

382. Bakris GL, Mulopulos BB, Tiwari S, Franklin C. Orphenadrine citrate: an effective alternative for muscle contraction headaches. Ill Med J 1982; 161:106–108.

383. Batterman RC. Methodology of analgesic evaluation: experience with orphenadrine citrate compound. Curr Ther Res 1965; 7:639–647.

384. Birkeland IW, Clawson DK. Drug combinations with orphenadrine for pain relief associated with muscle spasm. Clin Pharmacol Ther 1968; 9:639–646.

385. Cass LJ, Brederick WS. An evaluation of orphenadrine citrate in combination with APC as an analgesic. Curr Ther Res 1964; 6:400–408.

386. Gilbert MM. Efficacy of percogesic in relief of musculoskeletal pain associated with anxiety. Psychosomatics 1976; 17:190–193.

387. Gilbert MM. Analgesic/calmative effects of acetaminophen and phenyltoloxamine in treatment in treatment of simple nervous tension accompanied by headache. Curr Ther Res 1976; 20:53–58.

388. Gold RH. Treatment of low back syndrome with oral orphenadrine citrate. Curr Ther Res 1978; 23:271–276.

389. Hingorani K. Orphenadrine/paracetamol in backache - a double blind controlled trial. Br J Clin Pract 1971; 25:227–231.

390. Krabbe AA, Olesen J. Headache provocation by continuous intravenous infusion of histamine. Clinical results and receptor mechanism. Pain 1980; 8:253–259.

391. McGuinness BW. A double-blind comparison in general practice of a combination tablet containing orphenadrine citrate and paracetamol with paracetamol alone. J Intern Med Res 1983; 11:42–45.

392. Nanda RN. Cimetidine in the prophylaxis of migraine. Acta Neurol Scand 1980; 62:90–95.

393. Stambaugh JE, Lane C. Analgesic efficacy and pharmacokinetic evaluation of meperidine and hydroxyzine, alone and in combination. Cancer Invest 1983; 1:111–117.

394. Tervo T, Petaja L, Lepisto P. A controlled clinical trial of a muscle relaxant analgesic combination in the treatment of accute lumbago. Brit J Clin Pract 1976; 30:62–64.

395. Bruera E, Chadwick S, Brenneis C, Hanson J, MacDonald RN. Methylphenidate associated with narcotics for the treatment of cancer pain. Cancer Treatment Reports 1987; 71:67–70.

396. Kaiko RF, Kanner R, Foley KM, et al. Cocaine and morphine interaction in acute and chronic cancer pain. Pain 1987; 31:35–45.

397. Portenoy RK. Use of methylphenidate as an adjuvant to narcotic. Journal of Pain and Symptom Management 1989; 4(Suppl):2,4.

398. Ashley JJ. Chronic intractable pain. N Z Med J 1984; 97:23.

399. Bowsher D. A case of tabes dorsalis with tonec pulis and lightning pairs relieved by sodium valproate. J Neuro Neurosurg Psychiatry 1987; 50:239–41.

400. Caccia MR. Clonazepam in facial neuralgia and cluster headache. Clinical and electrophysiological study. Eur Neurol 1975; 13:560–563.

401. Emhjellen S, Skjelbred P. Clonazepam versus amitriptylin in patients with chronic orofacial pain. Pain 1990; S5:A78, S42.

402. Fishbain DA, Goldberg M, Rosomoff H, Steele-Rosomoff R, Jorge M, Abdel-Moty E. Clonazepam open clinical trial for chronic pain of myofascial pain syndrome origin refractory to pain unit treatment. American Psychiatric Association 144th Annual Meeting, New Orleans, NR538, 117, 1991.

403. Hering R, Kuritzky A. Sodium valproate in the treatment of cluster headache: an open clinical trial. Cephalalgia 1989; 9(3):195–8.

404. Mathew NT, Ali S. Valproate in the treatment of persistent chronic daily headache. An open label study. Headache 1991; 31:71–74.

405. Yajnik S, Singh GP, Singh G, Kumar M. Phenytoin as a coanalgesic in cancer pain. Journal of Pain and Symptom Management 1992; 7(4):209–13.

406. Bussone G, Leone M, Peccarisi C, et al. Double blind comparison of lithium and verapamil in cluster headache prophylaxis. Headache 1990; 30:411–7.

407. Chazot G, Chauplannaz G, Biron A, Schott B. Migraines: traitment par lithium. Nouv Presse Med 1979; 8;2836–2837.

408. Ekbom K. Lithium in the treatment of chronic cluster headache. Headache 1977; 17:39–40.

409. Kudrow L. Comparative results of prednisone, methysergide and lithium therapy in cluster headache. In: Green R, ed. Current concepts in migraine research, New York: Raven Press, 1978; 159–163.

410. Mathew NT. Clinical subtypes of cluster headaches and response to lithium therapy. Headache 1978; 18:26–30.

411. Medina JL, Fareed J, Diamond S. Blood amines and platelet changes during treatment of cluster headache with lithium and other drugs. Headache 1978; 19:112.

412. Medina JL. Cyclic migraine: a disorder responsive to lithium carbonate. Psychosomatics 1982; 23:625–637.

413. Nieper HA. The clinical application of lithium orotate. A two-year study. Agressologie 1978; 14:407–411.

414. Peatfield RC, Rose FC. Exacerbation of migraine by treatment with lithium. Headache 1981; 21:140–142.

415. Peatfield RC. Lithium in migraine and cluster headache: a review. Journal of the Royal Society of Medicine 1981; 74:432–436.

23

NEUROPSYCHIATRY OF SUICIDE

Yeates Conwell and Robin E. Henderson

Overview

Although the word "suicide" did not appear in regular use until the late 17th century, references to intentional self-destructive behavior are as old as recorded time (1). Sacred oriental writings suggest an ambivalent acceptance of suicide by Brahminism and Buddhism consistent with their philosophies of the acquisition of knowledge through the denial of life's passions. Mohammedanism vigorously condemned suicide, which was also rare in ancient Judaism. During Greek and Roman periods, suicide gained gradual acceptance, paralleled by growing autonomy of the individual expressed in the philosophies of Seneca, the Stoics, Cynics, and Epicureans. Suicide was initially embraced by early Christian martyrs. The church's subsequent antisuicide stance was initially articulated by St. Augustine, and later by Thomas Aquinas in the 13th century. Subsequent modification of those attitudes has continued through recent centuries, shaped by a broad range of social, religious, and cultural influences. Indeed, the phenomenon of self-destruction can be understood for any individual, as for any society, only in terms of the underlying influence of these and other numerous factors.

Great advances in the neurosciences in the last two decades have further shaped our understanding of suicide and self-injury in this decade. With greater understanding of brain-behavior relationships, we can also recognize the probable neurobiological bases for suicide. This chapter reviews the evidence that links suicide and self-injurious behaviors to central nervous system function. It first provides an overview of the epidemiology and demography of suicidal behaviors, as well as social and psychological risk factors. Following a review of animal models of self-injury, we consider the neurobiological studies of human populations that implicate specific neurochemical or neuroanatomical systems in the etiology of suicide. We will review the known associations between suicide and specific psychiatric, medical, and neuropsychiatric syndromes, and their implications for the diagnosis and treatment of patients at risk for self-injury.

Nosology

The terms used in the literature to describe suicidal behavior and the populations studied are often ill-defined and loosely applied, making the interpretation and generalization of findings difficult. Although the need for a more precise typology of aggressive and self-destructive behaviors in humans has been well recognized, no consensus has yet been reached (2). For example, a common system of classification is to distinguish people who commit suicide, those who make suicide attempts, and those with suicidal ideation. The relationships between these three groups are, however, a subject of active debate (3). Striking demographic differences between attempters and completers suggest that they are distinct but overlapping populations. Whereas the risk for completed suicide is highest for elderly males, the risk for attempted suicide is highest in young females. Yet the margins of overlap for those populations are indistinct. Suicidal ideation is common to both groups, but is common in the general population as well. Estimates of nonclinical populations found that from 50% to as high as 80% of individuals have considered suicide at some point in their lives (4). As an alternative typology, Farberow (5) has advocated distinguishing "direct" from "indirect" self-destructive behavior on the basis of conscious intent to do self-harm. Kreitman coined the term "parasuicide" (6), referring to all forms of intentional self-destructive behavior, which is in turn distinguished from "self-mutilation," self-harm without stated or apparent intent to die. Some authors have even suggested that deliberate self-harm, in the absence of suicidal intent, is sufficiently distinctive to warrant classification as a separate diagnostic syndrome (7).

In contrast to these "categorical" nosologies, Litman (8) and others (3) advocate classifying self-destructive behavior on a continuum of lethality, either of medical risk (lethality of implementation) or extent of the will to die (lethality of intent). Many variables of interest in neurobiological studies are continuous, such as the level of monoamine metabolites in the cerebrospinal fluid, while the populations studied are classified in categorical terms.

This chapter reviews only those behaviors that have conscious self-destructive intent, for which we use the terms "attempted" and "completed suicide." Our emphasis is stronger regarding completed suicides for two reasons. First, it is a more clearly defined behavior for which constructs such as lethality and impulsivity can be taken as associated variables rather than components of the definition. Second, much of the most compelling evidence of a neurobiological basis for suicide is derived from postmortem studies of suicide victims.

CLINICAL BACKGROUND
Epidemiology of Suicide

ATTEMPTED SUICIDE

The largest study to date of the prevalence of psychiatric illness in the general community is the Epidemiological Catchment Area (ECA) Study, in which over 18,000 individuals age 18 years and over from five representative communities across the United States were administered structured diagnostic interviews. Of the entire sample, 2.9% reported that they had attempted suicide at some time in their lives. By far those at highest risk for having made an attempt were individuals with a lifetime diagnosis of psychiatric disorder. Additional risk factors included female gender, being separated or divorced, and a lower socioeconomic status. Whites had significantly higher rates of suicide attempts than blacks, and with increasing age a smaller proportion had a past history of suicidal behavior (9). Other studies have estimated a prevalence of from 120 to 730 attempts per 100,000 population per year, compared to rates of approximately 12 per 100,000 per year for completed suicide.

Estimates of the ratio of attempts to completed suicides range from 8:1 to as high as 20:1 for the general population, varying markedly by age and gender. Parkin and Stengel (10) found, for example, only four attempts for each completed suicide victim age 60 years and over, whereas young white women have been estimated to make 200 attempts per completed suicide. In contrast to completed suicides, suicide attempts are more common in women than men at all ages.

Of those who attempt suicide, approximately two-thirds make no further attempt; 10–20% make an additional attempt within 1 year; 1–2% will complete suicide within the year of an attempt, and approximately 10–15% of suicide attempters will eventually take their own lives (11).

COMPLETED SUICIDE

Statistics regarding completed suicides in the United States are compiled from death certificates submitted by medical examiners and coroners from each state and the District of Columbia. There is general agreement that suicide rates are underreported, due to variations in the training and reporting practices of the responsible officials.

However, studies differ on the extent of this phenomenon and its implications (12). By comparing suicide rates with rates of death by undetermined manner and suicide combined, Speechley and Stavraky (13) estimated that the average potential underreporting for suicide in Canada was 17.5% for females and 12% for males. Adopting a similar strategy, Barraclough (14) compared rank order of suicide rates in 22 countries in 1968 with the rank order of combined rates for suicide plus undetermined deaths. Finding few differences, he concluded that although underreporting likely occurred in each nation, their differences in suicide rates could not simply reflect differences in methods of ascertainment. These and other studies (15, 16) suggest that underreporting of completed suicide is sufficiently random that it does not invalidate the observations made by epidemiologists in comparing rates between and within countries over time.

As Figure 23.1 illustrates, suicide rates in the United States have fluctuated greatly over the course of the 20th century. Period effects are phenomena occurring at a certain time that influence suicide rates in a population. Reproducible period effects include elevations in rates in the years during and immediately after a significant economic downturn, exemplified by the Great Depression; and decreasing rates during times of war (World Wars I and II). In the years following World War II, fluctuation in suicide rates has diminished considerably, a function of more uniform reporting practices and a larger database, stabilizing at a rate of approximately 12 per 100,000 per year. In 1992, at a rate of 12.0 per 100,000, there were over 30,000 suicide deaths in the United States. For the general population, suicide was the ninth leading cause of death. It was the third leading cause of death for young adults, and the 13th leading cause of death in the elderly (17).

Suicide rates differ dramatically by age, gender, and race. In the general population, rates rise through young adulthood to an initial peak of approximately 15 per 100,000 in the 35–44 year age group, plateau through midlife, and rise again to a high of 22.8 per 100,000 in 75–84-year-olds. Thus, in contrast to the popular perception of young adults as the group at highest risk, it is the elderly who kill themselves more frequently than any other age group.

In 1992 the suicide rate for white Americans was two times that for blacks (13.0 vs. 6.8 per 100,000). This differential is present at all ages across the life course, although the relative proportion changes. In young adulthood, rates for blacks approximate those for whites, whereas in late life whites are at approximately six times greater risk.

Figure 23.2 demonstrates the important role gender plays in determining suicide risk. At all ages males are at greater risk than females within each racial subgroup. Although women make approximately three times as many suicide attempts as men, the overall ratio of females to males in completed suicides is 1 to 4. This difference has been ascribed in large part to the males' choice of more violent, and hence potentially lethal, means. For example, approximately half of the suicides in the United States are

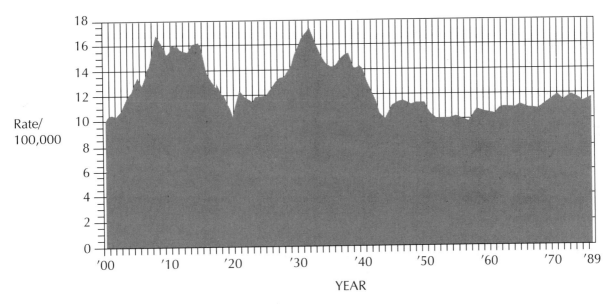

Figure 23.1. U.S. suicide rates over time (1900–1989).

SUICIDE RATES BY AGE, RACE AND GENDER
UNITED STATES–1992

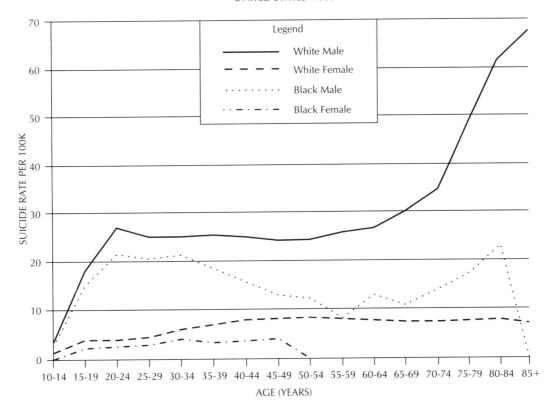

Source: National Center for Health Statistics

Figure 23.2. Suicide rates by race/sex.

committed by males using firearms (see Fig. 23.3). Although females also use firearms in substantial proportions, poisonings constitute a far greater proportion than for males.

In addition to period, age, race, and gender effects on suicide rates, epidemiologic studies have demonstrated potent cohort effects as well. Solomon and Hellon (18) were the first to apply cohort analysis to death records, demonstrating that suicide rates in Canada were birth-cohort-specific. That is, within any given birth cohort, suicide rates rise with age. Across the course of the 20th century, however, patterns of suicide rates for young adults and the elderly have differed greatly. Whereas rates for the population age 65 years and over have dropped substantially since a peak in 1930, rates rose over 300% between 1950 and 1980 for white males, ages 15 to 19 years, and 200% for males, ages 20 to 24 years. These changes have been ascribed to a variety of factors including, in the case of the elderly population, increased economic security resulting from the implementation of Social Security and Medicare legislation (19), and in the young adult population the more widespread use of alcohol and drugs (20). Beyond these factors, however, cohort effects are clearly operative, as demonstrated by Solomon and Hellon in Alberta, Canada (18) and Murphy and Wetzel (21) and Manton and colleagues (22) in the United States. However, studies in Great Britain (23) and Australia (24) have not supported the ability of a cohort's suicide rates in young adulthood to predict their risk in later years.

Although the overall suicide rate has remained stable, this complex interaction of period and cohort effects with other demographic factors has continued in the last decade to cause significant fluctuations in suicide rates in specific demographic subgroups. As reviewed by Meehan and colleagues (25) the following demographic groups experienced significant increases in rates between 1980 and 1986: white males, ages 65 years and over—23%; black males, age 65—42%; divorced males—38%.

Regional and national differences in suicide rates are worth noting as well because, like age and gender effects, they may shed light on the relative contribution of social, cultural, and perhaps biological underpinnings of suicide. As depicted in Figure 23.4, rates within the United States are lowest in the northeastern region. They increase as one moves south and west, peaking in the mountain region, and decreasing again in the Pacific states. Satisfactory explana-tions for these sometimes substantial differences have not been established.

Circumannual patterns have been identified in which rates characteristically peak in spring and early summer months, declining to a nadir in early winter. This pattern is present in a wide range of industrialized and agrarian nations (26). In addition, McCleary and colleagues (27) have demonstrated peaks in the number of suicides occurring in the United States on the first day of each week and in the first week of each month. More detailed analysis by age and sex, however, demonstrated these cycles occurring only in select subpopulations, supporting a combination of psychosocial and biological etiologic influences on suicide.

Comparison of rates across nations further underscores suicide's complex determinants. Table 23.1 lists rates per 100,000 population in a wide range of industrialized nations. Rates from other smaller and nonindustrialized nations are either unavailable or based on incomplete data. Stillion and colleagues (28) reviewed suicide rates by age and sex for the 12 countries that reported suicide statistics between 1983 and 1985, demonstrating remarkable consistency in age- and sex-specific patterns. Eleven of the 12 reporting countries showed suicide rates rising progressively with age in males. Only Poland showed a peak rate for males in midlife. Rates in women, however, showed more variability. In the United States, Australia, Denmark, Poland, and Sweden, rates for women peaked for the period from 45 to 54 years. In Canada and the United Kingdom, rates for women peaked somewhat later, from 55 to 64 years, while in the remaining five countries (Austria, France, Italy, Japan, and the Netherlands), the suicide rate for women, like men, peaked at age 65 years or older.

The large differences in suicide rates between countries and across ethnic subgroups within a country reflect the complex interplay of social, cultural, and religious influences. Particularly relevant to this chapter, however, is that fairly consistent associations between suicide rates, age, and gender that are expressed across cultures may suggest further

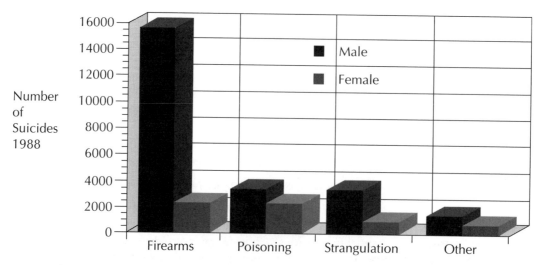

Figure 23.3. Suicide method by sex. Poisoning includes solid, liquid, and gas methods. Strangulation includes hanging and suffocation.

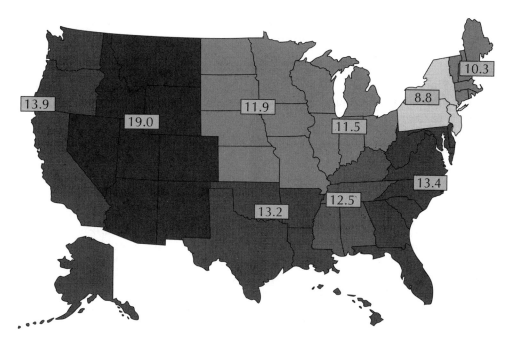

Figure 23.4. U.S. regional suicide rates; 1988 rate/100,000 population.

Table 23.1. Suicide Rates per 100,000 Population in Industrialized Nations

Hungary	39.9
Denmark	26.8
Finland	26.7
Austria	22.6
Belgium	21.0
France	20.9
Switzerland	20.7
Czechoslovakia	18.1
Japan	18.1
Sweden	17.3
Bulgaria	16.0
W. Germany	15.5
Norway	15.4
Australia	14.0
Canada	13.9
New Zealand	13.1
Poland	13.0
United States	12.5
Scotland	11.4
Netherlands	10.8
England	8.0
Portugal	7.9
Italy	7.6
Spain	6.6

support for the neurobiological hypotheses developed further below. Indeed, any adequate neurobiological model of suicide must account for gender and age effects.

Demographic Risk Factors

In addition to the epidemiologically defined suicide risk factors of age, gender, and race, a number of other demographic influences should be noted. A married conjugal status has been consistently associated with lower suicide risk, with those who are single, separated, divorced, or widowed at higher risk across the life course. Individuals widowed in young adulthood may be especially vulnerable (29), at greatest risk in the first year following loss of a spouse, with gradually decreasing risk thereafter (30).

As it has throughout history, religion continues to play a powerful role in determining suicide rates. Observing that rates are generally higher among Protestants than Catholics and Jews, Durkheim (31) suggested that this pattern reflects the possible influence of the doctrinal prohibitions of each religion against suicide. Indeed, those countries with a greater proportion of Catholics in the population tend to have lower suicide rates. In the U.S., Templer and Veleber (32) found an inverse relationship between the proportion of population who were Catholic and the suicide rate in each state. Others suggest, however, that it may be the degree of religious involvement, rather than the religion and its doctrines that is the vital factor (33).

The association between suicide and socioeconomic status is complex. Some studies have found a link between unemployment and suicide in the general population (34–36), while others have found that this association held only for men, and only on a national rather than regional level (37). Other studies have found no association, or even a negative correlation, between suicide rates and unemployment (15,38).

Stressful Life Events

In general, studies of suicide attempters have found that an increased number of stressful life events occur in the months preceding the self-destructive act (39,40). High rates of stressful events have been noted in the lives of completed suicides as well (41–43). More specifically, the nature of the stressful life events immediately preceding suicide differs as a function of both age and diagnosis. Job, financial, and interpersonal difficulties, often the result of psychiatric illness and substance abuse, are the events most commonly associated with suicide in young adulthood and middle age. The elderly most frequently commit suicide in the context of physical ill health and loss. Bereavement (29), retirement (44), and threatened loss of autonomy, such as functional disability or impending nursing home placement (45) are losses that commonly precede late-life suicide.

Physical Illness

Physical illness is a stressor far more often associated with suicide in the elderly than in younger populations. Sainsbury (15), for example, estimated that physical illness contributed to suicide in 10% of younger cases, 25% of cases in middle age, and 35% of elderly suicides. Others have made similar observations (46–49). However, few investigations have included an adequate control group with which to compare the prevalence of specific physical conditions in completed suicides. The concerns about physical ill health expressed by people in the days and weeks before they take their own lives are for some a reflection of distorted or delusional ideation rather than objectively evident organic disease (50). Murphy, for example, observed in 1,300 consecutive forensic autopsies a pattern in which suicide victims often believed that they had cancer, but in fact showed none (51).

Whitlock (52) found in a thorough review of the literature that reports of the prevalence of physical illness in completed suicide varied from 25–70% of cases, and that it appeared to be an important contributory cause of the patient's death in 10.9–51%. Malignant neoplasms and diseases of the central nervous system were overrepresented in suicide deaths (15). In his study of 35 completed suicides, ages 65 years and over, Barraclough (53) found physical illness in 56% of cases, considerably higher than in a matched control group of accident victims. Among psychiatric patients who completed suicide, Stenback and colleagues (54) found no greater physical illness than in nonsuicidal psychiatric patient controls. To measure the prevalence of physical illness in suicide victims against that of similar illnesses in the general population, Whitlock (52) compared the autopsy findings on 1,000 suicides with an epidemiological database of physical illnesses observed in general practice in Great Britain. He found that a significantly higher proportion of suicides suffered with diseases of the central nervous system (seizure disorders, cerebrovascular disease, dementia, visual deficits, multiple sclerosis, head injury, and cerebral tumor), peptic ulcer disease in males, cancer, and hepatic cirrhosis. Hypertension, cardiac disease, pulmonary, endocrine, and hematologic abnormalities showed no such association. Whitlock ascribed the findings for gastrointestinal disorders to their association with alcoholism. The literature regarding associations between specific psychiatric and neurological disorders most highly associated with suicide are reviewed in detail in the following section.

Family History of Suicide

It has long been recognized that suicidal behaviors tend to cluster in vulnerable families, suggesting a role for genetic factors in determining the behavior. Sainsbury, for example, (44) found that two percent of the deceased relatives of completed suicides had also died by that same means. Farberow and Simon (55) reported that 6% of suicide victims had a parent who had died by suicide. Psychiatric patients with a family history of suicide are at greater risk of suicidal behavior as well. Roy (56) found that a family history of suicide significantly increased the risk for a suicide attempt in patients with diagnoses of schizophrenia, major affective disorders, depressive neurosis, and personality disorders. Tsuang (57, 58) reported on the long-term follow-up of three subject groups: 525 patients with diagnoses of schizophrenia or manic-depressive illness; 160 patient controls admitted to the hospital for routine surgical procedures; and 5,721 of their first-degree relatives. They found significantly more suicides among patients than controls during the 30–40-year follow-up period, and a significantly greater risk of suicide in the relatives of patients than in the relatives of surgical controls. Furthermore, the relatives of patients who had committed suicide showed significantly higher risk for suicide than did those relatives of patients who did not commit suicide in the follow-up period. Notably, the increased risk was most pronounced for relatives of patients with affective illness, leaving open the question of whether the vulnerability was for the depressive disorder rather than suicide more directly. Scheftner et al. (59) followed 955 affectively disordered probands for 5 years, comparing the frequency of suicide in first-degree relatives of patients who committed suicide during the follow-up period with relatives of nonsuicidal patients. They found no significant difference either for completed or attempted suicides. Although the shorter follow-up period could explain these negative findings, they would also be expected if the transmissible vulnerability related to the affective disorder were common to both groups in this comparison.

Egeland and Sussex (60) saw in the Old-Order Amish community an opportunity to study familial patterns of suicide in the absence of several important confounding variables. The Amish are by tradition nonviolent, abstinent from drugs and alcohol, provide extensive community support throughout life, and have negligible unemployment. Meticulously kept records of multigenerational families enabled the researchers to ascertain all suicides in the community over a 100-year period. Ninety-two percent of the 26 documented suicides occurred in individuals with retrospectively diagnosed major affective illness. Furthermore, the suicides clustered in a distribution closely matching that of affective illness in these Amish pedigrees. Although this study suggested the role of inheritance for both suicide and major affective disorders, it could neither distinguish genetic from environmental influences, nor determine whether the heritability of suicide was distinct from that for affective illness.

Additional evidence for a genetic component to suicide

has been provided by twin studies that demonstrate a higher concordance for suicide among monozygotic than dizygotic twins (61). Again, however, separating the genetic predisposition to psychiatric illness from a genetic risk for suicide is problematic. Of 10 twin pairs concordant for suicide reported in the literature reviewed by Roy (62), all were monozygotic. In five of these twin pairs, however, the twins were also concordant for either depression or schizophrenia.

Twin studies are also unable to distinguish with confidence the effects of nature, or genetic predisposition, from nurture, or environmental influences. Although presumably raised under comparable conditions, identical twins may be subject to different social, environmental, and cultural influences than fraternal twins. Danish records of individuals adopted between the years 1925 and 1948 offered an opportunity to control for these confounds. Wender and colleagues (63) matched 71 adoptees with major or minor depressive disorders with 71 adoptive controls, and searched death records for indications of suicide in biological and adoptive relatives. They found that a significantly greater proportion of biological relatives of depressed adoptees had committed suicide than had biological relatives of controls. Schulsinger et al. (64) conducted a similar search for suicides in the biological and adoptive relatives of 57 adoptees who had themselves committed suicide and 57 nonsuicidal controls adoptees matched for sex, age, social class of adoptive parents, and time spent with biological parents. Twelve of 269 biological relatives of suicide adoptees (4.5%) had themselves committed suicide, a significantly greater proportion than of the biological relatives of control adoptees (0.7%). None of the adoptive relatives in either group had committed suicide. Given that proband adoptees had been reared separately from, and thus unexposed to, the environmental influences of their biological families, the data strongly favor a genetic determinant of suicide. However, given the well-established heritability of those psychiatric disorders most highly correlated with suicidal behavior, the available data cannot at this point distinguish a genetic factor for suicide that is distinct from a genetic predisposition to major mental disorders.

NEUROBIOLOGY OF SUICIDE

Having reviewed the life circumstances and demographic and social factors associated with suicide risk, and having seen preliminary evidence from genetic studies of a heritable component to suicide that may be independent of social and environmental factors, we now turn to a review of studies concerning the neurobiology of suicidal behavior. These include the consideration of relevant animal models of self-destruction, and data derived both pre- and postmortem in humans regarding specific neurochemical systems.

Animal Models

The development of animal models of psychiatric illness is an important objective for three reasons. Animal models allow investigators to control experimental factors and thus manipulate the system in ways that enable far more precise testing of hypotheses than is feasible in humans. Invasive studies that could not be conducted in people for obvious ethical reasons can be conducted in animals to both generate and test hypotheses concerning the mechanisms underlying disorders or behaviors, such as suicide. These same models can then be used to develop and test treatments and screening tools based on biological measures to identify individuals at high risk.

Although animal models may be useful for the development and testing of neurobiological hypotheses, their applicability to suicide research has clear limitations as well. For example, if one requires conscious intent to end one's life as a defining feature of suicide, then animal models of self-destructive behaviors may be of limited or no relevance (65). The migratory patterns of the Norwegian lemming are a case in point. Their plunge into the sea is commonly interpreted as self-destruction, while for many ethologists it is an incidental outcome of emigration away from an area of overcrowding (66). Hamilton (67) offers numerous similar examples from which he draws the conclusion that suicide-like behavior is in fact rare in animals and that where found, it probably has its basis in parental behavior or kin selection.

Self-sacrifice as an altruistic behavior is common among social insects and other animals. Crawley et al. (65) offer as an example the self-sacrifice of hymenoptera, including wasps, ants, and bees, in which members of the sterile soldier caste die after using their stinger once in the defense of the community. Similar soldiering behaviors are seen in other mammals, including primates and in the schooling of fish and birds. When considered as behaviors of each individual organism, they may have some relevance to our understanding of suicide. When seen, however, as constituents of a larger social organism, an individual's sacrifice has less immediate relevance to human suicide.

Stress-related behaviors in animals have more inherent similarity to self-destructive behaviors in humans. Frequently cited examples include self-mutilation in animals confined to small cages and removed from social stimuli. Bach-Y-Rita and Vero (68) compared confinement-induced self-injury in animals with self-destructive behavior in human prison populations. This similarity in behavior and social context can be taken as evidence to support noncognitive determinants of human self-injury (65).

Among laboratory models, learned helplessness in rats and social separation in primates elicit behaviors reminiscent of depression in humans, which respond in turn to known human antidepressant therapies (65). Each has an incidence of self-destructive behavior associated as well.

Although it is beyond the scope of this chapter, extensive studies concerning animal models of externally aggressive behavior may well be relevant to suicide in humans. Neurotransmitters that have been associated with aggression in animals include serotonin, γ-aminobutyric acid (GABA), pamine (DA), norepinephrine (NE), acetylcholine (ACh), cyclic nucleotides, and neurohormones (69). Indeed, the clinical correlate of altered neurotransmitter function in studies of the psychobiology of suicide in humans may be impulsiveness or aggression rather than self-destructive intent. Whether that aggression or impulse to injure is directed inwardly or externally may be determined by the dynamic balance of neurobiological systems (70), culture, and cognition (71–75). Animal models offer the opportunity to test hypotheses as they become better formulated by studies of self-destructive behavior in humans.

Neurochemical Systems and Suicide in Humans

Abnormalities in central serotonin function have been implicated in the pathobiology of depression for over 30 years. Based on the observation that reserpine, an alkaloid that depletes brain stores of monoamines, causes severe depression, and on the discovery of antidepressant drugs whose effects are mediated through augmentation of monoaminergic systems, noradrenergic (76) and serotonergic (77) hypotheses of affective illness have been proposed. Among the numerous studies that ensued from the formulation of these hypotheses, many researchers attempted to correlate abnormalities in monoamine function with specific depressive symptoms, including suicidality. These studies in turn lead to the rapidly expanding literature on the psychobiology of suicidal behavior, in which abnormalities of numerous neurochemical systems have been implicated. It is the serotonin (5HT) system that has received the most attention.

SEROTONIN

The serotonergic system in suicide can be studied in the brain tissue of victims obtained postmortem, in the cerebrospinal fluid of individuals who have attempted suicide, or those at high risk who are subsequently followed longitudinally until they attempt or complete suicide; in other peripheral tissues of living subjects, principally platelets; and through neuroendocrine challenge paradigms. Here we examine the evidence of a role for serotonin (5HT) in modulating suicidal behavior for each of these sources.

Postmortem Studies

Tissue levels of 5HT and 5HIAA. The first evidence linking neurochemical changes in the brain and suicidal behavior was provided by studies of 5HT and 5-hydroxyindoleacetic acid (5HIAA) in tissue obtained postmortem from suicide victims. Table 23.2 lists 13 studies in which indolamine and metabolite levels from a variety of brain regions were compared in suicides and controls. In five of these studies, investigators found no differences in 5HT levels between suicides and controls, (78–82), and in four no differences in 5HIAA could be demonstrated (81–84). 5HT levels were significantly decreased in specific brain regions of suicides in five studies, including brain stem (84, 85), raphe nuclei (86), the putamen (81), and in the hypothalamus of

victims with diagnoses other than schizophrenia (87). Only two studies showed significant reduction in 5HIAA levels in brains of suicides relative to controls. In both cases long postmortem intervals complicate interpretation (78, 80), as do the finding of elevated 5HT levels in the basal ganglia (87), and elevated 5HIAA levels in the amygdala (81) and hippocampus (88) of suicide victims.

At most, these studies suggest a trend for decreased indolamine and metabolite levels in brainstem nuclei of suicide victims. The inconsistency of findings may be attributed to the influence on monoamine levels of age, sex, postmortem interval, antemortem exposure to centrally active drugs, diurnal and seasonal variation, and the duration and nature of the agonal state (89). Lack of detail regarding diagnosis and treatment histories of subjects further limits the interpretation of these data.

Presynaptic receptor studies. As a methodology for studying neurochemical systems in suicide, the assay of receptor binding in postmortem tissue has great advantages over measurement of monoamine levels. In general, receptor binding is far less subject to the influences of postmortem interval and acute (but not chronic) antidepressant exposure. Presynaptically, the most intensively studied receptor has been the imipramine binding site, located on the nerve terminal and thought to be associated with the 5HT transport system (90). Thus, the amount and affinity of imipramine binding sites may reflect the number and functional status of 5HT nerve terminals.

Table 23.3 lists results of studies comparing measures of binding at the serotonin reuptake site in the brains of suicide victims and controls. Although the greatest number of studies found no difference in frontal cortex (88, 91–95) or other brain regions (88, 92, 93), others have found significant decreases in imipramine binding (82, 91, 96–98) in the brains of suicide victims. One study that showed greater imipramine binding in frontal cortex of suicides than controls ascribed this inconsistent finding to premorbid drug exposure in the suicide group (99). Other explanations offered for the inconsistent findings include the observation that imipramine is a relatively nonspecific ligand that binds to muscarinic and α-adrenergic receptors in addition to the serotonin reuptake site (90, 93).

Regional differences in neurochemical measures may also explain the variability between studies. Gross-Isseroff and colleagues (91) found increased imipramine binding in pyramidal and molecular cell layers of certain hippocampal fields and decreased imipramine binding in tissues of the claustrum, postcentral gyrus, and insular cortex. Similarly, Arató and colleagues (82, 97) found that in suicides imipramine binding was significantly greater in the left compared with the right frontal cortex, in marked contrast to controls in whom binding was greater on the right. Although others have failed to replicate this pattern of interhemispheric differences (93, 95), it serves to stress the need for specificity in future studies regarding not only descriptive characteristics of the population, but of the neuroanatomical region sampled as well.

Table 23.2. Studies Comparing Levels of 5HT and 5HIAA in Brains of Suicide Victims and Controls

Study	Subjects	Tissue	Findings
Crow et al., 1984 (83)	10 suicides (7 depressed) 9 depressives with natural deaths 20 Alzheimer's disease 19 controls	Frontal cortex	Nonsignificant trend for ↓ 5HIAA in suicides.
Bourne et al., 1968 (78)	23 suicides 28 controls	Brain stem	↓ 5HIAA in suicides No difference in 5HT.
Cochran et al., 1976 (79)	10 depressed suicides 9 alcoholic suicides 12 controls	33 brain regions	No difference in 5HT.
Beskow et al., 1976 (80)	23 suicides 62 controls	7 brain regions	No difference in 5HT. ↓ 5HIAA in suicides (no difference after controlling for PM interval).
Shaw et al., 1967 (85)	28 suicides 17 controls	Hindbrain	↓ 5HT in depressed suicides.
Cheetham et al., 1989 (81)	19 suicides 19 controls	Cortex Hippocampus Brain stem	↑ 5HIAA in amygdala of suicides. ↓ 5HT in putamen.
Pare et al., 1969 (84)	24 suicides 15 controls	Brain stem Hypothalamus Caudate	No difference in 5HIAA. ↓ 5HT in brain stem of suicides.
Owen et al., 1986 (88)	19 suicides 19 controls	Occipital and frontal cortex Hippocampus	↑ 5HIAA in hippocampus of suicides.
Owen et al., 1983 (104)	17 suicides 20 controls	Frontal cortex	No difference in 5HIAA.
Lloyd et al., 1974 (86)	5 suicides 5 controls	Raphe nuclei	↓ 5HT in nucleus dorsalis and centralis inferior.
Korpi et al., 1986 (87)	30 schizophrenics 14 nonschizophrenic suicides 29 normal controls	14 brain regions	↓ 5HT in hypothalamus of nonschizophrenic suicides.
Arató et al., 1987 (82)	13 suicides 14 controls	Frontal cortex Hippocampus	No difference in 5HT or 5HIAA.

Postsynaptic 5HT receptor binding studies. In addition to the 5HT reuptake site, five distinct 5HT receptors have been identified. Thus far two receptor types have been studied in victims of completed suicide, $5HT_1$ (and its $5HT_{1A}$ subtype) and $5HT_2$.

The $5HT_2$ receptor is located on the postsynaptic neuron, with its greatest density in frontal cortex projections of the ascending dorsal raphe nucleus. Based on the observation that the lesioning of serotonergic neurons in the raphe nuclei leads to upregulation of postsynaptic $5HT_2$ receptors and decreased imipramine binding presynaptically (100, 101), Stanley and Mann (96) predicted that, if the serotonin deficiency hypothesis is operative, then a similar pattern would be found in victims of completed suicide. They found that the density (B_{max}) of $5HT_2$ receptors was 44% greater in the frontal cortex of 11 suicide victims than controls matched for age, gender, and postmortem interval. As shown in Table 23.4, these results were subsequently replicated by some, but not all, groups. Mann and colleagues found a 28% increase in $5HT_2$ receptor binding in frontal cortex of 21 suicides compared with matched controls (102), and Arora

and Meltzer (103) found 35% greater B_{max} in suicides versus controls. This latter study, which also used ^{3}H-spiroperidol, found a 35% increase in an even larger group of suicide victims compared with controls, noting higher values in men than women, but no difference in $5HT_2$ binding between suicides who died by violent and nonviolent means. Four studies investigated this question using ^{3}H-ketanserin as the ligand, all of which failed to show a significant difference between suicide victims and controls in frontal cortex (83, 88, 104, 105).

Cheetham et al. (105) studied 19 suicides, ages 16–57 years, all of whom had documented depressive disorders. Although they found no difference in ketanserin binding between suicides and controls in the frontal cortex, they noted an inverse correlation between receptor density and age, and that $5HT_2$ receptor binding was significantly decreased in the hippocampus of depressed suicide victims who had not been treated with antidepressant medications compared to controls. They concluded that reports of increased $5HT_2$ binding in the frontal cortex of suicide victims may be due to drug treatments or to the quality of aggression rather than to depression per se. Other studies, however, have found increased 5HT$_2$ receptor binding in subjects with major depression who died from natural causes compared with controls (106), and Mann and colleagues note that chronic antidepressant therapies down-regulate 5HT$_2$ receptors (90). The meaning of these discrepant findings, therefore, remains unclear.

Three studies have used the technique of in vitro quantitative receptor autoradiography to compare receptor binding in suicides and controls. Gross-Isseroff and colleagues (107), using ^{3}H-ketanserin as the ligand, found decreased binding in the frontal cortex of victims of suicide, ages 50 years and younger compared to controls, whereas there was no such difference in subjects over age 50 years. Furthermore, they found differing patterns of age dependence of ketanserin binding in different brain regions. In the frontal cortex of controls and, to a lesser extent, suicides' age was inversely correlated with ketanserin binding. In the

Table 23.3. Studies Comparing Binding at the Serotonin Reuptake Site in Brains of Suicide Victims and Controls

Study	Subjects	Tissue	Findings
Crow et al., 1984 (83)	10 suicides (7 depressed) 9 depressives natural deaths 20 Alzheimer's disease 19 controls	Frontal cortex	[^{3}H]imipramine binding ↓ only in depressed suicides.
Owen et al., 1986 (88)	19 suicides 19 controls	Frontal cortex Occipital cortex Hippocampus	[^{3}H]imipramine binding; no difference between groups.
Gross-Isseroff et al., 1989 (91)	12 suicides 12 controls	Multiple cortical and subcortical regions	↑ [^{3}H]imipramine binding in specific cell layers of hippocampus fields. ↓ imipramine binding in postcentral and insular cortex and claustrum; no difference in prefrontal cortex or brain stem.
Arató et al., 1987 (82)	13 suicides 14 controls	Frontal cortex Hippocampus	[^{3}H]imipramine binding in frontal cortex of suicides L > R hemisphere. In controls R > L hemisphere; no difference in hippocampus.
Lawrence et al., 1990a (92)	22 suicides 20 controls	10 brain regions	No difference in [^{3}H]paroxetine binding in any region.
Lawrence et al., 1990b (93)	8 suicides 8 controls	Frontal cortex Putamen Substantia nigra	[^{3}H]paroxetine binding–no interhemispheric differences; no differences in either hemisphere between suicides and controls.
Meyerson et al., 1982 (99)	8 suicides 10 controls	Frontal cortex	↑ [^{3}H]imipramine binding in suicides.
Stanley et al., 1982 (98)	9 suicides 9 controls	Frontal cortex	↓ [^{3}H]imipramine binding in suicides.
Arora and Meltzer 1991 (95)	6 suicides 10 controls	Frontal cortex	No interhemispheric differences; no differences between suicides and controls.
Arora and Meltzer 1989 (94)	28 suicides 28 controls	Frontal cortex	[^{3}H]imipramine binding–no differences between groups.
Arató et al., 1991 (97)	23 suicides 23 controls	Frontal cortex	↑ [^{3}H]imipramine binding in left hemisphere of suicides vs. controls; ↓ binding in right hemisphere of suicides vs. controls; differences more pronounced in violent suicides.

Table 23.4. Studies Comparing 5HT2 Receptor Binding in Brains of Suicide Victims and Controls

Study	Subjects	Tissue	Findings
Owen et al., 1983 (104)	17 suicides 20 controls	Frontal cortex	[^{3}H]ketanserin binding; trend for ↓ in suicides.
Owen et al., 1986 (88)	19 suicides 19 controls	Frontal cortex Occipital cortex Hippocampus	[^{3}H]ketanserin binding; no difference at any site.
Mann et al., 1986 (102)	21 suicides 21 controls	Frontal cortex	Spiroperidol binding— ↑ in suicides.
Arora and Meltzer 1989 (103)	32 suicides 37 controls	Frontal cortex	[^{3}H]spiperone binding— ↑ in suicides (males > females; violent > nonviolent).
Gross-Isseroff et al., 1990 (107)	12 suicides 12 controls	Frontal cortex Hippocampus Other	[^{3}H]ketanserin binding— ↓ in frontal cortex of young suicides vs. controls; no difference for suicides > age 50 years vs. controls.
Stanley and Mann 1983 (96)	11 suicides 11 controls	Frontal cortex	[^{3}H]spiroperidol binding—in suicides.
Arango et al., 1992 (109)	13 suicides 13 controls	Prefrontal cortex Temporal	^{125}I-LSD binding ↑ in suicides in frontal cortex only.
Cheetham et al., 1988 (105)	19 suicides 19 controls	Frontal, temporal, and occipital cortex Amygdala Hippocampus	[^{3}H]ketanserin binding— ↓ in hippocampus; no difference in other regions.
Arango et al., 1990 (108)	11 suicides 11 controls	Prefrontal cortex Temporal cortex	^{125}I-LSD binding— ↑ in suicides in frontal cortex only.
Crow et al., 1984 (83)	10 suicides 9 depressives, natural deaths 20 Alzheimer's disease 19 controls	Frontal cortex	[^{3}H]ketanserin binding; no difference between groups.

hippocampal formation, however, young suicide victims had higher binding and older victims lower binding, than controls. Thus the impact of aging on 5HT$_2$ receptor function may differ between groups as a function of anatomical site.

In autoradiographic studies Arango and colleagues used the more specific 5HT$_2$ receptor ligand, I-125-lysergic acid diethylamide, to demonstrate significantly greater binding in the prefrontal, but not the temporal, cortex of suicides compared with controls (108, 109). They further demonstrated a laminar pattern in cortex, similar in both suicides and controls, in which binding was greatest in intermediate cell layers. The variability in these studies, therefore, can be accounted for by many factors, including variation in the specificity of ligands, age of subjects, and brain region studied, in addition to the effects previously noted of antemortem drug exposures, manner of death (violent vs. nonviolent; prolonged vs. brief agonal state), and other factors.

5HT$_1$ receptors have both pre- and postsynaptic subtypes, with highest density in areas of the hippocampus and basal ganglia receiving projections from the median raphe nucleus. Table 23.5 lists studies examining 5HT$_1$ receptor binding in brains of suicide victims and controls assayed by a variety of methods. Using ^{3}[H]-5HT, a number of studies have found no difference between suicides and controls in

frontal (83, 88, 102, 104, 110), occipital (88), or temporal cortex (110). However, Cheetham and colleagues (110) found a 20% decrease in ^{3}[H]-5HT binding in the hippocampus of suicides.

Using a selective 5HT$_{1A}$ receptor agonist, OH-DPAT, as a ligand, other groups have found no (110, 111), or equivocal differences between groups. Matsubara et al. (112), for example, found that suicides who died by nonviolent means had 25% higher 5HT$_{1A}$ receptor binding than did violent suicides or controls, possibly due to the effect on receptors of carbon monoxide poisoning and drugs taken in overdose, the principal means of death in the nonviolent group. They also reported that 5HT$_{1A}$ receptor binding was negatively correlated with age in male controls but not females, while no such relationship could be demonstrated for suicide victims of either sex.

In summary, evidence from studies in both suicide attempters and victims of completed suicide supports a potential role for abnormalities in central serotonin function in the expression of suicidal behavior. This evidence is derived from cerebrospinal fluid and brain tissue levels of 5HT and 5HIAA, imipramine binding and serotonin uptake, 5HT$_1$, 5HT$_{1A}$, and 5HT$_2$ receptor binding. In general, these findings are consistent with a decrease in presynaptic serotonin function, reflected in decreased serotonin levels, serotonin turnover, and presynaptic receptor

Table 23.5. Studies Comparing 5HT1 and 5HT1A Receptor Binding in Brains of Suicide Victims and Controls

Study	Subjects	Tissue	Findings
Owen et al., 1983 (104)	17 suicides 20 controls	Frontal cortex	[³H]5HT receptor binding; no difference between groups.
Owen et al., 1986 (88)	19 suicides 19 controls	Frontal cortex Occipital cortex Hippocampus	[³H]5HT receptor binding; no difference between groups.
Dillon et al., 1991 (111)	14 suicides 14 controls	Numerous cortical and subcortical brain regions	OH-DPAT binding; no difference between groups; negative correlation with age in males.
Matsubara et al., 1991 (112)	23 suicides 40 controls	Frontal cortex	OH-DPAT receptor binding; negative correlation with age in male controls, but not females or suicides of either sex; ↑ binding in nonviolent suicides.
Mann et al., 1986 (102)	21 suicides 21 controls	Frontal cortex	[³H]5HT receptor binding; no difference between groups.
Cheetham et al., (1990) 110	19 suicides 19 controls	Frontal cortex Temporal cortex Hippocampus	[³H]5HT receptor binding; ↓ in hippocampus of suicides; no difference in cortical regions.
Crow et al., 1984 (83)	10 suicides 9 depressives 20 Alzheimer's disease 19 controls	Frontal cortex	[³H]5HT receptor binding; no differences between groups.

binding, coupled with postsynaptic receptor upregulation as a compensatory response. Frontal cortex is the brain region most intensively studied, with few significant abnormalities reported in temporal cortex tissue. Cheetham and colleagues (105, 110) noted decrements in hippocampal $5HT_1$ and $5HT_2$ receptor binding in the absence of differences in these measures in the frontal cortex of depressed suicides and controls, leading them to suggest the need for further more detailed studies of this brain region as a mediator of suicidal behavior in affective illness.

Despite the weight of these findings, they are far from unanimous. The inconsistency between studies has been ascribed to many factors, including postmortem interval, season of the year, premorbid exposure to prescribed and illicit drugs, the manner of death (including its violent nature, which may be a central feature of the proported biological abnormality), age and sex of subjects, the specificity of ligands used, and regional differences within the brain (interhemispheric and intrahemispheric).

Cerebrospinal Fluid Studies

Because of the availability of brain tissue for postmortem analysis, cerebrospinal fluid (CSF) serotonin measures have not been studied in completed suicide. However, Stanley and colleagues (113) simultaneously sampled CSF 5HIAA drawn from the spinal cistern postmortem with levels of 5HIAA in the cerebral cortex. Demonstrating a strong correlation, they concluded that CSF metabolite concentrations are a valid reflection of brain serotonin activity. It is

with greater confidence, then, that the findings of many studies of serotonergic indices from the lumbar CSF of suicide attempters can be assumed to reflect brain function.

CSF sampling has the great advantage of easy accessibility. Furthermore, because the fluid is obtained from a living subject, simultaneous measurements of symptoms and behaviors can be made, and the subjects followed longitudinally to establish the predictive value of CSF measures. There are, nonetheless, numerous limitations to such studies that should be considered in their interpretation. As previously noted, suicide attempters are not uniformly representative of completed suicides. The subjects in CSF studies likely represent a heterogeneous group, only some of whom may share any postulated neurobiological profile with suicide completers. Studies frequently fail to define adequately the subjects' diagnoses or past history of suicidal behavior, and to distinguish adequately, at times, among suicidal ideation, low-lethality attempts, or high-lethality attempts.

Measuring CSF monoamines and metabolites is technically difficult because of numerous factors that influence their concentration. As reviewed by Åsberg and colleagues (114), these factors include age (increasing concentrations of 5HIAA with aging), sex (lower concentrations in men), body height, diet, level of physical activity prior to the lumbar puncture, the intervertebral space used and position of the subject, the amount of CSF drawn, the time of day and season of the year, and recent history of exposure to psychotropic medications. Given these cautions, a large and relatively consistent body of work offers support to the postmortem studies suggesting altered central serotonin function in suicide.

The first observation of an association between CSF serotonin measures and suicidal behavior was made during the course of investigations of CSF monoamines in major depression (115). Although some studies had found CSF 5HIAA levels to be decreased in depressed patients (116); other studies had found them to be no different (117) or greater than in controls (116). These mixed findings could potentially be explained by the technical difficulties in working with CSF monoamines. However, the consistent observation by investigators that a subgroup of 30–40% of depressives had diminished CSF 5HIAA levels led them to speculate that abnormalities in this neurotransmitter system reflected an etiologically distinct subgroup (118). Åsberg and colleagues (115) then noted that depressives with low CSF levels of 5HIAA had a higher incidence of suicide attempts. Of 68 patients with depressive illness in their study, 15 had made a suicide attempt during the index episode. Concentrations of CSF 5HIAA were bimodally distributed in the sample, with 40% of the low 5HIAA group having attempted suicide compared with 15% of patients with normal CSF 5HIAA levels. Furthermore, all suicide attempts by violent means clustered in the low 5HIAA group, two of whom subsequently killed themselves during the study period.

A number of subsequent studies have confirmed Åsberg's original finding, while others have failed to do so (see reference 114 for a representative review). Negative results may be explained by methodologic differences or by differences between patient groups. For example, two of the studies that found no association between CSF 5HIAA and suicidal behavior included substantial numbers of patients with bipolar disorders in their sample (117, 119). Although Roy-Byrne and colleagues (119) found no difference in mean CSF 5HIAA between patients with affective disorders with and without a past history of suicide attempts, separate analyses for unipolar and bipolar patients were more revealing. They found no difference between suicidal and nonsuicidal bipolars, but suicidal unipolar depressives tended to have lower CSF 5HIAA than the other groups. Ågren (120) also found a significant negative correlation between 5HIAA levels and a history of suicide attempts among unipolar depressives only, with no such difference evident for bipolar patients.

The frequent need for maintenance antidepressive medications in treated depressives makes follow-up studies of CSF monoamines in suicide attempters problematic. Nonetheless, the few available data suggest the possibility that low CSF 5HIAA is a trait rather than a state characteristic. VanPraag (121) found that in approximately 50% of patients, a low CSF 5HIAA concentration persisted after recovery from the depressive episode. Abnormal values have been associated with both past (115, 120, 122) and future (115, 123) attempts. Åsberg and colleagues (89) have suggested the existence of a subgroup of depressives whose CSF concentrations of 5HIAA are both lower and more

unstable over time than normal. Further reductions at times of illness exacerbation may augment suicide risk. Träskman and colleagues (123) reported on follow-up of 119 patients for whom CSF 5HIAA determinations had been made in research protocols from 1970 to 1978. Seven of these patients went on to commit suicide, six of whom had a past history of attempt. A 5HIAA level below the median for the entire patient group was a significant predictor of subsequent suicide. Among attempters, all six who went on to complete suicide had 5HIAA levels below the median. Subsequent reports support the notion that low CSF 5HIAA may be a useful indicator of subsequent attempted (124) or completed (114) suicide.

Diagnoses Other Than Depression

To further explore whether abnormalities in CSF 5HIAA in suicide attempters were a result solely of their mood disturbance rather than, for example, a dimension of psychopathology that crosses diagnostic boundaries, researchers expanded studies to include patients with a variety of psychiatric illnesses. Schizophrenics with a history of suicide attempts have lower levels of CSF 5HIAA than either controls or schizophrenics without history of suicidal behavior (125–128). In addition to depressives, Banki and colleagues found a significant association between recent suicide attempts and CSF 5HIAA levels in both patients with adjustment disorders and subjects with alcoholism. Although Roy and colleagues (129) found no such association with suicide attempts in alcoholics, very few of their subjects had made violent attempts. Also, a period of months to years between last attempt and testing was typical for these patients, suggesting that low CSF 5HIAA was not a trait marker in this sample.

In further support of the notion that CSF 5HIAA measures a dimension of psychopathology independent of affective disorder, Brown and colleagues (122) studied 22 young active duty military men with diagnoses of personality disorder in the absence of affective symptomatology. Subjects with a history of suicide attempt had lower CSF 5HIAA than those without such histories. In a subsequent study of 12 military men with borderline personality disorder and no affective illness, their findings were the same (130). In both studies, however, the authors went on to make associations between 5HIAA levels and measures of aggression and impulsivity, demonstrating a strong and significant inverse relationship. Subjects with more "impulsive" personality disorders, higher scores on a measure of lifetime history of aggression/impulsive behavior, and higher T scores on the psychopathic deviate scale of the MMPI, had lower levels of CSF 5HIAA.

These findings spurred other investigators to question whether similar correlations could be found in other subject groups with histories characterized by aggressiveness or impulsivity rather than suicidal behavior per se. Linnoila and colleagues (131) studied individuals with personality disorders incarcerated after violent acts. Dividing the group into "impulsive" and "nonimpulsive" offenders, they found significantly lower CSF 5HIAA concentrations in the former group. Some subjects, however, had a past history of suicide attempt; these individuals had the lowest metabolite levels. Subsequently Virkkunen and colleagues (132) compared CSF monoamine metabolite levels in normal controls with 20 habitually violent offenders and 20 arsonists, a group felt to represent an extreme of impulsivity relatively free from traits of aggressiveness and violence. 5HIAA levels were significantly lower in arsonists than comparison groups. Controls had the highest levels, with violent offenders showing intermediate levels of 5HIAA. The results were interpreted to support the hypothesis that poor impulse control is associated with low levels of monoamine metabolites. A 3-year follow-up study of 36 violent offenders and 22 arsonists subsequently demonstrated lower CSF 5HIAA levels at baseline in subjects who went on during the follow-up period to commit new violent offenses or arson (133). Again, interpretation of results is complicated by the fact that 27 of 58 subjects had a past history of a suicide attempt, 25 of whom fulfilled criteria for an alcohol abuse diagnosis (134). Based on the additional observation that CSF 5HIAA levels were significantly lower among the 35 subjects with alcoholic fathers than among those without, Linnoila and colleagues have suggested that low CSF 5HIAA, in addition to impulsivity, may be characteristic of type 2 alcoholism, explaining some of the inconsistency in the literature regarding associations between alcoholism, suicidality and CSF monoamine measures (135).

Other studies have demonstrated altered 5HT metabolism in aggressive patients with an XYY chromosomal pattern (136), murder-suicides (137), children and adolescents with disruptive behavior disorders (138), and individuals who had murdered a sexual partner (139). In this latter study the finding that CSF measures were significantly lower in crimes of passion than for other homicide offenders was taken as an indication of impulsivity in the former group.

Other Biological Measures of Serotonin Function

In addition to CNS tissue assays and CSF measures, a variety of other strategies have been employed to explore serotonin function in suicidal people.

Glucose Tolerance Test. In addition to measuring CSF 5HIAA in his populations of violent and impulsive offenders, Virkkunen and colleagues conducted glucose tolerance tests to demonstrate that the pattern of response differentiated impulsive from nonimpulsive groups (132, 140, 141). Subjects with antisocial personality disorder and intermittent explosive disorder demonstrated blood glucose nadirs significantly below that of controls. Arsonists similarly demonstrated a significantly lower nadir. They speculate that altered serotonin input to the suprachiasmatic nucleus alters regulatory mechanisms demonstrated in rat models to regulate insulin and hyperglycemic responses to oral or intravenous glucose loads (142).

Platelet Studies. Human platelets have long been recognized to have qualities of central presynaptic neurons (143). For example, platelet membranes contain serotonin reuptake sites and high-affinity binding of tritiated imipramine, enabling efforts to replicate findings from postmortem brain tissue in this easily accessible peripheral source. Although results have been mixed in studies of imipramine binding and serotonin uptake in platelets of major depressives (144), a number of investigators have found significant results in studies of depressed suicide attempters. Wägner and colleagues (145) found a trend for depressives who had made a violent suicide attempt to have higher platelet imipramine binding values than depressed nonattempters. Roy and colleagues (144) compared patients with affective disorders to controls, finding differences only between the women in each group. However, four of the 51 depressed patients committed suicide in 1-year follow-up. In retrospect, a past history of suicide attempt in combination with either decreased platelet imipramine binding or serotonin uptake appeared to place patients at especially high risk for future suicide. Nemeroff and colleagues (146) studied platelet imipramine binding in young and old controls, major depressives, and elderly with probable Alzheimer's disease. Depressives of all ages demonstrated decreased platelet imipramine binding relative to age-matched controls and patients with dementia, but the authors made no comments with regard to histories of suicidal behavior. Schneider and colleagues (147) found that decreased platelet imipramine binding distinguished dementia with agitation and delusions from controls and subjects with uncomplicated Alzheimer's disease. Although suicide was not the focus of this study, these findings validate the argument that agitation (or aggressiveness) is the psychopathological correlate of central serotonin dysfunction rather than suicide per se. In subsequent studies both positive (148) and negative (149) findings of association between platelet imipramine binding and suicidal behavior have been reported.

In addition to imipramine binding sites, human platelets also have $5HT_2$ receptors involved in the mediation of serotonin-amplified platelet aggregation (150). Biegon and colleagues (151) compared the platelets of suicidal males with controls and found increased $5HT_2$ receptors, while Pandey et al. (150) found significantly higher $5HT_2$ binding in a subgroup of depressives with recent attempts or serious ideation compared with nonsuicidal depressives and controls. McBride et al. (152) found a direct association among depressed attempters between $5HT_2$ receptor binding on platelets and lethality of suicidal behavior as well.

Studies of whole blood serotonin levels (153) and platelet serotonin levels (154), albeit questionable indicators of central serotonin function, offer some additional support for the association of decreased $5HT_2$ activity with suicide.

Neuroendocrine Studies. Altered levels of serotonin and metabolites in the CSF and peripheral tissues leave unresolved the question of where in this dynamic system the deficit lies. Presynaptic lesions may result in decreased

5HIAA due to diminished synthesis and release of serotonin, whereas increased presynaptic function could result in decreased turnover as a compensatory postsynaptic response. A variety of challenge paradigms have been designed that take advantage of the regulatory interaction between serotonin and neuroendocrine systems to test their integrity. Among the agents most frequently used are 5HT precursors and agonists.

Meltzer and colleagues (155) administered 5-hydroxy-tryptophan (5HTP) to 40 patients with major affective disorder, and measured the hypercortisolemic response. They observed a significant correlation between the degree of cortisol response and a past history of suicidal behavior and interpreted the finding to reflect postsynaptic $5HT_2$ receptor up-regulation in the hypothalamus.

Concerned with the possibility that cortisol response to 5HTP does not specifically reflect $5HT_2$ receptor function (156), Coccaro and colleagues chose fenfluramine as their challenge agent (157). Fenfluramine both augments the release and blocks the reuptake of endogenous stores of 5HT, resulting in increased serum prolactin levels in the peripheral circulation. They found that, compared with normal controls and male patients with no past history of suicidal behavior, subjects with either major depression or a personality disorder diagnosis who had a suicide attempt in the past demonstrated a significantly blunted prolactin response to fenfluramine infusion. They interpreted these findings to suggest an overall reduction in 5HT neurotransmission in the limbic-hypothalamic-pituitary axis in affective and/or personality disordered patients with a past history of parasuicide.

Only one group to date has used prolactin and cortisol responses to the 5HT uptake inhibitor, clomipramine, to explore this system (158). They found no association in 66 patients of mixed diagnoses between prolactin and cortisol responses and limited measures of suicidal ideation or behavior.

Summary

In summary, data from studies using a broad range of technologies and tissues support the existence of an association between suicidal behavior and functioning of the central serotonin system. The nature of that association, however, remains unclear for many reasons that together reflect the complexity of this issue. The methodologies are intricate, easily confounded by difficulties controlling the numerous variables that independently affect them. Researchers have been inconsistent in defining their patient groups, particularly with regard to the nature of the suicidal behavior they are attempting to correlate with the biological measure. Despite these limitations, it seems most likely that serotonin plays its role in suicidal behavior through the mediation of impulse control and aggression. Deficits in this system may predispose individuals to violent behavior, as has been demonstrated in animal models, under specific circumstances, such as the development of a co-morbid depressive disorder or individually significant stressful life circumstances. Whether the emergent behavior is destructive to self or others may depend in turn on complex interactions with other neurochemical systems, reviewed below.

DOPAMINE

The catecholamines, dopamine and norepinephrine, have received far less attention than serotonin in studies of suicidal behavior. Many authors have noted an association in the CSF between levels of 5HIAA and the dopamine metabolite, homovanillic acid (HVA). It is unclear whether that close correlation is due to a shared transport mechanism or to a functional connection between the parent amines (114). Several authors have reported low levels of CSF HVA paralleling decreases in 5HIAA in suicidal depressives (123, 159, 160). For example, Roy and colleagues (160) studied 27 patients with major depressive disorders, finding lower CSF HVA in those patients with a past history of suicide attempts. They then followed these patients for 5 years (124) and continued to find an association between decreased CSF HVA levels and further suicide attempts during the follow-up period. In fact, in some studies of depressed patients, the association has been stronger between suicide attempts and low CSF HVA than with low CSF 5HIAA (120, 161).

Some authors suggest that the association between central dopaminergic function and suicidal behavior is specific to affective illness (123). The failure by Ninan and colleagues (162) to find any difference in CSF HVA levels between suicidal and nonsuicidal schizophrenics supports this possibility.

Roy and colleagues (163) also measured the urinary output of dopamine metabolites in patients with major depression and normal controls, to explore whether DA dysregulation differentiated those with suicidal behavior. Not only did patients with a past history of suicide attempts have lower urinary outputs of DA metabolites than nonattempters or controls, but patients who made repeat attempts during the 5-year follow-up period had significantly lower values than other groups. In combination with CSF HVA levels in suicidal subjects, these data indicate that while decreased dopamine function may have little bearing on the expression of suicidal behavior in other diagnostic groups, it may signal vulnerability in patients with affective illness.

Few postmortem studies have addressed this issue. Neither Pare et al. (84) nor Beskow et al. (80) could demonstrate differences in any brain region in dopamine content between suicide victims and controls. Crow and colleagues (83) found an insignificant trend for suicides to have lower levels of HVA in frontal cortex than normal controls had, but no studies to date have examined dopamine receptor function in postmortem tissue.

Despite the lack of attention paid in the literature to the role of dopamine and suicidal behavior, several other lines of evidence suggest its potential importance. In reviewing the epidemiology of suicide, we noted the striking rise in rate

Table 23.6.   Studies Comparing Measures of β-Adrenergic Receptor Binding in Brains of Suicide Victims and Controls

Study	Subjects	Tissue	Findings
Arango et al., 1990 (108)	11 suicides 11 controls	Frontal cortex Temporal cortex	↑ ^{125}I-pindolol binding in prefrontal and temporal cortex in suicides.
Stockmeier and Meltzer 1991 (174)	22 suicides 22 controls	Frontal cortex	Dihydroalprenolol (DHA) binding; no difference between groups.
Meyerson et al., 1982 (99)	8 suicides 10 controls	Frontal cortex	DHA binding; no difference between groups.
DePaermentier et al., 1990 (176)	21 suicides 20 controls	9 brain regions	CGP12177 binding; ↓ in temporal and frontal cortex of suicides (violent > nonviolent).
Biegon and Israeli 1988 (173)	14 suicides 14 controls	Prefrontal cortex	DHA binding ↑ in suicides.
Mann et al., 1986 (102)	21 suicides 21 controls	Frontal cortex	DHA binding ↑ in suicides.
Crow et al., 1984 (83)	10 suicides 19 controls	Frontal cortex	DHA binding; no difference between groups.
Little et al., 1990 (175)	15 suicides 15 controls	Frontal cortex	^{125}I-pindolol binding ↓ in suicides.

with age in males. As in other monoaminergic systems, there are well-documented reductions in dopaminergic neurons, the function of receptors and uptake sites, and synthetic enzyme activity with increasing age (164–166). Furthermore, as discussed later in this chapter, suicide risk is elevated in both Huntington's and Parkinson's disease, disorders in which degenerative changes of the central dopaminergic systems have been implicated (167–170).

NOREPINEPHRINE/EPINEPHRINE

As for dopamine, there have been very few studies examining the noradrenergic system in suicide, and those that have been conducted provide equivocal results. Positive findings include the observation of an inverse correlation between CSF levels of the norepinephrine (NE) metabolite 3-methoxy-4-hydroxyphenylglycol (MHPG) and ratings of suicidal intent in unipolar and bipolar depressives (159), and arsonists and violent offenders (134). MHPG in the CSF is negatively correlated with a lifetime history of aggression in children and adolescents with disruptive behavior disorders (138) as well. In contrast, Brown and colleagues (122) found a significant positive correlation between CSF MHPG levels and aggression scores among 26 military recruits with personality disorders, and significantly higher levels in those with a past history of suicidal behavior than those who had not made a suicide attempt. These investigators were unable to replicate this finding, however, in a subsequent study of 12 men with borderline personality disorder but no depressive illness (130). Roy et al. (171) found no difference between depressives with and without suicide attempts in CSF, plasma, or urinary indices of noradrenergic function, but Ostroff and colleagues showed in two studies that a low ratio of urinary NE to epinephrine (E) was predictive of suicidal behavior in patients with mixed psychiatric diagnoses (70, 172).

Only a handful of studies have explored noradrenergic receptor function in postmortem tissue (Table 23.6). Of eight studies that used membrane preparations and/or autoradiography to measure β-adrenergic receptors, three studies reported significantly increased binding in the frontal cortex of suicides compared with controls (102, 108, 173). Arango et al. (108) found no apparent correlation with age, sex, or $5HT_2$ receptor binding in the same subject group. On the other hand, three studies found no difference (83, 99, 174), and one found decreased (175) β-receptor density in the frontal cortex of suicides compared with controls. Using the highly specific ligand H3CGP12177 in nine brain regions in drug-free depressed suicides and controls, DePaermentier et al. (176) found significantly decreased β-receptor binding in the temporal cortex of suicide victims. Dividing depressives into those with violent and nonviolent suicides, they found that the victims by violent means had significantly lower β-receptor binding in the frontal cortex than either controls or nonviolent suicides, while the nonviolent suicides had significantly lower β-receptor binding compared with controls in occipital and temporal cortex. There was no difference in subcortical structures. As with postmortem examination of other receptor populations, variation in results may be explained by differences in region studied, ligand specificity, and the extent to which the effects of age, postmortem interval, drug effects, and circadian rhythms were accounted for in study design.

Fewer studies have examined α_1-adrenergic receptor function (Table 23.7). Whereas one study using in vitro quantitative autoradiography with tritiated prazosin found significant decreased binding in the prefrontal cortex of suicides compared with controls (177), a second study with similar methodology found an increased binding specific to layers IV–V of the prefrontal cortex in suicides (178).

α_2-Adrenergic receptor function has been examined in suicide victims and controls by three groups. Finding no difference in iodoclonidine binding on autoradiography of the locus ceruleus of suicides and controls, Ordway and colleagues (179) concluded that if a difference exists in α_2-receptor binding, it must be in the terminal fields. Arango and colleagues (180), however, found no difference in any cortical layer in comparing suicides and controls, while Meana et al. (181) found increased α_2-receptor density in the frontal cortex, amygdala, and the head of the caudate for depressed suicides compared with controls. Unable to demonstrate any differences between schizophrenic suicides and controls, their findings suggest a role for noradrenergic receptor dysfunction in affective illness rather than suicidal behavior per se.

OTHER NEUROCHEMICAL SYSTEMS

Although not systematically investigated, a number of neurochemical systems other than monoamines have been implicated in suicidal behavior as well. In light of the proposed relationship of changes in cholinergic function to affective disorders (182), three groups have measured receptor ligand binding for ^{3}H-quinuclidinyl benzilate (QNB), a muscarinic antagonist, in the brains of suicide victims and controls. Using frontal cortex, Meyerson and colleagues (99) found a 47% increase in receptor binding in suicides compared with controls. Neither Kaufman et al. (183) nor Stanley (184) could replicate this finding in frontal cortex or other tissues. This discrepancy may be explainable by differences between studies in the proportion of suicide victims with affective disorder.

Although no data have been reported on function of the inhibitory neurotransmitter γ-aminobutyric acid (GABA) in suicide attempters, findings from a variety of studies suggest that it too plays a role in anxiety and affective disorders (185). As well, anxiety has been reported by some authors

(186) to be a powerful short-term predictor of completed suicide. Therefore, six studies have explored various aspects of the GABA system in the brains of suicide victims. None, however, has demonstrated a difference between suicides and controls in the function of GABA's principal synthetic (185) or degradative enzymes (187) in cortical sites, GABA receptor binding in cortex or hippocampus (188), or benzodiazepine receptor binding (to which the GABA receptor complex is linked) in subcortical tissue (189, 190). Korpi et al. (191) found no difference between suicides and controls in GABA levels by reversed-phase HPLC in frontal cortex or four other subcortical sites. Only Cheetham and colleagues (185) found a significant (18%) increase in benzodiazepine binding in the frontal cortex of depressed suicide victims compared with controls.

It is possible that abnormalities in GABA function may be more relevant to suicide in later life than in young adulthood and middle age. In comparing elderly depressed patients who died of natural causes with controls, Perry and colleagues (192) found a marked reduction in the GABA synthetic enzyme, glutamic acid decarboxylase (GAD), in elderly depressives, individuals who may be at higher suicide risk than any other demographic or diagnostic subgroup. Furthermore, GAD was markedly reduced in terminal illness, particularly when associated with hypoxia, a circumstance associated with much increased suicide risk.

In studies of neuropeptides, no difference was demonstrated in somatostatin immunoreactivity in the cortex of suicide victims and controls (193), whereas neuropeptide Y, which coexists in the brain with monoamines and GABA, was significantly reduced in the frontal cortex, temporal cortex, caudate of suicide victims compared with controls (194). A large body of literature has accumulated to suggest that disturbances of the endogenous opioid system may be involved in the pathophysiology of self-mutilatory be-

Table 23.7. Studies Comparing α_1- and α_2-Adrenergic Binding in Brains of Suicide Victims and Controls

Study	Subjects	Tissue	Findings
α_1-Receptor Studies			
Gross-Isseroff et al., 1990 (177)	12 suicides 12 controls	Prefrontal cortex Temporal cortex Amygdala Hippocampus Caudate	[^{3}H]prazosin binding ↓ in cortical regions and caudate of suicides.
Arango et al., 1989 (178)	10 suicides 10 controls	Prefrontal and temporal cortex	[^{3}H]prazosin binding ↑ in prefrontal cortex (layers IV–V) of suicides.
α_2-Receptor Studies			
Ordway et al., 1990 (179)	13 suicides 13 controls	Locus ceruleus	Iodoclonidine binding; no difference between groups.
Arango et al., 1990 (180)	12 suicides 12 controls	Prefrontal cortex	[^{3}H]clonidine binding; no difference between groups.
Meana et al., 1992 (181)	45 suicides 42 controls	7 brain regions	[^{3}H]clonidine binding ↑ in frontal cortex, amygdala, and caudate in depressed suicides; no difference in schizophrenic suicides.

haviors in individuals with mental retardation (195–198), Tourette's syndrome (199) Lesch-Nyhan syndrome (200) and patients with personality disorders (201, 202). Very few studies, however, have considered this issue in patients whose intent was clearly suicide. Frecska and colleagues (203) administered the opioid agonist, fentanyl, to 10 women with major depression and measured their prolactin secretory response. Although they found no difference between healthy volunteers and depressed patients, four of the depressed women showed the most blunted response, three of whom committed suicide within 1 year follow-up. Gross-Isseroff and colleagues (204) used quantitative auto-radiography to examine regional differences in μ-opioid receptors between the brains of 14 pairs of suicide victims and age- and sex-matched controls. Finding a significant increase in μ-receptor density in frontal and temporal cortical gyri in suicides, the authors speculate that greater postsynaptic receptor density is a compensatory response to diminished presynaptic release of endogenous peptides. They also noted significant age effects, most pronounced in temporal gyri, in which receptor binding was correlated with age in both suicides and controls.

A second postmortem study of the opiate system examined β-endorphin levels in the frontal and temporal cortex, caudate nucleus, hypothalamus, and thalamus in seven suicide victims and controls, showing both intergroup and interhemispheric differences (205). β-endorphin concentrations were decreased in the temporal and frontal cortex and caudate nucleus of suicides compared with controls. However, the reductions were observed only in samples taken from the left side of the brain. Suicide victims demonstrated a marked asymmetry in the distribution of β-endorphin, lower on the left side of the brain than on the right, a pattern that was not observed in controls. Although consistent with the findings of Gross-Isseroff et al. (204), lower β-endorphin levels may be due either to decreased production of the endogenous peptide or to a greatly increased turnover. These data suggest the need for studies that measure the integrity and function of neuropeptide containing neurons, as well as additional data concerning regional specificity and lateralization of neurochemical function as it relates to the regulation of mood and impulse.

Neuroendocrine Systems and Suicide

Although a wide range of neuroendocrine systems have been implicated in the pathophysiology of psychiatric illness, only two have been investigated in any detail with regard to their role in suicidal behavior: the hypothalamic-pituitary-thyroid axis, and the hypothalamic-pituitary-adrenal (HPA) axis.

THYROID AXIS

As reviewed elsewhere, individuals with depressive disorders have a blunted thyrotropin (TSH) response to the infusion of thyrotropin-releasing hormone (TRH) (206). Retrospective analysis in two studies has demonstrated an association between blunted TSH response and attempted (207) and completed suicide (208). In contrast, Banki and colleagues (128) found an augmented TRH response to TSH in suicidal vs. nonsuicidal psychiatric patients of mixed diagnoses. As with other neurobiological measures, the distinction between violent and nonviolent suicidal behavior may be important because a number of studies have found associations between thyroid axis abnormalities and suicide in those who used violent methods only (209–211).

HPA AXIS AND SUICIDE

Many lines of evidence suggest that disturbances of the HPA axis may be associated with suicide as well. The earliest observations were of elevated urinary excretion of cortisol (172) and 17-hydroxy corticosteroids in patients who attempted or completed suicide (212, 213). Others failed to find that relationship (214, 215). Elevated plasma cortisol has been associated with completed suicide at follow-up as well (216). In postmortem studies, CSF corticotropin releasing factor (CRF) levels were significantly higher (217) and CRF binding sites in the frontal cortex significantly reduced (218) in suicides compared with sudden death controls. Others have failed to show any difference between CSF cortisol or CRF levels in suicide attempters and depressed nonattempters or normal controls (219–222). Depressed mood and suicidal ideation are among the common manifestations of Cushings syndrome (223, 224) and corticosteroid administration (225). Braunig and colleagues found a higher frequency of suicidal ideation in patients with corticosteroid induced psychoses than in organic psychoses of other origins (226).

A number of groups have found that escape from dexamethasone suppression predicts suicidality (227–231), whereas others have failed to find that association (216, 232–235). Furthermore, failure of the dexamethasone suppression test (DST) to normalize has also been associated with subsequent completed suicide (236, 237).

Numerous explanations for the lack of clarity in these studies have been offered, including differences between studies of diagnostic composition, definition of suicidal behavior, and DST methodology. Age and gender may be factors as well. Although there are few overt changes in HPA axis functioning with normal aging (238, 239), subtle abnormalities of the axis's regulatory response emerge in stressful conditions or pathological states (240–242). For example, Stangl and colleagues (243) found that in two-thirds of 50 studies of the DST in major affective disorder, nonsuppressors were older than suppressors. Furthermore, in males, postdexamethasone cortisol was positively correlated with age in both depressives and normals, albeit at higher levels across the age spectrum in depressives. In females, on the other hand, only depressives showed the correlation between age and postdexamethasone cortisol. Unfortunately, no analyses were reported regarding the subjects' histories of suicidal behavior, and there are no reported studies of the DST response in suicidal elderly.

OTHER NEUROENDOCRINE SYSTEMS

Finally, preliminary evidence linking a number of other biological variables to suicidal behavior is noteworthy. Testosterone, long associated with aggression in both animal models and humans (244) has not been specifically measured in a population of suicide attempters or completers. Banki and colleagues (245) measured CSF magnesium levels in psychiatric patients and controls, finding that patients who had made suicide attempts by either violent or nonviolent means had significantly lower mean CSF magnesium levels, regardless of diagnosis, than nonsuicidal patients or controls. CSF magnesium and 5HIAA levels were highly correlated. Exploring the possibility of a "low melatonin syndrome" in patients with major depressive disorders, Beck-Friis and colleagues (246) found that patients with a past history of suicidal behavior had significantly higher mean nocturnal serum melatonin levels than did those without a past history of suicidal behavior. No other investigators have reported an association between melatonin and suicidal behavior, and the significance of this observation remains unclear. However, because serotonin is a precursor of melatonin, because melatonin may be involved in the regulation of a broad range of neuroendocrine functions, and because of the progressive decline in the ability of the pineal gland to produce this hormone into late life, this discrepancy between suicidal and nonsuicidal patients warrants further study.

An association between low serum cholesterol concentrations and suicide has been observed and provides one further example of the complex interplay of neurobiological factors in determining risk for self-injury. In a review of six randomized, controlled, primary prevention trials in which the serum cholesterol of middle-age subjects was lowered by diet, drugs, or both strategies, Muldoon and colleagues (247) found that while mortality from coronary heart disease was decreased, deaths from other causes were not. A subsequent Swedish study (248) linked that excess mortality to violent deaths, including suicide. In over 50,000 people followed for 20 years, mortality from injuries was strongly negatively correlated with baseline cholesterol level in men. Those individuals in the lowest quartile of the cholesterol distribution had a 4.2 times greater risk of suicide than other male subjects. No such relationship was observed for women. Complicating interpretation of the results, investigators had no information regarding the psychological state of their subjects. They also had no other potential confounds such as alcohol use and other parameters of nutritional state in the follow-up period, which may have been modified as a function of the development of affective or other psychopathology. In an effort to explain these observations, Engelberg (249)

postulated that a reduction in brain cell cholesterol may cause dysfunction at the serotonin reuptake site through alterations in membrane lipid viscosity. Lower presynaptic levels of 5HT would result, causing disruptions in mood and impulse control and suicidal behavior.

Interactions such as these at the neuronal level are likely to characterize biological abnormalities in suicide more generally. Monoaminergic, GABA-ergic, peptidergic, and neuroendocrine systems have complex interrelationships that are beyond the scope of this text. For example, as reviewed by Sulser (250), an intact serotonergic neuronal input is required for the proper functioning of β-adrenergic receptors. The secretion of cortisol and prolactin is regulated in part through stimulation of $5HT_1$ receptors (251), in addition to renin, vasopressin, and corticotropin (ACTH). As well, the HPA axis appears to modulate both serotonergic and catecholamine function (252), the relationships of which may be altered during episodes of illness (253). It is most likely, therefore, that the expression of suicidal behavior in an individual represents, in addition to psychological and social factors, subtle alterations in the balance of numerous neurochemical systems. These alterations in turn result from a wide range of intrinsic or extrinsic factors, such as genetic programming, the aging of neurotransmitter and hormonal systems, structural lesions, exposure to toxins, and nutritional influences. The impact of these factors on individual neurochemical or neuroanatomical systems determines whether the resulting violent behavior is directed outward toward others or inward toward the self.

SUICIDE IN NEUROPSYCHIATRIC DISORDERS

The study of suicide in specific neuropsychiatric disorders offers two potential benefits. First, it facilitates the identification of individuals at risk, and thus the more efficient and effective implementation of preventive strategies. Second, it offers the opportunity to learn even more about brain-behavior relationships and the neurobiological basis of suicidal behavior in particular.

Psychiatric Illness

In the course of this chapter we have reviewed a wide range of social, psychological, genetic, and potential neurobiological risk factors for suicidal behavior. None, however, is more potent than mental illness. In describing the association between emotional disorders and suicide, one must take two complementary approaches. Initially, studies of general population samples are made, in which retrospective psychiatric diagnoses are determined for all suicides occurring in a particular area and time period. While such studies are important in establishing the prevalence of particular diagnoses in a sample of completed suicides, they do not specify the risk inherent to a given psychiatric or neuropsychiatric disorder. These data must be derived from retrospective or prospective studies of particular diagnostic

Table 23.8. Psychological Autopsy Studies: Percent of Completed Suicides with Selected Diagnoses

Author	Affective Disorder	Substance Use Disorder	Schizophrenia	Axis II	No Diagnosis
Robins et al., 1959 (46) [N = 134]	45	25	2	—	6
Dorpat et al., 1960 (255) [N = 108]	30	27	12	9	0
Chynoweth et al., 1980 (48) [N = 135]	55	34	4	3	11
Barraclough et al., 1974 (256) [N = 100]	80	19	3	—	7
Rich et al., 1986 (20) [N = 283]	44	60	14	5	6
Conwell et al., 1991 (257) [N = 85]	55	42	8	18	11

groups. Each of these approaches is reviewed in the sections that follow.

STUDIES OF SUICIDE IN THE GENERAL POPULATION

Since the mid-1950s, over a dozen retrospective studies of suicide in the general population have been conducted worldwide (Table 23.8). Using a method known as the psychological autopsy, investigators construct a detailed picture of the victim's symptomatology, behaviors, and life circumstances in the weeks and months before death by reviewing records and conducting detailed interviews with knowledgeable informants (254). Psychiatric diagnoses established for victims in six of the most comprehensive of these studies are listed in Table 23.8 (20, 46, 48, 255–257). They differ in sample size, the years that they were conducted, and the criteria by which diagnoses were made. Nonetheless, all these investigations show a remarkable and important consistency in finding diagnosable psychopathology in 90% or more of cases. In general, affective disorders were most common, present in 30–80% of cases, closely followed by substance use disorders in 19–60% of cases. Schizophrenia was diagnosed in 2–14% of completed suicides in these studies.

To explore the marked variation in suicide rates as a function of age and sex (Fig. 23.2), a number of authors have examined differences between males and females who completed suicide. Rich and colleagues (258) compared 143 men and 61 women in their sample from the San Diego suicide study and found that women had a significantly greater mean age at death. There was no difference in the proportion in each group with a substance use disorder diagnosis. However, women were significantly more likely to have had a major depressive disorder. Men used firearms significantly more often and drugs or poison significantly less often as a means of death than did women.

A study of Åsgard (259) of 104 women who committed suicide in Sweden helps to further characterize gender differences in the psychopathology of victims. They found, for example, that 59% met criteria for a mood disorder in the last month of life, a percentage similar to that reported for men. Substance use disorders were present in only 12% of cases. They further found that 63% of their victims had made a suicide attempt at some time in their lives, 36% having done so in the year preceding death. Seventy-one percent

had a past history of psychiatric care, with almost 60% having received treatment in the last year of life. Unfortunately, there are no data on Swedish men with which to compare these figures.

A number of investigators have noted differences in the distribution of psychiatric diagnoses by age. Dorpat and Ripley (255) found schizophrenia to be the most common diagnosis in completed suicides under the age of 40 years, alcoholism most common between ages 40 and 60, and psychotic depression most common in suicides over the age of 60 years. Carlson (260) reanalyzed Robins's detailed case histories of suicides occurring in St. Louis in the 1950s (261) to show that affective disorder diagnoses were more common and alcoholism less frequent in those over 65 years than in younger victims. In a more contemporaneous sample, Rich and colleagues (20) found significantly more substance use disorders and antisocial personality in suicide victims age 30 years and younger than in the older cohort, who were more likely to be suffering from affective illness.

The examination of differences in psychiatric diagnosis by age in completed suicides was the principle objective of a psychological autopsy study by Conwell and colleagues (262). In 151 victims of completed suicide ages 21 to 92 years, multiple regression analyses were used to establish whether age, sex, or their interaction could predict specific diagnoses in suicide victims (unpublished data). They found that increasing age was a significant predictor of major depressive disorder. Younger age predicted schizophrenic illness, while female gender predicted anxiety and somatoform disorder diagnoses. Older victims were less likely to have been hospitalized for psychiatric care or to have ever been in mental health treatment. In those subjects with major depressive disorder, increasing age significantly predicted a single episode rather than recurrent illness. Finally, younger victims were significantly more likely to have multiple co-morbid diagnoses than their older counterparts, whose affective illness was much less likely to be complicated by substance abuse or dependence.

We now turn to more detailed consideration of suicide in specific diagnostic subgroups.

AFFECTIVE DISORDER

Suicide rates in patients with affective illness are far higher than in the general population. Miles (263) reviewed 30 studies in which patients with primary depressive disorders were followed longitudinally. In agreement with Guze and Robins (264), he concluded that approximately 15% of affected individuals will ultimately die by suicide. Several studies have attempted to calculate the rate of suicide in patients with depressive disorder. Pokorny (265) followed 4,800 male veterans for a mean of 5 years, during which time 67 took their own lives. Whereas the overall suicide rate was 279 per 100,000 per year, patients with affective illness diagnoses died by suicide at the rate of 695 per 100,000 per year. Again, age may be a factor. By linking psychiatric case register data with death certificates, Gardner and colleagues (266) calculated a suicide rate for psychiatric patients with a diagnosis of affective psychoses of 351 per 100,000. However, when they divided the population at age 55 years, younger depressives had a rate of 207 per 100,000 compared to a rate of 475 per 100,000 for older patients. Furthermore, they observed that while 2% of the patient population who attempted suicide went on to take their own lives within 1 year, 6% of attempters over age 55 completed suicide within the same time period. These data suggest that elderly people with affective illness may be at higher risk for suicide than both normal elderly and younger depressive individuals as well.

In an attempt to define the clinical characteristics unique to those depressed patients at highest risk for suicide, a number of studies have compared depressed completers with living patients. Barraclough and Pallis (267) found that depressed suicides studied by the psychological autopsy method were more likely to be male, single, and living alone than the comparison group of ambulatory patients with affective disorder diagnoses. Symptoms of insomnia, self-neglect, impaired memory, and a history of suicide attempts also were distinguishing features. Roy (268) matched psychiatric patients with recurrent depressions who were known to have committed suicide with depressed inpatients who had not taken their own lives, and found that significantly more of those who committed suicide had lived alone, suffered early parental loss, and had past histories of suicide attempts. Berglund and Nilsson (269) followed over 1200 psychiatric inpatients with severe affective illness for up to 27 years. Comparing male subjects who committed suicide during the follow-up period with those males who had not, they found an acute onset of illness, marital problems, and lower ratings for psychomotor retardation to distinguish the suicide group. Women completers with depressive disorders had a significantly higher frequency of attempted suicide than other women.

In apparent contrast, Fawcett and colleagues (270) did not find a history of suicide attempts to be a significant predictor of subsequent suicide in 954 patients with major affective disorder followed longitudinally for an average of 4 years. Instead, hopelessness, anhedonia, and mood cycling during the index episode differentiated the 25 patients who had died by suicide from the remainder. However, in a subsequent report after an average of 10 years of follow-up, 32 patients had died by suicide. The researchers divided the

sample into those who had died within 1 year of initial evaluation and those who had died 2–10 years later, in an effort to distinguish short- from long-term predictors. They found that short-term, but not long-term suicide, was associated with severe anhedonia and psychic anxiety, obsessive-compulsive features, global insomnia, acute alcohol intoxication, impairments in concentration, and panic attacks. Symptoms associated with long-term, suicide—2–10 years—were hopelessness, suicidal ideation, and a past history of suicide attempts. The authors suggest that recognition and intervention in short-term risk factors, such as severe anxiety and panic attacks, through appropriate pharmacotherapy, psychotherapy, and environmental manipulation may help to prevent imminent suicide.

Although consensus is lacking, there is no clear association between any subtype of affective illness and suicide. Whereas some studies have found patients with bipolar affective illness to be at lower risk than those with unipolar disorders (271, 272), others have found no difference in suicide rates between unipolar and bipolar patients (57, 273), or even higher risk in the bipolar type (274).

Roose and colleagues (275) found that delusionally depressed patients were overrepresented in suicides committed in an inpatient facility. Others, however, have found no increased risk for suicide in psychotic depressed patients in either short- (276) or long-term follow-up (277).

The posthospitalization period is the time of greatest risk for suicide in affective illness (263), decreasing progressively after the first several years postdischarge. Thirty-two percent of the suicides among patients followed longitudinally by Fawcett and colleagues occurred within 6 months of entry into their study, and 52% within 1 year. Hospital discharge, therefore, represents a time for special vigilance on the part of patients and their caretakers.

SCHIZOPHRENIA

Epidemiologic studies in the United States and other countries estimate that the prevalence of schizophrenia in the general population is approximately 1%. Yet approximately 5–10% of completed suicides carry that diagnosis. The implication that schizophrenics are at much increased risk for completed suicide has been confirmed in a number of long-term follow-up studies, most recently reviewed by Caldwell and Gottesman (278). Based on suicides in follow-up intervals from 4–40 years, suicide rates for schizophrenics have been estimated to be as high as 615 per 100,000 (279), more than 50 times greater than that of the general population. An estimated 10% of schizophrenics ultimately end their lives by suicide (57, 263).

Although some studies have indicated that the standardized mortality ratios for suicide are greater for schizophrenic women than men (280, 281), other investigators have noted a heavy preponderance of men among schizophrenic suicide victims (282–284).

Younger age appears to be a risk factor for suicide in schizophrenics. Breier and Astrachan (282) found the mean age of schizophrenic suicide victims of 30.3 years to be significantly less than that of schizophrenic patient controls, consistent with an earlier report by Roy (283). Similarly, schizophrenic suicide victims have been shown to be significantly younger than suicide victims with other diagnoses (285, 286). With increasing age, however, risk seems to diminish. In a record linkage study, Newman and Bland (287) found the highest risk for suicide among schizophrenic patients age 29 years or less, with a standardized mortality ratio of approximately 33. Between ages 30 and 49 years, however, relative risk decreased to 18 times that of the general population, while in schizophrenics age 50 to 69 years, risk was only seven times that of the general population. Others have reported similar trends, with the exception that peak risk for women occurs approximately 10 years later (281), consistent with their characteristically later onset of illness (288). Perhaps more relevant than age at death is the total duration of illness, which is similar for men and women—typically 5–10 years after initial diagnosis (282–284).

Like patients with other psychiatric disorders, the schizophrenic is at highest risk for suicide in the first weeks and months after admission and discharge from the hospital. In studies of suicide committed while in the hospital, schizophrenia is the most common diagnosis (278). Roy (289) reviewed seven studies revealing that up to 50% of schizophrenic patients who commit suicide do so in the first few weeks and months after discharge. Contrary to popular belief, suicide is less common in the acutely psychotic state than at a time when, as psychosis resolves, the patient is more vulnerable to a depressive syndrome. In such situations the proper diagnosis and treatment of depression, which may be difficult to differentiate from medication effects or the negative symptomatology of the psychotic process, are critical.

Other factors associated with risk of suicide in people with schizophrenia include unemployment and a relapsing, deteriorating course (283), particularly in individuals with higher levels of educational achievement (284), which result in feelings of inadequacy and hopelessness regarding their future (290). As with depressed patients, schizophrenics with a past history of serious attempts to take their lives also places them at greater risk for completed suicide (282, 290).

SUBSTANCE USE DISORDERS

Through long-term follow-up of hospitalized patients, Black (291) and others have clearly demonstrated that patients with alcohol and other drug abuse have excess mortality not only because of suicide but due to physical causes, accidental, and other violent deaths as well. Lindberg and Ågren (292), for example, found in 2–20-year follow-up that the relative risk of death from all causes was three times greater for male alcoholics, and over five times greater for female alcoholics, than the general Swedish population. Furthermore, male alcoholics were 7.9 times and female alcoholics 15.2 times more likely than expected to die by

suicide. Murphy and Wetzel (293) reviewed the literature in critical examination of the frequently quoted estimate that the lifetime risk of suicide and alcoholism was as high as 15%. They found this figure untenable based on suicide rates reported in both short- and long-term follow-up studies, and on the estimation that the alcoholic population at risk for suicide is approximately 5.6 million people in the United States. They calculated a lifetime risk for suicide of 2–3.4% in alcoholics in the United States and other Western countries with similar suicide rates, or 60 to 120 times higher than that of the nonpsychiatrically ill.

Whereas depression is more common among completed suicides with increasing age, substance use disorders are less prevalent. The most frequently cited reason for this observation is early mortality among alcoholics from other causes (294), leaving a smaller absolute number subject to suicide risk in later life. However, suicide rates among alcoholics may increase with age (266), with the duration of abusive drinking being an important variable. Murphy (295) calculated that the mean duration of alcoholism prior to death was 19.8 years for men and 12.3 years for women. However, alcoholics with an older age at death were more likely to have had a late onset of the disorder, and thus a duration of illness similar to that of younger alcoholic victims.

Far fewer data are available on the suicidal behavior and risk of other substance users. Allgulander and colleagues (296) noted four suicides among 40 patients with sedative hypnotic dependence in 4–6-year follow-up. Social deterioration and a prevalence of depressive symptoms were characteristic. Suicide rates for heroin addicts have been estimated to range from 82 to 350 per 100,000, with 2.5–7% dying by their own hand. These age-adjusted rates are five to 20 times greater than that for the general population. Susan Murphy and colleagues (297) found that 17.3% of 533 opiate addicts treated in a drug dependency unit had a past history of at least one suicide attempt. Marzuk and colleagues (298) recently reported that cocaine metabolites were detectable in over 20% of New York City suicide victims age 60 years and younger, with the highest prevalence (45.7%) in young Hispanic males. Seven percent of all cocaine-positive deaths in New York City in 1986 were suicides. In the San Diego Suicide Study, Fowler and colleagues (299) found that 30% of suicide victims under age 30 years had histories of cocaine use. The authors speculate that the striking rise in suicide rates in young adults over the last three decades is in part a consequence of increasing substance use over the same time period.

Because drug and alcohol abuse have such widespread effects both in the short and long term on the individual's physical health, social network, and psychological equilibrium, the mechanism of an association between suicide and substance abuse is obscure. Comorbidity is common. Data from the Epidemiologic Catchment Area (ECA) Study show that individuals with either an alcohol or drug use disorder were over seven times more likely than the rest of the population to have a second addictive disorder, and that 37% of those with alcoholism and 53% of those with other drug addictions, had a comorbid mental illness (300). Among alcoholics who completed suicide, Murphy found that 72% met criteria for a definite or probable major affective disorder (301). Citing five other studies that yielded qualitatively similar results, he speculates that the presence of depression in alcoholics is a major risk factor for suicide in that group.

Additional data from studies of alcoholics (302, 303) and other substance abusers (43, 304) have demonstrated that a disproportionate number of suicide victims with substance use disorders had experienced the loss of a close interpersonal relationship in the last 6 weeks of life. This concentration was markedly statistically different from suicides with major depressive disorders in the absence of substance use co-morbidity.

In a subsequent analysis, Murphy et al. (301) compared alcoholic suicides studied by the psychological autopsy method with data from living alcoholic controls. They identified seven features that appeared to be related to suicide: continued drinking, development of a major depressive episode, communication of suicidal intent, poor social supports, unemployment, living alone, and a serious intervening medical illness. Their findings underscored the need in the treatment of alcohol and drug abuse to achieve and sustain abstinence, diagnose and aggressively treat depressive symptoms, and to be especially alert for suicide at times of disruption and further impoverishment of the patient's social support network.

Biological factors require further clarification. Prolonged exposure to alcohol has been shown to produce progressive depressive symptoms, both in normals and in abusive drinkers (305). The toxic effects of alcohol on the central nervous system are well known. There is an inverse correlation between the length of abstinence from alcohol and CSF 5HIAA levels, and some indication that alcoholics have deficits in central 5HT function that chronic alcohol consumption serves only to further deplete those levels (306). Decreased tryptophan to total amino acid ratios have been demonstrated in a subgroup of alcoholics at risk for depression, suicide, and aggressive behavior (307) as well. Like major depressives, alcoholics have been shown to have a blunted ACTH response to CRF infusion, and to escape from dexamethasone suppression in the acute withdrawal (308).

OTHER PSYCHIATRIC DISORDERS

Structured diagnostic criteria for personality disorders and the diagnostic instruments with which to measure them have yet to be applied in a systematic way to psychological autopsy method. Hence, prevalence rates of character pathology in populations of suicide completers represent only estimates, ranging from 3–18%. However, longitudinal study of clinical populations has convincingly demonstrated an increased risk for premature death from suicide in patients with personality disorders (309, 291). Individuals with borderline personality disorder (310) and antisocial personality disorder (263, 311) appear to be at higher risk for subsequent suicide attempts and completed suicide than other character disorders.

Individuals with panic disorder (312), particularly if accompanied by another psychiatric illness (313) are significantly more likely to have a past history of suicide attempts than the general population. However, anxiety disorder diagnoses are rarely made in psychological autopsy studies. It remains unclear whether this discrepancy represents an artifact of the psychological autopsy methodology, obtaining information from informants, or whether suicide attempts in panic disorder signify less risk for subsequent completed suicide than does suicidal behavior in major depression, schizophrenia, or substance use disorders.

NEUROLOGICAL ILLNESS

The majority of studies that have focused upon completed suicide in neurological illness have been epidemiologically based, seeking to examine the prevalence and risk of suicide in known neurodegenerative disorders such as Huntington's disease and multiple sclerosis (MS). Increased suicide risk in these disorders relative to the general population is suggestive, in part, of a biological basis for the behavior (either primary or secondary). Supplementation of these data by clinicopathological-correlative studies, most often in the form of single case design, allows for more specific examination of structural or neurochemical brain abnormalities.

The neurological conditions in which suicide has been studied in greatest detail include Huntington's disease, multiple sclerosis, Parkinson's disease, epilepsy, and traumatic spinal cord injury. For the most part, these investigations have been retrospective, utilizing archival databases such as death certificates, hospital records, and federal or state disease rosters. Less frequently, the information gathered has been supplemented by seeking interviews with identified patients, or family members when the patient is deceased. On rare occasions, longitudinal research has been conducted, the goal of which has been to study the natural history of a specific disease. In such cases, evaluation of suicide and related behaviors has had a secondary or incidental focus. The study of attempted suicide in neurological illness has received less attention than completed suicide and can best be described, with the exception of the epilepsy literature, as anecdotal.

HUNTINGTON'S DISEASE

Huntington's disease (HD) is a neurodegenerative, autosomally dominant genetic disorder of adult onset. The major neuropathological changes include neuronal degeneration in the caudate nucleus, putamen, and associated pathways (314). In addition to progressive choreiform movement abnormalities, psychiatric sequelae, including mood disorder, personality change, and dementia are considered hallmark features of this disorder (315–317). Perhaps because of its clear neuropsychiatric nature, the cognitive and emotional symptoms, including suicide, have been of interest to study since the first description of this disease by George Huntington in 1872 (318). Early work focused upon case history, which included anecdotal reference to completed or attempted suicide. Two investigations were carried out to investigate the course, progression, and inherited transmission patterns of the disease. The first of these studies, conducted by Minski and Guttmann (319), was a comprehensive review of identified HD cases in England. Identified cases were followed up with personal interview, revealing that four subjects had attempted suicide. Psychiatric syndromes found in the group included schizophrenia, paranoid reaction, affective disorder, and alcoholism. The method of psychiatric diagnosis and the description of suicidal behavior were not clearly defined, nor was the relationship between suicidal behavior and psychiatric diagnosis explored.

Chandler's (320) survey of 761 HD individuals in Michigan found that 7.8% of male, and 6.4% of female deaths were suicides. Because subjects were not routinely followed until death, these figures may be underestimates. The authors concluded that suicide was an "important cause of death in non-institutionalized HD patients," especially in early onset cases (15–40 years).

To examine the sociopsychiatric consequences associated with HD, Dewhurst and colleagues (317) studied 102 HD patients and their families. They found 10 completed suicides, 11 individuals who had attempted suicide, and 13 "self-mutilators" among subjects with a HD diagnosis.

In a study designed to evaluate gender-related differences in psychopathology, Tamir et al. (321) retrospectively reviewed the clinical records of 32 psychiatrically hospitalized HD patients. The authors identified one of 13 women and eight of 19 men who were "depressed," with no men and three women who were "suicidal" during the time of hospitalization. They concluded that there was a greater prevalence of depression and suicidality in women, with greater "aggression" in men with HD. Methods and definition of psychiatric terms were not specified.

Of 199 patients with HD admitted to psychiatric departments in Norway during a 59-year period, one individual subsequently attempted and one completed suicide (322). When compared with non-HD psychiatric admissions, there was no evidence to suggest increased risk of completed suicide in the HD group.

The primary purpose of two studies was to examine the prevalence of completed suicide in HD. Schoenfeld et al., (323) conducted record reviews and family interviews for 506 cases of HD deaths in the New England area. Known cause of death could be established in 157 cases. Twenty suicides were identified, making it the third leading cause of death in this group. Making adjustments for age and gender in comparing their findings with the Massachusetts Census, the authors concluded that HD patients age 50 years and over were at eight times higher risk for suicide than the general population. There was no increased risk for HD patients in the younger age group.

Using the National HD Research Roster, Farrer (324) examined the proportion of deaths in 831 patients that were due to suicide, through a detailed questionnaire sent to families. Of 452 individuals identified as deceased, 25 had died of suicide, four times greater than would be expected in a general population sample. Of the suicide victims, 27.6% had attempted suicide at least once (18.5% of males, 22.2% of females). Interestingly, age at onset of HD was not correlated with completed suicide. However, suicide did tend to occur in early to middle stages of the illness. Cautions regarding this work include the lack of age and gender adjustment, as well as a relatively substantial dropout rate.

The advent of preclinical genetic testing has fostered examination of psychiatric sequelae, including suicidal behavior, in asymptomatic persons at risk for expression of the HD gene. Kessler (325) conducted semistructured interviews and administered multiple psychological symptom inventories in their investigation of attitudes toward predicative testing. Of 69 subjects, 37% reported a history of suicide attempts in family members, with 34% identified as having a family member who had been psychiatrically hospitalized. Eleven percent reported they would consider suicide if they tested positive. Similarly, 29% of 131 at risk individuals surveyed by Mastromauro and colleagues (326) stated that they would consider suicide if testing revealed that they carried the HD gene. These latter two studies highlight the psychological impact of the illness on an individual and his/her family (327), complicating efforts to correlate suicide with the brain lesions of HD.

Only two case studies of HD patients have attempted to correlate neurobiological measures with suicidal behavior. Albin (328) reported the results of immunohistochemical analysis, in conjunction with a structured family interview, of a 32-year-old presymptomatic (i.e., no movement abnormalities) woman whose death was attributable to suicide. Her history was also notable for two prior suicide attempts, beginning at age 21 years. Psychiatrically, she was diagnosed as having cyclothymia with superimposed major depression. Neurochemical analysis revealed selective impairment of striatal enkephalinergic neurons projecting to the globus pallidus. As well, substance P neurons projecting to the substantia nigra were of reduced density.

The second case study was reported by Lam et al. (329). It described a woman in her 30s who attempted suicide following positive genetic testing results. She, too, had multiple suicide attempts in the remote past, although no significant psychiatric symptoms had been reported for the last 13 years. PET scan results obtained prior to the index suicide attempt revealed diminished glucose metabolism in both caudate nuclei. As in the previous study, the relationship between suicidal behavior, other disease variables, and the observed neurochemical abnormalities is unclear but worthy of further pursuit.

In summary, multiple investigations of completed and attempted suicide in HD are suggestive of increased prevalence and risk in these patients, with most studies focusing on completed suicide. Calculated risk has varied significantly across studies, ranging from one to eight times that of normals, with the most consistent estimate approximately four times that of the general population. An increased incidence of other psychopathological symptoms is also consistently reported, although the co-morbidity of other psychiatric phenomena within the context of suicidal behavior has not been addressed. These findings must be considered with caution, given the diversity of populations and control groups utilized across studies, as well as the clear methodologic difficulties inherent to most investigations. Specific study of neuropathological abnormalities in relation to suicide in HD is in its infancy, with no research as yet conducted in which suicidal behavior serves as a primary focus.

MULTIPLE SCLEROSIS

Multiple sclerosis (MS) is a chronic demyelinating disease of the CNS, more common in females than males (1.7:1) (330). The course is progressive but unpredictable, and patients may have multiple periods of illness exacerbation and remission. Although there is a site preference for the periventricular white matter, particularly surrounding the anterior horns, lesions may occur virtually anywhere in the brain and spinal cord, causing considerable variability across patients with regard to neuropathological changes (330). Onset usually occurs in the 20s and 30s. Mental disorder, including depression, has long been associated with this disease (331). These symptoms may precede the onset of focal neurological abnormality, leading to misdiagnosis of primary psychiatric illness in some patients. To date, the most comprehensive evaluation of coexisting psychopathology in MS patients was conducted by Joffe (332). Through structured clinical interview and affective rating scales administered to 100 MS clinic patients, they reported a 42% lifetime prevalence of depressive illness, with 13% fulfilling criteria for a major depressive episode. Thirteen percent of patients received a diagnosis of bipolar affective disorder. The authors suggested that MS and affective disorder may share a common pathobiology, citing as additional evidence the lack of any correlation between level of functional disability and the presence of mood disorder. Unfortunately, suicidal behavior was not examined in this well-designed study. Given the high prevalence of depressive illness within the context of a chronic debilitating illness, the potential for suicide, and its rate in this population, is clearly of import.

Of four studies that attempted to establish the prevalence of suicide in patients with MS, all but one found patients to be at increased risk. Schwartz and Pierron (333), who examined death certificates only, found four suicides among 408 MS-related deaths in Michigan, a proportion of suicides (1%) no greater than is seen in the general population. Sadovnick et al. (334) found 18 of 119 deaths in MS patients for which a cause could be established were due to suicide, estimated to be a rate 7.5 times higher than expected.

The most recent and carefully conducted study was an epidemiologic investigation by Stenager and Stenager (335) of 6088 Danish patients with MS. Adjusting for age, gender, and effects of early mortality in MS from causes other than suicide, the expected suicide rate in this population was significantly lower than they observed (2.0% vs. 3.7%). The risk of suicide in MS was greatest for males, for individuals with disease onset prior to age 30, and for those diagnosed before age 40 years. Furthermore, in two studies of the physical illnesses found in victims of completed suicide, MS was present in numbers significantly greater than would be expected in the general population (52, 336).

Given the close association of affective illness with both MS and suicide, one would expect to find depressive symptomatology in a large proportion of MS patients who took their lives. Only one preliminary report has directly addressed this issue. Of 18 MS patient suicides investigated by psychological autopsy, 83% suffered with a major depressive episode (Berman, unpublished data).

There is no research with an MS population, to our knowledge, in which the focus is attempted suicide. One Greek study did examine a series of 50 outpatients with concurrent psychiatric and physical illness, referred following a suicide attempt (337). These subjects were compared to 85 suicide attempters without concurrent physical illness. Forty percent of the concurrent illness group suffered from neurological disease, of which MS represented 2%. Major affective illness was identified as the most common co-morbid psychiatric syndrome. The physical illness attempter group had a greater incidence of "organic" and "major" depression, were prone to more violent attempts, and had profiles "more similar to completers" than did the attempters without physical illness.

In summary, there is clear evidence to support the findings of increased suicide risk in this population, with estimates that 3.7–5.7% of MS patients take their own lives. Affective illness—primarily major depressive syndromes and bipolar illness—is also present in increased numbers, although the relation between mood disorder and suicidal behavior in this population has yet to be systematically studied. In addition, direct studies of brain abnormalities in MS patients with psychiatric symptoms are almost nonexistent, with no study focusing primarily upon either attempted or completed suicide.

PARKINSON'S DISEASE

Parkinson's disease (PD) is a progressive neurodegenerative disorder that affects the nigrostriatal system, resulting in movement abnormalities, including tremor, gait disturbance, rigidity, and bradykinesia. Sensory symptoms and cognitive phenomena, including dementia, may also be part of the disease (338). Primary PD, considered idiopathic in its etiology, commonly has onset in the 6th and 7th decade of life. It is surprising that suicidal behaviors have rarely been studied in PD because depressive disorders are estimated to occur simultaneously in 20–90% of cases, the majority of studies suggesting a 40–60% prevalence rate (339). Furthermore, PD is associated with degradation of both central dopaminergic and serotonergic function (340, 341), systems that the pre- and postmortem neurobiological evidence reviewed earlier suggests may be dysregulated in suicidal states. One study, the focus of which was to examine the prevalence of physical disease in victims of completed suicide, found PD present at a rate four times greater than expected based on the prevalence of PD in the general population (336).

In contrast, Hoehn and Yahr (342) reviewed clinical records and death certificates of 672 idiopathic PD cases. Of 340 deaths, only three were attributed to suicide. In 60 cases, cause of death could not be determined. While age, gender, and percent of deaths were compared with statistics for the general population of New York City for several causes of death, suicide was not included in the comparative analysis. No study, to our knowledge, has examined the prevalence of attempted suicide in PD.

EPILEPSY

Epilepsy is the term used to describe a heterogeneous group of disorders whose common feature is multiple seizure episodes. Single or multiple brain regions may be involved. Problems with use of epilepsy as a neurobiological model include the heterogeneity of symptoms, etiologies, and brain regions affected. Also, in the cases of childhood onset seizures, the degree to which early CNS insult may affect the developing brain is not well understood.

Comorbid psychological variables, including suicide risk, have been a topic of considerable interest in the literature. Depressive symptoms are common in epilepsy (343), and severe depressive illness has been estimated to occur in 19% of temporal lobe epileptics (344). As well, an increased prevalence of psychosis has been identified. It is not surprising, therefore, that estimates of suicide risk in individuals with epilepsy are three to four times higher than the general population (345).

The most comprehensive and methodologically sound study of completed suicide in epilepsy was conducted by White and associates (346). Evaluating the records of 2099 epilepsy patients admitted to a British epilepsy center, they concluded that suicide was among the chief causes of excess death in this population. Of 636 deaths that had occurred, 21 were by suicide, a rate 5.4 times greater than expected.

Mendez and Doss (347) studied the factors associated with four completed suicides that had occurred among 1611 epileptics seen in the neurology clinic. Three of the suicide victims were male, three were actively psychotic, and all four had a temporal lobe seizure focus.

Two major review articles have been published regarding completed suicide in epilepsy. Reviewing 16 studies, Barraclough (348) concluded that severe epileptics were at five times greater risk of suicide than the general population, with up to 25 times greater risk in individuals with temporal

lobe epilepsy. Matthews and Barabas (349), in their review of five studies, arrived at a similar estimate that approximately 5% of epileptics die by their own hand. Because the articles reviewed in both papers were diverse in their methodology and populations, the overall findings should be considered tentative.

Like completed suicide, attempted suicide rates among epileptics is very high. These individuals are estimated to be at four to five times greater risk of attempted suicide than the general population (343, 350). Factors distinguishing epileptic attempters from attempters with other diagnoses include recent alcohol use (350), psychotic symptomatology, borderline personality disorder, and a past history of impulsive attempts (345). Comparing 325 epileptics who had made suicide attempts with 166 nonattempter epileptic controls, Batzel and Dodrill (351) found an increased incidence of anxiety, "general psychopathology," and diminished ego strength on the Minnesota Multiphasic Personality Inventory (MMPI) profile of the suicide attempter group. No difference was found on the depression or schizophrenia subscales. Unfortunately, neither formal diagnoses nor specific symptoms were considered.

ACUTE SPINAL CORD TRAUMA

Investigation of suicidal behavior in traumatic spinal cord injury is of potential research interest for a variety of reasons. As with increased prevalence of completed suicide in other populations, the identification of risk factors is critical to effective diagnosis and treatment of vulnerable patients. Also, given that these static lesions are confined to the spinal cord, this group may represent a suitable control group when trying to establish neurobiological models of suicide in other neurological disease entities.

A series of rather large investigations have been conducted to investigate mortality and associated cause of death in spinal injury cases. Increased mortality in this group has been well established (352–354), as has increased frequency of death by suicide (353–358). Risk estimates ranging from two to six times that of the general population have been calculated (358), with the most methodologically sound investigations reporting a four- to fivefold increase (353, 354). Younger age (353, 354, 357) and quadriplegia (352–354) place patients with spinal cord injury at increased risk, particularly in the first few years following injury (352–354, 357).

Charlifue (358) compared 42 completed suicides with spinal cord lesions with a spinal-injured group matched for gender, age at injury, and lesion location. Preinjury variables associated with suicide included a history of alcohol, drug abuse, or depression. Postinjury variables of import included despondency, shame, apathy and helplessness, anger, alcohol abuse, destructive behaviors, and attempted suicide. Interestingly, 7% of completed suicides suffered their spinal cord injury during an attempt on their lives, whereas no control group patients acquired their injury in that manner. Judd and Brown (359) identified six suicides among 342 spinal cord patients occurring over a 5-year period. Clinical aspects common to the completed suicide group included male gender, "schizoid, depressive or narcissistic personality traits," alcohol or drug abuse, and the presence of "significant depression." These findings should be considered tentative, given their descriptive, nonempirical nature.

In summary, completed suicide in traumatic spinal cord injury patients appears to occur at a rate that is four to five times that of the general population when mortality and demographic factors are considered. Those at greatest risk include male quadriplegics in the first few years following injury. Although the prevalence of affective illness in this population has not been established, depressive symptomatology is common. Studies of attempted suicide in traumatic spinal injury have yet to be conducted.

OTHER NEUROLOGICAL DISORDERS

Cerebral neoplasms and cerebral vascular accidents (CVAs) are other neurological disorders of potential interest in the study of attempted suicide, particularly given the reportedly high incidence of depressive illness in the latter group (360). No focused research on attempted or completed suicide has been conducted in either of these groups of disorders, although anecdotal case illustrations are reported (331). Studies of the prevalence of specific physical illnesses in suicide have suggested a possible increased incidence of completed suicide in individuals with CNS neoplasms. In these studies, illness prevalence rates were compared to prevalence rates for the disease in the general population (52, 336). The results are less consistent for CVA, with one study reporting a higher rate of stroke in completed suicide (52), and another finding no suggestion of increased illness representation in a completed suicide population (336).

SUMMARY

Increased risk for suicide has been fairly well established in MS, epilepsy, and traumatic spinal cord injury, with probable increased risk associated with HD as well. The study of suicidal behavior in PD has been too limited to allow definite conclusions. Phenomenological description of specific suicidal behaviors in these disorders is scant.

The relative contributions of a high incidence of comorbid psychiatric sequelae, particularly depressive illness, has also been well documented. The degree to which depressive illness or other psychiatric phenomena such as psychosis serve to mediate suicidal behavior in neurological illness, vs. suicidal behavior existing as an independent disease-related behavior, is unclear. As well, comprehensive assessment of pertinent demographic and socioenvironmental variables such as age, gender, functional disability, and disease prognosis issues have not been adequately addressed.

Clearly, the development of systematic research that addresses and rigorously defines this comprehensive array of factors within specific neurological illnesses will represent an important step toward the development of neurobiological

Table 23.9. Summary of Risk Factors for Suicide

Older
Male
White
Living alone
History of suicide attempt(s)
Psychiatric illness
    affective disorder
    substance abuse/dependence
    schizophrenia
Medical illness
Neurological illness
    MS
    epilepsy
    traumatic spinal cord injury
    HD
Life stressors
    recent or threatened loss
Lack of available support
Inability to accept help

models of completed and attempted suicide. At the very least, the application of such carefully designed investigations will serve to provide greater clarity in the identification of pertinent risk factors for suicidal behavior in these disorders.

PREVENTION AND TREATMENT

Despite decades of research and progress in the recognition of risk factors for suicide, efforts to construct a useful and sufficiently sensitive and specific predictive scale have thus far failed (265, 361). Although many hope that the development of biological markers will greatly enhance our ability to identify individuals at risk, the body of knowledge we now possess can serve only in a nonspecific manner to enhance our clinical judgment (Table 23.9).

The subjective nature of suicidal thinking, along with the relatively low point prevalence of suicidal behavior, makes the phenomenon difficult to study. At the same time, the multiple causality of suicide suggests the possibility of intervention at numerous sites, any of which may be effective in resolving at least the immediate crisis. As a general rule, any intervention that decreases the subject's "intolerable psychological pain" (362) will diminish his/her suicide risk. The literature on the treatment of suicidal people is vast (363). For this text, however, we have structured a summary discussion using the terms of preventive medicine: *primary prevention*—those strategies concerned with preventing the occurrence of suicidal behavior or the development of the suicidal state; *secondary prevention*—the early recognition of the suicidal crisis, intervention to reduce its progression to complete suicide, and treatments that lead to its full resolution; and *tertiary prevention*—a term used in this context to signify interventions targeted at those who survive the death of a loved one by suicide, decreasing the psychiatric and social morbidity of this special "at-risk" group.

Primary Prevention

The definition of demographic and psychosocial risk factors for suicide suggest that interventions made at the level of social policy may have a beneficial effect on suicide rates. For example, if social isolation were diminished for depressed elders through more vigorous outreach and socialization programs, fewer may choose to end their lives. In young adult cohorts, drug abuse prevention programs should be expected to diminish rates of death by all violent means, including suicide.

Gun control is a third example for which more data are available to suggest benefits to suicide rates by education or legislative intervention. Sixty percent of people who die by suicide each year in the U.S. use a firearm to kill themselves. Almost 50% of all firearm-related deaths are suicides. Although the subject remains politically controversial, a number of recent studies have provided evidence to suggest that more restrictive gun control legislation would lower suicide rates. In a carefully conducted psychological autopsy study comparing adolescent suicide victims with psychiatric inpatients and normal controls, Brent and colleagues (364) found that the presence of a firearm in the home was significantly associated with completed suicide. The manner in which the gun was stored (e.g., in a locked place without ammunition) had no impact on the likelihood that it would be used for suicide. Sloan and colleagues (365) compared suicide rates between two locales with markedly different gun control regulations. Although risk of death from suicide did not significantly differ between the two regions, suicide by handguns was far higher in the region with less restrictive laws. Loftin, et al. (366) compared rates of gun related death in the District of Columbia before and after the adoption of restrictive hand gun policies and found a 25% decrease in firearm homicides and suicides after the law went into effect. There was no such drop in the surrounding metropolitan area, where the laws remain unchanged, and no compensatory increase in suicides by other means. Although it appears that access to means of suicide with greater potential lethality is associated with higher rates of completed suicide (367), there is ongoing debate about whether removal of more lethal means will lead only to substitution of other methods (365, 368).

Perhaps of greatest potential benefit, however, are efforts to educate the public and their health care providers about the warning signs of suicide and about its close association with treatable psychiatric illness. A great many myths about suicide are commonly held by the public. One such misconception is that, if a person truly wants to commit suicide, there is little that can be done to prevent him. Other myths are that people who threaten suicide will not follow through, or that discussing suicide with a depressed person may lead them to the act (11). Given these misconceptions, people may fail to recognize the need for intervention or understand its potential benefits.

In addition to education of the general public about suicide, suicidal elderly may particularly benefit from edu-

cation of health care professionals. Numerous studies have shown that up to 75% of elderly suicide victims had seen a physician in the last month of life (53, 369). However, physicians in general have limited knowledge of suicide risk (370) and often fail to recognize and adequately treat depressive disorders in primary care settings (371, 372). Given the association between affective illness and suicide, therefore, it is reasonable to conclude that a program to educate primary care providers on the recognition and aggressive treatment of affective disorders in late life would decrease suicide rates in that subgroup of the population. This hypothesis has been validated in one Swedish study (373).

Secondary Prevention

Secondary prevention efforts can be divided into those concerning assessment of individuals at risk and treatment interventions. Assessment relies heavily on the recognition of risk factors previously noted. As with any medical tool, however, risk factors are only as useful as the skill with which they are applied in any particular case. For more detailed discussions of assessment and interview techniques, the reader is referred to the many excellent texts in this area (362, 374).

Generally, assessment of an individual's suicidality must begin with a direct, yet sensitive, discussion with the patient about the nature and extent of his suicidal ideation, including the potential lethality of any plans the individual has considered. One should carefully define the nature and extent of the patient's social support network and the elements in their environment that may be mobilized to ameliorate a suicidal crisis. Most important, one must determine the patient's willingness and ability to work with his/her caretakers in finding alternative solutions to suicide.

In the presence of more highly developed suicidal ideation and planning, the absence of helpful supports in the patient's social network, and with resistance by the patient to available interventions, hospitalization may be lifesaving. In the great majority of cases, suicidal thoughts are transient, a symptom of illness that emerges at times of episodic crisis, and which resolves with treatment. Therefore, the maintenance of the individual's safety—even by involuntary hospitalization or restraint—will almost always lead, following appropriate treatment, to the resolution of suicidal thoughts. In less emergent situations, outpatient treatment may be a viable alternative, particularly if family and friends can be responsibly engaged in a supportive supervisory role.

Psychiatric consultation should be obtained for all suicidal patients to help assess the extent of risk and establish a psychiatric diagnosis and formulation. This latter element of the database includes a thorough assessment of the individual's intrapersonal (psychological/cognitive) resources, most prominent defense mechanisms, and the life stressors that have led to the current situation. With an understanding of these factors, one can better define with the patient the source of his/her intolerable pain, and thereby a means to ameliorate it. The wish for death is **always** ambivalently held by the suicidal person (362). As articulated by Edwin Shneidman, "The clinical rule is: Reduce the level of suffering, often just a little bit, and the individual will choose to live" (362, p. 5). This strategy, in addition to the maintenance of the patient's safety, is the short-term goal of treatment.

Having established the patient's safety and defused the acute suicidal crisis, one can afford to shift the focus of treatment to longer-term goals: the evaluation and treatment of psychiatric illness, resolution of conflicts, and augmentation of internal defenses and external supports so that the individual can cope more effectively with new and ongoing stressors in his/her life. The choice of treatment modalities, which depends of course on the specific needs of the patient, may include a wide range of effective somatic and/or psychological therapies.

Pharmacotherapeutic interventions are primarily directed at the psychiatric condition of which suicidal ideation and behavior may be symptomatic manifestations (161). Because it would be ethically wrong to withhold antidepressant therapies from affectively ill individuals at risk for suicide, and because of the low point prevalence of completed suicide, there are no controlled outcome studies to confirm the generally held clinical observation that antidepressants decrease suicide risk. Only electroconvulsive therapy (ECT) has been demonstrated to decrease suicidal outcomes in depressed patients followed prospectively (375–377). However, the emerging evidence that abnormalities in central serotonergic function underlie suicide suggests that selective serotonergic reuptake inhibitors or agonists may have a role in the treatment of the suicidal person independent from their antidepressant effects (378). Much more research is needed on the neurobiological correlates of suicidal behavior before specific recommendations can be formulated.

In addition to somatic therapies, the suicidal individual may respond to a range of psychological, cognitive, and behavioral treatment modalities (379), all of which have been thoroughly reviewed elsewhere (380).

TERTIARY PREVENTION

Despite the best efforts of all involved, suicides will continue to occur. Although empirical studies are few (381), there is a growing consensus that the grief following a death by suicide involves a complex combination of depression, guilt, and anger that is distinctive from "normal" bereavement. It is a grief that may place the survivor at increased risk for psychiatric morbidity and suicide mortality (382). Therefore, treatment should not end with the death of a patient by suicide. The important tasks that remain include attention to the impact of the suicide on the patient's survivors—family, friends, and health care providers, including the physician her/himself.

The recognition of survivors as a large group in need of recognition and services has led to the development of a broad network of self-help and support groups (383). As with almost every other aspect of suicide, however, there

remains a great need for carefully conducted, ethically sound, and clinically sensitive research. As we learn more about the differential roles played by social, psychological, and biological determinants, suicide may, like other illnesses, give up the mystery and stigma in which it is shrouded.

References

1. Farberow NL. Cultural history of suicide. In: Farberow NL, ed. Suicide in different cultures. Baltimore: University Park Press, 1975:1–15.
2. Eichelman B. Aggressive behavior: from laboratory to clinic: Quo vadit? Arch Gen Psychiatry 1992;49:488–492.
3. Linehan MM. Suicidal people: one population or two? In: Mann JJ, Stanley M, eds. Psychobiology of suicidal behavior. New York: New York Academy of Sciences, 1986:16–33.
4. Berman AL. Self-destructive behavior in suicide: Epidemiology and taxonomy. In: Roberts AR ed. Self-destructive behavior. Springfield: Charles C Thomas, 1975:5–20.
5. Farberow NL. Indirect self-destructive behavior: classification and characteristics. In: Farberow NL ed. The many faces of suicide. New York: McGraw-Hill, 1980:15–27.
6. Kreitman N. Parasuicide. London: John Wiley & Sons, 1977.
7. Pattison EM, Kahan J. The deliberate self-harm syndrome. Am J Psychiatry 1983;140:867–872.
8. Litman RE. Psychodynamics of indirect self-destructive behavior. In: Farberow N, ed. The many faces of suicide. New York: McGraw-Hill, 1980:28–40.
9. Mościcki EK, O'Carroll P, Rae DS, Locke BZ, Roy A, Regier DA. Suicide attempts in the epidemiologic catchment area study. Yale J Biol Med 1988;61:259–268.
10. Parkin D, Stengel E. Incidence of suicidal attempts in an urban community. Brit Med J 1965;2:133–138.
11. Fremouw WJ, de Perczel M, Ellis TE. Suicide risk: assessment and response guidelines. New York: Pergamon Press, 1990.
12. McCarthy PD, Walsh D. Suicide in Dublin: I. The under reporting of suicide and the consequences for national statistics. Brit J Psychiatry 1975;126:301–308.
13. Speechley M, Stavraky KM. The adequacy of suicide statistics for use in epidemiology and public health. Can J Public Health 1991;82:38–42.
14. Barraclough BM. Differences between national suicide rates. Brit J Psychiatry 1973;122:95–96.
15. Sainsbury P. Suicide in London. Maudsley Monograph No. 1. London: Chapman & Hall, 1955.
16. Atkinson MW, Kesselblank N, Dalgaard JB. The comparability of suicide rates. Brit J Psychiatry 1975;127:247–256.
17. National Center for Health Statistics. Advance report of final mortality statistics. Monthly vital statistics report. Hyattsville, MD: Public Health Service, 1994.
18. Solomon MI, Hellon CP. Suicide and age in Alberta, Canada, 1951 to 1977. Arch Gen Psychiatry 1980;37:511–513.
19. Busse EW. Geropsychiatry: social dimensions. In: Maletta GJ, ed. Survey reports on the aging nervous system. DHEW Publication No. 74-296; Washington, DC: U.S. Government Printing Office, 1974:195–225.
20. Rich CL, Young D, Fowler RC. San Diego suicide study: I. Young vs. old subjects. Arch Gen Psychiatry 1986;43:577–582.
21. Murphy GE, Wetzel RD. Suicide risk by birth cohort in the United States, 1949 to 1974. Arch Gen Psychiatry 1980;37:519–523.
22. Manton KG, Blazer DG, Woodbury MA. Suicide in middle age and later life: sex and race specific life table and cohort analyses. Gerontology 1987;42:219–227.
23. Murphy E, Lindesay J, Grundy E. 60 years of suicide in England and Wales: a cohort study. Arch Gen Psychiatry 1986;43:969–976.
24. Goldney RD, Katsikitis M. Cohort analysis of suicide rates in Australia. Arch Gen Psychiatry 1983;40:71–74.

25. Meehan PJ, Saltzman LE, Sattin RW. Suicides among older United States residents: Epidemiologic characteristics and trends. Am J Public Health 1991;81:1198–1200.
26. Chew K, McCleary R. The spring peak in suicides: a cross-national analysis. Soc Sci Med 1995;40:223–230.
27. McCleary R, Chew KSY, Hellsten JJ, Flynn-Bransford M. Age- and sex-specific cycles in United States suicides, 1973 to 1985. Am J Public Health 1991;81:1494–1497.
28. Stillion JM, McDowell EE, May JH. Suicide across the lifespan—premature exits. New York: Hemisphere Publishing Corp., 1989.
29. Kreitman N. Suicide, age, and marital status. Psychol Med 1988;18:121–128.
30. MacMahon B, Pugh TF. Suicide and the widowed. Am J Epidemiology 1965;81:23–31.
31. Durkheim E. Suicide. 1st ed. New York: The Free Press, 1966.
32. Templer DI, Veleber DM. Suicide rate and religion within the United States. Psychol Rep 1980;47:898.
33. Maris, R. Pathways to suicide: a survey of self-destructive behaviors. Baltimore: Johns Hopkins University Press, 1981.
34. Brenner M. Mental illness and the economy. Cambridge: Harvard University Press, 1973.
35. Boor M. Relationships between unemployment rates and suicide rates in eight countries, 1962–1976. Psych Rep 1980;47:1095–1101.
36. Platts S. Unemployment and suicidal behavior: a review of the literature. Soc Sci Med 1984;19:93–115.
37. Crombie IK. Trends in suicide and unemployment in Scotland, 1976–86. Br Med J 1989;298:782–784.
38. Walbran B, MacMahon B, Bailey AE. Suicide and unemployment in Pennsylvania, 1954–1961. Arch Environ Health 1965;10:1115.
39. Paykel ES, Prusoff BA, Myers JK. Suicide attempts and recent life events. Arch Gen Psychiatry 1975;32:327–333.
40. Cochran R, Robertson A. Stress in the lives of parasuicides. Soc Psychiatry 1975;10:161–171.
41. Conwell Y, Rotenberg M, Caine ED. Completed suicide at age 50 and over. J Am Geriatr Soc 1990;38:640–644.
42. Murphy GE, Armstrong JW, Hermele SL, Fischer JR, Clendenin WW. Suicide and alcoholism: interpersonal loss confirmed as a predictor. Arch Gen Psychiatry 1979;36:65–69.
43. Rich CL, Fowler RC, Fogarty LA, Young D. San Diego Suicide study: III. Relationships between diagnoses and stressors. Arch Gen Psychiatry 1988;45:589–592.
44. Sainsbury P. Suicide and depression. In: Coppen A, Walk A, eds. Recent developments in affective disorders: a symposium. Ashford, England: Headley Bros., 1968:1–13.
45. Loebel JP, Loebel JS, Dager SR, Centerwall BS, Reay DT. Anticipation of nursing home placement may be a precipitant of suicide among the elderly. J Am Geriatr Soc 1991;39:407–408.
46. Robins E, Murphy GE, Wilkinson RH, et al. Some clinical considerations in the prevention of suicide based on a study of 134 successful suicides. Am J Pub Health 1959;49:888–889.
47. Mackenzie TB, Popkin MK. Suicide in the medical patient. Intl J Psychiatry Med 1987;17:3–22.
48. Chynoweth R, Tonge JI, Armstrong J. Suicide in Brisbane—a retrospective psychosocial study. Aust N Z J Psychiatry 1980;14:37–45.
49. Dorpat TL, Anderson WF, Ripley HS. The relationship of physical illness to suicide. In: Resnik HPL, ed. Suicidal behaviors: diagnosis and management. Boston: Little, Brown & Co., 1968:209–219.
50. Conwell Y, Caine ED, Olsen K. Suicide and cancer in late life. Hosp Community Psychiatry 1990;41:1334–1339.
51. Murphy GK. Cancer and the coroner. JAMA 1977;237:786–788.
52. Whitlock FA. Suicide and physical illness. In: Roy A, ed. Suicide. Baltimore: Williams & Wilkins, 1986:151–170.
53. Barraclough BM. Suicide in the elderly. Br J Psychiatry 1971;6 (suppl):87–97.
54. Stenback A, Achte KA, Rimon RN. Physical disease, hypochondria and alcohol addiction in suicides committed by mental hospital patients. Brit J Psychiatry 1965;111:933–937.
55. Farberow NL, Simon MD. Suicide in Los Angeles and Vienna: an intercultural study of two cities. Public Health Rep 1969;84:389–403.
56. Roy A. Family history of suicide. Arch Gen Psychiatry 1983;40:971–974.
57. Tsuang MT. Suicide in schizophrenics, manics, depressives, and surgical controls: a comparison with general population suicide mortality. Arch Gen Psychiatry 1978;35:153–155.
58. Tsuang MT. Risk of suicide in the relatives of schizophrenics, manics, depressives, and controls. J Clin Psychiatry 1983;44:396–400.
59. Scheftner WA, Young MA, Endicott J, et al. Family history and five-year suicide risk. Br J Psychiatry 1988;153:805–809.
60. Egeland JA, Sussex JN. Suicide and family loading for affective disorders. JAMA 1985;254:915–918.
61. Roy A, Segal NL, Centerwall BS, Robinette CD. Suicide in twins. Arch Gen Psychiatry 1991;48:29–32.
62. Roy A. Genetics of suicide. Ann NY Acad Sci 1986;487:97–105.
63. Wender PH, Kety SS, Rosenthal D, Schulsinger F, Ortmann J, Lunde I. Psychiatric disorders in the biological and adoptive families of adopted individuals with affective disorders. Arch Gen Psychiatry 1986;43:923–929.
64. Schulsinger F, Kety SS, Rosenthal D, et al. A family study of suicide. In: Schou M, Stromgren E, eds. Origin, prevention, and treatment of affective disorders. New York: Academic Press, 1979:277–287.
65. Crawley JN, Sutton ME, Pickar D. Animal models of self-destructive behavior and suicide. Psychiatr Clin North Am 1985;8:299–310.
66. Clough GC. Lemmings and population problems. American Scientist 1965;53:199–212.
67. Hamilton WJ. Do nonhuman animals commit suicide? Behavioral and Brain Sciences 1980;3:278–279.
68. Bach-Y-Rita G, Vero A. Habitual violence: a profile of 62 men. Am J Psychiatry 1974;131:1015–1017.
69. Brown GL, Goodwin FK. Cerebrospinal fluid correlates of suicide attempts and aggression. In: Mann JJ, Stanley M, ed. Psychobiology of suicidal behavior. New York: New York Academy of Sciences, 1986:175–188.
70. Ostroff RB, Giller E, Harkness L, Mason J. The norepinephrine-to-epinephrine ratio in patients with a history of suicide attempts. Am J Psychiatry 1985;142:224–227.
71. Jones IH. Self-injury: toward a biological basis. Perspect Biol Med 1982;26:137–150.
72. Weiger WA, Bear DM. An approach to the neurology of aggression. J Psychiatr Res 1988;22:85–98.
73. Sheard MH. Testosterone and aggression. In: Sandler M, ed. Psychopharmacology of aggression. New York: Raven Press, 1979:111–121.
74. Sheard MH. Clinical pharmacology of aggressive behavior. Clin Neuropharmacol 1988;11:483–492.
75. Valzelli L. Psychobiology of aggression and violence. New York: Raven Press, 1981.
76. Schildkraut JJ. The catecholamine hypothesis of affective disorders: a review of supporting evidence. Am J Psychiatry 1965;122:509–522.
77. Lapin IP, Oxenkrug GF. Intensification of the central serotoninergic processes as a possible determinant of the thymoleptic effect. Lancet 1969;1:132–136.
78. Bourne HR, Bunney WE, Colburn RW, et al. Noradrenaline, 5-hydroxytryptamine, and 5-hydroxyindoleacetic acid in hindbrains of suicidal patients. Lancet 1968;2:805–808.
79. Cochran E, Robins E, Grote S. Regional serotonin levels in brain: a comparison of depressive suicides and alcoholic suicides with controls. Biol Psychiatry 1976;11:283–294.
80. Beskow J, Gottfries CG, Roos BE, Winblad B. Determination of monoamine and monoamine metabolites in the human brain: post mortem studies in a group of suicides and in a control group. Acta Psychiatr Scand 1976;53:7–20.
81. Cheetham SC, Crompton MR, Czudek C, Horton RW, Katona CLE, Reynolds GP. Serotonin concentrations and turnover in brains of depressed suicides. Brain Res 1989;502:332–340.

82. Arató M, Tekes K, Palkovits M, Demeter E, Falus A. Serotonergic split brain and suicide. Psychiatry Res 1987;21:355–356.

83. Crow TJ, Cross AJ, Cooper SJ, et al. Neurotransmitter receptors and monoamine metabolites in the brains of patients with Alzheimer-type dementia and depression, and suicides. Neuropharmacology 1984; 23:1561–1569.

84. Pare CMB, Yeung DPH, Price K, Stacey RS. 5-Hydroxytryptamine, noradrenaline, and dopamine in brainstem, hypothalamus, and caudate nucleus of controls and of patients committing suicide by coal-gas poisoning. Lancet 1969;2:133–135.

85. Shaw DM, Camps FE, Eccleston EG. 5-Hydroxytryptamine in the hind-brain of depressive suicides. Brit J Psychiatry 1967;113:1407–1411.

86. Lloyd KG, Farley IJ, Deck JHN, Hornykiewicz O. Serotonin and 5-hydroxyindoleacetic acid in discrete areas of the brainstem of suicide victims and control patients. Adv Biochem Psychopharmacol 1974; 11:387–397.

87. Korpi ER, Kleinman JE, Goodman SI, et al. Serotonin and 5-hydroxyindoleacetic acid in brains of suicide victims. Arch Gen Psychiatry 1986;43:594–600.

88. Owen F, Chambers DR, Cooper SJ, et al. Serotonergic mechanisms in brains of suicide victims. Brain Res 1986;362:185–188.

89. Åsberg M, Nordström P, Träskman-Bendz L. Cerebrospinal fluid studies in suicide: an overview. In: Mann JJ, Stanley M, eds. Psychobiology of suicidal behavior. New York: New York Academy of Sciences, 1986:243–255.

90. Mann JJ, Arango V, Marzuk PM, Theccanat S, Reis DJ. Evidence for the 5HT hypothesis of suicide: a review of post-mortem studies. Brit J Psychiatry 1989;155:7–14.

91. Gross-Isseroff R, Israeli M, Biegon A. Autoradiographic analysis of tritiated imipramine binding in the human brain post mortem: Effects of suicide. Arch Gen Psychiatry 1989;46:237–241.

92. Lawrence KM, DePaermentier F, Cheetham SC, Crompton MR, Katona CLE, Horton RW. Brain 5HT uptake sites, labelled with [^{3}H]paroxetine, in antidepressant-free depressed suicides. Brain Res 1990;526:17–22.

93. Lawrence KM, DePaermentier F, Cheetham SC, Crompton MR, Katona CLE, Horton RW. Symmetrical hemispheric distribution of [^{3}H]paroxetine binding sites in postmortem human brain from controls and suicides. Biol Psychiatry 1990;28:544–546.

94. Arora RC, Meltzer HY. [^{3}H]imipramine binding in the frontal cortex of suicides. Psychiatry Res 1989;30:125–135.

95. Arora RC, Meltzer HY. Laterality and [^{3}H]imipramine binding: studies in the frontal cortex of normal controls and suicide victims. Biol Psychiatry 1991;29:1016–1022.

96. Stanley M, Mann JJ. Increased serotonin-2 binding sites in frontal cortex of suicide victims. Lancet 1983;1:214–216.

97. Arató M, Tekes K, Tóthfalusi L, et al. Reversed hemispheric asymmetry of imipramine binding in suicide victims. Biol Psychiatry 1991;29:699–702.

98. Stanley M, Virgilio J, Gershon S. Tritiated imipramine binding sites are decreased in the frontal cortex of suicides. Science 1982;216:1337–1339.

99. Meyerson LR, Wennogle LP, Abel MS, et al. Human brain receptor alterations in suicide victims. Pharmacol Biochem Behav 1982;17:159–163.

100. Brunello N, Chauang DM, Costa E. Different synaptic location of mianserin and imipramine binding sites. Science 1982;215:1112–1115.

101. Roth BL, McLean S, Zhu XZ, et al. Characterization of two [^{3}H]ketanserin recognition sites in rat striatum. J Neurochem 1987;49:1833–1838.

102. Mann JJ, Stanley M, McBride PA, McEwen BS. Increased serotonin$_2$ and β-adrenergic receptor binding in the frontal cortices of suicide victims. Arch Gen Psychiatry 1986;43:954–959.

103. Arora RC, Meltzer HY. Serotonergic measures in the brains of suicide victims: 5HT$_2$ binding sites in the frontal cortex of suicide victims and control subjects. Am J Psychiatry 1989;146:730–736.

104. Owen F, Cross AJ, Crow TJ, et al. Brain 5HT$_2$ receptors and suicide [letter]. Lancet 1983;2:1256.

105. Cheetham SC, Crompton MR, Katona CLE, Horton RW. Brain 5-HT$_2$ receptor binding sites in depressed suicide victims. Brain Res 1988;443:272–280.

106. Yates M, Leake A, Candy JM, Fairbairn AF, McKeith IG, Ferrier IN. 5HT$_2$ receptor changes in major depression. Biol Psychiatry 1990; 27:489–496.

107. Gross-Isseroff R, Salama D, Israeli M, Biegon A. Autoradiographic analysis of [^{3}H]ketanserin binding in the human brain postmortem: effect of suicide. Brain Res 1990;507:208–215.

108. Arango V, Ernsberger P, Marzuk PM, et al. Autoradiographic demonstration of increased serotonin 5-HT$_2$ and β-adrenergic receptor binding sites in the brain of suicide victims. Arch Gen Psychiatry 1990;47:1038–1047.

109. Arango V, Underwood MD, Mann JJ. Alterations in monoamine receptors in the brain of suicide victims. J Clin Psychopharmacol 1992;12:8S–12S.

110. Cheetham SC, Crompton MR, Katona CLE, Horton RW. Brain 5-HT$_1$ binding sites in depressed suicides. Psychopharmacology 1990;102:544–548.

111. Dillon KA, Gross-Isseroff R, Israeli M, Biegon A. Autoradiographic analysis of serotonin 5-HT$_{1A}$ receptor binding in the human brain postmorten: effects of age and alcohol. Brain Res 1991;554:56–64.

112. Matsubara S, Arora RC, Meltzer HY. Serotonergic measures in suicide brain: 5-HT$_{1A}$ binding sites in frontal cortex of suicide victims. J Neural Transm 1991;85:181–194.

113. Stanley M, Traskman-Bendz L, Dorovini-Zis K. Correlations between aminergic metabolites simultaneously obtained from human CSF and brain. Life Sci 1985;37:1279–1286.

114. Åsberg M, Nordström P, Träskman-Bendz L. Biological factors in suicide. In: Roy A, ed. Suicide. Baltimore: Williams & Wilkins, 1986:47–71.

115. Åsberg M, Thorén P, Träskman L, Bertilsson L, Ringberger V. "Serotonin depression" — a biochemical subgroup within the affective disorders? Science 1976;191:478–480.

116. Koslow SH, Maas JW, Bowden CL, Davis JM, Hanin I, Javaid J. CSF and urinary biogenic amines and metabolites in depression and mania: a controlled, univariate analysis. Arch Gen Psychiatry 1983;40:999–1010.

117. Vestergaard P, Sørensen T, Hoppe E, Rafaelsen OJ, Yates CM, Nicolaou N. Biogenic amine metabolites in cerebrospinal fluid of patients with affective disorders. Acta Psychiatr Scand 1978;58:88–96.

118. VanPraag HM. Depression, suicide and the metabolism of serotonin in the brain. J Affect Disord 1982;4:275–290.

119. Roy-Byrne P, Post RM, Rubinow DR, Linnoila M, Savard R, Davis D. CSF 5HIAA and personal and family history of suicide in affectively ill patients: a negative study. Psychiatry Res 1983;10:263–274.

120. Ågren HL. Life at risk: markers of suicidality in depression. Psychiatric Developments 1983;1:87–104.

121. VanPraag HM. Significance of biochemical parameters in the diagnosis, treatment, and prevention of depressive disorders. Biol Psychiatry 1977;12:101–131.

122. Brown GL, Goodwin FK, Ballenger JC, Goyer PF, Major LF. Aggression in humans correlates with cerebrospinal fluid aminometabolites. Psychiatry Res 1979;1:131–139.

123. Träskman L, Åsberg M, Bertilsson L, Sjöstrand L. Monoamine metabolites in CSF and suicidal behavior. Arch Gen Psychiatry 1981;38:631–636.

124. Roy A, DeJong J, Linnoila M. Cerebrospinal fluid monoamine metabolites and suicidal behavior in depressed patients. Arch Gen Psychiatry 1989;46:609–612.

125. VanPraag HM. CSF 5HIAA and suicide in non-depressed schizophrenics [letter]. Lancet 1983;2:977–978.

126. VanPraag HM. (Auto)aggression and CSF 5HIAA in depression and schizophrenia. Psychopharmacol Bull 1986;3:669–673.

127. Ninan PT, vanKammen DP, Scheinin M, Linnoila M, Bunney WE, Goodwin FK. CSF 5-Hydroxyindoleacetic acid levels in suicidal schizophrenic patients. Am J Psychiatry 1984;141:566–569.

128. Banki CM, Arató M, Papp Z, Kurcz M. Biochemical markers in suicidal patients. Investigations with cerebrospinal fluid amine metabolites and neuroendocrine tests. J Affect Disord 1984;6:341–350.

129. Roy A, Lamparski D, DeJong J, Adinoff B, et al. Cerebrospinal fluid monoamine metabolites in alcoholic patients who attempt suicide. Acta Psychiatr Scand 1990;81:58–61.

130. Brown GL, Ebert MH, Goyer PF, et al. Aggression, suicide, and serotonin: relationships to CSF amine metabolites. Am J Psychiatry 1982;139:741–746.

131. Linnoila M, Virkkunen M, Scheinin M, Nuutilla A, Rimon R, Goodwin FK. Low cerebrospinal fluid 5-hydroxyindoleacetic acid concentration differentiates impulsive from non-impulsive violent behavior. Life Sci 1983;33:2609–2614.

132. Virkkunen M, Nuutila A, Goodwin FK, Linnoila M. Cerebrospinal fluid monoamine metabolite levels in male arsonists. Arch Gen Psychiatry 1987;44:241–247.

133. Virkkunen M, DeJon J, Bartko J, Goodwin FK, Linnoila M. Relationship of psychobiological variables to recidivism in violent offenders and impulsive fire setters: a follow-up study. Arch Gen Psychiatry 1989;46:600–603.

134. Virkkunen M, DeJong J, Bartko J, Linnoila M. Psychobiological concomitants of history of suicide attempts among violent offenders and impulsive fire setters. Arch Gen Psychiatry 1989;46:604–606.

135. Linnoila M, DeJon J, Virkkunen M. Family history of alcoholism in violent offenders and impulsive fire setters. Arch Gen Psychiatry 1989;46:613–616.

136. Bioulac B, Benezech M, Renaud B, Noel B, Roche D. Serotoninergic dysfunction in the 47, XYY syndrome. Biol Psychiatry 1980;15:917–923.

137. Lidberg L, Åsberg M, Sundqvist-Stensman UB. 5-Hydroxyindole-acetic acid levels in attempted suicides who have killed their children (letter). Lancet 1984;2:928.

138. Kruesi MJP, Rapoport JL, Hamburger S, et al. Cerebrospinal fluid monoamine metabolites, aggression, and impulsivity in disruptive behavior disorders of children and adolescents. Arch Gen Psychiatry 1990;47:419–426.

139. Lidberg L, Tuck JR, Åsberg M, Scalia-Tomba GP, Bertilsson L. Homicide, suicide and CSF 5-HIAA. Acta Psychiatr Scand 1985;71:230–236.

140. Virkkunen M. Reactive hypoglycemic tendency among habitually violent offenders: a further study by means of the glucose tolerance test. Neuropsychobiology 1982;8:35–40.

141. Virkkunen M. Reactive hypoglycemic tendency among arsonists. Acta Psychiatr Scand 1984;69:445–452.

142. Roy A, Virkkunen M, Linnoila M. Monoamines, glucose metabolism, aggression towards self and others. Intern J Neurosci 1988;41:261–264.

143. Stahl SM. The human platelet: a diagnostic and research tool for the study of biogenic amines in psychiatric and neurologic disorders. Arch Gen Psychiatry 1977;34:509–516.

144. Roy A, Everett D, Pickar D, Paul SM. Platelet tritiated imipramine binding and serotonin uptake in depressed patients and controls. Arch Gen Psychiatry 1987;44:320–327.

145. Wägner A, Åberg-Wistedt A, Åsberg M, Ekqvist B, Martensson B, Montero, D. Lower [3H]imipramine binding in platelets from untreated depressed patients compared to healthy controls. Psychiatry Res 1985;16:131–139.

146. Nemeroff CB, Knight DL, Krishnan RR, et al. Marked reduction in the number of platelet-tritiated imipramine binding sites in geriatric depression. Arch Gen Psychiatry 1988;45:919–923.

147. Schneider LS, Severson JA, Chui HC, Pollock VE, Sloane RB, Fredrickson ER. Platelet tritiated imipramine binding and MAO activity in Alzheimer's disease patients with agitation and delusions. Psychiatry Res 1988;25:311–322.

148. Marazziti D, DeLeo D, Conti L. Further evidence supporting the role of the serotonin system in suicidal behavior: a preliminary study of suicide attempters. Acta Psychiatr Scand 1989;80:322–324.

149. Theodorou AE, Katona CLE, Davies SL, et al. [3H]imipramine binding to freshly prepared platelet membranes in depression. Psychiatry Res 1989;29:87–103.

150. Pandey GN, Pandey SC, Janicak PG, Marks RC, Davis JM. Platelet serotonin-2 receptor binding sites in depression and suicide. Biol Psychiatry 1990;28:215–222.

151. Biegon A, Grinspoon A, Blumenfeld B, Bleich A, Apter A, Mester R. Increased serotonin 5-HT2 receptor binding on blood platelets of suicidal men. Psychopharmacology 1990;100:165–167.

152. McBride PA, Brown RP, Demeo M, et al. Platelet 5-HT2 receptors: depression and suicide. Chicago: Annual Meeting of the American Psychiatric Association, 1987.

153. Bräunig P, Rao ML, Fimmers R. Blood serotonin levels in suicidal schizophrenic patients. Acta Psychiatr Scand 1989;79:186–189.

154. VanKempen GMJ, Notten P, Hengeveld MW. Repeated measures of platelet MAO activity and 5-HT in a group of suicidal women. Biol Psychiatry 1992;31:529–530.

155. Meltzer HY, Perline R, Tricou BJ, Lowy M, Robertson A. Effect of 5-hydroxytryptophan on serum cortisol levels in major affective disorders: II. Relation to suicide, psychosis, and depressive symptoms. Arch Gen Psychiatry 1984;41:379–387.

156. Coccaro EF, Astill JL. Central serotonergic function in parasuicide. Prog Neuropsychopharmacol Biol Psychiatry 1990;14:663–674.

157. Coccaro EF, Siever LJ, Klar HM, et al. Serotonergic studies in patients with affective and personality disorders: correlates with suicidal and impulsive aggressive behavior. Arch Gen Psychiatry 1989;46:587–599.

158. Golden RN, Gilmore JH, Corrigan MHN, Ekstrom RD, Knight BT, Garbutt JC. Serotonin, suicide, and aggression: clinical studies. J Clin Psychiatry 1991;52:61–69.

159. Ågren H. Symptom patterns in unipolar and bipolar depression correlating with monoamine metabolites in the cerebrospinal fluid: II. Suicide. Psychiatry Res 1980;3:225–236.

160. Roy A, Ågren H, Pickar D, et al. Reduced CSF concentrations of homovanillic acid and homovanillic acid to 5-hydroxyindoleacetic acid ratios in depressed patients: relationship to suicidal behavior and dexamethasone nonsuppression. Am J Psychiatry 1986;143:1539–1545.

161. Montgomery SA, Montgomery D. Pharmacological prevention of suicidal behaviour. J Affect Disord 1982;4:291–298.

162. Ninan PT, vanKammen DP, Linnoila M. Letter to the editor. Am J Psychiatry 1985;142:148.

163. Roy A, Karoum F, Pollack S. Marked reduction in indexes of dopamine metabolism among patients with depression who attempt suicide. Arch Gen Psychiatry 1992;49:447–450.

164. Govoni S, Rius RA, Battaini F, Magnoni MS, Lucchi L, Trabucchi M. The central dopaminergic system: susceptibility to risk factors for accelerated aging. Gerontology 1988;34:29–34.

165. Morgan DG. The dopamine and serotonin systems during aging in human and rodent brain—a brief review. Prog Neuropsychopharmacol Biol Psychiatry 1987;11:153–157.

166. DeKeyser J, Ebinger G, Vauquelin G. Age-related changes in the human nigrostriatal dopaminergic system. Ann Neurol 1990;27:157–161.

167. Richfield EK, O'Brien CF, Eskin T, Shoulson I. Heterogeneous dopamine receptor changes in early and late Huntington's disease. Neurosci Lett 1991;132:121–126.

168. Farrer LA. Suicide and attempted suicide in Huntington disease: implications for preclinical testing of persons at risk. Am J Med Genet 1986;24:305–311.

169. Schoenfeld M, Myers RH, Cupples LA, Berkman B, Sax DS, Clark E. Increased rate of suicide among patients with Huntington's disease. J Neurol Neurosurg Psychiatry 1984;47:1283–1287.

170. Mayeux R. Depression in the patient with Parkinson's disease. J Clin Psychiatry 1990;51:20–23.

171. Roy A, Pickar D, DeJong J, Karoum F, Linnoila M. Suicidal behavior in depression: relationship to noradrenergic function. Biol Psychiatry 1989;25:341–350.
172. Ostroff R, Giller E, Bonese K, Ebersole E, Harkness L, Mason J. Neuroendocrine risk factors of suicidal behavior. Am J Psychiatry 1982;139:1323–1325.
173. Biegon A, Israeli M. Regionally selective increases in β-adrenergic receptor density in the brains of suicide victims. Brain Res 1988; 442:199–203.
174. Stockmeier CA, Meltzer HY. β-Adrenergic receptor binding in frontal cortex of suicide victims. Biol Psychiatry 1991;29:183–191.
175. Little KY, Duncan GE, Breese GR. Beta-adrenergic binding in suicide victims [Abstract]. Soc Neurosci Abstr 1990;16:140.
176. DePaermentier F, Cheetham SC, Crompton MR, Katona CLE, Horton RW. Brain β-Adrenoceptor binding sites in antidepressant-free depressed suicide victims. Brain Res 1990;525:71–77.
177. Gross-Isseroff R, Dillon KA, Fieldust SJ, Biegon A. Autoradiographic analysis of α₁-noradrenergic receptors in the human brain postmortem: effect of suicide. Arch Gen Psychiatry 1990;47:1049–1053.
178. Arango V, Hoffman L, Ernsberger P, Reis DJ, Mann JJ. Quantitative autoradiography of cortical α-adrenergic receptors in suicide victims. Soc Neurosci Abstr 1989;15:585.
179. Ordway GA, Widdowson PS, Streator-Smith K, Halaris AE. Neurochemistry of the human locus coeruleus in suicide and depression [Abstract]. Soc Neurosci Abstr 1990;16:140.
180. Arango V, Ernsberger P, Underwood MD, Mann JJ. Alpha₂-adrenergic binding is not altered in suicide [Abstract]. Soc Neurosci Abstr 1990;16:140.
181. Meana JJ, Barturen F, García, JA. α₂-Adrenoceptors in the brain of suicide victims: increased receptor density associated with major depression. Biol Psychiatry 1992;31:471–490.
182. Janowsky DS, el-Yousef MK, Davis JM, Sekerke HJ. A cholinergic-adrenergic hypothesis of mania and depression. Lancet 1972;2:632–635.
183. Kaufman CA, Gillin JC, Hill B, et al. Muscarinic binding and suicides. Psychiatry Res 1984;12:47–55.
184. Stanley M. Cholinergic receptor binding in the frontal cortex of suicide victims. Am J Psychiatry 1984;141:1432–1436.
185. Cheetham SC, Crompton MR, Katona CLE, Parker SJ, Horton RW. Brain GABAₐ/benzodiazepine binding sites and glutamic acid decarboxylase activity in depressed suicide victims. Brain Res 1988;460:114–123.
186. Fawcett J, Scheftner WA, Fogg L, et al. Time-related predictors of suicide in major affective disorder. Am J Psychiatry 1990;147:1189–1194.
187. Sherif F, Marcusson J, Oreland L. Brain gamma-aminobutyrate transaminase and monamine oxidase activities in suicide victims. Eur Arch Psychiatry Clin Neurosci 1991;241:139–144.
188. Cross JA, Cheetham SC, Crompton MR, Katona CLE, Horton RW. Brain GABAᵦ binding sites in depressed suicide victims. Psychiatry Res 1988;26:119–129.
189. Manchon M, Kopp N, Rouzioux JJ, Lecestre D, Deluermoz S, Miachon S. Benzodiazepine receptor and neurotransmitter studies in the brain of suicides. Life Sci 1987;41:2623–2630.
190. Stocks GM, Cheetham SC, Crompton MR, Katona CLE, Horton RW. Benzodiazepine binding sites in amygdala and hippocampus of depressed suicide victims. J Affect Disord 1990;18:11–15.
191. Korpi ER, Kleinman JE, Wyatt RJ. GABA concentrations in forebrain areas of suicide victims. Biol Psychiatry 1988;23:109–114.
192. Perry EK, Gibson PH, Blessed G, Perry RH, Tomlinson BE. Neurotransmitter enzyme abnormalities in senile dementia: choline acetyl transferase and glutamic acid decarboxylase in necropsy brain tissue. Journal Neurol Sci 1977;34:247–265.
193. Charlton BG, Wright C, Leake A, et al. Somatostatin immunoreactivity in postmortem brain from depressed suicides. Arch Gen Psychiatry 1988;45:597–598.
194. Widdowson PS, Ordway GA, Halaris AE. Neuropeptide Y concen-

trations in postmortem brain from victims of suicide and controls [Abstract]. Society of Neuroscience Abstracts 1990;16:140.
195. Kars H, Broekema W, Glaudemans-van Gelderen I, Verhoeven WMA, van Ree JM. Naltrexone attenuates self-injurious behavior in mentally retarded subjects. Biol Psychiatry 1990;27:741–746.
196. Sandman CA, Barron JL, Chicz-DeMet A, DeMet EM. Plasma β-endorphin levels in patients with self-injurious behavior and stereotype. Am J Ment Retard 1990;95:84–92.
197. Barrett RP, Feinstein C, Hole WT. Effects of naloxone and naltrexone on self-injury: a double-blind, placebo-controlled analysis. Am J Ment Retard 1989;93:644–651.
198. Taylor DV, Hetrick WP, Neri CL, Touchette P, Barron JL, Sandman CA. Effect of naltrexone upon self-injurious behavior, learning and activity: a case study. Pharmacol Biochem Behav 1991;40:79–92.
199. Bruun R, Kurlan R. Opiate therapy and self-harming behavior in Tourette's syndrome. Mov Disord 1991;6:184–185.
200. Richardson JS, Zaleski WA. Naloxone and self-mutilation. Biol Psychiatry 1983;18:99–101.
201. Coid J, Allolio B, Rees LH. Raised plasma metenkephalin in patients who habitually mutilate themselves. Lancet 1983;2:545–546.
202. Konicki PE, Schulz SC. Rationale for clinical trials of opiate antagonists in treating patients with personality disorders and self-injurious behavior. Psychopharmacol Bull 1989;25:556–563.
203. Frecska E, Arató M, Banki CM, et al. Prolactin response to fentanyl in depression. Biol Psychiatry 1989;25:692–696.
204. Gross-Isseroff R, Dillon KA, Israeli M, Biegon A. Regionally selective increases in μ opioid receptor density in the brains of suicide victims. Brain Res 1990;530:312–316.
205. Scarone S, Gambini O, Calabrese G, et al. Asymmetrical distribution of beta-endorphin in cerebral hemispheres of suicides: preliminary data. Psychiatry Res 1990;32:159–166.
206. Loosen PT, Prange AJ. Serum thyrotropin response to thyrotropin-releasing hormone in psychiatric patients: a review. Am J Psychiatry 1982;139:405–416.
207. Linkowski P, VanWettere JP, Kerkhofs M, Brauman H, Mendlewicz J. Thyrotropin response to thyrostimulin in affectively ill women: relationship to suicidal behavior. Brit J Psychiatry 1983;143:401–405.
208. Linkowski P, VanWettere JP, Kerkhofs M, Gregoire F, Brauman H, Mendlewicz J. Violent suicidal behavior and the thyrotropin-releasing hormone-thyroid-simulating hormone test: a clinical outcome study. Neuropsychobiology 1984;12:19–22.
209. Banki CM, Bissette G, Arató M, Nemeroff CB. Elevation of immunoreactive CSF TRH in depressed patients. Am J Psychiatry 1988;145:1526–1531.
210. Linkowski P, VanWettere JP, Kerkhofs M, Brauman H, Mendlewicz J. Thyrotrophin response to thyreostimulin in affectively ill women relationship to suicidal behaviour. Brit J Psychiatry 1983;143:401–405.
211. Prasad AJ. Neuroendocrine differences between violent and non-violent parasuicides. Neuropsychobiology 1985;13:157–159.
212. Bunney WE, Fawcett JA. Possibility of a biochemical test for suicidal potential. Arch Gen Psychiatry 1965;13:232–239.
213. Bunney WE, Fawcett JA, Davis JM, Gifford S. Further evaluation of urinary 17-hydroxy-corticosteroid in suicidal patients. Arch Gen Psychiatry 1969;21:138–150.
214. Levy B, Hansen E. Failure of the urinary test for suicidal potential. Arch Gen Psychiatry 1969;20:415–418.
215. Krieger G. Biochemical predictors of suicide. Diseases of the Nervous System 1970;31:478–482.
216. Krieger G. The plasma level of cortisol as a predictor of suicide. Dis Nerv Syst 1979;35:237–240.
217. Arató M, Banki CM, Bissette G, Nemeroff CB. Elevated CSF CRF in suicide victims. Biol Psychiatry 1989;25:355–359.
218. Nemeroff CB, Owens MJ, Bissette G, Andorn AC, Stanley M. Reduced corticotropin releasing factor binding sites in the frontal cortex of suicide victims. Arch Gen Psychiatry 1988;45:577–579.
219. Traskman L, Tybring G, Åsberg M, Bertilsson L, Lantto O, Schalling

D. Cortisol in the CSF of depressed and suicidal patients. Arch Gen Psychiatry 1980;37:761–767.

220. Arató M, Banki CM, Nemeroff CB, Bissette G. Hypothalamic-pituitary-adrenal axis and suicide. Ann N Y Acad Sci 1986;487:263-270.

221. Banki CB, Bissette G, Arató M, O'Connor L, Nemeroff CB. CSF corticotropin-releasing factor-like immunoreactivity in depression and schizophrenia. Am J Psychiatry 1987;144:873–877.

222. Kocsis JH, Kennedy S, Brown RP, Mann JJ, Mason B. Suicide and adrenocortical function. Psychopharmacol Bull 1986;22:650–655.

223. Starkman MN, Schteingart DE, Schork MA. Depressed mood and other psychiatric manifestations of Cushing's syndrome: relationship to hormone levels. Psychosom Med 1981;43:3–18.

224. Cohen SI. Cushing's syndrome: a psychiatric study of 29 patients. Br J Psychiatry 1980;136:120–124.

225. Lewis DA, Smith RE. Steroid-induced psychiatric syndromes: a report of 14 cases and a review of the literature. J Affect Disord 1983;5:319–332.

226. Braunig P, Bleistein J, Rao ML. Suicidality and corticosteroid-induced psychosis. Biol Psychiatry 1989;26:209–210.

227. Banki CM, Arató M. Amine metabolites and neuroendocrine response related to depression and suicide. J Affect Disord 1983;5:223–232.

228. Coryell W, Schlesser MA. Suicide and the dexamethasone suppression test in unipolar depression. Am J Psychiatry 1981;138:1120–1121.

229. Targum SD, Rosen L, Capodanno AE. The dexamethason suppression test in suicidal patients with unipolar depression. Am J Psychiatry 1983;140:877–879.

230. Robbins DR, Alessi NE. Suicide and the dexamethasone suppression test in adolescence. Biol Psychiatry 1985;20:107.

231. Carroll BJ, Greden JF, Feinberg M. Suicide, neuroendocrine dysfunction and CSF 5-HIAA concentrations in depression. In: Angrist B, Burrows GD, Lader ME, eds. Recent advances in neuropsychopharmacology. Elmsford: Pergamon Press, 1981:307–313.

232. Zimmerman M, Coryell W, Pfohl B. The validity of the dexamethasone suppression test as a marker for endogenous depression. Arch Gen Psychiatry 1986;43:347–355.

233. Schmidtke A, Fleckenstein P, Beckmann H. The dexamethasone suppression test and suicide attempts. Acta Psychiatr Scand 1989;79:276–282.

234. Ayuso-Gutierrez JL, Cabranes JA, Garcia-Camba E, Almoguera I. Pituitary-adrenal disinhibition and suicide attempters in depressed patients. Biol Psychiatry 1987;22:1409–1412.

235. Brown RP, Mason B, Stoll P, et al. Adrenocortical function and suicidal behavior in depressive disorders. Psychiatry Res 1986;17:317–323.

236. Yerevanian B, Olafsdottir H, Milanese E, et al. Normalization of the dexamethasone suppression test at discharge: its prognostic value. J Affect Disord 1983;5:191–197.

237. Greden JF, Albala AA, Haskett RF, et al. Normalization of the dexamethasone suppression test: a laboratory index of recovery from endogenous depression. Biol Psychiatry 1980;15:449–458.

238. Sapolsky RM, Armani M, Packan D, Tombaugh G. Stress and glucocorticoids in aging. Endocrinol Metab Clin North Am 1987;16:965–980.

239. Blackman MR. Pituitary hormones and aging. Endocrinol Metab Clin North Am 1987;16:981–995.

240. Desai D, March R, Watters JM. Hyperglycemia after trauma increases with age. J Trauma 1989;29:719–723.

241. Greenwald BS, Mathe AA, Mohs RC, Levy MI, Johns CA, Davis KL. Cortisol and Alzheimer's disease II: dexamethason suppression, dementia severity, and affective symptoms. Am J Psychiatry 1986;143:442–446.

242. Jacobs S, Mason J, Kosten T, Brown S, Ostfeld A. Urinary free cortisol excretion in relation to age in acutely stressed persons with depressive symptoms. Psychosom Med 1989;46:213–221.

243. Stangl D, Pfohl B, Zimmerman M, Coryell W, Corenthal C. The relationship between age and post dexamethasone cortisol: a test of three hypotheses. J Affect Disord 1986;11:185–197.

244. Olweus D, Mattsson Å, Schalling D, Löw H. Circulating testosterone levels and aggression in adolescent males: a causal analysis. Psychosom Med 1988;50:261–272.

245. Banki CM, Vojnik M, Papp Z, Balla KZ, Arató M. Cerebrospinal fluid magnesium and calcium related to amine metabolites, diagnosis, and suicide attempts. Biol Psychiatry 1985;20:163–171.

246. Beck-Friis J, Kjellman BF, Aperia B, et al. Serum melatonin in relation to clinical variables in patients with major depressive disorder and a hypothesis of a low melatonin syndrome. Acta Psychiatr Scand 1985;71:319–330.

247. Muldoon MF, Manuck SB, Matthews KM. Lowering cholesterol concentrations and mortality: a quantitative review of primary prevention trials. Brit Med J 1990;301:304–314.

248. Lindberg G, Råstam, Gullberg B, Eklund G. Low serum cholesterol concentration and short term mortality from injuries in men and women. BMJ 1992;305:277–279.

249. Engelberg H. Low serum cholesterol and suicide. Lancet 1992;339:727–729.

250. Sulser F. Serotonin-norepinephrine receptor interactions in the brain: implications for the pharmacology and pathophysiology of affective disorders. J Clin Psychiatry 1987;43:12–18.

251. Van de Kar LD. Neuroendocrine aspects of the serotonergic hypothesis of depression. Neurosci Biobehav Rev 1989;13:237–246.

252. Nausieda PA, Carvey PM, Weiner WJ. Modification of central serotonergic and dopaminergic behaviors in the course of chronic corticosteroid administration. Eur J Pharmacol 1982;78:335–343.

253. Rupprecht R, Rupprecht M, Rupprecht C, et al. Effects of glucocorticoids on plasma catecholamines in depression. Psychiatry Res 1989;29:187–198.

254. Beskow J, Runeson B, Åsgård U. Psychological autopsies: methods and ethics. Suicide Life Threat Behav 1990;20:307–323.

255. Dorpat TL, Ripley HS. A study of suicide in the Seattle area. Compr Psychiatry 1960;1:349–359.

256. Barraclough BM, Bunch J, Nelson B, et al. 100 cases of suicide—clinical aspects. Br J Psychiatry 1974;125:355–373.

257. Conwell Y. Suicide in the elderly. In: Schneider LS, Reynolds CF III, Lebowitz BD, Friedhoff AJ, eds. Diagnosis and treatment of depression in late life. Washington DC: American Psychiatric Press, Inc., 1994:397–418.

258. Rich CL, Ricketts JE, Fowler RC, Young D. Some differences between men and women who commit suicide. Am J Psychiatry 1988;145:718–722.

259. Åsgård U. A psychiatric study of suicide among urban Swedish women. Acta Psychiatr Scand 1990;82:115–124.

260. Carlson GA. More analysis of Eli Robins' data. Am J Psychiatry 1984;141:323.

261. Robins E. The final months. New York: Oxford University Press, 1981.

262. Conwell Y, Caine ED, Henderson RE, Flannery CJ, Forbes NT. Suicide and aging: psychological autopsy findings. American Psychiatric Association. New Orleans, May, 1991.

263. Miles CP. Conditions predisposing to suicide: a review. J Nerv Ment Dis 1977;164:231–246.

264. Guze SB, Robins E. Suicide and primary affective disorders. Br J Psychiatry 1970;117:437–438.

265. Pokorny AD. Prediction of suicide in psychiatric patients: a report of a prospective study. Arch Gen Psychiatry 1983;40:249–257.

266. Gardner EA, Bahn AK, Mack M. Suicide and psychiatric care in the aging. Arch Gen Psychiatry 1964;10:547–553.

267. Barraclough BM, Pallis DJ. Depression followed by suicide: a comparison of depressed suicides with living depressives. Psychol Med 1975;5:55–61.

268. Roy A. Suicide in recurrent affective disorder patients. Can J Psychiatry 1984;29:319–322.

269. Berglund M, Nilsson K. Mortality in severe depression: a prospec-

tive study including 103 suicides. Acta Psychiatr Scand 1987;76: 372–380.

270. Fawcett J, Scheftner W, Clark D, Hedeker D, Gibbons R, Coryell W. Clinical predictors of suicide in patients with major affective disorders: a controlled prospective study. Am J Psychiatry 1987;144: 35–40.

271. McGlashan TH. The Chestnut Lodge follow-up study: II. Long-term outcome of schizophrenia and the affective disorders. Arch Gen Psychiatry 1984;41:586–601.

272. Black DW, Winokur G, Nasrallah A. Suicide in subtypes of major affective disorder. Arch Gen Psychiatry 1987;44:878–880.

273. Weeke A, Vaeth M. Excess mortality of bipolar and unipolar manic-depressive patients. J Affect Disord 1986;11:227–234.

274. Morrison JR. Suicide in a psychiatric practice. J Clin Psychiatry 1982;43:348–352.

275. Roose SP, Glassman AH, Walsh BT, Woodring S, Vital-Herne J. Depression, delusions, and suicide. Am J Psychiatry 1983;140:1159–1162.

276. Wolfersdorf M, Keller F, Steiner B, Hole G. Delusional depression and suicide. Acta Psychiatr Scand 1987;76:359–363.

277. Coryell W, Tsuang MT. Primary unipolar depression and the prognostic importance of delusions. Arch Gen Psychiatry 1982;39: 1181–1184.

278. Caldwell CB, Gottesman II. Schizophrenia—a high risk factor for suicide: clues to risk reduction. Suicide Life Threat Behav 1992;22: 479–493.

279. Wilkinson DG. The suicide rate in schizophrenia. Br J Psychiatry 1982;140:138–141.

280. Allebeck P, Wistedt B. Mortality in schizophrenia: a ten-year follow-up based on the Stockholm County Inpatient Register. Arch Gen Psychiatry 1986;43:650–653.

281. Black DW, Winokur G, Warrack G. Suicide in schizophrenia: the Iowa record linkage study. J Clin Psychiatry 1985;46:14–17.

282. Breier A, Astrachan BM. Characterization of schizophrenic patients who commit suicide. Am J Psychiatry 1984;141:206–209.

283. Roy A. Suicide in chronic schizophrenia. Br J Psychiatry 1982;141: 171–177.

284. Drake RE, Gates C, Cotton PG, Whitaker A. Suicide among schizophrenics. Who is at risk? J Nerv Ment Dis 1984;172:613–617.

285. Langley GE, Bayatti NN. Suicide in Exe Vale Hospital, 1972-1981. Br J Psychiatry 1982;145:463–467.

286. Virkkunen M. Suicide in schizophrenia and paranoid psychosis. Acta Psychiatr Scand 1974;250(suppl):1–305.

287. Newman SC, Bland RC. Mortality in a cohort of patients with schizophrenia: a record linkage study. Can J Psychiatry 1991;36: 239–245.

288. Loranger AW. Sex difference in age at onset of schizophrenia. Arch Gen Psychiatry 1984;41:157–161.

289. Roy A. Suicide in schizophrenia. In: Roy A, ed. Suicide. Baltimore: Williams & Wilkins, 1986:97–112.

290. Warnes H. Suicide in schizophrenics. Diseases of the Nerv Syst 1968;29(suppl):35–40.

291. Black DW, Warrack G, Winokur G. The Iowa record linkage study. Arch Gen Psychiatry 1985;42:71–75.

292. Lindberg S, Ågren G. Mortality among male and female hospitalized alcoholics in Stockholm 1962-1983. Br J Addict 1988;83:1193–1200.

293. Murphy GE, Wetzel RD. The lifetime risk of suicide in alcoholism. Arch Gen Psychiatry 1990;47:383–392.

294. Goodwin DW. Alcohol in suicide and homicide. Quarterly Journal of Studies on Alcohol 1973;34:144–156.

295. Murphy GE. Suicide in alcoholism. New York: Oxford University Press, 1992.

296. Allgulander C, Borg S, Vikander B. A 4–6 year follow-up of 50 patients with primary dependence on sedative and hypnotic drugs. Am J Psychiatry 1984;141:1580–1582.

297. Murphy SL, Rounsaville BJ, Eyre S, Kleber HD. Suicide attempts in treated opiate addicts. Compr Psychiatry 1983;24:79–89.

298. Marzuk PM, Tardiff K, Leon AC, Stajic M, Morgan EB, Mann JJ. Prevalence of cocaine use among residents of New York City who committed suicide during a one-year period. Am J Psychiatry 1992;149:371–375.

299. Fowler RC, Rich CL, Young D. San Diego suicide study. II. Substance abuse in young cases. Arch Gen Psychiatry 1986;43:962–965.

300. Regier DA, Farmer ME, Rae DS, et al. Co-morbidity of mental disorders with alcohol and other drug abuse. JAMA 1990;264:2511–2518.

301. Murphy GE, Wetzel RD, Robins E, McEvoy L. Multiple risk factors predict suicide in alcoholism. Arch Gen Psychiatry 1992;49: 459–463.

302. Murphy GE, Robins E. Social factors in suicide. JAMA 1967;199: 303–308.

303. Murphy GE, Armstrong JW, Hermele SL, Fischer JR, Clendenin WW. Suicide and alcoholism: interpersonal loss confirmed as a predictor. Arch Gen Psychiatry 1979;36:65–69.

304. Duberstein PR. Interpersonal stressors, substance abuse, and suicide. J Nerv Ment Dis 1993;181:80–85.

305. Tamerin JS, Mendelson JH. The psychodynamics of chronic inebriation: observations of alcoholics during the process of drinking in an experimental group setting. Am J Psychiatry 1969;125:886–899.

306. Ballenger JC, Goodwin FK, Major LF, Brown GL. Alcohol and central serotonin metabolism in man. Arch Gen Psychiatry 1979;36: 224–227.

307. Branchey L, Branchey M, Shaw S, Lieber CS. Depression, suicide, and aggression in alcoholics and their relationship to plasma amino acids. Psychiatry Res 1984;12:219–226.

308. Buydens-Branchey L, Branchey MH, Noumair D, Lieber CS. Age of alcoholism onset. II. Relationship to susceptibility to serotonin precursor availability. Arch Gen Psychiatry 1989;46:231–236.

309. Babigian HM, Odoroff C. The mortality experience of a population with psychiatric illness. Am J Psychiatry 1969;126:470–480.

310. Pope HG, Jonas JM, Hudson JI, Cohen BM, Gunderson JG. The validity of DSM-III borderline personality disorder. Arch Gen Psychiatry 1983;40:23–30.

311. Maddocks PD. A five year follow-up of untreated psychopaths. Br J Psychiatry 1970;116:511–515.

312. Weissman MM, Klerman GL, Markowitz JS, Ouellette R, Phil M. Suicidal ideation and suicide attempts in panic disorder and attacks. N Engl J Med 1989;321:1209–1261.

313. Johnson J, Weissman MM, Klerman GL. Panic disorder, co-morbidity, and suicide attempts. Arch Gen Psychiatry 1990;47:805–808.

314. Vonsattel JP, Myers RH, Stevens TJ, Ferrante RJ, Bird ED, Richardson EP. Neuropathological classification of Huntington's disease. J Neuropathol Exp Neurol 1985;44:559–577.

315. Boll T, Heaton R, Reitan R. Neuropsychological and emotional correlates of Huntington's chorea. J Nerv Ment Dis 1974;158:61–69.

316. Heathfield KWG. Huntington's chorea. Brain 1967;90:203–232.

317. Dewhurst K, Oliver JE, McKnight AL. Socio-psychiatric consequences of Huntington's disease. Am J Psychiatry 1970;116: 255–258.

318. Huntington G. On chorea. Med Surg Reporter 1872;26:317–321.

319. Minski L, Guttmann E. Huntington's chorea: a study of thirty-four families. J Ment Sci 1938;84:21–96.

320. Chandler JH, Reed E, DeJong RN. Huntington's chorea in Michigan. III. Clinical observations. Neurology 1960;10:148–153.

321. Tamir A, Whittier J, Korenyi C. Huntington's chorea: a sex difference in psychopathological symptoms. Dis Nerv Sys 1969;30:103.

322. Saugstad L, Odegård O. Huntington's chorea in Norway. Psychol Med 1986;16:39–48.

323. Schoenfeld M, Myers RH, Cupples LA, Berkman B, Sax DS, Clark E. Increased rate of suicide among patients with Huntington's disease. J Neurol Neurosurg Psychiatry 1984;47:1283–1287.

324. Farrer LA. Suicide and attempted suicide in Huntington disease: implications for preclinical testing of persons at risk. Am J Med Genet 1986;24:305–311.

325. Kessler S, Field T, Worth L, Mosbarger H. Attitudes of persons at risk

for Huntington disease toward predictive testing. Am J Med Genet 1987;26:259–270.

326. Mastromauro C, Myers RH, Berkman B. Attitudes toward presymptomatic testing in Huntington disease. Am J Med Genetics 1987;26: 271–282.

327. Kessler S, Bloch M. Social system responses to Huntington's disease. Family Process 1989;28:59–68.

328. Albin RL, Young AB, Penney JB, et al. Abnormalities of striatal projection neurons and N-methyl-$_D$-aspartate receptors in presymptomatic Huntington's disease. N Engl J Med 1990;322:1293–1298.

329. Lam RW, Bloch M, Jones BD, et al. Psychiatric morbidity associated with early clinical diagnosis of Huntington disease in a predictive testing program. J Clin Psychiatry 1988;49:444–447.

330. Rao SM. Neuropsychology of multiple sclerosis: a critical review. J Clin Exper Neuropsychol 1986;8:503–542.

331. Stenager EN, Stenager E. Suicide and patients with neurologic diseases. Arch Neurol 1992;49:1296–1303.

332. Joffe RT, Lippert GP, Gray TA, Sawa G, Horvath Z. Mood disorder and multiple sclerosis. Arch Neurol 1987;44:376–378.

333. Schwartz ML, Pierron M. Suicide and fatal accidents in multiple sclerosis. Omega 1972;3:291–293.

334. Sadovnick AD, Eisen K, Ebers GC, Paty DW. Cause of death in patients attending multiple sclerosis clinics. Neurology 1991;41: 1193–1196.

335. Stenager EN, Stenager E, Koch-Henriksen N, et al. Suicide and multiple sclerosis: an epidemiological investigation. J Neurol Neurosurg Psychiatry 1992;55:542–545.

336. Stensman R, Sundqvist-Stensman U. Physical disease and disability among 416 suicide cases in Sweden. Scand J Soc Med 1988;16: 149–153.

337. Kontaxakis VP, Christodoulou GN, Mavreas VG, Havaki-Kontaxaki BJ. Attempted suicide in psychiatric outpatients with concurrent physical illness. Psychother Psychosom 1988;50:201–206.

338. Stacy M, Jankovic J. Clinical and neurobiological aspects of Parkinson's disease. In: Huber SJ, Cummings JL, eds. Parkinson's disease: neurobehavioral aspects. New York: Oxford University Press, 1992: 10–31.

339. Santamaria J, Tolosa E. Clinical subtypes of Parkinson's disease and depression. In: Huber SJ, Cummings JL eds. Parkinson's disease: neurobehavioral aspects. New York: Oxford University Press, 1992: 217–228.

340. Enna SJ. Brain serotonin receptors and neuropsychiatric disorders. Adv Exp Med Biol 1981;133:347–357.

341. Cash R, Raisman R, Ploska A, Agid Y. High and low affinity [^{3}H]imipramine binding sites in control and Parkinsonian brains. Eur J Pharmacol 1985;117:71–80.

342. Hoehn MM, Yahr MD. Parkinsonism: onset, progression, and mortality. Neurology 1967;17:427–442.

343. Mendez MF, Cummings JL, Benson DF. Depression in epilepsy. Arch Neurol 1986;43:766–770.

344. Currie S, Heathfield KWG, Henson RA, et al. Clinical course and prognosis of temporal lobe epilepsy: a survey of 666 patients. Brain 1972;94:173–190.

345. Mendez MF, Lanska DJ, Manon-Espaillat R, Burnstine TH. Causative factors for suicide attempts by overdose in epileptics. Arch Neurol 1989;46:1065–1068.

346. White SJ, McLean AEM, Howland C. Anticonvulsant drugs and cancer: a cohort study in patients with severe epilepsy. Lancet 1979;2:458–461.

347. Mendez MF, Doss RC. Ictal and psychiatric aspects of suicide in epileptic patients. Int J Psychiatry Med 1992;22:231–237.

348. Barraclough BM. The suicide rate of epilepsy. Acta Psychiatr Scand 1987;76:339–345.

349. Matthews WS, Barabas G. Suicide and epilepsy: a review of the literature. Psychosomatics 1981;6:515–524.

350. Hawton K, Fagg J, Marsack P. Association between epilepsy and attempted suicide. J Neurol Neurosurg Psychiatry 1980;43: 168–170.

351. Batzel LW, Dodrill CB. Emotional and intellectual correlates of unsuccessful suicide attempts in people with epilepsy. J Clin Psychology 1986;42:699–702.

352. Le CT, Price M. Survival from spinal cord injury. J Chron Dis 1982;35:487–492.

353. DeVivo MJ, Black KJ, Richards JS, Stover SL. Suicide following spinal cord injury. Paraplegia 1991;29:620–627.

354. Frisbie JH, Kache A. Increasing survival and changing causes of death in myelopathy patients. J Am Paraplegia Soc 1983;6:51–56.

355. Geisler WO, Jousse AT, Wynne-Jones M. Survival in traumatic transverse myelitis. Paraplegia 1977;14:262–275.

356. Geisler WO, Jousse AT, Wynne-Jones M, Breithaupt D. Survival in traumatic spinal cord injury. Paraplegia 1983;21:364–373.

357. Nyquist RH, Bors E. Mortality and survival in traumatic myelopathy during nineteen years, from 1946 to 1965. Paraplegia 1967; 5:22–47.

358. Charlifue SW, Gerhart KA. Behavioral and demographic predictors of suicide after traumatic spinal cord injury. Arch Phys Med Rehabil 1991;72:488–492.

359. Judd FK, Brown DJ. Suicide following acute traumatic spinal cord injury. Paraplegia 1992;30:173–177.

360. Robinson RG, Kubos KL, Starr LB, Rao K, Price TR. Mood disorders in stroke patients: importance of location of lesion. Brain 1984;107:81–93.

361. Goldstein RB, Black DW, Nasrallah A, Winokur G. The prediction of suicide: sensitivity, specificity, and predictive value of a multivariate model applied to suicide among 1906 patients with affective disorders. Arch Gen Psychiatry 1991;48:418–422.

362. Shneidman ES. Some essentials of suicide and some implications for response. In: Roy A, ed. Suicide. Baltimore: Williams & Wilkins, 1986:1–16.

363. McIntosh JL. Research on suicide: a bibliography. Westport: Greenwood Press, 1985.

364. Brent DA, Perper JA, Allman CJ, Moritz GM, Wartella ME, Zelenak JP. The presence and accessibility of firearms in the homes of adolescent suicides: a case-control study. JAMA 1991;266:2989–3029.

365. Sloan JH, Rivara FP, Reay DT, Ferris JAJ, Path MRC, Kellermann AL. Firearm regulations and rates of suicide: a comparison of two metropolitan areas. N Engl J Med 1990;322:369–373.

366. Loftin C, McDowall D, Wiersema B, Cottey TJ. Effects of restrictive licensing of handguns on homicide and suicide in the District of Columbia. N Engl J Med 1991;325:1615–1620.

367. Marzuk PM, Leon AC, Tardiff K, Morgan EB, Stajic M, Mann JJ. The effect of access to lethal methods of injury on suicide rates. Arch Gen Psychiatry 1992;49:451–458.

368. Rich CL, Young JG, Fowler RC, Wagner J, Black NA. Guns and suicide: possible effects of some specific legislation. Am J Psychiatry 1990;147:342–346.

369. Clark DC. Suicide among the elderly. Final report to the AARP Andrus Foundation, January 28, 1991.

370. Rockwell DA, O'Brien W. Physicians' knowledge and attitudes about suicide. JAMA 1973;225:1347–1349.

371. Knights EB, Folstein MF. Unsuspected emotional and cognitive disturbance in medical patients. Ann Intern Med 1977;87:723–724.

372. Nielsen AC, Williams TA. Depression in ambulatory medical patients. Arch Gen Psychiatry 1980;37:999–1004.

373. Rutz W, von Knorring L, Walinder J. Frequency of suicide on Gotland after systematic postgraduate education of general practitioners. Acta Psychiatr Scand 1989;80:151–154.

374. Maltsberger JT. Suicide risk—the formulation of clinical judgment. New York: New York University Press, 1986.

375. Avery D, Winokur G. Mortality in depressed patients treated with electroconvulsive therapy and antidepressants. Arch Gen Psychiatry 1976;33:1029–1037.

376. Avery D, Winokur G. Suicide, attempted suicide, and relapse rates in depression. Arch Gen Psychiatry 1978;35:749–753.

377. Huston PE, Locher LM. Manic-depressive psychosis. Course when

treated and untreated with electric shock. Arch Neurology Psychiatry 1948;60:37–48.

378. Montgomery SA, Montgomery DB, Green M, Bullock T, Baldwin D. Pharmacotherapy in the prevention of suicidal behavior. J Clin Psychopharmacol 1992;12:27S–31S.

379. Hirsch SR, Walsh C, Draper R. Parasuicide: a review of treatment interventions. J Affect Disord 1982;4:299–311.

380. Blumenthal SJ, Kupfer DJ, eds. Suicide over the life cycle: risk factors, assessment, and treatment of suicidal patients. 1st ed. Washington, DC: American Psychiatric Press, Inc., 1990.

381. Farberow NL, Gallagher DE, Gilewski MJ, Thompson LW. An examination of the early impact of bereavement on psychological distress in survivors of suicide. Gerontologist 1987;27:592–598.

382. Ness DE, Pfeffer CR. Sequelae of bereavement resulting from suicide. Am J Psychiatry 1990;147:279–285.

383. Appel YH, Wrobleski A. Self-help and support groups: mutual aid for survivors. In: Dunne EJ, McIntosh JL, Dunne-Maxim K, eds. Suicide and its aftermath: understanding and counseling the survivors. New York: WW Norton, 1987:215–233.

24

NEUROPSYCHIATRY OF AGGRESSION

Jeffrey L. Saver, Stephen P. Salloway, Orrin Devinsky, and David M. Bear

---

Human aggression is an urgent social and clinical problem. In the United States, homicide is the 12th leading cause of death and the second most common cause of mortality among young, healthy individuals (1, 2).

Aggression is an inescapable clinical challenge in diverse neuropsychiatric patient populations. Relatives of individuals with traumatic brain injury identify temper and irritability as major behavioral difficulties in 70% of patients (3). Ten to twenty percent of psychiatric inpatients commit acts of violence or assault during the 2 weeks prior to their admission (4–7), and 3–37% assault staff or patients during their hospitalization (8–11). Costs of inpatient care for assaultive patients are over 40% greater than for their nonassaultive counterparts (12).

Past attempts to understand and treat violent behavior have been thwarted by the outmoded dichotomy of nature versus nurture. Undoubtedly, sociocultural factors are critically important in the genesis of many aggressive behaviors. Epidemiological studies demonstrate that key environmental variables contributing to the development of repeatedly violent individuals include rearing in disordered households, physical and/or sexual abuse in childhood, and social deprivation (13–16).

However, every violent behavior, whether motivated by disturbed rearing or the highest political and religious ideals, requires a neurobiological substrate to orchestrate the complex array of perceptual, motor, and autonomic components of acts that constitute aggressive conduct. In humans, acquired brain lesions may disrupt the neural systems that ordinarily regulate hostile behavior. In some instances, individuals with focal brain injury may exhibit aggressive behavior that has no relevant developmental or environmental precipitant, or only minimal social provocation. More often, damage to neural circuits controlling aggression leads not to random acts of overt aggression, but to alterations in temperament and inappropriate choices of targets and settings for aggressive behavior. The recognition, diagnostic evaluation, and treatment of such patients are challenges facing the neuropsychiatrist and behavioral neurologist.

Neuropsychiatric investigations of aggression have been hampered by an overly simplified concept of "organicity."

Explicitly or implicitly, some authors have suggested that neurological impairment produces a unitary "organic aggression syndrome," possessing stable, invariant behavioral features independent of lesion type or location. The stereotypic organic aggression syndrome is often postulated to lower a general threshold for aggression or to result in episodic dyscontrol. This formulation is both simplistic and imprecise, obscuring fundamental evolutionary, neurochemical, neurophysiological, and clinical distinctions among discrete aggression-related neural circuits in the brainstem, diencephalon, limbic system, and neocortex.

As an alternative, this chapter outlines a multiregional, hierarchical model of the neural regulation of aggression that draws upon converging sources of evidence from evolutionary studies, ethology, neurophysiology, pharmacology, and clinical neuroscience. Recognizing multiple, hierarchical controls over hostile behavior affords the neuropsychiatrist a framework for identifying distinctive clinical syndromes of aggression due to brain injury, considering the differential diagnosis and diagnostic workup of patients, and implementing rational, pathophysiologically-directed treatment.

NEUROSCIENCE OF AGGRESSION

Biological Origins of Human Aggression

Clinicians confronted with aggressive patients tend to regard hostile behavior as a problem needing to be suppressed. However, aggression has important sociobiological functions. Like fear, hunger, sexual desire, and social cohesion, adaptive aggression is present throughout the order Mammalia, triggered by environmentally appropriate and highly specific stimuli (17–19). Agonistic behavior to obtain food, defend a territory, protect offspring, or win a mate is essential for the survival of the individual and for propagation of its genetic material.

Recent formulations of evolutionary theory suggest that competitive selection favors the development of closely regulated and intertwined aggressive and peacemaking behaviors (18, 20, 21). Within the primate and other lines of evolution, unregulated, wanton aggression would rapidly reduce support among an organism's conspecifics and impair

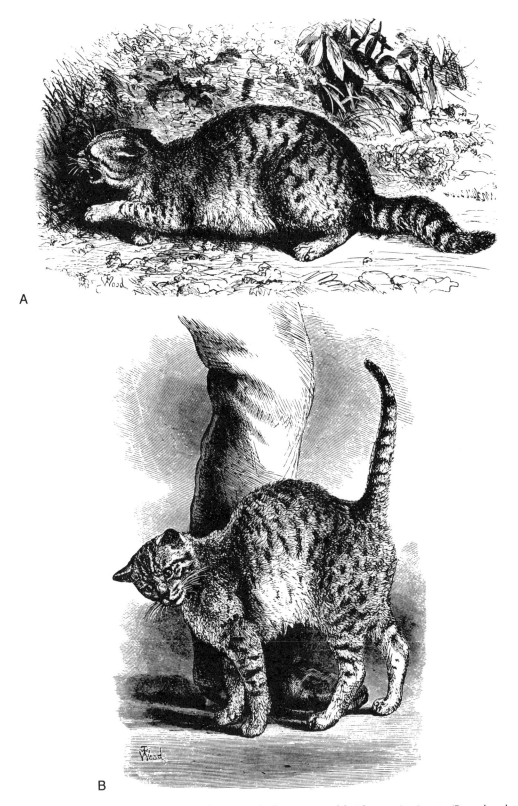

Figure 24.1. Aggression (**A**) and affection (**B**) signaled through opposing body postures and facial expression in cats. (Reproduced with permission from Darwin C. The expression of emotions in man and animals [1873]. Reprinted, London: Appleton, 1965.)

reproductive success. Conversely, uniformly submissive and avoidant behavior would prevent an organism from gaining access to needed resources. Selection pressures on social behavior naturally tend to foster "evolutionarily stable strategies" in which an organism may variably express either aggressive or affiliative behaviors, depending on the state of several variables at the time of a particular encounter with conspecifics, including its past interactions with that indi-

Table 24.1.   Behavioral Classification of Aggression[a]

Type	Eliciting Stimulus	Form
Predatory	Natural prey	Efficient, little affective display
Territorial	Boundary crossing	—
Intermale	Conspecific male	Ritualized responses
Fear-induced	Threat	Autonomic reactions, defensive behaviors
Maternal	Distress calls, threat to offspring	Initial attempts to avoid conflict
Irritable	Frustration, deprivation, pain	Hyperactivity, affective display
Instrumental	—	—

[a]Modified from Moyer KE. The psychobiology of aggression. New York: Harper & Row, 1976.

vidual, position in dominance hierarchies, age, strength, and the general availability of environmental resources (22–25). The need for a neural system to regulate aggression is greater in social animals than for species leading a solitary existence. In social primates, its expression is precisely controlled at multiple anatomical levels.

Concerning the outward display of emotion, natural selection has fostered principles of signaling among conspecifics that recur in invertebrates, dogs, cats, primates, and humans (26–28). Emotional displays are highly stereotyped, and opposing emotions are frequently conveyed by "antagonistic" postures, assuring accurate communication of an organism's emotional state. Darwin first suggested that human facial expressions originated from postures associated with adaptive actions among our mammalian forebears. He concluded that an expression of anger such as the sneer evolved from the baring of the canine teeth prior to a biting attack. Over time, assuming a fighting posture through body and facial musculature may come to signal the possibility of, rather than solely the enactment of, attack: inhibition of the neuronal assembly triggering an aggressive posture, and activation of neurons enabling opposing postures, can then convey the "antagonistic" emotion of friendliness or submissiveness (Fig. 24.1). In this way, a complex affective communication system can develop, hard-wired at its lowest neuronal level of implementation, but regulated by higher centers that moderate the timing and intensity of display, and may even allow feigning of aggressive or other emotional states.

An efficient neurobiological mechanism for regulating emotional expressions and modifying the probability of aggressive versus submissive responses would employ opposing neuromodulators to excite or inhibit groups of motoneurons that enact aggressive postures. The lobster provides an example of such a hormonal system that has been characterized in detail (29). Serotonin biases the organism to assume an aggressive or fighting stance (extension of major muscle groups), while octopamine promotes a submissive posture (flexion of major muscle groups).

The substantial role of subcortical neuromodulators, such as norepinephrine, acetylcholine, and serotonin, in modifying aggressive propensities in man likely developed from their phylogenetically ancient functions in promoting relevant peripheral skeletal postures and autonomic responses. The complex array of controls over aggression in social

primates, however, clearly could not be achieved by simple changes in levels of subcortical neuromodulators or peripheral neurohormones.

One source of the complexity of neural regulation of aggression in mammals is the existence of several distinct subtypes of aggressive behavior. In general, aggressive acts are triggered, targeted, promptly terminated, and specifically inhibited by various classes of environmental stimuli. Ethologists have identified several classes of aggressive behavior, each with a specific outward display and set of determining stimuli. Moyer's widely recognized classification scheme divides hostile behavior into predatory, territorial, inter-male, maternal, defensive, fear-induced, irritable, and instrumental subtypes (Table 24.1) (30). Each subtype is probably controlled by distinct, albeit somewhat overlapping, neuranatomical and neurochemical substrates (31–33). In various animal models, neuronal recording and lesion studies have identified important loci participating in neural networks controlling these discrete assertive behaviors (Table 24.2) (34). Evidence for broadly similar predatory and affective clustering of aggressive behaviors has been reported in psychiatric patients (35).

Neural Regulation of Aggression in Man—General Principles

While in simple organisms neurohormonal mediation of aggressive-submissive postures might suffice for regulating hostile behavior, in social mammals and especially in primates, the need for flexible and precise control of aggressive and other emotional behaviors has driven the evolution of hierarchic levels of intermediate and higher neural circuitry. In general, both somatic and nervous system evolution proceed not by replacing preexisting circuitry, but by modification and the addition of subtler levels of control over older structures (so-called "evolution by tinkering") (36). The human brain has developed through a progressive elaboration of neural elements surrounding the brainstem core found in less complex organisms. In the regulation of emotion, more recently evolved limbic, paralimbic, and neocortical components of the nervous system have established anatomical and physical controls over brainstem structures that implement autonomic, endocrine, and motoric somatic states (37, 38).

Discrete structures controlling drives exist at each level of the neuraxis, mediating between sensory and motor systems. Relatively simple protoreptilian nervous system regulatory mechanisms persist in the human brain at the level of the brainstem and hypothalamus. A second critical level of control in the mammalian brain is provided by the limbic structures, each of which projects directly to the hypothalamus. A third level, greatly expanded in higher primates, is the frontal neocortex, modulating both limbic and hypothalamic output. These levels are functionally distinctive, and each provides varying representations of the internal milieu and external environment; their differences may be clarified by a comparative analysis of their inputs (afferent circuitry), outputs (efferent circuitry), and functional organization (39). (See Chapter 7 on frontal and limbic neuroanatomy.)

Neurons controlling such basic drives as feeding and reproduction are closely associated at each anatomical site. Circuitry regulating aggression, which is often an instrumental response in the service of these basic drives, is

Table 24.2. Neuroanatomic Correlates of Aggression in Experimental Animals[a]

Triggers	Suppressors
Predatory offensive aggression	
Anterior hypothalamus	Prefrontal cortex
Lateral hypothalamus	Ventromedial hypothalamus
Lateral preoptic nuclei	Basolateral amygdala
Ventral midbrain tegmentum	Mammillary bodies
Ventral midbrain	
Ventromedial periaqueductal gray matter	
Inter-male (competitive) aggression	
Laterobasal septal nuclei	Dorsolateral frontal lobe
Centromedial amygdala	Olfactory bulbs
Ventrolateral posterior thalamus	Dorsomedial septal nuclei
Stria terminalis	Head of caudate
Fear-induced aggression	
Centromedial amygdala	Ventromedial hypothalamus
Fimbria fornix	Septal nuclei
Stria terminalis	Basolateral amygdala
Ventrobasal thalamus	Ventral hippocampus
Maternal-protective aggression	
Hypothalamus	Septal nuclei
Ventral hippocampus	Basolateral amygdala
Anterior hypothalamus	Frontal lobes
Ventromedial hypothalamus	Prefrontal cortex
Dorsomedial hypothalamus	Medial prepiriform cortex
Posterior hypothalamus	Ventromedial hypothalamus
Anterior cingulate gyrus	Head of caudate
Thalamic center median	Dorsomedian nucleus of thalamus
Ventrobasal thalamus	Stria terminalis
Ventral hippocampus	Dorsal hippocampus
Ventral midbrain tegmentum	Posterior cingulate gyrus
Ventromedial periaqueductal gray matter	Periamygdaloid cortex
Cerebellar fastigium	
Sex-related aggression	
Medial hypothalamus	Septal nuclei
Fimbria fornix (male)	Fimbria fornix (female)
Ventral hippocampus	Cingulate gyrus
	Dorsolateral amygdala

[a]Reproduced with permission from Treiman DM. Psychobiology of ictal aggression. Adv Neurol 1991;55:343.

localized in adjacent regions. Because of this anatomical propinquity, dysregulation of aggression caused by neurological injury is frequently accompanied by simultaneous abnormalities in feeding and sexual behavior, reflecting damage to adjacent neurons.

Brainstem Regulation of Aggression

Pontine and mesencephalic nuclei mediate fragments of aggressive displays. Inputs to the system include spinoreticular proprioceptive and nociceptive sensory circuits. Outputs incorporate pontine (facial) and descending motor centers, leading to stereotypic movements. Delgado evoked different fragments of aggressive facial expressions and vocalizations in subhuman primates with electrical stimulation in several upper brainstem nuclei, dissociated from offensive or defensive behavior (40). Other brainstem circuits contribute to somatomotor patterns for gestures and approach and avoidance behaviors (41). Medullary sympathetic and parasympathetic nuclei exert direct autonomic effects on cardiovascular, respiratory, and gastrointestinal peripheral organ systems. In humans, however, full-fledged aggression-related behavior patterns are not produced at the brainstem level. Response coordination and decision-making are carried out at higher processing stations. Consequently, brainstem lesions, although sometimes disturbing fragments of aggressive behavioral output, generally do not produce a syndrome of altered aggressivity.

One important exception is aggressive behavior arising from disruption of brainstem regulation of sleep-awake states, most notably rapid eye movement (REM) sleep behavior disorders. In normal individuals, during dreaming REM sleep, neurons in the vicinity of the locus ceruleus actively inhibit spinal motoneurons, suppressing motoric activity. As Jouvet and colleagues first demonstrated in the cat, bilateral pontine tegmental lesions may compromise REM sleep muscle atonia and permit the enactment of oneiric behaviors, frequently including biting and other attack conduct (42–44).

A similar parasomnia has recently been delineated in humans (45). Most commonly, middle-aged men will experience a violent dream in which they are attacked by animals or unfamiliar people. In response, the dreamer engages in vigorous, coordinated motor acts that are often violent in nature. Patients may jump off the bed, smash furniture, or attack their bed partner. Physical injuries are common to both the patient and spouse (46).

Although normal subjects wakened from REM sleep report an extremely diverse array of movements and activities fictively performed in dreams (47), violent actions comprise the overwhelming preponderance of behaviors actually enacted by individuals with the REM sleep behavior disorder. It may be speculated that aggressive responses orchestrated in the forebrain during REM dreaming must produce more powerful descending motor outputs than feeding, sexual, or other drive-related activities, and disproportionately override the partial residual muscle atonia in these patients. The REM sleep behavior disorder has been associated with diverse neurological and medical conditions in up to one-half of patients. Recently, it has been described as an accompaniment of PTSD. Ross et al. (47a) found muscle activation during REM sleep in many PTSD patients who underwent polysomnography.

A 68-year-old man evaluated by one of the authors (S.S.) reported an 8-year history of awakening several nights per month in the midst of a dream urge to strangle his children. On awakening, his hands were positioned as if he were grabbing their necks. On an overnight ferry to Italy, he attempted to strangle the man next to him and screamed, "Blood! Blood! Blood!" Polysomnographic study confirmed a REM sleep behavior disorder and clonazepam eliminated the sleep-related violence.

Hypothalamic Regulation of Aggression

The primate hypothalamus receives inputs conveying information regarding the internal state of the organism through chemoceptors, osmoceptors, and viscerosensory cranial nerves. In contrast to these rich sources of interoceptive data, the hypothalamus does not directly receive sensory input regarding the external world from primary sensory or association neocortex. Important outputs of the hypothalamus are to the pituitary gland through releasing factors and directly transported peptides, to the autonomic nervous system, for which it serves as "head ganglion," and to midbrain and spinal motor centers that coordinate stereotypic movements (48). In controlling biological drives, the decision-making apparatus of the hypothalamus employs a hard-wired antagonism of excitatory and inhibitory nuclei. Algebraic, neurophysiological comparison of chemically coded inputs lead to either graded and homeostatic or threshold, stereotypic, all-or-none responses. These characteristics are exemplified by the reciprocally active lateral versus medial hypothalamic centers controlling hunger and satiety respectively. In the rat, stimulation of the lateral hypothalamic area initiates feeding, and ablation can lead to starvation; stimulation of the ventromedial neurons abruptly terminates eating, and lesions result in obesity. These hard-wired systems lead to predictable responses independent of the animal's experience.

Extensive studies in animals suggest that the principle of threshold elicitation of stereotypic response also characterizes hypothalamic control of aggression (Fig. 24.2). Bard demonstrated in cats that when all neural structures rostral to the hypothalamus were destroyed, the decorticate animals periodically entered a state of "sham rage" (49). With little or no provocation, they exhibited a combination of hissing, piloerection, pupil dilation, and extension of the claws. Later studies pinpointed the posterior lateral hypothalamus as the responsible site; stimulation reliably elicited sham rage in animals who had undergone cortical ablation. In the intact feline or rodent brain, stimulation of the posterior lateral hypothalamus shortens the latency for species-specific predatory attack (50, 51). Attack behavior can similarly be

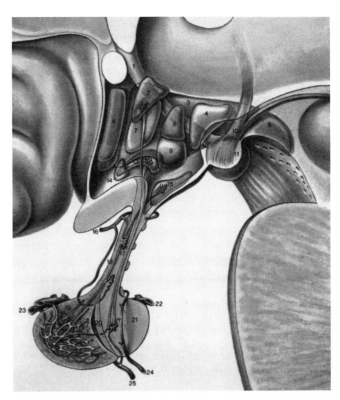

Figure 24.2. The hypothalamus and regulation of aggression. In cats, stimulation of the posterolateral hypothalamus facilitates aggression; ventromedial stimulation inhibits aggression. Stimulation of the lateral hypothalamic area (3) initiates feeding; stimulation of the ventromedial nucleus (9) abolishes eating. 1, Fornix; 2, Paraventricular nucleus; 3, Lateral hypothalamic area; 4, Posterior nucleus; 5, Ventral tegmental area; 6, Medial preoptic nucleus; 7, Anterior hypothalamic area; 8, Dorsomedial nucleus; 9, Ventromedial nucleus; 10, 11, Mammillary bodies; 12, Lateral preoptic nucleus; 13, Supraoptic nucleus; 14, Suprachiasmatic nucleus; 15, Infundibular nucleus. (Modified with permission from Nieuwenhuys R, Voogd J, Van Huijzen C. The human central nervous system: a synopsis and atlas. 3rd ed. Berlin: Springer-Verlag, 1988:297.)

facilitated by instilling acetylcholine and cholinomimetics into the lateral hypothalamus, promoting biting attacks of a cat upon a mouse or rat, or of a rat upon a mouse or frog, even by previously docile animals (52, 53). Injection of cholinergic antagonists will eliminate a biting attack, even in usually aggressive cats or rats.

Conversely, ventromedial hypothalamic stimulation may inhibit rather than facilitate aggression or can lead to a defensive posture (54). Ablation studies also suggest that the ventromedial area restrains hostile behavior, and its removal may permit the activity of regions that promote aggression to proceed unchecked. Bilateral ventromedial nucleus lesions increase the overall level of aggression in operated cats, and produce unprovoked attacks by previously friendly animals upon their caretakers (55).

Several case reports and small case series suggest a broadly similar role of the hypothalamus in human aggression (56–59). Neoplasms that destroy the ventromedial area bilaterally are associated with attacks on attendants reminiscent of animal aggression following ventromedial lesions. In Reeves and Plum's classic report, a 20-year-old woman developed bulimia and obesity, amenorrhea, diabetes insipidus, and a profound behavioral change. Over a 2-year period, she displayed outbursts of aggression characterized by indiscriminately scratching, hitting, or biting examiners who approached. She denied experiencing angry or vindictive internal feelings toward these individuals and frequently expressed surprise and regret for her attacks. The outbursts may have occurred more frequently when she had not eaten for several hours, suggesting the emergence of predatory-like aggression. Postmortem examination revealed a hamartoma that was destroying the ventromedial hypothalamus (56).

Another patient with bilateral hypothalamic lesions exhibited aggressive outbursts that appeared to be influenced by seasonal light levels, erupting more often in dark, winter months (57). These and other clinical cases suggest that in the human brain the hypothalamus plays an important role in the setting of a threshold for aggressive responses.

Amygdala and Temporolimbic Cortex Regulation of Aggression

In contrast to the hypothalamus, the amygdaloid complex is reciprocally connected with multiple cortical sensory systems capable of conveying highly processed information regarding the external world. Rich connections are established with a variety of both unimodal and polymodal sensory regions, such as the perirhinal cortex and the superior temporal sulcus, allowing convergence of information from visual, auditory, tactile, and gustatory cortices (60–62). Of particular note, the basolateral amygdala receives extensive projections from unimodal visual cortices in the inferotemporal cortex (such as area TE in primates) that are specialized for recognizing objects such as faces in central vision. Extensive intrinsic connections within the amygdala promote further coordination of sensory information.

Important outputs from the amygdala in primates are to the hypothalamus, through the stria terminalis and ventral amygdalofugal pathway, to brainstem centers controlling heart rate and respiration through the central nucleus projection pathway, and to the extrapyramidal motor system, especially the ventral striatum, also through the stria terminalis and ventral amygdalofugal pathway (Fig. 24.3) (61–63).

The amygdala appears to provide a critical link between sensory input processed in the cortical mantle to produce a model of external reality and hypothalamic and somatomotor centers evoking pain, fear, and other basic drive-related emotions (64). Many observations of animals and humans suggest that a fundamental function performed by the amygdaloid complex and related temporolimbic structures is linking perceived objects with appropriate emotional valences. The result is a qualitative steering of behavior rather than quantitative regulation of threshold. On the basis of prior experience, sensory-emotional associations direct consummatory behavior to appropriate targets in the external world.

The importance of the amygdaloid complex in the recall of the affective significance of stimuli is demonstrated by the

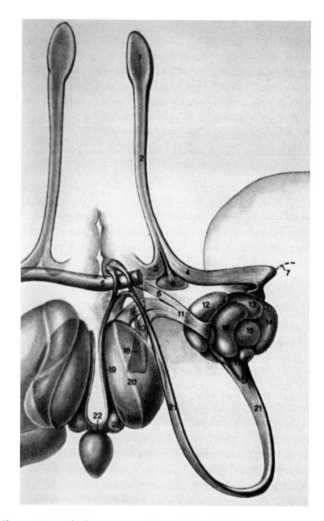

Figure 24.3. The human amygdala and selected subcortical efferents. 11, Ventral amygdalofugal pathway; 12–17, The amygdala; 12, Cortical nucleus; 13, Anterior nucleus; 14, Lateral nucleus; 15, Central nucleus; 16, Medial nucleus; 17, Basal nucleus; 18, Lateral hypothalamic area; 20, Medial thalamic nucleus; 21, Stria terminalis. (Modified with permission from Nieuwenhuys R, Voogd J, Van Huijzen C. The human central nervous system: a synopsis and atlas. 3rd ed. Berlin: Springer-Verlag, 1988:301.)

drive-object dysregulation of the Klüver-Bucy syndrome, observed in animals when the amygdala (and often overlying temporal neocortex) are removed bilaterally (65). Monkeys with such lesions move about in a continuous olfactory and oral exploration of their environment in which each object evokes the same response of tasting and sniffing as though the monkey had never encountered it previously. The animals fail to distinguish food from inedible objects and eat metal bolts and feces as readily as normal dietary items. Animals have difficulty distinguishing appropriate from inappropriate sexual partners; similarly lesioned cats will attempt copulation with chickens or other animals (66). These results suggest that lesioned animals cannot identify particular objects as being appropriate or inappropriate to satisfy hypothalamic drives (65–67).

The effects of bilateral amygdalectomy on aggressive behavior are consistent with such a hypothesis. Amygdala removal results in taming and placidity in most animals (65,

67). Objects that previously evoked signs of fear or provoked attack seem to lose their past associations. Monkeys no longer behave aggressively toward experimenters, becoming tame and easy to handle. Unilateral amygdalectomy with lesions of all commissural pathways produces taming when stimuli are presented to the operated hemisphere, but appropriate hostile responses when the stimuli are shown to the unoperated hemisphere (68). However, amygdalectomy in submissive monkeys has led to a maintained or increased level of aggression, consonant with the view that the fundamental effect of amygdalectomy on aggression is not a change in aggressive threshold, but a modification of previously acquired patterns of linking stimuli with aggressive responses (69, 70). Fundamentally appetitive drives, such as feeding and reproduction, are released onto inappropriate targets. An instrumental drive such as aggression is no longer elicited or suppressed according to past, learned responses of the animal.

In humans, extensive bilateral temporolimbic damage produces behavior that is similar to that of lesioned monkeys, frequently accompanied by amnesia, aphasia, and visual agnosia (Fig. 24.4) (71, 72). Patients may engage in indiscriminate oral and tactile exploration of their environment (hyperorality and hypermetamorphosis) and change their sexual preferences. Such individuals exhibit a flattened affect and report diminished subjective emotional responses to stimuli (73). Aggressive behaviors become uncommon, and apathy with lack of either strongly positive or negative responses become the rule. Placidity was noted in all 12 patients with the Klüver-Bucy syndrome in the series of Lilly et al. (74). One group performing bilateral amygdalotomies in aggressive patients reported that among 481 cases,

approximately 70% showed a reduction in either restlessness or destructiveness, and one-half of these remained placid even when purposefully provoked (75).

The first reported case of the Klüver-Bucy syndrome in humans well illustrates the characteristic clinical picture. A 19-year-old man underwent sequential left, followed by right temporal lobectomy for treatment of a refractory complex partial and generalized seizure disorder accompanied by frequent outbursts of violent behavior. Following the second operation, he demonstrated dramatic behavioral changes, including compulsive manual manipulation of objects in the environment, insatiable appetite, sexual exhibitionism with frequent masturbation, a severe retrograde and anterograde amnesia, and prosopagnosia. Most surprising to the reporting physicians was a new placidity and the disappearance of his previously aggressive behavior. "He no longer manifested the slightest rage reactions toward the nurses and doctors, upon whom, before the second operation, he used to rush as soon as they came into sight. The patient, on the contrary, now assumed an extremely childish and meek behavior with everyone and was absolutely resistant to any attempt to arouse aggressiveness and violent reactions in him" (76).

Related, modality-specific alterations in aggressive responding may appear when bilateral lesions may spare the amygdaloid complex but selectively interrupt pathways linking unimodal cortical sensory processing areas with the temporolimbic region. Stimuli presented solely within the sensory modality disconnected from the amygdala fail to evoke learned associations, but stimuli that may be processed through other sensory channels elicit normal responses. In the monkey, lesions that disconnect exclusively visual or

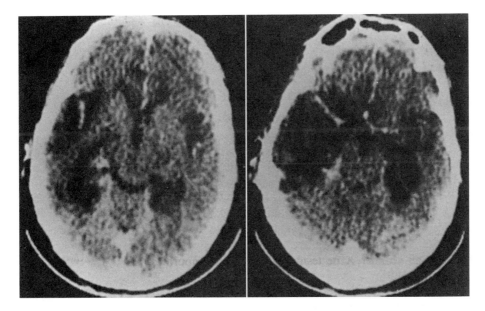

Figure 24.4. Hypoaggression (passivation) with bilateral temporolimbic lesions producing the Klüver-Bucy syndrome: A 42-year-old man with herpes simplex type II encephalitis. He was apathetic and indifferent to his troubles. Concurrently, he constantly manipulated and frequently mouthed objects; made sexual propositions to staff, especially men (prior to his illness he had been heterosexual); and exhibited severe anterograde amnesia and visual agnosia. Axial cranial CT images demonstrate large right-temporal and smaller left-mesial temporal hypodense lesions. (Reproduced from Bakchine S, Chain F, Lhermitte F. Rev Neurol 1986;142:126–132.)

tactile input to the temporal lobes result in isolated inability to discriminate food from non-food by sight or touch (77, 78).

Strategically placed structural lesions produce similar modality-specific limbic disconnection in humans (79, 80). Bauer et al. described a 39-year-old college graduate who suffered severe brain injury in a motorcycle accident. Computed tomography scans demonstrated bilateral cerebral hemorrhages in the inferior occipitotemporal region, interrupting visual input to polar and mesial temporolimbic structures. In addition to right hemiparesis, left hemidystonia, and prosopagnosia, he exhibited visual hypoemotionality—an isolated inability to react affectively to visual stimuli. A former assistant city planner, he was no longer moved by aesthetic differences between buildings. He stopped hiking because he now found natural scenery dull. He complained of total loss of emotional reaction to seeing attractive women in everyday encounters, and to erotic visual stimuli. However, he maintained a strong interest in music, to which he listened almost constantly. He could be sexually aroused by verbal-auditory stimuli and derived pleasure from touching and being touched. This modality-specific limbic disconnection extended to fear and aggressive responses. In laboratory testing, when exposed to a series of slides, he rated as neutral and unemotional threatening images such as a gun and a snake, which normal controls scored as negative and highly arousing (81).

An intriguing contrast to the behavioral alterations that result from removal of the temporal lobes is provided by far a more common clinical condition, temporal lobe epilepsy, in which abnormal neuronal excitability develops within temporolimbic cell populations. Although patients are rarely aggressive during ictal discharges, recent interest has focused on interictal behavioral alterations among patients with a long-standing temporal lobe focus.

Within the temporal lobe, the amygdaloid complex is particularly sensitive to the phenomenon of kindling, in which repeated stimulation of neurons leads to a progressive lowering of the threshold for discharge. Because many processing pathways converge on the amygdala, activity of epileptic foci throughout (and in fact beyond) the temporal lobe can affect amygdalar excitability. The resulting enhancement of amygdaloid activity may, in a general sense, be the converse of the decreased activity underlying Klüver-Bucy syndrome (82, 83).

In normal animals, individual amygdaloid neurons respond selectively to biologically significant food and social stimuli (84, 85). Kindling may lead to long-term changes in limbic physiology that alter and enhance aggressive and other emotional responses to both drive-related and neutral stimuli (86–89). Rather than losing previously acquired associations between sensory stimuli and drives, some temporal lobe epilepsy patients appear to forge new, fortuitous associations. Rather than a lack of emotional response to stimuli, they exhibit deepened and generalized affective associations (90).

Interictal behavioral changes consistent with the aforementioned model have been observed in a subset of patients with temporal lobe epilepsy. A cluster of interictal behaviors (the Geschwind syndrome) encompasses deepening emotions, a sensitivity to moral issues, often with religious and philosophical preoccupations, and hypergraphia—a tendency to write about these subjects at great length (91, 92).

As a consequence of strongly felt emotions, these individuals may become especially sensitive to slights or violations of principle, and experience intense anger. Strong moral and philosophical beliefs often preclude violent acts. However, if patients do act aggressively, their behavior typically is performed in clear consciousness and often followed by sincere regret. One patient with a nondominant temporal lobe focus attributed aggression to an "alternate personality" (93).

In an illustrative case, a 40-year-old man developed complex partial seizures in his 20s, characterized by fear followed by flushing, tachycardia, and loss of consciousness. He had suffered febrile seizures in childhood. Electroencephalography (EEG) showed bilateral temporal discharges, and pneumoencephalography demonstrated a dilated temporal horn of the left lateral ventricle.

His interictal behavior was remarkable for extreme seriousness with virtually no sense of humor and a sensitivity to infractions of minor military procedures. When fellow servicemen lightheartedly violated minor rules, he would attempt to reason with them. However, he became incensed by their failure to appreciate his concerns, and many brawls ensued. The patient was enraged when sentenced to a military stockade for 7 days, especially because his elaborate ethical justification for his actions was not taken seriously. To indicate his anger, he destroyed plumbing fixtures in his cell and subsequently threatened to kill the magistrate whom he believed had treated him unfairly.

Following release and neuropsychiatric treatment, his temper became better controlled as he developed strong religious and philosophical convictions that prohibited violence. Nonetheless, several years after overt violent behavior had ceased, he told an examiner, "I have more of a problem with anger than anybody I have ever met in my life." He described a constant internal tension between feelings of being treated unjustly and a sincere desire not to harm another individual. Other aspects of his behavior consistent with the interictal behavior syndrome included evangelical religiosity, extensive and detailed writing, and inappropriately prolonged encounters with fellow patients and caretakers (enhanced social cohesionviscosity) (93).

In another illustrative case, a 10-year-old girl had experienced a head injury with loss of consciousness, followed by episodes of déja vu and impaired consciousness beginning at age 14. Subsequently these simple and complex partial seizures progressed to secondarily generalized tonic-clonic convulsions. EEG demonstrated bilateral, independent temporal lobe spikes with right-sided predominance. She developed behavior changes of an interictal behavioral syndrome, including extensive writing of poetry and philosophical manuscripts, conversion from heterosexual to homosexual orientation, and irritability.

At age 15, she experienced the first of many dissociative episodes. She traveled a long distance from her home, identifying herself as "Chris," spoke with a harsh, masculine voice, and was threatening. Once she found herself lying in a park with a bloody stick in her hand next to the unconscious body of an unfamiliar man. On another occasion, she abruptly dissociated during psychotherapy and held a knife to her psychiatrist's throat for 3 hours. Later, when the main personality had regained control, her remorse was so profound that she presented the therapist with a vial of her own blood by way of an apology (93). Such dissociative episodes are interictal phenomena, and not seizures.

Prefrontal Cortical Regulation of Aggression

The dorsolateral prefrontal cortex receives extensive afferents from multiple posterior neocortical association areas, including dense connections with the inferior parietal lobule, a region intimately involved in surveying extrapersonal space for relevant stimuli. The orbitofrontal cortex is reciprocally connected to the rest of the neocortex principally via the dorsolateral convexity of the frontal lobe (94–96). Projections from the hypothalamus through the dorsal medial nucleus of the thalamus and from the rostral temporal lobe through the uncinate fasciculus potentially inform the frontal lobes of both internal (hypothalamus) and external (neocortical association to temporal lobe) stimuli of affective significance (39, 97).

The prefrontal cortex has direct outputs to the pyramidal motor system, the neostriatum, temporal neocortex, and the hypothalamus. Schematically, prefrontal cortices appear to integrate a current account of the outside world, the state of the internal milieu, and the recognition of drive-relevant objects with knowledge of learned social rules and previous experiences relating to reward and punishment. The prefrontal cortex may play a particularly important role in both working memory and social modeling, maintaining an abstract representation of the world that allows anticipation of the effects of one's actions upon other individuals and the likely consequences of such actions. The prefrontal cortices construct a behavioral plan that is consistent with experience and especially the rules of socialization, in order to optimize the satisfaction of biological drives.

The simplest summary of these complex functions in humans is judgment (39), which should not be simply equated with purely rational cost-benefit calculations that may be quite time-consuming and biologically uneconomical. Rather, it has been proposed that, in selecting among alternative response options, prefrontal cortices are guided by internal, somatic state markers, physiological cues that allow rapid choice of previously rewarded, effective options (98, 99).

Damage to the dorsal convexity in humans results in a diminution of long-term planning and a state of apathy or indifference (100). On formal neuropsychological testing, shifting of response set and the ability to apply strategy to problem solving are impaired (101, 102) (see also Chapter 19).

By contrast, damage to the orbital undersurface of the frontal lobe has classically been described as resulting in superficial, reflexive emotional responses to stimuli in the immediate environment (103). Patients are impulsive without foresight or consideration of the remote consequences of their actions. Orbital frontal lesions thus lead to episodes of transient irritability. Often a patient strikes out quickly after a trivial provocation, with little consideration of social prohibitions limiting aggressive behavior or untoward future consequences. The targets of aggression are categorically appropriate, but patients are unable to apply abstract rules that would override the immediate environmental provocation.

Numerous case reports illustrate the tendency of patients with orbitomedial frontal injuries to act impulsively, without regard to long-term consequences or sustained courses of action. Well known is the case of Phineas Gage, a railroad worker who suffered an injury primarily to the left orbitomedial frontal lobe when an explosion projected a tamping rod through his skull (100). Subsequently, Harlow reported, "he was no longer Gage." Previously a temperate, hardworking individual, he became "disrespectful," "irreverent," and "profane." He rejected attempts to restrain him from satisfying desires of the moment, but rapidly abandoned plans he made to achieve these desires.

In a recently described case, a middle-aged nurse suddenly lost interest in her work, domestic chores, and maternal responsibilities for two young children. A cranial magnetic resonance imaging (MRI) study demonstrated an extensive region of high-signal abnormality on T2-weighted images within subcortical white matter of the right frontal lobe, consistent with a new demyelinative lesion of multiple sclerosis (MS). She had previously experienced episodes of blurred vision, right-sided weakness, and truncal ataxia.

The patient was generally apathetic and expressed little spontaneous affection for her children or her own mother. She denied a depressed or dysphoric mood. She spent hours lying in bed, failing to report to work and inattentive to the needs of her family. When left undisturbed, she rarely displayed anger. However, questions from family members elicited sharp verbal retorts, often accompanied by attempts to physically push away the individual. She was particularly irritated by the cries of her young son and burned his arms with lighted cigarette butts on several occasions. When he fled from the room, she denied feeling angry and showed no concern for the serious injuries she had inflicted (104).

In addition to detailed single case studies, case series of murderers have demonstrated a high incidence of frontal structural abnormalities on CT and MRI, frontal hypofunction on PET, and abnormal neuropsychologic performance on frontal systems tasks (104a).

Combined Lesions of Temporal and Frontal Lobes

Some pathological processes may simultaneously damage the multiple levels of neural circuitry critical to the regulation of aggression (schematically summarized in Fig. 24.5). The

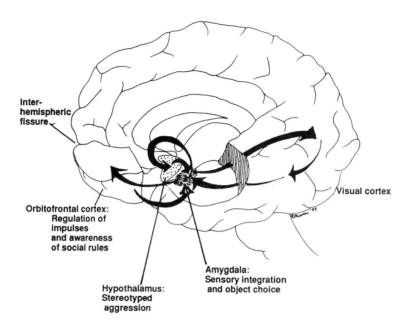

Figure 24.5. Cutaway view of the midsagittal aspect of the human brain sparing the posterior aspect of the left temporal and occipital lobes. Portions of the left orbitofrontal and temporal regions are exposed to display key sites and pathways in the hierarchical, multiregional neural system regulating aggressive behaviors.

orbitofrontal surface and rostral temporal poles are particularly susceptible in closed head injuries, and conjoint lesions in the same patient are not uncommon (105–107). Temporolimbic epilepsy is a frequent sequel of both closed and open head injury.

Aggressive behavioral syndromes may result that have features associated with dysfunction of several brain regions. For example, a patient may, as a result of brain trauma, develop a temporolimbic epileptic focus as well as a contusion of the orbital frontal cortex. Such a patient can display the deepened emotions and anger associated with the interictal behavior syndrome as well as a failure to inhibit or modulate hostile responses typical of a frontal lesion. In one reported case, a young man suffered severe brain injury in a motor vehicle accident. Imaging studies demonstrated enlargement of the frontal and temporal horns of both lateral ventricles and EEG abnormalities were recorded over the right frontotemporal area. The patient displayed intermittent apathy suggestive of frontal lobe damage, but also developed personality changes characteristic of the interictal behavior syndrome of temporal lobe epilepsy. He had outbursts of extremely violent behavior and eventually attempted to murder his parents and former girlfriend. When questioned regarding his aggression, the patient failed to appreciate that his behavior might be distressing to others (108). One serial murderer studied with MRI and CT scans had sustained bifrontal and left temporal injuries during a severe beating in childhood (104). Evidence for frontal and temporolimbic dysfunction in violent criminals was recently renewed by Raine and colleagues (104a). They demonstrated frontal lobe hypometabolism by PET scans in murderers found not guilty by reason of insanity.

Hemispheric Asymmetries in the Regulation of Aggression

Several lines of neuropsychological research suggest differences in left- and right-hemisphere specialization for the processing of emotion, including anger and aggression. The left hemisphere plays a greater role in decoding linguistically conveyed emotional information, and the right hemisphere is more important in processing nonverbal emotional cues, such as prosody and facial expression of emotion (109). Moreover, the right hemisphere may be more highly specialized for mediating emotional responses in general, and negative emotional responses such as fear and anger in particular. These conclusions are supported by studies of functional asymmetry for verbal versus nonverbal expression of affect, verbal versus nonverbal decoding of affects expressed by others, and asymmetric facial expression of affect in patients with unilateral stroke, other asymmetric neurological injuries, transient hemisphere inactivation during Wada testing, and in normal experimental subjects (110–118).

Neuropsychological studies in unselected populations of violent criminal offenders also support an important role of hemispheric specialization in the genesis of hostile behaviors. When neuropsychological deficits are observed in studies of violent groups, they tend to involve not only frontal-executive functions (119, 120), but also verbal comprehension, expressive speech, and other left-hemisphere language functions (121–124). These findings are consonant with a large number of studies in conduct-disordered and delinquent juveniles, indicating that the lowered IQ found in these groups frequently reflects disproportionately lowered verbal IQ (language—left hemisphere) compared to performance IQ (visuospatial—right hemisphere) (125–127).

Psychophysiological studies in violent offenders also show a trend toward left hemispheric dysfunction. Though plagued by methodological defects and not adequately addressing laterality, early studies of large samples of violent offenders suggested that a substantial proportion, about 50%, exhibit EEG abnormalities (128, 129). More recent studies employing computerized EEG spectral analysis have suggested that persistently violent behavior among psychiatric inpatients is linked to increased δ-band slow-wave activity in left frontotemporal derivations (130), although studies in other aggressive populations have not confirmed such an asymmetry (131). Divided visual field (132), dichotic listening (133, 134), skin conductance asymmetry (135), and lateral preference studies (136) additionally suggest subtle abnormalities of left hemispheric function in sociopathic individuals without overt neurological lesions. In one small series of subjects examined by positron emission tomography (PET), decreased blood flow and metabolism were observed in the left temporal lobe of all four institutionalized, sexually violent offenders studied, and left frontal hypometabolism in two of the four (137).

Different theorists have integrated the results of these and other laterality studies in violent individuals without overt structural brain lesions to propose that either left hemispheric (138, 139) or right hemispheric (140) networks play a predominant functional role in the regulation of aggression. In addition, subtle developmental hemispheric abnormalities underlie repeatedly aggressive behavior in a proportion of "functional" psychopaths. A broader view is that each hemisphere performs complementary processing related to hostile behavior, and functional abnormalities of either hemisphere may produce disturbed aggressive responding through distinctive mechanisms. Left-hemisphere dysfunction, implicated in a preponderance of studies, may lead to overt expression of negative affects mediated by the right hemisphere, diminished linguistic regulation over behavior, and adverse social encounters due to impaired verbal communication. Right-hemisphere dysfunction may lead to improper intrahemispheric decoding and encoding of prosody, facial expressions, or other nonverbal emotional responses, overreliance on semantic processing, and a different pattern of altered aggressivity.

Awareness of differential features of right- and left-hemisphere emotional functioning may be helpful for the neuropsychiatrist caring for patients with overt destructive or irritative lateralized brain lesions (141). For example, evidence suggests that the expression of interictal behavior syndromes related to temporolimbic epilepsy differs in patients with left versus right temporolimbic foci. In one study, an "ideative" cluster of attributes distinguished left temporolimbic epileptics, including religiosity, philosophical interest, paranoid concerns, and hypergraphia (92). Such patients may be more liable to plan and execute complex aggressive actions in response to perceived moral injustices. An "emotive" group of traits was associated with right temporolimbic epileptic discharges, including euphoria, sadness, overt aggressivity, and altered sexual behavior. Were

they to develop hostility, these patients would be more likely to display an impulsive, unreflective, immediate pattern of aggressive behavior (142).

Studies of patients who develop the alien hand syndrome from left medial frontal cortex or corpus callosum lesions may provide insight into different hemispheric control over aggression (143, 144). In subjects who have undergone callosal transection for control of intractable seizure disorders, hemifield presentation of visual stimuli have demonstrated that the isolated hemispheres may have contrasting emotional responses to the same eliciting stimuli (145–147). In a minority of patients, interhemispheric antagonism may be expressed in clinically apparent, even disabling, intermanual conflict. The dominant and nondominant hands pursue opposing goals, and in carrying out such basic manual tasks as eating, opening and closing doors, or washing, the nondominant hand may terminate an action that the dominant hemisphere has initiated.

Reeves and Roberts observed a commissurotomy patient who developed enduring postoperative difficulties in daily ablutions, dressing, and shopping. The left and right arms at times physically abused each other. The dominant left hemisphere verbally expressed antipathy toward the left arm and leg, considering them another hostile person (148). Though aggression in patients with alien hand syndromes is most often directed against the contralateral hemibody, reports of aggression toward others have been occasionally noted. The nondominant hemisphere most often initiates both types of aggressive responses, perhaps reflecting its lack of access to linguistic channels or, alternatively, a right-hemisphere bias toward aggressive responding. Careful studies of unilateral aggressive behavior in relation to varied stimuli might allow a more detailed profile of distinctive predilections of the right and left hemispheres.

Right-hemisphere parietofrontal lesions may impair an individual's ability to interpret and produce emotional gestures, prosody, and affect. This may produce an acquired "sociopathy," even in the absence of bifrontal lesions (99). Although the most frequently noted pattern of altered behavior after right-parietal cortical lesions is one of inappropriate cheerfulness and denial of illness (110, 140, 149), irritability and aggressive outbursts may also ensue. Former Supreme Court Justice William Douglas exhibited disturbed social judgment following a right-hemisphere stroke. While he retained sufficient linguistic and abstract reasoning ability to return to the bench, inappropriate social behaviors soon forced his retirement (150).

Neurochemistry of Aggression

There has been an explosion of knowledge regarding neurotransmitter-receptor systems that modulate aggressive behavior in animals and humans over the past decade. However, many studies have focused exclusively upon the effects of a specific neurotransmitter or receptor subtype on one or more aspects of violent or aggressive behavior. Integration of such fine-scale neurochemical data with the large-scale neurocognitive network data acquired in neuroanatomical and neurophysiological studies has been limited. Most experimental and clinical reports on "the neurochemistry of aggression" likely describe the effects of neuromodulators at peripheral, brainstem and hypothalamic sites, which can reduce or raise the individual's overall predisposition to aggression. Still lacking are studies that evaluate the multisynaptic integration of parallel-processed streams of complex sensory and limbic information that link amygdala, orbitofrontal, and other higher cortical centers. Quite likely, these networks are subserved by diverse messenger systems and not exclusively controlled by a single neurotransmitter. We also have insufficient understanding of the complex interactive effects that neurotransmitters and neurohormones exert upon one another, or the specific receptor subtypes mediating a particular response. However, because neurochemical studies provide the basis for pharmacological interventions in aggressive patients, data from such studies are of clinically invaluable.

The hypothalamus, amygdala, and frontal lobe are richly innervated by monoaminergic neurotransmitters, acetylcholine, and neuropeptides (151). This section highlights findings concerning the roles that serotonin, acetylcholine, norepinephrine, dopamine, γ-aminobutyric acid (GABA), and testosterone and other androgens play in mediating aggression. Particular attention is paid to serotonergic systems, which have been the subject of intense recent experimental and clinical investigation.

SEROTONIN

Animal and human studies suggest that serotonin is a critical modulator of aggressive behavior (152). Studies in humans have focused on serotonergic markers in suicidal patients and violent criminals. Some postmortem studies have found decreased levels of serotonin in subcortical and neocortical brain regions in patients completing violent suicide (153–155). However, serotonin is not uniformly decreased in the brains of suicidal patients. Variations in region of interest sampling, prior treatment, cause of death, and the matching of cases and controls are important reasons for conservative interpretation of these findings.

Several investigators have found increases in serotonin type 2($5HT_2$) (postsynaptic) receptor binding in the frontal cortex of violent suicides (156–161). However, at least two studies did not replicate these results (162, 163). The positive studies suggest that postsynaptic serotonin receptors are increased because of decreased presynaptic serotonergic activity. Violent juvenile delinquents had *decreased* platelet $5HT_2$ binding in one recent study (163a).

Cerebrospinal fluid (CSF) levels of 5-hydroxyindoleacetic acid (5-HIAA), a metabolite of serotonin, are decreased in patients attempting suicide and in violent criminal offenders (164). A stronger relationship has been reported between CSF 5-HIAA and suicidal behavior than suicidal ideation alone. Violent and impulsive self-injurious acts tend to have the strongest negative correlation with CSF 5-HIAA values, suggesting that low CSF 5-HIAA levels are not simply a

marker of depression and suicidal risk, but also of a tendency to aggressive and impulsive behavior. Several studies in criminal and interpersonally violent psychiatric populations support this view. Lowered CSF 5-HIAA levels were found in samples of impulsive fire setters (165) and individuals committing impulsive manslaughter (166). In a group of soldiers with behavior problems, there was a negative correlation between CSF 5-HIAA and aggressive behavior (167), and CSF 5-HIAA was reduced in a group of borderline patients with aggressive and suicidal behavior (168). Adolescent male rhesus macaque monkeys also show an inverse correlation between risk-taking and aggression in the wild, and CSF 5-HIAA (168a).

Neuroendocrine challenge studies have been utilized to probe serotonergic function in aggression. Serotonin administration in normals causes a release of prolactin. Suicidal depressed patients and patients with personality disorders who exhibit impulsive and aggressive behavior have a blunted prolactin response to fenfluramine, a releaser of presynaptic serotonin stores, and to M-CPP (m-chlorophenylpiperazine), a $5HT_2$ agonist (169, 170). This work suggests that suicidal and impulsive/aggressive patients have serotonergic hypoactivity. Patients with depression and suicidality demonstrated an increased release of cortisol to 5-hydroxytryptamine, suggesting hypersensitivity of other postsynaptic serotonin receptors in this group (171). Other workers have not found a significant correlation between neuroendocrine challenge abnormalities and suicidality (151).

Recent investigations of the relationship between serotonin and aggression have shifted to exploring agents that act at specific serotonergic receptor subtypes. Buspirone, a $5HT_{1A}$ agonist, produced a normal prolactin release when given intravenously to healthy male volunteers. This effect was blocked by the nonselective 5HT-receptor antagonist metergoline and by pindolol, a β-adrenergic and $5HT_1$ antagonist, in a dose-related fashion. Prolactin response to buspirone was inversely correlated with levels of "irritability" in patients with personality disorders, suggesting that decreased sensitivity of the $5HT_{1A}$ receptor may be responsible for components of impulsive-aggressive behavior in patients with personality disorders (172). Recently, Personen et al. reported amino acid substitutions in the 5HT-7 receptor gene among alcoholics with violent behavior.

Work in animal models of aggressive conduct supports and amplifies studies of serotoninergic systems in human populations. Eltoprazine, a $5HT_1$ agonist, reduces offensive (as opposed to defensive) aggression in several species. In the rat brain, eltoprazine binding is greatest in the dorsal subiculum, substantia nigra, ventral pallidum, and globus pallidus (173). Other $5HT_{1A}$ agonists, including buspirone, gepirone, and 8-OH-DPAT (8-hydroxy-2[di-n-propylamino] tetralin), reduce isolation-induced aggression in mice without causing sedation or incoordination (174). Soubrie suggests that serotonin increases the ability of an organism to arrange for and tolerate delay (175). Decreased serotonin leads to an increase of behaviors that are usually suppressed. Studies of isolation-induced aggression, shock-induced fighting, and muricidal and filicidal behavior have demonstrated an inverse relationship between serotonin functions and aggression in rats and mice (176–179). Other studies suggest that the response to manipulation of serotonin is more complex and species-specific (180). For example, a recent rat study found that agonists at $5HT_{1A}$, $5HT_{1B}$, and $5HT_2$ receptors all reduced offensive aggression, but only $5HT_2$ agonists reduced defensive aggression (180a).

Studies of naturally behaving animal populations support the findings from experimentally induced aggression paradigms. Domesticated silver foxes who easily tolerated human contact had a higher level of midbrain and hypothalamic serotonin than wild silver foxes bred in captivity (181). The domesticated foxes also had a reduced density of $5HT_{1A}$ receptor binding in the hypothalamus. Mice lacking the 5HT1p receptor exhibited enhanced aggressive behavior (178). Higley et al. found that rhesus monkeys with the highest CSF 5-HIAA and whole blood serotonin were socially dominant, while animals with decreased whole blood serotonin tended to be ostracized, and monkeys with the lowest CSF 5-HIAA were aggressive and socially deviant (182). Aggressive behavior was also associated with high levels of cortisol, suggesting greater stress. However, not all monkey studies have shown a significant correlation between 5-HIAA and aggression (183, 184).

Serotonin interacts with other neurotransmitter and neurohumoral systems in modulating impulsivity and aggression. For example, one group of investigators examined the effects of testosterone and serotonin administration on dominance and aggression in rats (185). In their model, male rats given testosterone became dominant. Quipazine, a serotonin agonist, blocked aggression in both naturally dominant and testosterone-induced dominant rats. Nonspecific serotonin antagonists blocked aggression only in testosterone-induced dominant males. This study begins to address the pharmacoselectivity of different forms of aggression and foreshadows an important future avenue for pharmacological research.

ACETYLCHOLINE

Some of the earliest work on the neurochemistry of aggression focused on acetylcholine. Electrical stimulation of the lateral hypothalamus in rats leads to predatory attack on mice in animals that previously had tolerated mice in their cage without attacking them (186). The attack terminates as soon as the electrical stimulation is discontinued. Applying carbachol, a cholinergic agonist, to the lateral hypothalamus provokes the sterotypic aggressive response, which can be blocked by atropine and facilitated by acetylcholinesterases (187). This cholinergic-induced predatory response is target-specific—directed only at the animal's usual prey—and without affective display. Electrical stimulation of the lateral or dorsal amygdala facilitates predatory attack through its connections to the lateral hypothalamus (188). Applying carbachol to the amygdala also induces a predatory response (189). Aggressive behavior following human exposure to cholinesterase inhibitors has been observed in several clinical case reports (59).

Despite well-documented experimentation, the cholinergic mediation of aggression and its clinical implications have been understudied in recent years. For example, the muscarinic receptor subtypes mediating hypothalamic aggression and cholinergic regulation of aggression in the frontal cortex have not been characterized in detail.

NOREPINEPHRINE AND DOPAMINE

Catecholamine systems are associated with aggressive behavior in several animal models and clinical populations. Peripherally administered norepinephrine (NE) enhances shock-induced fighting in rats (190). Alpha 2 receptor agonists increase rat aggressive behavior whereas clonidine decreases rodent aggressive behavior acutely (191). Long-term treatment with β-adrenergic blocking agents such as propranolol can decrease aggressive behavior in laboratory animals and in diverse neuropsychiatric patient groups with violent behaviors (33, 192, 193). Not all studies have found a correlation between increased CSF or frontal cortex NE and its metabolite 3-methoxy-4-hydroxyphenylglycol (MHPG) and aggressive behavior (194).

Fenwick suggests that central noradrenergic tracts originating in the locus coeruleus innervate a behavioral inhibitory system that projects widely to the hippocampus, septal region, and frontal lobes. Modulatory disturbances in central norepinephrine would then lead to impulsivity and episodic violence (195). Induction of sham rage in cats through electrical stimulation is associated with a fall in brainstem and forebrain NE. High decerebrate lesions that induce sham rage also produce a fall in NE (196, 197).

L-dopa can induce aggressive behavior in rodents and humans (198). Apomorphine, a potent dopamine agonist, can induce fighting in rats (199). Dopamine antagonists tend to reduce aggression but usually at doses that also slow motor and cognitive performance. A few studies have shown reduced levels of a dopamine metabolite, homovanillic acid, in suicidal patients (200, 201).

γ-AMINOBUTYRIC ACID (GABA)

Several lines of evidence suggest that GABA inhibits aggression in animals and humans. GABA injected into the olfactory bulbs in rats inhibits mouse killing (202). GABA antagonists can induce mouse killing behavior (201). Benzodiazepines and other agents that facilitate GABA can decrease isolation-induced fighting in mice (203–205), and attenuate aggression caused by limbic lesions (203, 206). Benzodiazepines most likely exert their antiaggressive effects by binding to sites on the GABA receptor (203). In humans, despite their tranquilizing and antiaggressive effect in the vast majority of patients, benzodiazepines rarely can lead to a transient increase in aggressive behavior ("paradoxical rage") (33).

TESTOSTERONE AND OTHER ANDROGENS

Testosterone is an important mediator of aggressive responding in diverse mammalian species. In rats, dominant males have higher levels of testosterone than submissive males. Prolactin levels rise after a fight in submissive males but not in dominant individuals. Cortisol rises in both groups, but cortisol is higher in the submissive group, suggesting that they experience a greater level of stress. Release of prolactin may be part of the serotonin response seen in defensive aggression (207). The lack of a prolactin response in offensive aggression could be due to inhibitory dopaminergic levels in dominant males. In vervet monkeys, increases in serum and salivary testosterone levels correlated with the number of aggressive encounters (208). Moyer suggested that androgens increased inter-male and irritable, but not predatory, sexual, fear-induced and maternal forms of aggression (209). An interaction between androgens and other neuromodulators such as the monoamine neuro-transmitters appears to govern aggressive responding. Testosterone-induced dominance in rats is reduced after treatment with 5HT1A, 1B, and 2A/2C receptor agonists.

Compelling evidence for the importance of androgens in mediating aggression comes from the literature on spotted hyenas (210–212). The spotted hyenas are among the most aggressive animals in the wild. They also have a very organized and highly nurturant clan society. Male and female hyenas are roughly equal in size. However, the colonies are dominated by the females in a tightly ranked hierarchy. Females are more aggressive, and adult males are usually not able to feed from a kill while the dominant females are eating. The female has a hypertrophied clitoris (the size of a male penis) with full erectile potential. The labia form a scrotum. The females' large body habits, androgenous genitalia, and aggressive behavior are related to the high circulating levels of androstenedione. This convergent hormonal-behavioral relationship in the hyena supports the association of androgens with aggression initially suggested by the observation that males enact aggressive behaviors more frequently than females in most mammalian species, including humans.

Human studies support an important link between circulating androgens and aggressive behavior. Elevated testosterone levels in adolescent boys correlate with low frustration tolerance and impatience (213). Boys with increased testosterone are more likely to respond aggressively when provoked. Increased levels of free testosterone have been measured in the saliva of incarcerated violent criminals (214). Victorious collegiate wrestlers show a greater rise in their serum testosterone than their defeated counterparts (215). Violent behaviors have been reported in individuals taking anabolic steroids for body-building programs (216). Archer's meta-analysis of reported studies demonstrated a strong positive correlation between testosterone levels and observer-rated aggressiveness (217). More recently, Bergman and Brismor showed that male alcoholics who abused other people had higher levels of testosterone and lower levels of cortisol than those who did not (217a). Loosen and colleagues (217b) showed that inhibiting gonadal function with a GnRH antagonist reduced outward-directed aggression.

It is important to note some common weaknesses in the data currently available on the neurochemistry of aggression:

1. Most studies on neurotransmitter and neurohormonal effects on aggression have been conducted on male animals and men. Endocrine and neurochemical factors influencing aggression in females have not been fully evaluated.
2. Caution must be employed when generalizing findings across species, and particularly when comparing responses between humans, other primates, and other mammalian orders. Many aggression-related neurotransmitters are conserved across species, but there are probably important variations in receptor subsystems. For example, the $5HT_{1B}$ receptor is found in rodents but so far has not been identified in man.
3. Precision in defining and measuring aggression, impulsivity, and irritability in many animal models and human is difficult to achieve. Also, many studies fail to recognize and fully clarify state-trait distinctions. The neurochemical substrates for responses related to rapidly shifting behavioral states and those related to enduring dispositional traits may differ.
4. Neuroendocrine challenge studies are subject to wide variability, depending on agent dosage, route of administration, and outcome measure.

Nonetheless, progress in basic investigations of the neurochemical and neuroendocrine mediators of aggression may set the stage for advances in the pharmacotherapeutics of violent disorders. As receptor subtypes involved in modulating specific aggressive behaviors are isolated, it becomes feasible to tailor pharmacological diagnostic probes and treatments to specific clinical settings. Once a better understanding of the individual neurochemical and neuroendocrine factors contributing to aggression is attained, interactions among the multiple agents operating convergently and divergently at hierarchial sites in the neuraxis to regulate hostile behavior may be more fully explored.

THE AGGRESSIVE PATIENT: A CLINICAL NEUROPSYCHIATRIC APPROACH

General Approach

The recognition that specific neurological lesions may lead to violent behavior in human beings, and that abnormalities at different levels of the neuraxis result in distinctive types of aggressive behavior, provides a guiding schema for the evaluation and treatment of inappropriately aggressive (and inappropriately hypoaggressive) individuals (Tables 24.3–24.5). In addition to emphasizing the need for careful neuropsychiatric evaluation of every violent patient, the hierarchical model for the regulation of aggression suggests important parameters that may help to characterize any aggressive act. The neuropsychiatrist should integrate information regarding the clinical manifestations of aggressive

Table 24.3.   Features that Distinguish Clinical Syndromes of Hyperaggression

Syndrome	Eliciting Stimulus	Provocation	Outbursts	Complex Plans	Memory for Acts	Remorse	Mode
Hypothalamic	Individuals who happen to be present	Basic drive (e.g., hunger); unprovoked	Yes	No	Yes	Yes	Simple kicking, biting, scratching; infrequently, throwing of readily available objects
Ictal	Any nearby individual or inanimate object	None	Yes	No	No	Yes	Random, undirected; wild swinging, kicking movements
Postictal	Caretakers	Attempts to restrain/protect patient	Yes	No	No	Yes	Disoriented, irritable; simple kicking, biting, scratching
Interictal	Individuals	Threat, including misinterpretation of trivial stimulus; perception of moral injustice	Occasional	Yes	Yes	Yes, may be intense	1) Morally driven; complex plans; may be enacted over long time period; may involve weapons; 2) Quick-tempered lashing out
Orbitofrontal	Individuals	Minor provocations	Yes	No	No	No	1) Irritable lashing out; 2) Rarely may carry out plan of minor-intermediate complexity

Table 24.4. Selected Differential Diagnosis of Syndromes of Hyperaggressivity

Syndrome	Diseases
Hypothalamic	Hamartoma
	Craniopharyngioma, Astrocytoma
	Parasomnias
Temporal lobe epilepsy	Mesial temporal sclerosis
	Glioma
	Vascular malformation
	Traumatic brain injury
Orbitofrontal systems	Traumatic brain injury
	Herpes simplex encephalitis
	Anterior communicating artery aneurysm
	Orbital meningioma
	Pick's disease
	Frontal dementia without specific histological features
	Huntington's disease
Combined frontotemporal	Traumatic brain injury
	Pick's disease
	Herpes simplex encephalitis
Multifocal or poorly localized	Attention deficit disorder
	Toxic-metabolic encephalopathies
	Vitamin B_{12} deficiency
	Multiple sclerosis
	Subcortical vascular dementia
	Alcohol, cocaine
Delusional cognition	Paranoid schizophrenia
	Endogenous depression (uni- or bipolar)
	Late-life paraphrenia
	Mania
	Alzheimer's disease
	Vascular dementia

Table 24.5. Differential Diagnosis of Syndromes of Hypoaggressivity

Syndrome	Diseases
Bilateral amygdalotemporal	Pick's disease
	Herpes simplex encephalitis
	Bilateral posterior cerebral artery infarction
	Traumatic brain injury
	Urbach-Wiethe disease
	Temporal lobectomy
Dorsolateral frontal systems	Subdural hematoma
	Glioma
	Progressive supranuclear palsy
	Anterior cerebral artery infarction

behavior, additional aspects of the history (particularly related to other drive-related behaviors), the neurological and psychiatric examinations, and structural and functional laboratory studies to classify patients among major syndromes of dysregulation and aggression.

Hypothalamic/Brainstem Syndromes

In patients with hypothalamic lesions, outbursts of violent behavior may be precipitated by internal or visceroceptive states, such as hunger, fatigue, light deprivation, or hormonal stimulation; alternatively, patients may exhibit a heightened general level of aggressivity. Most frequently,

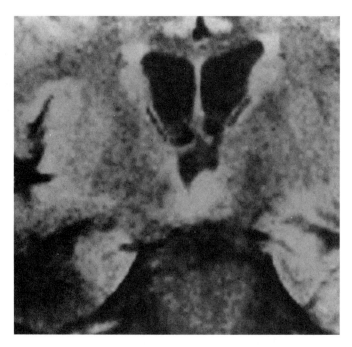

Figure 24.6. Aggression with hypothalamic lesion. A 19-year-old boy presented with several-year history of seizures of multiple types, including ictal laughter, aggressive behavior, and poor social adjustment. Coronal proton density weighted MRI scan demonstrates a 1-cm high-signal intensity mass in the substance of the hypothalamus, consistent with a hypothalamic hamartoma. (Reproduced with permission from Berkovic SF, Andermann F, Melanson D, et al. Ann Neurol 1988; 435.)

attacks are upon individuals who happen to be near the patient, without the formation of complex plans. Patients often have diminished insight into the reasons for their actions, although they recall and may demonstrate remorse for their actions. Subjects with hypothalamic lesions may demonstrate altered patterns of sleeping or eating, polydipsia, and polyuria, or deficient regulation of sex hormones, thyroid, or adrenocortical function. Heteronymous visual field impairments may be evident if lesions extend to involve the optic nerves, chiasm, or tracts. The workup of patients with suspected hypothalamic lesions should include MRI or other structural imaging of the region of the third ventricle, endocrine studies, and formal visual fields. The differential diagnosis includes benign and malignant tumors such as craniopharyngiomas and astrocytomas, which present with subacute alterations in behavior. Another etiology is hypothalamic hamartoma, which usually presents with a distinctive clinical profile. Patients in childhood have the onset of gelastic epilepsy (ictal laughter), sometimes accompanied by precocious puberty, along with interictal bouts of uncontrolled rage (Fig. 24.6) (218, 219).

In patients with brainstem and hypothalamic-mediated sleep-related disorders of violence, aggressive actions are generally nocturnal, associated with incomplete maintenance of REM or non-REM sleep states. The REM sleep behavior disorder predominantly occurs in middle-aged men. Violence most commonly occurs during a vivid and frightening dream, often is directed at a bed partner mistaken for a dream figure, and is unplanned, without the use of weapons. Affected patients are difficult to arouse from their dreaming state. Afterwards, they generally recall the dream material that provoked aggression, but report believing they were attacking animal or human oneiric figures rather than their furniture or spouse. They exhibit great remorse about their actions and, before a diagnosis is made, frequently self-treat their disorder by tying themselves in restraining devices at night (220).

The REM sleep disorder must be distinguished from other parasomnias that may be injurious to patient and spouse, such as somnambulism, sleep drunkenness, and sleep terrors, which arise out of non-REM sleep (221). Nocturnal seizures must also be excluded. The diagnostic workup in suspected cases includes a thorough history of sleep complaints from patient and bed partner, neurological and psychiatric examination, overnight polysomnographic study, and MRI. REM sleep behavior disorder has been associated with a variety of neurological conditions, including dementia, stroke, MS, and alcohol withdrawal. However, over 50% of cases are idiopathic. Pontine tegmental lesions, which might be expected from animal studies, are rare, possibly because pontine injury frequently produces devastating motor and arousal deficits that preclude expression of the disorder. Approximately 90% of patients exhibit sustained improvement when treated with clonazepam.

Temporolimbic Epilepsy Syndromes

Few topics in neuropsychiatry are more controversial than the relationship of aggression to epilepsy. Failure to adequately distinguish between aggressive actions in the ictal, postictal, and interictal periods has contributed greatly to the confusion regarding the relationship between temporolimbic epileptic foci and violent behavior.

Ictal aggression does occur, but with extreme rarity. An international consensus panel found that only seven of 5400 patients studied on video-EEG monitoring exhibited aggressive behavior during recorded seizures (222). Hostile behaviors ranged from physical violence directed toward inanimate objects to mild verbal or physical aggression directed toward a person. With the exception of two additional patients described by Weiser (223), few subsequent reports have unambiguously demonstrated aggressive acts during complex partial seizures documented on scalp or depth EEG recordings (224). When aggressive acts during complex seizures occur, they may appear without provocation or in response to an environmental stimulus, and are characterized by spontaneous, undirected aggression toward nearby objects or individuals (225, 226). The patient is amnestic for actions and often expresses remorse.

A much more common form of aggressive behavior in epilepsy is resistive violence during the postictal period. Following a complex partial seizure or, more frequently, a generalized convulsion, patients may be disoriented and confused. During this epoch, well-intended attempts at physical restraint can provoke aggression, which almost always ceases when restraint is withdrawn (107). The attacks generally involve striking out without the use of a weapon

or sometimes with objects that happen to be close at hand. Patients have no memory for their actions upon clearing of consciousness and will express dismay if they have injured others. Aggression immediately following the end of a seizure activity can also occur in the context of postictal psychosis, especially in patients with paranoid delusions and threatening hallucinations (107, 223).

Overt aggression related to the interictal behavior syndrome of temporolimbic epilepsy is unusual, because the heightened moral and religious values that are features of the syndrome preclude violent actions. However, in rare circumstances, intense emotional reactions to perceived injustice or threat can lead subjects to formulate and carry out complex plans of violent response. Attacks may be directed against a specific individual and could involve the use of a weapon. Not all hostile actions by these patients involve long-term planning—rarely, the intensity of feelings evoked in a particular situation might lead to an immediate response. Patients fully recall their actions, and often exhibit extreme remorse. Some individuals continue to feel their acts had ample moral justification (93).

In individuals with epilepsy, sedative antiepileptic medications such as barbiturates may contribute to hostile behaviors by impairing impulse control. Irritability, a common complaint among patients with poorly controlled partial and primary generalized seizures, may result from environmental factors, medications, or in relation to the underlying cerebral pathology or epileptogenic process.

In patients in whom ictal, postictal, or interictal aggression is suspected, history taking should first be directed at eliciting symptoms of simple or complex partial seizures. Although tonic-clonic convulsions and loss of consciousness will be easily recognized, focal manifestations of temporolimbic seizures may escape notice or be dismissed as psychological in origin (227). Noxious odors, epigastric pain, forced feelings of sadness or fear, sensations of familiarity and unfamiliarity, and other partial seizure phenomena should be directly inquired after.

These subjects should also be questioned for elements of the interictal behavior syndrome: hypergraphia, heightened philosophic concerns, change in sexual interest, deepened emotionality. Neurological examination is often normal, but may reveal asymmetric "soft signs" or infrequently a superior quadrantic visual field deficit (sometimes only noted with double simultaneous stimulation). An additional sign is unilateral facial weakness on spontaneous expression of emotion (228).

Routine scalp EEG may show interictal spikes or slow-wave abnormalities in the temporal region, but may miss physiological discharges occurring in deep, mesial temporal regions. Sleep-deprived and sleep recordings and the use of nasopharyngeal or sphenoidal leads may increase the yield of scalp recording. In selected cases, ambulatory EEG or long-term inpatient video-EEG monitoring with scalp and sphenoidal electrodes, or invasive subdural grids or depth electrodes may be necessary to establish the seizure focus.

CT and especially MRI are utilized to exclude slowly growing gliomas and other mass lesions. Volumetric MRI or careful visual analysis of the hippocampus and amygdala (seen best on T1-weighted coronal cuts) may aid in the diagnosis of mesial temporal sclerosis by demonstrating unilateral or bilateral atrophy. Metabolic imaging with PET or SPECT may show increased blood flow and hypermetabolism in mesial temporal structures during ictal discharges and decreased blood flow and hypometabolism interictally. PET is the more sensitive technique interictally; SPECT is more practical for capturing ictal events. Common etiologies of temporolimbic epilepsy include mesial temporal sclerosis, hamartomas, dysplasia, low-grade astrocytomas, oligodendrogliomas, vascular malformations, and traumatic brain injury.

Orbitofrontal Systems Syndromes

Patients with lesions in orbitofrontal cortices or associated subcortical structures such as the caudate nucleus may engage in directed acts of aggression (Fig. 24.7). However, they are often incapable of planning or executing a complex response that requires an extended sequence of actions. Failure to consider long-term and especially social consequences of violent outbursts is a salient feature. Frequently the patient engages in impulsive, unreflective responses to identifiable but trivial environmental provocations. In some patients, extended but inefficient rational analysis of social situations without guidance from somatic-emotional systems is observed (98). Patients remember their actions, but often lack remorse, and fail to link aggressive actions with

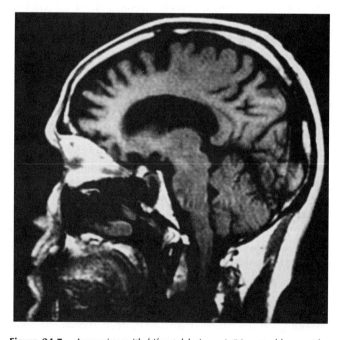

Figure 24.7. Aggression with bifrontal lesions. A 56-year-old man who, over 3 years, developed ritualistic behaviors, and became disinhibited and jocular. He exhibited inappropriate violent outbursts and persistent foul language. MRI demonstrates frontal lobar atrophy in an advanced "picket fence" pattern consistent with Pick's disease. Aggressive behavior eventually diminished with high doses of propranolol. However, the patient required being confined to a chair with a locking top and occasional treatment with neuroleptics.

punishment or other long-term adverse outcomes, contributing to repeated offenses (39).

The neurological exam may reveal anosmia due to damage to the olfactory nerves or tracts on the undersurface of the frontal lobes and release phenomena such as the grasp reflex (229). If the lesion is confined strictly to orbitofrontal cortices, subjects may show few deficits on conventional IQ tests, or even on neuropsychological tests explicitly concerned with frontal-executive function (230). When lesions trespass upon dorsolateral frontal territories, deficits in go-no-go testing, verbal and nonverbal fluency, and set-shifting may be evident (101). CT and especially MRI studies are helpful in screening for structural lesions. Common etiologies include traumatic brain injury, anterior communicating artery aneurysm rupture, anterior cerebral artery infarction, orbital meningioma, the frontal lobe dementias, and Huntington's disease.

Syndromes of Diffuse or Multifocal Brain Injury

Several medical conditions that produce aggression have effects on the brain that are diffuse or multifocal. A large body of neuropsychiatric literature has demonstrated the frequency of "minimal brain dysfunction" and poorly localized neurological "soft signs" in violent patients (231, 232). Elliot, for example, noted irregularly distributed perceptual, motor, sensory, reflex, and cognitive defects in 119 of 286 patients with a history of recurrent attacks of uncontrollable rage (233). Neurologic findings are common in violent individuals in juvenile reform school and on death row (234, 235). Attention deficit disorder (ADD) was significantly correlated with criminal and violent offenses in a prospective study (236). Not surprisingly, developmental or acute medical conditions producing scattered minor neurological impairments places an individual at higher risk of expressing aggressive impulses. Diffuse or multifocal brain insults are likely to affect one or several circuits within the multiregional, hierarchical aggression regulatory system. In addition, a history of being abused or reared in an unstable household is likely to interact synergistically with multifocal brain injuries. An individual who has learned a model of acting on impulse and possesses a limited repertoire of other response options is all the more likely to demonstrate diminished flexibility and inhibition of aggression after diffuse, especially frontal, injuries.

The clinical manifestations of aggression in these patients are heterogenous. However, the existence of a subgroup in whom dysregulation of aggression occurs almost uniformly without overt abnormalities on anatomic neuroimaging studies underscores the need for careful history taking, physical examination, and use of ancillary laboratory testing in all recurrently violent individuals. History of school difficulty, learning disability, hyperactivity, or head trauma associated with brief loss of consciousness or amnesia should be elicited. School records are helpful because patients may deny or minimize past academic or disciplinary problems. A clouded sensorium or subtle sensorimotor or visual impairments may be found on neurological examination. Etiologies of diffuse brain dysfunction with episodic violence include, in addition to ADD, toxic-metabolic encephalopathies (such as hyper- and hypoglycemia, B_{12} deficiency, and thiamine deficiency), MS, and subcortical vascular dementia.

Delusional Syndromes

Delusional individuals are prone to violent behavior. In these patients, aggression-related neural systems may, like the intellect, be placed in service of the psychosis. In a variety of neuropsychiatric disorders, including schizophrenia, endogenous depression, mania, Alzheimer's disease (AD), and other dementias, the presence of thought disorder and hallucinations, especially of persecutory type, increases the risk of violent outbursts (237–239). In a series of 181 subjects with probable AD, physical aggression was observed in 30% of patients; delusions and misidentifications frequently preceded violent outbursts (240). Dementia patients with paranoia and aggressive behavior have an increased rate of early institutionalization (241). Delusions are more likely to lead to aggression if frontal systems are also impaired.

The clinical approach to these patients is focused on the diagnosis and treatment of the underlying psychotic disorder. Etiologies of delusional disorders include paranoid schizophrenia, affective illness, late-life paraphrenia, AD, multi-infarct dementia, and subcortical dementias (Fig. 24.8) (242).

Treatment

Consideration of multiregional neural processing may guide selection of appropriate environmental and biological interventions to control aggression (Table 24.6).

Regular satisfaction of feeding drives and sleep-awake cycles may minimize hostile outbursts in patients with hypothalamic aggression. Much of our current pharmacological armamentarium for the treatment of violence is targeted on neuromodulators within the brainstem and hypothalamus, relying upon a pharmacologically induced bias against all types of aggressive responses. Brainstem structures, for example, are the likely sites of action for drugs that block β-adrenergic receptors (194, 243, 244), activate $5HT_1$ receptors (245), or enhance GABA activity. By raising the threshold for aggressive responding, such agents may have an ameliorative effect on aggression resulting from lesions at all levels of the neuraxis. Agents modulating muscarinic cholinergic receptors in the lateral hypothalamus might be systematically investigated for antiaggressive effects, based on observations that cholinomimetics directly instilled in the lateral hypothalamus elicit aggression. In one patient with lesions thought to disconnect hypothalamic circuitry from higher control, oral administration of a centrally active cholinergic antagonist dramatically suppressed aggressive, biting behavior (39).

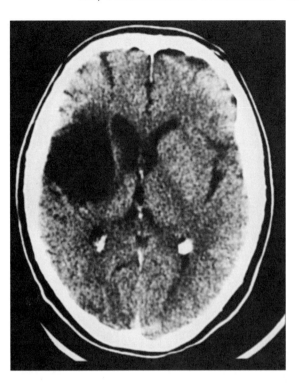

Figure 24.8. Aggression related to organic delusional syndrome. A 70-year-old right-handed man sustained a large right middle cerebral artery infarction, with residual left hemiparesis. Following the stroke, he believed that his wife was having an affair with a number of men in the neighborhood, aged 16–84. He attacked her in bed with his cane because he was convinced that she was sleeping with a covert sexual partner. The pathological jealousy (Othello) syndrome persisted for several years. Psychotherapy was not helpful. The intensity of jealous complaints and physical outbursts decreased on a combination of pimozide and sertraline.

Intervention at the temporolimbic level of control introduces additional considerations. Patients in whom a focal seizure disorder is diagnosed should be treated with agents effective for complex partial seizures, especially those such as carbamazepine and valproate, which have mood-stabilizing effects. Neuroleptics, which lower the seizure threshold, should be employed with caution. Avoiding restraint and providing gentle reassurance and reorientation in the postseizure period reduces postictal resistive violence. Patients whose clinical seizures remain refractory to antiepileptic therapy and who have well-defined unilateral foci are candidates for surgical resection. Temporal lobectomies or amygdala-hippocampectomies produce excellent seizure control in the preponderance of such patients and may have a beneficial effect upon aggression in patients whose epilepsy is associated with violent behaviors. Reduced aggression has been reported in more than 35% of violent epilepsy patients after temporal lobectomy (246).

Principles of pharmacological therapy for interictal aggression differ from those directed at reducing aggression levels in the hypothalamus. At the amygdalar level, the problem of timing is critical. To form appropriate sensory-emotional associations, the normal amygdala must be active in a brief time window to bind a specific stimulus or event with the hypothalamic signal of hunger or anger.

Table 24.6. Therapeutic Approaches to Aggressive Behavior

Clinical Setting of Aggression	Strategies	Specific Agents	Comment
Impulsive aggressive acts in setting of congenital brain abnormality (mental retardation) or diencephalic injury	1. Control of appetite, sleep, diurnal cues 2. β-adrenergic blocker 3. Selective serotonin reuptake inhibitors 4. Cholinergic (muscarinic) antagonists (?) 5. Avoid barbiturates, benzodiazepines, or sedatives	Propranolol Fluoxetine, sertraline, paroxetine Trihexyphenidyl	Hydrophilic β-blockers may have delayed (up to 4–6 weeks) onset of action. 5HT, agonists (e.g., eltoprazine) may have special utility. Anticholinergic agents of theoretic value but not systematically evaluated.
Aggression related to deepened affect or ideation of the interictal behavior syndrome of temporolimbic epilepsy (moralistic conviction)	1. Antiepileptic medications 2. Selective serotonin reuptake inhibitors 3. Reality-oriented psychotherapy 4. Avoid lithium carbonate (can compromise seizure control and worsen behavior)	Carbamazepine, valproic acid Fluoxetine, sertraline, paroxetine	Aggressive acts occur in clear consciousness as interictal, not ictal, events. Reality-oriented therapy may improve patient's understanding of deepened emotions and the need to control them.
Superficial (reflexive) aggression in response to transient environmental stimuli—signs of social disinhibition (prefrontal, dysexecutive personality syndrome)	1. Explicit and concrete social structure 2. Selective serotonin reuptake inhibitors 3. β-adrenergic blockers 4. Avoid barbiturates, benzodiazepines, or sedatives	Fluoxetine, sertraline, paroxetine Propranolol	The environment must supply cues that the patient cannot retain in "working memory." Avoid disinhibiting medications and alcohol.
Aggression prompted by hallucinations, delusions from underlying psychotic illness	1. Antipsychotic agents	Haloperidol, perphenazine, risperidone, clozapine	High-potency agents may be preferable as sedation can lead to disinhibition, increased paranoia. When used to treat chronic aggression, tardive dyskinesia risk may be increased. Akathesia may exacerbate paranoia.
Irritability related to manic or hypomanic states in bipolar illness or secondary mania	1. Mood stabilizers	Lithium carbonate Carbamazepine, valproic acid	Antipsychotic agents may also be necessary and are generally preferable to benzodiazepines, which may lead to behavioral disinhibition.
Acute violence or agitated aggression	1. Neuroleptics 2. Benzodiazepines	Haloperidol, thioridazine Lorazepam, diazepam	Exploit both sedative/hypnotic and antiaggressive properties of agents. Rare "paradoxical rage" with benzodiazepines.

Prolonged responses evoked by temporolimbic epileptic foci lead to an inappropriate broadening of the range of associated stimuli. Antiepileptic agents such as carbamazepine or valproic acid, which reduce prolonged, rapid discharges of neurons, may favor more selective, adaptive associations (247).

Recent studies have suggested that excitatory amino acid receptors, such as the class activated by N-methyl-D-aspartate (NMDA), may be critically involved in the associative process of long-term potentiation within the hippocampus and amygdala (248). Agents that modulate this response, such as selective NMDA-receptor blockers or nitric oxide synthetase inhibitors, merit investigation for antiaggressive and serenic properties in temporolimbic epileptic patients.

Processing within the orbitofrontal cortices represents an advanced stage of synaptic interaction occurring at the convergence of multiple streams of prior sensory evaluations. It is unlikely that a single neurotransmitter could be modulated to duplicate or restore prefrontal functions. Conversely, drugs that nonselectively inhibit neuronal function through inhibition of chloride channels or other mechanisms, such as ethanol, benzodiazepines, and barbiturates, exert a disproportionate effect upon prefrontal functioning, which is particularly dependent upon polysynaptic inputs. A paradox in the current psychopharmacology of aggression may be illuminated by considering the prefrontal effects of agents that simultaneously act at other levels of the neuraxis. Benzodiazepines, for example, have antiaggressive properties in many species and tranquilizing effects in man, likely mediated by their potentiating effects at GABA-ergic inhibitory receptors (249, 250). Yet these compounds are known to precipitate "paradoxical rage," the release of previously inhibited hostile responses (242, 251). A possible explanation is that benzodiazepines impair prefrontal processing through nonselective neuronal inhibition in a manner similar to ethanol intoxication (252). In some patients, the resulting loss of social insight and judgment more than offsets the general tranquilizing effects of these agents.

Serotonergic agents may also exert substantial effects upon prefrontal function. Serotonergic efferents from prefrontal cortices appear to serve an important role in the inhibition of impulsive responses. Lowered levels of 5-hydroxyindoleacetic acid and blunted responses to fenfluramine in impulsive aggressive individuals are consonant with this formulation (171), suggesting that serotonergic agents, especially those acting at $5HT_1$ receptors, may be beneficial to patients with orbitofrontal dysfunction. α_2 adrenergic agonists, such as clonidine and guafacine, have been shown to ameliorate frontal focused attention deficits and may thus be helpful to individuals with orbitofrontal derangements.

Supportive psychotherapy is helpful to many patients with temporolimbic and orbitofrontal aggression syndromes. Insight-oriented therapy is unlikely to be beneficial to the patient with prefrontal injury who may verbally comprehend a behavioral problem and propose solutions, but cannot reliably call on this knowledge to control behavior (98). Some patients with interictal behavior changes associated with temporal lobe epilepsy are amenable to insight psychotherapy, but many accept neither criticism nor advice (253). However, in our experience, by alerting patients to their intensified emotional responses, and capitalizing upon their heightened moral and religious sensitivities, a therapist may reduce their likelihood of aggressive actions.

CONCLUSIONS

The authors of this chapter recognize that many aggressive behaviors are neither maladaptive nor the result of neurological disease. Even when violent behavior and neurological lesions coexist, they may not be causally related. A violent lifestyle may lead to head trauma and neurological abnormalities that are the consequence, rather than the cause, of aggression.

While fully accepting these qualifications, we believe that neuropsychiatric care is enriched by recognizing both that a diverse array of neurological lesions that may contribute to violent behavior in human beings, and that abnormalities at different levels of the neuraxis produce distinctive subtypes of aggression. Future basic and clinical studies that consolidate and extend our understanding of the multiregional, hierarchical neural networks regulating aggression are urgently needed to refine diagnostic and therapeutic approaches to violent individuals.

References

1. Violence Prevention Panel. Prevention of violence and injuries due to violence. MMWR 1992;41:5–7.
2. Blum R. Contemporary threats to adolescent health in the United States. JAMA 1987;257:3390–3395.
3. McKinlay WW, Brooks DN, Bond MR, Martinage DP, Marshall MM. The short-term outcome of severe blunt head injury as reported by relative of the injured persons. J Neurol Neurosurg Psychiatry 1981;44:527–533.
4. Rossi AM, Jacobs M, Monteleone M, et al. Characteristics of psychiatric inpatients who engage in assaultive or other fear-inducing behaviors. J Nerv Ment Dis 1986;174:154–160.
5. Tardiff K. Characteristics of assaultive patients in private hospitals. Am J Psychiatry 1984;141:1232–1235.
6. Binder RL, McNiel DE. Effects of diagnosis and context on dangerousness. Am J Psychiatry 1988;145:728–732.
7. Karson CN, Bigelow LB. Violent behavior in schizophrenic inpatients. J Nerv Ment Dis 1987;175:161–164.
8. Larkin E, Murtagh S, Jones S. A preliminary study of violent incidents in a special hospital (Rampton). Br J Psychiatry 1988;153:226–231.
9. Cooper AJ, Mendonca JD. A prospective study of patient assaults on nurses in a provincial psychiatric hospital in Canada. Acta Psychiatr Scand 1991;84:163–166.
10. Davis S. Violence by psychiatric inpatients: a review. Hosp Community Psychiatry 1991;42:585–590.
11. McNiel DE, Binder RL. Clinical assessment of the risk of violence among psychiatric inpatients. Am J Psychiatry 1991;148:1317–1321.
12. Karson CN, Kashner TM. Assault increases the cost of care among inpatient veterans with schizophrenia. J Nerv Ment Dis 1991;179:702–704.

13. Widom CS. The cycle of violence. Science 1989;244:160–166.

14. Oliver JE. Successive generations of child maltreatment: the children. Br J Psychiatry 1988;153:543–553.

15. Glueck S, Glueck E. Unraveling juvenile delinquency. New York: Commonwealth Fund, 1980.

16. Pincus JH, Lewis DO. Episodic violence. Semin Neurol 1991;11:146–154.

17. Archer J. The behavioral biology of aggression. Cambridge: Cambridge University Press, 1988.

18. Huntingford FA, Turner AK. Animal conflict. London: Chapman and Hall Ltd, 1987.

19. Lore RK, Schultz LA. Control of human aggression: a comparative perspective. Am Psychol 1993;48:16–25.

20. Axelrod R. The evolution of cooperation. New York: Basic Books, 1984.

21. Maynard Smith J. The theory of games and the evolution of animal conflicts. J Theoret Biol 1974;47:209–221.

22. Silverberg J, Gray JP. Violence and peacefulness as behavioral potentialities of primates. In: Silverberg J, Gray JP, eds. Aggression and peacefulness in humans and other primates. New York: Oxford University Press, 1992:1–36.

23. de Waal FBM. Aggression as a part of primate social relationships. In: Silverberg J, Gray JP, eds. Aggression and peacefulness in humans and other primates. New York: Oxford University Press, 1992:37–56.

24. York A, Rowell T. Reconciliation following aggression in patas monkeys, *Erythrocebus patas*. Animal Behaviour 1988;36:502–509.

25. Benus RF, Bohus B, Koolhaas JM, van Oortmerssen GA. Heritable variation for aggression as a reflection of individual coping strategies. Experientia 1991;47:1008–1019.

26. Darwin C. The expression of emotion in man and animals (1873). Reprinted, London: Appleton, 1965.

27. Wilson EO. Sociobiology: the new synthesis. Cambridge: Harvard University Press, 1975.

28. Levenson RW, Ekman P, Friesen WV. Voluntary facial action generates emotion-specific autonomic nervous system activity. Psychophysiology 1990;27:363–383.

29. Kravitz EA. Hormonal control of behavior: amines and the biasing of behavioral output in lobsters. Science 1988;241:1775–1781.

30. Moyer KE. Kinds of aggression and their physiological basis. Commun Behav Biol 1968;2A:65–87.

31. Parmigiani S, Palanza P. Fluprazine inhibits intermale attack and predation, but not infanticide, in male mice. Neurosci Behav Rev 1991;15:511–513.

32. Nikulina EM. Neural control of predatory aggression in sill and domesticated animals. Neurosci Biobehav Rev 1991;15:545–547.

33. Sheard MH. Clinical pharmacology of aggressive behavior. Clin Neuropharmacol 1988;11:483–492.

34. Treiman DM. Psychobiology of ictal aggression. Adv Neurol 1991;55:341–356.

35. Vitiello B, Behar D, Hunt J, Stoff D, Ricciuti A. J Neuropsychiatr Clin Neurosci 1990;2:189–192.

36. Jacob F. Evolution and tinkering. Science 1977;196:293–314.

37. Derryberry D, Tucker DM. Neural mechanisms of emotion. J Consult Clin Psychol 1992;60:329–338.

38. MacLean PD. The triune brain in evolution: role in paleocerebral functions. New York: Plenum Press, 1990.

39. Weiger WA, Bear DM. An approach to the neurology of aggression. J Psychiatr Res 1988;22:85–98.

40. Delgado JMR. Social rank and radiostimulated aggressiveness in monkeys. J Nerv Ment Dis 1967;144:383–390.

41. Bechara A, van der Kooy D. The tegmental pedunculopontine nucleus; a brain-stem output of the limbic system critical for the conditioned place preferences produced by morphine and amphetamine. J Neurosci 1989;8:3400–3409.

42. Jouvet M, Delorme JF. Locus coeruleus et sommeil paradoxal. C R Soc Seances Soc Biol Fil 1965;159:895–899.

43. Jouvet M, Sastre J-P, Sakai K. Toward an etho-ethnology of dreaming. In: Karacan I, ed. Psychophysiological aspects of sleep. Park Ridge, NJ: Noyes Publishers, 1981:204–214.

44. Webster HW, Friedman L, Jones BE. Modification of paradoxical sleep following transections of the reticular formation at the pontomedullary junction. Sleep 1986;9:1–23.

45. Schenck CH, Mahowald MW. Polysomnographic, neurologic, psychiatric, and clinical outcome on 70 consecutive cases with the REM sleep behavior disorder (RBD). Cleve Clin J Med 1990;57:s10–s24.

46. Schenck CH, Milner DM, Hurwitz TD, Bundlie SR, Mahowald MW. A polysomnographic and clinical report on sleep-related injury in 100 adult patients. Am J Psychiatry 1989;146:1166–1173.

47. Porte H, Hobson JA. Fictive movement in sleep: REM vs NREM sleep reports. In: Chase MH, McGinty D, Crane G, eds. Sleep research. Los Angeles: University of California Press, 1986:82.

47a. Ross RJ, Ball WA, Dinges DF et al. Motor dysfunction during sleep in posttraumatic stress disorder. Sleep 17(8):723–732, 1994.

48. MacLean P. Brain evolution relating to family, play, and the separation call. Arch Gen Psychiatry 1985;42:405–417.

49. Bard P. A diencephalic mechanism for the expression of rage with special reference to the sympathetic nervous system. Am J Physiol 1928;84:490–515.

50. Wasman M, Flynn JP. Directed attack elicited from the hypothalamus. Arch Neurol 1962;6:220–227.

51. Kruck MR. Ethiology and pharmacology of hypothalamic aggression in the rat. Neurosci Biobehav Rev 1991;15:527–538.

52. Bandler RJ. Cholinergic synapses in the lateral hypothalamus for the control of predatory aggression in the rat. Brain Res 1970;20:409–424.

53. Smith DE, King MD, Hoebel BG. Lateral hypothalamic control of killing: evidence for a cholinoceptive mechanism. Science 1970;167:900–901.

54. Roberts WW. Escape learning without avoidance learning motivated by hypothalamic stimulation in cats. J Comp Physiol Psychol 1958;51:391–399.

55. Wheatley MD. The hypothalamus and affective behavior in cats: a study of experimental lesions with anatomic correlations. Arch Neurol Psych 1944;52:296–316.

56. Reeves AG, Plum F. Hyperphagia, rage and dementia accompanying a ventromedial hypothalamic neoplasm. Arch Neurol 1969;20:616–624.

57. Haugh RM, Markesbery WR. Hypothalamic astrocytoma: syndrome of hyperphagia, obesity and disturbances of behavior and endocrine and autonomic function. Arch Neurol 1983;40:560–563.

58. Tonkonogy JM, Geller JL. Hypothalamic lesions and intermittent explosive disorder. J Neuropsychiatr Clin Neurosci 1992;4:45–50.

59. Devinsky O, Kernan J, Bear DM. Aggressive behavior following exposure to cholinesterase inhibitors. J Neuropsychiatr Clin Neurosci (in press).

60. Van Hoesen GW. The differential distribution, diversity and sprouting of cortical projections to the amygdala in rhesus monkey. In: Beh-Ari Y, ed. The amygdaloid complex. Amsterdam: Elsevier, 1981:77–90.

61. Amaral DG, Price JL, Pitkänen, Carmichael ST. Anatomical organization of the primate amygdaloid complex. In: Aggleton JP, ed. The amygdala: neurobiological aspects of emotion, memory, and mental dysfunction. New York: Wiley-Liss, 1992:1–66.

62. Iwai E, Yukie M. Amydalofugal and amydalopetal connections with modality specific visual cortex area in macaques (*M.fuscata, M.mulatta, M.fascicularis*). J Comp Neurol 1987;261:362–387.

63. Harper RM, Frysinger RC, Trelease RB, et al. State-dependent alteration of respiratory cycle timing by stimulation of the central nucleus of the amygdala. Brain Res 1984;306:1–8.

64. Halgren E. Emotional neurophysiology of the amygdala within the context of human cognition. In: Aggleton JP, ed. The amygdala: neurobiological aspects of emotion, memory, and mental dysfunction. New York: John Wiley & Sons, 1992:191–228.

65. Klüver H, Bucy PC. Preliminary analysis of functions of the temporal

lobe in monkeys. Arch Neurol Psychiatry 1939;42:979–1000.

66. Schreiner L, Kling A. Behavioral changes following rhinencephalic injury in cat. J Neurophysiol 1953;16:643–659.

67. Kling AS, Brothers LA. The amygdala and social behavior. In: Aggleton JP, ed. The amygdala: neurobiological aspects of emotion, memory and mental dysfunction. New York: Wiley-Liss, 1992: 353–377.

68. Downer JL. Changes in visual gnostic functions and emotional behaviour following unilateral temporal pole damage in the "split-brain" monkey. Nature 1961;191:50–51.

69. Rosvold HE, Mirsky AF, Pribram KH. Influence of amygdalectomy on social behavior in monkeys. J Comp Physiol Psychol 1954;47: 173–178.

70. Dicks P, Myers RE, Kling A. Uncus and amygdala lesions: effects on social behavior in the free-ranging rhesus monkey. Science 1969;165: 69–71.

71. Aggleton JP. The functional effects of amygdala lesions in humans: a comparison with findings from monkeys. In: Aggleton JP, ed. The amygdala: neurobiological aspects of emotion, memory, and mental dysfunction. New York:Wiley-Liss, 1992:485–503.

72. Marlowe WB, Mancall EL, Thomas JJ. Complete Klüver-Bucy syndrome in man. Cortex 1975;11:53–59.

73. Jacobson R. Disorders of facial recognition, social behavior and affect after combined bilateral amygdalotomy and subcaudate tractotomy — a clinical and experimental study. Psychol Med 1986;16:439–450.

74. Lilly R, Cummings JL, Benson F, Frankel M. The human Klüver-Bucy syndrome. Neurology 1983;33:1141–1145.

75. Ramamurthi B. Stereotactic operation in behavior disorders. Amygdalotomy and hypothalamotomy. Acta Neurochir 1988; 44(suppl):152–157.

76. Terzian H, Dalle Ore G. Syndrome of Klüver and Bucy: reproduced in man by bilateral removal of temporal lobes. Neurology 1955;5: 373–380.

77. Horel JA. Recovery from the behavioral effects of occipital temporal disconnection. Anat Rec 1971;169:342–343.

78. Keating EG. Somatosensory deficit produced by parieto-temporal disconnection. Anat Rec 1971;169:353–354.

79. Bauer RM. Visual hypoemotionality as a symptom of visual-limbic disconnection in man. Arch Neurol 1982;39:702–708.

80. Habib M. Visual hypoemotionality and prosopagnosia associated with right temporal lobe isolation. Neuropsychologia 1986;24: 577–582.

81. Bauer RM, Bradley M, Lang PJ. Personal communication, 1993.

82. Bear DM. Temporal lobe epilepsy: a syndrome of sensory-limbic hyperconnection. Cortex 1979;15:357–384.

83. Gastaut H. Interpretation of the symptoms of psychomotor epilepsy in relation to physiologic data on rhinencephalic functions. Epilepsia 1954;3:84–88.

84. Iwai E, Yukie M, Watanabe J, et al. A role of amygdala in visual perception and cognition in macaque monkeys (M.fuscata and M.mulatta). Tohoku J Exp Med 1990;16(suppl):95–120.

85. Ono T, Nishijo H. Neurophysiological basis of the Klüver-Bucy syndrome: responses of monkey amygdaloid neurons to biologically significant objects. In: Aggleton JP, ed. The amygdala: neurobiological aspects of emotion, memory, and mental dysfunction. New York: Wiley-Liss, 1992:167–190.

86. Adamec RE. Partial kindling of the ventral hippocampus: identification of changes in limbic physiology which accompany changes in feline aggression and defense. Physiol Behav 1991;49:443–453.

87. Griffith N, Engel J Jr, Bandler R. Ictal and enduring interictal emotional disturbances in emotional behaviour in an animal model of temporal lobe epilepsy. Brain Res 1987;400:360–364.

88. Engel J Jr, Bandler R, Griffith NC, Caldecott-Hazard S. Neurobiological evidence for epilepsy-induced interictal disturbances. Adv Neurol 1991;55:97–111.

89. Siegel A. Aggression in epilepsy: animal models. In: Devinsky O, Theodore O, eds. Epilepsy and behavior. New York: Wiley-Liss, 1991, 389–404.

90. Bear DM, Schenck L, Benson H. Increased autonomic responses to neutral and emotional stimuli in patients with temporal lobe epilepsy. Am J Psychiatry 1981;38:843–845.

91. Waxman SG, Geschwind N. The interictal behavior syndrome of temporal lobe epilepsy. Arch Gen Psychiatry 1975;32:1580–1586.

92. Bear DM, Fedio P. Quantitative analysis of interictal behavior in temporal lobe epilepsy. Arch Neurol 1977;34:454–467.

93. Devinsky O, Bear DM. Varieties of aggressive behavior in temporal lobe epilepsy. Am J Psychiatry 1984;141:651–656.

94. Pandya DN, Dye P, Butters N. Efferent cortico-cortical projections of the prefrontal cortex in the rhesus monkey. Brain Res 1971;31: 35–46.

95. Leichnetz GR, Astruc J. Efferent connections of the orbitofrontal cortex in the marmoset (saguinus oedipus). Brain Res 1975;84:169–180.

96. Goldmann-Rakic PS. Topography of cognition: parallel distributed networks in primate association cortex. Ann Rev Neurosci 1988;11: 137–156.

97. Kievit J, Kuypers HGJM. Basal forebrain and hypothalamic connections to frontal and parietal cortex in the rhesus monkey. Science 1975;187:660–662.

98. Saver JL, Damasio AR. Preserved access and processing of social knowledge in a patient with acquired sociopathy due to ventromedial frontal damage. Neuropsychologia 1991;29:1241–1249.

99. Damasio AR, Tranel D, Damasio H. Somatic markers and the guidance of behavior: Theory and preliminary testing. In: Levin H, Eisenberg H, Benton A, eds. Frontal lobe function and dysfunction. New York: Oxford University Press, 1992.

100. Stuss DT, Benson DF. The frontal lobes. New York: Raven Press, 1986.

101. Milner B, Petrides M. Behavioural effects of frontal-lobe lesions in man. Trends Neurosci 1984;7:403–407.

102. Shallice T, Burgess PW. Deficits in strategy application following frontal lobe damage in man. Brain 1991;114:727–741.

103. Blumer D, Benson DF. Personality changes with frontal and temporal lobe lesions. In: Benson DF, Blumer D, eds. Psychiatric aspects of neurologic disease. New York: Grune & Stratton, 1975.

104. Bear D. Neurological perspectives on aggressive behavior. J Neuropsychiatr Clin Neurosci 1991;3(suppl):3–8.

104a. Raine A, Leucz T, Scerbo A. Antisocial behavior: neuroimaging, neuropsychology, neurochemistry, and psychophysiology. In: Ratey JJ, ed. Neuropsychiatry of Personality Disorders. Cambridge, MA: Blackwell Scientific, 1995;50–78.

105. Adams JH, Graham DI, Scott G. Brain damage in fatal non-missile head injury. J Clin Pathol 1980;33:1132–1145.

106. Levin HS, Amparo EG, Eisenberg HM, et al. Magnetic resonance imaging and computerized tomography in relation to the neurobehavioral sequelae of mild and moderate head injuries. J Neurosurg 1987;66:706–713.

107. Devinsky O. Behavioral neurology: 100 maxims. London: Edward Arnold, 1992.

108. Sabin TD, Mark VH. Boston City Hospital Grand Rounds: a case of intractable rage. Behav Med 1981;8:332–341.

109. Ross ED. Nonverbal aspects of language. Neurol Clin 1993;11:9–23.

110. Gainnoti G. Emotional behavior and hemispheric side of the lesion. Cortex 1972;8:41–45.

111. Landis T, Graves R, Goodglass H. Aphasic reading and writing: possible evidence for right hemisphere participation. Cortex 1982; 18:105–112.

112. Serafetinides EA, Hoare RD, Driver MV. Intracarotid sodium amylobarbitone and cerebral dominance for speech and consciousness. Brain 1965;88:107–130.

113. Sackheim HA, Gur RC, Savoy MC. Emotions are expressed more intensely on the left side of the face. Science 1978;202: 424–435.

114. Morrow L, Vrtunski P, Kim PB, Boller F. Arousal responses to emotional stimuli and laterality of lesion. Neuropsychologia 1981; 19:65–71.

115. Borod JC, Koff E, White B. Facial asymmetry in posed and

spontaneous expressions of emotions. Brain Cogn 1983;2:165–175.

116. Sackeim HA, Greenberg MS, Weiman AL, Gur RC, Hungerbuhler JP, Geschwind N. Hemispheric asymmetry in the expression of positive and negative emotions. Arch Neurol 1982;39:210–218.

117. Borod JC. Interhemispheric and intrahemispheric control of emotion: a focus on unilateral brain damage. J Consult Clin Psychol 1992;60:339–348.

118. Hauser MD. Right hemisphere dominance for the production of facial expression in monkeys. Science 1993;261:475–477.

119. Yeudall LT, Fromm-Auch D. Neuropsychological impairments in various psychopathological populations. In: Gruzelier J, Flor-Henry P, eds. Hemispheric asymmetries of function and psychopathology. New York: Elsevier, 1979:5–13.

120. Bryant ET, Scott ML, Golden CJ, Tori CD. Neuropsychological deficits, learning disability, and violent behavior. J Consult Clin Psychol 1984;52:323–324.

121. Brickman AS, McManus M, Grapentine WL, Alessi NE. Neuropsychological assessment of seriously delinquent adolescents. J Am Acad Child Psychiatry 1984;23:453–457.

122. Hart C. The relevance of a test of speech comprehension deficit to persistent aggressiveness. Personality and Individual Differences 1987;8:317–384.

123. Mungas D. Psychometric correlates of episodic violent behavior: a multi-disciplinary neuropsychological approach. Br J Psychiatry 1988;152:180–187.

124. Raine A, Scerbo A. Biologic theories of violence. In:Miller JS, ed. Neuropsychology of aggression. Boston: Kluwer Academic Publishers, 1991:1–25.

125. Quay HC. Intelligence. In: Quay HC, ed. Handbook of juvenile delinquency. New York: John Wiley & Sons, 1987:106–117.

126. Moffitt TE. The neuropsychology of juvenile delinquency: a critical review. In: Tonry M, Morris N, eds. Crime and justice: a review of the literature. Chicago: University of Chicago Press, 1990: 99–169.

127. Moffitt TE, Henry B. Neuropsychological studies of juvenile delinquency and juvenile violence. In: Miller JS, ed. Neuropsychology of aggression. Boston: Kluwer Academic Publishers, 1991:67–91.

128. Hill D, Pond DA. Reflections on 100 capital cases submitted for electroencephalography. J Ment Sci 1952;98:23–43.

129. Bach-y-Rita G, Lion JR, Climent CE, Ervin F. Episodic dyscontrol: a study of 139 violent patients. Am J Psychiatry 1971;127:1473–1478.

130. Convit A, Czobor P, Volavka J. Lateralized abnormality in the EEG of persistently violent psychiatric inpatients. Biol Psychiatry 1991; 30:363–370.

131. Milstein V. EEG topography in patients with aggressive violent behavior. In: Moffitt T, Mednick S, eds. Biological contributions to crime causation. Dordrecht: Martinus Nijhoff, 1988:40–52.

132. Hare RD, Jutai J. Psychopathy and cerebral asymmetry in semantic processing. Personality and Individual Differences 1988;9:329–337.

133. Nachson I. Hemispheric function in violent offenders. In: Moffitt TE, Mednick SE, eds. Biological contributions to crime causation. Dordrecht: Martinus Nijhoff, 1988:55–67.

134. Hare RD, McPherson LM. Psychopathy and perceptual asymmetry during verbal dichotic listening. J Abnorm Psychol 1984;93: 141–149.

135. Hare RD. Electrodermal and cardiovascular correlates of psychopathy. In: Hare RD, Schalling D, eds. Psychopathic behavior: approaches to research. New York, John Wiley & Sons, 1978:107–144.

136. Nachson I, Denno D. Violent behavior and cerebral hemisphere dysfunction. In: Mednick SA, Moffitt TE, Stack SA. The causes of crime: new biological approaches. Cambridge: Cambridge University Press, 1987:185–217.

137. Volkow ND, Tancredi L. Neural substrates of violent behavior: a preliminary study with positron emission tomography. Br J Psychiatry 1987;151:668–673.

138. Nachson I. Hemisphere dysfunction in psychopathy and behavior disorders. In: Myslobodsky M, ed. Hemisyndromes: Psychobiology, neurology, psychiatry. New York: Academic Press, 1983:389–414.

139. Nachson I. Neuropsychology of violent behavior: controversial issues and new developments in the study of hemisphere function. In: Miller JS, ed. Neuropsychology of aggression. Boston: Kluwer Academic Publishers, 1991:93–116.

140. Ellis LJ. Left- and mixed-handedness and criminality: explanations for a probable relationship. In: Coren S. Left-handedness. Amsterdam: Elsevier, 1990:485–507.

141. Bear DM. Hemispheric specialization and the neurology of emotion. Arch Neurol 1983;40:195–202.

142. McIntyre M, Pritchard PB, Lombroso CT. Left and right temporal lobe epileptics: a controlled investigation of some psychological differences. Epilepsia 1976:17:377–386.

143. Feinberg TE, Schindler RJ, Flanagan NG, Haber LD. Two alien hand syndromes. Neurology 1992;42:19–24.

144. Volpe BT. Observations of motor control in patients with partial and complete callosal section: implications for current theories of apraxia. In: Reeves AG, ed. Epilepsy and the corpus callosum. New York: Plenum Press, 1985:381–391.

145. Gazzaniga MS, Ledoux JE. The integrated mind. New York: Plenum Press, 1978.

146. Joseph R. The right cerebral hemisphere: emotion, music, visual-spatial skills, body-image, dreams and awareness. J Clin Psychol 1988;44:630–673.

147. Joseph R. Dual mental functioning in a 'split-brain' patient. J Clin Psychol 1988;44:770–779.

148. Reeves AJ. Behavioral changes following corpus callosotomy. Adv Neurol 1991;55:293–300.

149. Gasparrini WG, Satz P, Heilman K, et al. Hemispheric asymmetries of affective processing as determined by the Minnesota Multiphasic Personality Inventory. J Neurol Neurosurg Psychiatry 1978;41: 470–473.

150. Gardner H. Art, mind and brain: a cognitive approach to creativity. New York: Basic Books, 1984.

151. Fallon J, Gofi P. Distribution of monamines within the amygdala. In: Aggleton JP, ed. The amygdala: neurobiological aspects of emotion, memory, and mental dysfunction. New York: Wiley-Liss, 1992: 97–114.

152. Golden R, Gilmore J, Mark H, et al. Serotonin, suicide and aggression: clinical studies. J Clin Psychiatry 1991;52 (suppl 12):61–69.

153. Stanley M, Stanley B. Postmortem evidence for serotonin's role in suicide. J Clin Psychiatry 1990;51(suppl 4):22–28.

154. Stanley M, Virgilio J, Gershon S. Tritiated imipramine binding sites are decreased in the frontal cortex of suicides. Science 1982;216: 1337–1339.

155. Stanley M, Schalling D, Traskman-Bendz L, et al. Psychobiology of suicide, impulsivity and related phenomena. In: Meltzer H, ed. Psychopharmacology: the third generation of progress. New York: Raven Press, 1987:656–668.

156. Stanley M, Mann J. Increased serotonin-2 binding sites in frontal cortex of suicide victims. Lancet 1983;2:214–216.

157. Owen F, Cross AJ, Crow TJ, et al. Brain 5-HT receptors and suicide. Lancet 1983;2:1256.

158. Mann J, Stanley M, McBride P. Increased serotonin and beta-receptor binding in frontal cortices of suicide victims. Arch Gen Psychiatry 1986;43:954–959.

159. Ferrier I, McKeith I, Cross A. Postmortem neurochemical studies in depression. Ann N Y Acad Sci 1986;487:128–142.

160. Arora RC, Meltzer H. Serotonergic measures in the brains of suicide victims: 5-HT binding sites in the frontal cortex of suicide victims and control subjects. Ann J Psychiatry 1989;46:730–736.

161. Arango V, Ernsberger P, Marzuk P, et al. Autoradiographic demonstration of increased serotonin 5-HT$_2$ and β-adrenergic binding sites in the brains of suicide victims. Arch Gen Psychiatry 1990;47:1038–1047.

162. Cheetham S, Crompton M, Katona C, et al. Brain 5-HT2 receptors binding sites in depressed suicide victims. Brain Res 1988;443: 272–280.

163. Owen F, Chambers D, Cooper S. Serotonergic mechanisms in the

brains of suicide victims. Brain Res 1986;362:185–188.

163a. Blumensohn R, Ratzoni G, Weizman A, et al. Reduction in serotonin 5HT$_2$ receptor binding on platelets of delinquent adolescents. Psychopharmacology 1995;118(3):354–356.

164. Asberg M, Nordstrom P, Traskman-Bendz L. Cerebrospinal fluid studies in suicide: an overview. Ann N Y Acad Sci 1986;487:243–255.

165. Virkkunen M, DeJong J, Bartko J, et al. Psychobiological concomitants of history of suicide attempts among violent offenders and impulsive fire setters. Arch Gen Psychiatry 1989;46:604–608.

166. Linnoila M, Virkkunen M, Scheinin M, et al. Low cerebrospinal fluid 5-HIAA concentration differentiates impulsive from non-impulsive violent behavior. Life Sci 1983;33:2609–2614.

167. Brown G, Goodwin F, Ballenger J, et al. Aggression in humans correlates with cerebrospinal fluid metabolites. Psychol Res 1979;1:131–139.

168. Brown G, Ebert M, Goyer D, et al. Aggression, suicide and serotonin: relationship to CSF amine metabolites. Am J Psychol 1982;139:741–746.

168a. Mehlman PT, Higley JD, Faucher L, et al. Low CSF-5-H1AA concentrations and severe aggression and impaired impulse control in nonhuman primates. Amer J Psychiatry. 1994;151(10):1485–1491.

169. Coccaro E, Siever L, Klar H, et al. Serotonergic studies in patients with affective and personality disorders. Arch Gen Psychiatry 1989;46:587–599.

170. Coccaro E. Central serotonin and impulsive aggression. Br J Psychol 1989;155(suppl 8):52–62.

171. Meltzer H, Perline R, Tricov BJ, et al. Effect of hydroxytryptophan on serum levels in major affective disorders. Arch Gen Psychiatry 1984;41:379–387.

172. Coccaro E, Gabriel S, Siever L. Buspirone challenge: preliminary evidence for a role for central 5-HT$_{1A}$ receptor function in impulsive aggressive behavior in humans. Psychopharmacol Bull 1990;26:393–405.

173. Sijbesma H, Schipper J, deKloet E. Eltoprazine, a drug which reduces aggressive behavior, binds selectively to 5-HT$_1$ receptor sites in the rat brain. Eur J Pharmacol 1990;177:55–66.

174. White S, Kuchank R, Moyer J. Effects of serotonergic agents on isolation-induced aggression. Pharmacol Biochem Behav 1991;39:729–736.

175. Soubrie P. Reconciling the role of central serotonin neurons in humans and animal behavior. Behav Brain Res 1989;9:319–364.

176. Valzelli L, Bernasconi S. Aggressiveness by isolation and brain serotonin turnover changes in different strains of mice. Neuropsychobiology 1979;5:129–135.

177. Sewell R, Gallus J, Gault F, et al. P-chlorophenylalomine effects on shock-induced attack. Pharmacol Biochem Behav 1982;17:945–950.

178. Katz R. Role of serotonergic mechanisms in animal models of predation. Prog Neuropsychopharmacol 1980;4:219–231.

179. Copenhaver J, Schaloch R, Carver M. P-chlorophenylalomine-induced filicidal behavior in the female rat. Pharmacol Biochem Behav 1978;8:263–270.

180. Miczek K, Mos J, Oliver B. Serotonin, aggression and self-destructive behavior. Psychopharmacol Bull 1989;25:399–403.

180a. Muehlencamp F, Lucion A, Vogel WH. Effects of selective serotonin agonists on aggressive behavior in rats. Pharmacol Biochem Behav 1995;50(4):671–674.

181. Popova N, Voitenko N, Kulikov A, et al. Evidence for involvement of central serotonin in mechanism of domestication of silver foxes. Pharmacol Biochem Behav 1991;40:751–756.

182. Higley J, Mehlman P, Taub D, et al. Cerebrospinal fluid monoamine and adrenal correlates of aggression in free-ranging rhesus monkeys. Arch Gen Psychiatry 1992;49:436–441.

183. Yodyingyuad U, de lar Riva C, Abbott D, et al. Relationship between dominance hierarchy, CSF levels of amine transmitter metabolites. Neuroscience 1985;16:851–858.

184. Kraemer G. The primate social environment, brain neurochemical changes and psychopathology. Trends Neurosci 1985;8:339–340.

185. Bonson K, Winter J. Reversal of testosterone-induced dominance by the serotonergic agent quipazine. Pharmacol Biochem Behav 1992;42:809–813.

186. Bandler RJ. Cholinergic synapses in the lateral hypothalamus for the control of predatory aggression in the rat. Brain Res 1970;20:409–424.

187. Bandler RJ. Facilitation of aggressive behavior by direct cholinergic stimulation of the hypothalamus. Nature 1969;224:1035–1036.

188. Egger M, Flynn J. Effects of electrical stimulation of the amygdala in hypothalamically elicited attack behavior in cats. J Neurophys 1963;26:705–720.

189. Grossman SP. Chemically induced epileptiform seizures in the cat. Science 1963;142:409–411.

190. Stolk JM, Conner RL, Levine S, Barchas JD. Brain norepinephrine metabolism and shock-induced fighting behavior in rats. J Pharmacol Exp Ther 1974;190:193–209.

191. Sheard M. In: Usdin E, ed. Catecholamines: basic and clinical frontiers. New York: Pergamon Press, 1979:1690–1692.

192. Greendyke R, Kanter D, Schuster D, et al. Propanolol treatment of assaultive patients with organic brain disease. J Nerv Ment Dis 1986;174:290–294.

193. Mattes J. Comparative effectiveness of carbamazepine and propanolol for rage outbursts. J Neuropsychiatry 1990;2:159–164.

194. Stockmeier C, Metzer H. Beta-adrenergic receptor binding in frontal cortex of suicide victims. Biol Psychol 1991;29:183–191.

195. Fenwick P. Dyscontrol. In: Reynolds EH, Trimble MR, eds. Bridge between neurology and psychiatry. London: Churchill Livingstone, 1989, 263–287.

196. Gunne LM, Reis DJ. Changes in brain catecholemines associated with electrical stimulation of the amygdaloid nucleus. Life Sci 1963;11:804–809.

197. Reis DJ. The relationship between brain norepinephrine and aggressive behavior. Res Publ Assoc Res Nerv Ment Dis 1972;50:266–297.

198. Lammers AJJC, Van Rossum JM. Bizarre social behavior in rats induced by a combination of a peripheral decarboxylase inhibitor and dopa. Eur J Pharmacol 1968;5:103–106.

199. Serrault B. Psychopharamcologia 1970;18:271–287.

200. Traskman L, Asberg M, Bertilsson L, Sjostrand L. Monoamine metabolites in CSF and suicidal behavior. Arch Gen Psychol 1981;38:631–636.

201. Roy A, Agren H, Pickar D, et al. Reduced CSF concentrations of homovanillic acid and homovanillic acid to 5-hydroxyindoleacetic acid ratios in depressed patients: relationship to suicidal behavior and dexamethasone nonsuppression. Am J Psychol 1986;143:1539–1545.

202. Mandel P, Mack G, Kempf E. In: Jandler M, ed. Psychopharmacology of aggressive behavior. New York: Raven Press, 1979:95–110.

203. Malick JB, Sotia RD, Goldberg ME. A cooperative study of the effects of selected psychoactive agents upon three lesion-induced models of aggression in the rat. Arch Int Pharmacodyn Ther 1969;181:459–465.

204. Skolnick P, Reed G, Paul S. Benzodiazepine-receptor mediated inhibition of isolation-induced aggression in mice. Pharmacol Biochem Behav 1985;23:17–20.

205. Eichelman B. Neurochemical and psychopharmacologic aspects of aggressive behavior. In: Meltzer H, ed. Psychopharmacology: the third generation of progress. New York: Raven Press, 1987:697–704.

206. Puglesi-Allegra S, Mandel P. Psychopharmacology 1980;70:287–290.

207. Hormonal reactions to fighting in rat colonies: prolactin rises during defense, not during offense. Physiol Behav 1992;51:961–968.

208. Steldis H, Brammer G, Raleigh M, et al. Serum testosterone, male dominance and aggression in captive groups of vervet monkeys. Horm Behav 1985;19:154–163.

209. Moyer KE. The psychobiology of aggression. New York: Harper & Row, 1976.

210. Frank L. Social organization of the spotted hyena. II. dominance and reproduction. Animal Behavior 1986;34:1510–1527.
211. Frank LG, Glickman SE, Licht P. Fatal sibling aggression, precocial development and androgens in neonatal spotted hyenas. Science 1991;252:702–704.
212. Frank L, Davidson J, Smith E. Androgen levels in the spotted hyena: the influence of social factors. Journal of Zoology (London) 1985;206:525–531.
213. Olweus D, Mattsson A, Schalling D, et al. Circulating testosterone levels and aggression in adolescent males: a causal analysis. Psychosom Med 1988;50:261–272.
214. Dabbs JM, Frady R, Carr T, et al. Saliva testosterone and criminal violence in young adult prison inmates. Psychosom Med 1987;49:174–182.
215. Elias M. Serum cortisol, testosterone, and testosterone-binding globulin responses to competitive fighting in human males. Aggressive Behavior 1981;7:215–224.
216. Pope HG, Katz DL. Homicide and near homicide by anabolic steroid users. J Clin Psychiatry 1990;51:28–31.
217. Archer J. The influence of testosterone on human aggression. Br J Psychiatry 1991;82:1–28.
217a. Bergman B, Brismor B. Hormone levels and personality traits in abusive and suicidal male alcoholics. Alcohol Clin Exp Res 1994; 18(2):311–316.
217b. Loosen PT, Purdon SE, Pavlou JN. Effects on behavior of modulation of gonadal function in men with gonadotropin-releasing hormone antagonists. Am J Psychiatry 1994;151(2):271–273.
218. Berkovic SF, Andermann F, Melanson D, Ethier RE, Feindel W, Gloor P. Hypothalamic hamartomas and ictal laughter: evolution of a characteristic epileptic syndrome and diagnostic value of magnetic resonance imaging. Ann Neurol 1988;23:429–439.
219. Cascino GD, Andermann F, Berkovic SF, et al. Gelastic seizures and hypothalamic hamartomas: evaluation of patients undergoing chronic intracranial EEG monitoring and outcome of surgical treatment. Neurology 1993;43:747–750.
220. Mahowald MW, Bundlie SR, Hurwitz TD, Schenck CH. Sleep violence – forensic science implications: polygraphic and video documentation. J Forensic Sci 1990;35:413–432.
221. Mahowald MW, Schenck CH, Rosen GM, Hurwitz TD. The role of a sleep disorder center in evaluating sleep violence. Arch Neurol 1992;49:604–607.
222. Delgado-Escueta AV, Mattson RH, King L, et al. The nature of aggression during epileptic seizures. N Engl J Med 1981;305:711–716.
223. Weiser HG. Depth recorded limbic seizures and psychopathology. Neurosci Biobehav Rev 1983;7:427–440.
224. Treiman DM. Psychobiology of ictal aggression. Adv Neurol 1991;55:341–356.
225. Devinsky O, Vazquez B. Behavioral changes associated with epilepsy. Neurol Clin 1993;11:127–149.
226. Fenwick P. Aggression and epilepsy. In: Devinsky O, Theodore WH, eds. Epilepsy and behavior. New York: Wiley-Liss, 1991:85–96.
227. Blumer D, Benson DF. Psychiatric manifestations of epilepsy. In: Benson DF, Blumer D, eds. Psychiatric aspects of neurologic disease. New York: Grune & Stratton, 1975:151–170.
228. Remillard GM, Anermann F, Rhi-Sausa A, et al. Facial asymmetry in patients with temporal lobe epilepsy. Neurology 1977;27:109–114.
229. De Renzi E, Barbieri C. The incidence of the grasp reflex following hemispheric lesion and its relation to frontal damage. Brain 1992; 115:293–313.
230. Eslinger PJ, Damasio AR. Severe disturbance of higher cognition after bilateral frontal lobe ablation: patient EVR. Neurology 1985; 35:1731–1741.
231. Monroe RR. Brain dysfunction in aggressive criminals. Lexington, MA: Lexington Books, 1978.
232. Elliot FA. Violence. The neurologic contribution: an overview. Arch Neurol 1992;49:595–603.
233. Elliot FA. Neurological findings in adult minimal brain dysfunction and the dyscontrol syndrome. J Nerv Ment Dis 1982;170:680–687.
234. Lewis DO, Pincus JH, Glaser GH. Violent juvenile delinquents: psychiatric, neurological, psychological and abuse factors. J Am Acad Child Psychiatry 1979;18:307–319.
235. Lewis DO, Pincus JH, Feldman, et al. Psychiatric, neurological and psychoeducational characteristics of 15 death-row inmates in the United States. Am J Psychiatry 1986;143:838–845.
236. Satterfield JH, Hope CM, Schell AM. A prospective study of delinquency in 110 adolescent boys with attention deficit disorder and 88 normal adolescent boys. Am J Psychiatry 1982;139:795–798.
237. Cooper AJ, Mendonca JD. A prospective study of patient assaults on nurses in a provincial hospital in Canada. Acta Psychiatr Scand 1991;84:163–166.
238. Beck JC, White KA, Gage B. Emergency psychiatric assessment of violence. Am J Psychiatry 1991;148:1562–1565.
239. Davis S. Violence by psychiatric inpatients: a review. Hosp Community Psychiatry 1991;42:585–590.
240. Deutsch LH, Bylsma FW, Rovner BW, Steele C, Folstein MF. Psychosis and physical aggression in probable Alzheimer's disease. Am J Psychiatry 1991;148:1159–1163.
241. O'Donnell BF, Drachman DA, Barnes HJ, Peterson KE, Swearer JM, Lew RA. Incontinence and troublesome behaviors predict institutionalization in dementia. J Geriatr Psychiatry Neurol 1992;5:45–52.
242. Gorman DG, Cummings JL. Organic delusional syndrome. Semin Neurol 1990;10:229–238.
243. Yudofsky SC, Silver JM, Hales RE. Pharmacologic management of aggression in the elderly. J Clin Psychiatry 1990;51(suppl):22–28.
244. Ratey JJ, Sorgi P, O'Driscoll GA, et al. Nadolol to treat aggression and psychiatric symptomatology in chronic psychiatric inpatients: a double-blind, placebo-controlled study. J Clin Psychiatry 1992;53:41–46.
245. Coccaro EF, Siever LJ, Klar HM, et al. Serotonergic studies in patients with affective and personality disorders; correlates with suicidal and impulsive aggressive behavior. Arch Gen Psychiatry 1989;46:587–599.
246. Falconer MA. Reversibility by temporal-lobe resection of the behavioral abnormalities of temporal-lobe epilepsy. N Engl J Med 1973;289:451–455.
247. Bear DM. Behavioral changes in temporal lobe epilepsy; conflict, confusion, challenge. In: Trimble MR, Bolwig TG, eds. Aspects of epilepsy and psychiatry. New York: John Wiley & Sons, 1986:19–30.
248. Heinmann U, Hamon B. NMDA receptors become involved in synaptic transmission following kindling. Exp Brain Res 1986;65:1–10.
249. Quenzer LF, Feldman RS, Moor JW. Toward a mechanism of the anti-aggressive effects of chlordiazepoxide in rats. Psychopharmacologia 1974;34:81–94.
250. Salzman C, Soloman D, Miyawaki E, et al. Parenteral lorazepam versus parental haloperidol for the control of psychotic disruptive behavior. J Clin Psychiatry 1991;52:177–180.
251. Bond AJ. Pharmacological manipulation of aggressiveness and impulsiveness in healthy volunteers. Prog Neuropsychopharmacol Biol Psychiatry 1992;16:1–7.
252. Bushman BJ, Cooper HM. The effects of alcohol on human aggression: an integrative research review. Psychol Bull 1990;107:341–354.
253. Benson DF. The Geschwind syndrome. Adv Neurol 1991;55:411–421.

25

NEUROPSYCHIATRY OF MENTAL RETARDATION AND CEREBRAL PALSY

John J. Ratey and Maureen P. Dymek

The American Association on Mental Deficiency (AAMD) defines mental retardation as significantly subaverage intellectual functioning coupled with deficits in adaptive behavior and manifested during the developmental period (1). Despite the prevalence of mental retardation (estimated at 3% of our population) and its diverse biological and psychological manifestations, little has been done to promote neuropsychiatric intervention with this needy community.

The 1950s and 1960s witnessed some of the greatest advances in modern neuropsychiatry. This era encompassed the advent of neuroleptic agents, "miracle drugs" that were largely effective in curbing many of the seemingly resilient maladaptive behaviors of people with severe mental illness. With the demonstrated efficacy of neuroleptics in many psychotic populations, psychiatry became all too eager to prescribe these agents to patients with developmental disabilities. Neuroleptic overmedication became predominant among persons with retardation, often culminating in disastrous results. Untoward side effects, such as extreme sedation, tardive dyskinesia, tardive akathisia, and neuroleptic malignant syndrome, tortured many patients on antipsychotic medications. Numerous medical professionals failed to recognize the oppressive conditions that the neuroleptically-medicated patients with mental retardation had to endure. The consequences of this oversight were tragic for the field of psychiatry, generating extensive public criticism and dire legal implications.

Since the outcry against the abuse of neuroleptics among people with mental retardation in the 1970s, care of these clients has grown very political in nature. Treatments have been quantified and observable behaviors dissected. Individuals with developmental disabilities have become a primary population of behaviorists and educators. As a result, very positive changes have occurred in the care of individuals with mental retardation, humanizing the treatment process. However, the shift of medical practitioners away from the mentally retarded has been unfortunate for many reasons. The intellectual and social impairments, and the maladaptive behaviors central to mental retardation are often precipitated by neurotransmitter anomalies, anatomical defects, or degenerative diseases, many of which are treatable. Medical intervention could provide invaluable help for these clients.

Obviously, neuropsychiatry has much to offer in the habilitation of this population. Recent research has improved our understanding of the pathophysiology underlying much of mental retardation. Individuals with analogous cognitive and adaptive impairments are no longer being lumped together because of superficial similarities. The development of highly specific drugs, along with the wide range of diagnostic techniques made possible by technological advances, have improved our understanding of mental retardation. Accordingly, diverse interventions for the mentally retarded are available. This chapter outlines the importance of neuropsychiatry in mental retardation by highlighting many of the clinical, diagnostic, neuroscientific, and therapeutic variables associated with this population.

CLINICAL BACKGROUND

It is a common, although unfounded, belief that people with mental retardation form a homogeneous group of individuals with low intelligence and similar behavioral patterns. However, mental retardation is a term that encompasses a large and variable body of cognitive aptitude, emotional adjustment, and social development. Because of the complex classification scheme of mental retardation, behavioral variables range considerably, and it is difficult to typify an individual with mental retardation. However, when defined according to cognitive capability and respective etiology, this goal is attainable. We use this strategy here as we discuss the more common clinical presentations of the mentally retarded and identify some psychiatric problems to which the mentally retarded often are prone.

Levels of Retardation

Mental retardation is broken down into four categories: mild, moderate, severe, and profound. Although the diagnosis of mental retardation must be based on both intellectual ability and adaptive functioning, the salient factor this classification emphasizes is intelligence. Intelligence tests, such as the Wechsler Adult Intelligence Scale (WAIS) and the Stanford-Binet are the major indices of intellectual ability and serve to distinguish the extent to which retardation spans.

MILD MENTAL RETARDATION

According to standards set by the American Psychiatric Association (APA), those individuals with mild forms of mental retardation generally have IQ levels ranging from 55 to 70 (2). This group consists of about 2% of our general population and roughly 80% of the mentally retarded. Individuals with mild degrees of intellectual impairment often appear relatively normal during the childhood years. Their predicament usually becomes apparent in early adolescence, as the social and scholastic demands placed upon them increase. The mildly retarded typically are able to master essential school skills and by adulthood can achieve a satisfactory level of socially adaptive behavior.

Some cases of mild retardation are attributed to structural brain disease (discussed in next section); however, many cases seem to stem from normal intellectual variation or adverse sociocultural conditions (3, 4). Many of these functionally retarded individuals are marked by impoverished and deprived backgrounds and generally have no physical problems associated with their disorder.

MODERATE MENTAL RETARDATION

IQ levels in those diagnosed with moderate mental retardation stand in the range of 40–55 (2). This group is much smaller than that of the mildly retarded, comprising about 10–15% of retarded individuals. Moderate mental retardation is usually recognized early in life, when developmental milestones such as language are delayed. By adulthood, many of these individuals have fair verbal abilities, although their rate of learning remains slow. As a whole, those with moderate intellectual impairments acquire daily living and simple vocational skills and are able to function in society with guidance.

Causal factors pertaining to moderate mental retardation are less likely to be attributed to psychosocial or sociocultural factors than mild retardation. Biological factors are frequently implicated, and the neurogenic basis in many cases of moderate mental retardation is often evident through physiological abnormalities in the patient. Many times poor coordination and mild body deformities are present.

SEVERE MENTAL RETARDATION

IQ levels of the severely retarded individual range from 20–39 (2). The deficits present in these individuals are apparent at very young ages and range from severely defective speech quality to somatosensory deficits to motor handicaps. Severely retarded patients can sometimes develop limited levels of hygiene and self-help, but invariably will remain dependent upon the care of others. Most cases of severe retardation stem from biological phenomena.

PROFOUND MENTAL RETARDATION

The IQ level of profoundly retarded individuals is measured at or under 20 (2). With the exception of those individuals plagued with inborn errors of metabolism, the problems present in these individuals are often noticeable at birth, due to the presence of severe physical malformations and other obvious symptoms of abnormality. As with the severely retarded, gross central nervous system (CNS) pathology is almost always present. The profoundly retarded show multiple handicaps, severe deficits in adaptive skills, and are very resistant to learning.

Behavioral and Psychiatric Phenomenology

MILD AND MODERATE MENTAL RETARDATION

The mildly and moderately retarded once were thought of as a happy-go-lucky group, too simple-minded to be affected by emotional difficulty. The inadequacy of this view has become obvious in recent decades, with numerous studies indicating that these individuals are more susceptible to psychological problems than the general population. Research indicates that roughly 50–60% of mentally retarded individuals have mild psychological disturbances, and 10–15% are plagued by severe psychiatric disorders (5).

The degree of social and intellectual functioning greatly affects both frequency and type of mental illness in the mentally retarded. Individuals in the mild to moderate range of mental retardation are characterized by their simplistic cognitive schemes and heightened sensitivity to internal and external stimuli. Their thinking often utilizes a concrete approach and can be filled with perseverations and inflexibility. They usually have adequate verbal capacities and are generally adept at learning and performing well in simple activities and tasks. Because of their perceived capabilities, society often places unrealistically high expectations upon these individuals, which can leave them prone to failure. Their reduced capacity to withstand stress, paired with limited social and peer supports, and society's emphasis on intellect and competition leaves this population extremely vulnerable to psychological and behavioral disorders.

Elevated occurrences of personality disorders, adjustment reactions, and anxiety disorders in this group suggest a biological predisposition to overreact to stimuli and a high risk for personality disorganization secondary to minimal stress. Sands and Ratey (6) discuss this population's vulnerability to stimulus overloading, or "noise." Due to their limited cognitive capacity and resulting inability to filter stimuli, numerous situations, even ordinary ones, can be experienced as catastrophic. When internal or external stimuli are perceived as unpredictable or uncontrollable, as often happens with the mentally retarded, the resulting inner state becomes chaotic. As a consequence of situations that can be neither integrated or controlled, the individual retreats to a lower level of functioning and a more constricted form of organization. Attempts to escape from this distress and organize experience often result in impulsive or chaotic behavior, stereotypic responses, or withdrawal.

Serious psychiatric illness, such as schizophrenia and the bipolar and unipolar affective disorders, are also diagnosed in the mildly retarded. These disorders are difficult to gauge in this population because of their limited ability to understand and verbalize thoughts and feelings. In the verbally competent mild to moderate retardate, symptoms of schizophrenia are similar to the traditional symptoms found in normal populations and are likely to have paranoid and catatonic features (7). Characteristic features of affective disorders are also found readily among the retarded, although depression is commonly underdiagnosed. This may occur because the withdrawn and passive behavior patterns found in depression are falsely thought to be typical behaviors of mentally retarded individuals, and the nondisruptive nature of depression is likely to go unnoticed in large institutional settings.

Other behavior problems commonly found in this subgroup are aggression, hyperactivity, impulsivity, emotional lability, selective isolation, and temporary regression to primitive self-stimulatory activities. The source of these problems can be linked to psychological, environmental, and biological factors. Poor ego development and individuation, mixed with poor social skills and reduced stress tolerance, target the mildly or moderately retarded individual for behavior disturbances. Internal catalysts, such as physical illness or premenstrual syndrome often manifest themselves in forms of behavioral dyscontrol. Again, communication difficulties and limited verbal skills lead the retarded individual to express pain and discomfort in maladaptive and inappropriate ways. Organic conditions such as epilepsy can also lead to a high incidence of behavior problems. The increased levels of complex partial seizures in retarded populations leads to elevated occurrences of interictal behavior syndrome, a result of frequent seizures symptomized by emotional intensity, lability, and aggression.

SEVERE AND PROFOUND MENTAL RETARDATION

Individuals with severe and profound mental retardation are likely to have atypical behavior patterns, partially because of their nominal cognitive capabilities, and partially because of their multiple physical and physiological handicaps. The severe language dysfunction and gross CNS impairments commonly found in this group also contribute to seemingly abnormal behavior. Behaviors commonly associated with this level of retardation are characterized by stereotypy, hyperorality, aggression, and primitivism. Rudimentary use of sense modalities such as touch and position are common, as are autistic behaviors. Self-injurious behavior (SIB) is a widespread manifestation of the extreme forms of mental retardation, and often takes form as headbanging, eye-gouging, biting, scratching, self-pinching and rectal digging.

Severe psychiatric disorders such as schizophrenia are extremely difficult to characterize in this population. The lack of expressive ability severely hinders diagnosis because symptoms central to schizophrenia such as hallucinations and delusions are so verbally based. The behavioral disturbance may arise from the specific brain dysfunction that causes the intellectual subnormality. The high incidence of psychotic behavior in individuals plagued with phenylketonuria, and the centrality of aggression and SIB in Lesch-Nyhan syndrome are examples of psychiatric disorders that are secondary manifestations of an underlying genetic or metabolic disorder.

There are numerous reasons behind the maladaptive behaviors commonly seen in the seriously retarded. Many of these problematic behaviors are brought on by an inner tendency toward disorganization and an inability to order experience. Repetitive shouting, headbanging, or rocking, which are seen as grossly deviant or even psychotic behaviors, may merely be attempts to organize inner experience around a stereotypic, rhythmic action (6). Sometimes acting out operates on a reinforcement contingency, and is a purposeful attempt to receive attention, no matter how unpleasant it may be. Other times brain dysfunction and neurotransmitter anomalies are at the root of behavioral defects, as discussed in the following section.

GENETIC AND NEUROSCIENCE ISSUES

Because mental retardation is composed of such a vast number of symptomatologies, it follows that the etiologies of such disorders are proportionally complex. There are over 350 known disorders and conditions that generate mental retardation, varying among genetic and acquired factors. Mild mental retardation was once thought to be precipitated only through social and environmental factors; however, this seems to be a vast oversimplification. As medical technology becomes more advanced, many forms of mild intellectual impairments are being found to have a neurobiologic basis. Subtle but significant biological events such as chromosomal anomalies, genetic syndromes, prenatal and postnatal infections, exposure to perinatal risks, and maternal teratogens increasingly are implicated in mental retardation. This section delineates the medical and biological etiologies of mental retardation, and discusses the neuroscientific variables associated with these pathologies.

Biological and Medical Etiologies of Mental Retardation: Prenatal Causes

GENETIC FACTORS

Research on the genetic aspects of mental retardation has flourished over the past several decades. Advances in medical technology have elucidated our understanding of the mechanisms involved in genetic transmission, and thus have expanded our potential for diagnosis, prevention, and treatment of associated disorders.

Genetic factors are the single most common cause of mental retardation and can be partially implicated in up to 90% of cases (8). Syndromes of differing genetic origin are associated with distinct profiles of cognitive, emotional, and linguistic performance, as well as unique patterns of individual development. Chromosomal abnormalities, including Down syndrome and fragile X syndrome, and single gene disorders such as Cornelia de Lange syndrome are correlated with high levels of mental retardation. Hereditary precipitants of mental retardation are not always associated with a specific genetic syndrome and can be classified as normal intellectual variation.

Chromosomal Abnormalities

Chromosomal abnormalities are heritable mutations or variations of genetic material. Rare autosomal abnormalities such as Lesch-Nyhan syndrome, trisomy D, and *cri du chat* syndrome have been implicated in mental subnormality, as have aberrations of the sex chromosomes such as Turner's syndrome and Klinefelter's syndrome. The most widespread forms of chromosomal abnormalities implicated in mental retardation are fragile X syndrome and Down syndrome.

Fragile X syndrome. Fragile X syndrome (Martin-Bell syndrome; fra(X)) is the single most common chromosomal form of mental retardation. As the name implies, this syndrome is an X-linked disorder, wherein associated phenotypic traits are usually expressed in the male and carried by the female. The disorder is induced by a fragile site/gap on the long arm of the X chromosome. About 30% of females who carry numerous active, mutated X chromosomes actually show symptoms of mental retardation (9, 10). Heterozygous females may express mental retardation but do not show the characteristic physical traits found in males with fra(X).

There is a significant degree of phenotypic variability expressed in the disorder. Fragile X males usually are mentally retarded and have learning disabilities that may be characterized by defective speech and language patterns. Hyperactive behavior is common, as are autistic behaviors and major affective or schizoaffective disorders (11). In a small group of fra(X) patients studied, the following symptoms were noted: stereotypic behavior (65%), incoordination (59%), hyperactivity (47%), *grand mal* seizures (41%), and extensor plantar responses (41%) (12). Physical characteristics of the disorder common to males are macro-orchidism, abnormally structured large ears, large nose, prominent forehead, prognathism, and abnormal dermatoglyphics.

Down syndrome. Down syndrome (DS; trisomy 21) is a genetic aberration produced by extra material in the 21st chromosome, and its estimated presence is one in every 1000 live births (13). DS seems to have a familial link (high concordance in twins and families), and the occurrences show a linear increase with the mother's age. For mothers over 35, the risk is two to three times the normal rate; by the maternal age of 40, the risk is 1%; and by the age of 43, it doubles to 2% (14).

With few exceptions, individuals with DS are mentally retarded, usually to a mild or moderate degree. Intellectual and social handicaps are customarily paired with labored physical and emotional development. Historically, the literature has described these individuals as very sociable, affectionate, and amiable; and although this may be true, it is important to realize that they are susceptible to aggression, behavioral dyscontrol, and any other psychopathological conditions associated with mental retardation.

Specific physical features characterize the disorder, such as decreased muscle tone, thin and dry hair, small head, slanted and almond-shaped eyes, and small hands and feet. Neuroanatomical conditions such as decreased intracranial volume exhibiting smaller gyri and simple patterns, and an underdeveloped cerebellum have also been noted. By the age of 40, Down syndrome subjects exhibit neuropathologies that are strikingly similar to those found in the brains of patients with Alzheimer's disease (AD). Nearly all patients with DS develop neuropathic changes in tissue, such as neurofibrillary tangles and senile plaques, and show evidence of amyloid angiopathy. Furthermore, many DS patients develop the clinical manifestations of AD, showing similar cognitive decline and dementia (15, 16).

Single Gene Disorders

Single gene disorders, which are passed on through simple mendelian inheritance, account for approximately 15% of mental retardation. These disorders can be passed down generationally through either dominant or recessive mechanisms.

Autosomal-dominant syndromes. Autosomal-dominant syndromes can be passed down when either parent carries the disturbed genotype. All offspring of a parent with the mutant gene possess a 50% chance of inheriting the disorder. Alterations such as nonpenetrance and variable expressivity often modify the degree and type of phenotypic expression in autosomally dominant inheritance. Extent of gene expressivity in these conditions is extremely variable, and the severity and quality of the clinical manifestations vary greatly. Many autosomally dominant conditions are associated with increased risks of mental retardation, the most common of these being tuberous sclerosis, neurofibromatosis, Sturge-Weber syndrome, and Cornelia de Lange syndrome.

Cornelia de Lange syndrome is a disorder transmitted through a dominant inheritance (17–19) in which nearly all cases manifest mental retardation. The physical markers of the syndrome are short stature, facial and skeletal abnormalities, hirsutism, and associated gastrointestinal, cardiac, and genital abnormalities. Behaviorally, the disorder is characterized by attention seeking, transient aggression, hyperactivity, and noncompulsive self-injury. The vast majority of individuals with Cornelia de Lange syndrome are self-abusive (13). There is some evidence that these troublesome behaviors are caused by serotonergic dysfunction; one study reported low levels of cerebrospinal 5-hydroxyindeoleacetic acid (5-HIAA) in a case of Cornelia de Lange (20), while another study found serotonergic treatment to be effective in curbing self-injury in this population (21).

Autosomal-recessive syndromes. Autosomal-recessive inheritance necessitates that both parents carry the mutant gene, and the offspring must be homozygous-positive for the associated phenotype to be expressed. If the individual has only one mutant allele, he or she will not display the associated phenotype but will carry the mutant gene, and has a 50% chance of passing it onto his or her offspring.

Most autosomal-recessive syndromes associated with mental retardation are the relatively rare inborn errors of metabolism. In these disorders, many different metabolic pathways may be involved, such as those of the amino acids, carbohydrates, lipids, plasma proteins, and vitamins. Problems arise when the body does not have the capacity for certain normal metabolic processes. Generally, this leads to a build-up of toxic substance in the body, which may result in progressive loss of mental or neurological function. The degree of mental retardation with such disorders is rather severe. Detrimental effects of these disorders can sometimes be avoided by dietary modification or medication early in life. Examples of autosomal recessive inborn errors of metabolism implicated in mental retardation are phenylketonuria, congenital hypothyroidism, Tay-Sachs disease, galactosemia, Neiman-Pick disease, Gaucher's disease, and maple syrup urine disease.

PRENATAL CAUSES: ENVIRONMENTAL FACTORS

Numerous environmental components can alter fetal development, and because of the fragility of the central nervous system in utero, teratogenic effects are devastating to the fetus. Nongenetic prenatal causes of mental subnormality can be attributed to diverse maternal factors, caused by such various denominators as age, improper diet, physical injury, disease or infection, toxic states, and blood incompatibility. Any of these conditions can lead to prematurity, low birth weight, meningitis, congenital malformations, or a host of other climates detrimental to development of the individual.

Maternal Medical Problems

Many maternal infections play a sizable role in the genesis of mental retardation and neurological impairments in the offspring. Syphilis, rubella, toxoplasmosis, and cytomegalovirus are examples of infections that have the ability to diffuse through the placenta and enter the fetus. These bacterial and viral infections generally have a proclivity to settling in the CNS, eventually resulting in microcephaly, epilepsy, hydrocephalus, or cerebral calcification. More often than not, adverse maternal conditions are more detrimental to the baby than the mother. Toxemias are a group of diseases common in the last 3 months of pregnancy that may result in prematurity and anoxia to the fetus, with the end result being mental retardation. Prenatal infections such as polio, measles, mumps, chicken pox, and flu were once thought to cause mental retardation, but there has been no conclusive evidence supporting this theory. In addition to acute infections, chronic diseases in the mother leave the fetus susceptible to developing mental handicaps. Conditions such as kidney disease, diabetes mellitus, thyroid disease, and hypertension all predispose the baby to diverse neurological problems.

Various precautions can be made by a pregnant woman to decrease the chances of bearing a handicapped baby. She should take steps to ensure a diet that is enriched and balanced, avoid alcohol and tobacco, and take the fewest possible drugs and only those known to be safe. The expectant mother should attempt to diminish emotional stress and do all that she can to safeguard her own health. She should have access to good health care in case of emergency. Educational prevention programs can assist in significantly altering many of these factors. It has been stated that if preventive measures were utilized effectively, the current incidence of mental retardation could be cut nearly in half (22). Additionally, there are recognized treatments for many of these infections or diseases in the mother, such as antibiotics and vaccines, which may act to prevent the development of disorders in the child.

Maternal Intoxication

Many drugs ingested in pregnancy have teratogenic effects on the child, causing deviations in the CNS and other body systems, which often lead to mental retardation in the child. The developing brain is one of the most vulnerable organs in the human body and is especially so from the moment of conception to the second or third year of life. Many less than optimal conditions may leave the mother unaffected, but are devastating to the child. The teratogenic effects of chemical agents are caused by an interruption in the developmental stages of the body organs, particularly the CNS. Specific drugs that are especially harmful to the offspring are endocrine substances, alkylating agents, antibiotics, many psychotropic medications (hallucinogens, azodyes, thalidomide), and any drug that interferes with metabolism (antipurines, antipyrimidines, antiglutamines). Each agent generally produces a specific and distinguishing array of defects. Some widely used drugs, such as alcohol and tobacco, have been associated with specific syndromes of fetal malformation. Fetal alcohol syndrome often results in growth retardation, physical malformations, and mental subnormality.

The clinical manifestations found in the progeny of maternal drug users depend as much on the time in development when the drug was introduced as the specific agent itself. The CNS is susceptible to external factors during myelinization (7 months of pregnancy to the first few months after birth). Defective myelinization is associated with impaired intellectual development in the newborn; these effects may have long-lasting results. To be teratogenic, an agent must bear some specific relationship to the metabolic requirements of the growing embryo. Whether a tissue is affected depends upon the agent's mechanism of action, and whether it is relevant to developmental events in the tissue at the time of treatment. In general, the earlier a toxic drug affects the fetus, the more devastating the consequences are likely to be.

PERINATAL FACTORS

The perinatal stage begins at birth and occupies the first several days of life. Obstetric complications such as prolonged and difficult delivery, birth injury, anoxia, or maternal anesthesia have a considerable effect on the neonate, and are major causes of neurological and mental handicaps. Up to 18% of cases of mental retardation are attributed to difficulties encountered in the perinatal period (23, 24). Prematurity is a perinatal factor associated with mental retardation, although prematurity is an effect rather than a primary cause. Prematurity itself does not lead to mental retardation, but the factors leading to prematurity also may result in mental retardation. The premature infant is more likely to be born with problems and is more likely to develop them over time. Postmaturity, as with prematurity, does not lead to mental retardation directly, but those factors causing postmaturity may. With the increasing sophistication of birthing processes, the contribution of perinatal risk factors in mental retardation in future years is likely to decrease.

POSTNATAL FACTORS

Although postnatal factors are implicated less often than prenatal and perinatal conditions in mental retardation, many conditions in the first several years of life can lead to mental handicaps. Factors such as head trauma and ingestion of toxic substances are often implicated in postnatal brain damage, but postnatal injury due to infection is by far the most serious of these postnatal factors. Encephalitis and meningitis are two of the major forms of cerebral infection. These can have primary causes from specific infections such as bacterial meningitis or viral encephalitis, where brain damage is caused by direct infection and inflammation of brain tissue. On the other hand, these problems can be secondary reactions of other infectious agents in the body, such as herpes simplex infection, diphtheria, and rubella. When an infection directly invades and destroys brain cells, and inflammation of the brain is present, mental retardation is a common outcome. The degree of impairment imposed by such difficulty depends on a variety of factors, including the causative agent, the age of the affected individual, and the length and severity of the disease. Many of the detrimental outcomes of these diseases can be avoided by early diagnosis and treatment.

Neuropathologies in Syndromes of Retardation

Autopsy studies have shown that over 80% of moderate and severely mentally retarded individuals have structural brain damage. In recent years, many in vivo techniques have been developed to assess CNS function. Techniques that measure the chemistry of cerebrospinal fluid (CSF) offer hints as to the neurochemical makeup of the individual. Neuroimaging techniques, such as the computerized axial tomography (CT), magnetic resonance imaging (MRI), and positron emission tomography (PET), are able to identify deep-seated pathologies in the CNS, thereby aiding our understanding of the organic processes that underlie cognition and behavior.

Genetic syndromes of mental handicap, such as Down syndrome, phenylketunuria, and Lesch-Nyhan syndrome can be correlated with specific neuroanatomical abnormalities. Individuals with Down syndrome generally display a small cerebellum and occipital lobes, a narrow superior temporal gyrus, and a decreased total intracranial and gray plus white matter volume (25). The presence of senile plaques and neurofibrillary tangles in the cerebral cortex and limbic system are found in virtually all DS individuals over 40 years old (26–28). In addition to specific enzyme disturbances, substantial decreases in central cholinergic and adrenergic activity are common among these individuals. Brain glucose metabolism is also abnormal in DS. PET studies show that young DS individuals show hypermetabolism, while hypometabolism is exhibited in older DS persons with dementia (25, 29, 30).

Lesch-Nyhan syndrome is caused by an inborn error of metabolism that leads to mental retardation and severe compulsive self-mutilation. Several studies have found a low serotonin turnover in these individuals (31, 32), although dopamine and norepinephrine disturbances have also been noted. The literature reports reduced CSF levels of homovanillic acid (HVA; dopamine metabolite) in Lesch-Nyhan patients (33), in addition to low levels of 3-methoxy-4-hydroxyphenylethylene glycol (MHPG; norepinephrine metabolite) in the CSF of these individuals (32). It has been suggested that striatal dopamine D_1-receptor supersensitivity may be a mechanism involved in the self-mutilation of Lesch-Nyhan individuals (34), this hypothesis is in agreement with the findings that self-injury can be experimentally induced by dopamine agonists and curbed with selective D_1-receptor antagonists (35–37).

Other syndromes of mental retardation have been associated with specific cerebral abnormalities. Cerebral edema and diffuse neuronal degeneration have been noted in individuals where lead poisoning has induced mental retardation. Multiple small patchy granulomata and cortical necrosis are common effects of mental retardation secondary to maternal toxoplasmosis. Retardation secondary to rubella often ends in cerebrovascular damage, microcephaly, hydrocephalus, and spotty necrosis in the white matter and basal ganglia. In individuals where hypothyroidism has led to mental retardation, cortical atrophy and incomplete cerebral and endocrine system development are often found. Lowered levels of tyrosine and serotonin are common findings in individuals with phenylketunuria, while dopamine, opiate, and serotonin system dysfunction have been implicated in Prader-Willi syndrome.

Epilepsy

Epilepsy is a condition characterized by repetitive electrical seizures of the brain that are paired with disturbances of consciousness. These abnormal electrical impulses have various etiologies, including brain damage, disease, trauma, genetic defects, and metabolic disorders. The prevalence of epilepsy in the mentally retarded is much greater than that of the general population. Data suggest that 30% of mildly retarded individuals and 50% of severely retarded individuals have epilepsy (38). Another report estimates that up to 50% of institutionalized mentally retarded suffer from epileptic seizures (39). A general negative correlation between IQ and rates of epilepsy has also been noted (40). Epilepsy that is idiopathic is less likely to be associated with mental handicap or dementia than symptomatic epilepsy, which is associated with overt brain damage or neuropathic processes (41, 42).

NEUROPSYCHIATRIC CONDITIONS AND EPILEPSY

The condition of epilepsy coincides with a variety of neuropsychiatric complications. Many factors may lead to behavioral deterioration of the epileptic patient. Acquired neuropathologies in which the epileptic condition is secondary may induce behavior problems. Neuropathic changes that induce behavioral deterioration may be a direct byproduct of the electrical seizure activity itself (43–45). Deviant behaviors may be ictal, as a result of actual electrical discharge, or interictal, as a product of an interictal kindling syndrome. Interictal syndromes are characterized by changes in personality, behavior, and emotional expression. Interictal personality traits may develop in the chronic epileptic, and similar personality patterns can sometimes be noticed in epileptics with the same seizure foci. Depression is a common interictal emotional manifestation of epilepsy (46), as is schizophreniform psychosis. Some problems occurring in the epileptic patient may also be caused by side effects of

anticonvulsants, especially barbituates, that dull cognition, cause aggression, induce depression, or hyperactivity. For a more in depth review of behavioral syndromes associated with epilepsy see Chapter 33 of this book.

DIAGNOSTIC EVALUATION

When considering the diagnosis of the mentally retarded, the two main issues at hand are (a) the identification of mental retardation, and (b) the identification of psychiatric disorders in retarded individuals. This section discusses these procedures and delineates the techniques important in the diagnosis of mental retardation, the variables integral in attributing causal factors to mental retardation, and the issues surrounding psychiatric evaluation of the retarded individual.

Diagnosis of Mental Retardation

IDENTIFICATION OF MENTAL RETARDATION

Intellectual ability, adaptive behavior, and age of disorder onset are the three variables that must be considered in the definitive diagnosis of mental retardation. In order for a positive diagnosis to occur, the individual must have a significantly subaverage IQ and show deficits in adaptive functioning by the age of 18 years. IQ is regarded as significantly subaverage if it is calibrated to be at least two standard deviations below the mean (70 or below) on a standardized IQ test. The most valid measures of IQ have traditionally been the Stanford-Binet and the Weschler Intelligence Scale for children or adults. By categorizing the measure of intelligence into distinct subcomponents, these tests are sensitized to individual intellectual variation, thereby giving hints to differential diagnosis.

The significance of adaptive functioning is often overshadowed by intelligence in the diagnosis of retardation, but according to the American Association on Mental Deficiency (AAMD), it is of equal diagnostic importance (1, 47). The construct of adaptive behavior deals with the effectiveness of the individual in adapting to and coping with the dynamic and constantly changing demands of his or her environment. For behavior to be considered adaptive, the individual must be able to meet the standards of personal independence and social responsibility expected by his or her age and social group. Adaptive functioning is more subjective than intellectual capacity, and is therefore more difficult to assess. The Vineland Social Maturity Scale (VSMS) and the Adaptive Behavior Scale (ABS) are considered two of the most effective measures of adaptive level. The ABS gauges levels of daily living skills and the frequency of inappropriate behaviors, while the VSMS concentrates on personal maturity and independence.

DIFFERENTIAL DIAGNOSIS

Accurate diagnosis enables the clinician to better compose effective therapy for the problem in question. In most cases the mere labeling of mental retardation is not sufficient in a diagnostic evaluation. To facilitate a strong course of treatment and habilitation, causal factors of specific disorders should be examined, even if the assessment is speculative.

When considering etiological components, the diagnostician needs to determine if the problem is primarily neurobiological in origin, or of primary environmental origin. If there is a discrepancy of 15 points or more on the IQ test favoring verbal abilities, the etiology may be neurobiological, whereas if the performance scale significantly is higher than the verbal, it is more likely to be psychological (48). The presence of physical abnormalities and/or abnormal movements also point to a possible organic cause. Additionally, the evaluator should carefully map the pattern of the disorder to determine if the condition is static or degenerative. Finally, the complete symptomatology should be scrutinized to determine if the problem may fit into one of the many syndromes of retardation.

EVALUATIONS

The diagnostic evaluation of mental retardation must be thorough and should examine diverse functional systems of the whole person. Physical and neurological exams are essential, as are psychological testing and neuropsychological assessment. The physical exam may aid in identifying specific disorders such as fragile X syndrome, Down syndrome or hypothyroidism, which may be acting as precipitating forces to the intellectual and adaptive impairments. The neurological exam is performed to identify levels of attention, consciousness, and overall cognitive condition. In addition to a mental status exam, the comprehensive neurological workup includes an examination of the cranial nerves, the motor system, and sensory function. Findings of motor and sensory impairments may increase suspicion of structural brain disease. Psychological and neuropsychological assessment are additional important components of the evaluation. In the formulation of a diagnostic impression, the diagnostician should also take into account important historical features of the individual. Factors such as course and duration of pregnancy, labor and delivery, neonatal course, developmental milestones, medical conditions, traumatic events, school achievement, behavior problems, and family history all convey important information about the ontogeny of the disorder.

Biologically based tests are also utilized in the examination of a person with mental retardation. These tests often lead to a more precise differential diagnosis. Laboratory tests allow recognition of blood and chemical abnormalities that are associated with cognitive impairment. If a genetic disorder is suspected, a karyotype is useful in identifying chromosomal abnormalities. If a seizure disorder is indicated, the electroencephalogram (EEG) can be useful in the identification of epileptic patterns and seizure foci. X-rays are constructive in identifying cranial abnormalities, such as skull calcification. Neuroimaging techniques also assist in

effective diagnosis. See Table 25.1 for a complete list of syndromes.

Diagnosis of Psychopathology in Mental Retardation

The high rates of psychopathology in the mentally retarded attest to the importance of diagnosis and treatment of the dually diagnosed. In the past, differential diagnosis of emotional problems in the mentally retarded was based on quick, informal assessments made by the clinician. This practice led to a very low rate of reliability (49) and to the subsequent implementation of inappropriate therapeutic modalities.

Many diagnostic techniques that are used with nonretarded individuals generalize within the retarded population with great difficulty. The clinical interview and the *Diagnostic and Statistical Manual-4th ed.* (DSM-4), widely recognized as the cornerstones of psychiatric diagnosis, are of limited utility with the mentally retarded. Their compromised intellectual capacity and lack of insight, restrict the information obtained through interviewing techniques. Even the highest functioning retarded individuals have difficulty understanding and communicating their thoughts and feelings.

Sovner (50) describes four factors (intellectual distortion, psychosocial masking, cognitive disintegration, and baseline exaggeration) that contribute to the difficulty in distinguishing mental illness among retarded individuals. Intellectual distortion refers to diminished cognitive and communicative ability, which results in the individual's inability to understand and report subjective experiences and feelings. Psychosocial masking refers to the scant social skills and limited repertoire that may lead the clinician to apocryphal judgments with respect to the client's difficulties. Cognitive disintegration alludes to the inability of the retardate to cope with stressful situations and to the behavioral outbursts that may follow. Baseline exaggeration pertains to the tendency for behavior to be particularly uncontrolled during stressful times, which may lead to a misinterpretation of the actual problem during assessment (50).

The altered presentation of the mentally ill, mentally retarded individual may further cloud and confuse diagnosis. Mental illness in the retarded individual is often characterized by a lack of classic symptoms and general qualitative alteration of presentation in the intellectually impaired. A review of affective disorders in the mentally retarded describes the mania found in this population to be less infectious and clever than that found in nonretarded individuals (51). The authors also report that depression is likely to be characterized by aggression, withdrawal, and somatic complaints, rather than the classic depressive complaints and feelings of hopelessness that characterize this state in people without mental retardation. Accordingly, one study found that symptomatology of psychiatric illness was altered with IQ and ambulatory status. The authors con-

Table 25.1.   Thirty-five Important Syndromes with Multiple Handicaps[a]

Syndrome	Diagnostic Manifestations					
	Craniofacial	Skeletal	Other	Mental Retardation	Short Stature	Genetic Transmission
Aarskog syndrome	Hypertelorism, broad nasal bridge, anteverted nostrils, long philtrum	Small hands and feet, mild inter-digital webbing, short stature	Scrotal "shawl" above penis	+/-	+	X-linked semidominant
Apert's syndrome (acrocephalosyndactyly)	Craniosynostosis, irregular midfacial hypoplasia, hypertelorism	Syndactyly, broad distal thumb and toe		+/-		A, D[b]
Cerebral gigantism (Sotos syndrome)	Large head, prominent forehead, narrow anterior mandible	Large hands and feet	Large size in early life, poor coordination	+/-		?
Cockayne's syndrome	Pinched facies, sunken eyes, thin nose, prognathism, retinal degeneration	Long limbs with large hands and feet, flexion deformities	Hypotrichosis, photosensitivity, thin skin, diminished subcutaneous fat, impaired hearing	+	+	A, R
Cohen syndrome	Maxillary hypoplasia with prominent central incisors	Narrow hands and feet	Hypotonia, obesity	+	+/-	A, R
Cornelia de Lange syndrome	Synophrys (continuous eyebrows), thin down-turning upper lip; long philtrum, anteverted nostrils, microcephaly	Small or malformed hands and feet, proximal thumb	Hirsutism	+	+	?
Cri du chat syndrome	Epicanthic folds and/or slanting palpebral fissures, round facial contour, hypertelorism, microcephaly	Short metacarpals or metatarsals; four-finger line in palm	Cat-like cry in infancy	+	+	#5p-
Crouzon's syndrome (craniofacial dysostosis)	Proptosis with shallow orbits, maxillary hypoplasia, craniosynostosis					A, D
Down syndrome	Upward slant to palpebral fissures, midface depression, epicanthic folds, Brushfield spots, brachycephaly	Short hands, clinodactyly of 5th finger, four-finger line in palm	Hypotonia, loose skin on back of neck	+	+	21 Trisomy
Dubowitz syndrome	Small facies, lateral displacement of inner canthi, ptosis, broad nasal bridge, sparse hair, microcephaly		Infantile eczema, high-pitched hoarse voice	+/-	+	? A, R
Fetal alcohol syndrome	Short palpebral fissures, midfacial hypoplasia, microcephaly		+/- Cardiac defect, fine motor dysfunction	+	+	
Fetal hydantoin syndrome (Dilantin)	Hypertelorism, short nose, occasional cleft lip	Hypoplastic nails, especially 5th	Cardiac defect	+/-	+/-	
Goldenhar's syndrome	Malar hypoplasia, macrostomia, micrognathia, epibulbar dermoid and/or lipodermoid, malformed ear with preauricular tags	+/- Vertebral anomalies				?
Incontinentia pigmenti	+/- Dental defect, deformities of ears, +/- patchy alopecia		Irregular skin pigmentation in fleck, whorl, or spidery form	+/-		? D, X-linked ?, lethal in males
Laurence-Moon-Bardet-Biedl syndrome	Retinal pigmentation	Polydactyly, syndactyly	Obesity, seizures, hypogenitalism	+	+/-	A, R
Linear nevus sebaceus syndrome	Nevus sebaceus, face or neck		+/- Seizures	+	+/-	?
Lowe's syndrome (oculo-cerebrorenal syndrome)	Cataract	Renal tubular dysfunction	Hypotonia	+	+	X-linked recessive

Continued.

Table 25.1.   *(Continued)*

Syndrome	Diagnostic Manifestations					Genetic Transmission
	Craniofacial	Skeletal	Other	Mental Retardation	Short Stature	
Mobius syndrome (congenital facial diplegia)	Expressionless facies, ocular palsy	+/− Clubfoot, syndactyly		+/−	+/−	?
Neurofibromatosis	+/− Optic gliomas, acoustic neuromas	+/− Bone lesions, pseudarthroses	Neurofibromas, café-au-lait spots, seizures	+/−		A, D
Noonan's syndrome	Webbing of posterior neck, malformed ears, hypertelorism	Pectus excavatum, cubitus valgus	Cryptorchidism, pulmonic stenosis	+/−	+	?
Prader-Willi syndrome	+/− Upward slant to palpebral fissures	Small hands and feet	Hypotonia, especially in early infancy, then polyphagia and obesity; hypogenitalism	+	+	?
Robin complex	Micrognathia, glossoptosis, cleft palate					
Rubella syndrome	Cataract, retinal pigmentation, ocular malformations		Sensorineural deafness; patent ductus arteriosus; +/− Cardiac anomalies	+/−	+/−	?
Rubinstein-Taybi syndrome	Slanting palpebral fissures, maxillary hypoplasia, microcephaly	Broad thumbs and toes	Abnormal gait	+	+	?
Seckel syndrome	Facial hypoplasia, prominent nose, microcephaly	Multiple minor joint and skeletal abnormalities		+	+	A, R
Sjögren-Larsson syndrome		Spasticity, especially of legs	Ichthyosis	+	+	A, R
Smith-Lemli-Opitz syndrome	Anteverted nostrils and/or ptosis of eyelid	Syndactyly 2nd and 3rd toes	Hypospadias; cryptorchidism	+	+	A, R
Sturge-Weber syndrome	Flat hemangioma of face, most commonly trigeminal in distribution		Hemangiomas of meninges with seizures	+/−		?
Treacher-Collins syndrome (mandibulofacial dysostosis)	Malar and mandibular hypoplasia, downslanting palpebral fissures, defect of lower eyelid, malformed ears					A, D
Trisomy 18 syndrome	Microstomia, short palpebral fissures, malformed ears, elongated skull	Clenched hand, 2nd finger over 3rd; low arches on fingertips; short sternum	Cryptorchidism, congenital heart disease	+	+	18 Trisomy
Trisomy 13 syndrome	Defects of eye, nose, lip, ears, and forebrain of holoprosencephaly type	Polydactyly, narrow hyperconvex fingernails	Skin defects, posterior scalp	+	+	13 Trisomy
Tuberous sclerosis	Hamartomatous pink to brownish facial skin nodules	+/− Bone lesions	Seizures, intracranial calcification	+/−		A, D
Waardenburg syndrome	Lateral displacement of inner canthi and puncta		Partial albinism, white forelock, heterochromia or iris, vitiligo; +/− deafness			A, D
Williams syndrome	Full lips, small nose with anteverted nostrils, iris dysplasia	Mild hypoplasia of nails	+/− Hypercalcemia in infancy, supravalvular aortic stenosis	+	+	?
Zellweger cerebrohepatorenal syndrome	High forehead, flat facies		Hypotonia, hepatomegaly, death in early infancy	+	+	A, R

aFrom Smith DW. Patterns of malformation. In: Vaughan VC III, McKay RJ Jr, Behrman RE, eds. Nelson textbook of pediatrics. 11th ed. Philadelphia: WB Saunders, 1979:2035.
bA, autosomal; D, dominant; R, recessive.

cluded that the degree of motility and the level of intellectual impairment may play a role in determining the manifestations of underlying psychiatric disorders (52).

Because of the unique diagnostic challenges in assessing the mentally retarded, clinicians must learn to rely more on signs (disturbed behavior) and less on symptoms (verbally reported distress and dysfunction) (53). When dealing with the severely or profoundly retarded, clinicians must make judgments based on extended observations. Target behaviors should be objectively measured, and the context in which they occur scrutinized. This focus on observable behaviors may be useful in attributing causes to the behaviors as well as defining them, and should alleviate many of the problems encountered by relying on modes of verbal communication.

Clinicians should also consider the precipitating events of an emotional disturbance in a mentally retarded individual's life. With a diminished capacity to accurately interpret their surroundings, mentally retarded individuals are prone to overreacting during certain environmental situations. A behavioral deterioration may be related to a primary psychiatric disorder or to a change in the patient's environment. Thus, it is crucial to be aware of any changes in the mentally retarded individual's life (i.e., staff turnover, new housemates, illnesses in family members). Such events are likely to precipitate behavioral decompensation.

Several standardized assessments have been constructed to simplify psychiatric diagnosis in the mentally retarded. The most widely used tests are the Psychopathology Instrument for Mentally Retarded Adults (PIMRA) and the Reiss Screen for Maladaptive Behavior. These scales cover most major forms of psychopathology and have been proven effective in diagnosing mental illness in mentally retarded populations (49, 54). There has been some evidence that standardized psychopathology inventories, modified to include simplified language, may be effective in substantiating a diagnosis in mildly and moderately retarded individuals. One report reveals that modified versions of Beck's Depression Inventory and the Zung Self Rating Depression Scale were potent measures of depression in the mildly and moderately retarded (55).

THERAPY

The most effective treatment for mentally retarded individuals is multimodal, and takes into consideration the individual's strengths while minimizing weaknesses. Treatment planning that incorporates vocational programming, daily living and social skills training, and appropriate schooling is very beneficial to these individuals. The following pages specify a course of therapeutic intervention for persons with mental retardation that includes behavioral management and pharmacotherapy strategies, with an emphasis on soliciting adaptive behavior, and enhancing the quality of life.

Social Matrix

The social matrix largely informs and influences the behavioral repertoires and patterns on which an individual relies. Likewise, the patterns of behavior exhibited in the mentally retarded are influenced by their residential arrangements. For better or for worse, the residential arrangements of the mentally retarded dramatically shape and pattern their conduct. Until several decades ago, large institutions housed hundreds, even thousands of the cognitively impaired. This approach kept these individuals politely protected from the stresses of society (and less politely, kept society protected from the problems of the mentally retarded). However, this practice of segregation has been more damaging than protective to the individuals supposedly served by it. Human behavior is prone to shaping, and when the only visible role models are mentally retarded peers, imitated behaviors tend to be maladaptive ones, ones that are likely to be disruptive and noticeable in nature. One report reveals that the institutionalized retarded have higher rates of psychiatric disturbances than those mentally retarded individuals living in community residences (5). It has been suggested that mental illness leading to institutionalization can only partially account for this difference. The frequent lack of social skill training and independence programming found in large institutions preclude the cognitively impaired individuals from acquiring the coping strategies they so desperately need. Thus, they are left all the more vulnerable to deficient ego development and reduced stress tolerance, leading to psychiatric disturbance. Furthermore, many of the behavior problems seen in this population are expressions of emotional detachment and chronic affect hunger—problems induced by the impoverished social environments of large institutions (56).

The premise of segregation and institutionalization was based upon the assumption that the low cognitive functioning of the mentally retarded are static, unamenable to instruction or enrichment; therefore, the main goal of caring for these individuals was supervision rather than habilitation. Research in the past several decades, however, has proved this "untrainable" premise a fallacy. Studies consistently demonstrate that with proper instruction, mentally retarded individuals of all levels are capable of learning a wide variety of skills and behaviors (57–60). The power of this finding, coupled with abhorrent living conditions in large institutions and an increase in societal awareness of the mentally retarded have acted as an impetus to change the treatment course for this population.

Community residential programs, which operate on the foundation of normalization, are succeeding in many of the areas where institutions failed. Apparently, the recent trend toward community-based programs has prevented many symptoms of institutionalization with the younger mentally handicapped, and has significantly reduced the incidence of psychiatric complications (61). As opposed to large institutions that ignored the needs of the individual, community residential programs attempt to maximize culturally acceptable behavior by training the mentally retarded for integration into normal community modes, such as work, school, and social outlets. In these settings, their special needs are supported by a consistent set of caretakers who challenge and expand upon the talents they have. In this sense, the mentally retarded are treated in a more humane, less restrictive manner, allowing them to function independently or semi-independently. Stimulating living experiences may actually heighten intellectual proclivity, whereas a lack thereof can lower IQ (48). By placing higher (yet not unreasonable) expectations on these individuals, they are challenged and are less likely to fall into a negative spiral of failure. This move toward less restrictive settings has vastly improved the care of the mentally retarded, and has helped to set a trend that imparts "cure for a few, treatment for many, habilitation for all" (62).

Biopsychosocial Model

RATIONALE OF TREATMENT

The vast majority of mentally retarded individuals are mildly or moderately retarded and show little evidence of psychiatric or behavioral disorders. In most cases, habilitative programs in the areas of school, work, social, and daily living skills are the only therapeutic modalities called for. However, additional treatment is necessary for those individuals plagued by behavioral disturbances or dual diagnosis.

Psychiatric treatment traditionally has assumed that a specific symptomatology was based on one specific etiology, and therefore necessitated one uniform remedy. This linear model is a constrictive and ineffective rationale for treatment of the mentally retarded. Mental retardation is extremely heterogeneous in nature, with no clear symptomatic picture. In addition, mental retardation is causally linked to a variety of interrelated factors, which differ among individuals. Unquestioned acceptance of the linear model has resulted in a narrow and unconvincing range of psychiatric treatment options for this population.

As mentioned earlier, widespread neuroleptic overuse is a problem that can be traced back to this outdated medical model. In times of stress, many mentally retarded individuals tend to have a psychotic-like presentation characterized by disorganization, aggression, stereotypy, and bizarre behavior. Because these symptoms have an outward appearance of schizophrenia, the efficacy of neuroleptics in schizophrenic populations was generalized onto the mentally retarded: If neuroleptics can control disorganized, uncontrolled behavior in schizophrenics, it seemed logical that they would be equally effective in the mentally retarded. Neuroleptics became widely used in the mentally retarded as a prophylactic for disorganized, psychotic-like, violent behavior. Although neuroleptics can be effective in curbing inappropriate behaviors, they do so by globally sedating the individual so that all behaviors, both adaptive and maladaptive, are inhibited. Cognitive blunting and an exacerbation of behavioral dyscontrol can result from neuroleptic medication (63–65), along with the common extrapyramidal side effects of tardive dyskinesia and akathisia.

Fortunately, the outdated linear model of psychiatry is being replaced by the determination that active and effective treatment requires an integration of therapies. The biopsychosocial model of psychiatry takes into account the varying origins of problematic behavior and the plethora of variables that act to wax and wane respective illnesses. Effective treatment of mentally retarded individuals targets the abnormal physiology, the psychological suffering, the inconsistent environment, and the maladaptive behavioral repertoire (66). Treatment must take into account the dynamic interactions between biological mechanisms and external events. Instead of searching for a unitary global "cure" for all problems, concomitant symptoms may need to be addressed separately, as problems occurring together are often causally unrelated.

Modalities of Treatment

The two most commonly used treatment methods for the mentally retarded, behavioral and pharmacological, have historically been segregated and regarded as mutually exclusive. Behavior modification techniques have been considered the sole sphere of the educators and psychologists, and at the same time relatively ignored by much of the medical profession, whereas pharmacotherapy remained the sole working ground of the physicians. Unfortunately, by excluding efficacious modalities of therapy, this split has been detrimental to the patient. Many reports (67–69) have found a combination of behavior therapy and pharmacotherapy to be more effective than either modality alone in eliciting behavior change. One study reported this combined medical/behavioral model not only effective in producing desired behavior change in mentally retarded adults, but also in decreasing overall levels of psychotropic drug use (69). It is crucial to pay attention to the external environment of the mentally retarded individual as well as the pharmacological environment. Drugs that modify the microenvironment in a specific synaptic neighborhood of the brain may decrease the "noisy" state. The "noisy" state we are referring to is created by a variety of unpredictable stimuli internally experienced as a subjective feeling of being crowded and confused, which makes it difficult for mentally retarded individuals to tolerate and organize their experiences. Decreasing this state assists in the success of external programs such as behavioral management, learning therapies, and skill development. Thus, a neuropsychiatrist attuned to the multisystems approach is more likely to see beyond the one-drug, one-symptom model, increasing the likelihood of enhancing the life of the patient (70).

With regard to noise, when the internal environment is quieted, the mentally retarded individual is more capable of attenuating to the external environment in an adaptive fashion. When information from the external environment is processed accurately, without exaggeration, the individual possesses greater facilities, enabling him or her to function adaptively in the world. Obviously, neuropsychiatry must employ a multisystems approach that considers behavior and biology complementary rather than antagonistic (70), instead of focusing on the separation of these perspectives.

BEHAVIOR MODIFICATION

For the past three decades, behavioral approaches have been the most thoroughly researched and most widely used therapeutic intervention with the mentally retarded (71). Behavioral therapies stem from the belief that maladaptive behaviors result from environmental contingencies at work to promote these behaviors. Behavior modification techniques are effective treatments for many of the inappropriate learned behavior patterns found in the mentally retarded. The behavioral approach works to break down and objectively define specific behaviors, dissecting the contextual basis in which they occur. This functional analysis is often effective in unearthing the contingencies that are maintaining and reinforcing undesirable behaviors. With this knowledge, the clinician can devise new environments to reinforce desirable behaviors and extinguish those that are maladaptive. Reinforcement and feedback contingencies seem to be the technique of choice in replacing maladaptive behaviors with adaptive ones, although punishment, when implemented cautiously, is also effective in curbing serious problematic behaviors.

A number of studies have found operant learning contingencies to be effective in decreasing maladaptive while increasing adaptive behaviors in this population (72–75). Many studies also show that behavior modification techniques are effective in specifically curbing aggression in the mentally retarded. One evaluation (76) found positive reinforcement procedures to be effective in controlling aggression in the severely retarded. Studies have also supported the efficacy of behavioral techniques in reducing self-injurious behavior (77, 78).

Behavior modification is frequently an effective and benign treatment in controlling specific learned maladaptive behavior patterns. However, many behavioral and most psychiatric problems are related to physiological dysfunction and require biologically based management.

PHARMACOTHERAPY

The issue of pharmacotherapy with the mentally retarded has received a great deal of unfavorable attention in recent years. Factors that have kindled this viewpoint stem from tendencies toward chronic overmedication and the heightened sensitivity to psychotropic agents in this population. Neuroleptics have traditionally been the most common medication prescribed to the mentally retarded, and studies have consistently reported that between 45–55% of mentally retarded individuals receive antipsychotics (79). The overmedication of this population often reflects the numbers of individuals receiving drug therapy as well as high dosage levels (80). However, a review of related literature reports that low to moderate doses of neuroleptics are at least equally effective, and even superior to high doses in a majority of patients (81). The same study further details that lower doses are implicated in fewer unwanted side effects than high doses.

Biologically and cognitively, the mentally retarded tend to be especially sensitive to drugs and vulnerable to developing pronounced side effects. CNS malfunction and abnormality leave the brain less able to cope with drug therapy, and peripheral physiological deficits impair mentally retarded individuals' capacity for metabolic degradation (66). Neuroleptics have been implicated in detrimental neurological side effects in nonretarded people, and these effects become even more pronounced in mentally retarded populations. One study found tardive dyskinesia to be present in 34% of neuroleptically treated retarded individuals, and moreover found low IQ levels to be statistically related to the development of moderate to severe forms of tardive dyskinesia (82). Beyond the primary discomfort of these conditions, tardive dyskinesia and akathisia may agitate and frustrate the patient to a point of dyscontrol, thus indirectly exacerbating the behaviors the drugs were intended to control. In addition to movement problems, neuroleptics are commonly implicated in extreme sedation, cognitive dulling, and withdrawal. One study indicates that neuroleptics inhibit cognitive abilities and may actually harm the "mental fitness" of the individuals so treated (83). The reduced intellectual capacity further potentiates the cognitive side effects of neuroleptics in these patients.

In addition to neuroleptics, benzodiazepines have been especially deleterious with mentally retarded individuals. The disinhibiting side effects of benzodiazepines actually exacerbate many of the behaviors they are intended to control (84). In addition, addictive properties and inter-dose rebound are unfavorable effects that work to undermine the usefulness of the benzodiazepines.

Clearly, indiscriminate use of pharmaceuticals with the mentally retarded is harmful. However, in many instances, drugs are habilitative and therapeutic. Often, pharmacotherapy can effectively mitigate an underlying biochemical dysfunction, thereby altering the behavioral and cognitive manifestations of these anomalies.

Often, the most effective forms of pharmacological management employ different agents that concentrate on different effects. Pharmacotherapy must arise from differential diagnosis, and should employ specific agents that ameliorate the biochemical underpinnings of disturbed functioning respective to each patient. The optimal treatment program may require several agents, may employ doses considered homeopathic, may be used in conjunction with clinical observations of behavior, and is perfected over time in accord with research and experimentation (85). When employed carefully and cautiously, pharmacotherapy can be most beneficial in many mentally retarded individuals, minimizing side effects while maximizing desired effects (85).

Behavioral Dyscontrol

Behavioral dyscontrol is typically characterized by aggression, self-abuse, stereotypy, and agitation. Often these problems have organic etiologies and can be ameliorated with the proper medical interventions. Behavioral dyscontrol has been cited as the single most common indication for pharmacotherapy in the mentally retarded (7). Overarousal and serotonergic dysfunction are thought to be the most common biological determinants of these behaviors. The most effective treatments for these conditions have focused on replacing maladaptive behaviors with adaptive, using a combination of pharmacotherapy and behavioral interventions. When the proper steps are taken to differentially diagnose the causative forces behind a patient's maladaptive behaviors, and specific organic pathologies are suspected, and behavior therapy is unsuccessful, conservative pharmacotherapy becomes beneficial.

Noise and overarousal. Many behavior problems are secondary to a chronic noisy state of hyperarousal stemming from CNS pathology. The developmentally disabled are especially vulnerable to overarousal because of their inability to cognitively filter internal and external stimuli. This lack of filtering results in a noisy state of stimulus overload, which can actuate internal chaos, personal distortions, impulsivity, hypervigilance, physiological stress, and aggression (6, 86, 87). Such dyscontrol is often nothing more than an attempt to organize experience into a predictable pattern. These behaviors, especially aggression or the threat thereof, often prevent participation in habilitative programming and social interactions, thus constricting the quality of life and patient care. These forms of overarousal not only promote undesirable behaviors, but also impair memory, learning, and performance (88).

If overarousal is a precipitating force in behavioral dyscontrol, it follows that decreased arousal may increase tolerance and reduce behavioral outbursts. β-Blockers have been found to be a successful prescription for the related symptoms of behavioral dyscontrol. These agents have been efficacious in reducing anxiety and ameliorating outbursts in a variety of disadvantaged populations. Several studies have illustrated the efficacy of propranolol in reducing agitation and outbursts in individuals with traumatic brain injury (89), generalized cortical damage (90), organic dementia (91), autism (92), and in individuals with pervasive developmental disorders, conduct disorders, and intermittent explosive disorders (93). Propranolol has also been reported to down-regulate hyperarousal, subsequently reducing aggressive outbursts in the severely and profoundly retarded (94). In addition to propranolol, nadolol appears to initiate a gradual disappearance of inner restlessness and tension. Nadolol has reduced aggression and hostility secondary to hyperarousal in a group of patients that included mentally retarded adults who had been previously unresponsive in pharmacological trials (95). A review of controlled studies reported β-blockers to have an overall success rate of 83% in controlling aggression and self-injury in the mentally retarded (96).

As opposed to most anxiolytic medications that depress behavioral outbursts, β-blockers have shown little tendency to cause adverse cognitive side effects. This leads to a patient's heightened environmental integration and shifts the focus of care from protective to habilitative (88). In addition to their antianxiety effects, and low propensity for unwanted effects, β-blockers promote the emergence of habilitative behaviors, such as speech and socialization (97). Furthermore, adjunctive treatment with β-blockers may actually mediate behavioral teaching contingencies. Gaind and colleagues (98) showed that oxprenolol therapy prior to behavior modification techniques aided in the facilitation of desired behaviors.

Mechanisms responsible for the anxiolytic effects of β-blockers are still unclear, but have been attributed to dearousal in both peripheral and central systems. Pindolol and propranolol may in part act centrally to specifically block adrenergic receptors and exert nonspecific effects on dopaminergic and serotonergic systems. These drugs also have peripheral effects, which include interruption of adrenergic pathways, and down-regulation of autonomic activity, leading to lowered resting tension (6, 99). Nadolol seems to be as effective as propranolol and pindolol but does not cross the blood-brain barrier. Thus, it exerts its behavioral effects through peripheral mechanisms.

Serotonin. Abnormalities in serotonergic functioning have also been implicated in behavioral dyscontrol. Many studies have found correlations between decreased CSF levels of the serotonin metabolite 5-HIAA and impulsive aggression (100–104). These findings have given rise to a "low-serotonin syndrome" hypothesis of aggression and impulsive behaviors, which asserts that decreased central serotonin may be involved in precipitating impulsive aggression. Many effective biochemically based treatments for behavioral dyscontrol have focused on increasing serotonergic activity, using such agents as serotonin agonists and reuptake inhibitors. Tryptophan, a serotonin precursor, appears to have antiaggressive effects in schizophrenic populations (105). Further studies have found that a diet rich in serotonin is effective in reducing behavioral dyscontrol in the mentally retarded (106, 107).

Buspirone is a psychopharmaceutical that has demonstrated efficacy in lowering occurrences of destructive behaviors through serotonergic agonist mechanisms. Buspirone was originally marketed as an anxiolytic; however, we have postulated that its antiaggressive properties may be unrelated to its antianxiety effects (108). At low doses, buspirone seems to curb aggression directly, by exerting specific agonist effects on serotonin. In a controlled trial with mentally retarded patients, low-dose buspirone was efficacious in regulating behavioral dyscontrol and aggression. In another study, we documented that low-dose buspirone had a positive response in nine of 14 mentally retarded adults with maladaptive behaviors (109). We have also found buspirone to be effective in the amelioration of paramenstrual aggression in this population (110). Additional studies have established buspirone to be effective in curbing agitation and violence associated with dementia (111) and autism (112), disturbances that have been associated with serotonin underactivity.

The primary benefits of buspirone therapy include its nonsedating, specific properties. Buspirone appears to reduce episodic dyscontrol with no known sedative or addictive effects. In a study of persons with developmental disabilities, low-dose buspirone produced desirable behavioral effects, while concurrently improving cognitive task performance (113). Furthermore, buspirone does not interact with other CNS agents, such as anticonvulsants (114).

Additional serotonergic agents have shown promise in decreasing behavior and aggression outbursts. Serenics are a novel class of drugs that produce specific antiaggressive effects through serotonergic mechanisms (115). We have found eltoprazine, a newly developed serenic, to decrease behavioral dyscontrol and facilitate social behaviors in a mentally retarded adult (116). Fluoxetine, a serotonin reuptake inhibitor, has also demonstrated efficacy in the reduction of aggression and related behavioral dyscontrol in psychiatric populations (117–120). The possibility that serotonergic action plays a role in antiaggressive effects has also been proposed for clozapine (121, 122) and carbamazepine (123).

Other agents. Lithium carbonate has demonstrated efficacy in controlling behavior in mentally retarded individuals. Worrall and colleagues (124) were among the first to describe the antiaggressive properties of lithium in the mentally retarded. A more recent study demonstrated that lithium rapidly reduced aggressive behavior in 11 out of 15 mentally retarded adults (125). Sovner and Hurley (126) also report lithium to be effective in the treatment of chronic behavior disorders, including hyperactivity and aggression the mentally retarded. Lithium stabilizes membranes, regulating mood and thereby decreasing behavior outbursts. Lithium may also have serotonergic effects, which act to enhance its antiaggressive properties (127). Overall, lithium seems to be efficacious in rapidly curbing episodic dyscontrol in some retarded clients; however, the potential toxicity of this agent and its partial sedative effects prevent it from being the primary treatment of choice for behavioral dyscontrol.

Self-Injurious Behavior (SIB)

Self-abuse has been recognized as an exceedingly common problem in this population, manifesting itself in at least 10% of severely and profoundly retarded (52). As with most other acting-out behaviors, self-injury can be induced by both internal and external conditions. When environmental regulation fails to completely control SIB, the severity of the problem warrants pharmacotherapy. As with behavioral dyscontrol, self-injury may be mediated by hyperaroused states and serotonergic dysfunction. In circumstances of SIB precipitated by hyperarousal, β-blockers have been effective in the amelioration of self-abuse (128). Low levels of CSF 5HIAA have been found in self-mutilatory individuals (129), and the serotonergic agonist buspirone has been

reported to control self-injury in mentally retarded populations (130). Tryptophan and trazodone, serotonin enhancers, have also proved successful in treating self-injury (21).

Dopaminergic activity also has been repeatedly implicated in self-injury (32–36). The antagonism of D_1 and D_2 receptors in clozapine treatment has been shown to stop self-mutilatory behavior (122). Additionally, the inhibitory responses on self-mutilatory behavior of fluphenazine, a D_1, D_2 blocker has been reported (13). Self-injurious behavior has also been associated with opioid dysfunction. It has been suggested that enhanced opioid activity resulting in a generalized analgesic state may predispose certain mentally retarded individuals to self-injury (131). Opioid antagonists, such as naltrexone, have been shown to reduce SIB in certain mentally retarded individuals (132, 133).

Psychiatric Disorders

Schizophrenia. The dopamine hypothesis of schizophrenia asserts that psychotic symptoms are induced by excessive dopaminergic activity in the limbic cortex. Most antipsychotics traditionally work to centrally block dopamine receptors, assuaging psychotic symptoms. When a mentally retarded individual has been definitively diagnosed with psychotic symptoms, antipsychotic agents are clearly the treatment of choice. When prescribing an antipsychotic agent for a mentally retarded client, the clinician must be especially vigilant of cognitive side effects that dampen already low levels of intellectual functioning. Antipsychotics should not be used as a standing regimen for agitated or aggressive behavior.

When considering the wide array of antipsychotics, side-effect profiles can be a determining factor. Generally, low-potency neuroleptics, such as chlorpromazine and thioridazine, need to be taken in high doses to achieve a beneficial antipsychotic effect. These higher doses often lead to increased sedation. On the other hand, high-potency drugs, such as thiothixene and haloperidol, may be used in smaller doses and lead to less sedation, but their potency may be more likely to induce unwanted motor reactions. Thiothixene seems to have a more rapid onset and produces fewer undesirable cognitive effects than thioridazine in the schizophrenic mentally retarded (134). However, higher rates of extrapyramidal side effects may ensue with thiothixene administration (134). Haloperidol has also demonstrated efficacy over the low-potency neuroleptics in mentally retarded populations (135). Clozapine or risperidone should also be given consideration for the treatment of schizophrenic symptoms in this population because of their specificity compared with most other neuroleptics and lower rate of extrapyramidal effects.

Affective disorders. Mood disorders in the mentally retarded are rarely reported but are suspected to be relatively common (51). Specific depressive mechanisms have been attributed to the serotonergic and catecholinergic systems. In determining whether an affective disorder is biochemical in nature, the dexamethasone suppression test has demonstrated efficacy in identifying altered neuroendocrine function (136). Pharmacotherapy of endogenous affective disorders in the mentally retarded has produced positive results utilizing lithium, carbamazepine, and traditional antidepressants.

Lithium appears to be effective as a prophylactic therapy for both bipolar and unipolar affective disorders in mentally retarded populations. Lithium has demonstrated efficacy in controlling the duration of unipolar depression in 14 mentally retarded inpatients (137). Additional case studies demonstrate the efficacy of lithium in curbing both bipolar and unipolar affective disturbances in mentally retarded adults (138).

A number of studies promote the efficacy of carbamazepine in controlling affective disorders. Carbamazepine appears to be as effective as lithium in regulating mood (139); in one study, 60% of patients treated with carbamazepine for bipolar disorder showed significant improvement (140). Carbamazepine may be particularly effective in decreasing the frequency, severity, and duration of affective cycling in lithium nonresponders (141), and a combination of carbamazepine and lithium is effective in the control of cycling when noncombination therapy is ineffective (142). Carbamazepine usually takes several weeks to treat affective symptomatology. During this latency period, carbamazepine may induce behavioral deterioration. Freidman and colleagues (143) report that 13% of mentally retarded individuals treated with carbamazepine for nonepileptic disturbances displayed adverse behavioral effects. The same study reveals that carbamazepine is implicated in more behavioral side effects with the mentally retarded than with nonretarded populations. Valproate is emerging as an efficacious treatment for bipolar disorder in persons with MR, but controlled studies have yet to be done.

Antidepressants are generally regarded as the treatment of choice for cases of unipolar depression. Heterocyclic antidepressants appear to be effective in curbing depressive symptoms in the nonverbal severely and profoundly retarded, while displaying few serious untoward effects (144). Fluoxetine has also demonstrated specific antidepressant effects in mentally retarded adults and is reported to have a more favorable side effect profile than traditional antidepressants (145). Imipramine has demonstrated some efficacy in regulating depressive symptoms in the mentally retarded (146), although it can induce agitation, mania, and other unwanted effects in this population (143, 144).

Epilepsy

Seizure control has been one of the most dominant indications for pharmacological intervention in mentally retarded individuals. Carbamazepine and valproic acid are the safest and most effective anticonvulsants for persons with compromised cognitive functioning. Carbamazepine is the best choice for complex partial seizures, while valproic acid is also effective for absence seizures. For the most part, these two anticonvulsants have benign cognitive side effects, although valproic acid has been associated with some toxic effects. Carbamazepine is favorable when compared with most other anticonvulsants, although it has been implicated in causing memory impairments in some individuals (13). Anticonvulsants such as phenobarbital, phenytoin and clonazepam should be used with caution in this population. Phenytoin has shown negative influences on attention, memory, and overall test performance (13), and for these reasons should be avoided in mental retardation. Clonazepam, a benzodiazepine, should also be avoided because of its disinhibiting effects on behavior (13).

Conservative and thoughtful pharmacological approaches have numerous benefits in the habilitation of the mentally retarded. Technological advances are allowing the field to unearth many of the primary determinants that elicit mental retardation. These advances are further allowing us to directly target these defects through the development of novel pharmaceuticals. Through their specific mechanisms, these drugs can elicit desired effects and minimize unwanted reactions. Neuropsychiatry can no longer disregard mental retardation because many neuropsychiatric techniques, when used in a multimodal setting, allow for the fullest habilitation of the mentally retarded individual.

CEREBRAL PALSY

Cerebral palsy (CP) is a chronic and variable neurological disorder of movement and posture induced by a nonprogressive defect of the central nervous system. Cerebral palsy is an umbrella term used to cover a medley of conditions, including movement and balance problems, delays in physical development, floppy or tight muscles, abnormalities of vision, hearing, and speech, and seizure disorders. The factor that ties these symptoms together under the heading of CP is an abnormality of the immature brain, caused by prenatal, perinatal, or postnatal influences.

Mental retardation is found in 50–75% of cases of cerebral palsy (146). Learning disabilities and frequent social, emotional, and interfamilial problems may also be present. Recent figures have shown CP to have an incidence of 2.5 per 1000 live births (147), although the incidence varies among classification, with spasticity constituting at least 50% of the cases (146). Generally, patients have been considered to be equally distributed among the mild, moderate, and severely afflicted categories (148).

Classification

Cerebral palsy is classified according to the location of the neurological lesion, the severity of the damage, the number of limbs involved, and the kind of movement affected by the disorder. The four main classifications of CP are spastic, athetosis or dystonia, ataxia, and mixed types. The clinical presentation of cerebral palsy varies in symptomatology and etiology according to each classification.

SPASTICITY

Spasticity results from damage to the motor portion of the cerebral cortex and pyramidal tract, which is responsible for the initiation of voluntary movement. Spasticity accounts for over 50% of all cases of cerebral palsy (146). Spacticity is topographically subgrouped into diplegia and hemiplegia.

Diplegia

Spastic diplegia is the most common form of cerebral palsy in premature infants, resulting in 10–33% of the cases. This term refers to disabling of the limbs on both sides of the body, with the legs more severely affected than the arms. The result is abnormally stiff and resistant muscles, with locomotor development more impaired than manipulative skills. Mental subnormality is often concurrent and may cause retardation in social, language, and other areas of development.

Spastic diplegia is almost always congenital, with a large percentage of affected children born prematurely, with low birth weight (149). The fibers of the pyramidal tract leading to the legs are closest to the blood vessels surrounding the ventricles of the brain. In premature infants, cerebral hemorrhages are most likely to occur in this area, damaging the pyramidal tract (150).

Hemiplegia

Hemiplegia refers to the unilateral disturbance of the extremities, independent of whether the upper or the lower portions are affected. This disorder results in increased tendon reflexes, weakness, and difficulty with discrete finger movements. When the unaffected limbs are active, associated movements, particularly in the arm, occur. Mental retardation is less common in hemiplegic CP than in other forms, although the child's motor problems create educational difficulties even among the most intelligent (151).

Most cases of hemiplegic CP are congenital in origin, resulting from prenatal factors in about two-thirds of the cases, and perinatal brain damage in others (152–154). A higher incidence of right hemiplegia over left has been noted (151, 155), which may be due to the fact that 70% of deliveries occur in a left occipitoanterior position, leaving the left side of the skull more vulnerable to trauma during the birth.

ATHETOSIS (DYSKINETIC CEREBRAL PALSY)

Athetosis results from damage to the extrapyramidal tract, causing a form of CP in which fine-motor movements are affected and involuntary movements of the limbs are prominent. These involuntary movements often take the form of unwanted, sympathetic movements by several limbs of the individual during an attempt to make one controlled, purposeful movement. The full-blown effects of this disorder are often not apparent until the age of 2, when ability to control the use of muscles is fully developed.

The most common cause of athetosis is hypoxia; however, contributions are made by predisposing harmful prenatal influences. Three-quarters of children with dyskinetic CP are born at term (149).

ATAXIA

Ataxic cerebral palsy accounts for up to 10% of cases and may result from a cerebellar lesion. Ataxia is a condition in which coordination of movement and balance are disturbed. Delays are seen in developmental milestones such as sitting, reaching, and walking. Ataxic diplegia can be mistaken for mental retardation or neuromuscular disease due to similar delays in development and associated hyptonia. This form of CP differs from others in that its etiology is unknown in approximately 41% of the cases (153). Still, most of these cases are thought to be congenital. The rates of preterm delivery, low birth weight and growth retardation are consistent with the general population (149).

Causal Factors

Although many cases of cerebral palsy are of unknown origin, it is believed that 85% are prenatally induced. A recent ultrasound study of 512 premature infants provides evidence that many cases of CP result from brain damage that occurred at least 2 weeks before birth (147). In two national cohort studies, comparison of cases and controls showed no consistent differences in social and environmental factors, history of pregnancy, labor, or delivery, confirming the hypothesis that most cases are not associated with adverse obstetric factors. Significant differences were found in the incidence of respiratory and neurological symptoms in the neonatal period, confirming that neonatal neurological symptoms are associated with subsequent CP (156).

Prenatal influences such as central nervous system malformations, chromosomal aberrations, and congenital infections account for up to 75% of all CP cases (157). Untreated medical conditions, such as infections, rubella, toxoplasmosis, cytomegalovirus, encephalitis, meningitis, herpes, and AIDS have been linked to the pathology of CP; however, these account for only 6% of children with CP (158).

A potential hereditary basis for CP has been given substantial consideration in the past, although it has been linked to only a small percentage of the cases. The likelihood of genetic determination in spastic diplegia and quadripligia is approximately 10%; the risk is greater if the spasticity is symmetrical (159). In such cases, a genetic structural deficit in the pyramidal tract in the upper cervical area has been found (160). The genetic risk of athetoid and dystonic CP is unknown, but is probably similar to that of spastic CP. The highest likelihood of a genetically determined disorder is in the category of ataxia and ataxic diplegia (162, 163). Gustavon et al. (163) estimate that approximately one-third to one-half of these cases are genetically determined. Although there are examples of multiple cases of CP within a family, one must not assume genetic origin; multiple involvement may be explained by a pregnancy or birth history (146).

Neonatal asphyxia was once believed to be a direct link to cerebral palsy, but such difficulties rarely result in neurological deficit. In most cases, evidence for asphyxial damage is lacking, and it is now believed that asphyxia alone plays little or no role in the majority of CP cases (162).

Diagnosis

As with mental retardation, the differential diagnosis of cerebral palsy is especially important and somewhat difficult. The milestones of maturity are extremely delayed in both retardation and CP, and must be scrutinized to differentiate between the two. Early reflexes such as the Moro reflex and palmar grasp reflex extend beyond their normal time frame in the beginning stages of CP and can offer an important diagnostic cue to both parents and physicians (149). Effective diagnostic comparisons must be made not only between the patient's development and that of a normal child, but also between the function of the right and left limbs, and of the arms and legs. In this way, hemiplegic and diplegic CP may be suspected. Because the motor deficit in CP is one that evolves with maturity, assessments must be continually repeated to detect deterioration in function. Reassessment is also helpful in ensuring the consideration of appropriate treatment, schooling, and educational needs.

Treatment

Most treatment regimens attempt to facilitate the patient's movement to allow the patient to live a relatively normal life; no cure has been found because the disorder stems mostly from neonatal or perinatal damage to the brain. Because CP is a constantly evolving disorder, the most efficient treatment plan includes repeated assessments. A multidisciplinary approach, has shown great benefit, for it encompasses many of the problems experienced by the individual with CP.

Although there is debate about the value of physiotherapy in treating CP, most pediatricians believe there is some benefit. They recommend early rather than late onset of such treatment in hopes of preventing severe contractures and deformity, and promoting normal motor development. Other forms of therapy include treatment of vision and hearing deficits, feeding and speech therapy, and orthopaedic therapy (149).

Medications are also being considered as treatment options for the motor deficits of CP, especially in spastic forms. Baclofen has proved to be very effective in some hemiplegic and diplegic children in reducing spasticity and facilitating physiotherapy (165). Neurosurgery is currently a questionable option in the treatment of children with CP, at present showing very limited justification. According to Neville (166), some benefit has been shown to arise from a selective dorsal rhizotomy, the division of lumbar and sacral dorsal roots for the treatment of spastic cerebral palsy.

The assessment and treatment of psychiatric disorders in patients with CP follows the same guidelines as for mental retardation.

References

1. Grossman HJ. Manual of terminology and classification on mental retardation. Washington DC: American Association on Mental Deficiency, 1983.
2. American Psychiatric Association Task Force on Nomenclature and Statistics. Diagnostic and statistical manual on mental disorders. 3rd ed. (DSM III). Washington DC: American Psychiatric Association, 1980.
3. Munro JD. Epidemiology and the extent of mental retardation. Psychiatr Clin North Am 1986;9:591–623.
4. Richardson WP, Higgins AC. The handicapped children of Alamance County, North Carolina. Wilmington: Nemours Foundation, 1965.
5. Parsons JA, May JG, Menolascino FJ. The nature and incidence of mental illness in mentally retarded individuals. In: Menolascino FJ, Stark JA, eds. Mental illness in the mentally retarded. New York: Plenum Press: 1984.
6. Sands S, Ratey JJ. The concept of noise. Psychiatry 1986;49: 290–297.
7. Eaton LF, Menolascino FJ. Psychiatric disorders in the mentally retarded: types, problems, and challenges. Am J Psychiatry 1982; 139:1297–1303.
8. Steele MW. Genetics of mental retardation. In: Jacob I, ed. Mental retardation. Basel; Karger, 1982:27–37.
9. Turner G, Brookwell R, Daniel A, Selikowitz M, Zilibowitz M. Heterozygous expression of x-linked mental retardation and x-chromosome marker fra(x) (q27). N Engl J Med 1980;303: 662–664.
10. Knoll JH, Chudley AE, Gerrard JW. Fragile x-linked mental retardation. II. Frequency and replication pattern of fragile x (q28) in heterozygotes. Am J Hum Genet 1984;36:640–645.
11. Reiss AL, Feinstein C, Toomey KE, Goldsmith B, Rosenbaum K, Caruso MA. Psychiatric disability associated with the fragile x chromosome. Am J Med Genet 1986;23:393–401.
12. Finelli PF, Pueschel SF, Padre-Mendoza T, O'Brien MM. Neurological findings in patients with the fragile x syndrome. J Neurol Neurosurg Psychiatry 1985;48:150–153.
13. Gualtieri CT. Neuropsychiatry and behavioral pharmacology. New York: Springer-Verlag, 1991.
14. Ferguson-Smith MA. Recent developments in prenatal diagnosis: biomedical aspects. In: Hicks EK, Berg JM, eds. The genetics of mental retardation. Dordrecht: Kluwer Academic Publishers, 1988:3–14.
15. Lai F, Williams RS. A prospective study of Alzheimer disease in Down's syndrome. Arch Neurol 1989;46:849–853.
16. Lott IT, Lai F. Dementia in down syndrome: observations from a neurology clinic. Applied Research in Mental Retardation 1982;3: 233–239.
17. Robinson K, Wolfsberg E, Jones KL. Brachmann-de Lange syndrome: evidence for autosomal dominant inheritance. Am J Med Genet 1985;22:109–115.
18. Leavitt A, Nuhad D, Davis C. Cornelia de Lange syndrome in a mother and daughter. Clin Genet 1985;28:157–161.
19. Bankier A, Haan E, Birrell R. Letter: familial occurance of Brachman-de-Lange syndrome. Am J Med Genet 1986;25:163–165.
20. LaCourt GC, Arendt J, Cox J, Beguin F. Microcephalic dwarfism with associated low amniotic fluid 5-hydroxyindole -3-acetic acid (5-HIAA). Helvetica Paediatrica Acta 1977;32:149–154.
21. O'Neal M, Page N, Adkins WN, Eichelmann B. Tryptophan-trazodone treatment of aggressive behavior. Lancet 1986;2:859–860.
22. Menolascino FJ, Egger ML, eds. Medical dimensions of mental retardation. Lincoln: University of Nebraska Press, 1978.
23. Corbett JA, Harris R, Robinson R. Epilepsy. In: Wortis J, ed. Mental

retardation and developmental disabilities. New York: Bruner Mazel, 1977.

24. Koranyi EK. Mental retardation: medical aspects. Psychiatr Clin North Am 1986;9(suppl):635–645.

25. Shapiro MB, Haxby JV, Grady CL. Nature of mental retardation and dementia in Down's syndrome: study with PET, CT, and neuropsychology. Neurobiol Aging 1992;13:723–734.

26. Karlinski H. Alzhiemer's disease in Down's syndrome. J Am Geriatr Soc 1986;34:728–734.

27. Mann DMA. The pathological association between Down syndrome and Alzheimer disease. Mech Ageing Dev 1988;43:99–136.

28. Wisniewski KE, Wisniewski HM, Wen GY. Occurrence of neuropathological changes and dementia in Down's syndrome. Ann Neurol 1985;17:278–282.

29. Cutler NR. Cerebral metabolism as measured with positron emmission tomography (PET) and [$_{18}$F] 2-deoxy-D-glucose: healthy aging, Alzheimer disease and Down syndrome. Prog Neuropsychopharmacol Biol Psychiatry 1986;10:309–321.

30. Shapiro MB, Ball MJ, Grady CL, et al. Dementia in Down's syndrome: cerebral glucose utilization, neuropsychological assessment, and neuropathology. Neurology 1988;38:938–942.

31. Castells S, Chakrabarti C, Winsberg BG, Hurwic M, Perel JM, Nyhan WL. Effects of L-5 hydroxytryptophan on monoamine and amino acid turnover in the Lesch-Nyhan syndrome. J Autism Dev Disord 1979;9:95–103.

32. Jankovic J, Caskey TC, Stout JT, Butler IJ. Original articles: Lesch-Nyhan syndrome: a study of motor behavior and cerebrospinal fluid turnovers. Ann Neurol 1988;23:466–469.

33. Silverstein FS, Faye M, Johnston MV, Hutchinson RJ, Edwards NL. Lesch-Nyhan syndrome: CSF neurotransmitter abnormalities. Neurology 1985;6:907–911.

34. Goldstein M, Anderson LT, Reuben R, Dancis J. Self mutilation in Lesch Nyhan disease is caused by dopaminergic denervation. Lancet 1985;1:338–339.

35. Breese GR, Napier TC, Mueller RA. Dopamine agonist induced locomotor activity in rats treated with 6-hydroxydopamine at differing ages: functional supersensitivity of D1 dopamine receptors in neonatally lesioned rats. J Pharmacol Exp Ther 1985;234:447–455.

36. Casas-Brudge M, Almenar C, Gray IM, et al. Dopaminergic receptor supersensitivity in self mutilatory behavior of Lesch Nyhan disease. Lancet 1985;1:991.

37. Goldstein M, Kuga S. Dopamine agonist reduced compulsive biting behavior in monkeys: animal model for Lesch-Nyhan syndrome (Abstract). Social Neuroscience 1984;239:1.

38. Richardson SA, Katz M, Koller H, et al. Some characteristics of a population of mentally retarded young adults in a British city. J Ment Defic Res 1979;23:287–295.

39. Niedermeyer E. The epilepsies. In: Jakab I, ed. Mental retardation. Basel: Karger, 1982;211–239.

40. Roberts JKA. Neuropsychiatric complications of mental retardation. Psychiatr Clin North Am 1986;9:647–657.

41. Tarter RE. Intellectual and adaptive functioning in epilepsy. Diseases of the Nervous System 1972;33:763–770.

42. Ellenberg JH, Hirtz DG, Nelson KB. Do seizures in children cause intellectual deterioration? N Engl J Med 1986;314:1085–1088.

43. Meldrum BS, Brierly JB. Prolonged epileptic seizures in primates. Arch Neurol 1973;28:10–17.

44. Wasterlain CG. Effects of epileptic seizures on brain ribosomes: mechanism and relationship to cerebral energy metabolism. J Neurochem 1977;29:707–716.

45. Menini C, Meldrum BS, Riche D, Silva-Comte C, Stutzman JM. Sustained limbic seizures induced by intraamygdaloid kainic acid in the baboon: symptomatology and neuropathological consequences. Ann Neurol 1980;8:501–509.

46. Mendez MF, Cummings JL, Benson F. Depression in epilepsy. Arch Neurol 1986;43:766–770.

47. Huberty TJ, Koller JR, Brink TDT. Adaptive behavior in the definition of mental retardation. Except Child 1980;46:256–261.

48. Jakab I. Diagnosis and differential diagnosis of mental retardation. In: Jakab I, ed. Mental retardation. Basel: Karger, 1982;70–115.

49. Matson JL. Emotional problems in the mentally retarded: the need for assessment and treatment. Psychopharmacol Bull 1985;21:258–261.

50. Sovner R. Limiting factors in the use of DSM-III criteria with mentally ill mentally retarded persons. Psychopharmacol Bull 1986;22:1055–1059.

51. Sovner R, Hurley AD. Do the mentally retarded suffer from affective illness? Arch Gen Psychiatry 1983;40:61–67.

52. Matson JL, Coe DA, Gardner WI, Sovner R. A factor analytic study of the diagnostic assessment for the severely handicapped scale. J Nerv Ment Disord 1991;179:553–557.

53. Reudrich S, Menolascino FJ. Dual diagnosis of mental retardation and mental illness: an overview. In: Menolascino FJ, Stark JA, eds. Handbook of mental illness in the mentally retarded. New York: Plenum Press, 1984.

54. Reiss S. Assessment of a man with dual diagnosis. Ment Retard 1992;30:1–6.

55. Kazdin AE, Matson JF, Senatore V. Assessment of depression in mentally retarded adults. Am J Psychiatry 1983;140:1040–1043.

56. Donaldson JY, Menolascino FJ. Past, current, and future roles of child psychiatry in mental retardation. J Am Acad Child Adolesc Psychiatry 1977;16:38–52.

57. Azrin NH, Armstrong PM. The "mini meal": a method of teaching eating skills to the profoundly retarded. Ment Retard 1973;2:9–13.

58. Azrin NH, Foxx RM. A rapid method of toilet training the institutional retarded. J Appl Behav Anal 1971;4:89–99.

59. Matson JL. Use of independence training to teach shopping skills to mildly mentally retarded adults. Am J Ment Defic 1981;86:178–183.

60. Twardosz S, Baer DM. Training two severely retarded adolescents to ask questions. J Appl Behav Anal 1973;6:665.

61. Balthazar EE, Stevens HA. The emotionally disturbed mentally retarded. Englewood Cliffs, NJ: Prentice-Hall, 1975.

62. Menolascino FJ, Eaton LF. Future trends in mental retardation. Psychiatry Human Development 1980;10:156–169.

63. Yesavage JA. Correlates of dangerous behavior by schizophrenics in hospital. Psychiatry Res 1984;18:225–231.

64. Yudofsky S, Silver J, Schneider S. Pharmacologic treatment of aggression. Psychiatric Annals 1987;17:397–407.

65. Ratey J, Sorgi P, Polakoff S. Nadolol as a treatment for akathisia. Am J Psychiatr 1985;142:640–642.

66. Crabbe HF. A guidebook for the use of psychotropic medication in persons with mental illness and mental retardation. State of Connecticut Department of Mental Retardation, 1989.

67. Greenberg I, Altman JL, Cole JO. Combination of drugs with behavior therapy. In: Greenblatt M, ed. Drugs in combination with other therapies. New York: Grune & Stratton, 1975;242–258.

68. Fielding LT, Murphy RJ, Reagan MW, Peterson TL. An assessment program to reduce drug use with the mentally retarded. Hosp Community Psychiatry 1980;31:771–773.

69. Schalock RL, Foley JW, Toulouse A, Stark JA. Medication and programming in controlling the behavior of mentally retarded individuals in community settings. Am J Ment Defic 1985;849:503–509.

70. Ratey JJ, Gualtieri CT. Neuropsychiatry and mental retardation. In: Ratey J, ed. Mental retardation: developing pharmacotherapies. Washington DC: American Psychiatric Press, 1991:1–17.

71. Rever M. Mental retardation. Psychiatr Clin North Am 1992:15:511–522.

72. Appolloni T, Cooke SA, Cooke TP. Establishing a normal peer as a behavior model for developmentally delayed toddlers. Percept Mot Skills 1976;43:1155–1165.

73. Azrin NH, Wesolowski MD. Theft reversal: an overcorrection procedure for eliminating stealing by retarded persons. J Appl Behav Anal 1974;7:577–581.

74. Azrin NH, Wesolowski MD. Eliminating habitual vomiting in a

retarded adult by positive practice and correction. J Behav Ther Exp Psychiatry 1975;6:145–148.

75. Deitz SM, Slack DJ, Schwartsmueller EB, et al. Reducing inappropriate behavior in special classrooms by reinforcing average interresponse times: interval DRL. Behav Ther 1978;9:37–46.

76. Vukelich R, Hake DF. Reduction of dangerously aggressive behavior in a severely retarded resident through a combination of positive reinforcement procedures. J Appl Behav Anal 1971;4:215–225.

77. Altman K, Haavik S, Cook J. Punishment of self-injurious behavior in natural settings using aromatic ammonia. Behav Res Ther 1978;16:85–96.

78. Baumeister AA, Baumeister AA. Suppression of repetitive self-injurious behavior by contingent inhalation of aromatic ammonia. Autism and Childhood Schizophrenia 1978;8:71–77.

79. Aman MG, Singh NN. Pharmacological Intervention. In: Matson JL, Mulick JA, eds. Handbook of mental retardation. Elmsford, NY: Pergamon Press, 1983:317–337.

80. White JR. Changing patterns of psychoactive drug use with the mentally retarded. N Z Med J 1983;96:686–688.

81. Baldessarini RJ, Cohen BM, Teicher MH. Significance of neuroleptic dose and plasma level in the pharmacological treatment of psychoses. Arch Gen Psychiatry 1988;45:79–91.

82. Gualtieri CT, Schroeder SR, Hicks RE, Quade D. Tardive dyskinisia in young mentally retarded individuals. Arch Gen Psychiatry 1986;43:335–340.

83. Strauss WH, Klieser E. Cognitive disturbances in neuroleptic therapy. Acta Psychiatr Scand 1990;82(suppl 358):56–57.

84. Ayd FJ. Buspirone update: comparison with the benzodiazepines. International Drug Therapy Newsletter 1985;20.

85. Mandell AJ. From mollecular biological simplification to more realistic central nervous system dynamics: an opinion. In: Judd J, Grove P, eds. Psychiatry: psychobiological foundations of clinical psychiatry, vol 4. New York: Basic Books, 1986;209–218.

86. Glass GV, Singer JE. Urban stress: experiments on noise and social stressors. New York: Academic Press, 1972.

87. Miller JG. Information overload in psychopathology. American Journal of Psychotherapy 1959;133:627–634.

88. Ratey JJ, Lindem KJ. Beta blockers as primary treatment for aggression and self-injury in the developmentally disabled. In: Ratey J, ed. Mental retardation: developing pharmacotherapies. Washington DC: American Psychiatric Press, 1991;51–82.

89. Elliot FA. Propranolol for the control of belligerent behaviors following acute brain damage. Ann Neurol 1977;1:489–491.

90. Yudofsky S, Williams D, Gorman J. Propranolol in the treatment of rage and violent behaviors in patients with chronic behavioral syndrome. Am J Psychiatry 1981;138:218–220.

91. Greendyke R, Kanter D, Schuster D, et al. Propanolol in the treatment of assaultive patients with organic brain disease: a double blind, crossover, placebo controlled study. J Nerv Ment Disord 1986;5:290–294.

92. Ratey J, Mikkelsen E, Sorgi P, et al. Autism: treatment of aggressive behaviors. J Clin Psychopharmacol 1987;7:35–41.

93. Williams DT, Mehl R, Yudofsky S, et al. The effects of propranolol on uncontrolled rage outbursts in children and adolescents with organic brain disfunction. J Am Acad Child Adolesc Psychiatry 1982;2:125–135.

94. Ratey JJ, Morrill R, Oxenkrug G. Use of propranolol for provoked and unprovoked episodes of rage. Am J Psychiatry 1983;140:1356–1357.

95. Ratey JJ, Sorgi P, Lindem K, et al. Nadolol to treat aggression and psychiatric symptomatology in chronic psychiatric inpatients: a double blind placebo controlled study. J Clin Psychiatry 1992;53:41–46.

96. Reudrich SL, Grush L, Wilson J. Beta adrenergic blocking medications for aggressive and self injurious mentally retarded persons. Am J Ment Retard 1990;95:110–119.

97. Ratey J, Bemporad J, Sorgi P, et al. Brief report: open trial effects of

98. Gaind R, Suri AK, Thompson J. Use of beta blockers as an adjunct in behavioral techniques. Scott Med J 1984;20:284–286.

99. Koella W. CNS related effects of β-Blockers with special reference to mechanisms of action. Eur J Clin Pharmacol 1985;28(suppl):55–63.

100. Linnoila M, Virkkunen M, Scheinin M, Nuutila A, Rimon R, Goodwin FK. Low cerebrospinal fluid 5-hydroxyinoleacetic acid concentration differentiates impulsive from nonimpulsive violent behavior. Life Sci 1983;33:2609–2614.

101. Linnoila M, DeJong J, Virkkunen M. Family history of alcoholism in violent offenders and impulsive fire setters. Arch Gen Psychiatry 1987;46:613–616.

102. Linnoila M, Virkkunen M. Aggression, suicidality and serotonin. J Clin Psychiatry 1992;53(suppl):46–51.

103. Asberg M, Traskman L, Thoren P. 5-HIAA in the cerebrospinal fluid: a biochemical suicide predictor? Arch Gen Psychiatry 1976;33:93–97.

104. Brown G, Ebert M, Goyer P, et al. Aggression, suicide and serotonin, Am J Psychiatry 1982;139:741–746.

105. Morand C, Young SN, Ervin FN. Clinical response of aggressive schizophrenics to oral tryptophan. Biol Psychiatry 1989;18:575–578.

106. Gedye A. Dietary increase in serotonin reduces self injurious behavior in a Down's syndrome adult. J Ment Defic Res 1990;34:195–203.

107. Gedye A. Buspirone alone or with a serotonergic diet reduced aggression in a developmentally disabled adult. Biol Psychiatry 1991;30:88–91.

108. Ratey J, Sovner R, Parks A, Rogentine K. The use of buspirone in the treatment of aggression and anxiety in mentally retarded patients: a multiple baseline placebo controlled study. J Clin Psychiatry 1991;52:159–164.

109. Ratey JJ, Sovner R, Mikkelsen E, Chmielinski HE. Buspirone therapy for maladaptive behavior and anxiety in developmentally disabled persons. J Clin Psychiatry 1989;50:382–384.

110. Colella R, Ratey J, Glaser A. Paramenstrual aggression in a mentally retarded adult ameliorated by buspirone. Int J Psychiatry Med 1992;22:351–355.

111. Tiller JG. Short term buspirone treatment in disinhibition with dementia. Lancet 1989;1:1169.

112. Realmutto GM, August GJ, Garfinkel BD. Clinical effect of buspirone in autistic children. J Clin Psychopharmacol 1989;9:122–124.

113. Ratey JJ, O'Driscoll GA. Buspirone as a habilitative drug for patients with a dual diagnosis. Fam Pract Recert 1989;11(suppl):39–45.

114. Ratey JJ, Komry V, Gaffar K, Leveroni CL, Miller AC. Low dose buspirone to treat agitation and maladaptive behavior in the brain injured: two case reports. J Clin Psychopharmacol 1992;12:362–364.

115. Olivier B, Mos J, Hartog J, Rasmussen D. Serenics. Drug News Perspectives 1990;3:261–271.

116. Ratey JJ, Leveroni CL, Aney J. Eltoprazine to treat aggression. J Clin Psychopharmacol, submitted for publication.

117. Norden MJ. Fluoxetine in borderline personality disorder. Biol Psychiatry 1989;13:885–893.

118. Stark P, Fuller RW, Wong DT. The pharmacological profile of fluoxetine. J Clin Psychiatry 1985;46:7–13.

119. Coccaro EF, Astil JL, Herbert J, Schut AG. Fluoxetine treatment of impulsive aggression in DSM IIIR personality disorder patients. J Clin Psychopharmacol 1990;10:373–375.

120. Cornelius JR, Soloff PH, Perel JM, Ulrich RF. Fluoxetine trial in borderline personality disorder. Psychopharmacol Bull 1990;26:151–154.

121. Ratey J, Leveroni C, Kilmer D, Guthiel C, Swartz B. The effects of clozapine on severely aggressive inpatients on a difficult to manage unit of a state hospital J Clin Psychiatry, in press.

122. Criswell HE, Mueller RA, Breese GA. Clozapine antagonism of D-1 and D-2 dopamine receptor mediated behaviors. Eur J Pharmacol 1989;159:141–147.

123. Pratt JA, Jenner P, Johnson A. Anticonvulsant drugs after plasma

tryptophan concentrations in epileptic patients: implications for anti-epileptication and mental function. J Neurol Neurosurg Psychiatry 1984;47:1131–1133.

124. Worrall EP, Moody JP, Naylor GJ. Lithium in nonmanic depressives: antiaggressive effect and red blood cell lithium values. Br J Psychiatry 1975;126:464–468.

125. Dale PG. Lithium therapy in aggressive mentally subnormal patients. Br J Psychiatry 1980;137:464–474.

126. Sovner R, Hurley A. Management of chronic behavior disorders in mentally retarded adults with lithium carbonate. J Nerv Ment Dis 1981;169:191–195.

127. Coccaro EF, Astil JL, Szeeley PJ, Malkowicz DE. Serotonin in personality disorder. Psychiatr Ann 1990;20:587–592.

128. Polakoff S, Sorgi P, Ratey J. The treatment of impulsive and aggressive behaviors with nadolol. J Clin Psychopharmacol 1986;6:125–126.

129. Simeon D, Stanley B, Frances A, et al. Self mutilation in personality disorders: psychological and biological correlates. Am J Psychiatry 1992;149:221–226.

130. Ratey J, Sovner R, Mikkelsen E, Chmielinski H. Buspirone therapy of maladaptive behavior and anxiety in developmentally disabled persons. J Clin Psychiatry 1989;50:382–384.

131. Herman BH. Effects of opioid receptor antagonists in the treatment of autism and self injurious behavior. In: Ratey J, ed. Mental retardation: developing pharmacotherapies. Washington DC: American Psychiatric Press, 1991:107–138.

132. Herman BH, Hammock MK, Egan J, et al. Naltrexone induces dose dependent decreases in self-injurious behavior. Soc Neurosci Abstr 1985;11:468.

133. Sandman CA. β-endorphin disregulation in autistic and self-mutilatory behavior: a neurodevelopmental hypothesis. Synapse 1988;2:193–199.

134. Menolascino FJ, Wilson J, Golden CJ, Ruedrich SL. Medication and treatment of schizophrenia in persons with mental retardation. Ment Retard 1986;24:277–283.

135. Ucer E, Kreger C. A double blind study comparing haloperidol with thioridizine in emotionally disturbed mentally retarded children. Curr Ther Res 1969;11:202–205.

136. Carroll BJ, Feinberg M, Greden JF. A specific laboratory test for the diagnosis of melancholia. Arch Gen Psychiatry 1981;138:143.

137. Naylor GJ, Donald JM, LePoidevin D, et al. A double blind trial of long term lithium therapy in mental defectives. Br J Psychiatry 1974;124:52–57.

138. Rivinus TM, Harmatz JS. Diagnosis and lithium treatment of affective disorders in the retarded: five case studies. Am J Psychiatry 1979;136:551–554.

139. Lerer B, Moore N, Meyendorff E, et al. Carbamazepine versus lithium in mania: a double blind study. J Clin Psychiatry 1987;48:89–93.

140. Post RM, Uhde TW, Joffe, et al. Anticonvulsant drugs in psychiatric illness: new treatment alternatives and theoretical implications. In: Trimble MR, ed. The psychopharmacology of epilepsy. Chicester, England: John Wiley & Sons, 1985.

141. Post RM, Uhde TW, Ballenger JC, Squillace KM. Prophylactic efficacy of carbamazepine in manic-depressive illness. Am J Psychiatry 1983;140:1602–1604.

142. Lipinski JF, Pope HG. Possible synergistic action between carbamazepine and lithium carbonate in the treatment of three acutely manic patients. Am J Psychiatry 1982;139:948–949.

143. Friedman DL, Kastner T, Plummer AT, Ruiz MQ, Henning D. Adverse behavioral effects in individuals with mental retardation and mood disorders treated with carbamazepine. Am J Ment Retard 1992;96:541–546.

144. Langee HR, Conlon M. Predictors of response to antidepressant medications. Am J Ment Retard 1992;97:65–70.

145. Howland RH. Fluoxetine treatment of depression in mentally retarded adults. J Nerv Ment Dis 1992;180:202–205.

146. Field CJ, Aman MG, White AJ, Vaithianathan C. Single subject study of imiprimine in a mentally retarded woman with depressive symptoms. J Ment Defic 1986;30:191–198.

147. Aman MG, White AJ, Vaithianathan C, Teehan CJ. Preliminary study of imipramine in profoundly retarded residents. J Aut Dev Dis 1986;16:263–273.

148. Scherzer A, Tscharnuter I. Early diagnosis and therapy in cerebral palsy. New York: Marcel Dekker, 1990.

149. Skolnick A. New ultrasound evidence appears to link prenatal brain damage, cerebral palsy. JAMA 1991;265.

150. Franco S, Andrews B. Reduction of cerebral palsy by neonatal intensive care. Pediatr Clin North Am 1977;24:639.

151. Batshaw ML. Your child has a disability: a complete sourcebook of daily and medical care. Boston: Little, Brown & Co., 1991.

152. Eiben RM, Crocker AC. Cerebral palsy within the spectrum of developmental disabilities. In: Thompson et al, eds. Comprehensive management of cerebral palsy. New York: Grune & Stratton, 1983.

153. Crothers B, Paine RS. The natural history of cerebral palsy. Oxford: Oxford University Press, 1959.

154. Hagberg B, Hagberg O, Olow I. The changing panorama of cerebral palsy in Sweden 1954–1970. II. Analysis of the various syndromes. Acta Pediatri Scand 1975;64:193–200.

155. Goutiéres F. Role of circulatory disturbances in the genesis of some prenatal encephalopathies. Paper presented at EFNCS 5th Conference, Brussels, 1979.

156. Michaelis R, Rooschutz B, Dopfer R. Prenatal origin of congenital spastic hemipareses. Early Hum Dev 1985;4:243–255.

157. Ingram TTS. Pediatric aspects of cerebral palsy. Edinburgh: Churchill Livingstone, 1964.

158. Emond A, Golding J, Peckham C. Cerebral palsy in two national cohort studies. Arch Dis Child 1989;64:848–852.

159. Coorssen E, Msall ME, Duffy LC. Multiple minor malformations as a marker for prenatal etiology of cerebral palsy. Dev Med Child Neurol 1991;33:730–736.

160. Naeye RL, Peters EC, Bartholomew M, Lanis R. Origins of cerebral palsy. Am J Dis Child 1989;143:1154–1161.

161. Hughes I, Newton R. Genetic aspects of cerebral palsy. Dev Med Child Neurol 1992;34:80–86.

162. Silver J. Familial spastic paraplegia with amyotrophy of the hands. Ann Hum Genet 1966;30:69.

163. Gustavon KH, Hagberg B, Sanner G. Identical syndromes of cerebral palsy in the same family. Acta Paediatr Scand 1969;58:330–340.

164. Freeman JM, Nelson KB. Intrapartum asphyxia and cerebral palsy. Pediatrics 1988;82:240–249.

165. Milla PJ, Jackson ADM. A controlled trial of baclofen (Lioresal) in children with cerebral palsy. J Int Med Res 1977;5:398.

166. Neville BGR. Selective dorsal rhizotomy for spastic cerebral palsy. Dev Med Child Neurol 1988;30:395–398.

26

AUTISM AND PERVASIVE DEVELOPMENTAL DISORDERS

Deborah Fein, Stephen Joy, Lee Anne Green, and Lynn Waterhouse

Pervasive developmental disorders (PDD) generally and infantile autism in particular have been the focus of a great deal of research and clinical speculation. In part, this intense interest relates to the perplexing pathogenesis and devastating consequences of the disorder. Equally compelling are the issues raised by the disorder concerning human sociability. A full understanding of autism would contribute substantially to developmental neuropsychology, and to the neurology of social behavior. The present review examines: (*a*) the historical development of the concept of autism/PDD; (*b*) diagnostic criteria; (*c*) findings and theories relative to its cognitive, emotional, and behavioral characteristics; (*d*) epidemiology, including prevalence and genetics; (*e*) the boundaries of the autism/PDD concept and its co-morbidity with other neuropsychiatric conditions; (*f*) associated biomedical conditions; (*g*) neuroanatomical findings; (*h*) neurophysiological findings; (*i*) neurochemical findings; (*j*) clinical assessment; and (*k*) pharmacological and psychological/educational treatments.

HISTORICAL DEVELOPMENT OF THE CONCEPT OF AUTISM

PDD is the current term for what is probably a group of related neurodevelopmental disorders characterized by a similar behavioral profile; others have labeled this cluster of conditions "autistic spectrum disorders" (1). The relationship between autism and PDD is confusing. Technically, autism is a diagnostic category under the broader heading of PDD. In clinical practice, PDD is often used to describe children who have mild autism, high-functioning autism or an incomplete set of autistic features. DiLalla and Rogers (2) found that autistic children can best be discriminated from PDD children by degree of social impairment. The validity of non-autistic PDD syndromes is explored by Szatmari (1). Autism was first described by Leo Kanner (3) and became known as infantile autism or autistic disorder. The concept has expanded since that date, and the term "Kanner autism" is sometimes used to refer to cases presenting with symp-

toms similar to those of Kanner's original sample; such cases are a subset of PDD. Kanner's original description remains influential, and there is a tendency in the literature to assume that persons with "Kanner autism" represents the "nuclear" or "core" form of PDD, an assumption that may or may not be warranted (4).

Kanner (3) presented case studies of 11 children (eight male, three female). He identified three fundamental characteristics common to the entire group:

1. "Extreme autistic aloneness" (p. 242) — an inability to enter into affective contact with others;
2. Failure to use language in a communicative fashion (muteness, literalness, echolalia and/or pronoun reversal); and
3. "Anxiously obsessive desire for the maintenance of sameness" (p. 245), with the children showing distress at any change in their usual routines.

Related to these factors were a severely limited repertoire of spontaneous activities and an associated tendency to repeat the same actions in a ritualized manner. Kanner argued that their extreme need for constancy led to a skillful enjoyment of inanimate physical objects.

Two more characteristics asserted by Kanner were normal intellectual potential (based mainly on their "intelligent physiognomies") and good physical health, though the case descriptions include neurological abnormalities (4). Kanner concluded: "These children have come into the world with innate inability to form the usual, biologically provided affective contact with people, just as other children come into the world with innate physical or intellectual handicaps" (p. 250).

Kanner's judgment obviously was flawed with regard to the intelligence of persons with autism, a majority of whom function in the mentally retarded range. Otherwise, his clinical description has held up remarkably well over half a century of research.

The major trend in thinking about autism during the two decades following Kanner's original paper must be regarded as an unfortunate digression. Influenced by popular psychodynamic ideas, several authors (5–7) claimed that autism was caused by pathological parenting. Kanner (8) himself came to believe that lack of parental warmth contributed to the genesis of the disorder (the famous "refrigerator parent" hypothesis). Margaret Mahler's (9, 10) writings on autistic and "symbiotic" psychoses of childhood figured prominently in this trend, though as Hobson (11) has pointed out, Mahler accepted the notion of a constitutional deficit in the child, which she identified as an inability to use the mother as a "beacon of emotional orientation." Although Mahler's clinical observations anticipated later research on social referencing, her views led researchers away from neurodevelopment. The erroneous attribution of responsibility to the parents—termed the "pernicious hypothesis" by Rimland (12)—can be understood only in the context of mainstream general psychiatry of that period, which usually minimized biological formulations.

A shift toward neurodevelopmental theories began in the 1960s. Researchers outlined a variety of models of autism positing impairment in: (*a*) allocating attention to coordinate new stimuli with memories (12); (*b*) vestibular mediation of perceptual processes (13); and (*c*) left-hemisphere mediated linguistic abilities (14). Today, those advocating a primary cognitive deficit (15, 16) and those favoring a primary social/affective deficit (17, 18) agree that the basic PDD deficit stems from a neurological dysfunction.

Differential diagnosis was a conceptual problem for early autism research. Some clinicians believed that autism was a variant of or precursor of schizophrenia. Not until the 1970s was there an awareness that psychotic disorders beginning in infancy must be regarded as separate from those with onset in later childhood, adolescence, or adulthood (19, 20). Autistic-like disorders virtually always begin before age 3, while schizophrenic-like disorders almost never begin before age 7 (19). This realization revitalized interest in infantile autism as a distinct nosologic entity, leading to the development of more operationally precise diagnostic criteria (10–22) and a reconceptualization of the syndrome as a pervasive developmental disorder, under which label it was incorporated by the American Psychiatric Association in the 3rd edition of their Diagnostic and Statistical Manual of Mental Disorders (DSM-III) (23).

DIAGNOSTIC CRITERIA

The first sets of systematic diagnostic criteria for autism appeared in 1978 (20, 21).

Rutter (20) proposed four essential criteria: Onset before the age of 30 months; Impaired social development out of keeping with the child's intellectual level; Delayed and deviant language development out of keeping with the child's intellectual level, and Insistence on sameness, as shown by stereotyped behavioral patterns, abnormal preoccupations, or resistance to change.

The diagnosis was limited to cases with onset before age 30 months in order to differentiate maximally between autism and other symptomatically similar disorders such as Heller's syndrome and Asperger's syndrome. Rutter recognized that some cases of autism arise at slightly older ages, but unfortunately, the 30-month guideline became a rigid rule in DSM-III. He emphasized that social impairment in autism often lessens after early childhood, though more subtle social ineptitude persists.

Ritvo and Freeman (21) outlined slightly different criteria for autism, which were adopted by the National Society for Autistic Children: Disturbances of development rate and/or sequences; Disturbances of response to sensory stimuli; Disturbances of speech, language-cognition, and nonverbal communication; and Disturbances of the capacity to appropriately relate to people, events, and objects.

Age of onset was stated to be typically before 30 months of age, but the system is descriptive and has no fixed, requisite criteria. Associated features were said to include mood lability without identifiable cause; failure to appreciate real danger; inappropriate fears; self-injurious behaviors; mental retardation; and abnormal electroencephalograms (EEGs) with or without seizures.

Ritvo and Freeman placed strong emphasis on sensory abnormalities. They described abnormalities of every sensory modality: visual (prolonged staring, absence of eye contact); auditory (nonresponse or overresponse to sounds); tactile (over- or underresponse to pain or temperature change); vestibular (whirling and preoccupation with spinning objects); olfactory/gustatory (repetitive sniffing); and proprioceptive (posturing or hand flapping). All of these behaviors are seen in many autistic children (a very low sensitivity to painful stimulation is, for example, a common finding). Whether they reflect an underlying deficit in sensory modulation is not known, and most sets of diagnostic criteria have not included sensory abnormalities as an essential feature. The Ritvo and Freeman (21) criteria identify a somewhat different set of children as autistic from those that Rutter (20) lists.

Lorna Wing and colleagues took an empirical approach to the diagnosis, investigating a population of mentally handicapped children with deficits in social relatedness, communicative language, and repertoire of interests and behaviors. They identified three subgroups based on social behavior: aloof, passive, and active-but-odd (24, 25).

Two aspects of Wing et al.'s work are relevant to diagnosis. First, they broadened the concept of PDD. Previously, researchers and clinicians had focused on Kanner's criteria. Wing et al. started with the fundamental, universally accepted symptom areas of autism, and used them as the basis of classification. Hence, any child with serious impairment in social, communicative, and imaginative/behavioral function, disproportionate to any general mental retardation, would be deemed part of the autistic spectrum, even if his or her presentation differed slightly from that of the prototypical Kanner-type autistic.

Second, Wing et al. described social behaviors associated with different types of functioning at different developmental stages. Behaviors of the "aloof" group, for example, most closely approximate Kanner autism, with aberrant self absorption and lack of interaction with others. Those in the "passive" group, tolerate interactions with others but do not initiate them. Those in the "active-but-odd" group initiate interactions with others, but their social bids tend to be awkward and one-sided, consisting of an attempt to draw the other person into their own sphere of interest. Subgroup membership can change with development in the direction of greater sociability. Some "aloof" young children grow into "passive" or "active-but-odd" older children. However, "active-but-odd" young children are unlikely to become either "passive" or "aloof."

In DSM-III (23), infantile autism, now listed under the general heading of PDDs, was diagnosed on the basis of a monothetic criterion set (i.e., in which every major feature had to be present in order for the diagnosis to be made). The DSM-III criteria (23) were as follows: onset before 30 months of age; pervasive lack of responsiveness to other people (autism); gross deficits in language development; if speech is present, peculiar speech patterns such as echolalia; bizarre responses to various aspects of the environment, e.g., resistance to change; absence of delusions, hallucinations, loosening of associations, and incoherence as in schizophrenia.

Because failure to meet any one of these six criteria rules out a diagnosis of infantile autism, it is not surprising that the use of DSM-III criteria yielded lower prevalence rates of autism. In DSM-III, older children and adults who no longer met all diagnostic criteria were assigned a new, separate diagnosis: Infantile Autism Residual State. DSM-III also included a category termed "Childhood-Onset PDD," which applied to few cases and was open to cases with diverse behavioral presentations and prognoses (e.g., Heller's syndrome or Asperger's syndrome). DSM-III also included a category for "atypical" cases, which in some samples outnumbered those diagnosed as autistic.

Substantial changes were made in the revision of DSM-III (DSM-III-R [22]). The purely monothetic criteria were replaced by a partially polythetic, and more fully operationalized, criterion set developed by Wing et al. (25).

DSM-III-R criteria required that at least eight of the following 16 items are present, including at least two items from set A, one from B, and one from C: A. Qualitative impairment in reciprocal social interaction: marked lack of awareness of the existence or feelings of others; no or abnormal seeking of comfort at times of distress; no or impaired imitation; no or abnormal social play; gross impairment in ability to make peer friendships; B. Qualitative impairment in verbal and nonverbal communication and in imaginative activity: no mode of communication, markedly abnormal nonverbal communication; Absence of imaginative activity; marked abnormalities in the production of speech; marked abnormalities in the form or content of speech; marked impairment in the ability to initiate or sustain a conversation with others, despite adequate speech; C. Markedly restricted repertoire of activities and interests: stereotyped body movements; persistent preoccupation with parts of objects; marked distress over changes in trivial

aspects of environment; Unreasonable insistence on following routines in precise detail; Markedly restricted range of interests and a preoccupation with one narrow interest. DSM-III-R (26) established only three diagnostic classifications for severe childhood psychopathology: Autistic Disorder (AD); Pervasive Developmental Disorder Not Otherwise Specified (PDDNOS); and, Schizophrenia with Onset in Childhood (SOC). DSM-III-R eliminated COPDD because it lacked research and clinical validity (27), and replaced Atypical PDD with PDDNOS to conform to the terminology established in DSM-III-R for all clinical remainder categories (27). The DSM-IV (28) followed DSM-III-R categories for AD and PDDNOS, but added three diagnostic categories to parallel the World Health Organization's International Classification of Diseases Tenth Edition (ICD-10) PDD diagnostic subgroups Rett Syndrome, Other Childhood Disintegrative Disorder, and Asperger's Syndrome (29). DSM-IV Pervasive Developmental Disorders includes the following subgroups:

299.00 Autistic Disorder;
299.80 Rett's Disorder;
299.10 Other Childhood Disintegrative Disorder;
299.80 Asperger's Disorder; and,
299.80 Pervasive Developmental Disorder Not Otherwise Specified (including Atypical Autism).

It is important to note that Rett's Disorder, PDDNOS, and Atypical Autism (identified within PDDNOS), all carry the same diagnostic code (299.80). Diagnosticians thus actually code the PDDNOS remainder category (299.80) when they diagnose Rett's Disorder, Asperger's Disorder, or Atypical Autism.

This is not true for ICD-10 PDD subgroups (29):
F84.0 Childhood Autism;
F84.1 Atypical Autism;
F84.2 Rett Syndrome;
F84.3 Other Childhood Disintegrative Disorder;
F84.4 Overactive Disorder Associated with Mental Retardation and Stereotyped Movements;
F84.5 Asperger's Syndrome; and,
F84.8 Other.
F84.9 Unspecified

DSM-IV (28) and ICD-10 (29) provide 12 parallel polythetic diagnostic criteria for Autistic Disorder and Childhood Autism. Six symptoms must be present, four of which are specified. At least two symptoms must come from a subset of four impaired social skills (nonverbal interactional behavior, friendship, joint attention, and reciprocity). One must come from a subset of four impaired communication skills (delayed or absent language, given speech—abnormal conversation, perseverative speech, and abnormal play), and at least one of the six must come from a subset of four abnormal activities (obsessive interests, rigid rituals, stereotypies, and preoccupation with parts of objects).

A study comparing DSM-III, DSM-III-R, and ICD-10 diagnoses of autism with diagnoses determined by latent class analysis found that ICD-10 best fit the latent diagnostic standard (30). This latent class model, however, indicated that the latent standard was best approximated "by the sensitivity of DSM-III-R criteria and the specificity of the two other systems (DSM-III and ICD-10)" (30, p. 220).

A study comparing DSM-III, DSM-III-R, DSM-IV, and ICD-10 autism and non-autistic PDD (31) reported that all four diagnostic systems identified autistic groups that were significantly lower in IQ and adaptive functioning, and expressed significantly more autistic symptomatology than the four systems' non-autistic PDD groups. However, all four non-autistic PDD groups expressed a pattern of autistic characteristics nearly identical to the pattern found for autism.

It is true that "it has been difficult to develop a methodology for the evaluation and comparison of diagnostic criteria in psychiatry" (30, p. 220). ICD-10 and DSM-IV criteria for autism have included reliable diagnostic items and are consonant with clinical judgment. However, the external validity of these diagnoses (e.g., association with brain imaging or genetic findings) has yet to be determined.

BEHAVIORAL, COGNITIVE, AND EMOTIONAL CHARACTERISTICS

This section presents a selective review of research findings concerning behavioral, cognitive, and emotional characteristics of autism/PDD, and of current theories regarding the nature of the basic deficits that may play etiological roles in the development of autistic symptomatology. Some of these theories postulate neural mechanisms that might account for the supposed "core" deficits, but none of these models offers sufficiently clear pathways between aberrant behaviors and the neurochemical and neuroanatomical findings discussed in a later section.

Method

The study of differential deficit in autistic individuals poses the problem of identifying appropriate control groups. Normal children of similar chronological age (CA) will score higher than autistic children on any standard measure. Normal children matched for mental age (MA) are a better choice, but will not control for general effects of psychopathology or for years of experience. Normal MA matches will be younger chronologically than the autistic children, so their sensory-motor systems may be too immature to be comparable. Psychiatric patients with non-PDD diagnosis also are likely to outperform autistic subjects on most measures. Mentally retarded controls may be matched with autistic individuals on both CA and MA, and are the most frequently used comparison group. Mental retardation, though, is an even more heterogeneous classification than PDD: persons with mental retardation may have little in common beyond their general cognitive delay. Sometimes this heterogeneity is reduced by using a mentally retarded sample of known, homogeneous etiology such as Down syndrome. Even this, however, limits inference. Most individuals with Down syndrome are highly social (above their MA, in many cases), and this will skew comparisons with autistic samples. Another comparison population is children with developmental language disorders, because they have verbal and nonverbal skill patterns similar to those of autistic children. The choice of the control group obviously will affect the areas in which autistic individuals appear relatively impaired. Some studies utilize more than one comparison group to offset the problems with each alternative. Other researchers study only autistic individuals with IQs above the retarded range. Although it is difficult to assemble samples meeting this criterion, it is a useful strategy in that it allows for the study of autism uncomplicated by global intellectual impairment. The generalizability of results to the whole autistic spectrum, however, will be limited.

Another problem for research design is that because autistic individuals by definition have a specific deficit in language skill, their verbal IQs tend to be substantially lower than their nonverbal IQs. In most comparison samples (language disorders being an exception), verbal and nonverbal mental levels do not differ equally. As a consequence, if a control group is matched to the autistic group on verbal IQ, then the autistic group will tend to be more capable overall because of their superior visuospatial skills. If a control group is matched on nonverbal IQ, it will be superior because of its greater language competence. Some forms of PDD, such as Asperger's syndrome, however, do not display this verbal-nonverbal IQ discrepancy.

In practice, all of the comparison groups just described are used, as are a variety of matching strategies. This must be kept in mind when comparing research findings across studies.

Core Deficits in Autism

Social impairment is a universally recognized core deficit in autism. It differs qualitatively from the impairments seen in other developmental or behavioral disorders. The many specific types of social deficits in autism are well-documented. As indicated by DSM criteria, autism is marked by a general inability to form relationships, failure to use nonverbal communicative behaviors such as eye contact, lack of reciprocity, lack of awareness of others, and failure to share experiences with others (28). Other well-recognized impairments in the social domain are difficulties with affection, giving and seeking comfort, awareness of social rules, social imitation, attachment and symbolic play (32).

The most fundamental of social deficits in autism is that of impairment in basic face-to-face interaction skills. The difficulty has been described as a failure in reciprocity and in adaptation to the changing demands of social encounters, given an inherent disorganization and uneven development of social skills (33). In general, studies show that autistic children cannot orchestrate the give and take of social interactions, including conversation and play (34). Abnormalities are present in joint attention behaviors, and in both initiations and responses to others, extending to the realm of peer play (35, 36). These symptoms appear to vary depending on the interactive partner and setting involved (34, 37), as well as on a cognitive level (34, 35) and severity of symptoms (35). In sum, findings suggest that the autistic child is unlikely to initiate interactions, but is more likely to respond in adult-initiated situations (34, 38). In situations in which free play was observed, autistic children were found to engage in play much less frequently, and at a developmental level much lower than peers of similar intellectual ability (39). When symbolic play is modeled, autistic children appear to be able to engage in a higher, albeit relatively deficient, level of play. When vigorously encouraged and elicited, normal levels of play have emerged in high-functioning autistic children (40). This is consistent with the recent findings of a large scale study in which symbolic play deficits in high functioning autistic children seemed more related to motivation than to capacity (41). A recent review of studies since 1964 affirms deficits in play relative to intellectual level and tendencies for sensorimotor play to the exclusion of symbolic play (42). A review of attachment studies (43) conclude that while attachment is not absent in autistic children, there is a high proportion of insecure and avoidant attachment styles as well as a delayed development of attachment. Autism also involves specific deficits in perception of others mental states, perception of others' emotional states, pragmatic aspects of communication, and possibly executive functions and long-term verbal memory. Autistic individuals typically function better on visuospatial than on verbal tasks, though this is not universally the case. Visual discrimination learning, motor learning, rote learning, and short-term declarative memory also appear to be areas of relative strength. (See Prior [44], Sigman et al. [45] and Green et al. [46] for general reviews of cognitive functioning in autism.)

A small subset of autistic individuals display islands of exceptional ability against a background of widespread cognitive impairment (so-called savant syndrome). Rimland and Fein (47) and Treffert (48) have described autistic savant abilities: music and musical memory, spatial memory, decoding written material, and calculations. Rimland and Fein summarized three theories to explain savant skills:

1. Overdevelopment of skills from perseverative attention;
2. Rededication of cortical association areas to pattern recognition (49); and
3. Hyperfunction of the hippocampus.

The emerging consensus on a cognitive profile of PDD does not include an agreement as to which deficits are casual and which are epiphenomenal. Currently, the most influential theories focus on social cognition. A major debate is whether the affective or representational aspect of social cognition is primary. This reflects a fundamental question that goes far beyond autism: is human emotion a result of cognitive evaluation or does it depend on the operation of phylogenetically older neural systems independent of cog-

nition (50–54)? Affective primacy in autism has been proposed by Fein, Waterhouse and their associates (11, 50) and by Hobson (55). Representational primacy has been claimed by Leslie, Baron-Cohen, and Frith (15).

Kanner (3) proposed an innate, presumably biologically determined, social deficit as the basis of autism. In the ensuing decades, the affective deficits continued to occupy center stage in autism theory, but parents were postulated as causing the disorder. When the concept of a neurological basis reemerged (12), the field turned away from both the discredited and notion that cold parents created autism and the logically unrelated but historically associated idea that the core dysfunction in autism was affective. Measurement tools have also constrained exploration on affective deficits. Almost the entire technology of neuropsychological assessment relates to cognitive functions. Language use, declarative memory, visuoconstructional skills, and pattern recognition can be measured reliably, but ratings of social behavior and affective responses have not been standardized. Researchers have used the available measurement instruments that were available, whether or not they addressed the behaviors of impairments most relevant to understanding the phenomenology of autism.

Deficits in Attention

Observations of unusual responses to stimuli led researchers to investigate attentional abnormalities in autism. Autistic individuals are found to be overselective in their attention to stimuli, such that their focus of attention is abnormally narrow (56, 57). They also have difficulties in shifting attention between modalities (58), and in shifting spatial attention (59). Autistic children are able to sustain their attention at a level appropriate for their mental age, if given tangible reinforcements (60), and high-functioning autistic adolescents and adults have been found to be impaired on some attention tests (61).

Several early cognitive theories of autism focused on abnormalities in mechanism related to attention. Rimland (12) proposed that the autistic child failed to associate incoming stimuli with established memory. In this model, autistic social deficit arises from a failure to link the presence of mother with the memory of the biological rewards she has brought. Rimland hypothesized that this deficit might result from a hypoactive or underaroused reticular formation. Hutt et al. (62) developed a related but opposite theory: autistic children, they suggested, have a hyperactive or overaroused reticular formation, and gate out all stimuli that threaten to further arouse them. Both of these theories accounted for many of the known perceptual and behavioral peculiarities of autism, though in different ways. For example, Rimland saw motor stereotypies as a method of increasing arousal; Hutt and colleagues saw them as a method of reducing arousal by screening out extrinsic stimuli. Current theories also invoke neurologically-based attentional dysregulation as the cause of perseverative behavior and social deficits in autism (63–65) (see more extensive discussion of Courchesne's work). Kinsbourne (65) and Dawson and Lewy (64) have suggested that hypersensitivity to novelty and overactivation of brainstem mechanisms of arousal causes narrowed attentional focus and stimulus overselectivity in autistic children. This could result in deployment of mechanisms for de-arousal such as stereotypies and avoidance of social stimuli.

Language Deficits

Many aspects of verbal functioning are impaired in autistic children, many of whom are entirely mute. Studies examining cognitive profiles in autism are uniform in finding that verbal skills are performed at a lower level than nonverbal skills (66–68). Verbal autistic children generally are able to acquire normal grammatical morphology and syntax, although onset is delayed (66, 69). Some autistic children learn grapheme-phoneme correspondence, enabling them to write and to decode words for reading (66); in fact, early acquisition of written (but not spoken) language often marks high-functioning autism (66). However, language comprehension is significantly impaired relative to expression, and deficits in the semantic and pragmatic aspects of language are common (66). Autistic children generally do not rely on meaning when comprehending or expressing acquired morphemes, grammatical structures and vocabulary (66, 70). They are also deficient in interactive communication, including conversational behavior, nonverbal communication and speech prosody (24, 69). Even when language is relatively spared, there are usually deficits in comprehending complex language and in formulating complex output (61, 66). In these functions, even high-functioning autistic children are more deficient than are children with language disorders (66).

Rutter (14) argued that deficits in language-mediated functions are independent of social impairment and may play a casual role in the disorder. Later, Rutter (71) suggested that the language deficit might be only a special case of a more general impairment in the perception and expression of meaningfully patterned stimuli. McCann (72) related Rutter's ideas to hemispheric lateralization research and suggested that autism might result from left temporal lobe dysfunction. This model accounts for language impairment co-occurring with relatively good visual-motor abilities, and is consistent with some of the neuroimaging literature. Fein et al. (73), however, argued that the model is inadequate, pointing out that: autistic language is most impaired in prodosy and pragmatics, which may suggest right-hemisphere dysfunction and that language deficits are widely variable, and perceptual processes are by no means always preserved. (See Caplan's chapter on language for details of the distinctions among linguistic processes.)

Deficits in "Theory of Mind"

Recently the cognitive approach to autism has appeared in a new form: Baron-Cohen et al. (15) suggested that autistic children lack a theory of mind, that is, they lack the ability to form mental representations of another's mental representations. In this view, the inability to represent the internal states of others leads to the autistic child's range of difficulty with others. Pretend play, pragmatic communication, and empathy, which are impaired in autism, require one to symbolize the surrounding world and be aware that other people have their own subjective frame of reference. In its strongest form (74) this theory holds that the autistic child has a dysfunctional brain module subserving theory of mind. This theory, although controversial, has resulted in a great deal of research over the past 5–10 years, and has been revised recently to accommodate a great deal of neurobiological research. Autistic children have been shown to be impaired on a variety of experimental tasks requiring theory of mind for successful solutions (15, 75–82).

While the theory of mind model account for some autistic behaviors and cognitive deficits, it is flawed as a primary casual factor. One line of criticism is phylogenetic: if a theory of mind were crucial for affiliative social behavior, then a species lacking a theory of mind should not be affiliative. This is manifestly not the case. Another line of criticism is ontogenetic (83): if autism begins with a failure to develop theory of mind, then social behaviors that emerge prior to theory of mind should be undisturbed, and deficits in social behaviors hypothesized to be dependent upon theory of mind should be universal in autism. Klin et al. (83) explored these questions in a study of 29 autistic children and 29 age and IQ matched controls, using the Vineland Adaptive Behavior Scales (84) to assess social development. Not only did some autistic children display higher-level social behaviors, but many social behaviors that emerge before eight months of age significantly discriminated between autistic subjects and controls. Ozonoff et al. (85) found that not all high-functioning autistic children failed theory of mind measures, and that Asperger's Syndrome subjects were unimpaired on theory of mind tasks. Other studies have shown that theory of mind performance is highly correlated with mental development, verbal ability, age, and IQ (86, 87) and that adequately controlling these factors (88) or reducing the complexity of the task (89, 90) eliminates group differences. These findings suggest that although autistic children may be selectively impaired on theory of mind tasks, their failure to develop a theory of mind is not the cause of autism.

Other Social/Cognition Deficits

Fein et al. (11) suggested that autism originates in a developmental failure of neural systems governing social-emotional functioning. They pointed out that although social and cognitive development ordinarily are highly correlated and presumably interdependent, they can be dissociated in disorders of development. Within the PDD population, for example, degree of autistic social impairment is not highly correlated with IQ or other cognitive measures. Autistic individuals with higher IQs may manifest their social deficit in less disruptive or less salient ways, but it is still apparent. The opposite pattern — social development superior to cognitive functions — is seen in Down syndrome. This double dissociation suggests a complex source of sociability. Fein et al. (11) also argues that there is no single cognitive deficit that is universal in autism, nor is there any single cognitive deficit found in autism that is not also found among non-PDD populations. They also proposed that none of the reported cognitive deficits adequately explains the frequently observed autistic aloofness, or disinterest for people, during the first year of life. Fein et al. suggest, on the contrary, that infants who fall short of a minimum level of social reciprocity may be unable to experience shared attention or communicative intent, and as a result will fail to develop symbolic play or proper language functions.

Recent research into social/affective communication in PDD has been influenced by Hobson (18, 55, 91). Hobson's initial studies (55, 91) explored the hypothesis that autistic children should be more impaired in emotional recognition than their cognitive deficit would warrant. Hobson compared autistic children with several matched control groups for their ability to recognize facial, gestural, and vocal expressions of four basic emotions: happy, unhappy, angry, and scared. Subjects were also tested for recognition of movements, sounds, and contexts of inanimate objects (e.g., automobiles). All subjects obtained maximal scores on the object recognition task, but the autistic children alone were severely impaired on the emotion recognition measures. There were two methodological problems with Hobson's early studies. The emotion and object recognition tasks were not of equal difficulty, and controls were matched with autistic subjects on nonverbal mental age, so the effects of differential verbal skills were not adequately controlled (92). Hobson et al. (93) addressed these problems in an expanded study. The autistic sample continued to show a significantly greater discrepancy between their "object" and "affect" scores, but their performance on the affect recognition task was now not significantly lower than that of the controls. Thus, his original findings was only partly replicated.

Several investigators have attempted to replicate and extend Hobson's findings. Tantam et al. (94) found autistic children impaired relative to age and performance-IQ-matched controls on an affect recognition task, a finding that also applies to high-functioning autistic adults (95). Braverman et al. (96) found that PDD children were impaired relative to MA-matched controls on an affect-matching task, and that the autistic children performed significantly less well on affect and face matching than on object matching. PDD children also are selectively impaired at matching emotion with appropriate contexts (75) and at responding to affective stimuli (83). These findings do not seem to reflect a deficit in recognition of faces as such (76). They are, however, influenced by verbal mental age. Like Hobson et al. (93), Prior et al. (77) reported an insignificant difference between the emotion recognition scores of autistic children and those of psychiatric controls matched for verbal MA, while

Ozonoff et al. (78) reported a significant emotion perception deficit relative to nonverbal MA-matched controls, which shrank to insignificance relative to a verbal MA-matched control group. The extent to which emotion perception depends on verbal development remains uncertain: perhaps the experimental measures require more verbal processing than does everyday affective responsiveness.

Autistic subjects also seem to be impaired in the expression of emotion. Yirmiya et al. (79) coded the affect expressions of autistic children and several control groups, using Izard's (84) system for rating facial expressions. The autistic children displayed less facial affect, especially positive affect, than the other groups, but more incongruous, difficult-to-interpret expressions. MacDonald et al. (95) reported that high-functioning autistic adults displayed impaired emotional expressiveness, and noted that although no single measure discriminated individual autistic subjects from controls, a composite multitask score of socioemotional communication correctly classified 18 of 20 subjects as autistic or nonautistic.

Fine et al. (85) studied the extent to which high-functioning autistic, Asperger syndrome, and psychiatric control subjects employed intonation (prosody) in a meaningfully communicative fashion. High-functioning autistic subjects used communicative intonation less than the other groups, but made greater use of noncommunicative patterns of intonation. Asperger's syndrome subjects differed only slightly from controls in their use of different types of intonation, though they seemed to often use intonation inappropriately. Because autistic individuals are able to perceive patterns of vocal stress and to produce them on request, their failure to do so appropriately in conversation suggests an inability to map these vocal patterns onto appropriate verbal contexts.

Memory Deficits

Other theoretical models of autistic cognition have been proposed. Boucher and Warrington (97) and Delong (98) have noted similarities between the behavior of autistic children and that of animals with hippocampal lesions: increased general activity, motor stereotypies, reduced exploration of the environment, reduced responsiveness to novel stimuli when familiar stimuli are present, perseveration and impaired active error reduction in learning and memory tasks. Hippocampal lesions in adult humans can produce an amnesic syndrome involving specific deficits in long-term declarative memory formation, with short-term memory, procedural memory, and visual-spatial abilities grossly intact; the latter functions are also areas of relative strength among autistic individuals. These authors hypothesized that autism might be a kind of developmental amnesic syndrome. In their original study, Boucher and Warrington (97) tested high-functioning autistic children and several control groups. Visual and auditory memory of the autistic subjects resembled that of amnesic adults: retention was impaired when measured by free recall, but not when measured by cued recall. However, only a subset of them showed memory deficits, and autistic subjects were unimpaired at learning paired associations of unrelated words. A number of subsequent studies (44, 45, 99-103) have examined memory in autistic subjects, either as a primary or incidental issue. They have not shown a consistent pattern of memory deficits, while as expected, autistic subjects have shown worse performance than controls on various specific measures. The most specific finding is that visual and rote auditory memory tend to be spared, while verbal memory for semantically organized material such as stories is quite impaired (61, 73, 104). Anecdotally many high-functioning autistic individuals show hyperamnesia for specific kinds of material including spatial arrays, routes, music and events (47), a fact that "amnesia" theories of autism must be able to explain.

Executive Function Deficits

Rumsey and Hamburger (105) compared high-functioning autistic adult males with matched normal controls on a battery of neuropsychological tests. Perceptual and motor skills, visuomotor integration, and memory functions failed to discriminate between the groups, nor was there evidence of lateralized dysfunction, but two tests of executive function, the Wisconsin Card Sort Test and the Trail-Making Test, revealed significant impairment in the autistic subjects. These tests require subjects to formulate problem-solving strategies and to respond flexibly to changing task demands; successful performance is thought to be mediated by frontal cortical systems. A later study (106) replicated this result. Szatmari et al. (107) also reported significant impairment using the Wisconsin Card Sort Test in a study of high-functioning autistic individuals. Like Szatmari, Berger et al (108) found that set shifting was a better predictor of social adjustment than was IQ, in high-functioning autistic adolescents, and in younger autistic children, executive functions had a relationship to social communication independent of verbal ability (109).

Based on these findings, Ozonoff et al. (99) have hypothesized that executive functions are selectively impaired in autism. These authors pointed out that the perseverative, inflexible behavior displayed by autistic subjects, and their frequently observed impulsivity and social ineptitude, are consistent with the presence of executive function deficits, as shown by patients with prefrontal lesions. To explore this idea, they tested high-functioning autistic children and psychiatric controls matched for age and IQ on a number of tasks, including "theory of mind" measures, emotion perception tasks, and executive function test (99, 110). The autistic group was impaired on all three sets of tests, and the executive function measures were the best discrimination between groups. The control group actually made more errors in failure to maintain set, while the autistic subjects made many more perseverative errors. Autistic performance on these tasks did not improve on follow-up (111). Autistic deficits in

set shifting and in planning were also demonstrated by Hughes et al. (112).

Ozonoff et al. (99) reported that Asperger's syndrome subjects performed adequately on theory of mind tasks but showed executive function deficits. The authors hypothesized that theory of mind and executive functions might be mediated by proximate brain regions, and might often be damaged together, or else that executive functions and theory of mind both rely on some more fundamental system. They suggested widespread damage to the prefrontal cortex as likely anatomical substrate. Given the scarcity of studies of this brain region in autism, and the largely negative findings on those that exist (113), this remains highly speculative. The picture is complicated by the fact that separate components of executive functioning may be uncorrelated (110, 112) and that autistic subjects appear unimpaired on some aspects of executive function, especially inhibitory functions (110, 114). Nevertheless, executive function deficits in autism deserve further investigation.

Discussion

Waterhouse and Fein (50) considered obstacles to developing a satisfactory comprehensive theory of autism, and they suggested possible "solutions" in the absence of complete knowledge of the neurobiology of social behavior. One suggestion was to accept that the heterogeneity apparent in autism theory may parallel an actual heterogeneity in the autistic population. Cognition, affect, and behavior are widely variable in PDD; so are the associated medical conditions and other neurological findings in the disorder. It is possible that there are multiple neural subsystems involved in social behavior, that these subsystems operate as parts of a complex, integrated whole, and that disruption of any one of these elements can lead to some form of PDD. If a dysfunctional brain region is involved in another function (e.g., perception, language, or verbal memory), the subset of PDD patients with damage to that specific brain locus also would display impairment in the cognitive functions subserved by that anatomical site.

DEVELOPMENTAL COURSE AND PROGNOSIS

Autism is a developmental disorder and cannot be described from a purely cross-sectional perspective. The typical Kanner autistic lacks interest in human relationships, lacks communicative language, expresses a strong need for environmental constancy, and engages in stereotyped behaviors; yet this presentation is most characteristic of the preschool years. Even during this period, there are often signs of increasing social relatedness (e.g., differential attachment to caregivers [45]) and diminishing behavioral peculiarities. During middle childhood, autistic children often master daily living skills and make some accommodation to demands made by other people, while their ritualized behaviors and idiosyncratic preoccupations tend to diminish (115). School behavior may come to resemble that of hyperactive and/or retarded children, rather than continuing to conform to "classic" autistic patterns.

Adolescence can be a difficult time. Besides the frequent onset of seizures during this period, a number of PDD children regress behaviorally as adolescents. Paradoxically, one of the most difficult aspects of life for many adolescents with autism is their increasing interest in close personal relationships during these years (115). Higher-functioning individuals (e.g., those with Asperger's syndrome) are especially prone to psychological problems, as they realize the extent of their ineptitude in the realm of social interaction. Their feelings of helplessness may engender depressed moods or clinical depression. On a more positive note, both social and language skills usually do continue to develop during adolescence, and increased interest in relating to other people can make psychosocial intervention easier.

Paul (115) summarized the results of seven long-term follow-up studies of autism (87, 116–121) stating that about half of all autistic adults remain in residential care. Many of those not in residential treatment continue to be dependent on caregivers. No more than one in five achieves truly independent living, including gainful employment; of these, many no longer meet diagnostic criteria for PDD, though social peculiarities often persist, and neither close friendships nor sexual relationships are common.

The two most important predictors of good outcome in autism are IQ and language function. The presence of associated neurological disorders is a strong negative prognostic indicator. Individuals with IQs below 60 rarely achieve any independence; those with IQs in the normal or near-normal range have a reasonably good chance of becoming at least partially independent (121, 122). Language development obviously is related to IQ, but apparently makes an independent contribution to the prediction of long-term outcome. In particular, the emergence of communicative speech by age 5 is thought to be a critical indicator. According to Paul (115), there is a subset of PDD children whose speech is limited but who go on to improve socially; these children are characterized by relatively high IQ and good receptive language skills. Recent follow-up studies (104) generally support these findings. Both IQ and adaptive behavior measures are as stable over time among autistic subjects as among other children. There seems to be a relatively low correlation between intelligence and the presence or absence of maladaptive behaviors (123). Recent evidence (73) suggests that there may be two distinct subgroups of autism varying in level of function, with the higher functioning group improving over time and the lower group showing stable or declining functioning. Other studies support this bifurcation of outcome (124, 125).

Given that only those autistic children with fairly high IQ and some of language can be expected to do well over the long term, and given that only a subset of these children will in fact enjoy good outcomes, there has been interest in identifying outcome predictors within the high-functioning autistic population. Szatmari et al. (107) in a follow-up study of such subjects, showed that even within this group IQ was a good predictor of adaptive behavior in adulthood, as was childhood performance on a test of nonverbal problem solving. Venter et al. (126), in a similar follow-up study of high-functioning autistic children, also found verbal IQ to be the single best predictor of achievement and social adaptation in early adulthood, followed by other language measures and nonverbal IQ.

EPIDEMIOLOGY

Prevalence

Long-standing convention places the prevalence of Kanner autism between two and four per 10,000 children (127). Based on the concept of an autistic spectrum on which Kanner autism accounts for half of all cases of PDD, the estimated prevalence for all PDD is in the range or four to eight per 10,000 children.

In recent years, however, prevalence estimates have increased. This may be attributable to any combination of the following factors: (a) improved procedures for identifying cases; (b) more lenient diagnostic practice; (c) actual increases in the proportion of individuals with the disorder; or (d) changes in the conceptualization of the disorder. All of these factors may have affected one or the other of the recent epidemiological surveys, but it seems likely that the actual prevalence of PDD has been greater than previously believed all along.

In an epidemiological study of mentally retarded children with deficits in social relatedness, communication, and behavior, Wing and Gould (24) found that although the prevalence of Kanner autism was in the four per 10,000 range, the prevalence of individuals with the Wing triad of deficits was in the range of 21 per 10,000. Similar diagnostic criteria applied in a Swedish population (128) also resulted in an estimated prevalence of 21 per 10,000 population. Neither of these studies included individuals displaying the triad of deficits who did not also have mental retardation.

Gillberg's research has provided a good perspective on the changing figures for PDD prevalence, as his team has conducted three epidemiological surveys over the course of a decade (129–131), and so are in a position to look for the sources of the increase. In their earliest study, the prevalence of autism (diagnosed according to Rutter [20] and DSM-III criteria) was 2.0 per 10,000 children (another 1.9 per 10,000 were described as PDD but not classically autistic). Four years later, these figures became respectively 4.7 and 2.8 per 10,000. In their most recent study (131), the prevalence of autism was reported to be 7.8 per 10,000, plus 3.4 per 10,000 fulfilling criteria for autistic spectrum disorders. The autistic-like conditions described in these studies were symptomatically very similar to autism, but either had a relatively late age of onset or some atypical symptom such as severe, frequent seizures of early onset. The total prevalence estimate from the last study, 11.2 per 10,000, agrees well with the results of a recent Canadian epidemiological survey (132), which found a rate of 10.1 per 10,000.

Gillberg (4) has claimed that part of the increased rate of autistic conditions in the Gothenburg area of Sweden is attributable to a large number of cases among the children of new immigrants from distant, especially tropical, countries, possibly due to maternal health problems during pregnancy. The remainder of the increase is accounted for by cases who either have severe to profound mental retardation or who have normal-range intelligence. Gillberg has suggested that these populations previously were unlikely to be identified as autistic. Only with increasing sensitivity to the clinical phenomenology of the disorder did diagnostic practice begin consistently to look for evidence of PDD among institutionalized retardates or superficially intact children. (The prevalence of classic Kanner autism, which is associated with moderate mental retardation, has not increased over the years.)

Sex Ratio

PDDs are more common among males than among females. This is a universal finding dating back to Kanner's original clinical sample. Gillberg (4) has reported that the male : female ratio in broadly defined PDD is between 2.0:1 (133) and 2.9:1 (130). The preponderance of males is greater in narrowly defined Kanner autism, with sex ratios ranging from 2.6:1 to 5.7:1, and greater still in Asperger's syndrome, with sex ratios ranging from 7.1:1 to 10:1 across studies. The male : female ratio appears to be lower only when individuals with severe and profound retardation are included (113).

Genetic Contributions

The proportion of families with two autistic children is greater than would be expected based on chance, and reports of twins concordant for autism have appeared frequently (134). However, there have been few controlled family studies and twin studies, so that it has been difficult to make a convincing case for familial patterns of autistic conditions (135). It is clear that at least some cases of autism have a genetic substratum (136–138).

Smalley et al. (138) reviewed six family studies (138–143), two of which (141, 143) also included twin studies, and a number of case studies of twin pairs with at least one autistic proband. The family studies revealed a pooled sibling incidence rate of 2.7% (24 of 886 siblings), which is 270 in 10,000, whereas the estimated prevalence range of autism in the general population is 4–20 in 10,000. Examined individually, all six studies yielded highly similar results. A more recent history study (144) corroborates this figure (3.0%). An epidemiological survey in Utah (145) found a somewhat higher level of sibling risk (4.5%), though still consistent with earlier studies.

For purposes of genetic counseling, Ritvo et al. (146)

noted that the recurrence risk of autism (the probability of any given sibling born after an autistic child also being autistic) was 8.6%, somewhat higher than the sibling concordance rate. If the autistic child was female, recurrence risk increased to 14.5%, while recurrence risk after a male autistic birth was only 7.0%.

The picture from twin studies is less clear, though all sources agree that the risk for monozygotic (MZ) twins is far greater than that for dizygotic (DZ) twins. Folstein and Rutter (141) reported concordance rates of 36% and 0% for same-sex MZ and DZ twin pairs, respectively, while Ritvo et al. (143) reported rates of 96% and 24% in a sample that included mixed-sex pairs. The aggregate of single-case studies yielded an 82% concordance for MZ twins and a 22% for DZ twins. The true population figures are, however, probably lower, because these results have been inflated by ascertainment bias. Individual case reports are more likely to be submitted and published when there is a positive finding, and in controlled studies there is a greater chance that families with two autistic members will be brought to the attention of the researchers, because a report on either proband will lead to investigation of the family. Furthermore, Ritvo et al. (143) specifically solicited families with multiple cases, undoubtedly leading to some overrepresentation of concordant twin pairs (138). Smalley et al. (138) suggested an adjusted concordance rate of 64% for MZ twin pairs and 9% for DZ twin pairs. A recent population-based twin study conducted in Scandinavia (147), limited to same-sex pairs, found 10 of 11 MZ twin pairs (91%) concordant for autism as compared with none of the 10 DZ twin pairs, a finding closely parallel to those of Ritvo et al. (143) or the case studies reviewed by Smalley et al. (138). Similarly, Bailey and colleagues (148) reported a 60% concordance rate for autism in 25 MZ twins, and no concordance in 20 DZ twins. The concordance rate for a broader phenotype of autistic-like social and/or cognitive disorders, however, was 92% for MZ twins, and 10% for DZ twins.

Despite minor discrepancies among these twin studies, all investigations support the hypothesis of a genetic contribution to autism.

Because of the early age of onset of autistic conditions and the extremely low fertility of persons with full-blown autism, it is not surprising that no adoption studies have been attempted.

Mental retardation and learning disability occur among siblings of autistic probands more frequently than among siblings of Downs syndrome probands (149). Piven et al. (144) found that 15% of the siblings of autistic probands had a history of learning disability, including disorders of language and academic skills. Folstein and Rutter (141) reported that six of seven nonautistic patients had some form of cognitive deficit. Minton et al. (142) found an elevated incidence (7%) of mental retardation in the siblings of autistic probands, and also reported that performance IQ was higher than verbal IQ in siblings, indicating a neuropsychological profile similar to that often found in autistic individuals. On the other hand, neither Freeman et al. (150) nor Szatmari et al. (151) found elevated rates of clinically significant cognitive impairment among the siblings or parents of their autistic probands. Aggregating results of seven studies of the cognitive functioning of siblings of autistic probands, Smalley et al. (138) reported a 16.5% rate of cognitive impairment. Bolton et al. (152) recently reported that in autistic probands with speech, the number of the proband's autistic symptoms was significantly correlated with the number of relatives who expressed some milder aspect of autism. The correlation did not appear in the families of autistic individuals without speech (152).

"The issue of whether family members, especially parents, of autistic children are typified by social deficits is emotionally charged. Perfectionism, lack of interest in interpersonal relationships, and an excessive focus on intellectual interests was a casual hypothesis (153) that was not supported by objective, quantified evidence (154). Yet the absence of a casual link does not rule out a mild genetic covariation, and several studies (152, 155–157) have found an elevated incidence of subclinical autistic-like traits among first-degree relatives of autistic probands. Clinicians should not be surprised to find social communication deficits in a subset of patients' relatives, but should not assign any casual significance to these traits."

Links between autism and affective illness have been reported. In Piven et al.'s (144) family history study, 10 of 67 adult siblings of autistic individuals had been treated for a mood disorder. Autistic individuals have been treated for mood disorders, including bipolar disorder (158). Lainhart and Folstein (159), in a recent review of 17 published cases of autistic individuals with affective disorder, found a 50% rate of positive family history for affective disorder, and found that its occurrence appears to be rare in patients that are high functioning. They also highlighted that it is difficult to make a diagnosis of a mood disorder given that its presentation can differ drastically from that seen in nonautistic individuals. Asperger's syndrome, a mild subtype of PDD, has also been linked to affective illness (160), including bipolar disorder (155), as well as possible links between autism, Asperger's syndrome, and schizoaffective disorder (161).

Attempts have been made to find morphological, biochemical, and DNA markers in autism. There is no morphological profile characteristic of autism, but elevated rates of minor physical anomalies (MPAs) are found in some samples. Smalley et al. (138) reviewed five studies that compared the frequencies of MPAs in autistic subjects versus controls (162–166). In every study, a higher percentage of autistic subjects displayed anomalies. Links et al (164) noted that MPAs are frequently seen in autistic individuals with low IQs , and hypothesized that high MPA counts indicate nonfamilial forms of autism. Minor physical anomalies may not be a useful marker for familial autism, but still prove useful in genetic research as an exclusion criterion for

probands unlikely to have relatives with autistic-spectrum disorders.

No DNA marker for autism has been identified. Spence et al. (167) found only one marginally significant marker. This marker was in the ABO blood group on chromosome 9: it was found only in families with at least one affected female. Hérault et al. (168) compared five polymorphism markers in a sample of 50 autistic children and 50 controls, and found that the HRAS marker B3/B3 homozygous genotype was significantly less frequent in autistic children than in controls. Because the HRAS gene (chromosome 11p15.5) codes for the *ras* protein which is active in neuron development, the researchers hypothesize that it may be the basis of autism. A partial trisomy of chromosome 15 was identified by Gillberg et al. (169) in six unrelated boys, five of whom had autism and one with profound retardation. All had at least moderate mental retardation, all manifested gaze avoidance, and most were hypotonic. Duplication of chromosome 15q11-13 also has emerged as a possible factor in case studies (170, 171). Hotopf and Bolton (172) and Ghaziuddin, Sheldon, Venkataraman, and Tsai (173) also have reported case studies of autism with partial tetrasomy 15. Hotopf and Bolton (172) offered several interpretations of this finding, hypothesizing autism as having a heterogeneous genetic basis, and alternatively, that autism may have a consistent genetic basis in an overlapping partial tetrasomy of chromosome 15.

The mode of transmission of the gene or genes responsible for vulnerability to autism remains unknown. The preponderance of evidence weighs against autosomal-dominant or recessive, including X-linked, transmission (138). This principal hypothesis at present is that the diathesis is a polygenic, multifactorial trait, with a number of different genes contributing additively to a dimension of vulnerability. Pickles and colleagues (174) have argued for three epistatic loci as a plausible genotypic basis for autism. They have proposed a continuum of possible gene-to-phenotype effects ranging from independent genes for each component of autistic symptomatology (e.g., one for social impairment, one for cognitive impairment, one for perseverative abnormalities) to each gene affecting all symptoms (174, p.725).

As in other areas of PDD research, the issues of subtyping and establishing the boundaries of the PDD construct complicate efforts to model familial patterns. If mild phenotypic variants of the PDD genotype continue to go undetected, genograms will be incomplete. In addition, if certain as-yet undifferentiated subtypes of autism represent discrete disorders, with their own modes of transmission, the mixture of different disorders within autism will confound investigations of causality.

BOUNDARY CONDITIONS AND COMORBIDITY

Comorbidity is the co-occurrence of two discrete disorders in a single individual. If two disorders occur together with a frequency greater than that predicted by chance (i.e., by multiplying the base rates of the disorders), then it may be concluded that they are somehow related. The nature of this relationship is correlational; one cannot assume that one disorder causes the other, or that a single underlying factor causes both. Both hypotheses merit further investigation.

The assessment of comorbidity is complicated when one or both of the disorders lacks clearly defined boundaries. In such cases, it is possible that the two syndromes represent two aspects of a single disease process. As a practical matter, co-morbidity cannot be ascertained when hierarchical diagnostic rules are applied. For example, if epilepsy were designated as a diagnostic entity superordinate to autism, such that the presence of seizures precluded a diagnosis of PDD, then clinical research would indicate zero overlap between the two conditions. The same would apply where autism was the superordinate category, e.g., if a PDD diagnosis ruled out consideration of Tourette's Disorder. Thus, any discussion of comorbidity is inextricably intertwined with the issue of boundary conditions. Moreover, prevalence will vary depending on the narrowness of defining criteria, including the number and nature of any diagnosis regarded as superordinate.

As noted earlier, it is generally acknowledged that "Kanner autism" is but one of a heterogeneous group of subtly differing overlapping clinical pictures. Kanner autism could be the "core" disorder, and the other forms could be variants, but there is no a priori reason to accept this proposition. Alternatively, it is possible that: (a) a common etiology may lead to any of a number of more or less clearly demarcated outcomes, perhaps depending on the specific brain regions affected by a CNS insult; and/or, (b) the autism syndrome may represent a final common pathway for a number of different pathological events, such as viral infections, toxic conditions, or genetically programmed neurodevelopmental deviations. Attempts to subtype the PDD spectrum are important, and need not take as their starting point the assumption that Kanner autism is the prototypical disorder. Furthermore, there is no logical border between indemnification of subtypes, on the one hand, and identification of comorbid conditions on the other. We must recognize that at our present state of knowledge the outer boundaries of the PDD spectrum (as well as boundaries within the spectrum) remain uncertain.

In our view, autism/PDD is a clinical diagnosis that should be made whenever a patient's symptoms meet diagnostic criteria, regardless of any associated conditions. Autism is a syndrome, like mental retardation: it is applied to persons with a wide range of etiologies or co-morbid disorders. If, for example, a patient displays autistic symptoms, moderate mental retardation, and the fragile X abnormality, all three diagnosis should be made: failure to do so would impoverish the clinical portrayal of that patient. Diagnosis of associated conditions will also contribute to knowledge concerning the relationship of the disorders.

DISORDERS WIDELY REGARDED AS BELONGING TO THE PDD SPECTRUM

Heller's Syndrome (Disintegrative Disorder)

One variant form of autism is the condition known as infantile dementia (175), disintegrative psychosis (19, 156), or Heller's syndrome. The disorder is characterized by 2 or more years of essentially normal development followed by marked regression into a stare seemingly indistinguishable from autism, including the loss of already-acquired social abilities and linguistic competence. The validity of this diagnostic category remains controversial. DSM-III (23) included the diagnosis Childhood-Onset Pervasive Developmental Disorder (COPDD). Cases of Heller's syndrome could be diagnosed as COPDD; however, so could cases of many other subtypes of PDD. DSM-III-R (26) deleted this diagnosis, though encouraging clinicians to note "childhood onset" of PDD when applicable. ICD-10 (29) includes disintegrative disorder as a discrete diagnosis in the PDD spectrum. The disorder is also listed in the DSM-IV (28).

Heller's syndrome is poorly understood. The one point of agreement is that it is very rare. Fewer than 100 cases have been documented in the literature. Burd et al. (176), for example, surveyed North Dakota and found that, of 59 children and adolescents diagnosable with PDD, only two met criteria for Heller's syndrome. Both were severely impaired and failed to improve. Evans-Jones and Rosenbloom (156) reported on 10 cases from the Liverpool area, eight of whom showed a static course of severe impairment after onset of the disorder. On follow-up over a decade later (177), six remained mute; another had learned only two words; only two had progressed to the point of making short statements (one was lost to follow-up). Volkmar and Cohen (178) identifies 10 cases in a group of 135 autistic children. All had reached the point of speaking in sentences before regressing. At the time of the study, the subjects were in their teens and 20s. Most had severe retardation, four remained entirely mute, and all but one were in residential placements. They had IQs lower than those of comparison groups of PDD cases, and they exhibited stereotypies, self-injury, and aggression.

The validity of disintegrative disorder remains in doubt. Kurita (179) reviewed the 60 known cases and concluded that the case for its nosologic validity was insufficient. Volkmar (153), on the other hand, reviewed 77 cases (including those reported by Kurita) and argued for the distinctiveness of the syndrome, primarily by reason of its later age of onset (mean age was 3.36 years, with wide variability).

It has been argued that Heller's syndrome should not be regarded as a developmental disorder (154), because its defining feature is a behavioral regression than failure to develop (hence "disintegrative disorder"). Yet the syndrome clearly involves developmental processes gone awry, and although termed " disintegrative" it is included as a pervasive developmental disorder in ICD-10.

In summary, Heller's syndrome is indistinguishable from autism on cross-sectional inspection. Onset (by definition) is later, and the prognosis appears to be uniformly poor, though not worse than poor-outcome autism. It is not clear that it is a discrete clinical entity. The syndrome could represent the extreme tail of the distribution of age of onset of PDD. (As Kurita (157) pointed out, up to a third of autistic children may progress to the point of speaking at least a few words before the disorder develops.) The label may be useful as a marker of poor prognosis, and deserves further investigation. This will undoubtedly be facilitated by the inclusion of childhood Disintegrative Disorder in DSM-IV. The diagnostic criteria are: apparently normal development for at least the first 2 years after birth; loss of previously acquired skills (before age 10 years) (in at least two of the following areas: expressive or receptive language, social skills or adaptive behavior, bowel or bladder control, play, motor skills); impairment in at least two of the following: social interaction, communication or restricted, repetitive, and stereotyped patterns of behavior, interests, and activities. (taken from DSM-IV) (APA) (28)

Rett's Syndrome

Another autistic spectrum condition is Rett's syndrome, which is unusual among developmental disorders because it apparently affects only females. First described by Andreas Rett in 1966, the syndrome remained largely unknown to the English-speaking world until Hagberg et al. (180) described 35 cases in the *Annals of Neurology*. Diagnostic criteria (181) and developmental stages (182) were soon proposed, and interest in the syndrome has since expanded. A recent review (183) cited over 100 sources without claiming to be exhaustive; another review (184) asserted that over 200 papers on Rett's syndrome have been published.

Like disintegrative disorder, Rett's syndrome is characterized by a period of apparently normal development (6–18 months) followed by profound deterioration of social and psychomotor skills accompanying a progressive cerebral atrophy. The classic symptom involves loss of purposeful use of the hands, accompanied by the development of complex stereotypic hand movements.

Rett's syndrome follows a clear longitudinal course with four well-defined stages (182). Stage one, referred to as "early-onset stagnation," typically lasts several months. The child shows reduced interest in her playing, may begin showing odd hand waving behaviors at times, and head growth decelerates. There may be reductions in her communicative abilities and eye contact.

Stage two, the "rapid destructive stage," can take place in a few weeks or several months. Cases of especially rapid onset may be mistaken for toxic reactions or encephalitic conditions. During this phase, the classic Rett presentations (hand wringing, hand clapping, and hand washing) appear, and purposeful hand use is lost. Other motor abilities are better preserved, but the child will be clumsy, with ataxia and apraxia. Breathing is often irregular, and hyperventilation

may occur. Cognitively, the child displays severe dementia. Seizures sometimes develop. Behaviorally, classic autistic symptomatology is present.

Stage three, the "pseudostationary" period, usually lasts several years. There is some cognitive recovery, and autistic symptoms diminish markedly. With the increased emotional contact of this period, the child's presentation is better described as showing severe mental retardation than as autistic-like. However, gross motor skills often deteriorate further, with gait apraxia and jerky movements of the trunk common. Seizures are present in about 70% of cases, and abnormal EEGs are apparently universal.

The final stage, termed "late motor deterioration," begins anywhere from age 5 through late adolescence. Epileptic symptoms diminish and emotional contact with caregivers improves. Growth is retarded, but puberty occurs at the normal age. There is progressive wasting away and weakness of muscle, combined with spasticity: severe scoliosis and trophic foot disturbances are common, and most Rett's syndrome sufferers become wheelchair-bound.

The estimated prevalence of Rett's syndrome is between one in 15,000 (181) and one in 12,000 (185) live female births. Thus, Rett's syndrome may account for a quarter or more of all cases of PDD in females. Because Rett's syndrome is (at different stages) easily mistaken for Kanner autism, cerebral palsy, mental retardation of unknown origin, or encephalopathy, diagnosis may be difficult.

The etiology of Rett's syndrome remains unknown. Killian (186) suggested an X-linked chromosomal mutation lethal to males. Wahlstrom (187) suggested an inherited X-linked trait combined with a spontaneous mutation at the same site on the other X chromosome. Research on the neuropathology of Rett's syndrome has just begun. Several studies have found neurochemical aberrations (188, 189). Recent neurological and management research has been reviewed by Braddock, Braddock and Graham (190).

Rett's syndrome has been included in DSM-IV under the PDD heading with the following criteria (184): apparently normal prenatal and perinatal development, apparently normal psychomotor development through the first 5 months after birth, normal head circumference at birth; then deceleration of head growth between ages 5 and 48 months, loss of previously acquired purposeful hand skills between ages 5 and 30 months with the subsequent development of stereotyped hand movements, loss of social engagement early in the course (although often social interaction develops later), appearance of poorly coordinated gait or trunk movement, and severely impaired expressive and receptive language development with severe psychomotor retardation (28).

There is consensus that Rett's syndrome is a distinct nosologic entity. However, the relative homogeneity of its presentation and course suggests that a unitary biomedical etiology will be found to underlie all cases. Logically, this would remove Rett's syndrome from the Axis I domain of behaviorally-defined syndromes and place it on Axis III as a physical disorder.

Asperger's Syndrome

Another condition that may belong on the autistic spectrum is Asperger's syndrome (191). Where the syndrome described by Heller and Rett are severe variants of PDD, Asperger's syndrome is a milder variant, with normal or near-normal IQ and relatively good language skills. Asperger's syndrome also appears to be more common than Rett's or Heller's syndrome, with an estimated prevalence between 10 and 26 cases per 10,000 population (192).

Like Rett's syndrome, Asperger's syndrome was little known in the English-speaking world for many years. Early reports (193, 194) attracted little attention, and it was not until the 1980s that the syndrome began to be referred to with any frequency. An influential article by Wing (195) undoubtedly contributed to this trend. Asperger's syndrome too, has been included in DSM-IV.

There have been many descriptions of Asperger's syndrome (191, 195–198). Children with Asperger's syndrome typically are brought to clinical attention soon after they enter school. In early childhood, their behavior is odd but often not so unusual as to impel the parents to seek psychiatric advice. Anecdotal evidence suggests that these children often are slow to walk. Speech, too, may be delayed, but improves rapidly once begun. Parents report some as having first spoken in complete sentences. There may be language problems such as pronoun reversal, but these are more transient than in cases of Kanner autism. Imaginative play is apt to be impoverished, as in autism, but stereotypies are less common. Instead, the insistence on sameness takes the form of special interests. Children with Asperger's syndrome usually have one or two topics (such as trains or weather) to which they are passionately devoted, largely to the exclusion of all else. Often the same general topic continues to captivate them for many years. Occasionally these develop into useful careers.

Once children with Asperger's syndrome enter school, their deficits soon become apparent. Single-minded pursuit of their own interests, on their own schedule, conflicts with the demands of the structured classroom. Academic performance will be variable. Persons with Asperger's syndrome tend to excel in subjects requiring rote memorization, but tend to fail when problem-solving or higher-order conceptualization are needed. In elementary grades, this may entail high grades in reading and spelling, but poor performance in arithmetic.

Individuals with Asperger's syndrome are not socially withdrawn, but their attempts at social interaction are awkward and odd. Often they try to tell others about their special subjects, without regard for the responses of the other person. Their speech tends to be stilted and pedantic, with flat or exaggerated prosody and gesture. They have great difficulty understanding or following the rules of games, and tend to be clumsy. These characteristics are conducive to social isolation and peer rejection in school.

Persons with Asperger's Syndrome crave and pursue social contact and are keenly aware of the consequences of their social deficits. Sexual frustration is a major clinical issue in adolescence and adulthood, as is their frequent failure to achieve occupational goals in keeping with their academic work. They often seek clearly stated rules of conduct to guide them in their interactions, but their clumsy, rigid enactment of these "rules" seldom succeeds in winning them friends. Depression is a frequent complication, and there is evidence of a genetic link between Asperger's syndrome and affective disorders (155, 160, 199, 200). Unless school difficulties are extreme, or other psychiatric conditions develop, persons with Asperger's syndrome may not be brought to clinical attention. Tantam (201, 202) suggests that many patients with lifelong social isolation combined with eccentric behavior and interests may have Asperger's syndrome.

The majority of persons with Asperger's syndrome are scrupulously law-abiding, but a small subset do engage in rather bizarre antisocial actions, including cases of poisoning people, setting fire to occupied buildings, or assaulting people without apparent provocation (160, 191, 203–206). Often these actions are related to special interests of the attacker. Asperger construed these behaviors as motivated by spitefulness, which seems incompatible with an autistic lack of awareness of others' feelings. Frith (196) suggested that it is their very lack of empathy that underlies these behaviors. They are not motivated to hurt others, but if the pursuit of their interests calls for actions that might harm another person, they do not inhibit the behavior.

Kanner and Asperger worked independently and simultaneously, each describing what he believed to be a unique disorder, yet the two syndromes share unmistakable family resemblance, and most authors assume that the syndromes are related (198, 206). Some, however (207, 208), conceive of Asperger-type cases as schizoid personalities. There is, however, no evidence linking Asperger's syndrome with schizophrenia (202). Nagy and Szatmari (209) described a group of children meeting criteria for Schizotypal Personality Disorder who also could be diagnosed as Asperger's syndrome cases. Szatmari has regarded these cases as exemplifying autistic-spectrum disorders.

Is Asperger's syndrome a discrete diagnostic entity, or simply very high-functioning autism? Szatmari et al. (210) compared cases of Asperger's syndrome, high-functioning autism, and non-PDD psychiatric controls on a neuropsychological battery. Asperger's syndrome and high-functioning autism were indistinguishable. High-functioning autistic subjects did less well on the Wisconsin Card Sort Test and the Similarities test of the WISC-R, while Asperger's syndrome cases did less well on a pegboard task using their nondominant hand, but these differences, while statistically significant, did not allow for accurate group classification. Similarly, in a follow-up study of Asperger's syndrome and high-functioning autism, Szatmari et al. (211) found no qualitative differences between the groups, though high-functioning autistic subjects were more socially impaired and had more restricted interests, while Asperger's syndrome cases had more associated psychiatric problems. However, Ozonoff et al. (85) have reported cognitive differences between high-functioning autistic subjects and Asperger subjects matched for mental age: Asperger cases had higher verbal IQs and verbal memory than did the high-functioning autistic cases, and also performed better on "theory of mind" tests.

In sum, there are two differences between Asperger's syndrome and autism. First, autistic individuals perform well on visuospatial tasks and have severe language impairments; patients with Asperger's syndrome exhibit the opposite profile. These opposite skill profiles cannot easily be reconciled with the idea of a close relationship between the disorders. However, Asperger's syndrome does not involve normal use of language: pragmatic interactive skills are lacking. The second key difference is the motoric clumsiness often found in Asperger's syndrome. Tantam (205) noted that Asperger patients with the fewest gross neurological impairments exhibit the most clumsy behavior. He suggested that their clumsiness may reflect their many attempts to imitate the behavior of others. Clumsiness is less evident on self-taught tasks. The apparent motor deficit may be a manifestation of impaired imitation.

Several sets of diagnostic criteria were developed by investigators of Asperger's syndrome (192, 197, 212) before the disorder was finally included in ICD-10 and DSM-IV. One study (213) suggests that the ICD-10 criteria are more restrictive than are those unofficial criteria, chiefly because the diagnosis is disallowed in cases where language development is delayed. This presumably also holds true for the DSM-IV criteria, which are as follows: (a) Qualitative impairment in social interaction, as manifested by at least two of the following: Marked impairment in the use of multiple nonverbal behavior; Failure to develop peer relationships appropriate to developmental level; Lack of spontaneous seeking to share enjoyment, interests, or achievements with other people; or Lack of social or emotional reciprocity; (b) Restricted repetitive and stereotyped patterns of behavior, interests, and activities, as manifested by at least one of the following: Encompassing preoccupation with one or more stereotyped and restricted patterns of interest that is abnormal either in intensity or focus; Apparently inflexible adherence to specific, nonfunctional routines or rituals, stereotyped and repetitive motor mannerisms, or Persistent preoccupation with parts of objects; (c) The disturbance causes clinically significant impairment in social, occupational, or other important areas of functioning; (d) There is no clinically significant general delay in language; (e) There is no clinically significant delay in cognitive development or in the development of age-appropriate self-help skills, adaptive behavior (other than in social interaction), and curiosity about the environment in childhood (28).

Non-verbal (Social-Emotional) Learning Disabilities

Shea and Mesibov (214) have noted the lack of a clear boundary between high-functioning autism and severe learning disabilities, and family studies have suggested that certain milder cognitive and social disabilities may be part of the PDD spectrum. The classification of learning disabilities continues to be fraught with controversy. One distinction of possible value involves linguistic or academic skill disorders versus disturbances of social development. Discussion of dyslexia is beyond the scope of this chapter, but the less familiar social or nonverbal developmental disorders deserve mention because of their sometimes striking resemblance to the core disturbances of autism (215).

Gillberg's group (216, 217) studied children with a combination of "deficits in attention, motor control, and perception" (DAMP) and found that many of them also exhibited the triad of deficits in social relatedness, communication, and behavioral repertoire/imaginative activity typical of PDD children. Some met diagnostic criteria for Asperger's syndrome.

Based on the right (nondominant) cerebral hemisphere's apparent role in the comprehension and expression of emotion, visuospatial skills, and directed attention (see Chapter 18 of this volume), other researchers have sought to identify children with specific deficits in these functions. Thus, different authors speak of "developmental learning disabilities of the right hemisphere" (218), "right-hemisphere deficit syndrome" (219), and "social-emotional learning disability" (220, 221). Weintraub and Mesulam (218), for example, studied 14 cases, all of whom tended to avoid eye contact, none of whom used gesture normally, and only two of whom made proper use of prosody. The cases resembled high-functioning autism or Asperger's syndrome.

Rourke (222, 223) used a psychometric approach to identify a subgroup of learning disabled children with a syndrome he labels "nonverbal learning disability" (NLD). These children displayed a pattern of cognitive strengths and weaknesses opposite to dyslexia. Children with NLD were reported to be strong in phoneme-grapheme matching, rote verbal learning, and related psycholinguistic skills, but were impaired on visuospatial and nonverbal problem-solving tasks, including arithmetic. Rourke found psychomotor and tactile-perceptual deficits as well. Based on the awkward social behavior of NLD subjects, which includes disturbances in affect comprehension, gestural communication, and prosody, Rourke (223) suggested that the NLD syndrome represents the mild end of the autistic spectrum. Follow-up studies suggest that, as in Asperger's syndrome, persons with NLD tend to be stymied by the complex social demands of adult life, failing to find employment commensurate with their formal education and often lapsing into depression (223). Weintraub and Mesulam's (218) sample showed a similar pattern of difficulty with arithmetic, social isolation, and proneness to depression.

The justification for including Asperger's syndrome and right-hemisphere developmental disorder in the PDD spectrum is their autistic-like social impairment. Also, although both groups are competent in syntax and semantics, their language use nevertheless is impaired. Their communication has peculiar "one-way" quality: they speak only of their own interests, regardless of feedback. Their words often do not seem to be grounded in reality, but rather to exist on a purely abstract, mentalistic level.

DISORDERS NOT USUALLY REGARDED AS PART OF THE PDD SPECTRUM

Tourette's Syndrome and Obsessive-Compulsive Disorder

Tourette's syndrome is characterized by the presence of both motor and vocal tics, persisting for at least 1 year and typically following a chronic course (see Chapter 35 of this volume). Often as the disorder develops, the tics become increasingly complex and apparently meaningful. Some complex tics resemble the rituals and stereotypies found in autism and PDD. For example, common complex motor tics include seemingly ritualized walking behavior and self-injurious behaviors like self-biting; common complex vocal tics include repetition of phrases out of context. Studies have suggested that Tourette's syndrome and other chronic tic disorders are strongly influenced by genetic factors, and are associated with obsessive-compulsive disorder (OCD) (also reviewed in Chapter 35).

Tourette's syndrome is not regarded as a PDD spectrum disorder. Individuals with tic disorders are not impaired in social relatedness. Onset of Tourette's syndrome is later than autism (age 7 is the mean). Realmuto and Main (224) reported a single case of co-morbid autism and Tourette's syndrome but argued that the coincidence of the two disorders is at a chance level (20 cases per 100,000,000 population). One problem with this view is that autism, beginning earlier in life and usually more severe, is likely to overshadow the presence of Tourette's syndrome in all but the most extreme cases of the latter.

Other case reports of co-morbidity have been reported (25), including instances of Tourette's syndrome co-morbid with Asperger's syndrome (225). Cases also exist where Tourette-like symptoms occured in autism (226) or Asperger's syndrome (227) after long-term treatment with neuroleptics, but the significance of these reports is uncertain, as similar effects of neuroleptic administration have been observed in the absence of PDD (228).

It now appears likely that there is a relationship between at least some forms of PDD and Tourette's syndrome. Burd et al. (229) found Tourette's syndrome or chronic motor tics in 25% of a sample of 59 PDD patients, and noted that those who developed Tourette's syndrome tended to have higher IQ and better language skills, suggesting that the presence of tics might be associated with high-functioning autism and might even be a positive prognostic indicator. Comings and Comings (230) found 16 cases with a history of PDD in a sample of 1400 Tourette's syndrome patients, a proportion far exceeding that expected by chance, with an additional three cases where the proband had a near relative diagnosed with autism. Similarly, Sverd (231) has reported 13 cases of PDD with Tourette's syndrome or chronic motor tics from his clinical practice, a number well exceeding the total number of co-morbid cases expected by chance in his catchment area. A majority of Sverd's cases, too, were high-functioning autistic individuals. There also is evidence linking Tourette's syndrome with Asperger's syndrome (232).

In summary, clinicians will rarely have difficulty with the differential diagnosis of PDD and Tourette's syndrome, but may fail to identify cases where tics develop in individuals previously diagnosed with PDD. Because tics, unlike autistic symptoms, frequently respond to drug treatment, it is important not to allow the diagnosis of PDD to exclude the diagnosis of Tourette's syndrome. On a nosological level, the association of the two syndromes deserves further investigation and may provide useful clues to the pathogenesis of both conditions.

Given that Tourette's syndrome is linked with OCD, the association between PDD and Tourette's syndrome suggests the likelihood of a PDD-OCD connection. If complex motor tics can be difficult to distinguish from stereotypies, and complex vocal tics from delayed echolalia or stereotyped language, the distinction between autistic behaviors and OCD symptoms is even less clear. In OCD, unlike Tourette's syndrome, the behaviors are performed voluntarily, albeit under internally mediated pressure (Tourette's syndrome sufferers, too, feel mounting pressure when they resist their tics). Classically, OCD symptoms are differentiated from so-called psychotic ones largely by virtue of their ego-dystonic nature: the person resists engaging in them, and has insight into their senselessness. These criteria, however, frequently are not met by children with OCD (and sometimes not even by adults); DSM-IV no longer requires insight for the diagnosis of OCD in children. Obviously, there will be cases where distinguishing between an "overvalued idea" and preoccupation with a special interest will be a difficult and probably unreliable procedure. The boundary between PDD and OCD is an area of interest for future research.

Childhood Schizophrenia

The issue of a possible connection between PDD and childhood schizophrenia has a long history. At one time the two disorders were widely believed to be related (233), but the different age of onset and different symptomatology of the disorders (19, 234, 235) have clearly indicated otherwise. Kolvin (19) found delusions, hallucinations, blunted or incongruent affect, and loose associations to be more common in cases with onset after age 5 (i.e., childhood schizophrenia). He found gaze avoidance, odd preoccupations, disinterest in people, impoverished play, stereotypies, echolalia, and overactivity to be more common in cases with onset before age 3 (i.e., infantile autism).

Green et al. (236) verified these findings in a study that used DSM-III diagnostic criteria for the two disorders. Several studies (19, 236, 237) have found childhood schizophrenia to involve less intellectual impairment than infantile autism. In addition, Howells and Guirguis (238) found the schizophrenic symptomatology to be highly stable over a 20-year period.

Still, the notion of a close link between PDD and schizophrenia persists. Reports have been published of the two disorders occurring in the same individual. Petty et al. (239) described four cases of adult schizophrenia in persons with a history of infantile autism. Cantor (240-242), suggested that Kanner autism represents a particularly severe form of schizophrenic disturbance. Tantam (160) found that three subjects in his sample of 85 adults with a history of Asperger's syndrome could be considered schizophrenic, a figure slightly in excess of that which would be predicted by chance. Volkmar and Cohen (243) conducted a chart review of 163 adolescents and adults who had been diagnosed with infantile autism, finding only one case with a definite diagnosis of schizophrenia. It seems reasonable to conclude, barring future evidence to the contrary, that a pathogenetic link between PDD and schizophrenia is unlikely.

Developmental Receptive Language Disorder

Another problematic differential diagnosis is that between PDD and the class of developmental dysphasias (or childhood aphasias), termed Developmental Receptive Language Disorder in DSM-III-R (25). (See Chapter 31 of this volume for detailed accounts of language disorders.) Language disturbance is, after all, one of the cardinal features of infantile autism, and has even been posited to be the core deficit (14). The existence of PDD with apparently excellent command of language (as in Asperger's syndrome) militates against this position, except that even in these cases the pragmatic use of language seems to be markedly impaired. The most useful distinguishing characteristic is that children with receptive language disorders usually possess normal interpersonal relatedness and an interest in communicating with others via gestures, facial expressions, and intonation. At the same time, some children with deficient or absent comprehension of language do exhibit social deficits.

Bartak et al. (244) compared 19 autistic, 23 dysphasic, and five "mixed" diagnosis children, matched for nonverbal intelligence. They found that aberrant behavior in the past or present discriminated effectively between the groups, as did the nature of both past and current language behavior. Autistic subjects did less well on the Similarities, Comprehension, and Picture Arrangement subtests of the WISC, and were less able to comprehend the meaning of gestural communication. These findings suggest that differentiating between PDD and developmental dysphasia is relatively straightforward; however, about 20% of the sample could not clearly be classified as belonging to either diagnostic group. These subjects appeared to be autistic on some variables and dysphasic on others. Furthermore, the use of discriminant function analysis in single samples, as was done here, generally leads to an overestimate of the discriminability of two subgroups for the overall population. Cross-validation on a different sample is required before one may speak with confidence of the degree to which the groups may be differentiated.

Clarification of the distinction between PDD and developmental receptive language disorder will require large-scale longitudinal studies of children diagnosed with one or the other disorder, including assessment of changing status over the course of development. Such a study is currently underway by a group of investigators headed by Dr. Isabelle Rapin; extensive analyses of differences between autistic children and children with language disorders in development and in preschool functioning will be forthcoming soon. Results indicate somewhat different patterns of early language development; delay of comprehension milestones was more differentiating than delay of expressive milestones. Within the group of expressive milestones, delay in appearance of Wh-questions and connected sentences was most discriminating. Regression of language skills was also much more typical of the autistic spectrum than of language disorders. On formal language testing, somewhat different patterns of language skills appear; degree of deficit in comprehension is the single most differentiating feature of language, with the children with autism showing worse comprehension than the children with language disorders. The children with autism were also much less able to use meaning to assist in recall of verbal material. Although the children with language disorders were virtually normal in their pretend play, the high-functioning autistic children seemed able to engage in this kind of play but were unwilling or unable to sustain it.

Seizure Disorders

The link between autism and seizures dates back to Kanner's first sample of 18 children, two of whom went on to develop epileptic conditions. Estimates of the prevalence of seizures in autism range from one-quarter (245) to one-third (104) of autistic individuals. If autistic patients without seizures, but with abnormal EEGs, are added, then about half of all persons with autism exhibit epileptoid conditions. A biomodal distribution of age of seizure onset is frequently observed: infancy and adolescence are both high-risk periods. Seizures occur more often in individuals with lower IQ.

Tuchman et al. (246) reviewed a series of 314 autistic cases, and found a prevalence of epilepsy of 14%, but some individuals had not yet reached adolescence. Major risk factors for epilepsy were severe mental deficiency and motor deficit. Perinatal maternal disorder, a difficult perinatal course, and family history of epilepsy were not risk factors. The most frequent types of seizures were generalized tonic-clonic and atypical absence, followed by myolonic and partial seizures, followed by atonic seizures and infantile spasms.

Two other studies, one clinic-based (247) and one population based (248), have provided information about seizures in autism. Volkmar and Nelson (247) found that 21% of the 194 autistic patients evaluated had seizure histories, with onset occurring either in early childhood or adolescence. Because many of the subjects had not yet passed the peak risk years (mean age was 14.1), the adjusted lifetime co-morbidity estimate was 29%. Those with full-scale IQs below 50 were particularly likely to develop seizures (84.1%), and females were slightly more likely than males to suffer from seizures. Olsson et al. (248) found that 20% of prepubertal autistic children and 41% of prepubertal PDD children were experiencing seizures. Although autistic symptoms preceded seizures in all of the infantile autism cases, onset of seizure activity actually preceded the development of autistic symptoms in several autistic-like PDD cases. This supports the hypothesis, consistent with clinical observations, that early-onset seizures can play a causal role in the development of autistic-like behavior (249). If this is true, seizure disorders should be added to the list of medical conditions known to predispose to PDD.

ASSOCIATED BIOMEDICAL CONDITIONS

No single known biomedical condition plays a casual role in all cases of PDD, but a number of conditions have been connected with some cases of the disorder. It is uncertain whether the association of autism with a given medical condition is causal or a coincidence, but the possibility exists that some known medical disorders are capable of causing PDD. This could shed some light on the pathogenesis of autistic spectrum disorders generally. In addition, from a clinical perspective it is important to note any associated conditions whose presence might moderate the symptoms and/or course of PDD.

Gillberg (4) lists 16 medical conditions that have been linked with autism in at least two different studies: fragile X syndrome, marker chromosome syndrome, tuberous sclerosis, neurofibromatosis (but see Mouridsen et al. [250]), hypomelanosis of Ito (see Zappella [251], Smalley et al. [252], and Hunt and Shepherd [253]), Goldenhar's syndrome, Rett's syndrome, Moebius's syndrome, phenylketonuria (PKU), lactic acidosis, hypothyroidism, rubella embryopathy, herpes encephalitis, CMV infection, Williams syndrome, and Duchenne muscular dystrophy.

How commonly such conditions are comorbid with PDD is uncertain. Ritvo et al. (254) reported that 12% of their autistic subjects had associated medical disorders, but Gillberg's group (255), who conducted a thorough neurobiological workup on their sample, found that 37% had specific medical conditions. Gillberg (4) posited that if only the more standard diagnostic tests had been performed, the prevalence would have been 18%. PDD was frequently linked with the neurocutaneous disorders: tuberous sclerosis, neurofibromatosis, or hypomelanosis of Ito. Rutter et al. (256) estimate that 10% of all cases of autism have known biomedical causes, but add that this figure will be higher if profoundly retarded or "atypical" cases are included.

Two broad classes of medical conditions have been identified in autism/PDD: (*a*) those with a genetic basis (such as tuberous sclerosis or fragile X); and (*b*) those traceable to pre-, peri-, or postnatal insults or infections (such as rubella embryopathy or herpes encephalitis). Genetic conditions may represent familial traits or spontaneous mutations. A full discussion of all such conditions is beyond the scope of this chapter, but examples of each group are discussed in the sections that follows.

Genetic Syndromes

Of all the chromosomal abnormalities associated with PDD, the fragile X syndrome (fra(x)) has attracted the most interest. The fra(x) syndrome itself is a recent discovery. Although Martin and Bell (257) reported a form of X-linked mental retardation conforming to what is now recognized as the fra(x) phenotype in 1943, it was not until 1969 that Lubs (258) identified a chromosomal marker in four males with mental retardation in a single family. Reports of other families with the same cytogenetic marker came slowly, but by the late 1970s fra(x) syndrome was a widely recognized diagnostic entity. Estimates of the prevalence of fra(x) have been creeping upward as screening techniques improve. According to Sherman (259), prevalence of fra(x) with mental retardation is four to eight in 10,000 males, and two to six in 10,000 females. Because fra(x) is not always associated with mental retardation, its actual prevalence must be somewhat higher.

The classic fra(x) phenotype (260) involves large, prominent ears, a long, narrow face, and (in males, especially post pubertally) macroorchidism; at least 80% of all cases show one or more of these features. Other common characteristics include strabismus, hypotonia, tactile defensiveness, and recurrent otitis media. At least half of all fra(x) males are hyperactive as youngsters, and attentional deficits are universal. One in six fra(x) males develop seizures. In general, males are much more severely affected by fra(x) than are females, many of whom are very mildly affected. This, of course, is typical of X-linked traits, but fra(x) also displays a paradoxical pattern of transmission that cannot be accounted for by classic genetics (259).

Autism and autistic features are common in this population. Brown et al. (261) combined data from a number of studies and found fra(x) in 7.7%; in their own multisite sample, fra(x) was found in 13.1% of the males with autism. Similarly, Hagerman (260) suggested that 5–10% of all autistic individuals had the fra(x) anomaly, and that 15–30% of those with fra(x) syndrome are autistic. Some studies question the strength of the PDD-fra(x) connection. Einfeld et al. (262) found the rate of occurrence of fra(x) in autism to be no higher than in a mentally retarded sample matched for IQ. Similarly, Payton et al. (263) reported a rate of 2.4% in a sample of 85 autistic males. Piven et al. (264) also found a relatively low rate (2.7%) of fra(x) in a sample of 75 autistic individuals, but argued that the rate was high enough to be clinically significant. Bailey et al. (265) also found a fairly low rate, (1.6%) of fra(x) in several groups of autistic patients. The wide variability in rates of fra(x) among autistic individuals may be attributable not only to different diagnostic criteria for autism but to diagnostic thresholds for fra(x) expression that range from 1–4% (of X chromosomes) (136). Also, a large minority of known fra(x) gene carriers fail to express the anomaly at all (259).

The fra(x) PDD pattern is fairly distinctive (260). Compared with other autistic patients, fra(x) patients are less likely to show echolalia but more likely to display perseverative speech. Hand flapping, hand biting, and hyperactivity are more common in fra(x) than in other forms of PDD. The most interesting distinguishing characteristic of fra(x) "autism" is that fra(x) cases generally are not aloof; rather, they are interested in social interactions, but experience intense social anxiety. Cohen et al. (266) studied gaze patterns in fra(x) males and non-fra(x) autistic males, and found that although the non-fra(x) subjects tended to ignore parent-initiated eye contact, the fra(x) subjects were highly sensitive to eye contact but found it aversive. Nonautistic fra(x) males also display gaze avoidance while making a social approach (267).

The neuropsychological performance characteristic of fra(x) syndrome was reviewed by Pennington et al. (268). Among males, IQ is most often in the 35–50 range; there is some evidence of a decline in IQ at puberty. Reading tends to be a relative strength, and mathematics, a relative weakness. Long-term memory is better than short-term memory. Findings with respect to visual-motor skills are mixed. Receptive language skills are superior to language production. Articulation difficulties reminiscent of developmental dyspraxia are common, as is cluttered speech. Spontaneous speech is often repetitive, incoherent, and littered with interjections. Prosody tends to be deviant: "jocular" and "litany-like" patterns are described.

Females are much more variable in functioning. Carrier females are relatively unaffected. Although fra(x)-positive females have a mean IQ of about 85, most of those with IQs above 85 still evince cognitive impairments. Typically, verbal skills are superior to visual-spatial skills, and arithmetic abilities are particularly poor. The cognitive profiles of fra(x)-positive individuals resemble those of autistic spectrum disorders and nonverbal learning disabilities (268).

Another genetic condition, albeit a very rare one, merits brief mention: Joubert's syndrome, an autosomal-recessive trait whose major feature is agenesis of the cerebellar vermis. Mental retardation, abnormal eye movements, poor muscle tone, ataxia, and tongue protrusion are typical. Fewer than 100 cases have been described, and little is known about the behavioral or neuropsychological profiles that may characterize Joubert syndrome, but given recent findings of underdeveloped cerebellar vermis in autistic patients (269) and fragile X syndrome (270), one would predict autistic features in Joubert's syndrome patients. Holroyd et al. (271) report on two cases of Joubert's syndrome, one of whom met full criteria for infantile autism while the other manifested partial autism. These preliminary, findings are consistent with recent neuroanatomical research in autism.

Teratogenic Factors

Given the presumed connections between autistic symptoms and CNS dysfunction, and between central nervous system (CNS) dysfunction and prenatal, perinatal, and neonatal insults, quite possibly some cases of autism might be traceable to neurological damage acquired during gestation, delivery, or the first hours of life.

There is a high prevalence of autism and autistic-like features among children who suffered congenital rubella. Chess (272) reported that 18 of 243 with congenital rubella displayed autistic symptoms, 10 of whom had a form of autism. This represents a prevalence rate more than 100 times that in the population at large. Chess (273) followed up on these children when they were 8 and 9 years of age; all but one of those previously judged autistic were reevaluated. Six had made a full recovery, but four other children had begun to exhibit autistic features in their interim. The high recovery rate suggested to Chess that the autistic-like illness was part of a chronic infection running its course.

Such clear-cut casual connections between specific gestational or obstetrical conditions and autism are rarely found. However, a majority of studies of possible perinatal insult (140, 274–277) have found that autism is associated with difficult pregnancies and deliveries, though this finding is not universal (278, 279). It is likely that the obstetrical problems are secondary to fetal abnormalities, rather than causal (280, 281).

Finegan and Quarrington (275) found that autistic children, but not their siblings, had a high incidence of various obstetrical problems: breech delivery, low birth weight, low Apgar scores, elevated bilirubin, and respiratory distress syndrome. Deykin and MacMahon (140) obtained similar findings in a considerably larger sample. Prenatally, maternal accidents or heavy bleeding were several times more common among the autistic subjects: emergency cesarean sections and hemorrhage were the most powerful discriminators. At birth, many more autistic children were slow to cry and/or were of low birth weight. Two limitations of this study should be noted: (a) diagnostic criteria for autism were very loose; and (b) the autistic children (unlike controls) were predominantly male, and male children in general have mothers with a higher incidence of pregnancy and birth complications than female children. Gillberg and Gillberg (276) corrected for the latter problem in a population-based study that examined the obstetrical records of autistic children and sex-matched controls. They also developed an objective checklist of possible complications and derived a reduced optimality score. Twelve (48%) of the autistic subjects had scores above those of all but one (95%) of the control group. Both prenatal and neonatal scores discriminated effectively between the groups. Bleeding during pregnancy and signs of clinical dysmaturity were the best discriminators between groups. Other problems, such as severe maternal infection, generalized edema during pregnancy, and low Apgar scores, were also more common among the autistic children. Only those autistic children with reduced optimality in the prenatal period showed reduced optimality perinatally or as neonates, so peri- and neonatal problems may be signals of nonoptimal pregnancy rather than independent risk factors.

Mason-Brothers et al. (279) found that maternal bleeding and influenza-like symptoms were less frequent in mothers who had more than one autistic child. Finally, Bryson et al. (274) used an expanded version of Gillberg and Gillberg's reduced optimality scale to compare autistic children from their epidemiological study with several control groups. Reduced optimality scores were significantly greater for the autistic sample than for the controls. Autistic children showed delayed crying, respiratory distress syndrome, and anemia as neonates. Maternal bleeding was a significant risk factor for autism. However, reduced optimality scores characterized only 25% of the autistic group.

These results must be set against other, negative findings (278, 279). Still, the preponderance of evidence converges to support the hypothesis that certain pregnancy and birth complications may cause some cases of autism.

NEUROANATOMICAL FINDINGS

Studies of neuroanatomical abnormalities in autism have relied upon postmortem neuropathologic examinations and imaging techniques such as computerized tomography (CT) and magnetic resonance imaging (MRI). These methods have produced inconsistent findings and have uncovered great variability within the autistic population (282–285).

The cerebral cortex has not been found to be consistently abnormal in autistic subjects (285–289). Individual malformations have been reported, however, including cerebral lipidosis (290), microgyria and schizencephaly (291), slight enlargement of parieto-occipital regions in the right hemisphere (292), and slightly lower counts of glia in the primary auditory cortex of the left hemisphere, and of auditory association cortex pyramidal neurons in the right hemisphere (287).

Neuroanatomical studies with autistic patients have provided some evidence for involvement of hippocampus and amygdala. In an early pneumoencephalographic study, Hauser, DeLong and Rosman (293) noted temporal horn enlargement that was most prominent in the area in which the hippocampus should protrude into the ventricle. In a postmortem investigation, Baumen and Kemper (286) found that the hippocampus and selected nuclei of the amygdala showed abnormally increased cell packing density and diminished neuron size. Baumen and Kemper's (286, 294) neuroanatomical investigations have also revealed six consistent cases of limbic pathology, including abnormalities of the entorhinal cortex, anterior cingulate gyrus, septal nuclei, and mamillary bodies, all of which appeared to have occurred 30 weeks' gestation. A case study of a child with temporal lobe tumor also implicated the amygdala and hippocampus, when he was found to display autistic-like behaviors that persisted after a substantial loss of surrounding tissue sustained during tumor extraction (295). A recent case study also reported 2 boys with autistic regression which appeared with limbic lesions and epilepsy (296).

Fein and Waterhouse (297, 298) have suggested that a primary impairment in autism is assignment of affective significance to social and novel stimuli, stemming from dysfunction of amygdala and related limbic structures. Similar ideas have been suggested by Bachevalier (299), Brothers (300) and Fotheringham (301).

Many studies of the cerebellum have produced findings of neuroanatomical differences between the autistic and normal brain (302). Purkinje and granule cell loss within cerebellar tissue of autistic subjects has been observed by several researchers (286, 289, 303), and both total cerebellum size and cerebellum hemisphere size as measured from MRI have been found to be reduced in autistic subjects as compared with normal controls (304, 305). When compared with normal and neurologically disordered subjects, autistic individuals have been found to show hypoplasia of neocerebellar vermal lobules VI and VII (269, 305). More recently, re-analysis of cerebellar vermal data revealed hypoplastic *and* hyperplastic subtypes in autism (302). The vermal lobules VI and VII have been implicated in auditory startle response and heart rate response (306), both of which have been found to be abnormal in autistic subjects (307, 308). The association between neocerebellar vermal hypoplasia and autistic symptomology is supported by findings related to the genetic disorder described earlier, namely, Joubert's syndrome, which marked by underdevelopment of the cerebellar vermis. Again children with Joubert's syndrome display symptoms such as social-communicative deficits, stereotypic behavior, perseveration, and a restricted and unusual range of interests (271). The hypoplasia of vermal lobules VI and VII has been proposed to result from a circumscribed loss of Purkinje and granule cells during prenatal or early postnatal neural genesis and migration (309). Measurement with the use of MRI, including scans of the midsagittal area of the ventral pons, led some researchers to conclude that cerebellar hypoplasia is a product not of deficient input or output, but rather of pathological development within the cerebellum itself (310). Courchesne (311) has hypothesized that damage to the neocerebellum disrupts the coordination of rapid shifts of selective attention, causing stimulus overselectivity, restriction of activities, and impaired concept formation. All of these effects are thought to ultimately impair social interchange in autism. Patients with cerebellar damage were found to have similar impairment to autistic patients in rapid attention shifting (312), however, this finding cannot be taken as evidence that cerebellar abnormality is responsible for autistic symptoms. In fact, Cieselski (313) found that cerebellar vermal abnormality is not specific to autism and that its associated sequelae are not consistently "autistic" in nature. The involvement of neocerebellar vermal hypoplasia in autism was also challenged when studies revealed no differences in cerebellar lobules between young autistic subjects and controls (314, 315).

Generally, studies of neuroanatomical deficits in autistic

patients have produced a wide variety of findings, proving great variability among the autistic population. Some neuroanatomical theories of autism have implicated the brainstem, hippocampus, limbic system and cerebellum. Currently, the most consistent findings appear to be of abnormalities in the cerebellum, and in the hippocampus, amygdala and other limbic nuclei.

NEUROPHYSIOLOGICAL INVESTIGATIONS

Studies of the neurophysiology of autism generally attempt to assess deficits in sensory-perceptual functioning, information processing, and their neuroanatomical substrates through the use of methods that rely mainly on the measurement of metabolic or electrical activity.

Cerebral Activity: Glucose Metabolism and Cerebral Blood Flow

A study investigating correspondence between metabolic and neuroanatomical imaging methods found that 11 of 13 autistic cases showed consistency across methods, in which 4 of the 13 had metabolic abnormality corresponding with abnormal structural imaging results (316).

Based on neuroanatomical findings of cerebellar deficits, Heh and colleagues (317) assessed function of the cerebellum through positron emission tomography (PET) measurement of regional glucose metabolic rate (rGMR). No significant regional deficiencies were found; however, all autistic subjects displayed glucose utilization rates greater than or equal to rates of normal subjects. This finding was consistent with earlier findings of diffuse, whole brain glucose hypermetabolism in the absence of regional deficiencies in autistic subjects (318). Another study involving auditory processing tasks, however, found neither any evidence of global glucose hypermetabolism nor any differences between autistic and normal subjects with respect to regional cerebral blood flow and oxygen consumption (319). More recent studies show that young autistic adults fail to show the hemispheric assymetry in both cortical and specific regional GMR found for normals during testing state and attention tasks, as well as abnormally high GMR in varying regions (320, 321).

Recent studies of regional cerebral blood flow (rCBF) using single photon emission computerized tomography (SPECT) in autistic children have shown the frontal hypoperfusion characteristic of much younger children, that normalizes with maturation; this led the authors to conclude that frontal development is delayed in autism (322). Deutsch (323) cautions, however, that hypofunction of the frontal lobes, as measured by CBF or GMR, is not specific to autism and may be secondary to other pathology. The evidence appears to suggest that frontal hypofunction observed in autism and other disorders is a reflection of disruptions in mental activity that are actually caused by other pathologies. CBF studies have also shown diminished CBF in the temporal lobes, and reversal of normal hemispheric

temporo-occiptal asymmetry in response to auditory stimuli, while others find a total absence of regional abnormalities (324–326).

A recent preliminary study using ^{31}P nuclear magnetic resonance spectroscopy (NMRS) in dorsal prefrontal cortex of high-functioning autistic males revealed low levels of high-energy phosphate and membrane phospholipid, and high levels of membrane metabolites, correlating with low scores on neuropsychological measures and language tests (327). These findings were taken as an indication of membrane hypermetabolism and hyposynthesis in autism.

Retinal Function

The introduction of electroretinography to the study of autism was based on a potential animal model with a genetic syndrome involving both depletion of cerebellar Purkinje cells and retinal dysfunction (328). In measuring currents produced in the retina by flashes of light, the electroretinogram (ERG) can provide assessment of retinal dysfunction through readings of b-wave amplitudes, which were found in a pilot study to be significantly lower in 48% of autistic subjects (328). Originally attributed to maturational delay or retinal abnormality (328), subnormal b-wave amplitudes were later hypothesized to result from dopaminergic dysfunction, as b-wave amplitudes arise in an area of the retina in which dopamine is the main neurotransmitter (329). Subnormal b-wave readings were further suggested to be rooted in the aberrant production of melatonin, which is involved in the regulation of dopamine (330).

Cerebral Electrical Recording

Cerebral electrical recordings have enabled investigators to identify deficits in sensory processing from waves derived from EEGs and, more specifically, event-related brain potentials (ERPs). Studies have found general abnormalities in basic EEG readings in autistic subjects, including irregular activity and desynchronous rhythms, but have failed to establish specific patterns of pathology (331).

Ornitz and Ritvo (13) discovered through analysis of auditory-evoked responses (AERs) that autistic children under age 5 failed to display normal inhibition of sensory responses during the oculomotor burst phase of REM: the relative amplitude of wave N2, which reflects basic sensory response, was abnormally increased. This suppressed inhibition of sensory response was believed to relate to autistic children's impaired perception of sensory input, and was hypothesized to stem from vestibular system dysfunction (13). Autistic subjects were also found to have diminished phasic oculomotor activity during REM sleep in response to vestibular stimulation, further suggesting vestibular and REM disorganization (332).

These findings, combined with clinical observations of spinning and of unresponsiveness to stimuli, led to studies of the vestibular responses of autistic children, which have been found to be abnormal (297, 333–336). Several researchers have demonstrated that autistic children show a suppression of post-rotatory nystagmus, a vestibularly-induced oculomotor response (333, 335, 336). Autistic children generally have been found to have abnormally low oculomotor output in response to vestibular stimulation in the presence of visual stimulation (335). Recent studies have found prolonged time constants of the nystagmus response to acceleration and deficiencies in recorded nystagmus beats (297). Ornitz and colleagues (297, 336) have concluded that abnormalities in nystagmus response may be caused by dysfunction of the vestibular nuclei in the brainstem.

Brainstem dysfunction was a prevalent hypothesis in autism research in the 1960s and 1970s (12, 13, 297, 332, 334, 336, 337). Brainstem dysfunction has been found in a subgroup of autistic subjects, in the form of abnormalities on brainstem auditory-evoked potentials, including higher inter-trial ERP variability, and delayed latencies for waves I, III, IV, and V, especially at lower stimulus intensities (338–347). Studies finding no brainstem dysfunction using evoked potential techniques appear to have tested older children with higher IQs.

The physiological substrate of perceptual and cognitive processing is thought to be reflected in middle to longer latency components, or waves, of the ERP. Models of autism as a disorder of attention and information processing have implicated frontal cortex, basal ganglia (348) and the limbic system (348, 349). Findings from many evoked potential studies offer tentative support for these models (341, 350–358). High-functioning autistic subjects of varying ages have usually shown abnormally small amplitudes for the long-latency, auditory-evoked wave P3b, which is thought to reflect the cognitive processes of detection and classification of target stimuli (341, 350–354, 357, 359). Dawson and colleagues (354) found P3 amplitudes diminished in response to phonetic, but not musical stimuli at central-cortical and left-hemisphere recording sites. Interestingly, the P3 amplitude has been found in autistic subjects to be higher in response to affective-prosodic stimuli than to linguistic-prosodic stimuli (360).

Studies have sought to distinguish deficits in voluntary, selective attention from sensory-perceptual dysfunction in autistic subjects have examined wave component Nc and the negative difference waves known as auditory Nd and N270. These components involve frontal neural activity and are thought to reflect uncued self-generated attention. Investigators have found abnormally small amplitudes of component Nc (353, 361), and total absences of wave Nd and N270 (350) in autistic subjects. Investigations of orientation and processing of novel stimuli in autism have revealed diminished amplitude for components A/Pcz/300 and A/Pcz/800, which are thought to reflect the physiological process of detection of unexpected and novel "biological significant" stimuli (351, 361).

Other neurophysiological studies have found disrupted patterns of normal hemispheric lateralization (362–365), including diminished left-hemisphere EEG α-attenuation

(366) and right temporoparietal ERP N1 amplitude augmentation (367) in response to phonetic processing.

Results have suggested that although autistic individuals seem to be able to attend to stimuli sufficiently to complete tasks and are apparently neither hypersensitive nor oblivious to novelty as was suspected, they may possess abnormal mechanisms for that processing and selection of stimuli. These perhaps compensate for frontal cortical dysfunction (350, 351, 353, 361).

Summary of Neurophysiological Findings

Neurophysiological studies of autism have found tentative support for inefficient metabolism, sensory processing deficits, abnormalities in retinal function, indicating dopaminergic involvement, and vestibular dysfunction, suggesting brainstem pathology. The largest body of physiological evidence for brain dysfunction has been generated from studies of ERPs. Auditory-evoked ERPs have revealed delays in basic brainstem auditory processing for a subgroup of autistic patients. Attenuated longer-latency ERPs in autistic subjects have suggested disruptions in attention and information processing. Overall, findings may suggest a disruption of brainstem systems, which has been tentatively supported by some neuroanatomical findings (286, 294, 304). The failure of many other studies to find corroborating anatomical evidence for brainstem disruption may reflect a limitation of this line of research: given both the complexity of the nervous system and the network of neurochemical systems, it is possible that abnormalities may be present anywhere in a given neurochemical pathway and thus not even visible as a gross microscopic lesion. The most reasonable expectation of neuropathology may be one that is based upon a neurochemical hypothesis.

NEUROCHEMICAL CORRELATES OF AUTISM

Studies of the neurochemical correlates of autism have focused mainly on the assessment of blood and cerebrospinal fluid (CSF) levels of primary neurotransmitters and peptides. CSF levels of transmitter metabolites directly reflect abnormalities in central metabolism and thus are usually thought to be stronger indicators of CNS vulnerabilities (368). Aberrations in synthesis, metabolism, and receptor function have been hypothesized as being responsible for the diverse symptomology associated with autism. The neurochemical studies that have explored these possibilities vary greatly with respect to the size and composition of their autistic and control samples. Caution is thus advised when comparing and interpreting their findings.

Serotonin

The neurochemical exploration of autism began with the investigation of the monoamine neurotransmitter serotonin (5HT)(369), which has been implicated in the brain's regulation of many functions relevant to PDD, including learning, memory, sensory, and motor processes (370). Existing research has failed to characterize the precise relationship between 5HT and autism, as both central and peripheral 5HT disruptions have been implicated.

Studies of serotonergic abnormalities have measured 5HT in whole blood and plasma, and its principal metabolite 5-hydroxyindoleacetic acid (5HIAA) in urine and CSF. The occurrence of higher levels of whole blood, plasma, and platelet 5HT in autistic children relative to normal controls, a phenomenon referred to as hyperserotonemia, is the most solidly documented neurochemical finding in autism research. Numerous studies have been demonstrated that approximately 30% of the autistic children exhibit hyperserotonemia (371). Hyperserotonemia appears to be a familial phenomenon, as 5HT levels are correlated between autistic children and their family members (372–374). In fact, approximately 40% of hyperserotonemic autistic patients have been found to have family members that also show hyperserotonemia (375). Hyperserotonemia has been suggested as a marker for familial genetic liability for autism/PDD, because 5HT levels have been found to be higher in autistic children who have siblings with PDD symptomology than in those with normal siblings (376). Although hyperserotonemia forms a consistent subgroup of autism, it is not unique to autism: it has been found in other behavior disorders (377) and mental retardation (369, 378-380). Moreover, hyperserotonemia has not been linked to any specific behavioral or cognitive profiles within autism (381).

The precise cause of hyperserotonemia in autism is unknown. Some researchers have investigated the role of $5HT_{1A}$ receptor binding inhibition in creating excess blood 5HT. Examination of circulating autoantibodies against the $5HT_{1A}$ receptor found no correlation between inhibition of 5HT cortical membrane binding and elevated 5HT levels for autistic patients (382), and immunoglobulins isolated from plasma of autistic children showed no apparent differences in inhibition of binding of a $5HT_{1A}$ agonist in hippocampal membrane compared to controls (383).

While central 5HT disruption has been hypothesized by many researchers, blood 5HT levels can only safely be interpreted as reflections of peripheral mechanisms. Because platelet 5HT accounts for over 99% of whole-blood 5HT levels, hyperserotonemia may be a reflection of abnormal platelet 5HT mechanisms (373), whether in disruptions in uptake and release, greater platelet storage ability, or increased platelet number or size (384, 385).

Investigations of platelet uptake and release in autism have yielded conflicting findings. Relatively decreased uptake was found in subjects with autistic features and mental retardation (386, 387), but other studies have found no decreases (388–391) or increased uptake (392, 393). It is important to remember that there is great individual variability in platelet 5HT uptake (394). An investigation of the imipramine binding site, thought to label the 5HT uptake site, revealed no differences between autistic and normal subjects (395). Platelet 5HT efflux in autistic individuals was found to be twice as rapid as normal (388,

396). Later investigations, however, did not replicate this finding (389, 391). Studies of platelet 5HT receptor binding sites have also yielded conflicting results: both normal and reduced numbers of sites have been found in autistic subjects (397, 398).

Serotonin receptors located on the blood platelet may serve as models for 5HT neuronal receptor function. As central 5HT receptors are known to modulate 5HT-potentiated platelet aggregation, disruptions in platelet aggregation magnitude may indicate systemic 5HT receptor dysfunction (397). Investigations of platelet function have suggested abnormalities in platelet aggregation in autistic subjects, including decreased plasma β-thromboglobulin and platelet factor 4, slight trends for decreased aggregability in response to adenosine disphosphate (ADP) and collagen, higher ADP threshold concentrations (399, 400), and subnormal 5HT-induced increases in ADP-induced aggregation (397).

Hyperserotonemia could be caused by increased synthesis or decreased metabolism of 5HT; however, there is no consistent evidence for this in autism. Launay and colleagues (401) investigated several of the possible causes of hyperserotonemia, including decreased platelet 5HT release, increased platelet uptake, decreased metabolism and increased synthesis: only metabolism and synthesis were found to be disrupted. Changes in platelet monoamine oxidase (MAO), which breaks 5HT down into 5HIAA, were found to have no effect on urine 5HIAA levels (401), which suggested disrupted 5HT metabolism. (Platelet levels of MAO in autistic patients have been consistently found to be no different from those of normal individuals [389, 402, 403]). High levels of free plasma tryptophan (chemical precursor for 5HT) and radiochromatographic findings both suggested overactive 5HT synthesis. Increased peripheral 5HT synthesis will also be reflected by urine levels of 5HIAA (404). However, while high 5HT urine levels have been found in one study (405), urinary 5HT and 5HIAA are more often found to be normal (380, 406, 407). Urine 5HIAA has not been found to correlate with blood 5HT, which suggests that synthesis may not in fact be disrupted.

Central 5HT dysfunction in autism has been investigated through examination of CSF levels of 5HIAA. Studies of CSF 5HIAA levels have revealed no consistent, significant differences between normal and autistic subjects. 5HIAA was found to be relatively lower in one study of children with PDD, yet no different from the controls in later investigations (403, 408, 409). These findings suggest that the hyperserotonemia observed in autistic individuals may reflect a purely peripheral mechanism.

Clinical trials with fenfluramine have provided evidence for involvement of central serotonergic systems in autism: however, its mechanism is unclear. By blocking 5HT uptake, fenfluramine acts to increase synaptic levels of 5HT. After chronic administration, fenfluramine can result in the reduction of 5HT blood levels up to 57% in autistic children (410). Several studies have revealed ameliorative effects of fenfluramine on autistic symptomology, usually in the form of decreased hyperactivity, stereotypies, and inattentiveness (410–419). Although fenfluramine has been expected to improve cognitive and social functioning in addition to motor behavior, the results of clinical trails have been generally conflicting. Several recent investigations (420, 421) have found no improvements in either motor, social, or intellectual features, while Ekman et al. (422) found improvement only in motor functioning, and Stern et al. (423) found insignificant improvements in cognitive and language skills. A nationwide multicenter study by the UCLA Neuropsychiatric Institute found fenfluramine had greatest effect on motor disturbances in autistic subjects with low baseline peripheral 5HT levels and high baseline performance IQs (415). Although these findings support the idea of a modulatory role of 5HT in autistic symptomology, some difficulties arise with this thinking. If excessive 5HT is in fact directly related to autistic symptomology, fenfluramine should be more efficacious in reducing autistic symptoms in patients with high 5HT levels. However, fenfluramine appears to be *less* effective with this subgroup. Furthermore, research has shown that fenfluramine-induced changes in 5HT levels do not always coincide with changes in autistic symptoms (424). This suggests that hyperserotonemia may not directly contribute to autistic symptomology, and/or that central serotonergic dysfunction may not be related to hyperserotonemia.

Some animal laboratory studies have provided evidence for involvement of elevated central 5HT in autistic-like behaviors, such as restricted range of activity and avoidance of novel situations (425–427), inhibited startle response (428, 429), and disrupted attachment behavior (430, 431). The basic literature is filled with demonstrations of many different behavioral functions of 5HT, many of which do not contribute to our understanding of its relationship to autism. The lack of concordance among laboratory and clinical studies underscores the need for a coherent guiding theory for the role of 5HT in autism.

Dopamine

The catecholamine dopamine has been implicated in such functions as stimulus-reward mechanisms, selective attention, motor activity, and cognition (385). The are several primary dopaminergic systems within the brain that are of particular interest in relation to autism. The nigrostriatal dopaminergic system, which is known to modulate sensorimotor integration and response coordination and selection (432), arises in the substantia nigra of the midbrain and projects to the basal ganglia, limbic and cortical structures, including the caudate and putamen. The mesolimbic system originates in the ventral tegmental area of the midbrain and projects to the nucleus accumbens. It is believed to modulate motivational behavior. Damasio and Maurer (348) hypothesized that abnormalities in dopaminergic input from the mesolimbic and nigrostriatal pathways might account for some autistic symptoms, specifically the unusual motoric features such as stereotypies. This model was later refined, targeting the pathway that arises in the brainstem and projects to mesolimbic structures as the locus of dopaminergic overactivity (433, 434). Coleman and Gillberg (433) have implicated this pathway in the interpersonal-perceptual deficits of autism. The nigrostriatal system has been found to modulate stereotypies (435) and may contribute to the unusual motor behaviors of autism.

Observations of hypothalamic dysregulation (436) and hyposensitive hypothalamic dopamine receptors in individuals with autistic features (437) may also implicate a third dopaminergic system, which arises in the hypothalamus and projects to the pituitary gland. Although this system is known to regulate the hormone prolactin, its contribution to the autistic syndrome is unclear.

As in serotonin research, investigation of the role of dopamine in autism has concentrated mainly on measurement of the neurotransmitter and its principal metabolite (homovanillic acid) in plasma, platelets, urine, and CSF. Attempts to assess plasma and platelet dopamine and urinary homovanillic acid (HVA) have yielded conflicting results that generate evidence for both augmented and depressed levels (438–445), including elevations of both free and conjugated HVA (446). Aside from urinary HVA, the majority of which is believed to originate in the brain, most plasma and urinary dopamine and HVA appear to originate peripherally (404). As such, plasma and urine levels are usually not considered to be as reliably reflective of central dopamine activity in the brain as CSF levels of HVA (385).

Gillberg and colleagues (408, 447) found elevated CSF levels of HVA that were correlated with a degree of autistic symptomology. This finding failed to replicate, however (409, 448). Probenecid administration is sometimes used to block the transport of metabolites out of CSF, to permit more reliable assessment of transmitter metabolism. Using this method, Cohen and colleagues (403, 449) found a subgroup of autistic children with severe symptoms of motor overactivity and stereotypies to have elevated CSF HVA when compared to autistic subjects without these behaviors. Further investigation of abnormalities in dopaminergic function is warranted, both the existing neurochemical evidence for dopaminergic dysfunction in autism is conclusive.

Clinical pharmacological trials have provided more consistent evidence for the role of dopamine in autism. Neuroleptics, which act as dopamine antagonists, have been found to inhibit the symptoms of autism in children, while the dopamine agonists, which have stimulant properties, may exacerbate the symptoms (450). One to two months of treatment with the neuroleptics pimozide (451) or haloperidol (452, 453), or 6 months of treatment with haloperidol (454) improved abnormal speech patterns, social unrelatedness, stereotypies, and inattention/hyperactivity. Conversely, experimental trials with amphetamines such as dextroamphetamine resulted in the exacerbation of the same symptoms (455). The correlation between expression of symptoms and level of dopaminergic activity suggests some causal role for dopamine in autism.

Laboratory research has uncovered relationships between dopamine and autistic-like symptoms. The mesolimbic and mesocortical DA pathways have been found to be involved with incentive reward mechanisms (456–460). Accordingly, the self-stimulatory activities, absence of interest in conventionally gratifying pursuits, and relative resistance to conditioning present in autistic children may reflect mesolimbic and mesocortical DA pathway disruption. Laboratory administration of dopamine agonists to animals induces stereotypies and self-stimulation, while administration of selected dopamine antagonists to mice results in reduction of stereotypies (461–463). Chronic administration of the dopamine agonist amphetamine to mice has resulted in self-injurious behavior and disruption of normal social relations (464). These effects are parallel to those seen in clinical pharmacological trials with autistic children. In general, a number of clinical medication trials and animal studies suggest possible hyperactivity of the dopaminergic system in autism.

Norepinephrine and Epinephrine

The catecholamines norepinephrine (NE) and epinephrine (E) function as hormones and neurotransmitters, and both have been found to be involved in the regulation or arousal, attention, activity level, anxiety, responses to stress, memory, and learning. Assessment of NE and E activity has been through measurement of CSF levels of NE's primary metabolite, 3-methoxy-4-hydroxy-phenylglycol (MHPG) and plasma, platelet, and urine levels of NE, E, and MHPG. The findings are inconsistent. Increases have been found among autistic subjects in plasma NE (402, 442, 443) and platelet NE (443), but not in plasma MHPG (465, 466). Plasma NE levels are thought to reflect central activity, because they correlate highly with levels of CSF MHPG (467, 468). But although studies have shown increased plasma levels of NE in autistic subjects, CSF MHPG has not been found to be significantly different from normal controls (385, 408). The source of this contradiction is unclear. Findings for urine levels are also opposite to expectations of increase, given plasma findings: decreases in NE, E, and MHPG (466, 469) have been found. Similarly, plasma measurement of dopamine-β-hydroxylase (DBH), the enzyme that synthesizes NE from DA, has yielded mixed results: both depressed levels (402) and no differences from normal controls have been reported (440, 470, 471). A more recent study found disruptions in levels of catecholamine metabolites but no association with genetic markers coding for enzymes involved in catecholamine synthesis (472). Other investigators recently found no abnormalities in plasma and urine MHPG or urinary excretion rates of NE, E, and vanillylmandelic acid (VMA), leading them to conclude there is no apparent adrenergic/noradrenergic dysfunction in autism (473).

Peptides

Observations of the similarities between the symptoms of opiate addiction and autism (471) and the role of opioids in the attenuation of the emotional perception of pain have led some researchers to implicate endorphins in autism. Elevated endorphin levels are hypothesized to contribute to the development of autistic symptoms, particularly deficits in attachment and social interaction and self-injurious behaviors caused by elevated pain threshold (471, 474). The endogenous opioids appear to be strong candidates as modulators of socioemotional mechanisms. This is because they are distributed in areas of the brain known to integrate sensation and emotion (430, 475). Their role in emotional behavior has been supported by relevant animal models.

Peripheral levels of β-endorphin are understood to have an inverse, negative feedback relationship with central opioid activity, in which excesses in brain opioids are expected to be reflected by low plasma levels (476). Such has been the finding from several investigations of opioid levels in autism, which have demonstrated low plasma endorphin levels (477, 478) and increased CSF endorphin levels (479, 480). Plasma measurement of β-endorphin via radioimmunoassay reveals variable immunoreactivity dependent upon the use of C-versus N-terminally directed antisera (481). Nonautistic self-injuring individuals also display low plasma and high CSF opioid levels (479), which suggests that impairment of the opioid system may contribute to the autistic syndrome primarily through disruption of pain and reinforcement mechanisms.

Clinical pharmacological trials with opiate antagonists naloxone and, more reliably, naltrexone have proven somewhat successful in improving autistic symptomology (482). Studies of naloxone and naltrexone administration have demonstrated decreases in the frequency of self-injurious behavior; decreases in stereotypic motor behavior, decreases in hyperactivity and increases in social and communicative behaviors (483–494). Recent open and double blind studies of naltrexone report successful treatment of symptoms, and claim that naltrexone acted to lower abnormally high levels of β-endorphin (495). In general, these results suggest that endogenous opioid activity affects global components of the autistic syndrome. Or, perhaps reducing obsession with self-injurious behavior merely permits the emergence and development of socially acceptable behaviors. From the clinical perspective, the utility of opiate antagonist treatments for autistic children appears to be fairly well supported.

Animal literature offers additional support for the role of the opioid system in both the motoric and social symptomology of autism. Prenatal exposure to high levels of β-endorphin has been reported to result in disruptions of cognitive and developmental processes and adult sociosexual behavior (496, 497). Animals have been observed to exhibit "autistic-like" symptoms after administration of exogenous opiate agonists, including absence of normal distress upon separation from mothers (430), decreased affiliative behaviors, and high pain threshold (474, 498). Blockade of opioid receptors through administration of opiate antagonists resulted in the reversal of all these behaviors as well as exacerbation of distress vocalizations (474, 499), although this effect has been observed to vary slightly, depending on the age of the subject, time of administration, and type of opioid receptor involved (430).

Another peptide that has been implicated in the syndrome of autism is oxytocin (OT) (500), a centrally and peripherally active neurohormone that is produced mainly in the hypothalamus and is known to modulate affiliative behaviors among animals (501). Oxytocin levels have been found to be positively associated with aspects of human attachment as well, including mother-infant bonding, sexual relations, and socially extroversive personalities (500). Autistic social deficits may result from hypoactive central oxytocin.

Like β-endorphin, administration of OT will decrease separation-distress vocalizations in pups; this suggests a hypothesis of overactive OT in autism (502). Oxytocin is also known to be inhibited by β-endorphin (503), which is positively associated with autistic symptomology (471, 474, 476). Preliminary analyses from our study, the first to explore OT in autism, suggest that autistic children have significantly *lower* levels of OT than normal controls, however there is significant within-group variability, as well as substantial overlap between each group (504). There is also evidence for the involvement of pituitary peptides, indicated by findings of social behavioral improvements following administration of synthetic ACTH (505). This finding, and recent findings that autistic children appear to overproduce melatonin into the morning hours (506), fit Chamberlain and Herman's (482) hypothesis that melatonin hypersecretion produces increased 5HT and decreased β-endorphin in autism.

Recently, investigations of amino acids in autism have revealed abnormally low levels of platelet aspartic acid, glutamine, glutamic acid and GABA, as well as elevated tyrosine and diminished cysteine, which may be linked to dopamine and opioid dysfunction, respectively (507, 508).

Summary of Neurochemical Findings

To summarize further investigations and more refined methodology are needed to clarify the status of neurochemical involvement in autism. Research in this area has been limited by small and heterogeneous samples, inconsistent methodology, the uncertainty of peripheral assessment, technological limitations, and lack of sufficient control over variables such as presence of medication, intellectual abilities, circadian rhythms, age, and diagnostic overlap. The most consistent finding among autistic patients is hyperserotonemia in approximately 30% of the autistic population, which has been suggested to result from abnormal platelet function. Clinical evidence for sero-

tonergic dysfunction in autism derived from pharmacological trials with fenfluramine, which reduces plasma 5HT levels up to 57%, and has typically been found to result in improvements in stereotypies and hyperactivity. Fenfluramine has uncertain effects on social and cognitive skills. Serotonergic dysfunction is not unique to autism: hyperserotonemia has been found in other patient populations as well. Studies of the opioids have found fairly consistent support for some role in the autistic syndrome; opioid dysfunction is linked to self-injurious behavior, and perhaps to social deficits as well. Findings regarding plasma and CSF opioid levels have been in agreement with each other, and clinical administration of the opiate antagonist naltrexone has resulted in improvements in self-injurious behavior, stereotypies, hyperactivity, and social and communicative behaviors. There are also animal models that support opioid involvement in cognitive development, affiliative behavior, and tolerance for painful stimuli.

Despite neuroanatomical evidence for deficits in the structures associated with various dopamine pathways, the support for disrupted dopaminergic activity in autistic subjects is limited. Administration of dopamine antagonists to autistic children has resulted in the amelioration of abnormal motor behavior and social deficits. This finding tentatively supports the presence of dopaminergic hyperactivity in autism. However, direct assessment of plasma, platelet, and urine levels of dopamine has yielded contradictory findings, which may suggest that this method of measurement may be inadequate or misleading in the determination of dopaminergic involvement in autism.

Promising directions for research include the role of oxytocin, which has been associated with affiliative behavior, and integrative models such as that of Chamberlain and Herman (482), which implicates a cascade of effects of the neuromodulator melatonin, and offers a clear and comprehensive linkage between chemical and clinical features.

Clearly, neurochemical abnormalities are present, but variability with which they are expressed within the autistic population and the degree to which findings appear to contradict one another have prevented the confirmation of causal factors. Furthermore, it appears that attempts to delineate core features of "pure" autism and focus on one single factor of origin may be futile. The variability in cognitive and behavioral features and neuroanatomical and neurochemical deficits suggest that autism is best understood as a spectrum. Symptoms of mental retardation and unusual or restricted social and motor behaviors appear in many variant patterns. These variations may be best understood as resulting from combinations of disruptions to CNS morphology and/or neurochemistry. The complexity of the nervous system and its genetic determinants provide a vast number of opportunities for deviation in structures and processes. Research to date has modeled only a small portion of this complexity.

CLINICAL ASSESSMENT
Medical Assessment

Issues in assessment, referrals, and management of children with autism and related syndromes are reviewed in a number of recent publications (433, 509–515). In brief, the developmental history and behavioral and mental status examinations are the basis for the diagnosis of autism or PDD.

Once a diagnosis or tentative diagnosis of PDD or autism is made, assessments in specific areas should be done. The child's hearing must be assessed thoroughly and definitively (511, 513). In any case where behavioral assessment of hearing is not considered reliable, the child should be referred for brainstem-evoked-response audiology.

Individuals with autism are subject to a wide variety of motor impairments, especially stereotypies, hypotonia, and apraxia, as well as frank movement disorders (516, 517). A complete motor examination may reveal remediable conditions.

Medical and family history and physical exam may suggest specific etiologies, such as hydrocephalus, or a genetic or neurocutaneous syndrome. The genetic syndrome most often reported in association with autism is fragile X syndrome (261), although other investigators conclude that fragile X is no more common in autistic retarded males than in the wider population of retarded males (263). Examination of the child's physiognomy can suggest the diagnoses of Williams syndrome, Prader-Willi syndrome, or other neurobehavioral entities, and can dictate referral to a clinical geneticist. Allen et al. (511) have concluded that in general, screening for abnormalities in amino acids, organic acids, or other metabolites in blood and urine, in the absence of a specific indication for such testing, has a very low yield.

Gillberg (513), however, has claimed that a high proportion of autistic individuals have associated conditions that can be uncovered by extensive medical investigation. He proposed the investigation of fragile X syndrome, tuberous sclerosis, and neurofibromatosis, hypomelanosis of Ito, Rett's syndrome, Möbius's syndrome, Williams syndrome, Cornelia de Lange syndrome, Laurence-Moon-Biedl syndrome, mucopolysaccharidosis, and the Coffin-Lowry syndrome. Gillberg (513) suggested that other conditions worth investigating include PKU, rubella, lactic acidosis, congenital toxoplasmosis, CMV infection, herpes encephalitis, hydrocephalus, hypothyroidism, infantile spasms, and purine and calcium disorders. Gillberg (513, 515) also recommended a specific regimen of laboratory analyses. This includes blood work (chromosomes, phenylalanine, uric acid, lactic acid, pyruvic acid, and herpes titer), urine studies (metabolic screen, uric acid, calcium), CSF examination for protein, EEG, and CT or MRI to look for evidence of tuberous sclerosis, infection, neurofibromatosis, and hypomelanosis of Ito. Gillberg (518), and Coleman (519) review recommended medical work-ups for autistic patients.

Epilepsy is one neurological disorder that is often found in association with the autistic behavioral syndrome (248, 249). Rates of seizures from 11–42% have been reported (246). Adolescent onset of seizures is more common in autism than in other developmental syndromes (520, 521). Tuchman et al. (246) found agreement between the clinical diagnosis of epilepsy, and epileptiform EEGs, and concluded that EEGs may be useful in determining whether unusual stereotyped behaviors represent seizure activity. In young autistic children without stereotypies or seizures, EEGs may be useful in cases with regressive loss of previously acquired language skills. When EEGs are performed, they should include sleep EEG (511).

The use of routine CT or MRI remains controversial (511). Although the likelihood of finding an abnormality is low, and although a discovered abnormality is not likely to have treatment implications, the routine screening of autistic children with brain imaging is a common practice. Gillberg (513) recommends it as part of a standard medical workup of autistic children.

Psychiatric evaluation includes assessment for co-morbid psychiatric disorders, including attention deficit, hyperactivity disorder, depression, psychosis, anxiety, and OCD. Family issues and interpersonal conflicts also should be assessed. Neurological assessment includes sufficient neurocognitive assessment to determine whether retardation is present. Rapin (522), found that neurologists missed the diagnosis of mental retardation in about 25% of children shown to have mental retardation by formal testing. IQ testing in autistic children has been shown to have the same predictive validity and stability as for normal children (523). Therefore, formal testing of intellectual function would be preferable to reliance on a clinical impression based on incomplete neurocognitive assessment.

Neuropsychological Assessment

Children and adolescents with autism or PDD should also have periodic neuropsychological assessments. These are necessary for describing the child's current level and profile of cognitive abilities, which will have implications for educational programs and long-range goals. Periodic re-evaluations are also necessary to monitor the child's progress, to detect any deterioration that might signal the onset of negative medical or psychological events, and to evaluate the success of programs. Procedures and issues in neuropsychological evaluations of autistic children are reviewed by Wainwright et al. (524).

These evaluations should be done by a trained neuropsychologist experienced with autistic or PDD children. Multiple sessions at the office, home, or school may be necessary to complete evaluation. With difficult children, the school can be an excellent place for testing, because the children are accustomed to working there and the teachers aid compliance. Whenever possible, a neuropsychological evaluation should thoroughly assess cognition in the areas of language (vocabulary, syntax, and pragmatics), visuospatial skills, abstract thinking and problem solving, memory, attention, and social cognition. Language, in particular, must be very thoroughly assessed. Usually a neuropsychologist can administer a complete language assessment. If not, a referral to a speech and language pathologist is advisable. Many clinicians would argue that such a referral is warranted in any case.

Watson and Marcus (525) reviewed a series of tests for use with young autistic children, including the Bayley Mental Scale of Infant Development, Merrill-Palmer Test of Mental Abilities, McCarthy Scales of Children's Abilities, Wechsler tests, and the Kaufman Assessment Battery for Children. Additional tests that are frequently used, and that are appropriate for this population, include the Leiter International Performance Scale (526), the Stanford-Binet (4th ed.), and the Differential Ability Scales (527). The neuropsychologist should also adapt testing procedures to optimize the individual child's attention and comprehension, such as giving simultaneous visual/auditory input, simplified language input, periodic shifts of task, and individualized reinforcers. Limiting factors on achievement should be specified; individual children may handicapped by lack of motivation, interfering behaviors, language difficulties, or poor attention.

Behavioral Assessment

Thorough behavioral description is as important as assessment of cognition. This may be done by a neuropsychologist, psychiatrist, or other developmental, behavioral, or pediatric specialist. A profile of the individual's adaptive abilities should be included in the behavioral assessment. One clinical/psychoeducational approach to assessment of functional skills at home and in the classroom is described by Mesibov et al. (528). A standardized instrument for the assessment of adaptive skills is the revised Vineland Adaptive Behavior Scales (529); it has been shown to be a powerful, highly descriptive, well-normed instrument that works well with autistic children (530). It provides age equivalents and standard scores for communication, daily living, and socialization skills, and motor scores for younger children. Because autistic children have more intradomain scatter in development than other children (531), it behooves the clinician to examine individual developmental items passed and failed by the child. Autistic children will often have their lowest age equivalent scores in the socialization domain. Daily living scores reflect self-help activities taught at home or at school, so particularly low scores in this domain may suggest that the child has not been pushed to capacity, or is particularly deficient in motivation to master these skills. Deficits in motor ability may also affect daily living skills.

Play is an area of adaptive skill that warrants special attention. The development of play in normal children proceeds from simple sensory-motor play, to functional play, to the emergence of symbolic play, which then follows development along several lines of increasing abstraction and complexity (532, 533). Particular impairment of symbolic play has been shown to characterize autistic children (534–538). Results of these investigations suggest that spontaneous free play is infrequent and immature in autism, but that modeling can elicit free play in high-functioning autistic children, who are nevertheless generally uninterested in symbolic play activities. The clinician assessing play should be familiar with the development of play in normal children, and with procedures for the elicitation of play. The clinician should judge the degree of play deficit relative to the child's mental age and not chronological age.

A clear description of problem behaviors is important. Behaviors central to the syndrome (such as social incapacity and resistance to change), those associated with the syndrome (such as self-injury and abnormal motor behaviors), and those ancillary to it (such as hyperactivity, aggressiveness, and passivity) should be noted. Many instruments exist to document abnormal behaviors in autism; reviews of such instruments are found in Parks (539) and Powers (540). The Autism Diagnostic Interview (541) and the Autism Diagnostic Observation Schedule (542) are a pair of companion instruments for interviewing an informant, and for direct interview of the autistic individual. These instruments are reliable and have good coverage of clinical content. However, administration of these instruments is quite lengthy, and training of examiners is required.

Often neglected in the description of problem behaviors is the analysis of antecedent conditions and consequences of the behaviors. These may clarify the role or function of the behavior for the particular autistic individual, and may suggest changes in stimulus conditions and reinforcements to ameliorate problem behaviors, as well as to foster positive behaviors. Such behavioral assessment procedures are reviewed by Powers (540).

Family Assessment

Assessments of strengths, resources, and needs of families coping with autism is described in detail in Schopler and Mesibov (543) and by Harris (544). Harris reviewed family assessment instruments and has outlined the application of the McCubbin and Patterson (545) framework for assessment of the family, in which the clinician assesses personal financial resources, educational attainment, physical and emotional health, and psychological characteristics, family cohesion and adaptability, and social support from the extended family, neighbors, and community. Harris (544) also describes how to arrive at the proper balance between focus on the child's difficulties and the family's handling of the problems.

TREATMENT

Pharmacological Treatments

Pharmacological treatment for autism is reviewed in several recent publications (513, 546–553). Gualtieri reviews many treatments for co-morbid conditions, including epilepsy, self-injurious behavior and compulsions. Holm and Varley (550) cautioned that many studies of pharmacological effectiveness are anecdotal, use inadequately defined populations, use inadequate instruments for measuring change, lack control groups, or report statistically but not clinically significant changes. Harty (549) argued that although pharmacological therapies do not fundamentally alter the natural course or core symptoms of autism, they can be useful in reducing aberrant behaviors.

While attention difficulties and hyperactivity are often prominent in the clinical picture of autism, the autistic child's behavior usually does not improve with stimulant medications. Exacerbation or initiation of stereotypies and psychosis has in fact been reported in autistic children placed on stimulants. Therefore, Holm and Varley (554) concluded that stimulant medication is therapeutic for a few autistic children; these tend to be high-functioning autistic children with symptoms of attention deficit. Harty (555) recommended trials of stimulants for hyperactive autistic children without stereotypies.

Research on the use of anxiolytics with anxious or sleep-disturbed autistic individuals is sparse. Harty (555) reported that agents such as buspirone will reduce agitated behavior in some autistic children.

The use of neuroleptics, especially haloperidol, is controversial. While some researchers have reported positive effects (556), others (1) dispute its efficacy. Holm and Varley (554) concluded that while haloperidol may have beneficial effects on agitation, hyperactivity, aggression, stereotypies and liability, it is less effective in improving social relationships and language. They advised that the risk of tardive dyskinesia (which occurs in 20% of treated autistic individuals) be weighed carefully. Clozapine, an atypical neuroleptic, has received favorable review for its effectiveness (557). Beta-blockers have been reported to be useful in managing impulsive, aggressive and self-abusive behavior in autistic adults (558). Ratey et al (558) have hypothesized that β-blockers reduce a chronic state of hyperarousal. Lipinski et al. (559) suggested that β-blockers may act by ameliorating akathisia induced by long-term neuroleptic administration. Other drugs considered to be effective with self-injury include fluoxetine, domipramine, buspirone, and opiate antagonists, especially when combined with behavioral therapy (560, 561). The opiate blockers naltrexone and nalaxone have been found to have beneficial effects on self-injury, and also on social withdrawal and stereotypies (494, 495, 561–563). Harty (549) has reviewed the differences between the two classes of agents and the symptoms targeted by each.

Tricyclic antidepressants have not been subjected to careful study in the autistic population, but clinicians sometimes prescribe them, especially to autistic individuals who have a close relative who had depression that was responsive to tricyclics. Holm and Varley (550) note that although tricyclics appear to improve language and social responsiveness in some autistic persons, many show adverse behavioral reactions, and aggravation of seizures is possible (512). Lithium carbonate has also been tried in autistic children (158, 564); some children experienced amelioration of agitation and aggression. DeLong and Aldershof (564) reported that high-functioning, perseverative children with hyperactivity unresponsive to stimulants, and a family history of bipolar disorder, are most likely to respond well.

Recently, studies (565-569) have obtained encouraging results using clomipramine, a tricyclic compound that acts preferentially on the serotonergic system and that is widely used in treatment of OCD. Two of these (565, 568) found clomipramine superior to desipramine, using a crossover design and a double blind comparison. Social relatedness improved, while aggression and ritualistic behaviors diminished. A recent open trial found reductions in adventitious movements and compulsions (567) and case reports also indicate similar improvements (569). Similarly, case reports have begun to appear on the use of selective serotonin reuptake inhibitors such as fluoxetine in autism (570, 571), including autism co-morbid with depression (572), with trichotillomania (573), with self-injury (560) and with OCD (574). One study (575) found that fluoxetine led to clinical improvement in many subjects, though some subjects experienced undesirable side effects such as agitation. These results are encouraging (and consistent with findings of serotonin abnormalities in autism), but are preliminary and therefore mainly of heuristic significance.

The much more numerous studies on the effectiveness of fenfluramine were reviewed in detail by Holm and Varley (550). The cumulative results are inconsistent, but more studies show positive change than not. In general, where there is an effect, behaviors related to hyperactivity and stereotypies appear to show more consistent improvement than cognition, language, or social relatedness. Holm and Varley cautioned that many parents and clinicians have felt that the benefits were transitory, and Leventhal et al (576) recently reported no substantial advantage to using fenfluramine for autism, particularly its social deficits.

Nutritional treatments, reviewed by Holm and Varley (550) and by Raiten (577), have also been recommended by a variety of autism researchers and clinicians (578–581). Holm and Varley (550) criticized these studies in methodological grounds and cited evidence that large doses of vitamins such as B_6 may not be as safe as had been supposed. Kozlowski (582) asserts that megavitamins are by no means a proven success in the treatment of behavioral problems in mentally retarded autistic children. Folate has been tried with boys with fragile X syndrome (583), showing positive effects on behavior. However, Lowe et al (584) found no positive effects of folate on an unselected group of autistic children. A preliminary crossover trial of supplemental ascorbic acid found improvements in severity of symptoms over 10 weeks of treatment (585). Rimland's ongoing publication, *Autism Research Review International,* (Autism Research Institute, 4182 Adams Avenue, San Diego, CA 92116), periodically reviews nutritional studies, and advocates specific regimens of vitamins and minerals.

Antiepileptic drugs generally are given for control of documented seizure disorders in autistic children, and not for the control of behavior. There is no firm evidence for their effectiveness in improving behavior, although some anecdotal evidence exists for improvement of depression and irritability (549, 550). Recently, treatments with a synthetic form of the pituitary peptide ACTH (ORG 2766) resulted in improvements in play, social interaction and ratings of social withdrawal (586).

In sum, treatment is as individual as the presentation of autistic symptoms. Clinicians prescribing medication must monitor effects closely and be open to many alternate options.

Behavioral and Educational Treatments

The major treatments for autism are special education and behavioral programming. Early and extensive work on language, social interaction, preacademic and academic skills, and self-help skills are the autistic child's best hope for a positive outcome. There is a very extensive body of literature dating back 30 years on various aspects of behavior modifications and other nonpharmacological interventions for autism, but it is beyond the scope of this chapter to review this literature in detail. In brief, there are different approaches to intervention, but no large-scale controlled study exists to compare their efficacy. The methodological and practical problems inherent in attempting such a study seems almost insurmountable. Representatives of two such approaches are the developmental program of Rogers and Lewis (587) in Denver, and the behavioral program of Lovaas (588) at UCLA. In the Rogers and Lewis approach, the child is stimulated to take the next step in relatedness, language, and conceptual knowledge, and social knowledge, and social interaction is made as reinforcing as possible. In the Lovaas approach, the child is the recipient of intensive behavior modification from a very early age. Lovaas (588–590) has reported that 47% of children in his program attained normal intellectual and academic functioning by first grade. Others, however urge caution in accepting the full extent of Lovaas' claims (591). There is good evidence that behavioral methods are the treatment of choice for problem behaviors, such as self-injury (592, 593), while more naturalistic methods, such as play groups with typical peers, may effectively stimulate play and social development (594, 595).

Intellectual, language, and social status before treatment certainly contribute major variance to outcome; children with higher levels of communication, language, IQ, and social skills will have better outcomes in any type of program. It is probable that certain types of children may do better with certain types of programs; for example, some clinicians refer children with severe social withdrawal, poor compliance, or poor attention to behavioral programs, while referring children with odd but related social behavior and some degree of compliance and attention to more developmental or language-based programs. In the absence of any empirical data concerning which type of autistic child does well in which type of program, the clinician is forced to make referral based on clinical judgment of the child and knowledge of available local resources. Information is lacking concerning which type of special education or behavioral treatment is most effective for which type of autistic child, but there is general agreement that early aggressive intervention optimizes chances for better outcome. There is a growing trend to refer autistic children for language and/or behavioral and other therapies as early as possible, family and community resources permitting (596). One specific early intervention approach is the option method, which is critically received by Jordan and Powell (597).

At school age, there is a strong recent trend toward "inclusion" or "integration" in which the autistic child is placed, with or without an aide, into a "normal" public school class, sometimes with "pull-out" time for special services. Although there is ample evidence that autistic children's social interaction benefits from exposure to normal role models and peers who initiate and reinforce social interaction (555, 598, 599), it is too soon to tell whether the cohort of autistic children placed in mainstream settings will be able to cope with the increasingly complex social and academic activities of the later grade-school years. An intermediate solution also on the ascent is the integrated classroom, especially in preschool, in which typical and atypical children are mixed in roughly equal proportions. These classrooms look very promising to the clinical observer, but large-scale follow-up data on their success are not yet available.

As part of the child's special education, and perhaps in addition to it, the child should receive aggressive language therapy. Except for children with severe articulatory dysfunction, this should focus more on the semantic and pragmatic use of language than on articulation and syntax. Prizant and Wetherby (596) discussed the analysis of the communicative functions of autistic utterances, and have outlined a very pragmatically oriented approach to language therapy. Evidence shows that teaching functional communication skills not only increases interactive possibilities but may actually decrease problem behaviors (600). Teaching of specific, pivotal social skills not only increases the occurrence of these skills, but also generalizes to other social behaviors and to ratings of overall social appropriateness (601). Many autistic children suffer from a variety of motor delays and impairments, and may benefit from physical and/or occupational therapy. One approach, again lacking in well-controlled experimental validation, but adhered to by many clinicians and parents, is the sensory integration school of occupational therapy, described by Cook (554).

A recent development in the treatment of autism is facilitated communication. In this approach, a "facilitator" assists the autistic individual to communicate via a letter board or keyboard, by pulling the individual's hand away from the board, and sometimes by helping the individual to form a pointing gesture. This approach seems to be based on the notion that a severe motor apraxia interferes with the autistic individual's capacity to express him or herself; the facilitator breaks the perseverative motor movements that prevent intentional movements. This treatment has led to claims of remarkable success, with autistic children, adolescents, and adults thought to be nonverbal and severely retarded communicating via facilitation at a cognitively normal level. As of this writing, several controlled experiments have been done, in which the autistic individual is exposed to information to which the facilitator has no access, and then is questioned about this information. So far, findings are negative; the studies show that the autistic individuals cannot communicate via facilitation at a level very discrepant from their usual verbal and nonverbal communicative capacity, unless the facilitator can influence the communication consciously or unconsciously (602–605). Updates on this research can be found in Rimland's *Autism Research Review International.*

Finally, physicians, psychologists, and other clinicians must help families to obtain other necessary services, such as respite care, extended day programs, and summer programs to prevent the behavioral and cognitive regression that can occur within 2 months of unstructured time. They may also be able to suggest appropriate leisure activities, such as gymnastics, swimming, or play or social groups, that can provide constructive ways to spend after school hours and opportunities for social interaction with typical children, and can promote self-esteem.

Prescription with therapies and services for the autistic individual must always include sensitivity to the often devastating effect of the disability on the family. Harris (544), Scopler and Mesibov (606) and Konstantareas (556) describe frameworks for assessing, and for helping families to cope with their disabled member. Harris (544) and Konstantareas (556) have discussed how to recognize and try to address family stress, without undue attention to family dynamics that may imply adherence to the outdated notion that family pathology causes the autistic condition. Social support from other affected families, and keeping abreast of the latest developments in treatment and other research, can help families manage their affected children and their own emotional reactions. The Autism Society of America (8601 Georgia Ave., Suite 503, Silver Spring, MD 20910) publishes a regular newsletter with much information useful to parents; another good resource for parents and professionals on recent developments in autism is Rimland's newsletter *Autism Research Review International.*

SUMMARY AND CONCLUSIONS

Pervasive Developmental Disorder is a psychiatric diagnostic category that encompasses the autistic spectrum of disorders: autism, Asperger's syndrome, Disintegrative Disorder, and Rett's Syndrome. All children diagnosed with PDD will have serious social impairments. Most will have some form of cognitive impairment, from profound retardation to rigidity of executive functions. Many will evince

signs of neurological impairment, such as motor dysfunction, seizures, and abnormal EEGs. Very few will make a satisfactory near-normal adjustment in adult life, despite intense educational treatment programs and sensitive pharmacological therapy.

Clinical practice rests on assessment: neurological, medical, psychiatric, behavioral, neuropsychological, and language evaluations are crucial to treatment and management.

Future understanding of autism depends on a much needed change in research strategy. Despite evidence from all domains of research that autism is not a unitary disease entity, most investigations of the autistic spectrum are designed to search for a single cause for the entire spectrum, whether it be genetic, neuroanatomical, neurophysiological, or psychological. Future research programs that are designed to explore various causal mechanisms within one design framework will have a better chance to improve our understanding of the autistic spectrum of disorders.

The core deficit of the spectrum is social impairment. Neuroscience has begun exploration of the neurobiology of social behavior. Advances in our understanding of brain systems that serve sociability will also help us to understand the nature of the autistic spectrum.

References

1. Szatmari P. The validity of autistic spectrum disorders: a literature review. J Autism Dev Disord 1992;22:583–600.
2. DiLalla DL, Rogers SJ. Domains if the Childhood Autism Rating Scale: relevance for diagnosis and treatment. J Autism Dev Disord 1994;24:115–128.
3. Kanner L. Autistic disturbances of affective contact. Nervous Child 1943;2:217–250.
4. Gillberg C. Autism and autistic-like conditions: subclasses among disorders of empathy. J Child Psychol Psychiatry 1992;33:813–842.
5. Bene E. A Rorschach investigation into the mothers of autistic children. Br J Med Psychol 1958;38:226–227.
6. Bettelheim B. The empty fortress–infantile autism and the birth of the self. New York: The Free Press, Collier-MacMillan, 1967.
7. Despert J. Some considerations relating to the genesis of autistic behavior in children. Am J Orthopsychiatry 1951;12:366–371.
8. Eisenberg L, Kanner, L. Early infantile autism: 1943-55. Am J Orthopsychiatry 1956;26:55–65.
9. Mahler M. On child psychosis and schizophrenia: autistic and symbiotic infantile psychoses. Psychoanalytic Study if the Child 1952;7:286–305.
10. Mahler M, Gosliner B. On symbiotic child psychosis: genetic, dynamic and restitutive aspects. Psychoanal Study Child 1955;10:195–212.
11. Hobson RP. On psychoanalytic approaches to autism. Am J Orthopsychiatry 1990;60:324–336.
12. Rimland B. Infantile autism: the syndrome and its implications. New York: Appleton-Century-Crofts, 1964.
13. Ornitz E, Ritvo E. Perceptual inconstancy in early infantile autism. Arch Gen Psychiatry 1968;18:76–98.
14. Rutter M. Concepts of autism: a review of research. J Child Psychol Psychiatry 1968;9:1–25.
15. Baron-Cohen S, Leslie A, Frith U. Does the autistic child have a "theory of mind"? Cognition 1985;21:37–46.
16. Ozonoff S, Pennington B, Rogers, S. Executive function deficits in high-functioning autistic individuals: relationship to theory of mind. J Child Psychol Psychiatry 1991;32:1081–1105.
17. Fein D, Pennington B, Markowitz P, Braverman M, Waterhouse L. Toward a neuropsychological model of infantile autism: are the social

deficits primary? J Am Acad Child Adolesc Psychiatry 1986;25: 198–212.

18. Hobson RP. Beyond cognition: a theory of autism. In: Dawson G. ed. Autism: nature, diagnosis, and treatment. New York: Guilford.

19. Kolvin I. Studies in the childhood psychoses: I. Diagnostic criteria and classification. Br J Psychiatry 1971;118:318–384.

20. Rutter M. Diagnosis and definition of childhood autism. J Autism Childhood Schizophrenia 1978;8:139–384.

21. Ritvo E, Freeman B. National Society for Autistic children definition of the syndrome of autism. J Autism Childhood Schizophrenia 1978;8:162–169.

22. Schopler E. Diagnosis and definition of autism. J Autism Childhood Schizophrenia 1978;8:167–169.

23. American Psychiatric Association. Diagnostic and Statistical Manual of Mental Disorders, 3rd ed. (DSM-III). Washington, DC, 1980.

24. Wing L, Gould J. Severe impairments of social interaction and associated abnormalities in children: epidemiology and classification. J Autism Dev Disord 1979;9:11–29.

25. Wing L, Attwood A. Syndromes of autism and atypical development. In: Cohen D, Donnellan A, eds. Handbook of autism and pervasive developmental disorder. New York: John Wiley & Sons, 1987.

26. American Psychiatric Association. Diagnostic and Statistical Manual of Mental Disorders, 3rd Ed. Revised (DSM-III-R). Washington DC, 1987.

27. Waterhouse L, Wing L, Spitzer R, Siegel B. Pervasive developmental disorders: From DSM-III-R. J Autism Dev Disord 1992;22: 525–549.

28. American Psychiatric Association. Diagnostic and Statistical Manual of Mental Disorders (4th ed.) Washington DC, 1994.

29. World Health Organization: mental disorders: the ICD-10 classification of mental and behavioral disorders. Diagnostic criteria for research. Geneva, Switzerland 1993.

30. Szatmari P, Volkmar F, Walter S. Evaluation of diagnostic criteria for autism using latent class models. J Am Acad Child Adolesc Psychiatry, 1995;34:216–222.

31. Waterhouse L, Morris R, Allen D, Dunn M, Fein D, Feinstein C, Rapin I, Wing L. Diagnosis and classification in autism. J Autism Develop Disord (in press).

32. Mundy P, Sigman M. The theoretical implications of joint-attention deficits in autism. Devel Psychopathol 1989;1:173–183.

33. Howlin P. An overview of social behavior in autism. In: E Schopler, G Mesibov (eds.), Social Behavior in Autism 1992. New York: Plenum Press, 1986.

34. Hauck M, Fein D, Waterhouse L, Feinstein C. Social initiations by autistic children to adults and other children. J Autism Devel Disord, in press.

35. Stone W, Caro-Martinez L. Naturalistic observations of spontaneous communications in autistic children. J Autism Develop Disord 1990;20:437–453.

36. Stone W, Lemanek K. Parental report of social behaviors in autistic preschoolers 1990;20:513–522.

37. Volkmar F. Social development. In: Cohen D, Donnellan A (eds), Handbook of Autism and Pervasive Developmental Disorders. New York: John Wiley & Sons, 1987.

38. Kasari C, Sigman M, Yirmiya N. Focused on social attention of autistic children in interactions with familiar and unfamiliar adults: a comparison of autistic, mentally retarded, and normal children. Development Psychopathology 1993;5:403–414.

39. Riquet CB, Taylor ND, Benroya S, Klein LS. Symbolic play in autistic, Downs and normal children of equivalent mental age. J Aut Dev Dis 1981;11:439–448.

40. Lewis V, Boucher J. Spontaneous, instructed and elicited play in relatively able autistic children. Br J Devel Psychol 1988;6:325–339.

41. Wainwright L, Fein D. Play. In: Rapin I (ed.) Preschool children with inadequate communication: developmental language disorder; autism, mental deficiency. Clinics in Developmental Medicine, in press.

42. Roeyers H, Van Berckelaer O. Play in autistic children. Communication Cognition 1994;27:349–359.

43. Rogers SH, Ozonoff S, Maslin-Cole C. Developmental aspects of attachment behavior in young children and pervasive developmental disorder. J Am Acad Child Adolesc Psychiatry; 32:1274–1282.

44. Prior M. Cognitive abilities and disabilities in infantile autism: a review. J Abnorm Child Pscho 1979;7:357-380.

45. Sigman M, Ungerer J, Mundy P, Sherman T. Cognition in autistic children. In: Cohen D, Donnellan A, Paul R, eds. Handbook of autism and pervasive developmental disorder. New York: John Wiley & Sons, 1987.

46. Green LA, Fein D, Joy S, Waterhouse L. Cognitive functioning in autism: an overview. In: E Schopler, G Mesibov (eds.) Learning and Cognition in Autism 1994; New York: Plenum Press.

47. Rimland B, Fein D. Special talents of autistic savants. In: Obler L, Fein D, eds. The exceptional brain: neuropsychology of talent and special abilities. New York: Guilford, 1988. pp. 474–485.

48. Treffert D. The idiot savant: a review of the syndrome. Am J Psychiatry 1988;145:563–572.

49. Waterhouse L. Speculations on the neuroanatomical substrate of special talents. In: Obler L, Fein D, eds. The exceptional brain: neuropsychology of talent and special abilities. New York: Guilford, 1988. pp. 493–509.

50. Waterhouse L, Fein D. Social or cognitive or both? Crucial dysfunctions in autism. In: Gillberg C, eds. Diagnosis and treatment of autism. New York: Plenum, 1989.

51. Lazarus R. Thoughts on the relationship between emotion and cognition. Am Psychol 1982;37:1019–1024.

52. Lazarus R. On the primacy of cognition. Am Psychol 1984;39: 124–129.

53. Zajonc R. Feeling and thinking: preferences need no inferences. Am Psychol 1980;35:151–175.

54. Zajonc R. On the primacy of affect. Am Psychol 1984;39:117–123.

55. Hobson RP. The autistic child's appraisal of expressions of emotion. J Child Psychol Psychiatry 1986;27:321–342.

56. Lovaas OI, Schreibman L, Koegel R, Rehm R. Selective responding by autistic children to multiple sensory input. J Abnor Psychol 1971;77:211–222.

57. Fein D, Tinder P, Waterhouse L. Stimulus generalization in autistic and normal children. J Child Psychol Child Psychiatry 1979;20: 325–335.

58. Courchesne E, Townsend J, Akshoomoff N, Saitoh O, et al. Impairment in shifting attention in autistic and cerebellar patients. Behav Neurosci 1994;105:848–865.

59. Townsend J, Courchesne E, Eggs B. Visual attention deficits in autistic adults with cerebellar and partial abnormalities. Society for Neuroscience Abstracts 1992;18:332.

60. Garretson H, Fein D, Waterhouse L. Sustained attention in autistic children. J Autism Devel Disord 190;20:101–114.

61. Minshew NJ, Goldstein G, Muenz LR, Payton JB. Neuropsychological functioning nonmentally retarded autistic individuals. J Clin Exper Neuropsychol 1992;14:749–761.

62. Hutt S, Hutt C, Lee D, Ounsted D. A behavioral and electroencephalographic study of autistic children. J Psychiatric Research 1965;3: 181–197.

63. DeLong Gr. Autism, amnesia, hippocampus and learning. Neurosci Behav Rev 1992;16:63–70.

64. Dawson G, Lewy A. Arousal, attention and the socioemotional impairments of individuals with autism. In: Dawson G, ed. Autism: nature, Diagnosis and treatment. New York: Guilford, 1989.

65. Kinsbourne M. Cerebral-brainstem relations in infantile autism. In: Dawson G, ed. Autism: nature, Diagnosis and Treatment. New York: Guilford Press, 1989.

66. Rapin I. Preschool children with inadequate communication: developmental language disorder, autism, mental deficiency. Clinics in Developmental Medicine, in press.

67. Sandberg AD, Nydern A, Gillberg C, Hjelmquist E. The cognitive profile in infantile autism: a study of 70 children and adolescents using the Griffiths Mental Developmental Scale. Br J Psychol 1993;84: 365–373.

68. Carpentieri SC, Morgan SB. Brief report: a comparison of patterns of cognitive functioning of autistic and nonautistic retarded children on the Stanford-Binet—Fourth Edition. J Autism Devel Disord 1994;24:215–223.

69. Waterhouse L, Fein D. Language skills in developmentally disabled children. Brain Language 1982;15:307–333.

70. Tager-Flusberg H. A psycholinguistic perspective on language development in the autistic child. In Dawson G, ed. Autism: nature, Diagnosis and Treatment. New York: Guilford Press, 1989.

71. Rutter M. The description and classification of infantile autism. In: Churchill D, Alpern G, DeMyer M, eds. Infantile autism: proceedings of the Indiana University Colloquium. Springfield, IL: Charles C Thomas, 1971.

72. McCann B. Hemispheric asymmetries and early infantile autism. J Autism Dev Disord 1981;11:401–411.

73. Fein D, Humes M, Kaplan E, Lucci D, Waterhouse L. The question of left hemisphere dysfunction in infantile autism. Psychol Bull 1984;95:258–281.

74. Leslie AM, Thaiss L. Domain specificity in conceptual development: neuropsychological evidence. Cognition 1992;43:225–251.

75. Fein D, Lucci D, Braverman M, Waterhouse L. Comprehension of affect in context in children with pervasive developmental disorders. J Child Psychol Psychiatry 1992;33:1157.

76. Volkmar F, Sparrow S, Rende R, Cohen D. Facial perception in autism. J Child Psychol Psychiatry 1989;30:591–598.

77. Prior M, Dahlstrom B, Squires T. Autistic children's knowledge of thinking and feeling states in other people. J Child Psychol Psychiatry 1990;31:587–601.

78. Ozonoff S, Pennington B, Rogers S. Are there emotion perception deficits in young autistic children? J Child Psychol Psychiatry 1990;31:343–361.

79. Yirmiya N, Kasari C, Sigman M, Mundy P. Facial expressions of affect in autistic, mentally retarded and normal children. J Child Psychol Psychiatry 1989;30:725–735.

80. Happe FGE. An advanced test of theory of mind: understanding of story characters' thoughts and feelings by able autistic, mentally handicapped, and normal children and adults. J Autism Devel Disord 1994;24:129–154.

81. Tager-Flusberg H, Sullivan K. Predicting and explaining behavior: a comparison of autistic, mentally retarded and normal children. J Child Psychol Psychiatry Allied Disciplines 1994;35:1059–1075.

82. Baron-Cohen S, Goodhart F. The seeing-leads-to-knowing deficit in autism: the Pratt and Bryant probe. Br J Devel Psychol 1994;12:397–401.

83. Hertzig M, Snow M, Sherman M. Affect and cognition in autism. J Am Acad Child Adoles Psychiatry 1989;28:195-199.

84. Izard C. The face of emotion. New York: Appleton-Century-Crofts, 1971.

85. Fine J, Bartolucci G, Ginsberg G, Szatmari P. The use of intonation to communicate in pervasive developmental disorders. J Child Psychol Psychiatry 1991;32:771–782.

86. Happe FGE, Francesca GE. Wechsler IQ profile and theory of mind in autism: a research note. J Child Psychol Psychiatry Allied Disciplines 1994;35:1461–1471.

87. Brown J. Adolescent development of children with infantile psychosis. Seminar in Psychiatry 1969;1:79–89.

88. Fombonne E, Siddons F, Achard S, Frith U, et al. Adaptive behavior and theory of mind in autism. European Child Adolesc Psychiatry 1994;3:176–186.

89. Tager-Flusberg H, Sullivan K. A second look at second-order belief attribution in autism. J Autism Devel Disord 1994;24:577–586.

90. Reed T. Performance of autistic and control subjects on three cognitive perspective-taking tasks. J Autism Devel Disord 1994;24:53–66.

91. Hobson RP. The autistic child's appraisal of expressions of emotion: a further study. J Child Psychol Psychiatry 1986;27:671–680.

92. Hobson R. Methodological issues for experiments on autistic individuals' perception and understanding of emotion. J Child Psychol Psychiatry 1991;32:1135–1158.

93. Hobson R, Ouston J, Lee A. Emotion recognition in autism: coordinating faces and voices. Psychol Med 1988;18:911–923.

94. Tantam D, Monaghan L, Nicholson H, Stirling J. Autistic children's ability to interpret faces: a research note. J Child Psychol Psychiatry 1989;30:623–630.

95. MacDonald H, Rutter M, Howlin P, et al. Recognition and expression of emotional cues by autistic and normal adults. J Child Psychol Psychiatry 1989;30:865–877.

96. Braverman M, Fein D, Lucci D, Waterhouse L. Affect comprehension in children with pervasive developmental disorders. J Autism Dev Disord 1989;19:301–315.

97. Boucher J, Warrington E. Memory deficits in early infantile autism: some similarities to the amnesic syndrome. Br J Psychol 1976;67:73–87.

98. DeLong GR. Autism, amnesia, hippocampus and learning. Neurosci Biobehav Rev 1992;16:63–70.

99. Ozonoff S, Rogers S, Pennington B. Asperger's syndrome: evidence of an empirical distinction from high-functioning autism. J Child Psychol Psychiatry 1991;32:1107–1122.

100. Boucher J. Immediate free recall in early childhood autism: another point of behavioral similarity with the amnesic syndrome. Br J Psychol 1981;72:211–215.

101. Boucher J. Memory for recent events in amnesic children. J Autism Dev Disord 1981;11:293–302.

102. Minshew N, Goldstein G. Is autism an amnesic disorder? Evidence from the California Verbal Learning Test. Neuropsychol 1993;7:209–216.

103. Delis D, Kramer J, Kaplan E, Ober B. California Verbal Learning Test. San Antonio, TX: Psychological Corporation, 1987.

104. Gillberg C, Steffenburg S. Outcome and prognostic factors in infantile autism and similar conditions: a population-based study of 46 cases followed through puberty. J Autism Dev Disord 1987;17:273–287.

105. Rumsey J, Hamburger S. Neuropsychological findings in high-functioning men with infantile autism, residual state. J Clin Ex Neuropsychol 1988;10:210–221.

106. Rumsey J, Hamburger S. Neuropsychological divergence of high-level autism and severe dyslexia. J Autism Dev Disord 1990;20:155–168.

107. Szatmari P, Bartolucci G, Bremner R, Bond S, Rich S. A follow-up study of high-functioning autistic children. J Autism Dev Disord 1989;19:213–225.

108. Berger HJ, VanSpaendonck KP, Horstink MW, Buytenhuijs EL, et al. cognitive shifting as a predictor of progress in social understanding in high-functioning adolescents with autism: a prospective study. J Autism Dev Disord 1993;23:341–359.

109. McEvoy RE, Rogers SJ, Pennington BF. Executive function and social communication deficits in young autistic children. J Child Psychol Psychiat Allied Disciplines 1993;34:563–578.

110. Ozonoff S, Strayer DL, McMahon WM, Filloux F. Executive function abilities in autism and Tourette syndrome: an information processing approach. J Child Psychol Psychiat Allied Disciplines 1994;35:1015–1032.

111. Ozonoff S, McEvoy RE. A longitudinal study of executive function and theory of and development in autism. Devel Psychopathology 1994;6:415–431.

112. Hughes C, Russell J, Robbins TW. Evidence for executive dysfunction in autism. Neuropsychologia 1994;32:477–492.

113. Wing L. Sex ratios in early childhood autism and related conditions. Psychiatry Res 1981;5:129–137.

114. Jarrold C, Boucher J, Smith PK. Executive function deficits and the pretend play of children with autism: a research note. J Child Psychol Psychiat Allied Disciplines 1994;35:1473–1482.

115. Paul R. Natural history. In: Cohen D, Donnellan A, Paul R, eds. Handbook of autism and pervasive developmental disorder. New York: John Wiley & Sons 1987.

116. Creak M. Childhood psychosis: a review of 100 cases. Br J Psychiatry 1963;109:84–89.

117. DeMyer M, Barton S, DeMyer W, Norton J, Allen J, Steele R.

Prognosis in autism: a follow-up study. J Autism Childhood Schizophrenia 1973;3:199–246.

118. Eisenberg L. The autistic child in adolescence. Am J Psychiatry 1956;112:607–613.

119. Kanner L. Follow-up of 11 autistic children originally seen in 1943. J Autism Childhood Schizophrenia 1971;1:119–145.

120. Lotter V. Social adjustment and placement of autistic children in Middlesex: a follow-up. J Autism Childhood Schizophrenia 1974;4: 11–32.

121. Rutter M, Greenfield D, Lockyer L. A five to fifteen year follow-up of infantile psychosis: II. Social and behavioral outcome. Br J Psychiatry 1967;113:1183–1199.

122. Gonzales NM, Murray A, Shay J, Campbell M, et al. Autistic children on follow-up: change of diagnosis. Psychopharmacology Bulletin 1993;29:353–358.

123. Freeman B, Rahbar B, Ritvo E, Bice T, Yokota A, Ritvo R. The stability of cognitive and behavioral parameters in autism: a twelve-year prospective study. J Am Acad Child Adoles Psychiatry 1991; 30:479–482.

124. Kobayashi R, Murata T, Yoshinaga K. A follow-up study of 201 children with autism in Kyusha and Yamaguchi areas, Japan. J Autism Dev Disord 1992;22:395–411.

125. Waterhouse L, Fein D. Longitudinal trends in cognitive skills for children diagnosed as autistic and schizophrenic. Child Development 1984;55:236–248.

126. Venter A, Lord C, Schopler E. A follow-up study of high-functioning autistic children. J Child Psychol Psychiatry 1992;33:489–507.

127. Lotter V. Epidemiology of autistic conditions in young Children: I. Prevalence. Social Psychiatry 1966;1:124–137.

128. Gillberg C, Persson U, Grufman M, Temner U. Psychiatric disorders in mildly and severely mentally retarded urban children and adolescents: epidemiological aspects. Br J Psychiatry 1986;149:68–74.

129. Gillberg C. Infantile autism and other childhood psychoses in a Swedish urban region. Epidemiological aspects. J Child Psychol Psychiatry 1984;25:377–403.

130. Steffenburg S, Gillberg C. Autism and autistic like conditions in Swedish rural and urban areas: a population study. Br J Psychiatry 1986;149:81–87.

131. Gillberg C, Steffenburg S, Schaumann H. Is autism more common now than ten years ago? Br J Psychiatry 1991;158:403–409.

132. Bryson S, Clark B, Smith I. First report of a Canadian epidemiological study of autistic syndromes. J Child Psychol Psychiatry 1988;29: 433–445.

133. Cialdella P, Mamelle N. An epidemiological study of autism in a French department (Rhone): a research note. J Child Psychol Psychiatry 1989;30:433–445.

134. Rutter M. Psychotic disorders in early childhood. In: Coppen A, Walk A, eds. Br J Psychiatry, Special Publication No. 1. Ashford, Kent, Headley Brothers, 1967.

135. Hanson D, Gottesman I. The genetics, if any, of infantile autism and childhood schizophrenia. J Autism Childhood Schizophrenia 1976; 6:209–234.

136. Folstein S, Piven J. Etiology of autism: genetic influences. Pediatrics 1991; (Suppl) 88:767–773.

137. Folstein S, Rutter M. Autism: familial aggregation and genetic implications. J Autism Dev Disord 1988;18:3–30.

138. Smalley S, Asarnow R, Spence A. Autism and genetics: a decade of research. Arch Gen Psychiatry 1988;45:953–961.

139. Baird T, August G. Familial heterogeneity in infantile autism. J Autism Dev Disord 1985;15:315–321.

140. Deykin E, MacMahon B. Pregnancy, delivery, and neonatal complications among autistic children. Am J Dis Child 1980;134: 860–864.

141. Folstein S, Rutter M. Infantile autism: a genetic study of 21 twin pairs. J Child Psychol Psychiatry 1977;18:297–321.

142. Minton J, Campbell M, Green W. Cognitive assessment of siblings of autistic children. J Am Acad Child Adolesc Psychiatry 1982;21: 256–261.

143. Ritvo E, Freeman B, Mason-Brothers A, Mo A, Ritvo A. Concordance for the syndrome of autism in 40 pairs of afflicted twins. Am J Psychiatry 1985;142:74–77.

144. Piven J, Gayle J, Chase G, Fink B, Landa R, Wzorek M, Folstein S. A family history in the adult siblings of autistic individuals. J Am Acad Child Adolesc Psychiatry 1990;29:177–183.

145. Ritvo E, Freeman B, Pingree C, et al. The UCLA-University of Utah epidemiologic survey of autism: prevalence. Am J Psychiatry 1989; 146:194–199.

146. Ritvo E, Jorde L, Mason-Brothers A, et al. The UCLA-University of Utah epidemiologic survey of autism: recurrence risk estimates and genetic counseling. Am J Psychiatry 1989;146:1032–1036.

147. Steffenburg S, Gillberg C, Hellgren L, et al. A twin study of autism in Denmark, Finland, Iceland, Norway and Sweden. J Child Psychol Psychiatry 1989;30:405–416.

148. Bailey A, Le Couteur A, Gottesman I, Bolton P, Simonoff E, Yuzda E, Rutter M. Autism as a strongly genetic disorder: evidence from a British twin study. Psychological Medicine, 1995;25:63–77.

149. August G, Stewart M, Tsai L. The incidence of cognitive disabilities in the siblings of autistic children. Br J Psychiatry 1981;138: 416–422.

150. Freeman B, Ritvo E, Mason-Brothers A, et al. Psychometric assessments of first-degree relatives of 62 autistic probands in Utah. Am J Psychiatry 1989;146:361–364.

151. Szatmari P, Jones M, Tuff L, Bartolucci G, et al. Lack of cognitive impairment in first-degree relatives of children with pervasive developmental disorders. J Am Acad Child Adolesc Psychiatry 1993;32:1264–1273.

152. Bolton P, MacDonald H, Pickles A, Rios P, Goode S, Crowson M, Bailey A, Rutter M. A case-control family history study of autism. J Child Psychol Psychiatry 1994;35:877–900.

153. Volkmar F. Childhood Disintegrative Disorder: issues for DSM-IV. J Autism Dev Disord 1992;22:625–642.

154. Corbett J, Harris R, Taylor E, Trimble M. Progressive disintegrative psychosis of childhood. J Child Psychol Psychiatry 1977;18: 211–219.

155. Delong G, Dwyer J. Correlation of family history with specific autistic subgroups: Asperger's syndrome and bipolar affective disease. J Autism Dev Disord 1988;18:593–600.

156. Evans-Jones L, Rosenbloom L. Disintegrative psychosis in childhood. Dev Med Child Neurol 1978;20:462–470.

157. Kurita H. Infantile autism with speech loss before the age of thirty months. J Am Acad Child Psychiatry 1985;24:191–196.

158. Steingard R, Biederman J. Lithium responsive manic like symptoms in two individuals with autism and mental retardation. J Am Acad Child Adolesc Psychiatry 1987;26:632–635.

159. Lainhart JE, Folstein SE. Affective disorders in people with autism: a review of published cases. J Autism Dev Disord 1994;24: 587–601.

160. Tantam D. Asperger syndrome in adulthood. In: Frith U, ed. Autism and Asperger syndrome. Cambridge, UK: Cambridge University Press, 1991. pp. 147–183.

161. Gillberg C, Gillberg I, Steffenburg S. Siblings and parents of children with autism: a controlled population based study. Devel Med Child Neurology 1992;34:389–398.

162. Campbell M, Geller B, Small A, Petti T, Ferris S. Minor physical anomalies in young psychotic children. Am J Psychiatry 1978;135: 573–575.

163. Gualtieri C, Adams A, Shen C, Loiselle D. Minor physical anomalies in alcoholic and schizophrenic adults and hyperactive and autistic children. Am J Psychiatry 1982;139:640–643.

164. Links P, Stockwell M, Abichandani F, Simeon J. Minor physical anomalies in childhood autism: I. Their relationship to pre- and perinatal complications. J Autism Dev Disord 1980;10: 273–292.

165. Steg J, Rapaport J. Minor physical anomalies in normal, neurotic, learning disabled, and severely disturbed children. J Autism Childhood Schizophrenia 1975;5:299–307.

166. Walker H. Incidence of minor physical anomaly in autism. J Autism Dev Disord 1977;7:165–176.

167. Spence M, Ritvo E, Marazita M, Funderburk S, Sparkes R, Freeman B. Gene mapping studies with the syndrome of autism. Behav Gene 1985;15:1–13.

168. Hérault J, Martineau J, Petit E, Perrot, Sauvage D, Barthélémy C, Mallet J, Müh JP, LeLord G. Genetic markers in autism: association study on short arm of Chromosome 11. J Autism Devel Disord 1994;24:233–235.

169. Gillberg C, Steffenburg S, Wahlstrom J, et al. Autism associated with marker chromosome. J Am Acad Child Adolesc Psychiatry 1991;30:489–494.

170. Bundy S, Hardy C, Vickers S, Kilpatrick M, et al. Duplication of the 15q11-13 region in a patient with autism, epilepsy and ataxia. Devel Med Child Neurology 1994;36:736–742.

171. Baker P, Piven J, Schwartz S, Patil S. Duplication of chromosome 15q11-13 in two individuals with autistic disorder. J Autism Devel Disord 1994;24:529–535.

172. Hotopf M, Bolton P. A cases of autism associated with partial tetrasomy 15. J Autism Devel Disord 1995;25:41–49.

173. Ghaziuddin M, Sheldon S, Venkataraman S, Tsai L. Autism associated with tetrasomy 15: a further report. European Child Adolesc Psychiatry, 1993;2:226–230.

174. Pickles A, Bolton P, MacDonald H, Bailey A, Le Couteur A, Sim CH, Rutter M. Latent-class analysis of recurrence risks for complex phenotypes with selection and measurement error: a twin and family history study of autism. Am J Human Genetics 1195;57:717–726.

175. Hulse W. Dementia infantilis. J Nerv Ment Dis 1954;119:471–477 (translation of T. Heller's 1930 article).

176. Burd L, Fisher W, Kerbeshian J. Childhood onset pervasive developmental disorder. J Child Psychol Psychiatry 1988;29:155–163.

177. Hill A, Rosenbloom L. Disintegrative psychosis of childhood: teenage follow-up. Dev Med Child Neuro 1986;28:34–40.

178. Volkmar F, Cohen D. Disintegrative disorder or "late onset" autism. J Child Psychol Psychiatry 1989;30:717–724.

179. Kurita H. The concept and nosology of Heller's syndrome: review of articles and report of two cases. Jpn J Psychiatry Neurol 1988;42:785–793.

180. Hagberg B, Aicardi J, Dias K, Ramos O. A progressive syndrome of autism, dementia, ataxia, and loss of purposeful hand use in girls: Rett's syndrome: report of 35 cases. Ann Neurol 1983;14:471–479.

181. Hagberg B, Goutieres F, Hanefeld F, Rett A, Wilson J. Rett syndrome: criteria for inclusion and exclusion. Brain Dev 1985;7:372–373.

182. Hagberg B, Witt-Engerstrom I. Rett syndrome: a suggested staging system for describing impairment profile with increasing age towards adolescence. Am J Med Genet 1986;24(Suppl 1):47–59.

183. Van Acker R. Rett syndrome: a review of current knowledge. J Autism Dev Disord 1991;21:381–406.

184. Tsai L. Is Rett syndrome a subtype of pervasive developmental disorders? J Autism Dev Disord 1992;22:551–561.

185. Kerr A, Stephenson J. A study of the natural history of Rett syndrome in 23 girls. Am J Med Genet 1986;24:77–83.

186. Killian W. On the genetics of Rett syndrome: analysis of family and pedigree data. Am J Med Genet 1986;24(Suppl 1):369–376.

187. Wahlstrom J. Genetic implications of Rett's syndrome. Brain Dev 1985;7:573–574.

188. Wenk G, O'Leary M, Nemeroff C, Bissette G, et al. Neurochemical alterations in Rett's syndrome. Developmental Brain Research 1993;74:67–72.

189. Matsuishi T, Urabe F, Percy AK, Komori H, et al. Abnormal carbohydrate metabolism in cerebrospinal fluid in Rett's syndrome. J Child Neurology 1994;9:26–30.

190. Braddock SR, Braddock BA, Graham JM. Rett's syndrome: an update and review for the primary pediatrician. Clinical pediatrics 1993;32:613–626.

191. Asperger H. "Autistic psychopathy" in childhood. Frith U, trans. In: Frith U, ed. Autism and Asperger syndrome. Cambridge, UK: Cambridge University Press, 1991 (original article published 1944). pp. 37–92.

192. Gillberg I, Gillberg C. Asperger syndrome–some epidemiological considerations: a research note. J Child Psychol Psychiatry 1989;30:631–638.

193. Van Krevelen D. The psychopathology of autistic psychopathy. Acta Paedopsychiatr 1962;29:22–31.

194. Van Krevelen D. Early infantile autism and autistic psychopathy. J Autism Childhood Schizophrenia 1971;1:82–86.

195. Wing L. Asperger's syndrome: a clinical account. Psychol Med 1981;11:115–129.

196. Frith U. Asperger and his syndrome. In: Frith U, ed. Autism and Asperger syndrome. Cambridge, UK: Cambridge University Press, 1991. pp. 1–36.

197. Tantam D. Asperger's Syndrome (annotation). J Child Psychol Psychiatry 1988;29:245–255.

198. Wing L. The relationship between Asperger's syndrome and Kanner's autism. In: Frith U, ed. Autism and Asperger syndrome. Cambridge, UK: Cambridge University Press, 1991. pp. 93–121.

199. Gillberg C. Asperger's syndrome and recurrent psychosis–a case study. J Autism Dev Disord 1985;15:389–397.

200. Gillberg C. Clinical and neurobiological aspects of Asperger syndrome in six family studies. In: Frith U, ed. Autism and Asperger syndrome. Cambridge, UK: Cambridge Press, 1991. pp. 22–146.

201. Tantum D. Lifelong eccentricity and social isolation: I. Psychiatric, social, and forensic aspects. Br J Psychiatry 1988;153:777–782.

202. Tantum D. Lifelong eccentricity and social isolation: II. Asperger's syndrome or schizoid personality disorder? Br J Psychiatry 1988;153:783–791.

203. Baron-Cohen S. An assessment of violence in a young man with Asperger's syndrome. J Child Psychiatry 1988;29:351–360.

204. Mawson D, Grounds A, Tantam D. Violence and Asperger's syndrome: a case study. Br J Psychiatry 1985;147:566–569.

205. Wolff S, Cull A. Schizoid personality and antisocial conduct: a retrospective case note study. Psychol Med 1986;16:677–687.

206. Bowman, E. Asperger's Syndrome and autism: the case for a connection. Br J Psychiatry 1988;152:377–382.

207. Wolff S, Barlow A. Schizoid personality in childhood: a comparative study of schizoid, autistic and normal children. J Child Psychol Psychiatry 1979;20:29–46.

208. Wolff S, Chick J. Schizoid personality in childhood: a controlled follow-up study. Psychol Med 1980;10:85–100.

209. Nagy J, Szatmari P. A chart review of schizotypal personality disorders in children. J Autism Dev Disord 1986;16:351–367.

210. Szatmari P, Tuff L, Finlayson A, Bartolucci G. Asperger's syndrome and autism: neurocognitive aspects. J Am Acad Child Adolesc Psychiatry 1990;29:130–136.

211. Szatmari P, Bartolucci G, Bremner R. Asperger's syndrome and autism: comparison of early history and outcome. Dev Med Child Neurol 1989;31:709–720.

212. Szatmari P, Bremner R, Nagy J. Diagnostic criteria for Asperger's syndrome: a review of clinical features. Can J Psychiatry 1989;34:559–560.

213. Ghaziuddin M, Tsai L, Ghaziuddin N. A comparison of the diagnostic criteria for Asperger syndrome. J Autism Dev Disord 1992;22:643–649.

214. Shea V, Mesibov G. Brief report: the relationship of learning disabilities and higher-level autism. J Autism Dev Disord 1985;15:425–435.

215. Semrud-Clikeman M, Hynd G. Right hemisphere dysfunction in nonverbal learning disabilities: social, academic, and adaptive functioning in adults and children. Psychol Bull 1990;107:196–209.

216. Gillberg C. Perceptual, motor and attentional deficits in Swedish primary school children: some child psychiatric aspects. J Child Psychol Psychiatry 1983;25:377–403.

217. Gillberg C, Rasmussen P, Carlstrom C, Svenson B, Waldenstrom E.

Perceptual, motor and attentional deficits in six year old children: epidemiological aspects. J Child Psychol Psychiatry 1982;23:131–144.

218. Weintraub S, Mesulam M. Developmental Learning disabilities of the right hemisphere: emotional, interpersonal, and cognitive components. Arch Neurol 1983;40:463–468.

219. Voeller K. Right-hemisphere deficit syndrome in children. Am J Psychiatry 1986;143:1004–1009.

220. Denckla M. The neuropsychology of social-emotional learning disabilities. Arch Neurol 1983;40:461–462.

221. Morris M. Social-emotional learning disability [Abstract]. J Exp Clin Neuropsychol 1992;14:369.

222. Rourke B. The syndrome of nonverbal learning disabilities: developmental manifestation in neurological disease, disorder, and dysfunction. The Clinical Neuropsychologist 1988;2:293–330.

223. Rourke, B. Nonverbal learning disabilities: the syndrome and the model. New York: Guilford Press, 1989.

224. Realmuto G, Main B. Coincidence of Tourette's disorder and infantile autism. J Autism Dev Disord 1982;12:367–372.

225. Kerbeshian J, Burd L. Asperger's syndrome and Tourette syndrome: the case of the pinball wizard. Br J Psychiatry 1986;148:731–736.

226. Stahl S. Tardive Tourette's syndrome in an autistic patient after long-term neuroleptic administration. Am J Psychiatry 1980;137:1267–1269.

227. Littlejohns C, Clarke D, Corbett J. Tourette-like disorder in Asperger's syndrome. Br J Psychiatry 1990;156:430–433.

228. Klawans H, Nausieda P, Goetz C, Tourette-like symptoms following chronic neuroleptic therapy. Adv Neurol 1982;35:415–418.

229. Burd L, Fisher W, Kerbeshian J, Arnold M. Is development of Tourette disorder a marker for improvement in patients with autism and other pervasive developmental disorders? J Am Acad Child Adolesc Psychiatry 1987;26:162–165.

230. Comings D, Comings B. Clinical and genetic relationships between autism- pervasive developmental disorder and Tourette syndrome: a study of 19 cases. Am J Med Genet 1991;39:180–191.

231. Sverd J. Tourette syndrome and autistic disorder: a significant relationship. Am J Med Genet 1991;39:173–179.

232. Marriage K, Miles T, Stokes D, Dave M. Clinical and research implications of the co-occurrence of Asperger's and Tourette's syndromes. Australian New Zealand J Psychiatry 1993;27:666–674.

233. Bender L. Childhood schizophrenia: clinical study of 100 schizophrenic children. Am J Orthopsychiatry 1947;17:40–56.

234. Kolvin I, Ounsted C, Humphrey M, McNay A. Studies in the childhood psychoses: II. The phenomenology of childhood psychoses. Br J Psychiatry 1971;118:385–395.

235. Rutter M. Childhood schizophrenia reconsidered. J Autism Childhood Schizophrenia 1972;2:315–337.

236. Green W, Campbell M, Hardesty A, et al. A comparison of schizophrenic and autistic children. J Acad Child Psychiatry 1984;23:399–409.

237. Eggers C. Course and prognosis of childhood schizophrenia. J Autism Childhood Schizophrenia 1978;8:21–35.

238. Howells J, Guirguis W. Childhood schizophrenia 20 years later. Arch Gen Psychiatry 1984;41:123–128.

239. Petty L, Ornitz E, Michelman J, Zimmerman E. Autistic children who become schizophrenic. Arch Gen Psychiatry 1984;41:129–135.

240. Cantor S. Childhood schizophrenia. New York: Guilford Press, 1988.

241. Cantor S, Evans J, Pearce J, Pezzot-Pearce T. Childhood schizophrenia: present but not accounted for. Am J Psychiatry 1982;139:758–762.

242. Tanguay P, Cantor S. Schizophrenia in children. J Am Acad Child Psychiatry 1986;25:591–594.

243. Volkmar F, Cohen D. Co-morbid association of autism and schizophrenia. Am J Psychiatry 1991;148:1705–1707.

244. Bartak L, Rutter M. Cox A. A comparative study of infantile autism and specific developmental receptive language disorders: III. Discriminant function analysis. J Autism Childhood Schizophrenia 1977;7:383–396.

245. Rutter M. The development of infantile autism. Psychol Med 1974;4:147–163.

246. Tuchman RF, Rapin I, Shinnar S. Autistic and dysphasic children. II. Epilepsy. Pediatrics 1991;88:1219–1225.

247. Volkmar F, Nelson D. Seizure disorders in autism. J Am Acad Child Adolesc Psychiatry 1990;29:127–129.

248. Olsson I, Steffenburg S, Gillberg C. Epilepsy in autism and autistic-like conditions: a population-based study. Arch Neurol 1988;45:666–668.

249. Gillberg C, Schaumann H. Epilepsy presenting as infantile autism? Two case studies. Neuropediatrics 1983;14:206–212.

250. Mouridsen S, Anderson L, Sorenson S, Rich B, et al. Neurofibromatosis in infantile autism and other types of childhood psychosis. Acta Pedopsychiatrica 1992;55:15–18.

251. Zappella M. Autism and hypomelanosis of Ito in twins. Devel Med Child Neurology 19932;35:826–832.

252. Smalley S, Tanguay P, Smith M, Guitierrez G. Autism and tuberous sclerosis. J Autism Devel Disord 1194;22:339–355.

253. Hunt A, Shepherd C. A prevalence study of autism in tuberous sclerosis. J Autism Devel Disord 1194;23:323–339.

254. Ritvo E, Jorde L, Mo A, Ritvo A. The UCLA-University of Utah Epidemiological survey of autism: the etiologic role of rare diseases. Am J Psychiatry 1990;147:1614–1621.

255. Steffenburg S. Neuropsychiatric assessment of children with autism: a population-based study. Dev Med Child Neurol 1991;33:495–511.

256. Rutter M, Bailey A, Bolton P, LeCouteur A. Autism and known medical conditions: myth and substance. J Child Psychol Psychiatry 1994;35:311–322.

257. Martin J, Bell J. A pedigree of mental defect showing sex-linkage. J Neurol Psychiatry 1943;6:154–157.

258. Lubs H. A marker X chromosome. Am J Hum Genet 1969;21:31–244.

259. Sherman S. Epidemiology. In: Hagerman R, Silverman A, eds. Fragile X syndrome: diagnosis, treatment,, and research. Baltimore: Johns Hopkins University Press, 1991.

260. Hagerman R. Physical and behavioral phenotype. In: Hagerman R, Silverman A, eds. Fragile X syndrome: diagnosis, treatment, and research. Baltimore: Johns Hopkins University Press, 1991.

261. Brown W, Jenkins E, Cohen I, et al. Fragile X and autism: a multicenter survey. Am J Med Genet 1986;26:643–664.

262. Einfeld S, Molony H, Hall. Autism is not associated with the fragile X syndrome. Am J Med Genet 1989;34:187.

263. Payton JB, Steele M, Wenger S, Minshew N. The fragile X marker and autism in perspective. J Am Acad Child Adolesc Psychiatry 1989;28:417–421.

264. Piven J, Gayle J, Landa R, Wzorek M, Folstein S. The prevalence of fragile X in a sample of autistic diagnosed using a standardized interview. J Am Acad Child Adolesc Psychiatry 1991;30:825–830.

265. Bailey A, Bolton P, Butler L, LeCouteur A, et al. Prevalence of the fragile X anomaly amongst autistic twins and singletons. J Child Psychol Psychiatry 1993;34:673–688.

266. Cohen I, Vietze P, Sudhalter V, Jenkins E, Brown W. Parent-child dyadic gaze patterns in fragile X males and fragile x females with autistic disorder. J Child Psychol Psychiatry 1989;30:845–856.

267. Cohen I, Fisch G, Sudhalter V, et al. Social gaze, social avoidance and repetitive behavior in fragile X males: a controlled study. Am J Ment Retard 1988;92:436–446.

268. Pennington B, O–Connor R, Sudhalter V. Toward a neuropsychology of fragile X syndrome. In: Hagerman R, Silverman A, eds. Fragile X syndrome: diagnosis, treatment, and research. Baltimore: Johns Hopkins University Press, 1991.

269. Courchesne E, Yeung-Courchesne R, Press GA, Hesselink JR, Jernigan TL. Hypoplasia of cerebellar vermal lobules IV and VII in autism. N Eng J Med 1988;318:1349–1354.

270. Reiss A, Patel S. Kumar A, Freund L. Neuroanatomical variations of the posterior fossa in men with the fragile X (Martin -Bell) syndrome. Am J Med Genet 1988;31:407–414.

271. Holroyd S, Reiss A, Bryan N. Autistic features in Joubert syndrome: a genetic disorder with agenesis of the cerebellar vermis. Biol Psychiatry 1991;29:287–294.

272. Chess S. Autism in children with congenital rubella. J Autism Childhood Schizophrenia 1971;1:33–47.

273. Chess S. Follow-up report on autism in congenital rubella. J Autism Childhood Schizophrenia 1977;7:69–81.

274. Bryson S, Smith I, Eastwood D. Obstetrical suboptimality in autistic children. J Am Acad Child Adolesc Psychiatry 1988;27:418–422.

275. Finegan J, Quarrington B. Pre-, peri, and neonatal factors and infantile autism. J Child Psychol Psychiatry 1979;20:119–128.

276. Gillberg C, Gillberg IC. Infantile autism: a total population study of reduced optimality in the pre-, peri, and neonatal period. J Autism Dev Disord 1983;13:153–166.

277. Mason-Brothers A, Ritvo E, Guze B, et al. Pre-, peri, and postnatal factors in 181 autistic patients from single and multiple incidence families. J Am Acad Child Adolesc Psychiatry 1987;26:39–42.

278. Levy S, Zoitak B, Saelens T. A comparison of obstetrical records of autistic and nonautistic referrals for psychoeducational evaluations. J Autism Dev Disord 1988;18:573–581.

279. Mason-Brothers A, Ritvo E, Pingree C, et al. The UCLA-University of Utah epidemiologic survey of autism: prenatal, perinatal, and postnatal factors. Pediatrics 1990;86:514–519.

280. Coleman M. Second trimester of gestation: a time of risk for classical autism? Developmental Brain Dysfunction 1994;7:104–109.

281. Bolton P, MacDonald H, Pickles A, Rios P, et al. A case-control family history study of autism. J Child Psychol Psychiatry 1994;34:877–900.

282. Gaffney GR, Tsai LY. Magnetic resonance imaging of high level autism. J Autism Dev Disord 1987;17:433–438.

283. DaMasio H, Maurer RG, DaMasio AR, Chui HC. Computerized tomographic scan findings in patients with autistic behavior. Arch Neurol 1980;37:504–510.

284. Gillberg C, Svendsen P. Childhood psychosis and computed tomographic brain scan findings. J Autism Dev Disord 1983;13:19–32.

285. Prior MR, Tress B, Hoffman WL, Boldt D. Computed tomographic study of children with classic autism. Arch Neurol 1984;41:482–484.

286. Bauman NM, Kemper T. Histoanatomic observations of the brain in early infantile autism. Neurology 1985;35:866–874.

287. Coleman, P, Romano J, Lapham L, Simon W. Cell counts in cerebral cortex of an autistic patient. J Autism Dev Disord 1985;15:245–256.

288. Creasey H, Rumsey JM, Schwartz M, Duara R, Rapport SI. Brain morphometry in autistic men as measured by volumetric computed tomography. Arch Neurol 1986;43:669–672.

289. Williams RS, Hauser SL, Purpura DP, DeLong GR, Swisher CN. Autism and mental retardation: neuropathologic studies performed on four retarded persons with autistic behavior. Arch Neurol 1980;37:749–753.

290. Darby JK. Neuropathologic aspects of psychosis in children. J Autism Childhood Schizophrenia 1976;6:339–352.

291. Piven J, Berthier ML, Starkstein SR, et al. Magnetic resonance imaging evidence for a defect of cerebral cortical development in autism. Am J Psychiatry 1990;147:734–739.

292. Hier DB, LeMay M, Rosenberger PB. Autism and unfavorable left-right asymmetries of the brain. J Autism Dev Disord 1979;9:153–159.

293. Hauser SL, DeLong, Rosman NP. Pneumographic findings in the infantile autism syndrome: a correlation with temporal lobe disease. Brain 1975;98:667–688.

294. Bauman M, Kemper T. Limbic and cerebellar abnormalities: consistent findings in infantile autism. J Neuropathol Exp Neurol 1988;47:369.

295. Hoon AH, Reiss Al. The mesial-temporal lobe and autism: case report and review. Dev Med Child Neurol 1992;34:252–265.

296. Deonna T, Ziegler AL, Moura-Serra J, Innocenti G. Autistic regression in relation to limbic pathology and epilepsy: report of two cases. Developmental Med Child Neurology 1993;35:166–176.

297. Fein D, Waterhouse L. Infantile autism: delineating the key deficits. Paper presented at a meeting of the International Neuropsychology Symposium, North Berwick, Scotland 1985.

298. Waterhouse L, Fein D, Modahl C. Neurofunctional mechanisms I autism. Psychological Review. in press.

299. Bachevalier J. Medial temporal lobe structure and autism: a review of clinical and experimental findings. Neuropsychologia 1994;32:627–648.

300. Brothers L. A biological perspective on empathy. Am J Psychiatry 1989;146:10–19.

301. Fotheringham JB. Autism and its primary psychological and neurological deficit. Canadian J Psychiatry 1991;36:686–692.

302. Courchesne E, Townsend J, Saito O. The brain in infantile autism: posterior fossa structures are abnormal. Neurology 1994;44:214–223.

303. Ritvo ER, Freeman BJ, Scheibel AB, et al. Lower purkinje cell counts in the cerebella of four autistic subjects: initial findings of the UCLA-NSAC autopsy research report. Am J Psychiatry 1986;143:862–866.

304. Gaffney GR, Tsai LY, Kuperman S, Minchin S. Cerebellar structure in autism. Am J Disabled Child 1987;141:1330–1332.

305. Murakami JW, Courchesne E, Press GA, Yeung-Courchesne R, Hesselink, JR. Reduced cerebellar hemisphere size and its relationship to vermal hypoplasia in autism. Arch Neurol 1989;46:689–694.

306. Leaton R, Supple WF. Cerebellar vermis: essential for long-term habituation of the acoustic startle response. Science 1986;232:513–515.

307. Courchesne E. A neurophysiological view of autism. In: Schopler E, Mesibov GB, eds. Neurobiological issues in autism. New York: Plenum, 1987:285–324.

308. Kootz JP, Cohen DJ. Modulation of sensory intake in autistic children: cardiovascular and behavioral indices. J Am Acad Child Psychiatry 1981;20:692–701.

309. Courchesne, E. Neuroanatomical systems involved in infantile autism. In: Dawson G, ed. Autism: new perspectives on diagnosis, nature and treatment. New York: Guilford Press, 1989:119–143.

310. Hsu M, Yeung-Courchesne R, Courchesne E, Press, GA. Absence of magnetic resonance imaging evidence of pontine abnormality in infantile autism. Arch Neurol 1991;48:1160–1163.

311. Courchesne E, Townsend JP, Ashkoomoff NA, et al. A new finding: impairment in shifting attention in autistic and cerebellar patients. In: Broman SH, Grafman J, eds. Atypical deficits in developmental disorders: implication for brain function. New Jersey: Lawrence Erlbaum, 1994. pp. 101–137.

312. Courchesne E, Townsend J, Aksoomoff N, Saitoh O, et al. Impairment in shifting attention in autistic and cerebellar patients. Behav Neurosci 1994;108:848–865.

313. Ciesielski KT, Knight JE. Cerebellar abnormality in autism: a nonspecific effect of early brain damage. Acta Neurobiologiae Experimentalis 1994;54:151–154.

314. Ritvo ER, Garber HJ. Cerebellar hypoplasia and autism. N Eng J Med 1988;319:1152.

315. Kleiman MD, Neff S, Rosman NP. The brain in infantile autism: are posterior fossa structures abnormal? Neurology 1992;43:753–760.

316. Schifter T, Hoffman JM, Hatten HP, Hanson MW. Neuroimaging in infantile autism. J Child Neurology 1994;9:155–161.

317. Heh CWC, Smith R, Wu J, et al. Positron emission tomography of the cerebellum in autism. Am J Psychiatry 1989;146:242–245.

318. Rumsey JM, Duara R, Grady C, et al. Brain metabolism in autism: resting cerebral glucose utilization rates as measured with positron emission tomography. Arch Gen Psychiatry 1985;42:448–455.

319. Herold S, Frackowiak RSJ, LeCouteur A, Rutter M, Howlin P. Cerebral blood flow and metabolism of oxygen and glucose in young autistic adults. Psychol Med 1988;18:823–831.

320. Siegel BV, Asarnow RB, Tanguay P, Call JD, et al. regional cerebral glucose metabolism and attention in adults with a history of childhood autism. J Neuropsychiat Clin Neurosci 1992;4:406–414.

321. Buschsbaum MS, Siegel BV, Wu JC, Hazlett E, et al. Brief report: attention performances in autism and regional brain metabolic rate assessed by positron emission tomography. J Autism Dev Dis 1992;22:115–125.

322. Zilbovicius M, Garreau B, Samson Y, Remy P, et al. Delayed maturation of the frontal cortex in childhood autism. Am J Psychiatry 1995;152:248–252.

323. Deutsch G. The nospecificity of frontal dysfunction in disease and altered states: cortical blood flow evidence. Neuropsychiatry, Neuropsychol Behav Neurology 1992; 5:301–307.

324. Garreau B, Zilbovicius M, Guerin P, Samson Y, et al. Effects of auditory stimulation on regional cerebral blood flow in autistic children. Developmental Brain Dysfunction 1994;7:119–128.

325. Zilbovicius M, Garreau B, Tzourio N, Mazoyer B, et al. Regional cerebral blood flow in childhood autism: a SPECT study. Am J Psychiat 1992;149:924–930.

326. Gillberg IC, Bjure J, Uvebrant P, Vestergren E, et al. SPECT in 31 children and adolescents with autism and autistic-like conditions. European Child Adolesc Psychiatry 1993;2:50–59.

327. Minshew NJ, Goldstein G, Dombrowski SM, Panchalingam K, et al. A preliminary -sup-3-sup1P MRS study of autism: evidence for undersynthesis and increased degradation of brain membranes. Biological Psychiatry 1993;33:762–773.

328. Ritvo ER, Creel D, Realmuto G, et al. Electroretinograms in autism: a pilot study of b-wave amplitudes. Am J Psychiatry 1988;145:229–232.

329. Castrogiovanni P, Marazziti D. ERG b-wave amplitude and brain dopaminergic activity. Am J Psychiatry 1989;146:1085–1086.

330. Yuwiler A, Ritvo ER. "ERG b-wave amplitude and brain dopaminergic activity": reply. Am J Psychiatry 1989;146:1086.

331. Hutt S, Hutt C, Lee D, Ounsted D. A behavioral and electroencephalographic study of autistic children. J Psychiatr Res 1965;3:181–197.

332. Ornitz, EM, Forsythe AB, de la Pena A. Effect of vestibular and auditory stimulation on the REM's sleep in autistic children. Arch Gen Psychiatry 1973;29:786–791.

333. Colbert G, Koegler RR, Markham CH. Vestibular dysfunction in childhood schizophrenia. Arch Gen Psychiatry 1959;1:600–617.

334. Ornitz EM. Vestibular dysfunction in schizophrenia and childhood autism. Comparative Psychiatry 1970;11:159–173.

335. Ornitz EM, Brown MB, Mason A, Putnam NH. Effect of visual input on vestibular nystagmus in autistic children. Arch Gen Psychiatry 1974;31:369–375.

336. Ritvo ER, Ornitz EM, Eviatar A, et al. Decreased post-rotatory nystagmus in early infantile autism. Neurology 1969;19:653–658.

337. Ornitz, EM, Ritvo ER, Brown MB, La Franchi S, Parmelee T, Walter RD. The EEG and rapid eye movement during REM sleep in normal and autistic children. Electroencephalogr Clin Neurophsyiol 1969;26:167–175.

338. Gillberg C, Rosenhall U, Johansson E. Auditory brainstem responses in childhood psychosis. J Autism Dev Disord 1983;13:181–194.

339. Fein D, Skoff B, Mirsky AF. Clinical correlates of brainstem dysfunction in autistic children. J Autism Dev Disord 1981;11:303–315.

340. Narita T, Koga Y. Neuropsychological assessment of childhood autism. Adv Biol Psychiatry 1987;16:156–170.

341. Novick B, Vaughn HG, Kurtzberg D, Simon R. An electrophysiologic indication of auditory processing defects in autism. Psychiatry Res 1980;3:107–114.

342. Rosenblum SM, Arick JR, Krug DA, Stubbs EG, Young NB, Pelson RO. Auditory brainstem evoked responses in autistic children. J Autism Dev Disord 1980;10:215–225.

343. Skoff B, Mirsky A, Turner D. Prolonged brainstem transmission time in autism. Psychiatry Res 1980;2:157–166.

344. Student M, Sohmer H. Evidence from auditory nerve and brainstem evoked responses for an organic brain lesion in children with autistic

345. Tanguay PE, Edwards RM, Buchwald J, Schwafel J, Allen V. Auditory brainstem evoked responses in autistic children. Arch Gen Psychiatry 1982;39:174–180.

346. Thivierge J, Bedard C, Cote R, Maziade M. Brainstem auditory evoked response and subcortical abnormalities in autism. Am J Psychiatry 1990;147:1609–1613.

347. Wong V, Wong SN. Brainstem auditory evoked potential study in children with autistic disorder. J Autism Dev Disord 1991;21:329–340.

348. Damasio A, Maurer R. A neurological model for childhood autism. Arch Neuro 1978;35:777–786.

349. DeLong GR. A neuropsychological interpretation of infantile autism. In: Schopler E, Rutter M, eds. Autism: a reappraisal of concepts and treatment. New York: Plenum, 1978:207–218.

350. Cieselski KT, Courchesne E, Elmasian R. Effects of focused selective attention tasks on event-related potentials in autism and normal individuals. Electroencephalogr Clin Neurophysiol 1990;75:207–220.

351. Courchesne E, Kilman BA, Galambos R, Lincoln AJ. Autism: processing of novel auditory information assessed by event-related brain potentials. Electroencephalogr Clin Neurophysiol 1984;59:238–248.

352. Courchesne E, Lincoln AJ, Kilman BA, Galambos R. Event related brain potentials of the processing of novel visual and auditory information in autism. J Autism Dev Disord 1985;15:55–76.

353. Courchesne E, Lincoln AJ, Yeung-Courchesne R, Elmasian R, Grillon C. Pathophysiologic findings in nonretarded autism and receptive developmental language disorder. J Autism Dev Disord 1989;19:1–18.

354. Dawson G, Finley C, Phillips S, et al. Reduced P3 amplitude of the event-related brain potential: its relationship to language ability in autism. J Autism Dev Disord 1988;18:493–504.

355. Martineau J, et al. Effects of vitamin B6 on average evoked potentials in infantile autism. Biol Psychiatry 1981;16:627–641.

356. Oades RD, Walker MK, Geffen LB, Stern LM. Event-related potentials in autistic and healthy children on an auditory choice reaction time task. Int J Psychophysiol 1988;6:25–37.

357. Novick B, Kurtzberg D, Vaughn HG. An electrophysiologic indication of defective information storage in childhood autism. Psychiatry Res 1979;1:101–108.

358. Verbaten R, Van Engeland H. Autism: psychofysiologisch benaderd (Autism: psychophysiologic assessment) [Abstract]. Psycholoog 1988;23:289–295.

359. Niwa S, Ohta M, Yamazaki M. P300 and stimulus evaluation process in autistic subjects. J Autism Dev Disord 1983;13:33–42.

360. Erwin RJ, Van Lancker D, Guthrie D, et al. P3 responses to prosodic stimuli in adult autistic subjects. Electroencephalogr Clin Neurophysiol 1991;80:561–571.

361. Courchesne E, Courchesne RY, Hicks G, Lincoln AJ. Functioning of the brainstem auditory pathway in non-related autistic individuals. Electroencephalogr Clin Neurophysiol 1985;61:491–501.

362. Tanguay PE, Ornitz EM, Forsythe AB, Ritvo ER. Rapid eye movement (REM) activity in normal and autistic children during REM sleep. J Autism Childhood Schizophrenia 1976;6:275–288.

363. Dawson G, Warrenburg S, Fuller P. Hemisphere functioning and motor imitation in autistic persons. Brain Cogn 1983;2:346–354.

364. Ogawa T, Sugiyama A, Ishiwa S, Suzuki M, Ishihara T, Sato K. Ontogenic development of EEG-asymmetry in early infantile autism. Brain Dev 1982;4:439–449.

365. Small JG. EEG and neurophysiological studies of early infantile autism. Biol Psychiatry 1975;10:385–397.

366. Dawson G, Warrenburg S, Fuller P. Cerebral lateralization in individuals diagnosed as autistic in early childhood. Brain Lang 1982;15:353–368.

367. Dawson G, Finley C, Phillips S, Galpert L. Hemispheric specialization

and the language abilities of autistic children. Child Dev 1986;57: 1440–1453.

368. Sedvall G, Fyrö, B., Gillberg, B. et al. Relationships in healthy volunteers between concentration of monoamine metabolites in cerebrospinal fluid and family history of psychiatric morbidity. Br J Psychiatry 1980;136:366–374.

369. Schain RJ, Freedman DX. Studies on 5-hydroxyindoleamine metabolism in autistic and other mentally retarded children. J Pediatr 1961;58:315–320.

370. Ciarenello RD, Vanderberg SR, Anders TF. Intrinsic and extrinsic determinants of neuronal development: relation to infantile autism. J Autism Dev Disord 1982;12:115–145.

371. Anderson GM, Freedman DX, Cohen DJ, et al. Whole blood serotonin in autistic and normal subjects. J Child Psychol Psychiatry 1987;28:885–900.

372. Kuperman S, Beeghly J, Burns T, Tsai L. Serotonin relationships of autistic probands and their first-degree relatives. J Acad Child Adolesc Psychiatry 1985;24:186–190.

373. Cook EH, Leventhal BL, Freedman DX. Free serotonin in plasma: autistic children and their first degree relatives. Biol Psychiatry 1988;24:488–491.

374. Cook EH, Leventahl BL, Heller W, Metz J, Wainwright M, Freedman DX. Autistic children and their first-degree relatives: relationship between serotonin and norepinephrine levels and intelligence. J Neuropsychiatry Clin Neurosci 1990;2:268–274.

375. Leventhal BL, Cook EH, Morford M, Ravitz A, Freedman DX. Relationships of whole blood serotonin and plasma norepinephrine within families. J Autism Dev Disord 1990;20:499–511.

376. Piven J, Tsai G, Nehme E, Coyle JT, Chase GA, Folstein SE. Platelet serotonin, a possible marker for familial autism. J Autism Dev Disord 1991;21:51–59.

377. Takahashi S, Kanai H, Miyamoto Y. Reassessment of elevated serotonin levels in blood platelet in early infantile autism. J Autism Childhood Schizophrenia 1976;6:317–326.

378. Hanley HG, Stahl SM, Freedman DX. Hyperserotonemia and amine metabolites in autistic and retarded children. Arch Gen Psychiatry 1977;34:521–531.

379. Pare CMB, Sandler M, Stacey RS. 5-Hydroxyindoles in mental deficiency. J Neurol Neurosurg Psychiatry 1960;23:341–346.

380. Partington MW, Tu JB, Wong CY. Blood serotonin levels in severe mental retardation. Dev Med Child Neurol 1973;15:616–627.

381. Hoshino Y, Yamamoto T, Kaneko M. Blood serotonin and free tryptophan concentrations in autistic children. Neuropsychobiology 1984;11:22–27.

382. Yuwiler A, Shih JC, Chen CH, Ritvo ER, et al. Hyperserotoninemia and antiserotonin antibodies in autism and other disorders. J Autism Devel Disord 1992;22:33–45.

383. Cook EH, Perry BD, Dawson G, Wainwright MS, et al. Receptor inhibition by immunoglobulins: specific inhibition by autistic children, their relatives and control subjects. J Autism Devel Disord 1993;67–78.

384. Anderson GM, Horne WC, Chatterjee D, Cohen DJ. The hyperserotonemia of autism. Ann N Y Acad Sci 1990;600:331–342.

385. Young JG, Kavanagh ME, Anderson GM, Shaywitz BA, Cohen DJ. Clinical neurochemistry of autism and associated disorders. J Autism Dev Disord 1982;12:147–165.

386. Sanker DVS. Biogenic amine uptake by blood platelets and RBC in childhood schizophrenia. Acta Paedopsychiatr 1970;37:174–182.

387. Sanker DVS. Uptake of 5-hydroxytryptamine by isolated platelets in childhood schizophrenia and autism. Neuropsychobiology 1977;3:234–239.

388. Boullin DJ, Coleman M, O–Brien RA. Abnormalities in platelet 5-hydroxy-tryptamine efflux in patients with infantile autism. Nature 1970;226:371–372.

389. Boullin DJ, Freeman BJ, Geller E, Ritvo E, Rutter M, Yuwiler A. Toward the resolution of conflicting findings. J Autism Dev Disord 1982;12:97–98.

390. Lucas AR, Warner K, Gottlieb JS. Biological studies in childhood schizophrenia: serotonin uptake by platelets. Biol Psychiatry 1971;3:123–128.

391. Yuwiler A, Ritvo E, Geller E, Glousman R, Schneiderman G, Matsuno D. Uptake and efflux of serotonin from platelets of autistic and nonautistic children. J Autism Dev Disord 1975;5:83–98.

392. Katsui T, Okuda M, Usuda S, Koizumi T. Kinetics of sub-3-serotonin uptake by platelets in infantile autism and developmental language disorder (including five pairs of twins). J Autism Dev Disord 1986;16:69–76.

393. Rotman A, Caplan R, Szekely GA. Platelet uptake of serotonin in psychotic children. Pyschopharmacology 1980;67:245–248.

394. Halbreich U, Rojansky N, Zander KJ, Barkai A. Influence of age, sex and diurnal variability on imipramine receptor binding and serotonin uptake in platelets of normal subjects. J Psychiatr Res 1991;25:7–18.

395. Anderson GM, Minderaa RB, van Bentem PPG, Volkmar FR, Cohen DJ. Platelet imipramine binding in autistic subjects. Psychiatry Res 1984;11:133–141.

396. Boullin DJ, Coleman M, O–Brien RA, Rimland B. Laboratory predictions of infantile autism based on 5-hydroxy-tryptamine efflux from blood platelets and their correlation with the Rimland E-2 score. J Autism Childhood Schizophrenia 1971;1:63–71.

397. McBride PA, Anderson GM, Hertzig ME, et al. Serotonergic responsivity in male young adults with autistic disorder. Arch Gen Psychiatry 1989;46:205–212.

398. Perry BD, Cook EH, Leventhal BL, Wainwright MS, Freedman DX. Platelet 5-HT-sub-2 receptor binding sites in autistic children and their first-degree relatives. In: Proceedings of the American Academy of Child and Adolescent Psychiatry. New York, 1989:67–68.

399. Saffai-Kutti S, Denfors I, Kutti J, Wadenvik H. In vitro platelet function in infantile autism [Abstract]. Folia Haematol (Leipz) 1988;(Suppl):897–901.

400. Saffai-Kutti S, Kutti J, Gillberg C. Impaired in vivo platelet reactivity in infantile autism. Acta Paediatr Scand 1985;74:799–800.

401. Launay JM, Ferrari P, Haimart M, et al. Serotonin metabolism and other biochemical parameters in infantile autism. Neuropsychobiology 1988;20:1–11.

402. Lake C, Ziegler M, Murphy D. Increased Norepinephrine levels and decreased dopamine-beta-hydroxylase activity in primary autism. Arch Gen Psychiatry 1977;34:553–566.

403. Cohen DJ, Caparulo BK, Shaywitz BA, Bowers, MB. Dopamine and serotonin metabolism in neuropsychiatrically disturbed children. Arch Gen Psychiatry 1977;34:545–550.

404. Volkmar FR, Anderson GM. Neurochemical perspectives on infantile autism. In: Dawson G, ed. Autism: new perspectives on diagnosis, nature and treatment. New York: Guilford Press, 1989:209–224.

405. Herault J, Martineau J, Perrot-Beaugerie A, Jouve J, et al. Investigation of whole blood and urine monoamines in autism. European Child Adolesc Psychiatry 1993;2:211–220.

406. Anderson GM, Minderaa RB, Cho SC, Bolkmar FR, Cohen DJ. The issue of hyperserotonemia and platelet serotonin exposure: a preliminary study. J Autism Dev Disord 1989;19:349–351.

407. Minderaa RB, Anderson GM, Volkmar FR, Akkerhuis GW, Cohen DJ. Urinary 5-hydroxyindoleacetic acid and whole blood serotonin and tryptophan in autistic and normal subjects. Biol Psychiatry 1987;22:933–940.

408. Gillberg C, Svennerholm L, Hamilton-Hellberg C. Childhood psychosis and monoamine metabolites in spinal fluid. J Autism Dev Disord 1983;13:383–396.

409. Narayan M, Srinath S, Anderson GM, Meundi DB. Cerebrospinal fluid levels of homovanillic acid and 5-hydroxyindoleacetic acid in autism. Biological Psychiatry 1993;33:630–635.

410. Ritvo ER, Freeman BJ, Yuwiler A, et al. Fenfluramine treatment of autism: UCLA collaborative study of 81 patients at nine medical centers. Psychopharmacol Bull 1986;22:133–140.

411. Aman MG, Kern PA. Review of fenfluramine in the treatment of the developmental disabilities. J Am Acad Child Adolesc Psychiatry 1990;28:549–565.

412. August GJ, Raz N, Baird TD. Fenfluramine response in high and low functioning autistic children. J Am Acad Child Adolesc Psychiatry 1987;26:342–346.

413. Campbell M, Deutsch SI, Perry R, Wolsky BB, Paliz M. Short-term efficacy and safety of fenfluramine in hospitalized preschool-age autistic children: an open study. Psychopharmacol Bull 1986;22:141–147.

414. Campbell M, Perry R, Polonsky B. Brief report: an open study of fenfluramine in hospitalized young autistic children. J Autism Dev Disord 1986;46:495–506.

415. Du Verglas G, Banks SR, Guyer KE. Clinical effects of Fenfluramine in children with autism: a review of the research. J Autism Dev Disord 1988;18:297–308.

416. Geller E, Ritvo ER, Freeman BJ, Yuwiler A. Preliminary observations on the effect of fenfluramine on blood serotonin and symptoms in three autistic boys. N Eng J Med 1982;307:165–169.

417. Groden G, Groden J, Dondey M, et al. Effects of fenfluramine on the behavior of autistic individuals. Res Dev Disabil 1987;8:203–211.

418. Ritvo ER, Freeman BJ, Yuwiler A, et al. Study of fenfluramine in outpatients with the syndrome of autism. J Pediatr 1984;105:823–828.

419. Ritvo ER, Freeman BJ, Geller E, Yuwiler A. Effects of fenfluramine on 14 outpatients with the syndrome of autism. J Am Acad Child Adolesc Psychiatry 1983;22:549–558.

420. Duker PC, Welles K, Seys D, Rensen H, et al. Brief report: effects of fenfluramine on communicative, stereotypic and inappropriate behaviors of autistic-type mentally handicapped individuals. J Autism Dev Disord 1991;21:355–363.

421. Sherman J, Factor DC, Swinson R, Darjes RW. The effects of fenfluramine (hydrochloride) on the behaviors of autistic children. J Autism Dev Disord 1989;19:533–543.

422. Ekman G, Miranda-Linne F, Gillberg C, et al. Fenfluramine treatment of twenty children with autism. J Autism Dev Disord 1989;19:511–532.

423. Stern LM, Walker MK, Sawyer M, et al. A controlled crossover trial of fenfluramine in autism. J Child Psychol Psychiatry 1990;31:569–585.

424. Duker PC, Welles K, Seys D, Rensen H, et al. Brief report: effects of fenfluramine on communicative, stereotypic and inappropriate behaviors of autistic-type mentally handicapped individuals. J Autism Devel Disord 1991;21:355–363.

425. Pucilowski O, Plaznik A, Kostowski W. Aggressive behavior inhibition by serotonin and quipazine injected into the amygdala in the rat. Behav Neural Biol 1985;43:58–68.

426. Shepard RA, Buxton DS, Boadhurst PL. Beta-adrenoceptor antagonists may attenuate hyponeophagia in the rat through serotonergic mechanism. Pharmacol Biochem Behav 1982;16:741–744.

427. Gately PF, Poon SL, Segal DS, Geyer MA. Depletion of brain serotonin by 5, 7-dihydroxytryptamine alters the response to amphetamine and the habituation of locomotor activity in rats. Psychopharmacology 1985;87:400–405.

428. Davis M, Kehne JH, Commissaris RL. Antagonism of apomorphine-enhanced startle by alpha 1-adrenergic antagonists. Eur J Pharmacol 1985;108:233–241.

429. Kuperman S, Beeghly JHL, Burns TL, Tsai LY. Association of serotonin concentration to behavior and IQ in autistic children. J Autism Dev Disord 1987;17:133–140.

430. Panksepp J, Sivy SM, Normansell LA. Brain opioids and social emotions. In: Reite M, Field T, eds. The psychobiology of attachment and separation. New York: Academic Press, 1985.

431. Herman BH, Panksepp J. Ascending endorphin inhibition of distress vocalization. Science 1981;221:1060–1062.

432. Freed CR, Yamomato BK. Regional brain dopamine metabolism: a marker for the speed, direction and posture of moving animals. Science 1985;229:62–65.

433. Coleman M, Gillberg C. The biology of the autistic syndromes. New York: Praeger, 1985.

434. Maurer RG, DaMasio AR. Childhood autism from the point of behavioral neurology. J Autism Dev Disord 1982;12:195–205.

435. Broderick PA, Gardner EL, Van Praag HM. In vivo electrochemical and behavioral evidence for specific neural substrates modulated differentially by encephalon in rat stimulant stereotypy and locomotion. Biol Psychiatry 1984;19:45–54.

436. Meltzer HY, Busch D, Fang VS. Hormones, dopamine and schizophrenia. Psychoneuroendocrinology 1981;6:17–36.

437. Deutsch SI, Campbell M, Sachar EJ, Green WH, David R. Plasma growth hormone response to oral 1-dopa in infantile autism. J Autism Dev Disord 1985;15:205–212.

438. Barthelemy C, Bruneau N, Cottet-Eymard JM, et al. Urinary Free and conjugated catecholamines and metabolites in autistic children. J Autism Dev Disord 1988;18:583–591.

439. Boullin DJ, O–Brien RA. Uptake and loss of sup-14-C-dopamine by platelets from children with infantile autism. J Autism Dev Disord 1972;12:97–98.

440. Garnier C, Comoy E, Barthelemy C, et al. Dopamine-beta-hydroxylase (DBH) and homovanillic acid (HVA) in autistic children. J Autism Dev Disord 1986;16:23–29.

441. Garreau B, Barthelemy C, Domenech J, et al. Disturbances in dopamine metabolism in autistic children: results of clinical tests and urinary dosages on homovanillic acid (HVA). Acta Psychiatr Belg 1980:80:249–265.

442. Iskrangkun PP, Newman HAI, Patel ST. Potential biochemical markers for infantile autism. Neurochem Pathol 1986;5:51–70.

443. Launay JM, Bursztje C, Ferrari P, et al. Catecholamines metabolism in infantile autism: a controlled study of 22 autistic children. J Autism Dev Disord 1987;17:333–347.

444. Minderaa RB, Anderson GM, Volkmar FR, Akkerhuis GW, Cohen DJ. Neurochemical study of dopamine functioning in autistic and normal subjects. J Am Acad Child Adolesc Psychiatry 1989;28:190–194.

445. Piggot LR. Overview of selected basic research in autism. J Autism Dev Disord 1979;9:199–218.

446. Garreau B, Barthelemy C, Jouve J, et al. Urinary homovanillic acid levels of autistic children. Dev Med Child Neurol 1988;30:93–98.

447. Gillberg C, Svennerholm L. CSF monoamines in autistic syndromes and other pervasive developmental disorders of early childhood. Br J Psychiatry 1987;151:89–94.

448. Ross DL, Klykylo WM, Anderson GM. Cerebrospinal fluid indoleamine and monoamine effects of fenfluramine treatment of infantile autism. Ann Neurol 1985;15:394.

449. Cohen DJ, Shaywitz BS, Johnson WT, Bowers M. Biogenic amines in autistic and atypical children: cerebrospinal fluid measures of homovanillic acid a 5-hydroxyindoleacetic acid. Arch Gen Psychiatry 1974;34:845–853.

450. Mikkelsen E. Efficacy of neuroleptic medication in pervasive developmental disorders of childhood. Schizophren Bull 1982;8:320–328.

451. Naruse H, Nagahata M, Nakane Y, Shirahashi K, Takesada M, Yamazaki K. A multi-center double-blind trial of pimozide (Orap), haloperidol and placebo in children with behavioral disorders, using crossover design. Acta Paedopsychiatr 1982;48:173–184.

452. Anderson GM, Campbell M, Adams P, Small AM, Perry R, Shell J. The effects of haloperidol on discrimination learning and behavioral symptoms in autistic children. J Autism Dev Disord 1989;19:227–239.

453. Campbell M, Anderson LT, Meier M, et al. A comparison of haloperidol and behavior therapy and their interaction in autistic children. J Am Acad Child Adolesc Psychiatry 1978;17:640–655.

454. Perry R, Campbell M, Adams P, et al. Long-term efficacy of haloperidol in autistic children: continuous verses discontinuous drug administration. J Am Acad Child Adolesc Psychiatry 1989;28:87–92.

455. Campbell M, Fish B, David R, Shapiro T, Collins P, Koh C. Response to triiodothyronine and dextroamphetamine: a study of preschool schizophrenic children. J Autism Childhood Schizophrenia 1972;2: 343–358.

456. Beninger RJ, Mason ST, Phillips AG, Fibinger HC. The use of conditioned suppression to evaluate the nature of neuroleptic-induced avoidance deficits. J Pharmacology Experimental Therapeutics 1980; 213:623–627.

457. Beninger RJ, Mason ST, Phillips AG, Fibinger HC. The use of extinction to investigate the nature of neuroleptic-induced avoidance deficits. Psychopharmacology 1980;69:11–18.

458. Goeders NE, Smith JE. Cortical dopaminergic involvement in cocaine reinforcement. Science 1983;221:773–775.

459. Hand TH, Franklin KB. 6-OHDA lesions of the ventral tegmental area block morphine-induced but not amphetamine-induced facilitation of self-stimulation. Brain Res 1985;328:233–241.

460. Hoffman DC, Beninger RJ. The effects of pimozide on the establishment of conditioned reinforcement as a function of the amount of conditioning. Psychopharmacology 1985;87:454–460.

461. Lyon M, Robbins T. The action of central nervous system drugs: a general theory concerning amphetamine effects. In: Current developments in psychopharmacology, vol. 2. Spectrum Publications. 1975:80–163.

462. McKim WA. Drugs and behavior. New Jersey: Prentice-Hall, 1986.

463. Yurek DN, Randall PK. Simultaneous catalepsy and apomorphine-induced stereotypic behavior in mice. Life Sci 1985;37:1665–1673.

464. Carranza AJ. Behavioral changes induced by the chronic administration of amphetamines. Foreign Psychiatry 1973;2:42–47.

465. Young JG, Cohen DJ, Kavanagh ME, Landis JD, Shaywitz BA, Maas JW. Cerebrospinal fluid, plasma, and urinary MHPG in children. Life Sci 1981;28:2837–2845.

466. Minderaa RB, Anderson GM, Volkmar FR, Harcherik D, Akkerhuis GW, Cohen DJ. Plasma levels of 3-methoxy-4-hydroxyphenylglycoll (MHPG) and urinary excretion of norepinephrine, epinephrine, and MHPG in autistic and normal subjects. Unpublished manuscript, 1988.

467. Roy A, Picker D, De Jong J, et al. Norepinephrine and its metabolites in cerebrospinal fluid, plasma, and urine: relationship to hypothalamic-pituitary-adrenal axis function in depression. Arch Gen Psychiatry 1988;45:849–857.

468. Ziegler MG, Wood JH, Lake CR, Kopin IJ. Norepinephrine and 3-methoxy-4-hydroxyphenyl glycol gradients in human cerebrospinal fluid. Am J Psychiatry 1977;134:565–568.

469. Young JG, Donald CJ, Caparulo BK, et al. Decreased 24 hour urinary MHPG in childhood autism. Am J Psychiatry 1979;136:1055–1057.

470. Coleman M, Campbell M, Freedman LS, Roffman M, Ebstein RP, Goldstein M. Serum dopamine-beta-hydroxylase levels in Down's syndrome. Clin Gene 1974;5:312–315.

471. Kalat JW. Letter to the editor: speculations on similarities between autism and opiate addiction. J Autism Childhood Schizophrenia 1978;8:447–479.

472. Martineau J, Herault J, Petit E, Guerin P, et al. Catecholaminergic metabolism and autism. Devel Medicine Child Neurology 1994;36: 688–697.

473. Menderaa RB, Anderson GM, Volkmar FR, Akkerhuis GW, et al. Noradrenergic and adrenergic functioning in autism. Biological Psychiatry 1994;36:237–241.

474. Herman BH, Panksepp J. Effects of morphine and naloxone on separation distress and approach attachment: evidence for opiate mediation of social affect. Pharmacol Biochem Behav 1978;9: 213–220.

475. Watson SJ, Barchas JD, Li CH. Beta-lipotropin: localization in cells and axons in rat brain by immunocytochemistry. Proc Nat Acad Sci USA 1977;74:5155–5158.

476. Sahley TL, Panksepp J. Brain opioids and autism: an updated analysis of possible linkages. J Autism Dev Disord 1987;1:201–216.

477. Weizman R, Gil-Ad I, Dick J, et al. Low plasma immunoreactive

478. Weizman R, et al. Humoral endorphin blood levels in autistic, schizophrenic and healthy subjects. Psychopharmacology 1984;82: 368–370.

479. Gillberg C, Terenius L, Lonnerholm G. Endorphin activity in childhood psychosis: spinal fluid levels in 24 cases. Arch Gen Psychiatry 1985;42:780–783.

480. Ross DL, Klykylo WM, Hitzeman R. Reduction of elevated CSF beta-endorphin by fenfluramine in infantile autism. Pediatr Neuro 1987;3:83–86.

481. LeBoyer M, Bouvard MP, Recasens C, Philippe A, et al. Difference between plasma N-and C-terminally directed b-endorphin immunoreactivity in infantile autism. Am J Psychiatry 1994;151:1797–1801.

482. Chamberlain RS, Herman BH. A novel model linking dysfunctions in brain melatonin, proopiomelanocortin peptides, and serotonin in autism. Biol Psychiatry 1990;28:773–793.

483. Barrett RP, Feinstein C, Hole WT. Effects of naloxone and naltrexone on self-injury: a double-blind, placebo-controlled analysis. Am J Men Retard 1989;93:644–651.

484. Bernstein GA, Hughes JR, Mitchell JE, Thompson T. Effects of narcotic antagonists on self-injurious behavior: a single case study. J Am Acad Child Adolesc Psychiatry 1987;26:886–889.

485. Herman BH, Hammock MK, Arthur-Smith A, et al. Naltrexone decreases self-injurious behavior in children. Ann Neurol 1987;22: 550–552.

486. LeBoyer M, Bouvard MP, Dugas M. Effects of naltrexone on infantile autism. Lancet 1988;I:715.

487. Panksepp J, Lensing P. A synopsis of a open-trial of naltrexone treatment of autism with four children. J Autism Dev Disord 1991;21:243–249.

488. Sandman CA, Datta PC, Barron J, et al. Naloxone attenuates self-abusive behavior in developmentally disabled clients. Applied Research in Mental Retardation 1983;4:5–11.

489. Sandman CA. β-endorphin disregulation in autistic and self-injurious behavior: a neurodevelopmental hypothesis. Synapse 1988;2: 193–199.

490. Sandyk R. Naloxone abolished self-injuring in a mentally retarded child. Ann Neurol 1985;17:520.

491. Walters A, Barrett RP, Feinstein C, et al. A case report of naltrexone treatment of self-injury and social withdrawal in autism. J Autism Dev Disord 1990;20:169–176.

492. Campbell M, Adams P, Small AM, Tesch LH, Curren E. Naltrexone in infantile autism. Psychopharmacol Bull 1988;24:135–139.

493. Herman BH, Hammock MK, Arthur-Smith et al. Role of opioid peptides in autism: effects of acute administration of naltrexone. Society of Neuroscience Abstracts 1986;14:465.

494. Panksepp J, Lensing P, LeBoyer M, Bouvard MP. Naltrexone and other potential new pharmacological treatments of autism. Brain Dysfunction 1991;4:281–300.

495. LeBoyer M, Bouvard MP, Launay JM, Recasens C, et al. Opioid excess hypothesis of autism: clinical trails with naltrexone. Encephale 1993;95–102.

496. Sandman C. The opiate hypothesis in autism and self injury. J Child Adolesc Psychopharmacol 1991;1:237–248.

497. Meyerson BJ. Influence of early β-endorphin treatment on the behavior and reaction to β-endorphin in the adult male rat. Psychoneuroendocrinology 1985;10:135–147.

498. Tikal K, Svoboda J. Stress-induced spontaneous social isolation and its influencing in rats. Acta Nervosa Superior 1985;27: 30–31.

499. Panksepp J, Meeker R, Bean NJ. The neurochemical control of crying. Pharmacol Biochem Behav 1980;12:437–443.

500. Modahl C, Fein D, Waterhouse L, Newton N. Does oxytocin deficiency mediate social deficits on autism? Letter to the editor. J Autism Dev Disord 1992;22:449–451.

β-endorphin levels in autism. J Am Acad Child Adolesc Psychiatry 1988;27:430–433.

501. Insel TR. Oxytocin—a neuropeptide for affiliation: evidence from behavioral, receptor autoradiographic, and comparative studies. Psychoneuroendocrinology 992;17:3–35.

502. Panksepp J. Oxytocin effects on emotional processes: separation distress, social bonding, and relationships to psychiatric disorders. Annals of the New York Academy of Sciences 1992;652:243–252.

503. Bicknell RJ, Leng G, Lincoln DW, Russell JA. Nalaxone excites oxytocin neurons in the supraoptic nucleus of lactating rats after chronic morphine treatment. J Physiol 1988;396:297–317.

504. Modahl C, Green L, Fein D, Waterhouse L, Feinstein C, Morris M. Oxytocin levels in autistic and normal children. Manuscript in preparation.

505. Buitelaar JK, Vanengeland H, deKogel KH, deVries H, et al. The use of adrenocorticotrophic hormone (4-9) analog ORG 2766 in autistic children: effects on the organization of behavior. Biological Psychiatry 1992;31:1119–1129.

506. Ritvo ER, Ritvo R, Yuwiler A, Brother A, et al. Elevated daytime melatonin concentrations in autism; A pilot study. European Child Adolesc Psychiatry 1993;2:75–78.

507. Rolf LH, Haarmann FY, Grtemeyer KH, Kehrer H. Serotonin and amino acid content in platelets of autistic children. Acta Psychiatrica Scandinavica 1993;87:312–316.

508. Visconti P, Piazzi S, Posar A, Santi A, et al. Amino acids and infantile autism. Developmental Brain Dysfunction 1994;86–92.

509. Rapin I. Children with inadequate language development: management guidelines for otolaryologists. Int J Pediatr Otorhinolaryngol 1988;16:189–198.

510. Klein SK, Rapin I. Clinical assessment of pediatric disorders of higher cerebral function. Curr Probl Pediatr 1990;20:111–160.

511. Allen DA, Rapin I, Wiznitzer M. Communication disorders of preschool children: the physician's responsibility. Devel Behav Pediatrics 1988;9:164–170.

512. Minshew N, Payton JB. New perspectives in autism, part 2: the differential diagnosis and neurobiology of autism. Curr Probl Pediatr 1988;988:615–694.

513. Gillberg C. Medical work-up in children with autism and Asperger syndrome. Brain Dysfunction 1990;3:249–260.

514. Steffenburg S. Comprehensive neuropsychiatric assessment in autism. A population-based study. Dev Med Child Neurol 1991;33:495–511.

515. Gillberg C, Coleman M. In: MacKeith, ed. The biology of the autistic syndromes. 2nd ed. New York: Praeger, 1992.

516. Bauman ML. Motor dysfunction in autism. In: Joseph AB, Young RR, eds. Movement disorders in neurology and psychiatry. Boston: Blackwell Scientific Publications, 1992. pp. 658–662.

517. Rossi PG, Visconti P, Posar A. Stereotypies in autistic children. J Movement Disorders 1992;7(Suppl 1):166.

518. Gillberg C. Autism and related behaviors. 9th World Conference of the International Association for the Scientific Study of Mental Deficiency. J Intellectual Disability Research 1993;37:343–372.

519. Coleman M. Clinical review: medical differential diagnosis and treatment of the autistic syndrome. European Child Adolesc Psychiatry 1993;2:161–168.

520. Rutter M, Bartak L. Causes in infantile autism: some considerations from recent research. J Autism Childhood Schizophrenia 1971;1:20–32.

521. Deykin E, MacMahon B. The incidence of seizures among children with autistic symptoms. Am J Psychiatry 1979;136:1310–1312.

522. Fein D, Dunn M, Morris R. Neuropsychological findings in CNS/INS study. Paper presented to the International Neuropsychological Society, Galveston, 1993.

523. Lord C, Schopler E. Intellectual and developmental assessment. In: Schopler E, Mesibov G, eds. Diagnosis and assessment in autism. New York: Plenum Press, 1980.

524. Wainwright L, Fein D, Waterhouse L. Neuropsychological assessment of children with developmental disabilities. In: Amir N, Rapin I, Branski D, eds. Pediatric neurology: behavior and cognition of the child with brain dysfunction. Basel: Karger, 1991. pp. 146–163.

525. Watson LR, Marcus LM. Diagnosis and assessment of preschool children. In: Schopler E, Mesibov G, eds. Diagnosis and Assessment of Autism. New York: Plenum Press, 1988. pp. 271–301.

526. Leiter RG. The Leiter International Performance Scale (Research Publication No. 13). Honolulu: The University of Hawaii, 1936.

527. Elliott C. Differential Ability Scales. San Antonio: The Psychological Corporation, 1990.

528. Mesibov GB, Troxler M, Boswell S. Assessment in the classroom. In: Schopler E, Mesibov G, eds. Diagnosis and assessment of autism. New York: Plenum Press, 1988. pp. 261–270.

529. Sparrow S, Balla D, Cicchetti D. Vineland Adaptive Behavior Scales. Circle Pines, MN: American Guidance Service, 1984.

530. Klin A, Volkmar F, Sparrow S. Autistic social dysfunction: some limitations of the theory of mind hypothesis. J Child Psychol Psychiatry 1992;33:861–876.

531. Van Meter L, Fein D, Morris R. Social behavior in autism: an analysis of intrasubtest scatter on the Vineland Adaptive Behavior Scales [Abstract]. J Clin Exp Neuropsychol 1992;14:390.

532. McCune-Nicolich L. Toward symbolic functioning: structure of early pretend games and potential parallels with language. Child Dev 1981;52:785–797.

533. Rubin KH, Fein G, Vandenberg B. Play. In: Mussen P, Hetherington E, eds. Handbook of child psychology. New York: John Wiley & Sons, 1983.

534. Lewis V, Boucher J. Spontaneous, instructed and elicited play in relatively able autistic children. Br J Dev Psychol 1988;6:325–339.

535. Mundy P, Sigman M, Ungerer J, Sherman T. Nonverbal communication and play correlates of language development in autistic children. J Autism Dev Disord 1987;17:349–364.

536. Riquet, Taylor, Benroya and Klein, 1981.

537. Ungerer J, Sigman M. Symbolic play and language comprehension in autistic children. J Aca Child Psychiatry 1981;20:318–337.

538. Wainwright L, Fein D. Free play in autistic language disordered and mentally deficient children. Paper presented before the International Neuropsychological Society, Galveston, 1993.

539. Parks SL. Psychometric instruments available for the assessment of autistic children. In: Schopler E, Mesibov G, eds. Diagnosis and assessment in autism. New York: Plenum, 1988. pp. 123–136.

540. Powers M. Behavioral assessment of autism. In: Schopler E, Mesibov G, eds. Diagnosis and Assessment in Autism. New York: Plenum, 1988.

541. LeCouteur A, Rutter M, Lord C, et al. Autism diagnostic interview: a standard investigator-based instrument. J Autism Dev Disord 1989;19:363–387.

542. Lord C, Rutter M, Good S, Heemsbergen J. Autism diagnostic observation schedule: a standardized observation of communication and social behavior. J Autism DevDisord 1989;19:185–212.

543. Schopler E, Mesibov G, eds. Neurobiological issues in autism. New York: Plenum, 1987.

544. Harris S. Family assessment in autism. In: Schopler E, Mesibov G. eds. Diagnosis and assessment in autism. New York: Plenum, 1988. pp. 199–210.

545. McCubbin J, Patterson J. Stress and the family. Vol. I: Coping with normative transitions. New York: Brunner/Mazel, 1983.

546. Campbell M, Anderson L, Small A. Pharmacotherapy in autism: a summary of research at Bellevue/New York University. Brain Dysfunction 1990;3:299–307.

547. Campbell M, Kafantaris V, Malone RP, et al. Diagnostic and assessment issues related to pharmacotherapy for children and adolescents with autism. Behav Modif 1991;15:326–354.

548. Campbell M, Spencer EK. Psychopharmacology in child and adolescent psychiatry: a review of the past five years. J Am Acad Child Adolesc Psychiatry. 1988;27:269–279.

549. Harty JR. Pharmacotherapy in infantile autism. Focus on Autistic Behavior 1990;5:1–15.

550. Holm VA, Varley CK. Pharmacological treatment of autistic children. In: Dawson G, ed. Autism: nature, diagnosis, and treatment. New York: Guilford Press, 1989. pp. 386-404.

551. McDaniel KD. Pharmacologic treatment of psychiatric and neurodevelopmental disorders in children and adolescents I. Clinical Pediatrics 1986;2:143–146.

552. McDaniel KD. Pharmacologic treatment of psychiatric and neurodevelopmental disorders in children and adolescents II.

553. McDaniel KD. Pharmacologic treatment of psychiatric and neurodevelopmental disorders in children and adolescents III.

554. Cook D. A sensory approach to the treatment and management of children with autism. Focus on Autistic Behavior 1990;5:1–19.

555. McGee G, Almeida M, Sulzer-Azaroff B, Feldman R. Promoting reciprocal interactions via peer incidental teaching. J Appl Behav Anal 1992;25:117–126.

556. Konstantareas M. A psychoeducational model for working with families of autistic children. J Marital Family Therapy 1990;16:59–70.

557. Rapoport JL. Clozapine and child psychiatry. J Child Adolesc Psychopharm 1994;4:1–3.

558. Ratey J, Mikkelson E, Sorgi P, et al. Autism: the treatment of aggressive behaviors. J Clin Psychopharmacol 1987;7:35–41.

559. Lipinski J, Keck P, McElroy SL. B-adrenergic antagonists in psychosis: is improvement due to treatment of neuroleptic-induced akathesia? J Clinical Psychopharmacol 1988;8:409–416.

560. Gualtieri T. Italian J Intellectual Impairment 1992;5:127–136.

561. Rothenberger A. Psychopharmacological treatment of self-injurious behavior in individuals with autism. Acta Paedopsychiatrica Int'l J Child Adolesc Psychiat 1993;56:99–104.

562. Campbell M, Adams P, Small A, Tesch L, Curren E. Naltrexone in infantile autism. Psychopharmacol Bull 1988;24:135–139.

563. Sandman C, Barron J, DeMet E, Chicz-DeMet A, Rothenberg S, Zea F. Opioid peptides and perinatal development: is β-endorphin a natural teratogen? Ann N Y Acad Sci 1990;579:91–108.

564. DeLong G, Aldershof A. Long-term experience with lithium treatment in childhood: correlation with clinical diagnosis. J Am Acad Child Adoles Psychiatry 1987;26:389–394.

565. Gordon C, Rapoport J, Hamburger S. Differential responses of seven subjects with autistic disorder to clomipramine and desipramine. Am J Psychiatry 1992;149:363–366.

566. McDougle C, Price L, Volkmar F, et al. Clomipramine in autism: preliminary evidence of efficacy. J Am Acad Child Adolesc Psychiatry 1992;31:746–750.

567. Brasic JR, Barnett JY, Kaplan D, Sheitman BB, et al. Clomipramine ameliorates adventitious movements and compulsions in prepubertal boys with autistic disorder and severe mental retardation. Neurology 1994;44:1309–1312.

568. Gordon CT, State RC, Nelson JE, Hamburger SD, et al. A double-blind comparison of clomipramine, desipramine, and placebo in the treatment of autistic disorder. Archives of Gen Psychiat 1993;50:441–447.

569. McDouble CJ, Price LH, Volkmar FR, Goodman WK, et al. Clomipramine in autism: preliminary evidence of efficacy. J Amer Acad Child Adolesc Psychiat 1992;31:746–750.

570. Mehlinger R, Scheftner W, Poznanski E. Fluoxetine and autism. J Am Acad Child Adolesc Psychiatry 1990;29:985.

571. Todd R. Fluoxetine in autism. Am J Psychiatry 1991;148:1089.

572. Ghaziuddin M, Tsai L, Ghaziuddin N. Fluoxetine in autism with depression. J Am Acad Child Adolesc Psychiatry 1991;30:508–509.

573. Hamdan-Allen G. Brief report: Trichotillomania in an autistic male. J Autism Dev Disord 1991;21:79–82.

574. McDougle C, Price L, Goodman W. Fluvoxamine treatment of coincident autistic disorder and obsessive-compulsive disorder: a case report. J Autism Dev Disord 1990;20:537–543.

575. Cook E, Rowlett R, Jaselskis C. Fluoxetine treatment of children and adults with autistic disorder and mental retardation. J Am Acad Child Adolesc Psychiatry 1992;31:739–745.

576. Leventhal BL, Cook EH, Morford M, Ravitz AJ, et al. Clinical and neurochemical effects of fenfluramine in children with autism. J Neuropsychiatry Clin Neurosci 1993;5:307–315.

577. Raiten D. Nutrition and developmental disabilities: a clinical assessment. In: Schopler E, Mesibov G, eds. Diagnosis and assessments of autism. New York: Plenum, 1988. pp. 211–223.

578. Rimland B. Controversies in the treatment of autistic children: vitamin and drug therapy. J Child Neurol 1988;3(Suppl):67–72.

579. Rimland B, Callaway E, Dreyfus P. The effects of high doses of vitamin B6 on autistic children: a double-blind crossover study. Am J Psychiatry 1978;135:472–475.

580. LeLord G, Muh J, Barthelemy C, Martineau J, Garreau B, Callaway E. Effects of pyridoxine and magnesium on autistic symptoms: initial observations. J Autism Dev Disord 1981;11:219–230.

581. Martineau J, Barthelemy C, Garreau B, LeLord G. Vitamin B6, magnesium, and combined B6-Mg: therapeutic effects in childhood autism. Biol Psychiatry 1985;20:476–478.

582. Kozlowski BW. Megavitamin treatment of mental retardation in children: a review of effects on behavior and cognition. J Child Adolesc Psychopharmacol 1992;2:307–320.

583. Hagerman R, Jackson A, Levitas A, et al. Oral folic acid versus placebo in the treatment of males with the fragile X syndrome. Am J Med Genet 1986;23:241–262.

584. Lowe T, Cohen D, Miller S, Young J. Folic Acid and B12 in autism and neuropsychiatric disturbances of childhood. J Am Acad Child Adolesc Psychiatry 1981;20:104–111.

585. Dolske MC, Spollen J, McKay S, Lancashire E, et al. A preliminary trial of ascorbic acid as supplemental therapy for autism. Progress in Neuro-Psychopharmacology Biological Psychiatry 1993;117:765–774.

586. Buitelaar JK, VanEngeland H, deKogel K, deVries H et al. The adrenocorticotrophic hormone (4-9) analog ORG 2766 benefits autistic children: report on a second controlled clinical trial. J Amer Child Adolesc Psychiat 1992;31:1149–1156.

587. Rogers S, Lewis H. An effective day treatment model for young children with pervasive developmental disorder. J Am Acad Child Adolesc Psychiatry 1989;28:207–214.

588. Lovaas OI. Behavioral treatment and normal educational and intellectual functioning in young autistic children. J Consult Clin Psychol 1987;55:3–9.

589. Lovaas OI. The development of a treatment-research project for developmentally disabled and autistic children. J Applied Behav Analysis 1993;26:617–630.

590. McEachin JJ, Smith T, Lovaas OI. Long-term outcome for children with autism who received early intensive behavioral treatment. Am J Mental Retardation 1993;97:359–372.

591. Kazdin AE. Replication and extension of behavioral treatment of autistic disorder. Amer J Mental Retardation 1993;97:377–379.

592. LeBlanc R. Educational management of self-injurious behavior. Acta Paedopsychiatrica Int–l J Child Adolesc Psychiatry 1993;56:91–98.

593. Howlin P. Behavioral techniques to reduce self-injurious behavior in children with autism. Acta Paedopsychiatrica Int–l J Child Adolesc Psychiatry 1993;56:75–84.

594. Wolfberg PJ, Schuler AL. Integrated play groups: a model for promoting the social and cognitive dimensions of play in children with autism. J Autism Dev Disord 1993;23:467–489.

595. McGee GG, Paradis T, Feldman RS. Free effects of integration on levels of autistic behavior. Topics in Early Childhood Special Education 1993;13:57–67.

596. Prizant B, Wetherby A. Providing services to children with autism (ages 0–2 years) and their families. Topics in Language Disorders 1988;9:1–23.

597. Jordon R, Powell SD. Reflections on the option method as a treatment for autism. J Autism Devel Disord 1993;23:682–685.

598. Lord D, Hopkins J. The social behavior of autistic children. J Autism Dev Disord 1986;16:449–462.

599. Odom S, Strain P. Comparison of peer initiation and teacher antecedent interventions. J Applied Behavior Analysis 1986;19:59–71.

600. Day HM, Horner RH, O–Neill RE. Multiple functions of problem behaviors: assessment and intervention. J Applied Behav Analysis 1994;27:279–289.

601. Koegel RL, Frea WS. Treatment of social behavior in autism through the modification of pivotal social skills. J Applied Behav Analysis 1993;26:369–377.

602. Hudson A, Melita B, Arnold N. Brief report: a case study assessing the validity of facilitated communication. J Autism Dev Disord 1993;23:165–173.

603. Smith M, Belcher R. Brief report: facilitated communication with adults with autism. J Autism Dev Disord 1993;23:175–183.

604. Mundy P, Adreon D. Commentary: Facilitated communication: attitude, effect, and theory. J Pediatric Psychol 1994;19:677–680.

605. Regal RA, Rooney JR, Wandas T. Facilitated communication: an experimental evaluation. J Autism Devel Disord 1994;24:345–355.

606. Schopler E, Mesibov G, eds. The effects of autism on the family. New York: Plenum, 1984.

27

TRANSIENT DISORDERS OF MEMORY AND CONSCIOUSNESS

Michael D. Kopelman

Differentiating transient amnesic states or disturbances of consciousness from psychogenic phenomena, and authentically "hysterical" or "unconscious" from simulated or "factitious" disorders, can be notoriously difficult. The present chapter considers the clinical features of syndromes likely to be significant in such instances, the underlying neurobiological and neuropsychological basis of memory disorders, diagnostic evaluation, and management.

CLINICAL SYNDROMES OF SIGNIFICANCE

Transient Global Amnesia

Hodges and Ward (1) recently defined transient global amnesia (TGA) as "a witnessed amnesia, occurring in clear consciousness, without focal signs or other signs of epilepsy, resolving within twenty-four hours." In a combined retrospective and prospective study, these authors obtained 114 cases, between the ages of 39 and 82, of whom 61% were male. The duration of the amnesia ranged between 15 minutes and 12 hours (mean = 4.2 hours), and 15% of the sample reported multiple episodes. In the preceding 24 hours, 10% had experienced either headache or nausea, and 14% had experienced a stressful life event, while in others the attack was preceded by a medical procedure or severe exercise. The repetitive questioning, previously described in this syndrome (2), was a characteristic feature, but no patients reported a loss of the sense of personal identity. In 25% of the sample, there was a past history of migraine, which was considered to have a possible etiological role; and in 7% of the sample, the episode was subsequently attributed to undiagnosed epilepsy. However, there was no association with either a past history of vascular disease, clinical signs suggestive of vascular pathology, or known risk factors for vascular disease: this pattern was quite different from that obtained in a sample of patients who had had transient ischemic attacks (TIAs). In short, the underlying etiology of the attacks was unclear in 60–70% of the sample.

Several authors have argued that transient dysfunction in the limbic-hippocampal circuits may be the physiological basis of the TGA syndrome (1). Stillhard et al. (3) reported severe bitemporal hypoperfusion during an episode of TGA using single photon emission computed tomography (SPECT). Following recovery from the episode, cerebral perfusion returned to normal. Similarly, Evans et al. (4) reported bilateral hypoperfusion in the posteromedial temporal lobes on SPECT during an episode of TGA in a 55-year-old woman, which had recovered to normal 7 weeks later. Fujii et al. (5) used positron emission tomography (PET) to study four patients with TGA within 3 months of the episode, and compared the findings in these patients with those in seven cases of transient ischemic attacks (TIAs). Regional cerebral blood flow (rCBF) and oxygen metabolism were better preserved in the TGA patients than in the TIA patients in each area of the brain examined; and the only abnormality in a TGA patient was a slight reduction of rCBF in the right basal ganglia and frontal cortex of a single patient.

Hodges and Ward (1) administered neuropsychological tests to five patients during their acute episode of memory loss. As expected, all these patients showed profound anterograde amnesia on tests of both verbal and nonverbal memory. Performance on retrograde memory tests was variable. Three out of five patients showed impairments on a test requiring the recognition of famous faces from earlier decades; the other two patients performed within the "normal" range for this test. Similarly, on a test requiring the subjects to produce autobiographical memories to specific cue-words, one of three patients administered this task performed normally. In short, although anterograde memory is always severely impaired, the effect of a TGA episode upon retrograde memory is variable. In addition, Hodges and Oxbury (6) followed up a subgroup of the total series of 114 patients over 6 months, and they found that there were mild, residual impairments on verbal anterograde and retrograde memory tests in comparison with the performance of an age- and IQ-matched comparison group.

In general, these findings are consistent with those obtained in other large-scale studies of TGA (7–9). However, Kritchevsky and colleagues (10, 11) found that complete recovery on neuropsychological tests of memory had occurred within 1 month of the acute episode, consistent with clinical expectations.

Transient Epileptic Amnesia

Epileptic seizures give rise to amnesia, and they may be associated with epileptic automatisms or postictal confusional states (see chapter on epilepsy in this volume). Where an automatism arises, there is always bilateral involvement of the limbic structures involved in memory formation, including the hippocampal and parahippocampal structures bilaterally, as well as the mesial diencephalon (12). Hence, amnesia for the period of automatic behavior is always present and is usually complete (13).

More likely to be missed is the phenomenon that Kapur (14) has termed transient epileptic amnesia (TEA). This refers to that minority of cases of TGA, in whom various authors have implicated epilepsy as the "cause" of the syndrome (1, 7–9). The main predictive factors for an epileptic basis to such attacks, where epilepsy has not previously been diagnosed, are the existence of multiple attacks and their relatively brief duration. In the Hodges and Warlow (15) series, all four subjects who had had multiple attacks, lasting 1 hour or less, were subsequently found to have an epileptic basis for the disorder. Other authors have corroborated this finding (9, 14). Standard electroencephalograms (EEGs) and computerized tomography (CT) scans may be normal, and the epileptic basis to the disorder may be revealed only on a sleep EEG (16). The only PET study of such cases found no abnormality 6 months after commencement of treatment with an anticonvulsant (16).

Kapur and colleagues (17) have reported a residual interictal retrograde amnesia, in the presence of only minor anterograde memory impairment, in a single case study of a patient with this syndrome. Their patient showed spike waves in the left temporal lobe and occasional spike discharges in the right temporal region (more precise detail was not given). By contrast, Kopelman and colleagues (16) found a moderate degree of residual, anterograde memory impairment in their patient with only minimal evidence of retrograde memory loss. This latter finding was consistent with the evidence of independent, bilateral foci on sleep EEG in the medial temporal lobes of this patient. Presumably, the difference between the two case studies results from small differences in the precise sites of the underlying foci.

Head Injury

Head injury can, of course, produce a discrete or transient episode of memory loss, and, if it is severe, it can give rise to persistent memory and general cognitive impairment. In the former case, it gives rise to the familiar pattern of memory loss, consisting of a brief period of retrograde amnesia (RA), which may last only a few seconds or minutes, a longer period of posttraumatic amnesia (PTA), and islets of

preserved memory within the amnesic gap (18, 19). Occasionally, PTA may occur without any RA, although this is more common in cases of penetrating lesions (20, 21). Sometimes there is a particularly vivid memory for images or sounds occurring immediately before the injury, on regaining consciousness, or during a lucid interval between the injury and the onset of PTA (18, 19).

As is well known, the duration of PTA is assumed to reflect the degree of underlying diffuse brain pathology. Rotational forces, such as those in a car accident, are particularly likely to produce axonal tearing and generalized cognitive impairment. The length of PTA is predictive of eventual cognitive outcome (22), psychiatric outcome (20), and social outcome (22, 23). However, these relationships are weaker than is often assumed, and unfortunately, the duration of PTA is often not adequately documented in the medical records. There appears to be a relationship with age, in that older subjects tend to have a longer PTA and more serious deficits at a given PTA (23), whereas in subjects under 30, PTA is sometimes found to be less effective as a predictor of subsequent memory impairment (24). In addition, contusion to the frontal and anterior temporal lobes is a common consequence of head injury. Recently, two sets of authors have attributed a disproportionate degree of retrograde memory loss, associated with only a mild degree of anterograde memory impairment, to damage in these structures (25, 26).

Following a mild head injury, a neurotic (posttraumatic) syndrome sometimes ensues, in which forgetfulness is a prominent complaint, as well as anxiety, irritability, poor concentration, and various somatic complaints. The etiology of this syndrome remains controversial, but it is clear that the symptoms commonly persist long after the settlement of any compensation issues (27–29). In more severe head injury, the ability to learn new material is the slowest cognitive function to recover, and the pattern of residual memory deficit resembles, in many respects, that of a classical amnesic syndrome (22, 30).

Alcoholic Blackouts

Goodwin et al. (31) described discrete episodes of "memory loss for significant events," which occurred in 64% of a sample of 100 hospitalized alcoholics. These "blackouts" were always accompanied by prolonged alcohol abuse and severe intoxication. Commonly, they were also associated with state-dependent phenomena. Three gradations of alcohol-induced memory impairment have been documented:

1. *State-dependent effects,* in which subjects cannot remember events or facts when sober, which they recall easily when they are intoxicated again—for example, where they have hidden their money or drink.
2. *Fragmentary blackouts,* in which subjects become aware of their memory loss on being told of an event later: there are "islets" of preserved memory, and the amnesia

tends to recover partially through time by a shrinking of the amnesic gap, similar to that which occurs in head injury.

3. *En bloc blackouts,* in which subjects become abruptly aware of the memory gap (e.g., on waking up), and there is a sense of lost time: the amnesia has a definite starting point, islets of preserved memory are rare, and the memories are very seldom recovered.

Alcoholic blackouts are related to the peak plasma level of alcohol and may be somewhat more common in binge drinkers. There is no evidence that they are an ictal phenomenon, but hypoglycemia may be a contributory factor. It seems likely that the blackouts involve a shutdown of the same limbic-diencephalic structures as are implicated in TGA.

The diagnosis of an alcoholic blackout can be important in medicolegal cases, in which a defendant may claim amnesia for his or her offense, as noted later in this chapter.

Sleepwalking

Sleepwalking occurs most commonly in childhood and adolescence and occasionally arises in adult life, especially when precipitated by fatigue, mental stress, sleep deprivation, drugs or alcohol, or a change in the sleeping environment (32–35). Most often it occurs within 2 hours of falling asleep, and this also applies if the subject is awakened in the middle of the night. Episodes usually last only a few minutes. A substantial number of studies in the medical and legal literature report cases of violent attacks during sleepwalking, often involving strangulation or attempted strangulation and the use of available implements as weapons, with a sleeping partner as the victim (33, 34). Most commonly in these case reports, there has not been any previous hostility between the offender and the victim, and the behavior is entirely out of character.

Characteristically, episodes of violence accompanying sleepwalking terminate in the subject appearing confused on awakening, recalling very little detail of any accompanying dream, but being aware of a sense of acute dread or terror in such a dream (so-called "night terrors"; 36). This arises because sleepwalking and night terrors characteristically occur in stage four of slow-wave sleep, shortly before a transition to rapid eye movement (REM) sleep. Later in the night, dreams and possibly nightmares occur in association with REM sleep, and on awakening from these, there is little or no confusion and the subject can recall his or her dreams very well. Until recently, English law regarded offenses committed during sleepwalking as a form of "sane automatism" (34, 35), alongside offenses perpetrated during an abnormal state of mind as a result of the accidental or involuntary administration of an external agent (e.g., hypoglycemia induced by an overdose of insulin, but not voluntary intoxication with alcohol). A sane automatism is regarded as unlikely to recur and, if accepted by the Court, results in an acquittal. However, the status of sleepwalking offenses has changed (in English law), and they are now

classified as examples of insane automatism (34, 35), alongside offenses resulting from recurrent brain disease, such as epilepsy. If upheld by the Court, an insane automatism results in a psychiatric placement, and, for many offenses, this will mean a secure hospital (34, 35). Although it is more logical to include sleepwalking in the "recurrent disease" group, the literature suggests that violent attacks during sleepwalking are very unlikely to recur (33).

Post-Electroconvulsive Therapy

This is an iatrogenic form of transient amnesia, and it is useful to remember that anticholinergic agents (37, 38) and benzodiazepines (39, 40) can also give rise to transient amnesia. However, the adverse effects of electroconvulsive therapy (ECT) on memory are generally much more severe, and were noted from an early stage (41).

Squire and his colleagues (42, 43) have found that subjects tested within a few hours of ECT show a retrograde impairment for information from the preceding 1–3 years, and a pronounced anterograde deficit on both recall and recognition memory tests. Other authors have corroborated these findings (44, 45). There is general agreement that, 6–9 months after completion of a course of ECT, memory performance on objective tests returns to normal, apart from a persistent loss of material acquired within a few hours of the convulsions (42–46). However, complaints of memory impairment may persist, and can still be evident 3 years or more after the course of ECT (46). Squire and Slater (46) found that the complaints focused upon the period for which there had been an initial retrograde and anterograde amnesia, as determined by neuropsychological tests, even though that memory loss was no longer evident on formal assessment. Freeman et al. (47) reported that those subjects who complain most do, in fact, perform poorer on objective tests than do those who do not complain, but Squire and Slater (46), using similar tests, did not find this. On the contrary, both Squire and Slater (46) and Frith et al. (45) found that the "complainers" were the patients who, on other criteria, had recovered least well from their depression.

Neuropsychological studies have found that verbal memory appears to be particularly sensitive to disruption. Unilateral ECT to the nondominant hemisphere produces considerably less memory impairment than bilateral ECT (42), making it important to identify the nondominant hemisphere by a valid procedure (48). Various recent studies have attempted to minimize memory disruption by either changes in premedication or concomitant administration of other substances: the agents employed have included glycopyrrolate, physostigmine, thyroxine, nimodipine, vasopressin, naloxone, dexamethasone, ACTH, and caffeine infusion (49–57). In general, these agents have produced little or no benefit, and the most effective methods of avoiding memory deficit consist of electrode placement either over the frontal rather than the temporal lobes (58) or over the nondominant temporal lobe (42, 59).

Posttraumatic Stress Disorder

The posttraumatic stress disorder (PTSD) syndrome is characterized by a brief period of numbness, followed by (*a*) intrusive thoughts and memories about the traumatic experience, including nightmares; (*b*) phobic anxiety and avoidance phenomena; and (*c*) a variety of other somatic and anxiety symptoms, including poor concentration, hyperacuity, and depressed mood (60).

In short, unlike the characteristic features of a head injury, the intrusive and sometimes very vivid memories predominate. However, there may be instances of frank memory loss, distortions, or even frank confabulations or delusional memories. For example, in the Herald of Free Enterprise disaster at Zeebruge, one patient described holding onto the hand of his wife, after he had clambered up onto the side of the ship, while she remained in the water unable to move: he could not remember anything else until he "came round" on dry land. Another victim was convinced he had tried to rescue a close friend while still on board ship, when it was clearly apparent (from the accounts of other witnesses) that the close friend had not been seen by the victim from the moment the ship had turned over.

However, these cases are, of course, confounded by metabolic factors—most of the passengers on the Herald of Free Enterprise, which turned over in the North Sea in midwinter, were suffering from profound or more moderate degrees of hypothermia. Similarly, the victims of head injury, road accidents, or severe burns, while describing unequivocal PTSD symptoms, could have their memory loss explained in terms of brain injury or other related factors. Nevertheless, even where evidence for neurological factors is minimal, there are similarities between the concurrence of vivid, intrusive memories and periods of memory loss in PTSD, which resemble the classic phenomena of head injury (18). Moreover, PTSD victims can show deficits in current anterograde memory on formal learning tasks, when tested many years after the original trauma and after physical factors have been controlled for (61). Psychological factors may contribute to the memory loss; and what remains to be satisfactorily explained is why certain memories are vividly and intrusively recalled, while others cannot be retrieved.

At a physiological level, Charney et al. (62) have argued that the amygdala is particularly important in the conditioning and extinction of sensory and cognitive associations to the original trauma and the subsequent activation of traumatic memories. They postulated that the noradrenergic, dopaminergic, endogenous opiate, and NMDA receptor systems all make important contributions in modulating these responses.

Psychogenic Fugue

A "fugue state" is an example of a psychogenic, global amnesia. It refers, in essence, to a syndrome consisting of a sudden loss of all autobiographical memories and the sense of self or personal identity, usually associated with a period of wandering, for which there is a subsequent amnesic gap upon recovery (63). Fugue states usually last a few hours or days only, and they appear to have occurred more commonly earlier in the century, particularly in wartime (64).

A review of the earlier literature on psychogenic fugue states (63) suggested that three main factors predisposed individuals to such episodes. First, fugue states are always preceded by a severe, precipitating stress such as marital or emotional discord (65), bereavement (66), financial problems (65), a criminal charge (67), or stress during wartime (68, 69). Secondly, depressed mood is an extremely common antecedent for a psychogenic fugue state. Berrington et al. (70) wrote that: "in nearly all fugues, there appears to be one common factor, namely a depressive mood. Whether the individual in the fugue is psychotic, neurotic, or even psychopathic, a depression seems to start off the fugue." For example, Schacter et al.'s (66) patient was in a depressed mood because he had just attended the funeral of his grandfather, of whom he had been particularly fond. In fact, many patients in a fugue have been contemplating suicide just before the episode or do so following recovery from it (71, 72). For example, Abeles and Schilder (71) described a woman who deserted her husband for another man: after a week, she determined to return to her family, but as she descended into the railway underground station, she was contemplating suicide. The authors tersely reported that "instead amnesia developed." The third factor that commonly precedes a fugue state is a history of a transient, neurological amnesia. Stengel (72) reported that 10% of his sample had a history of epilepsy, and Berrington et al. (70) reported that 16 of their 37 cases had previously experienced a severe head injury, and three additional cases had suffered a head injury of unknown severity. In brief, it appears that patients who have experienced a previous, transient organic amnesia and who have become depressed and/or suicidal are particularly likely to go into a fugue in the face of a severe, precipitating stress.

A confounding factor, however, is that several authors have noted that some of their patients appeared to be somewhat unreliable personalities with a possible legal motive for wanting to claim amnesia (67, 70, 72). Kopelman (63) gave the example of a man who reported about 10 or 12 fugue episodes, several of which were well documented in medical records, and who also had a past history of depression and suicide attempts as well as transient amnesia following epileptic seizures and ECT. Unfortunately, this gentleman claimed amnesia for a period of a few hours, during which he was involved in a motor accident while driving when disqualified, without any insurance, while under the influence of alcohol, making assessment (for a medicolegal report) particularly difficult.

The multiple personality syndrome (73) could be perceived as an extreme instance of a fugue state, when the subject is shifting constantly between one personality and another (or many others). However, it is seldom diagnosed in the United Kingdom, and its precise diagnostic status remains unclear.

Amnesia for Offenses

This is an example of a situation-specific, psychogenic memory loss; and it is claimed much more commonly than are fugue states, although it attracts less media attention. Various studies have reported that amnesia is claimed by between 25 and 45% of offenders convicted of homicide (74–76). Approximately 8% of perpetrators of other violent crimes also claim amnesia (76), and a small percentage of nonviolent offenders do so in cases of shoplifting, theft, or even embezzlement (77).

A very small percentage of these cases claim their amnesia in association with evidence of a frank neurological or metabolic disorder, such as an epileptic automatism or postictal confusional state, head injury, hypoglycemia, or sleepwalking. In these instances, the presence of amnesia is essential to establish the existence of an automatism. If present, English law allows the case to be argued for a sane automatism (if the consequence of an external force or agent) or an insane automatism (if the result of an internal brain disease), as discussed earlier. Other jurisdictions have rules allowing for related notions—e.g., the concept of "temporary insanity." However, in the vast majority of offenders claiming amnesia, no evidence of organic brain disease will be found (75, 76). In these latter instances, amnesia for an offense is most commonly associated with:

1. States of extreme emotional arousal, particularly in homicide cases, in which the offense has usually been unpremeditated, and the victim is often closely related to the offender—a lover, wife, close friend or family member;
2. Alcohol abuse and intoxication, in which there is commonly a history of chronic alcohol abuse as well as severe intoxication at the time of the offense. Other drugs are sometimes also implicated. The offense is not necessarily homicide, and any victim is not necessarily related to the offender;
3. Florid psychotic states or depressed mood: in a small minority of cases, the alleged offender appears to have been floridly psychotic and to have given a delusional account of what occurred, quite at odds with what was witnessed by other observers. In such instances, the offender may occasionally confess to a crime he or she has not actually committed (76), and the memory loss is probably best regarded as either a paramnesia or a delusional memory.

In many other cases, including the homicide cases just mentioned, depressed mood appears to be a common accompaniment of amnesia for criminal offense, just as it often appears to be associated with psychogenic fugue states.

Many commentators consider that the amnesia claimed for offenses must consist of deliberate simulation in many instances. Against this theory is the high number of offenders who, while claiming amnesia, have reported their own crime or failed to take measures to avoid their capture (76–81). This makes an account of amnesia as simulation to avoid punishment seem less plausible. Secondly, it is known by many lawyers that amnesia per se, in the absence of any organic factor, does not carry any legal implications. Nevertheless, their clients continue to plead amnesia, even in instances where recall of what actually happened would be helpful to their cause. Thirdly, it should be noted that some of the factors that have been associated with amnesia in offenders overlap with those that have been implicated in cases of impaired recall by the eyewitnesses or victims of crime—notably, violent crime, extreme emotional arousal, and alcohol intoxication (82–86).

NEUROBIOLOGY AND NEUROPSYCHOLOGY OF MEMORY IMPAIRMENT

Neurobiology

Contemporary accounts of the neurologically based amnesia syndrome view the disorder as resulting from damage to structures in either the diencephalon, the medial temporal lobes, the basal forebrain, or the frontal lobes (87–89).

Diencephalic amnesia was classically described in the account by Victor et al. (90) of patients with the Wernicke-Korsakoff syndrome. Those authors attributed the amnesic deficit to small lesions in the dorsal medial nuclei of the thalamus, because these were implicated in every case in which a persistent memory impairment resulted, whereas mammillary body lesions were seen in five cases who had a classic Wernicke episode, without any residual memory loss. However, subsequent studies, in which there has been a careful assessment of both premorbid neuropsychological function and pathological changes at autopsy, have found damage restricted to the mammillary bodies, the mammillo-thalamic tract, and a small portion of the anterior thalamus, with the medial dorsal nuclei of the thalamus being spared (91, 92). Consistent with this, two cases of traumatic amnesia have recently been attributed to lesions in the mammillary bodies (93, 94). In addition, a review of CT scan findings in patients, in whom thalamic infarction had produced amnesia, indicated that the anterior nuclei, rather than the dorsal medial nuclei, were critical for memory formation (95).

The role of the medial temporal lobes in amnesia has been evident since Scoville and Milner's (96) report of nine patients, who had had bilateral medial temporal lobectomy, who showed variable degrees of amnesia, according to the extent of the hippocampi removed. Milner's (97, 98) descriptions of patient HM, who was one of the three most severely affected cases in this sample, established the neuropsychological nature of the amnesia produced—a severe anterograde amnesia, with a retrograde memory loss covering approximately the 3 years preceding the operation. More recently, Zola-Morgan et al. (99) have described a patient with a more moderate degree of anterograde memory loss (and a retrograde loss of approximately 2 years), resulting from a series of anoxic and ischemic episodes. When this patient came to postmortem, it was found that he had only very small lesions, encompassing the CA1 fields of the hippocampi bilaterally, suggesting that this is a critical region for memory formation.

The role of the basal forebrain in memory has been implicated only more recently. There are reports of relatively focal lesions in this brain region producing anterograde amnesia without retrograde amnesia (100–103). Animal lesion studies have obtained findings consistent with this (104, 105), but their importance is that basal forebrain cholinergic neurons are severely depleted in Alzheimer's disease (106, 107), providing a putative explanation for the severe memory deficit in this disorder (38).

Until recently, it was believed that isolated frontal lobe lesions produced only mild anterograde and/or retrograde memory impairment (108), and that the frontal lobes might be important only for specific aspects of memory processes, such as the recall of contextual information, awareness of memory impairment, and the organization of memory processes (109). More recently, increasing attention has been paid to the severe memory deficits that arise in at least some patients with focal frontal lesions, including a deficit in retrieving autobiographical or retrograde memories and the occurrence of florid or "spontaneous" confabulation (110–112).

Neuropsychology

There is extensive neuropsychological literature on the deficits produced by brain lesions. In general, primary or "working" memory, the priming phenomenon, and procedural memory (for skills) are all well preserved in the presence of severe amnesia (87–89). By definition, there is a severe deficit in so-called "explicit" memory—the conscious recollection of incidents and events, although the rate of forgetting new information, once learning has been accomplished, may be surprisingly normal (113–116). In addition, there is a variable degree of retrograde memory loss and a variable degree of involvement of semantic memory (knowledge of facts, concepts, and language).

Many authors have attempted to differentiate discrete patterns of memory impairment resulting from diencephalic and temporal lobe lesions—for example, patients with temporal lobe lesions might forget faster than patients with diencephalic lesions (113, 114, 117). However, most of these findings have not been upheld, including the purported difference in forgetting rates (115, 118). In addition, various authors have argued that lesions in separate memory systems underlie anterograde and retrograde amnesia, respectively (119–121). Although there is general agreement on the lesion sites that produce anterograde amnesia, there is more controversy regarding which sites are critical for retrograde memory loss. Frontal dysfunction (112, 122) or anterior temporal lobe pathology (25, 26) are the most frequently implicated regions.

The underlying basis of the amnesic deficit has been attributed at varying times to faulty consolidation (97, 98), a pure retrieval deficit (123), an impairment in encoding semantic information (124), and a particular deficit in encoding and retrieving the contextual components of information (88, 125). This issue remains essentially unresolved, and various attempts to model amnesic deficits using connectionist neural networks are currently underway (see also the chapter by Squire).

DIAGNOSTIC EVALUATION

Diagnostic procedures depend very much on what any referral information suggests about the underlying nature of the amnesic disorder. More detailed accounts of the assessment of the amnesic syndrome are given elsewhere (19, 88) as is a discussion of the assessment of dementing disorders (126).

Where a transient amnesia occurs, both the clinical history and the neuropsychological evaluation can be helpful. For example, repetitive questioning suggests the TGA syndrome or an acute confusional state; multiple episodes of TGA suggest an epileptic basis; and loss of the sense of personal identity suggests a psychogenic amnesia. Precipitating life stresses can be misleading because they commonly precede TGA (1, 9, 16). The rate and clinical circumstances of the onset of the memory loss are important to establish; and it is always important to obtain corroborative evidence by interviewing informants, examining medical records, or scrutinizing legal documents where applicable. The subject's initial complaint of amnesia can be revealing—how long after an accident, trauma, or offense it occurred, and how consistent the description has been thereafter. Any past history of head injury, epilepsy, hypoglycemia, or other relevant organic disorder should, of course, be obtained. Medical examination may reveal physical stigmata of alcohol or drug abuse, and blood and urine analysis, EEG, and a CT or MRI scan are often required.

In cases of transient organic amnesia, the neuropsychological pattern of the memory disorder during the acute episode, as well as any residual deficit thereafter, conforms with the well-described pattern in the organic amnesic syndrome discussed earlier (1, 11, 16). In cases of transient, psychogenic amnesia, the neuropsychological pattern of deficit may be much more variable. Sometimes there are islets of preserved memory within the amnesic gap, akin to that which occurs in a head injury (65, 66), although the subject may adopt a detached attitude to these memory fragments, describing them as "strange and unfamiliar" (127). In many cases, semantic knowledge remains intact, e.g., foreign languages, the names of streets, towns, and famous people (65, 66, 128), whereas in others it is also implicated (65, 71, 127, 129). Similarly, performance at verbal learning tests has been reported as unaffected (71, 128), mildly impaired (66), or more severely impaired (81). Memory for skills is often preserved (127), but in the Padola hearing in 1959 (75), retention of a rudimentary knowledge of aerodynamics and of other skills (e.g., solving jigsaw puzzles) was taken as evidence against an organic amnesia—a frankly erroneous interpretation in light of contemporary findings of preserved procedural memory in organic amnesia (87, 88). Sometimes memory retrieval may be facilitated by chance cues in the environment (66, 71, 129), but deliberate cueing is often unsuccessful (65, 127, 128).

Various neuropsychological tests have been developed, that purport to differentiate psychogenic from neurobiologically based memory loss, and hysterical amnesia/unconscious forgetting from simulated or "factitious" memory loss. In general, the basis of these various experimental procedures is that "simulators" or "fakers" will fail at relatively easy test items on specific memory tasks, where patients with either a neurobiological or hysterical amnesia would succeed. For example, Brandt et al. (130) suggested that simulators score below chance on recognition memory tests; and Wiggins and Brandt (131) argued that they show relatively poor recognition memory compared with recall performance. Wiggins and Brandt (131) also suggested that simulators show normal primacy and recency effects, whereas the latter may be absent in some patients with organic amnesia. Schacter (132, 133) predicted that simulators may fail to show normal priming effects on memory tasks, a prediction that was recently confirmed by Horton et al. (134) in a laboratory study. Furthermore, Schacter (133) produced experimental evidence indicating that simulators show abnormally low "feelings-of-knowing," in that they say that neither cueing, recognition testing, nor additional time would help their performance, unlike subjects who genuinely cannot remember test material. With regard to tests of retrograde memory, Wiggins and Brandt (131) argued that simulators show abnormally poor performance on tests of autobiographical memory and produce more implausible responses, while manifesting relatively mild impairment on tests of public event memory, or anterograde memory. Failure at the easiest item on Ravens Progressive Matrices has also been interpreted as evidence of a simulated amnesia (135).

Although many of these techniques are promising (136), they are by no means foolproof. Kopelman et al. (128) described a patient in whom there was independent evidence that she was at least partially simulating her amnesia. This patient performed extremely well at all anterograde memory tasks, including recognition memory and word-completion priming tasks. On the other hand, she did show a disproportionate impairment of retrograde memory, particularly involving autobiographical memories, with an aberrant temporal gradient (indicating a strong "recency effect"). Moreover, she showed impaired "feelings-of-knowing" on a recognition memory test for the names of people and places that she had known before the onset of her amnesia. In brief, this patient's anterograde memory performance was entirely normal; but her disproportionate autobiographical memory loss was indicative of a psychogenic etiology, and her impaired feelings-of-knowing were suggestive of simulation.

MANAGEMENT

The management of these disorders depends, of course, on the underlying diagnosis. In TGA, there must be an investigation for any underlying migrainous or epileptic source, and, if found, treatment should be conducted accordingly. Consistent with this, anticonvulsant therapy in so-called "transient epileptic amnesia" has proved effective (16). The management of acute and chronic head injury is discussed in many texts elsewhere (22) as well as the use of strategies to overcome memory impairments (137). In alcoholic blackouts, subjects need to be "dried out" and warned of the long-term medical, cognitive, and personality effects of severe intoxication, although clinical management is notoriously ineffective (138). In sleepwalking, post-ECT amnesia, and PTSD, an explanation of the underlying syndrome is an important first step in management, and in the latter two disorders, the effective treatment of any residual depression is critical. In psychogenic fugue, the underlying stressors or precipitants need to be identified, and treatment of any underlying depression is paramount. Amnesic offenders will usually be seen for the preparation of a medicolegal report. Treatment of any depression or psychosis, is, of course, essential.

CONCLUSIONS

The present chapter has reviewed transient disorders of memory and consciousness, although the assessment and management of specific conditions will vary, our increasing understanding of the neurobiology and neuropsychology of organic amnesia provides a core of knowledge against which to compare individual disorders as well as individual patients. Not only do transient, organic disorders implicate the same brain structures as are known to be involved in chronic or persistent memory disorders—for example, in TGA, epileptic automatisms, and almost certainly TEA, but the pattern of neuropsychological deficit is similar. In psychogenic amnesia, brain lesions are assumed not to be involved, but there is at least suggestive evidence that, where the neuropsychological deficit is very discrepant with what would be expected in organic amnesia, the disorder is more likely to result from simulation or fabrication, rather than from authentic hysterical or unconscious processes.

Acknowledgment

The author is grateful to Miss C. Hook for patiently typing the manuscript and the support of the West Lambeth Community Care Trust.

References

1. Hodges JR, Ward CD. Observations during transient global amnesia: a behavioural and neuropsychological study of five cases. Brain 1989;112:595–620.
2. Whitty C, Stores G, Lishman WA. Amnesia in cerebral disease. In: Whitty CWM, Zangwill OL, eds. Amnesia. 2nd ed. London and Boston: Butterworths, 1977.
3. Stillhard G, Landis T, Schiess A, Regard M, Sialer G. Bitemporal hypoperfusion in transient global amnesia: 99m-Tc-HM-PAO SPECT and neuropsychological findings during and after an attack. J Neurol Neurosurg Psychiatry 1990;53:339–342.
4. Evans J, Wilson B, Wraight PW, Hodges JR. Neuropsychological and SPECT scan findings during and after transient global amnesia: evidence for the differential impairment of remote episodic memory. J Neurol Neurosurg Psychiatry (in press).

5. Fujii K, Sadoshima S, Ishitsuka T, Kusuda K, Kuwabara Y, Ichiya Y, Fujishima M. Regional cerebral blood flow and metabolism in patients with transient global amnesia: a positron emission tomography study. J Neurol Neurosurg Psychiatry 1989;52:622–630.

6. Hodges J, Oxbury SM. Persistent memory impairment following transient global amnesia. J Clin Exp Neurol 1990;12:904–920.

7. Heathfield KWG, Croft PB, Swash, M. The syndrome of transient global amnesia. Brain 1973;96:729–736.

8. Fisher CM. Transient global amnesia. Arch Neurol 1982;39:605–608.

9. Miller JW, Petersen RC, Metter EJ, Millikan CH and Yanagihara T. Transient global amnesia: clinical characteristics and prognosis. Neurology 1987;37:733–737.

10. Kritchevsky M, Squire LR, Zouzounis JA. Transient global amnesia: characterization of anterograde and retrograde amnesia. Neurology 1988;38:213–219.

11. Kritchevsky M, Squire LR. Transient global amnesia: evidence for extensive, temporally graded retrograde amnesia. Neurology 1989;39:213–218.

12. Fenton GW. Epilepsy and automatism. Bri J Hosp Med 1972;7:57–64.

13. Knox SJ. Epileptic automatism and violence. Med Sci Law 1968;8:96–104.

14. Kapur N. Transient epileptic amnesia: a clinically distinct form of neurological memory disorder. In: Markowitsch HJ, ed. Transient global amnesia and related disorders. Lewiston, NY: Hogrefe and Huber, 1990.

15. Hodges J, Warlow CP. The aetiology of transient global amnesia. Brain 1990;113:639–657.

16. Kopelman MD, Panayiotopoulos CP, Lewis P. Transient epileptic amnesia differentiated from "fugue": neuropsychological, EEG and PET findings. J Neurol Neurosurg Psychiatry (in press).

17. Kapur N, Young A, Bateman D, Kennedy P. Focal retrograde amnesia: a long term clinical and neuropsychological follow-up. Cortex 1989;25:387–402.

18. Russell WR, Nathan PW. Traumatic amnesia. Brain 1946;69:280–300.

19. Lishman WA. Organic psychiatry: the psychological consequences of cerebral disorder. 2nd ed. Oxford: Blackwell Scientific Publications Ltd, 1987.

20. Lishman WA. Brain damage in relation to psychiatric disability after head injury. Bri J Psychiatry 1968;114:373–410.

21. Newcombe F. Missile wounds of the brain. Oxford: Oxford University Press, 1969.

22. Brooks N, ed. Closed head injury: psychological, social and family consequences. Oxford: Oxford University Press, 1984.

23. Russell WR, Smith A. Post-traumatic amnesia in closed head injury. Arch Neurol 1961;5:4–29.

24. Brooks N. Memory and closed head injury. J Nerv Ment Dis 1972;155:350–355.

25. Kapur N, Ellison D, Smith M, McLellan L, Burrows EH. Focal retrograde amnesia following bilateral temporal lobe pathology: a neuropsychological and magnetic resonance study. Brain 1992;116:73–86.

26. Markowitsch HJ, Calabrese P, Haupts M, Durwen HF, Liess J, Gehlen W. Searching for the anatomical basis of retrograde amnesia. J Clin Exp Neuropsychol 1993;15:947–967.

27. Merskey H, Woodforde JM. Psychiatric sequelae of minor head injury. Brain 1972;95:521–528.

28. Miller E. The long-term consequences of head injury: a discussion of the evidence with special reference to the preparation of legal reports. British Journal of Social and Clinical Psychology 1979;18:87–98.

29. Tarsh MJ, Royston C. A follow-up study of accident neurosis. Br J Psychiatry 1985;146:178–125.

30. Baddeley AD, Harris JE, Sunderland A, Watts K, Wilson B. Closed head injury and memory. In: Levin H, ed. Neurobehavioural recovery from head injury. Oxford: Oxford University Press, 1987.

31. Goodwin DW, Crane JB, Guze SE. Phenomenological aspects of the alcoholic "blackout." Br J Psychiatry 1969;115:1033–1038.

32. Kales A, Soldatos CR, Caldwell AB, et al. Somnambulism. Arch Gen Psychiatry 1980;37:1406–1410.

33. Howard C, d'Orbán PT. Violence in sleep: medico-legal issues and two case reports. Psychol Med 1987;17:915–925.

34. Fenwick P. Automatism, medicine and the law. Psychological Medicine Monograph, Supplement 17, Cambridge University Press, 1990.

35. Fenwick P. Brain, mind and behaviour: some medico-legal aspects. Br J Psychiatry 1993;163:565–573.

36. Kales JD, Kales A, Soldatos CR, Caldwell AB, Charney DS, Martin ED. Night terrors. Arch Gen Psychiatry 1980;37:1413–1417.

37. Kopelman MD. The cholinergic neurotransmitter system in human memory and dementia: a review. Q J Exp Psychol 1986;38A;535–573.

38. Kopelman MD, Corn TH. Cholinergic "blockade" as a model for cholinergic depletion: a comparison of the memory deficits with those of Alzheimer-type dementia and the alcoholic Korsakoff syndrome. Brain 1988;111:1079–1110.

39. Curran HV. Tranquillising memories: a review of the effects of benzodazepines on human memory. Biol Psychol 1986;23:179–213.

40. Curran HV. Benzodiazepines, memory and mood: a review. Psychopharmacology 1991;105:1–8.

41. Janis IL, Astrachan M. The effects of electroconvulsive treatments on memory efficiency. J Abnorm Soc Psychol 1951;46:501–511.

42. Squire LR. ECT and memory loss. Am J Psychiatry 1977;134:997–1001.

43. Squire LR, Cohen NJ, Nadel L. The medial temporal region and memory consolidation: a new hypothesis. In: Weingartner H, Parker E. Memory consolidation. Hillsdale, NJ: Erlbaum Associates, 1984.

44. Weeks D, Freeman CPL, Kendall RE. ECT, 3: enduring cognitive deficits. Br J Psychiatry 1980;137:26–37.

45. Frith CD, Stevens M, Johnstone EC, Deakin JFW, Lawler P, Crow TJ. Effects of ECT and depression on various aspects of memory. Br J Psychiatry 1983;142:610–617.

46. Squire LR, Slater PC. ECT and complaints of memory dysfunction: a prospective three-year follow-up study. Br J Psychiatry 1983;142:1–8.

47. Freeman CPL, Weeks D, Kendell RE. Electroconvulsive therapy. Br J Psychiatry 1980;137:8–37.

48. Kopelman MD. Speech dominance, handedness and electro-convulsions. Psychol Med 1982;12:667–670.

49. Stern RA, Nevels CT, Shelhorse ME, Prohaska ML, Mason GA, Prange AJ. Antidepressant and memory effects of combined thyroid hormone treatment and electroconvulsive therapy: preliminary findings. Biol Psychiatry 1991;30:623–627.

50. Cohen MR, Swartz CM. Absence of nimodipine premedication effect on memory after electroconvulsive therapy. Neuropsychobiology 1991;24:165–168.

51. Coffey CE, Figiel GS, Werner RD, Saunders WB. Caffeine augmentation of ECT. Am J Psychiatry 1990;147:579–585.

52. Mattes JA, Pettinati HM, Stephens S, Robin SW, Willis KW. A placebo-controlled evaluation of vasopressin for ECT-induced memory impairment. Biol Psychiatry 1990;27:289–303.

53. Sommer BR, Satlin A, Friedman L, Cole JO. Glycopyrrolate versus atropine in post-ECT amnesia in the elderly. J Geriatr Psychiatry Neurol 1989;2:18–21.

54. Levin Y, Elizur A, Korczyn AD. Physostigmine improves ECT-induced memory disturbances. Neurology 1987;37:871–875.

55. Nasrallah HA, Varney N, Coffman JA, Bayless J, Chapman S. Opiate antagonism fails to reverse post-ECT cognitive deficits. J Clin Psychiatry 1986;47:555–556.

56. Horne RL, Pettinati HM, Menken M, Sugerman AA, Varga E, Wilson GF. Dexamethasone in electroconvulsive therapy: efficacy for depression and post-ECT amnesia. Biol Psychiatry 1984;19:13–27.

57. d'Elia G, Frederiksen SO. ACTH4-10 and memory in ECT-treated

and untreated patients. I. Effect on consolidation. Acta Psychiatr Scand 1980;62:418–428.

58. Lawson JS, Inglis J, Delva NJ, Rodenburg M, Waldron JJ, Letemendia FJ. Electrode placement in ECT: cognitive effects. Psychol Med 1990;20:335–344.

59. Sackheim HA, Prudic J, Devanand DP, et al. Effects of stimulus intensity and electrode placement on the efficacy and cognitive effects of ECT. N Engl J Med 1993;328:839–846.

60. Raphael B, Middleton W. After the horror. Br Med J 1988;296:1142–1143.

61. Bremner JD, Scott TM, Delaney RC, et al. Deficits in short-term memory in post-traumatic stress disorder. Am J Psychiatry 1993;150:1015–1019.

62. Charney DS, Deutch AY, Krystal JH, Southwick SM, Davis M. Psychobiologic mechanisms of post-traumatic stress disorder. Arch Gen Psychiatry 1993;50:294–305.

63. Kopelman MD. Amnesia: organic and psychogenic. Br J Psychiatry 1987;150:428–442.

64. Hunter IML. Memory. Harmondsworth: Penguin, 1964.

65. Kanzer M. Amnesia: a statistical study. Am J Psychiatry 1939;96:771–716.

66. Schacter DL, Wang PL, Tulving E, Freeman M. Functional retrograde amnesia: a quantitative case study. Neuropsychologia 1982;20:523–532.

67. Wilson G, Rupp C, Wilson WW. Amnesia. Am J Psychiatry 1950;106:481–485.

68. Sargant W, Slater E. Amnesic syndromes in war. Proc R Soc Lond 1941;34:757–764.

69. Parfitt DN, Gall CMC. Psychogenic amnesia: the refusal to remember. Journal of Mental Science 1944;90:511–527.

70. Berrington WP, Liddell DW, Foulds GA. A reevaluation of the fugue. J Ment Sci 1956;102:281–286.

71. Abeles M, Schilder P. Psychogenic loss of personal identity. Arch Neurol Psychiatry 1935;34:587–604.

72. Stengel E. On the aetiology of the fugue states. Journal of Mental Science 1941;87:572–599.

73. Fahy TA. The diagnosis of multiple personality disorder: a critical review. Br J Psychiatry 1988;153:597–606.

74. O'Connell BA. Amnesia and homicide. British Journal of Delinquency 1960;10:262–276.

75. Bradford J, Smith SM. Amnesia and homicide: the Padola case and a study of thirty cases. Bull Am Acad Psychiatry Law 1979;7:219–231.

76. Taylor PJ, Kopelman MD. Amnesia for criminal offences. Psychol Med 1984;14:581–588.

77. Kopelman MD. Crime and amnesia: a review. Behavioral Sciences and the Law 1987;5:323–342.

78. Hopwood JS, Snell HK. Amnesia in relation to crime. Journal of Mental Science 1933;79:27–41.

79. Leitch A. Notes on amnesia in crime for the general practitioner. Medical Press 1948;219:459–463.

80. Gudjonsson GH, MacKeith J. A specific recognition deficit in a case of homicide. Med Sci Law 1983;23:209–219.

81. Gudjonsson GH, Taylor PJ. Cognitive deficit in a case of retrograde amnesia. Br J Psychiatry 1985;147:715–718.

82. Kuehn LL. Looking down a gun barrel: person perception and violent crime. Percept Mot Skills 1974;39:1159–1164.

83. Clifford BR, Scott J. Individual and situational factors in eyewitness testimony. J Appl Psychol 1978;63:852–859.

84. Yuille JC, Cutshall JL. A case study of eye-witness memory of a crime. J Appl Psychol 1986;71:291–301.

85. Deffenbacher K. Eyewitness research: the next ten years. In: Gruneberg M, Morris P, Sykes R, eds. Practical aspects of memory, vol 1. Chichester: Wiley, 1988.

86. Yuille JC. The effects of alcohol and marijuana on eyewitness recall. Paper presented at Conference on Practical Aspects of Memory, Swansea, UK, 1987 (unpublished).

87. Squire LR. Memory and brain. Oxford: Oxford University Press, 1987.

88. Mayes AR. Human organic memory disorders. Cambridge: Cambridge University Press, 1988.

89. Baddeley AD. Human memory: theory and practice. Hove and London: Lawrence Erlbaum Associates, 1990.

90. Victor M, Adams RD, Collins GH. The Wernicke-Korsakoff Syndrome. 1st ed. Philadelphia: FA Davis, 1971.

91. Mair WGP, Warrington EK, Weiskrantz L. Memory disorder in Korsakoff's psychosis; a neuropathological and neuropsychological investigation of two cases. Brain 1979;102:783.

92. Mayes AR, Meudell PR, Mann D, Pickering A. Location of lesions in Korsakoff's syndrome: neuropsychological and neuropathological data on two patients. Cortex 1988;24:367–388.

93. Squire LR, Amaral DG, Zola-Morgan S, Kritchevsky M, Press G. Description of brain injury in the amnesic patient N.A. based on magnetic resonance imaging. Exp Neurol 1989;105:23–35.

94. Dusoir H, Kapur N, Byrnes DP, McKinstry S, Hoare RD. The role of diencephalic pathology in human memory disorder: evidence from a penetrating paranasal injury. Brain 1990;113:1695–1706.

95. Von Cramon DY, Hebel N, Schuri U. A contribution to the anatomical basis of thalamic amnesia. Brain 1985;108:997–1008.

96. Scoville WB, Milner B. Loss of recent memory after bilateral hippocampal lesions. J Neurol Neurosurg Psychiatry 1957;20:11–21.

97. Milner B. Amnesia following operation on the temporal lobes. In: Whitty CWM, Zangwill O, eds. Amnesia. 1st ed. London: Butterworths, 1966.

98. Milner B. Disorders of learning and memory after temporal lobe lesions in man. Clin Neurosurg 1972;19:421–426.

99. Zola-Morgan S, Squire LR, Amaral DG. Human amnesia and the medial temporal region: enduring memory impairment following a bilateral lesion limited to field CA1 of the hippocampus. J Neurosci 1986;6:2950–2967.

100. Damasio AR, Graff-Radford NR, Eslinger PJ, Damasio H, Kassell N. Amnesia following basal forebrain lesions. Arch Neurol 1985;42:263–271.

101. Damasio AR, Eslinger PJ, Damasio H, van Hoesen GW, Cornell S. Multimodal amnesic syndrome following bilateral temporal and basal forebrain damage. Arch Neurol 1985;42:252–259.

102. Salazar AM, Grafman J, Schlesselman S, et al. Penetrating war injuries of the basal forebrain: neurology and cognition. Neurology 1986;36:459–465.

103. Phillips S, Sangalang V, Sterns G. Basal forebrain infarction—a clinicopathological correlation. Arch Neurol 1987;44:1134–1138.

104. Irle E, Markowitsch HJ. Basal forebrain-lesioned monkeys are severely impaired in tasks of association and recognition memory. Ann Neurol 1987;22:735–743.

105. Arendt T, Allen Y, Sindon J, et al. Cholinergic-rich brain transplants reverse alcohol-induced memory deficits. Nature 1988;332:448–450.

106. Rossor MN, Iversen LL, Reynolds GP, Mountjoy CQ, Roth M. Neurochemical characteristics of early and late onset types of Alzheimer's disease. Bri Med J 1984;288:961–964.

107. Mann DMA, Yates PO, Marcyniuk B. Some morphometric observations on the cerebral cortex and hippocampus in presenile Alzheimer's disease, senile dementia of Alzheimer type, and Down's syndrome in middle age. J Neurol Sci 1985;69:139–159.

108. Schacter DL. Memory, amnesia and frontal lobe dysfunction. Psychobiology 1987;15:21–36.

109. Shimamura AP, Janowsky JS, Squire LR. What is the role of frontal lobe damage in amnesic disorders? In: Levin HS, Eisenberg HM, Benton AL, eds. Frontal lobe function and dysfunction, New York: Oxford University Press, 1991.

110. Baddeley AD, Wilson B. Amnesia, autobiographical memory, and confabulation. In: Rubin, DC, ed. Autobiographical memory. Cambridge: Cambridge University Press, 1986.

111. Kopelman MD. Frontal dysfunction and memory deficits in the alcoholic Korsakoff syndrome and Alzheimer-type dementia. Brain 1991;114:117–137.

112. Della Sala S, Laiacona M, Spinnler H, Trivelli C. Impaired

autobiographical recollection in some frontal patients. Neuropsychologia 1993;31:823–840.

113. Huppert FA, Piercy M. Dissociation between learning and remembering in organic amnesia. Nature 1978;275:317–318.

114. Squire LR. Two forms of human amnesia: an analysis of forgetting. J Neurosci 1981;1:635–640.

115. Kopelman MD. Rates of forgetting in Alzheimer-type dementia and Korsakoff's syndrome. Neuropsychologia 1985;23:623–638.

116. Martone E, Butters N, Trauner D. Some analyses of forgetting of pictorial material in amnesic and demented patients. J Clin Exp Neuropsychol 1986;8:161–178.

117. Parkin AJ. Memory and amnesia: an introduction. Oxford: Basil Blackwell, 1987.

118. McKee RD, Squire LR. Equivalent forgetting rates in long-term memory for diencephalic and medial temporal lobe amnesia. J Neurosci 1992;12:3765–3772.

119. Shimamura AP, Squire LR. Korsakoff's syndrome: a study of the relation between anterograde amnesia and remote memory impairment. Behav Neurosci 1986;100:165–170.

120. Kopelman MD. Remote and autobiographical memory, temporal context memory, and frontal atrophy in Korsakoff and Alzheimer patients. Neuropsychologia 1989;27:437–460.

121. Parkin A. Recent advances in the neuropsychology of memory. In: Weinman J, Hunter J, eds. Memory: neurochemical and abnormal perspectives, London: Harwood Academic Publishers, 1991:141–162.

122. Kopelman MD. The "new" and the "old": components of the anterograde and retrograde memory loss in Korsakoff and Alzheimer patients. In: Squire LR, Butters N, eds. The neuropsychology of memory. 2nd ed. New York: Guilford, 1992.

123. Warrington EK, Weiskrantz L. Amnesic syndrome: consolidation or retrieval? Nature 1970;228:628–630.

124. Butters N, Cermak LS. Alcoholic Korsakoff's syndrome: an information-processing approach to amnesia. New York and London: Academic Press, 1980.

125. Huppert FA, Piercy M. Recognition memory in amnesic patients: effect of temporal context and familiarity of material. Cortex;1976;12:3–20.

126. Morris RG, Kopelman MD. The neuropsychological assessment of dementia. In: Crawford J, McKinlay W, Parker D, eds. A handbook of neuropsychological assessment. London: Lawrence Erlbaum, 1992:295–321.

127. Coriat IH. The Lowell case of amnesia. J Abnorm Psychol 1907;2:93–111.

128. Kopelman MD, Christensen H, Puffett A, Stanhope N. The great escape: a neuropsychological study of psychogenic amnesia. Neuropsychologia 1993.

129. Kopelman MD. The assessment of psychogenic amnesia. In: Baddeley A, Wilson B, Watts F, eds. Handbook of memory disorders. New York: John Wiley & Sons, 1993.

130. Brandt J, Rubinsky E, Lassen G. Uncovering a malingered amnesia. Ann N Y Acad Sci 1985;444:502–503.

131. Wiggins EC, Brandt J. The detection of simulated amnesia. Law and Human Behavior 1988;12:57–78.

132. Schacter DL. Amnesia and crime: how much do we really know. Am Psychol 1986;41:286–295.

133. Schacter DL. On the relation between genuine and simulated amnesia. Behavioral Sciences and the Law 1986;4:47–64.

134. Horton KD, Smith SA, Barghout NK, Connolly DA. The use of indirect memory tests to assess malingered amnesia: a study of metamemory. J Exp Psychol General 1992;121:326–351.

135. Gudjonsson GH, Shackleton H. The pattern of scores on Raven's matrices during "faking bad" and "non-faking" performance. Br J Clin Psychol 1986;25:35–41.

136. Brandt J. Detecting amnesia's imposters. In: Squire LR, Butters N, eds. Neuropsychology of memory. 2nd ed. New York and London: Guilford, 1992.

137. Wilson B. The rehabilitation of memory, London: Guilford, 1987.

138. Vaillant GE, Milofsky FS. Natural history of male alcoholism: 4: Paths to recovery. Arch Gen Psychiatry 1982;39:127–133.

28

SOMATIZATION AND CONVERSION DISORDERS

Maria A. Ron

CLINICAL BACKGROUND

Symptoms suggestive of neurological dysfunction without a known physiological explanation and for which a psychogenic etiology is presumed fall under the diagnosis of *conversion disorder* or hysterical neurosis, conversion type. In the *Diagnostic and Statistical Manual of Mental Disorders* (DSM-IV), conversion is classified as a somatoform disorder. According to the DSM-IV, the diagnosis of conversion disorder can be made only if the neurological disturbance is not intentionally produced and only in the presence of clear *psycho*pathological mechanisms.

The concept of conversion or hysterical neurosis has not been immune to the changes in nosology that have occurred over the centuries. Several comprehensive reviews are available on this subject (1–3). A crucial role for unconscious motives in the genesis of symptoms was emphasized by Breuer and Freud (4), who postulated that a traumatic experience—usually of sexual content—was rendered innocuous by being transformed into a somatic symptom. The resolution of this unconscious conflict is known as primary gain. The advantages the person experiences when assuming the sick role, the so-called secondary gain are important in maintaining the symptoms that were initiated for primary gain. Some of the neurological abnormalities exhibited by patients with conversion disorders (e.g., mutism, sensory and motor disturbances) were considered to be symbolically linked to the initial traumatic psychological conflict. Others (e.g., pseudoseizures) were more difficult to link to specific conflicts; these were not initially thought to represent conversion disorders.

The diagnostic criteria for conversion, the legacy of the psychoanalytical era, often are difficult to establish, detracting from their clinical usefulness. In some patients relevant psychological factors, even if present, may become apparent only after recovery. Most likely, the degree of insight will vary from patient to patient, partially related to the duration of the illness and the patient's contact with doctors and other health professionals.

A number of other psychological features of different predictive value have also been considered relevant in making the diagnosis. Of these features, the presence of a previous history of somatization, associated psychopathology, emotional distress before the onset, and the availability of a "model" for the choice of symptom appear to have some diagnostic value (5), but their presence may be difficult to establish in a given patient. Others, such as "la belle indifference," a feeling of unconcern or detachment from the problem, histrionic personality, and disturbed sexuality, add little to the diagnostic accuracy. The interpretation of classical symptoms of hysteria such as hypochondriasis, secondary gain, and la belle indifference should be cautious. The same care has to be exercised when dealing with neurological signs such as a nonanatomical distribution of sensory loss and "give-way" weakness, which may also be seen in anxious patients with well-documented organic disease. In a study of 30 consecutive patients with clear organic pathology admitted to a neurological ward (6), at least one of these symptoms or signs was present in all the patients, and most had more than one. The relevance of these diagnostic criteria for the management of these patients is equally limited. Strong arguments have been advanced (7, 8) to exclude them from future diagnostic classifications. However, conversion disorder and dissociative/conversion disorder are still to be found in current diagnostic classifications (DSM-IV and ICD-10).

Conversion disorder is not a clearly demarcated diagnosis; it overlaps with somatization disorder or *Briquet's syndrome,* a narrowly defined, chronic syndrome that encompasses recurrent and fluctuating symptoms pertaining to many systems. Briquet's syndrome is predominantly diagnosed in women, begins before the age of 30, and, as in the case of conversion disorder, is often associated with depression and other psychiatric disturbances (9). The neurological symptoms of these patients are similar to those of conversion disorder, but the differences between the two categories concern chronicity and severity. Varying degrees of overlap are also present with other somatoform disorders such as hypochondriasis. In this chapter the distinction between conversion and somatization disorders is neither possible nor useful. Rather, they are considered as part of a continuum. The labels *conversion disorder* and *hysteria* will be used interchangeably.

Conversion disorders can be episodic, as in pseudoepileptic seizures, or more persistent, as in some cases of motor or sensory disturbance. The neurological manifestations are protean and have been comprehensively reviewed (10, 11) as has their relevance in clinical practice (12). Pseudoepileptic seizures, motor and sensory disturbances, fugues, amnesic states, and blindness are among the commonest. Many of these syndromes are discussed in greater detail in this chapter and in Chapter 27 by Michael Kopelman.

Validity of the Diagnosis

Doubts about the validity of the diagnosis of conversion disorder have often been expressed. The diagnostic difficulties stem from the vagueness of the diagnostic criteria and the lack of objective laboratory tests to support the diagnosis. The influential follow-up study of Slater (13) provided considerable ammunition to the critics of the diagnosis. In his study more than two-thirds of those patients who had been given the diagnosis of hysteria some years earlier had demonstrable organic pathology at follow-up. Major psychiatric illness was also apparent in about half of those without organic pathology. Other early studies reached similar conclusions (14–17). These reports, which introduced a necessary note of caution, have led in turn to the neglect of psychogenic mechanisms in the causation of physical symptoms, although the concept of hysteria has proved more resistant to extinction than its critics had anticipated. The very high incidence of organic pathology reported in early follow-up studies is likely to reflect the inaccuracies of the neurological diagnosis at a time when modern brain imaging was not available and when the nosological status of conditions such as dystonia was far less clear. The diagnosis still remains difficult in conditions such as rare movement disorders or difficult-to-observe intermittent symptoms, where the diagnosis is largely clinical. In addition, many of these studies assumed that the presence of organic pathology or other psychiatric diseases was incompatible with the diagnosis of conversion disorder.

As can be expected, the diagnosis of hysteria is more stable when the symptoms are chronic and involve many different systems, as is the case in Briquet's syndrome. A long-term follow-up study (15) found this diagnosis to be stable in 80% of those diagnosed between 6–12 years earlier. On the other hand, the retrospective validity of the diagnosis was much lower; thus, only a third of those newly diagnosed had the same diagnosis when seen some years previously.

Psychiatric Comorbidity

Association with other psychiatric diagnoses, especially depression, is common. The prevalence rates for major depression in conversion disorder have been reported as high as 52% (18) and 94% (19), and a lifetime prevalence of 50% for depression and of 20% for panic disorder have been reported (20). In the last-cited study the lifetime prevalence rates for affective disorder were lower (18% for depression) in those with less chronic symptoms limited to the nervous system. The strong association between conversion and depression raises the possibility that affective disorder may be a predisposing factor for the development of conversion symptoms and not simply a reaction to disability or psychological stressors.

Psychiatric symptoms, however, are frequently overlooked in these patients who are often unable to communicate psychic distress by conventional means. This lack of awareness of inner feelings and attitudes, known as a-lexithymia, appears to be a crucial determinant in the somatic presentation of psychiatric illness.

Incidence and Prevalence

Given the difficulties in establishing the diagnosis, it is not surprising that the estimates of the frequency of conversion disorder vary widely, depending on the setting, socioeconomic features of the cohort, and thoroughness of the investigations performed to exclude organic pathology. A low prevalence (under 1%) has been reported (21) in a psychiatric population, while a recent postal survey (22) suggests that about 20% of patients seen by British neurologists have symptoms for which an organic explanation is not forthcoming, and the proportion is even greater for those admitted to a neurological ward. These rates are in agreement with those found in a cross-sectional survey of neurologic patients (23), which reported a prevalence of 17.3% for primary psychiatric illness presenting with neurological symptoms. This group included patients with conversion, anxiety, and somatization disorder. Another study of 133 women admitted to a neurological ward (24) found that symptoms could be satisfactorily explained as a result of organic pathology in only a third, psychological factors being solely responsible for the neurological symptoms in a quarter. In the rest, both neurological and psychiatric etiologies were considered to be relevant. This study highlighted the difficulties experienced by clinicians trying to find a suitable psychiatric diagnosis for many of these patients. Thus, psychiatric labels were found to be inappropriate for a fifth of these patients in whom organic pathology could not be found. A more recent study of consecutive acute neurological admissions in Denmark (25) reported an adequate organic explanation for only 40 out of 100 patients.

Reports on the prevalence of Briquet's syndrome have also varied. One of the early studies of the syndrome (26) found a prevalence of 1–2% in a group of American women in the puerperium, but the common occurrence of affective symptoms after childbirth is likely to have artificially inflated the prevalence rate. A much lower prevalence (4/1000) was reported in an American household study (27) that also included men. In the United Kingdom, the prevalence was considered to be around 2/1000 in a general practice setting that included women aged 16–25 (28). The use of different classification systems (DSM and ICD), and the variations in the two health care systems, are likely to account for these transatlantic discrepancies.

The influence of socioeconomic factors in the prevalence of the diagnosis was recognized by Briquet in his treatise (29), where he listed low social class, migration, and situational difficulties as predisposing to hysteria. The same factors have again been highlighted in an epidemiological study (30) that used a strict definition requiring the presence of multiple symptoms pertaining to several systems. The prevalence of conversion disorder was significantly higher (0.7%) for Puerto Ricans living in Puerto Rico when compared with non-Hispanic whites in Los Angeles (0.06%), while Mexicans living in Los Angeles occupied an intermediate position. These differences, which reflect class differences among the three groups, disappeared when socioeconomic class and education were controlled.

The changing prevalence of conversion disorder as a reflection of changing social and cultural conditions has also received attention in underdeveloped countries. In a recent survey of the changing prevalence of psychiatric diagnoses in rural India (31), two villages were studied in 1972 and again in 1987. In the first village, with a largely Moslem population, the diagnosis of hysteria had declined from 32 to 2.5/1000, and in the second village, of mixed Moslem and Hindu population, from 17 to 5/1000 at the time of the second survey. This decline in the rates of hysteria was proportionally greater for women and was accompanied in both villages by a parallel increase in the frequency of depression, leaving the overall rate of psychiatric morbidity unchanged. These dramatic changes were attributed to the improvement in education and socioeconomic conditions that had occurred in the years between the two surveys. A similar decline in the frequency of the diagnosis, which in past centuries was subsumed together with hypochondriasis and dyspepsia into the category of "nervous disorders," has also been documented in Western countries from the 17th to mid-19th centuries (32).

Genetics of Conversion Disorder

The contribution of genetic studies to the understanding of hysteria is limited. Higher concordance rates have been reported for monozygotic twins (33), although the difference with dizygotic twins failed to reach statistical significance, and shared environmental factors may have accounted for these differences. The same applies to the increased risk reported in relatives, particularly in women, of those with conversion disorder (15, 34). Of greater interest are adoption studies (35, 36), which have reported an increased prevalence of anxiety neurosis, alcohol abuse, and criminality among the relatives of those with somatoform disorders. It remains to be established whether this psychiatric comorbidity is specific to this group of disorders or whether it also applies to other conditions.

Association with Organic Brain Disease

The association of brain disease and hysteria has been recognized for a long time and has always been a fertile ground for controversy. For some (13), the presence of organic disease meant that the diagnosis of hysteria was incorrect, and passionate pleas were made to abolish it. This stance seems appropriate in patients in whom investigations are inconclusive and in whom careful reassessment is mandatory before the final diagnosis is reached, but current opinion has veered towards the view that both diagnoses often coexist and that the presence of organic pathology may have a central role in the causation of some conversion symptoms (12). An association between symptoms of conversion and head injury was highlighted long ago (37) in a series of patients from United Kingdom and Australian centers. In many of the patients reported in this study, the head injury was mild and it had occurred some time before conversion symptoms manifested themselves. The same association has been reported more recently by neurologists (38) who found evidence for organic pathology in about half of those with conversion symptoms who were consecutive referrals to a neurological center. However, the prevalence of organic disease in conversion disorder appears to be much lower (3%) in patients admitted to psychiatric hospitals (39).

The presence of organic pathology may both predispose and provide a model for conversion symptoms. Clearly, the interaction between the two is a complex one, best exemplified in the case of epilepsy, where epileptic seizures and pseudoseizures may occur together in as many as a quarter of all people with epilepsy (40). The role played by brain pathology in these patients is suggested by the greater incidence of pseudoseizures in epileptics who had sustained brain damage during childhood and in those with cognitive impairment or antiepileptic drug levels in the toxic range (41). At the same time, the importance of primary psychiatric factors is exemplified by the common coexistence of other mental disorders in these patients and their relatives (42).

The incidence of conversion symptoms in other neurological diseases is less well known, and no comparative studies are available. Claims have been made that this association is also common in multiple sclerosis (MS) (43), but recent studies have failed to substantiate this. The prevalence and incidence of mental disorders in MS are considerably higher than in those with similar physical disability but without brain damage (44), but this was accounted for by the presence of depression and anxiety disorders. In this study, control subjects with the same degree of disability resulting from nonneurological disease, actually were more likely to demonstrate histrionic behavior than MS patients. Furthermore, psychiatric morbidity in MS was more closely related to environmental factors than to the severity of brain disease as detected by magnetic resonance imaging (MRI). The possibility remains that certain types of brain damage carry a greater risk of developing conversion symptoms. Tentatively it may be suggested that brain damage acquired early in life and leading to cognitive impairment may confer greater vulnerability. The possibility that damage to specific brain structures may have a preferential effect in the causation of conversion symptoms is worth considering, although conclusive evidence is lacking. Frontal lobe damage leading to impairment of attentional mechanisms and executive functions could, in theory, facilitate dissociative mechanisms. This hypothesis deserves systematic investigation in future studies of dissociation and conversion.

NEUROSCIENCE BACKGROUND

Pathophysiological Mechanisms of Conversion Symptoms

The pattern of disability in conversion disorder does not follow that of known neurological disease but reflects the patient's notion of dysfunction, mimicking neurological symptoms to a variable degree. This key fact has led to the belief that some "central" mechanism such as an altered state of awareness or dissociation may be a common and necessary facilitator for the generation of such disparate symptoms. Such theories are based on the fact that symptoms of conversion may be induced or removed during hypnosis, a state of apparently altered consciousness considered to be similar to dissociation. Early studies (45) using electroencephalography (EEG) or event-related potentials (ERP) found little evidence to suggest that hypnosis differs significantly from the normal wakeful state. However, more recent studies reviewed by Spiegel (46) suggest that subtle neurophysiological changes may occur during hypnosis, or in those easily hypnotized, and that these changes may be important in explaining dissociative states.

These changes relate mainly to the ability of some subjects to increase or decrease the amplitude of the ERP to sensory stimuli, depending on the cognitive tasks employed during hypnosis (e.g., the suggestion of numbness results in decreased amplitude, while that of pleasant stimuli results in the opposite response). ERP changes appear to be more marked in the late components (P300), but may also be detected earlier (P100). These studies suggest that attentional mechanisms may be implicated in hypnosis and dissociation, but it is important to remember that with very few exceptions these changes have not been documented in patients with conversion disorder. Corticofugal inhibition of afferent stimulation at the level of the brainstem reticular formation, resulting in an inability to integrate afferent information and in a lack of awareness of specific body parts has been suggested as a possible mechanism (37, 47). It seems more likely that anterior attentional systems involved in focusing (anterior cingulate) and arousal (frontal lobes) may be implicated (46). Preliminary evidence suggests that attentional changes may also be present in conversion disorder, and a study (48) has reported enhanced ERP amplitude to irrelevant stimuli in conversion patients compared with controls.

The role of neurotransmitters in mediating attentional changes in hypnosis and dissociation remains to be determined. The dopaminergic system, with its predominant distribution in the basal ganglia and frontal cortex, is an obvious candidate. Spiegel (46) has reported a significant correlation between the levels of homovanillic acid (HVA) in the the cerebrospinal fluid (CSF), a dopamine metabolite, and hypnotizability. However the relevance of these findings to conversion disorder is unclear, and it seems likely that other neurotransmitter systems will also be implicated.

Conversion symptoms appear to be more common on the left side of the body, especially in the case of sensory symptoms (49, 50). This finding has led some workers to postulate a prominent role for the nondominant hemisphere. A parallel has been drawn with the unilateral unawareness and neglect found in patients with right-sided parietal lesions (50). In patients with hemiplegia due to cortical stroke, unawareness of disease is more often observed on the left side of the body, and is often accompanied by a flatness of affect, reminiscent of the "belle indifference."

The similarity between complex partial seizures and dissociative states, and the occasional occurrence of the two in the same patients, has lead to speculation about their having a common mechanism (51). Following this line of thought, a role for the nondominant hemisphere has been suggested by Mesulam (52), who reported the presence of EEG abnormalities in the nondominant temporal lobes of patients with multiple personalities or with the illusion of possession. He postulated that in these patients, who did not have clinical manifestations of epilepsy, the disordered brain activity may have resulted in a dissociative state. A similar report of two patients with multiple personalities (53) expands on Mesulam's hypothesis by postulating an imbalance of activation between the two hemispheres, with greater EEG activation of the left hemisphere, which was reversed after recovery. This theory implies the presence of an unexplained individual vulnerability, because the vast majority of patients with right-hemisphere disease do not exhibit dissociative symptoms. In addition, EEG abnormalities do not appear to be more common in those with other manifestations of conversion disorder. Furthermore, the rarity of the multiple personality syndrome and the limitations of EEG as a measure of hemispheric activity dictate caution in interpreting these claims and in extrapolating them to the more common manifestations of conversion disorder.

Psychophysiological studies have not been very successful in shedding light on the mechanisms of hysteria. High levels of arousal have been reported in those with chronic symptoms of conversion (54), while normal levels appear to be present during the acute stages (56), suggesting a puzzling variability of arousal in different stages of conversion. More recently, magnetic stimulation of the motor cortex in patients with hysterical arm weakness has demonstrated normal latency and amplitude of responses (56). It remains to be determined whether patients with motor conversion symptoms show abnormalities in the readiness potential, a negative shift that precedes a self-initiated action. This preparatory "unconscious" cerebral activity, which lasts for 500 msec or more, is followed by the conscious intention to perform an action, at which time a veto on activity can be exerted voluntarily (57). Studies of this kind may give important insights into the underlying mechanisms of some conversion symptoms, but are unlikely to provide a comprehensive explanation.

Attentional disturbances and other neurophysiological changes may operate only when the symptom first appears and may be secondary to other psychological processes best explained in terms of the sick role or learning theory. Kendell (58) provides a lucid account of the interplay of these various factors by suggesting that patients may adopt the sick role (59) or exhibit abnormal illness behavior (60) when the demands of life are too onerous. To some the sick role becomes attractive only in exceptional circumstances, when demands are abnormally great (e.g., soldiers at war, pending litigation). For most of those seen in ordinary clinical practice, the sick role becomes attractive when the normal demands of life become too difficult to cope with because of limited emotional resources or because the care and attention of others is available only when they are ill. This learned behavior is in part determined by cultural factors and childhood experiences and is reinforced by the advantages of the sick role.

The choice of symptom is usually determined by the previous experiences of illness in the individual patient or others, and the resemblance to neurological illness depends on the medical sophistication of the patient. In many cases symptoms can be considered a magnification of normal sensations or physiological symptoms such as those resulting from hyperventilation (61). In other cases the process of morbid magnification can be triggered by the presence of usually mild organic symptoms when the patient fails to make the connection between the stimulus that causes physiological arousal and the ensuing symptom that comes to be seen as primary (62, 63). This psychological approach has the advantage of bypassing the uncertainty of whether the patient is aware that the symptoms are feigned and makes allowances for variations in the level of self-awareness likely to occur with time and therapeutic intervention.

SYNDROMES OF SIGNIFICANCE

The manifestations of conversion disorder are protean (10, 11), and several of them may cluster in the same patient. Pseudoepileptic seizures, motor and sensory disturbances, fugues, amnesic states, and blindness are among the commonest. Some of these manifestations (pseudoseizures, amnesic states) are reviewed elsewhere in this book. In this chapter only ophthalmological (blepharospasm), motor symptoms (tremor and gait disturbances) and childhood presentations of conversion disorder are discussed in detail. The investigation and treatment of these syndromes follow the same format outlined below, but some salient points are mentioned when dealing with the specific syndromes.

Ophthalmological Presentations

The ophthalmological presentations of conversion disorder have been extensively reviewed (64). The frequency of these presentations has been estimated at 1/600 of those admitted to ophthalmological wards (65), but less severe cases probably are much more common. A variety of ophthalmological symptoms can be seen in conversion disorders, but sensory symptoms are more frequent than motor ones. Thus, amblyopia, field defects, diplopia, pain, hypesthesia, and dysesthesia are seen more often than pupillary abnormalities, ptosis, hyperlacrimation, problems of convergence and accommodation, nystagmus, and strabismus. As with other manifestations of conversion disorder, ophthalmological symptoms vary in their resemblance to organic disease, depending on the patient's sophistication and medical knowledge. Presentations such as bilateral blindness with normal pupillary reactions are almost certainly a conversion symptom, but greater caution is needed in interpreting other findings such as tubular, spiral or star-shaped visual fields, which can be observed in suggestible or tired patients with organic pathology. At the other end of the spectrum, symptoms such as monocular diplopia and central scotomata are far more likely to have an ophthalmological or neurological cause.

Among the ocular motor symptoms, *blepharospasm* deserves special mention because it is a common clinical complaint and because over the years its nosological status has changed from that of an hysterical symptom to that of a probable neurological disorder. Blepharospasm can occur in a number of neurological conditions such as Parkinson's disease, supranuclear palsy, multisystem atrophy, Huntington's disease, and Wilson's disease. It is also known to occur following encephalitis lethargica or administration of cytotoxic drugs and neuroleptics. More recently it has been recognized as part of Meige's disease, a syndrome of orofacial dyskinesia, probably hyperdopaminergic in origin. Blepharospasm also occurs as a consequence of ocular pathology (e.g., uveitis and keratitis), but idiopathic blepharospasm is the most common type.

Idiopathic blepharospasm is nearly twice as common in women and usually starts in the sixth decade. Dystonic symptoms, usually in the craniocervical region, have been described in three-quarters of these patients, together with a history of movement disorder in first-degree relatives in approximately a quarter (66). The association with other dystonic features and the low prevalence of psychiatric morbidity (around 12%) have led to the current views that favor its inclusion among the dystonic disorders of organic etiology. Further support for organicity has derived from electrophysiological studies showing abnormalities in the electrically induced blink reflex, suggesting dysfunction in descending basal ganglia pathways. On the other hand, even if a strong case can be made to consider organic factors as important in causing blepharospasm, as with many other neurological conditions, psychological factors may play a role in the manifestations and severity of the symptom.

The diagnosis of conversion disorder in patients with

ophthalmological symptoms follows the same lines as for other presentations. Clinical observation is of paramount importance, and often the discrepancy between the disability claimed by the patient and the ability to perform everyday tasks is a clue to the diagnosis. In all cases a careful clinical and laboratory examination to detect organic pathology is mandatory. This should include the testing of visual acuity, visual fields, color vision, and pupillary reactions, and clinical examination of the fundi. The search for intracranial pathology will make it necessary to perform imaging studies in many cases. In cases of blindness, preserved visual evoked responses are of particular value. Many ways of "tricking" the patient to display abnormalities incompatible with neurophysiological mechanisms have been described, but caution has to be exercised in the interpretation of these findings.

Movement Disorders

The diagnosis of conversion disorder is often difficult in those exhibiting abnormal movements. This difficulty stems from the fact that the diagnosis of many of the systems is based on clinical, impressionistic criteria, seldom backed by objective laboratory tests. Detailed description of tremors and other involuntary movements has occupied many distinguished neurologists. Over a century ago, Gowers (67) had already provided a cogent description of hysterical tremor, which still forms the basis of its differential diagnosis. He described the variable frequency and amplitude of hysterical tremor as compared with that of organic conditions such as Parkinson's disease. He also noted the delayed activation of hysterical tremor that may appear only after the affected limb has been kept in a fixed position for a few minutes, and its frequent disappearance when the attention of the patient is diverted. A more recent study (68) examined the features of psychogenic tremor in those patients in whom psychiatric treatment resulted in the disappearance of symptoms, or in whom the association with other psychiatric disorders made the diagnosis of hysteria highly probable. In this study patients exhibited tremor both at rest and during movement with a variable frequency and amplitude, but distraction resulted in cessation of the tremor. Head tremors were uncommon, other neurological features were absent, and there was no response to conventional pharmacological treatment. A high rate psychiatric co-morbidity, multiple somatic complaints, a history of previously undiagnosed physical symptoms, and involvement in litigation were frequently reported in these patients.

A variety of motor disorders, usually involving loss of power and coordination, are common in conversion disorder. *Hysterical paralysis* usually affects global movements rather than muscle groups, and patients may be able to use the same muscle groups to perform a different movement. A changing passive resistance ("give-way" weakness) is frequently observed during testing, and the strength of the affected limb can often be ascertained indirectly by asking the patient to lift the normal leg and observing whether the normal response of pushing down with the contralateral heel

is present (Hoover's sign). Unilateral changes in deep tendon reflexes, spasticity, and extensor plantar responses are indicative of organic disease, but their absence does not rule it out. Muscle wasting and contractures are very uncommon in these patients, but have been described in a few (10, 69). *Gait disorders* (astasia-abasia) are particularly frequent and have been observed in a quarter of those with neurological symptoms of conversion (69), commonly in association with other hysterical symptoms such as visual field loss, aphonia, and tremor.

It is important to remember when dealing with motor disorders that a mixture of organic and nonorganic symptoms may coexist in the same patient. This makes a detailed neurological assessment and appropriate investigations mandatory. Equally useful is to keep in mind that most organic movement disorders are made worse by anxiety and that improvement in the severity of motor symptoms when the patient is unaware of being observed is not diagnostic of hysteria.

Conversion Disorder in Childhood

Conversion disorders are very rare in children before the age of 6 (70), but their frequency increases with age. It has been estimated that up to 10% of those presenting to child psychiatric clinics may receive this diagnosis (71), although this rate nearly doubles in pediatric inpatients referred to psychiatrists (70). Pseudoseizures, motor and sensory symptoms are the commonest presentations. As in adults, multiple somatic symptoms are often present, especially in older children, and they may coexist with organic pathology, with the combination of pseudoseizures and epilepsy particularly common. In young children, conversion disorders are equally frequent in both sexes, but by adolescence, females predominate in a ratio of 3:1 (72).

Psychiatric comorbidity of conversion disorder in childhood and adolescence appears to be less frequent than in adults. Mild emotional disturbances have been observed in less than half of these children (71), and good premorbid adjustment is the rule. Sexual abuse or bereavement appear to be important factors in only a minority. The same lack of overt psychopathology has been observed in the families, with significant disturbances present in less than a quarter (73). On the other hand, sociocultural factors appear to be particularly relevant when children and adolescents with conversion disorder are compared to other children with different psychiatric diagnoses (72). In the last-cited study, migrant families of low socioeconomic status were overrepresented in the conversion group. The parents of these children, and particularly the fathers, had also experienced significantly more neurological, medical, and psychiatric illness than the other parents.

The same psychopathological mechanisms postulated to explain hysteria in adults are likely to apply to conversion disorder in children and adolescents. Symptoms are often a way of escaping an otherwise untenable situation and in childhood, even more than in adult life, an ally, usually a family member, is required to allow and promote the sick role. Symptoms again reflect the experience children had of illness in themselves or their relatives. The need for this sophisticated interplay has been suggested as the reason why hysterical symptoms do not occur in very young children (74). Given that depression is less common in children with conversion disorder than in adults, the facilitatory role of affective illness is less obvious. The prognosis of conversion disorder in childhood is good, with recovery rates of between 60–85% (71, 73), depending on the acuteness of the symptoms.

DIAGNOSTIC EVALUATION

The first step in making the diagnosis is to perform a detailed and comprehensive *neurological and psychiatric evaluation*. This is best achieved when close collaboration exists between psychiatrists and neurologists (12). The features of the symptoms should be elicited from the patient and informants, paying special attention to the similarities and differences with known neurological disorders. This should be followed by documenting a previous history of similar complaints or unexplained physical symptoms. Useful hints about the way to interview this patient and to gain compliance have been discussed by Creed and Guthrie (75). The neurological examination will highlight possible inconsistencies between the patient's complaints and the deficits that may not conform to known physiological patterns. Maneuvers aimed at tricking the patients into making mistakes believed to be indicative of nonorganicity should be interpreted with great care, as tired or anxious subjects with organic pathology can also be very suggestible.

The aims of the psychiatric evaluation are twofold: first, to detect abnormalities in the current mental state; and second, to elicit psychological issues relevant to the presenting symptoms. The frequent psychiatric comorbidity of conversion disorder should be kept in mind at all times, so that associated psychiatric disorders can be detected and treated. The exploration of relevant psychological stresses is often difficult and may require several interviews before the patient is able to disclose significant events or even begin to realize their significance. For this reason, the absence of clear psychopathological mechanisms should not be an exclusion criterion when making the diagnosis.

The appropriate neurological investigations will vary, depending on the presenting symptom, and are described in the chapters dealing with the neurologic disorder being mimicked. In many cases a thorough clinical examination is sufficient, while in others extensive laboratory tests, including electrophysiological and imaging studies, will be required. Many of these tests can be performed in ambulatory patients, but admission to the hospital for observation often clarifies complex problems in a way other costly investigations may fail to do. Equally important is the need to limit the number of investigations to those that are strictly necessary. This often requires careful discussion with pa-

tients and relatives who may be relentless in the pursuit of organic pathology and often unwilling to entertain a psychological explanation for the symptoms.

In a few cases the diagnostician may be aided by the use of *intravenous amytal* to interview the patient under sedation to access otherwise inaccessible psychopathology. This technique was introduced in the 1930s, and its current uses have been extensively reviewed (76). It has proved valuable mainly in emergency settings to elicit traumatic experiences in the stuporous or mute patient. The procedure for the amytal interview involves the slow intravenous administration of the drug until the sedation threshold is reached (usually after a dose of 150–350 mg). At this point drowsiness, rapid horizontal nystagmus, and slurring of speech appear. This level of sedation should ideally be maintained during the interview, which should be conducted as any other psychiatric interview. Affect-laden material should be approached gradually, and the patient should be assured that only those questions that were asked during standard interviews will be asked while under the effects of the drug. The diagnostic value of amytal in patients with motor symptoms is less clear (10). A dramatic improvement or worsening argues in favor of hysterical or organic causes, respectively, but minor motor changes are inconclusive.

In the United Kingdom, hypnosis is rarely used in the diagnosis and treatment of these patients. This is in no small measure due to the uncertainty of its physiological mechanisms (1), and to the fact that it involves a submissive patient/doctor relationship objectionable to many physicians. At best, its applications and results are similar to those achieved with amytal, but without the ease of the amytal procedure, which does not require patient susceptibility.

THERAPY

Once the investigations have ruled out the presence of neurological disease or revealed the extent of its contribution, the patient needs to be told about the findings and further investigations must be avoided. This first step, critical in establishing a therapeutic relationship, often is time-consuming. The therapist must show a considerable knowledge of neurological and psychiatric aspects of the patient's illness to maintain credibility and obtain the patient's cooperation with treatment. At the same time it is necessary to avoid a confrontation about the psychological nature of the illness (21). Usually it is much easier to deal with psychological problems by inquiring about the social and psychological consequences of being ill than to directly address social and psychological causes of the illness.

At an early stage in the management, the treatment of the associated psychiatric symptoms should be initiated. Depression or anxiety disorders should be treated with conventional drug therapy and/or cognitive-behavioral therapy. The use of analgesics and benzodiazepines, common in these patients, should be restricted and carefully monitored, because drug abuse often occurs. An improvement in the mental state often facilitates the treatment of the conversion symptoms and fosters the therapeutic alliance. At this stage further exploration and modification of interpersonal or environmental factors that may perpetuate the sick role should be tackled.

Treatment of the conversion symptoms often is based on behavioral programs tailored to the patients, usually including physiotherapy and a cognitive component aimed at modifying the patient's interpretation and attitude toward the symptoms. A useful review of these therapeutic strategies is provided by Bass and Benjamin (77). In many cases these programs can be carried out on an outpatient basis, but in severe cases inpatient treatment with a detailed and comprehensive treatment plan is required.

Intravenous amytal has a limited role in the *treatment* of hysterical symptoms. Considerable success was initially claimed in psychiatric casualties during World War II (78), but it remains unclear whether the removal of the symptoms was permanent. In the case of patients with hysterical paralysis, suggestion and passive movement of the affected limb are recommended, with continuation of exercise into the wakeful state. In the experience of the author, intravenous amytal is more useful in restoring memory in those with hysterical amnesia than in removing paralysis. The use of amytal should be seen as an adjunct to treatment, and failures to restore function may be expected to occur even if the diagnosis is not in doubt. A videotape recording of the interview has the added usefulness of being able to demonstrate to the patient the normality of the affected limbs, speech, memory, or other symptoms, and can used as an encouraging first step in a more comprehensive treatment program. Hypnosis, for those familiar with the technique, can be used for similar purposes, but at least in the United Kingdom, appears to be unpopular currently.

The treatment of conversion disorders in children and adolescents follows these same principles (79). In this group treatment should move at a pace the family can handle, and a punitive approach toward the child should be avoided. Hospital admission, if necessary, does not need to last until symptoms disappear, as improvement usually continues after discharge from hospital. The role of psychotropic medication in children with conversion disorders is not clearly defined, but the need to treat any psychiatric co-morbidity should always be kept in mind.

Patients with chronic conversion symptoms present a more difficult problem, and the goals of treatment may have to be limited to alleviating physical and mental disability and avoiding iatrogenic damage. The principles of treatment likely to be useful in these cases have been extensively discussed (80). One physician, usually but not necessarily a psychiatrist, should take charge of the treatment, to avoid multiple consultations. Visits to the doctor should be planned at regular intervals rather than as emergencies to avoid the use of physical symptoms as the primary means of getting medical attention. During consultations psychological problems should be explored and the patient helped to make connections between them and the physical symptoms. Coexisting psychiatric problems are in this way easier

to detect and treat, and the use of analgesics and psychotropic drugs can be monitored.

The *outcome of treatment* has seldom been monitored over long periods, and the variety of approaches adopted in the few available studies makes comparisons difficult. Acute conversion symptoms are regarded as having better prognosis. Striking improvements have been reported with simple supportive measures in patients with hysterical paraplegia or quadriplegia following minor trauma (81), and in those with acute gait disturbances (69).

A follow-up study of 220 patients with predominantly limb weakness and pseudoseizures (21) reported an overall recovery rate of 40%, with some improvement in a further 29% of patients. The treatment varied from patient to patient, but usually involved psychotherapy and psychotropic medication. Younger, male patients with acute symptoms following mechanical trauma fared better, while those in whom emotional disturbances were prominent or had expressed a desire to retire from work were less likely to have recovered. The type of symptom, on the other hand, had little prognostic significance. Similar results have been reported in groups of patients with visual symptoms followed up a year later (65). Twenty of 41 patients had improved significantly, while in the rest the symptoms remained unchanged. Symptom substitution had occurred in some of those in whom ophthalmological symptoms had improved. Once again, younger patients had a better prognosis, and most of those who recovered did so while still in the hospital. Loss of visual acuity with or without visual field impairment had a better prognosis than isolated field defects. The reasons for this are unclear, but it has been suggested (58) that intermittent symptoms (e.g., pseudoseizures) or those causing little functional impairment (e.g., sensory loss, visual field defects) may be more resistant to treatment than more disabling, continuous symptoms (e.g., paralysis or blindness). A recent follow-up study (82) including a variety of conversion disorder patients, other than pseudoseizures has again emphasized that simple reassurance and supportive measures during hospital admission may lead to a favorable long term prognosis. In this study, as in previous ones, acute symptoms were the ones most likely to improve.

It remains to be determined whether a given therapeutic regime has a greater chance of succeeding than another, and which components of complex treatments are particularly effective. The good prognosis of acute symptoms and their response to minimal, nonspecific intervention suggests that patient-related factors may be very important, at least in the early stages. It is also useful to remember that insight into the cause of the symptoms is not a prerequisite for improvement. Indeed, one study (72) found that only four of 29 recovered patients had given psychological difficulties as the reason for their symptoms when they were asked years later.

When treatment fails, attempts to minimize the cost of these patients to the health system may still be worthwhile. Such an approach, focused on advising referring physicians on how to manage these patients to avoid unnecessary consultations (61) has been an encouraging cost-cutting exercise. Unfortunately, monetary savings were not accompanied by reduction of symptoms or by an increase in patients' satisfaction with treatment.

References

1. Merskey H. The analysis of hysteria. Balliere Tindall 1979:7–45.
2. Ey H. History and analysis of the concept. In: Roy A, ed. Hysteria. New York: John Wiley & Sons, 1982:3–19.
3. Mace CJ. Hysterical conversion. I: History. Br J Psychiatry 1992;161: 369–377.
4. Breuer J, Freud S. Studies on hysteria. Standard edition, vol 2. London: Hogarth Press, 1905.
5. Lazare A. Conversion symptoms. N Engl J Med 1981;305:745–748.
6. Gould R, Miller BL, Goldberg MA, Benson DF. The validity of hysterical signs and symptoms. J Nerv Ment Dis 1986;174: 593–597.
7. Cloninger CR. Diagnosis of somatoform disorders. A critique of DSM-III. In: Tischler GL, ed. Diagnosis and classification in psychiatry. A critical appraisal of DSM-III. New York: Cambridge University Press, 1987:243–259.
8. Miller E. Defining hysterical symptoms. Psychol Med 1988;18: 275–277.
9. Guze SB, Perley MJ. Observations on the natural history of hysteria. Am J Psychiatry 1963;119:960–965.
10. Pincus J. Hysteria presenting to the neurologist. In: Roy A, ed. Hysteria. New York: John Wiley & Sons, 1982:131–143.
11. Weintrub MI. Hysterical conversion reaction: a clinical guide to diagnosis and treatment. Jamaica, New York: Medical and Scientific Books, 1983.
12. Ron MA. Somatization in neurological practice. J Neurol Neurosurgery and Psychiatry. 1994;57:1161–1164.
13. Slater E. Diagnosis of hysteria. Br Med J 1965;1:1395–1399.
14. Gatfield PD, Guze SB. Prognosis and differential diagnosis of conversion reactions: a follow up study. Diseases of the Nervous System 1962;23:623-631.
15. Guze SB, Cloninger CR, Martin RL, et al. A follow up and family study of Briquet's syndrome. Br J Psychiatry 1986;149:17–23.
16. Raskin M, Talbott JA, Meyerson AT. Diagnosed conversion reactions: predictive value of psychiatric criteria. JAMA 1966;197:530–534.
17. Stefansson JG, Messina JA, Meyerowitz S. Hysterical neurosis, conversion type: clinical and epidemiological considerations. Acta Psychiatr Scand 1976;53:119–138.
18. Zocolillo M, Cloninger CR. Somatization disorder: psychological symptoms, social disability and diagnosis. Compr Psychiatry 1986;27: 65–73.
19. Liskow B, Penick EC, Powell BJ, et al. In-patients with Briquet's syndrome: presence of additional psychiatric syndromes and MMPI results. Compr Psychiatry 1986;27:461–470.
20. Tomasson K, Kent D, Coryel lW. Somatization and conversion disorders: comorbidity and demographics at presentation. Acta Psychiatr Scand 1991;84:288–293.
21. Krull F, Schifferdecker M. Inpatient treatment of conversion disorder: a clinical investigation of outcome. Psychother Psychosom 1990;53: 161–165.
22. Mace CJ, Trimble MR. "Hysteria", "functional" or "psychogenic"? A survey of British neurologists preferences. J R Soc Med 1991;84: 471–475.
23. Schiffer RB. Psychiatric aspects of clinical neurology. Am J Psychiatry 1983;140:205–207.
24. Creed F, Firth D, Timol M, Metcalfe R, Pollock S. Somatization and illness behaviour in a neurology ward. J Psychosom Res 1990;34: 427–437.
25. Ewald H, Rogne T, Ewald K, Fink P. Somatization in patients newly admitted to a neurological department. ACTA Psychiatrica Scandinavica 1994;89:174–179.
26. Farley J, Woodruff A, Guze S. The prevalence of hysteria and conversion symptoms. Br J Psychiatry 1968;114:1121–1125.
27. Weissman MM, Myers JK, Harding PS. Psychiatric disturbance in a US urban community:1975–76. Am J Psychiatry 1984;135: 459–462.
28. Deighton CM, Nicol AR. Abnormal illness behaviour in young women in a primary care setting: is Briquet's syndrome a useful category? Psychol Med 1985;15:515–520.
29. Mai FM, Merskey H. Briquet's treatise on hysteria. A synopsis and commentary. Arch Gen Psychiatry 1980;37:1401–1405.
30. Escobar JI, Canino G. Unexplained physical complaints. Psychopathology and epidemiological correlates. Br J Psychiatry 1989; 154 (Suppl):24–27.
31. Nandi DN, Benerjee G, Nandi S, Nandi P. Is hysteria on the wane? A community survey in West Bengal. India: Br J Psychiatry 1992;160: 87–91.
32. Hare E. The history of "nervous disorders" from 1600 to 1840, and a comparison with modern views. Br J Psychiatry 1991;159:37–45.
33. Torgersen S. Genetics of somatoform disorders. Arch Gen Psychiatry 1986;43:502–504.
34. Ljungberg L. Hysteria: a clinical, prognostic and genetic study. Acta Psychiatr Neurol Scand 1957;32 (Suppl) 1957.
35. Cloninger CR, Sigverdsson S, von Knorring AL, et al. An adoption study of somatoform disorders. Arch Gen Psychiatry 1984;41: 863–871.
36. Sigvardsson S, Knorring AL, Bohman M, et al. Adoption study of somatoform disorders. I: The relationship of somatization to psychiatric disability. Arch Gen Psychiatry 1984;41:853–859.
37. Whitlock FA. the aetiology of hysteria. Acta Psychiatr Scand 1967; 43:144–162.
38. Marsden CD. Hysteria. A neurologist's view. Psychol Med 1986;16: 277–286.
39. Roy A. Hysteria: a case note study. Can J Psychiatry 1979;24: 157–160.
40. Scott DF. Recognition and diagnostic aspects of nonepileptic seizures. In: Riley TL, Roy A, eds. Pseudoseizures. Baltimore: Williams & Wilkins, 1982.
41. Fenton G. Epilepsy and hysteria. Br J Psychiatry 1986;149:28–37.
42. Roy A. Hysterical fits previously diagnosed as epilepsy. Psychol Med 1977;7:271–273.
43. Langworthy OR. A survey of the maladjustment problems in multiple sclerosis and the possibilities of psychotherapy. Proceedings of the Association for Research in Nervous and Mental Diseases 1950;28: 598–611.
44. Ron MA, Logsdail SJ. Psychiatric morbidity in multiple sclerosis: a clinical and MRI study. Psychol Med 1989;19:887–895.
45. Halliday AM, Mason AA. The effect of hypnotic anaesthesia on cortical responses. J Neurol Neurosurg Psychiatry 1964;27:300–312.
46. Spiegel D. Neurophysiological correlates of hypnosis and dissociation. J Neuropsychiatry Clin Neurosci 1991;3:440–445.
47. Ludwig AM. Hysteria. A neurobiological theory. Arch Gen Psychiatry 1972;27:771–777.
48. James L, Evian G, Kraiuhin C, Meares R. Selective attention and auditory event-related potentials in somatization disorder. Compr Psychiatry 1989;30:84–89.
49. Galin D, Diamond R, Braff D. Lateralization of conversion symptoms: more frequent on the left. Am J Psychiatry 1977;134:578–580.
50. Stern DB. Handedness and the lateral distribution of conversion reactions. J Nerv Ment Dis 1977;164:122–128.
51. Schenk L, Bear D. Multiple personality and related dissociative phenomena in patients with temporal lobe epilepsy. Am J Psychiatry 1981;138:1311–1316.
52. Mesulam MM. Dissociative states with abnormal temporal lobe EEG. Arch Gen Psychiatry 1981;38:176–181.
53. Flor-Henry P, Tomer R, Kumpula I, Koles ZJ, Yeudall LT. Neurophysiological and neuropsychological study of two cases of multiple personality syndrome and comparison with chronic hysteria. Int J Psychophysiol 1990;10:151–161.

54. Lader MH, Sartorius N. Anxiety in patients with hysterical conversion symptoms. J Neurol Neurosurg Psychiatry 1968;31:490–497.

55. Meares R, Horvath T. Acute and chronic hysteria. Br J Psychiatry 1972;121:653–657.

56. Schriefer TN, Mills KR, Murray NMF, et al. Magnetic brain stimulation in functional weakness. Muscle Nerve 1987;10:643.

57. Libet B, Gleason CA, Wright EW, Pearl DK. Time of conscious intention to act in relation to onset of cerebral activity (readiness potential). Brain 1983;106:623–642.

58. Kendell RE. A new look at hysteria. Medicine 1972;30:1780–1783.

59. Mechanic D. The concept of illness behaviour. Journal of Chronic Disease 1962;15:189–194.

60. Parsons T. The social system. New York: Free Press, 1951.

61. Smith GR, Monson RA, Ray DC. Patients with multiple unexplained symptoms. Arch Intern Med 1986;146:69–72.

62. Sharpe M, Bass C. Pathophysiological mechanisms in somatization. International Review of Psychiatry 1992;4:81–97.

63. Tyrer PJ. Relevance of bodily feelings in emotion. Lancet 1973;1:915–916.

64. Weller M, Wiedemann P. Hysterical symptoms in ophthalmology. Doc Opthalmol 1989;73:1–33.

65. Sletteberg O, Bertelsen T, Hovding G. The prognosis of patients with hysterical visual impairment. Acta Ophthalmol 1989;67:159–163.

66. Grandas F, Elston J, Quinn N, Marsden CD. Blepharospasm: a review of 264 patients. J Neurol Neurosurg Psychiatry 1988;51:767–772.

67. Gowers WR. Diseases of the nervous system. Philadelphia: Blakiston, Son and Co., 1888.

68. Koller W, Lang A, Vetere-Overfield B, et al. Psychogenic tremors. Neurology 1989;39:1094–1099.

69. Keane JR. Hysterical gait disorders. Neurology 1989;39:586–589.

70. Maloney MD. Diagnosing hysterical conversion reactions in children. J Pediatr 1980;97:1016–1020.

71. Leslie SA. Diagnosis and treatment of hysterical conversion reactions. Arch Dis Child 1988;63:505–511.

72. Steinhausen HC, Aster M, Pfeiffer E, Gobel D. Comparative studies of conversion disorders in childhood and adolescence. J Child Psychol Psychiatry 1989;30:615–621.

73. Grattan-Smith P, Fairley M, Procopis P. Clinical features of conversion disorder. Arch Dis Child 1988;63:408–414.

74. Taylor DC. Hysteria, play-acting and courage. Br J Psychiatry 1986;149:37–41.

75. Creed F, Guthrie E. Techniques for interviewing the somatizing patient. Br J Psychiatry 1993;162:467–471.

76. Perry JC, Jacobs D. Overview: clinical applications of the amytal interview in psychiatric emergency settings. Am J Psychiatry 1982;139:552–559.

77. Bass C. Benjamin S. The management of chronic somatization. Br J Psychiatry 1993;162:472–480.

78. Lambert C, Rees WL. Intravenous barbiturates in the treatment of hysteria. Br Med J 1944;2:70–73.

79. Garralda ME. A selective review of child psychiatric syndromes with a somatic presentation. Br J Psychiatry 1992;161:759–773.

80. Bass CM, Murphy MR. Somatization disorder: critique of the concept and suggestions for future research. In: Bass CM, ed. Somatization: physical and psychological illness. Oxford: Blackwell Scientific Publications, 1990:301–333.

81. Apple DF. Hysterical spinal paralysis. Paraplegia 1989;27:428–431.

82. Couprie W, WJ Dicks EFM, Rooijmand HGM, van Gijn J. Outcome in conversion disorder: a follow up study. J Neurol Neurosurg Psychiatry 1995;58:750–752.

29

NEUROBIOLOGY OF DRUG ABUSE

Edythe D. London, Steven J. Grant, Michael J. Morgan, and Stephen R. Zukin

Drug abuse has important social and legal dimensions; however, from a biological standpoint, abuse potential is an attribute of a drug, and it derives from the reinforcing properties of the drug. Drugs of abuse comprise a chemically heterogeneous group that represents a very small percentage of all drugs. The neurobiology of substance abuse encompasses both drug-specific mechanisms in brain, and commonalities of action, that explain how such diverse compounds share the property of abuse liability. This chapter reviews biological aspects of the acute and chronic effects of drug abuse. Information about neurochemical and anatomical substrates of these effects is presented with a discussion of the techniques used to elucidate them. Clinical aspects of drug abuse are the subject of the following chapter.

RECEPTORS: INITIAL TARGETS FOR ACTIONS OF ABUSED DRUGS

Given the complexity of brain circuitry, it is unlikely that an action of a drug at a single target per se could produce the constellation of behaviors, such as reward, conditioning, and compulsive self-administration, that characterize addiction. Nonetheless, despite the propagation of pharmacological effects to locations that are remote from the initial loci of action, drugs of abuse interact with specific neuronal receptors (Table 29.1). A considerable and rapidly expanding body of data concerns these central target sites at which drugs of abuse initiate their effects.

Dopamine Receptors and the Dopamine Transporter

Although drugs of abuse generally do not interact directly with dopamine (DA) receptors, as shown below, activation of the mesolimbic DA system is critically important to the rewarding effects and perhaps to other behavioral actions of these drugs. Therefore, it is useful to review the following discussion on DA receptors and the DA transporter.

DOPAMINE RECEPTORS

Over a decade ago, biochemical studies revealed heterogeneity among DA receptors. All subtypes of DA receptors belong to a class of receptors that manifest relatively slow (seconds) responses, consistent with a modulatory function (1). Whereas activation of the D_1 receptor subtype stimulates adenylate cyclase activity, stimulation of D_2 receptors either inhibits or has no effect on adenylate cyclase (2–4). Both D_1 and D_2 receptors are coupled to adenylate cyclase by guanine nucleotide regulatory proteins (G proteins). The D_1 receptor is coupled via a G_s subtype, and D_2 via a G_i subtype. In addition, both synergistic and opposing interactions between D_1 and D_2 receptors occur (5–7). A proposal that the D_2 receptor gene is a marker for vulnerability to substance abuse has created considerable controversy. (8–10).

The classification of DA receptors into more than two receptor subtypes was questioned for many years (4, 11). Nonetheless, molecular biological approaches have now established that there are at least five subtypes: two subtypes of D_1 receptors and three subtypes of D_2 receptors (12–16). The two products of D_1 receptor genes are known as D_{1A} and D_{1B}; the D_{1B} gene in rats may be homologous to the D_5 receptor gene identified in humans (17). The D_{1B}/D_5 receptor appears to have a higher affinity for DA than the D_{1A} receptor (18). The D_2 receptor gene family includes D_3 and D_4 receptors. All of these receptor genes have considerable amino acid sequence homology, and they belong to a superfamily of receptors with seven membrane spanning regions. The major differences in the amino acid sequences of the receptors occur in the intracellular portions believed to be responsible for the G-protein coupling to adenylate cyclase.

Neurochemical markers for DA receptor subtypes exhibit differential distributions in the brain (13, 15, 19–21). DA receptors were initially mapped in the brain by assay of binding in dissected regions (22); the findings were extended using light microscopic autoradiography (23–26). The development of hybridization probes for receptor RNA and antibodies against nonhomologous receptor protein segments has allowed a more precise mapping of new receptor subtypes. The highest levels of D_{1A} receptors are found in dopaminergic terminal fields, including the striatum, nucleus accumbens and olfactory tubercle, in the forebrain; lower densities occur in the cortex, amygdala,

Table 29.1. Receptors for Drugs of Abuse

Prototype Compounds	Chemical/ Pharmacological Classification	Receptor	Receptor Family	Drug Effect	Endogenous Ligands of Drug Binding Sites
Morphine	Opiate alkaloid	μ-opiate receptor	G protein-coupled receptors	Inhibits adenylate cyclase	Enkephalins, Endorphins, Morphine (?)
Δ^9-Tetrahydro-cannabinol	Cannabinoid	Cannabinoid receptor	G protein-coupled receptors	Inhibits adenylate cyclase	Anandamid (?)
Diazepam	Benzodiazepine	Benzodiazepine site of $GABA_A$ receptor complex	Ligand-gated anion channels	Enhances GABA effect; increases Cl^- influx	Diazepam binding inhibitor ?
Phencyclidine (PCP)	Arylcyclohexylamine (dissociative anesthetic)	PCP site within channel of NMDA receptor complex	Ligand-gated cation channels	Blocks channel; noncompetitive NMDA antagonist	?
Nicotine	Alkaloid	Nicotinic cholinergic receptor	Ligand-gated cation channels	Activates nicotinic receptor	Acetylcholine
Cocaine	Alkaloid (psychomotor stimulant)	DA transporter	Na^+/Cl^--dependent neurotransmitter transporters	Blocks DA uptake	Dopamine ?
Amphetamine	Psychomotor stimulant	DA terminal (DA transporter monoamine oxidase)	Na^+/Cl^--dependent neurotransmitter transporters	Promotes DA release	?
Lysergic acid diethylamide	Hallucinogen	$5HT_2$-serotonin receptor	Second messenger coupled receptor	Partial agonist; increases phosphoinositol hydrolysis	Serotonin

hypothalamus, and thalamus. In these regions, the receptors are located primarily on postsynaptic neurons (27, 28). Although D_1 receptors are about 10-fold more abundant than D_2 receptors in the cortex of most species, including primates, the electrophysiological effects of DA in rats have a profile more consistent with D_2 receptor interactions (29–31). There is evidence that D_1 and D_2 receptors may be located on different functional subsets of pyramidal cells in the primate prefrontal cortex (32). In primate and human cortex, staining for antibodies against the D_{1a} receptor has been found at extrasynaptic locations on spines of pyramidal cell dendrites (33). Extrasynaptic DA receptors in both the cortex and striatum may have an important role in regulating input from afferents that use excitatory amino acids as transmitters (33, 34). Such extrasynaptic receptors may be important to the actions of drugs of abuse, since they enhance DA output, thereby increasing the overflow of DA out of the synaptic cleft (34). The D_{1B} receptor, in contrast, is confined primarily to limbic regions, mainly the mammillary nuclei and hippocampus, with little or no presence in the striatum (15, 19–21).

D_2 receptors are not only expressed in high concentrations in postsynaptic neurons localized to DA terminal regions, but unlike other DA receptors, they are also located presynaptically on both axonal terminals and somato dendritic portions of dopaminergic neurons (13, 15, 19–21, 27, 28). The presynaptic D_2 receptors are referred to as autoreceptors (35–37). Autoreceptors are not unique to dopaminergic neurons, but are found in all monoamine-containing systems, on cholinergic neurons, and perhaps on other chemically defined neurons. The D_2 DA autoreceptor, exerts inhibitory feedback onto dopaminergic neurons. As concentrations of DA rise in the synapse, autoreceptors inhibit firing rates, decrease transmitter release, and inhibit transmitter synthesis. Not all dopaminergic neurons contain autoreceptors. In the rat, a subpopulation of dopaminergic neurons projecting to the medial portions of the prefrontal cortex lack release or impulse-modulating autoreceptors (37, 38). In human and nonhuman primate brains, a larger proportion of DA neurons lack autoreceptors. A recent report indicated that virtually all dopaminergic neurons in the ventral tegmental area (VTA) in human and monkey brains fail to express D_2 autoreceptors (39).

Both D_3 and D_4 receptors are much less abundant than D_1 and D_2 receptors, with concentrations about one-tenth those of the other receptors (13, 15, 21, 27, 28). The distribution of the D_3 receptor may be especially relevant to the actions of drugs of abuse. D_3 receptors are found primarily in mesolimbic DA terminal regions, such as nucleus accumbens, amygdala, and olfactory tubercle, with much lower concentrations in dorsal striatal regions, such as the caudate-putamen. There is also evidence that D_3 receptors are autoreceptors on a subpopulation of dopaminergic neurons (40). The distribution of the D_4 receptor has not been mapped in detail, but this receptor may be more concentrated in the frontal cortex and amygdala (16).

Substantial interest in the D_4 receptor has been prompted by the finding that the atypical antipsychotic drug clozapine, is a relatively selective ligand for this receptor, and that D_4 receptors have a higher concentration in postmortem striatal tissue from schizophrenic patients than in controls (41, 42).

DOPAMINE TRANSPORTER

It has been known for over three decades that cocaine and other drugs could block the reuptake of DA and other amine and indoleamine transmitters into their synaptic terminals (35). The development of new ligands that are highly selective for the DA transporter has permitted detailed study of the binding properties of the transporter (43–46). The exact steps in the transport mechanism are not known at this time, although translocation of DA across the membrane is ion-dependent. It has been suggested that ionic gradients for Cl^- and Na^+ may provide the driving force for DA translocation. There also appears to be more than one binding site on the transporter, suggesting that different drugs that inhibit DA uptake may have differential influences on transporter functions (47).

The DA transporter has been sequenced and cloned (48, 49). It is a membrane-bound protein consisting of 12 membrane-spanning regions and a large extracellular loop with the C- and N-terminal strands located in the intracellular domain (44, 45). Although only one gene for the DA transporter has been identified, there is evidence for different molecular forms of the transporter (44, 45). The structure of the DA transporter is similar to that of transporters for norepinephrine (NE) and serotonin (5-hydroxytryptamine, 5HT), suggesting that these molecules form a superfamily of proteins analogous to the G-protein-linked receptor superfamily (50).

The distribution of the DA transporter has been studied using receptor autoradiography, in situ hybridization, and specific antibodies; 45, 50a, 51). Ligands for the DA transporter have also been used for positron emission tomography (PET) and single photon emission computed tomography (SPECT) (52, 53). In binding studies, the DA transporter is found in nearly all of the DA terminal fields, with the highest concentration in the striatal DA terminal fields, including the ventral striatal components (nucleus accumbens and olfactory tubercle) (45). Lower concentrations are found in other DA terminal areas, such as the cerebral cortex and amygdala. Moderate concentrations are found in the regions containing DA neurons, with the substantia nigra having higher concentrations than the VTA. In contrast, in situ hybridization reveals detectable amounts of DA transporter messenger RNA (mRNA) only in dopaminergic cell bodies (54). Consistent with the data from ligand binding studies, dopaminergic neurons in the VTA contain lower concentrations of DA transporter mRNA than neurons in the substantia nigra. Some regions, such as the retina, olfactory bulb, and arcuate nucleus that are known to contain DA neurons, have virtually no detectable levels of DA transporter mRNA. This pattern has been confirmed in a preliminary immunohistochemical study (50a).*

OPIATE RECEPTORS

About 20 years ago, biochemical evidence of the existence of stereospecific binding sites for opiates in the brain emerged from several laboratories (55–57). These sites bound opiate agonists and antagonists in a rank order of affinities consistent with the analgesic potencies of the drugs. In a chronic spinal dog preparation, Martin and co-workers demonstrated distinct physiological profiles for the prototypical opiate compounds morphine, ketocyclazocine and SKF 10, 047 (*N*-allylnormetazocine). They proposed that these disparate profiles reflected selective interactions of the drugs with corresponding distinct μ, κ, and σ opiate receptors (58, 59). Because the effects of σ opiates were subsequently demonstrated to be unaffected by naltrexone (60), the σ receptor is no longer classified as an opiate receptor (61). At least some of the behavioral properties of SKF 10,047 and related compounds are mediated through phencyclidine (PCP)-like action at the *N*-methyl-D-aspartate (NMDA) receptor (reviewed in 62). Of the distinct families of endogenous opioid neuropeptides, the dynorphins interact preferentially with κ receptors (63). Because of the preferential interaction of the enkephalins with a receptor type having properties distinct from those of μ or κ receptors, the existence of a δ receptor was postulated (64). In addition, subtypes of μ and κ receptors have been identified (reviewed in 65). All opiate receptor subtypes inhibit adenylate cyclase and increase potassium conductance (66).

The validity of classifying opioid receptors into μ, δ, and κ classes with distinct patterns of ligand selectivity, stereospecificity (67, 68), and neuroanatomical distribution has now been confirmed by molecular cloning of brain μ (69, 70), δ (71–73) and κ (73) receptors. All of the cloned receptors manifest structures consistent with members of the family of G protein-coupled receptors. An additional opioid receptor clone, apparently lacking subtype specificity, has been obtained from human placenta (74). Naturally occurring opioid peptides lack absolute specificity for any single class of opiate receptor; their behavioral effects, therefore, represent a summation of their actions at μ, δ, and κ receptors. Pharmacological determination of the predominant receptor type governing the effects of a particular opiate can be guided by criteria, such as sensitivity of its effects to the prototypical opiate antagonist naloxone, its ability to act as a discriminative stimulus in experimental animals trained to distinguish injections of highly subtype-specific opiates from inactive treatments, or its binding affinity in membrane preparations labeled with a highly subtype-specific radioligand (75). Opiates that acting preferentially at μ or δ receptors display reinforcing properties in animal models

and human subjects, whereas those acting preferentially at κ receptors tend to lack reinforcing properties and to induce dysphoria (76).

The anatomical distribution of opioid receptors has been the subject of numerous autoradiographic studies of rodent brain (77, 78). These studies have shown that μ, δ, and κ receptors display sharply different distribution patterns in the CNS. High levels of μ receptors, labeled with the μ-selective radioligand [D-Ala^2, methyl-Phe^4, Gly^5-ol]-enkephalin (DAMGO) occur (in approximate rank order) in striatal "patches" and "streaks," accessory olfactory bulb, nucleus accumbens, ventral subiculum and dentate gyrus of the hippocampal formation, amygdala, central gray, superior and inferior colliculi, geniculate bodies, thalamic nuclei, and substantia nigra. By contrast, high levels of δ receptors, labeled with the selective δ radioligand [^{3}H][D-Pen^2,D-Pen^5]-enkephalin ([^{3}H]DPDPE), are found in nucleus accumbens, external plexiform layer of olfactory bulb, olfactory tubercle, striatum, amygdala, and layers of I-II and V-VI of cortex. The distribution pattern of κ receptors, labeled with [^{125}I]dynorphin (1–8) in the presence of specific blockers of μ and δ receptors, reveals a narrower range of densities than those of μ and δ receptors, with high densities in the tail of the striatum, hypothalamus (medial preoptic area, suprachiasmatic nucleus), globus pallidus, and nucleus accumbens (79). Opiate receptors in sensory and accessory sensory brain areas presumably mediate the analgesic effects of opiate drugs, while limbic, extrapyramidal, and hypothalamic/neuropituitary opiate receptors may be associated with reinforcing, motor, and endocrine effects of opiates, respectively.

Nicotinic Acetylcholine Receptor

The actions of nicotine are mediated by receptors for the natural transmitter acetylcholine in the central and peripheral nervous systems. Cholinergic receptors are classified as either muscarinic or nicotinic, depending upon their sensitivities to the natural alkaloids muscarine and nicotine. Nicotinic cholinergic receptors (nAChRs) represent a class of heterogeneous receptors, including those found in the electric organ (electroplax) of *Torpedo* skeletal muscle, autonomic ganglia, and the brain. Unlike muscarinic receptors, which are coupled to G proteins (1), nAChRs, (which give a faster response to agonists), are rapidly responding ligand-gated sodium ion (Na$^+$) channels. The four subunits of the nAChR belong to a ligand-gated channel superfamily that also includes the GABA$_A$ subtype of the γ-aminobutyric acid (GABA) receptor, and the glycine receptor (80).

The availability of radioligands that can bind with high affinity to central nicotinic receptors has allowed the mapping of the distribution of nAChR in the brain (81). Quantitative in vitro autoradiographic studies of [^{3}H]nicotine to slices of rat brain have shown densest labeling in the interpeduncular nucleus and medial habenula; dense labeling in thalamic nuclei, brain areas related to sensory function, and the cerebral cortex; moderate labeling of the molecular layer of the dentate gyrus, and subiculum; sparse

---

*Freed C, Revay R, Vaughan R, Kriek E, Grant S, Uhl G, Kuhar M. Dopamine transporter immunoreactivity in rat brain. J Comp Neurol, in press.

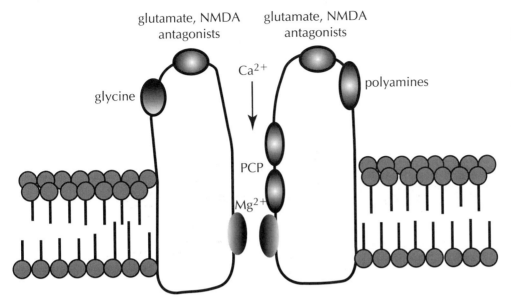

glutamate, NMDA antagonists

glutamate, NMDA antagonists

Ca^{2+}

glycine

polyamines

PCP

Mg^{2+}

Figure 29.1. Schematic diagram of the NMDA receptor. The receptor is a polymeric complex that gates a nonselective cation channel. It bears binding sites for agonists (glutamate and NMDA). Competitive antagonists also can bind to these sites. A strychnine-insensitive binding site for the coagonist glycine (Gly) has been characterized, as have sites for various modulators, including H^+ and polyamines. PCP and Mg^{2+} bind within the channel to block to influx of Ca^{2+}. (Modified from Kameyama T, Nebeshima T, Domino EF, eds. NMDA receptor related agents: biochemistry, pharmacology, and behavior. Ann Arbor: NPP Books, 1991.)

specific binding in the hypothalamus and caudate-putamen; and no detectable specific binding in Ammon's horn of the hippocampus or in the periaqueductal gray matter (82).

A series of critical studies of nAChR from *Electrophorus* and *Torpedo* electric organs rendered it the best characterized neurotransmitter receptor a decade ago (83, 84). This work was advanced by characterization of nAChR in detergent extracts (85–87) and its subsequent purification (88–91). Additional critical information was derived from knowledge of the subunit composition (92–95) and primary structure of the subunits (93, 96).

Purified nAChR from Torpedo has been characterized as a glycoprotein, composed of four subunits that surround the cationic channel (83, 84). The subunits are assembled into a transmembrane pentamer formed from two α subunits and one each of the β, γ, and δ subunits. Nicotine and other agonists (such as acetylcholine, carbamylcholine, and methylcarbamylcholine) bind to the α subunits. A group of structurally unrelated drugs, including mecamylamine, PCP, chlorpromazine, and local anesthetics, act as noncompetitive inhibitors by interacting at sites within the channel. Prolonged exposure to agonists or allosteric effectors cause decrements in the response amplitude of the receptor. This process is termed "desensitization."

Detailed information about the composition of mammalian nAChRs has been revealed through molecular biological investigations that have allowed cloning and sequence analysis of the various subunits. The genes encoding rat neuronal nAChR subunits have been designated α_2–α_5 and β_2–β_4 on the basis of the primary structure of the encoded proteins (97–100, 101–103). The subunits can combine to form functional receptors, as demonstrated in *Xenopus* oocytes, into which mRNA encoding the β_2 subunit is injected in combination with mRNA encoding α_2, α_3, or α_4 subunits (97, 103). Furthermore, in situ hybridization studies have revealed that while the β_2 gene and the α_2 subunit genes, as a group, are expressed in most regions of

the brain, each gene is localized to a unique but partially overlapping set of neuronal structures (104).

N-Methyl-D-Aspartate Receptor

A stereo-specific brain receptor site for PCP and related drugs was demonstrated biochemically in 1979 (105, 106). Considerable biochemical, neuroanatomical, functional, and clinical evidence indicates that this receptor represents the central target site at which PCP-type drugs initiate their unique effects (107, 108). The rank order of potencies of drugs in eliciting PCP-like behavioral effects correlates highly with the potencies of the drugs in inhibiting specific binding of radioligands for the PCP receptor and in inhibiting NMDA receptor-mediated increases in calcium (Ca^{2+}) conductances in electrophysiological assays (109). The PCP receptor is located within the ion channel gated by the NMDA class of glutamate receptors. Thus, binding of PCP-type ligands block the channel and act as uncompetitive NMDA receptor antagonists.

The major excitatory neurotransmitter of the central nervous system (CNS), L-glutamate, acts at a minimum of four types of receptors named for their selective agonists, which are: NMDA, kainate, α-amino-3-hydroxy-5-methyl-4-isoxazole propionic acid (AMPA), and *trans*-1-amino-cyclopentyl-1, 3-decarboxylate (ACPD). The NMDA receptor gates a Ca^{2+}/Na^+ ion channel. Receptor activation is regulated at a number of sites and requires the binding of two molecules of L-glutamate to the agonist sites (110, 111) as well as the presence of glycine (112) (Fig. 29.1).

Distinct NR1 and NR2 NMDA receptor subunits, with limited homology to one another, have been cloned and sequenced (113, 114). The native receptors appear to exist as NR1–NR2 heteromers. NR1 occurs as various splice variants that confer pharmacological differences. At least four different NR2 subunits have been described. Although NR1 can self-assemble upon expression to form channels

Figure 29.2. Schematic diagram of the GABA-benzodiazepine receptor. The receptor is a polymeric complex that gates a Cl^- channel. It bears binding sites for GABA and agonistic drugs, such as muscimol and for a variety of drugs (benzodiazepines, barbiturates, and convulsants such as picrotoxin). In addition, the activity of the receptor is modulated through the actions of endogenous neurosteroids, such as pregnenolone sulfate, dehydroepiandrosterone sulfate, and desoxycorticosterone sulfate.

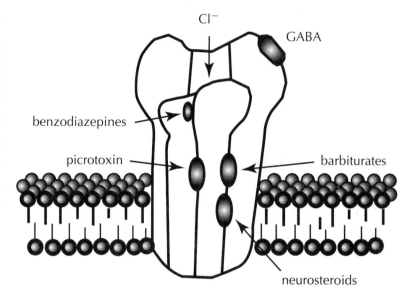

with properties of the NMDA complex, NR1–NR2 heteromers form channels of far greater efficiency, with the type of NR2 subunit primarily dictating the properties of the channel. High levels of NR1 mRNA are found in the majority of neurons, while neuroanatomical distributions of NR2 mRNAs are highly patterned and localized (115).

γ-Aminobutyric Acid Receptor

A molecular target of benzodiazepines, barbiturates, and ethanol, the γ-aminobutyric acid ($GABA_A$) receptor is an inhibitory ligand-gated receptor-channel complex, consisting of distinct α, β, and γ subunits surrounding a central pore. Each subunit exists in multiple isoforms, indicating several thousand possible distinct structures for the $GABA_A$ receptor (116).

The $GABA_A$ complex comprises multiple functional domains (Fig. 29.2). The GABA recognition site binds up to two molecules of agonist, resulting in conformational shifts that permit anion flow through the channel (117). Ligand binding to the benzodiazepine recognition site enhances the affinity of GABA for its own recognition site, and thus alters the sensitivity of the entire complex to agonist. Ligands for the benzodiazepine site can be divided into three groups on the basis of their effects. Clinically utilized anxiolytic, sedative, and anticonvulsant benzodiazepines (such as diazepam), classified as agonists of the benzodiazepine binding site, increase the sensitivity of the complex to GABA. Inverse agonists, such as the β-carbolines, decrease the sensitivity of the complex to GABA, thus exerting anxiogenic effects (118). Antagonists, such as flumazenil, lack significant intrinsic effect, upon agonist sensitivity of the receptor complex, but can block the effects of benzodiazepine agonists or of inverse agonists (119).

Barbiturates also enhance $GABA_A$ receptor function, acting at a domain of the complex independent of the benzodiazepine binding site. While at lower concentrations

barbiturates act primarily by potentiating the effects of GABA, at higher doses they may activate the channel even in the absence of GABA (120).

Ethanol represents the third type of drug that has abuse liability and that interacts with the $GABA_A$ receptor. In CNS-derived tissues, ethanol potentiates GABA-activated chloride (Cl^-) currents in a dose-dependent manner (121). The neurosteroids, dehydroepiandrosterone sulfate (122, 123) and pregnenolone sulfate (124), act as negative allosteric modulators of $GABA_A$ receptor function, whereas tetrahydroprogesterone and tetrahydrodeoxycorticosterone manifest allosteric GABA-agonistic features (125, 126). These observations suggest that such steroids may serve as endogenous regulators of $GABA_A$ receptor function. The rate and type of neurosteroidogenesis may be regulated in part by binding of an endogenous peptide termed the diazepam binding inhibitor, to mitochondrial benzodiazepine receptors on glial cells (127).

Cannabinoid Receptor

The active principle of marijuana, Δ^9-tetrahydrocannabinol (Δ^9-THC) (128), proved a challenging probe for a CNS recognition site because of its extreme hydrophobicity (129). Identification of the cannabinoid receptor was facilitated by demonstration of cannabinoid enantioselectivity (130) and by synthesis of a series of novel cannabinoids (131). These developments made it possible to demonstrate that cannabinoids inhibit adenylate cyclase activity in rank order, correlating with their physiological effects (132, 133). One of the new cannabinoids, radiolabeled, was found to bind to a unique site that displayed biochemical and neuroanatomical characteristics consistent with those of a receptor coupled to a G protein (134–136). A complementary DNA (cDNA), SKR6, isolated from a rat cerebral cortex library, was found to code for a 473-amino acid protein structurally belonging to the family of G-protein-coupled receptors. This protein was classified as a cannabinoid receptor on the basis of ligand selectivity and anatomical distribution of mRNA that codes for this receptor(137).

As had been the case with opiates, characterization of a specific cannabinoid receptor raised the question of the existence of endogenous ligands. Recently, a novel derivative of arachidonic acid, arachidonylethanolamide (anandamide), isolated from porcine brain, was identified as a ligand of the cannabinoid receptor (138) and was proven to exert cannabinoid-like behavioral effects (139). Anandamide has been shown to function as a partial agonist of the cannabinoid receptor in an electrophysiological assay (140).

THEORIES OF ADDICTION AND THE SELF-ADMINISTRATION PARADIGM

Until the mid-1950s, it was widely assumed that addictive behavior was uniquely human and was defined primarily by drug withdrawal syndromes. According to this physical dependence model, drug abusers were driven by predisposing internal states, and were soon trapped in a cycle of self-administration, tolerance, physical dependence, and readmintration. Thus, the drug abuser was believed to be motivated primarily by a desire to avoid the negative consequences of withdrawal. By the 1930s, it had been found that monkeys could be made physically dependent if they were forced to consume a drug, but they had never been observed to make themselves physically dependent simply as a result of free access to the drug (141). It was believed that animals were not capable of learning the association between an injection and subsequent relief (15 to 20 minutes later) from withdrawal symptoms (142). These findings and interpretation resulted in considerable skepticism about the possibility of developing an animal model of drug abuse.

During the 1950s, researchers began to find evidence that laboratory animals would learn to perform behavior that resulted in drug injections. This work was boosted by the development of technology that allowed intravenous delivery of drug infusions to the freely moving animal. Reflecting the influence of the physical dependence doctrine, early studies of drug self-administration in animals were performed in subjects that had been made physically dependent by repeated injections of morphine prior to experimentation. The animals were then placed in an operant chamber and were given the opportunity to self-administer morphine via an intravenous catheter. They quickly learned to self-administer morphine under these conditions, and it soon became apparent that they were responding to the drug infusion as if it were a positive reinforcer (143). In subsequent studies, animals self-administered doses of morphine that were too low to produce physical dependence (144). They also self-administered stimulants, such as cocaine, and no obvious withdrawal syndrome upon cessation of stimulant use had been described (145, 146). Further studies demonstrated that animals even self-administered certain abused substances without any previous experience of having received the drug (147). Studies such as these had

an immense impact on the concept of motivation underlying drug abuse in humans, and have resulted in a shift in emphasis away from the physical dependence model toward the view that drug abuse is largely driven by the motivation to seek and experience the incentive (rewarding or reinforcing) properties of abused drugs.

In addition to the roles played by negative and positive primary reinforcement in drug addiction, secondary reinforcement has recently been found to play a significant role. Secondary reinforcers or incentives are otherwise neutral stimuli present in the environment that become associated with drug-taking after repeated administration through a process of incentive learning. Once acquired, secondary reinforcement can become an extremely powerful source of motivation for drug-seeking behavior. Indeed, the recent incentive-sensitization theory, posits that after incentive learning has occurred, "wanting" a drug (drug craving) can become more important than "liking" a drug (drug reward) in determining drug-seeking behavior (148). The authors of this theory cite the example of cigarette smoking in experienced smokers, in which the intensity of cravings for cigarettes (produced by abstinence and/or the presence of secondary reinforcers) appears to be out of proportion to the reward produced by smoking. They also cite a report that low doses of opiates, which produce no subjective effects, can maintain response in human volunteers with histories of intravenous opiate abuse (149) as evidence that drug taking can become independent of positive subjective effects.

Brain Reward Systems

One of the most basic principles of behavior is the "law of effect," which states that behaviors that lead to a desired outcome are repeated (150, 151). These outcomes are referred to as "reinforcers." A precise definition of the term "reinforcer" has been difficult to formulate and is beyond the scope of this review. In general, however, a reinforcer is an event that facilitates learning. In the literature on animal research, reinforcers are often events or objects that satisfy biological needs; for humans, reinforcers can also be objects (rewards) that produce pleasurable (hedonic) subjective experiences.

The terms "reward" or "hedonic," used by physiological psychologists, are not synonymous with the term "reinforcement." For example, when animals are trained on a conditioned emotional response, in which they acquire an association between a tone and a withdrawal response produced by mild footshock, the posttraining, noncontingent consumption of sucrose (152), or a brief application of intense foot-shock (153), have identical memory improving effects. Thus, both rewarding and aversive events can produce reinforcement. Rewarding events can produce positive reinforcement and aversive events can produce negative reinforcement. Furthermore, in the paradigm just outlined, memory is not improved by posttraining consumption of saccharine solutions in concentrations that are equally preferred to those of retention-improving sucrose solutions (152, 154). Thus, equally rewarding events do not necessarily produce the same degree of reinforcement, and the property of being rewarding is neither necessary nor sufficient for reinforcement to occur. The difference between reinforcement and reward, and the more subtle distinction between positive reinforcement and reward, has resulted in some confusion in the literature concerning the neuroanatomical and neurochemical substrates of these phenomena.

The notion that the brain contains circuits that mediate reward or pleasure is central to our current understanding of the neural basis of drug abuse. The identification of the specific neural systems involved in reward originated with the work of Olds and Milner (155), who discovered that laboratory animals will avidly self-administer electrical stimulation delivered via electrodes to specific deep regions of the brain. This finding was of great significance for several reasons. First, this apparently rewarding brain stimulation acted as a positive reinforcer that could be used to selectively strengthen any behavior linked contingently to it. Second, only a limited number of sites were found to support brain stimulation reward (156). This observation suggested that there are anatomically specific circuits in the brain that mediate reward or pleasure (157). Third, subsequently it was found that rewarding brain stimulation could elicit natural consummatory responses (158–162). Thus, rewarding electrical stimulation appeared to activate the same neural systems that are involved in natural reward and motivation. Finally, only a few years after the original discovery of brain stimulation reward, it was found that drugs that are abused by humans facilitated brain stimulation reward when administered to animals (163). This finding suggested that drugs of abuse influence the same brain reward system that is activated by electrical stimulation or by natural rewards. In fact, the acute enhancement of brain reward mechanisms by abusable drugs is now considered to constitute their single most important property, and provides the basis for the hypothesis that abused substances produce reward by acting at specific neural systems. The remainder of this section reviews evidence concerning the neuroanatomy of brain reward systems derived from two main paradigms: self-administration and electrical brain stimulation reward.

Self-Administration Paradigm

The self-administration procedure generally utilizes the intravenous route of administration, although many others, including oral, intramuscular, and intracerebral routes, have been used. Animals, surgically implanted with chronic indwelling catheters, are placed in operant chambers and are given the opportunity to press a lever that causes delivery of the drug through the catheter. Typically rhesus monkeys and rats are used, although many other species, such as squirrel monkeys, baboons, dogs, cats, pigs, and mice, have also been used successfully (164). Such operant conditioning procedures have demonstrated that abusable drugs have positive reinforcing properties that are very similar to those of natural

rewards, such as food and water. Unlike natural rewards, however, the drugs can also have nonspecific effects on motor activity and, under certain reinforcement schedules, can accumulate in the body to cause changes in responding over time.

The most striking feature of drug self-administration is how closely the classes of drugs that are self-administered by animals correspond with those that are abused by humans. With ratio schedules of operant reinforcement, laboratory animals have been observed to respond for amphetamine (165, 166), cocaine (165), methamphetamine (166), methylphenidate (167), nicotine (168), caffeine (169), opiates (170), ethanol (171), nicotine (164), barbiturates (173), benzodiazepines (174), PCP (175, 176), and THC (172). With interval schedules of reinforcement, responding for cocaine (142), opiates (177), ethanol (178), barbiturates (173, 179, 180), and other abusable substances has been demonstrated. The list of drugs that are self-administered is remarkable because it is comprised of compounds that differ markedly in their chemical structure and in their spectra of pharmacological activity. Perhaps even more significant is the observation that laboratory animals will not self-administer drugs from the myriad of other classes available. Many drugs, including opioid antagonists, neuroleptics, and tricyclic antidepressants, either do not maintain self-administration in animals (181, 182) or stimulate voluntary termination of drug infusion (183, 184). These results suggest that drugs that are self-administered must share some underlying commonalities distinguishing them from the much larger number of drugs that are not self-administered.

Furthermore, drugs that have not been found to support self-administration in animals are, almost without exception, not abused by humans. Lysergic acid diethylamide (LSD) is one of the few exceptions. It is not self-administered by laboratory animals and is, in fact, actively avoided by rhesus monkeys (164, 183). This disparity between animal and human drug self-administration may be partly explained by a peculiarly human urge to seek altered states of consciousness. Nevertheless, the fact that most drugs, other than hallucinogens, that are abused by humans are also self-administered by animals provides general support to the hypothesis that drug self-administration in animals is a reliable predictor of potential abuse liability in humans.

Intravenous drug self-administration behavior in animals is maintained across a wide range of doses (184a). Although specific patterns of intake vary with drug class, generally the rate of drug self-administration is inversely related to the dose or duration of the drug effect. Low to intermediate drug doses result in increases in the rate of responding, but higher doses decrease response rate. It has been a long-standing assertion that this pattern of responding results from attempts by the subject to titrate blood levels of the drug (184b). Thus, according to this hypothesis, when the dose per injection is increased, decline in drug concentration in blood occurs at a slower rate and results in longer inter-injection intervals and decreased rates of responding.

Conversely, when the injection dose is decreased, blood levels of the drug fall more rapidly, shortening inter-injection intervals and increasing rates of responding.

NEURAL SUBSTRATES OF DRUG SELF-ADMINISTRATION REWARD

Systemic Pharmacological Challenge

Pharmacological challenge is one approach that has been used in an attempt to elucidate the neurochemical substrates of drug-induced reward. This technique involves the non-contingent coadministration of an agonist or an antagonist of a particular neurotransmitter and an examination of the effect of this manipulation on drug self-administration responding. The rationale for challenge with an agonist of a particular neurotransmitter is that if the neurotransmitter facilitates reward, the agonist should substitute for the self-administered drug and it should temporarily decrease self-administration of the drug. Conversely, challenge with an antagonist should produce a selective increase in responding to compensate for the reduced effectiveness of the self-administered drug. However, higher doses would further reduce rewarding efficacy of the self-administered drug and would therefore reduce responding.

Examples of such pharmacological challenge paradigms can be drawn from studies of cocaine self-administration. For example, treatment with bromocriptine, a DA receptor agonist, decreased cocaine self-administration in the rat (185). In contrast, pretreatment with low doses of a variety of DA receptor antagonists, including pimozide (186, 187), α-flupenthixol (187, 188), haloperidol (187), perphenazine (189), and chlorpromazine (187), increased the rate of responding by rats for intravenous cocaine. When a high dose of a DA receptor antagonist was given, the rate of responding was reduced, suggesting that the reinforcing effects of cocaine were attenuated (186). In subsequent experiments, SCH 23390 and spiperone, antagonists that are relatively selective for D_1-like and D_2-like DA receptors, respectively, increased the rate of responding for cocaine on a fixed-ratio schedule of reinforcement at doses of up to 10 mg/kg, and reduced the rate at higher doses (190). In the same study, both drugs decreased the highest ratio completed in rats self-administering cocaine on a progressive ratio. These findings suggested that both D_1-like and D_2-like DA receptors contribute to the reinforcing effects of cocaine.

One major problem that is encountered with pharmacological challenges of self-administration relates to the non-specific pharmacological effects of the coadministered drug. Thus, a compound might affect the ability of an animal to press a lever or a bar for drug injection by stimulating or inhibiting motor activity generally, rather than by selectively increasing or reducing the rewarding properties of the self-administered drug. Confounding by such nonspecific effects must be guarded against by ensuring that the dose of the drug that is used to challenge self-administration responding has minimal effects on performance.

Lesion Studies

Another approach has been used to map the neuroanatomical and neurochemical substrates of reward associated with systemic self-administration of various abusable drugs. This method examines the effect of selective lesions of specific neurotransmitter systems on drug responding. Particular neurotransmitter systems can be rendered dysfunctional by surgery (e.g., knife cuts), electrolytic lesions, thermocoagulative lesions, or by treatment with neurotransmitter-specific toxins, such as 6-hydroxydopamine (6-OHDA). Effects of the loss of contribution of a particular neurotransmitter system on drug self-administration can then be investigated.

Lesion studies have provided considerable information about the localization of central sites that are important to drug-induced reward. Such studies have demonstrated that the mesolimbic DA system plays a critical role (Fig. 29.3). The cell bodies of this system originate in the VTA. They project rostrally to the nucleus accumbens and to more anterior regions, including the amygdala, olfactory tubercle, and prefrontal cortex. Selective lesions of the nucleus accumbens, produced by the catecholamine-specific neurotoxin 6-OHDA, disrupt self-administration of cocaine (191–193) and amphetamine (194). Both drugs act presynaptically to augment concentrations of intrasynaptic DA. Similarly, selective 6-OHDA lesions of the VTA disrupt self-administration of cocaine (195, 196). In contrast, self-administration of the direct DA receptor agonist apomorphine, which acts at postsynaptic sites in the mesolimbic DA system, is unaffected by such lesions (191, 195). Furthermore, 6-OHDA lesions of other brain regions have not been found to affect cocaine self-administration (191, 192, 197).

Interpretation of some of the earlier of these findings (191) was complicated because 6-OHDA produces lesions of both DA and NE systems. Later studies employed pretreatment with desmethylimipramine to prevent depletion of NE, however, and found similar reductions in cocaine self-administration (192).

Another concern related to the anatomical specificity of 6-OHDA lesions of the nucleus accumbens because such lesions deplete DA and NE in more anterior structures. This issue was addressed by examining the effect of kainic acid lesion of the nucleus accumbens on cocaine self-administration. Kainic acid selectively destroys cell bodies but preserves the fibers of passage to, in this case, more anterior regions, such as the olfactory tubercle, amygdala, and prefrontal cortex. Placement of kainic acid lesions in the nucleus accumbens significantly reduced responding for cocaine, but did not affect catecholamine levels in more anterior structures (195). Thus, the studies employing kainic acid and those employing 6-OHDA lesions provided compelling evidence that the nucleus accumbens plays a critical role in self-administration of psychomotor stimulants by laboratory mammals.

Lesion studies have also demonstrated that the mesolimbic DA system is critical for the self-administration of other

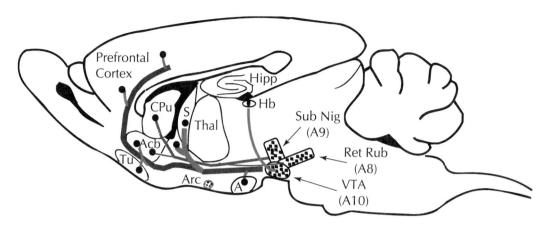

Figure 29.3. Chemical neuroanatomy of (rat) DA systems relevant to drug abuse. Cell bodies of DA-containing neurons are indicated by dotted regions. The mesocorticolimbic dopaminergic pathway (heavy stippling) has been specifically implicated in the rewarding properties of drugs. The mesocorticolimbic DA system consists of projections from dopaminergic neurons found mainly in the VTA (A10) to the nucleus accumbens (Acb), olfactory tubercle (Tu), bed nucleus of the stria terminalis and septum (S), amygdala (A), lateral habenula (Hb), and portions of the prefrontal cortex. The nigrostriatal system (light stippling) consists of dopaminergic neurons in the substantia nigra (A9) that project primarily to the dorsal portions of the caudate and putamen (CPu). DA neurons in the retro-rubral (Ret Rub) region (A8) contributes to both systems. The tuberoinfundibular DA neurons (A12) in the arcuate nucleus (Arc) are of interest because of their regulation of neuroendocrine function, such as inhibition of prolactin release. (Modified from Cooper JR, Bloom FE, Roth RH, eds. The biochemical basis of neuropharmacology. 6th ed. New York: Oxford University Press, 1991.)

classes of abusable drugs. Selective 6-OHDA lesions of this system have been found to disrupt self-administration of heroin and morphine (198–201). Therefore, the mesolimbic DA system appears to comprise a common neuronal substrate that mediates both opioid and psychomotor stimulant reward (202–204).

In addition, the ventral pallidum appears to play a role in mediating reward produced by self-administration of cocaine as well as opioids. This region receives afferent projections from the nucleus accumbens (205). Lesions produced by injections of ibotenic acid—which, like kainic acid, is an axon-sparing excitotoxin—into the ventral pallidum of rats reduce cocaine and heroin self-administration behavior maintained on a fixed-ratio schedule of reinforcement (206). At the same time, they decrease the highest ratio sustained in progressive-ratio procedures. These findings suggest that a circuit involving the nucleus accumbens and ventral pallidum may be a common pathway in stimulant and opioid reward.

Intracranial Self-Administration of Drugs

Challenge of the systemic self-administration of drugs by the coadministration of selective agonists and antagonists for particular receptors, or by production of selective lesions, has considerably advanced our knowledge of the neural bases of reward. Nonetheless, both of these techniques are inherently indirect. A more direct method of exploring the neural systems underlying self-administration reward involves microinjection of abusable substances into the brain itself. The rationale behind this technique is straightforward. If there are discrete brain circuits that mediate drug reward, then animals should self-administer abusable drugs directly into these regions of the brain, and not into other regions that are not involved in reward. In practice, however, many meth-

odological problems are encountered. Some of these are associated with slow infusion rates of drugs and minute injection volumes; both of these conditions are necessary to minimize nonspecific neuronal responses. Furthermore, problems similar to those encountered with systemic self-administration of drugs also arise. Therefore, it is not always possible to conclude that a brain region is not involved in reward simply because it does not support self-administration. It may be that the dose of drug in question is activating competing behaviors that can inhibit responding and mask the reward behavior.

Studies using the intracranial self-administration procedure have shown that animals will voluntarily self-administer microinjections of amphetamine into the nucleus accumbens and the prefrontal cortex (orbitofrontal cortex of the rhesus monkey) (207–209) but not into other brain regions. Cocaine is also voluntarily self-administered into the prefrontal cortex (210). Morphine is self-administered into the VTA (211, 212), lateral hypothalamus (213), and nucleus accumbens (215), all of which are either nuclei or terminal projection regions of the mesolimbic DA system. Other synthetic and endogenous opioids are also self-administered intracranially into the mesolimbic system. Fentanyl is self-administered into the VTA (216), metenkephalin is self-administered into the nucleus accumbens (217), and the metenkephalin analogue D-ala^2-metenkephalinamide is self-administered into the lateral hypothalamus (218).

A variant of the intracranial microinjection procedure has provided further evidence that the mesolimbic DA system plays a critical role in opioid self-administration, although the periaqueductal gray also appears to be involved. In these studies, intravenous self-administration of opioids was challenged with an intracranially administered quaternary opioid antagonist. Microinjection of diallyl-normorphinium bromide into the VTA, but not into other brain regions, produced dose-dependent increases in rates of responding for heroin self-administration (219). In contrast, administration of methylnaloxonium chloride, at a low dose, into the nucleus accumbens increased heroin self-administration, whereas injections into the VTA were not effective (220). These results support a role of the mesolimbic DA system in opioid reward, but they imply that opioid receptors in the VTA are not essential in this regard. The first evidence that opiate receptors in the vicinity of the periaqueductal gray may play a role in intravenous self-administration of opioid drugs derives from the observation that intracranial micro-injections of methylnaltrexone into this brain region produced dose-related increases in responding for heroin, but not for cocaine, by rats on a continuous reinforcement schedule (221). In the same study, microinjections of methylnaltrexone in the nucleus accumbens also increased responding for heroin, confirming the involvement of this DA terminal region in opiate self-administration.

Self-Administration of Direct and Indirect Dopaminergic Agonists

There is now a considerable body of evidence that implicates DA as a critical neurochemical substrate of drug self-administration reward. The most obvious is that the psychomotor stimulants amphetamine and cocaine, indirect DA agonists that prolong the actions of DA in the synaptic cleft, are avidly self-administered by laboratory animals. Further support for the latter feature of this theory is provided by reports that laboratory animals also avidly self-administer direct DA receptor agonists, such as apomorphine and piribedil (222–226), as well as DA reuptake blockers, such as bupropion, mazindol, nomifensine, and GBR 12909 (167, 227–234), which prolong the action of DA in the synaptic cleft.

It has been known for two decades that cocaine blocks the reuptake of DA in the brain (235). Although cocaine also blocks the reuptake of NE and serotonin, the potencies of a series of cocaine analogues in self-administration studies in monkeys were highly correlated with potencies of the same compounds in inhibiting binding to uptake sites for DA but not to NE or 5HT uptake sites (43). This observation indicated that the rewarding properties of cocaine were due to interaction of the drug with the DA transporter.

Self-Administration of Nicotine

In addition to the evidence implicating dopaminergic neurotransmission in the self-administration of direct and indirect dopaminergic agonists, studies of nicotine self-administration provide support for the view that nicotine-induced reward requires intact functioning of the mesolimbic DA system. Rats given D_1- and D_2-selective DA receptor antagonists have reduced self-administration of nicotine (236, 237). In selective lesioning studies, rats subjected to injections of 6-OHDA into the nucleus accumbens show reductions of DA in the nucleus accumbens, the caudate-putamen, and the olfactory tubercle, as compared with levels in sham-injected control rats (238, 239). When lesioned in this manner, rats showed reduced self-administration of nicotine over a 10-day acquisition period in one study (238), and over a 3-week period of testing in a continuous reinforcement schedule in other studies (236, 239).

Neurochemical evidence supports the feasibility of a role for mesolimbic DA in reinforcement due to nicotine. Nicotinic receptors are present in the midbrain area containing the substantia nigra and the VTA (82) and in the terminal fields (nucleus accumbens, olfactory tubercle) of the mesolimbic DA system (104, 240–242). Systemic nicotine increases the firing rate of neurons in the VTA, and intracellular recording from presumed DA-containing cells of the VTA in vitro reveals that nicotine directly depolarizes the neurons (243–245). Likewise, studies on intact rats demonstrate that systemic nicotine stimulates the regional cerebral metabolic rate for glucose (rCMRglc), an index of local brain function, in the VTA (246). Nicotine stimulates DA release from slices of the nucleus accumbens (247) and increases the concentration of extracellular DA in the nucleus accumbens, as measured by in vivo microdialysis (248–250).

Electrical Brain Stimulation Reward Paradigm

Since the seminal discovery by Olds and Milner that laboratory animals will self-administer electrical stimulation to specific brain regions (155), the electrical brain stimulation reward paradigm and relationships between the type of reward it produces and drug and natural rewards have been well researched. The technique of intracranial self-stimulation (ICSS) involves surgically implanting chronic indwelling stimulating electrodes into specific brain nuclei of animals and training the animals to self-administer the rewarding electrical stimulation by pressing a bar or a lever. Generally, animals learn rapidly to press the lever for brain stimulation, with very little prompting, and then they maintain extremely high levels of responding. In fact, the reward derived from the electrical stimulation of certain brain regions can be sufficiently powerful that animals ignore natural rewards or endure pain to receive it.

Human studies of the effects of electrical stimulation of the brain have confirmed that stimulation of certain brain regions can produce intense feelings of euphoria (251). Thus, the reward produced by electrical self-stimulation of the brain is an extremely potent phenomenon that is only matched by that produced by the most avidly self-administered drugs.

Furthermore, a notable common feature of drugs, such as opiates, stimulants, barbiturates, benzodiazepines, PCP, alcohol, and marijuana, which are self-administered systemically by laboratory animals, is that they enhance brain stimulation reward (203, 204, 252–254). In addition, when coadministered, abusable substances from different pharmacological classes have synergistic effects on brain stimulation reward thresholds (255, 256). These findings provide support for the hypothesis that abused drugs activate the same reward system that is activated by electrical stimulation of specific anatomical sites in the brain.

CHARACTERISTICS OF INTRACRANIAL SELF-STIMULATION

A detailed discussion of all of the characteristics of ICSS is beyond the scope of this review (see 254). Nonetheless, it is important to discuss some characteristics that, at first glance, appear to distinguish responding for ICSS from responding for either abusable drugs or natural rewards. In the case of simple operant schedules of reinforcement for abusable drugs or natural rewards, termination of reward elicits a temporary increase in responding. This increase characterizes the frustrative, nonreward response phase that precedes extinction. In the case of conventional ICSS, however, termination of the stimulation results in an almost instantaneous extinction of responding. Furthermore, drugs that are believed to block the rewarding properties of brain stimulation depress the rate of ICSS or lead to extinction of the response. In contrast, as has been noted earlier, the administration of a pharmacological antagonist of a drug generally produces a compensatory increase in self-administration responding.

The apparent differences between the characteristics of ICSS and other types of reward have puzzled investigators and have been taken by some as evidence that the neural substrates underlying these types of reward are dissociable. An alternative hypothesis is that these discrepancies are artifacts that arise from differences between the kinetics of brain stimulation and other types of reward. Thus, even the most rapidly acting drugs, such as heroin or cocaine, have a time course of action that is at least an order of magnitude longer than that of a maximally effective train of brain stimulation. Furthermore, animals respond reliably for drug reward even when the time course of the effect of a single dose lasts for many minutes or even hours (257, 258).

The latter hypothesis has been investigated in an important series of studies in which drug kinetics were modeled with frequency-modulated trains of brain stimulation (259). Under these conditions, animals self-administer brain stimulation in a manner that closely resembles drug self-administration. Termination of stimulation results in a frustrative nonreward increase in lever-pressing followed by a slow decline and ultimate cessation of responding. Similarly, treatment with drugs that block reward produces an increase in responding. This recent work suggests that brain stimulation reward is not as easily distinguishable from pharmacological and natural rewards as it was once believed to be. Further direct support for the hypothesis that ICSS activates, albeit indirectly, the same neural substrates acted upon by abusable drugs and natural rewards is provided by neuroanatomical investigations of brain stimulation reward.

NEUROANATOMICAL AND NEUROCHEMICAL SUBSTRATES

Shortly after his discovery of ICSS, Olds found that brain-stimulation reward is strongly attenuated by drugs that block catecholaminergic transmission (157, 260). He subsequently identified the medial forebrain bundle (MFB) in the region of the lateral hypothalamus as a highly effective locus for ICSS (156). In the mid 1960s, the use of histofluorescence microscopy, then a newly developed technique for mapping neurotransmitter systems, demonstrated that most ICSS-positive sites in the MFB were proximal to the mesotelencephalic DA system. This anatomical correspondence led to investigations of the effects of pharmacological manipulations of dopaminergic neurotransmission on brain stimulation reward. By the end of the 1980s, extensive research suggested that DA is the most important catecholamine involved in reward produced by stimulation of the MFB (261). The main evidence for this conclusion was that low doses of specific DA antagonists mimicked the effect of decreasing the intensity of rewarding brain stimulation, while higher doses eliminated ICSS. Microinjections of DA antagonists into various sites have shown that the relevant site of dopaminergic action for ICSS is the nucleus accumbens (262–266).

There are two major dopaminergic systems in the MFB. They are the nigrostriatal system, which terminates in the caudate-putamen, and the mesolimbic system, which innervates several forebrain regions, including the nucleus accumbens, the olfactory tubercle, the ventral pallidum, and parts of the frontal cortex (see Fig. 29.3) (267). The discovery of dopaminergic pathways in the MFB led many investigators in the 1960s to assume that these must be the paths activated by rewarding MFB stimulation. However, the axons of dopaminergic neurons in the MFB are unmyelinated. Although the stimulation most commonly used at the time was a 60-HZ sine wave current, which is capable of stimulating unmyelinated fibers, it was known that animals would work to receive pulses of stimulation of 0.1 msec or shorter durations, and measurements of refractory period have suggested that such short pulses stimulate mostly myelinated fibers (268–271). More recent studies confirm that the neurophysiological properties of the primary MFB substrate that is directly activated by electrical brain stimulation reward do not match those of the mesotelecephalic DA system (272–274). Instead, rewarding electrical stimulation appears primarily to activate a nondopaminergic, myelinated, caudally projecting fiber system whose neurons have absolute refractory periods of 0.4 to 1.2 msec.

To explain the inconsistency between the physiological properties of dopaminergic neurons and those activated by rewarding stimulation, it was proposed that directly stimulated, non-DA "first-stage" neurons synapse with "second-stage" dopaminergic neurons in the midbrain tegmentum and stimulate ascending DA pathways indirectly (204, 275). The neurochemistry of the "first-stage," myelinated, caudally projecting fiber system remains an open question. There is some evidence that at least some of these neurons may be cholinergic. Cholinergic neurons in the pedunculopontine and laterodorsal tegmental nucleus make synaptic contact with dopaminergic neurons (276–279). The axons with the shortest refractory periods (0.4–0.7 msec) are blocked by peripherally injected atropine (280). However, axons with longer refractory periods (0.7–1.2 msec) are insensitive to this manipulation (281).

Effects of intracranial microinjections of abusable drugs on electrical brain stimulation reward suggest that these substances produce reward by direct actions on a small subset of "second-stage" dopaminergic, unmyelinated axons (261, 282). Studies using this paradigm have demonstrated that neural substrates for the enhancement of brain stimulation reward by amphetamine lie within the nucleus accumbens and neostriatal forebrain terminal projections of mesotelencephalic dopaminergic neurons (283). Similarly, the substrate for the enhancing effect of morphine on brain stimulation reward was localized to cell body regions of the mesotelencephalic DA system, including the posterior hypothalamus, and less consistently, the VTA (284). Finally, microinjection of haloperidol, a DA-receptor antagonist, into the nucleus accumbens and other dopaminergic neostriatal projection sites inhibits brain stimulation reward. This finding provides more general support for the view that the mesotelencephalic DA system plays an essential role in electrical brain stimulation reward (285).

Virtually all substances that are self-administered by animals have the effect of increasing basal neuronal firing and/or basal neurotransmitter release in brain circuits that are relevant to reward. The use of in vivo brain microdialysis and in vivo brain voltammetry have demonstrated that monoamines in general, and the neurotransmitter DA in particular, participate in the neurochemical actions of abused drugs. Enhancement of extracellular mesotelencephalic DA has been reported after administration of amphetamine (286, 287), cocaine (287, 288), opiates (289), ethanol (290), nicotine (248, 250), barbiturates (291), PCP (287, 292), and Δ^9-THC (293, 294). Although benzodiazepines are self-administered as well, neurochemical evidence does not support the view that this class of abused drugs increases the activity of dopaminergic neurons (295–299). This common feature among all drugs that are self-administered by animals provides the basis for the theory that drug self-administration activates the same reward circuits as those activated by electrical brain stimulation reward, and that the mechanisms involve an important dopaminergic component.

Aside from the wealth of information pointing to a major role for DA in reward secondary to the administration of drugs of abuse, pharmacological interventions have demonstrated an involvement of serotonergic systems as well. Treatments that would be expected to enhance serotonergic tone *reduce* self-administration of drugs of abuse. For example, pretreatment with L-tryptophan, a precursor of 5HT (300), or feeding with a diet enriched in tryptophan

(301), attenuated amphetamine self-administration. Administration of fluoxetine, an inhibitor of 5HT uptake (302, 303), or quipazine, a 5HT receptor agonist (300), also reduced amphetamine self-administration in rats. Fluoxetine likewise reduced the self-administration of ethanol (304) and cocaine (305) in rats. Another 5HT uptake inhibitor, zimelidine, reduced morphine intake in dependent rats (306) and reduced ethanol consumption in humans (307). Furthermore, the potencies of amphetamine and related phenethylamines in operant drug self-administration studies were inversely correlated with their potencies in inhibiting [^{3}H]paroxetine binding to the 5HT transporter (308). This finding supported the view that inhibition of 5HT uptake opposes reinforcing effects of amphetamine and related drugs. In addition to these studies of self-administration, a serotonergic role in drug-induced reward also was shown using the conditioned place preference paradigm. In this regard, ICS 205-930 and MDL 72222, specific antagonists of 5HT$_3$ receptors, reduced place preference produced by morphine and nicotine, but not amphetamine, in rats (309). These results indicated an involvement of 5HT$_3$ receptors in the reinforcing properties of morphine and nicotine.

Another system that has been implicated in drug abuse-related reward is glutamatergic transmission involving the NMDA subtype of glutamate receptor. When 2-amino-5-phosphonovaleric acid, an antagonist of the NMDA receptor, was microinfused into the nucleus accumbens of rats trained to lever-press for intravenous cocaine or heroin, the intake of cocaine, but not of heroin was increased (310). Thus, it appeared that blocking glutamatergic transmission at NMDA receptors of the nucleus accumbens reduced the rewarding value of cocaine but not of heroin.

Lastly, a role of Ca^{2+} in the rewarding properties of both morphine and cocaine has been implied by studies in which dihydropyridine Ca^{2+} channel antagonists reduced self-administration of both cocaine and morphine in mice (311). The effects of the Ca^{2+} antagonists may be related to the DA system, as impulse-driven release of DA is dependent upon Ca^{2+}, and removal of Ca^{2+} from the perfusion medium abolishes cocaine-stimulated increases in extracellular DA in the nucleus accumbens (287). Human studies support the view that Ca^{2+} antagonists interfere with positive affective responses that may be related to reward. In this regard, verapamil reduced morphine-elevated scores on the morphine-Benzedrine group subscale of the Addiction Research Center Inventory while potentiating the effect of morphine to elevate pain threshold (312). These results support the view that Ca^{2+} has a differential role in mediating or influencing actions of opioids.

Dopamine in Natural Reward

The view that DA is a mediator of drug-induced reward is consonant with the literature implicating brain DA in the maintenance of positively rewarded behaviors in general. The techniques employed to generate these findings include systemic treatment of animals with DA agonist and antagonist drugs, microinjections into specific brain loci, microdialysis, and selective lesioning of the DA system.

Free-feeding, operant feeding, and stimulation of the perifornical lateral hypothalamus all increase DA turnover in the nucleus accumbens, as measured by microdialysis in rats (313). DA-agonist drugs increase rates of operant responding by rats for food, water, or rewarding brain stimulation, whereas DA-receptor antagonists reduce responding at doses below those that would reduce appetite or general motor activity (314, 315). For example, when the effects of DA receptor antagonists on water-rewarded operant lever-pressing and on nonconditioned water intake were studied in parallel, the drugs were more potent in attenuating lever-pressing than in affecting consummatory water intake (316, 317). Destruction of DA terminals in the nucleus accumbens and olfactory tubercle disrupted schedule-induced drinking (318). In developing rat pups, treatment either with SCH 23390, a D_1-like DA-receptor antagonist, or with raclopride, a D_2-like DA-receptor antagonist, was more potent in reducing intake of sucrose in an independent ingestion test than in a test in which sucrose was continually infused into the mouth in developing rats (319). Therefore, both D_1-like and D_2-like DA receptors appear to be important to sucrose reward.

Studies of conditioned reinforcement also suggest a role of DA, particularly in the nucleus accumbens, in supporting reward. Microinjections of *d*-amphetamine into the nucleus accumbens elicit dose-dependent, selective enhancement of responding for conditioned reinforcement, whereas injections into other striatal regions produce effects that are ineffectual, nonreproducible, or not selective for conditioned reward (320). Additional experiments designed to elucidate the neurochemical specificity of the effect of intra-accumbens *d*-amphetamine on conditioned reinforcement show that DA, but not NE, microinjected into the nucleus accumbens selectively increases responding for conditioned reinforcement, and that injections into the caudate-putamen are ineffective (321).

Neurochemical evidence for the effects of natural rewards on dopaminergic activity has been obtained from postmortem studies of the striata of rats that responded over 30 minutes for water (322), and of the nucleus accumbens and striatum following 1 hour of feeding by food-deprived rats. However, observations that the type of food ingested can influence the response, measured in terms of DA metabolism, argues against an exclusive role of reward or motor processes in determining dopaminergic responses. Using in vivo microdialysis, it was shown that either free-feeding or lever-pressing for food reward produced an increase in extracellular DA followed by an increase in homovanillic acid (HVA, a metabolite of DA) in the nucleus accumbens but not in the ventral striatum (313). A subsequent study, employing linear sweep voltammetry at electrodes implanted intracranially, demonstrated that 30-minute sessions of responding for food reward increased uric acid and then HVA in the caudate-putamen, with a similar effect on HVA

in the nucleus accumbens (323). Thus, it appears that an increase of DA metabolism accompanies food-induced reward.

LONG-TERM EFFECTS OF DRUGS OF ABUSE ON THE CENTRAL NERVOUS SYSTEM

The long-term consequences of chronic drug administration are defining features of drug abuse and addiction. The most prominent and persistent of these effects include alterations in the magnitude of the response to the drug, effects that emerge upon cessation of drug taking, and responses to environmental cues that become associated with drug-taking. Over the past decade, there has been substantial progress in our understanding of the neuronal mechanisms by which drugs act to effect these consequences.

The term "neuroadaptation" is now commonly used to describe the neural mechanisms underlying alteration in magnitude of drug effect, as both decreases (tolerance) and increases (sensitization) in the response can accompany chronic exposure to a drug. The emergence of withdrawal symptoms when the drug is no longer present is thought to reflect the consequences of such enduring neuroadaptations. In addition, a distinction has been made between neuroadaptive mechanisms that occur at receptors, which are the primary sites of drug action (within-system changes), and the secondary consequences that are propagated throughout the target neuronal networks (between-system changes) (324).

Tolerance, or a diminution in the response to a given dose of the drug, is the classic consequence of chronic drug administration. Although the development of tolerance to a particular drug, by definition, requires that higher doses of drug are needed to obtain the same level of effect, the presence of tolerance to a particular drug does not necessarily imply a potential for abuse of the drug. In fact, the ability to produce tolerance is a nearly universal property of all drugs (325). For example, tolerance develops rapidly to antihistamines, yet these agents are not commonly considered to be drugs of abuse. Furthermore, tolerance is not a unitary phenomenon. The mechanisms underlying tolerance are varied, and tolerance can develop differentially to various actions of a drug (326). For example, individuals who use opioid drugs and are highly tolerant to respiratory depressant actions still manifest opioid-induced miosis and experience constipation (327).

Classical pharmacology attributed tolerance to altered availability of a drug at the relevant receptor site (bioavailability) or to changes in the receptor (328). Altered bioavailability constitutes the simplest mechanism of neuroadaptation. In this case, tolerance can result from reduced absorption, increased metabolism or excretion, or impaired distribution of the drug (e.g., through reduced blood flow). With chronic use of some drugs of abuse, these mechanisms contribute appreciably to the development of tolerance. The induction of hepatic microsomal enzymes by alcohol and barbiturates provides a prototypical example of metabolic tolerance (327). Nonetheless, altered bioavailability is not a primary reason for tolerance to most drugs of abuse.

Repeated exposure to a drug can also lead to an increase in the response to the drug. This phenomenon is termed "sensitization" or "reverse tolerance." Sensitization has been increasingly emphasized in neurobiological hypotheses of addiction, and it is thought to contribute to the escalation of drug-taking or relapse after a period of abstinence (148, 329, 330). For example, locomotor activity tends to increase with repeated administration of psychomotor stimulants or opioids. The neurobiological substrates of sensitization are not characterized as well as those of tolerance, and may involve complex interactions between multiple neuronal systems (330, 331). There is evidence in rodents that increased bioavailability contributes to enhancement of the locomotor effects of cocaine (331a, 331b).

Long-term changes in the specific receptors that are the targets of the drugs of abuse have proven to be complex. Both up- and down-regulation of receptor function accompanying chronic drug exposure have been documented. In addition to changes at the ligand-binding site, alterations can also occur along signal transduction pathways. (In fact, at the cellular level, adaptation to a particular drug may depend on the signal transduction mechanism used by the receptor to which the drug binds.) Tolerance to drugs that act on receptors linked to second messengers (e.g., opioids and stimulants) appears to involve modulation of signal transduction mechanisms, with little or no change in ligand-binding affinity or receptor density. On the other hand, tolerance to drugs, such as nicotine and sedative-hypnotics, which act on ionotropic receptors, appears to involve a paradoxical increase in ligand binding associated with functional desensitization of the relevant receptor. Some common mechanisms may contribute to tolerance produced by drugs of abuse that belong to different chemical classes. Evidence for this view derives from observations of cross-tolerance (i.e., the phenomenon observed when one drug induces tolerance to another one). Such cross-tolerance has been observed, for example, between nicotine and ethanol (332, 333).

The presence of a withdrawal syndrome was long considered to be the defining feature of addiction (327). It is currently thought that the cellular mechanisms underlying tolerance and withdrawal are often related. The specific features of a given withdrawal syndrome are often expressions of a rebound from the homeostatic adaptations associated with the development of tolerance. The cellular mechanisms underlying withdrawal symptoms induced by opioids are best understood, and less is known about the basis of withdrawal from psychostimulants and sedative-hypnotics.

Opioids

Over the past two decades, substantial progress has been made in resolving the cellular mechanisms underlying opioid tolerance and dependence. It is now believed that adapta-

tions involving changes in signal transduction pathways, rather than in the binding sites of receptors, mediate tolerance and dependence (334). As proof for this hypothesis, no consistent relation has been found between physical dependence and the number or affinity of opioid binding sites or the level of endogenous opioids in the brain (335). Nonetheless, tolerance and dependence may rely on specific opioid receptors or subtypes (336). It has been proposed that subtypes of μ receptors make independent contributions to analgesic tolerance and physical dependence. Administration of naloxonazine, an antagonist at the μ_1-receptor subtype, concurrently with morphine, prevents the development of analgesic tolerance, but not the expression of withdrawal signs (337). This finding implies that analgesic tolerance is caused by changes in μ_1-receptors, whereas physical withdrawal involves another type of μ receptor. However, CXBK mice, which are deficient in μ_1 receptors, exhibit a less severe withdrawal syndrome than C57BL/6 mice, suggesting that μ_1 receptors make a partial contribution to the expression of opioid withdrawal (338). Finally, cellular changes occurring in a specific neuronal system may be responsible for adaptations to only one aspect of opioid action. For example, local injection of morphine into the VTA supports self-administration of morphine, but does not lead to the development of physical dependence (339).

TOLERANCE

Cellular adaptive changes to chronic opioid administration have been best characterized in the signal transduction pathways activated by μ receptors on noradrenergic neurons in the locus ceruleus (LC). The effects of opioids on these neurons have been studied intensively because of their critical contribution to the expression of opioid withdrawal symptoms (66, 334, 340–342). Most of the noradrenergic cell bodies in the brain are found in the LC, a nucleus adjacent to the floor of the fourth ventricle at the pontine-medullary junction (343, 344). Both μ and κ receptors are found in this nucleus. The somata of LC neurons contain μ opioid receptors (78, 328), and these receptors are thought to mediate the direct effects of opiates on LC neurons (78, 328). In contrast, κ receptors are probably located on the presynaptic terminals, since κ agonists attenuate excitatory input without altering spontaneous firing rates (345, 346).

Acute administration of morphine or selective μ-opioid agonists produces dose-dependent decreases in the spontaneous activity of LC neurons (340, 342, 347–351). These decreases are blocked by specific μ antagonists, such as β-chlornaltrexamine and β-funaltrexamine, as well as by prototypical opiate antagonists, such as naloxone and naltrexone (342, 351, 352). Intracellular studies indicate that the decrease in impulse activity is accompanied by a hyperpolarization generated by an increased outward K^+ conductance and a decreased slow inward cation current (66, 340, 342, 351, 353). Opiate receptors are coupled to both

Figure 29.4. Sequence of cellular events underlying development of tolerance to opiates in (LC) neurons. **A.** Upon acute administration, opiates decrease the spontaneous firing rate of LC neurons through activation of G proteins associated with the μ-opioid receptor. One G protein (G_i) decreases cAMP synthesis, and the fall in cAMP levels results in a closing of nonspecific cation channels, which contribute to the pacemaker potentials that regulate spontaneous firing. Another G protein (G_o) directly opens K^+ ion channels, and this action hyperpolarizes the cell. Decreased cAMP synthesis impacts upon other biochemical processes, including DNA transcription, which is reduced. **B.** After chronic administration of opiates, the G proteins are desensitized, leading to a decrease in K^+ conductance, but a net up-regulation of the cAMP synthesis and inward cation current. Other proteins dependent on cAMP phosphorylation are also up-regulated, as is expression of immediate early genes (e.g., c-fos). When the tonic opioid levels drop, as during abstinence or antagonist-precipitated withdrawal, these adaptive changes leave the neuron in a state of increased excitability. This state is responsible for the hyperactivity seen in these neurons during withdrawal. Clonidine can normalize firing, as the α_2 receptor is coupled to the same set of G proteins as the μ-opioid receptor. See text for details. (Modified from Nestler EJ. Molecular mechanisms of drug addiction. J Neurosci 1992;12:2439–2450.)

ACUTE OPIATE ACTION IN THE LC

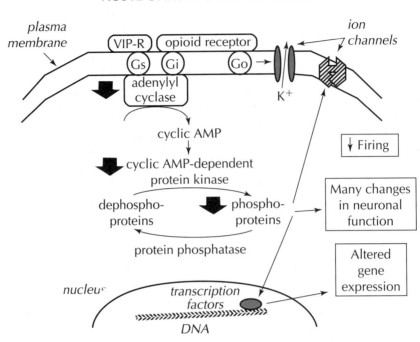

CHRONIC OPIATE ACTION IN THE LC

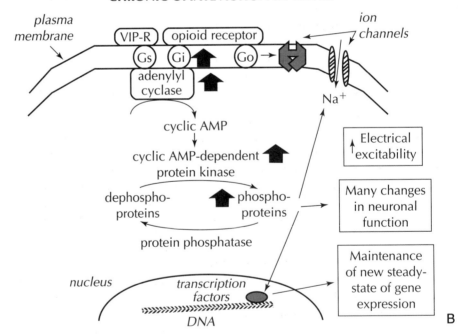

conductances through G proteins that inhibit the synthesis of cyclic adenosine monophosphate (cAMP) (Fig. 29.4*A*) (66, 340, 353–356).

Neurons in the LC develop tolerance to opioids in rats chronically treated with morphine. After 3–5 days of chronic treatment, spontaneous firing rates of LC neurons are no longer suppressed and are equivalent to those in drug-naive animals (351, 352, 354). Larger doses of opiates are then required to suppress firing (351, 352). This tolerance appears to result from the uncoupling of opiate binding sites

from their associated signal transduction pathways (334, 356, 357) (Fig. 29.4*B*). "Uncoupling" compensates for continued occupation of the opiate receptors. In support of this hypothesis, chronic opiate treatment inactivates G_i-proteins through ribosylation of adenosine diphosphate (ADP), which produces a net up-regulation of cAMP synthesis and restores protein kinase A activity to pre-drug levels (356, 358, 359). As predicted from earlier studies of whole brain (360, 361), cAMP levels in the LC increase above pre-drug levels during precipitated withdrawal (362).

The inactivation of the G proteins during chronic opiate treatment probably reflects changes in gene regulation. Acute administration of opiates decreases the expression of the immediate early genes, c-fos and c-jun. Conversely, expression of these genes increases several-fold during naltrexone-induced withdrawal (334). Because the time course for gene regulation is much longer than the decrease in spontaneous activity of the cell in response to acute opiates, decreased expression of these immediate early genes may play a role in adaptation of the cells to chronic treatment.

In addition to opioids themselves, other endogenous substances modulate tolerance to the chronic effects of morphine. The NMDA receptor, and the novel neuronal messenger, nitric oxide (NO), have both been implicated in the development of tolerance. Coadministration of either an NMDA-receptor antagonist (363) or an inhibitor of NO synthetase (364) blocks the development of analgesic tolerance to morphine. Preliminary studies have also found that inhibition of NO synthesis blocks the development of tolerance to morphine at the cellular level (365). When rats were given an inhibitor of NO synthase during chronic morphine treatment, LC neurons in brain slices of morphine-dependent animals were as sensitive to challenge doses of either morphine or the μ-specific agonist DAMGO as neurons from animals who had never received morphine. The direct effects of opioids on LC neurons are mediated exclusively through μ receptors; thus, cellular effects are consistent with the ability of NO synthesis inhibitors to block tolerance to μ and not to κ-receptor agonists (366). The molecular bases of these modulatory effects are not known. It has been proposed that the modulatory actions of NMDA receptors and NO may be causally linked because NMDA cytotoxicity apparently depends on synthesis of NO (367). NO may be critical to the ribosylation of G proteins, a process that has been proposed as the molecular mechanism of tolerance for μ receptors (see previous discussion). This hypothesis is supported by a recent study showing that NO promotes ADP ribosylation (368).

PHYSICAL WITHDRAWAL

The classic hallmark of addiction to opioid drugs is the emergence of a well-defined cluster of physiological signs and symptoms, the "physical" withdrawal syndrome, upon the discontinuation of opioid drug use. The appearance of this syndrome indicates that the organism depends on the presence of the opioid for normal physiological functioning. The severity of the syndrome is dependent on the dosage and duration of use. When the withdrawal syndrome is precipitated by administration of an opioid antagonist, it has a more rapid onset and is more severe than the syndrome produced by "spontaneous" withdrawal. Otherwise spontaneous and precipitated withdrawal are qualitatively similar, and it is commonly acknowledged that they involve identical neural mechanisms (369).

The opioid withdrawal syndrome is quite similar across species, although the exact time course and specific constellation of signs and symptoms are different. The general characteristics of the physical withdrawal syndrome resemble those of influenza, and they are similar in humans and animals (141, 327, 370, 371). Behavioral and physiological signs include pronounced secretory activity (lacrimation, rhinorrhea, sweating), piloerection (goose pimples), mastication (teeth chattering and chewing), elevated heart rate, blood pressure, respiratory rate, and body temperature, irritability, tremors and "wet dog shakes," and gastrointestinal disturbances (intestinal spasms, nausea, and diarrhea). Subjective symptoms in humans include agitation and anxiety, dysphoria, drug craving, aches in joints and muscles, loss of appetite, and insomnia. In humans, the symptoms begin to appear 8–12 hours after the last dose of an opioid agonist, depending on the pharmacokinetics of the individual drug (327). The syndrome reaches a peak over the next 48–72 hours, and is virtually absent by 7–10 days. In rodents, the time course is more rapid (370). Also, opioid withdrawal in rodents includes increased locomotor activity, escape behavior (digging, jumping), and ptosis.

With the development of selective antagonists, it has become possible to assess the differential contribution made by specific opioid receptor subtypes to physical dependence. Because morphine and other commonly abused opioids are primarily μ agonists, it is not suprising that physical dependence appears to be primarily mediated by μ-opioid receptors (372), as are the reinforcing effects of heroin (373). Substantially higher doses of κ and δ antagonists are required to elicit even a mild withdrawal syndrome compared with doses of selective μ antagonists (372).

Although many brain areas, including thalamic, hypothalamic, limbic, and hindbrain areas, are activated during the physical withdrawal from opiates (374), it is now generally acknowledged that hyperactivity of noradrenergic innervations in the CNS contributes substantially to the expression of many of the physical symptoms seen during opiate withdrawal (341, 375). This hypothesis is based on both preclinical animal research and clinical treatment research.

The most compelling evidence for a noradrenergic role in opiate withdrawal is that pharmacological suppression of noradrenergic activity attenuates morphine withdrawal in both animals and humans (341, 376–378). Systemic and local (intracerebral) administration of clonidine, a specific α_2 adrenergic receptor agonist that decreases the spontaneous activity of LC neurons, attenuate both the increase in LC firing due to withdrawal (340, 348) and most of the accompanying physiological signs (377–380).

LC neurons actually become hyperactive during antagonist precipitated withdrawal, as evidenced by increased impulse activity, transmitter release, and metabolite levels (380–385). The hyperactivity is correlated with the intensity of the physical signs (340, 348, 382, 386). Behaviorally, the effects of electrical or pharmacological stimulation of the LC, the major source of noradrenergic innervation in the CNS, resemble opiate withdrawal (387). Opiate withdrawal can be induced by local injections of naloxone (380) or of methylnaloxium, a quaternary derivative of naloxone that has more limited diffusion, directly into the LC (388). In fact, a pattern of widely distributed increases in rCMRglc, similar to that observed after systemic injection of naloxone in morphine-dependent rats (374), is obtained by intracerebral injections of methylnaloxonium directly into the LC (Kimes et al., submitted). Finally, lesions of the LC greatly attenuate the withdrawal behaviors precipitated by intraventricular injection of opiate antagonists (389).

The hyperactivity associated with withdrawal is generated by a rebound of the mechanisms that underlie the development of tolerance (Fig. 29.4*B*). Following cessation of chronic opiate administration (abstinence) or blockade of opiate receptors by naloxone (precipitated withdrawal), cAMP levels rise as the down-regulated G_i proteins cease to inhibit up-regulated adenylate cyclase (360–362). Since cAMP normally inactivates an outward K^+ channel and activates an inward cation conductance, the rise in cAMP levels during withdrawal produces a net depolarization of the neuron and a profound increase in firing rates (352, 354, 357). These cellular mechanisms account for the ability of cAMP and pharmacological agents that elevate cAMP to increase the spontaneous firing rate of LC neurons, and to mimic the behavioral signs of opiate withdrawal (quasi-morphine withdrawal syndrome) (357, 360, 381, 385, 386, 390).

Withdrawal hyperactivity probably involves altered afferent input as well as intrinsic changes in LC neurons. Intraventricular administration of the nonselective glutamate antagonist kynurenic acid blocks the withdrawal-induced activation of LC neurons (391), and systemic administration of antagonists for either NMDA or non-NMDA glutamate receptors attenuates withdrawal behaviors (363, 392). Increased release of glutamate and aspartate adds excitatory drive to LC neurons during withdrawal (393), but opioids do not change the sensitivity of excitatory amino acid receptors on LC neurons (385, 394). Since the nucleus paragigantocellularis (Pgi) in the ventrolateral medulla is the most prominent source of excitatory input to the LC, hyperactivity of these neurons during opioid withdrawal could be the source of increased excitatory drive (395). Lesions of the Pgi attenuate, but do not completely abolish, the increase in basal firing rates after induced withdrawal (391). It is not known whether neurons in the Pgi become hyperactive during opioid withdrawal. Chronic morphine treatment does produce changes in the levels of cAMP in the Pgi (334), but unlike the LC and other regions, the Pgi does not show an increase in c-fos expression, indicative of cellular activation during opioid withdrawal, (396). This discrepancy suggests that increased neuronal activity in other regions, such as the prefrontal cortex, which provide excitatory amino acid input to the LC, may contribute to withdrawal-induced hyperactivity in the LC (396).

There have been observations that coadministration of MK-801, a noncompetitive NMDA receptor antagonist, or of 5,7-dichlorokynurenic acid, an antagonist at the glycine coagonist site of the NMDA receptor, during chronic morphine treatment attenuated a behavioral sign (jumping) of precipitated withdrawal. These findings suggest that NMDA receptor activation is involved in the development of opiate dependence (363, 392). Acute administration of either a competitive or noncompetitive NMDA receptor antagonist immediately prior to precipitating withdrawal also attenuated withdrawal behaviors, but was less effective than subchronic treatment (363, 397). However, the attenuation of withdrawal behaviors after acute administration of noncompetitive NMDA antagonists may be the result of nonspecific motoric effects of these drugs (363, 398). This interpretation is consistent with the inability of acute administration of either competitive and noncompetitive NMDA antagonists to block the withdrawal-associated hyperactivity of LC neurons (397), even though LC neurons do contain NMDA receptors (399, 400). Alternatively, it is possible that the relevant NMDA receptors are located on neurons in regions that receive primary or secondary projections from the LC.

Recently, inhibition of NO synthesis was shown to attenuate the behavioral signs of opioid withdrawal (18, 401–403). This observation reflects the evidence reviewed previously proposing a critical role for NO in the development of morphine tolerance at both the behavioral and cellular level. At this time, it is not known whether inhibition of NO prevents LC hyperactivity during opioid withdrawal, or if the actions of NO are mediated at some other brain site. Furthermore, the dense collection of NO synthase-containing neurons in the laterodorsal tegmental (LDT) nucleus, immediately adjacent to the LC is a likely source of NO that might diffuse to act in the LC (404). If the LDT is the source of NO input to the LC, a cholinergic involvement in opioid withdrawal would be implicated because all NO synthase-containing neurons in the LDT are cholinergic (404, 405). This view would support previous studies implicating the ascending brainstem cholinergic systems in opioid withdrawal (406, 407).

AFFECTIVE ASPECTS OF WITHDRAWAL

Opioid withdrawal also has an affective component that represents a rebound from reinforcing effects of opioids, much as classic physical withdrawal signs represent the converse of acute physiological effects of opioids (e.g., diarrhea as the opposite of constipation) (331). Dysphoria is a prominent part of opioid withdrawal in human subjects (377, 408). Opioid withdrawal interferes with motivational states, as seen by reductions in the performance of operant schedules for food reward (409). Opioid withdrawal also acts as a negative unconditioned stimulus in conditioning paradigms. Presentation of a normally preferred tastant solution (e.g., saccharine) during induction of opioid withdrawal results in taste aversion conditioning (i.e., persistent avoidance of the tastant upon later presentations) (410). The place-conditioning paradigm has also been used to demonstrate that opioid withdrawal induces a negative affective state (411). Place conditioning consists of repeatedly administering of a drug in a distinctive physical environment. If the subjects then chooses to spend more time in that environment, it is taken as an index of the reinforcing properties of a drug. The finding that subjects will avoid an environment where they have undergone opioid withdrawal (place aversion) indicates that the environment was associated with an unpleasant experience.

Although it is possible that these changes in motivated behaviors are generated by peripheral mechanisms (e.g., gastrointestinal disturbance), they appear to be separate from the physiological malaise associated with classic physical withdrawal. Much lower doses of naloxone are required to affect motivated behaviors than to cause expression of classic withdrawal signs (412). Place aversion associated with opioid withdrawal can be produced by intraventricular administration but not by subcutaneous administration of methylnaloxonium (411). Because methylnaloxonium does not readily cross the blood-brain barrier, the results indicate that affective components of withdrawal are generated by central mechanisms and are not due to peripherally mediated physiological malaise.

The nucleus accumbens appears to play a critical role in the affective components of withdrawal, complementary to its role in opioid reinforcement. Local injection of methylnaloxonium disrupts performance on operant schedules for food reward and produces place-aversion conditioning (154, 413). In contrast to local injections of methylnaloxonium into the locus ceruleus, the affective withdrawal signs induced by nucleus accumbens injections are not accompanied by expression of physical signs of withdrawal (154). Furthermore, clonidine is less effective in alleviating dysphoria than other signs in humans during opioid withdrawal (377).

The cellular substrate of opioid withdrawal in the nucleus accumbens is not as well characterized as in the LC, but may involve similar mechanisms (334). Chronic morphine produces a desensitization of G proteins and an increase in adenylate cyclase activity in the nucleus accumbens, similar to that seen in the LC (414). Brain regions other than the nucleus accumbens do not manifest these changes. The mechanism of opioid action in the nucleus accumbens is more complex than in the LC. In contrast to the situation in the LC, where opioids act primarily through postsynaptic μ receptors, presynaptic μ and δ receptors located on cortical afferents are primarily responsible for the electrophysiological effects of opioids within the nucleus accumbens (372). Opioid-induced changes in other transmitter systems, especially in dopaminergic afferents, also influence activity of nucleus accumbens neurons (415, 416). For example, there are reports indicating that whereas DA release in the nucleus accumbens decreases (384, 417, 418), acetylcholine release increases during opioid withdrawal.

In conclusion, expression of opioid withdrawal is not a unitary phenomenon. There are at least two distinct components, each mediated through distinct neural systems. Classic physical withdrawal signs involve a μ receptor-

mediated hyperactivity of brain noradrenergic neurons. In contrast, affective and motivational aspects of opioid withdrawal are probably mediated by the same mesolimbic system regions involved in opioid reinforcement (e.g., nucleus accumbens).

Sedative-Hypnotics

TOLERANCE

Continued use of sedative-hypnotic drugs (e.g., benzodiazepines, barbiturates, ethanol, aldehydes) produces tolerance to their sedative, anti-convulsant and anxiolytic effects (420–422). However, tolerance develops differentially to each of these effects. Tolerance to the sedative and anticonvulsive effects develops within days. Whether tolerance occurs to the anxiolytic effects is still unclear. Tolerance to the anxiolytic effects have been difficult to demonstrate, especially in the clinical setting except under specific experimental conditions (420, 423). This finding suggests that different neuronal mechanisms could be responsible for tolerance to these individual effects. The discovery of various specific binding sites associated with GABA receptors suggests that the primary consequence of chronic administration of sedative-hypnotic drugs, such as benzodiazepines and barbiturates (which bind to these sites), involves alterations in the GABA-benzodiazepine-ionophore receptor complex. These changes are best understood with respect to the benzodiazepine family.

After repeated administration, benzodiazepines produce less potentiation of the electrophysiological inhibition by GABA of cerebellar Purkinje cells (424) and of serotonergic neurons in the dorsal raphe (425, 426). The diminution in effect does not appear to reflect changes in benzodiazepine receptors. Decreases in the number of benzodiazepine binding sites—but not their affinity—after chronic benzodiazepine treatment were found by some investigators (427–430), but others observed little or no changes in benzodiazepine binding (425, 431, 432). These discrepancies may result from differences in the specific drug administered (e.g. diazepam, lorazepam, alprazolam, or flurazepam), in routes of administration (oral vs. injected), or in dose levels.

Chronic administration of benzodiazepines does not alter responses to benzodiazepines per se, but induces a reduction in the actions of GABA. This view is based on observations that both GABA-potentiated benzodiazepine binding (425) and electrophysiological responses to direct application to GABA alone are diminished after chronic benzodiazepine treatment (426, 433). These changes occur whether drugs are injected intermittently (425) or delivered continuously (426). The decreased electrophysiological response to GABA is associated with decreases GABA-stimulated Cl^- flux (434), even though chronic benzodiazepine treatment does not decrease the number of GABA receptor-linked Cl^- channels (435). Consistent with the development of GABA subsensitivity, the threshold for seizures induced by bicuculline, a convulsant that binds to the GABA$_A$ receptor complex, was reduced during chronic benzodiazepine treatment (436).

These alterations in GABA sensitivity, however, are not seen in all neurons responsive to benzodiazepines. Neurons in the substantia nigra pars reticulata, which also use GABA as a transmitter, exhibit tolerance to benzodiazepine administration but no changes in GABA sensitivity (437–439), and cerebellar Purkinje cells do not exhibit decreases in GABA-stimulated Cl$^-$ influx (434).

The development of GABA-ergic subsensitivity may be due to changes in the molecular composition of the GABA-benzodiazepine-ionophore complex. Although chronic benzodiazepine treatment fails to alter the total number of GABA binding sites or the high-affinity component of GABA binding, the affinity for GABA increases at low-affinity GABA binding sites (440). This change may involve alterations in the protein structure of the receptor complex. Chronic, but not acute, administration of benzodiazepines decreases the expression of mRNA that codes for the α_1 subunit of the GABA receptor complex (441). Changes in the protein structure of the receptor complex are consistent with the time-dependent nature of the changes in GABA sensitivity (436). GABA subsensitivity does not start to develop until after a week of chronic treatment, but it persists for at least 5 days after discontinuation of drug administration.

Based on this combination of electrophysiological and biochemical data, some researchers have argued that subsensitivity to GABA underlies tolerance to benzodiazepines. In turn, this subsensitivity is due to conversion of low-affinity GABA binding sites to a desensitized state that exhibits higher affinity (442). Since nicotinic receptors also exhibit a paradoxical increase in binding coupled to a functional desensitization, this pattern may represent a general neuroadaptive mechanism underlying tolerance in the superfamily of ionotropic receptors.

Tolerance to other sedative-hypnotic drugs may also involve changes to the GABA-benzodiazepine receptor complex. This mechanism is most likely the basis of cross-tolerance between these drug classes (443, 444). It has been suggested that chronic ethanol and barbiturate administration reduces the coupling between the Cl$^-$ channel and the GABA and benzodiazepine binding sites. In this regard, barbiturates and ethanol open the Cl$^-$ ionophore of the GABA$_A$ receptor directly (445–447). Similar to treatment with benzodiazepines, chronic administration of barbiturates or ethanol induces a functional subsensitivity of the receptor complex by reducing GABA- or benzodiazepine-stimulated Cl$^-$ influx (431, 447, 448). Unlike benzodiazepines, however, chronic ethanol increases the number of ionophore binding sites (measured using t-butylbicyclophosphorothionate as the ligand) (448). A study in which mice were made tolerant to ethanol showed that chronic ethanol decreases the ability of a benzodiazepine agonist (flunitrazepam) to potentiate Cl$^-$ influx induced by the GABA agonist muscimol, but did not cause [^{3}H]SR, 95531

(2- (3'-carbethoxy-2'propyl) -3-amino-6-p-methoxyphenyl-pyridazinium bromide) binding to low-affinity GABA$_A$ receptors (449). These results suggest that chronic ethanol treatment reduces the coupling between the benzodiazepine agonist site and the Cl$^-$ channel of the GABA$_A$ receptor. This phenomenon may be related to the development of tolerance to or dependence to ethanol.

Tolerance to ethanol also involves direct changes in the function of the NMDA receptor (450). Acutely, ethanol decreases NMDA receptor function (445, 451), probably through an action within the ion channel (451, 452). There is evidence that ethanol modulates a specific molecular subtype of the NMDA receptor that is located in the hippocampus, but not in the septum (453). Chronic exposure to ethanol produces up-regulation of NMDA receptors, in contrast to the subsensitivity ethanol induces in the GABA receptors (445, 454). Enhanced NMDA receptor function may mediate cell death that can occur during chronic ethanol use (450, 455). Changes in NMDA receptors during chronic ethanol treatment may also be involved in conditioned drug effects (456).

DEPENDENCE AND WITHDRAWAL

It is now well-accepted that withdrawal syndromes can be produced by abrupt cessation of treatment with any anxiolytic/sedative drug (420–422, 457, 458). Drugs in this class produce withdrawal syndromes that are qualitatively similar, but not identical (459). Because characterization of the benzodiazepine withdrawal syndrome has led to recognition of common cellular substrates underlying withdrawal from this diverse class of drugs, (457, 458, 458a) the following section focuses on benzodiazepine withdrawal as prototypical of the response to abstinence from chronic treatment with sedative-hypnotics.

Behaviorally, the predominant symptoms are the converse of the primary effects of the sedative-hypnotics. They include anxiety, increased locomotor activity, insomnia, tremors, and convulsions (460–467). As with opioid withdrawal, the severity of the syndrome is dependent on the dose, duration of use, and especially the rate of elimination of the drug (458, 463, 468–470).

Recognition of a benzodiazepine withdrawal syndrome was hampered by its relatively slow temporal development. For nearly 20 years after the clinical introduction of the benzodiazepines, the existence of a benzodiazepine withdrawal syndrome was questioned, even though withdrawal from other anxiolytic/sedative drugs (e.g., barbiturates and ethanol) was well-known (420, 421, 458, 471, 472). Barbiturate and ethanol withdrawal symptoms appear soon after discontinuation of drug use, even after short-term use of moderate doses (459, 460, 466). Benzodiazepine withdrawal symptoms can take several days or weeks to emerge, although faster onsets have been noted after very long durations of use (464, 473). This delayed development of symptoms has been attributed to the slow decline in plasma levels of most benzodiazepines in humans, even when drug administration is abruptly discontinued (457, 474). Thus, the full severity of benzodiazepine withdrawal was not seen until specific antagonists that could displace benzodiazepines from their receptors were developed (461, 462, 468, 470, 475, 476). Similarly, the introduction and widespread use of shorter-acting benzodiazepines (e.g., lorazepam and triazolam) with more rapid elimination rates accelerated the acceptance of the concept of a benzodiazepine withdrawal syndrome (457, 458).

The neurobiological substrates of anxiolytic/sedative withdrawal are not as well established as those that mediate opioid withdrawal, but development of a persistent subsensitivity to GABA appears to be the most proximal factor. Again, chronic exposure to anxiolytic/sedative drugs has the common effect of decreasing the sensitivity of receptors to GABA. Thus, during chronic administration the normally potentiating effects of benzodiazepines or barbiturates on the action of GABA are offset by the attenuated response to the transmitter itself; however, the subsensitivity persists for days after benzodiazepines are no longer present in the brain (436, 477). Since GABA is the primary inhibitory transmitter in the CNS, the net GABA-ergic subsensitivity increases general excitability of the nervous system. This postulated release from inhibition is consistent with the appearance of anxiety, seizures, and other behavioral signs of CNS hyperexcitability associated with withdrawal from anxiolytic/sedative drugs.

Withdrawal from ethanol also involves increased NMDA receptor function, in addition to changes in GABA-ergic function (445). Upon discontinuation of ethanol treatment, up-regulated NMDA receptors exacerbate the overall neural hyperexcitability, including the seizure activity associated with ethanol withdrawal (448, 454). Stimulation of NMDA receptors also mediates the increase in c-fos expression that accompanies ethanol withdrawal (478).

Although anxiolytic/sedative withdrawal could reflect a global increase in excitability throughout the neuroaxis, individual behavioral signs probably reflect hyperactivity in specific brain systems. A variety of cortical and subcortical sites exhibit significant alterations in glucose metabolism during mild diazepam withdrawal (479, 480). Interestingly, the pattern of glucose utilization was not entirely consistent with the known distribution of benzodiazepine receptors, suggesting that some regions were activated transsynaptically (480, 481). In some cases, reasonable connections between specific withdrawal signs and individual brain structures can be made. It is widely accepted that decreased GABA-ergic function in the hippocampus and cerebral cortical regions leads to seizures (35, 482). Likewise, the amygdala is thought to be critically involved in fear and anxiety has high concentrations of benzodiazepine receptors and putative benzodiazepine-like peptides (127, 481). On the other hand, dysfunction in any number of the myriad regions implicated in sleep and arousal may contribute to the insomnia associated with anxiolytic/sedative withdrawal (483, 484).

Hyperactivity of the central noradrenergic system may also contribute to the anxiolytic/sedative abstinence syndrome, although evidence for noradrenergic involvement is less well established in this situation than it is for opioid withdrawal. The potential involvement of noradrenergic systems in withdrawal from opiates and anxiolytic/sedative drugs may explain the commonalities between the two withdrawal syndromes. These include gastrointestinal distress (decreased food intake, retching, and vomiting), weight loss, wet dog shakes, increased startle responses, vocalizations, and piloerection (370, 461, 463, 465, 469, 476). Both antagonist-precipitated withdrawal from diazepam in primates (476) and discontinuation of chronic use of diazepam by humans (485) increase the concentrations of NE metabolites in the brain. Furthermore, activation of the noradrenergic system by yohimbine exacerbates benzodiazepine withdrawal (486). There also is evidence for noradrenergic hyperactivity during withdrawal from barbiturates and alcohol (487). Firing rates of LC neurons increased during ethanol withdrawal, and this hyperactivity is mediated through up-regulated NMDA receptors (488). These changes may not be simply correlative, as lesions of the noradrenergic system diminish the effects of benzodiazepine withdrawal on the firing rate of neurons in the cerebellum (442).

A noradrenergic role in sedative-hypnotic withdrawal was predicted from the hypothesis that hyperactivity of brain noradrenergic systems contributes to anxiety states, especially panic in humans (489). Acute administration of diazepam decreases the firing rate of noradrenergic neurons in the LC of rats (490, 491), attenuates the behavioral effects of LC stimulation in primates (489, 492), and decreases the concentrations of noradrenergic metabolites in human subjects (493). Alcohol and barbiturates also decrease central noradrenergic activity (421, 494, 495), and lesions of noradrenergic neurons decrease tolerance to barbiturates (496, 497). Conversely, inverse agonists at the benzodiazepine receptor increase firing rates of LC neurons (498) and mimic the behavioral effects of LC stimulation (383, 489, 499).

If hyperactivity of the noradrenergic system is involved in withdrawal from anxiolytic/sedative drugs, treatment that reduces noradrenergic activity should attenuate this withdrawal syndrome as it does the opioid abstinence syndrome. A preliminary clinical study demonstrated that clonidine decreased the severity of withdrawal from alcohol (500) and the time required for tapered withdrawal from alprazolam (501). Furthermore, consistent with the known anticonvulsant actions of clonidine (502), preliminary studies in monkeys indicated that clonidine attenuated seizures associated with benzodiazepine withdrawal (G. Redmond, personal communication). In contrast, preclinical studies in rats have not shown a consistent action of clonidine against sedative-hypnotic withdrawal (503–505).

It is likely that non-noradrenergic transmitter systems contribute to the withdrawal syndrome as well. However, the functional contributions of serotonergic or dopaminergic systems to anxiolytic/sedative withdrawal have not been well characterized (418, 506–509).

STIMULANTS

The existence and nature of long-term consequences of chronic stimulant use have been subjects of considerable research over the past decade. The prototypical stimulants are amphetamine and cocaine. As recent research on stimulant abuse has been driven largely by the widespread abuse of cocaine, especially in the form of "crack," this section focuses on the sequelae of chronic cocaine use on brain function; however, many of the findings can be generalized to other stimulants, such as amphetamine, which act as indirect aminergic agonists (510, 511). In addition, changes in the mesolimbic DA system will be emphasized because this system is the primary target of stimulant action.

The long-term consequences of psychostimulant abuse differ from those of other abused drugs, such as opioids and sedative/hypnotics. In addition to the psychological problems engendered by addiction, the detrimental consequences of prolonged use of these drugs include cardiovascular pathology (hypertension, cardiac infarctions, arrhythmias, and neuropathy) (512–515), hepatotoxicity (516), neurotoxicity (517–519), seizures (520), and psychopathology (paranoid psychosis) (512, 518, 521). On the other hand, long-term use of stimulants does not invariably lead to tolerance, nor does cessation of chronic use produce clear withdrawal signs.

TOLERANCE AND SENSITIZATION

After repeated administration of stimulants, the response to a challenge dose of the drug can either be attenuated (tolerance) or enhanced (sensitization). Classically, tolerance was thought to underlie the progressive increase in drug intake associated with addiction. As the response to a drug diminishes, larger amounts of the drug would have to be taken to obtain the same level of effect. Some cellular and behavioral effects of stimulants, such as induction of immediate early genes or discriminative stimulus properties, do exhibit tolerance (522–525). Nonetheless, long-term use of stimulants is now recognized to lead to an enhancement of other effects of these drugs. These effects include increased locomotor activity and seizure susceptibility (520, 526–528). Because sensitization can persist long after discontinuation of drug administration, it has been proposed that sensitization is the basis not only for the pathological consequences of long-term stimulant use but also for other essential features of addiction (e.g., craving and relapse)(39, 148, 529).

It is unclear whether tolerance or sensitization develops to the rewarding effects of stimulants. Tolerance to the subjective and cardiovascular effects of cocaine in human subjects was reported to occur within hours after a single dose, but it dissipated by the next day (530). On the other hand, studies in animals suggest that pre-exposure to stimulants produces sensitization to the reinforcing effects of these drugs (531–533).

One difficulty in assessing the chronic effects of stimulants is that the same drug effect can show tolerance under one set of experimental conditions but exhibit sensitization under a different set of conditions (531). Sensitization of locomotor activity depends critically on the treatment regimen, including dosage and intervals between drug administration (522). For example, if the drug is administered intermittently, locomotor activity exhibits sensitization, but if the drug is continuously infused, tolerance occurs (534). The interval between the last administration of the drug and the challenge dose is also an important factor. Tolerance is more evident during the first 24–72 hours after the last drug administration, especially when high doses are used, whereas sensitization can take several days to emerge (535). The differential development between sensitization and tolerance can also be influenced by psychological variables, such as method of drug administration (noncontingent vs. self-administered) or environmental stimuli associated with drug administration (conditioned cues) (23, 531, 533, 536, 537).

Initial hypotheses regarding the long-term effects of stimulants assumed that tolerance would develop as the release and metabolism of DA outpaced its synthesis and the presynaptic stores of DA became depleted (35, 538). The blockade of DA reuptake into the presynaptic terminal would eliminate a major source of releasable transmitter. Under normal conditions, D_2-like dopaminergic autoreceptors located on dopaminergic cell bodies, dendrites, and axons, limit increases in intrasynaptic DA levels by inhibiting impulse activity and transmitter release (539). Increases in intrasynaptic DA levels would stimulate these presynaptic autoreceptors, resulting in an inhibition of transmitter synthesis and impulse-dependent transmitter release. The combination of these regulatory mechanisms was expected to counteract the rise in intrasynaptic DA levels by diminishing overall neurotransmission and, thus, was expected to produce tolerance. These adaptive mechanisms were long cited as the basis for tolerance to the euphorigenic effects of stimulants and the rapid escalation in doses of stimulants self-administered by addicts (540). What was not taken into account was the fact that the homeostatic mechanisms themselves could be altered by continued use of a stimulant.

Recognizing that increased dopaminergic transmission in the mesolimbic system was responsible for the behaviors that exhibit sensitization (e.g., locomotor activity), researchers hypothesized that sensitization is due to a progressive enhancement of the ability of stimulant drugs to increase the levels of synaptic DA in the nucleus accumbens (287, 289, 291). Because of the extensive scope of this rapidly developing topic, only a sample of recent studies are discussed here. The reader is directed to recent reviews for a more comprehensive treatment (329, 330, 520, 531, 533, 535, 537, 541, 542).

Despite the apparent simplicity of the hypothesis that synaptic DA is augmented by chronic stimulant use, the empirical results have not yielded a clear picture. Evidently, whether sensitization to cocaine-induced increases in extracellular DA is measurable depends on whether the absolute concentration of DA—or rather the change in DA concentration relative to basal levels—is assayed (543). Whereas rats treated with saline for 10 days exhibited larger increases in extracellular DA in the nucleus accumbens in response to a challenge dose of cocaine, absolute DA concentrations in response to cocaine challenge were larger in rats that had received the subchronic cocaine treatment. These results reflected an elevation in basal levels of extracellular DA in the cocaine-treated rats. Furthermore, the increase in basal level of extracellular DA and in the levels of DA assayed after cocaine challenge were no longer present a week after discontinuation of daily cocaine treatments, even though sensitization of locomotor responses persisted for several weeks after the final dose of cocaine. A similar pattern of effect on extracellular DA was observed in the VTA (544). Both basal levels of DA in this cell body region and the relative increase in extracellular DA evoked by a challenge dose of cocaine were elevated the day after discontinuation of daily cocaine administration; however, as in the terminal regions, the enhancing effects on DA levels were no longer present 2 weeks after discontinuation of daily cocaine, despite persistence of sensitization of locomotor responses to cocaine.

Paradoxically, sensitization of the increase in extracellular DA levels produced by cocaine may be inversely related to the dose of daily cocaine during the pretreatment period (545). When rats were pretreated with half the dose of cocaine used in the studies just cited, the relative increase in extracellular DA in the nucleus accumbens in response to a challenge dose of cocaine was enhanced, and the enhancement was correlated with sensitization of locomotor activity. However, when the daily dose of cocaine was increased to the amount used in these same studies, enhancement of the increase in DA levels by cocaine challenge the day after discontinuation of daily cocaine was less than in the control group, even though an alteration in basal DA levels, as seen in the previous studies, was not observed. In contrast, higher daily doses of cocaine did produce more sensitization of the locomotor responses. Furthermore, the DA response to cocaine challenge continued to increase rather than diminish over a 21-day period in both of the cocaine-treated groups.

Although the process of sensitization does not depend on a single mechanism (546), it is believed that sensitization is initiated by an action on dopaminergic neurons. Repeated injection of amphetamine directly into the VTA of rats is sufficient to produce sensitization to a subsequent systemic administration of amphetamine or cocaine (547). This finding suggests that changes in the dopaminergic cell bodies mediate sensitization (535). Following repeated administration of cocaine or amphetamine, these drugs have a decreased ability to inhibit the firing rate of dopaminergic neurons due to a decrease in the sensitivity of the autoreceptors (548–550). Therefore, the net increase in DA output at the terminal regions would increase because the accumulation of synaptic DA would be less effective in exerting inhibitory feedback through the autoreceptors. A correlation between behavioral sensitization and molecular changes in dopaminergic neurons has also been reported. The functional significance of these changes is not clear (414,

551, 552) because the molecular effects (e.g., changes in DA autoreceptor sensitivity and G protein ribosylation in the VTA) are fairly transient and cannot account for the persistence of sensitization (548, 551). Also, increased inhibitory feedback from terminal regions appears to contribute more than activation of somatodendritic autoreceptors to the inhibition of DA impulse activity by acute amphetamine and cocaine (553).

It is now believed that persistent changes in DA terminal regions are responsible for the maintenance of sensitized responses, but that dopaminergic transmission may contribute only minimally to the sensitized response once sensitization is established. Chronic injections of amphetamine directly into the VTA can induce sensitization to a subsequent systemic administration of amphetamine (547), but a challenge dose of amphetamine injected directly into the VTA does not elicit a sensitized response (554). In contrast, a sensitized response is seen if the challenge injection is made directly into the nucleus accumbens (554). At present, the two most likely alternative interpretations are that adaptations occurring either in the presynaptic dopaminergic terminals or at nondopaminergic neurons or terminals could be critical to sensitization. Changes in the number of presynaptic DA transporters do not seem to be well correlated with the degree of sensitization (555, 556). On the other hand, electrophysiological studies have shown that neurons in the nucleus accumbens become supersensitive to DA, and that this supersensitivity is mediated by D_1 receptors (549, 557). Unlike the changes in the autoreceptors on DA cell bodies, the D_1 supersensitivity can persist for several weeks. Alterations in other DA receptors have yet to be characterized.

If sensitization is caused by changes in nondopaminergic neurons, other transmitters must be involved in maintaining sensitization. Endogenous opioids appear to contribute to sensitization, and there is evidence for cross-sensitization between stimulants and opioids (558). Coadministration of naltrindole, a δ-opioid antagonist, with cocaine blocks sensitization (559). In addition, repeated doses of cocaine increase the expression of precursors for opioid peptides in the striatum (525). Excitatory amino acid transmitters, most likely originating from cortical inputs to the striatum and nucleus accumbens, are also involved in sensitization. Coadministration of the noncompetitive NMDA-receptor antagonist dizocilpine prevents the development of behavioral sensitization (560, 561). Dizocilpine also prevents development of autoreceptor desensitization in dopaminergic neurons and D_1 receptor supersensitivity in nucleus accumbens neurons associated with sensitization (562). Finally, it is likely that the direct effects of stimulants on noradrenergic and serotonergic systems are also important contributors to the chronic effects of these drugs (563–565).

STIMULANT WITHDRAWAL

The epidemic of cocaine use during the last two decades has provided overwhelming evidence for the addictive properties of cocaine and other psychostimulants. Unlike withdrawal syndromes from opioids and sedative-hypnotic drugs, abstinence from cocaine and other psychostimulants is believed to be characterized primarily by emotional and motivational disturbances (566).

The description of a cocaine abstinence syndrome by Gawin and Kleber (566, 567) has provided a provocative heuristic framework for both clinical and preclinical research. Based on clinical interviews of an outpatient population, these authors proposed that cocaine withdrawal consists of three distinct temporal phases, each marked by progressive changes in mood and drug craving. The first stage ("crash") is analogous to an alcohol "hangover." The "crash" phase lasts for 1–4 days after cessation of cocaine use and is characterized by exhaustion and intense craving for cocaine. The true withdrawal syndrome was considered to start about a week after the last dose of cocaine and to last for 1–10 weeks, during which there was a high probability of relapse. This phase is marked by a subtle dysphoric syndrome, consisting of decreased activity, loss of motivation, increased boredom, and anhedonia, punctuated by episodes of drug craving. If abstinence is maintained for 1–2 months, mood, although somewhat labile, begins to normalize. This normalization of mood represents the beginning of a protracted extinction phase, during which the craving response to cues gradually decreases if abstinence is maintained, although intermittent episodes of drug craving and relapse can occur.

While this description of cocaine withdrawal has substantial intuitive appeal, it has been difficult to validate these phases under controlled conditions. Data from a sample of six inpatients suggested no consistent disturbances in mood (anxiety or depression) during a 22-day detoxification period, but there was a sharp increase in craving for cocaine 1–2 weeks after admission (568). However, two subsequent studies using a larger sample of subjects failed to demonstrate a phasic pattern of "crash" and "withdrawal" (566, 567). In a 28-day residential study, mood disturbances and drug craving were highest upon admission and declined steadily over the succeeding 4-week period (569). Furthermore, mood disturbances were relatively mild. Cocaine abusers and normal control subjects exhibited similar sleep patterns throughout the study period (i.e., cocaine addicts did not exhibit definite sleep disturbances), and there were no consistent cardiovascular or other physiological alterations during the study period. Three independent residential studies confirmed that mood disturbances and drug craving decrease sharply over the first week of abstinence and normalize over the next 3 weeks, although there was electroencephalographic evidence of protracted sleep disturbances (570–572).

The failure to observe discrete phases of cocaine withdrawal, especially with respect to craving, in these residential studies may be related to differences between inpatient and outpatient settings. In particular, these findings have led to an emphasis on the importance of environmental stimuli (e.g., people, places, and paraphernalia) related to drug use

in triggering craving (566, 567, 570, 573–575). Even though craving is central to descriptions of stimulant withdrawal, and is a major factor in relapse, the neural basis of craving is currently unknown (566, 567, 573, 574). One problem with this line of investigation is that craving does not have a widely accepted definition or physiological measure (573, 576–578). The subjective nature of craving has impeded the development of animal models that could be used to assess the physiological basis for craving (579). Recently, Robinson and Berridge (148) have argued that sensitization of an incentive-motivational system centered in the mesolimbic DA system may serve as the neural basis of craving. Although only a heuristic model, it would be consistent with the evidence for increased dopaminergic activity during presentation of cues that predict delivery of cocaine or food rewards (580–582).

Despite difficulties in demonstrating a distinct clinical cocaine abstinence syndrome, there has been substantial progress in characterizing neuronal phenomena following chronic use of stimulants. Cocaine and other psychostimulants exert their acute behavioral effects through enhancement of dopaminergic transmission, particularly in the mesolimbic system. Accordingly, behavioral changes seen upon abstinence from cocaine and other psychostimulants were presumably the result of depletion of DA and/or a down-regulation of dopaminergic neurotransmission (566, 567, 583). However, neurochemical evidence for dopaminergic depletion has been difficult to demonstrate in clinical studies (568, 570, 583). A recent postmortem binding study reported reductions in the number of DA transporter sites in the prefrontal cortex of cocaine users, but these changes may have been due to residual cocaine present at the time of death (584).

Evidence for altered dopaminergic function has been found in PET studies of abstinent cocaine abusers. A transient decrease in availability of D_2-like DA receptors labeled with $[^{18}F]N$-methylspiroperidol in the striatum was observed during the first week of abstinence, but labeling of these receptors was at control levels when assayed during the subsequent month (585). In one report, similar transient alterations were seen when glucose metabolism was assayed in PET scans of abstinent cocaine users (586). Compared to non-cocaine using controls, rCMRglc of cocaine users was higher during the first week of cocaine abstinence in the basal ganglia and a ventral medial portion of the prefrontal cortex — areas that receive dopaminergic projections. However, there was no difference in rCMRglc in any region between subjects who had been abstinent for 2 weeks and non-cocaine using controls. In contrast, a subsequent study from the same group reported that cocaine users who had been abstinent for 1–6 weeks had lower rCMRglc in dorsal prefrontal regions than non-cocaine using controls (587). This difference in rCMRglc was still present in a subset of subjects who were retested after 3–4 months of abstinence.

More substantial evidence has been obtained from animal studies. Behavioral changes consistent with a down-regulation of the DA system have been noted in animal studies during the first few hours to days of abstinence. There is behavioral evidence for increased anxiety and anhedonia during cocaine withdrawal, but these effects normalize within several days (588, 589). A more general disruption of operant responding, which persists for up to 2 weeks and is, perhaps indicative of motivational dysregulation, also occurs (590).

Direct evidence for progressive changes in dopaminergic transmission during each of the proposed phases of cocaine withdrawal has been obtained from animal studies. Although acute administration of cocaine produced selective stimulation of rCMRglc in extrapyramidal motor and limbic regions (591, 592), immediately after 12 hours of self-administration by rats, there is a decrease in rCMRglc in the mesolimbic and anterior striatal regions, including the nucleus accumbens, olfactory tubercle, amygdala, septum, limbic cortex (cingulate and piriform cortices) and rostral caudate-putamen (593). Decreases also occurred in motor, somatosensory, and auditory regions of the neocortex. The decrements in rCMRglc were inversely correlated to the amount of self-administered cocaine. Spontaneous firing rates of DA neurons in the VTA were increased during the first day after 1–2 weeks of cocaine or amphetamine administration (550, 594, 595). The increased impulse activity was attributed to a subsensitivity of inhibitory autoreceptors. In a different study, autoreceptor subsensitivity was also seen in DA neurons of the substantia nigra, but the subsensitivity was not accompanied by changes in the spontaneous firing rates (596). The increase in extracellular DA levels, observed 24 hours after the cessation of chronic cocaine administration in one study, is consistent with an increase in firing rate (543). However, three other studies reported that basal extracellular levels of DA measured by in vivo dialysis in the nucleus accumbens were normal during the early stages of withdrawal (545, 597, 598). The discrepancy between increased impulse activity and normal extrasynaptic DA levels could be explained by enhanced clearance of synaptic DA due to an increase in the number of DA transporters or enhancement of their efficiency. An elevation in DA transporter binding sites was recently reported in one study (599), but three other studies found that the number of DA transporter binding sites in the nucleus accumbens was unchanged either immediately after or up to 3 days after cessation of chronic cocaine administration in rats or mice (555, 556, 600). However, a recent report of an increase in the velocity of DA transport and turnover rate in rats, revealed a functional activation of the DA transporter at 24 hours after cessation of chronic cocaine administration, that persisted for at least 2 weeks (601). An increase in the efficiency of the transporter would presumably lead to a normalization of synaptic DA levels.

Studies of postsynaptic receptor densities during the early phases of abstinence have also yielded equivocal results. A decrease in the number of D_1-DA receptors in rats, was observed 2 hours after the final cocaine dose in one study (602), but not at 4 hours in a second study (603). Paradoxically, electrophysiological studies have found that

neurons of the nucleus accumbens exhibit an enhanced response to DA and D_1 agonists the day after cessation of 2 weeks of cocaine treatment (549, 557). An increase in the number of D_2 receptors in the striatum, but a decrease in the nucleus accumbens, immediately after 2 weeks of cocaine administration, have also been observed (604). As with the induction of sensitization (see previous discussion), differences in the method of cocaine administration may underlie the discrepant findings related to cocaine withdrawal. In most of the studies cited, cocaine was noncontingently administered by the experimenters one or more times during the day. However in other studies, rats self-administered cocaine (593, 599, 602) or were given a cocaine infusion continuously (596, 603).

About 1 week after the last cocaine administration, more reliable alterations in the dopaminergic function can be detected, but these changes do not clearly support a pattern of either dopaminergic hypoactivity or hyperactivity (583, 605). There is a marked decline in the number of DA transporter sites in the nucleus accumbens but not in the more dorsal portions of the striatal complex (555, 556, 599, 600, 606). This decline is accompanied by a decrease in expression of mRNA for the transporter in ventral tegmental DA neurons, but not in DA neurons of the substantia nigra (606). Although a decline in transporter binding should result in less DA reuptake and thus in an elevation of extracellular DA concentrations, most studies have found either normal (545, 606–608) or decreased DA levels in the nucleus accumbens 1 week after abstinence (598, 609). The lack of elevated DA levels may be due to a persistent increase in the velocity of turnover or transport (584). The reduction in the spontaneous activity of DA neurons in the VTA along with normalized autoreceptor sensitivity would further compensate for increased DA release (595, 596). Despite a reduction in the number of D_1 receptors (602, 603), neurons in the nucleus accumbens continue to exhibit a paradoxical increase in electrophysiological responses to D_1 agonists. In contrast, D_2-receptor density in the nucleus accumbens is normal, as is the response to D_2-receptor agonists.

The picture that emerges from the contradictory changes during this period is a progressive restabilization of the interactive mechanisms that regulate dopaminergic neurotransmission. Consistent with the clinical model, many of these changes persist for several weeks. For example, the reduction in DA transporter binding in the rat nucleus accumbens persists up to 2 months after the final dose of cocaine (556). The increased sensitivity of nucleus accumbens neurons to D_1 agonists also is present after 2 months of abstinence (557).

Nicotine

TOLERANCE

The effects of repeated administration of nicotine involve a variety of physiological and behavioral functions. Chronic administration of nicotine produces tolerance, although evidence for sensitization to the effects of nicotine has also been obtained in animal studies. Furthermore, it is now clear that deprivation of nicotine, in subjects that have been exposed chronically to the drug, also leads to the emergence of withdrawal signs, indicating dependence upon the drug. The mechanisms for producing these effects appear to involve cellular adaptation rather than dispositional changes.

Tolerance to the chronic effects of nicotine has been demonstrated in human investigations (610). In addition, studies in animals have demonstrated a rapid development of tolerance, albeit incomplete, to many of the effects of nicotine (611). Reversible tolerance to some of the effects of nicotine can develop in a matter of minutes (612). Tolerance is not explained by pharmacokinetics. In this regard, human studies demonstrated higher blood levels of nicotine, despite a diminution in heart rate acceleration and subjective responses to a second intravenous infusion of nicotine given 1 or 2 hours after the first infusion (613).

In rodents, nicotine produces biphasic effects, including a depression in locomotor activity, followed by stimulation. Both of these phenomena have been used to characterize the effects of chronic or subchronic treatment with nicotine on the response to an acute nicotine challenge. The initial depression of spontaneous motor activity by nicotine was used to demonstrate tolerance to this central effect of nicotine (614, 615). In rats given nicotine for about a month, motor activity, measured using a T maze, as well as several parameters of exploratory activity showed tolerance to a nicotine challenge that was presented 24 hours after withdrawal (616). Tolerance to the depressant effects of nicotine on motor behavior in rats persisted 80 days after withdrawal (615). Frequent dosing with nicotine was not required for the production of tolerance to the depressant effect on locomotor behavior, as it developed when nicotine was given once every 3 days, and a single administration of nicotine produced acute tolerance 2 hours later (617).

Another central effect of nicotine that shows the development of tolerance is hypothermia. Tolerance to the hypothermic effect of a challenge dose of nicotine was seen in mice that were treated subchronically (4 days) with nicotine three times per day (618). At times after nicotine challenge when cerebral nicotine levels were the same in mice given the subchronic treatment as in naive mice, naive mice showed maximum hypothermia but pretreated mice showed none. These data provided no support for a pharmacokinetic explanation of nicotine tolerance, and suggested a cellular mechanism. Other experiments in which tolerance to hypothermia in rats was attenuated by the concomitant administration of mecamylamine pointed to a mechanism of tolerance that involves central nicotinic receptors (619).

SENSITIZATION

Whereas tolerance has been the predominant effect of chronic nicotine on nicotine-induced hypothermia and suppression of locomotor activity, chronic nicotine enhances behavioral activation, which follows the early suppression of locomotor behavior by nicotine. Such stimulation has been observed 20–80 minutes after a nicotine challenge in rats given repeated administration of low doses of nicotine (620).

DEPENDENCE AND WITHDRAWAL

Observations of long-term neurochemical changes in the brain following chronic administration of nicotine are consistent with the view that nicotine can produce physical dependence. Acceptance of the view that nicotine produces such dependence derives from observations of withdrawal signs and symptoms in human subjects that were previously exposed chronically and then deprived of cigarettes or smokeless tobacco products (621, 622). The syndrome is characterized by anxiety, irritability, difficulty in concentration, sleep disturbances, increases in appetite, and craving for tobacco (622, 623). Abstinence from chronic treatment with 4 mg nicotine gum produces more signs and symptoms than withdrawal from 2 mg nicotine gum, and more severe symptoms are seen after withdrawal from cigarettes than from 4 mg gum (624).

The greater severity of the withdrawal syndrome following abstinence from cigarette smoking as compared with chewing of nicotine gum likely reflects differences in the bioavailability of nicotine administered by the two routes. Unlike nicotine gum, which provides a more constant concentration of the drug in the bloodstream, cigarette smoking produces rapid peaks in the arterial concentration of nicotine (625, 626).

Because the signs and symptoms of withdrawal are similar, whether subjects are withdrawn from tobacco or from nicotine gum (627, 628), it appears that nicotine is the active ingredient in tobacco that produces dependence. Other evidence attributing dependence from the consumption of tobacco products to nicotine could include production of withdrawal signs by antagonists of nAChRs activation and amelioration of withdrawal signs by the administration of nicotine. In this regard, results of studies in which mecamylamine was used to test whether antagonism of nAChRs would produce signs and symptoms of withdrawal have been equivocal (629–631). On the other hand, nicotine gum alleviates some of the symptoms of withdrawal (632-636). These include anxiety, irritability, and decreased ability to concentrate, but not craving for tobacco. Therefore, although interaction with nAChRs appears to be a key feature in the production and amelioration of dependence upon nicotine, long-term changes in nonnicotinic neurotransmitter systems, such as endogenous opioids, may also play a role in the behavioral response to nicotine abstinence.

NEUROCHEMICAL MECHANISMS IN LONG-TERM EFFECTS OF NICOTINE

Studies on the effects of chronic or subchronic nicotine on the binding of radioligands to nAChRs in the brain have supported the view that nAChR is at least one of the cellular targets that contributes to the long-term changes in behavioral responses to nicotine. Despite some discrepancies in reports on the effects of chronic nicotine on the binding of radioligands to nAChR in different regions of the rodent brain, the findings generally indicate that chronic nicotine produces up-regulation of nAChRs, particularly in the cerebral cortex (637–641).

Alterations in nAChRs produced by chronic treatment with nicotine in parallel with changes in the behavioral response to the drug have implicated nAChR as critical in neuroadaptive mechanisms. For example, a 14-day nicotine treatment regimen produced tolerance to the acute effects of nicotine on body temperature and locomotor depressant activity in rats and also increased the binding of [^{3}H]acetylcholine (in the presence of an antagonist to block muscarinic sites) in the midbrain and hippocampus (639). This observation suggested that the tolerance was related to up-regulation of nAChRs in the brain. However, in the same study, chronic nicotine treatment had no effect on the binding of [^{3}H]nicotine in the brain, suggesting that the two radioligands used labeled different sites.

In another study, repeated administration of nicotine for 5 days enhanced both the behavioral stimulant effects of nicotine in rats and the binding of [^{3}H]acetylcholine to nAChRs, measured in postmortem brain tissue (642). By 21 days after the last exposure to nicotine in the same study, both the behavioral effect as well as the effect on [^{3}H]acetylcholine binding were no longer seen, suggesting that the two effects were functionally linked. Ksir et al. (642) have suggested several interpretations of the augmentation of the stimulant properties of nicotine by chronic administration of the drug. One view purports that the depressant and stimulant effects of nicotine are caused by actions of the drug at different receptor types, and that stimulation is "unmasked" when tolerance develops to the depressant actions. Another interpretation is that biochemical events in the brain lead to sensitization. Subsequently, Ksir (643) showed that repeated administration of 0.03–0.3 mg/kg/day (but not 0.01 mg/kg/day) of nicotine enhanced the behavioral stimulant effect of nicotine and also increased the binding of [^{3}H]acetylcholine in the brain. The parallelism in the behavioral and biochemical responses indicated again that these two phenomena were linked. However, in the same study, rats that received 1.6 mg/kg nicotine twice daily showed no increase in behavioral stimulation due to a test dose of nicotine, although receptor binding was increased even more than at the lower doses of nicotine. The authors suggested that the dissociation between receptor up-regulation and the behavioral response to repeated high-dose treatment with nicotine could reflect actions on multiple receptor types, additional tolerance mechanisms, and prolonged receptor desensitization.

The finding of an increased density of nAChRs in animals treated with nicotine chronically or subchronically does little to explain the mechanism for an alteration in the behavioral response. One theory of neuroadaptational change in

response to chronic nicotine involves desensitization of cholinergic mechanisms (644). In this model of neuroadaptation, a desensitized receptor can bind drug, but the binding is not coupled with a biological response (644). Current information about nAChR is consistent with this model because exposure to an agonist (such as nicotine) induces a conformational change in the receptor, leading to increased affinity but reduced sensitivity.

Aside from the focus on nAChR as the prime mediator of long-term adaptational changes to chronic nicotine, non-cholinergic systems also have been implicated. For example, evidence for opioid involvement in the response to nicotine withdrawal derives from the use of a rodent model of the nicotine abstinence syndrome (645). The model employs continuous, subcutaneous infusion of nicotine tartrate via osmotic minipump. After termination of nicotine infusion, a syndrome emerges, characterized by teeth chatter, chewing, gasps, writhes, body shakes, ptosis, and seminal ejaculation. These signs, which are similar to those seen in opiate withdrawal, are reversible by administration of nicotine. In rats that are treated with continuous nicotine infusion, the withdrawal syndrome can also be elicited by the injection of naloxone, and morphine can reduce spontaneous abstinence signs observed after termination of nicotine infusion (646). These findings support the view that changes in endogenous opioid systems are involved in nicotine dependence.

Unlike cocaine, amphetamine, and opioids, behavioral sensitization after chronic nicotine does not appear to involve potentiation of the mesolimbic dopaminergic transmission. Despite the ability of nicotine to activate DA impulse activity and to increase extracellular DA in the nucleus accumbens, these effects are not enhanced by repeated administration of nicotine (244, 248, 250, 647). Behavioral sensitization to nicotine may involve direct effects on neurons of the nucleus accumbens or actions on cortically projecting DA neurons (647, 648), or changes in other monoaminergic neurons (649).

Some studies of the chronic effects of nicotine have involved metabolic mapping with 2-deoxy-D-[1-^{14}C] glucose method. One of these experiments has provided an example of a dissociation between the behavioral response to chronic nicotine administration and a biochemical marker in the brain (650). When rats were subjected to a twice daily regimen of subcutaneous nicotine injection for 10 days, the percentage of animals manifesting certain behaviors after the nicotine injection either increased (Straub tail, hyperkinesia, tremor) or did not change (ataxia) over the 10-day period. In contrast, none of the 45 brain regions showed evidence of sensitization to the stimulant effects of nicotine on rCMRglc, but tolerance to nicotine challenge was seen in the metabolic responses of the VTA, some components of visual pathways, the cerebellum, and vestibular nuclei. In part, the discrepancies between the behavioral and neurochemical findings in this study may be due to involvement of brain regions, other than those that showed tolerance, in the behavioral responses to nicotine that were enhanced by

Figure 29.5. Pseudocolor transforms of PET scan images, showing rCMRglc, in three levels of brain, under two conditions. As compared with the response to placebo (**top**), morphine produced a generalized decrease in rCMRglc (**bottom**). Units of cerebral glucose metabolism (mg/100 g/min) are indicated on the color scale.

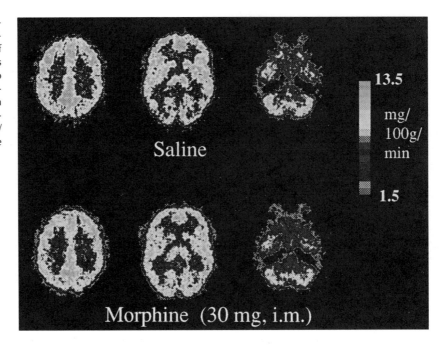

repeated administration. In addition, because rCMRglc is an indication of activity in a heterogeneous population of neurons within a region, it may not discriminate an enhanced response to nicotine in a discrete neurochemical system within the region. One other study on the effects of chronic nicotine on rCMRglc was performed in rats (651). Using a subcutaneous infusion method (osmotic minipumps), this study showed stimulation of rCMRglc in regions that previously showed stimulation in response to acute nicotine. There was no evidence of tolerance, although a challenge dose was not given to test for tolerance.

CONCLUSION

The last two decades have seen remarkable advances in our understanding of the mechanism of action and drug abuse. Receptor pharmacology has provided major insights about the initial sites of drug action in the brain. It is now recognized that drugs of abuse act on classic receptors or transporter molecules associated with specific neurotransmitter systems. Starting with the first assays of opiate-receptor binding, using radiolabeled naloxone in the 1970s, relevant receptors for every major drug of abuse have been identified in the brain. The impact of chronic administration of drugs of abuse on receptor function has become characterized in increasing detail, which has explained tolerance and other long-term drug effects at a cellular level. Furthermore, rapid advances in molecular biological techniques have allowed the cloning of these receptive molecules, with elucidation of their amino acid sequences.

Equally important are advances in our understanding of how receptor-mediated events influence neural systems, and how effects in these systems produce the behavioral manifestations of addiction. One critical feature of drugs of abuse is their rewarding properties, which are required for the

initiation and maintenance of drug use. It is now well established that the mesolimbic DA system serves as a common substrate for this phase of addiction. On the other hand, a plethora of evidence has implicated noradrenergic systems in the physical aspects of withdrawal. The neurobiological substrates of other aspects of the addictive process, such as sensitization, conditioning, and predisposition, are not characterized as well. Current investigations are uncovering mechanisms that include involvement of serotonergic, glutamatergic, and other neurotransmitter systems in these processes.

Until now, most of the major advances in our understanding of substance abuse has been derived from investigations of laboratory animals. The challenge for the future is to verify and to extend this work in human investigations. Noninvasive techniques, such as PET, for imaging brain function with biochemical and anatomical resolution, will be paramount in this effort. The availability of PET has already facilitated investigations of the biological correlates of drug-induced alterations of mood and feeling state. Studies of volunteers with histories of polysubstance abuse have shown that doses of either morphine or cocaine that produce positive affect, as measured by standard rating scales, also produce widespread reductions of cerebral glucose utilization (652, 653) (Figs. 29.5 and 29.6). In fact, a wide variety of substances that are self-administered reduce cerebral glucose metabolism, as measured by PET in human volunteers. In addition to morphine and cocaine, this group of substances includes alcohol (654, 655), amphetamine (656), barbiturates (657), and benzodiazepines (658, 659). It has been hypothesized that this action of drugs of abuse is related to the euphorigenic properties of these drugs and may result from effects on dopaminergic neurotransmission (660). Ultimately, the anatomical resolution and subcortical definition provided by PET will be combined with the exquisite

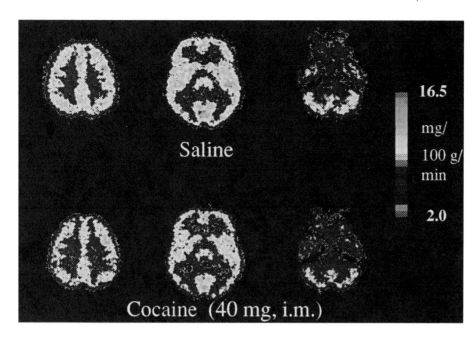

Figure 29.6. Pseudocolor transforms of PET scan images showing rCMRglc in three levels of brain under two conditions. As compared with the response to placebo (**top**) cocaine produced a generalized decrease in rCM-Rglc (**bottom**). Units of cerebral glucose metabolism (mg/100 g/min) are indicated on the color scale.

time resolution of electrophysiological measures, such as cortical-evoked-potential mapping, to provide a meaningful picture of the acute and chronic cerebral mechanisms of substance abuse.

Acknowledgment

The authors are grateful for the outstanding work and dedication of Mrs. Cindy Ambriz, who did extensive library and editorial work and prepared the manuscript.

References

1. Strange PG. The structure and mechanism of neurotransmitter receptors. Implications for the structure and function of the central nervous system. Biochem J 1988;249:309–318.
2. Creese I, Sibley DR, Hamblin MW, Leff SE. The classification of dopamine receptors: relationship to radioligand binding. Annu Rev Neurosci 1983;6:43–71.
3. Kebabian JW, Calne DB. Multiple receptors for dopamine. Nature 1979;277:93–96.
4. Stoof JC, Kebabian JW. Two dopamine receptors: biochemistry, physiology and pharmacology. Life Sci 1984;35:2281–2296.
5. Carlson JJ, Bergstrom DA, Walters JR. Stimulation of both D_1 and D_2 dopamine receptors appears necessary for full expression of postsynaptic effects of dopamine agonists: a neurophysiological study. Brain Res 1987;400:205–218.
6. Walters JR, Bergstrom DA, Carlson JH, Chase TN, Braun AR. D_1 dopamine receptors activation required for postsynaptic expression of D_2 agonist effects. Science 1987;236:719–722.
7. Clark D, White FJ. Review: D1 dopamine receptor-the search for a function: a critical evaluation of the D1/D2 dopamine receptor classification and its functional implications. Synapse 1987;1:347–388.
8. Blum K, Noble EP, Sheridan PJ, et al. Allelic association of human dopamine D_2 receptor gene in alcoholism. JAMA 1990;263:2055–2260.
9. Smith SS, O'Hara BF, Persico A, et al. Genetic vulnerability to drug abuse. The D_2 dopamine receptor Taq B1 restriction fragment length polymorphism appears to move frequently in polysubstance abusers. Arch Gen Psychiatr 1992;49:723–727.
10. Gejman PV, Ram A, Gelernter J, et al. No structural mutation in the dopamine D_2 receptor gene in alcoholism or schizophrenia. JAMA 1994;271:204–208.
11. Seeman P, Grigoriadis D. Dopamine receptors in brain and periphery. Neurochem Int 1987;10:1–25.
12. Sokoloff P, Giros B, Martres M-P, Bouthenet M-L, Schwartz J-C. A new dopamine receptor: the gain falls mainly in the brain. Discovery of a third dopamine receptor stimulates new studies of neurotransmitter systems and signal transduction pathways in the brain. J NIH Res 1990;2:59–62.
13. Schwartz J-C, Giros B, Martres M-P, Sokoloff P. The dopamine receptor family: molecular biology and pharmacology. Semin Neurosci 1992;4:99–108.
14. Van Tol HHM, Bunzow JR, Guan H-C, et al. Cloning of the gene for a human dopamine D_4 receptor with high affinity for the antipsychotic clozapine. Nature 1991;350:610–614.
15. Gingrich JA, Caron MG. Recent advances in the molecular biology of dopamine receptors. Annu Rev Neurosci 1993;16:229–321.
16. Van Tol HHM. The dopamine-D_4 receptor. In: Niznik HB, ed. Dopamine receptors and transporters. Pharmacology, structure, and function. New York: Marcel Dekker, 1994;189–204.
17. Grandy DK, Zhang Y, Bouvier C, et al. Multiple human D5 dopamine receptor genes: a functional receptor and two pseudogenes. Proc Natl Acad Sci U S A 1991;88:9175–9179.
18. Sunahara RK, Guan H-C, O'Dowd BF, et al. Cloning of the gene for a human dopamine D_5 receptor with higher affinity for dopamine that D_1. Nature 1991;350:614–619.
19. Joyce JN, Murray A. Distribution of dopamine D_1- and D_2-like dopamine receptors in human brain. In: Niznik HB, ed. Dopamine receptors and transporters. pharmacology, structure, and function. New York: Marcel Dekker, 1994;345–381.
20. Van Tol HHM. Immunocytochemical localization of D_1 and D_2 receptors in rat brain. In: Niznik HB, ed. Dopamine receptors and transporters. Pharmacology, structure, and function. New York: Marcel Dekker, 1994;383–400.
21. Meador-Woodruff JH, Mansour A, Saul J, Watson SJ, Jr. Neuroanatomical distribution of dopamine receptor messenger RNAs. In: Niznik HB, ed. Dopamine receptors and transporters. Pharmacology, structure, and function. New York: Marcel Dekker, 1994;401–418.
22. Snyder SH, Creese I, Burt DR. The brain's dopamine receptor: labeling with [^{3}H]dopamine and [^{3}H]haloperidol. Psychopharmacol Commun 1975;1:663–673.
23. Hollt V, Schubert P. Demonstration of neuroleptic sites in mouse brain by autoradiography. Brain Res 1978;151:149–153.

24. Kuhar MJ, Murrin LC, Malouf AT, Klemm N. Dopamine receptor binding *in vivo:* the feasibility of autoradiographic studies. Life Sci 1978;22:203–210.

25. Murrin LC, Kuhar MJ. Dopamine receptors in the rat frontal cortex: an autoradiography study. Brain Res 1979;177:279–285.

26. Palacios JM, Niehoff DL, Kuhar MJ. 3H-Spiperone binding sites in brain: Autoradiographic localization of multiple receptors. Brain Res 1981;213:277–289.

27. Madras BK, Fahey MA, Canfield DR, Spealman RD. D_1 and D_2 dopamine receptors in caudate-putamen of nonhuman primates (*macaca fascicularis*). J Neurochem 1988;51:934–943.

28. Beckstead RM. Association of dopamine D_1 and D_2 receptors with specific cellular elements in the basal ganglia of the cat: the uneven topography of dopamine receptors in the striatum is determined by intrinsic striatal cells, not nigrostriatal axons. Neuroscience 1988;27:851–863.

29. Richfield EK, Young AB, Penney JB. Comparative distributions of dopamine D-1 and D-2 receptors in the cerebral cortex of rats, cats, and monkeys. J Comp Neurol 1989;286:409–426.

30. Lidow MS, Goldman-Rakic PS, Gallager DW, Rakic P. Distribution of dopaminergic receptors in the primate cerebral cortex: quantitative autoradiographic analysis using [^{3}H]raclopride, [^{3}H]spiperone and [^{3}H]SCH23390. Neuroscience 1991;40:657–671.

31. Sesack SR, Bunney BS. Pharmacological characterization of the receptor mediating electrophysiological responses to dopamine in the rat medial prefrontal cortex: a microiontophretic study. J Pharmacol Exp Ther 1989;248:1323–1333.

32. Goldman-Rakic PS. Dopamine-mediated mechanisms of the prefrontal cortex. Semin Neurosci 1992;4:149–159.

33. Smiley JF, Levey AI, Ciliax BJ, Goldman-Rakic PS. D_1 dopamine receptor immunoreactivity in human and monkey cerebral cortex: predominant and extrasynaptic localization in dendritic spines. Proc Natl Acad Sci USA 1994;91:5270–5274.

34. Grace AA. Phasic versus tonic dopamine release and the modulation of dopamine system responsibility: a hypothesis for the etiology of schizophrenia. Neuroscience 1991;41:1–24.

35. Cooper JR, Bloom FE, Roth RH, eds. The biochemical basis of neuropharmacology. 6th ed. New York: Oxford University Press, 1991.

36. Bunney BS, Sesack SR, Silva NL. Midbrain dopaminergic systems: neurophysiology and electrophysiological pharmacology. In: Meltzer HY, ed. Psychopharmacology: the third generation of progress. New York: Raven Press, 1994:113–126.

37. Weinrieb RM, O'Brien CP. Persistent cognitive deficits attributed to substance abuse. Neurol Clin 1993;11:663–691.

38. Chiodo LA, Bannon MJ, Grace AA, Roth RH, Bunney BS. Evidence for the absence of impulse-regulating somatodendritic and synthesis-modulating nerve terminal autoreceptors on subpopulations of mesocortical dopamine neurons. Neuroscience 1984;12:1–16.

39. Meador-Woodruff JH, Damask SP, Watson SJ, Jr. Differential expression of autoreceptors in the ascending dopamine systems of the human brain. Proc Natl Acad Sci U S A 1994;91:8297–8301.

40. Sokoloff P, Giros B, Martres M-P, Bouthenet M-L, Schwartz J-C. Molecular cloning and characterization of a novel dopamine receptor (D_3) as a target for neuroleptics. Nature 1990;347:146–150.

41. Seeman P. Dopamine receptor sequences. Therapeutic levels of neuroleptics occupy D_2 receptors, clozapine occupies D_4. Neuropsychopharmacology 1992;7:261–284.

42. Seeman P, Guan H-C, Van Tol HHM. Dopamine D4 receptors elevated in schizophrenia. Nature 1993;365:441–445.

43. Ritz MC, Lamb RJ, Goldberg SR, Kuhar MJ. Cocaine receptors on dopamine transporters are related to self-administration of cocaine. Science 1987;237:1219–1223.

44. Kuhar MJ, Carroll FI, Boja J, et al. A cocaine receptor: properties and significance. In: Korenman SG, Barchas JD, eds. Biological basis of substance abuse. New York: Oxford University Press, 1993:70–80.

45. Boja JW, Vaughan R, Patel A, Shaya EK, Kuhar MJ. The dopamine transporter. In: Niznik HB, ed. Dopamine receptors and transporters. Pharmacology, structure, and function. New York: Marcel Dekker Inc., 1994:611–644.

46. Boja JW, McNeill RM, Lewin AH, Abraham P, Carroll FI, Kuhar MJ. Selective dopamine transporter inhibition by cocaine analogs. NeuroReport 1992;3:984–986.

47. Dersch CM, Akunne HC, Partilla JS, et al. Studies of the biogenic amine (amine) transporters. I. Dopamine reuptake blockers inhibit [^{3}H]mazindol binding to the dopamine transporter by a competitive mechanism: preliminary evidence for different binding domains. Neurochem Res 1994;19:201–208.

48. Shimada S, Kitayama, S, Lin C-L, et al. Cloning and expression of a cocaine-sensitive dopamine transporter complementary DNA. Science 1991;254:576–578.

49. Pacholczyk T, Blakely RD, Amara SG. Expression cloning of a cocaine and antidepressant-sensitive human noradrenaline transporter. Nature 1991;350:350–354.

50. Uhl GR. Neurotransmitter transporters (plus): a promising new gene family. Trends Neurosci 1992;15:265–268.

50a. Freed C, Revay R, Vaughan R, Krick E, Grant S, Uhl G, Kuhar M. Dopamine transporter immunoreactivity in rat brain. J Compr Neurol, in press.

51. Kaufman MJ, Spealman RD, Madras BK. Distribution of cocaine recognition sites in monkey brain: I. In vitro autoradiography with [^{3}H]CFT. Synapse 1991;9:177–187.

52. Scheffel U, Dannals RF, Wong DF, Yokoi F, Carroll FI, Kuhar MJ. Dopamine transporter imaging with novel, selective cocaine analogs. NeuroReport 1992;3:969–972.

53. Wong DF, Yung B, Dannals RF, et al. *In vivo* imaging of baboon and human dopamine transporters by positron emission tomography using [^{11}C]WIN 35,428. Synapse 1993;15:130–142.

54. Cerruti C, Walther DM, Kuhar MJ, Uhl GR. Dopamine transporter mRNA expression is intense in rat midbrain neurons and modest outside midbrain. Mol Brain Res 1993;18:181–186.

55. Simon EJ, Hiller JM, Edelman I. Stereospecific binding of the potent narcotic analgesic [^{3}H]etorphine to rat brain homogenate. Proc Natl Acad Sci USA 1973;70:1947–1949.

56. Terenius L. Stereospecific interaction between narcotic analgesics and a synaptic plasma membrane fraction of rat brain cortex. Acta Pharmacol Toxicol (Copenhagen) 1973;32:317–320.

57. Pert CB, Snyder SH. Opiate receptor: demonstration in nervous tissue. Science 1973;179:1011–1014.

58. Martin WR, Eades CG, Thompson JA, Huppler RE, Gilbert PE. The effects of morphine- and nalorphine-like drugs in the nondependent and morphine-dependent chronic spinal dog. J Pharmacol Exp Ther 1976;197:517–532.

59. Gilbert PE, Martin WR. The effects of morphine- and nalorphine-like drugs in the nondependent, morphine-dependent and cyclazocine-dependent chronic spinal dog. J Pharmacol Exp Ther 1976;198:66–82.

60. Vaupel DB. Naltrexone fails to antagonize the σ effects of PCP and SKF 10,047 in the dog. Eur J Pharmacol 1983;92:269–274.

61. Quirion R, Chicheportiche R, Contreras PC, et al. Classification and nomenclature of phencyclidine and *sigma* receptor sites. Trends Neurosci 1987;10:444–446.

62. Zukin RS, Zukin SR. The σ receptor. In: Pasternak GW, ed. The opiate receptors. Clifton: Humana, 1988:143–163.

63. Chavkin C, James IF, Goldstein A. Dynorphin is a specific endogenous ligand of the κ opioid receptor. Science 1982;215:413–415.

64. Itzhak Y. Multiple opioid binding sites. In: Pasternak GW, ed. The opiate receptors. Clifton: Humana Press, 1988:95–142.

65. Pasternak GW. Pharmacological mechanisms of opioid analgesics. Clin Neuropharmacol 1993;16:1–18.

66. North RA, Williams JT, Suprenant A, Christie MJ. μ and σ receptors belong to a family of receptors that are coupled to potassium channels. Proc Natl Acad Sci U S A 1987;84:5487–5491.

67. Zukin SR, Brady KT, Slifer BL, Balster RL. Behavioral and

biochemical steroselectivity of *sigma* opiate/PCP receptors. Brain Res 1984;294:174–177.

68. Zukin SR. Differing stereospecificities distinguish opiate receptor subtypes. Life Sci 1982;31:1307–1310.

69. Chen Y, Mestek A, Liu J, Hurley JA, Yu L. Molecular cloning and functional expression of a μ-opioid receptor from rat brain. Mol Pharmacol 1993;44:8–12.

70. Wang JB, Imai Y, Eppler CM, Gregor P, Spivak CE, Uhl GR. μ opiate receptor: cDNA cloning and expression. Proc Natl Acad Sci U S A 1993;90:10230–10234.

71. Evans CJ, Keith DE, Jr., Morrison H, Magendzo K, Edwards RH. Cloning of a *delta* opioid receptor by functional expression. Science 1992;258:1952–1955.

72. Kieffer BL, Befort K, Gaveriaux-Ruff C, Hirth CG. The delta-opioid receptor: Isolation of a cDNA by expression cloning and pharmacological characterization. Proc Natl Acad Sci U S A 1992;89:12048-12052.

73. Yasuda K, Raynor K, Kong H, et al. Cloning and functional comparison of κ and σ opioids receptors from mouse brain. Proc Natl Acad Sci U S A 1993;90:6736–6740.

74. Xie G-X, Miyajima A, Goldstein A. Expression cloning of cDNA encoding a seven-helix receptor from human placenta with affinity for opioid ligands. Proc Natl Acad Sci U S A 1992;89:4124–4128.

75. Zukin RS, Zukin SR. The case for multiple opiate receptors. Trends Pharmacol Sci 1984;7:160–164.

76. Simon EJ. Opiates: neurobiology. In: Lowinson JH, Ruiz P, Millman RB, Langrod JG, eds. Substance abuse. A comprehensive textbook. Baltimore: Williams & Wilkins, 1992:195–204.

77. Mansour A, Khachaturian H, Lewis ME, Akil H, Watson SJ. Anatomy of CNS opioid receptors. Trends Neurosci 1988;11:308–314.

78. Knapp RJ, Hunt M, Wamsley JK, Yamamura HI. CNS receptors for opioids. In: London ED, ed. Imaging drug action in the brain. Boca Raton: CRC Press, 1993:119–176.

79. Sharif NA, Hughes J. Discrete mapping of brain *mu* and *delta* opioid receptors using selective peptides: quantitative autoradiography, species differences and comparison with *kappa* receptors. Peptides 1989;10:499–522.

80. Tobin AJ, Khrestchatisky M. Gene expression in the mammalian nervous system. In: Siegel G, Agranoff B, Albers RW, Molinoff P, eds. Basic neurochemistry. Raven Press: New York, 1989:417–428.

81. Clarke PBS, Pert CB, Pert A. Autoradiographic distribution of nicotine receptors in rat brain. Brain Res 1984;323:390–395.

82. London ED, Waller SB, Wamsley JK. Autoradiographic localization of [³H]nicotine binding sites in the rat brain. Neurosci Lett 1985;53:179–184.

83. Changeux J-P, Devillers-Thiéry A, Chemouilli P. Acetylcholine receptor: an allosteric protein. Science 1984;225:1335–1345.

84. Changeux J-P, Giraudat J, Dennis M. The nicotinic acetylcholine receptor: molecular architecture of a ligand-regulated ion channel. Trends Pharmacol Sci 1987;8:459–465.

85. Changeux JP, Kasai M, Lee CY. Use of a snake venom toxin to characterize the cholinergic receptor protein. Proc Natl Acad Sci U S A 1970;67:1241–1247.

86. Miledi R, Molinoff P, Potter LT. Isolation of the cholinergic receptor protein of *Torpedo* electric tissue. Nature 1971;229:554–557.

87. Changeux JP. The acetylcholine receptor: an allosteric membrane protein. Harvey Lect 1979-80;75:85–254.

88. Olsen RW, Meunier JC, Changeux JP. Progress in the purification of the cholinergic receptor protein from *electrophorus electricus* by affinity chromatography. FEBS Lett 1972;28:96–100.

89. Karlin A, Cowburn D. The affinity-labeling of partially purified acetylcholine receptor from electric tissue of *Electrophorus*. Proc Natl Acad Sci USA 1973;70:3636–3640.

90. Chang HW. Purification and characterization of acetylcholine receptor-I from *Electrophorus electricus*. Proc Natl Acad Sci USA 1974;71:2113–2117.

91. Meunier JC, Sealock R, Olsen R, Changeux JP. Purification and properties of the cholinergic receptor protein from *Electrophorus electricus* electric tissue. Proc Natl Acad Sci U S A 1974;45:371–394.

92. Weill CL, McNamee MG, Karlin A. Affinity-labeling of purified acetylcholine receptor from *Torpedo californica*. Biochem Biophys Res Commun 1974;61:997–1003.

93. Raftery MA, Hunkapiller MW, Strader CD, Hood LE. Acetylcholine receptor: Complex of homologous subunits. Science 1980;208:1454–1456.

94. Raftery MA, Vandlen R, Michaelson D, et al. The biochemistry of an acetylcholine receptor. J Supramol Struct 1974;2:582–592.

95. Reynolds JA, Karlin A. Molecular weight in detergent solution of acetylcholine receptor from *Torpedo californica*. Biochem 1978;17:2035–2038.

96. Devillers-Thiéry A, Changeux JP, Paroutaud P, Strosberg AD. The amino-terminal sequence of the 40,000 molecular weight subunit of the acetylcholine receptor protein from *Torpedo marmorata*. FEBS Lett 1979;104:99–105.

97. Wada K, Ballivet M, Boulter J, et al. Functional expression of a new pharmacological subtype of brain nicotinic acetylcholine receptor. Science 1988;240:330–334.

98. Boulter J, Evans K, Goldman D, et al. Isolation of a cDNA clone coding for a possible neural nicotinic acetylcholine receptor α-subunit. Nature 1986;319:368–374.

99. Goldman D, Deneris E, Luyten W, Kochhar A, Patrick J, Heinemann S. Members of a nicotinic acetylcholine receptor gene family are expressed in different regions of the mammalian central nervous system. Cell 1987;48:965–973.

100. Deneris ES, Connolly J, Boulter J, et al. Primary structure and expression of β₂: a novel subunit of neuronal nicotinic acetylcholine receptors. Neuron 1988;1:45–54.

101. Deneris ES, Boulter J, Swanson LW, Patrick J, Heinemann S. β₃: a new member of nicotinic acetylcholine receptor gene family is expressed in brain. J Biol Chem 1989;264:6268–6272.

102. Boulter J, O'Shea-Greenfield A, Duvoisin RM, et al. α₃, α₅, and β₄: three members of the rat neuronal nicotinic acetylcholine receptor-related gene family form a gene cluster. J Biol Chem 1990;265:4472–4482.

103. Boulter J, Connolly J, Deneris E, Goldman D, Heinemann S, Patrick J. Functional expression of two neuronal nicotinic acetylcholine receptors from cDNA clones identifies a gene family. Proc Natl Acad Sci U S A 1987;84:7763–7767.

104. Wada E, Wada K, Boulter J, et al. Distribution of *alpha₂*, *alpha₃*, *alpha₄*, and *beta₂* neuronal nicotinic receptor subunit mRNAs in the central nervous system: A hybridization histochemical study in the rat. J Comp Neurol 1989;284:314–335.

105. Zukin SR, Zukin RS. Specific [³H]phencyclidine binding in rat central nervous system. Proc Natl Acad Sci U S A 1979;76:5372–5376.

106. Vincent JP, Kartalovski B, Geneste P, Kamenka JM, Lazdunski M. Interaction of phencyclidine ("angel dust") with a specific receptor in rat brain membranes. Proc Natl Acad Sci U S A 1979;76:4678–4682.

107. Javitt DC, Zukin SR. The role of excitatory amino acids in neuropsychiatric illness. Journal of Neuropsychiatry and Clinical Neurosciences 1990;2:44–52.

108. Javitt DC, Zukin SR. Recent advances in the phencyclidine model of schizophrenia. Am J Psychiatry 1991;148:1301–1308.

109. Zukin SR, Zukin RS. Phencyclidine. In: Lowinson JH, Ruiz P, Millman RB, Langrod JG, eds. Substance abuse. A comprehensive textbook. Baltimore: Williams & Wilkins, 1992:290–302.

110. Javitt DC, Frusciante MJ, Zukin SR. Rat brain N-methyl-D-aspartate receptors require multiple molecules of agonist for activation. Mol Pharmacol 1990;37:603–607.

111. Benveniste M, Mayer ML. Kinetic analysis of antagonist action at N-methyl-D-aspartic acid receptors. Two binding sites each for glutamate and glycine. Biophys J 1991;59:560–573.

112. Kleckner NW, Dingledine R. Requirement for glycine in activation of NMDA-receptors expressed in *Xenopus* oocytes. Science 1988;241:835–837.

113. Moriyoshi K, Masu M, Ishii T, Shigemoto R, Mizuno N, Nakanishi S. Molecular cloning and characterization of the rat NMDA receptor. Nature 1991;354:31–37.

114. Monyer H, Sprengel R, Schoepfer R, et al. Heteromeric NMDA receptors: molecular and functional distinction of subtypes. Science 1992;256:1217–1221.

115. Seeburg PH. The molecular biology of mammalian glutamate receptor channels. Trends Neurosci 1993;16:359–365.

116. Burt DR, Kamatchi GL. GABA$_A$ receptor subtypes: from pharmacology to molecular biology. FASEB J 1991;5:2916–2923.

117. Macdonald RL, Twyman RE. Kinetic properties and regulation of GABA$_A$ receptor channels. In: Narahashi T, ed. Ion channels, vol 3. New York: Plenum Press, 1992:315–343.

118. Doble A, Martin IL. Multiple benzodiazepine receptors: no reason for anxiety. Trends Pharmacol Sci 1992;13:76–81.

119. Luddens H, Wisden W. Function and pharmacology of multiple GABA$_A$ receptor subtypes. Trends Pharmacol Sci 1991;12:49–51.

120. Bormann J. Electrophysiology of GABA$_A$ and GABA$_B$ receptor subtypes. Trends Neurosci 1988;11:112–116.

121. Weight FF, Aguayo LG, White G, Lovinger DM, Peoples RW. GABA- and glutamate-gated ion channels as molecular sites of alcohol and anesthetic action. In: Biggio G, Concas A, Costa E, eds. GABAergic synaptic transmission. New York: Raven Press, 1992:335–347.

122. Demirgören S, Majewska MD, Spivak CE, London ED. Receptor binding and electrophysiological effects of dehydroepiandrosterone sulfate, an antagonist of the GABA$_A$ receptor. Neuroscience 1991;45:127–135.

123. Majewska MD, Demirgören S, London ED. Binding of pregnenolone sulfate to rat brain membranes suggest multiple sites of steroid action at the GABA$_A$ receptor. Eur J Pharmacol 1990;189:307–315.

124. Majewska MD, Demirgören S, Spivak CE, London ED. The neurosteroid dehydroepiandrosterone sulfate is an allosteric antagonist of the GABA$_A$ receptor. Brain Res 1990;526:143–146.

125. Harrison NL, Majewska MD, Harrington JW, Barker JL. Structure-activity relationships for steroid interaction with the g-aminobutyric acid$_A$ receptor complex. J Pharmacol Exp Ther 1987;241:346–353.

126. Majewska MD, Harrison NL, Schwartz RD, Barker JL, Paul SM. Steroid hormone metabolites are barbiturate-like modulators of the GABA receptor. Science 1986;232:1004–1007.

127. Costa E, Guidotti A. Diazepam binding inhibitor (DBI): a peptide with multiple biological actions. Life Sci 1991;49:325–344.

128. Gaoni Y, Mechoulam R. Isolation, structure, and partial synthesis of an active constituent of hashish. Journal of American Chemistry Society 1964;86:1646–1647.

129. Garrett ER, Hunt CA. Physiochemical properties, solubility, and protein binding of Δ^9-tetrahydrocannabinol. J Pharm Sci 1974;63:1056–1064.

130. Martin BR, Balster RL, Razdan RK, Harris LS, Dewey WL. Behavioral comparisons of the stereoisomers of tetrahydrocannabinols. Life Sci 1981;29:565–574.

131. Johnson MR, Melvin LS. The discovery of nonclassical cannabinoid analgetics. In: Mechoulam R, ed. Cannabinoids as therapeutic agents. Boca Raton: CRC Press, 1986:121–145.

132. Howlett AC, Johnson MR, Melvin LS, Milne GM. Nonclassical cannabinoid analgesics inhibit adenylate cyclase: development of a cannabinoid receptor model. Mol Pharmacol 1988;33:297–302.

133. Little PJ, Compton DR, Johnson MR, Martin BR. Pharmacology and stereoselectivity of structurally novel cannabinoids in mice. J Pharmacol Exp Ther 1988;247:1046–1051.

134. Devane WA, Dysarz FA, III., Johnson MR, Melvin LS, Howlett AC. Determination and characterization of a cannabinoid receptor in rat brain. Mol Pharmacol 1988;34:605–613.

135. Herkenham M, Lynn AB, Little MB, et al. Cannabinoid receptor localization in brain. Proc Natl Acad Sci USA 1990;87: 1932–1936.

136. Herkenham M, Lynn AB, Johnson MR, Melvin LS, de Costa BR, Rice KC. Characterization and localization of cannabinoid receptor in rat brain: a quantitative *in vitro* autoradiographic study. J Neurosci 1991;11:563–583.

137. Matsuda LA, Lolait JS, Brownstein M, Young AC, Bonner TI. Structure of a cannabinoid receptor and functional expression of the cloned cDNA. Nature 1990;346:561–564.

138. Devane WA, Hanus L, Breuer A, et al. Isolation and structure of a brain constituent that binds to the cannabinoid receptor. Science 1992;258:1946–1949.

139. Fride E, Mechoulam R. Pharmacological activity of the cannabinoid receptor agonist, anandamide, a brain constituent. Eur J Pharmacol 1993;231:313–314.

140. Devane WA, Hille B. Anandamide, an endogenous cannabinoid, inhibits calcium currents as a partial agonist in N18 neuroblastoma cells. Mol Pharmacol 1993;44:498–503.

141. Seevers MH. Opiate addiction in the monkey I. Methods of study. J Pharmacol Exp Ther 1935;56:147–156.

142. Goldberg SR, Kelleher RT. Behavior controlled by scheduled injections of cocaine in squirrel and rhesus monkeys. J Exp Anal Behav 1976;25:93–104.

143. Thompson T, Schuster CR. Morphine self-administration, food-reinforced, and avoidance behaviors in rhesus monkeys. Psychopharmacologia 1964;5:87–94.

144. Schuster CR. Psychological approaches to opiate dependence and self-administration by laboratory animals. Fed Proc 1970;29:1–5.

145. Pickens R, Thompson T. Cocaine-reinforced behavior in rats: effects of reinforcement magnitude and fixed-ratio size. J Pharmacol Exp Ther 1968;161:122–129.

146. Thompson T, Pickens R. Stimulant self-administration by animals: some comparisons with opiate self-administration. Fed Proc 1970;29:6–12.

147. Gardner EL. Brain reward mechanisms. In: Lowinson JH, Ruiz P, Millman RB, Langrod JG, eds. Substance abuse. A comprehensive textbook. Baltimore: Williams & Wilkins, 1992:70–99.

148. Robinson TE, Berridge KC. The neural basis of drug craving: an incentive-sensitization theory of addiction. Brain Res Rev 1993;18:247–291.

149. Lamb RJ, Preston KL, Schindler CW, et al. The reinforcing and subjective effects of morphine in post-addicts: a dose-response study. J Pharmacol Exp Ther 1991;259:1165–1173.

150. Thorndike EL, ed. Animal intelligence. New York: MacMillan, 1911.

151. Skinner BF, ed. The behavior of organisms: an experimental analysis. New York: Appleton-Century-Crofts, 1938.

152. Messier C, White NM. Contingent and non-contingent actions of sucrose and saccharin reinforcers: effects on taste preference and memory. Physiol Behav 1984;32:195–203.

153. White N, Legree P. Effect of post-training exposure to an aversive stimulus on retention. Physiological Psychology 1984;12:233–236.

154. Stinus L, Le Moal M, Koob GF. Nucleus accumbens and amygdala are possible substrates for the aversive stimulus effects of opiate withdrawal. Neuroscience 1990;37:767–773.

155. Olds J, Milner P. Positive reinforcement produced by electrical stimulation of septal area and other regions of rat brain. J Comp Physiol Psychol 1954;47:419–427.

156. Olds ME, Olds J. Approach-avoidance analysis of rat diencephalon. J Comp Neurol 1963;120:259–295.

157. Olds J. Pleasure centers in the brain. Sci Am 1956;195:105–116.

158. Miller NE. Motivational effects of brain stimulation and drugs. Fed Proc 1960;19:846–853.

159. Margules DL, Olds J. Identical "feeding" and "rewarding" systems in the lateral hypothalamus of rats. Science 1962;135:374–375.

160. Hoebel BG, Teitelbaum P. Hypothalamic control of feeding and self-stimulation. Science 1962;132:375–377.

161. Coons EE, Levak M, Miller NE. Lateral hypothalamus: learning of food-seeking response motivated by electrical stimulation. Science 1965;150:1320–1321.

162. Hoebel BG. Feeding and self-stimulation. Ann N Y Acad Sci 1969;157:758–778.

163. Killam KF, Olds J, Sinclair J. Further studies on the effects of centrally acting drugs on self-stimulation. J Pharmacol Exp Ther 1957;119:157

164. Yokel RA. Intravenous self-administration: response rates, the effects of pharmacological challenges, and drug preference. In: Bozarth MA, ed. Methods of assessing the reinforcing properties of abused drugs. New York: Springer-Verlag, 1987:1–33.

165. Goldberg SR. Comparable behavior maintained under fixed-ratio and second-order schedules of food presentation, cocaine injection or d-amphetamine injection in the squirrel monkey. J Pharmacol Exp Ther 1973;186:18–30.

166. Yokel RA, Pickens R. Self-administration of optical isomers of amphetamine and methylamphetamine by rats. J Pharmacol Exp Ther 1973;187:27–33.

167. Johanson CE, Schuster CR. A choice procedure for drug reinforcers: cocaine and methylphenidate in the rhesus monkey. J Pharmacol Exp Ther 1975;193:676–688.

168. Goldberg SR, Spealman RD, Goldberg DM. Persistent behavior at high rates maintained by intravenous self-administration of nicotine. Science 1981;214:573–575.

169. Deneau G, Yanagita T, Seevers MH. Self-administration of psychoactive substances by the monkey. Psychopharmacologia 1969;16:30–48.

170. Weeks JR. Experimental morphine addiction: method for automatic intravenous injections in unrestrained rats. Science 1962;138:143–144.

171. Woods JH, Ikomi F, Winger G. The reinforcing property of ethanol. In: Roach MK, McIsaac WM, Creaven PJ, eds. Biological aspects of alcohol. Austin: University of Texas Press, 1971:371–388.

172. Deleted.

173. Davis JD, Lulenski GC, Miller NE. Comparative studies of barbiturate self-administration. Int J Addict 1968;3:207–214.

174. Findley JD, Robinson WW, Peregrino L. Addiction to secobarbital and chlordiazepoxide in the rhesus monkey by means of a self-infusion preference procedure. Psychopharmacologia 1972;26:93–114.

175. Balster RL, Johanson CE, Harris RT. Phencyclidine self-administration in the rhesus monkey. Pharmacol Biochem Behav 1973;1:167–172.

176. Pilotto R, Singer G, Overstreet D. Self-injection of diazepam in naive rats: effects of dose, schedule and blockade of different receptors. Psychopharmacology (Berl) 1984;84:174–177.

177. Woods JH, Schuster CR. Reinforcement properties of morphine, cocaine, and SPA as a function of unit dose. Int J Addict 1968;3:231–237.

178. Carney JM, Llewellyn ME, Woods JH. Variable interval responding maintained by intravenous codeine and ethanol injections in the rhesus monkey. Pharmacol Biochem Behav 1977;5:577–582.

179. Winger G, Stitzer ML, Woods JH. Barbiturate-reinforced responding in rhesus monkeys: comparisons of drugs with different durations of action. J Pharmacol Exp Ther 1975;195:505–514.

180. Kelleher RT. Characteristics of behavior controlled by scheduled injections of drugs. Pharmacol Rev 1975;27:307–323.

181. Hoffmeister F, Goldberg SR. A comparison of chlorpromazine, imipramine, morphine and d-amphetamine self-administration in cocaine-dependent rhesus monkeys. J Pharmacol Exp Ther 1973;187:8–14.

182. Collins RJ, Weeks JR, Cooper MM, Good PI, Russell RR. Prediction of abuse liability of drugs using IV self-administration by rats. Psychopharmacology (Berl) 1984;82:6–13.

183. Hoffmeister F, Wuttke W. Psychotropic drugs as negative reinforcers. Pharmacol Rev 1976;27:419–428.

184. Kandel DA, Schuster CR. An investigation of nalorphine and perphenazine as negative reinforcers in an escape paradigm. Pharmacol Biochem Behav 1977;6:61–71.

184a. Herming RI, Jones RT, Benowitz NL, Mines AH. How a cigarette is smoked determines blood nicotine levels. Clin Pharmacol Ther 1983;33:84–90.

184b. Yokel RA, Pickens R. Drug levels of d and l-amphetamine during intravenous self-administration. Psychopharmacologia 1974;34:255–264.

185. Hubner CB, Koob GF. Bromocriptine produces decreases in cocaine self-administration in the rat. Neuropsychopharmacology 1990;3:101–108.

186. de Wit H, Wise RA. Blockade of cocaine reinforcement in rats with dopamine receptor blocker pimozide, but not with the noradrenergic blockers phentolamine or phenoxybenzamine. Can J Psychol 1977;31:195–203.

187. Roberts DCS, Vickers G. Atypical neuroleptics increase self-administration of cocaine: an evaluation of a behavioural screen for antipsychotic activity. Psychopharmacology (Berl) 1984;82:135–139.

188. Ettenberg A, Pettit HO, Bloom FE, Koob GF. Heroin and cocaine intravenous self-administration in rats: mediation by separate neural systems. Psychopharmacology (Berl) 1982;78:204–209.

189. Johanson CE, Kandel DA, Bonese K. The effects of perphenazine on self-administration behavior. Pharmacol Biochem Behav 1976;4:427–433.

190. Hubner CB, Moreton JE. Effects of selective D_1 and D_2 dopamine antagonists on cocaine self-administration in the rat. Psychopharmacology (Berl) 1991;105:151–156.

191. Roberts DCS, Koob GF, Klonoff P, Fibiger HC. Extinction and recovery of cocaine self-administration following 6-hydroxydopamine lesions of the nucleus accumbens. Pharmacol Biochem Behav 1980;12:781–787.

192. Roberts DCS, Corcoran ME, Fibiger HC. On the role of ascending catecholaminergic systems in intravenous self-administration of cocaine. Pharmacol Biochem Behav 1977;6:615–620.

193. Pettit HO, Ettenberg A, Bloom FE, Koob GF. Destruction of dopamine in the nucleus accumbens selectively attenuates cocaine but not heroin self-administration in rats. Psychopharmacology (Berl) 1984;84:167–173.

194. Lyness WH, Friedle NM, Moore KE. Destruction of dopaminergic nerve terminals in nucleus accumbens: effect on d-amphetamine self-administration. Pharmacol Biochem Behav 1979;11:553–556.

195. Zito KA, Vickers G, Roberts DCS. Disruption of cocaine and heroin self-administration following kainic acid lesions of the nucleus accumbens. Pharmacol Biochem Behav 1985;23:1029–1036.

196. Roberts DCS, Koob GF. Disruption of cocaine self-administration following 6-hydroxydopamine lesions of the ventral tegmental area in rats. Pharmacol Biochem Behav 1982;17:901–904.

197. Roberts DCS, Zito KA. Interpretation of lesion effects on stimulant self-administration. In: Bozarth MA, ed. Methods of assessing the reinforcing properties of abused drugs. New York: Springer-Verlag, 1987:87–103.

198. Glick SD, Cox RD. Dopaminergic and cholinergic influences on morphine self-administration in rats. Res Commun Chem Pathol Pharmacol 1975;12:17–24.

199. Bozarth MA, Wise RA. Heroin reward is dependent on a dopaminergic substrate. Life Sci 1981;29:1881–1886.

200. Bozarth MA. Neural basis of psychomotor stimulant and opiate reward: evidence suggesting the involvement of a common dopaminergic system. Behav Brain Res 1986;22:107–116.

201. Spyraki C, Fibiger HC, Phillips AG. Attenuation of heroin reward in rats by disruption of the mesolimbic dopamine system. Psychopharmacology (Berl) 1983;79:278–283.

202. Wise RA. Action of drugs of abuse on brain reward systems. Pharmacol Biochem Behav 1980;13:213–223.

203. Wise RA. The dopamine synapse and the notion of "pleasure centers" in the brain. Trends Neurosci 1980;3:91–95.

204. Wise RA, Bozarth MA. Brain reward circuitry: four circuit elements "wired" in apparent series. Brain Res Bull 1984;12:203–208.

205. Zaborszky L, Alheid GF, Alones VE, Oertel WH, Schmechel DE, Heimer L. Afferents of the ventral pallidum studies with a combined immunohistochemical-anterograde degeneration method. Soc Neurosci Abstr 1982;8:218.

206. Hubner CB, Koob GF. The ventral pallidum plays a role in mediating cocaine and heroin self-administration in the rat. Brain Res 1989; 508:20–29.

207. Phillips AG, Mora F, Rolls ET. Intracerebral self-administration of amphetamine by Rhesus monkeys. Neurosci Lett 1981;24: 81–86.

208. Monaco AP, Hernandez L, Hoebel BG. Nucleus accumbens: site of amphetamine self-injection: comparison with lateral ventricle. In: Chronister RB, DeFrance JF, eds. The neurobiology of the nucleus accumbens. Brunswick: Haer Institute for Electrophysiological Research, 1981:33–342.

209. Hoebel BG, Monaco AP, Hernandez L, Aulisi EF, Stanley BG, Lenard L. Self-injections of amphetamine directly into the brain. Psychopharmacology (Berl) 1983;81:158–163.

210. Goeders NE, Smith JE. Cortical dopaminergic involvement in cocaine reinforcement. Science 1983;221:773–775.

211. Bozarth MA, Wise RA. Intracranial self-administration of morphine in to the ventral tegmental area in rats. Life Sci 1981;28:551–555.

212. Bedford JA, Bailey LP, Wilson MC. Cocaine reinforced progressive ratio performance in the rhesus monkey. Pharmacol Biochem Behav 1978;9:631–638.

213. Stein EA, Olds J. Direct intracerebral self-administration of opiates in the rat. Soc Neurosci Abstr 1977;3:302

214. Haverkos HW. Kaposi's sarcoma and nitrite inhalants. In: Bridge TP, Mirsky AF, Goodwin FK, eds. Psychological, neuropsychiatric, and substance abuse aspect of AIDS: advances in biochemical psychopharmacology. New York: Raven Press, 1988:165–172.

215. Olds ME. Reinforcing effects of morphine in the nucleus accumbens. Brain Res 1982;237:429–440.

216. van Ree JM, de Wied D. Involvement of neurohypophyseal peptides in drug-mediated adaptive responses. Pharmacol Biochem Behav (suppl 1) 1980;13:257–263.

217. Goeders NE, Lane JD, Smith JE. Self-administration of methionine enkephalin into the nucleus accumbens. Pharmacol Biochem Behav 1984;20:451–455.

218. Olds ME, Williams KN. Self-administration of D-Ala²-Met-enkephalinamide at hypothalamic self-stimulation sites. Brain Res 1980;194:155–170.

219. Britt MD, Wise RA. Ventral tegmental site of opiate reward: antagonism by a hydrophilic opiate receptor blocker. Brain Res 1983;258:105–108.

220. Vaccarino FJ, Bloom FE, Koob GF. Blockade of nucleus accumbens opiate receptors attenuates intravenous heroin reward in the rat. Psychopharmacology (Berl) 1985;86:37–42.

221. Corrigall WA, Vaccarino FJ. Antagonist treatment in nucleus accumbens or periaqueductal grey affects heroin self-administration. Pharmacol Biochem Behav 1988;30:443–450.

222. Gill CA, Holz WC, Zirkle CL, Hill H. Pharmacological modification of cocaine and apomorphine self-administration in the squirrel monkey. In: Denker P, Radouco-Thomas C, Villeneuve A, eds. Proceedings of the tenth congress of the collegium internationale Neuro-Psychopharmacologicum. New York: Pergamon Press, 1978: 1477–1484.

223. Yokel RA, Wise RA. Amphetamine-type reinforcement by dopaminergic agonists in the rat. Psychopharmacology (Berl) 1978;58: 289–296.

224. Woolverton WL, Goldberg LI, Ginos JZ. Intravenous self-administration of dopamine receptor agonists by rhesus monkeys. J Pharmacol Exp Ther 1984;230:678–683.

225. Baxter BL, Gluckman MI, Stein L, Scerni RA. Self-injection of apomorphine in the rat: positive reinforcement by a dopamine receptor stimulant. Pharmacol Biochem Behav 1974;2:387–391.

226. Davis WM, Smith SG. Catecholaminergic mechanisms of reinforcement: direct assessment by drug self-administration. Life Sci 1977; 20:483–492.

227. Winger G, Woods JH. Comparison of fixed-ratio and progressive-ratio schedules of maintenance of stimulant drug-reinforced responding. Drug Alcohol Depend 1985;15:123–130.

228. Risner ME, Silcox DL. Psychostimulant self-administration by beagle dogs in a progressive-ratio paradigm. Psychopharmacology (Berl) 1981;75:25–30.

229. Corwin RL, Woolverton WL, Schuster CR, Johanson CE. Anorectics: effects on food intake and self-administration in rhesus monkeys. Alcohol Drug Res 1987;7:351–361.

230. van der Zee P, Koger HS, Gootjes J, Hespe W. 1,4-dialk-(en)ylpeperazines as selective and very potent inhibitors of dopamine uptake. Eur J Med Chem 1980;15:363–370.

231. Heikkila RE, Manzino L. Behavioral properties of GBR 12909, GBR 13609 and GBR 13098: specific inhibitors of dopamine uptake. Eur J Pharmacol 1984;103:241–248.

232. Woods JH, Katz JL, Medzihradsky F, Smith CB, Winger GD. Evaluation of new compounds for opioid activity: 1982 annual report. NIDA Res Monogr 1983;43:457–511.

233. Wilson MC, Schuster CR. Mazindol self-administration in the rhesus monkey. Pharmacol Biochem Behav 1976;4:207–210.

234. Bergman J, Madras BK, Johnson SE, Spealman RD. Effects of cocaine and related drugs in nonhuman primates. III. Self-administration by squirrel monkeys. J Pharmacol Exp Ther 1989;251:150–155.

235. Heikkila RE, Cabbat FS, Manzino L, Duvoisin RC. Rotational behavior induced by cocaine analogs in rats with unilateral 6-hydroxydopamine lesions of the substantia nigra: dependence upon dopamine uptake inhibition. J Pharmacol Exp Ther 1979;211: 189–194.

236. Corrigall WA. Regulation of intravenous nicotine self-administration–dopamine mechanisms. In: Adlkofer F, Thurau K, eds. Effects of nicotine on biological systems. Basel: Birkhauser Verlag, 1991:423–432.

237. Corrigall WA, Coen KM. Selective dopamine antagonists reduce nicotine self-administration. Psychopharmacology (Berl) 1991;104: 171–176.

238. Singer G, Wallace M, Hall R. Effects of dopaminergic nucleus accumbens lesions on the acquisition of schedule induced self injection of nicotine in the rat. Pharmacol Biochem Behav 1982;17: 579–581.

239. Corrigall WA, Franklin KBJ, Coen KM, Clarke PBS. The mesolimbic dopaminergic system is implicated in the reinforcing effects of nicotine. Psychopharmacology (Berl) 1992;107:285–289.

240. Clarke PBS, Pert A. Autoradiographic evidence for nicotine receptors on nigrostriatal and mesolimbic dopaminergic neurons. Brain Res 1985;348:355–358.

241. Deutch AY, Holliday J, Roth RH, Chun LLY, Hawrot E. Immunohistochemical localization of a neuronal nicotinic acetylcholine receptor in mammalian brain. Proc Natl Acad Sci U S A 1987;84: 8697–8701.

242. Swanson LW, Simmons DM, Whiting PJ, Lindstrom J. Immunohistochemical localization of neuronal nicotinic receptors in the rodent central nervous system. J Neurosci 1987;7:3334–3342.

243. Calabresi P, Lacey MG, North RA. Nicotinic excitation of rat ventral tegmental neurones *in vitro* studied by intracellular recording. Br J Pharmacol 1989;98:135–140.

244. Grenhoff J, Aston-Jones G, Svensson TH. Nicotinic effects on the firing pattern of midbrain dopamine neurons. Acta Physiol Scand 1986;128:351–358.

245. Clarke PBS, Hommer DW, Pert A, Skirboll LR. Electrophysiological actions of nicotine on substantia nigra single units. Br J Pharmacol 1985;85:827–835.

246. London ED, Connolly RJ, Szikszay M, Wamsley JK, Dam M. Effects of nicotine on local cerebral glucose utilization in the rat. J Neurosci 1988;8:3920–3928.

247. Rowell PP, Carr LA, Garner AC. Stimulation of [³H]dopamine release by nicotine in rat nucleus accumbens. J Neurochem 1987;49: 1449–1454.

248. Imperato A, Mulas A, Di Chiara G. Nicotine preferentially stimulates dopamine release in the limbic system of freely moving rats. Eur J Pharmacol 1986;132:337–338.

249. Mifsud J-C, Hernandez L, Hoebel BG. Nicotine infused into the

nucleus accumbens increases synaptic dopamine as measured by *in vivo* microdialysis. Brain Res 1989;478:365–367.

250. Nisell M, Nomikos GG, Svensson TH. Systemic nicotine-induced dopamine release in the rat nucleus accumbens is regulated by nicotinic receptors in the ventral tegmental area. Synapse 1994; 16:36–44.

251. Heath RG, Gallant DM. Activity of the human brain during emotional thought. In: Heath RG, ed. The role of pleasure in behavior. New York: Harper & Row, 1964:83–106.

252. Izenwasser S, Kornetsky C. Brain-stimulation reward: a method for assessing the neurochemical bases of drug-induced euphoria. In: Watson RR, ed. Drugs of abuse and neurobiology. Boca Raton: CRC Press, 1992:1–21.

253. Esposito RU, Kornetsky C. Opioids and rewarding brain stimulation. Neurosci Biobehav Rev 1978;2:115–122.

254. Esposito RU, Porrino LJ, Seeger TF. Brain stimulation reward: measurement and mapping by psychophysical techniques and quantitative 2-[^{14}C]deoxyglucose autoradiography. In: Bozarth MA, ed. Methods of assessing the reinforcing properties of abused drugs. New York: Springer-Verlag, 1987:421–445.

255. Seeger TF, Carlson KR. Amphetamine and morphine: additive effects on ICSS threshold. Soc Neurosci Abstr 1981;7:974

256. Hubner CB, Bain GT, Kornetsky C. Morphine and amphetamine: effect on brain stimulation reward. Soc Neurosci Abstr 1983; 9:893

257. Weeks JR, Collins RJ. Factors affecting voluntary morphine intake in self-maintained addicted rats. Psychopharmacologia 1964;6: 267–279.

258. Pickens R. Self-administration of stimulants by rats. Int J Addict 1968;3:215–221.

259. Lepore M, Franklin KBJ. Modelling drug kinetics with brain stimulation: Dopamine antagonists increase self-stimulation. Pharmacol Biochem Behav 1992;41:489–496.

260. Olds J, Travis RP. Effects of chlorpromazine, meprobamate, pentobarbital and morphine on self-stimulation. J Pharmacol Exp Ther 1960;128:397–404.

261. Wise RA, Rompre PP. Brain dopamine and reward. Annu Rev Psychol 1989;40:191–225.

262. Robertson A, Mogenson GJ. Evidence for a role for dopamine in self-stimulation of the nucleus accumbens of the rat. Can J Psychol 1978;32:67–76.

263. Stellar JR, Kelley AE, Corbett D. Effects of peripheral and central dopamine blockade on lateral hypothalamic self-stimulation: evidence for both reward and motor deficits. Pharmacol Biochem Behav 1983;18:433–442.

264. Stellar JR, Corbett D. Regional neuroleptic microinjections indicate a role for nucleus accumbens in lateral hypothalamic self-stimulation reward. Brain Res 1989;477:126–143.

265. Mora F, Sanguinetti AM, Rolls ET, Shaw SG. Differential effects of self-stimulation and motor behaviour produced by microintracranial injections of a dopamine-receptor blocking agent. Neurosci Lett 1975;1:179–184.

266. Kurumiya S, Nakajima S. Dopamine D$_1$ receptors in the nucleus accumbens: involvement in the reinforcing effect of tegmental stimulation. Brain Res 1988;448:1–6.

267. Ungerstedt U. Stereotaxic mapping of the monoamine pathways in the rat brain. Acta Physiol Scand 1971;367(suppl):1–48.

268. Deutsch JA. Behavioral measurement of the neural refractory period and its application to intracranial self-stimulation. J Comp Physiol Psychol 1964;58:1–9.

269. Gallistel CR. Self-stimulation: failure of pretrial stimulation to affect rats' electrode preference. J Comp Physiol Psychol 1969;69: 722–729.

270. Gallistel CR. The incentive of brain-stimulation reward. J Comp Physiol Psychol 1969;69:713–721.

271. Gallistel CR, Rolls E, Greene D. Neuron function inferred from behavioral and electrophysiological estimates of refractory period. Science 1969;166:1028–1030.

272. Gallistel CR. Self-stimulation in the rat: quantitative characteristics of the reward pathway. J Comp Physiol Psychol 1978;92:977–998.

273. Gallistel CR, Shizgal P, Yeomans JS. A portrait of the substrate for self-stimulation. Psychol Rev 1981;88:228–273.

274. Shizgal P, Bielajew C, Corbett D, Skelton R, Yeomans J. Behavioral methods for inferring anatomical linkage between rewarding brain stimulation sites. J Comp Physiol Psychol 1980;94:227–237.

275. Gallistel CR. Self stimulation. In: Deutsch JA, ed. The physiological basis of memory. New York: Academic Press, 1983:269–349.

276. Beninato M, Spencer RF. The cholinergic innervation of the rat substantia nigra: A light and electron microscopic immunohistochemical study. Exp Brain Res 1988;72:178–184.

277. Clarke PBS, Hommer DW, Pert A, Skirboll LR. Innervation of substantia nigra neurons by cholinergic afferents from pedunculopontine nucleus in the rat: neurochemical and electrophysiological evidence. Neuroscience 1987;23:1011–1019.

278. Gould E, Woolf NJ, Butcher LL. Cholinergic projections to the substantia nigra from the pedunculopontine and lateral dorsal tegmental nuclei. Neuroscience 1989;28:611–623.

279. Scarnati E, Prioria A, Campana E, Pacitti C. A microiniontophoretic study of the nature of the putative synaptic neurotransmitter involved in the pedunculopontine substantia nigra pars compacta excitatory pathway in the rat. Exp Brain Res 1986;62:470–478.

280. Gratton A, Wise RA. Hypothalamic reward mechanism: two first-stage fiber populations with cholinergic component. Science 1985;227:545–548.

281. Yeomans JS. Two substrates for medial forebrain bundle self-stimulation: Myelinated axons and dopamine axons. Neurosci Biobehavioral Rev 1989;13:91–98.

282. Wise RA, Bozarth MA. Brain substrates for reinforcement and drug self-administration. Prog Neuropsychopharmacol Biol Psychiatry 1981;5:467–474.

283. Broekkamp CLE, Pijnenburg AJJ, Cools AR, Van Rossum JM. The effect of microinjections of amphetamine into the neostriatum and the nucleus accumbens on self-stimulation behaviour. Psychopharmacologia 1975;42:179–183.

284. Broekkamp CL, van den Bogaard JH, Heijnen HJ, Rops RH, Cools AR, Van Rossum JM. Separation of inhibiting and stimulating effects of morphine on self-stimulation behaviour by intracerebral microinjections. Eur J Pharmacol 1976;36:443–446.

285. Broekkamp CLE, Van Rossum JM. The effect of microinjections of morphine and haloperidol into the neostriatum and the nucleus accumbens on self-stimulation behaviour. Arch Int Pharmacodyn Ther 1975;217:110–117.

286. Zetterström T, Sharp T, Marsden CA, Ungerstedt U. *In vivo* measurement of dopamine and its metabolites by intracerebral dialysis: changes after *d*-amphetamine. J Neurochem 1983;41:1769–1773.

287. Carboni E, Imperato A, Perezzani L, Di Chiara G. Amphetamine, cocaine, phencyclidine and nomifensine increase extracellular dopamine concentrations preferentially in the nucleus accumbens of freely moving rats. Neuroscience 1989;28:653–661.

288. Bradberry CW, Roth RH. Cocaine increases extracellular dopamine in rat nucleus accumbens and ventral tegmental area as shown by *in vivo* microdialysis. Neurosci Lett 1989;103:97–102.

289. Di Chiara G, Imperato A. Drugs abused by humans preferentially increase synaptic dopamine concentrations in the mesolimbic system of freely moving rats. Proc Natl Acad Sci USA 1988;85: 5274–5278.

290. Imperato A, Di Chiara G. Preferential stimulation of dopamine release in the nucleus accumbens of freely moving rats by ethanol. J Pharmacol Exp Ther 1986;239:219–228.

291. Di Chiara G, Imperato A. Preferential stimulation of dopamine release in the nucleus accumbens by opiates, alcohol, and barbiturates: studies with transcerebral dialysis in freely moving rats. Ann N Y Acad Sci 1986;473:367–381.

292. Hernandez L, Auerbach S, Hoebel BG. Phencyclidine (PCP) injected in the nucleus accumbens increases extracellular dopamine and

serotonin as measured by microdialysis. Life Sci 1988;42: 1713–1723.

293. Chen J, Paredes W, Li J, Smith D, Lowinson J, Gardner EL. Δ⁹-Tetrahydrocannabinol produces naloxone-blockable enhancement of presynaptic basal dopamine efflux in nucleus accumbens of conscious, freely-moving rats as measured by intracerebral microdialysis. Psychopharmacology (Berl) 1990;102:156–162.

294. Chen J, Paredes W, Lowinson J, Gardner EL. Δ⁹-Tetrahydrocannabinol enhances presynaptic dopamine efflux in medial prefrontal cortex. Eur J Pharmacol 1990;190:259–262.

295. Imperato A, Puglisi-Allegra S, Zocchi A, Scrocco MG, Casolini P, Angelucci L. Stress activation of limbic and cortical dopamine release is prevented by ICS 205-930 but not by diazepam. Eur J Pharmacol 1990;175:211–214.

296. Zetterström T, Fillenz M. Local administration of flurazepam has different effects on dopamine release in striatum and nucleus accumbens: a microdialysis study. Neuropharmacology 1990;29: 129–134.

297. Finlay JM, Damsma G, Fibiger HC. Benzodiazepine-induced decreases in extracellular concentrations of dopamine in the nucleus accumbens after acute and repeated administration. Psychopharmacology (Berl) 1992;106:202–208.

298. Fuxe K, Agnati LF, Bolme P, Hökfelt T, Lidbrink P, Ljungdahl A, Perez de la Mora M, Ogren SO. The possible involvement of GABA mechanisms in the action of benzodiazepines on central catecholamine neurons. In: Costa E, Greengard P, eds. Mechanism of action of benzodiazepines. New York: Raven Press, 1975:45–59.

299. Ishiko J, Inagaski C, Takaori S. Effects of diazepam, nitrazepam and brotizolam on dopamine turnover in the olfactory tubercle, nucleus accumbens and caudate nucleus of rats. Jpn J Pharmacol 1983;33: 706–708.

300. Lyness WH. Effect of L-tryptophan pretreatment on *d*-amphetamine self administration. Substance and alcohol actions/misuse 1983;4: 305–312.

301. Cone EJ, Risner ME, Neidert GL. Concentrations of phenethylamine in dog following single doses and during intravenous self administration. Res Commun Chem Pathol Pharmacol 1978; 22:211–232.

302. Yu DSL, Smith FL, Smith DG, Lyness WH. Fluoxetine-induced attenuation of amphetamine self-administration in rats. Life Sci 1986;39:1383–1388.

303. Leccese AP, Lyness WH. The effects of putative 5-hydroxytryptamine receptor active agents on *d*-amphetamine self-administration in controls and rats with 5,7-dihydroxytryptamine median forebrain bundle lesions. Brain Res 1984;303:153–162.

304. Zabik JE, Roache JD, Sidor R, Nash JF, Jr. The effects of fluoxetine on ethanol preference in the rat. Pharmacologist 1982;24:204.

305. Carroll ME, Lac ST, Asencio M, Kragh R. Fluoxetine reduces intravenous cocaine self-administration in rats. Pharmacol Biochem Behav 1990;35:237–244.

306. Rockman GE, Amit Z, Bourque C, Brown ZW, Ögren SO. Reduction of voluntary morphine consumption following treatment with zimelidine. Arch Int Pharmacodyn 1980;244:124–129.

307. Naranjo CA, Sellers EM, Roach CA, Woodley DV, Sanchez-Craig M, Sykora K. Zimelidine-induced variations in ethanol intake in non-depressed drinkers. Clin Pharmacol Ther 1984;35: 374–381.

308. Ritz MC, Kuhar MJ. Relationship between self-administration of amphetamine and monoamine receptors in brain: comparison with cocaine. J Pharmacol Exp Ther 1989;248:1010–1017.

309. Carboni E, Acquas E, Leone P, Di Chiara G. 5HT₃ receptor antagonists block morphine- and nicotine- but not amphetamine-induced reward. Psychopharmacology (Berl) 1989;97:175–178.

310. Pulvirenti L, Maldonado-Lopez R, Koob GF. NMDA receptors in the nucleus accumbens modulate intravenous cocaine but not heroin self-administration in the rat. Brain Res 1992;594:327–330.

311. Panksepp J, Herman BH, Vilberg T, Bishop P, DeEskinazi FG. Endogenous opioids and social behavior. Neurosci Biobehavioral Rev 1978;4:473–487.

312. Vaupel DB, Lange WR, London ED. Effects of verapamil on morphine-induced euphoria, analgesia and respiratory depression in humans. J Pharmacol Exp Ther 1993;267:1386–1394.

313. Hernandez L, Hoebel BG. Feeding and hypothalamic stimulation increase dopamine turnover in the accumbens. Physiol Behav 1988;44:599–606.

314. Robbins TW. Behavioural determinants of drug action: Rate-dependence revisited. In: Cooper SJ, ed. Theory in psychopharmacology. London: Academic Press, 1981:1–63.

315. Fibiger HC, Phillips AG. Mesocorticolimbic dopamine systems and reward. In: Kalivas PW, Nemeroff CB, eds. The mesocorticolimbic dopamine system. Bethesda: New York Academy of Science, 1988: 206–215.

316. Ljungberg T. Blockade by neuroleptics of water intake and operant responding for water in the rat: anhedonia, motor deficit, or both?. Pharmacol Biochem Behav 1987;27:341–350.

317. Ljungberg T. Effects of the dopamine D-1 antagonist SCH 23390 on water intake, water-rewarded operant responding and apomorphine-induced decrease of water intake in rats. Pharmacol Biochem Behav 1989;33:709–712.

318. Negus SS, Dykstra LA. κ Antagonist properties of buprenorphine in the shock titration procedure. Eur J Pharmacol 1988;156: 77–86.

319. Tyrka A, Gayle C, Smith GP. Raclopride decreases sucrose intake of rat pups in independent ingestion test. Pharmacol Biochem Behav 1992;43:863–869.

320. Kelley AE, Delfs JM. Dopamine and conditioned reinforcement: I. Differential effects of amphetamine microinjections into striatal subregions. Psychopharmacology (Berl) 1991;103:187–196.

321. Cador M, Taylor JR, Robbins TW. Potentiation of the effects of reward-related stimuli by dopaminergic-dependent mechanisms in the nucleus accumbens. Psychopharmacology (Berl) 1991;104: 377–385.

322. Heffner TG, Luttinger D, Hartman JA, Seiden LS. Regional changes in brain catecholamine turnover in the rat during performance on fixed ratio and variable interval schedules of reinforcement. Brain Res 1981;214:215–218.

323. Joseph MH, Hodges H. Lever pressing for food reward and changes in dopamine turnover and uric acid in rat caudate and nucleus accumbens studied chronically by *in vivo* voltammetry. J Neurosci Methods 1990;34:143–149.

324. Pert CB, Hill JM, Ruff MR, et al. Octapeptides deduced from the neuropeptide receptor-like pattern of antigen T4 in brain potently inhibit human immunodeficiency virus receptor binding and T-cell infectivity. Proc Natl Acad Sci U S A 1986;83:9254–9258.

325. Browne RG, Welch WM. Stereoselective antagonism of phencyclidine's discriminative properties by adenosine receptor agonists. Science 1982;217:1157–1159.

326. Nies AS. Principles of therapeutics. In: Gilman AG, Rall TW, Nies AS, Taylor P, eds. The pharmacological basis of therapeutics. New York: Pergamon Press, 1990:62–83.

327. Jaffe JH. Drug addiction and drug abuse. In: Gilman AG, Rall TW, Nies AS, Taylor P, eds. The pharmacological basis of therapeutics. New York: Pergamon Press, 1990:522–573.

328. Goodman RR, Adler BA, Pasternak GW. Regional distribution of opioid receptors. In: Pasternak GW, ed. The opiate receptors. Clifton: Humana, 1988:197–228.

329. White FJ, Wolf ME. Psychomotor stimulants. In: Pratt JA, ed. The biological bases of drug tolerance. London: Academic Press, 1991: 153–197.

330. Wolf ME, White FJ, Hu X-T. Behavioral sensitization to MK-801 (dizocilpine): neurochemical and electrophysiological correlates in the mesoaccumbens dopamine system. Behav Pharmacol 1993;4: 429–442.

331. Koob GF, Bloom FE. Cellular and molecular mechanisms of drug dependence. Science 1988;242:715–723.

331a. Falk JL, Fang MA, Lau CE. Chronic oral cocaine self-administration: pharmacokinetics and effects or spontaneous and discriminative motor functions. J Pharmacol Exp Ther 1991;257:457–465.

331b. Reith ME, Benuck M, Lajtha A. Cocaine disposition in the brain after continuous or intermittent treatment and locomotor stimulation in mice. J Pharmacol Exp Ther 1991;243:281–287.

332. Collins AC, Burch JB, de Fiebre CM, Marks MJ. Tolerance to and cross tolerance between ethanol and nicotine. Pharmacol Biochem Behav 1988;29:365–373.

333. Burch JB, de Fiebre CM, Marks MJ, Collins AC. Chronic ethanol or nicotine treatment results in partial cross-tolerance between these agents. Psychopharmacology (Berl) 1988;95:452–458.

334. Nestler EJ. Molecular mechanisms of drug addiction. J Neurosci 1992;12:2439–2450.

335. Loh HH, Smith AP. Molecular characterization of opioid receptors. Annu Rev Pharmacol Toxicol 1990;30:123–147.

336. Wüster M, Schulz R, Herz A. Opioid tolerance and dependence: re-evaluating the unitary hypothesis. Trends Pharmacol Sci 1985; 64–67.

337. Ling GSF, MacLeod JM, Lee S, Lockhart SH, Pasternak GW. Separation of morphine analgesia from physical dependence. Science 1984;226:462–464.

338. Suzuki T, Hayashi Y, Misawa M. The role of mu_1 receptor in physical dependence on morphine using the mu receptor deficient CXBK mouse. Life Sci 1992;50:849–856.

339. Bozarth MA, Wise RA. Anatomically distinct opiate receptor fields mediate reward and physical dependence. Science 1984;224:516–517.

340. Aghajanian GK, Wang Y-Y. Common α_2- and opiate effector mechanisms in the locus coeruleus: intracellular studies in brain slices. Neuropharmacology 1987;26:793–799.

341. Redmond DE, Jr., Krystal JH. Multiple mechanism of withdrawal from opioid drugs. Annu Rev Neurosci 1984;7:443–478.

342. Williams JT, North RA. Opiate-receptor interactions on single locus coeruleus neurones. Mol Pharmacol 1984;26:489–497.

343. Grant SJ, Redmond DE, Jr. The neuroanatomy and pharmacology of the nucleus locus coeruleus. In: Lal H, Fielding S, eds. Psychopharmacology of clonidine. N.Y.: Alan R. Liss, 1981:5–27.

344. Foote SL, Bloom FE, Aston-Jones G. Nucleus locus coeruleus: new evidence of anatomical and physiological specificity. Physiology 1983;63:844–900.

345. Pinnock RD. A highly selective kappa-opioid receptor agonist, CI-977, reduces excitatory synaptic potentials in the rat locus coeruleus in vitro. Neuroscience 1992;47:87–94.

346. McFadzean I, Lacey MG, Hill RG, Henderson G. Kappa opioid receptor activation depresses excitatory synaptic input to rat locus coeruleus neurons in vitro. Neuroscience 1987;20:231–239.

347. Korf J, Bunney BS, Aghajanian GK. Noradrenergic neurons: morphine inhibition of spontaneous activity. Eur J Pharmacol 1974;25:165–169.

348. Aghajanian GK. Tolerance of locus coeruleus neurones to morphine and suppression of withdrawal response by clonidine. Nature 1978;276:186–187.

349. Bird SJ, Kuhar MJ. Iontophoretic application of opiates to the locus coeruleus. Brain Res 1977;122:523–533.

350. Strahlendorf HK, Strahlendorf JC, Barnes CD. Endorphin-mediated inhibition of locus coeruleus neurons. Brain Res 1980;191:284–288.

351. Andrade R, Vandermaelen CP, Aghajanian GK. Morphine tolerance and dependence in the locus coeruleus: single cell studies in the brain slices. Eur J Pharmacol 1983;91:161–169.

352. Christie MJ, Williams JT, North RA. Cellular mechanisms of opioid tolerance: studies in single brain neurons. Mol Pharmacol 1987;32:633–638.

353. North RA, Williams JT. On the potassium conductance increased by opioids in rat locus coeruleus neurones. J Physiol (Lond) 1985;364:265–280.

354. Aghajanian GK, Wang Y-Y. Pertussis toxin blocks the outward currents evoked by opiate and α_2 agonists in locus coeruleus neurons. Brain Res 1986;371:390–394.

355. Pepper CM, Henderson G. Opiates and opioid peptides hyperpolarize locus coeruleus neurons in vitro. Science 1980;209:394–396.

356. Childers SR. Opioid receptor-coupled second messenger systems. Life Sci 1991;48:1991–2003.

357. Wang Y-Y, Aghajanian GK. Intracellular GTPγS restores the ability of morphine to hyperpolarize rat locus coeruleus neurons after the blockade by pertussis toxin. Brain Res 1987;436:396–401.

358. Nestler EJ, Erdos JJ, Terwilliger R, Duman RS, Tallman JF. Regulation of G-proteins by chronic morphine in the rat locus coeruleus. Brain Res 1989;476:230–239.

359. Nestler EJ, Tallman JF. Chronic morphine treatment increases cyclic AMP-dependent protein kinase activity in the rat locus coeruleus. Mol Pharmacol 1988;33:127–132.

360. Collier HOJ. Cellular site of opiate dependence. Nature 1980;283:625–629.

361. Collier HOJ, Francis DL. Morphine abstinence is associated with increased brain cyclic AMP. Nature 1975;255:159–162.

362. Duman RS, Tallman JF, Nestler EJ. Acute and chronic opiate-regulation of adenylate cyclase in brain: specific effects in locus coeruleus. J Pharmacol Exp Ther 1988;246:1033–1039.

363. Trujillo KA, Akil H. Inhibition of morphine tolerance and dependence by the NMDA receptor antagonist MK-801. Science 1991;251:85–87.

364. Kolesnikov YA, Pick CG, Pasternak GW. N^G-nitro-l-arginine prevents morphine tolerance. Eur J Pharmacol 1992;221:399–400.

365. Highfield DA, Grant SJ, Revay RS. Nitric oxide modulates opioid tolerance in LC neuronal activity in vitro. Soc Neurosci Abstr 1993;19:1460

366. Kolesnikov YA, Pick CG, Ciszewska G, Pasternak GW. Blockade of tolerance to morphine but not to k opioids by a nitric oxide synthase inhibitor. Proc Natl Acad Sci USA 1993;90:5162–5166.

367. Dawson VL, Dawson TM, London ED, Bredt DS, Snyder SH. Nitric oxide mediates glutamate neurotoxicity in primary cortical cultures. Proc Natl Acad Sci U S A 1991;88:6368–6371.

368. Zhang J, Dawson VL, Dawson TM, Snyder SH. Nitric oxide activation of poly(ADP-Ribose) synthetase in neurotoxicity. Science 1994;263:687–689.

369. Geary WA, II, Wooten GF. Similar functional anatomy of spontaneous and precipitated morphine withdrawal. Brain Res 1985;334:183–186.

370. Bläsig J, Hetz A, Reinhold K, Zieglgänsberger S. Development of physical dependence on morphine in respect to time and dosage and quantification of the precipitated withdrawal syndrome in rats. Psychopharmacologia 1973;33:19–38.

371. Tatum AL, Seevers MH, Collins KH. Morphine addiction and its physiological interpretation based on experimental evidences. J Pharmacol Exp Ther 1929;36:447–464.

372. Jiang ZG, North RA. Pre- and postsynaptic inhibition by opioids in rat striatum. J Neurosci 1992;12:356–361.

373. Negus SS, Henriksen SJ, Mattox A, et al. Effect of antagonists selective for $mu, delta,$ and $kappa$ opioid receptors on the reinforcing effects of heroin in rats. J Pharmacol Exp Ther 1993;265:1245–1252.

374. Kimes AS, London ED. Glucose utilization in the rat brain during chronic morphine treatment and naloxone-precipitated morphine withdrawal. J Pharmacol Exp Ther 1989;248:538–545.

375. Koob GF, Maldonado R, Stinus L. Neural substrates of opiate withdrawal. Trends Neurosci 1992;15:186–191.

376. Bowen WD, Kirschner BN, Newman AH, Rice KC. σ receptors negatively modulate agonist-stimulated phosphoinositide metabolism in rat brain. Eur J Pharmacol 1988;149:399–400.

377. Charney DS, Sternberg DE, Kleber HD, Heninger GR, Redmond DE, Jr. The clinical use of clonidine in abrupt withdrawal from methadone. Effects on blood pressure and specific signs and symptoms. Arch Gen Psychiatry 1981;38:1273–1277.

378. Taylor JR, Elsworth JD, Garcia EJ, Grant SJ, Roth RH, Redmond DE, Jr. Clonidine infusions into the locus coeruleus attenuate behavioral and neurochemical changes associated with naloxone-precipitated withdrawal. Psychopharmacology (Berl) 1988;96:121–134.

379. Klonoff DC, Andrews BT, Obana WG. Stroke associated with cocaine use. Arch Neurol 1989;46:989–993.

380. Esposito E, Kruszewska A, Ossowska G, Samanin R. Noradrenergic and behavioural effects of naloxone injected in the locus coeruleus of morphine-dependent rats and their control by clonidine. Psychopharmacology (Berl) 1987;93:393–396.

381. Valentino RJ, Wehby RG. Locus ceruleus discharge characteristics of morphine-dependent rats: effects of naltrexone. Brain Res 1989;488:126–134.

382. Swann AC, Elsworth JD, Charney DS, et al. Brain catecholamine metabolites and behavior in morphine withdrawal. Eur J Pharmacol 1983;86:167–175.

383. Crawley JN, Ninan PT, Pickar D, et al. Neuropharmacological antagonism of the β carboline-induced "anxiety" response in rhesus monkeys. J Neurosci 1985;5:477–485.

384. Silverstone PH, Done C, Sharp T. In vivo monoamine release during naloxone-precipitated morphine withdrawal. Neuroreport 1993;4:1043–1045.

385. Kogan JH, Nestler EJ, Aghajanian GK. Elevated basal firing rates and enhanced responses to 8-Br-cAMP in locus coeruleus neurons in brain slices from opiate-dependent rats. Eur J Pharmacol 1992;211:47–53.

386. Rasmussen K, Beitner-Johnson D, Krystal JH, Aghajanian GK, Nestler EJ. Opiate withdrawal and the rat locus coeruleus: behavioral, electrophysiological, and biochemical correlates. J Neurosci 1990;10:2308–2317.

387. Grant SJ, Aston-Jones G, Redmond DE, Jr. Responses of primate locus coeruleus neurons to simple and complex sensory stimuli. Brain Res Bull 1988;21:401–410.

388. Maldonado R, Stinus L, Gold LH, Koob GF. Role of different brain structures in the expression of the physical morphine withdrawal syndrome. J Pharmacol Exp Ther 1992;261:669–677.

389. Maldonado R, Koob GF. Destruction of the locus coeruleus decreases physical signs of opiate withdrawal. Brain Res 1993;605:128–138.

390. Valentino RJ, Aston-Jones G. Activation of locus coeruleus neurons in the rat by a benzazocine derivative (UM 1046) that mimics opiate withdrawal. Neuropharmacology 1983;22:1363–1368.

391. Rasmussen K, Aghajanian GK. Withdrawal-induced activation of locus coeruleus neurons in opiate-dependent rats: attenuation by lesions of the nucleus paragigantocellularis. Brain Res 1989;505:346–350.

392. Cappendijk SL, de Vries R, Dzoljic MR. Excitatory amino acid receptor antagonists and naloxone-precipitated withdrawal syndrome in morphine-dependent mice. Eur Neuropsychopharmacol 1993;3:111–116.

393. Aghajanian GK, Kogan JH, Moghaddam B. Opiate withdrawal increases glutamate and aspartate efflux in the locus coeruleus: an *in vivo* microdialysis study. Brain Res 1994;636:126–130.

394. Oleskevich S, Clements JD, Williams JT. Opioid-glutamate interactions in rat locus coeruleus neurons. J Neurophysiol 1993;70:931–937.

395. Saper CB. Function of the locus coeruleus. Trends Neurosci 1987;10:343–344.

396. Hayward MD, Duman RS, Nestler EJ. Induction of the *c-fos* proto-oncogene during opiate withdrawal in the locus coeruleus and other regions of rat brain. Brain Res 1990;525:256–266.

397. Murase S, Nisell M, Grenhoff J, Svensson TH. Decreased sensory responsiveness of noradrenergic neurons in the rat locus coeruleus following phencyclidine or dizocilpine (MK-801): role of NMDA antagonism. Psychopharmacology (Berl) 1992;109:271–276.

398. Rasmussen K, Fuller RW, Stockton ME, Perry KW, Swinford RM, Ornstein PL. NMDA receptor antagonists suppress behaviors but not norepinephrine turnover or locus coeruleus unit activity induced by opiate withdrawal. Eur J Pharmacol 1991;197:9–16.

399. Trujillo KA, Akil H. The NMDA receptor antagonist MK-801 increases morphine catalepsy and lethality. Pharmacol Biochem Behav 1991;38:673–675.

400. Shiekhattar R, Aston-Jones G. NMDA-receptor mediated sensory responses of brain noradrenergic neurons are suppressed by *in vivo* concentrations of extracellular magnesium. Synapse 1992;10:103–109.

401. Kimes AS, Vaupel DB, London ED. Attenuation of some signs of opioid withdrawal by inhibitors of nitric oxide synthase. Psychopharmacology (Berl) 1993;112:521–524.

402. Vaupel DB, Kimes AS, London ED. Comparison of 7-nitroindazole with other nitric oxide synthase inhibitors as attenuators of opioid withdrawal. Psychopharmacology (Berl) 1995;118:361–368.

403. Adams ML, Kalicki JM, Meyer ER, Cicero TJ. Inhibition of the morphine withdrawal syndrome by a nitric oxide synthase inhibitor, N^G-nitro-L-arginine methyl ester. Life Sci 1993;52:PL245–PL249.

404. Hope BT, Michael GJ, Knigge KM, Vincent SR. Neuronal NADPH diaphorase is a nitric oxide synthase. Proc Natl Acad Sci USA 1991;88:2811–2814.

405. Dawson TM, Bredt DS, Fotuhi M, Hwang PM, Snyder SH. Nitric oxide synthase and neuronal NADPH diaphorase are identical in brain and peripheral tissues. Proc Natl Acad Sci USA 1991;88:7797–7801.

406. Fanelli RJ, Dersch CM, London ED. Effects of subchronic morphine on choline acetyltransferase and muscarinic binding in the rat brain. Res Commun Subst Abuse 1985;6:189–192.

407. Buccafusco JJ. Inhibition of the morphine withdrawal syndrome by a novel muscarinic antagonist (4-DAMP). Life Sci 1991;48:749–756.

408. Kanof PD, Handelsman L, Aronson MJ, Ness R, Cochrane KJ, Rubinstein KJ. Clinical characteristics of naloxone-precipitated withdrawal in human opioid-dependent subjects. J Pharmacol Exp Ther 1992;260:355–363.

409. Gellert VF, Sparber SB. A comparison of the effects of naloxone upon body weight loss and suppression of fixed-ratio operant behavior in morphine-dependent rats. J Pharmacol Exp Ther 1977;201:44–54.

410. Manning FJ, Jackson MC, Jr. Enduring effects of morphine pellets revealed by conditioned taste aversion. Psychopharmacology (Berl) 1977;51:279–283.

411. Hand TH, Koob GF, Stinus L, Le Moal M. Aversive properties of opiate receptor blockade: evidence for exclusively central mediation in naive and morphine-dependent rats. Brain Res 1988;474:364–368.

412. Higgins GA, Sellers EM. Antagonist precipitated opioid withdrawal in rats: evidence for dissociation between physical and motivational signs. Pharmacol Biochem Behav 1994;48:1–8.

413. Koob GF, Wall TL, Bloom FE. Nucleus accumbens as a substrate for the aversive stimulus effects of opiate withdrawal. Psychopharmacology (Berl) 1989;98:530–534.

414. Terwilliger RZ, Beitner-Johnson D, Sevarino KA, Crain SM, Nestler EJ. A general role for adaptations in G-proteins and the cyclic AMP system in mediating the chronic actions of morphine and cocaine on neuronal function. Brain Res 1991;548:100–110.

415. Hakan RL, Henriksen SJ. Systemic opiate administration has heterogenous effects on activity recorded from nucleus accumbens neurons *in vivo*. Neurosci Lett 1987;83:307–312.

416. Hakan RL, Henriksen SJ. Opiate influences on nucleus accumbens neuronal electrophysiology: dopamine and non-dopamine mechanisms. J Neurosci 1989;8:3538–3546.

417. Pothos E, Rada P, Mark GP, Hoebel BG. Dopamine microdialysis in the nucleus accumbens during acute and chronic morphine, naloxone-precipitated withdrawal and clonidine treatment. Brain Res 1991;566:348–350.

418. Rossetti ZL, Hmaidan Y, Gessa GL. Marked inhibition of mesolimbic dopamine release: a common feature of ethanol, morphine, cocaine and amphetamine abstinence in rats. Eur J Pharmacol 1992;221:227–234.

419. Rada P, Pothos E, Mark GP, Hoebel BG. Microdialysis evidence that acetylcholine in the nucleus accumbens is involved in morphine withdrawal and its treatment with clonidine. Brain Res 1991;561:354–356.

420. File SE, Pellow S. Behavioral pharmacology of minor tranquilizers. In: Balfour DJK, ed. Psychotropic drugs of abuse. New York: Pergamon Press, 1990:147–172.

421. Pohorecky LA, Brick J. Pharmacology of ethanol. In: Balfour DJK, ed. Psychotropic drugs of abuse. New York: 1990:189–281.

422. Okamoto M, Boisse NR. Sedative-hypnotic tolerance and physical dependence. Trends Pharmacol Sci 1981;2:9–13.

423. Tallman JF, Gallager DW. The GABA-ergic system: a locus of benzodiazepine action. Annu Rev Neurosci 1985;8:21–44.

424. Waterhouse BD, Moises HC, Yeh HH, Geller HM, Woodward DJ. Comparison of norepinephrine- and benzodiazepine-induced augmentation of Purkinje cell response to γ-aminobutyric acid (GABA). J Pharmacol Exp Ther 1984;228:257–267.

425. Gallager DW, Lakoski JM, Gonsalves SF, Rauch SL. Chronic benzodiazepine treatment decreases postsynaptic GABA sensitivity. Nature 1984;308:74–77.

426. Gallager DW, Malcolm AB, Anderson SA, Gonsalves SF. Continuous release of diazepam: electrophysiological, biochemical and behavioral consequences. Brain Res 1985;342:26–36.

427. Miller LG, Woolverton S, Greenblatt DJ, Lopez F, Roy RB, Shader RI. Chronic benzodiazepine administration. IV. Rapid development of tolerance and receptor downregulation associated with alprazolam administration. Biochem Pharmacol 1989;38:3773–3777.

428. Rosenberg HC, Chiu TH. Regional specificity of benzodiazepine receptor down-regulation during chronic treatment of rats with flurazepam. Neurosci Lett 1981;24:4–52.

429. Chiu TH, Rosenberg HC. Reduced diazepam binding following chronic benzodiazepine treatment. Life Sci 1978;23:1153–1158.

430. Rosenberg HC, Chiu TH. Decreased ^{3}H-diazepam binding is a specific response to chronic benzodiazepine treatment. Life Sci 1979;24:803–808.

431. Allan AM, Baier LD, Zhang X. Effects of lorazepam tolerance and withdrawal on GABA-$_A$ receptor-operated chloride channels. J Pharmacol Exp Ther 1992;261:395–402.

432. Lamb RJ, Griffiths RR. Effects of Ro 15-1788 and CGS 8216 in diazepam-dependent baboons. Eur J Pharmacol 1987;143:205–212.

433. Wilson MA, Gallager DW. GABAergic subsensitivity of dorsal raphe neurons *in vitro* after chronic benzodiazepine treatment *in vivo*. Brain Res 1988;473:198–202.

434. Marley R, Gallager DW. Chronic diazepam treatment produces regionally specific changes in GABA-stimulated chloride influx. Eur J Pharmacol 1989;159:217–223.

435. Heninger C, Gallager DW. Altered gamma-aminobutyric acid/benzodiazepine interaction after chronic diazepam exposure. Neuropharmacology 1988;27:1073–1076.

436. Gonsalves SF, Gallager DW. Time course for development of anticonvulsant tolerance and GABAergic subsensitivity after chronic diazepam. Brain Res 1987;405:94–99.

437. Wilson MA, Gallager DW. Effects of chronic diazepam exposure on GABA sensitivity and on benzodiazepine potentiation of GABA-mediated responses of substantia nigra pars reticulata neurons of rats. Eur J Pharmacol 1987;136:333–343.

438. Wilson MA, Gallager DW. Responses of substantia nigra pars reticulata neurons to benzodiazepine ligands after acute and prolonged diazepam exposure. II. Modulation of firing rate. J Pharmacol Exp Ther 1989;248:886–891.

439. Wilson MA, Gallager DW. Responses of substantia nigra pars reticulata neurons to benzodiazepine ligands after acute and prolonged diazepam exposure. I. Modulation of γ-aminobutyric acid sensitivity. J Pharmacol Exp Ther 1989;248:879–885.

440. Gallager DW, Rauch SL, Malcolm AB. Alterations in a low affinity GABA recognition site following chronic benzodiazepine treatment. Eur J Pharmacol 1984;98:159–160.

441. Heninger C, Saito N, Tallman JF, et al. Effects of continuous diazepam administration on GABA-A subunit mRNA in rat brain. J Mol Neurosci 1990;2:101–107.

442. Bell J, Bickford-Wimer PC, de la Garza R, Egan M, Freedman R. Increased central noradrenergic activity during benzodiazepine withdrawal: an electrophysiological study. Neuropharmacology 1988;27:1187–1190.

443. Morrow AL, Suzdak PD, Karanian JW, Paul SM. Chronic ethanol administration alters g-aminobutyric acid, pentobarbital, and ethanol-mediated ^{36}Cl-uptake in cerebral cortical synaptoneurosomes. J Pharmacol Exp Ther 1988;246:158–164.

444. Gray PL, Taberner PV. Evidence for GABA tolerance in barbiturate-dependent and withdrawn mice. Neuropharmacology 1985;24:437–444.

445. Sanna E, Harris RA. Recent developments in alcoholism: neuronal ion channels. Recent Dev Alcohol 1993;11:169–186.

446. Im WB, Blakeman DP. Correlation between γ-aminobutyric acid$_A$ receptor ligand-induced changes in *t*-butylbicyclophosphoro [^{35}S]thionate binding and ^{36}Cl-uptake in rat cerebrocortical membranes. Mol Pharmacol 1991;39:394–398.

447. Saunders PA, Ho IK. Barbiturates and the GABA-A receptor complex. Prog Drug Res 1990;34:261–286.

448. Sanna E, Serra M, Cossu A, et al. Chronic ethanol intoxication induces differential effects on GABA$_A$ and NMDA receptor function in the rat brain. Alcohol Clin Exp Res 1993;17:115–123.

449. Buck KJ, Harris RA. Benzodiazepine agonist and inverse agonist actions on GABA-$_A$ receptor-operated chloride ion channels. II. Chronic effects of ethanol. J Pharmacol Exp Ther 1990;253:713–719.

450. Wu PH, Mihic SJ, Liu JF, Le AD, Kalant H. Blockade of chronic tolerance to ethanol by the NMDA antagonist, (+)-MK-801. Eur J Pharmacol 1993;231:157–164.

451. Weight FF, Lovinger DM, White G. Alcohol inhibition of NMDA channel function. Alcohol Alcohol Suppl 1991;1:163–169.

452. Snell LD, Tabakoff B, Hoffman PL. Radioligand binding to the N-methyl-D-aspartate receptor/ionophore complex: alterations by ethanol *in vitro* and by chronic *in vivo* ethanol injections. Brain Res 1993;602:91–98.

453. Criswell HE, Simson PE, Duncan GE, et al. Molecular basis for regionally specific action of ethanol on gamma-aminobutyric acid A receptors: generalization to other ligand-gated ion channels. J Pharmacol Exp Ther 1993;267:522–537.

454. Tabakoff B, Hoffman PL. Ethanol, sedative hypnotics, and glutamate receptor function in brain and cultured cells. Behav Genet 1993;23:231–236.

455. Davidson MD, Wilce P, Shanley BC. Increased sensitivity of the hippocampus in ethanol-dependent rats to toxic effect of N-methyl-D-aspartic acid *in vivo*. Brain Res 1993;606:5–9.

456. Szabo G, Tabakoff B, Hoffman PL. The NMDA receptor antagonist dizocilpine differentially affects environment-dependent and environment-independent ethanol tolerance. Psychopharmacology (Berl) 1994;113:511–517.

457. Tyrer P. Dependence as a limiting factor in the clinical use of minor tranquilizers. In: Balfour DJK, ed. Psychotropic drugs of abuse. New York: Pergamon Press, 1990:173–188.

458. Griffiths RR, Sannerud CA. Abuse of and dependence on benzodiazepines and other anxiolytic/sedative drugs. In: Meltzer HY, ed. Psychopharmacology: the third generation of progress. New York: Raven Press, 1987:1535–1541.

458a Tall JF, Gallager DW. The GAB-ergic system: a locus of benzodiazepine action. Annu Rev Neurosci 1985;8:21–44.

459. Martin WR, McNicholas LF, Cherian S. Diazepam and pentobarbital dependence in the rat. Life Sci 1982;31:721–730.

460. Wulff MH. The barbiturate withdrawal syndrome. A clinical and electroencephalographic study. Electroencephalogr Clin Neurophysiol 1960;Suppl 14:1–173.

461. Lukas SE, Griffiths RR. Precipitated withdrawal by a benzodiazepine receptor antagonist (Ro 15-1788) after 7 days of diazepam. Science 1982;217:1161–1163.

462. Emmett-Oglesby M, Spencer DG, Jr., Lewis MW, Elmesallamy F, Lal H. Anxiogenic aspects of diazepam withdrawal can be detected in animals. Eur J Pharmacol 1983;92:127–130.

463. Martin WR, Sloan JW, Wala EP. Precipitated abstinence in the diazepam-dependent rat. Pharmacol Biochem Behav 1993;46:683–688.

464. Winokur A, Rickels K, Greenblatt DJ, Snyder PJ, Schatz NJ. Withdrawal reaction from long-term, low-dosage administration of

diazepam. A double-blind, placebo-controlled case study. Arch Gen Psychiatry 1990;37:101–105.

465. Miczek KA, Vivian JA. Automatic quantification of withdrawal from 5-day diazepam in rats: ultrasonic distress vocalizations and hyper-reflexia to acoustic startle stimuli. Psychopharmacology (Berl) 1993;110:379–382.

466. Essig CF. Barbiturate withdrawal in white rats. Int J Neuropharmacol 1966;5:103–107.

467. Essig CF. Clinical and experimental aspects of barbiturate withdrawal convulsions. Epilepsia 1967;8:21–30.

468. Lukas SE, Griffiths RR. Precipitated diazepam withdrawal in baboons: effects of dose and duration of diazepam exposure. Eur J Pharmacol 1984;100:163–171.

469. Ryan GP, Boisse NR. Experimental induction of benzodiazepine tolerance and physical dependence. J Pharmacol Exp Ther 1983;226:100–107.

470. McNicholas LF, Martin WR. The effect of a benzodiazepine antagonist, Ro 15-1788, in diazepam dependent rats. Life Sci 1982;31:731–737.

471. Balfour DJK. Nicotine as the basis of the smoking habit. In: Balfour DJK, ed. Psychotropic drugs of abuse. New York: Pergamon Press, 1990:453–481.

472. Dituri B, Gilman LH. Withdrawal symptoms of barbiturate addiction: a little-known syndrome. J Phila Gen Hosp 1951;2:2–5.

473. Pevnick JS, Jasinski DR, Haertzen CA. Abrupt withdrawal from therapeutically administered diazepam. Report of a case. Arch Gen Psychiatry 1978;35:995–998.

474. Greenblatt DJ, Shader RI. Pharmacokinetics of antianxiety agents. In: Meltzer HY, ed. Psychopharmacology: the third generation of progress. New York: Raven Press, 1987:1377–1386.

475. Rosenberg HW, Chiu TH. An antagonist-induced benzodiazepine abstinence syndrome. Eur J Pharmacol 1982;81:153–157.

476. Grant SJ, Golloway MP, Maynor R, et al. Precipitated diazepam withdrawal elevates noradrenergic metabolism in primate brain. Eur J Pharmacol 1985;107:127–132.

477. Gonsalves SF, Gallager DW. Spontaneous and Ro 15-1788-induced reversal of subsensitivity to GABA following chronic benzodiazepines. Eur J Pharmacol 1985;110:163–170.

478. Morgan PF, Nadi NS, Karanian J, Linnoila M. Mapping rat brain structures activated during ethanol withdrawal: role of glutamate and NMDA receptors. Eur J Pharmacol 1992;225:217–223.

479. Ableitner A, Wüster M, Herz A. Specific changes in local cerebral glucose utilization in the rat brain induced by acute and chronic diazepam. Brain Res 1985;359:49–56.

480. Marietta CA, Eckardt MJ, Zbicz KL, Weight FF. Cerebral glucose utilization during diazepam withdrawal in rats. Brain Res 1990;511:192–196.

481. Young WS, III, Kuhar MJ. Radiohistochemical localization of benzodiazepine receptors in rat brain. J Pharmacol Exp Ther 1980;212:337–346.

482. Rall TW, Schleifer LS. Drugs effective in the therapy of the epilepsies. In: Gilman AG, Rall TW, Nies AS, Taylor P, eds. The pharmacological basis of therapeutics. New York: Pergamon Press, 1990:436–462.

483. Hobson JA, Lydic R, Baghdoyan HA. Evolving concepts of sleep cycle generation: from brain centers to neuronal populations. Behav Brain Sci 1986;9:371–448.

484. Steriade M, McCarley RW, ed. Brainstem control of wakefulness and sleep. New York: Plenum Press, 1990.

485. Nutt D, Molyneux S. Benzodiazepines, plasma MHPG and *alpha-2* adrenoceptor function in man. Int Clin Psychopharmacol 1987;2:151–157.

486. Idemudia SO, Mathis DA, Lal H. Enhancement of a diazepam withdrawal symptom by bicuculline and yohimbine. Neuropharmacology 1987;26:1739–1743.

487. Wilkins JN, Gorelick DA. Clinical neuroendocrinology and neuro-pharmacology of alcohol withdrawal. Recent Dev Alcohol 1986;4:241–263.

488. Engberg G, Hajos M. Alcohol withdrawal reaction as a result of adaptive changes of excitatory amio acid receptors. Naunyn Schmiedebergs Arch Pharmacol 1992;346:437–441.

489. Redmond DE, Jr. Studies of the nucleus locus coeruleus in monkeys and hypotheses for neuropsychopharmacology. In: Meltzer HY, ed. Psychopharmacology: the third generation of progress. New York: Raven Press, 1987:967–983.

490. Grant SJ, Huang YH, Redmond DE. Benzodiazepines attenuate single unit activity in the locus coeruleus. Life Sci 1980;27:2331–2236.

491. Simon PE, Weiss JM. Peripheral, but not local or intracerebroventricular, administration of benzodiazepines attenuates evoked activity of locus coeruleus neurons. Brain Res 1989;490:236–242.

492. Redmond DE, Jr., Huang YH. New evidence for a locus coeruleus-norepinephrine connection with anxiety. Life Sci 1979;25:2149–2162.

493. Duka T, Ackenheil M, Noderer J, Doenicke A, Dorow R. Changes in noradrenaline plasma levels and behavioural responses induced by benzodiazepine agonists with the benzodiazepine antagonist Ro 15-1788. Psychopharmacology (Berl) 1986;90:351–357.

494. Aston-Jones G, Foote SL, Bloom FE. Low doses of ethanol disrupt sensory responses of brain noradrenergic neurones. Nature 1982;296:857–860.

495. Pohorecky LA, Brick J. Activity of neurons in the locus coeruleus of the rat: inhibition by ethanol. Brain Res 1977;131:174–179.

496. Osmanovic SS, Shefner SA. Enhancement of current induced by superfusion of GABA in locus coeruleus neurons by pentobarbital, but not ethanol. Brain Res 1990;517:324–329.

497. Verbanck PMP, Seutin V, Massotte L, Dresse A. Differential effects of picrotoxin and RO 15-1788 on high and low ethanol concentrations on rat locus coerules *in vitro*. Eur J Pharmacol 1992;211:15–21.

498. Grant SJ, Mayor R, Redmond DE, Jr. Effects of alprazolam, a novel triazolobenzodiazepine on locus coeruleus unity activity. Soc Neurosci Abstr 1984;10:952.

499. Insel TR, Ninan PT, Aloi J, Jimerson DC, Skolnick P, Paul SM. A benzodiazepine receptor-mediated model of anxiety. Studies in nonhuman primates and clinical implications. Arch Gen Psychiatry 1984;41:741–750.

500. Wilkins AJ, Jenkins WJ, Steiner JA. Efficacy of clonidine in treatment of alcohol withdrawal state. Psychopharmacology (Berl) 1983;83:78–80.

501. Fyer AJ, Leibowitz MR, Gorman JM, et al. Effects of clonidine on alprazolam discontinuation in panic patients: a pilot study. J Clin Psychopharmacol 1994;8:270–274.

502. Papanicolaou J, Summers RJ, Vajda FJE, Louis WJ. The relationship between α_2-adrenoceptor selectivity and anticonvulsant effect in a series of clonidine-like drugs. Brain Res 1982;241:393–397.

503. Baldwin HA, Hitchcott PK, File SE. Evidence that the increased anxiety detected in the elevated plus-maze during chlordiazepoxide withdrawal is not due to enhanced noradrenergic activity. Pharmacol Biochem Behav 1989;34:931–933.

504. Siegel EG, Bonfiglio JF. Investigation of clonidine and lofexidine for the treatment of barbiturate withdrawal in mice. Vet Human Toxicol 1985;27:503–595.

505. Kunchandy J, Kulkarni SK. Reversal by *alpha-2* agonists of diazepam withdrawal hyperactivity in rats. Psychopharmacology (Berl) 1986;90:198–202.

506. Gil E, Colado I, Lopez F, Ferbadez-Briera A, Fernandez-Lopez A, Calvo P. Effects of chronic treatment with ethanol and withdrawal of ethanol on levels of dopamine, 2,4-dihydroxyphenylacetic acid and homovanillic acid in the striatum of the rat. Influence of benzodiazepines, barbiturate and somatostatin. Neuropharmacology 1992;31:1151–1156.

507. Nutt DJ, Cowen PJ. Diazepam alters brain 5HT function in man: implications for the acute and chronic effects of benzodiazepines. Psychol Med 1987;17:601–607.

508. Ida Y, Roth RH. The activation of mesoprefrontal dopamine neurons

by FG 7142 is absent in rats treated chronically with diazepam. Eur J Pharmacol 1987;137:185–190.

509. Rastogi RB, Lapierre YD, Singhal RL. Evidence for the role of brain norepinephrine and dopamine in "rebound" phenomenon seen during withdrawal after repeated exposure to benzodiazepines. J Psychiatr Res 1976;13:65–75.

510. Creese I, ed. Stimulants: neurochemical, behavioral, and clinical perspectives. New York: Raven Press, 1983.

511. Cho AK, Segal DS, eds. Amphetamine and its analogs. Psychopharmacology, toxicology, and abuse. San Diego: Academic Press, 1994.

512. Doweiko HE. ed. Concepts of chemical dependency. 2nd ed. Belmont: Brooks/Cole Publishing Company, 1993.

513. Gillis RA, Quest JA, Wilkerson RD. Mechanisms responsible for cardiovascular disorders associated with cocaine abuse. In: Lakoski JM, Galloway MP, White FJ, eds. Cocaine: pharmacology, physiology, and clinical strategies. Boca Raton: CRC Press, 1992: 371–390.

514. Nademanee K. Cardiovascular effects and toxicities of cocaine. J Addict Dis 1992;11:71–82.

515. Gould L, Gopalaswamy C, Patel C, Betzu R. Cocaine-induced myocardial infarction. N Y State J Med 1985;11:660–661.

516. Roberts SM, James RC, Harbison RD. Cocaine-induced heptotoxicity. In: Lakoski JM, Galloway MP, White FJ, eds. Cocaine: pharmacology, physiology, and clinical strategies. Boca Raton: CRC Press, 1992:15–33.

517. Gibb JW, Hanson GR, Johnson M. Neurochemical mechanisms of toxicity. In: Cho AK, Segal DS, eds. Amphetamine and its analogs. Psychopharmacology, toxicology, and abuse. San Diego: Academic Press, 1994:269–296.

518. Ellison GD. Paranoid psychosis following continuous amphetamine or cocaine: Relationship to selective neurotoxicity. In: Korenman SG, Barchas JD, eds. Biological basis of substance abuse. New York: Oxford University Press, 1993:355–371.

519. Marshall JF, O'Dell SJ, Weihmuller FB. Dopamine-glutamate interactions in methamphetamine-induced neurotoxicity. J Neural Transm Gen Sec 1993;91:241–254.

520. Post RM, Weiss SRB, Pert A. Sensitization and kindling effects of chronic cocaine administration. In: Lakoski JM, Galloway MP, White FJ, eds. Cocaine: pharmacology, physiology, and clinical strategies. Boca Raton: CRC Press, 1992:115–161.

521. Angrist B. Psychoses induced by central nervous system stimulants and related drugs. In: Creese I, ed. Stimulants: neurochemical, behavioral, and clinical perspectives. New York: Raven Press, 1983:1–30.

522. Wood DM, Emmett-Oglesby MW. Characteristics of tolerance, recovery from tolerance and cross-tolerance for cocaine used as a discriminative stimulus. J Pharmacol Exp Ther 1986;237: 120–125.

523. Bhat RV, Cole AJ, Baraban JM. Chronic cocaine treatment suppresses basal expression of *zif268* in rat forebrain: *in situ* hybridization studies. J Pharmacol Exp Ther 1992;263:343–349.

524. Hope B, Kosofsky B, Hyman SE, Nestler EJ. Regulation of immediate early gene expression and AP-1 binding in the rat nucleus accumbens by chronic cocaine. Proc Natl Acad Sci USA 1992;89: 5674–5678.

525. Daunais JB, McGinty JF. Acute and chronic cocaine administration differentially alters striatal opioid and nuclear transcription factor mRNAs. Synapse 1994;18:35–45.

526. Segal DS, Mandell AJ. Long-term administration of d-amphetamine: progressive augmentation of motor activity and stereotypy. Pharmacol Biochem Behav 1974;2:249–255.

527. Post RM, Rose H. Increasing effects of repetitive cocaine administration in the rat. Nature 1976;260:731–732.

528. Downs AW, Eddy NB. The effect of repeated doses of cocaine on the rat. J Pharmacol Exp Ther 1932;46:199–202.

529. Segal DS, Schuckit MA. Animal models of stimulant-induced psychosis. In: Creese I, ed. Stimulants: neurochemical, behavioral, and clinical perspectives. New York: Raven Press, 1983:131–167.

530. Fischman MW, Schuster CR, Hatano Y. A comparison of the subjective and cardiovascular effects of cocaine and lidocaine in humans. Pharmacol Biochem Behav 1983;18:123–127.

531. Stewart J, Badiani A. Tolerance and sensitization to the behavioral effects of drugs. Behav Pharmacol 1993;4:289–312.

532. Horger BA, Shelton K, Schenk S. Preexposure sensitizes rats to the rewarding effects of cocaine. Pharmacol Biochem Behav 1990;37: 707–711.

533. Kalivas PW, Sorg BA, Hooks MS. The pharmacology and neural circuitry of sensitization to psychostimulants. Behav Pharmacol 1993;4:315–334.

534. Reith MEA, Benuck M, Lajtha A. Cocaine disposition in the brain after continuous or intermittent treatment and locomotor stimulation in mice. J Pharmacol Exp Ther 1987;243:281–287.

535. Kalivas PW, Stewart J. Dopamine transmission in the initiation and expression of drug- and stress-induced sensitization of motor activity. Brain Res Rev 1991;16:223–244.

536. Kalivas PW, Barnes CD, eds. Sensitization in the nervous system. Caldwell: Telford Press, 1988.

537. Segal DS, Kuczenski R. Behavioral pharmacology of amphetamine. In: Cho AK, Segal DS, eds. Amphetamine and its analogs. Psychopharmacology, toxicology, and abuse. San Diego: Academic Press, 1994:115–150.

538. Mandell AJ, Knapp S. Acute versus chronic effects of psychotropic drugs: Adaptive responses in brain amine systems and their clinical implications. Evidence for multiphasic presynaptic adaptation: studies with cocaine and lithium. Psychopharmacol Bull 1977;13: 40–42.

539. Roth RH, Wolf ME, Deutch AY. Neurochemistry of midbrain dopamine systems. In: Meltzer HY, ed. Psychopharmacology: the third generation of progress. New York: Raven Press, 1987:81–94.

540. Mandell AJ. Neurobiological barriers to euphoria. American Scientist 1993;61:565–573.

541. Galloway MP. Neuropharmacology of cocaine: effects on dopamine and serotonin systems. In: Lakoski JM, Galloway MP, White FJ, eds. Cocaine: pharmacology, physiology, and clinical strategies. Boca Raton: CRC Press, 1992:163–190.

542. Zahniser NR, Peris J. Neurochemical mechanisms of cocaine induced sensitization. In: Lakoski JM, Galloway MP, White FJ, eds. Cocaine: Pharmacology, physiology, and clinical strategies. Boca Raton: CRC Press, 1992:229–260.

543. Weiss F, Paulus MP, Lorang MT, Koob GF. Increases in extracellular dopamine in the nucleus accumbens by cocaine are inversely related to basal levels: effects of acute and repeated administration. J Neurosci 1992;12:4372–4380.

544. Weber E, Sonders M, Quarum M, McLean S, Pou S, Keana JFW. 1,3-Di(2-[5-³H]tolyl)guanidine: a selective ligand that labels σ-type receptors for psychotomimetic opiates and antipsychotic drugs. Proc Natl Acad Sci USA 1986;83:8784–8788.

545. Kalivas PW, Duffy P. Time course of extracellular dopamine and behavioral sensitization to cocaine. I. Dopamine axon terminals. J Neurosci 1993;13:266–275.

546. Wise RA, Leeb K. Psychomotor-stimulant sensitization: a unitary phenomenon? Behav Pharmacol 1993;4:339–349.

547. Kalivas PW, Weber B. Amphetamine injection into the ventral mesencephalon sensitizes rats to peripheral amphetamine and cocaine. J Pharmacol Exp Ther 1988;245:1095–1102.

548. Ackerman JM, White FJ. A10 somatodendritic dopamine autoreceptor sensitivity following withdrawal from repeated cocaine treatment. Neurosci Lett 1990;117:181–187.

549. White FJ, Henry DJ, Hu X-T, Jeziorski M, Ackerman JM. Electrophysiological effects of cocaine in the mesoaccumbens dopamine system. In: Lakoski JM, Galloway MP, White FJ, eds. Cocaine: pharmacology, physiology, and clinical strategies. Boca Raton: CRC Press, 1992:261–294.

550. White FJ, Wang RY. Electrophysiological evidence for A10 dopamine autoreceptor subsensitivity following chronic d-amphetamine treatment. Brain Res 1984;309:283–292.

551. Striplin CD, Kalivas PW. Correlation between behavioral sensitiza-

tion to cocaine and G protein ADP-ribosylation in the ventral tegmental area. Brain Res 1992;579:181–186.

552. Nestler EJ, Guitart X, Beiter-Johnson D. Second-messenger and protein phosphorylation mechanisms underlying opiate and cocaine addiction. In: Korenman SG, Barchas JD, eds. Biological basis of substance abuse. New York: Oxford University Press, 1993:49–69.

553. Einhorn LC, Johansen PA, White FJ. Electrophysiological effects of cocaine in the mesoaccumbens dopamine system: studies in the ventral tegmental area. J Neurosci 1988;8:100–112.

554. Perugini M, Vezina P. Amphetamine administered to the ventral tegmental area sensitizes rats to the locomotor effects of nucleus accumbens amphetamine. J Pharmacol Exp Ther 1994;270:690–696.

555. Koff JM, Shuster L, Miller LG. Chronic cocaine administration is associated with behavioral sensitization and time-dependent changes in striatal dopamine transporter binding. J Pharmacol Exp Ther 1994;268:277–282.

556. Pilotte NS, Sharpe LG, Kuhar MJ. Withdrawal of repeated intravenous infusions of cocaine persistently reduces binding to dopamine transporters in the nucleus accumbens of Lewis rats. J Pharmacol Exp Ther 1994;269:963–969.

557. Henry DJ, White FJ. Repeated cocaine administration causes persistent enhancement of D_1 dopamine receptor sensitivity within the rat nucleus accumbens. J Pharmacol Exp Ther 1991;258:882–890.

558. Cunningham ST, Kelley AE. Evidence for opiate-dopamine cross-sensitization in nucleus accumbens: studies of conditioned reward. Brain Res Bull 1992;29:675–680.

559. Heidbreder C, Goldberg SR, Shippenberg TS. Inhibition of cocaine-induced sensitization by the γ-opioid receptor antagonist naltrindole. Eur J Pharmacol 1993;243:123–127.

560. Wolf ME, Jeziorski M. Coadministration of MK-801 with amphetamine, cocaine or morphine prevents rather than transiently masks the development of behavioral sensitization. Brain Res 1993;613:291–294.

561. Gur RC, Gur RE, Resnick SM, Skolnick BE, Alavi A, Reivich M. The effect of anxiety on cortical cerebral blood flow and metabolism. J Cereb Blood Flow Metab 1987;7:173–177.

562. Wolf ME, White FJ, Hu X-T. MK-801 prevents alterations in the mesoaccumbens dopamine system associated with behavioral sensitization to amphetamine. J Neurosci 1994;14:1735–1745.

563. White FJ, Hu X-T, Henry DJ. Electrophysiological effects of cocaine in the rat nucleus accumbens: microintophoretic studies. J Pharmacol Exp Ther 1993;266:1075–1084.

564. Lakoski JM, Black ER, Moday HJ. Electrophysiological effects of cocaine on serotonin neuronal systems. In: Lakoski JM, Galloway MP, White FJ, eds. Cocaine: pharmacology, physiology, and clinical strategies. Boca Raton: CRC Press, 1991:295–311.

565. Harris GC, Williams JT. Sensitization of locus ceruleus neurons during withdrawal from chronic stimulants and antidepressants. J Pharmacol Exp Ther 1992;261:476–483.

566. Gawin FH, Kleber HD. Abstinence symptomatology and psychiatric diagnosis in cocaine abusers: clinical observations. Arch Gen Psychiatry 1986;43:107–113.

567. Gawin FH. Cocaine addiction: psychology and neurophysiology. Science 1991;251:1580–1586.

568. Martin SD, Yeragani VK, Lodhi R, Galloway MP. Clinical ratings and plasma HVA during cocaine abstinence. Biol Psychiatry 1989;26:356–362.

569. Weddington WW, Brown BS, Haertzen CA, et al. Changes in mood, craving, and sleep during short-term abstinence reported by male cocaine addicts: a controlled, residential study. Arch Gen Psychiatry 1990;47:861–868.

570. Satel SL, Price LH, Palumbo JM, et al. Clinical phenomenology and neurobiology of cocaine abstinence: a prospective inpatient study. Am J Psychiatry 1991;148:1712–1716.

571. Flowers Q, Elder IR, Voris J, Sebastian PS, Blevins O, Dubois J. Daily cocaine craving in a 3-week inpatient treatment program. J Clin Psychol 1993;49:292–297.

572. Kowatch RA, Schnoll SS, Knisely JS, Green D, Elswick RK. Electroencephalographic sleep and mood during cocaine withdrawal. J Addict Dis 1992;11:21–45.

573. Ehrman RN, Robbins SJ, Childress AR, O'Brien CP. Conditioned responses to cocaine-related stimuli in cocaine abuse patients. Psychopharmacology (Berl) 1992;107:523–529.

574. Kosten TR. Can cocaine craving be a medication development outcome? Am J Addict 1992;1:230–238.

575. Kranzler HR, Bauer LO. Bromocriptine and cocaine cue reactivity in cocaine-dependent patients. Br J Addict 1992;87:1537–1548.

576. Koob GF, Stinus L, Le Moal M, Bloom FE. Opponent process theory of motivation: neurobiological evidence from studies of opiate dependence. Neurosci Biobehav Res 1989;13:135–140.

577. Newlin DB. A comparison of drug conditioning and craving for alcohol and cocaine. Recent Dev Alcohol 1992;10:147–164.

578. Kozlowski LT, Mann RE, Wilkinson DA, Poulos CX. "Cravings" are ambiguous: ask about urges or desires. Addict Behav 1989;14:443–445.

579. Markou A, Weiss F, Gold LH, Caine SB, Schulteis G, Koob GF. Animal models of drug craving. Psychopharmacology (Berl) 1993;112:163–182.

580. Gratton A, Wise RA. Drug- and behavior-associated changes in dopamine-related electrochemical signals during intravenous cocaine self-administration in rats. J Neurosci 1994;14:4130–4146.

581. Schultz W. Activity of dopamine neurons in the behaving primate. Semin Neurosci 1992;4:129–138.

582. Schultz W, Romo R. Dopamine neurons of the monkey midbrain: contingencies of responses to stimuli eliciting immediate behavioral reactions. J Neurophysiol 1990;63:607–624.

583. Dackis CA, Gold MS. New concepts in cocaine addiction: the dopamine depletion hypothesis. Neurosci Biobehavioral Rev 1985;9:469–477.

584. Hitri A, Casanova MF, Kleinman JE, Wyatt RJ. Fewer dopamine transporter receptors in the prefrontal cortex of cocaine users. Am J Psychiatry 1994;15:1074–1076.

585. Volkow ND, Fowler JS, Wolf AP, et al. Effects of chronic cocaine abuse on postsynaptic dopamine receptors. Am J Psychiatry 1990;147:719–724.

586. Volkow ND, Fowler JS, Wolf AP, et al. Changes in brain glucose metabolism in cocaine dependence and withdrawal. Am J Psychiatry 1991;148:621–626.

587. Volkow ND, Hitzemann R, Wang G-J, et al. Long-term frontal brain metabolic changes in cocaine abusers. Synapse 1992;11:184–190.

588. Wood DM, Lal H. Anxiogenic properties of cocaine withdrawal. Life Sci 1987;41:1431–1436.

589. Markou A, Koob GF. Postcocaine anhedonia: an animal model of cocaine withdrawal. Neuropsychopharmacology 1991;4:17–26.

590. Carroll ME, Lac ST. Cocaine withdrawal produces behavioral disruptions in rats. Life Sci 1987;40:2183–2190.

591. London ED, Wilkerson G, Goldberg SR, Risner ME. Effects of *l*-cocaine on local cerebral glucose utilization in the rat. Neurosci Lett 1986;68:73–78.

592. Porrino LJ, Domer FR, Crane AM, Sokoloff L. Selective alterations in cerebral metabolism within the mesocorticolimbic dopaminergic system produced by acute cocaine administration in rats. Neuropsychopharmacology 1988;1:109–118.

593. Hammer RP, Jr., Pires WS, Markou A, Koob GF. Withdrawal following cocaine self-administration decreases regional cerebral metabolic rate in critical brain reward regions. Synapse 1993;14:73–80.

594. Henry DJ, Greene MA, White FJ. Electrophysiological effects of cocaine in the mesoaccumbens dopamine system: repeated administration. J Pharmacol Exp Ther 1989;251:833-839.

595. Ackerman JM, White FJ. Decreased activity of rat A10 dopamine

neurons following withdrawal from repeated cocaine. Eur J Pharmacol 1992;218:171–173.

596. Zhang H, Lee TH, Ellinwood EH, Jr. The progressive changes of neuronal activities of the nigral dopaminergic neurons upon withdrawal from continuous infusion of cocaine. Brain Res 1992;594:315–318.

597. Pettit HO, Pan H, Parsons LH, Justice JBJ. Extracellular concentrations of cocaine and dopamine are enhanced during chronic cocaine administration. J Neurochem 1990;55:798–804.

598. Parsons LH, Smith AD, Justice JB, Jr. Basal extracellular dopamine is decreased in the rat nucleus accumbens during abstinence from chronic cocaine. Synapse 1991;9:60–65.

599. Wilson JM, Nobrega JN, Carroll ME, et al. Heterogeneous subregional binding patterns of ^{3}H-WIN 35,428 and ^{3}H-GBR 12,935 are differentially regulated by chronic cocaine self-administration. J Neurosci 1994;14:2966–2979.

600. Sharpe LG, Pilotte NS, Mitchell WM, De Souza EB. Withdrawal of repeated cocaine decreases autoradiographic [^{3}H]mazindol-labelling of dopamine transporter in rat nucleus accumbens. Eur J Pharmacol 1991;203:141–144.

601. Meiergerd SM, McElvain JS, Schenk JO. Effects of cocaine and repeated cocaine followed by withdrawal. Alterations of dopaminergic transporter turnover with no changes in kinetics of substrate recognition. Biochem Pharmacol 1994;47:1627–1634.

602. Laurier LG, Corrigall WA, George SR. Dopamine receptor density, sensitivity, and mRNA levels are altered following self-administration of cocaine in the rat. Brain Res 1994;634:31–40.

603. Neisewander JL, Lucki I, McGonigle P. Time-dependent changes in sensitivity to apomorphine and monoamine receptors following withdrawal from continuous cocaine administration in rats. Synapse 1994;16:1–10.

604. Goeders NE, Kuhar MJ. Chronic cocaine administration induces opposite changes in dopamine receptors in the striatum and nucleus accumbens. Alcohol Drug Res 1987;7:207–216.

605. Gawin FH, Kleber HD. Evolving conceptualizations of cocaine dependence. Yale J Biol Med 1988;61:123–136.

606. Cerruti C, Pilotte NS, Uhl G, Kuhar MJ. Reduction in dopamine transporter mRNA after cessation of repeated cocaine administration. Brain Res Mol Brain Res 1994;22:132–138.

607. King GR, Kuhn C, Ellinwood EH, Jr. Dopamine efflux during withdrawal from continuous or intermittent cocaine. Psychopharmacology (Berl) 1993;111:179–184.

608. Kalivas PW, Duffy P. Time course of extracellular dopamine and behavioral sensitization to cocaine. II. Dopamine perikarya. J Neurosci 1993;13:276–284.

609. Robertson MW, Leslie CA, Bennett JP, Jr. Apparent synaptic domaine deficiency induced by withdrawal from chronic cocaine treatment. Brain Res 1991;538:337–339.

610. Larson PS, Silvette H. eds. Tobacco: experimental and clinical studies, Suppl I. Baltimore: Williams & Wilkins, 1968.

611. Marks MJ, Stitzel JA, Collins AC. Time course study of the effects of chronic nicotine infusion on drug response and brain receptors. J Pharmacol Exp Ther 1985;235:619–628.

612. Benowitz NL, Porchet H, Jacob P, III. Nicotine dependence and tolerance in man: pharmacokinetic and pharmacodynamic investigations. In: Nordberg A, Fuxe K, Holmsted B, Sundwall A, eds. Progress in brain research, vol 79. Amsterdam: Elsevier, 1989:279–287.

613. Porchet HC, Benowitz NL, Sheiner LB. Pharmacodynamic model of tolerance: application to nicotine. J Pharmacol Exp Ther 1988;244:231–236.

614. Morrison CF, Stephenson JA. The occurrence of tolerance to a central depressant effect of nicotine. Br J Pharmacol 1972;46:151–156.

615. Stolerman IP, Fink R, Jarvik ME. Acute and chronic tolerance to nicotine measured by activity in rats. Psychopharmacologia 1973;30:329–342.

616. Falkeborn Y, Larsson C, Nordberg A. Chronic nicotine exposure in rat: a behavioural and biochemical study of tolerance. Drug Alcohol Depend 1981;8:51–60.

617. Stolerman IP, Bunker P, Jarvik ME. Nicotine tolerance in rats; role of dose and dose interval. Psychopharmacologia 1974;34:317–324.

618. Mansner R, Alhava E, Klinge E. Nicotine hypothermia and brain nicotine and catecholamine levels in the mouse. Med Biol 1974;52:390–398.

619. Horstmann M. Influence of mecamylamine and atropine on tolerance development to nicotine hypothermia in rats. J Pharm Pharmacol 1984;36:770–771.

620. Clarke PBS, Kumar R. The effects of nicotine on locomotor activity in non-tolerant and tolerant rats. Br J Pharmacol 1983;78:329–337.

621. U.S. Department of Health and Human Services. Benowitz NL, Grunberg NE, Henningfield JE, Lando HA, eds. The health consequences of smoking: nicotine addiction. A report of the Surgeon General. Washington, D.C.: U.S. Department of Health and Human Services, Public Health Service, Centers for Disease Control, Center for Health Promotion and Education, Office on Smoking and Health; DHHS Publication No. (CDC) 88-8406, 1988.

622. Hughes JR, Higgins ST, Hatsukami D. Effects of abstinence from tobacco: a critical review. In: Kozlowski LT, Annis HM, Cappell HD, et al., eds. Research advances in alcohol and drug problems, vol 10. New York: Plenum Press, 1990:317–398.

623. Hughes JR, Gust SW, Skoog K, Keenan RM, Fenwick JW. Symptoms of tobacco withdrawal: a replication and extension. Arch Gen Psychiatry 1991;48:52–59.

624. Hatsukami DK, Skoog K, Huber M, Hughes J. Signs and symptoms from nicotine gum abstinence. Psychopharmacology (Berl) 1991;104:496–504.

625. Henningfield JE, London ED, Benowitz NL. Arterio-venous differences in plasma concentrations of nicotine after cigarette smoking. JAMA 1990;263:2049–2050.

626. Henningfield JE, Stapleton JM, Benowitz NL, Grayson RF, London ED. Higher levels of nicotine in arterial than in venous blood after cigarette smoking. Drug Alcohol Depend 1993;33:23–29.

627. West RJ, Russell MA. Effects of withdrawal from long-term nicotine gum use. Psychol Med 1985;15:891–893.

628. Hughes JR, Hatsukami DK, Skoog KP. Physical dependence on nicotine in gum. A placebo substitution trial. JAMA 1986;255:3277–3279.

629. Stolerman IP, Goldfarb T, Fink R, Jarvik ME. Influencing cigarette smoking with nicotine antagonists. Psychopharmacologia 1973;28:247–259.

630. Tennant FS, Jr., Tarver AL, Rawson RA. Clinical evaluation of mecamylamine for withdrawal from nicotine dependence. NIDA Res Monogr 1984;49:239–246.

631. Nemeth-Coslett R, Henningfield JE, O'Keeffe MK, Griffiths RR. Effects of mecamylamine on human cigarette smoking and subjective ratings. Psychopharmacology (Berl) 1986;88:420–425.

632. Jarvis MJ, Raw M, Russell MAH, Feyerabend C. Randomized control trial of nicotine chewing gum. Br Med J (Clin Res Ed) 1982;285:537–540.

633. Hughes JR, Hatsukami DK, Pickens RW, Krahn D, Malin S, Luknic A. Effect of nicotine on the tobacco withdrawal syndrome. Psychopharmacology (Berl) 1984;83:82–87.

634. Schneider NG, Jarvik ME. Nicotine vs. placebo gum in the alleviation of withdrawal during smoking cessation. Addict Behav 1984;9:149–156.

635. West RJ, Jarvis MJ, Phil M, Russell MAH, Carruthers ME, Feyerabend C. Effect of nicotine replacement on the cigarette withdrawal syndrome. Brit J Addict 1984;79:215–219.

636. Gross J, Stitzer ML. Nicotine replacement: ten-week effects on tobacco withdrawal symptoms. Psychopharmacology (Berl) 1989;98:334–341.

637. Schwartz RD, Kellar KJ. Nicotinic cholinergic receptor binding sites in the brain: regulation in vivo. Science 1983;220:214–216.

638. Ksir C, Hakan R, Hall DP, Jr., Kellar KJ. Exposure to nicotine

enhances the behavioral stimulant effect of nicotine and increases binding of [³H]acetylcholine to nicotinic receptors. Neuropharmacology 1985;24:527–531.

639. Larsson C, Nilsson L, Halén A, Nordberg A. Subchronic treatment of rats with nicotine: effects on tolerance and on [³H]acetylcholine and [³H]nicotine binding in the brain. Drug Alcohol Depend 1986;17:37–45.

640. Marks MJ, Burch JB, Collins AC. Genetics of nicotine response in four inbred strains of mice. J Pharmacol Exp Ther 1983;226:291–301.

641. Nordberg A, Wahlström G, Arnelo U, Larsson C. Effect of long-term nicotine treatment on [³H]nicotine binding sites in the rats brain. Drug Alcohol Depend 1985;16:9–17.

642. Price RW, Brew B, Sidtis J, Rosenblum M, Scheck AC, Cleary P. The brain in AIDS: central nervous system HIV-1 infection and AIDS dementia complex. Science 1988;239:586–592.

643. Ksir C, Hakan RL, Kellar KJ. Chronic nicotine and locomotor activity: influences of exposure dose and test dose. Psychopharmacology (Berl) 1987;92:25–29.

644. Ochoa ELM, Li L, McNamee MG. Desensitization of central cholinergic mechanisms and neuroadaption to nicotine. Mol Neurobiol 1990;4:251–287.

645. Malin DH, Lake JR, Newlin-Maultsby P, et al. A rodent model of nicotine abstinence syndrome. Pharmacol Biochem Behav 1992;43:119–184.

646. Malin DH, Lake JR, Carter VA, Cunningham JS, Wilson OB. Naloxone precipitates nicotine abstinence syndrome in the rat. Psychopharmacology (Berl) 1993;112:339–342.

647. Tassin JP, Vezina P, Trovero F, Blanc G, Herve D, Glowinski J. Cortico-subcortical interactions in behavioral sensitization: differential effects of daily nicotine and morphine. Ann NY Acad Sci 1992;654:101–116.

648. Hakan RL, Hart C, Eyl C. Specific neurophysiological effects of systemic nicotine on neurons in the nucleus accumbens. Synapse 1993;15:191–197.

649. Grenhoff J, Svensson TH. Pharmacology of nicotine. Br J Addict 1989;84:477–492.

650. London ED, Fanelli RJ, Kimes AS, Moses RL. Effects of chronic nicotine on cerebral glucose utilization in the rat. Brain Res 1990;520:208–214.

651. Grünwald F, Schröck H, Theilen H, Biber A, Kuschinsky W. Local cerebral glucose utilization of the awake rat during chronic administration of nicotine. Brain Res 1988;456:350–356.

652. London ED, Broussolle EPM, Links JM, et al. Morphine-induced metabolic changes in human brain: studies with positron emission tomography and [fluorine 18]fluorodeoxyglucose. Arch Gen Psychiatry 1990;47:73–81.

653. London ED, Cascella NG, Wong DF, et al. Cocaine-induced reduction of glucose utilization in human brain. A study using positron emission tomography and [fluorine 18]fluorodeoxyglucose. Arch Gen Psychiatry 1990;47:567–574.

654. de Wit H, Metz JT, Gatley J. Relationship between mood and regional metabolism after a moderate dose of ethanol. J Cereb Blood Flow Metab 1989;9:S325

655. Volkow ND, Hitzemann R, Wolf AP, et al. Acute effects of ethanol on regional brain glucose metabolism and transport. Psychiatry Res 1990;35:39–48.

656. Wolkin A, Angrist B, Wolf A, et al. Effects of amphetamine on local cerebral metabolism in normal and schizophrenic subjects as determined by positron emission tomography. Psychopharmacology (Berl) 1987;92:241–246.

657. Theodore WH, DiChiro G, Margolin R, Fishbein D, Porter RJ, Brooks RA. Barbiturates reduce human cerebral glucose metabolism. Neurology 1986;36:60–64.

658. Buchsbaum MS, Wu J, Haier R, et al. Positron emission tomography assessment of effects of benzodiazepines on regional glucose metabolic rate in patients with anxiety disorder. Life Sci 1987;40:2393–2400.

659. Foster NL, VanDerSpek AFL, Aldrich MS, et al. The effect of diazepam sedation on cerebral glucose metabolism in Alzheimer's disease as measured using positron emission tomography. J Cereb Blood Flow Metab 1987;7:415–420.

660. London ED, Morgan MJ. Positron emission tomographic studies on the acute effects of psychoactive drugs on brain metabolism and mood. In: London ED, ed. Imaging drug action in the brain. Boca Raton: CRC Press, 1993:265–280.

661. Kameyama T, Nabeshima T, Domino EF, eds. NMDA receptor related agents: biochemistry, pharmacology and behavior. Ann Arbor: NPP Books, 1991.

30

NEUROPSYCHIATRY OF ALCOHOL AND DRUG ABUSE

Walter Ling, Peggy Compton, Richard Rawson, and Donald R. Wesson

Although addiction medicine draws its membership from a diverse group of medical specialties, a chapter in substance abuse is especially fitting for a textbook in neuropsychiatry. Substance dependence and abuse are clinically defined in behavioral terms, and their description and classification constitute a formal part of the current psychiatric disease nomenclature. The generic disease of substance dependence and abuse, the clinical syndromes of substance intoxication and withdrawal, and the substance-induced psychiatric syndromes, many of which resemble primary psychiatric disorders, clinically fall within the realm of psychiatry. On the other hand, neurologists see some of the most dramatic and devastating complications of addictive diseases, ranging from trauma to strokes, seizures, and the neurological manifestations of acquired immunodeficiency syndrome (AIDS). Indeed, few medical events rival the drama of a patient's ostensible instant recovery from heroin-induced coma after administration of naloxone, or the tragedy of severe head injury resulting from a drunk driving accident. Moreover, some medications used by neurologists for treatment of chronic painful neurological disorders, such as chronic headache and painful neuropathies, may contribute to the development of an independent substance abuse disorder.

Thus, apparently, substance dependence and abuse should be an area of common interest for neurologists and psychiatrists and, in particular, for neuropsychiatrists. Unfortunately, the area of common interest often becomes an area of mutual neglect. Few psychiatrists involved in the treatment of substance abuse disorders do in fact see the catastrophic neurological complications from drug abuse, and few neurologists who treat neurological complications are involved in the management of the underlying addictive disorder beyond recovery of the acute neurological illness. The goal of this chapter is to provide for psychiatrically trained neuropsychiatrists some understanding of the neurological syndromes related to substance abuse, and for neurologically trained neuropsychiatrists, some understanding of the pharmacological and nonpharmacological approaches to treating the underlying substance-related disorders.

We begin with some definitions of terms, followed by a discussion of the general approach to patient assessment, and formal clinical diagnosis with laboratory confirmations. We next discuss specific neuropsychiatric syndromes induced by alcohol, cocaine, other stimulants, opiates, sedative-hypnotics, and hallucinogens, and the pharmacological management of the three major classes of drugs of abuse, opiates, cocaine, and alcohol. We then address some specific problems of neuropsychological function relating to drug abuse, issues of comorbidity, human immunodeficiency virus (HIV) disease and pain, and consideration of their implications for pharmacological and nonpharmacological treatment strategies.

It is not our intent to write a neurological primer for psychiatrists or a psychiatric primer for neurologists; instead, the focus is on the more commonly seen neuropsychiatric syndromes of interest to both groups. Some of these are common knowledge, such as those related to acute and chronic alcohol abuse. Others have been more recently described, such as seizures and strokes in cocaine and other stimulant abusers. We have decided not to include any discussion relating to caffeine and nicotine dependence, even though both are listed in the American Psychiatric Association's *Diagnostic and Statistical Manual,* 4th ed. (DSM-IV), and we touch only lightly on the neurological manifestations of AIDS, mainly to serve as a reminder that AIDS, deserving full treatment in its own right, is an increasingly common medical complication among substance abusers.

DEFINITION OF TERMS

Drug abuse: Broadly defined, this term refers to the use of a drug for nonmedicinal purposes, with intent to affect consciousness, distinct from *misuse,* which implies inappropriate medicinal use (e.g., for the wrong indication, at the wrong dose, or for the wrong amount of time). The term *drug abuse* is deeply embedded in cultural and social values and often implies social disapproval or illegality. The use of alcohol in any amount is prohibited in Muslim cultures, whereas the use of marijuana and other hallucinogens for religious purposes is quite acceptable in many Native American tribal cultures. Contemporary American psychiatry views abuse as a maladaptive pattern of use, leading to recurrent, significant adverse physical, legal, occupational, and/or social consequences. It is thus embedded within the larger context of dependence, though not necessarily less serious. The diagnosis of substance dependence preempts the diagnosis of abuse in the same drug class.

Dependence: This term includes both psychic dependence, characterized by compulsive drug-seeking behavior, and physical dependence, characterized by the presence of withdrawal symptoms upon abrupt discontinuation of the drug. Physical dependence is best understood in terms of the body's adjustment to a new level of homeostasis during the period of drug use. This new state of equilibrium manifests itself by symptoms of withdrawal when the drug is discontinued or when its action is reversed by administration of specific antagonists, as exemplified by naloxone-precipitated opiate withdrawal.

Addiction: This term refers to a state of physical and psychic dependence, although it can refer to psychic dependence alone when physical dependence is not apparent.

Tolerance: Tolerance is the body's compensatory response to the effect of the drug and refers to the decreased response to drug effects such that an increasingly larger dose is required to achieve the same effect. It is closely related to physical dependence and can be of several types. *Metabolic tolerance* refers to increased disposition of the drug from increased metabolism with decreased availability of the drug at its site of action. *Cellular tolerance* refers to diminished response without concomitant reduction in drug concentration or availability. *Functional tolerance* refers to the compensatory changes due to receptor mechanisms, whereas *behavioral tolerance* refers to the clinical ability to compensate for drug effects. Tolerance invariably leads to the need for larger doses of a drug to achieve the same effect but it is unclear at present how tolerance relates to drug craving and drug seeking.

CLINICAL ASSESSMENT OF PATIENTS

Patient assessment can serve clinical, administrative, research, or medical-legal purposes. In general, the goals of assessment include detecting substances of abuse, formulating diagnoses, establishing the severity of the disorder and the baseline status of the patient for purposes of treatment planning, monitoring treatment progress, and formulating a prognosis.

Clinical evaluation should lead toward formal diagnosis with laboratory confirmation. It should also consider the context within which the assessment is made. An assessment performed in a general medical setting may differ from one performed for admission to a substance abuse treatment program.

Substance abuse disorders are underrecognized in general medical and neuropsychiatric practices. This is suggested by the high incidence of substance abuse disorders noted in surveys of general medical and neuropsychiatric patients, in contrast to hospital chart reviews, which show a rather low documentation of these disorders (1–4). Failure of recognition, however, may only partially explain underreporting substance abuse disorders. Indeed, most physicians are aware that substance abuse is one of the most frequently encountered problems in their practice but may be reluctant to report it because of the current structure of medical care and reimbursement.

Although the general approach to assessing drug abuse disorders follows traditional lines of history taking and physical and mental status examinations supported by laboratory tests, the circumstance under which evaluation takes place merits special consideration. This is because it can greatly influence the patient's attitude toward the process of evaluation and the information to be gathered.

An empathetic, nonjudgmental attitude on the part of the evaluator is necessary but does not come easily for many physicians, whose training has by and large exposed them to the most medically frustrating aspects of drug abuse. The term "addict" itself conjures up images of the most undesirable of patients. Physicians therefore need to be aware of their own attitude toward the addict. A nonjudgmental attitude encourages self-disclosure and makes it easier to establish a working relationship. Patients referred from a medical service are likely to be apprehensive and are often embarrassed by the referral. The addict's seeming lack of candor in disclosing information should not automatically be interpreted as resistance, denial, or lack of motivation. Sometimes patients are simply too embarrassed by the implications of the referral. Or, there may be a genuine and not totally groundless fear of losing a job or professional licensure. Addicts are by and large ambivalent but not necessarily in denial about their disease. The nature of addictive disease is such that it often cuts the patient off from all social contacts. The addiction itself becomes the only meaningful relationship left in life, and this is not easy for the addict to give up. Also, some patients simply are unable to cooperate or remember details of events because they are still under the influence of drugs or have suffered from their chronic effects.

Patient interviews should be conducted in private. Sensitivity to the patient's need to avoid feelings of shame and guilt promote candid disclosure. The interview should not be interrupted by phone calls or beepers. It is not that addicts need special consideration. It is simply that many physicians do not give addicts the same due consideration given to other patients with illnesses that cause potential embarrassment and shame. By ensuring privacy, the physician shows respect and sensitivity, essential first steps toward establishing a therapeutic rapport.

Patients should be assured at the outset of the confidential nature of the information they are about to give. Their understanding of the confidentiality will enhance the validity of the information obtained. Physicians should be aware that substance abuse treatment information is, under the law, treated with a degree of confidentiality more stringent than general medical information (5).

Although the general approach to patient inquiry needs to be empathetic, the questioning itself should be direct and straightforward. It is better to use simple language and avoid street terms, unless one is certain of the meaning. Misuse of street terms tends to give the addict a feeling of superiority over the physician, which may in turn encourage manipulative behavior. Most addicts will give a reliable enough history if some allowances are made and if inquiry is limited to factual information without dwelling excessively on reasoning and motivation. Keep in mind that addicts often rationalize as a defense mechanism against their own sense of guilt and shame; their explanations are mostly for themselves and they do not expect the inquirer to believe them. It is sufficient, for instance, in exploring legal complications, to ascertain how many times the patient has gone to jail and for what charges, without being too concerned with matters of justice. An addict will often volunteer a reason, such as bad luck or prejudice from the legal system, while admitting the fact of incarceration. There is no need to echo the patient's sentiment or contradict the patient's claims.

Remember that addicts do not always want to deny or minimize the extent of their drug problems. A man referred by his employee assistance program (EAP) may well want to minimize his drinking, but heroin addicts seeking detoxification commonly exaggerate the size of their habits.

The history is the cornerstone of clinical evaluation. Begin with the suspected drug of abuse that brought the patient to medical attention and explore each commonly abused drug systematically, one at a time. Keep in mind local fads that may be unique for the population under evaluation. For some drugs of abuse, even the history of use on a single occasion may be considered abuse. For others, like alcohol, the pattern and extent of use determines if abuse or dependence is present. Because substance abuse and dependence disorders are clinically defined as maladaptive patterns of use, it is important to explore such issues as amount of use, presence of withdrawal on cessation of use, amount of time spent in procurement and use, past attempts to control or cut down, neglect of social responsibility, and continuous use in the face of adverse physical and social consequences.

For each drug class, age of first use and age of first regular use or intoxication must be determined. Most drug abusers begin their careers in their early teens. Late adult onset of drug or alcohol abuse suggests presence of a coexisting or preexisting psychiatric disease, in particular an affective disorder.

Past periods of heavy use and periods of abstinence, and the surrounding life circumstances that may give clues to events precipitating relapse or motivation for abstinence, should also be ascertained. This information can also aid in planning treatment. The pattern of use during the 3–4 weeks prior to evaluation, including the amount and time of last use, should be explored in detail. This information is crucial in deciding whether a period of hospitalization will be necessary to establish abstinence because withdrawal from certain substances, such as alcohol, sedative-hypnotics, and other central nervous system (CNS) depressants, may have serious medical complications. The present illness should be supplemented with a detailed review of systems, past history, family history, and social and occupational history. Whenever possible, an independent source should be sought to confirm the information obtained. Even when an addict wants to be candid, he or she is likely to distort out of habit.

Screening for substance abuse disorders in a general medical or neuropsychiatric context differs from evaluating patients seeking treatment. In the former, the subject matter can sometimes be approached by means of a questionnaire such as the Michigan Alcohol Screening Test (MAST) (6) or the CAGE (a four-item screener) (7) for alcoholism or the Drug Abuse Screening Test for other drugs of abuse. These instruments are easy to administer and ensure that busy clinicians do not omit important questions. However, these instruments lack the flexibility of a live interview; they tend to be constructed around a specific drug and miss the local fads. The mechanical application of a questionnaire can detract from the process of building a therapeutic rapport. In practice, these instruments are of greatest value to supplement general medical and psychiatric evaluations for the clinician whose practice does not focus on addictive disease. For clinicians who devote a substantial portion of time to the practice of addiction medicine, the points covered by these instruments come almost second nature to general history taking, and their use is unnecessary.

The history should be supplemented by careful observation and a thorough physical examination. Common physical findings of injection drug abuse include fresh needle marks and old scars, thrombosed veins, abscesses and congested nasal mucosa, enlarged liver, and local lymph nodes. Spider nevi and gynecomastia are common in alcoholism, as are cardiac murmur or arrhythmia in cocaine addiction. Signs of intoxication or withdrawal may be present, depending on the time of the last "fix." The mental status examination should include observation for any unusual behaviors or mannerisms, speech, orientation, attention, concentration, thought content, simple calculation, recent and remote memory. The patient's response and behavior during history taking and physical examination usually give sufficient clues to the mental status, but sometimes it is useful to employ a standardized cognitive screening test such as the Mini-Mental State Examination (8). Formal neurocognitive evaluation is usually reserved for patients suspected of having drug-induced dementia. Taken together, these components of patient evaluation should lead naturally to a formal diagnosis.

CLINICAL DIAGNOSIS

The formal diagnosis of drug-related neuropsychiatric syndromes, covered under Substance-Related Disorders in DSM-IV (9), contains three distinct but related diagnostic categories: (*a*) the generic diagnosis of substance depen-

Table 30.1. DSM-IV Criteria for Substance Dependence and Substance Abuse

Dependence (three or more in a 12-month period)	Abuse (one or more in a 12-month period)[a]
Tolerance (marked increase in amount; marked decrease in effect)	Recurrent use resulting in failure to fulfill major role obligations at work, home, or school
Characteristic withdrawal symptoms/substance taken to relieve withdrawal	Recurrent use in physically hazardous situations
Substance taken in larger amount and for longer period than intended	Recurrent substance-related legal problems
Persistent desire or repeated unsuccessful attempt to quit	Continued use despite persistent or recurrent social or interpersonal problems caused or exacerbated by substance
Much time/activity to obtain, use, recover	
Important social, occupational, or recreational activities given up or reduced	
Use continues despite knowledge of adverse consequences (e.g., failure to fulfill role obligation, use when physically hazardous)	

[a]Symptoms must never have met criteria for substance dependence for this class of substance.

dence and substance abuse (Substance Use Disorders); (*b*) the clinical syndromes directly related to intoxication and withdrawal (Substance-induced Disorders); and (*c*) the drug-induced psychiatric disorders phenomenologically related to other specific psychiatric disorders (Substance-induced Mental Disorders).

Substance dependence and substance abuse are characterized by a cluster of cognitive, behavioral, and physiological symptoms occurring within a specific time frame. Central to substance dependence are compulsive drug-seeking behavior and continuing drug use despite adverse consequences, with or without tolerance and withdrawal, whereas substance abuse emphasizes repeated use under hazardous conditions and/or despite harmful consequences, in an individual who does not meet criteria for dependence on the substance.

Table 30.1 lists the salient features of substance dependence and substance abuse. For dependence, three of seven criteria must be met within a 12-month period, and for abuse, one of four criteria must be met and the individual must not be dependent on the substance. Most neurological complications related to substance use disorders fall outside the primary concerns of psychiatry and are only briefly mentioned in DSM-IV as associated general medical conditions.

Laboratory Testing

Several laboratory tests serve important functions in the evaluation and treatment of substance-related disorders.

Screening for drugs of abuse is invaluable in investigating patients suspected of drug overdose, confirming the diagnosis of drug dependence for planning and initiating treatment, differentiating drug-induced psychopathology from syndromes of other causes, detecting multiple drugs of abuse, monitoring compliance and treatment progress, and detecting relapse. Results of drug testing can also be a powerful tool in counseling and, in some circumstances, such as in the military and in the workplace, an effective deterrent for drug use (10). Drug testing has been used

for other purposes outside the therapeutic setting. It is commonly used for screening of prospective employees, detecting drug use by workers in certain professions, monitoring compliance for parolees and probationers, prosecuting suspected drunk drivers, excluding athletes from competitions, confirming or disputing information given in employment or insurance applications, and investigating certain unexplained or suspicious deaths.

Drug testing can be performed on several body fluids and tissues, including blood, urine, saliva, sweat, and hair. By far the most commonly used is urine because of the large amounts of drugs and metabolites excreted in the urine and because urine is easily obtained. Unfortunately, addicts, for a variety of reasons, do not want their use of drugs made known and resort to many ways of "cheating" on urine tests. This has necessitated direct observation for urine collection, which has become one of the most demeaning aspects of substance abuse treatment. The problem has increased over the years as more women have entered into treatment.

Direct observation for urine collection may be obviated, however, by using a collection device incorporating a temperature-sensitive strip to register the temperature of the urine at the time of collection. Because the temperature of freshly voided urine falls within a narrow range, this device is virtually tamper-proof (11, 12).

Routine use of blood for drug testing is not practical because of the need for venipuncture and because drug concentrations are often too low for routine lab detection. Drug testing technology using saliva, sweat, and hair has not yet reached general clinical utility.

Several test methods are available for drug screening. They vary in sensitivity, specificity, and cost, and each has its own advantages and disadvantages. Thin-layer chromatography (TLC), the least expensive, is also the least sensitive. Its primary advantage besides cost is that a single test can detect multiple drugs. It is highly suitable for detecting high-dose drug use of recent origin, as in cases of suspected overdose in emergency rooms where the types of drugs may be unknown but the need to detect low levels of drugs is not an issue. TLC is also widely used for routine therapeutic monitoring of patients on methadone maintenance. Because of the low sensitivity, TLC tends to give false-negative results. It is not suitable, therefore, for use to detect illicit drugs of high potency, such as fentanyl, LSD, or some of the designer drugs. Many labs confirm results of TLC by an alternative method and, alone, TLC is insufficient for forensic purposes.

Several immunoassay methods are available, based on antigen-antibody interactions. These include the enzyme multiplied immunoassay test (EMIT), radioimmunoassay (RIA) and fluorescent polarization immunoassay (FPIA). These methods are highly sensitive, and the tests are quick and quite easy to perform. Unfortunately, though, they can test for only one drug at a time; thus, a drug that is not thought of is not detected. However, because no extraction is required for these tests, they lend themselves to automation for large-volume testing.

More highly sophisticated assay methods using gas-liquid chromatography (GLC) and gas chromatography with mass spectrometry (GC/MS) are available in some laboratories. These tests give the best sensitivity and specificity but are also costly and labor-intensive. They are used mainly to confirm results of less expensive tests.

Interpreting results of drug screening is no simple matter for the clinician. The detectability of a drug depends not only on its characteristics but also on a host of other factors, including the size of the dose, the frequency of its use, the time of the last use, the time of the sample collection, the metabolites of the drug, and, of course, the type of body fluid used for testing and the sensitivity and specificity of the analytic methods. For the busy clinician, the best strategy is to become acquainted with the personnel of the local lab, become familiar with their general methodology, and find out what a comprehensive panel means, so that if a particular drug of abuse is suspected that does not appear on the panel, a specific request can be made. Most laboratory directors are quite responsive to questions and special requests. It may be helpful to have available a copy of the lab's report forms listing the drugs contained in its routine comprehensive panel, information about other drug tests the lab can perform, and knowledge about the sensitivity of the tests and the cutoff level where results are reported as positive or negative (13).

In addition to drug screening, a number of other laboratory tests are useful in evaluation and treatment of substance-related disorders. A simple breath test can estimate a γ-glutamyl blood alcohol level. Increased serum γ-glutanyl transferase (GGT), absent other evidence of liver disease or the use of hepatotoxic prescription drugs, is a fairly sensitive indicator of heavy drinking in alcoholics, although it does not distinguish alcoholic liver disease from other forms of liver disease, and its specificity for heavy alcohol consumption diminishes in the presence of chronic hepatitis. A high aspartate aminotransferase (AST) can also indicate alcohol abuse, and the ratio of mitochondrial AST to total AST can differentiate chronic alcoholics from other patients

(14). Changes in GGT and AST levels are more useful when taken in conjunction with changes in mean corpuscular volume (MCV), which increases after a period of heavy drinking (15). These laboratory findings tend to reverse with abstinence and can be used serially to monitor treatment progress. Other laboratory changes, such as increased uric acid, increased triglycerides, and decreased BUN also suggest alcohol abuse, and they too tend to return toward normal with abstinence.

Injection drug abusers commonly show elevated liver enzymes that, under treatment, improve or become stable. In the absence of acute clinical liver disease, these elevated enzymes should not be cause for withholding substance abuse intervention. Any indication of active hepatitis, which, unfortunately, is also very common among addicts, requires appropriate evaluation and treatment. Recent advances in neurobiology of drugs of abuse and in neuroimaging techniques (see Chapter 29) have allowed the visualization of many acute and chronic drug effects in the living human brain. Such advances offer exciting possibilities in the development of new medications to treat substance-related disorders and may help define subgroups of patients who may respond preferentially to different therapeutic interventions. Meanwhile, an unexpected clinical bonus has been realized from sharing with the patient the colorful and intriguing pictures from these neuroimaging studies. Patients are often fascinated by them and are motivated to enter or remain in treatment because they show drug-related brain dysfunction.

CLINICAL SYNDROMES

Some clinical syndromes, like acute alcohol intoxication and withdrawal, result directly from the effects of the drug on the CNS; others, like seizures and strokes in stimulant abusers, may result from the drug's direct effect on the CNS or be secondary to drug effects on the cardiovascular system. Still others, like meningitis, brain abscess, peripheral neuropathy, and AIDS, arise from more distal factors relating to the use of contaminated needles and from the addict's high-risk life-style.

Each class of drugs of abuse can produce a number of neuropsychiatric syndromes. Alcohol, for example, leads to intoxication, withdrawal, seizures, and dementia. On the other hand, each syndrome can be produced by more than one class of drugs of abuse. For example, seizures can result from acute stimulant abuse or from withdrawal from alcohol or sedative-hypnotics. Consequently, without adequate information, making a differential diagnosis can be difficult.

Clinical syndromes can be organized from the perspective of the class of drugs of abuse or from the perspective of the clinical syndromes they produce. The following sections present the more commonly seen clinical syndromes associated with each major class of drugs of abuse, followed by tables summarizing each one by drug class and clinical syndrome. Table 30.2 shows the common syndromes seen with each class of drugs of abuse.

Table 30.2. Neuropsychiatric Syndromes Associated with Drug Abuse

Syndrome	Drug-related Etiology
Seizure	Alcohol intoxication
	Cocaine, CNS stimulant toxicity
	Alcohol, sedative-hypnotic withdrawal
Stroke	Cocaine, CNS stimulant intoxication, and toxicity
	Opiate toxicity
	Alcohol abuse
	Intravenous drug use
Coma	Opiate toxicity
	Alcohol, sedative-hypnotic toxicity
	Drug-induced stroke or seizure
	Life-style-related (head trauma, hypoglycemia)
Delirium	Cocaine, CNS stimulant intoxication
	Alcohol, sedative-hypnotic withdrawal
CNS infection	Intravenous drug use
Peripheral neuropathy	Alcohol abuse
	Injection drug use

Neuropsychiatric Syndromes by Drug Class

ALCOHOL

Alcohol is the most commonly used psychoactive drug in the United States. Recent estimates indicate that 88% of all Americans over the age of 18 have used alcohol at some point in their lives, and 50% report drinking on at least one occasion in the past 30 days (16). Its popularity is due, in no small part, to its legal and sanctioned status, making it readily available at a relatively low cost to virtually all Americans of drinking age. It is safe to say that one of the most frequently occurring neurological syndromes in our society is alcohol intoxication, followed closely (in terms of both prevalence and time) by uncomplicated alcohol withdrawal, or "hangover."

Nearly 14% of the adults in the U.S. population meet diagnostic criteria for alcohol abuse or dependence at some point in their lives (17). Approximately 10,000,000 Americans over the age of 21 are classified as heavy drinkers, defined as drinking five or more drinks per occasion on five or more occasions in the past 30 days (16). Alcohol-related neurological syndromes occur in relationship to the last drink consumed, as well as to drinking over a lifetime, and differ markedly among individuals and between persons who are physically dependent and those who are not.

Alcohol Intoxication

At low doses, alcohol acts primarily as a CNS intoxicant, whereas at high doses, its sedative and anesthetic actions predominate (18–20). Thus, neurological syndromes associated with acute alcohol ingestion vary with alcohol dose (Table 30.3). Individual response to acute alcohol ingestion is highly variable and dependent upon the amount of alcohol ingested, the rate at which blood levels of alcohol rise, individual tolerance to the psychological and physical effects

of alcohol, genetic factors that determine the responsiveness of the nervous system to the effects of alcohol, mood state of the individual while drinking, and the setting or environment in which the drinking occurs. Gastric metabolism of alcohol is decreased in women, which effectively increases their blood-alcohol levels (21).

Alcohol acutely depresses the integrating and inhibitory functions of the cerebral cortex and reticular activating system (22, 23). Miller and Gold (24) refer to this effect as a "descending paralysis," affecting the cortex first, then the limbic system, and finally the brainstem. The action of alcohol in the CNS is nonspecific, which accounts in part for the high doses (23) needed to achieve, relative to other psychoactive drugs, comparable levels of intoxication (25). The sensitivity with which neurotransmitter systems respond to alcohol appears to have a genetic basis (26–31).

The average adult metabolizes 7–10 grams (1 oz.) of alcohol per hour (32–34). Once this clearance rate is exceeded, blood-alcohol levels begin to rise and CNS manifestations of intoxication occur. Blood-alcohol level (BAL), a commonly used measure of intoxication, accurately reflects the CNS effects of alcohol in nontolerant persons. Severity of intoxication at a given blood level is typically greater when BAL is rising as opposed to falling. At BALs between .01–.10%, mild declines in coordination and cognition are experienced, and individuals present with disinhibited behavior, euphoric mood, and decreased anxiety. At concentrations slightly above this level, persons are notably intoxicated, demonstrating dysarthria, ataxia, poor coordination, decreased sensory function, impaired judgment and psychomotor skills, decreased attention span, and mood swings. At .20%, individuals are severely intoxicated, manifesting nausea and vomiting, diplopia, gross motor incoordination, incoherence and confusion (35–38).

Other neurological findings in alcohol intoxication reflect CNS stimulation, and include facial flushing, increased heart rate, increased respiratory rate, and hyperreflexia (23, 34, 37, 39). Behavior may be boisterous, belligerent, or dysphoric. Examination of the eyes and third cranial nerve reveal mydriatic or normal-sized pupils, sluggish pupillary light reflex, nystagmus and diplopia, redness of sclera, corneal glazing, and nonconvergence (40). With increasing alcohol dependence, individuals become tolerant to its intoxicating effects and no longer complain of getting drunk when they drink. Alcoholics have been shown to perform quite well on psychomotor or cognitive tasks at BALs between .20–.30% (41). Marked intoxication is rarely noted in alcoholics at this level of blood alcohol.

Memory disturbances are common with alcohol intoxication (42). Anterograde amnesia has been demonstrated at BALs as low as .04%. During an alcohol blackout, a classic example of anterograde amnesia, the intoxicated individual appears alert, is able to ambulate, carry on conversation, and perform previously learned tasks. No impairment of long-term memory or immediate recall is noted. Upon becoming sober, however, the person has total and permanent amnesia for the period. These amnestic episodes are self-limiting, rarely lasting longer than 48 hours, and can occur both in persons dependent and not dependent on alcohol. They tend to occur when the slope of increasing BAL over time is steep, and at BALs of greater than .25% (43–45). Anterograde memory function is usually recovered fully once the individual is sober, but the chance of incurring residual memory deficits increases with the chronicity of alcohol abuse (44, 46).

At higher BALs, the depressant and anesthetic actions of alcohol predominate. At .30%, individuals become stuporous, and by .40%, they may lose consciousness, thus protecting themselves from further increases in BAL. A BAL of .50–.70% results in coma, respiratory depression, and eventual death (20, 36). Typically, the chronic alcoholic is protected from alcohol overdose by his or her extreme tolerance to the depressant effects of the drug, although Mendelson and Mello (34) report no elevation in the lethal dose of alcohol for alcoholics, and severe respiratory depression can occur with chronic alcohol intoxication.

Coma induced by high-dose alcohol is a metabolic coma characterized by an absence of focal neurological signs and a fluctuating level of consciousness. The patient is typically unresponsive but may show a purposeful motor response with vigorous or painful stimulation. Respirations are depressed and noisy, pupils are normal to dilated and react to light sluggishly, and hypothermia is common, further depressing neurological response (47).

Alcohol frequently plays a role in overdose of other drugs, especially CNS depressants. In one study, three-quarters of comatose patients admitted to the emergency room tested positive for alcohol, 65% of them having a BAL greater than .08% (48). In another study of suspected drug overdose in 492 patients, serum toxicology was positive for alcohol in 50% of the sample, and 38% had BAL of .10% or greater (49). Alcohol increases the overdose potential of other psychoactive drugs because of its sedative effects as well as its disinhibitory effects on behavior.

Alcohol Withdrawal

As with intoxication, the nature and course of alcohol withdrawal depends on whether or not the individual is alcohol-dependent (Table 30.4). Alcohol withdrawal is characterized by rebound effects in those physiological systems that were initially modified by its ingestion. Alcohol withdrawal results in adrenergic hyperactivity at the level of the cortex, limbic system, and brainstem (50, 51).

Uncomplicated alcohol withdrawal or "hangover" is commonly experienced by the nonalcohol-dependent individual after an occasion of heavy drinking (52). It is characterized by tremulousness, mild autonomic hyperactivity, nausea and vomiting, photophobia, malaise, irritability, and vascular headache. The syndrome typically occurs 4–6 hours after the last drink, and subsides within 48 hours (53). It appears to be, in part, genetically determined. Sons of alcoholics have been shown to suffer a more severe hangover than control males drinking the same amount of alcohol (54).

For the individual physically dependent on alcohol, sudden abstinence or a significant decrease in alcohol intake precipitates a withdrawal syndrome of varying severity (37, 55). CNS hyperstimulation results from both decreased inhibitory and increased excitatory neurotransmission (50). In their classic work, Victor and Adams (38) described an early and late stage of acute withdrawal in alcoholics, which, although temporally related, do not necessarily co-occur. The severity of withdrawal correlates partially with chronicity of alcoholism and the degree of tolerance (56), the genetic predisposition of the individual (28), the number and severity of prior withdrawal experiences, and age (56, 57). The history of a severe withdrawal is one of the best predictors of the severity of the subsequent withdrawal syndrome (58). The entire acute withdrawal syndrome typically subsides within 5–7 days.

Alcoholic tremulousness, alcoholic hallucinosis, and withdrawal seizures appear within 6–24 hours after the last drink. Although described as if progressive in nature, their sequence and interdependence are inconsistent (20, 37, 38, 46, 59). Most alcoholics experience the mildest of these syndromes, *alcoholic tremulousness,* as BAL drops to between .10–.20% (20, 37). This is similar to uncomplicated withdrawal in the nondependent individual, but with a somewhat greater amount of autonomic excitation and the potential for mild and transient hallucinations. Postural tremors of the distal upper extremities and tongue, mild tachycardia, headache, irritability, anxiety, anorexia, insomnia, moderate diaphoresis, hyperreflexia, and systolic hypertension are common (34, 38, 59). Typically, this is the extent of alcohol withdrawal for the alcohol-dependent individual; only 10% of alcoholics progress to more severe withdrawal symptomatology (34, 38).

Table 30.3. Neurological Syndromes Associated with Acute Alcohol Ingestion

Syndrome	Blood-alcohol Concentration (g/100 mL[a])	Neurological Findings
Intoxication	.02–.25	Dysarthria, vestibular and cerebellar impairment (ataxia, impaired balance, poor coordination), hyperreflexia, autonomic excess; sluggish pupillary response, nystagmus, diplopia, nonconvergence; impaired judgment, impaired cognition, decreased attention span, emotional lability, anterograde amnesia.
Overdose	.30–.90	Stupor to coma, fluctuating level of consciousness, absence of focal neurological signs, depressed respirations, normal to dilated pupils, sluggish pupillary response.

[a]Blood levels for nontolerant individuals.

Table 30.4. Neurological Syndromes Associated with Alcohol Withdrawal

Syndrome	Alcohol Dependent ?	Time Since Last Drink	Duration	Neurological Findings
Uncomplicated withdrawal	no	4–6 hours	24–48 hours	Tremors, vascular headache, photophobia, mild autonomic excitation, irritability
Acute withdrawal: Early stage Alcohol tremulousness	yes	6–24 hours	24–48 hours	Tremors, headache, irritability, anxiety, mild to moderate autonomic excitation, hyperreflexia, potential transient hallucinations, clear sensorium
Alcoholic hallucinosis				Vivid, threatening, auditory hallucinations, clear sensorium, tremors, moderate autonomic excitation
Withdrawal seizures				Generalized tonic-clonic seizures, occurring in groups of two to six, without EEG focus, postictal confusion and disorientation
Acute withdrawal: Late stage Alcohol withdrawal delirium	yes	36–72 hours	24–72 hours	Profound disorientation, fluctuating level of consciousness, poor remote and immediate memory, visual, auditory or tactile hallucinations, gross tremor, dilated pupils, extreme autonomic hyperactivity
Protracted withdrawal	yes	2–3 weeks	6–24 months	Autonomic dysfunction, sleep disturbance, EEG changes, impaired short-term memory, fatigue

Alcoholic hallucinosis, in which the individual experiences vivid, typically auditory, and often threatening hallucinations, also occurs in early withdrawal (60, 61). The individual's level of consciousness and orientation does not change dramatically, and hallucinations are recognized as such (62, 63). There is mixed evidence that hallucinosis can become chronic, persisting for weeks to years after late-stage alcohol withdrawal, although an underlying schizophrenia needs to be ruled out (60, 63).

Alcohol withdrawal seizures also take place during the early stage of withdrawal, often within several hours after the last drink. They are characteristically generalized tonic-clonic seizures, occurring in groups of two to six (34, 38, 59), with 90% occuring within the first 48 hours of alcohol abstinence (51, 64–66). They are more likely to occur in individuals with previous alcohol withdrawal seizures, an effect some authors have likened to the "kindling" effects of epileptic seizures (67). Of the persons who suffer withdrawal seizures, 88% have less than five such episodes. Rarely does status epilepticus develop (34, 58, 68). These individuals are not epileptic and have normal EEGs (66, 69–71).

Management of these seizures must include ruling out structural diseases and other causes of seizures. Treatment should consider the entirety of the alcohol withdrawal syndrome because other signs of full-blown withdrawal usually develop quickly. Thiamine, 100 mg intravenously, should be part of the initial fluid and electrolyte management. There is no convincing evidence, however, to warrant prophylactic anticonvulsants to prevent alcohol withdrawal seizures (72, 73).

The late stage of alcohol withdrawal syndrome, known as alcohol withdrawal delirium or, more commonly, delirium tremens (DTs), occurs 36–72 hours after the last drink. It is relatively rare, occurring in about 5% of alcoholics (34). Seizure activity increases the likelihood of late-stage withdrawal; between 12–33% of alcoholics who experience seizures upon withdrawal develop DTs (34, 64). Its presence suggests concomitant medical problems, such as pneumonia, subdural hematoma, pancreatitis, fractures, liver disease, or malnutrition.

Alcohol withdrawal delirium is characterized by extreme autonomic hyperactivity, profound disorientation, gross disturbances of recent and remote memory, fluctuating levels of consciousness, incoherence, and confusion (63). The individual is agitated and restless, with terrifying visual, auditory, and tactile hallucinations that cannot be differentiated from reality. Autonomic hyperactivity is evidenced by hyperventilation, tachycardia (commonly 130–150 beats per minute), hypertension (greater than 150/100), hyperthermia (38°–39.5°C), pronounced diaphoresis, facial flushing, gross tremor, and dilated pupils. The development of profuse diarrhea and hyperpyrexia (temperature over 40°C) portend vascular collapse and death (58). Mortality rates of alcohol withdrawal delirium range from 5–15% (74).

Although the most severe withdrawal symptoms for alcoholics occur within the first week of abstinence, there is increasing evidence that persons continue to suffer residual effects of chronic CNS intoxication for weeks to years after their last drink. This is referred to as protracted abstinence, and appears to follow acute withdrawal from many drugs of abuse (e.g., opiates, cocaine) (75). The syndrome is characterized by the persistence of mild to moderate subjective feelings of discomfort or distress, which may play an important role in relapse. The syndrome, which varies considerably across individuals, appears to slowly clear with continued abstinence. The most commonly reported neurological finding associated with protracted alcohol abstinence is some degree of autonomic dysfunction (irregular respirations, labile blood pressure, and pulse), which may persist for up to 2 years (76). Sleep disturbances, electroencephalogram (EEG) changes, impaired short-term memory, fatigue, tremor, and increased muscle tension may persist from 6–24 months after abstinence (46, 77, 78). More importantly, depression and anxiety also tend to persist.

SYNDROMES ASSOCIATED WITH CHRONIC ALCOHOL ABUSE

These syndromes (Table 30.5) typically present after at least a decade of heavy drinking and, in many cases, are permanent conditions, improving only slightly (if at all) with continued abstinence (63, 79). Acute intoxication and withdrawal in persons who continue to drink often complicate the clinical picture.

Wernicke's Encephalopathy

The onset of Wernicke's encephalopathy is typically abrupt, but may develop over several days to weeks, and often is accompanied by drowsiness, headache, nausea, and vomiting. The so-called "classic triad" of ataxia, encephalopathy, and ophthalmoplegia were present in only one-third of persons for whom Wernicke's lesions were found on autopsy; conversely, lesions have been found in a number of patients who were asymptomatic during life (79, 80). Profound confusion and disorientation may be confounded by withdrawal delirium (63). Oculomotor palsies of the third and sixth cranial nerves are common, as is horizontal or vertical nystagmus. Pupils react sluggishly and may be unequal. Ataxia is typically cerebellar, evident in the gait and lower extremitites, with the upper extremities and speech being relatively spared (81). Ataxia may be aggravated by peripheral polyneuropathy and cerebellar degeneration, which are common in Wernicke's encephalopathy (125). Untreated, Wernicke's encephalopathy will progress to stupor and coma. Fortunately, it is responsive to parenteral thiamine therapy, with improvement noted (especially ocular symptoms) within days to weeks (63). If memory deficits persist, a diagnosis of alcohol amnestic disorder must be considered. Alcohol appears to interact with thiamine deficiency to accelerate the progression of neurological dysfunction (83, 84), although genetic factors also play a role, which explains why only a subset of malnourished thiamine-deficient alcoholics develop Wernicke's encephalopathy and why there are large individual differences. Recent evidence suggests that measurement of serum thiamine monophosphate may be a more accurate indicator of chronic alcoholism compared with measurement of free thiamine and thiamine diphosphate, and may help identify patients predisposed to Wernicke's encephalopathy (85).

Alcohol Amnestic Disorder

More commonly known as Korsakoff's psychosis, alcohol amnestic disorder appears to result from cumulative effects of Wernicke's encephalopathy, hence the term "Wernicke-Korsakoff syndrome" (79, 81). Alcohol amnestic disorder is primarily a gross memory disorder of both anterograde and retrograde function, although anterograde deficits predominate. Frequently the sufferer cannot retain new information for more than a few seconds. Intelligence, language, and speech are unaffected and sensorium is clear. Related to profound memory deficits, the patient is usually disoriented to time and place, confabulates to reconstruct forgotten events, and may perseverate. These patients are typically unaware of and unconcerned about their amnesia. The sufferer becomes emotionally flat, inattentive, placid, and apathetic (63, 79, 86). Typically, drinking is stopped spontaneously, which can result in mild memory improvement to complete recovery in 20% of cases. Based on the observation of relative deficit of noradrenaline metabolites in the cerebrospinal fluid (CSF) of a small number of alcoholic Korsakoff syndrome patients, McEntee and Mair treated two small groups of such patients with clonidine and reported improvement of memory performance after 2 weeks of treatment. O'Carroll and associates, in a subsequent study, however, failed to replicate the results (87–90).

Alcoholic Dementia

The diagnosis of alcoholic dementia is made when slowly progressive but stable cognitive dysfunction, attributed to metabolic or organic disease, is noted in alcoholics with extensive drinking histories (79, 91). Current thought is that the dementia relates to the neuropathology of Wernicke's encephalopathy, in that these lesions are commonly found upon autopsy of persons diagnosed with alcoholic dementia (79, 92, 93). Factors to which alcohol dementia have been linked include nutritional deficits, history of head trauma, and direct alcohol neurotoxicity (94–97). Conflicting evidence exists on the correlation between the dementia and frontal lobe atrophy and ventricular enlargement noted on magnetic resonance imaging (MRI) and computed tomography (CT) examination of alcoholics' brains.

Table 30.5. Neurological Syndromes Associated with Chronic Alcohol Abuse[a]

Syndrome	Neurological Findings
Wernicke's encephalopathy	Mental confusion, oculomotor disturbances, gait ataxia, may present with headache, nausea, and vomiting
Alcohol amnestic disorder	Pronounced anterograde and retrograde amnesia, confabulation, perseveration, placid, emotionally flat
Alcoholic dementia	Stable cognitive dysfunction of unknown origin, sensorium clear, aphasia absent, heterogeneous presentation
Cerebellar degeneration	Gait and upper extremity ataxia, bilateral cerebellar incoordination, absence of oculomotor disturbances
Polyneuropathy	Distal, bilateral sensory and lower motor neuron deficits, decreased reflexes, and atrophy of affected areas

[a]All patients report a 10+ year history of heavy alcohol intake.

Table 30.6. Clinical Syndromes of Cocaine Intoxication and Withdrawal

Clinical Syndromes	Clinical Findings	Other Associated Features
Intoxication	euphoria or affective blunting; sociability; hypervigilance; anxiety; tremor; stereotyped movement; dyskinesia and dystonia; impaired judgment	tachycardia; papillary dilation; elevated or lowered blood pressure; sweating or chills; nausea and vomiting; weight loss; psychomotor agitation or retardation; muscle weakness; respiratory depression; cardiac arrhythmia; confusion; seizure
Withdrawal	Phase 1: "crash;" depression; fatigue; craving; anxiety; suspiciousness; paranoia; exhaustion; sleep Phase 2: dysphoria; anhedonia; craving (cue-induced) Phase 3: intermittent craving	

Presenting symptoms are heterogeneous, but typically a progressive lack of interest in the environment and the appearance of oneself, impaired judgment, attention deficits, and slowed thought processes are noted. Symptomatology resembles frontal lobe dysfunction, but emotional lability and grandiosity are absent. Unlike most dementias, there is no disruption of language or loss of primary motor and sensory function. Cognitive deficits typically center in the areas of nonverbal intelligence and visuospatial abilities. Memory deficits are present, but never to the extent noted in alcohol amnestic disorder (98–100). Sensorium is typically clear and aphasia is not present. If the patient continues to drink, alcoholic dementia will progress. DTs exacerbate its course. Slight improvement, absence of progression, and even complete recovery have been reported in abstinent persons (63).

Cerebellar Degeneration

Degeneration of the Purkinje cells in the cerebellar cortex has been noted in certain alcoholics (79). Symptoms related to these lesions tend to develop subacutely over a period of months and worsen with an uneven trajectory as drinking continues. Symptoms include gait ataxia, and may be accompanied by upper extremity ataxia and dysarthria. Cerebellar incoordination is typically bilateral (35, 101). Unlike Wernicke's encephalopathy, oculomotor and mental deficits are absent, although Victor et al. (79) present evidence that alcoholic cerebellar degeneration represents the same disease process. The cerebellum is noted to have high thiamine turnover rates, and stance and gait may respond to thiamine therapy, implicating thiamine deficiency as a possible etiology (102, 103). As with alcoholic dementia, mild improvement of symptoms is reported with abstinence.

Neuropathy

Inadequate nutrition has been shown to play an important role in the development of polyneuropathy in alcoholics, perhaps related to general vitamin B deficiencies as opposed to thiamine deficiency specifically (79, 94, 102). Alcohol-induced neurotoxic effects on axonal transport may be a contributing factor as well. Alcoholic neuropathy tends to

progress gradually and affects sensory and motor nerves more than autonomic nerves. Deficits are distal, bilateral, and asymmetrical, in a glove and stocking distribution, and affect all sensory modalities. Motor weakness, atrophy, and absent or decreased distal deep tendon reflexes signify lower motor neuron deficit (35). Improvment occurs with more adequate nutrition in conjunction with abstinence.

Head Trauma

Alcohol abuse, common among patients with traumatic brain injuries (TBIs), affects the morbidity and recovery of these patients. Behavior disinhibition, prone to occur in such patients, is exaggerated by alcohol (104, 105), and even moderate amounts of alcohol can profoundly affect their balance, reaction time, and cognitive functions (106, 107). Moreover, alcohol lowers the seizure threshold in these patients, who are already at risk from their brain injury (108). Recognition and management of alcohol abuse should be an integral part of managing patients with TBI (109, 110).

COCAINE

Although the neuropsychiatric sequelae of cocaine abuse were well-described over 70 years ago (111), the cocaine epidemic of the 1980s, combined with the switch to the potent smoked (alkaloidal) form, or "crack," have resulted in better clinical description of the intoxication, withdrawal, and cerebrovascular syndromes associated with cocaine use (Table 30.6) (112, 113). In 1991, over 24,000,000 Americans reported having at some time used cocaine, with approximately one in 10 of these reporting cocaine use in the past month. Of the recent cocaine users, over one-quarter had used crack cocaine in the past month (114). Approximately 0.2% of the U.S. population has met dependence or abuse criteria for cocaine at some point over their lifetime (17). The more dramatic neurological complications of cocaine abuse tend be related to acute cocaine toxicity, whereas withdrawal-related neurological symptoms appear to be relatively mild. Neurological impairment related to long-term use is less well defined and may be evident as frontotemporal dysfunction (115), cerebral atrophy (116), or subtle neuropsychological deficits.

Cocaine Intoxication

The acute effects of cocaine use are dependent on dose and route of administration, and are often confounded by concurrent use of marijuana, heroin, alcohol, or other CNS depressants. Oral ingestion of cocaine hydrochloride results in a delayed onset (10–30 minutes) and prolonged duration (45–90 minutes) of action, with relatively low peak plasma levels; intranasal use results in similar peak plasma levels, but with a more rapid onset (2–3 minutes) and shorter duration (30–45 minutes) of drug effects. Smoking and intravenous use result in rapid onset of cocaine effects, within 5–45 seconds, lasting between 5–20 minutes, with peak plasma levels five to 10 times those achieved by oral and intranasal routes (117).

The plasma half-life of cocaine, whichever route of administration, is between 40–60 minutes. Benzoylecgonine, the primary metabolite of liver enzymatic degradation, is itself a potent CNS stimulant. Cocaine is detectable in the urine for up to 36 hours following use, while benzoylecgonine may be present in heavy users for up to 3 weeks.

At low doses, cocaine produces euphoria and a sense of enhanced self-image. Users report increased energy and mental acuity, heightened sensory (including sexual) awareness and self-confidence, and diminished appetite. The euphoric "rush" following intravenous or crack cocaine use is described as intense and orgasmic, lasting from seconds to several minutes. The sympathomimetic effects of cocaine result in increased motor activity and tremor, and increased heart rate, blood pressure, and temperature. At higher doses, taken by chronic users to counteract tolerance to cocaine's euphoric effects, psychological symptoms tend to be more dysphoric and physiological symptoms more indicative of sympathetic overactivity. Anxiety, affective instability, and suspiciousness accompany tachycardia, hypertension and tachypnea.

Psychotic disorders associated with cocaine abuse range from delusional disorders to schizophrenia-like symptoms, and are characterized by anxiety, paranoia, agitation, and impaired judgment, with relative sparing of general cognitive function (117, 118). Cocaine-induced delusions are commonly persecutory, jealous, or somatic, with the latter including parasitosis or cocaine "bugs." These psychoses correlate with high cocaine plasma levels and are believed to be the result of sustained dopamine release. Symptoms gradually resolve as plasma levels fall, and clear within 24 to 48 hours in relatively inexperienced cocaine users, and in several days to weeks in chronic abusers. Increasingly, a hyperarousal delirium syndrome has been noted secondary to cocaine use, characterized by sudden onset of disturbances in perception and attention, disorientation, and cognitive impairment (119). The delirium, theorized to be a variant of neuroleptic malignant syndrome (120) following a prolonged cocaine binge, is frequently accompanied by extremely violent behavior (121). Untreated, the delirium can progress to include hyperthermia, mydriasis, autonomic instability, and fatal respiratory collapse.

Cocaine-induced seizures have been well described (122–125) and are believed to arise from lowered seizure threshold by the local anesthetic effects of the drug, although cerebral anoxia may also play a role (121, 126, 127). Seizures typically occur immediately after or within hours of cocaine use and are more likely to occur when cocaine is injected intravenously or smoked as crack. Most often seizures develop in persons with no history of convulsive disorders. Although chronic cocaine use has been implicated as having a "kindling" effect (128) on seizure activity, seizures are not uncommon in first-time cocaine users. Typically, these seizures are single and generalized and not associated with lasting neurological deficits. Multiple or focal seizures suggest underlying brain pathology and other substance abuse. Rarely, cocaine-induced partial complex seizures with clouded sensorium and stereotyped movements are misdiagnosed as cocaine psychosis (129). Individuals with preexisting convulsive disorders and women are most vulnerable to cocaine-induced seizures (125). Status epilepticus and death have occurred when large amounts of cocaine are ingested, as happens when latex cocaine-filled condoms rupture in the body of "body packers" (130). Death from cocaine-related seizures are believed to result from cardiac arrhythmias (121) and hyperthermia (131), mechanisms quite apart from underlying cocaine-induced seizures.

Cerebrovascular accidents (CVAs) in cocaine abusers result from specific effects of cocaine on the cerebral vasculature in combination with the sympathomimetic effects of cocaine on vascular tone. It has been estimated that the relative risk for stroke among drug abusers after controlling for other stroke risk factors is 6.5 (132), making drug abuse the most common cause of stroke in persons under the age of 35; cocaine abuse accounts for the overwhelming majority of these events (133). Also, cocaine abusers frequently abuse alcohol, which itself is a risk factor for stroke.

The majority of cocaine-related strokes have sudden onset and occur within 72 hours of cocaine use. Hemorrhagic and ischemic strokes occur with approximately equal frequency in cocaine abusers compared with the general population, where infarcts predominate (121), and there is some evidence that the use of alkaloidal cocaine is more likely to result in ischemic strokes than the use of cocaine hydrochloride (134). In almost half of the hemorrhagic strokes, underlying vascular abnormalities (saccular aneurysms and arteriovenous malformations) are present; in the remainder of cases, thalamic and basal ganglia bleeds are common (135). Cocaine-induced hypertension is believed to be the primary cause of intracerebral and subarachnoid hemorrhage.

The mechanisms responsible for ischemic CVAs in cocaine abusers remain unclear, but several possible mechanisms have been described. Vasospasm of the cerebral vessels may be induced by the catacholaminergic effect of cocaine, deranged cerebral autoregulation related to sudden changes in perfusion pressure, increased release of serotonin, or the vasoconstrictive effects of cocaine's primary metabolite,

Table 30.7. Syndromes of Opiate Intoxication and Withdrawal[a]

Syndrome (onset and duration)	Characteristics
Opiate intoxication	Conscious, sedated, "nodding"; mood normal to euphoric; pinhole pupils; history of recent opiate use
Acute overdose	Unconscious; pinhole pupils; slow, shallow respirations
Opiate withdrawal	
Anticipatory[b] (3–4 hours after last "fix")	Fear of withdrawal; anxiety; drug craving; drug-seeking behavior
Early (8–10 hours after last "fix")	Anxiety; restlessness; yawning; nausea; sweating; nasal stuffiness, rhinorrhea; lacrimation; dilated pupils; stomach cramps; drug-seeking behavior
Fully developed (1–3 days after last "fix")	Severe anxiety; tremor; restlessness; piloerection;[c] vomiting, diarrhea; muscle spasms;[d] muscle pain; increased BP; tachycardia; fever, chills; impulse-driven drug-seeking behavior
Protracted abstinence (may last up to 6 months)	Hypotension; bradycardia; insomnia; loss of energy, appetite; stimulus-driven opiate cravings

[a]The times given in the table refer to heroin. Withdrawal will develop more slowly with long-acting opiates.
[b]Anticipatory symptoms begin as the acute effects of heroin begin to subside.
[c]The piloerection has given rise to the term "cold turkey."
[d]The sudden muscle spasms in the legs have given rise to the term "kicking the habit."

benzoylecgonine (113, 121, 127, 134, 136, 137). Increased platelet responsivity and cardiogenic emboli are other possible causes of occlusion (121, 138). Cocaine-induced cerebral hypoperfusion, specifically in the frontal lobe and other superficial cortical areas, contribute to these ischemic events. Transient ischemic attacks have also been reported in cocaine abusers (139, 140), many of which escape medical attention due to their spontaneous resolution.

Cocaine Withdrawal

Physiological dependence on cocaine is evidenced by the development of tolerance to its euphorigenic effects, and by emergence of distinct withdrawal phenomena within a few hours of last cocaine use. Withdrawal symptoms are commonly recognized following heavy and prolonged cocaine use, although a substantial number of individuals dependent on cocaine have few clinically evident withdrawal symptoms on cessation of use (141). Symptoms characteristic of cocaine withdrawal attributed to acute dopamine depletion and receptor up-regulation include dysphoric mood, fatigue, vivid, unpleasant dreams, insomnia or hypersomnia, increased appetite, and either psychomotor agitation or retardation. Muscle pains, chills, twitching, and tremors have also been reported (142). However, the most serious problems associated with cocaine withdrawal are suicidal ideation and suicide attempts, associated with profound withdrawal depression.

Three phases of cocaine abstinence have been described (143). The first phase, commonly referred to as the "crash," occurs within hours of last cocaine use and lasts 3–4 days. Agitation, anorexia, and intense cocaine craving appear early in the crash, but are quickly replaced with fatigue, hypersomnolence, and hyperphagia as craving subsides. Depression persists throughout this first phase. During the second phase which occurs over the next 8–10 weeks, patients experience an early return to normalized mood and sleep pattern with little cocaine craving, although as the anhedonia, anergia, anxiety, and craving for cocaine gradually intensify, patients are at high risk for relapse. The third, or final extinction

phase occurs with continued cocaine abstinence. During this period, the risk of relapse decreases as mood and hedonic response normalize, although cocaine craving continues to emerge intermittently, especially in the presence of conditioned cues. Such craving, resembling protracted alcohol and opiate withdrawal syndromes, can persist indefinitely.

Cocaine- and Stimulant-induced Movement Disorders

Cocaine has been reported to induce chorea, dystonia, choreoathetoid movements, akathisia, buccolingual dyskinesia, eye blinking and lip smacking (144, 145). These movements, referred to as "crack dancing" within certain drug-using communities, have typical onset within two hours of use and appear to be self-limited, although follow-up data are sparse and a few appear to persist. They are similar to those previously described with amphetamine abuse (146, 147) and have recently been associated with norpseudoephedrine use (148). Most likely these symptoms result from accumulated high levels of dopamine in the synaptic cleft within the basal ganglia.

OPIATES

The extent to which Americans abuse opiates is difficult to quantify because the majority of opiates ingested are legally dispensed for analgesic use; illicit use of street opiates accounts for a relatively small proportion of the total amount of opiates consumed. Recent estimates indicate that over 6% of the U.S. population has used analgesics for nonmedical reasons, while less than 2% report having used heroin in the past year (16). The lifetime prevalence of persons meeting diagnostic criteria for opiate dependence has been estimated to be 0.7%, with 0.1% meeting dependence criteria within the past 6 months (17).

As with alcohol, syndromes commonly associated with opiate use are temporally related to the last opiate use and chronicity of use (Table 30.7). The duration of opiate intoxication and onset of withdrawal varies with the pharmacological half-life of the particular opiate. For example, heroin and meperidine have relatively short half-lives, and withdrawal symptoms from these opiates can emerge within 8 hours of drug abstinence. Tolerance and physical dependence develop quite rapidly after repeated opiate exposure; mild physical dependence has been demonstrated after short-term postoperative opiate analgesic administration. Tolerance, however, does not develop uniformly to all opiate effects; notable tolerance develops to the analgesia, euphoria, sedation, and respiratory depression, and little to the gastrointestinal, pupillary and endocrine effects (149). Cross-tolerance to the CNS effects of opiates exists across opiate medications.

Opiate Intoxication

The CNS effects of opiates include analgesia, drowsiness, changes in mood, and mental clouding. Respiratory depression, miosis, nausea and vomiting, and cough reflex suppression are other opiate effects mediated centrally (150). Acute subjective effects vary, depending on whether the individual is in pain, is dependent upon opiates, or is without either pain or addiction. In normal, pain-free individuals, the acute effects of opiates are frequently described as unpleasant, and include nausea, vomiting, inability to concentrate, lethargy, and reduced visual acuity. For those experiencing pain, analgesia is the predominant response and is accompanied by drowsiness, pruritis and, occasionally, euphoria. For drug-free ex-addicts, mental clouding is less severe and euphoria is pronounced, typically peaking with the "rush" following intravenous injection.

Opiate overdose occurs when the respiratory depressant effects result in a decreased level of consciousness. Despite the notable tolerance opiate addicts develop to opiate respiratory depression, overdose is not uncommon, partly because tolerance is not complete and partly because addicts tend to combine opiates with alcohol or other CNS depressants. Pinhole pupils, slow, shallow respirations, and coma are the classic triad of acute opiate overdose. If hypoxia persists, pulmonary edema, hypotension, and cardiovascular collapse occur, and eventually death supervene. Establishment of an airway and intravenous administration of naloxone, an opiate antagonist, are the key elements of treatment for opiate overdose (151).

Opiate Withdrawal

CNS hyperexcitability characterizes the opiate withdrawal syndrome. The severity of withdrawal depends on the degree of physical dependence, the particular opiate used, the health and personality of the addict, and the setting in which the withdrawal occurs (149, 151). Early symptoms include lacrimation, rhinorrhea, yawning and sweating, with progression of symptoms to include dilated pupils, anorexia, gooseflesh, restlessness, irritability, and tremor. In fully developed opiate withdrawal, increased irritability, insomnia, marked anorexia, violent yawning, severe sneezing, lacrimation, nausea, vomiting, diarrhea, weakness, pronounced depressed mood, tachycardia, and hypertension are

noted. Fluid and electrolyte imbalance occur with prolonged anorexia, vomiting, diaphoresis and diarrhea, although rarely does opiate withdrawal require medical intervention. The most common outcome of opiate withdrawal is relapse to opiate use.

As with alcohol, a protracted abstinence syndrome has been described in drug-free opiate addicts, emerging after the patient has been completely detoxified and lasting from weeks to months. Although subtle, the symptoms of protracted abstinence, including hypotension, hyperalgesia, and poor stress tolerance, have been identified as important reasons for relapse following opiate withdrawal (150).

Neuropsychiatric Syndromes Associated with Opiate Abuse

Opiates themselves do not directly cause either neuropathology or psychopathology; rather it is the common routes of administration (subcutaneous and intravenous), the adulterants used to cut or prepare abused opiates (e.g., quinine, lead, chloroquine, MPTP) (152, 153), and the life-style associated with illicit opiate use that account for the majority of neurological complications of opiate abuse. Other than those associated with HIV infection and AIDS (see later discussion of HIV), the majority of infective neurological complications of intravenous drug use are those that accompany endocarditis, which is typically right-sided with tricuspid valve involvement (154). Infectious material filtered in the pulmonary tree are circulated systemically when arteriovenous shunts develop secondary to pulmonary hypertension, and can result in intraparenchymal and extraparenchymal abscess of the brain and spinal cord, meningitis, embolic cerebral infarction, diffuse vasculitis, and septic aneurysm (139, 155). Other neurological complications of infectious origin in street opiate addicts include hepatitis, encephalopathy, CNS syphilis, tetanus, and botulism (156).

A neurological complication of noninfective origin associated with parenteral opiate use is cerebral or spinal embolic stroke as the result of relatively insoluble foreign materials or adulterants being injected directly into the vasculature along with opiate drugs (139); other possible causes of cerebral infarction in opiate addicts include hypoperfusion with opiate overdose, and allergic or toxic vasculitis (157). Hemorrhagic strokes in heroin addicts follow hypertension secondary to nephropathy, or clotting derangements secondary to liver disease. Peripheral neuropathy may occur due to nerve damage at common injection sites or pressure palsies during overdose (158, 159), and fibrotic myositis has resulted from repeated needle trauma and local toxic responses (160).

SEDATIVE-HYPNOTICS

The sedative-hypnotics include a chemically diverse group of medications (Table 30.8) that relieve anxiety, produce sedation, and induce sleep. Although it is estimated that over 8,000,000 Americans report having used sedatives for nonmedical purposes, most sedative-hypnotics are not primary drugs of abuse. Some of the short-acting barbiturates

Table 30.8. Chemical Classification of Drugs Used for Hallucinogenic Effects

Chemical Class	Drugs	Common or Street Names
Indoles	Lysergic acid diethylamide	LSD, acid
	Dimethyltryptamine	DMT
	Psilocybin and psilocin	magic mushrooms
Phenethylamines	Mescaline	
	2,5-dimethoxy-4-methylamphetamine	DOM
	3,4-methylenedioxyamphetamine	MDA
	3,4-methylenedioxymethylamphetamine	MDMA, XTC, Ecstasy
	3,4-methylenedioxyethylamphetamine	Eve

are injected for the "rush" or taken orally to produce a state of disinhibition similar to alcohol, while benzodiazepines are often used by substance abusers to relieve opiate withdrawal, to augment the effects of methadone, or to ameliorate the adverse effects of cocaine or methamphetamine. Unlike other drugs of abuse, most sedative-hypnotics are manufactured by legitimate pharmaceutical companies and diverted to the illicit street-drug market through medical channels.

Sedative-Hypnotic Intoxication

Most people do not find the subjective effects of sedative-hypnotics pleasant or appealing beyond their therapeutic effects (i.e., relief of anxiety or facilitation of sleep), while persons predisposed to addiction find the effects of sedative-hypnotics reinforcing (161). The acute effects of sedative-hypnotics consist of slurred speech, incoordination, ataxia, sustained nystagmus, impaired judgment, and mood lability. In large amounts, sedative-hypnotics produce progressive respiratory depression and coma. The amount of respiratory depression produced by the benzodiazepines is much less than that produced by the barbiturates and other sedative-hypnotics.

Sedative-Hypnotic Withdrawal

Barbiturates produce tolerance and physical dependence, which can be induced within several days of continuous infusion of anesthetic doses. The withdrawal syndrome from sedative-hypnotics is similar to the withdrawal syndrome from alcohol. Signs and symptoms include anxiety, tremors, nightmares, insomnia, anorexia, nausea, vomiting, postural hypotension, seizures, delirium, and hyperpyrexia. The syndrome is qualitatively similar for all sedative-hypnotics; however, the time course depends upon the particular drug. With short-acting sedative-hypnotics (e.g., pentobarbital, secobarbital, meprobamate, oxazepam, alprazolam, and triazolam), withdrawal symptoms typically begin 12–24 hours after the last dose and peak in intensity between 24–72 hours. Symptoms may develop more slowly in patients with liver disease or in the elderly because of decreased drug metabolism. With long-acting drugs (e.g., phenobarbital, diazepam, and chlordiazepoxide), withdrawal symptoms peak on the 5th–8th day.

During untreated sedative-hypnotic withdrawal, the EEG may show paroxysmal bursts of high-voltage, slow-frequency activity that precede the development of seizures. The withdrawal delirium may include confusion and visual and auditory hallucinations. Some patients may have only delirium or only seizures, while some may have both. Benzodiazepines can also produce a protracted withdrawal syndrome in some patients, after cessation of long-term therapeutic use.

HALLUCINOGENS

Hallucinogens are a chemically diverse group of compounds that produce perceptual distortion and prominent visual hallucinations. Perceptual changes include depersonalization, derealization, illusions, and synesthesias, in which sensory stimuli in one sense produce changes in another, e.g., a beating drum is seen as a flashing light. Many drugs, like nicotine or atropine, can produce visual hallucinogens as a facet of high-dose toxicity and, in some cultures, are ritualistically used for their hallucinations effects. The hallucinogenic drugs considered here are those commonly used by drug abusers in the United States. Hallucinogens do not produce physical dependence, and, because tolerance to the psychological effects develops rapidly, they are typically used episodically.

Hallucinogens are used for a variety of reasons, ranging from a means of spiritual quest to enhancing enjoyment of dancing, or simply to experience the alterations of perception. Recently, MDMA has enjoyed popularity at dances (called raves) in the United States (162) and England (163, 164). In the 1960s, LSD was the most commonly used hallucinogen, while MDMA seems to be more popular in the 1990s. Although 8.2% of the U.S. population report having used a hallucinogen (16), less than 0.3% have ever met diagnostic criteria for dependence. The true prevalence of use is difficult to determine because most users do not come to medical attention.

Hallucinogen Intoxication

The effects of hallucinogens depend on the drug, the dose, the setting, and the circumstances of use. Typically, CNS effects include dilated pupils, tachycardia, sweating, palpitations, and tremors. Experienced hallucinogenic users accept these signs and symptoms as an expected part of the drug experience, although novice users sometimes find the symptoms frightening. Perceptual alterations associated with intoxication include changes in mood, intensification of perceptions, depersonalization, and derealization. Hallucinations are usually visual, but auditory and tactile hallucinations sometimes occur. When users become frightened by the content of the hallucinations or by paranoid ideation, they may become acutely anxious and are said to have a "bad trip." These "bad trips" rarely come to medical attention because experienced users are skilled at "talk-down" techniques, which usually take the form of reassurance or redirecting attention to another topic or image. The combined effects of perceptual distortion, impaired judgment, and excitation sometimes result in serious adverse consequences. For instance, users may fall off a building not because of suicidal ideation, but because they believe they can fly.

Neuropsychiatric Syndromes Associated with Hallucinogen Abuse

Sporadic case reports suggest that LSD can cause significant vasospasm and stroke (165). Subarachnoid hemorrhage has been reported in association in MDMA abuse (166). MDA and MDMA have been implicated in degeneration of serotonergic neurons in animals, but the clinical significance is uncertain (167). Neuropsychological impairment has been reported in heavy users of MDMA (168).

"Flashbacks" are transient recurrences of perceptual alterations like those that occurred under the influence of the hallucinogen. Perceptual alterations may include flashes of color, peripheral field images, after-images, halos, or macropsia and micropsia. Flashbacks may last seconds to several minutes and may be triggered by other drugs, anxiety or fatigue. Flashbacks can occur up to 5 years or more after abstinence. The person is aware that the perceptual alteration is a drug effect. LSD and MDMA can cause flashbacks and have also been reported to induce panic disorder (169–172) and chronic paranoid psychosis (173, 174).

MARIJUANA

Marijuana intoxication has been demonstrated to impair learning and short-term memory (175, 176) and the performance of complex motor tasks (177–179). However, it is fairly well established that chronic marijuana use produces no notable neurological impairment. In an extensive review of the literature, Wert and Raulin (180) found no significant differences between volunteer and heavy user samples and normal controls on CT scan or EEG measures, nor upon detailed neurological examination. Furthermore, the majority of studies reviewed provided no evidence that chronic marijuana use resulted in diminished psychological or neuropsychological performance (181). Yet the authors caution that undetected subtle neurological impairments may exist, and these may become more pronounced with

age, noting that few of the subjects studied were over the age of 35.

It is pertinent to add that the cannabinoids found in marijuana have been reported to have both antiepileptic and antispasmodic activity. Prior to the 1937 passage of the Marijuana Tax Act, cannabis was listed in the *National Formulary and Pharmacopoeia* for these clinical indications, and was available in over 28 different pharmaceuticals (182). Although virtually never used today as an antiepileptic agent, animal data have provided evidence that the cannabinoid cannabidiol depresses epileptiform electrophysiological responses with little to no development of tolerance to these effects (183–186). In a small placebo-controlled clinical trial with 15 patients with epilepsy refractory to traditional anticonvulsant pharmacotherapy, improvement was noted in 85% of patients receiving 200–300 mg of cannabinoid daily as compared with only one patient on placebo (187).

There is much anecdotal but little published evidence for the use of marijuana as an antispasmodic agent for the treatment of muscle spasms that occur with spinal cord injury and multiple sclerosis (MS) (188), which is attributed to the inhibitory effects of the tetrahydrocannabinol cannabinoid (THC) on polysynaptic reflexes (189). In one small double-blind clinical trial (190), nine patients with MS-related spasticity were treated with two doses of THC or placebo on three separate occasions. Both THC doses (5 mg and 10 mg) significantly improved spasticity as measured by deep tendon reflex tone, resistance to stretch, and the presence of abnormal reflexes. Clinical populations frequently report self-medicating with marijuana to lessen muscle spasticity, and support recent efforts to make THC more readily available to clinicians and patients (191).

Specific Neuropsychiatric Syndromes Associated with Drug Abuse

Just as a particular drug of abuse can result in a number of neuropsychiatric syndromes, a particular neuropsychiatric syndrome can be associated with a number of drugs of abuse. The most common neuropsychiatric syndromes that occur across drug classes include seizure, stroke, coma, delirium, CNS infection, and peripheral neuropathies. When patients present these complaints for medical care, it is essential to rule out primary neurological diseases and to include long-term drug abuse treatment in the total care plan.

SEIZURES

Seizures are sudden alterations in cerebral function produced by excessive discharge of groups of neurons in the brain. They can be generalized or focal, depending on whether the entire brain or localized brain areas are involved; not uncommonly seizures begin focally and quickly progress to generalized seizures as neuronal discharge spreads throughout the brain. Generalized seizures are the most frequent type encountered in drug abusers, and are characterized by loss of consciousness, loss of motor control, incontinence and tonic-clonic jerking of the extremities. Generalized seizures typically last between 1–5 minutes. Those that recur without the patient regaining consciousness in between seizures or continue unabated for greater than 5 minutes are termed status epilepticus, which requires immediate anticonvulsant pharmacotherapy, although cocaine-induced status epilepticus may be refractory to standard anticonvulsant agents. Focal seizures in drug abusers suggest the presence of a focal lesion, such as brain abscess or stroke.

Clinical experience suggests that seizures are much more common among drug abusers than in the general population. Drug-related seizures occur most frequently between the ages of 25–40 years. Diagnosis of drug-related seizures, usually made on the basis of patient history or witness report, can be difficult unless the incidents are observed, because addicts may feign seizures to obtain disability status or medications, and EEGs, while helpful when abnormal, may be normal between seizures.

Drug intoxication or withdrawal should not automatically be assumed to be the cause of seizures in drug abusers. Brain abscess, embolic stroke, and meningitis, all common complications of drug abuse, may first manifest as generalized or focal seizure activity, as may neurological diseases of non-drug abuse origin. Other causes of seizures must be considered, especially in patients whose seizures cannot temporally be related to drug use. When drug-related seizures seem likely, it should be determined whether they arise from intoxication or occur during withdrawal (Table 30.9).

STROKE

Strokes are a sudden, focal disruption of brain function produced by interruption of blood flow to brain tissue. They can be ischemic, occurring from obstruction of blood flow, or hemorrhagic, resulting from rupture and bleeding within the cerebrovasculature. In either case, neurons distal to the blood flow interruption become anoxic and die. Hemorrhagic strokes also induce vasospasm of nearby vessels, further aggravating cerebral anoxia. The nature, severity, and duration of neurological deficit following stroke varies with the location, size, and number of affected vessels; strokes originating in the circle of Willis can result in massive motor and sensory deficits, coma, or death, whereas multiple infarcts in small vessels may result in less obvious deficits that may become evident only upon careful neurological or neuropsychological testing. Deficits arising from embolic stroke may be transient (lasting less than 24 hours) if the embolus dissolves or if collateral blood flow is sufficient to prevent infarct.

The relationship between drug abuse and stroke has been recognized for over a decade (155) and abuse of drugs has been identified as a predisposing factor in 47% of stroke patients under the age of 35 (132). Stroke in cocaine abusers is likely to be hemorrhagic and related to drug-induced hypertensive bleeds in cerebral vessels with underlying weakness, such as aneurysms or AVMs (127, 139). Strokes in alcoholics also tend to be hemorrhagic secondary to hypertension from chronic alcohol abuse (192). Stroke in opiate abusers, on the other hand, is likely to be ischemic and related to inadequate cerebral perfusion during opiate overdose (274). Intravenous use of any drug puts individuals at risk for ischemic stroke due to emboli arising from an infected heart valve or foreign particulate matter injected into the bloodstream with the drug (139, 193) (Table 30.10).

COMA

Coma can complicate opiate, alcohol, and sedative hypnotic overdose due to profound respiratory depression and direct CNS effects associated with toxic levels of these drugs, singly or in combination. In opiate overdose, the respiratory rate is extremely low, and cyanosis may be present. Pupils are typically pinholes bilaterally, unless hypoxia is severe, in which case they will be fixed and dilated. Blood pressure falls as hypoxia persists, body temperature is low, the skin is cool and clammy, and the muscle tone is hypotonic. Pulmonary edema and shock commonly complicate opiate-induced coma, and respiratory failure is the typical cause of death (194). The maintenance of an adequate airway and administration of naloxone result in dramatic improvment, which can occur even in the presence

Table 30.9. Seizure Activity Associated with Drugs of Abuse

Drug Class	Intoxication	Withdrawal	Early Abstinence
Alcohol	Infrequent; may potentiate seizures in patients with underlying seizure disorder	Common	Infrequent; seizure threshold may be lowered
Opiates	May occur with meperidine and propoxyphene use	Absent, except in case of newborn	Rare; seizure threshold may be lowered in persons with intoxication seizures
Cocaine	Common	Absent	Rare; seizure threshold may be lowered in persons with intoxication seizures
Sedative hypnotics	Rare; these agents act as anticonvulsants	Common in abrupt withdrawal	Infrequent; seizure threshold may be lowered
Hallucinogens	Rare	Absent	Absent

Table 30.10. Causes of Cerebral Embolism in Intravenous Drug Abusers

Cause	Mechanism
Injection of particulate matter into the carotid artery	While attempting to inject into the jugular vein, abuser accidentally punctures carotid artery, sending particulate matter directly into cerebral circulation.
Reverse blood flow across patent foramen ovale	Recurrent embolization of particulate matter in lungs causes pulmonary hypertension, shunting venous blood to left ventricle and directly into cerebral circulation.
Formation of arteriovenous shunts in lung	Recurrent embolization of particulate matter in lungs produces granulomas and arteriovenous shunts in lung tissue, introducing venous blood into the arterial circulation to the brain.
Endocarditis	Repeated injection of infectious matter into the venous circulation results in friable right-sided heart valve tissue. Valvular emboli reach arterial circulation and brain via patent foramen ovale or pulmonary arteriovenous shunts described above.

of alcohol or sedative hypnotics, because of antagonism of opiate-induced respiratory depression.

The coma from toxic levels of barbiturates or alcohol is similar, with very slow or Cheyne-Stokes respirations, and low body temperature. Deep tendon reflexes are generally preserved, and the Babinski sign is often positive. Pupils are constricted but remain reactive unless hypoxia is severe. Death results from severe hypotension and shock, renal failure, or pulmonary complications. Treatment is primarily supportive, consisting of airway maintenance, adequate supply of oxygen, and maintenance of blood pressure with intravenous fluid and dopamine administration. If drug ingestion occurred within 24 hours, gastric lavage may be initiated; rarely hemodialysis may be indicated (195).

Overdosage of benzodiazepines alone does not cause coma; however, alcohol increases the absorption of benzodiazepines and potentiates its CNS depression (195). Other causes of coma in drug abusers include direct neurological sequelae from drug use (e.g., stroke, seizure) and from risky life-style and health behaviors (e.g., hypoglycemia, head trauma).

DELIRIUM

The delirium that accompanies cocaine intoxication and alcohol withdrawal is typical of delirium of neurological or metabolic origin. Clinical features include inattention, rambling irrelevant speech, clouded sensorium, disorientation, hallucinations, memory impairment, disturbances of the sleep-wake cycle, and psychomotor activity. Typically, substance-induced delirium is accompanied by hyperthermia, psychomotor hyperactivity or agitation, and auditory or tactile hallucinations that are recognized by the patient as such until delirium becomes severe. Transient paranoid psychosis, brief panic attacks, and marked physical agitation (including violent behavior) have been reported with delirium associated with cocaine intoxication (119, 196–198).

Management of substance-induced delirium includes provision of a calm, quiet, dimly lit, reassuring environment. Restraints, which should be used sparingly and only when the patient's safety cannot be assured, can lead to symptom escalation in some cases. Benzodiazepines are the pharmacotherapy of choice for substance-induced delirium; short-

acting agents are preferred for cocaine-induced delirium and longer-acting ones for the delirium associated with alcohol withdrawal (199).

CENTRAL NERVOUS SYSTEM INFECTION

The immunosuppression that accompanies cocaine and opiate abuse, apart from that associated with HIV disease, puts intravenous users of these drugs at high risk for neurological infections. Direct injection of pathogens, which are harbored on the heart valves in endocarditis and subsequently carried into the CNS as infective emboli, or as disseminated sepsis, can result in brain and epidural abcess (200) and meningitis. Subarachnoid hemorrage occurs from rupture of mycotic aneurysms (201, 202). Users who inject into the jugular vein are at particular risk for vertebral osteomyelitis (200, 203, 204), with secondary epidural and extradural spine infections. Common bacterial and fungal pathogens include hemolytic streptococci, *Staphylococcus aureus* (205–208), *Pseudomonas* (209–211) and *Candida* (212), although more exotic organisms have also been identified (213, 214).

PERIPHERAL NEUROPATHY

Peripheral neuropathy in substance abusers can result from direct trauma to the nerve from injection of toxic adulterants, from local infection due to contaminated paraphernalia, or from pressure palsies during periods of unconsciousness, or heavy sleep from intoxication (159). The disorder affects both motor and sensory nerves and is characterized by pain, weakness, and numbness. Alcohol neuropathies tend to be bilateral and symmetrical, affecting the distal limbs most profoundly. Neuropathies from trauma, traction, and pressure tend to be focal and affect nerves prone to pressure, like radial nerves in "Saturday night palsy" and brachial plexopathy from traction.

PHARMACOLOGICAL TREATMENT OF DRUG ABUSE

Management of the neuropsychiatric complications of drug abuse include treatment of the underlying addiction, which often begins with management of withdrawal symp-

Table 30.11. Opiate Addiction Pharmacotherapies

Medication	Drug Class	Indication	Clinical Action
Methadone	Opiate agonist	Maintenance therapy; Detoxification	Suppress withdrawal; block effects of subsequently administered opiates
LAAM	Opiate agonist	Maintenance therapy	Suppress withdrawal; block effects of subsequently administered opiates
Buprenorphine[a]	Partial opiate agonist	Maintenance therapy; Detoxification	Suppress withdrawal; block effects of subsequently administered opiates; produce less physical dependence than full agonists
Naltrexone	Opiate antagonist	Postdetoxification	Block effects of subsequently administered opiates
Clonidine	α_2-Adrenergic agonist	Withdrawal	Suppress withdrawal-induced noradrenergic hyperactivity

[a]Not yet FDA-approved for the treatment of opiate dependence.

toms accompanying abstinence. Although psychosocial and psychoeducational therapies have remained critical components to the overall recovery program, pharmacological strategies have assumed an increasingly important role in the management of opiate, cocaine, and alcohol abuse and dependence. Pharmacotherapy can be short term, narrowly focused, using specific medications for targeted clinical manifestations, such as benzodiazepines for alcohol withdrawal and naloxone for acute opiate overdose; or it can be more sustained and long term with more distal and global outcome implications. Treatment goals differ from the perspective of the physician, the patient, and the society. The physician wants the addict to stop using drugs and get healthier; the patient wants to avoid physical "sickness" from withdrawal and hassles from law enforcement, though not necessarily to stop using drugs; society wants crimes reduced, neighborhoods made safe, and addicts converted from tax eaters to taxpayers. These divergent goals can lead to frustration and disappointment when patients and clinicians fail to appreciate each others' expectations.

It is also important to distinguish pharmacological efficacy from clinical efficacy. Because pharmacotherapy primarily affects physiology, only certain changes can be attributed to the direct effects of the medication. For example, in substituting methadone for heroin, the prevention of withdrawal and blockade of the effects of subsequently administered street heroin can be attributed to the direct pharmacological effects of methadone. Retention in treatment and reduction in craving and in drug use can also be reasonably linked to methadone's pharmacological effects, though less directly. Reduction in criminal activities and increase in employment, while no less important clinical outcomes, are nonetheless more distal effects of methadone substitution and subject to many intervening events. Pharmacological efficacy cannot always be directly translated into clinical efficacy. Naltrexone, for instance, completely blocks the effects of heroin and is therefore pharmacologically highly efficacious, but it has only limited clinical efficacy because few addicts want to take it. On the other hand, clinical efficacy can only be attributed to medication effects where pharmacological efficacy has been shown.

Opiate Pharmacotherapies

Pharmacotherapy for opiate dependence includes treatment of acute overdose, detoxification, and long-term substitution (Table 30.11). Naloxone, a highly potent, virtually pure opiate antagonist, is the specific treatment for acute opiate overdose, characterized by slow, shallow respiration, pinhole pupils, and coma. The response is both dramatic and immediate. The patient, who moments earlier appeared virtually dead, awakens after an intravenous injection of 0.4–0.8 mg of naloxone, even before the needle is completely withdrawn from the injection site. This response is so specific that anything short of a clear reversal of coma should arouse suspicion of irreversible coma from severe, prolonged anoxia, mixed overdose, overdose from nonopiates, or presence of serious underlying neurological complications. A transient response should suggest overdose from long-acting opiates like L-alpha acetyl methadol (LAAM) or methadone. Coma may return in these patients after the effects of naloxone wears off. Such patients require a longer period of observation or hospitalization overnight. Because of its short duration of action, naloxone may need to be given repeatedly or administered by an intravenous drip.

Opiate Detoxification (Gradual Withdrawal)

Methadone and clonidine are the two most commonly employed medications for opiate detoxification. A synthetic full opiate agonist, methadone effectively suppresses the symptoms of opiate withdrawal and can be conveniently administered once daily in an oral preparation, usually diluted with juice. The starting dose for detoxification of street heroin addicts is usually 30–40 mg. After several days of stabilization, the dose is tapered to zero over 2–3 weeks. In practice, because methadone is a schedule II narcotic under strict legal control and generalist physicians are prohibited by law from prescribing a narcotic for treatment of opiate addiction, methadone detoxification is available only in specially licensed outpatient methadone clinics.

The failure rate for patients treated in outpatient methadone detoxification is very high, in part because continued exposure to street drugs triggers intense craving, which often leads to relapse, and in part because the treatment period allowable under the law is too short to achieve abstinence and psychosocial stabilization. For many years, detoxification was limited to 21 days, beyond which administration of methadone moved the patient into maintenance treatment, which is governed by its own set of rules and regulations. Although the FDA now allows detoxification to be extended to 180 days, many states still have not adopted these changes.

Clonidine, an α-adrenergic agonist marketed for treatment of hypertension, suppresses the physiological manifestation of opiate withdrawal related to rebound sympathetic hyperactivity. It is not a scheduled medication and is therefore available to physicians in general. Although it has not received FDA approval for the treatment of opiate withdrawal, it has been used for this purpose extensively, and several dosing strategies have been described (149). Its major drawbacks are orthostatic hypotension and sedation, which limit the amount of medication that can be safely administered. Also, clonidine suppression of opiate withdrawal symptoms is incomplete. It has little effect on craving, and ancillary medication is often needed for aches and pains and for insomnia.

There is no reason to believe that LAAM, approved for maintenance treatment of opiate dependence, would not be suitable for opiate detoxification. However, as a schedule II narcotic, it shares all the administrative constraints of methadone. Buprenorphine, under intense study but not yet approved for general use, may be a very useful medication for detoxification, especially if the naloxone combination dosage form is successfully developed, allowing its use outside the context of specially licensed clinics.

The severity of opiate withdrawal depends not only on the degree of dependence but also on environmental influences. Experiences from therapeutic communities and other closed environments suggest that most opiate addicts can undergo withdrawal in a supportive closed environment without much need for medication. The physical symptoms of withdrawal clear rapidly, and the process can be expedited with ancillary medications. The withdrawal process is physiologically benign; thus, drastic measures are unnecessary. However, there is a high rate of relapse after patients leave the controlled environment. Hence, the major challenge in opiate detoxification is to find a medication that can be used, without unnecessarily burdensome legal constraints, by general physicians in their office practice while their patients live and work in the real world.

OPIATE MAINTENANCE

Two relatively long-acting opiate agonists, methadone and LAAM, are currently available for chronic maintenance treatment for opiate dependence. Buprenorphine, a partial agonist, may become available soon. Naltrexone, an orally effective, long-acting antagonist, has been available for over a decade for the prevention of relapse but has enjoyed only limited clinical success.

Methadone

Methadone maintenance is the prototype for opiate substitution pharmacotherapy, having been administered in specially licensed clinics for more than 30 years. It is a full opiate agonist that, when administered orally, suppresses the emergence of withdrawal symptoms in opiate-dependent individuals and blocks the effects of subsequently administered opiates for up to 72 hours (215, 216). Methadone has a slower onset and longer duration of action than heroin and other short-acting, abused opiates and thus does not provide a reinforcing "rush" upon administration. Most patients can be effectively maintained with once-daily dosing and, because of its blocking action at the μ-opiate receptor, addicts no longer need to use drugs to counteract or avoid withdrawal. Because it is orally administered, secondary reinforcements related to needle use are obviated. Methadone maintenance frees patients from having to engage in illegal and risky activities (including intravenous drug use) to obtain and use opiates and provides them the opportunity to participate in rehabilitative activities. High-dose methadone maintenance (70–90 mg/day) has proven more effective than low-dose maintenance in reducing injection drug use, which in turn is important in reducing HIV transmission among the drug-abusing population (217–219).

Methadone maintenance is available to addicts only in specially licensed clinics. Federal and state regulations govern virtually every aspect of its practice, including, among other things, criteria for admission, limits on dosing, requirements of urine testing, and special requirements on confidentiality of patient treatment information.

LAAM

A derivative of methadone, LAAM was first synthesized by German scientists in 1948. Its slow onset and long duration of action, unique among the group of related compounds, suggested the presence of active metabolites. This finding was subsequently confirmed by laboratory and human studies. Shortly after its discovery, Fraser and Isbell (220), in a series of studies with past addicts and addicts maintained on morphine, showed that orally administered LAAM produced euphoria, pupillary constriction, and constipation, and cross-substituted for morphine, preventing the emergence of abstinence in subjects maintained on 240 mg daily morphine in dosing intervals up to 96 hours. Clinical interest in LAAM as a maintenance treatment for opiate addiction emerged in the late 1960s with the growing success of methadone maintenance.

During the course of some 27 studies, in both open and double-blind clinical trials, LAAM was tested in over 4000 patients (221). Its efficacy in reducing illicit opiate use and keeping patients in treatment, as well as its safety with chronic administration, were demonstrated convincingly. The accumulated evidence allowed for drafting of labeling information, which was tested in a 12-week labeling assessment study involving 623 patients in 26 methadone clinics across the country (222). Again, LAAM's safety and efficacy were confirmed and, on 7/9/93, the FDA approved LAAM for treatment of opiate dependence, making it the first available opiate substitution alternative to methadone in over 3 decades.

LAAM is a synthetic opiate agonist, with actions qualitatively similar to morphine, a prototype μ-agonist that affects the CNS and smooth muscles. Its principal actions, to which tolerance develops over time, are analgesia and sedation. An abstinence syndrome, similar to that observed with other opiates but with slower onset, less intensity, and a more protracted course, occurs on cessation after chronic administration. After oral administration, LAAM is well absorbed in the gastrointestinal tract. It is metabolized by N-demethylation to nor-LAAM and dinor-LAAM, both potent opiate agonists, with the former being three to six times more active than methadone and the latter about equivalent to methadone. Opiate activities, representing the combined effects of the parent drug and its active metabolites, begin in 1–2 hours, peak at 4–8 hours, and last up to 72 hours. It is widely distributed throughout the body and, unlike methadone, is excreted largely in the feces as nor-LAAM and dinor-LAAM. Less than 20% is excreted in the urine, mostly as conjugates.

The slow onset and long duration of action confers on LAAM a unique pharmacological profile that offers both pharmacological and logistic advantages in opiate maintenance pharmacotherapy. Its slow onset of action makes it less subject to abuse, greatly decreases its street value and, thus, minimizes its risk for street diversion. Its long duration of action provides a more stable blood level and allows for three times a week dosing. Thus, clinics can serve larger numbers of patients by reducing the amount of paperwork and manpower needed for daily dosing preparation and record keeping (220, 223–227).

Any patient suitable for methadone maintenance can be similarly treated with LAAM, although LAAM may be particularly appealing to those who have difficulty attending clinics on a daily basis, find methadone's duration of action too short due to rapid metabolism, or find methadone's effects too sedating because LAAM appears to have less sedative effect than methadone. Patients fearing methadone's stigmatization may also find LAAM an attractive alternative.

Because LAAM is also a schedule II narcotic, its use is governed by regulations similar to methadone. It is currently not recommended for pregnant women or patients under 18 years of age, and no take-home doses are allowed. Further clinical experience should allow for reconsideration of these issues in the near future.

Buprenorphine

Derived from the opium alkaloid thebaine, buprenorphine is a potent partial agonist at the μ receptor and a weak antagonist at the κ receptor. As a result, its agonist activities, like analgesia and respiratory depression, have a ceiling effect even at full receptor occupancy. Due to its κ antagonist effect, it is devoid of psychomimetic effects. Buprenorphine is 20 to 30 times more potent than morphine on a weight basis, its equivalent parenteral analgesic dose being 0.3 mg. It blocks the effect of subsequently administered full agonists and precipitates withdrawal in patients maintained on full agonists. Buprenorphine binds tightly to its receptors and, with its slow dissociation, confers a long duration of action and poor irreversibility by naloxone. It is poorly absorbed after oral administration and has a large first-pass effect. On the other hand, it is relatively well absorbed sublingually, bypassing the first-pass effect and having approximately two-thirds of the bioavailability of intramuscular administration.

Buprenorphine is widely distributed throughout the body, with the highest concentration seen in the liver, kidneys, lungs, and heart. It possesses high affinity to brain tissue relative to plasma concentration, which peaks about 90 minutes after sublingual administration. Its terminal half-life of approximately 45 hours and 10-day requirement to reach steady state account for the slow onset of withdrawal symptoms after cessation of dosing. Buprenorphine is highly bound to α- and κ-globulin. It is metabolized by conjugation and N-dealkylation, and is predominantly excreted by fecal route as buprenorphine conjugate, N-dealkylbuprenorphine and its conjugate, with renal excretion accounting for less than 5% of the administered drug in 48 hours.

Unlike LAAM and methadone, buprenorphine remains an investigational pharmacotherapy for opiate dependence, although it is approved in the United States for analgesic use. Its unique activities at the opiate receptors and its potential benefit for treatment of opiate addicts were first noted by Jasinski and colleagues (228), who demonstrated that daily doses of 8 mg sublingual buprenorphine blocked the effects of subsequently administered morphine and did not appear to induce significant physical dependence. Mello and Mendelson showed that buprenorphine suppresses heroin self-administration by opiate-dependent primates and humans (229–231).

Two controlled clinical trials have compared the effectiveness of buprenorphine and methadone in maintenance treatment. In the first study, 8 mg buprenorphine over 17 weeks of treatment was found to be significantly better than 20 mg of methadone in retaining patients in treatment and in reducing opiate use. It was not significantly different from the 60-mg methadone group on the same measures (232). The second study compared 2 mg and 6 mg of buprenorphine to 30 mg and 65 mg of methadone over 24 weeks. Drug use decreased in all groups, but was greater in the methadone groups and least in the 2-mg buprenorphine group.

A year-long study conducted at the Los Angeles Addiction Treatment Research Center compared 8 mg of sublingual buprenorphine to 30 mg and 80 mg of methadone in 225 addicts. The 8-mg buprenorphine patients performed comparably to patients on 30 mg of methadone, but both groups performed more poorly than the 80-mg methadone group. Findings from a subsequent dose ranging study suggest that the median doses for adequate clinical stabilization may be closer to the 12–16 mg range (233). A National Institute on Drug Abuse (NIDA) sponsored 12-site multi-center study comparing 1, 4, 8, and 16 mg buprenorphine has also been completed.

Altogether, these clinical studies are expected to provide sufficient data for buprenorphine's new drug application for the treatment of opiate dependence. Efforts have currently been directed toward development of a dosage formula, perhaps in combination with an antagonist, that will be useful in a wide range of clinical settings. When available, buprenorphine, with its relatively low physical dependence and wide patient acceptance, may be an ideal initial medication for treatment of opiate addiction. It offers the addicts and the clinicians the widest treatment options. Patients can be started on buprenorphine with ease and, after a period of stabilization, those patients who do well and desire to discontinue can be tapered off the medication with or without a period of antagonist follow-up treatment. Those who are doing well but want to continue treatment with buprenorphine can remain on a daily dosing schedule or choose to be dosed at less frequent intervals (234, 235). Patients with a higher level of physical dependence, whose needs cannot be met by buprenorphine due to its ceiling effect, can be transferred to one of the full agonists, LAAM and methadone.

Naltrexone

Produced by *N*-allyl substitution of naloxone with the cyclopropyl-methyl group of cyclazocine, naltrexone combines the relatively pure antagonist property of the former with the long duration of action of the latter and comes close to being the ideal opiate antagonist. It is absorbed quickly, after a single oral dose of 50 mg, reaching peak plasma concentration within an hour and lasting for up to 24 hours. At doses of 150 mg, it provides blockade for subsequently administered opiates for up to 72 hours and needs, therefore, to be given only once every 3 days. It produces no euphoria or dysphoria, is not addicting, has no street value, and is not abused by addicts. Clinical studies in the 1970s and early 1980s demonstrated its value as an adjunct to treatment of opiate dependence (236, 237). It was approved by the FDA in 1984 and had been available under the trade name Trexan, until recently when, after being approved for use in alcohol relapse prevention, its trade name was changed to ReVia (see discussion that follows).

Within the context of opiate maintenance pharmacotherapy, naltrexone has only found limited success. One major drawback relates to its potent and virtually pure antagonist property that precipitates acute abstinence in patients with any degree of physical dependence. It cannot, therefore, be administered to addicts until detoxification is complete, which, unfortunately, has generally been very difficult or impossible for the majority of cases. Detoxification in an inpatient setting, assisted by ancillary medication and other mea-

sures, has been somewhat more successful. Buprenorphine in this context may also prove to be a useful adjunct (238).

Another drawback of naltrexone is its low patient acceptance, perhaps also because of its lack of appreciable agonist activity. Patients often discontinue the medication after only a short time and, because naltrexone has no reinforcing property, patients rarely, if ever, return to treatment on their own. Certain subgroups of patients, such as physicians and other professionals, do considerably better with naltrexone treatment compared with street addicts (239). The reasons for the discrepancy are not always clear, but the first group generally has a great deal more to lose, and they are under considerable outside pressure. Quite possibly, naltrexone works best when there is significant external motivation, like the threat of loss of job or professional license.

COCAINE PHARMACOTHERAPIES

Although a recent survey of addiction medicine physicians found that over 70% reported prescribing medications to cocaine-addicted patients to manage acute and chronic cocaine withdrawal (240), no FDA-approved pharmacotherapy for cocaine addiction currently exists. This prevails despite the large number of medications that have been empirically evaluated as cocaine treatment agents over the last decade. In a recent review, Tennant and colleagues listed over 30 such agents, the majority of which were reported to have some degree of utility on various outcome measures, yet demonstration of replicable, clinically significant reductions in cocaine use or improved treatment outcomes is lacking (241). Reflected in this literature is the desperation on the part of researchers and clinicians to find an agent that is clearly effective in treating cocaine dependence (Table 30.12).

The reinforcing psychostimulant effects of cocaine are attributed to its actions on several neurotransmitter systems, notably dopamine, serotonin, and norepinephrine. Cocaine withdrawal, a significant precipitator of relapse, is believed to arise from neurobiological adaptations in these systems as a result of chronic cocaine use. The primary outcome of the withdrawal is a relative paucity of dopamine by virtue of dopamine receptor up-regulation. The majority of pharmacotherapeutic agents evaluated thus far for the treatment of cocaine dependence are those that either block cocaine's reinforcing effects at the dopamine receptor or increase the availability of dopamine within the mesolimbic pathway to minimize withdrawal discomfort, cocaine craving, and dysphoria (Table 30.13). These agents, which increase the availability of dopamine and decrease withdrawal severity, include dopamine receptor antagonists, which make cocaine use less rewarding, dopamine-receptor agonists, dopamine-reuptake and degradation inhibitors, and dopamine releasers and precursors.

As with dopamine, the reuptake of serotonin is also blocked with acute cocaine use, and relative serotonin depletion appears to play a part in the withdrawal syndrome. Thus, medications that block the serotonin receptor have been used in attempts to attenuate cocaine reinforcement, and functional serotonin agonists have been used to minimize the severity of withdrawal (Table 30.14). Because of the limited demonstrated efficacy of medications acting singly within the dopamine or serotonin systems, multiple alternate mechanisms, including concurrent serotonergic and dopaminergic therapy, stimulant substitution, and antiepileptic drug therapy, are also being explored.

ALCOHOL PHARMACOTHERAPIES

Pharmacotherapy, apart from the treatment of medical complications and psychiatric co-morbidity, may be directed toward treatment of acute intoxication, acute withdrawal, or relapse prevention.

Intoxication

In theory, the intoxicating effect of alcohol can be reduced or reversed by inhibiting its absorption, antagonizing its effect at the receptor sites, altering or counteracting its physiological effects, or enhancing its elimination from the body. In practice, the search for a sobering agent has been singularly unsuccessful (242). Contrary to popular belief, caffeine and other stimulants do not reverse the intoxicating effects of alcohol, nor do they increase elimination of alcohol from the body. Ingestion of large amounts of fructose does modestly increase alcohol metabolism but has not proven to be clinically useful (243). Thus far, neither γ-aminobutyric acid (GABA) antagonists nor reverse agonists have been shown to block the effects of alcohol (244).

Acute Alcohol Withdrawal

Treatment of acute withdrawal has enjoyed considerably more success. Most currently employed medications for suppression of withdrawal are benzodiazepines. Some examples are diazepam, in doses of 5–20 mg orally every 4–6 hours; chlordiazepoxide, 25–100 mg orally every 4–6 hours, and oxazepam, 15–60 mg orally every 4–6 hours. Benzodiazepines of long duration of action and slow elimination are, in general, preferable. An added advantage of benzodiazepines is that they are also anticonvulsants and

Table 30.12. Miscellaneous Cocaine Dependence Pharmacotherapies

Drug Class	Medication	Mechanism of Action	Clinical Indication
Calcium channel blocker	Nifedipine, nimodipine	Decrease neurotransmission of dopamine and serotonin	Decrease reinforcing effects of cocaine
Norepinephrine reuptake inhibitor	Maprotiline	Increase availability of norepinephrine at receptor	Decrease severity of withdrawal
Stimulant	Methamphetamine, pemoline, diethylproprion, methylphenidate	Mimic cocaine by releasing or blocking the reuptake of dopamine, serotonin	Substitute for cocaine; suppress withdrawal
Antiepileptic	Carbamazepine, valproate	Block the development of cocaine-induced kindling, theorized to contribute to craving and anxiety with cocaine abstinence	Decrease severity of withdrawal
Mixed	Phentermine and fenfluramine	Combination of dopaminergic and serotonergic activity	Decrease severity of withdrawal
Alcohol dependence pharmacotherapy	Disulfiram	Toxic response with alcohol ingestion	Reduce alcohol-related cocaine use

Table 30.13. Cocaine Dependence Pharmacotherapies with Activity within the Dopamine System

Drug Class	Medication	Mechanism of Action	Clinical Indication
Dopamine receptor antagonist	Flupenthixol	Block dopamine receptor	Decrease reinforcing effects of cocaine
Dopamine reuptake inhibitor	Buproprion, mazindol, diethylproprion, desipramine, imipramine	Increase dopamine availability at receptor	Decrease severity of withdrawal
Dopamine precursor	L-tyrosine, L-dopa	Increase synthesis of dopamine, making more available at receptor	Decrease severity of withdrawal
Dopamine receptor agonist	Bromocriptine, pergolide	Substitute for dopamine at receptor	Decrease severity of withdrawal
MAO inhibitor	Selegiline, phenelzine	Reduce enzymatic degradation of dopamine, making more available at receptor	Decrease severity of withdrawal
Dopamine releaser (see also stimulant substitution agents)	Amantadine	Increase presynaptic dopamine release	Decrease severity of withdrawal

Table 30.14. Cocaine Dependence Pharmacotherapies with Activity within the Serotonin System

Drug Class	Medication	Mechanism of Action	Clinical Indication
Serotonin receptor antagonist	Buspirone, ondansetron	Block serotonin receptor	Decrease reinforcing effects of cocaine
Serotonin reuptake inhibitor	Fluoxetine, sertraline	Increase availability at receptor	Decrease severity of withdrawal
Serotonin precursor	L-tryptophan	Increase synthesis of serotonin, making more available at receptor	Decrease severity of withdrawal

may prevent emergence of alcohol withdrawal seizures. Where psychotic symptoms or extreme agitation occur, however, an antipsychotic medication such as haloperidol may need to be used. Seizures complicating withdrawal require separate consideration and are dealt with elsewhere. Clonidine, an α-adrenergic agonist has been useful in reducing the neurophysiological effects of withdrawal, as has propranolol, which counteracts the tachycardia, anxiety and tremor of acute withdrawal (245–247).

Relapse Prevention

Pharmacological strategies for relapse prevention have involved medications that produce an adverse reaction when alcohol is consumed and medications that modify craving and consumptive behavior. Disulfiram (Antabuse) irreversibly inactivates acetaldehyde dehydrogenase, a step in alcohol metabolism. This leads to the accumulation of acetaldehyde when alcohol is consumed and the appearance of the disulfiram-alcohol reaction, characterized by flushing, throbbing headache, nausea, vomiting, thirst, sweating, palpitation, chest pain, tachycardia, confusion, agitation, and, when severe, respiratory depression and cardiovascular collapse (248). The reaction can occur with blood-alcohol levels as low as 50–100 mg/100ml and last from 30–60 minutes. The dosage used ranges from 125–1000 mg per day, although most patients are treated with 250–500 mg daily. Alcoholics have characterized disulfiram as a "3-day insurance policy" because it takes about that long for the medication to be eliminated from the body after last dose. Some patients, however, are able to drink even while taking disulfiram without experiencing any disulfiram/alcohol reaction, whereas others are so sensitive that inadvertent use of over-the-counter medications, toiletries such as after-shave lotions, and foods that contain small amounts of alcohol may bring on a reaction. Patients must be cautioned, therefore, about the use of these while on disulfiram.

Calcium carbamide, a more selective acetylaldehyde dehydrogenese inhibitor, has more rapid onset of action than disulfiram and shorter duration of action (249). Nitrefazole, an antitrichomonal, also can induce acetaldehyde reaction. It has long duration of action, and a single dose of 800 mg lasts up to 6 days. However, it has serious toxic effects and, like calcium carbamide, is not available in the United States (250).

Medications that decrease alcohol craving and consumption aim at manipulating the brain neurotransmitter systems mediating reward, mood, and appetite behavior. Bromo-

criptine, a dopamine agonist, has been reported to reduce alcohol intake (251), as has acamprosate, a synthetic GABA agonist (252). Modest success has been reported with serotonin uptake inhibitors. Alcohol consumption decreases anywhere from 10% to about 25% in heavy drinkers (253–258). Most studies, however, involved small numbers of patients and lacked rigorous controls. Most recently, naltrexone, the narcotic antagonist developed originally for relapse prevention of opiate dependence, has received FDA approval as a recommended adjunct to alcohol relapse prevention in the context of comprehensive treatment programs. Although the exact mechanisms of naltrexone's action in preventing alcohol relapse is unknown, in animal studies it has been demonstrated empirically to reduce alcohol consumption (259). Two recent double-blind placebo-controlled human studies have shown that patients receiving naltrexone in the context of comprehensive treatment programs have lower rates of relapse, fewer drinking episodes, and longer time to relapse, and are less likely to suffer full-blown relapse when they "slip" (260). If they drank, they were less likely to resort to heavy drinking, they consumed fewer drinks on their drinking days, and they stayed in treatment longer (261).

Based on these clinical studies, the FDA has approved naltrexone, with the new trade name ReVia, for the treatment of alcoholism, the first medication so approved since disulfiram.

SPECIAL ISSUES

Comorbidity of Psychiatric Illnesses in Substance Abuse

A substantial body of literature has accumulated documenting the frequency of coexisting substance use disorders among different diagnostic categories of psychiatric patients. The identification and management of substance-abusing patients with coexistent psychopathology require an awareness of the characteristics of specific substance abuse disorders, and how these characteristics are manifested in the context of psychiatric illness.

Neuropsychiatric effects of psychoactive substances are most clearly manifested in intoxication and withdrawal syndromes. Yet a patient's cognitive development, interpersonal relationships, perception of self and others, and personality organization can be profoundly influenced by the use of psychoactive drugs. Consequences of substance abuse include the development of socially deviant, irresponsible, self-damaging, and antisocial patterns of behavior. Clearly, one of the challenges in diagnosing substance use disorders among psychiatric patients is to distinguish symptoms that are the result of psychiatric illness from those resulting from substance abuse or dependence. For example, the paranoia that occurs during and following extended stimulant abuse is difficult to distinguish from some forms of schizophrenia. Similarly, the socially and morally deviant behaviors associated with long-term drug dependence disorders overlap those of antisocial personality disorder.

The distinction between behaviors associated with psychiatric illness and psychoactive substance abuse is further obscured by the complex temporal relationship between these two classes of disorders. According to Meyer (262), psychopathology can be a risk factor or modifier of an addictive disorder. It can occur in the course of chronic intoxication or emerge as a consequence, and persist into the period of remission. Over time, psychopathology and addictive disorders can become meaningfully linked. Finally, each can occur independent of the other. A large amount of literature has established some important patterns of coexistence between psychopathology and addictive disorders.

COMORBIDITY OF MENTAL HEALTH AND SUBSTANCE USE DISORDERS IN THE GENERAL POPULATION

In the Epidemiologic Catchment Areas (ECA) study (17), the lifetime prevalence in the United States for coexisting mental health and substance dependence disorders was 32.7%. Mental health disorders, other than those that are alcohol- or drug-related, were diagnosed in 22.5% of the sample, while alcohol abuse or dependence was found in 13.5%, and drug abuse/dependence was found in 6.1% of the sample.

These rates are substantially higher in some special populations. In a sample of prisoners, 82.1% were found to have coexistent mental health and substance abuse/dependence disorders, with alcoholism prevalent in 56.2% and substance abuse/dependence prevalent in 53.7%. Likewise, among a homeless population in Los Angeles, the lifetime prevalence of mental health disorders other than substance abuse was 68.8% and lifetime substance abuse disorders was 62.9%.

Alcoholism

The rate of alcoholism in the 1990 ECA report was virtually unchanged from a similar study completed in 1984, in which 13.5% of the population were diagnosed with alcoholism. In both of these reports, alcoholism was the single most prevalent lifetime diagnosis given across all categories of psychiatric diagnoses. The frequency of secondary mental health diagnoses among alcoholics (36.6%) almost doubles the rate for mental disorders in the general population (19.9%), and the prevalence of other drug disorders (21.5%) in the alcoholic population is nearly six times the rate (3.7%) of drug disorders in nonalcoholics. Table 30.15 illustrates the relationship between alcoholism and other drug dependence disorders and the incidence of comorbid psychiatric disorders. The 36.6% rate of mental health disorders in alcoholics is 2.3 times the rate found in nonalcoholics. The odds ratios of 1.9 and 1.5 for affective and anxiety disorders, respectively, reflect the relatively high prevalence of these disorders in nonalcoholics. In contrast, although the prevalence of antisocial personality disorder is similar to the prevalence of affective and anxiety disorders (14.3%) in alcoholics, the odds ratio is 21 times the nonalcoholic group.

One of the most consistent epidemiological findings is the greater prevalence of alcohol dependence and abuse disorders in men compared with women. Moreover, while 44% of male alcoholics have a secondary psychiatric diagnoses, 65% of the female alcoholics were found to have concurrent diagnoses. The sex difference is particularly noteworthy with regard to depression. For male alcoholics, the rate of co-occurring depression is 5%, only slightly higher than for men in the general population (3%). For female alcoholics, the co-occurrence of depression is 19%, much greater than the incidence of depression among women in the general population (7%). For the majority of men (70%), alcoholism precedes the onset of depression, while for the majority of women (66%), depression precedes the onset of alcoholism (263).

Also noteworthy is the frequent co-occurrence of alcoholism and antisocial personality. Alcoholics with antisocial personality reported a longer history of alcoholism, and an earlier onset and greater severity of alcohol symptoms (263). The rebellious, delinquent, uncooperative behavior that characterizes antisocial personality contributes to the treatment resistance of some alcohol dependent patients with antisocial traits.

Drug Dependence

The prevalence of mental disorders among patients with drug abuse/dependence disorders is 53.1%, or 4.5 times the rate in the non-drug-abusing or dependent population. Similarly, the prevalence of alcohol abuse or dependence among drug abusers is 47.3%, or 7.1 times the rate in the non-drug-abusing/dependent population. In combination, the prevalence of any mental or alcohol disorder among drug abusers is 71.6%, or 6.5 times the non-drug-abusing/dependent population (17).

As with alcohol disorders, the rate of antisocial personality in the drug-dependent population is much higher (17.8%) than that found in non-drug-dependent groups, with an odds ratio of 13.4. This is differentially associated with different categories of drug use. For cocaine users, the rate of antisocial personality is 42.7%, or 29.2 times that of non-cocaine users; for opiate users, it is 36.7%, or 24.3 times that of non-opiate users; and for marijuana users it is 14.7%, or 8.3 times that of the non-marijuana-using group.

Table 30.15. Prevalence of Alcohol and Drug Dependence Disorders and Other Comorbid Psychiatric Disorders[a]

Comorbid Disorder	Any Alcohol		Any Other Drug		Marijuana		Cocaine		Opiates		Barbiturates		Amphetamines		Hallucinogens	
	%	OR	%	OR	%	OR	%	OR	%	OR	%	OR	%	OR	%	OR
Any mental	36.6	2.3	53.1	4.5	50.1	3.8	76.1	11.3	65.2	6.7	74.7	10.8	62.9	6.2	69.2	8.0
Schizophrenia	3.8	3.3	6.8	6.2	6.0	4.8	16.7	13.2	11.4	8.8	8.0	5.9	5.5	3.9	10.0	7.4
Any affective	13.4	1.9	26.4	4.7	23.7	3.8	34.7	5.9	30.8	5.0	36.4	6.6	32.7	5.7	34.3	5.8
Any anxiety	19.4	1.5	28.3	2.5	27.5	2.3	33.3	2.9	31.6	2.8	42.9	4.5	32.7	2.9	46.0	5.0
Antisocial personality	14.3	21.0	17.8	13.4	14.7	8.3	42.7	29.2	36.7	24.3	30.3	19.0	24.5	14.3	28.5	15.6
Alcohol abuse or dependence			47.3	7.1	45.2	6.0	84.8	36.3	65.9	12.8	71.3	16.9	61.7	11.1	62.5	10.9

[a]Adapted from Regier et al., 1990 (17).

Among marijuana users, the prevalence of alcohol abuse/dependence is 45.2%, or 6 times the nonuser group. Among opiate, amphetamine, and hallucinogen users, the rate of alcohol abuse or dependence ranges between 62–66%. However, among those diagnosed with cocaine disorders, the rate of alcohol abuse/dependence is 84.8%, or 36.3 times the rate of noncocaine-abusing groups. This strong relationship between cocaine abuse/dependence and alcohol abuse/dependence complicates treatment because patients are typically unaware of the severity and significance of their alcohol disorder (17).

Marijuana users, compared with users of "harder" drugs, have relatively low psychiatric comorbidity, whereas cocaine users have the highest comorbidity rate.

COMORBIDITY IN TREATMENT-SEEKING POPULATIONS: TREATMENT IMPLICATIONS

The co-occurrence of mental disorders and substance abuse disorders is substantially higher among patients who have sought treatment for either category of disorder than among untreated populations. One possible explanation for this observation is that the presence of a co-occurring disorder may exacerbate the symptoms of the other disorder and thus increase the probability of seeking treatment. Overall, the prevalence rates for psychiatric disorders among substance abusers in treatment were three times that of the general population (17). In one group of patients presenting for substance-abuse treatment, 68% had a concurrent non-substance-abuse psychiatric diagnosis and 43% had two or more (264).

Treatment for these patients is complicated by the fact that clinicians are typically trained to treat substance abuse disorders *or* psychiatric disorders. Consequently, treatment for comorbid disorders has generally been sequential rather than simultaneous. Clinicians who work with substance abusers often rely on a chemical dependency model of treatment that sees substance abuse as a lifelong affliction, while other psychopathologies, even those that preceded drug use, are viewed as part of the addiction disease process (265). In this perspective, the cure for addiction and its concomitant problems, including psychiatric disorders, is believed to be abstinence. Clinicians who rely solely on this perspective are often unprepared when abstinence unmasks psychiatric symptoms that need attention (265). Conversely, clinicians who treat individuals with psychiatric disorders often see alcoholism or drug dependence as simply an attempt to treat an underlying disorder; this "self-medication" hypothesis implies that successful treatment of the psychiatric disorder will eliminate the addiction. Raskin and Miller (266) note that the opposite is usually true: treatment of psychiatric disorders may only be possible once the addiction is under control. In general, treating individuals with comorbid diagnoses requires a broad conceptualization of addiction and psychopathology, encompassing the interactive and integral nature of the disorders.

Alcoholics

Only 25% of the men and 20% of the women in a sample of 321 hospitalized alcoholics did not meet current criteria for co-occurring psychiatric diagnoses. Among males, the most common co-occurring diagnosis was antisocial personality (49%), followed by substance abuse (38%) and major depression (32%). Among female alcoholics, the most common concurrent diagnoses were major depression (52%), phobias (44%), substance abuse (38%), and antisocial personality (20%) (267). The presence of a coexisting psychiatric disorder has an important effect on the course and severity of the alcohol abuse/dependence disorder. Alcoholics with additional psychopathology generally begin alcohol use and experience intoxication at an earlier age, and their alcoholism progresses more rapidly than those without concurrent psychopathology (267). Moreover, the severity of psychiatric illness has proven more predictive of treatment outcome for alcoholism than the severity of the alcoholism itself (268). Depression secondary to chronic alcohol abuse typically remits after 2 weeks of abstinence without the use of antidepressants (269). More long-lasting depression, however, which is often treated with antidepressant medication, has been associated with positive long-term outcomes in alcoholics, particularly female alcoholics (78, 270, 271). Yet alcoholics with co-morbid persistent depression are at high risk for suicide—particularly those who are unable to achieve abstinence. In a 2-year follow-up of 127 alcoholics with depression, 9% of those whose alcoholism did not remit had committed suicide (272).

Among treatment-seeking alcoholics, agoraphobia is found to co-occur twice as often, and social phobia nine times as often, as would be expected in community samples (273). Many anxiety symptoms predate alcoholism (273–276), worsen after drinking starts (277), and decline with increasing years of abstinence (78). Treatment of anxiety in alcoholics should employ educative, supportive, and cognitive-behavioral approaches (278) that emphasize that alcohol is not an effective anxiolytic (273).

The presence of antisocial personality has been associated with poor treatment outcome in alcoholics. It is believed that early onset of antisocial behavior and substance abuse contribute to poor social adjustment, which, in turn, leads to poor treatment outcome (267). In a prospective study of alcoholic women, a primary diagnosis of antisocial personality disorder predicted mortality at 11-year follow-up (279). However, antisocial personality does not necessarily predict poor outcome (272). In another study, alcoholics with antisocial personality showed comparable improvement in drinking and psychosocial functioning in comparison to alcoholics with and without other co-morbid psychiatric disorders, although those with antisocial personality did show higher levels of unemployment at 1-year follow-up.

Treatment of comorbid substance abuse disorders must be incorporated into all alcoholism treatment, as polysubstance abuse is the rule rather than exception. Patients must be taught that the use of other substances increases the risk of alcohol relapse.

Opiate Addicts

A current or lifetime diagnosis of antisocial personality, alcoholism, phobias, and anxiety is common in treatment-seeking opiate addicts, with specific rates varying with the treatment population. In traditional urban settings, rates of antisocial personality range from 27–35% (280, 281), while Croughan et al. (282) identified antisocial personality in 67% of opiate addicts in court-ordered treatment. Opiate addicts seeking treatment appear to have a lower lifetime prevalence of alcohol abuse (21%) (282) than those not in treatment (60–65%). The lifetime prevalence rate of anxiety disorders ranges between 11–16% (280, 281).

The high prevalence of depression among opiate addicts requires specific interventions. Rounsaville et al. (281) reported that patients who were diagnosed with a major or minor depression at intake were more likely to use illicit drugs during the following 6 months than those without such a diagnosis. Furthermore, 10% of the nondepressed addicts were subsequently diagnosed over the 6-month follow-up period as having a depressive disorder (281, 283). Dackis and Gold (284) refer to a "post-detoxification depression" and suggest that tricyclic antidepressants may be helpful. Alcohol abuse is also a common source of morbidity in opiate addicts, often in association with depression that needs specific intervention.

Cocaine and Stimulant Addicts

In a recent study of 298 cocaine addicts seeking treatment, 56% had a psychiatric diagnosis in addition to cocaine dependence/abuse (285), with a 61% lifetime prevalence of affective disorder, including 31% for major depression. These findings are consistent with those reported by Weiss and colleagues (286), who found that 38% of cocaine abusers in treatment had a co-morbid axis I diagnosis, 16% had an axis II diagnosis of antisocial personality, and over one-fourth had a current affective disorder, of which 9% were major depressive, 11% cyclothymic, and 5% bipolar. The rate of current anxiety disorders among cocaine abusers in treatment ranges from 2–16% (285, 286).

These investigators also found a lifetime prevalence rate of alcoholism among cocaine abusers in treatment at approximately 60% (285). The CNS depressant effects of alcohol was thought to counteract anxiogenic, insomniac, or dysphoric effects of cocaine (265, 285). Carroll et al. (287) compared cocaine addicts with and without an alcohol use disorder. They found that although both groups were equally likely to be drug dependent at 1-year follow-up, those diagnosed with alcohol abuse at intake were significantly more likely to be diagnosed with alcoholism at follow-up.

Cocaine abuse is also prevalent among treatment-seeking schizophrenics (288), and seems to worsen the course of schizophrenia. These individuals may be seen less frequently in substance abuse treatment settings because clinicians tend to treat overt schizophrenic symptoms first, but schizophrenics who use cocaine do require more psychiatric hospitalizations than their non-cocaine-abusing counterparts (289).

Almost 50% of stimulant abusers report affective symptoms during withdrawal. Depressive symptoms tend to decrease or remit within 2–4 weeks of abstinence (278, 286) and psychotropic medications have been used to reduce symptoms. Although it is commonly believed that individuals use cocaine in an attempt to self-medicate depression, the data suggest that the majority of patients with cyclothymia or bipolar disorder used cocaine when they were feeling "endogenously high" rather than when feeling depressed (286).

Although uncommon, cocaine and other stimulants can induce panic attacks that persist after individuals become abstinent (196, 265, 290). These attacks have been reported to improve after treatment with clonazepam or carbamazepine (291).

Marijuana and Hallucinogen Abusers

For individuals with a genetic predisposition to schizophrenia, potent hallucinogens may induce psychosis at an earlier age or precipitate a psychosis that might have otherwise remained dormant (292). Negrete et al. (293) compared schizophrenics who were active users of marijuana with those who had used marijuana in the past and those who had never used marijuana, and found that active users were more likely to demonstrate positive symptoms of schizophrenia.

Marijuana use has also been associated with acute anxiety states, including panic reactions (294). Patients with panic disorder who smoke marijuana report marijuana to be much more anxiogenic than do depressed patients or non-patient controls (295); this finding is interesting because marijuana is typically reported to have anxiolytic properties. Marijuana use among patients with panic disorder does not usually come to medical attention, mainly because these individuals tend to spontaneously cease use when they discover that marijuana increases anxiety (295).

NEUROPSYCHOLOGICAL CORRELATES OF SUBSTANCE ABUSE

In the final analysis, an altered neuropsychological state is the desired effect of drug abuse. Thus, it hardly seems surprising that chronic use of these drugs shows altered performance on neuropsychological testing. Specific abnormal findings in motor dexterity, sensory processing, attention and concentration, language, visuospatial analysis, verbal and nonverbal memory, abstraction and problem-solving skills have been demonstrated with chronic alcohol, cocaine, opiate, and polysubstance abuse. The temporal relationships between neuropsychological findings, drug use, and abstinence have significant implications for treatment and recovery.

Although neuropsychological impairments have frequently been demonstrated in chronic substance abusers, relating specific findings to the use of a particular drug has been difficult. Polydrug abuse is common, and typically there are other confounding factors, such as head injury, nutritional deficits, liver disease, concurrent psychiatric and medical illness (notably HIV disease), and impoverished family and social environments, all of which can affect neuropsychological functioning. Demographic factors are also at play in neuropsychological performance. For example, older alcoholics are generally more impaired than younger alcoholics (296), and educational differences among subjects may result in erroneous conclusions about neuropsychological abilities (297). Although brain function is known to be less lateralized in females than in males, few studies have explored the influence of gender on substance abuse and neuropsychological function (298–301).

NEUROPSYCHOLOGICAL FINDINGS IN SUBSTANCE ABUSERS

Alcohol

The preponderance of information gathered over the past 20 years regarding neuropsychological functioning in substance abusers has been derived from studies of alcoholics. These studies typically utilize recently detoxified (between 1 week and 2 months sober) alcoholic males compared with matched nonalcoholic samples. Deficits in abstraction and problem-solving abilities, learning and memory, and perceptual motor tasks are the three most frequently described areas of impairment (302–304) and appear to correlate with the lifetime amount of alcohol consumed (305).

In comparison to nonalcoholics, alcoholics have greater difficulty with the Wisconsin Card Sorting Task, reflecting lack of persistence, reduced flexibility of thought, and increased difficulty with maintaining a cognitive set (306). Similar deficits in alcoholics have been described in other measures of abstraction and problem solving, including the Category Test (303, 307), the Levine Hypothesis Testing Task (296), the Shipley Institute of Living Abstraction Scale (303, 308), the Raven Progressive Matrices (309), and the Stroop Color Naming Test (310). Glenn and Parsons (306) describe decreased efficiency and accuracy in problem-solving and abstraction ability using a composite measure derived from the WAIS-R Block Design Task, the Booklet Category Test, the Shipley Abstracting Scale, the Levine Hypothesis Test, and the Conceptual Levels Analogy Test.

Impaired visual learning and memory in recently detoxified alcoholics have been noted on the Rey-Osterreith Complex Figure Task (310) and the Visual Reproduction and Symbol-Digit Paired Associates Test of the Wechsler Memory Scale (304). Nonverbal deficits have been reported more consistently than verbal deficits, although Ryan and Butters (311) claim that with appropriate testing of verbal paired associates, verbal learning and memory impairment discriminate alcoholics from nonalcoholics. Verbal deficits have been noted in the recall of short stories on the Wechsler Memory Scale–Logical Memory Subtest (304) and on learning word lists over repeated trials in the Rey Auditory Verbal Learning Test (310). In combined measures of verbal and visual memory (a composite score derived from Face-name Paired Associate and Wechsler Memory Scale–Logical Memory and Visual Reproduction Subtests), efficiency and accuracy were significantly lessened in alcoholics, compared with nonalcoholics (300). Grant and Reed (303) found that alcoholics retain their capacity for learning but that more time and effort are required to master new material.

Recently detoxified alcoholics also demonstrate impaired perceptual motor functioning. They perform poorer than nonalcoholics on the Trail Making Test, a timed task that requires individuals to connect a series of numbers or letters sequentially (303, 307). Additionally, their performance is inferior to controls on the Tactual Performance Test (312), the WAIS Digit Symbol Test (304), the Grooved Pegboard Test (304), and on an investigator-devised computerized visual spatial task (312).

Cocaine

Despite the cocaine epidemic of the 1980s and 1990s, a recent review of the literature by Berry and colleagues (313) found only five controlled studies on the neuropsychological sequelae of cocaine abuse. These preliminary studies describe mild to moderate levels of neuropsychological impairment in short-term memory and attention in chronic, heavy cocaine abusers. Deficits persisting for 6 months or more were specifically linked to cocaine-induced cerebral hypoperfusion in frontal, periventricular, and temporoparietal areas, in a sample of cocaine abusers with an average use history of 2½ years (314).

Ardila et al. (315) assessed multiple areas of function in 37 freebase cocaine abusers who had used crack cocaine for more than a year and, at the time of testing, had been drug-free for almost 1 month. When compared with normative data, these subjects were found to be at least one standard deviation below the mean on indices of short-term memory (Wechsler Memory Scale–Logical Memory and Wechsler Memory Scale–Associative Learning) and attention (WISC-Digit Symbol). Lifetime cocaine use inversely affected performance on tasks of attention (Wechsler Memory Scale–Digit Span) and nonverbal memory (Rey-Osterreith Complex Figure) and was found to be a summative indicator of memory function (Wechsler Memory Scale–Memory Quotient). A pattern of cognitive decline was demonstrated with prolonged use, with short-term memory and attention being most sensitive to cocaine abuse.

O'Malley et al. (316) also reported mild cognitive impairment among chronic (average of 4 years regular use) cocaine abusers. They compared neuropsychological performance in 20 cocaine abusers, abstinent for an average of 23.6 (S.D. = 15) days, with two normal, age- and education-matched control groups. Subjects were found to have deficits in short-term memory (adaptation of the Wechsler Memory Scale–Logical Memory), abstracting ability (Category Test), and attention (Symbol-Digit Modalities Test, WAIS-R-Arithmetic). The amount and recency of cocaine use was related to performance on a test of verbal memory (adaptation of Wechsler Memory Scale–Logical Memory). On the summary index of the Neuropsychological Screening Battery, 50% of the cocaine abusers were identified as "mildly impaired," compared with 15% of the controls.

Similarly, Volkow et al (317) examined 20 freebase or injection cocaine users, with a 6-month history of use, within 3 days of admission to an inpatient detoxification facility. Impaired concentration and decreased ability to solve arithmetic problems and to perform backward number repetition were identified on mental status examination. In a study of neuropsychological functioning in 33 abstinent (mean = 59 days) crack cocaine abusers, persistent short-term verbal memory disturbances were evident in comparison with an age- and education-matched sample of nonco-caine abusers (318).

Neuropsychological assessment in recently abstinent cocaine abusers may be complicated by depression, which accompanies acute cocaine withdrawal. To explore the influence of cocaine withdrawal depression on neuropsychological performance, Berry et al. (313) compared the psychological functioning of 16 cocaine abusers, at three and 154 days after admission to an inpatient treatment facility, to 21 age- and education-matched community volunteers. Scores on the Beck Depression Inventory were used as co-variates to control for the effects of depression on test performance. At both time points, the cocaine abusers performed more poorly than controls on memory tasks (Rey-Osterreith Complex Figure delayed recall, Rey Auditory-Verbal Learning Test), visuospatial abilities (Rey-Osterreith Complex Figure Copy), psychomotor speed (Digit Symbol WAIS-R Subtest), and concentration (Paced Auditory Aerial Addition Test), and little improvement was noted over the testing interval. Thus, impairment did not appear attributable to withdrawal-related depression.

Opiates

Uniquely, long-term opiate abusers seem not to suffer neuropsychological deficits, although empirical literature is sparse. Bruhn and Maage (319) examined 87 polysubstance-abusing male prisoners, categorizing them on the basis of patterns and amount of drug use over time. Twenty subjects were identified as marijuana, hallucinogen, and amphetamine users, and 22 were identified as marijuana, hallucinogen, amphetamine, and opiate users; assuming differences between the groups could be attributed to opiate use. No differences between the groups were found. In fact, intelligence and all neuropsychological battery test scores were within the average range. Rounsaville et al. (320) compared

72 opiate addicts, 69% of whom were actively using street drugs or were on methadone maintenance, to a group of 60 epileptics and to 20 normal subjects matched demographically. No relationship was found between past or current opiate use and neuropsychological functioning; however, all three groups demonstrated mild impairment on tasks of attention (Trails A and B, Digit Symbol), visual scanning (Visual Search), and motor abilities (Grooved Pegboard). Guerra et al. (321) compared attention, memory, and verbal fluency in 93 opiate addicts, pre- and 1-week postdetoxification, to a group of matched controls. Although the addict group was significantly more impaired than the control group prior to detoxification, no differences between groups were detected at the second time point.

These findings are in contrast to the results of a study by Grant et al. (322) that compared 152 polysubstance abusers to control samples of psychiatric patients and non-drug-using, nonpsychiatric patient volunteers. Subjects with a history of opiate abuse were significantly more likely to be identified as impaired on a blind clinical neuropsychological rating, although the potential effects of polysubstance abuse on performance could not be ruled out. Pakesch et al. (323), comparing 31 opiate addicts with 50 volunteer controls, found the addicts scored significantly below controls on visual memory recall (Benton Visual Retention Test). Apparently, neuropsychological deficit in opiate addicts requires further investigation controlling for the effects of polysubstance abuse, opiate maintenance therapy, length of abstinence, and HIV status.

Polysubstance Abuse

Polysubstance abuse has been the norm for at least the past 20 years, especially when alcohol is considered, while users of a single substance have become rare. Consequently, neuropsychological deficits noted in most drug abusers today result from a combination of substances. The Collaborative Neuropsychological Study of Polydrug Users (322, 324) continues to provide the bulk of our current knowledge on the neuropsychological effects of polysubstance abuse. In general, perceptual-motor deficits were present in one-third of the chronic polysubstance abusers present, but no definitive data were obtained regarding abstracting and language skills.

Grant and Judd (324) studied 66 "heavy" polysubstance abusers attending an outpatient drug treatment program. All subjects had used drugs daily for at least 1 year, and 53% had used three or more substances on a regular basis. After 3 weeks of treatment, but not necessarily abstinence, 45% of the subjects were found to have mild to moderate impairment in abstraction and perceptual-motor tasks. These impaired subjects were more likely to report a history of heavy CNS depressant and alcohol use and heavy use of four or more psychoactive drugs. At 5-month follow-up, available data on 45% of the original sample indicated that eight of these subjects continued to evidence cognitive deficits.

Grant et al. (322) examined 151 polydrug abusers who had been in treatment for 21–30 days. Thirty-seven percent demonstrated impairment on the Halstead-Reitan Battery, compared with 26% of psychiatric patients and 8% of non-drug-using, nonpsychiatric patient controls; language and perceptual-motor deficits were identified, with degree of impairment positively correlated to use of CNS depressants and opiates. At 3-month follow-up, 34% of the polysubstance-abusing sample remained impaired. The authors concluded that CNS depressants and/or opiates may have long-term, slowly reversible effects. Carlin et al. (80), using the same sample of 151 polysubstance abusers, found the impaired abusers to be older (mean 28.7 years) than the nonimpaired abusers (mean 23.6 years), and more likely to be categorized by the investigators as "self-medicators" who used drugs regularly and in isolation. Unimpaired abusers tended to be "social/recreational" users who binged or showed compulsive patterns, but used generally within a social context.

Bruhn and Maage (319) compared 87 male prisoners, categorized according to their history of polydrug use, to a non-drug-using sample. IQ and neuropsychological findings were within normal range in both groups. Although polysubstance-abusing subjects had used various drugs between 1–8 years, verification and duration of abstinence were not provided, and the possibility that protracted abstinence in the prison setting, with concurrent neuropsychological recovery, accounted for the negative findings.

In a more recent assessment of polysubstance abusers, Sweeney et al. (325) identified neuropsychological deficits in a sample of 100 patients consecutively admitted to a 4–6 week detoxification and rehabilitation program, tested 7 days after detoxification. The effects of education were not taken into account. Verbal abstraction skills were assessed with the WAIS Similarities and WAIS Vocabulary Subtests. Performance on the Similarities Test was superior to performance on the Vocabulary Test, an unexpected finding because the Vocabularies Subtest is believed to be less sensitive to brain injury and a better indicator of premorbid functioning. The authors replicated their finding on another sample of 100 consecutively admitted polysubstance abusers and concluded that vocabulary testing might be more sensitive than similarities testing to chronic drug effects.

Fals-Stewart (326) assessed the cognitive skills of 112 polysubstance abusers 30 days after admission to an inpatient unit. Twenty-seven percent of the subjects were reported to be cognitively impaired according to a rating derived from the Halstead-Reitan Battery. Scores on a brief neuropsychological battery (the Brain Age Quotient) identified 23% of the subjects as globally impaired, but specific domains of brain function were not delineated.

In summary, neuropsychological impairment in polysubstance abusers cannot be predicted by what is known about impairments unique to specific drugs of abuse. The interaction of combined drugs may produce deficit patterns specific to the individual's drug use history.

Substance Abusers with HIV Disease

Substance abusers who administer drugs parenterally, support their drug use via sex work, or engage in high-risk sexual behavior while intoxicated are at significantly increased risk of infection by HIV, which is independently associated with neuropsychological deficits (327, 328). The neurocognitive decline associated with HIV disease, referred to as AIDS dementia complex, can occur at any time during the course of the disease, although detection in asymptomatic patients remains the subject of debate. The AIDS dementia complex involves many of the same neurological deficits noted with chronic substance abuse, including problems with verbal memory, attention, concentration, psychomotor speed, cognitive flexibility, and, in some cases, nonverbal skills and memory (329, 336).

Exploring neuropsychological decline in symptomatic and asymptomatic HIV seropositive and HIV seronegative substance abusers "in recovery" (drug history and length of time abstinent not detailed) (331), Wellman (1991) found deficits in attention, short-term memory, and abstraction in HIV-seropositive subjects, symptoms that do not usually emerge until later in the disease process. She attributed the escalated neuropsychological impairment in substance abusers, compared with available data on gay men, to the effects of chronic drug use. In a 4-year prospective study of neuropsychological function in HIV-seronegative and symptomatic and asymptomatic HIV-seropositive methadone-maintained patients, Siberstein and colleagues (332) assessed 121 subjects (51% of the baseline sample) over a 47-month period (some of the more impaired subjects were lost over the lengthy testing interval). Subtle cognitive decline was noted in the seropositive group in visual motor (Halstead-Reitan Trail Making Test, Parts A and B) and psychomotor (Digital Finger-Tapping Test) performance compared with the seronegative group. HIV-seropositive substance abusers, whether symptomatic or not, appear to have more neuropsychological impairment than substance abusers without the virus.

Concha and colleagues (333) examined the effects of chronic drug use on neuropsychological test performance in HIV-seropositive (not CDC-staged) and seronegative cocaine and heroin users over the course of three semiannual evaluations; retention rate for all three visits was 65%. Performance was not significantly affected by HIV status or drug use frequency, either recent and lifetime, with age and educational background being more powerful predictors of neuropsychological function. Similarly, Selnes and colleagues (334) found that a cohort of asymptomatic HIV-seropositive injection drug abusers did not evidence more neuropsychological impairment over the course of 1-year follow-up than HIV seronegative intravenous drug-using controls. They also found the effects of age and education to be better predictors of neurocognitive status, and concluded that HIV disease does not portend increased neuropsychological impairment in substance-abusing samples.

Unfortunately, none of these studies included a non-drug-abusing control group. To assess the influence of long-term drug abuse in the development of cognitive deficits in HIV-seropositive persons, Pakesh and colleagues (323) compared neuropsychological assessment in symptomatic (classified in CDC groups III and IV), HIV-seropositive opiate and polysubstance abusers, HIV-seronegative opiate and polysubstance abusers, and healthy control subjects (323). Both groups of substance abusers performed more poorly than controls on multiple tasks of short-term memory and concentration, but HIV seropositivity had no effect on neuropsychological performance. The authors concluded that the effects of chronic substance abuse on cognitive performance are so significant that they mask effects detectable in HIV-seropositive non-drug-abusing populations.

Utilizing a different population to explore the effects of drug and alcohol use on neuropsychological performance, Bornstein and colleagues (330) studied a sample of HIV-infected asymptomatic gay men. Subjects were classified on the basis of meeting DSM-III-R criteria for substance abuse, substance dependence, or not meeting diagnostic criteria. The three groups performed comparably, with no effects attributable to recency and severity of drug use.

DURATION OF IMPAIRMENT

The vast majority of studies assessing neuropsychological functioning in substance abusers have been limited to individuals in the first 2 months of abstinence. Becker and Kaplan (335) suggest that, although much recovery occurs within the first few months of abstinence, the recovery process continues with sustained abstinence and, depending upon the domain of function assessed, complete recovery of function may be experienced by some individuals. Utilizing a cross-sectional design, Brandt et al. (336) tested alcoholic subjects who had been sober for 1–2 months, 12–36 months, and more than 5 years. Complete recovery of verbal short-term memory occurred in the 5-year group, although recovery of nonverbal short-term memory was incomplete in that same group. Assessment with the Symbol–Digit Paired Associate Task and the Embedded Figures Test revealed no recovery of perceptual processing. Grant and Reed (297) administered the Halstead-Reitan Neuropsychological Test Battery to a group of alcoholics, 18 months and 42 months after sobriety, and found that 23% of the long-term abstinent alcoholics had improved significantly over the testing interval, compared with 7% of the age- and education-matched comparison group.

In a recent National Institute on Drug Abuse technical review on the residual behavioral effects of abused drugs, Reed and Grant (337) cited available literature as indicative of possible long-term, slow recovery from neuropsychological impairment, especially among alcoholics, but also among polysubstance abusers. The researchers proposed an "Intermediate-Duration Neurobehavioral Disorder Associated with Substance Abuse," with definitive diagnosis based on improvement in neurobehavioral testing with drug abstinence or reduced consumption.

A methodological problem inherent in assessing persistence of substance abuse-related deficits is the stability and consistency of neuropsychological test scores over time in a population subject to the variable effects of drug intoxication, withdrawal, motivation, and compliance. Richards and colleagues (338) found good test-retest reli- ability on a large number of neuropsychological assessments over a mean test interval of 10.4 days with a small sample of parenteral substance abusers. Tests of verbal memory (the Selective Reminding Test) and motor functioning (the Perdue Pegboard) were less reliable in this same group over the testing interval.

IMPAIRMENT PRECEDING SUBSTANCE ABUSE

It has been estimated that 45–70% of patients seeking treatment for alcohol abuse manifest neuropsychological deficits (339–341). However, neurotoxic effects of chronic alcohol abuse do not invariably result in neuropsychological impairment, and researchers have investigated the possibility that premorbid neuropsychological functioning may predispose certain individuals to substance-induced neuropsychological deficits. Parsons (342) found a substantial minority of alcoholics to be neuropsychologically unimpaired and suggested that alcoholics with a family history of alcoholism are more likely to perform poorly in studies of cognitive-perceptual functioning than those without. Miller and Gold (343) also believe that neurophysiological performance reflects premorbid constitutional features of cognitive style (344).

Certain measures of attention (particularly the Continuous Performance Test), as noted by Pogge et al (345), discriminate between adolescents who abuse alcohol and those who do not. Poor attention was associated not only with early alcohol abuse, but also with the clinical diagnosis of attention deficit disorder (ADD), suggesting that ADD may be a risk factor for alcoholism. Substance abusers who met the diagnostic criteria of antisocial personality also performed more poorly than substance abusers without that diagnosis on a composite index of cognitive functioning (Brain Age Quotient) and memory (Wechsler Memory Scale Verbal and Nonverbal Memory) (346), indicating that antisocial personality may predict neuropsychological deficits in abstinent substance abusers. Rodriguez (347) showed that when opiate and polydrug abusers with antisocial personality were excluded, the effect of family history of alcoholism on cognitive deficits in substance abusers disappeared. Parsons (342), in a series of studies, showed that alcoholics who relapsed after detoxification were more neuropsychologically impaired on intake than those who maintained abstinence, suggesting that relapsers may be somewhat more impaired initially.

The role of premorbid neuropsychological deficits in the development of substance use disorders remains an area of much empirical interest. Hesselbrock and colleagues (348) caution that the current evidence supporting cognitive deficits as risk factors for the development of alcoholism is not strong, and that future studies should focus on specific versus general measures of neuropsychological functioning. These studies should consider the different subtypes of alcoholics for whom the predictive strength of neuropsychological functioning as a risk factor in the development of substance abuse may vary.

IMPLICATIONS FOR TREATMENT AND RECOVERY

Neuropsychological impairment in treatment-seeking substance abusers necessitates consideration of how these impairments affect treatment and recovery. Becker and Kaplan (335) recommend that interventions with newly abstinent drug abusers should minimize cognitively demanding approaches. Complex skill training and vocational and educational interventions should not be introduced until several weeks of abstinence have been achieved.

The degree of neuropsychological impairment may be a significant predictor of treatment outcome. Substance abusers with cognitive deficits are at greater risk for relapse than those without (342, 349). Gregson and Taylor (350), in a sample of male alcoholics, demonstrated that a composite memory-based measure of cognitive efficiency strongly predicted relapse, with those more cognitively efficient having lower relapse rates, despite less involvement with the 12-step recovery program. Leber et al. (351) found a positive correlation between performance on neuropsychological testing and counselor-assessed clinical progress in therapy in two groups of alcoholic men. Kupke and O'Brien (352) found that alcoholics whose behavior was identified by treatment staff as "problematic" and not conducive to inpatient treatment had difficulties with psychomotor speed, problem solving, tactual-motor integration, elementary reasoning, memory and visuospatial analysis, and synthesis. In a large sample (n = 495) of substance abusers entering a drug-free therapeutic community, measures of diffuse cognitive impairment (WAIS Block Design and Digit–Symbol Subtests) predicted poor treatment retention, a finding attributed to the high level of complex information presented at treatment admission, upon which subsequent treatment performance was based (353). Chastian et al. found a demographically-derived estimate of premorbid IQ to be positively related to opiate abstinence of more than 1 year, and to an overall shorter addiction career. Smith and McCrady (354) found alcoholics with higher abstraction skills (Shipley Institute of Living Scale) better able to acquire and implement drink refusal skills in test situations, and to stay involved in outpatient aftercare.

In general, substance abusers with less neuropsychological compromise, whether predating or resulting from substance abuse, are better able to benefit from treatment interventions and achieve successful outcomes than those with greater neuropsychological compromise.

SUMMARY

Predictable patterns of neuropsychological impairment frequently accompany chronic substance abuse, with specific deficits varying according to the drug of abuse. The interaction of HIV disease with substance abuse complicates neuropsychological presentation, although does not appear to predict increased severity or scope of impairment. Although there is evidence that neuropsychological deficits may predispose individuals to substance use disorders, or make them more susceptible to the neurotoxic effects of drugs of abuse, there is also evidence that certain deficits may clear slowly with continued abstinence. Neuropsychological assessment upon treatment entry can help structure treatment interventions and can predict the patient's ability to remain abstinent. Despite a wealth of research literature on neuropsychological correlates of substance abuse, questions remain about individual differences in the development of impairment, the link between deficits and drug effects, and the time necessary for neuropsychological recovery. Advances in and standardization of measurement techniques, as well as increased emphasis on demographics, individual drug use history, and premorbid neuropsychological capacity, will contribute to better understanding of the relationship between substance abuse and neuropsychological function.

PAIN AND SUBSTANCE ABUSE

Substance abusers frequently develop painful conditions from the adverse effects of abused drugs. In addition to the direct toxic effects of the drugs themselves, trauma and infection are common causes of acute and chronic pain in substance abusers. Pain in the patient with a history of substance abuse must be managed appropriately to minimize suffering and promote health, and to establish a trusting relationship between the patient and the clinician, a crucial step to initiating or sustaining recovery from substance abuse.

Opiates provide one of the best pain relief options available to clinicians. Unfortunately, these medications have a clear abuse liability, and clinicians often are reluctant to provide them in sufficient amounts to their patients for fear of iatrogenic addiction (355–357). These fears are magnified in the case of patients with a past or current history of substance abuse (358). The fear of "feeding the addiction" or triggering a relapse tends to outweigh concerns about managing discomfort. Moreover, current legislation governing prescription of opiates to known substance abusers puts prescribing physicians at considerable risk of prosecution.

Strategies for management of pain in the substance abuser vary according to whether the pain is acute or chronic, and whether the patient is currently abusing opiates or other drugs, on opiate maintenance, or in drug-free recovery (359). Assessment of patterns of pain and opiate use provides the clinician with information on whether use patterns resemble those of abuse, pseudoaddiction, or appropriate pain self-medication.

Acute Versus Chronic Pain

Acute pain is typically sudden in onset, well localized, and easily recalled and described by the patient. Its duration is time-limited and generally brief (typically less than 1 week), and it may occur in a single episode (e.g., appendicitis) or be recurrent in nature (e.g., migraine headaches). The origin of the pain is usually obvious and can be attributed to dysfunction in a specific organ or to systemic disease. It is associated with signs of sympathetic hyperactivity and immobilization or guarding of the affected body region. The primary psychological response to acute pain is anxiety, with noticeable concern for determining its origin and seeking relief. Acute pain is extremely responsive to opiate analgesia, which may be the only intervention required to provide the patient adequate relief (360).

Chronic pain may or may not be preceded by an episode of acute pain. It can be of malignant (e.g., cancer) or nonmalignant (e.g., back pain) origin, and may last for months to years. It is typically described as constant, but may fluctuate in intensity. Psychological responses to chronic pain tend to be depression and insomnia, both of which can intensify the perception of pain. Opiate analgesics, although generally quite effective in managing chronic pain, are usually prescribed in combination with nonsteroidal analgesics and nonpharmacological interventions, especially if the pain is nonmalignant in origin.

Concern for the development of opiate abuse in non-substance-abusing persons receiving opiate analgesia is unfounded. In both single-episode and recurrent acute pain, the risk of iatrogenic addiction is low because the duration of opiate treatment is short and typically in response to intense pain. Patients with recurrent acute pain may be at slightly higher risk of developing abuse behaviors because of their increased access to opiate analgesics over prolonged periods, but empirical evidence of this occurrence is lacking. Evidence of opiate abuse is generally not a clinical issue in patients with chronic malignant or cancer-related pain, as maximum relief of discomfort and avoiding opiate toxicity are overriding concerns. Conversely, for persons with chronic pain of nonmalignant origin, opiates have not been generally considered a first-line strategy for pain management, and alternate, frequently nonpharmacological strategies are emphasized. As clinicians have learned more about chronic nonmalignant pain syndromes, it is increasingly recognized that opiate maintenance may be required to provide adequate relief (361, 362). Under these circumstances, development of tolerance and subsequent withdrawal upon opiate discontinuation, characteristics of physical dependence, should not be confused with substance abuse (See Chapters 21 and 22).

Pain in Addicted Patients

Pain management strategies for persons with a history of substance abuse depend on whether the history is remote or current, and whether the primary drug of abuse is an opiate or a nonopiate substance. For persons in drug-free recovery from opiate addiction, clinicians must recognize that pain (but not necessarily opiate analgesia) is a risk factor for relapse, and therefore aggressive attempts must be made to provide relief. The fear of relapse is likely to be strong in such patients. The clinician must be especially supportive and reinforce with the patient the distinction between use of opiate analgesics in the context of pain and their use in the absence of pain. The patient should be encouraged to intensify or reinitiate participation in recovery activities (e.g., 12-step meetings, relapse prevention sessions). Certainly the use of nonopiate analgesics and nonpharmacological strategies is indicated, but their effectiveness may be less than adequate, and provision of an opiate analgesic may be necessary. Ineffective pain management and the accompanying high levels of anxiety can induce craving for the drug(s) that had provided relief for the patient in the past.

Tapering of opiate analgesics as pain diminishes should proceed at a more gradual rate with the recovering addict than with opiate-naive patients to minimize the emergence of withdrawal symptoms. Use of mixed opiate agonist-antagonists (e.g., buprenorphine) may be preferable to full agonist analgesics, because the level of physical dependence may be less, and subjective feelings of withdrawal (which may induce opiate craving) will be minimized. Once completely withdrawn from opiates, the patient may be offered opiate antagonist maintenance therapy (e.g., naltrexone) for a short period of time to prevent relapse.

Patients, and even street addicts, on an opiate maintenance treatment (e.g., LAAM or methadone), require higher opiate analgesic doses than those required by opiate-naive patients because of tolerance. For patients receiving LAAM or methadone treatment, maintenance opiate medication should be continued at the usual dose, and not considered as contributing to analgesic requirement (363–367). Maintenance medications, chronically administered to prevent withdrawal and to block the psychoactive effects of subsequently administered opiates, have no demonstrated efficacy to provide analgesia. Instead, patients maintained on opiates for the treatment of addiction may have decreased tolerance to standard painful stimuli (368). An effective maintenance dose of a long-acting opiate, like LAAM or methadone, should be prescribed for opiate abusers not in treatment, and again, should be considered distinct from opiates prescribed to provide analgesia. Because opiate maintenance treatment is highly regulated, under current laws clinicians anticipating needing to treat such patients with opiates beyond 2–3 weeks should seek consultation early with an expert in opiate maintenance pharmacotherapy.

Mixed opiate agonist-antagonists or full antagonists cannot be used in opiate-dependent persons because they precipitate withdrawal, further diminish pain tolerance (369) and increase analgesic need. For patients with a remote or current history of opiate addiction, oral opiate analgesics with slow onset to minimize psychoactive effects are preferred. Prescription of the patient's identified opiate of abuse should be avoided. Any evidence that visitors may be supplying the patient with illicit opiates should trigger a review of the adequacy of pain relief or presence of withdrawal instead of punishing or policing the patient as a matter of automatic response.

Guidelines for managing acute pain in known or suspected substance abusers have been developed by the Agency for Health Care Policy and Research Guideline Panel (370). During an episode of acute pain, detoxification should never be attempted. Remember that pain relief is the priority; discussion of drug treatment options can follow once pain is adequately managed. With chronic nonmalignant pain, detoxification may be warranted to get baseline assessments of pain, addiction and analgesic need, and, where possible, should be initiated in an inpatient environment where both pain and withdrawal can be actively assessed and managed. Detoxified chronic pain patients anecdotally report less pain relative to that experienced prior to detoxification. Once the patient is opiate-free, the clinician and patient can explore controlled opiate maintenance as an option to effectively manage pain.

A similar strategy can be implemented for patients with a current or past history of abusing substances other than opiates. A past history of drug abuse, regardless of specific drug, predisposes the patient to becoming addicted to another drug (opiates). If opiate dependence is not an issue, mixed opiate agonist-antagonists and partial agonists may minimize the risk of physical dependence (371). Benzodiazepines should be avoided to augment analgesia in persons with a current or remote history of alcohol, sedative-hypnotic, or CNS depressant abuse, as should stimulants in persons with a history of cocaine or CNS stimulant abuse.

Table 30.16 provides a scheme for assessing the risk of opiate abuse in patients with a history of substance abuse, based upon their pain and opiate addiction history. Even if the patient's risk for opiate abuse is high or readily evident, the use of opiate analgesics is not necessarily contraindicated. Opiates may be necessary to provide effective pain relief. The intensity of monitoring by the clinician should be adjusted accordingly.

PATTERNS OF ANALGESIC USE

It is often necessary to determine if a patient with chronic nonmalignant pain is using opiate analgesics in an abusive or addictive manner. True substance abuse behaviors in the chronic pain patient often preclude adequate pain management and place the physician at significant legal risk for prescribing opiates to an opiate addict. Distinguishing between substance abuse and pain behaviors is complicated by the fact that pain patients who appropriately use opiate analgesics can meet DSM-IV diagnostic criteria for substance dependence.

Table 30.17 provides clinical features that further distinguish pain patients from addicts. It is necessary to rule out pseudoaddiction in pain patients manifesting addictive behaviors. Patients whose pain is not being effectively managed may evidence drug-seeking behaviors in legitimate attempts to achieve relief (e.g., utilizing multiple physicians or obtaining opiates from street sources). For this reason, it is important to ensure that all patients have achieved adequate analgesia before assuming that drug-seeking behaviors are indicative of addiction.

The clinician treating the substance abuser on opiate maintenance for analgesia must anticipate that relapse to abuse can and does occur, especially early in treatment. Relapse is an expected outcome of attempts to stop drug use in substance abuse treatment and, in this context, should be viewed as an integral part of the substance abuser's attempt to recover. When treating for either the pain or the substance abuse, it is counterproductive to threaten the patient with withholding opiate analgesics when a relapse is detected. Rather, relapse must be treated aggressively, as such, in the context of chronic pain.

The following guidelines are abstracted from those offered by Portenoy and Payne (360) on the management of opiate maintenance for chronic nonmalignant pain. They are applicable for all patients, including those with a history of substance abuse:

1. Opiate maintenance should be considered only after all other reasonable attempts at analgesia have failed;
2. A single practitioner should take primary responsibility for treatment;
3. After drug selection, doses should be given on a round-the-clock basis;
4. The initial goal is partial analgesia; failure to achieve at least partial analgesia within the first few weeks of maintenance at relatively low initial doses (acknowledg-

Table 30.16.   Risk of Opiate Abuse Based on Type of Pain and Opiate Addiction History[a]

Addiction Status	Acute, Single-Episode Pain	Chronic Malignant Pain	Acute Recurrent Pain	Chronic Nonmalignant Pain
No history of addiction	0	0	+	+
History of opiate addiction, recovering	+	+	+	+ +
Currently on opiate maintenance (methadone, LAAM)	+	+ +	+ +	+ + +
Currently using illicit opiates	+ + +	+ + +	+ + + +	+ + + +

[a]0 = no risk of abuse.
+ = little concern; abuse is a remote possibility.
+ + = moderate level of concern; abuse is a distinct possibility.
+ + + = high level of concern; abuse is a likely outcome.
+ + + + = abuse exists; carefully monitor use of opiates.

Table 30.17.   Clinical Features that Distinguish Pain Patients and Addicts

Clinical Features	Pain Patients	Addicts
Compulsive use	rare	common
Craving	rare	common
Obtain or purchase drugs from nonmedical sources	rare	common
Illegal activities to procure drugs	absent	common
Escalation of opiate dose without medical instruction	rare	common
Supplement with other opiate drugs	unusual	frequent
Demands specific opiate agent	rare	common
Ability to stop opiates when effective alternative treatments available	successful	usually unsuccessful
Requires unusually high dose	rare	common
Preference for specific routes of administration	no	yes
Able to regulate use according to supply	yes	no

Table 30.18.   Common Neurological Complications of HIV

	Central Nervous System	Peripheral Nervous System[a]
HIV neurotoxicity	AIDS dementia (subacute encephalitis, AIDS encephalopathy) Vacuolar myelopathy	Distal symmetric polyneuropathy Progressive lumbosacral polyradiculopathy Mononeuropathy multiplex Chronic inflammatory polyneuropathy Autonomic neuropathy
Secondary opportunistic infections	Cerebral toxoplasmosis Cryptococcal meningitis Progressive multifocal leukoencephalopathy Herpes simplex virus encephalitis Neurosyphillis Cytomegalovirus encephalitis *Mycobacterium tuberculosis* Varicella zoster virus encephalitis or vasculitis	Herpes zoster radiculitis Toxoplasmosis myopathy Varicella zoster neuropathy Cytomegalovirus neuropathy

[a]Additionally, toxic neuropathy or myopathy may arise as side effects from therapeutic drugs (e.g., vincristine, isoniacid, dapsone, AZT).

ing tolerance) may indicate that the pain is not responsive to opiate maintenance therapy;

5. Emphasis should be given to capitalize on improved analgesia by gains in physical and social functioning;
6. In addition to daily dose, patients should be permitted to escalate dose in small amounts transiently on days of increased pain, under tightly controlled conditions;
7. Exacerbations in pain not effectively treated by transient, small increases of dose should be treated in the hospital;
8. Patients must be seen and drugs prescribed at frequent intervals; and
9. Evidence of drug hoarding, drug diversion, or relapse should be immediately addressed with substance abuse treatment interventions.

A past or current history of substance abuse does not preclude the use of opiate analgesics to provide pain relief. A clear understanding of the differences between physical dependence and addictive behaviors, and of the abuse potential of opiates in the context of pain, enables clinicians to effectively address the challenging problem of pain in substance abusers. Clinicians should keep in mind that a chronic pain patient with an addictive disorder does not have one insurmountably hopeless condition but two difficult yet treatable medical illnesses.

HIV AND THE NERVOUS SYSTEM

Use of contaminated paraphernalia and the sharing of dirty needles puts the intravenous (i.v.) drug user at an inordinate risk of contracting the HIV virus. This risk is increased, especially for women, when unsafe sexual behaviors are engaged in to support the drug habit.

HIV infection has a wide range of effects on the central and peripheral nervous systems. The virus appears to invade the nervous system early (perhaps even before seroconversion occurs) (372), and is currently one of the most common causes of neurological disorders (predominantly dementia, myelopathy, and neuropathy) in young persons (373). Furthermore, neurological complications may result not only from secondary opportunistic infections and malignancies, but from the neurodegenerative effects of the virus itself (Table 30.18). Cells in the nervous system, including macrophages, microglia, astrocytes, oligodendrocytes, and neurons can be directly infected with HIV, although by different mechanisms from those identified in lymphocyte infection (374). Centrally, basal ganglia and temporolimbic brain structures are specifically susceptible, although secondary viral coinfections can produce cerebral vessel vasculitides, which can in turn lead to strokes and multi-infarcts in other brain areas.

A number of psychiatric complications may also arise as a result of HIV infection. Most commonly, these include anxiety and depression, which are primarily reactive responses to the diagnosis itself, and dementia and delirium, which relate directly to the systemic or CNS disease (375). This symbiotic relationship between the effects of i.v. drug use and HIV infection presents an important clinical challenge for the health care provider who is treating HIV-infected substance abusers. Distinction must be made between the neurological and psychological findings associated with HIV and those related to the chronic effects of substance abuse so that appropriate therapies can be instituted.

Acknowledgment

Preparation of this manuscript supported by NIDA grant R18 DA6082 to Friends Medical Research Center, Inc. The authors gratefully acknowledge the assistance of Mrs. Sandy Dow and of Mindy Blum, Ph.D.

References

1. Beresford TD, Lowe D, Hall RC, Adduci R, Goggans FC. Alcoholism in the general hospital. Psychiatr Med 1984;2:139–148.
2. Moore RD, Bone LR, Geller G, Mamon JA, Stokes EJ, Lavine DM. Prevalence, detection and treatment of alcoholism in hospitalized patients. JAMA 1989;261:403–407.
3. Cleary PD, Miller M, Bush PT, Warburg MM, Delbanco TL, Aronson ND. Prevalence and recognition of alcohol abuse in the primary care population. Am J Med 1988;85:466–471.
4. Buchsbaum DG, Buchanan RG, Schnoll SH, Lawton MJ. Screening for alcohol abuse using C.A.G.E. scores and likelihood ratios. Ann Intern Med 1991;115:744–777.
5. State Methadone Maintenance Guidelines. Center for Substance Abuse Treatment U.S. Department of Health and Human Services, 1992:337–369.
6. Selzer ML. The Michigan Alcoholism Screening Test: the quest for a new diagnostic instrument. Am J Psychol 1971;127:1653–1658.
7. Ewing J. Detecting alcoholism: the CAGE questionnaire. JAMA 1984;252:1905–1907.
8. Folstein M, Folstein S, McHugh P. The Mini-Mental State Examination. J Psychiatr Res 1975;12:189–198.
9. American Psychiatric Association. Diagnostic and statistical manual of mental disorders, 4th ed., revised. Washington, D.C., 1994.
10. Willette E. Drug testing programs. In: Hanks RI, Chiang NC, eds. Urine testing for drugs of abuse. NIDA Research Monograph #73. Washington, DC: Government Printing Office, 1986:5–12.
11. Person N, Ehrenkranz J. Evaluation of urine temperature methods to screen urine specimens for drug testing. Clin Chem 1989;35:1181–1189.
12. Herridge P, Ehrenkranz J, Pottash A, Gold M. The clinical laboratory. In: Sederer L, ed. Inpatient psychiatry. Baltimore: Williams & Wilkins 1991:338–359.
13. Council on Scientific Affairs. Scientific issues in drug testing. JAMA 1987;257:3110–3114.
14. Nalpas B, Vassault A, Le Guillou A, et al. Serum activity of mitochondrial aspartate aminotransferase: a sensitive marker of alcoholism with or without alcohol hepatitis. Hepatology 1984;4:893.
15. Bernadt MW, Taylor C, Mumford J, Smith B, Murray RM. Comparison of questionnaire and laboratory tests in the detection of excessive drinking and alcoholism. Lancet 1982;1:525.
16. NIDA. National household survey on drug abuse: main findings. Rockville, MD: National Institute of Drug Abuse, 1991.
17. Regier DA, Farmer ME, Rae DS, et al. Comorbidity of mental disorders with alcohol and other drug abuse. Results from the epidemiologic catchment area (ECA) study. JAMA 1990;264:2511–2518.
18. Kalant H, Woo N. Electrophysiological effects of ethanol on the nervous system. Pharmacol Ther 1981;14:431.
19. Majchrowicz E. Biologic properties of ethanol and the biphasic nature of the ethanol withdrawal syndrome. In: Tarter RE, Van Thiel DH, eds. Alcohol and the brain: chronic effects. New York: Plenum, 1985:315–338.
20. Rubino FA. Neurologic complications of alcoholism. Psychiatr Clin North Am 1992;15:359–372.
21. Frezza M, DiPadova C, Pazzato G, Terpin M, Barona E, Lieber CS. High blood alcohol levels in women: the role of decreased gastric alcohol dehydrogenase activity and first pass metabolism. N Engl J Med 1990;322:95–99.
22. Delin CR, Lee TH. Drinking and the brain: current evidence. Alcohol 1992;27:117–126.
23. Victor M. The effects of alcohol on the nervous system: clinical features, pathogenesis and treatment. In: Liever CS, ed. Medical and nutritional complications of alcoholism. New York: Plenum, 1992:413–457.
24. Miller NS, Gold MS. Alcohol. New York: Plenum 1991.
25. Light WJH. The neurobiology of alcohol abuse. Springfield, IL: Charles C Thomas, 1986.
26. Crabbe JC, Feller DJ, Terdal ES, Merrill CD. Genetic components of ethanol responses. Alcohol 1990;7:245–248.
27. Crabbe JC, Harris RA. The genetic basis of alcohol and drug actions. New York: Plenum Press, 1991.
28. Crabbe JC, Phillips TJ, Cunningham CL, Belnap JK. Genetic determinants of ethanol reinforcement. Ann N Y Acad Sci 1992;654:302–310.
29. Harris RA, Allan AM. Alcohol intoxication: ion channels and genetics. Faseb J 1989;3:1689–1695.
30. Kiianmaa K, Helevuo K. The alcohol tolerant and alcohol nontolerant rat line selected for differential sensitivity to ethanol: a tool to study mechanisms of the actions of ethanol. Ann Intern Med 1990;22:283–287.
31. Palmer MR. Neurophysiological mechanisms in the genetics of ethanol sensitivity. Soc Biol 1985;32:241–254.
32. Fernandez-del Moral R, Dawid-Milner S, Diaz-Calvia JE. Pharmacology of acute alcoholic intoxication. Rev Esp Fisiol 1989;45[Suppl]:337–346.
33. Jaffe J. Drug addiction and drug abuse. In: Gilman AG, Rolf TW, Nies AS, Taylor P, eds. Goodman and Gilman's Pharmacological bases of therapeutics. 8th ed. New York: Pergammon Press, 1990;1:522–523.
34. Mendelson JH, Mello NK. The diagnosis and treatment of alcoholism. New York: McGraw-Hill, 1979.
35. Charness ME, Simon RP, Greenberg DA. Ethanol and the nervous system. N Engl J Med 1989;321:442–454.
36. Little HJ. Mechanisms that may underlie the behavioral effects of ethanol. Prog Neurobiol 1991;36:171–194.
37. Majchrowicz E. Biologic properties of ethanol and the biphasic nature of the ethanol withdrawal syndrome. In: Tarter RE, Van Thiel DH, eds. Alcohol and the brain: chronic effects. New York: Plenum, 1985:315–338.
38. Victor M, Adams RD. The effects of alcohol on the nervous system. Res Publ Assoc Nerv Ment Dis 1953;32:526–573.
39. Naranjo CA, Bremner KE. Behavioral correlates of alcohol intoxication. Addiction 1993;88:25–35.

40. Tennant F. The rapid eye test to detect drug abuse. Postgrad Med 1988;84:108–114.
41. Mello NK, Mendelson JH. Alcohol and human behavior. In: Iversen LL, Eversen SD, Snyder SH, eds. Handbook of psychopharmacology. New York: Plenum, 1978;7:235–317.
42. Tamerin JS, Weiner S, Poppen R, Steinglass P, Mendelson JH. Alcohol and memory: amnesia and short-term memory function during experimentally induced intoxication. Am J Psychiatry 1971;127:1659–1664.
43. Goodwin DW, Othmer E, Halikas JA, Freemon F. Loss of short-term memory as a predictor of the alcoholic "blackout." Nature 1971;227:201–202.
44. Goodwin DW. Blackouts and alcohol induced memory dysfunction. In: Mello NK, Mendelson JH, eds. Recent advances in studies of alcoholism. Bethesda: NIMH, 1971:508–536.
45. Sweeney DF. Alcohol versus mnemosyne – blackouts. J Subst Abuse Treat 1989;6:159–162.
46. Gallant DM. Alcoholism: a guide to diagnosis, intervention and treatment. New York: WW Norton Company, 1987.
47. Taylor WA, Slaby AE. Acute treatment of alcohol and cocaine emergencies. Recent Dev Alcohol 1992;10:179–191.
48. Holt S, Steward IC, Dixon JW, Elton RW, Taylor TV, Little K. Alcohol and the emergency service patient. Br Med J 1980;281:638–640.
49. Kellermann AL, Fihn SD, LoGerfo JP, Copass MK. Impact of drug screening in suspected overdose. Ann Emerg Med 1987;16:1206–1216.
50. Nutt DJ, Glue P. Neuropharmacological and clinical aspects of alcohol withdrawal. Ann Intern Med 1990; 22:275–281.
51. Turner RC, Lichstein PR, Peden JG, Busher JT, Waivers LE. Alcohol withdrawal syndromes: a review of pathophysiology, clinical presentation, and treatment. J Gen Intern Med 1989;4:432–444.
52. Gauvin DV, Youngblood BD, Holloway FA. The discriminative stimulus properties of acute ethanol withdrawal (hangover) in rats. Alc Clin Exp Res 1992;16:336–341.
53. Missouri Medicine. Alcohol consumption and hangover. Mo Med 1990;87:875–876.
54. Newlin DB, Pretorius MB. Sons of alcoholics report greater hangover symptoms than sons of nonalcoholics: a pilot study. Alcohol Clin Exp Res 1990;14:713–716.
55. Rubino C, Butters N. Cognitive effects in alcohol abuse. In: Kissin B, Begleiter H, eds. The biology of alcoholism. New York: Plenum, 1982;6:485–538.
56. Edwards G. Withdrawal symptoms and alcohol dependence: fruitful mysteries. Br J Addict 1990;85:447–461.
57. Maier DM, Pohorecky LA. The effects of repeated withdrawal episodes on subsequent withdrawal severity in ethanol-treated rats. Drug Alcohol Depend 1989;23:103–110.
58. Cushman P. Delirium tremens: update on an old disorder. Postgrad Med 1987;5:117–122.
59. Alpert MA. Modern management of delirium tremens. Hospital Medicine 1990;26:111–136.
60. Glass IB. Alcoholic hallucinosis: a psychiatric enigma. Brit J Addict 1989;84:29–41.
61. Surawicz FG. Alcoholic hallucinosis: a missed diagnosis. Can J Psychiatry 1980;25:57–63
62. McMicken DB. Alcohol withdrawal syndromes. Emerg Med Clin North Am 1990;8:805–819.
63. Strub RL, Black FW, eds. Neurobehavioral disorders: a clinical approach. Philadelphia: FA Davis, 1988.
64. Gillman MA, Lichtigfeld FJ. The drug management of severe alcohol withdrawal syndrome. Postgrad Med J 1990;66:1005–1009.
65. Romach MK, Seller EM. Management of the alcohol withdrawal syndrome. Ann Rev Med 1991;42:323–340.
66. Young GP. Seizures in the alcoholic patient. Emerg Med Clin North Am 1990;8:821–833.
67. Lechtenberg R, Worner TM. Total ethanol consumption as a seizure risk factor in alcoholics. Acta Neurol Scand 1992;85:90–94.
68. Lowenstein DH, Alldredge BK. Status of epilepticus at an urban public hospital in the 1980s. Neurology 1993;43:483–488.
69. Krauss GL, Niedermeyer E. Neuropharmacology of cocaine and ethanol dependence. Recent Dev Alcohol 1992;10:201–233.
70. Loiseau P, Duche B, Loiseau J. Classification of epilepsies and epileptic syndromes in two different samples of patients. Epilepsia 1991;32:303–309.
71. Verma NP, Policheria H, Buber BA. Prior head injury accounts for the heterogeneity of the alcohol-epilepsy relationship. Clin Electroencephalogr 1992;23:147–151.
72. Alldredge BK, Lowenstein DH, Simon RP. Placebo-controlled trial of intravenous diphenylhydrate for short-term treatment of alcohol withdrawal seizures. Am J Med 1989;87:645–648.
73. Hillborn M, Tokola R, Kuusela V, et al. Prevention of alcohol withdrawal seizures with carbamazepine and Valproic acid. Alcohol 1989;6:223–226.
74. Thompson WL, Johnson AD, Maddrey WL. Diazepam and paraldehyde for treatment of severe delirium tremens. Ann Intern Med 1975;82:175–180.
75. Satel SL, Kosten TR, Schuckit MA, Fischman MW. Am J Psychiatry 1993;150:695–704.
76. Kissin B. Biologic investigations in alcohol research. J Stud Alcohol 1979;8:146–181.
77. Alling C, Balldin M, Bokstrom K, Gottfries CJ, Karlsson I. Studies on duration of a late recovery period after chronic abuse of ethanol. Acta Psychiatr Scand 1982;66:384–397.
78. De Soto CB, O'Donnell WE, Allred LJ, Lopes CE. Symptomatology in alcoholics at various stages of abstinence. Alcohol Clinic Exp Res 1985;9:505–512.
79. Victor M, Adams RD, Collins GH eds. The Wernicke-Korsakoff syndrome and related neurologic disorders due to alcoholism and malnutrition. Philadelphia: FA Davis, 1989.
80. Carlin AS, Strauss FF, Adams KM, Grant I. The prediction of neuropsychological impairment in polydrug abusers. Addict Behav 1978;3:5–12.
81. Greenberg DA, Diamond I. Wernicke-Korsakoff syndrome. In: Tarter RE, Van Thiel DH, eds. Alcohol and the brain: chronic effects. New York: Plenum, 1986:295–314.
82. Reuler JB, Girard DE, Cooney TG. Wernicke's encephalopathy. N Engl J Med 1985;312:1035–1040.
83. Zimitat C, Kril J, Harper CG, Nixon PF. Progression of neurological disease in thiamin-deficient rats is enhanced by ethanol. Alcohol 1990;7:493–501.
84. Manzo L, Locatelli C, Candura SM, Costa LG. Nutrition and alcohol neurotoxicity. Neurotoxicology 1994;15:555–566.
85. Tallaksen CM, Bohmer T, Bell H. Blood serum thiamin and thiamin phosphate esters concentrations in patients with alcohol dependence syndrome before and after thiamin treatment. Alcohol Clin Exp Res 1992:16:320-325.
86. Irle E, Kaiser P, Naumann-Stoll G. Differential patterns of memory loss in patients with Alzheimer's disease and Korsakoff's disease. Int J Neurosci 1990;52:67–77.
87. O'Carroll RE, Moffoot A, Ebmeier KP, Murray C, Goodwin GM. Korsadoff's syndrome, cognition and clonidine. Psychol Med 1993;23:341–347.
88. McEntee WJ, Mair RG. Memory impairment in Korsakoff's psychosis: a correlation with brain noradrenergic activity. Science 1978;202:905–907.
89. McEntree WJ, Mair RG. Memory enhancement in Korsakoff's psychosis by clonidine: further evidence for a noradrenergic deficit. Ann Neurol 1980;7:466–470.
90. McEntree WJ, Miar RG, Langlais PJ. Neurochemical pathology in Korsakoff's psychosis: implications for other cognitive disorders. Neurology 1984;34:648–652.
91. Benson DF, Cummings JL. A scheme to differentiate the dementias. In: Jeste DV, ed. Neuropsychiatric dementias. Washington, DC: American Psychological Association, 1986:1–25.
92. Akai J. Anatomo-pathological studies on alcohol dementia: a review

and up to date research. Drug Alcohol Depend 1991;26:134.

93. Cutting J. The relationship between Korsakoff syndrome and "alcoholic dementia." Br J Psychiatry 1978;132:240–245.

94. Blusewicz MJ. Neuropsychological correlates of chronic alcoholism and aging. J Nerv Ment Dis 1977;165:348–356.

95. Goldstein G. Dementia associated with alcoholism. In: Tarter RE, Van Thiel DH, eds. Alcohol and the brain: chronic effects. New York: Plenum, 1985:283–294.

96. Page RD, Shaub LH. Intellectual functioning in alcoholics during six months abstinence. J Stud Alcohol 1977;38:1240–1248.

97. Victor M, Banker BQ. Alcohol and dementia. In: Katzman R, Terry RD, Bick KL, eds. Alzheimer's disease: senile dementia and related disorders. New York: Raven Press 1978:149–170.

98. Jones B, Parsons OA. Impaired abstraction ability in chronic alcoholics. Arc Gen Psychiatry 1971;24:431–457.

99. Tarter R. An analysis of cognitive deficits in chronic alcoholics. J Nerv Ment Dis 1973;157:138–147.

100. Tarter R, Alterman A. Neuropsychological deficits in chronic alcoholics: etiological considerations. J Stud Alcohol 1984;45:1–9.

101. Neiman J, Lang AE, Fornazzari L, Carlen PL. Movement disorders in alcoholism: a review. Neurology 1990;40:741–746.

102. Butterworth RF, D'Amour M, Bruneau J, Herous M, Brisette S. Role of thiamine deficiency in the pathogenesis of alcoholic peripheral neuropathy and the Wernicke-Korsakoff syndrome: an update. In: Palmer TN, ed. Alcoholism: a molecular perspective. New York: Plenum, 1991:269–277.

103. Graham JR, Woodhouse D, Read FH. Massive thiamine dosage in an alcoholic with cerebellar degeneration. Lancet 1971;11:107.

104. Karol RL, Halla PD. Brain injury and alcohol: a workbook for making decisions after injury. Minneapolis: Thompson and Company, 1987.

105. Elliot FA. Neuroanatomy and neurology of aggression. Psychol Ann 1987;17:385–387.

106. Corthell DW, Tooman M. Twelfth Institute on Rehabilitation issues: rehabilitation of traumatic brain injury. Stout, WI: Research and Training Center, University of Wisconsin. Stout 1985.

107. Bombardier CH. Alcohol use and traumatic brain injury. West J Med 1995;162:150–151.

108. Heikkinen ER, Ronty HS, Tolonen U, Pyhtinen J. Development of posttraumatic epilepsy. Sterotact Funct Neurosurg 1990; 54–55:25–33.

109. Solomon DA, Sparadeo F. The effects of substance abuse on persons with traumatic brain injury. Neurorehabilitation 1992;2:16–26.

110. Langley MJ, Lindsay WP, Lam CS, Priddy DA. Programme development. A comprehensive alcohol abuse treatment programme for persons with traumatic brain injury. Brain Inj 1990;4:77–86.

111. Mayer E. The toxic effects following the use of local anesthetics. JAMA 1924;82:876–878.

112. Mendoza R, Miller BL, Mena I. Emergency room evaluation of cocaine-associated neuropsychiatic disorders. In: Galantar M. ed. Recent developments in alcoholism, vol. 10. New York: Plenum, 1992:73–87.

113. Levine SR, Brust JCM, Futrell N, et al. Cerebrovascular complications of the use of the crack form of alkaloidal cocaine. N Eng J Med 1990;323:699–704.

114. National household survey on drug abuse: population estimates. Rockville, MD: National Institute on Drug Abuse, 1991.

115. Pascual-Leone A, Dhuna A, Anderson DC. Longterm neurological complications of chronic, habitual cocaine abuse. Neurotoxicology 1991;12:393–400.

116. Pascual-Leone A, Dhuna A, Anderson DC. Cerebral atrophy in habitual cocaine abusers: a planimetric CT study. Neurology 1991; 41:34–38.

117. Gold MS. Cocaine (and crack): clinical aspects. In: Lowinson JH, Ruiz P, Millman RB, eds. Substance abuse: a comprehensive textbook. 2nd ed. Baltimore: Williams & Wilkins, 1992:205–221.

118. Mendoza R, Miller BL. Neuropsychiatric disorders associated with cocaine use. Hosp Community Psychiatry 1992;43:677–678.

119. Wetli CV, Fishbain DA. Cocaine-induced psychosis and sudden death in recreational cocaine users. J Forensic Sci 1985;30:873–879.

120. Kosten TR, Kleber HD. Rapid death during cocaine abuse: a variant of the neuroleptic malignant syndrome? Am J Drug Alcohol Abuse 1988;14:335–346.

121. Karch SB. The pathology of drug abuse. Boca Raton, FL: CRC Press, 1993.

122. Allredge BK, Lowenstein DH, Simon RP. Seizures associated with recreational drug abuse. Neurology 1989;39:1037–1039.

123. Chong-Kwong M, Lipton RB. Seizures in hospitalized cocaine users. Neurology 1989;39:425–427.

124. Kramer LD, Locke GE, Ogunyemi A, Nelson L. cocaine-related seizures in adults. Am J Drug Alcohol Abuse 1990;16:309–317.

125. Pascual-Leone A, Dhuna A, Altafullah I, Anderson DC. Cocaine-induced seizures. Neurology 1990;40:404–407.

126. Root RK, Rowbotham M. Neurologic aspects of cocaine abuse. West J Med 1988;149:442–448.

127. Rowbotham MC, Lowenstein DH. Neurologic consequences of cocaine use. Am Rev Med 1990;41:417–422.

128. Post RM, Kopanda RT. Cocaine, kindling, and psychosis. Am J Psychiatry 1976;133:327–334.

129. Merriam A, Medalia A, Levine B. Partial complex status epilepticus associated with cocaine abuse. Biol Psychiatry 1988;23:515–518.

130. Wetli C, Mittleman RE. The "body packer syndrome" – toxicity following ingestion of illicit drugs packaged for transportation. J Forensic Sci 1981;26:492–500.

131. Catravas JD, Waters IW. Acute cocaine intoxication in the conscious dog: studies on the mechanism of lethality. J Pharmacol Exp Ther 1981;217:350–356.

132. Kaku DA, Lowenstein DH. Emergence of recreational drug abuse as a major risk factor for stroke in young adults. Ann Intern Med 1990;113:821–827.

133. Sloan MA, Kittner SU, Rigamonti D, et al. Occurrence of stroke associated with use/abuse of drugs. Neurology 1991;41:1358–1364.

134. Levine SR, Brust JCM, Futrell N, et al. A comparative study of the cerebrovascular complications of cocaine: alkaloidal versus hydrochloride–a review. Neurology 1991;41:1173–1177.

135. Brust JCM. Neurological aspects of substance abuse. Boston: Butterworth-Heinemann, 1993.

136. Madden J, Powers R. Effects of cocaine and cocaine metabolites on cerebral arteries in vitro. Life Sci 1990;47:1109–1114.

137. Levine S, Washington J, Jefferson M, et al. "Crack" cocaine associated stroke. Neurology 1987;37:1849–1853.

138. Tongna G, Tempesta E, Tongna AR, Dolci N, Cebo B, Caprino L. Platelet responsiveness and biosynthesis of thromboxane and prostacyclin in response to in vitro cocaine treatment. Haemostasis 1985;15:100–107.

139. Kokkinos J, Levine SR. Stroke. Neurol Clin 1993;II:577–590.

140. Mendoza RP, Miller BL. Mena I. Emergency room evaluation of cocaine-associated neuropsychiatric disorders. In: Galanter M, ed. Recent developments in alcoholism, vol 10: alcohol and cocaine: similarities and differences. New York: Plenum, 1992.

141. Substance related disorders. In: Diagnostic and statistical manual of mental disorders. 4th ed. Washington, DC: American Psychiatric Association, 1994.

142. Brower KJ, Paredes A. Cocaine withdrawal [editorial]. Arch Gen Psychiatry 1987;44:297.

143. Gawin FH, Kleber HD. Abstinence symptomatology and psychiatric diagnosis in cocaine abusers. Arch Gen Psychiatry 1986a; 43:107–113.

144. Daras M, Koppel BS, Atos-Radzion E. Cocaine-induced choreoathetoid movements ("crack dancing"). Neurology 1994;44:751–752.

145. Habal R, Sauter D, Olowe O, Daras M. Cocaine and chorea. Am J Emerg Med 1991;9:618–620.

146. Lundh H, Tunving K. An extrapyramidal choreiform syndrome caused by amphetamine addiction. J Neurol Neurosurg Psychiatry 1981;44:728–730.

147. Rhee KJ, Albertson TE, Douglas JC. Choreoathetoid disorder

associated with amphetamine-like drugs. Am J Emerg Med 1988;6:131–133.

148. Thief A, Dressler D. Dyskinesias possibly induced by norpseu-doephedrine. J Neurol 1994;241:167–169.

149. Ling W, Wesson DR. Drugs of abuse-opiates. West J Med 1990;152:565–572.

150. Jaffe JH, Martin WR. Opioid analgesics and antagonists. In: Gilman AG, Rall TW, Nies AS, Taylor P, eds. Goodman and Gilman's The pharmacological basis of therapeutics. 8th ed. New York: McGraw-Hill 1993:21.

151. Jaffe JH. Opiates: clinical aspects. In: Lowinson JH, Ruiz JH, Millman RB, Langrod JG, eds. Substance abuse: a comprehensive textbook. 2nd ed. Baltimore: Williams & Wilkins 1992:186–194.

152. Brust JCM, Richter RW. Quinine amblyopia related to heroin addiction. Ann Intern Med 1971;74:84.

153. Dalessandro-Gandolfo L, Macci A, Biolcati G, et al. Inconsueta modaity d'intossicazione da piombo. Presentazione di un caso. Recenti Prog Med 1989;80:140.

154. Novick DM. The medically ill substance abuser. In: Lowinson JH, Ruiz P, Millman RB, Langrod JG, eds. Substance abuse: a comprehensive textbook. 2nd ed. Baltimore: Williams & Wilkins 1992:657–674.

155. Caplan L, Hier D, Banks G. Current concepts of cerebrovascular disease stroke: stroke and drug abuse. Stroke 1982;13:869–872.

156. Brust JCM. Neurological aspects of substance abuse. Boca Raton, FL: CRC Press, 1993.

157. Caplan LR, Hier DB, Banks G. Stroke and drug abuse. Stroke 1982;13:869.

158. Ammueilaph R, Boongird P, Leechawengwongs M, Vejjajiva A. Heroin neuropathy. Lancet 1973;1:1517.

159. Ritland D, Butterfield W. Extremity complications of drug abuse. Am J Surg 1973;126:639.

160. Chen SS, Chien CH, Yu HS. Syndrome of deltoid and gluteal fibrotic conracture: an injection myopathy. Acta Neurol Scand 1988;78:167.

161. Griffiths RR, Roache JD. Abuse liability of benzodiazepines: a review of human studies evaluation subjective and/or reinforcing effects. In: Smith DE, Wesson DR, eds. The benzodiazepines: current standards for medical practice. Hingham, MA: MTP Press, 1985:209–225.

162. Randall T. "Rave" scene, ecstasy use, leap Atlantic. JAMA 1992;268:1506.

163. Randall T. Ecstasy-Fueled "rave" parties become dances of death for english youths. JAMA; 268:1505–1506.

164. Henry JA. Ecstasy and the dance of death. Br Med J 1992;305:5–6.

165. Sobel J, Espinas O, Friedman, S. Carotid artery obstruction following LSD capsule ingestion. Arch Intern Med 1971;127:290–291.

166. Gledhill JA, Moore DF, Bell D, Henry JA. Subarachnoid haemorrhage associated with MDMA abuse [letter]. J Neurol Neurosurg Psychiatry 1993;56:1036–1037.

167. Allen RP, McCann UD, Ricaurte GA. Persistent effects of (±) 3,4-methylenedioxymethamphetamine (MDMA), (ecstasy) on human sleep. Sleep 1993;16:560–564.

168. Krystal JH, Price LH, Opsahl C, Ricaurte GA, Hininger GR. Chronic 3,4-methylenedioxymethamphetamine (MDMA) use: effects on mood and neuropsychological function. Am J Drug Alcohol Abuse 1992;18:331–341.

169. Creighton FJ, Black DL, Hyde CE. "Ecstasy" psychosis and flashbacks. Br J Psychiatry 1991;159:713–715.

170. Pallanti S, Mazzi D. MDMA (ecstasy) precipitation of panic disorder. Biol Psychiatry 1992;32:91–95.

171. McCann UD, Ricaurte GA. MDMA (ecstasy) and panic disorder: induction by single dose. Biol Psychiatry 1992;32:950–953.

172. Whitaker-Azmitia PM, Aronson TA. "Ecstasy" (3,4-methylenedioxymethamphetamine)-induced panic. Am J Psychiatry 1989;146:119.

173. Winstock AR. Chronic paranoid psychosis after misuse of 4,3-methylenedioxymethamphetamine. Br Med J 1991;302:1150–1151.

174. Schifano F. Chronic atypical psychosis associated with 3,4-methylenedioxymethamphetamine ("ecstasy") abuse. Lancet 1991;338:1335.

175. Varma VK, Malhotra AK, Dang R. Cannabis and cognitive functions: a prospective study. Drug Alcohol Depend 1988;21:147–152.

176. Schwartz RH, Gruenewald PJ, Klitzner M, Fedio P. Short-term memory impairment in cannabis-dependent adolescents. Am J Dis Child 1989;143:1214–1219.

177. Leirer VO, Yesavage JA, Morrow DG. Marijuana carryover effects on aircraft pilot performance. Aviat Space Environ Med 1991;62:221–227.

178. Janowsky DS, Meacham MP, Blaine JD, Schoor M, Bozzetti LP. Simulated flying performance after marijuana intoxication. Aviat Space Environ Med 1976;47:124–128.

179. Leirer VO, Yesavage JA, Morrow DG. Marijuana, aging and task difficulty effects on pilot performance. Aviat Space Environ Med 1989;60:1145–1152.

180. Wert RC, Raulin ML. The chronic cerebral effects of cannabis use. I. Methodological issues and neurological findings. Int J Addict 1986;21:605–628.

181. Wert RC, Raulin ML. The chronic cerebral effects of cannabis use. II. Psychological findings and conclusions. Int J Addict 1986;21:629–642.

182. Mikuriya TH, ed. Marijuana: medical papers 1939–1972. Oakland, CA: Medi-Comp Press, 1973.

183. Turkanis SA, Karler R. Electrophysiologic properties of the cannabinoids. J Clin Pharmacol 1981;21:449S–463S.

184. Karler R, Turkanis SA. The cannabinoids as potential antiepileptics. J Clin Pharmacol 1981;21:437S–448S.

185. Consroe P, Martin A, Singh V. Antiepileptic potential of cannabidiol analogs. J Clin Pharmacol 1981;21:428S–436S.

186. Lemberger L. Potential therapeutic usefulness of marijuana. Annu Rev Pharmacol Toxicol 1980;20:151–172.

187. Carlini EA, Cunha JM. Hypnotic and antiepileptic effects of cannabidiol. J Clin Pharmacol 1981;21:417S–427S.

188. Doyle E, Spence AA. Cannabis as a medicine? Br J Anaesth 1995;74:359–360.

189. Dagirmangian R, Boyd ES. Some pharmacological effects of two tetrahydrocannabinols. J Pharmacol Exp Ther 1962;135:25–33.

190. Petro DJ, Ellenberger C. Treatment of human spasticity with delta⁹-tetrahydrocannabinol. J Clin Pharmacol 1981;21:413S–416S.

191. Grinspoon L, Bakalar JB. Marihuana as medicine. A plea for reconsideration. JAMA 1995;273:1875–1876.

192. Gorelick DA. Seretonin uptake blockers and the treatment of alcoholism. In: Galanter ed. Alcoholism treatment research, vol. 7. New York: Plenum, 1989:267.

193. Lerner PI. Neurological complications of infective endocarditis. Med Clin North Am 1985;69:385–398.

194. Jaffe JH, Martin WR. Opioid analgesics and antagonists. In: Gilman AG, Rall TW, Nies AS, Palmer T, eds. Goodman and Gilman's The pharmacological basis of therapeutics. 8th ed. New York: McGraw-Hill, 1993:485–521.

195. Rall TW. Hypnotics and sedatives. In: Gilman AG, Rall TW, Nies AS, Palmer T, eds. Goodman and Gilman's The pharmacological basis of therapeutics. 8th ed. New York: McGraw-Hill, 1993:345–382.

196. Aronson TA, Craig TJ. Cocaine precipitation of panic disorder. Am J Psychiatry 1986;143:643–645.

197. Gawin FH, Ellinwood Jr EH. Cocaine and other stimulants. Actions, abuse, and treatment. N Engl J Med 1988;318:1173–1182.

198. Gold MS, Washton AM, Dackis CA. Cocaine abuse: neurochemistry, pharmacology, and treatment. NIDA Res Monogr 1985;61:130–150.

199. Litten RZ, Allen JP. Pharmacological therapies of alcohol addiction. In: Miller NS, Gold MS, eds. Pharmacological therapies for drug and alcohol addictions. New York: Marcel Dekker, 1995:127–141.

200. Koppel BS, Tuchman AJ, Mangiardi JR, Daras M, Weitzner I. Epidural spinal infection in intravenous drug abusers. Arch Neurol 1988;45:1331–1337.

201. Amine AB. Neurosurgical complications of heroin addiction: brain abscess and mycotic aneurysm. Surg Neurol 1977;7:385.

202. Gilroy J, Andaya L, Thomas VJ. Intracranial mycotic aneurysms and subacute endocarditis in heroin addiction. Neurology 1973;23:1193.

203. Holzman RS, Bishko F. Osteomyelitis in heroin addicts. Ann Intern Med 1971;75:693–696.

204. Siao PTC, McCabe P, Yagnik P. Nocardial spinal epidural abscess. Neurology 1989;39:996.

205. Cherubin CE. The medical sequelae of narcotic addition. Ann Intern Med 1967;67:23.

206. Gattell JM, Miro JM, Para C, Garcia-San Miguel J. Infective endocarditis in drug addicts. Lancet 1984;1:228.

207. Hubbell G, Cheitlin MD, Rapaport E. Presentation, management, and follow-up of infective endocarditis in drug addicts. Am Heart J 1981;138:85.

208. Louria DB, Hensle T, Rose J. The major medical complications of heroin addiction. Ann Intern Med 1967;67:1.

209. Jabbari B, Pierce JF. Spinal cord compression due to Pseudomonas in a heroin addict. Neurology 1977;27:1034.

210. Kasplan SS. Pseudomonas disc space infection in an occasional heroin user. Ariz Med 1974;31:916.

211. Reyes MP, Palutke WA, Wylin RF, et al. *Pseudomonas* endocarditis in the Detroit Medical Center, 1969-1972. Medicine 1973;52:173.

212. Harris PD, Yeoh CB, Breault J, et al. Fungal endocarditis secondary to drug addiction. Recent concepts in diagnosis and therapy. J Thorac Cardiovasc Surg 1972;6:980.

213. Pollack S, Magtader A, Lange M. Neisseria subflava endocarditis. Case report and review of the literature. Am J Med 1984;76:752.

214. Vartian CV, Shlaes DM, Padhye AA, Ajello L. Wangiella dermatitides endocarditis in an intravenous drug user. Am J Med 1985;78:703.

215. Dole VP, Nyswander ME. A medical treatment for diacetyl-morphine (heroin) addiction. JAMA 1965;193:646.

216. Dole VP, Nyswander ME, Kreek MJ. Narcotic blockade. Arch Intern Med 1966;118:304–309.

217. Ball JC, Lange WR, Myers CP, Friedman SR. Reducing the risk of AIDS through methadone maintenance treatment. J Health Soc Behav 1988;29:214–226.

218. Cooper JR. Methadone treatment and acquired immunodeficiency syndrome. JAMA 1989;262:1664–1668.

219. Des Jarlais DC, Friedman SR, Hopkins W. Risk reduction for acquired immunodeficiency syndrome among intravenous drug users. Ann Intern Med 1985;103:755–759.

220. Fraser HF, Isbell H. Actions and addiction liabilities of alpha-acetylmethadols in man. J Pharmacol Exp Ther 1952;105:458–465.

221. Blaine JD, Renault PF. Clinical use of LAAM. Ann N Y Acad Sci 1978;311:214–231.

222. Fudala PJ, Vocci F, Montgomery A, Collins J. Unpublished, LAAM New Drug Application submission, 1993.

223. Levine R, Zaks A, Fink M, Freedman AM. Levomethadyl acetate: prolonged duration of opioid effects, including cross-tolerance to heroin. In: Blaine JD, Renault PF, eds. Rx:3x week LAAM, alternative to methadone 1976. NIDA Res Monogr 8, Rockville, MD: NIDA.

224. Ling W, Blaine JD. The use of LAAM in treatment. In: Dupont RL, Goldstein A, O'Donnell J, eds. Handbook on drug abuse Washington, DC: U.S. Government Printing Office, 1976.

225. Ling W, Charuvastra VC, Kaim SC, Klett CJ. Methadyl acetate and methadone maintenance treatments for heroin addicts: a Veterans Administration cooperative study. Arch Gen Psychiatry 1976;33:709–720.

226. Ling W, Klett CJ, Gillis R. A cooperative clinical study of methadyl acetate. Arch Gen Psychiatry 1978;35:345–353.

227. Tennant FS, Rawson RA, Pumphrey E, Seecof R. Clinical experience with 959 opioid-dependent patients treated with levo-alpha-acetylmethadol (LAAM). J Subst Abuse Treat 1986;3:195–202.

228. Jasinski DR, Pevnick JS, Griffith JD. Human pharmacology and abuse potential of the analgesic buprenorphine. Arch Gen Psychiatry 1978;35:501–516.

229. Mello NK, Bree MP, Mendelson JH. Comparison of buprenorphine and methadone effects on opiate self-administration in primates. J Pharmacol Exp Ther 1983;225:378–386.

230. Mello MK, Mendelson JH. Buprenorphine suppresses heroin use by heroin addicts. Science 1980;27:657–659.

231. Mello MK, Mendelson JH, Kuehnle JC. Buprenorphine effects on human heroin self-administration: an operant analysis. J Pharmacol Exp Ther 1982;223:30–39.

232. Johnson RE, Jaffe JH, Fudala PJ. A controlled trial of buprenorphine treatment for opioid dependence. JAMA 1992;267:2750–2755.

233. Ling W, Charuvastra C, Kintaudi K, Wesson DR. Buprenorphine for opiate dependence: two ongoing clinical trials. Fifty-fifth Annual Scientific Meeting of College on Problems of Drug Dependence, Toronto, Canada, 1993.

234. Fudala PJ, Jaffe JH, Dax CM, Johnson RE. Use of buprenorphine in the treatment of opioid addiction II. Physiologic and behavioral effects of daily and alternate day administration and abrupt withdrawal. Clin Pharmacol Ther 1990;47:525–534.

235. Resnick RB, Pycha C, Galanter M. Buprenorphine maintenance: reduced dosing frequence. Fifty-fifth Annual Meeting of the College on Problems of Drug Dependence, Toronto, Canada, 1993.

236. Martin WR, Jasinski DR, Mansley PA. Naltrexone, an antagonist for the treatment of heroin dependence. Arch Gen Psychiatry 1973;28:784–791.

237. Report of the National Research Council Committee on Clinical Evaluation of Narcotics Antagonists. Clinical evaluation of naltrexone treatment of opiate dependent individuals. Arch Gen Psychiatry 1978;35:335–340.

238. Kosten TR, Kleber HD. Buprenorphine detoxification from opioid dependence: a pilot study. Life Sci 1988;42:635–641.

239. Ling W, Wesson DR. Naltrexone treatment for addicted health-care professionals: a collaborative private practice experience. J Clin Psychiatry 1984;45:46–48.

240. Halikas JA, Nugent SM, Crosby RD, Carlson GA. 1990–1991 survey of pharmacotherapies used in the treatment of cocaine abuse. J Addict Dis 1993;12:129–139.

241. Meyers RE. New pharmacotherapies for cocaine dependence revisited. Arch Gen Psychiatry 1992;49:900–904.

242. Gorelick DA. Overview of pharmacological treatment approaches for alcohol and other drug addiction: intoxication, withdrawal, relapse prevention. Psychiatr Clin North Am 1993.

243. Seller EM, Kalant H. Alcohol intoxication and withdrawal. N Engl J Med 1976;294:757–762.

244. Tabakoff B, Hoffman PL. Adaptive responses to ethanol in the central nervous system. In: Goedde HE, Agarwal DP, eds. Alcoholism: biomedical and genetic aspects. New York: Pergamon Press, 1989; 99–112.

245. Litten RZ, Allen JP. Pharmacotherapies for alcoholism. Promising agents and clinical issues. Alcoholism 1991;15:620–633.

246. Wilkins AJ, Jerkins WJ, Steiner JA. Efficacy of clonidine in treatment of alcohol withdrawal state. Psychopharmacology 1983;81:78–80.

247. Sellers EM, Zilm DH, Degani NC. Comparative efficacy of propranolol and chlordiazepoxide in alcohol withdrawal. J Stud Alcohol 1977;38:2096–2108.

248. Peachy JE, Annis HM. Pharmacologic treatment of chronic alcoholism. Psychiatry Clin North Am 1984;7:745–756.

249. Peachy JE, Annis HM, Bornstein ER, et al. Calcium carbimide in alcoholism treatment. Part 1: a placebo-controlled, double-blind clinical trial of short-term efficacy. Br J Addict 1989;84:877–887.

250. Sellers EM, Kalant H. Alcohol intoxication and withdrawal. Medical Intelligence 1976;294:757–762.

251. Borg V. Bromocriptine in the prevention of alcohol abuse. Acta Psychiatr Scand 1983;68:100–110.

252. Zeise ML, Kasparov S, Capogna M, Zieglgansberger W. Acamprosate (calciumacetylhomotaurinate) decreases postsynaptic potentials in the rat neocortex: possible involvement of excitatory amino acid receptors. Eur J Pharmacol 1993;231:47–52.

253. Gorelick DA. Serotonin uptake blockers in the treatment of alcoholism. Recent Dev Alcohol 1989;7:267–281.

254. Naranjo C, Sellers E, Sullivan J, Woodley D, Sanchez-Craig, Sykora K. Zimelidine-induced variations in alcohol intake by nondepressed heavy drinkers. Clin Pharmacol Ther 1984;35:374–381.

255. Naranjo C, Sellers E, Sullivan J, Woodley M, Kadlec K, Sykora K. The serotonin uptake inhibitor citalopram attenuates ethanol intake. Clin Pharmacol Ther 1987;41:266–274.

256. Naranjo C, Sullivan J, Kadlec K, Woodley D, Sykora K. Differential effects of biqualine on alcohol intake and other consummatory behaviors. Clin Pharmacol Ther 1989;46:301–309.

257. Naranjo C, Kadlec K, Sanhueza P, Woodley-Remus D, Kennedy R, Sellers E. Fluoxetine differently alters alcohol intake and other consummatory behaviors in problem drinkers. Clin Pharmacol Ther 1990;47:490–498.

258. Gorelick DA, Parendes A. Effect of fluoxetine on alcohol consumption in male alcoholics. Alcohol Clin Exp Res 1992;16:261–265.

259. Tabakoff B, Hoffman PL. Alcohol: neurobiology. In: Lowinson JH, Ruiz P, Millman RB, et al., eds. Substance abuse: a comprehensive textbook. 2nd ed. Baltimore: Williams & Wilkins 1992:152–185.

260. O'Malley SS, Jaffe AJ, Chang G, Schottenfeld RS, Meyer RE, Rounsaville B. Naltrexone and coping skills therapy for alcohol dependence. A controlled study. Arch Gen Psychiatry 1992; 49:881–887.

261. Volpicelli JR, Alterman AI, Hayashida M, O'Brien CP. Naltrexone in the treatment of alcohol dependence. Arch Gen Psychiatry 1992;49:876–880.

262. Meyer RE. How to understand the relationship between psychopathology and addictive disorders: another example of the chicken and the egg. In: Meyer RE, ed. Psychopathology and addictive disorders. New York: Guilford, 1986:3–16.

263. Helzer JE, Pryzbeck TR. The co-occurrence of alcoholism with other psychiatric disorders in the general population and its impact on treatment. J Stud Alcohol 1988;49:219–224.

264. Ross HE, Glaser FB, Germanson T. The prevalence of psychiatric disorders in patients with alcohol and other drug problems. Arch Gen Psychiatry 1988;45:1023–1031.

265. Beeder AB, Millman RB. In: Lowinson JH, Ruiz P, Millman RB, Langrod JG, eds. Substance abuse: a comprehensive textbook. 2nd ed. Baltimore: Williams & Wilkins, 1992:51.

266. Raskin VD, Miller NS. The epidemiology of the comorbidity of psychiatric and addictive disorders: a critical review. J Addict Dis 1993;12:45–57.

267. Hesselbrock MN, Meyer RE, Keener JJ. Psychopathology in hospitalized alcoholics. Arch Gen Psychiatry 1985;42:1050–1055.

268. McLellan AT, Luborsky L, Woody GE, O'Brien CP, Druley KA. Predicting response to alcohol and drug abuse treatments: role of psychiatric severity. Arch Gen Psychiatry 1983;40:620–625.

269. Dackis CA, Gold MS, Pottash ALC, Sweeney DR. Evaluating depression in alcoholics. Psychiatry Res 1986;17:105–109.

270. Pettinati HM, Sugerman AA, Maurer HS. Four year MMPI changes in abstinent and drinking alcoholics. Alcohol Clin Exp Res 1982;6:487–494.

271. Rounsaville BJ, Dolinsky ZS, Babor TF, Meyer RE. Psychopathology as a predictor of treatment outcome in alcoholics. Arch Gen Psychiatry 1987;44:505–513.

272. Hasin DS, Endicott J, Keller MB. RDC alcoholism in patients with major affective syndromes: two-year course. Am J Psychiatry 1989;146:318–323.

273. Kushner MG, Sher KJ, Beitman BD. The relationship between alcohol problems and the anxiety disorders. Am J Psychiatry 1990;147:685–695.

274. Lydiard RB, Brady K, Ballenger JC, Howell EF, Malcolm R. Anxiety and mood disorders in hospitalized alcoholic individuals. Am J Addict 1992;1:325–331.

275. Merikangas KR, Leckman JF, Prusoff BA, Pauls DL, Weissman MM. Familial transmission of depression and alcoholism. Arch Gen Psychiatry 1985;42:367–372.

276. Weiss KJ, Rosenberg DL. Prevalence of anxiety disorder among alcoholics. J Clin Psychiatry 1985;46:3–5.

277. Miller NS. Comorbidity of psychiatric and alcohol/drug disorders: interactions and independent status. J Addict Dis 1993;12:5–16.

278. Anthenelli RM, Schuckit MA. Affective and anxiety disorders and alcohol and drug dependence: diagnosis and treatment. J Addict Dis 1993;12:73–87.

279. Smith EM, Cloninger CR, Bradford S. Predictors of mortality in alcoholic women: a prospective follow-up study. Alcohol Clin Exp Res 1983;7:237–243.

280. Khantzian EJ, Treece C. DSM-III psychiatric diagnosis of narcotic addicts: recent findings. Arch Gen Psychiatry 1985;42:1067–1071.

281. Rounsaville BJ, Weissman MM, Crits-Christoph, Wilber C, Kleber H. Diagnosis and symptoms of depression in opiate addicts: course and relationship to treatment outcome. Arch Gen Psychiatry 1982a;39:151–156.

282. Croughan JL, Miller PH, Wagelin D, Whitman BY. Psychiatric illness in male and female narcotic addicts. J Clin Psychiatry 1982;43:225–228.

283. Rounsaville BJ, Weissman MM, Kleber H, Wilber C. Heterogeneity of psychiatric diagnosis in treated opiate addicts. Arch Gen Psychiatry 1982b;39:161–166.

284. Dackis CA, Gold MS. Opiate addiction and depression: cause or effect? Drug Alcohol Depend 1983;11:105–109.

285. Rounsaville BJ, Anton SF, Carroll K, Budde D, Prusoff BA, Gawin F. Psychiatric diagnoses of treatment-seeking cocaine abusers. Arch Gen Psychiatry 1991;48:43–51.

286. Weiss RD, Mirim SM, Griffin ML, Michael JL. Psychopathology in cocaine abusers: changing trends. J Nerv Ment Dis 1988;176:719–725.

287. Carroll KM, Rounsaville BJ, Bryant KJ. Alcoholism in treatment-seeking cocaine abusers: clinical and prognostic significance. J Stud Alcohol 1993;54:199–208.

288. McLellan AT, Druly KA. Non-random relation between drugs of abuse and psychiatric diagnosis. J Psychiatr Res 1977;13:179–184.

289. Brady K, Anton R, Ballenger JC, Lydiard RB, Adinoff B, Selander J. Cocaine abuse among schizophrenic patients. Am J Psychiatry 1990;147:1164–1167.

290. Geracioti TD, Post RM. Onset of panic disorder associated with rare use of cocaine. Biol Psychiatry 1991;29:403–406.

291. Louie AK, Lannon RA, Ketter TA. Treatment of cocaine-induced panic disorder. Am J Psychiatry 1989;146:40–44.

292. Ungerleider JT, Pechnick RN. Hallucinogens. In: Lowinson JH, Ruiz RB, Millman RB, Langrod JG, eds. Substance abuse: a comprehensive textbook. 2nd ed. Baltimore: Williams & Wilkins, 1992.

293. Negrete JC, Knapp WP, Douglas DE, Smith WB. Cannabis affects the severity of schizophrenic symptoms: results of a clinical survey. Psychol Med 1986;16:515–520.

294. Grinspoon L, Bakalar JB. Marijuana. In: Lowinson JH, Ruiz RB, Millman RB, Langrod JG, eds. Substance abuse: a comprehensive textbook. 2nd ed. Baltimore: Williams & Wilkins, 1992.

295. Szuster RR, Pontius EB, Campos PE. Marijuana sensitivity and panic anxiety. J Clin Psychiatry 1988;49:427–429.

296. Klisz DK, Parsons OA. Hypothesis testing in younger and older alcoholics. J Stud Alcohol 1977;38:1718–1729.

297. Grant I, Reed R. Neuropsychology of alcohol and drug abuse. In: Alterman AI, ed. Substance abuse and psychopathology. New York: Plenum, 1985:289–341.

298. Fabian MS, Parsons OA, Sheldon MD. Effects of gender and alcoholism on verbal and visuo-spatial learning. J Nerv Ment Dis 1985;172:16–20.

299. Fabian MS, Parsons OA, Silberstein JA. Impaired perceptual-cognitive functioning in women alcoholics: cross-validated findings. J Stud Alcohol 1981;42:217–229.

300. Glenn SW, Parsons OA. Neuropsychological efficiency measures in male and female alcoholics. J Stud Alcohol 1992;53:546–552.

301. Hewett LJ, Nixon SJ, Glenn SW, Parsons OA. Verbal fluency deficits in female alcoholics. J Clin Psychol 1991;47:716–720.

302. Grant I, Alcohol and the brain. Neuropsychological correlates. J Consult Clin Psychol 1987;545:310–324.

303. Grant I, Reed R. Neuropsychology of alcohol and drug abuse. In: Alterman AI, ed. Substance Abuse and Psychopathology. New York: Plenum Press, 1985:289–341.

304. Patterson BW, Sinha R, Williams HL, Parsons OA, Smith LT, Schaeffer KW. The relationship between neuropsychological and late component evoked potential measures in chronic alcoholics. Int J Neurosci 1989;49:319–327.

305. Williams CM, Skinner AEG. The cognitive effects of alcohol abuse: a controlled study. Br J Addict 1990;85:911–917.

306. Ron MA, Acker W, Lishman WA. Morphological abnormalities in the brains of chronic alcoholics: a clinical and computerized axial tomographic study. Acta Psychiatr Scand 1980;62:41–46.

307. Parsons OA, Farr SD. The neuropsychology of alcohol and drug abuse. In: Filskov SB, Boll TB, eds. Handbook of clinical neuropsychology. New York: John Wiley & Sons, 1981:320–365.

308. Donovan D, Queisser H, O'Leary MR. Group embedded figures as a predictor of cognitive impairment among alcoholics. Int J Addict 1976;11:125–139.

309. Jones B, Parsons OA. Impaired abstraction ability in chronic alcoholics. Arch Gen Psychiatry 1971;24:431–457.

310. Tuck RR, Jackson M. Social, neurological and cognitive disorders in alcoholics. Med J Aust 1991;155:225–229.

311. Ryan C, Butters N. Cognitive effects in alcohol abuse. In: Kissin B, Begleiter H, eds. The biology of alcoholism. New York: Plenum, 1982;6:485–538.

312. Gurling HMD, Curtis D, Murray RM. Psychological deficit from excessive alcohol consumption: evidence from a co-twin control study. Brit J Addict 1991;86:151–155.

313. Berry J, Van Gorp WG, Herzberg DS, Hinkin C, Boone K, Steinman L, Wilkins JN. Neuropsychological deficits in abstinent cocaine abusers: preliminary findings after two weeks of abstinence. Drug Alcohol Depend 1993;32:231–237.

314. Strickland TL, Mena I, Villaneueva-Meyer J. Cerebral perfusion and neuropsychological consequences of chronic cocaine use. J Neuropsychiatry Clin Neurosci 1993;5:419–427.

315. Ardila A, Rosselli M, Strumwasser S. Neuropsychological deficits in chronic cocaine abusers. Int J Neurosci 1991;57:73–79.

316. O'Malley SO, Adamse M, Heaton RK, Gawin FH. Neuropsychological impairment in chronic cocaine abusers. Am J Drug Alcohol Abuse 1992;18:131–144.

317. Volkow ND, Mullani N, Gould KL, Alder S, Krajewski K. Cerebral blood flow in chronic cocaine abusers: a study with positron emission tomography. Br J Psychiatry 1988;152:641–648.

318. Manschreck TC, Schner ML, Weisstein CC, et al. Freebase cocaine and memory. Compr Psychiatry 1990;31:369–375.

319. Bruhn P, Maage N. Intellectual and neuropsychological functioning in young men with heavy and long-term patterns of drug abuse. Am J Psychiatry 1975;132:397–401.

320. Rounsaville BJ, Jones C, Novelly RA, Kleber H. Neuropsychological functioning in opiate addicts. J Nerv Ment Dis 1982;170:209–216.

321. Guerra D, Sole A, Cami J, Tobena A. Neuropsychological performance in opiate addicts after rapid detoxification. Drug Alcohol Depend 1987;20:261–270.

322. Grant I, Adams KM, Carlin AS, Rennick PM, Judd LL, Schooff K. The collaborative neuropsychological study of polydrug users. Arch Gen Psych 1978;35:1063–1074.

323. Pakesh G, Loimer N, Grunberger J, Pfersmann D, Linzmayer L, Mayerhofer S. Neuropsychological findings and psychiatric symptoms in HIV-1 infected and noninfected drug users. Psychiatry Res 1992;41:163–177.

324. Grant I, Judd L. Neuropsychological and EEG disturbances in polydrug users. Am J Psychiatry 1976;133:1039–1042.

325. Sweeney JA, Meisel L, Walsh VL, Castrovinci D. Assessment of cognitive functioning in poly-substance abuser. J Clin Psychol 1989;45:346–351.

326. Fals-Stewart W, Schafer J. Using subtests of the brain age quotient to screen for cognitive deficits among substance abusers. Percept Mot Skills 1992;75:244–246.

327. Navia BA, Jordan BD, Price RW. The AIDS dementia complex, I: clinical features. Ann Neurol 1986;19:517–524.

328. Navia BA, Price RW. The acquired immunodeficiency syndrome complex as the presenting or sole manifestation of human immunodeficiency virus infection. Arch Neurol 1987;44:65–69.

329. Fernandez F, Ruiz P. Neuropsychiatric complications of HIV infection. In: Lowinson J, Ruiz P, Millman RB, eds. Substance abuse: a comprehensive textbook. 2nd ed. Baltimore: Williams & Wilkins, 1992:775–787.

330. Bornstein RA, Fama R, Rosenberger P, et al. Drug and alcohol use and neuropsychological performance in asymptomatic HIV infection. J Neuropsychiatry Clin Neurosci 1992;5:254–259.

331. Wellman MC. Neuropsychological impairment among intravenous drug users in pre-AIDS stages of HIV infection. Intern J Neurosci 1992;64:183–194.

332. Silberstein CH, O'Dowd MA, Chartock P, et al. A prospective four-year follow-up of neuropsychological function in HIV seropositive and seronegative methadone-maintained patients. Gen Hosp Psychiatry 1993;15:351–359.

333. Concha M, Graham NMH, Muñoz A, et al. Effect of chronic substance abuse on the neuropsychological performance of intravenous drug users with a high prevalence of HIV-1 seropositivity. Am J Epidemiol 1992;36:1338–1348.

334. Selnes OA, McArthur JC, Royal III W, et al. HIV-1 infection and intravenous drug use: longitudinal neuropsychological evaluation of asymptomatic subjects. Neurology 1992;42:1924–1930.

335. Becker JT, Kaplan RF. Neurophysiological and neuropsychological concomitants of brain dysfunction in alcoholics. In: Meyers RE, ed. Psychopathology and addictive disorders. New York: Guilford, 1986:1–25.

336. Brandt J, Butters N, Ryan C, Bayog R. Cognitive loss and recovery in long-term alcohol abusers. Arch Gen Psychiatry 1983;40:435–442.

337. Reed RJ, Grant I. The long-term neurobehavioral consequences of substance abuse: conceptual and methodological challenges for future research. NIDA Res Monogr 101: Residual effects of abused drugs on behavior 1990:10–56.

338. Richards M, Sano M, Goldstein S, Mindry D, Todak G, Stern Y. The stability of neuropsychological test performance in a group of parenteral drug users. J Subst Abuse Treat 1992;9:371–377.

339. Eckardt MJ, Martin PR. Clinical assessment of cognition in alcoholism. Alcohol Clin Exp Res 1986;10:123–127.

340. Parsons OA, Leber WR. The relationship between cognitive dysfunction and brain damage in alcoholics: causal, interactive or epiphenomenal? Alcohol Clin Exp Res 1981;5:326–343.

341. Tabakof B, Petersen RC. Intramural research program of the National Institute on Alcohol Abuse and Alcoholism. Br J Addict 1988;83:495–504.

342. Parsons OA. Do neuropsychological deficits predict alcoholics' treatment course and posttreatment recovery? In: Parsons OA, Butters N, Nathan PE, eds. Neuropsychology of alcoholism: implications for diagnosis and treatment. New York: Guilford, 1987:273–290.

343. Miller L. Predicting relapse and recovery in alcoholism and addiction: neuropsychology, personality, and cognitive style. J Subst Abuse Treat 1991;8:277–291.

344. Miller NS, Gold MS. Alcohol. New York: Plenum, 1991:280.

345. Pogge DL, Stokes J, Harvey PD. Psychometric vs. attentional correlates of early onset alcohol and substance abuse. J Abnorm Child Psychol 1992;20:151–162.

346. Malloy P, Noel N, Longabaugh R, Beattie M. Determinants of neuropsychological impairment in antisocial substance abusers. Addict Behav 1990;15:431–438.

347. Rodriguez M. Cognitive functioning in male polydrug abusers with and without family history of alcoholism. Percept Mot Skills 1993;77:484–488.

348. Hesselbrock V, Bauer LO, Hesselbrock MN, Gillen R. Neuropsycho-

logical factors in individuals as high risk for alcoholism. Recent Dev Alcohol 1991;9:21–39.

349. Yohman JR, Parsons OA, Leber WR. Lack of recovery in male alcoholics' neuropsychological performance one year after treatment. Alcohol Clin Exp Res 1985;9:114–117.

350. Gregson RAM, Taylor GM. Prediction of relapse in men alcoholics. J Stud Alcohol 1977;38:1749–1760.

351. Leber WR, Parsons OA, Nichols N. Neuropsychological test results are related to ratings of men alcoholics' therapeutic progress: a replicated study. J Stud Alcohol 1985;46:116–121.

352. Kupke T, O'Brien W. Neuropsychological impairment and behavioral limitations exhibited within an alcohol treatment program. J Clin Exp Neuropsychol 1985;7:292–304.

353. Fals-Stewart W, Schafer J. Fals-Stewart W, Schafer J. The relationship between length of stay in drug-free therapeutic communities and neurocognitive functioning. J Clin Psychol 1992;48:539–543.

354. Smith DE, McCrady BS. Cognitive impairment among alcoholics: impact on drink refusal skill acquisition and treatment outcome. Addict Behav 1991;16:265–274.

355. Morgan JP. American opiophobia: customary underutilization of opioid analgesics. Advances in Alcohol and Substance Abuse 1986;5:163–173.

356. Melzack R. The tragedy of needless pain. Sci Am 1990;262:27–33.

357. Friedman DP. Perspectives on the medical use of drugs of abuse. Journal of Pain and Symptom Management 1990;5(suppl 1):S2–S5.

358. Perry SW. Irrational attitudes toward addicts and narcotics. Bull N Y Acad Med 1985;61:706–727.

359. Wesson DR, Ling W, Smith DE. Prescription of opioids for treatment of pain in patients with addictive disease. Journal of Pain and Symptom Management 1993;8:428–435.

360. Portenoy RK, Payne R. Acute and chronic pain. In: Lowinson J, Ruiz P, Millman RB, eds. Substance abuse: a comprehensive textbook. 2nd ed. Baltimore: Williams & Wilkins, 1992.

361. Portenoy RK. Chronic opioid therapy in nonmalignant pain. Journal of Pain and Symptom Management 1990;5(suppl 1):S46–S62.

362. Portenoy RK, Foley KM. Chronic use of opioid analgesics in non-malignant pain: report of 38 cases. Pain 1986;25:171–186.

363. Hicks RD. Pain management in the chemically dependent patient. Hawaii Med J 1989;48:491–495.

364. Lamkis D, Kleber HD. Pain management of the methadone-dependent patient. Drugs in Patient Care VIII [letter] 1980;5.

365. Senay EC, Becker CE, Schnoll SH. Management of addicts in the general hospital. Emergency treatment of the drug abusing patient for treatment staff physicians. Rockville, MD:1980:35–39.

366. Rubenstein RB, Spira I, Wolff WI. Management of surgical problems in patients on methadone maintenance. Am J Surg 1976;131:566–569.

367. Kantor TG, Cantor R, Tom E. A study of hospitalized surgical patients on methadone maintenance. NIDA Res Monogr 1981;34:243–249.

368. Compton M. Cold pressor pain tolerance in opiate and cocaine abusers: correlates of drug type and use status. Journal of Pain and Symptom Management, in press.

369. Tilson HA, Rech RH, Stolman S. Hyperalgesia during withdrawal as a means of measuring the degree of dependence in morphine dependent rats. Psychopharmacology 1973;28:287–300.

370. U.S. Department of Health and Human Services. Acute pain management: operative or medical procedures and trauma. Rockville: Agency for Health Care Policy and Research, 1992.

371. Hughes JR, Bickel WK, Higgins ST. Buprenorphine for pain relief in a patient with drug abuse. Am J Drug Alcohol Abuse 1991;17:451–455.

372. Johnson RT. Pathogenesis of HIV infections. American Academy of Neurology Annual Courses, vol. 5: Infections, emergency, critical care 1993;140:169–177.

373. McArthur JC. HIV-associated CNS syndromes. American Academy of Neurology Annual Courses, vol. 5: Infections, emergency, critical care 1993;140:15–29.

374. Gonzales-Scarano F. Basic Biology of HIV-1. American Academy of Neurology Annual Courses, vol. 5: Infections, emergency, critical care 1993;140:3–14.

375. Perry S. Treatments of psychiatric complications. American Academy of Neurology Annual Courses, vol. 5: Infections, emergency, critical care 1993;140:133–143.

31

Language and Neuropsychiatry

David Caplan

This chapter presents an overview of language disorders in adults from a cognitive (psycholinguistic) point of view. There are several reasons for this perspective. First, the initial challenge clinicians face is to describe and classify patients' language disorders. Advances in linguistics and psycholinguistics now allow for a coherent framework within which to undertake this descriptive and classificatory effort. Second, the presence of certain types of language impairments has value for inferring the localization of lesions and their etiology. Third, when therapeutic efforts are directed at the functional language disorder, it is useful for the clinician to recognize how these efforts are structured.

This chapter presents models of normal function and descriptions of impairments, beginning with a description of the normal language system, and reviewing essential features of the language code and its processing in the usual tasks of language use (speech, auditory comprehension, reading, and writing). Aspects of methodology are then outlined, including psycholinguistic techniques, an approach to the diagnosis of language disorders, and neurological observations. This is followed by a synopsis of recent work that describes neurogenic language disorders in terms of disturbances of linguistic representations and psycholinguistic processes. This psycholinguistic approach is compared with a more traditional clinical approach to characterizing language disorders based upon "aphasic syndromes." Language disorders in psychiatric disorders are then discussed. The chapter concludes with a discussion of models of the functional neuroanatomy of language. This chapter is only a review of the literature in these areas; readers who are interested in more detailed accounts should consult the primary sources cited here and the references therein.

LANGUAGE STRUCTURE, LANGUAGE PROCESSING, AND FUNCTIONAL COMMUNICATION

Human language has many different facets. It can be vehicle for communication of information, a medium for artistic expression, a method for expression of emotions, a means for developing thought, or it can serve other functions. However, in its essence, language is a code, one whose structural properties makes it capable of serving this wide range of functions.

A code can convey virtually any sort of information, in almost any form. DNA consists of a series of nucleotides, and it conveys information about the structure of RNA, which in turn "codes" for the structure of proteins found in cells. Morse code consists of a set of sequences of dots and dashes that represent the letters of the alphabet. A military code may consist of a sequence of numbers that represent characters and words in a language.

Language is a very particular and fairly complicated code. It consists of a set of forms that are called *linguistic representations*. Different types of linguistic representations convey different aspects of meaning. These linguistic representations are organized into *levels* of the language code. The basic levels of the code are *simple words* (the *lexical level*,) *words with internal structure* (the *word-formation level*,) *sentences* (the *sentential level*,) and *discourse* (the *discourse level*). When we use language to speak, write, listen, or read, we simultaneously make use of all the types of linguistic representations in the language code. The result is that what we produce or perceive has a very complex structure that conveys a wide range of semantic information.

Structure of Language

The lexical level of language consists of simple words. The basic form of a simple word (or lexical item) consists of a phonological representation that specifies the segmental elements (phonemes) of the word and their organization into metrical structures such as syllables (1). The form of a word can also be represented orthographically (see Henderson [2], for a discussion of orthographic representational systems). Simple words are assigned to different syntactic categories, such as *noun, verb, adjective, article, preposition*, etc. The semantic values associated with the lexical level primarily consist of concepts and categories in the nonlinguistic world. Simple words tend to designate concrete objects, abstract concepts, actions, properties, and logical connectives.

The word-formation level of language allows words to be formed from other words. In English, word formation can take place via affixation (morphology) and compounding (3).

There are two basic types of morphological affixation in English—derivation and inflection. Derivational morphological processes allow the meaning associated with a simple lexical item to be used as a different syntactic category without coining a large number of new lexical forms that would have to be learned (e.g., *destroy → destruction;* [4]). Derivational affixes fall into at least three classes. Latinate suffixes attach to Latinate words; they tend to affect the sound patterns of the words they attach to (e.g., *destroy → destruction*). Anglo-Saxon affixes attach to Anglo-Saxon roots and to derived words formed by Latinate suffixation (e.g., *happy → happiness; receive → receptive → receptiveness*). Prefixes attach fairly freely. Derivational suffixes determine the syntactic category of a complex word (e.g., *happiness* is a noun, not an adjective). Inflectional morphological processes play roles in encoding syntactic relationships (e.g., subject-verb agreement: *destroy → destroys*). Inflectional suffixes attach after all derivational suffixes have been attached and do not affect the sound pattern or syntactic category of the words they attach to.

Compounding is productive in English. Most content words (nouns, verbs, and adjectives) can form compounds; function words (articles, prepositions, pronouns, auxiliary verbs, etc.) rarely do. Compounding affects stress; most compounds have stress on the first element (e.g., *light'house-keeper,* with stress on *light',* refers to the keeper of a lighthouse; *light house'keeper,* with stress on *house',* refers to a housekeeper who is light). Compound words have the syntactic category of their final element (e.g., *washbasin* is a noun not a verb). In compounding, the initial elements qualify the sense of the final element (e.g., a *horsefly* is a fly found on horses, not a horse that flies).

The sentential level of language consists of syntactic structures—hierarchical sets of syntactic categories (e.g., noun phrase, verb phrase, sentence, etc. [5–7])—into which words are inserted. The meaning of a sentence, known as its propositional content, is determined by the way the meanings of words combine in syntactic structures. Propositions convey aspects of the structure of events and states in the world. These include who did what to whom (thematic roles), which adjectives go with which nouns (attribution of modification), which words in a set of sentences refer to the same items or actions (the reference of pronouns and other anaphoric elements), and so on. For instance, in the sentence *The big boy told the little girl to wash herself,* the agent of *told* is "the big boy" and its theme is "the little girl;" "big" is associated with "boy" and "little" with "girl"; and "herself" refers to the same person as "girl." Sentences are a crucial level of the language code because the propositions they express make assertions about the world. These assertions can be entered into logical systems and can be used to add to an individual's knowledge of the world.

The propositional meanings conveyed by sentences are entered into higher-order structures that constitute the discourse level of linguistic structure (8, 9). Discourse includes information about the general topic under discussion, the focus of a speaker's attention, the novelty of the information in a given sentence, the temporal order of events, causation, among other things. The structure and processing of discourse involves many nonlinguistic elements and operations, such as search through semantic memory, logical inferences, as well as a more purely linguistic structure. For instance, consider the following set of sentences:

John and Henry went to Peter's last night. They were very glad they did. They raved about the dessert all the next day.

The reader infers that John and Henry ate dinner at Peter's. This is an inference that is based on information that is outside the language system. On the other hand, the reader takes the word *They* in the second sentence to refer to John and Henry, not John and Peter, or Henry or Peter, or all three men. This assignment is probably based on the fact that *They* and *John and Henry* are both noun phrases in the subject positions of their sentences—a linguistic fact.

Prosodic information—intonational contours—are also linguistic representations that determine aspects of discourse meaning. Phrases and sentences receive intonational contours that partially reflect syntactic structures (e.g., there tends to be a drop in pitch at the end of most sentences) and partially reflect discourse considerations. Prosody can determine whether a sentence is a statement or a question (the illocutionary force of a sentence) and whether an element conveys new or old information in a discourse. Many other linguistic devices—variation in the order of words, the use of repeated noun phrases, ellipsis, etc.—determine aspects of discourse meaning. A complex interplay between linguistic and nonlinguistic domains thus characterizes discourse structure. Information conveyed by the discourse level of language serves as a basis for updating an individual's knowledge of the world and for reasoning and planning action.

Our brief discussion of the interaction of general knowledge and linguistic structures in determining aspects of the semantics of discourse raises the question of the boundary between linguistic information and other types of knowledge. This boundary is not always easy to draw. For instance, consider the vocal expression of emotional state. Not only do speakers convey messages based on the meanings of the words, sentences, and discourse structures they produce, they also convey their emotional state (happiness, anger, sadness). Linguists do not include emotional state as a semantic value that is represented by the language system, but it is possible that future development of linguistic theory will allow for a better understanding of how emotional state affects aspects of speech production, and that forms and meanings related to emotional state will be incorporated into a broader theory of linguistic representations. Here we focus on those structures and semantic values that are broadly accepted as part of the language code.

Language Processing

The different forms of the language code are computed by a set of processors, or "components" of a language processing system, each dedicated to activating particular elements of the code. Considerable research has gone into the characterization of the components of the language processing system. It is far beyond the scope of this chapter to review this literature in depth. The reader is referred to Caplan (10) and the references cited there for an introduction to this research. Here we limit ourselves to a brief description of some of the general properties of the language processors and their organization.

One important characteristic of the language processing system is that each processor accepts only particular types of representations as input and produces only specific types of representations as output. For instance, the processor that activates syntactic structures from auditory input may use as input many features derived from the speech signal – the syntactic categories of the words presented to it, intonational contours, etc. but it probably does not make use of all aspects of the meanings of words in this process. Fodor (11) uses the term "encapsulation" to refer to this property of components of the language processing system. Similarly, the output of this processor is a syntactic structure – it is not a representation of the logical entailments of a sentence. Fodor (11) uses the term "domain specificity" to refer this property. A major research area is to determine the input and output representations that are paired by the operation of different language processors, whose operations range from conversion of the acoustic signal to speech sounds, through visual word recognition, spelling, the determination of sentence structure, structuring discourse, and others.

Information processing models of language are expressed as flow diagrams (often called "functional architectures") that indicate the sequence of operations of the different components that perform a language-related task. These models become extremely detailed and complex when all of the operations and components used in a task are specified. For our present purposes, it is adequate to identify the major components of the language processing system as those processors that activate units at the lexical, word-formation, sentential, and discourse levels of the language code in the usual tasks of language use – speech, auditory comprehension, reading, and writing. This approach to defining language processing components groups together different operations that all activate a similar type of linguistic representation in a given task into a single processor.

The major components of the language processing system that can be identified at this level of detail for simple words are listed in Table 31.1, and for the word formation and sentence levels in Table 31.2. Figure 31.1 presents a model indicating the sequence of activation of components of the lexical processing system. Figure 31.2 presents a similar model of the processing system for word formation and sentences. These tables and figures are based upon the results of experimental psychological research in both normal subjects and patient populations (see 2, 10, 12, 13, and the references cited there for introductions to aspects of this research).

Tables 31.1 and 31.2 and Figures 31.1 and 31.2 outline the way information – in this case, sets of related linguistic representations – flows through the tasks of speaking, understanding spoken language, reading, and writing. The model depicted in these tables and figures simplifies this information flow in three ways. First, it does not specify the nature of the operations in each of the major components of the system. Second, it does not fully convey the extent to which the components of the system operate in parallel. Third, it does not convey the extent of feedback among the components of the system. Despite these simplifications, the model captures enough aspects of information processing in the language system to constitute an adequate starting place for a psycholinguistic approach to language disorders.

There is more to a psychological model of language processing than merely specifying the flow of information through the system. A complete model of the language processing system must also specify the operating characteristics of the components of the system. The following points describe some of the more important aspects of these features (10, 13, 14).

First, most processors are obligatorily activated when their inputs are presented to them. For instance, if we attend to a sound that happens to be the word *elephant,* we must hear and understand that word; we cannot hear this sound as just a noise (15).

Second, language processors generally operate unconsciously. The unconscious nature of most of language processing can be appreciated by considering that when we listen to a lecture, converse with an interlocutor, read a novel, or engage in some other language-processing task, we usually have the subjective impression that we are extracting another person's meaning and producing linguistic forms appropriate to our intentions without being aware of the details of the sounds of words or sentence structure.

Third, components of the system operate remarkably quickly and accurately. For instance, it has been estimated on the basis of many different psycholinguistic experimental techniques that spoken words are usually recognized less than 125 msec after their onset; i.e., while they are still being uttered (16, 17). Similarly, normal word production in speech requires searching through a mental word production "dictionary" of over 20,000 items, but still goes on at the rate of about three words per second with an error rate of about one word misselected per million and another one word mispronounced per million (13). The speed of the language processing system as a whole occurs because of the speed of each of its components, but also is achieved because of the massively parallel functional architecture of the system, which leads to many components of the system being simultaneously active.

Fourth, the operation of each component of the language processing system can be thought of as requiring "processing resources." One can appreciate the need for processing resources by trying to understand the sentence, *The mouse that the dog that the cat scratched bit ran away*. It is relatively easy to understand each pair of relative clauses *(The mouse that the dog bit ran away and The dog that the cat scratched bit the mouse)*, but putting them all together exceeds the processing capacity of the sentence comprehension mechanism. Researchers have developed a number of theories of processing resources and their role in language and cognitive tasks (12, 18–20). Intuitively, one might think of each psycholinguistic operation as a machine, such as an old grist mill that demands power; the machine works efficiently above a certain level of power availability and is limited by the amount of power available. It is unclear whether there are separate pools of processing resources for each language processing component or for language processing as whole,

or whether language processing can "borrow" resources from other systems if it needs to.

Fifth, the operations of the language processing system are regulated by a variety of control mechanisms. These control mechanisms include both ones internal to the language processor itself and those that are involved in other aspects of cognition. The first category—language-internal control mechanisms—probably consists of a large number of operations that schedule psycholinguistic operations on the basis of the ongoing nature of a given psycholinguistic task. The second category of control mechanisms—those that are related to cognitive processing outside the language system—determine what combinations of processors become active in order to accomplish different tasks such as reading, repeating what one has heard, or taking notes on a lecture. Control mechanisms from outside the language

Table 31.1. **Summary of Components of the Language Processing System for Simple Words**

Component	Input	Operation	Output
Auditory-oral modality input-side			
Acoustic-phonetic processing	Acoustic waveform	Matches acoustic properties to phonetic features	Phonological segments (phonemes, allophones, syllables)
Auditory lexical access	Phonological units	Activates lexical items in long-term memory on basis of sound; selects best fit to stimulus	Phonological forms of words
Lexical semantic access	Words (represented as phonological forms)	Activates semantic features of words	Word meanings
Output-side			
Phonological lexical access	Word meanings ("lemmas")	Activates the phonological forms of words	Phonological form of words
Phonological output planning	Phonological forms of words (and nonwords)	Activates detailed phonetic features of words (and nonwords)	Phonetic values of phonological segments; word stress patterns
Articulatory planning	Phonetic values	Specifies articulatory movements	Neural commands for articulation
Wrtten modality input-side			
Written lexical access	Abstract letter identities	Activates orthographic forms of words	Orthographic forms of words
Written lexical semantic access	Orthographic forms of words	Activates semantic features of words	Word meanings
Output-side			
Accessing lexical orthography from semantics	Word meanings	Activates orthographic forms of words	Orthographic forms of words
Accessing lexical orthography from lexical phonology	Phonological representations of words	Activates orthographic forms of words from their phonological forms	Orthographic form of words
Accessing sublexical orthography from sublexical phonology	Phonological units (phonemes, other units)	Activates orthographic units corresponding to phonological units	Orthographic units in words and nonwords
Accessing lexical phonology from lexical orthography	Orthographic form of words	Activates phonological forms of words from their orthographic forms	Phonological forms of words
Accessing sublexical phonology from sublexical orthography	Orthographic units (graphemes, other units)	Activates phonological units corresponding to orthographic units	Phonological units in words and nonwords

Table 31.2. Summary of Components of the Language Processing System for Derived Words and Sentences (Collapsed Over Auditory-Oral and Written Modalities)

Component	Input	Operation	Output
Processing affixed words			
Input-side			
Morphological analysis	Word forms	Segments words into structural (morphological) units; activates syntactic features of words	Morphological structure; syntactic features
Morphological comprehension	Word meaning; morphological structure	Combines word roots and affixes	Meanings of morphologically complex words
Output-side			
Accessing affixed words from semantics	Word meanings; syntactic features	Activates forms of affixes and function words	Forms of affixes and function words
Sentence Level Processing			
Input-side			
Lexicoinferential comprehension	Meanings of simple and complex words; world knowledge	Infers aspects of sentence meaning on basis of pragmatic plausibility	Aspects of propositional meaning (thematic roles; attribution of modifiers)
Parsing and syntactic	Word meanings; syntactic features	Contructs syntactic representation and combines it with word meanings	Aspects of comprehension of propositional meaning
Heuristic sentence comprehension	Syntactic categories of words	Constructs simplified syntactic structures; combines word meanings in these structures	Aspects of propositional meaning
Output-side			
Construction of functional level representation	Messages	Activates content words and assigns thematic roles and other aspects of propositional meaning	Content words; thematic roles; other aspects of meaning
Construction of positional level representation	Content words; syntactic frames; discourse features	Activates syntactic frames in conjunction with function words; inserts phonological forms of content words into syntactic frames	Surface forms of sentences
Phonological output planning	Surface forms of sentences	Combines lexical phonological and sentence-level phonological information	Phonetic values; stress and intonation

system are also involved in deploying and shifting attention (20, 21), searching through knowledge stored in memory, matching motivations to actions, and similar tasks. These control mechanisms are utilized on all levels of the language code. We exercise control over the entire language processing system when we decide whether to use language to convey our thoughts and intentions, and when we decide to pay attention to a particular linguistic input. We exercise control over the choice of vocabulary elements in our speech on the basis of our estimation of our listeners' ability to understand different sets of words. We control the rate of our speech and the formality of the vocabulary and syntax we

choose. We enunciate differently for different listeners. We can place emphatic stress on any part of the sound of a word, if we think we need to (as in: "I said 'bat the ball,' not 'pat the ball' "). It is through the use of these control mechanisms that we use the language code for different purposes.

Functional Communication, Language Processing, and Communication Disorders

Functional communication involving the language code occurs when people inform others, ask for information, or use language for other specific purposes. The use of language

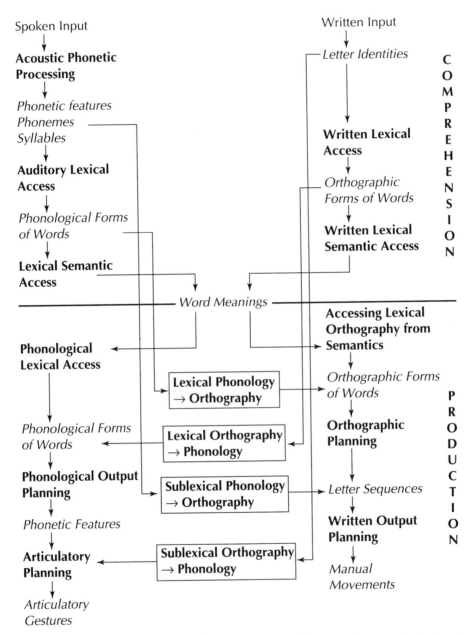

Figure 31.1 Diagrammatic representation of the sequence of activation of components of the processing system for single words. Processing components are presented in boldface; representations are presented in italics. Arrows represent the flow of information from one processing component to another. (Reprinted with permission from Caplan D. Toward a psycholinguistic approach to acquired neurogenic language disorders. American Journal of Speech-Language Pathology 1993;2:54–83.)

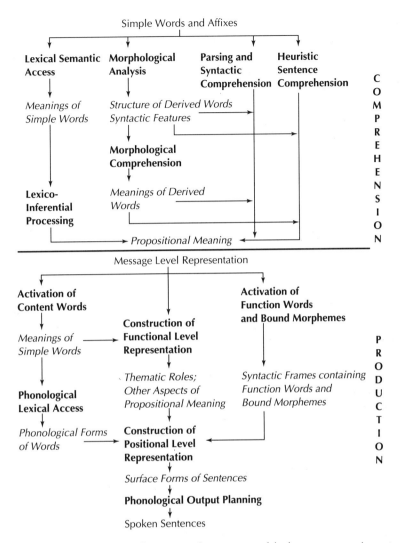

Figure 31.2 Diagrammatic representation of the sequence of operation of components of the language processing system for morphologically complex words and sentences. Processing components are presented in boldface; representations are presented in italics. Arrows represent the flow of information from one processing component to another. (Reprinted with permission from Caplan D. Toward a psycholinguistic approach to acquired neurologic language disorders. American Journal of Speech-Language Pathology 1993;2:59–83.)

is thus a special instance of intentional action (9). As noted before, language processors are used in different combinations to accomplish different language-related tasks in the service of these goals.

Language can be used for as simple a purpose as warning a person about a danger (e.g., the shout, "Watch out!") or as complex a purpose as explaining the benefits and risks of particular investments or deliberately attempting to mislead someone. As the intentions and motivations of the language user become more complex, functional communication is progressively more affected by disturbances of the language code and its processors. Thus, though "high-level" language-impaired patients may be able to function well in many settings, their language impairments can cause substantial functional limitations. The language code is a remarkably powerful code with respect to the semantic meanings it can encode and convey, and psycholinguistic processors are astonishingly fast and accurate. Without this code and the

ability to use it quickly and accurately, one's functional communicative powers are extremely limited, no matter how elaborate one's intentions and motives. This is the situation in which many patients who have disorders affecting the language code and the processors dedicated to its use find themselves.

Most patients' complaints regarding language tend to center on impairments of the use of language for functional communication. The clinician may attempt to assess language-based functional communication, must realize that this function is multifactorially determined. There is no simple, one-to-one relationship between impairments of elements of the language code or of psycholinguistic processors, on the one hand, and abnormalities in accomplishing the goals of language use, on the other. Patients adapt to their language impairments in many ways, some of which are remarkably effective at maintaining at least some aspects of functional communication: conversely, individuals with (or without) neurological disease who have intact language processing mechanisms may fail to communicate effectively.

It is possible and valuable to identify disturbances of elements of the language code or psycholinguistic processors in many patients who have functional communicative disturbances. To do so, it is necessary to use tests that identify such disturbances. Clinical tests are partly based upon an understanding of the structure of the language code, and partly upon methods that have been used to investigate language processing in normals. A brief description of these methods follows.

OVERVIEW OF PSYCHOLINGUISTIC, CLINICAL, AND NEUROLOGICAL METHODS

Experimental Studies of Language Processing and Language Disorders

Research on normal language processing has focused on the study of the obligatory, unconscious psycholinguistic processes just outlined. Techniques that have been used to study these processes have undergone considerable development over the past 20 years. Early psycholinguistic techniques made considerable use of what are now called "off-line" methods—methods that did not measure psycholinguistic operations at the time they were occurring, such as recall of the content of sentences or passages. By the mid-1960s, researchers had begun to use methods that required a subject to make responses to ongoing language stimuli and to respond to a stimulus in a way that does not require conscious consideration of the representation under investigation. The localization of extraneous noises (clicks) in a sentence (22), monitoring for phonemes (23), and other techniques were among the earliest experimental approaches to "on-line" psycholinguistic processing. More complex tasks mark subsequent on-line methods. For instance, Seidenberg and Tanenhaus (24) and Swinney (25) had subjects listen to a passage and simultaneously indicate whether a visually presented letter string was a word or not (a so-called visual lexical decision task) to investigate the time-course of activation of the meanings of ambiguous words and the relationship of this process to context. Techniques such as self-paced reading—a task in which subjects press a key to call up subsequent words or passages—and performance of psycholinguistic tasks under dual-task conditions or when stimulus input is made more difficult to perceive—as in rapid serial visual presentation (RSVP)—have been used to explore the locus of increases in processing load in sentence comprehension (26, 27). Researchers have been concerned with the "ecological validity" of these complex tasks. This has been approached by measuring dependent variables in more natural tasks, such as monitoring the loci and durations of eye fixations during reading (28).

Most of the studies of language impairments use off-line measures of language performance. In most of these studies,

the test is untimed, the dependent variable is accuracy and at times error type, and the interest of the study lies in what linguistic representations a patient can and cannot deal with in what tasks. These studies give us valuable data regarding the major dissociations found in patients with respect to their abilities to process language. They are the most common type of study of psycholinguistic impairments in contemporary cognitive neuropsychological research. So-called "double dissociations," in which one patient performs normally on one task and abnormally on a second and a second patient shows the opposite pattern, provide important evidence for the existence of separate processors, each involved in only one of the two tasks (12). Contemporary research in the area of neurogenic language disorders consists largely of the study of single cases, in whom a large number of tests can be administered and the results used to establish one or more specific deficits (10, 12).

On-line methods have begun to be applied to the study of language disorders. Some of the earliest on-line studies of language processing were in schizophrenia (29, 30), but these were not followed up. On-line techniques have been used more recently to study patients with neurological diseases (14, 31–33). The use of these techniques in patient populations is technically difficult, but valuable, because it can give quite different views of language processing than those that emerge from off-line studies.

Clinical Assessments of Language

A detailed experimental evaluation of every patient is not feasible. An achievable goal of a psycholinguistic assessment of a patient is to specify the types of linguistic representations (simple words, word formation, sentences, discourse) that are processed abnormally in each of the four major language-related tasks (speech, auditory comprehension, reading, writing). For each level of the code, the assessment specifies whether the disturbance affects linguistic forms (e.g., phonemes, syntactic structures) and/or the semantic meanings associated with those forms. It also attempts to identify selective impairments affecting each type of representation in each of these tasks and the overall level of functioning of the patient with respect to each linguistic representation in each task. This effort will lead to a description of the patient's language disorder in relation to the major components of the language processing system. In most cases, more than one disorder will be identified in a patient with a language impairment.

Existing aphasia batteries, like the Boston Diagnostic Aphasia Examination (34, 35); the Western Aphasia Battery (36, 37); the PICA (38), and more specific tests, like the Wepman (39); the Peabody Picture Vocabulary Test (40); the Boston Naming Test (41); and varieties of the Token Test (42), do not provide a systematic exploration of the levels of the language code that are disturbed in a given language processing task. New tests to screen patients psycholinguistically are beginning to be developed (43). What follows is a description of a language examination that can identify the major primary disturbances of language processing in a patient (10, 44).

The test begins with an informal assessment of whether the patient understands what is said and whether he or she is able to express ideas in a comprehensible form. Problems in speech production are noted, such as limited production of nouns and verbs, errors in function words, phonemic paraphasias and neologisms, and abnormal articulation and prosody. Next, the examiner assesses the patient's ability to recognize pictures, by presenting pictures of objects and asking yes/no questions about his or her physical and functional properties. If a patient does not demonstrate an ability to understand pictures, further testing is based only on tests that do not make use of pictures.

On the comprehension side, *phoneme discrimination* is tested by randomly presenting pairs of syllables, half identical (e.g., /ba/-/ba/) and half minimally different (e.g., /fa/-/va/); the patient must say which are the same and which different. *Word recognition* is tested by randomly presenting real simple words (e.g., *cattle, true*) and nonwords (e.g., *voot, efebant*) and asking the patient to indicate which are real and which are not. *Single word comprehension* is tested in two ways. The first is by asking questions about words, assessing the patient's knowledge of both physical and functional properties of objects (e.g., *Does a horse have hoofs or paws?; Is a chisel used for cooking or making furniture?*). The second is by word-picture matching (assuming the patient has done well on the test of picture recognition). Foils are from the same semantic category as the target and be visually similar to the target (e.g., the word *chisel* paired with pictures of a chisel and a screwdriver). Objects in the categories of tools, animals, and foods are tested. *Recognition of complex words* is tested by randomly presenting real complex words (e.g., *decision, runs*) and stimuli that are nonwords because of an illegal combination of a stem and an affix (e.g., *decidation, runned*) and asking the patient to say which are real and which are not. *Comprehension of morphologically complex words* is tested by asking the patient to match a complex word to one of two others, where the match depends upon understanding the affix (e.g., Does *official* mean *executive* or *execution?*). Sentence comprehension is assessed by having the patient match a sentence to one of two pictures. Both lexical foils (e.g., *The cake was eaten by the boy,* matched to a correct picture and a picture showing a cake being eaten by a girl) and syntactic foils (*The man was pushed by the woman* matched to the correct picture and one of a man pushing a woman) are used. Both active sentences (*The boy ate the cake*) and passive forms (*The cake was eaten by the boy*) are tested in both these conditions.

On the production side, *word production* is tested by picture naming. The items to be named come from the categories of tools, animals, and foods, and include words that are one syllable and three or more syllables in length. Tests of the ability to repeat long and short words and nonwords are administered. Errors of word and nonword production are classified as omissions, semantic errors, phonemic paraphasias, apraxic speech, and dysarthric speech. Tests of the ability to recognize that the word for two pictures are homophones (e.g., a pair of eyeglasses and a set of drinking glasses) provide information about a patient's ability to access the forms of words despite a speech production impairment. *Production of morphologically complex words* is tested by having the patient change a word to fit a sentence context (e.g., Change *courage* to fit in the sentence: *If a man is brave, we say he is* _____ .). *Sentence production* is tested by having the patient describe a picture, mentioning all the items in it and beginning with a particular item. For instance, the patient is required to describe a picture of a man pushing a bicycle, beginning with the word for bicycle; this forces him to use a complex syntactic form, such as the passive sentence, *The bicycle is being pushed by the man.* The ability to produce various syntactic forms is noted.

Testing written language proceeds along the same lines. In addition to the factors just described, the regularity of the mapping from orthography to phonology and vice versa is varied in stimuli used in lexical decision, reading aloud, and spelling tests.

If tests such as these are administered, three steps must be taken to relate abnormal performance on these tasks to disturbances of components of the language processing system.

First, the clinician must be able identify abnormal performance on each task. Doing this depends upon the availability of norms and Z-scores for tests of this sort, which are being developed for some psycholinguistic batteries. In the interim, clinicians will be forced to develop their own experience with tests of this sort, on the basis of which they can determine whether a particular level of performance is consistent with a patient's education, age, socioeconomic background, and other factors.

Second, the clinician must determine that major nonlinguistic factors are not affecting performance. Neuropsychological evaluations can help rule out disturbances of nonlinguistic factors as the basis for a patient's abnormal performance. In addition, the clinician can compare a patient's performance across similar tests. For example, if a patient can do a lexical decision task with simple words but not with words with morphologically complex structures (matched for length, frequency, and other relevant factors), it is likely that he or she has a specific problem with processing morphologically complex words, not with the lexical decision task itself.

Finally, the clinician must be able to interpret a pattern of performance on a series of tests as an indication of what language processing components are affected. The examiner can attribute a *primary* deficit in a particular processing component to a patient if (and only if): (*a*) his performance on the test(s) that requires that component is abnormal, and (*b*) the linguistic input to that component is intact (as judged by performance on other subtests). Thus, for instance, the auditory lexical access component may be considered to be the locus of an independent deficit if (and only if): (*a*) performance on an auditory lexical decision test is abnormal and (*b*) performance on a phonemic discrimination test is

Table 31.3.   Deficits in Auditory Comprehension, Defined by Performances on Psycholinguistic Tests[a]

Deficient Component	Pattern of Performance on Subtest
Word level	
Acoustic-phonetic processing	*Abnormal performance on the phonemic discrimination test*
Auditory lexical access	Normal performance on phonemic discimination test
	Abnormal performance on the lexical decision task with words
Lexical semantic access	Normal performance on the phonemic discrimination test
	Normal performance on the lexical decision task with words
	Abnormal performance on any lexical comprehension test
Affixed word level	
1. *Morphological analysis*	Normal lexical access
	Abnormal performance on lexical decision for affixed words
2. *Morphological comprehension*	Normal lexical decision for affixed words
	Abnormal performance on any test of affixed word comprehension
Sentence level	
1. *Lexicoinferential comprehension*	Normal lexical semantic access and morphological comprehension
	Abnormal comprehension of constrained sentences
2. *Parsing and syntactic comprehension*	Normal lexical semantic access and morphological comprehension
	Normal performance on constrained sentence comprehension
	Abnormal performance on semantically unconstrained syntactically complex sentence comprehension

[a]Subtests on which the subject must perform normally are indicated in plain type. Subtests on which abnormal performance is a prerequisite for the assignment of a particular deficit are italicized.

normal. It is inappropriate to conclude that a patient has a *primary* deficit in recognizing words if he or she cannot discriminate phonemes. The examiner can make the diagnosis of a *secondary* deficit in a language processing component when both performance on the test(s) that requires that component and performance on the subtests that assess processing of linguistic structures needed for the operation of the deficit component are abnormal. Thus, the auditory lexical access component can be considered to be the locus of a deficit that is secondary to a disturbance of acoustic-phonetic processing if: (*a*) performance on the auditory lexical decision test is abnormal, and (*b*) performance on the phonemic discrimination test is also abnormal. In general, a patent's performance must be compared across several subtests to come to a decision as to which component of the language processing system is impaired. The interpretation of the major patterns of performance on the tests described above in terms of deficits in psycholinguistically defined language processors is listed in Tables 31.3–31.5.

Neurological Observations

Until the mid-1970s, the vast majority of what was known about the neural basis for language was based on the correlation of language deficits with brain lesions described at autopsy. Clearly, this database is limited for many reasons: only a few individuals whose language has been studied have come to autopsy; autopsies can be performed years after a language impairment is described and new and unrelated central nervous system (CNS) pathology can occur in the interim; pathological changes give limited insight into the neural basis of on-line language processing disorders.

With the advent of computerized tomography (CT) and magnetic resonance imaging (MRI), clinical-neuroradiological correlations have greatly expanded the database relevant to localization of language processing. Modern work with MRI has led to computer-assisted image analysis programs that are capable of identifying the contours of a lesion and computing volumes of lesions and other cerebral structures (45). These programs can also be used to provide information regarding the localization of lesions, both by nonlinear scaling of images to fit a template in which regions of interest have been established and on the basis of any local landmarks that are preserved in the image (46, 47). Positron emission tomography (PET) with radiolabeled deoxyglucose and single proton emission computed tomography (SPECT) have been used to identify regions of cerebral hypometabolism in patients, for correlation with language deficits (48, 49). The regions of hypometabolism so identified are typically much larger than those in which necrosis is visible on CT or MRI.

Functional neuroimaging has recently emerged as a potentially powerful new way to provide data regarding the localization of language processors in normal subjects. The basis of the approach is to identify local increases in cerebral blood flow that accompany cognitive functions by comparing blood flow differences in suitably designed cognitive tasks (50–52). These increases reflect increases in neurophysiological activity associated with performing a cognitive operation PET with radiolabeled oxygen, the imaging technique most extensively used so far in these studies, requires approximately 60–90 seconds of uptake time, during which a subject must perform a given task, and has a spatial resolution of several mm. Functional magnetic

Table 31.4. Deficits in Oral Production, Defined by Performances on Psycholinguistic Tests[a]

Deficient Component	Pattern of Performance on Subtest
Word level	
Accessing lexical phonological forms (from semantics)	Normal performance on picture comprehension screen
	Abnormal performance on naming task
	Abnormal performance on homophone judgment task
Phonological output planning	Normal performance on picture comprehension screen, homophone judgment, phonemic discrimination, auditory, and written lexical decision
	Phonemic paraphasias in naming, repetition, and oral reading tasks
Affixed word level	
Accessing affixed words (from semantics)	Naming and repetition adequate for the patients' oral production of words to be recognized
	Abnormal production of complex words in morphology production task
Sentence level	
Expression of thematic roles	Normal word production in isolation
	Normal performance on affixed word production
	Failure to produce word sequences that convey correct thematic roles on sentence production task
Construction of syntactic structures	Normal word production in isolation
	Normal performance on affixed word production
	Failure to produce complex structures (e.g., passives) on sentence production task
Insertion of function words into syntactic structures	Normal word production in isolation
	Normal performance on affixed word production
	Agrammatism and/or paragrammatism on sentence production task
Insertion of content words into syntactic structures	Normal word production in isolation
	Normal performance on affixed word production
	Anomia and/or phonemic paraphasias in content words on sentence production task

[a]Subtests on which that the subject must perform normally are indicated in plain type. Subtests on which abnormal performance is a prerequisite for the assignment of a particular deficit are italicized.

Table 31.5. Deficits in Written Single Word Processing, Defined by Performances on Psycholinguistic Tests[a]

Deficient Component	Pattern of Performance on Subtest
Comprehension of written words	
Written lexical access	*Abnormal performance on the written lexical decision task*
Written lexical semantic access	Normal performance on the written lexical decision task
	Abnormal performance on any written lexical comprehension task
Production of written words	
Accessing lexical orthography from semantics	Normal performance on picture comprehension screen
	Normal writing of words to dictation
	Abnormal performance on written picture-naming task
Accessing lexical orthography from lexical phonology	Normal auditory lexical access
	Normal writing of nonwords to dictation
	Abnormal (regularized) writing of irregular words to dictation
Accessing sublexical orthography from sublexical phonology	Normal phoneme discrimination
	Normal writing of words to dictation
	Abnormal writing of nonwords to dictation
Reading single words	
Accessing lexical phonology from lexical orthography	Normal written lexical access
	Normal regular word reading and nonword reading
	Abnormal (regularized) reading of irregular words
Accessing sublexical phonology from sublexical orthography	Normal oral naming
	Normal word reading
	Abnormal nonword reading

[a]Subtests on which the subject must perform normally are indicated in plain type. Subtests on which abnormal performance is criteria for the assignment of a particular deficit are italicized.

resonance imaging (fMRI) appears promising as well. fMRI provides much better spatial and temporal resolution than PET and affords the opportunity to compare the results of identifying a rCBF correlate of cognitive processes (a "positive" correlation) with those of identifying the structural or metabolic correlates of a deficit in a cognitive function (a "negative" correlation).

Measurement of electrophysiological events associated with language processing has also increased in sophistication, both with respect to measurement and localization of event-related potentials, and with respect to the design of psycholinguistic experiments (53–55). Intracortical recordings in response to language stimuli have been undertaken during neurosurgical operations for focal epilepsy (56). Intraoperative cortical stimulation, pioneered by Penfield and Roberts (57), has been used by Ojemann and others to study the localization of several aspects of language processing (58). The technique has been extended to the preoperative situation, through the use of grids of electrodes positioned in the subdural space (59). This allows patients to be tested more extensively than is possible in the operating suite, and has led to more reliable information about the localization of aspects of language processing.

With this background, let us turn to a description of disorders of language processing.

NEUROGENIC DISORDERS OF PSYCHOLINGUISTIC PROCESSING IN ADULTS

Diseases of the CNS frequently result in disturbances of the ability to use the language code. These disorders are commonly referred to as "aphasia." *Primary* aphasic disturbances affect the operation of one or more of the components of the language processing system directly. An example of a primary aphasic disturbance is an inability to construct aspects of the syntactic structure of a sentence after having recognized the words in the sentence. *Secondary* aphasic disturbances arise when disruptions of other cognitive functions lead to interference with the normal operation of one or more of the components of the language processing system. An example of a secondary aphasic disturbance is so-called "neglect dyslexia," in which a disturbance of reading results from a disturbance of visual processing in part of the visual field (12). The boundary between the two is sometimes difficult to draw, but it may be important to attempt to do so for both diagnostic and therapeutic reasons in some patients. In this review, the focus is on primary psycholinguistic disturbances, beginning with those that affect single words, and then turning to word formation, sentences, and discourse. Etiological and localization considerations in connection with each type of disorder are provided here as well.

One final issue must be addressed. To this point in the presentation, I have presented an outline of the structure of the language code and a description of some basic characteristics of its processing. A description of the language disorder of a patient in psycholinguistic terms must specify the linguistic structures and pyscholinguistic processes that are disturbed in a patient. However, in addition, it must also specify the nature of the aphasiological impairments that affect these structures and processors. Suggestions have been made that certain impairments represent loss of representations and others are due to inability to access representations (see discussion of lexical semantic impairments, that follows). Moreover, this dichotomy does not suffice to capture all the impairments that occur. Aphasic impairments can lead to omission of structures, substitutions of one structure for an other, perseveration on a structure, blending of two or more structures into one, and other overt disturbances. We know very little about the basic aphasiological mechanisms underlying such impairments. In what follows, I describe the different aphasic impairments that affect different linguistic structures and psycholinguistic processors; relating these impairments to an adequate theory of the psychopathological mechanisms that produce aphasic disturbances remains a future goal.

Disturbances of Word Meanings

Most recent research on disturbances of word meanings in patients has focussed on words that refer to objects. Disturbances of word meanings cause poor performance on word-picture matching and naming tasks (60). However, the combination of deficits in word-picture matching and naming may be caused by separate input- and output-side processing disturbances that affect word recognition and production (61). Simultaneous deficits in naming and word-picture matching are more likely to result from a disturbance affecting concepts when (*a*) the patient makes many semantic errors in providing words to pictures and definitions, (*b*) he or she has trouble with word picture matching with semantic but not phonological foils, (*c*) he or she fails on categorization tasks with pictures, and (*d*) the same words are affected in production and comprehension tasks (62).

It has been argued that brain damage may affect either the storage or the retrieval of word meanings in semantic memory. Shallice (12, 63) Warrington and Shallice (64), and Warrington and McCarthy (65) have suggested that there are five hallmarks of the loss of items in semantic memory:

1. Consistent production of semantic errors on particular items across different inputs (pictures, written word, spoken words);
2. Relative preservation of superordinate information as opposed to information about an item's features;
3. Relative preservation of information about higher frequency items;
4. Improvement of performance by priming and cueing; and
5. No effect of the rate at which a task is performed upon performance. Disorders of retrieval of items and information from semantic memory are characterized by

the opposite effects of these variables on performance. However, these suggestions remain controversial ([10, 66]).

Warrington and her colleagues have described patients whose semantic impairments they say are of one or the other of these types. Some patients with storage disorders have had temporal lobe lesions secondary to herpes encephalitis, and others have had degenerative disease, probably dementia of the Alzheimer's Type (DAT) (32, 67–69). Access disorders have been suggested in patients with strokes in various parts of the perisylvian cortex (64, 70).

Disorders affecting processing of semantic representations for objects may be specific to certain types of inputs. Warrington (60) first noted a discrepancy between comprehension of words and pictures in two patients with signs of dementia. Bub, Black, Hampson, and Kertesz (71) have analyzed a stroke patient, M.P., who showed very poor comprehension of written and spoken words but quite good comprehension of pictures. These impairments have been taken as reflections of disturbances of "verbal" and "visual" semantic systems, though this interpretation is debated (72).

Semantic disturbances may also be category-specific. Several authors have reported a selective semantic impairment of concepts related to living things and foods compared to man-made objects (69, 73–75). The opposite pattern has also been found (65, 70). Selective preservation and disruption of abstract versus concrete concepts, and of nominal versus verbal concepts, have also been reported (76–79).

Milberg and his colleagues (33, 80) have described stroke patients who cannot match words to pictures or name objects, but who show "priming" effects in lexical decision tasks (that is, they are faster at saying that a stimulus is a word when it is preceded by a related word). The fact that priming occured in these patients suggests that they are able to appreciate the relations between words unconsciously, even when they cannot indicate understanding of word meaning in conscious, controlled tasks like word-picture matching. Milberg and his colleagues have suggested that this picture arises in patients with fluent aphasias and posterior lesions. Chertkow et al. (32) have demonstrated "hyperpriming" in DAT patients for words that have degraded semantic representations. Swinney, Zurif, and Nicol (81) have shown that some patients who appear to understand words well may show abnormalities in tasks that examine unconscious processing of the meanings of words. Swinney et al. and Milberg et al. have suggested that this pattern is more likely to be seen in patients with nonfluent aphasia and more anterior perisylvian lesions.

Disturbances of Spoken Word Production

Disturbances affecting the oral production of single words are extremely common in patients with language impairments. There are three basic disturbances affecting word production (other than semantic deficits). They affect accessing the forms of words from concepts, planning the form of a word for articulation, and articulation itself.

A disturbance in activating word forms from concepts is a very common consequence of stroke in the perisylvian region. It is manifest by an inability to produce a word from a semantic stimulus (a picture or a definition), coupled with intact processing at the semantic and phonological levels (determined by answering questions about pictures, picture categorization tests, and repetition). The form of a patient's errors is not a good guide to whether he or she has an impairment at this level of the production process, because disturbances in accessing word forms may appear in a variety of ways, ranging from pauses to neologisms (complex sequences of sounds that do not form words) and semantic paraphasias (words related to the meaning of the target item). Rarely, patients show an inability to name objects presented in one modality only, even though they demonstrate understanding of the concept associated with that object when it is presented in that modality: e.g. "optic aphasia" (82–84) and "auditory aphasia" (85). Because basic perceptual mechanisms appear to be intact in these patients, these modality-specific naming disorders are taken to reflect a failure to transmit information from modality-specific semantic systems to the processor responsible for activating the forms of words.

Disturbances of a patient's ability to convert the representation of the sound of a word into a form appropriate for articulatory production are usually manifest as phonemic paraphasias (substitutions, omissions, and misorderings involving phonemes and/or syllables). Three features of a patient's performance suggest a disturbance in word sound planning. First, some phonemic paraphasias are closely related to target words (e.g., /befenit/ for /benefit/) (86). Second, some patients make multiple attempts that come closer and closer to the correct form of a word (87). Third, some patients make similar phonological errors in word repetition, word reading, and picture naming. Because the form of a word is presented to the output system in very different ways in these three tasks, the errors in such patients most likely arise in the process of planning the form of the word that is suitable for articulation (88). These characteristics of errors, however, are not specific for articulatory planning disorders (89).

Linguistic factors frequently affect phonemic errors. Patients with sound planning problems tend to be more affected on longer words and on words with consonant clusters (90, 91). The frequency of occurrence of a word in the language has a variable effect upon the occurrence of these types of errors (92, 93). Planning disturbances only rarely affect function words compared with nouns, verbs, and adjectives (94). Some patients have trouble planning the sounds of words only when words are inserted into sentences, making phonemic paraphasias in sentence production but not naming or repetition tasks (95). In these cases, the errors probably arise when words are inserted into syntactic structures.

Patients often have disturbances of articulation itself, as

shown by abnormalities in the acoustic waveform produced by a patient (96, 97) and in the movement of the articulators in speech (98–100). Investigators have identified two major disturbances of articulation—dysarthria and apraxia of speech. Dysarthria is marked by hoarseness, excessive nasality, and imprecise articulation, and has been said to not be significantly influenced by the type of linguistic material that the speaker produces or by the speech task (101, 102). Apraxia of speech is marked by difficulty in initiating speech, searching for a pronunciation, better articulation for automatized speech (e.g., counting) than volitional speech, abnormal prosody, omissions of syllables in multisyllabic words, and simplification of consonant clusters (often by adding a short neutral vowel sound between consonants) (103, 104). Both dysarthria and apraxia of speech result in sounds that are perceived as distorted (105, 106). Apraxia of speech often coexists with dysarthria or with the production of phonemic paraphasias, and the relations between these disorders and the empirical basis for distinguishing one from another are the subject of active research.

Lexical phonological access disorders and phonemic paraphasias occur following lesions in all areas of the perisylvian language zone. Apraxia of speech and dysarthria arise after lesions in the anterior portions of the language zone; dysarthria also occurs with subcortical hemispheric lesions as well as lesions in the pons. Most basal ganglia lesions affect articulation (e.g., Parkinson's disease produces a low-volume, rapid speech with articulatory distortions; Huntington's disease and Wilson's disease produce characteristic disturbances affecting the production of phonemic quality as well as prosody). Cerebellar lesions affect the timing of speech, leading to a so-called "scanning" speech pattern.

Disturbances of Recognition of Auditorily Presented Simple Words

Disturbances affecting auditory comprehension of simple words have been attributed to impairments of semantic concepts, as discussed earlier, and/or to an inability to recognize spoken words. The latter disturbances have, in turn, been thought to have two possible origins: disturbances affecting the recognition of phonemes in the acoustic signal, and disturbances affecting the ability to recognize words despite good acoustic-phonetic processing.

Disturbances of acoustic-phonetic processing may affect the ability to discriminate or to identify phonemes (107). It is unclear, however, whether these disturbances lead to problems in recognizing or understanding spoken words. Several studies suggest that they do (108–111), but other researchers have found weak correlations between comprehension capacities and phoneme discrimination capacities in patients with language impairments (112–114). Blumstein et al. (113) specifically concluded that phonemic processing disturbances could not be the main reason for Wernicke's aphasics' disturbances of auditory comprehension, as had been suggested by Luria (115). Disorders of phonemic processing have been documented following strokes in all portions of the perisylvian language zone (97, 113).

Many researchers believe that patients can have disturbances of spoken word recognition despite good acoustic-phonetic processing. Such a disturbance was originally postulated by Wernicke (116). However, there is no clear case of a patient who has intact acoustic-phonetic processing and who cannot recognize spoken words. The patient whose deficit comes closest to this is a case described by Berndt and Mitchum (117) whose acoustic-phonetic processing was intact but who could not identify spoken nonsense words (e.g., *bez*) as nonwords. However, this patient correctly identified and interpreted real words. Tyler (14) presents the most extensive set of detailed case studies yet available using on-line methods of observation of patients who have been tested for their abilities to recognize spoken words.

In most cases, single word comprehension problems are probably multifactorial in origin, and result from a complex interaction of acoustic-phonetic disturbances, disturbances in recognizing spoken words, and disturbances affecting word meanings (118).

Disturbances of phoneme discrimination and identification have been documented following lesions in all areas of the perisylvian cortex, and other patients with lesions in all areas of this cortex have had no impairments on tests of these functions (113). The lesions responsible for "pure word deafness"—an inability to understand spoken words that is much greater than any difficulty with written word comprehension—tend to be bilateral and to involve posterior perisylvian regions, especially the temporal lobes (109, 119). However, the stage of word processing that is affected in patients with this syndrome is not well characterized.

Repetition of Single Words

Repetition of a word can be carried out in three ways (120):(*a*) "nonlexically"—by repeating sounds without recognizing the word (as if one were imitating a foreign language); (*b*) "lexically"—by recognizing the stimulus as a word and uttering it without understanding it; and (*c*) "semantically"—by understanding the word and reactivating its form from its meaning. Any of these routes to repetition may be disturbed. For instance, Morton (121) described a patient who could only repeat by the semantic route; this patient made many semantic paraphasias in repetition and could not repeat nonwords. McCarthy and Warrington (122) have documented a double dissociation between good performance on repetition tasks that maximize semantic processing and those that minimize such processing. Patients with relatively isolated disturbances affecting the repetition of nonwords have been described (123), reflecting disruption of the nonlexical route. In most cases, patients have a more complicated picture, with lexical status (whether a stimulus is a word or a nonword), word frequency, and stimulus length affecting performance differently in different patients (88, 124, 125). The classic localization of a repetition disorder is in the arcuate fasciculus connecting the temporal and frontal lobes, but repetition can be affected by lesions throughout the perisylvian cortex.

Disturbances of Processing Morphologically Complex Words

Disturbances of word formation can arise in either word recognition and comprehension or in word production.

On the input side, researchers have observed that some patients who make derivational paralexic errors (e.g., *write → wrote; fish → fishing; directing → direction*) in the oral reading of complex words have particular difficulty with the recognition and analysis of written morphologically complex words compared to morphologically simple words (126–129). A patient with a disturbance affecting the auditory processing of words with inflectional but not derivational morphology has been described (130).

Disturbances affecting morphological processing also appear in single word production tasks. Goodglass and Berko (131) described patients with difficulties in producing plural, possessive, and third-person singular forms of nonwords. Because this disorder arose with nonwords that the patients were given by the experimenters, the impairment may have affected the ability to produce morphological forms. Miceli and Caramazza (132) described a patient with a disturbance affecting the production of morphologically complex words, and Badecker and Caramazza (133) have shown that such disturbances can arise in patients who perform well on tasks that require recognition and comprehension of written morphologically complex words.

Disturbances affecting the production of morphologically complex words are most commonly seen in sentence production, where they are known as "agrammatism" and "paragrammatism." These disorders are described in the section that follows.

Too few cases with disturbances affecting word formation for isolated words have been described for any clear pattern to emerge regarding the localization of the responsible lesions.

Disorders of Sentence Production

Disturbances at the sentence production level are the inevitable results of disturbances affecting the production of simple or complex words. In addition, many patients have problems in the sentence planning process itself. Agrammatism and paragrammatism are impairments affecting the ability to produce function words and morphological elements (see earlier discussion) and may arise only in sentence production and not when a patient produces words in isolation (134).

The most noticeable deficit in agrammatism is the widespread omission of function words and affixes with better production of common nouns (135). This disparity is always seen in the spontaneous speech of patients termed agrammatic, and often occurs in their repetition and writing as well. The class of words that are affected in agrammatism has been described in both a psychological and a linguistic framework. According to the psychological account, the words that are affected in agrammatism are those that belong to the "closed class" of vocabulary elements—articles, prepositions, and other words in categories to which an adult speaker does not add new elements. The linguistic approach to the characterization of agrammatism has been explored by Kean (136), Rizzi (137), Grodzinsky (138, 139) and others, who have proposed definitions of the elements that agrammatic patients tend to omit in terms of linguistic theories. Patients in whom substitutions of these elements predominate, and whose speech is fluent, are called "paragrammatic" (140). Recent observations have emphasized the fact that these two patterns co-occur in many patients (141–143). They may result from a single underlying deficit that has different surface manifestations (138, 144).

Agrammatism and paragrammatism vary considerably, with different sets of function words and bound morphemes being affected or spared in different cases (135, 145). In some patients, there seems to be some systematicity to the pattern of errors. For instance, English agrammatic patients frequently produce infinitives (e.g., *to walk*) and gerunds (e.g., *walking*) because these are the basic forms in the verbal system (146). In other cases, substitutions are closely related to the correct target (145). Agrammatics' errors also tend to follow the tendencies seen in normal subjects with respect to errors that "strand" affixes (e.g., *I am going to school → I am schooling to go*), and the "sonorance hierarchy" that establishes syllabic forms as easier to produce than simple consonants (131, 134, 136, 143, 146). Agrammatics generally produce real words, which makes for different patterns of errors in different languages that differ with respect to whether or not they require inflections to appear on a word (138, 145). In almost all cases, errors do not violate the word formation processes of the language. This suggests that most agrammatic and paragrammatic patients retain some knowledge of the rules of word formation.

Agrammatic patients usually produce only very simple syntactic structures. Goodglass et al. (147) documented the syntactic constructions produced by one agrammatic patient and found virtually no syntactically well-formed utterances. All the agrammatic patients studied in a large contemporary cross-language study showed some impoverishment of syntactic structure in spontaneous speech (135). The failure to produce complex noun phrases and embedded verbs with normal frequency were the most striking features of the syntactic simplification shown by these patients. Ostrin, Schwartz, and Saffrin (148) described four patients who could produce either a determiner and a noun (*the man*) or an adjective and a noun (*old man*), but not both (*the old man*). Because the patients produced either phrase on different attempts, Ostrin et al. concluded that they could not produce adequately complex syntactic structures for the thoughts they had in mind. In a second study of the repetition abilities of six agrammatic subjects, Ostrin and Schwartz (149) found that the patients tended to reproduce the order of nouns and verbs in the presented sentence, but made many syntactic errors, such as producing *The bicycle is riding by the boy* for *The bicycle is being ridden by the boy*. They argued that these performances resulted from an incomplete memory trace of the thematic roles of the noun phrases in the presented sentence (who was accomplishing or receiving an action).

The ability to express the thematic roles of noun phrases requires the ability to use verbs. McCarthy and Warrington (150) described an agrammatic patient in whom a category-specific degradation of the meaning of verbs resulted in almost no production of verbs in speech and limited the ability to convey thematic roles of nouns. However, in a study by Miceli, et al. (76), patients' inabilities to produce verbs were only partially responsible for the shortened phrase length found in their speech. It thus appears that, in some patients, a disturbance affecting the ability to produce verbs affects the production of a normal range of syntactic structures. In others, at least some syntactic structures are built, despite poor verb production. Yet other patients cannot produce normal syntactic structures, despite relatively good verb production.

Several studies suggest that syntactic errors in sentence production differ in paragrammatic and agrammatic patients (151–153). Butterworth and Howard (151) described five paragrammatic patients who each produced many "long and complex sentences, with multiple interdependencies of constituents." Patients with primarily paragrammatic errors tend to produce many types of syntactic error, including errors in tag questions, illegal noun phrases in relative clauses, and illegal use of pronouns to head relative clauses (151); A type of error that has often been noted in paragrammatism is a "blend," in which the output seems to reflect a conflation of two different ways of saying the same thing (e.g., *They are not prepared to be of helpful*, a combination of *They are not prepared to be helpful* and *They are not prepared to be of help* ([151]). Von Stockert (154, 155). found that paragrammatic patients solved anagram tasks according to syntactic constraints while agrammatic patients solved them using semantic constraints. Because of the evidence that paragrammatic patients retain some ability to use syntactic structures, Butterworth (151, 156, 157) has argued that the syntactic and morphological errors in paragrammatism result from the failure of these patients to monitor their speech production processes and their output.

The various disturbances that affect sentence production usually occur simultaneously. A complex disturbance that results from the combination of the deficits in producing syntactic forms, disturbances in accessing and planning word forms, and impairments in producing morphologically complex words, is known as "jargonaphasia" (158, 159).

Agrammatism is classically associated with Broca's aphasia, which classically has been related to lesions of Broca's area — the pars triangularis and pars opercularis of the third frontal convolution. However, Broca's aphasia typically is a consequence of larger lesions that include, but are not restricted to, Broca's area (160). Vanier and Caplan (161) have documented considerable variability in the exact localization of strokes within language zone associated with agrammatic speech. Paragrammatism is thought to follow more posterior lesions than agrammatism; detailed deficit-lesion correlational studies equivalent to those that have been done for agrammatism have not yet been reported for paragrammatism.

Many patients have difficulty producing prosodic aspects of speech. These disturbances may be secondary to motor output disorders (104, 162, 163) or associated with other sentence production disorders (164, 165). However, these disturbances may occur in isolation. Shapiro and Danly (166) reported that patients with anterior and central right-hemisphere lesions had a variety of disturbances of prosody in sentence production. These patterns occured regardless of the emotion associated with a sentence, and thus are different from the aprosodias related to emotional display described after right-hemisphere disease described by other authors (167). Shapiro and Danly argued that they reflect a primary disturbance of production of intonation in right-hemisphere-damaged patients, which differs as a function of lesion location in the hemisphere.

Disorders of Sentence Comprehension

The greatest amount of work in the area of disturbances of sentence comprehension has involved patients whose use of syntactic structures to assign meaning is not normal. Caramazza and Zurif (168) were the first researchers to show that some patients have selective impairments of this ability. These researchers described patients who could match sentences such as *The apple the boy is eating is red* but not *The girl the boy is chasing is tall* to one of two pictures. The difference between the two sentences is that a listener can understand who is doing what to whom in the first sentence simply by understanding the words in the sentence, and realizing that, in the real world, boys eat apples and not *vice versa*, whereas understanding the second sentence requires assigning its syntactic structure because both boys and girls are capable of chasing one another.

Disorders of syntactic comprehension have since been examined in considerable detail (169–175). Patients may have very selective disturbances affecting the use of particular syntactic structures or elements to determine the meaning of a sentence. For example, two patients we studied showed a double dissociation in their abilities to understand sentences with reflexive elements (*himself*) and pronouns (*him*) (170). Some patients can understand very simple syntactic forms, such as active sentences (*The man hugged the woman*), but not more complex forms, such as passive sentences (*The woman was hugged by the man*) (176). Many of these patients use strategies such as assigning the thematic role of agent to a noun immediately before a verb to understand semantically reversible sentences, leading to systematic errors in comprehension of sentences such as *The boy who pushed the girl kissed the baby*. Other patients have virtually no ability to use syntactic structure. Most of these patients appear to rely upon inferences based upon their knowledge of the real world and their ability to understand some words in a sentence (174). Some patients can assign and interpret syntactic structures unconsciously but not use these structures in a conscious, controlled fashion. For instance, Tyler (175) reported a patient whose on-line word-monitoring performances indicated that he was sensitive to certain syntactic anomalies, but who could not make judgments regarding these same anomalies at the end of a sentence.

Linebarger and her colleagues (172, 177) have reported that some patients who have syntactic comprehension problems (who cannot match reversible sentences to pictures, for instance) can make judgments as to whether a sentence is grammatical or not. For instance, some patients can indicate that the utterance *The woman was watched the man* is ill-formed and the utterance *The woman was watched by the man* is acceptable. These same patients could not match sentences such as *The woman was watched by the man* to one of two pictures. These researchers have interpreted these results as an indication that some patients can construct syntactic structures but not use them to determine propositional meaning, a so-called "mapping" problem (178).

Many researchers have claimed that sentence comprehension disturbances can result from limitations in verbal short-term memory (STM) (179). Verbal short-term memory appears to be a specialized memory system in which small amounts of verbal material are maintained for seconds to a minute or so (179, 180). However, some patients with short-term memory impairments have been described who have excellent sentence comprehension abilities (181, 182). For example, a patient of ours with a short-term memory span of two to three items showed excellent comprehension of syntactically complex sentences, even under speeded response conditions (183). Though many patients with STM limitations have trouble in comprehension tasks, the relationship of these STM disorders to sentence comprehension impairments remains unclear (184).

Many patients who have difficulty with sentence comprehension tasks are agrammatic Broca's aphasics, a fact that has led several researchers to suggest that Broca's area is responsible for syntactic processing (185, 186). Grodzinsky (139) presents a more specific hypothesis regarding the syntactic operations carried out in this brain region. However, as noted earlier, lesions in patients with Broca's aphasia and in the subset of Broca's aphasics with expressive agrammatism often extend well beyond Broca's area (49, 160) and may even spare Broca's area, as judged by CT scan data (161). Tramo, Baynes and Volpe (187) documented syntactic comprehension impairments in three patients with Broca's aphasia, of which two had anterior and one had a posterior lesion. One study identified the dominant inferior parietal lobe as the main location of lesions that produced impairments in sentence comprehension while sparing comprehension of single words (188). Our own work has found no correlation between lesion site within the dominant perisylvian cortex and the severity of a syntactic comprehension deficit (189, 190). Sentence comprehension disorders are thus associated with lesions throughout the perisylvian cortex.

Disorders of Discourse Processing

Patients with disturbances affecting the word and sentence level of language processing would also be expected to have impairments of processing at the level of discourse. However, though aphasic patients do have some trouble with discourse structures, the ability to process discourse is often preserved to a surprising degree in aphasic patients.

Stachowiak, et al. (191) found that aphasic subjects performed at the same level as both the right-hemisphere affected patients and the normal controls in matching the last sentence in a text with one of five pictures that depicted the literal meaning of the sentence, the figurative meaning of the sentence, or a lexical foil. Brookshire and Nicholas (192) reported a similar finding regarding the retention of main ideas and details in discourses on the part of aphasic patients. Wegner et al. (193) reported that 10 aphasic patients performed less well than 10 control subjects in verifying details than they did in verifying main ideas in coherent paragraphs. Huber and Gleber (194) reported that aphasic patients, patients with right-hemisphere damage and normal controls performed similarly in several respects on both a sentence-ordering and a picture-ordering task. Though the aphasic patients were more impaired than controls in arranging sentences, none of the groups found it more difficult to arrange low-cohesion sentence sets than high-cohesion sentence sets. Armus and her colleagues (195) have provided evidence that despite their linguistic deficits, aphasic patients retain knowledge of "scripts" — knowledge of the structure of events that plays a part in understanding discourse.

These studies indicate that, although aphasic patients have some impairments relative to control subjects in tasks that require comprehending and retaining aspects of discourse structure, these subjects perform very well on tasks that require that they extract main ideas and topics from discourses. Huber and Gleber (194) concluded that all these groups of subjects construct discourse level representations on the basis of propositional content, and do not rely on "microstructural" features of sentences to build such structures. Stachowiak et al. (191) and Waller and Darley (196) proposed that aphasics can comprehend spoken discourse through a process of contextualization that involves recruiting internal knowledge structures that guide a listener's semantic construction of a discourse. Contextualization may be possible in aphasic patients, even on the basis of very little lexical and propositional information, and may be able to compensate for disorders in basic linguistic abilities.

Recent studies have documented disturbances affecting the comprehension of discourse in patients without other language impairments. The most extensive studies of this type have been carried out in right-handed patients with right-hemisphere lesions (mostly strokes). These patients have been shown to fail to draw certain types of inferences from discourse.

Brownell et al. (197–199) found that patients with right-hemisphere lesions did not choose the correct punchline of a joke, but rather chose non sequitur endings more often than normal controls. The authors suggested that this implied that these patients knew that the ending of a joke should be surprising, but had less ability than normals to make it coherent with the first part of a joke. Brownell et al. (200) described patients with right-hemisphere lesions who had difficulty revising their first inference when they were presented discourses in which the inference that might be drawn from a single sentence should be changed because of the remaining discourse. Brownell et al. (201) showed that the discourse comprehension deficits of patients with right-hemisphere lesions tend to result from an inability to employ affect and world knowledge effectively, rather than from linguistic deficits. Their study showed that these patients made less use of speaker mood, and marginally less use of plausibility, than did normal control subjects. In contrast, the patients with right-hemisphere lesions made appropriate use of an anaphoric pronoun in establishing discourse coherence. These results have led to the view that the right hemisphere is responsible for aspects of the processing of discourse.

Disorders of Reading (Alexia)

The contemporary study of acquired dyslexias has focused on impairments in the ability to read single words aloud. Neuropsychologists have described disorders of three separate and partially independent routines in the brain for converting a written word into its spoken form: The first pathway (routine 1) involves recognizing a word visually, gaining access to its meaning, and then activating the sound of the word from its meaning. The second pathway (routine 2) translates the orthography of the entire word directly into a pronunciation, without first contacting the meaning. Finally, routine 3 decomposes the word into orthographic segments (graphemes and other spelling units), and derives a pronunciation by assigning each of them a spoken (phonemic) value.

Certain patients ("phonological alexics") lose the operation of routine 3, which acts on subword units to assemble a response, leaving available routines 1 and 2, which deal with entire words (202). The patient with damage to routine 3 is impaired in the reading aloud of nonwords, whereas legitimate words are read correctly (127). Other reading disorders appear to be the outcome of severe damage to both routines 2 and 3. Patients with this pattern or impairment, termed "deep dyslexics" (203), are unable to pronounce written nonwords (indicating severe impairment to routine 3), but also make semantic paralexias (e.g., they read *chair* as *table*) and are poor at reading abstract words aloud compared to concrete words. The failure to read nonwords combined with the presence of semantic errors and the influence of a semantic variable on the ability to read a written word aloud is consistent with the interpretation that the patient has lost the use of the routine from subword units to sound and is forced to use a defective routine from the visual description of the word through meaning to pronunciation. Yet other dyslexic readers—"surface dyslexics" (204) have lost the ability to use both the semantically mediated reading route (routine 1) and the whole-word reading route (routine 2) but retain the translation of subword units into sound (routine 3). These patients can still read words aloud that obey regular correspondences between spelling and sound (e.g., *hint, mint, stint,* etc.), but not those that do not (e.g., *pint*). Finally, some patients with dementia show the ability to use the whole-word reading route (routine 2) without the benefit of semantics (routine 1). These patients can read irregularly spelled words correctly that they do not understand (77).

The fact that a patient has difficulties in reading words and/or nonwords aloud does not necessarily imply that he or she does not recognize or understand a printed word. Some patients have a severe disturbance of reading aloud known as "letter-by-letter reading" because they name each letter in a word in sequence before attempting (often with incomplete success) to pronounce the word. These patients can take many seconds to pronounce a printed word. Several of these patients have been tested for their abilities to recognize and comprehend words that are presented for short periods of time—far less than the seconds needed for them to read the words aloud. Bub et al. (31) reported that one such patient could recognize words and familiar letter strings as visual patterns, and Shallice and Saffran (205) and Coslett and Saffran (206) have shown that other patients with this reading disturbance can extract at least some semantic information from words presented in this fashion. These performances suggest that some reading problems arise after words have been recognized, and also that some alexic subjects, like the patients with disturbances affecting auditory-oral processing described above, may retain abilities to recognize and understand words of which they are not aware.

The classic lesion localization in pure alexia ("alexia without agraphia") is in the left occipital lobe and deep white matter, and is thought to disconnect language areas in the left hemisphere from visual input to the right (207, 208). In addition to this dysconnection, other left-hemisphere lesions cause the different forms of alexia. Deep dyslexics tend to have large lesions, and it has been suggested that their reading partially results from right-hemisphere mechanisms (209). Surface dyslexics also have fairly large lesions, perhaps most often involving temporal lobe structures (210). Lesions in phonological dyslexia have not been adequately described. Letter-by-letter readers (also termed "pure alexics") have been described with lesions affecting the left parietal lobe.

Disorders of Writing (Agraphia)

The acquired dyslexias have their counterparts in the acquired agraphias. Patients with phonological agraphia are severely impaired in their ability to spell or write nonsense words, but are capable of very good performance on legitimate words, even words that are low in frequency and contain unusual spelling patterns (e.g., *leopard*) (211–215). The deficit in these cases appears to lie in the ability to convert sublexical phonological units to orthographic units (graphemes and letters). The converse impairment—an inability to access the written forms of whole words with preserved ability to convert sublexical phonological units to orthographic units, termed surface agraphia or lexical agraphia—has also been described (216–218). A third disturbance, known as "asemantic writing" consists of the inability to write spontaneously but the retained ability to write to dictation (219). This suggests that the contents of the visual word-form system can be addressed from spoken input but not from the meaning of a word.

These disorders of writing can be strikingly different from patients' reading performances. For instance, the patient J.C. (220) was unable to write nonsense words to dictation, but read these items aloud without difficulty; R.G., studied by Beauvois and Désrouesné (202), produced numerous misspellings when attempting to write orthographically irregular or ambiguous words but accurately read the majority of legitimate words perfectly. These dissociations have led researchers to infer that "the orthographic knowledge necessary for word recognition in reading is different from the orthographic knowledge necessary for correct spelling in writing" (202), but Bub et al. (221) have a different viewpoint that sees these differences as due to different access mechanisms.

The abstract graphemic representation of familiar and unfamiliar words is ultimately converted by the writing mechanism into a sequence of rapid movements that generate letters on the page (222). According to Caramazza, et al. (223), a specialized working memory device is needed to maintain the graphemic code in a buffer zone while the spatial identity of each letter is chosen at the next processing stage. Caramazza et al. report a patient, L.B., who made the same kind of errors in writing, oral spelling, and typing, a result that suggests that the disturbance arose while these items were in the planning buffer, and *before* the programming and execution of a particular motor act began.

Written production takes place by generating the spatial form of each letter in the correct order. Ellis (222) refers to these letter forms as allographs. A few agraphic cases have been documented where the impairment is plainly confined to the retrieval of elements in the allographic code. In these patients, adequate knowledge of the word's orthography can be demonstrated, because oral spelling is carried out extremely well. When tested, other methods of forming a printed word that do not require a written response (typing or use of block letters) may also yield a high degree of accuracy. Writing, however, is characterized by numerous errors of omission, substitution, reversals, and insertions (124, 224–226). The agraphia is not merely a disturbance in the production of a graphic motor pattern, because the patients can write single letters to dictation, and their writing of words, though flawed, is clearly legible.

Finally, the motor schema for a letter appears to distinguish between the movements denoting the shape of a letter and the parameters that govern scale factors like magnitude and orientation (227). Cases of apractic agraphia reveal a loss of the motor programs necessary for producing letters. Written characters are poorly formed and may be indecipherable (228, 229), though even severely affected patients maintain the distinction between cursive and printed letters, and between upper and lower case (230). Evidence indicates that the disturbance need not be associated with limb apraxia (229, 231). Certain patients with right-hemisphere damage have no difficulty constructing written letters or words, but they exceed the correct number of strokes on letters needing repetitive movements (222).

Natural History of Language Disorders

As expected, etiology is the primary factor determining the evolution of an aphasic impairment. Most research into the natural history of language impairments has focused on the evolution of aphasic "syndromes" (37). We shall discuss these syndromes later, indicating that they are all heterogeneous with respect to primary language processing deficits. This severely limits the implications of these studies for the natural history of disorders of individual language processors. However, these studies as well as clinical experience suggest that there are two broad phases of aphasic symptomatology following acute necrotic lesions. In the acute phase, patients tend to be severely affected. Symptomatology varies widely—for instance, speech output may range from mutism to jargon—and often suggests major disturbances in control mechanism (e.g., perseveration is frequently present). In the chronic phase of evolution of such lesions, patients tend to show quite stable deficits that are often highly restricted, of the sort reviewed earlier. Both clinical experience and experimental investigations of patients with long-standing aphasia indicate that considerable recovery can occur following such lesions.

The role of speech-language therapy in the management of aphasic patients is well established, but controversy exists about the effectiveness of such intervention in improving specific psycholinguistic functions (232). There are few adequate studies of this subject, and the results of these studies are contradictory. New approaches to therapy based on a psycholinguistic analysis of deficits and making use of new technologies have met with some success (233, 234). (Saffran, Schwartz, Fink, Myers, and Martin, 1992; Byng, 1988).

Overview

This synopsis of primary language processing deficits emphasizes their selectivity. It should be noted, however, that most aphasic patients have many impairments. In addition, many patients have language processing deficits that are secondary to disturbance of either other language processors or of other cognitive systems. Most notably,

Table 31.6.   The Classic Aphasic Syndromes Affecting Auditory-Oral Language Functions[a]

Syndrome	Clinical Manifestations	Postulated Functional Deficit	Usual Lesion Location
Syndromes attributed to disturbances of cortical centers			
Broca's aphasia	Major disturbance in speech production with sparse, halting speech, often misarticulated, frequently missing function words and bound morphemes	Disturbances in the speech planning and production mechanisms	Primarily posteior aspects of the 3rd frontal convolution and adjacent inferior aspects of the precentral gyrus
Wernicke's aphasia	Major disturbance in auditory comprehension; fluent speech with disturbances of the sounds and structures of words (phonemic, morphological, and semantic paraphasias)	Disturbances of the permanent representations of the sound structures of words	Posterior half of the first temporal gyrus and possibly adjacent cortex
Anomic aphasia	Disturbance in the production of single words, most marked for common nouns with variable comprehension problems	Disturbances of the concepts and/or the sound patterns of words	Inferior parietal lobe or connections between parietal lobe and temporal lobe
Global aphasia	Major disturbance in all language functions	Disruption of all language processing components	Large portion of the perisylvian association cortex
Syndromes attributed to disruptions of connections between centers			
Conduction aphasia	Disturbance of repetition and spontaneous speech (phonemic paraphasias)	Disconnection between the sound patterns of words and the speech production mechanism	Lesion in the arcuate fasciculus and/or cortico-cortical connections between temporal and frontal lobes
Transcortical motor aphasia	Disturbance of spontaneous speech similar to Broca's aphasia with relatively preserved repetition	Disconnection between conceptual representations of words and sentences and the motor speech production system	White matter tracts deep to Broca's area
Transcortical sensory aphasia	Disturbance in single word comprehension with relatively intact repetition	Disturbance in activation of word meanings despite normal recognition of auditorily presented words	White matter tracts connecting parietal lobe to temporal lobe or in portions of inferior parietal lobe
Isolation of the language zone	Disturbance of both spontaneous speech (similar to Broca's aphasia) and comprehension, with some preservation of repetition	Disconnection between concepts and both representations of word sounds and the speech production mechanism	Cortex just outside the perisylvian association cortex and/or white matter beneath perisylvian cortex

[a]Modified from Benson DF, Geschwind N. Aphasia and related cortical disturbances. In: Baker AB, Baker LH, eds. Clinical neurology. New York: Harper & Row, 1971.

disorders of attention and memory surface in language as well as in other functional spheres. The delineation of primary language processing impairments is often a difficult undertaking.

This review also underscores the relative paucity of information about the specific neural localization of lesions that cause most specific deficits. We return to this issue in our discussion of the functional neuroanatomy of language.

APHASIC SYNDROMES AND THE CLASSIFICATION OF LANGUAGE DISORDERS

Physicians often describe patients with language impairments in terms of syndromes, such as Broca's aphasia, Wernicke's aphasia, conduction aphasia, among others. These syndromes are listed in Table 31.6. Given the widespread use of this approach to description and classification of patients with language impairments, it is important to understand how it differs from the psycholinguistic approach.

The major difference between the syndrome-oriented and psycholinguistic approaches to language disorders is that the syndrome-oriented approach assigns each patient to one and only one aphasic group, whereas the psycholinguistic approach allows a patient to be assigned any number of independent language processing impairments. The attempt to assign each patient into a single group leads to a variety of problems.

First, in order to assign each patient to a single group, the syndromes must be defined in such a way as to allow for disturbances of more than a single language-processing component to exist in a given syndrome. The solution that this approach takes to this problem is to define aphasic syndromes very broadly, and to have the relative degree of impairment of different language processing components define membership in a group. For instance, Benson and Geschwind (235) describe Broca's aphasia as follows:

> The language output of Broca's aphasia can be described as nonfluent. It is sparse, dysprosodic, and poorly articulated; it is made up of very short phrases and it is produced with effort, particularly in initiation of speech. The output consists primarily of substantive words, i.e., nouns, action verbs, or significant modifiers. The pattern of short phrases lacking prepositions is often termed "telegraphic speech". . . Comprehension of spoken language is much better than speech but varies, being completely normal in some cases and moderately disturbed in others. (p. 7)

The abnormalities that determine that a patient is a Broca's aphasic are only related to each other at a very general level of description of the language processing system—that of speech production. The definition of the syndrome ignores finer distinctions. For instance, the symptoms of "dysprosodic" speech, "poorly articulated" speech, and "short phrases lacking prepositions" are likely to reflect disturbances of different language processors (the components related to assignment of prosody, to specifying the articulatory gestures for phonemes, and to construction of syntactic forms, respectively). Moreover, Benson and Geschwind indicate that auditory comprehension can also be affected in this syndrome, as long as its impairment is not as severe as any expressive language disturbance. Because of these features of the classic syndromes, we cannot use a diagnostic label such as Broca's aphasia to convey information even about what language-related functions are affected in a patient, let alone about which levels of the language code are impaired in a particular task in a patient. All we can tell is that one task is better performed than another, and that the abnormalities that will be found in a given task fall into a specified but broad range.

A consequence of the overly broad nature of the classic syndromes is that, in practice, many syndromes are identified by a checklist of symptoms that does not establish unique criteria for membership in a group. As Benson (236)

indicates, any of the aforementioned symptoms may be absent in a case of Broca's aphasia. Schwartz (237) pointed out that the actual application of these criteria has led to grouping together many patients with no symptoms in common. The reverse is also frequently encountered: patients are often not uniquely classifiable. The criteria for inclusion of patients in different aphasic groups overlap (the presence of phonemic paraphasias is noted in several categories; anomia is mentioned in almost all categories), so that a patient who shows only or chiefly these symptoms cannot be uniquely classified. Most applications of the clinical taxonomy result in frequent disagreement as to a patient's classification (238) and/or to a large number of "mixed" or "unclassifiable" cases (239).

The syndrome-oriented approach is often said to receive support from the correlation of the classic aphasic syndromes with lesion sites in the brain. However, as the previous review of the neural correlates of language processing deficits reveals, the data relating impairments in specific language processing components to lesion localization within the perisylvian cortex are weak. In addition, there is evidence for variability of localization of specific processing components across the population. This variability entails that identifying a specific processing deficit in a patient would, at most, only lead to a probabilistic localization of the patient's lesion within the perisylvian cortical region.

If language processing components occupy different parts of the perisylvian cortex in different people, what is the basis for the correlations between the classic syndromes and lesions in specific areas of the perisylvian cortical area? One possible explanation is that the classic syndromes reflect the co-occurence of variable combinations of language processing deficits with motor speech impairments (18, 44). If a patient has many and/or severe language function deficits, he or she has either a global aphasia, if motor speech mechanisms are affected, or one of the types of classic Wernicke's aphasia, if motor speech mechanisms are not involved. If he or she has only a few and/or minor language function deficits, the patient has one of the "nonfluent" aphasias, such as Broca's aphasia, "aphemia," or transcortical motor aphasia (if there are motor speech impairments), or one of the minor "fluent" aphasias, such as anomia, conduction aphasia or transcortical sensory aphasia, (if there are no motor speech impairments). It is entirely possible that the localizing value of the classic syndromes is related to the invariant location of the motor system, while language processing components are themselves quite variable in their localization in different individuals. This would imply that the correlation between the classic aphasic syndromes and lesion sites provides no reason to think that these syndromes are associated with disturbances of particular language processors.

In contrast to the traditional, syndrome-oriented approach to language disorders, the psycholinguistic approach consists of identifying the disturbances in the major components of the language processing system that are present in each patient. In this approach to taxonomy, a patient is likely to have more than one deficit (e.g., a patient can have a disturbance of the nonlexical reading route, a separate disturbance in auditory comprehension of derived words, and a third disturbance in producing the form of sentences orally). Depending on the level of detail in which language impairments are described, there may be hundreds of primary language processing impairments. From a practical point of view, however, a very detailed taxonomy based upon specific deficits is unrealistic. For many clinical purposes, an adequate way to approach a psycholinguistic taxonomy of aphasic impairments is at the level of detail presented here—the level that identifies language processing components with the sets of related operations responsible for activating the major forms of the language code and their associated meanings in the usual language tasks of speaking, comprehending auditorily presented language, writing, and reading. Most researchers in the field now believe that very little is gained by retaining the more global and less precise traditional nomenclature to describe a patient when an adequate psycholinguistic characterization of a patient's deficit is available.

PSYCHIATRIC DISEASE AND LANGUAGE DISORDERS

Psychiatric diseases are increasingly understood to be conditions that primarily affect neurological functions such as synaptic transmission and secondary messenger systems in neurons. Some psychiatric disturbances are thought to represent reactions to life events and/or acquired behavioral and emotional repertoires that are maladaptive in the patient's present setting. These latter disorders are thus complex instances of learning. Most psychiatric diseases probably are due to variable combinations of these two mechanisms, with correspondingly complex neurological bases.

Language disorders have not been studied as thoroughly in psychiatric disease as in neurological disease. The psychiatric disease whose effects on language are best documented is schizophrenia. Early descriptions of schizophrenic patients often noted language abnormalities, some of which (e.g., "clang associations") could well reflect disturbances of language processors (240, 241). The older literature is difficult to interpret, however, because some of the patients included in these studies may well have had structural neurological disease, such as purely temporal lobe strokes, that could not be diagnosed at the time. However, contemporary studies, in which the diagnosis of schizophrenia is well established, have also shown linguistic abnormalities in these patients. Abnormalities most clearly affect the lexical and discourse levels of language, as well as certain aspects of verbal memory. They do not appear to affect the processing of syntactic form in sentence comprehension, but may do so in sentence production. There are no data available regarding word formation in schizophrenia, to my knowledge.

At the single word level, Faber and Reichstein (242) reported that schizophrenic patients with formal thought disorders performed less well than controls on the repetition of words and phrases, responsive naming, body-part naming, and picture naming subtests of the Boston Diagnostic Aphasia Examination (34). These patients did well on a test of spoken word comprehension. The pattern suggests a problem with accessing lexical phonological representations from semantics and/or with planning speech production. Kwapil et al. (243) found increased semantic priming for schizophrenics in a lexical decision task, and suggested that this may reflect differences in associational processing in schizophrenics and other groups. This suggestion is consistent with the findings, mentioned previously, that hyperpriming has been demonstrated in patients with Alzheimer's disease (AD), where it has been related to loss of semantic knowledge about specific words (32). However, an electrophysiological measure of lexical semantic process—the amplitude of the N400 wave of the visual event-related potential (ERP)—has been shown to be normal in schizophrenics (244). The exact mechanism underlying the increased associative priming found in schizophrenics remains to be explored.

At the sentence level, Faber and Reichstein (242) and Morice and McNicol (245) found that schizophrenics did less well than normals on the Token Test (42). The Token Test requires a subject to manipulate blocks of different sizes, shapes, and colors in response to commands. The Token Test has been considered a test of syntactic processing, but its syntactic processing demands are relatively slight and its verbal memory demands are high. Other researchers (29, 30) have demonstrated the integrity of syntactic processing in schizophrenics using a click-localization task. This task, developed by Garrett (246) in pioneering work in the early days of modern psycholinguistic research, requires a subject to locate an extraneous noise in a sentence; subjects tend to displace such noises ("clicks") to the nearest major syntactic boundary. Rochester et al. (29) and Carpenter (30) found that schizophrenics do the same, providing evidence for intact unconcious processing of syntactic structure in auditory comprehension.

Sentence production has been studied fairly extensively in schizophrenia. Most studies report simplification of syntactic structure in the spontaneous speech of these patients. Morris and McNicol (245) reported lower rates of production of reduced relative clauses and fewer complex embedded structures in free speech samples of schizophrenic patients. Thomas et al. (247) reported a computer-assisted analysis of spontaneous speech of acute and chronic schizophrenic patients and controls for complexity, integrity, and fluency, and found that the patients performed worse than controls on all three measures. The measures of complexity and integrity reflect the patients' use of syntactic structures. Thomas et al. (247) found that chronic patients performed less well than acute patients. In a companion article, King et al. (248) reported a decline in performance of schizophrenic patients on these measures, but not in the performance of manic or control subjects, retested after a 3-year interval. Some schizophrenic patients appear to have quite severe speech disorders. Chaika (249) described six major abnormalities in the speech of a single patient: lexical phonological access disorders; lexical associations driving lexical production; repetition of phonological segments; repetition of lexical items; syntactic errors; and failure to note the presence of errors. Fromkin (250) pointed out that all these types of errors occur in the speech of normal subjects, but the frequency of these types of errors in the speech of Chaika's patient greatly exceeded that in normal speech. Production of linguistic intonational contours has been reported to be normal in schizophrenia, but these patients are impaired in the use of prosody to convey emotional state (251).

The discourse level of language has also been shown to be abnormal in schizophrenia. Rochester and Martin (252) undertook an analysis of the speech of schizophrenic patients with and without thought disorders, and controls, which included detailed measurements of cohesion and different types of reference in three types of speech production situations—an interview, the description of cartoons, and the production of a narrative description of a presented passage. The authors found that it was possible to classify subjects correctly on the basis of 11 variables derived from these measures, of which five were most valuable: the presence of additional elements in narratives; the pattern of initiation of groups and the presence of bridging in cartoon descriptions; and the use of generic referential terms in narratives and interviews. Wykes and Leff (253) analyzed the spontaneous speech of schizophrenic and manic patients for the number and type of cohesive links between elements in a discourse, based on Halliday and Hasan's (254) model of cohesion in text, and found significantly more cohesive ties in the manic patients' speech. Knight and Sims-Knight (255) showed that schizophrenics are less capable than normals of recognizing sentences that integrated ideas in a presented discourse.

These studies document a wide range of language abnormalities in schizophrenia. Although some of these abnormalities may be secondary to other cognitive impairments in these patients, some are likely to be primary disturbances of psycholinguistic processors. Schizophrenia, like many nonfocal neurological conditions such as AD, appears to affect a variety of aspects of language processing. As with "neurological" disease, schizophrenia does not always affect language, and some of the language processing abnormalities found in schizophrenia appear to be mild. However, many abnormalities of language are identifiable in individual schizophrenic patients. More research into this condition and other diseases is necessary to identify the full range of language impairments in psychiatric disease.

FUNCTIONAL NEUROANATOMY OF LANGUAGE PROCESSING

The first step in understanding the neural basis for a function has traditionally been to identify the areas of the brain where that function takes place. Subsequently, the cellular and subcellular mechanisms involved in accomplishing that function have been explored. In the case of language, for which there are no animal models, the second of these stages of investigation is virtually nonexistent. There are data, however, on the gross functional neuroanatomy of the brain for language.

Clinical studies (256–261) indicate that the association cortex in the region of the sylvian fissure is responsible for language processing in the auditory-oral modality. This region includes the posterior half of the pars triangularis and the pars opecularis of the third frontal convolution (Broca's area), the association cortex in the opercular area of the pre- and postcentral gyri, the supramarginal and angular gyri of the parietal lobe, the first temporal gyrus from the supramarginal gyrus to a point lateral to Heschl's gyrus (Wernicke's area), and possibly a portion of the adjacent second temporal gyrus. In addition, language disorders have been described in association with electrocortical stimulation of the lingular gyrus (262, 263). On the basis of present knowledge, there is no other cortical area that can be confidently thought to subserve language functions.

The perisylvian region of the brain appears to be specialized for language in the auditory-oral modality. The role of the perisylvian association cortex as the substrate for language in the auditory-oral modality does not vary as a function of major endogenous biological factors, such as sex, or an important environmental phenomenological factor, literacy. Language in the visual-gestural modality in deaf individuals also is based in the perisylvian cortex, though it may recruit more superior regions of cortex in frontal and parietal lobes as well (264). Written language is a secondary development that depends on instruction. It appears to involve areas of the brain that are more closely associated with visual processing.

The supplementary motor area is the only other cortical structure that has been suggested to play a role in language processing. However, its primary function in language tasks appears to be to initiate vocalization, not to activate linguistic representations through subserving a component of the language processing system per se (265).

Several subcortical nuclei have also been suggested to play a role in language. These include the thalamus, the caudate, and possibly parts of the striatum (266, 267). White matter tracts are thought to play important roles in transmitting the products of computations in one cortical area to another (208) and to lower motor centers (268). We shall discuss the roles of these different portions of the hemispheres in turn.

Although these areas of the cerebral hemispheres are those in which lesion-deficit correlational studies and activation studies implicate in language processing, there are effects on language of a wide variety of lesions. Again, most of these effects are probably secondary to disturbances of other cognitive functions, especially attention and memory.

However, some probably represent impairments of language processors, as in certain schizophrenic patients. The existence of these impairments suggests one of two conclusions: either these conditions affect perisylvian cortex, or some aspects of language processing involve neural systems outside this region in some individuals. More must be known about the neuropathology of these conditions before the implications of these data are clear.

Cortical Structures and Language

Two general classes of theories of the relationship of portions of the perisylvian association cortex to components of the language processing system have been developed, one based on "holist" or distributed views of neural function (160, 269–272) and one based on localizationist principles (115, 116, 208, 256, 273–278).

HOLIST THEORIES

The basic tenet of holist/distributed theories of the functional neuroanatomy for language is that linguistic representations are distributed widely and that specific stages of linguistic processing recruit widely scattered areas of perisylvian association cortex. Lashley (279, 280) identified two functional features of holist/distributed models that determine the effects of lesions upon performance: equipotentiality (every portion of a particular brain region can carry out a specific function in every individual) and mass action (the larger the neuronal pool that carries out a particular function, the more efficiently that function is accomplished). The features of equipotentiality and mass action jointly entail that lesions of similar sizes anywhere in a specified brain region have equivalent effects upon function, and that the magnitude of any functional deficit is directly proportional to the size of a lesion in this specified area. More recently, models of lesions in parallel distrubuted processing (PDP) simulations of language and other cognitive functions have provided a mathematical basis for these properties of these systems (281).

The first line of evidence supporting holist theories consists of the ubiquity of general factors in accounting for the performance of aphasic patients. For instance, factor analyses of the performances of groups of patients both on general aphasia tests (35, 282) and on tests of specific language abilities (189) almost always result in first factors (usually accounting for more than half of the variance in performance) that are roughly equally weighted for most of the subtests used to test the population. Such factors are usually taken to reflect disruption of a single factor that affects performance on all measures, such as a limited amount of mental resources available for psycholinguistic computations. The existence of such factors would be the immediate consequence of a system in which functions were disruptable by lesions in a variety of locations, and they have therefore been widely taken as evidence for a distributed basis for language functions. A second finding supporting holist theories is the frequent observation of so-called "graceful degradation" of performance within specific language domains after brain damage. An example of such degradation is the strong tendency of certain dyslexic patients to read irregularly spelled words according to a regularization strategy (e.g., *pint* is read with a short *i*), a

tendency that is inversely proportional to the frequency of the word (217). Graceful degradation reflects the preservation of the simplest (in many cases, the most commonly occurring) aspects of language processing after brain damage. Modern work with PDP models, which provide formal models of holist concepts, indicate that such patterns of performance can arise following focal lesions in systems in which information is represented and processed in massively parallel, distributed, forms (281, 283). A third source of empirical support for holist theories comes from the finding of an effect of lesion size on the overall severity of functional impairments in several language spheres (188, 284–286). This would follow from the principle of mass action (279). These results therefore are consistent with some form of holism in the neural basis for linguistic representations and processes.

Against the complete adequacy of any holist model is the finding that multiple individual language deficits arise in patients with small perisylvian lesions, often in complementary functional spheres. For example, studies of acquired dyslexia have documented patients who cannot read by a whole-word route (i.e., by using the entire form of a written word to gain access to the mental representation of that word (287) and others who cannot read by the application of spelling-sound correspondences at the letter and grapheme level (202). Double dissociations of this sort abound in the contemporary psycholinguistic aphasiological literature (5, 75, 288). They indicate that the mode of organization of language in the brain must be one that allows focal lesions to disrupt specific aspects of psycholinguistic processing, not simply a mode of organization that produces complexity effects and degrades gracefully. Though some selective disruptions of function can occur when "lesions" are produced in simulated language processing systems that operate in PDP models (289, 290), to date no mechanism of lesioning a distributed neural system has been shown to produce the range of specific patterns of language breakdown observed in patients.

LOCALIZATIONIST THEORIES

Though many localizationist models exist, the "connectionist" model of language representation and processing in the brain revived by Geschwind and his colleagues (208) in the 1960s and 1970s probably remains the best-known localizationist model of the functional neuroanatomy of language, at least in medical circles in North America. This model is based upon observations of aphasic patients and the interpretation of those observations that were first made over a century ago (16, 273–275). It was revived by Geschwind in almost identical form in the 1960s and 1970s (208, 291–293), and has been stated with only minor modifications to the present (186, 294).

The basic connectionist model of auditory-oral language processing postulates three basic centers for language processing, all in cerebral cortex. The first center, located in Wernicke's area, stores the permanent representations for the sounds of words (what psycholinguists would now call a "phonological lexicon"). The second, located in Broca's area, houses the mechanisms responsible for planning and programming speech. These localizations are thought to evolve from the relationship of these areas of the brain to primary sensory and motor regions. The third center, diffusely localized in cortex in the 19th century models, stores the representations of concepts. Geschwind proposed that the inferior parietal lobule—the supra-marginal and angular gyri—is the site at which the fibers projecting from somesthetic, visual, and auditory association cortices all converge, and that as a consequence of this convergence, associations between word sounds and the sensory properties of objects can be established in this area. Geschwind argued that these associations are critical aspects of the meanings of words and that their establishment is a prerequisite of the ability to name objects.

Language processing in this model involves the activation of linguistic representations in these cortical centers and the transfer of these representations from one center to another, largely via white matter tracts. For instance, in auditory comprehension, the representations of the sound patterns of words are accessed in Wernicke's area following auditory presentation of language stimuli. These auditory representations of the sounds of words in turn evoke the concepts associated with words in the "concept center." Accessing the phonological representation of words and the subsequent concepts associated with these representations constitutes the function of comprehension of auditory language. In spoken language production, concepts access the phonological representations of words in Wernicke's area, which are then transmitted to the motor programming areas for speech in Broca's area. In most versions of this model, the proper execution of the speech act also depends upon Broca's area receiving input directly from the concept center. Repetition, reading, and writing involve similar sequences of activation of centers via connections.

The principal evidence in favor of this model is said to be the occurrence of specific syndromes of language disorders that can be accounted for by lesions of these centers and the connections between them, shown in Table 31.3. Our previous discussion of these syndromes indicates that it is impossible to base a theory of the localization of language processing components on the localization of these syndromes. In addition to this basic problem with the psychological data, there are many inadequacies in the neurological aspects of the published data. Lesion sites are often only reported for patient groups, not individual patients (37), precluding the investigation of variability in lesion sites across patients in these reports.

Lesions have often been described in very general terms (258, 295). The techniques used to localize lesions are often imprecise and have at times been inconsistently applied to imaging data (296). Beyond these technical problems, the correlations between lesion sites and aphasic syndromes are far from perfect, even in vascular cases, and they become less reliable in other neurological conditions (37). As early as

1908, François Moutier documented large numbers of stroke patients with lesions in Broca's area without Broca's aphasia and patients with the syndrome with lesions elsewhere (297, 298). Recent work has confirmed the failure of small Broca's area lesions to produce Broca's aphasia (299), leading to various modifications of the simplest version of the connectionist localizationist model (300). The variability in lesions associated with Wernicke's aphasia has been strikingly documented in a recent review (Bogen and Bogen, 1976) (301). The use of PET scanning to define lesions shows large, overlapping areas of hypometabolism in association with each of the clinical aphasic syndromes (48, 49, 302), leading to uncertainty regarding the areas of functionally abnormal brain responsible for each.

Lesion-deficit correlations have been studied in patients with more specific functional impairments than are captured by the classic aphasic syndromes, and have often not been consistent with the classic connectionist model. For instance, the localization of lexical semantic representations and processing in the temporal lobe contrasts with the Geschwind (208) hypothesis that these functions are based in parietal lobe. Thus, to the extent that they exist, many, if not all, of the claims of the classic connectionist model regarding language localization are almost certainly wrong. However, deficit-lesion correlations do suggest localization of some language processors; much more work is needed to establish the exact nature of these localizations with confidence.

Functional neuroimaging based on PET has recently been used to study the regions of cortex that are activated during the performance of a number of language tasks by normal subjects (50, 52). On the basis of these studies, a number of localizations have been suggested: visual word recognition in dominant peristriate cortex (50); auditory word recognition in temporal lobe (52); the lexicons (303) and lexical semantic functions in frontal cortex (52, 304); rehearsal in Broca's area (305). The dominant inferior parietal lobe has shown little activation in language tests to date, perhaps because of some degree of insensitivity of the technique. The PET activation results are generally compatible with the results of deficit-lesion correlations (a notable point of debate is the role of the frontal lobe in lexical semantics).

There is considerable evidence for individual variability in the effects of lesions at particular sites upon components of the language processing system. Blumstein et al. (113) reported no differences in phoneme discrimination in natural speech real word stimuli in 25 patients as a function of lesion site (anterior and posterior). Basso and her colleagues (112) reported a similar result using synthetic speech stimuli in 50 aphasic patients with left-hemisphere perisylvian lesions. Blumstein et al. (113) reported equal rates of disturbed and retained abilities to discriminate and identify synthetic stop consonants in 16 aphasic patients with either anterior or posterior lesions. A series of papers by Knopman and his associates documented considerable individual variability in localization of the lesions responsible for the comprehension of single words (188, 284–286).

Similar disturbances in the production of morphological forms have been described in patients with agrammatism (with more anterior lesions) and paragrammatism (with more posterior lesions (145)). Knopman's work also documents variability in the lesion sites associated with aspects of sentence comprehension (118). Caplan and his colleagues (189, 190) reported great variability in lesion sites in patients with different degrees and types of syntactic comprehension deficits, and in CT lesion sites in patients with a particular form of acquired dyslexia—"surface dyslexia" (210) and agrammatism (161). In other work (e.g., the production of phonemic errors by conduction and Broca's aphasics in spontaneous speech [306], picture naming [90], and repetition and reading [91]), the data are at least suggestive of individual variability in the effects of lesions. Electrocortical stimulation studies (58, 307) have found complete or partial interference in tests of phoneme discrimination, picture naming, sentence comprehension, and other language functions after stimulation in many parts of the perisylvian association cortex. Some early results from PET studies that suggest that interindividual variability is found using PET functional neuroimaging, though it is not as pronounced as the deficit-lesion correlational studies suggest. The reasons for this discrepancy are not yet clear.

Overall, the picture that is beginning to emerge is that different components of the language processing system are localized in different parts of the perisylvian neocortex. There is considerable evidence for some individual differences in localization, but the extent of this phenomenon is not yet clear. Several features of the effects of lesions—graceful degradation and complexity effects—are consistent with parallel distributing processing models of language; one possibility is that at least some language processors make use of this mode of representation and computation.

Subcortical Structures and Language

WHITE MATTER TRACTS

There are conflicting reports regarding the language disorders that follow white matter lesions. According to some reports, the aphasic syndromes that follow white matter lesions do not differ from those that occur with perisylvian cortical lesions, and the classic aphasic syndromes correlate with subcortical lesion sites (176, 267, 308). A study by Basso and her colleagues (309), however, reports that the language disorders seen with subcortical CT lesions are not easily classified as any of the standard aphasic syndromes, that language disturbances of all sorts occur with lesions in all subcortical areas, and that total sparing of language functions can follow lesions in identical subcortical areas. The literature on language disorders in multiple sclerosis (MS) has stressed the relative sparing of language functions in this disease (310). However, this may be because MS lesions do not affect white matter tracts in a manner needed to interrupt language processes. Knowledge of the white matter tracts that carry linguistic information

from one processor to another and to effector motor systems remains limited.

GRAY MATTER NUCLEI

Several studies report aphasic disturbances following strokes in the thalamus, caudate, and parts of the striatum (266, 299, 308). It is likely that at least some aphasic symptoms seen after deep gray matter lesions reflect the effects of disturbances in other cognitive functions upon language. For instance, the fluctuation between neologistic jargon and virtual mutism seen after some thalamic lesions corresponds to a more general fluctuation between states of delirium and near-akinetic mutism (299). This outcome most likely reflects the effects of some thalamic lesions upon arousal, alerting, and motivational functions, some of which are seen in the sphere of language. Intraoperative stimulation studies of the interference with language functions following dominant thalamic stimulation also suggest that the language impairments seen in at least some thalamic cases are due to disturbances of attentional mechanisms (58). However, many language impairments associated with subcorticval lesions are likely to be primary.

Perhaps the most important consideration regarding language disorders following subcortical lesions is the question of whether they result from altered physiological activity in the overlying cortex, not from disorders of the subcortical structures themselves. The availability of patients with focal strokes that are visible only subcortically on CT scans, in whom metabolic scanning is used to assess lesion site and size in both cortical and subcortical structures, provides an opportunity to investigate the role that both cortical and subcortical structures play in language. There is a perfect correspondence in published cases between the presence or absence of cortical hypometabolism or hypoperfusion and the presence or absence of aphasic impairments in patients with focal strokes visible only subcortically on CT scans (311, 312). Moreover, studies correlating the degree of hypometabolism measured cortically and subcortically with the degree of language impairment indicate a much higher correlation of language impairments with the indices of cortical hypometabolism (313–316). There is not a single published case in which an aphasia has been documented in a patient in whom metabolic scanning, blood flow studies, and physiological measures have all shown normally functioning perisylvian association cortex. The conclusion that is suggested by this pattern is that subcortical structures play no essential role in core language processes themselves, but are essential parts of complex neural systems, whose cortical regions are responsible for psycholinguistic computations. This remains an unsettled issue in the functional neuroanatomy of language.

Lateralization of Language Processes

In about 98% of familial strong right-handers, the left perisylvian association cortex accomplishes most if not all language processing functions at the word, word formation, and sentence level (256, 317, 318). In individuals with anomalous dominance (handedness) profiles (319–321), these psycholinguistic functions are far more likely to involve the corresponding regions of the right hemisphere (256, 257, 322), with different likelihoods of right- and left-hemispheric involvement in language functions in different subgroups within this population (323). The data on differential lateralization as a function of sex are controversial (324). Processing of discourse appears to involve the right hemisphere in right-handed subjects (197). Linguistic aspects of prosody are likely to be affected by right-hemisphere disease (164, 165).

Many aphasic syndromes that follow either left- or right-hemisphere lesions in subjects with anomalous dominance are often mild. To the extent that they reflect disturbances of isolated components of the language processing system, their occurrence indicates that many individual language processing components can be located in either hemisphere. Whether these language processing components are located in a given hemisphere in isolation from others can be resolved only by studies that establish whether remaining intact language components are based in the intact portions of the lesioned hemisphere or in the undamaged hemisphere of patients with mild aphasias. In some cases (325), intracarotid amytal injections (Wada studies) indicate that the latter appears to be the case. This would suggest separate control of lateralization for individual language processing components, but very few data are available on this point.

There are intriguing similarities between the phenomena of localization and lateralization of language. In both cases the location of a particular language processing component appears to vary across the adult population as a whole. But in both situations, however, there are central tendencies with respect to the location of particular language processing components. There appear to be preferred sites for particular language processing functions within the perisylvian region, and there is a strong preference for language processing components to be left-hemisphere based. In the case of lateralization, these central tendencies are strongly affected by handedness profiles. It is possible that these features result from commonalities in the genetically controlled mechanisms that determine the neural substrate responsible for particular language processing operations.

CONCLUSION

I have presented a view of language disorders that is based upon linguistic theory and psycholinguistic models. The beginnings of a detailed functional neuroanatomy of language processing are emerging from deficit-lesion correlations and functional neuroimaging studies that make use of this approach. Research using available and foreseeable psycholinguistic and neurolinguistic techniques is likely to continue to deepen our understanding of language disorders

and of the way the human brain supports language functions.

Acknowledgments

The preparation of this chapter was partially supported by a grant from NINDS (NS29101). Parts of this chapter have appeared in other publications (10, 44, 325).

References

1. Halle M, Vergnaud, JR. An essay on stress. Cambridge, MA: MIT Press, 1987.
2. Henderson L. Orthography and word recognition in reading. London: Academic Press, 1982.
3. Anderson SR. Where's morphology? Linguistic Inquiry 1982;13: 571–612.
4. Williams E. X features. In: Tavakolian S, ed. Language acquisition and linguistic theory. Cambridge, MA: MIT Press, 1981.
5. Chomsky N. Aspects of the theory of syntax. Cambridge, MA: MIT Press, 1965.
6. Chomsky N. Lectures on Government and Binding. Dordrecht, 1981.
7. Chomsky N. Knowledge of language. New York: Praeger, 1986.
8. Van Dijk TA, Kintsch W. Strategies of discourse comprehension. New York: Academic Press, 1983.
9. Grosz BJ, Pollack ME, Sidner CL. Discourse. In: Posner M, ed. Foundations of Cognitive Science. Cambridge, MA: MIT Press, 1989:437–468.
10. Caplan D. Language: structure, processing and disorders. Cambridge, MA: MIT Press (Bradford Books), 1992.
11. Fodor, JA. The modularity of mind. Cambridge, MA: MIT Press, 1983.
12. Shallice T. From neuropsychology to mental structure. Cambridge, MA: Cambridge University Press, 1988a.
13. Levelt WJM. (1989). Speaking: from intention to articulation. Cambridge, MA: MIT Press, 1989.
14. Tyler, LK. Spoken language comprehension: an experimental approach to disordered and normal processing. Cambridge, MA: MIT Press, 1992.
15. Marslen-Wilson WD. Functional parallelism in spoken word-recognition. Cognition 1987;25:71–102.
16. Marslen-Wilson WD, Welsh A. Processing interactions and lexical access during word recognition in continuous speech. Cognitive Psychology 1978;10:29–63.
17. Tyler LK, Wessels J. Quantifying contextual contributions to word-recognition processes. Perception and Psychophysics 1983;34: 409–420.
18. Caplan D. Neurolinguistics and linguistic aphasiology. Cambridge, England: Cambridge University Press, 1987a.
19. Just MA, Carpenter PA. A capacity theory of comprehension: individual differences in working memory. Psychol Rev 1992;99(1): 122–149.
20. Kahneman D. Attention and effort. Englewood Cliffs, NJ: Prentice Hall, 1973.
21. Treisman A, Gelade G. A feature integration theory of attention. Cognitive Psychology 1980;12:97–136.
22. Garrett MF. The analysis of sentence production. In: Bower G, ed. Psychology of learning and motivation, vol. 9. New York: Academic Press, 1975:137–177.
23. Foss DJ. Some effects of ambiguity upon sentence comprehension. Journal of Verbal Learning and Verbal Behavior 1970;9:699–706.
24. Seidenberg MS, Tanenhaus MK. Orthographic effects on rhyme monitoring. J Exp Psychol Hum Learn Mem 1979;5(6):546–554.
25. Swinney DA. Lexical access during sentence comprehension: (Re)consideration of context effects. Journal of Verbal Learning and Verbal Behavior 1979;18:645–659.

26. King J, Just MA. Individual differences in syntactic processing: the role of working memory. J Mem Lang 1991;30:580–602.

27. Waters G, Caplan D, Hildebrandt N. Working memory and written sentence comprehension. In: Coltheart M, ed. Attention and performance XII: the psychology of reading. London: Lawrence Erlbaum, 1987:531–555.

28. Ferreira F, Henderson JM. Use of verb information in syntactic parsing: Evidence from eye movements and word-by-word self-paced reading. J Exp Psychol Learn Mem Cogn 1990;16:555–568.

29. Rochester SR, Harris J, Seeman MV. Sentence processing in Schizophrenic listeners. J Abnorm Psychol 1973;82:350–356.

30. Carpenter MD. Sensitivity to syntactic structure: good versus poor premorbid schizophrenics. J Abnorm Psychol 1976;85:41–50.

31. Bub D, Black S, Howell J. Word recognition and orthographic context effects in a letter-by-letter reader. Brain Lang 1989;36:357–376.

32. Chertkow H, Bub D, Seidenberg MS. Priming and semantic memory loss in Alzheimer's Disease. Brain Lang 1989;36:420–446.

33. Milberg W, Blumstein SE. Lexical decision and aphasia: evidence for semantic processing. Brain Lang 1981;14:371–385.

34. Goodglass H, Kaplan E. The assessment of Aphasia and Related Disorders. Philadelphia: Lea & Febiger, 1972.

35. Goodglass H, Kaplan E. The Assessment of aphasia and related disorders. 2nd ed. Philadelphia: Lea & Febiger, 1982.

36. Kertesz A, Poole E. The aphasia quotient: the taxonomic approach to measurement of aphasic disability. Can J Neurol Sci 1974;1:7–16.

37. Kertesz A. Aphasia and associated disorders: taxonomy, localization, and recovery. New York: Grune & Stratton, 1979.

38. Porch BE. The Porch index of communicative ability: administration, scoring and interpretation. Palo Alto, CA: Consulting Psychologists 1971.

39. Wepman, JM. Auditory Discrimination Test. Chicago: Language Research Associates, 1958.

40. Dunn LM. Expanded Manual for the Peabody Picture Vocabulary Test. Circle Pines, Minn.: American Guidance Service, 1965.

41. Kaplan E, Goodglass H, Weintraub S. The Boston Naming Test. Boston: Veterans Administration, 1976.

42. DeRenzi E, Vignolo LA. The Token Test: a sensitive test to detect receptive disturbances in aphasics. Brain 1962;85:665–678.

43. Kay J, Lesser R, Coltheart M. Psycholinguistic assessments of language processing in aphasia (PALPA). East Sussex, U.K.: Lawrence Erlbaum Associates Ltd., 1992.

44. Caplan D. Toward a psycholinguistic approach to acquired neurogenic language disorders. American Journal of Speech-Language Pathology 1993;2:59–83.

45. Kennedy DN, Filipek PA, Caviness VS. Semi-automated image segmentation in multi-slice magnetic resonance images. Proceedings Soc of the Magnetic Resonance Medicine 1987;6:378.

46. Damasio H, Damasio AR. Lesion Analysis in Neuropsychology. New York: Oxford University Press, 1989.

47. Filipek PA, Kennedy DN, Caviness VS. A method of morphometric analysis of the human brain based upon magnetic resonance imaging. Ann Neurol 1988;24:356.

48. Metter EJ, Kempler D, Jackson CA, Hanson WR, Mazziotta JC, Phelps ME. Cerebral glucose metabolism: differences in Wernicke's, Broca's, and conduction aphasia. Clinical Aphasiology 1986;16:97–104.

49. Metter EJ, Kempler D, Jackson CA, Hanson WR, Mazziotta JC, Phelps ME. Cerebral glucose metabolism in Wernicke's, Broca's, and conduction aphasia. Arch Neurol 1989;46:27–34.

50. Petersen SE, Fox PT, Posner MI, Mintun M, Raichle ME. Positron emission tomographic studies of the cortical anatomy of single-word processing. Nature 1988;331:585–589.

51. Petersen SE, Fox PT, Snyder AZ, Raichle ME. Activation of extrastriate and frontal cortical areas by visual words and word-like stimuli. Science 1990;249:1041–1044.

52. Posner MI, Peterson SE, Fox PT, Raichle ME. Localization of cognitive operations in the human brain. Science 1988;240:1627–1631.

53. Gevins AS, Bressler SL, Cutillo BA, et al. Effects of prolonged mental work on functional brain topography. Electroencephal Clin Neuropsychol 1990;76:339–350.

54. Gevins AS, Cutillo BA, Bressler SL, Morgan NH, White RM, Illes J, Greer DS. Event related covariances during a bimanual visuomotor task. II. Preparation and feedback. Electroencephal Clin Neuropsychol 1989;74:147–160.

55. Gevins AS, Morgan NH, Bressler SL, et al. Human neuroelectric patterns predict performance accuracy. Science 1987;235:580–585.

56. Ojemann G, Fried I, Lettich E. Electrocorticographic (ECoG) correlates of language. I. Desynchronization in temporal language cortex during object naming. Electroencephal Clin Neurophysiol 1989;73:453–463.

57. Penfield W, Roberts L. Speech and brain mechanisms. Princeton, NJ: Princeton University Press, 1959.

58. Ojemann G. Brain organization for language from the perspective of electrical stimulation mapping. Behav Brain Sci 1983;6:189–230.

59. Uematsu S, Lesser R, Fisher R, et al. Resection of the epileptogenic area in critical cortex with the aid of a subdural electrode grid. Stereotac Func Neurosurg 1990;54:34–45.

60. Warrington EK. The selective impairment of semantic memory. Q J Exp Psychol 1975;27:635–657.

61. Howard D, Orchard-Lisle V. On the origin of semantic errors in naming: evidence from the case of a global aphasic. Cognitive Neuropsychology, 1984;1:163–190.

62. Hillis A, Rapp B, Romani C, Caramazza A. Selective impairment of semantics in lexical processing. Cognitive Neuropsychology 1990;7:191–243.

63. Shallice T. Specialisation within the semantic system. Cognitive Neuropsychology 1988b;5:133–142.

64. Warrington EK, Shallice T. Semantic access dyslexia. Brain 1979;102:43–63.

65. Warrington EK, McCarthy R. Categories of knowledge: further fractionation and an attempted integration. Brain 1987;110:1273–1296.

66. Caramazza A, Hillis AE, Rapp BC, Romani C. The multiple semantics hypothesis: Multiple confusions? Cognitive Neuropsychology 1990;7:161–189.

67. Bayles KA, Boone DR, Tomoeda CK, Slauson TJ, Kaszniak AW. Differentiating Alzheimer's patients from the normal elderly and stroke patients with aphasia. Journal of Speech and Hearing Disorders 1989;54:74–87.

68. Bayles KA, Tomoeda CK. Confrontation and generative naming abilities of dementia patients. In: Brookshire RHB, ed. Proceedings of the clinical aphasiology conference Minneapolis, MN: BRK Publishers, 1983:304–315.

69. Chertkow H, Bub D, Caplan D. Two stages in semantic memory processing: evidence from dementia. Cognitive Neuropsychology 1992;9:327–365.

70. Warrington EK, McCarthy R. Category specific access dysphasia. Brain 1983;106:859–878.

71. Bub DN, Black S, Hampson E, Kertesz A. Semantic encoding of pictures and words: Some neuropsychological observations. Cognitive Neuropsychology 1988;5:27–66.

72. Riddoch MJ, Humphreys GW. Visual object processing in optic aphasia: a case of semantic access agnosia. Cognitive Neuropsychology 1987;4(2):131–185.

73. Sartori G, and Job R. The oyster with four legs: a neuropsychological study on the interaction of visual and semantic information. Cognitive Neuropsychology 1988;5:105–132.

74. Silveri MC, Gainotti GB. Interaction between vision and language in category specific semantic impairment for living things. Cognitive Neuropsychology 1988;5:677–709.

75. Warrington EK, Shallice T. Category specific semantic impairments. Brain 1984;107:829–853.

76. Miceli G, Silveri M, Villa G, Caramazza A. On the basis for the agrammatic's difficulty in producing main verbs. Cortex 1984;20:207–220.

77. Schwartz MF, Marin OSM, Saffran EM. Dissociations of language function in dementia: a case study. Brain Lang 1979;7:277–306.

78. Warrington EK. Neuropsychological studies of verbal semantic systems. Philos Trans R Soc Lond 1981;B295:411–423.

79. Zingeser LB, Berndt RS. Grammatical class and context effects in a case of pure anomia: Implications for models of lexical processing. Cognitive Neuropsychology 1988;4:473–516.

80. Blumstein SE, Milberg W, Shrier R. Semantic processing in aphasia: evidence from an auditory lexical decision task. Brain Lang 1982;17:301–315.

81. Swinney D, Zurif E, Nicol J. The effects of focal brain damage on sentence processing: An examination of the neurological organization of a mental module. J Cogn Neurosci 1989;1:25–37.

82. Lhermitte F, Beauvois MF. A visual-speech disconnexion syndrome: report of a case with optic-aphasia, agnosic alexia and colour agnosia. Brain 1973;96:695–714.

83. Beauvois, MF (1982). Optic aphasia: A process of interaction between vision and language. Philos Trans R Soc Lond Biol 298, 35–47.

84. Beauvois MF, Saillant B, Meininger V, Lhermitte F. Bilateral tactile aphasia: a tactoverbal dysfunction. Brain 1978;101:381–401.

85. Denes G, Semenza C. Auditory modality-specific anomia: evidence from a case of pure word deafness. Cortex 1975;11:401–411.

86. Lecours AR, Lhermitte F. Phonemic paraphasias: linguistic structures and tentative hypotheses. Cortex 1969;5:193–228.

87. Joanette Y, Keller E, Lecours AR. Sequence of phonemic approximations in aphasia. Brain Lang 1980;11:30–44.

88. Caplan D, Vanier M, and Baker C. A case study of reproduction conduction aphasia: I. Word production. Cognitive Neuropsychology 1986;3:99–128.

89. McNeill D, Levy ET, Pedelty LL. Speech and gesture, In: Hammond GE, ed. Cerebral control of speech and limb movements. North Holland: Elsevier Science Publishers 1990:203–255.

90. Kohn SE. The nature of the phonological disorder in conduction aphasia. Brain Lang 1984;23:97–115.

91. Nespoulous JL, Joanette Y, Beland R, Caplan D, Lecours AR. Phonological disturbances in aphasia: Is there a "markedness" effect in aphasic phonemic errors? In: Rose FC, ed. Progress in aphasiology: advances in neurology. New York: Raven Press, 1984.

92. Garrett MF. Production of speech: Observations from normal and pathological language use. In: Ellis AW ed. Normality and pathology in cognitive functions. London: Academic Press 1982:19–75.

93. Pate DS, Saffran EM, Martin N. Specifying the nature of the production impairment in a conduction aphasic: a case study. Language and Cognitive Processes 1987;2:43–84.

94. Buckingham HW. Linguistic aspects of lexical retrieval disturbances in the posterior fluent aphasias. In: Whitaker H, ed. Studies in neurolinguistics, vol. 4. New York: Academic Press, 1979.

95. Kohn SE. The nature of the phonemic string deficit in conduction aphasia. Aphasiology 1989;3:209–239.

96. Blumstein S, Alexander MP, Ryalls JH, et al. On the nature of the foreign accent syndrome: a case study. Brain Lang 1987;31:215–244.

97. Blumstein S, Cooper WE, Zurif EB, Caramazza A. The perception and production of voice-onset time in aphasia. Neuropsychologia 1977b;15:371–383.

98. Itoh S, Sasanuma S, Hirose H. Abnormal articulatory dynamics in a patient with apraxia of speech: X-ray microbeam observation. Brain Lang 1980;11:66–75.

99. Itoh M, Sasanuma S, Tatsumi IF, Murakami S, Fukusako Y, Suzuki T. Voice onset time characteristics in apraxia of speech. Brain Lang 1982;17:193–210.

100. Schonle TW, Grabe K, Wenig P, Hohne J, Schroder J, Conrad B. Electromagnetic articulography: use of alternating magnetic fields for tracking movements of multiple points inside and outside the vocal tract. Brain Lang 1987;31:26–35.

101. Darley FL. Forward. In: Berry WR, ed. Clinical dysarthria. San Diego: College Hill Press, 1983.

102. Ansell BM, McNeil MR, Hunker CJ, Bless DM. The frequency of verbal and acoustic adjustments used by cerebral palsied dysarthric adults when faced with communicative failure. In: Berry WR, ed. Clinical dysarthria San Diego: College Hill Press, 1984:85–106.

103. Bowman CA, Hodson BW, Simpson RK. Oral apraxia and aphasic misarticulation. In: Brookshire RH, ed. Clinical aphasiology. Minneapolis: BRK. Publishers, 1980.

104. Kent R, and Rosenbek J. Prosodic disturbance and neurological lesion. Brain Lang 1982;15:259–291.

105. Odell K, McNeil MR, Rosenbek JC, Hunter L. Perceptual characteristics of consonant production by apraxic speakers. Journal of Speech and Hearing Disorders 1990;55:345–359.

106. Odell K, McNeil MR, Rosenbek JC, Hunter L. Perceptual characteristics of vowel and prosody production in apraxic, aphasic, and dysarthric speakers. J Speech Hear Res 1991;34:67–80.

107. Blumstein S, Cooper WE, Zurif EB, Caramazza A. The perception and production of voice-onset time in aphasia. Neuropsychologia 1977;15:371–383.

108. Albert ML, Bear D. Time to understand: a case study of word deafness with reference to the role of time in auditory comprehension. Brain 1974;97:373–384.

109. Auerbach SH, Allard T, Naeser M, Alexander MP, Albert ML. Pure word deafness: analysis of a case with bilateral lesions and a defect at the pre-phonemic level. Brain 1982;105:271–300.

110. Caramazza A, Berndt RS, Basili AG. The selective impairment of phonological processing: a case study. Brain Lang 1983;18:128–174.

111. Saffran EM, Marin O, Yeni-Komshian G. An analysis of speech perception and word deafness. Brain Lang 1976;3:209–228.

112. Basso A, Casati G, Vignolo LA. Phonemic identification defect in aphasia. Cortex 1977;13:85–95.

113. Blumstein SE, Baker E, Goodglass H. Phonological factors in auditory comprehension in aphasia. Neuropsychologia 1977a;15:19–30.

114. Miceli G, Gainotti G, Catagirone C, Masullo C Some aspects of phonologica impairment in aphasia. Brain Lang 1980;11:159–169.

115. Luria AR. The working brain. New York: Basic Books, 1973.

116. Wernicke C. The aphasic symptom complex: a psychological study on a neurological basis. Boston Studies in the Philosophy of Science 1974;4: 34–97.

117. Berndt RS, Mitchum CC. Auditory and lexical information sources in immediate recall: evidence from a patient with a deficit to the phonological short-term store. In: Vallar G, and Shallice T, eds Neuropsychological impairments of short-term memory. Cambridge: Cambridge University Press 1990:115–144.

118. Goodglass H, Gleason JB, Hyde MR. Some dimensions of auditory language comprehension in aphasia. J Speech Hear Res 1970;13:595–606.

119. Praamstra P, Hagoort P, Maassen B, Crul T. Word deafness and auditory cortical function: a case history and hypothesis. Brain 1991;114:1197–1225.

120. Marshall JC. Routes and representations in the processing of written language. In: Keller E, Gopnik M, ed., Motor and sensory processes of language Hillsdale, NJ: Lawrence Erlbaum 1987:237–256.

121. Morton J. Two auditory parallels to deep dyslexia. In: Coltheart M, Patterson K, Marshall JC, ed. Deep dyslexia. London: Routledge, 1980:189–197.

122. McCarthy RA, Warrington EK. A two-route model of speech production: evidence from aphasia. Brain 1984;107:463–485.

123. Caramazza A, Miceli G, Villa G. The role of the (output) phonological buffer in reading, writing and repetition. Cognitive Neuropsychology 1986;3: 37–76.

124. Bub D, Black S, Howell J, Kertesz A. Speech output processes and reading. In: Coltheart M, Sartori G, Job R, ed. The cognitive neuropsychology of language. London: Lawrence Erlbaum, 1987:79–110.

125. Miller D, Ellis AW. Speech and writing errors in "neologistic jargonaphasia": A lexical activation hypothesis. In: Coltheart M, Sartori G, ed. The cognitive neuropsychology of language. London: Erlbaum, 1987.

126. Badecker W, and Caramazza A. The analysis of morphological errors in a case of acquired dyslexia. Brain Lang 1987;32:278–305.

127. Funnell E. Ideographic communication and word class effects in aphasia. unpublished Ph.D. thesis, University of Reading, England, 1983.

128. Job R, Sartori G. Morphological decomposition: Evidence from crossed phonological dyslexia. Q J Exp Psychol 1984;36A:435–458.

129. Patterson KE. Derivatonal errors. In: Coltheart M, Patterson KE, Marshall JC, ed. Deep dyslexia London: Routledge, 1980:286–306.

130. Tyler LK, Cobb H. Processing bound grammatical morphemes in context: the case of an aphasic patient. Language and cognitive processes 1987;2:245–262.

131. Groundglass H, Berko J. Agrammatism and inflectional morphology in English. J Speech Hear Res 1960;3:257–267.

132. Miceli G, Caramazza A. Dissociation of inflectional and derivational morphology. Brain Lang 1988;35:24–65.

133. Badecker W, Caramazza A. Lexical morphological and it role in the writing process: evidence from a case of acquired dysgraphia. Cognition 1990;35:205–234.

134. Nespoulous JL, Dordain M, Perron C, et al. Agrammatism in sentence production without comprehension deficits: Reduced availability of syntactic structures and/or of grammatical morphemes? A case study. Brain Lang 1988;33:273–295.

135. Menn L, Obler L, Goodglass H. A cross-language study of agrammatism. Philadelphia: John Benjamins, 1990.

136. Kean ML, The linguistic interpretation of aphasic syndromes: agrammatism in Broca's aphasia, an example. Cognition 1977;5:9–46.

137. Rizzi L. Two notes on the linguistic interpretation of Broca's Aphasia. In: Kean ML, ed. Agrammatism London: Academic Press. 1985: 153–164.

138. Grodzinsky Y. The syntactic characterization of agrammatism. Cognition 1984;16:99–120.

139. Grodzinsky Y. Theoretical perspectives on language deficits. Cambridge, MA: MIT Press, 1990.

140. Goodglass H, Geschwind N. Language disorders (aphasia). In: Carterette EC, Friedman, ed. Handbook of Perception New York: Academic Press 1976.

141. Goodglass H, Menn L. Is agrammatism a unitary phenomenon? In: Kean ML, ed. Agrammatism London: Academic Press, 1985:1–26.

142. Heeschen C. Agrammatism vs. paragrammatism: a fictitious opposition. In: Kean ML ed. Agrammatism London: Academic Press 1985:207–248.

143. Menn L, Obler LK. Cross-language data and theories of agrammatism. In: Menn L, Obler LK, ed. Agrammatic Aphasia: A cross-language narrative sourcebook Philadelphia: John Benjamins 1990: 1369–1389.

144. Caplan D. In defense of agrammatism. Cognition 1986;24:263–276.

145. Miceli G, Silveri MC, Romani C, Caramazza A. Variation in the pattern of omissions and substitutions of grammatical morphemes in the spontaneous speech of so-called agrammatic patients. Brain Lang 1989;36:447–492.

146. Lapointe S. Some issues in the linguistic description of agrammatism. Cognition 1983;14:1–39.

147. Goodglass H, Gleason JB, Bernholtz N, Hyde MR. Some linguistic structures in the speech of a Broca's aphasic. Cortex, 1972;8: 191–212.

148. Ostrin RK, Schwartz MF, Saffrin EM. The influence of syntactic complexity in the elicited production of agrammatic aphasics. Paper Presented at the Annual Meeting of the Academy of Aphasia, Minneapolis, MN, 1983.

149. Ostrin R, Schwartz MF. Reconstructing from a degraded trace: a study of sentence repetition in agrammatism. Brain Lang 1986;28: 328–345.

150. McCarthy R, Warrington EK. Category specificity in an agrammatic patient: the relative impairment of verb retrieval and comprehension. Neuropsychologia 1985;23:709–727.

151. Butterworth B, Howard D. Paragrammatisms. Cognition 1987;26: 1–38.

152. Caplan D, Kellar L, Locke S. Inflection of neologisms in aphasia. Brain 1972;95:169–172.

153. Ellis A, Miller D, Sin G. Wernicke's aphasia and normal language processing: a case study in cognitive neuropsychology. Cognition 1983;15:111–144.

154. von Stockert TR. Recognition of syntactic structure in aphasic patients. Cortex 1972;8:322–334.

155. von Stockert TR, Bader L. Some relations of grammar and lexicon in aphasia. Cortex 1976;12:49–60.

156. Butterworth B. Speech errors: old data in search of new theories. In: Cutler A, ed. Slips of the tongue in language production. Mouton: The Hague, 1982.

157. Butterworth BL. Jargon aphasia: Processes and strategies. In: Newman S, Epstein R, ed. Current Perspectives in Dysphasia Edinburgh: Churchill Livingstone 1985.

158. Buckingham HW, Kertesz A. Neologistic jargon aphasia. Amsterdam: Swets and Zeitlinger, 1976.

159. Lecours AR, and Rouillon F. Neurolinguistic analysis of jargon aphasia and jargon agraphia. In H Whitaker H, Whitaker, ed. Studies in neurolinguistics, vol. 2, New York: Academic Press, 1976.

160. Mohr JP, Pessin MS, Finkelstein S, Funkenstein H, Duncan GW, Davis KR. Broca aphasia: pathologic and clinical. Neurology 1978;28:311–324.

161. Vanier M, Caplan D. CT scan correlates of agrammatism. In LM and L and Obler ed. Agrammatic aphasia. Amsterdam: Benjamins 1990:97–114.

162. Monrad Krohn GH. Prosody or altered "melody of language." Brain 1947;70:405–423.

163. Ryalls JH. Note. Intonation in Broca's aphasia. Neuropsychologia 1982;20(3):355–360.

164. Danly M, Cooper W, Shapiro B. Fundamental frequency, language processing, and linguistic structure in Wernicke's aphasia. Brain Lang 1983;19:1–24.

165. Danly M, Shapiro B. Speech prosody in Broca's aphasia. Brain Lang 1982;16:171–190.

166. Shapiro B, Danly M. The role of the right hemisphere in the control of speech prosody in propositional and effective context. Brain Lang 1985;25:19–36.

167. Ross E, Mesulam M. Dominant language functions of the right hemisphere? Prosody and emotional gesturing. Arch Neurol 1979; 36:144–148.

168. Caramazza A, Zurif EB. Dissociation of algorithmic and heuristic processes in language comprehension: evidence from aphasia. Brain Lang 1976;3:572–582.

169. Caplan D, Futter C. Assignment of thematic roles to nouns in sentence comprehension by an agrammatic patient. Brain Lang 1986;27:117–134.

170. Caplan D, Hildebrandt N. Disorders of syntactic comprehension. Cambridge MA: Bradford Books, 1988.

171. Hildebrandt N, Caplan D, Evans K. The man left without a trace: a case study of aphasic processing of empty categories. Cognitive Neuropsychology 1987;4:257–302.

172. Linebarger MC, Schwartz MF, Saffran EM. Sensitivity to grammatical structure in so-called agrammatic aphasics. Cognition, 1983; 13:361-392.

173. Martin RC, Wetzel WF, Blossom-Stach C, Feher E. Syntactic loss versus processing deficit: an assessment of two theories of agrammatism and syntactic comprehension deficits. Cognition 1989;32: 157–191.

174. Schwartz M, Saffran E, Marin O. The word order problem in agrammatism I: Comprehension. Brain Lang 1980;10:249–262.

175. Tyler LK. Real-time comprehension processes in agrammatism: a case study. Brain Lang 1985;26:259–275.

176. Cappa SF, Cavalotti G, Guidotti N, Papagno C, Vignolo LA. Subcortical aphasia: two clinical-CT scan correlation studies. Cortex 1983;19:227–241.

177. Linebarger MC. Neuropsychology of sentence parsing. In: Caramazza A, ed. Cognitive Neuropsychology and Neurolinguistics: Ad-

vances in Models of Cognitive Function and Impairment Hillsdale, NJ: Lawrence Erlbaum, 1990:55–122.

178. Schwartz MF, Linebarger MC, Saffran EM. The status of the syntactic deficit theory of agrammatism. In: Kean ML, ed. Agrammatism. New York: Academic Press, 1985:83–124.

179. Baddeley AD. Working memory. New York: Oxford University Press, 1986.

180. Baddeley AD. The psychology of memory. New York: Basic Books, 1976.

181. Butterworth B, Campbell R, Howard D. The uses of short-term memory: a case study. Q J Exp Psychol 1986;38:705–737.

182. McCarthy R, Warrington EK. Understanding: A function of short-term memory? Brain 1987;110:1565–1578.

183. Waters GS, Caplan D, Hildebrandt N. On the structure and function role of auditory-verbal short-term memory in sentence comprehension: a case study. Cognitive Neuropsychology, 1991;2:81–126.

184. Caplan, D, Waters, GS . Short-term memory and language comprehension: a critical review of the neuropsychological literature. In: Vallar G, and Shallice T, ed. Neuropsychological Impairments of Short-Term Memory. Cambridge: Cambridge University Press. 1990:337–389.

185. Mesulam MM. Large-scale neurocognitive networks and distributed processing for attention, language, and memory. Ann Neurol 1990;28:597–613.

186. Damasio A. Aphasia. New Engl J Med 1992;326:531–539.

187. Tramo MJ, Baynes K, Volpe BT. Impaired syntactic comprehension and production in Broca's aphasia: CT lesion localization and recovery patterns. Neurology 1988;38:95–98.

188. Selnes OA, Knopman D, Niccum N, Rubens AB, Larson D. CT scan correlates of auditory comprehension deficits in aphasia: a prospective recovery study. Neurology 1983;13:558–566.

189. Caplan D, Baker C, Dehaut F. Syntactic determinants of sentence comprehension in aphasia. Cognition 1985;21:117–175.

190. Caplan D. Discrimination of normal and aphasic subjects on a test of syntactic comprehension. Neuropsychologia 1987b;25:173–184.

191. Stachowiak FJ, Huber W, Poeck K, Kerschensteiner M. Text comprehension in aphasia. Brain Lang 1977;4:177–195.

192. Brookshire RH, Nicholas LE. Comprehension of directly and indirectly stated main ideas and details in discourse by brain-damaged and non-brain-damaged listeners. Brain Lang 1984;21:21–36.

193. Wegner ML, Brookshire RH, Nicholas LE. Comprehension of main ideas and details in coherent and noncoherent discourse by aphasic and nonaphasic listeners. Brain Lang 1984;21:37–51.

194. Huber W, Gleber J. Linguistic and nonlinguistic processing of narratives in aphasia. Brain Lang 1982;16:1–18.

195. Armus SR, Brookshire RH, Nicholas LE. Aphasic and non-brain-damaged adults' knowledge of scripts for common situations. Brain Lang 1989;36:518–528.

196. Waller M, Darley L. The influence of context on the auditory comprehension of paragraphs by aphasic subjects. J Speech Hear Res 1978;21:732–745.

197. Brownell HH, Michel D, Powelson JA, Gardner H. Surprise but not coherence: sensitivity to verbal humor in right hemisphere patients. Brain Lang 1983;18:20–27.

198. Brownell HH, Gardner H. Neuropsychological insights into humour. In: Durant J, Miller J, ed. Laughing Matters Essex: Longman Scientific 1988:17–34.

199. Bihrle AM, Brownell HH, Powelson JA, Gardner H. Comprehension of humorous and non-humorous materials by left and right brain-damaged patients. Brain Cogn 1986;5:399–411.

200. Brownell HH, Potter HH, Bihrle AM, Gardner H. Inference deficits in right brain-damaged patients. Brain Lang 1986;27:310–321.

201. Brownell HH, Carroll JJ, Rehak A, Wingfield A. The use of pronoun anaphora and speaker mood in the interpretation of conversational utterances by right hemisphere brain-damaged patients. Brain Lang 1992;43:121–147.

202. Beauvois MF, Désrouesné J. Phonological alexia: three dissociations. J Neurol Neurosurg Psychiatry 1979;42:1115–1124.

203. Coltheart M, Patterson KE, Marshall JC. Deep dyslexia. London: Routledge, 1980.

204. Patterson KE, Marshall JC, Coltheart M. Surface dyslexia: neuropsychological and cognitive studies of phonological reading. Hillsdale, NJ: Lawrence Erlbaum Associates, 1985.

205. Shallice T, Saffran EM. Lexical processing in the absence of explicit word identification; evidence from a letter-by-letter reader. Cognitive Neuropsychology 1986;3:429–458.

206. Coslett HB, Saffran EM. Evidence for preserved reading in 'pure alexia'. Brain 1989;112:327–359.

207. Dejerine J. Sur en case de cecite verbale avec agraphie, suivi d'autopsie. Compte Rendu des Seances de la Societe de Biologie 1891;3:197–201.

208. Geschwind N. Disconnection syndromes in animals and man. Brain 1965;88:237–394, 585–644.

209. Saffran EM, Schwartz MF, Marin O. The word order problem in agrammatism II: Production. Brain Lang 1980;10:263–280.

210. Vanier M, Caplan D. CT scan correlates of surface dyslexia. In: Patterson V, Marshall JC, Coltheart M, ed. Surface dyslexia. London: Erlbaum, 1985:511–525.

211. Shallice T. Phonological agraphia and the lexical route in writing. Brain 1981;104:412–429.

212. Bub D, Kertesz A. Evidence for lexicographic processing in a patient with preserved written over oral single word naming. Brain 1982a;105:697–717.

213. Baxter DM, Warrington EK. Neglect dysgraphia. J Neurol Neurosurg Psychiatry 1983;46:1073–1078.

214. Baxter DM, Warrington EK. Category-specific phonological dysgraphia. Neuropsychologia 1985;23:653–666.

215. Roeltgen DP, Heilman KM. Lexical agraphia: further support for the two system hypothesis of linguistic agraphia. Brain 1984;107:811–827.

216. Beauvois MF, Désrouesné J. Lexical or orthographic agraphia. Brain 1981;104:21–49.

217. Bub D, Cancelliere A, Kertesz A. Whole-word and analytic translation of spelling-to-sound in a non-semantic reader. In: Patterson KE, Coltheart M, Marshall JC, ed. Surface dyslexia. London: Lawrence Erlbaum 1985;15–34.

218. Hatfield FM, Patterson KE. Phonological spelling. Q J Exp Psychol 1983;35A:451–468.

219. Patterson KE. Lexical but nonsemantic spelling? Cognitive Neuropsychology 1986;3:341–367.

220. Bub D, Kertesz A. Deep agraphia. Brain Lang 1982b;17:146–165.

221. Bub D, Black S, Behrmann M. Are there two orthographic lexicons? Evidence from a case of surface dyslexia. Academy of Aphasia, Nashville, TN, 1986.

222. Ellis AW. Spelling and writing (and reading and speaking). In: Ellis AW, ed. Normality and pathology in cognitive function. London: Academic Press. 1982.

223. Caramazza A, Miceli G, Villa G, Romani C. The role of the grapheme buffer in spelling: evidence from a case of acquired dysgraphia. Cognition 1987;26:59–85.

224. Rosati G, De Bastiani P. Pure agraphia: a discrete form of aphasia. J Neurol Neurosurg Psychiatry 1979;42:266–269.

225. Kinsbourne M, Rosenfield DB. Agraphia selective for written spelling: an experimental case study. Brain Lang 1974;1:215–225.

226. Rothi LJ, Heilman KM. Alexia and agraphia with spared spelling and letter recognition abilities. Brain Lang 1981;12:1–13.

227. Van Galen GP, Teulings HL. The independent monitoring of form and scale factors in handwriting. Acta Psychologia 1983;54:9–22.

228. Margolin DI, Binder L. Multiple component agraphia in a patient with atypical cerebral dominance: an error analysis. Brain Lang 1984;22:26–40.

229. Coslett HB, Rothi LJ, Valenstein E, Heilman K. Dissociations of writing and praxis: Two cases in point. Brain Lang 1986;28:357–369.

230. Margolin DI. The neuropsychology of writing and spelling: semantic,

phonological, motor and perceptual processes. Q J Exp Psychol 1984;36A:459–489.

231. Baxter DM, Warrington EK. Ideational agraphia: A single case study. J Neurol Neurosurg Psychiatry 1986;49:369–374.

232. Wertz RT, Weiss DG, Aten JL, et al. Comparison of clinic, home and deferred language treatment for aphasia: a Veterans Administration cooperative study. Arch Neurol 1986;43:553–568.

233. Saffran EM, Schwartz MF, Find R, Myers J, Martin N. Mapping therapy: an approach to remediating agrammatic sentence comprehension and production. Bethesda, MD: National Institutes of Health 1992:77–90.

234. Byng S. Sentence comprehension deficit: theoretical analysis and remediation. Cognitive Neuropsychology 1988;5:629–676.

235. Benson DF, Geschwind N. Aphasia and related cortical disturbances. In: Baker AB, Baker LH, eds., Clinical neurology. New York: Harper & Row, 1971.

236. Benson DF. Aphasia, alexia and agraphia. London: Churchill Livingstone, 1979.

237. Schwartz M. What the classical aphasia categories can't do for us, and why. Brain Lang 1984;21:1–8.

238. Holland AL, Fromm D, Swindell CS. The labeling problem in aphasia: an illustrative case. Journal of Speech Hear Disorders 1986;51:176–180.

239. Lecours AR, Lhermitte F, Bryans B. Aphasiology. London: Balliere Tindall, 1983.

240. Bleuler E. Dementia praecox. New York: International Universities Press. Translated by Zinkin J, 1950.

241. Kraepelin E. Dementia praecox and paraphrenia. Translated by Barclay RM, Edinburgh: E. S. Livingston, 1919.

242. Faber R, Reichstein MB. Language dysfunction in Schizophrenia. Br J Psychiatry 1981;139:519–522.

243. Kwapil T, Hegley D, Chapman L, Chapman J. Facilitation of word recognition by semantic priming in schizophrenia. J Abnorm Psychol 1990;99:215–221.

244. Koyama S, Nageishi Y, Shimokochi M, et al. The N400 component of event-related potentials in schizophrenic patients: A preliminary study. Electroencephal Clin Neurophysiol 1991;78:124–132.

245. Morice R, McNicol D. The comprehension and production of complex syntax in Schizophrenia. Cortex 1985;21:567–580.

246. Garrett MF. Syntactic structures and judgments of auditory events. Unpublished doctoral dissertation, University of Illinois, 1965.

247. Thomas P, King K, Fraser WI, Kendell RE. Linguistic performance in schizophrenia: a comparison of acute and chronic patients. Br J Psychiatry 1990;156:204–210.

248. King K, Fraser WI, Thomas P, Kendell RE. Re-examination of the language of psychotic subjects. Br J Psychiatry 1990;156; 211–215.

249. Chaika E. A linguist looks at "schizophrenic" language. Brain Lang 1974;1:257–276.

250. Fromkin VA. A linguist looks at "A linguist looks at 'schizophrenic language'". Brain Lang 1975;2:498–503.

251. Murphy D, Cutting J. Prosodic comprehension and expression in schizophrenia. J Neurol, Neurosurg, Psychiatry 1990;53:727–730.

252. Rochester S, Martin J. Crazy Talk. New York: Plenum Press, 1979.

253. Wykes T, Leff J. Disordered speech: differences between manics and schizophrenics. Brain Lang 1982;15:117–124.

254. Halliday MAK, Hasan R. Cohesion in english. London: Longman, 1976.

255. Knight RA, Sims-Knight JE Integration of linguistic ideas in Schizophrenics. J Abnorm Psychol, 1979;88:191–202.

256. Luria AR. Traumatic aphasia. Mouton: The Hague, 1970.

257. Russell WR, Esper MLE. Traumatic aphasia. London: Oxford University Press, 1961.

258. Basso A, Lecours AR, Moraschini S, Vanier M. Anatomoclinical correlations of the aphasias as defined through computerized tomography: exceptions. Brain Lang 1985;26:201–29.

259. Weisenberg T, McBride K. Aphasia. Commonwealth Fund, New York, 1935.

260. Brown J. Aphasia, apraxia, and agnosia – clinical and theoretical aspects. Thomas, Springfield, IL: Charles C Thomas, 1972.

261. Pick A. Aphasia. In: Brown J, ed. and transl. Springfield, IL: Charles C Thomas, 1973.

262. Luders H, Lesser RP, Hahn J, Dinner DS, Morris H, Resor S, Harrison M. Basal temporal language area demonstrated by electrical stimulation. Neurology 1986;36:505–510.

263. Burnstine TH, Lesser RP, Hart JJ, et al. Characterization of the basal temporal language area in patients with left temporal lobe epilepsy. Neurology 1990;40:966–970.

264. Bellugi U. Mapping brain functions for language: evidence from language in a different modality. Paper presented at the 31st Annual Meeting of the Academy of Aphasia, Tucson, AZ, 1993.

265. Masdeu JC, Schoene WC, Funkenstein H. Aphasia following infarction of the left supplementary motor area: a clinicopathological study. Neurology 1978;28:1220–1223.

266. Damasio A, Damasio H, Rizzo M, Varney N, Gersch F. Aphasia with nonhemmorhagic lesions in the basal ganglia and internal capsule. Arch Neurol 1982;39:15–20.

267. Naeser MA, Alexander MP, Helm-Estabrooks N, Levine HL, Laughlin S, Geschwind N. Aphasia with predominantly subcortical lesion sites: description of three capsular/putaminal aphasia syndromes. Arch Neurol 1982;39:2–14.

268. Naeser MA, Palumbo CL, Helm-Estabrooks N, Stiassny-Eder D, Albert ML. Severe nonfluency in aphasia: role of the medial subcallosal fasciculus and other white matter pathology in recovery of spontaneous speech. Brain 1989;112:1–38.

269. Jackson JH. On affections of speech from disease of the brain. Brain 1878;1:304–30; 2:203–222; 323–56.

270. Freud S. On Aphasia, Deuticke: Leipzig, 1891.

271. Marie P. Révision de la question de l'aphasie: la troisième circonvolution frontale gauche ne joue aucun rôle spécial dans la fonction du langage. Semaine Médicale 1906;26:241–7.

272. Head H. Aphasia and kindred disorders of speech. Cambridge, MA: Cambridge University Press, 1926.

273. Broca P. Rémarques sur le siège de la faculté de la parole articulée, suives d'une observation d'aphémie (perte de parole). Bulletin de la Societé d'Anatomie 1861;36:330–57.

274. Dejerine JJ. Contribution à l'étude anatomo-pathologique et clinique des différentes variétés de cécité verbale. Mémoire Societé Biologique 1892;4:61-90.

275. Lichtheim L. On aphasia. Brain 1885;7:433–484.

276. Henschen SE. Klinische und anatomische beitrage zür pathologie des gehirns. Stockholm: Nordische Bokhandler, 1920.

277. Neilson JM. Agnosia, apraxia, aphasia. New York: Holber, 1936.

278. Damasio H, Damasio AR. The anatomical basis of conduction aphasia. Brain 1980;103:337–350.

279. Lashley KS. Brain mechanisms and intelligence. University of Chicago Press, Chicago, 1929.

280. Lashley KS. In search of the engram. Symp Soc Exp Biol 1950;4: 454–482.

281. McClelland JL, Rumelhart DE. Amnesia and distributed memory. In: McClelland JL, Rumelhart DE, eds. Parallel Distributed Processing. Cambridge, MA: MIT Press, 1986:503–528.

282. Schuell H. Minnesota test for the differential diagnosis of aphasia. Minneapolis: University of Minnesota Press, 1957.

283. Seidenberg M, McClelland J. A distributed, developmental model of word recognition and naming. Psychol Rev 1989;96:523–568.

284. Knopman DS, Selnes OA, Niccum N, Rubens AB. Recovery of naming in aphasia: relationship to fluency comprehension and CT findings. Neurology 1984;34:1461–70.

285. Knopman DS, Selnes OA, Niccum N, Rubens AB, Yock D, Larson D. A longitudinal study of speech fluency in aphasia: CT correlates of recovery and persistent nonfluency. Neurology 1983;33:1170–78.

286. Selnes OA, Niccum N, Knopman D, Rubens AB. Recovery of single word comprehension: CT scan correlates. Brain Lang 1984;21: 72–84.

287. Shallice T, McCarthy R. Phonological Reading: from patterns of

impairment to possible procedures, In: Patterson K, Coltheart M, Marshall JC, eds. Surface dyslexia. London: Lea & Febiger, 1985: 335–360.

288. Warrington EK, Shallice T. The selective impairment of auditory-verbal short-term memory. Brain 1969;92:885–96.

289. Wood C. Implications of simulated lesion experiments for the interpretation of lesions in real nervous systems. In: Arbib MA, Caplan D, Marshall JC, eds. Neural Models of Language Processes. New York: Academic Press, 1982:485–509.

290. Gordon B. Confrontation naming: computational model and disconnection simulation. In: Arbib MA, Caplan D, Marshall JC, eds. Neural Models of Language Processes. New York: Academic Press, 1982: 511–529.

291. Geschwind N. The organization of language and the brain. Science, 1970;170:940–999.

292. Geschwind N. Aphasia. N Engl J Med 1971;284:654–656.

293. Geschwind N. Language and the brain. Sci Am 1979;241:180–199.

294. Damasio A, Geschwind N. The neural basis of language. Annu Rev Neurosci 1984;7:127–147.

295. Naeser MA, Hayward RW. Lesion localization in aphasia with cranial computed tomography and the Boston diagnostic aphasia examination. Neurology 1978;28:545–551.

296. Kertesz A, Sheppard A, MacKenzie R. Localization in transcortical sensory aphasia. Arch Neurol 1982;39:475–478.

297. Moutier F. L'Aphasie de Broca. Paris: Steinheil, 1908.

298. Lecours, AR, Joanette Y. Francois Moutier, or "From folds to folds". Brain Cogn 1984;3:198–230.

299. Mohr JP, Watters WC, Duncan GW. Thalamic hemorrhage and aphasia. Brain Lang 1975;2:3–17.

300. Levine DN, Sweet E. The neuropathological basis of Broca's aphasia and its implications for the cerebral control of speech. In: Arbib MA, Caplan D, Marshall JC, eds. Neural models of Language processes. New York: Academic Press, 1982:29–326.

301. Bogen JE, Bogen GM. Wernicke's region: where is it? Ann N Y Acad Sci 1976;280:834–843.

302. Metter EJ, Riege WH, Hanson WR, Camras LR, Phelps ME, Kuhl DE. Correlations of glucose metabolism and structural damage to language function in aphasia. Brain Lang 1984;21:187–207.

303. Howard D, Patterson K, Wise R, et al. The cortical localization of the lexicons: positron emission tomography evidence. Brain 1992;115: 1769–1782.

304. Chertkow H, Bub D, Waters, GS Evans A. Separate effects of instructions and stimuli on cerebral blood flow on O^{15} tomographic transmission. Neurology, 1993;43:A189.

305. Zatorre RJ, Evans AC, Meyer E, Gjedde A. Lateralization of phonetic and pitch discrimination in speech processing. Science 1992;256: 846–849.

306. Blumstein S. A phonological investigation of aphasic speech. Mouton: The Hague, 1973.

307. Ojemann G, Ojemann J, Lettich E, Berger M. Cortical language localization in left, dominant hemisphere, J Neurosurg 1989;71: 316–326.

308. Alexander MP, Naeser MA, Palumbo CL. Correlations of subcortical CT lesion sites in aphasia profiles. Brain 1987;110:961–991.

309. Basso A, Della Sala S, Farabola M. Aphasia arising from purely deep lesions. Cortex 1987;23:29–44.

310. Rao SM. Neuropsychology of multiple sclerosis: a critical review. J Clin Exp Neuropsychol 1986;8:503–542.

311. Perani D, Vallar G, Cappa S, Messa C, Fazio F. Aphasia and neglect after subcortical stroke. A clinical/cerebral study. Brain 1987;110: 1211–1229.

312. Olsen TS, Bruhn P, Oberg RGE. Cortical hypertension as a possible cause of subcortical aphasia. Brain 1986;109:393–410.

313. Metter EJ, Riege WH, Hanson WR, Jackson CA, Kempler D, VanLancker D. Subcortical structures in aphasia: an analysis based on (F-18)-fluorodoxyglucose positron emission tomography, and computed tomography. Arch Neurol 1988;45:1229–1234.

314. Metter EJ, Riege WH, Hanson WR, et al. Comparison of metabolic rates, language and memory, and subcortical aphasias. Brain Lang 1983;19:33–47.

315. Kempler D, Metter EJ, Jackson CA, et al. Disconnection and cerebral metabolism: the case of conduction aphasia. Arch Neurol 1988;45: 275–279.

316. Metter EJ, Kempler D, Jackson CA, et al. Cerebellar glucose metabolism and chronic aphasia. Neurology 1987;37:1599–1606.

317. Milner B, Branch C, Rasmussen T. Observations on cerebral dominance. In: A. de Reuck, O'Conner M, eds. Disorders of language London: Churchill, Livingstone, 1964:200–214.

318. Milner B. Hemispheric Specialization: Its scope and limits, In: Schmidt FO, Warden FG, eds. The neurosciences: third study program. Cambridge, MA: MIT Press, 1974:75–89.

319. Geschwind N, Galaburda AM. Cerebral lateralization: biological mechanism, associations and pathology i-iii: a hypothesis and a program for research. Arch Neurol 1985;42:428–459, 421–452, 634–654.

320. Geschwind N, Galaburda AM. Cerebral lateralization: biological mechanisms, associations and pathology. Cambridge MA: MIT Press, 1987.

321. Annett M. Left, right, hand and brain: the right shift theory. London: Erlbaum, 1985.

322. Goodglass H, Quadfasel FA. Language laterality in the left-handed aphasics. Brain 1954;77:521–548.

323. Subirana A. The relationship between handedness and language function. Int J Neurol 1964;4:215–234.

324. McGlone J. Sex differences in human brain asymmetry: a critical survey. Behavioral and Brain Sciences 1980;3:215–263.

325. Caplan D. (in press). Language and the brain. In: Gernsbacher MA, ed. Handbook of psycholinguistics Academic Press.

326. Kinsbourne M. The minor cerebral hemisphere as a source of aphasic speech. Arch Neurol 1971;25:302–306.

327. Beauvois MF, Désrouésne, J. Phonological alexia: three dissociations. J Neurol Neurosurg Psychiatry 1979;42:1115–1124.

32

NEUROPSYCHIATRIC ASPECTS OF SEXUAL DYSFUNCTION

R. Taylor Segraves

Sexual function is an integral part of most of our patients' lives; therefore, some evaluation of sexual function should be part of a comprehensive medical evaluation. Unfortunately, this component often is omitted from psychiatric and neurological evaluations. This omission occurs in spite of the high prevalence of sexual problems in the general population (1, 2), medical outpatient populations (3–6), neurological patients (7), and certain psychiatric patients (8). Clearly, neurologists and neuropsychiatrists should be able to evaluate these disorders.

Because sexual behavior is multidimensional, assessing sexual function must consider biological as well as psychological variables. Within the field of psychiatry, there has been an emphasis on the interpersonal and intrapsychic determinants of sexual behavior. Except for a small number of investigators, very few biological psychiatrists have shown a major interest in sexual disorders. A similar situation exists within the field of neurology.

This chapter reviews a new and somewhat neglected area of neuropsychiatry—the neuropsychiatry of sexual dysfunction. Basic neurophysiology of sexual behavior is reviewed briefly first. This is followed by a discussion of drug effects on sexual behavior and by a review of sexual dysfunction occurring in association with neuropsychiatric disorders. The chapter concludes with a brief review of evaluation and treatment of sexual disorders.

NEUROPHYSIOLOGY OF THE HUMAN SEXUAL RESPONSE

Sexual physiology of the male has been more widely studied than that of the female. Accordingly, our knowledge of male sexual neurophysiology is more advanced than our knowledge of female physiology. Reflex vasodilation of the genital vasculature in response to sexual stimuli is responsible both for male penile erection and female lubrication (9, 10). Decreased vascular resistance in the penile corpora appears to be the major factor causing penile corpora vascular engorgement and penile erection (11). The smooth muscle of the corpora cavernosa is predominately innervated by adrenergic fibers, although cholinergic fibers are also present (12). α-Adrenergic impulses appear to maintain the penis in a nontumescent state (13). It is unclear whether a parallel innervation exists in the human female.

Neuroanatomical studies have demonstrated a dual innervation of the genitals in both sexes—sympathetic innervation from the T12–L4 segments of the spinal cord and parasympathetic innervation from the S2–S4 cord segments (14, 15). Stimulation of the sacral parasympathetic fibers has been shown to elicit penile erection in many species, and ablation of these nerves interferes with reflexogenic erections. These fibers are thought also to mediate the lubrication response in females. The postganglionic neurotransmitter in these parasympathetic fibers is unclear but does not appear to be acetylcholine.

The sympathetic outflow from the T12–L4 area contains both vasodilator and vasoconstrictor fibers. The exact nature of the contribution of these fibers to erection and lubrication is unclear. Some investigators have proposed that the sympathetic fibers mediate erections produced by erotic imagery and thoughts (e.g., psychogenic erections) as opposed to erections produced by tactile stimulation (e.g., reflexogenic reactions) (16). Presumably, a parallel mechanism exists in human females.

Stimulation and ablation experiments in laboratory animals, including mammals, have identified cerebral areas mediating erection. The major areas that elicit penile erection upon stimulation include the medial septopreoptic region and the medial part of the medial dorsal nucleus of the thalamus. Other areas involved in penile erection include septal projections of the hippocampus, the anterior cingulate gyrus, the mamillothalamic tract, and the mamillary bodies (17–19). The cerebral representation of vaginal lubrication is unknown.

Orgasm can be conceptualized as the sensory experience of a series of spinal cord reflexes. These reflexes are triggered when a series of sensory stimuli reach threshold values (20, 21). In the male, sensory impulses eliciting the ejaculatory reflex travel in the pudendal nerve to the sacral cord. Once a threshold value is reached, contractions of the vas deferens, seminal vesicles, and prostatic smooth muscle occur, resulting in the ejaculate being delivered into the pelvic urethra. Stimulation of the urethral bulb by the inflowing ejaculate elicits reflex closure of the bladder neck, preventing retrograde ejaculation, and rhythmic contractions of the perineal muscles and urethral bulb resulting in expulsion of the ejaculate (22).

Efferent fibers mediating ejaculation arise from the thoracolumbar cord, travel in the hypogastric nerve, and synapse with short adrenergic fibers that innervate the organs involved in orgasm. These fibers appear to be mainly α-adrenergic fibers, although these organs are also innervated by cholinergic fibers (23). Presumably, sensory impulses from the pudendal nerve to the sacral cord also are relayed cranially to the thalamus and sensory cortex, resulting in the experience of orgasm.

Female orgasm also appears to be a genital reflex. Sensory impulses travel to the sacral cord in the pudendal nerve, and efferent fibers innervate the ovary, fallopian tubes, vaginal musculature, and uterus. Rhythmic contractions of these structures appear to be mediated by α-adrenergic fibers, although the female sexual organs also have a cholinergic innervation.

Animal research has identified both subcortical and cortical structures associated with the ejaculatory reflex (24). In the monkey, ejaculation can be elicited by stimulation of the anterior thalamus and preoptic area (17). In both the human male and female, direct stimulation of the septal region of the brain has been reported to produce sexual orgasm (25, 26). Using deep recording electrodes, researchers have demonstrated that sexual orgasm in the human is accompanied by electrical discharges in the septal area (27).

Sensory representation of genital sensations appear to be localized in the paracentral lobule. Penfield and Rasmussen (28) reported that stimulation of the posterior part of the postcentral gyrus produced genital sensations, and epileptics with lesions in the paracentral lobule reported genital sensations as part of the aura (29).

Current evidence suggests that central dopamine and serotonin pathways are involved in sexual behavior. Animal studies have demonstrated that drugs that increase brain dopaminergic activity lower thresholds for ejaculatory and erectile reflexes (30). Infusions of dopamine agonists into the medial preoptic region and into the lumbar cord augment male sexual behavior (31, 32). Male patterns of sexual behavior are increased by drugs that lower brain serotonin levels (33–34). Other studies have demonstrated that destruction of central nervous system serotonergic fibers in the medial forebrain bundle facilitates ejaculation in laboratory animals (35).

From the preceding review of the neurophysiology of sexual behavior, it is clear that various neurological lesions could interfere with sexual behavior. These include lesions in the brain, cord, and peripheral nerves. It is also clear that many commonly prescribed drugs—especially psychiatric and hypotensive drugs that affect monoamine neuromodulators—might alter both central nervous system function and sexual behavior.

PSYCHIATRIC DRUGS AND SEXUAL BEHAVIOR

Within the last decade, physicians have become increasingly aware that many commonly prescribed drugs adversely affect sexual functioning. Although the list of drugs with adverse sexual side effects is quite extensive, the worst offenders are psychiatric drugs and drugs used to treat arterial hypertensive disease (36).

Antipsychotic drugs have been reported to cause disturbances in libido, ejaculatory impairment, female anorgasmia, and erectile failure (37, 38) Current evidence suggests that interference with orgasm is secondary to α-adrenergic blockade and that interference with libido and erectile capacity is probably secondary to central dopamine blockade (39). Case reports and clinical series have documented diminished libido with chlorpromazine, thioridazine, thiothixine, fluphenazine, and haloperidol (37). Erectile failure has been reported with chlorpromazine (40), pimozide (41), thiothixine (42), thioridazine (43–45), sulpiride (46), haloperidol (47), and fluphenazine (48). Many of these same neuroleptics have been reported to interfere with ejaculatory function (14). One controlled double-blind study of the effect of neuroleptics on sexual function in the human by Tennett and colleagues (49) found that low doses of benperidol (1.25 mg) and chlorpromazine (125 mg) had no effect on erectile function. When a patient complains of sexual dysfunction due to an antipsychotic drug, changing the patient to a different neuroleptic such as loxapine or molindone (with lesser alpha-adrenergic effects) may resolve the sexual problem.

Although benzodiazepines probably do not have adverse effects on erectile function (14), there is evidence that these drugs cause ejaculatory delay and may be used to treat premature ejaculation (50–55). If ejaculatory delay is a serious difficulty, buspirone might be substituted for the offending agent.

There have been case studies showing that lithium carbonate may cause erectile impairment (56). This has been confirmed in a double-blind placebo-controlled trial using therapeutic doses in men with affective disorder (57). Valproate might be considered as an alternative to lithium in bipolar patients who experience erectile failure on lithium.

Antidepressants have been reported to have a variety of sexual side effects. Heterocyclics, monoamine oxidase inhibitors, and SSRIs including imipramine, desipramine, nortriptyline, amitriptyline, doxepin, protriptyline, amoxapine, trazodone, maprotiline, tranylcypromine, phenelzine, bupropion, and fluoxetine (58) reportedly have caused diminished libido. The only controlled double-blind study of antidepressant effects on libido found that both phenelzine and imipramine decrease libido (59).

Treatment approaches for antidepressant-induced low libido include the coadministration of 7.5–15 mg of neostig-

Table 32.1.   Psychiatric Drugs Reported to Cause Erectile Dysfunction

Imipramine	Amoxapine
Desipramine	Trazodone
Nortriptyline	Maprotiline
Amitriptyline	Tranylcypromine
Doxepin	Phenelzine
Protriptyline	Isocarboxazid
Clomipramine	Lithium carbonate
Chlorpromazine	Thioridazine
Pimozide	Sulpiride
Thiothixene	Haloperidol
Fluphenazine	

Table 32.2.   Psychiatric Drugs Reported to Cause Orgasm Disturbances

Fluoxetine	Amitryptyline
Sertraline	Doxepin
Paroxetine	Protriptyline
Imipramine	Clomipramine
Desipramine	Amoxapine
Nortriptyline	Trazodone
Tranylcypromine	Maprotiline
Phenylzine	Alprazolam
Isocarboxazid	Chlordiazepoxide
Lorazepam	Thioridazine
Chlorpromazine	Mesoridazine
Chlorprothixine	Fluphenazine
Perphenazine	Thiothixene
Trifluoperazine	Haloperidol

mine prior to coitus (60), the coadministration of yohimbine with fluoxetine (61), or the substitution of bupropion because this drug has a very low incidence of sexual side effects (62). The mechanism by which antidepressant drugs influence libido is unclear. A similarly large group of antidepressants have been reported to cause erectile problems. Only one controlled study has documented an adverse effect of antidepressant drugs on erectile function (58). Kowalski and colleagues (63), in a double-blind placebo-controlled study, found that both amitriptyline and mianserin decreased erectile capacity as measured by nocturnal penile tumescence. It appears that substitution of bupropion may be an effective intervention for antidepressant-induced erectile impairment (62). Anorgasmia and delayed ejaculation have been reported with phenelzine (64), amoxapine (65), amitriptyline (66), clomipramine (67), imipramine (68), fluoxetine (69), trazodone (70), and sertraline (71). Double-blind studies have confirmed the effects of phenelzine, imipramine, and clomipramine on orgasm (58). Increased serotonergic activity may be a mechanism by which antidepressant drugs inhibit orgasm (72). Antidepressant-induced anorgasmia has been reported to be reversed by the use of bethanechol (73), cyproheptadine (74), and yohimbine (75). Drug substitution with desipramine or bupropion has also been reported to be effective (58).

It is noteworthy that spontaneous orgasm has been reported with clomipramine (76) and fluoxetine (77). There has also been a case report of trazodone being successfully used to treat male erectile disorder (78). Psychiatric drugs that have been reported to cause erectile and ejaculatory problems are listed in Tables 32.1 and 32.2.

HYPOTENSIVE AGENTS

Antihypertensive drugs are another class of drugs that have been found to frequently interfere with sexual function. Current evidence indicates that any clinician encountering a patient with sexual dysfunction should immediately inquire about drug usage and to suspect hypotensive agents as a possible etiologic agent. These drugs have been reported to interfere with erection, ejaculation, orgasm, and libido. The reader is referred elsewhere (5, 14, 39, 37) for more extensive reviews of this literature.

Diuretics are frequently utilized in the management of mild hypertension and were previously thought to be devoid of sexual side effects. Current evidence suggests that hydrochlorothiazide, chlorthalidone, and spironolactone may decrease libido as well as cause erectile problems (79–82). Spironolactone's antilibidinal effects may be related to its antiandrogen effect (83). The mechanism by which other diuretics influence sexual behavior is unclear. Antihypertensive drugs with central antiadrenergic effects, such as methyldopa and reserpine, have been reported to cause diminished libido, erectile failure, and ejaculatory impairment (37, 39). Current evidence also suggests that β-blockers may be associated with erectile failure (84, 85). The available evidence suggests that β-blockers that are more lipophilic are more likely to cause sexual dysfunction than those that are more hydrophilic, although impotence has been reported with atenolol, a hydrophilic β-blocker. Sexual problems appear to be less frequent with pindolol, metoprolol, and nadolol. Impotence has been reported as a side effect of timolol eye drops, which are systemically absorbed (86). Ejaculatory problems appear to be quite common with guanethidine, bethanidine, labetolol, and nifedipine (36). Among antihypertensive drugs, the angiotensin-converting-enzyme inhibitors, such as captopril, enalapril, and lisinopril, appear to lack sexual side effects.

OTHER DRUGS

Controlled studies indicate that cimetidine can cause decreased libido and erectile failure (87). Other H_2-receptor antagonists, such as ranitidine, appear to have this side effect less often. The mechanism for this phenomenon is unclear, since cimetidine has both antiandrogenic effects and ganglion-blocking effects. Controlled studies have also found decreased libido and erectile problems associated with long-term use of digoxin (88, 89). Antiepileptic drugs have been reported to decrease libido. Phenobarbital and primidone have been reported to have more adverse effects than phenytoin and carbamazepine (90). It is difficult to evaluate these reports because epilepsy may affect libido independent of drug effects. The reader is referred elsewhere for more extensive information concerning the effects of drugs on sexual function (36). Neuroendocrine issues in epilepsy are discussed in Chapter 12.

ENDOCRINE FUNCTION AND SEXUAL BEHAVIOR

In humans, normal endocrine function is necessary for reproduction. In subprimate mammals, sexual behavior is clearly hormonally dependent. In humans, the precise relationship between sexual behavior and endocrine function has not been established, with the relationship being less well understood for women. The tremendous influence of social learning on human sexuality contributes to the difficulty in determining endocrine effects on human sexual behavior.

In the human male, evidence concerning the relationship between endocrine function and sexual behavior can be obtained from studies of men who have been surgically castrated, men prescribed antiandrogens, and in hypogonadal men receiving androgen replacement therapy. Bilateral orchidectomy is used to treat sexual offenders in some countries, and as a palliative treatment for some neoplasms. Studies of patients following bilateral orchidectomy reveal a dramatic loss of libido, usually followed by an inability to ejaculate in most patients (91–93). However, a small number of patients remain sexually active for years past castration (94). The effects of castration are generally reversed by the administration of exogenous androgen. Some castrated males subsequently develop erectile problems. It has been hypothesized that these problems are secondary to attempted coitus in the presence of low libido and do not reflect a direct effect of androgen deficiency on erectile function (6). Studies of the effects of estrogenic compounds medroxyprogesterone and cyproterone acetate have shown that these drugs markedly diminish libido without interfering with erectile capacity (91). In men with a disease state of hypogonadism, it has been shown that androgen therapy restores libido and seminal emission (95). Thus, evidence from three different sources of information indicates that androgen levels are closely linked to seminal emission and sexual drive in the human male. Current evidence suggests that a certain minimal level of androgen is necessary for sexual function but that excess androgen above these levels has minimal or no effects.

In many subprimates, female sexual activity is restricted to estrus and is clearly related to estrogen or progesterone levels. In primates, the relationship between sexual activity and endocrine variables is more obscure. Current evidence suggests that estrogen levels are essential to vaginal epithelial integrity and lubrication, whereas androgen levels may be related to libido. Most of the evidence concerning endocrine effects on female sexual behavior consists of studies of sexual behavior across the menstrual cycle, with the use androgen therapy, and during hormonal replacement therapy.

A number of investigators have studied sexual activity across the menstrual cycle and in relationship to cyclic changes of progesterone and estradiol. A variety of measures, including coital frequency, self-rating of libido, and arousability to sexual stimuli as measured by vaginal plethysmography have been utilized (91). To date, there are no consistent data relating cyclic changes in estrogens or progesterone during the menstrual cycle and sexual activity. There is some evidence that sexual libido and arousability may be related serum androgen levels (96–100). In the past, androgen therapy was used for a number of medical conditions, and increased libido was noted as a side effect of this therapy (91). Some clinicians have reported using androgen therapy to treat hypoactive sexual desire disorders; others have reported that antiandrogens lower libido in females. The strongest evidence relating androgens to female libido has been reported by the McGill University research group. In a number of controlled studies (101, 102) they showed that estrogen-androgen preparations are superior to estrogen and placebo in restoring sexual function to patients with surgical menopause.

Hyperprolactinemia has been reported to be associated with decreased libido in both sexes (91). Male patients may also complain of erectile problems. In many cases, bromocriptine therapy will restore normal function.

NEUROLOGICAL DISEASE AND SEXUAL DYSFUNCTION

A number of neurological diseases have been reported to be associated with sexual dysfunction and should be considered in the differential diagnosis of a patient with sexual difficulties. In diseases causing peripheral neuropathies, the mechanism is usually clear. In diseases affecting the brain, the specific mechanisms usually are unclear.

Multiple Sclerosis

A number of different investigators have established that multiple sclerosis can cause decreased libido, decreased arousal, decreased sexual sensations, and decreased orgasmic capacity in both sexes, as well as decreased erectile response in male patients (103–107). Estimates of the frequency of sexual problems in such patients have ranged widely, from 26–90% (7, 103). Sexual life in such patients can be altered by various mechanisms, including neuropathological lesions in the brain as well as in the cord. In this regard, hypersexuality has been reported in a multiple sclerosis patient with frontal and temporal lesions (108). Psychosocial factors may also contribute to altered sexual function.

Diabetes Mellitus

Diabetes mellitus is known to be associated with erectile failure and to a lesser extent with ejaculatory disturbance (109–115). Decreased erectile function in diabetic males has been confirmed by nocturnal penile tumescence studies (116, 117) and by laboratory-based erotic stimulation studies (118). These sexual difficulties are suspected to be secondary to peripheral neuropathy of the autonomic nervous system (119, 120) although one investigator has suggested that cerebral dysregulation of autonomic nervous system activity may be responsible (121). Kolodny (122) reported that diabetic women had an increased frequency of acquired orgasmic dysfunction; however, numerous other investigators have failed to replicate this finding (123). Decreased vaginal lubrication in insulin-dependent diabetics has been consistently reported (124–126). One exception is a study by Schreiner-Engel and colleagues at the Mount Sinai School of Medicine (127). In this study, type I (insulin-dependent) diabetics had minimal evidence of sexual impairment whereas type II diabetics suffered both sexual and relationship discord. This finding is discrepant from many other studies and may reflect the interaction of psychosocial variables with the disease process. For example, it is postulated that some of the sexual impairment in type II diabetes may be secondary to the emotional consequences of a late-onset disease.

Spinal Cord Injury

One of the most common causes of neurogenic sexual difficulty in males is spinal cord injury. Although certain general statements can be made concerning site of the lesion and the resulting sexual impairment, there is some inconsistency in the literature. In most series, the location and completeness of the series are deduced by clinical examination, thus allowing for incorrect assignment of the level of lesion and the presence of partial communication between the brain and the partially severed cord. Complete cervical and high thoracic cord lesions are extremely destructive to ejaculatory function (128). Depending on the level of the cord lesion, reflexogenic erections to local stimuli or psychogenic erections to psychic stimuli may be intact. Reflexogenic erections occur most often in patients with complete upper motor lesions, especially in men with cervical lesions. Psychogenic erections are intact most often with lower motor neuron lesions below T9.

There is relatively little information concerning sexual behavior in female patients with cord lesions. Comarr and Vigue (129) could not correlate sexual function with any given level of cord lesion, although Berard (130), in his investigation of 15 cord-injured women, concluded that orgasm was impossible if the lesion was below T12, because of decreased sensation.

Damage to Autonomic Nervous System

A number of surgical procedures interfere with autonomic nervous system innervation of the pelvic organs and result in sexual impairment. These procedures include sympathectomies (131), retroperitoneal lymphadenectomy (132), abdominoperitoneal resection (133), anterior resection of the rectum (134), aortoiliac surgery (135, 136), and radical retropubic and transvesical prostatectomy (137). Most of these same procedures have been reported to cause orgasm disorders in female patients (138).

Seizure Disorder

Both ictal and intraictal sexual abnormalities have been noted in patients with epilepsy (139). Ictal sexual manifestations, such as sexual emotions, genital sensations, and sexual automatisms are somewhat rare and appear to be more common during partial complex seizures (140). Sexual auras are reported to have a temporal lobe origin (141–143), although the origin of other ictal sexual behavior is less clear.

Interictal sexual abnormalities are more common than ictal sexual abnormalities. Although hypersexuality (144) and paraphilia (145–147) have been reported, hyposexuality is the more common finding (148–154). Sexual abnormalities appear to be more common in patients with partial complex seizures (139). Partial complex seizures of temporal lobe origin are more commonly associated with sexual abnormalities than seizures from extratemporal foci (154), although there are examples of altered sexuality from extratemporal foci (153). Several different factors might explain altered sexual behavior in patients with epilepsy: "These include social and psychological factors, disruption of normal limbic function by epileptic discharges, altered pituitary and gonadal hormones, and alteration of behavior and hormones by AEDs" (139, p. 541).

Judging the importance of these factors in a given case can be quite difficult. However, in most cases the degree of alteration of pituitary and gonadal dysfunction associated with the epilepsy itself is insufficient to explain the degree of hyposexuality observed (90, 155). Some of the hyposexuality observed in some epileptics might be explained by the effects of antiepileptic drugs on endocrine function (156, 157). Testosterone exists in three forms in the serum: a free form, which is biologically active; a form loosely bound to albumin; and an inactive form, which is tightly bound to sex hormone-binding globulin. A number of antiepileptic drugs, notably carbamazepine, decrease the amount of free testosterone. Low levels of free testosterone appear to be related to decreased libido. Unfortunately, androgen replacement therapy has been only moderately successful in improving libido in men with epilepsy.

Other Neurological Diseases

A number of clinicians have noted a high frequency of sexual problems in patients with Parkinson's disease (158, 159). However, Lipe and colleagues (160) reported that the degree of sexual impairment in patients with Parkinson's disease is no higher than that in patients with arthritis. This suggests that the impairment may be due to chronic illness in general, and not specific to the disease process of Parkinson's disease. *Hyper*sexuality has repeatedly been reported in parkinsonian patients treated with dopaminergic drugs (161).

Another syndrome frequently associated with a decreased frequency of sexual activity is cerebral vascular accident (162–164). Although some investigators report that most men who were sexually active prior to stroke resume sexual activity, other investigators have found more devastating effects on sexual behavior (165–168). There are several potential mechanisms for the decrease in sexual activity, including hypotensive medications, partner reaction, immobility, and deformity. There is minimal evidence regarding specific brain regions infarcted and the likelihood of resulting sexual impairment. An important exception is the report of Monga and colleagues of *hyper*sexuality after stroke involving the temporal lobe close to the amygdaloid nucleus (169).

Similarly, most studies of brain trauma patients have documented hyposexuality (170, 171); however, hypersexuality has been noted after injury to the temporal lobes and to the dorsal septal region (172, 173). Damage to the hypothalamopituitary region of the brain by tumor results in decreased libido, which appears to be correlated with the degree of hypogonadism (174). Erectile failure has been reported to be common in patients with Alzheimer's disease (175). One case of hypersexuality in Huntington's chorea has been reported (176).

PSYCHIATRIC DISORDERS AND SEXUAL DYSFUNCTION

Recently, the prevalence of sexual disorders in various psychiatric diseases was reviewed (177). A number of investigators have documented the loss of libido and decreased sexual function in the presence of depressive disorder (178–180). Loss of libido is a common symptom in both dysthymia and major depression (181). After age 70, loss of libido is less indicative of depression primarily because loss of libido is common among nondepressed elderly (182, 183). As well as loss of libido, major depression may also be associated with decreased ability to attain and maintain penile erections (184, 185). Interestingly, Schreiner-Engel and Schiavi (186) reported that nondepressed patients with low sexual desire had an elevated lifetime prevalence rate of affective disorders. They hypothesized that there may be a common etiology to hypoactive sexual desire disorder and depressive disorders. During manic episodes, an increase in sexual thoughts, conduct, and number of sexual partners may occur. Some of the hypersexuality seen in manic patients can be a reflection of premorbid personality (177).

As Offit concluded in her summary of the evidence concerning sexuality and schizophrenia, "The literature is quite inconsistent about changes in sexual behavior among schizophrenics" (177, p. 2255). Part of this inconsistency may relate to changing diagnostic criteria and to alternative assessments of sexual behavior. Several well-conducted studies (187, 188) using good methodology have reported decreased sexual interest and activity among patients with schizophrenia.

Information concerning sexual behavior in other psychiatric disorders is scarce. Women with anorexia nervosa appear to have markedly diminished sexual activity and interest (189). There is little evidence linking any specific personality disorder with sexual difficulties, apart from the high frequency of sexual identity issues in young adults with borderline personality disorder. Patients with sensitivity to rejection (190) and a predisposition to anxiety and depression may be more likely to develop sexual problems (191).

NEUROPSYCHIATRIC EVALUATION OF SEXUAL DYSFUNCTION

A critical part of the evaluation of any sexual complaint is a careful history. The clinician needs to document the precise difficulty, the associated symptoms, its onset and course, and consider if the difficulty is secondary to another psychiatric disorder, such as affective disorder. One needs to ascertain gender identity and sexual preference for partners as well as assessing whether the problem appears secondary to relationship discord or life stress. One also needs to carefully delineate whether the disorder is generalized or partner-specific. It is unusual for biogenic sexual problems to be partner-specific. Thus, a history of a partner-specific difficulty is presumptive evidence of a psychogenic difficulty.

In cases of hypoactive sexual desire disorders, one needs to inquire closely regarding the frequency of romantic daydreams and sexual thoughts. A high frequency of sexual daydreams suggests that the problem is not biogenic. One also needs to inquire about masturbatory frequency and the preferred masturbatory fantasy. Obviously, a high frequency of masturbatory behavior or an aberrant sexual fantasy life would suggest that the problem is not biogenic. If one determines that the decreased desire is present in all contexts, one would have a greater suspicion that the problem might be biogenic and would evaluate androgen and prolactin levels.

Deficient sexual arousal as evidenced by decreased vaginal lubrication as an isolated complaint is almost always caused by atrophic vulvovaginitis, related to estrogen deficiency. Psychogenic arousal disorder in the female almost always occurs in conjunction with hypoactive sexual desire disorder (192).

Diagnostic evaluation of male erectile disorder can be quite complex. A careful sexual history should be a major part of the evaluation. The presence of full erections upon awakening is highly suggestive of a psychogenic erectile problem (193). To date there is minimal evidence that psychometric assessment aids in the differential diagnosis of biogenic from psychogenic erectile disorder (194). A global screening procedure to measure erectile capacity is to monitor nocturnal erections with a nocturnal penile tumescence (NPT) study (195, 196). The clinician needs to be aware of a number of possibly confounding influences, including affective disorder, aging, hypoandrogenic states, and hypoactive desire states. Barring these limitations, a large amount of normative data allow the clinician to judge deviancy from these values given normal sleep parameters. Alternative nonlaboratory approaches include snap gauges and portable nocturnal erection monitors (e.g., Rigiscan). The lack of sleep monitoring limits the diagnostic accuracy of these approaches. Another general screening procedure is the visual sexual stimulation method. In this procedure, the erectile response to erotica is monitored (197). The reliability, validity, sensitivity and specificity of this approach has not been established.

A variety of procedures can be used to test the integrity of the vascular system. Penile blood pressure, strain gauge plethysmography, and pulse wave assessment all have been employed; however, all of these procedures only assess hemodynamics in the flaccid penis. Intracorporal injection of papaverine/phentolamine or prostaglandin E_1 can be used to assess functional integrity of the penile vasculature. Unfortunately, it is not clear how much vascular disease must be present to cause diminution of the pharmacologically induced erection. A decreased response provides suggestive but not definitive evidence of vasculogenic impotence (195). More invasive procedures include cavernosometry and cavernosography (198, 199). To date, lack of standardization limits the usefulness of these procedures.

Most of the procedures currently available to assess integrity of the neurological components of erection primarily assess the pudendal nerve. Bulbocavernosus reflex latency testing consists of recording the EMG response of the bulbocavernosus muscle to electrical stimulation of the dorsal nerve of the penis. Absent or prolonged reflex latency indicates pathology within the reflex arc (200). A variation of this procedure is to stimulate the prostatic urethra, testing for autonomic neuropathy. Other procedures include measuring dorsal nerve conduction velocity, the threshold for perception of vibratory sensations in the penis, and somatosensory evoked potentials evoked by penile stimulation. All of the procedures can detect neurological abnormalities. However, the absence of adequate normative data limits the interpretation of these findings (195). In other words, it is unclear what values are clearly indicative of neurogenic impotence.

Premature ejaculation rarely has an organic cause, with the possible exception of acquired premature ejaculation as an early manifestation of multiple sclerosis. If the patient complains of retarded ejaculation, one can distinguish between retrograde ejaculation and an ejaculatory orgasm by examination of the postorgasm-spun urine sample. Anything that interrupts the orgasmic reflex arc can interfere with both male and female orgasmic function. Acquired orgasm disorder in the absence of marital discord mandates a search for treatable biogenic causes. Numerous drugs can cause orgasmic dysfunction. Also, numerous neuropathies (e.g., diabetes mellitus, multiple sclerosis, alcoholic neuropathy) and surgical procedures (e.g., aortoiliac surgery, lumbar sympathectomy, retroperitoneal lymphadenectomy) can cause anorgasmia. Severe hypogonadism in the male can result in anorgasmia. The sensory part of the orgasmic reflex arc could theoretically be measured by somatosensory evoked potentials or by the threshold for vibratory sensation.

To my knowledge, these procedures have not been used for that purpose.

PSYCHOLOGICAL TREATMENT OF SEXUAL DISORDERS

The psychological treatment of sexual dysfunction is based on techniques introduced by behavioral psychologists and then elaborated by Masters and Johnson (201). To briefly summarize, these techniques focus on attitude change and anxiety reduction. Sexual activity is structured such that there is the progressive experience of emotional and sexual intimacy at a pace tolerable to both partners. Preferably, the couple is seen together on a once-a-week basis. Either a dual-sex therapy team or a solo therapist of either sex may be used. More detailed descriptions of this treatment approach can be found elsewhere (177, 201, 202).

PHARMACOLOGICAL TREATMENT OF SEXUAL DISORDERS

Currently, there is evidence that both premature ejaculation and iatrogenic erectile disorder may respond to pharmacological interventions. Clinicians have reported successfully using low doses of thioridazine (203, 204), monoamine oxidase inhibitors (205), lorazepam (52), and clomipramine (206) in the treatment of premature ejaculation. One double-blind placebo-controlled study (207) has demonstrated that 25–50 mg clomipramine taken 6 hours prior to coitus extends the time to ejaculation by 6–8 minutes in men with premature ejaculation.

Current evidence suggests that yohimbine is effective in reversing certain cases of idiopathic erectile dysfunction (208). In a 10-week, double-blind partial cross-over study of yohimbine in the treatment of psychogenic erectile problems, Reid and colleagues (209) found yohimbine to be clearly superior to placebo. Two other studies (210, 211) of yohimbine have found it to be effective in the treatment of idiopathic erectile dysfunction. Current evidence suggests that yohimbine has its mechanism of action in the central nervous system. Direct injection of yohimbine into the corpora cavernosa does not induce erection, whereas intracerebral injection increases various parameters of sexual behavior in laboratory animals (208).

There is suggestive evidence that dopaminergic drugs and/or opioid-receptor blockers may prove useful in the treatment of human sexual disorders. Anecdotal evidence suggests that dopaminergic drugs such as levodopa and pergolide may increase libido (14). A number of independent investigators (212–214) have demonstrated in controlled studies that apomorphine administered subcutaneously in the arm elicits penile erections. In an open trial, Lal and associates (215) reported that oral bromocriptine is effective in men with impotence who previously demonstrated an erectile response to injected apomorphine. Unfortunately, side effects from apomorphine render it unsuitable as a treatment for erectile problems. There have been two controlled studies (216, 217) of the efficacy of levodopa in the treatment of erectile problems. Unfortunately, the results of these studies were contradictory. Although it is well known that opiate abuse may diminish libido, there are relatively few studies of the effects of opioid antagonists on sexual function. Charney and Heninger (218) reported that infusion of 1/mg/kg solution of naloxone resulted in partial penile erections in normal volunteers. In a placebo-controlled study of the efficacy of naltrexone in the treatment of erectile dysfunction, Fabbri et al. (219) reported that 50 mg of naltrexone significantly improved erectile function.

NEUROPSYCHIATRY OF GENDER IDENTITY AND SEXUAL PREFERENCE

The origins of gender identity and sexual orientation have been a subject of intense debate within the scientific community (220). Early sexologists such as Kraft-Ebing (221) argued that homosexuality must be innate, and numerous investigations have attempted to find evidence to support this viewpoint (222–224). In the 20th century, the work by John Money and his colleagues (225, 226) has been very influential in the United States. From studies of psychosexual development in children with ambiguous sexual development, it was concluded that gender identity is predominately determined by sex of rearing prior to age 2½ years. By contrast, Gunter Donner (227) suggested that a neuroendocrine predisposition for homosexuality might be based on the effects of prenatal androgen deficiency on the developing hypothalamus. This theory was largely ignored by many American sexologists. A major challenge to the concept of the predominant influence of rearing on sexual identity and orientation came from the work of Imperato-McGinley and associates (228) on the psychosexual development of children with 5-α-reductase deficiency. Genetic male children with this disorder are raised as females and then assume masculine roles at puberty. Although others (229) have questioned whether these children are raised unambiguously as females early in life, the work by this group rekindled interest in the search for biological etiologies to gender identity and sexual orientation. A fascinating series of recent reports suggests that sexual orientation may have biological correlates. However, most of these findings to date have not been verified by other investigations. Biological correlates of gender identity have received somewhat less study.

Prior to considering the biological factors that influence gender identity and sexual orientation, it is important to review basic definitions and to emphasize the complexity of this subject. For the human, gender identity may be defined as the persistent belief that one is male, female, or ambivalent. Current evidence suggests that sex assignment by parents plays a major role in determining gender identity. Gender role may be defined as behavior that society designates as masculine or feminine. Current evidence suggests that gender role behavior is influenced by gonadal

hormones during development (230). Sexual orientation refers to the erotic responsiveness of one individual to others of the same or opposite sex. The complexity of the area can be comprehended if one considers the situation where a genetic male raised by his parents as a male, but who has a behavior pattern that society defines as extremely feminine or effeminate. Such a male raised in a subculture that rigidly defines sex-specific behavior patterns might have difficulty being accepted as masculine by his peers or as an attractive love object by the opposite sex. A similar male raised in a different subculture might have considerably less difficulty. One can further complicate the situation by assuming that one parent encouraged role-discrepant behavior and gender identity, whereas the other did not. Clearly, the interaction between psychological and biological factors could be exceedingly complex to unravel because the manifestation of these early influences may not be evident until adult life.

Three basic strategies have been employed in the investigation of biological correlates of gender identity and sexual orientation. These can be labeled as heritability, neuroendocrine, and neuroanatomical studies. The neuroendocrine and neuroanatomical studies are based on animal models of the effects of prenatal hormones on sexual behavior and sexual differentiation of the brain.

Heritability

A number of twin studies have suggested approximately a 50% concordance rate for homosexuality in monozygotic twins (220). Most of these studies are deficient in terms of sample size or lack systematic sampling of a well-specified population. Bailey and Pillard (231, 232) have recently published their work concerning concordance for homosexuality in co-twins. In a study of male homosexuality, probands were solicited in a homophile publication by advertising for homosexual or bisexual men with either co-twins or adoptive brothers. Probands were asked to rate the sexual orientation of the co-twin or adoptive brother. Fifty-two percent of the 56 monozygotic co-twins were either homosexual or bisexual as compared with 22% of the 54 dizygotic co-twins and 11% of the 57 adoptive brothers. A similar methodology was employed in the study of the heritability of sexual orientation in women. In this study, 48% of monozygotic co-twins were homosexual or bisexual as compared with 16% of dizygotic co-twins and 6% of adoptive sisters. Somewhat similar findings were reported by Whitam and colleagues in 1993 (233). All of these studies can be criticized for not having a representative sample of the homosexual population. More recently, Hamer and co-workers (234) reported a pedigree and linkage analysis on 114 families of homosexual men. Index subjects, recruited from an HIV clinic and local homophile organizations, were asked to rate the sexuality of their fathers, sons, brothers, uncles, and male cousins. The highest rates of homosexuality were found in brothers, maternal uncles, and the sons of maternal aunts, suggesting that some instances of homosexuality might be male-limited and maternally inherited. To test this, they recruited families in which there were two homosexual brothers, no more than one lesbian relative, and no indication of direct father-to-son transmission of homosexuality. The sample for the linkage analysis consisted of 40 pairs of homosexual brothers together with mothers or siblings, if available. This study found a significant correlation between sexual orientation and the inheritance of genetic markers on chromosomal region X_q 28. The authors state that confirmation of their results is essential.

The available evidence is strongly suggestive of a genetic contribution to sexual orientation. The twin studies, in spite of possible sampling bias, are consistent in their findings. Pedigree studies must also be confirmed. To this author's knowledge, there have been no genetic studies of gender identity.

Neuroendocrine Studies

Most of these studies are based on the assumption that one can extrapolate from animal studies to sexual behavior in man. The underlying model differentiates the organizational aspects (enduring effects on the developing brain) from the activating (reversible) aspects of hormones. The basic assumption is that male heterosexuality, female homosexuality, and female-to-male transsexualism all result from prenatal exposure to high levels of testicular hormones. Male homosexuality, female heterosexuality, and male-to-female transsexualism are postulated to result from lower levels of prenatal testicular hormones, thus retaining a female pattern of brain organization. Studies of gender identity and sexual orientation in syndromes involving prenatal androgen insensitivity or deficiency in males and studies of females with syndromes involving androgen excess have, by and large, not produced evidence consistent with the prenatal hormonal hypothesis (220). The other major approach has been to study hormonal feedback mechanisms. The underlying assumption in these studies is that androgens have an organizing effect on the developing brain, abolishing the ability of estrogen to exert positive feedback on luteinizing hormone (LH) release. Thus, if male homosexuality or male-to-female transsexualism is associated with a deficiency of prenatal androgenization, then these groups should demonstrate more positive feedback than heterosexuals. Several studies (235, 236) found that male homosexuals had LH responses to estrogen stimulation that were intermediate between those of women and those of heterosexual men. Similar findings were reported in male-to-female transsexuals. Subsequent studies have failed to find differences in the neuroendocrine regulation of LH secretion between transsexuals, homosexuals, and heterosexuals (237).

Neuroanatomical Studies

LeVay (238) reported that heterosexual men, as compared with heterosexual females and homosexual men, have greater volume of the third interstitial nucleus of the anterior hypothalamus. Byne and Parsons (220) criticized this study on several grounds, the most important of which is that all of the brain tissue in homosexuals were from men who died of complications of AIDS. The other major issues of note are the small sample size (19 homosexual men, 16 heterosexual men, and 8 women) and the absence of replication. Byne and Parsons (220) also pointed out that there is no evidence that this area of the hypothalamus plays a critical role in generation of male-typical sexual behavior.

There has also been a report that the suprachiasmatic nucleus of the hypothalamus is larger in homosexual than heterosexual men (239). The meaning of this report is unclear because the size of this nucleus does not vary between men and women, and there is no evidence that this nucleus regulates sexual behavior (232). This study has not been confirmed by an independent laboratory.

Allen and Gorski (240) recently reported that the anterior commissure is larger in its midsagittal area in women and homosexual men than in heterosexual men. This study also has not been replicated. This is especially important because the only other study of sex differences in the anterior commissure found a tendency for it to be larger in men than in women (232).

CONCLUSION

It is clear that our understanding of the neuropsychiatry of sexual dysfunction is in its infancy. One factor hindering the development of a coherent model of the biological basis of sexual behavior is that the requisite knowledge base is spread across numerous disciplines. The adverse effects of both hypotensive and psychiatric drugs on sexual behavior as well as the effects of specific neurological lesions on sexual behavior can be seen as an opportunity to deduce probable neurochemical and neuroanatomical substrates for such behavior. The shortage of literature concerning biological treatment of sexual dysfunction attests to the need for further exploration. Fortunately, there is growing awareness that events and structures within the central nervous system are intimately associated with human sexual behavior. It is the hope of this author that the field of neuropsychiatry will incorporate the study of human sexual behavior within its purview.

References

1. Frank E, Anderson C, Rubinstein D. Frequency of sexual dysfunction in normal couples. N Engl J Med 1978;299:111–115.
2. Nettelbladt P, Uddenberg N. Sexual dysfunction and sexual satisfaction in 58 married Swedish men. Psychomatic Research 1979;23:141–147.
3. Slag MF, Mortem JE, Elson MK. Impotence in medical clinical outpatients. JAMA 1983;249:1736–1740.
4. Segraves RT, Schoenberg NW. Diagnosis and treatment of erectile problems: current status. In: RT Segraves, NW Schoenberg, eds. Diagnosis and treatment of erectile disturbances: a guide for clinicians. New York: Plenum, 1985:1–22.
5. Papadopoulos C. Sexual aspects of cardiovascular disease. New York: Praeger, 1989.

6. Bancroft J. Human sexuality and its problems. London: Churchill Livingstone, 1983.
7. Lundberg PO, Brattberg A, Hulter, B. Sexual dysfunction in patients with neurological and neuroendocrine disorders. In: Bezemer W, Cohen-Kettenis P, Slob K, van Son-Schooner N, eds. Sex matters. Amsterdam: Excerpta Medica, 1992:281–284.
8. Hawton K. Sexual dysfunctions and psychiatric disorders. In: Bezemer W, Cohen-Kettenis P, Slob K, van Son-Schooner N, eds. Sex matters. Amsterdam: Excerpta Medica, 1992:79–84.
9. Kaufman SA. The gynecologic evaluation of female excitement disorders. In: Kaplan HS, ed. The evaluation of sexual disorders: psychological and medical aspects. New York: Brunner/Mazel, 1983:122–127.
10. Rivard DJ. Anatomy, physiology, and neurophysiology of male sexual function. In: Bennett AH, ed. Management of male impotence. Baltimore: Williams & Wilkins, 1982:1–25.
11. Melman A. Neural and vascular control of education. In: Rosen RC, Leiblum SR, eds. Erectile disorders: assessment and treatment. New York: Guilford, 1992:55–71.
12. Benson GS, McConnell J, Lipshultz LI, Corrine JN, Wood J. Neuromorphology and neuropharmacology of the human penis. J Clin Invest 1980;65:605–612.
13. Sjostrand NO, Klinge E. Principal mechanisms controlling penile retraction and protrusion in rabbits. Acta Physiol Scand 1979;106:199–214.
14. Segraves RT. Effects of psychotropic drugs on human erection and ejaculation. Arch Gen Psychiatry 1989;46:275–284.
15. Kaufman SA. The gynecologic evaluation of female orgasm disorders. In: Kaplan HS, ed. The evaluation of sexual disorders: psychological and medical aspects. New York: Brunner/Mazel, 1983:117–121.
16. Bors E, Comarr AE. Neurological disturbances of sexual function with special reference to 529 patients with spinal cord injury. Urological Survey 1960;10:191–222.
17. MacLean PD. Brain mechanisms of primal sexual functions and related behavior. In: Sandler M, Gessa GL, eds. Sexual behavior: pharmacology and biochemistry. New York: Raven Press, 1975:1–12.
18. Dua S, MacLean PD. Localization for penile erection in medial frontal lobe. Am J Physiol 1964;207:1425–1434.
19. MacLean PD, Ploog DW. Cerebral representation of penile erection. J Neurophysiol 1962;25:29–55.
20. Bell C. Autonomic control of reproduction circulatory and other factors. Pharmacol Rev 1972;24:657–736.
21. Reckler JM. The urologic evaluation of ejaculatory disorders (male orgasm disorders, RE and PE). In: Kaplan HS, ed. The evaluation of sexual disorders: psychological and medical aspects. New York: Brunner/Mazel, 1983:139–149.
22. Kleeman FJ. The physiology of the internal urinary sphincter. J Urol 1970;104:549–554.
23. Robinson PM. A cholinergic component in the innervation of the longitudinal smooth muscle of the guinea pig vas deferens. J Cell Biol 1969;41:462–476.
24. Blumer D, Walker EA. The neural basis of sexual behavior. In: Besson DF, Blumer D, eds. Psychiatric aspects of neurologic disease. New York: Grune & Stratton, 1975:199–217.
25. Heath RG. Electrical self-stimulation of the brain in man. Am J Psychiatry 1963;120:571–577.
26. Heath RG. Brain function and behavior. J Nerv Ment Dis 1975;160:159–175.
27. Heath RG. Pleasure and brain activity in man: deep and surface electroencephalograms during orgasm. J Nerv Ment Dis 1972;154:3–18.
28. Penfield W, Rasmussen T. The cerebral cortex of man. New York: MacMillan, 1950.
29. Smith BH, Khatri AM. Cortical localization of sexual feeling. Psychosomatics 1979;20:771–776.
30. Gessa GL, Tagliamonte A. Role of brain monoamines in male sexual behavior. Life Sci 1974;14:425–436.
31. Foreman MM, Hall JL. Effects of D_2-dopaminergic receptor stimulation on male rat sexual behavior. J Neural Transm 1987;68:153–170.
32. Hasen S. Spiral control of sexual behavior: effects of intrathecal administration of lisuride. Neurosci Lett 1982;33:329–332.
33. Tucker TC, Ale SE. Serotonin and sexual behavior. In: Wheatley D, ed. Psychopharmacology and sexual disorders. New York: Oxford University Press, 1983:22–49.
34. Whalen RE, Luttge WG. Para-chlorophenylalanine methylester: an aphrodisiac. Science 1970;169:1000–1001.
35. Rodriquez M, Castro R, Hernandez G, Mas M. Different roles of catecholaminergic and serotoninergic neurons of the medial forebrain bundle on male rat sexual behavior. Physiol Behav 1984;33:5–11.
36. Segraves RT, Madsen R, Carter CS, Davis JM. Erectile dysfunction with pharmacological agents. In: Segraves RT, Schoenberg HW, eds. Diagnosis and treatment of erectile disturbances: a guide for clinicians. New York: Plenum Press, 1985:23–64.
37. Segraves RT. Drugs and desire. In: Leiblum SR, Rosen RC, eds. Sexual desire disorders. New York: Guilford Press, 1988:313–347.
38. Segraves RT. Sexual side-effects of psychiatric drugs. Int J Psychiatry Med 1988;18:243–252.
39. Segraves RT, Segraves KB. Aging and drug effects on male sexuality. In: Rosen SR, Leiblum SR, eds. Erectile disorders: assessment and treatment. New York: Guilford Press, 1992:96–138.
40. Greenberg HR. Inhibition of ejaculation by chlorpromazine. J Nerv Ment Dis 1971;152:364–366.
41. Ananth J. Impotence associated with pimozide. Am J Psychiatry 1982;139:1374.
42. Charalampous KD, Freemesser GF, Maleu J, Flord K. Loxapine succinate: a controlled double-blind study in schizophrenia. Current Therapeutics and Research 1974;16:829–837.
43. Sandison RA, Whitelaw E, Currie JDC. Clinical trials with Mellaril (TPZI) in the treatment of schizophrenia. Journal of Mental Science 1960;106:732–741.
44. Haider I. Thioridazine and sexual dysfunctions. International Journal of Neuropsychiatry 1966;2:255–257.
45. Witton K. Sexual dysfunction secondary to Mellaril. Diseases of the Nervous System 1962;23:175.
46. Weizman A, Maoz B, Treves I, Asher I, Ben-David M. Sulpiride-induced hyperprolactinemia and impotence in male psychiatric outpatients. Prog Neuropsychopharmacol Biol Psychiatry 1985;9:193–198.
47. Meco G, Falachi P, Casacchia M, et al. Neuroendocrine effects of haloperidol decanoate in patients with chronic schizophrenia. In: Kemal D, Ragagni G, eds. Chronic treatments in neuropsychiatry. New York: Raven Press, 1985:88–93.
48. Bartholomew AA. A long-acting phenothiazine as a possible agent to control deviant sexual behavior. Am J Psychiatry 1968;124:917–922.
49. Tennett G, Bancroft J, Cass J. The control of deviant sexual behavior by drugs: a double-blind controlled study of benperidol, chlorpromazine, and placebo. Arch Sex Behav 1974;3:261–271.
50. Riley AJ, Riley EJ. The effect of single dose diazepam on female sexual response induced by masturbation. Sexual and Marital Therapy 1986;1:49–53.
51. Hughes JM. Failure to ejaculate with chlordiazepoxide. Am J Psychiatry 1964;121:610–611.
52. Segraves RT. Treatment of premature ejaculation with lorazepam. Am J Psychiatry 1987;144:1240.
53. Uhde TW, Tancer ME, Shea CA. Sexual dysfunction related to alprazolam treatment of social phobia. Am J Psychiatry 1988;145:531–532.
54. Sangal R. Inhibited female orgasm as a side-effect of alprazolam. Am J Psychiatry 1985;142:1223–1224.
55. Munjack DJ, Crocker B. Alprazolam-induced ejaculatory inhibition. Journal of Clinical Psychopharmacology 1986;6:57–58.
56. Blay SL, Ferraz MPT, Calil HM. Lithium-induced male sexual impairment: two case reports. J Clin Psychiatry 1982;43:497–498.

57. Vinarova E, Uhlir O, Stika L. Side-effects of lithium administration. Activitas Nervosa Superior (Praha) 1972;14:105–107.

58. Segraves RT. Sexual dysfunction complicating the treatment of depression. J Clin Psychiatry (Monograph Series) 1992;1 (vol. 10):75–79.

59. Harrison WM, Rabkin JG, Ehrhardt AA, et al. Effects on antidepressant medication on sexual function: a controlled study. Journal of Clinical Psychopharmacology 1986;6:144–149.

60. Kraupl-Taylor F. Loss of libido in depression (Letter). Br Med J 1972;1:305.

61. Jacobsen FM. Fluoxetine-induced sexual dysfunction and an open trial of yohimbine. J Clin Psychiatry 1992;53:119–122.

62. Gardner EA, Johnston JA. Bupropion: an antidepressant without sexual pathophysiological action. Journal of Clinical Psychopharmacology 1985;5:24–29.

63. Kowalski A, Stanley RO, Dennerstein L, et al. The sexual side-effects of antidepressant medication: a double-blind comparison of two antidepressants in a non-psychiatric population. Br J Psychiatry 1985;147:413–418.

64. Hollander MH, Ban TA. Ejaculation retardation due to phenelzine. Psychiatric Journal University Ottawa 1980;4:233–234.

65. Schwarcz G. Case report of inhibition of ejaculation and retrograde ejaculation as side effects of amoxapine. Am J Psychiatry 1982;139: 233–234.

66. Nininger JE. Inhibition of ejaculation by amitriptyline. Am J Psychiatry 1978;135:750–751.

67. Monteiro WO, Noshirvani HF, Marks IM, et al. Anorgasmia from clomipramine in obsessive-compulsive disorder: a controlled trial. Br J Psychiatry 1987;151:107–112.

68. Glass RM. Ejaculatory impairment from both phenelzine and imipramine, with tinnitus from phenelzine. Journal of Clinical Psychopharmacology, 1981;3:152–154.

69. Goldbloom DS, Kennedy SH. Adverse interaction of fluoxetine and cyproheptadine in two patients with bulimia nervosa. J Clin Psychiatry 1991;52:261–262.

70. Jones SD. Ejaculatory inhibition with trazodone. Journal of Clinical Psychopharmacology 1984;4:279–281.

71. Reimherr FW, Chouinard G, Cohn CK. Antidepressant efficacy of sertraline: a double-blind, placebo and amitriptyline-controlled multicenter comparison study in outpatients with major depression. J Clin Psychiatry 1990;51(Suppl B):18–27.

72. Zajecka J, Fawcett J, Schaff M, et al. The role of serotonin in sexual dysfunction: fluoxetine-associated orgasm dysfunction. J Clin Psychiatry 1991;52:66–68.

73. Segraves RT. Reversal by bethanechol of imipramine-induced ejaculatory dysfunction (Letter). Am J Psychiatry 1987;144:1243–1244.

74. Steele TE, Howell EF. Cyproheptadine for imipramine-induced anorgasmia (Letter). Journal of Clinical Psychopharmacology 1986; 6:326–327.

75. Price J, Grunhaus LJ. Treatment of clomipramine-induced anorgasmia with yohimbine: a case report. J Clin Psychiatry 1990;51:32–33.

76. McLean JD, Forsythe RG, Kapkin IA. Unusual side effects of clomipramine associated with yawning. Can J Psychiatry 1983;28: 569–570.

77. Modell JG. Repeated observations of yawning, clitoral engorgement, and orgasm associated with fluoxetine administration. Journal of Clinical Psychopharmacology 1989;9:63–65.

78. Lal S, Rios O, Thavundayil JX. Treatment of impotence with trazodone: a case report. J Urol 1990;143:819–820.

79. Fletcher A, Bulpitt C. Antihypertensive medication and sexual dysfunction. In: Bezemer W, Cohen-Kettenis P, Slob K, van Son-Schooner N, eds. Sex matters. Amsterdam: Excerpta Medica, 1992:265–273.

80. Yendt RE, Gray GF, Garcia DA. The use of thiazides in the prevention of renal calculi. Can Med Assoc J 1970;102:614–620.

81. Curd JD, Borhani, NO, Blaszkowski TP, Zimbaldi N, Fotiv S, Williams W. Long-term surveillance for adverse effects of antihypertensive drugs. JAMA 1985;253:3263–3268.

82. Spark RF, Melby JC. Aldosteronism in hypertension. Ann Intern Med 1968;69:685–691.

83. Loriaux DL, Menard R, Taylor A, Pita JC, Santen R. Spironolactone and endocrine dysfunction. Ann Intern Med 1976;85:630–636.

84. Kostis JB, Rosen RC, Holzer BC, Randolph C, Taska LS, Miller MH. CNS side effects of centrally-active antihypertensive agents: a prospective, placebo-controlled study of sleep, mood state, cognitive and sexual function in hypertensive males. Psychopharmacology 1990;102:163–170.

85. Croog SH, Levine S, Sudilovsky A, Baume RM, Clive J. Sexual symptoms in hypertensive patients: a clinical trial of antihypertensive medications. Arch Intern Med 1988;148:788–794.

86. Fraunfelder FT, Meyer SM. Sexual dysfunction secondary to topical ophthalmic timolol. JAMA 1985;253:3092–3093.

87. Jensen RT, Collen MJ, Pandol SJ, et al. Cimetidine-induced impotence and breast changes in patients with gastric hypersecretory states. N Engl J Med 1983;308:883–887.

88. Neri A, Aygen M, Zuckerman Z, Bahany C. Subjective assessment of sexual dysfunction of patients on long-term administration of digoxin. Arch Sex Behav 1980;9:343–347.

89. Neri A, Zuckerman Z, Aygen M, Lidor Y, Kaufman H. The effect of long-term administration of digoxin or plasma androgens and sexual dysfunction. J Sex Marital Ther 1987;13:58–63.

90. Mattson RH, Cramer JA. Epilepsy, sex hormones, and antiepileptic drugs. Epilepsia 1985;26 (Suppl 1):540–551.

91. Segraves RT. Hormones and libido. In: Leiblum SR, Rosen, RC, eds. Sexual desire disorders. London: Guilford, 1988:271–312.

92. Luttge WB. The role of gonadal hormones in the sexual behavior of the rhesus monkey and human: a literature survey. Arch Sex Behav 1971;1:61–68.

93. Davidson JM, Rosen RC. Hormonal determinants of erectile function. In: Rosen, RC, Leiblum SR, eds. Erectile disorders: assessment and treatment. New York: Guilford, 1992:72–95.

94. Bremer J. Asexualization: a follow-up study of 244 cases. New York: MacMillan, 1959.

95. Luisi M, Franchi F. Double-blind comparison study of testosterone undecanoate and mesterolone in hypogonadal male patients. J Endocrinol Invest 1980;3:305–308.

96. Schreiner-Engel P, Schiavi RC, Smith H, White D. Sexual arousability and the menstrual cycle. Psychosom Med 1981;43:199–214.

97. Backstrom T, Sanders D, Leask R, Davidson D, Warner P, Bancroft J. Mood sexuality, hormones, and the menstrual cycle. II Hormone levels and their relationship to the premenstrual syndrome. Psychosom Med 1983;45:503–507.

98. Bancroft J, Sanders D, Davidson D, Warner P. Mood, sexuality, hormones and the menstrual cycle. III. Sexuality and the role of androgens. Psychosom Med 1983;45:509–516.

99. Sanders D, Warner P, Backstrom T, Bancroft J. Mood, sexuality, hormones and the menstrual cycle. I. Changes in mood and physical state: description of subjects and method. Psychosom Med 1983;15: 487–501.

100. Persky H, Lief HI, Strauss D, Miller WR, O'Brien CP. Plasma testosterone level and sexual behavior of couples. Arch Sex Behav 1978;7:157–173.

101. Sherwin BB, Gelfand MM. Differential symptom response to parental estrogen and/or androgen administration in the surgical menopause. Am J Obstet Gynecol 1985;151:153–160.

102. Sherwin BB, Gelfand MM, Brender W. Androgen enhances sexual masturbation in females: a prospective crossover study of sex steroid administration in the surgical menopause. Psychosom Med 1985;47: 339–351.

103. Ivers R, Goldstein N. Multiple sclerosis: a current appraisal of signs and symptoms. Proc Mayo Clin 1963;38:457–466.

104. Vas C. Sexual impotence and some autonomic disturbances in men with multiple sclerosis. Acta Neurol Scand 1969;45:166–182.

105. Lilius H, Valtoren E, Wilkstrom J. Sexual problems in patients suffering from multiple sclerosis. Journal Chronic Disease 1976;29: 643–647.

106. Szasz G, Paty D, Maurice WL. Sexual dysfunctions in multiple sclerosis. Ann N Y Acad Sci 1984;436:443–452.

107. Valleroy ML, Kraft GH. Sexual dysfunction in multiple sclerosis. Arch Phys Med Rehabil 1984;65:125–128.

108. Huns R, Shubsachs AP, Taylor PJ. Hypersexuality, fetishism and multiple sclerosis. Br J Psychiatry 1991;158:280–281.

109. Jensen, SB. Diabetic sexual dysfunction: a comparative study of 160 insulin treated diabetic men and women and an age-matched control group. Arch Sex Behav 1981;10:493–504.

110. Nathan D, Singer DE, Godine JE. Insulin dependent diabetes in older patients. Am J Med 1986;81:837–842.

111. McCulloch DK, Campbell IW, Wu FC, Prescott RJ, Clarke BF. The prevalence of diabetic impotence. Diabetiologia 1980;18:279–283.

112. Fairburn CG, Wu FCW, McCulloch DK, et al. The clinical features of diabetic impotence: a preliminary study. Br J Psychiatry 1982;140:447–452.

113. Kolodny RC, Kahn CB, Goldstein HH, Barnett DM. Sexual dysfunction in diabetic men. Diabetes 1973;23:306–309.

114. Fairburn CG, McCulloch DK, Wu FC. The effects of diabetes on male sexual function. Clinics in Endocrinology and Metabolism 1982;11:749–767.

115. McCulloch DK, Young RJ, Prescott RJ, Campbell IW, Clarke BF. The natural history of impotence in diabetic men. Diabetologia 1984;26:437–440.

116. Schiavi RC, Fisher C, Quadland M, Glover A. Nocturnal penile tumescence evaluation of erectile function in insulin-dependent diabetic men. Diabetologia 1985;28:90–94.

117. House WC, Pendleton L. Sexual functioning in male diabetics with impotence problems. Sexual and Marital Therapy 1988;3:205–212.

118. Bancroft J, Bell C, Ewing DJ, McCulloch DK, Warner P, Clarke BF. Assessment of erectile function in diabetic and non-diabetic impotence by simultaneous recording of penile diameter and penile arterial pulse. J Psychosom Res 1985;29:315–334.

119. Karacan I. Diagnosis of erectile impotence in diabetes mellitus. Ann Intern Med 1980;92 (part 2):334–337.

120. Quadri R, Veglio M, Flecchia D, et al. Autonomic neuropathy and sexual impotence in diabetic patients. Andrologia 1989;21:346–352.

121. Nofzinger EA, Schmidt HS. An exploration of central dysregulation of erectile function as a contributing cause of diabetic impotence. J Nerv Ment Dis 1990;178:90–95.

122. Kolodny RC. Sexual dysfunction in diabetic females. Diabetes 1971;20:557–559.

123. Prather RC. Sexual dysfunction in the diabetic female: a review. Arch Sex Behav 1988;17:277–284.

124. Jensen SB. Sexual dysfunction in younger insulin-treated diabetic females. Diabete Metab 1985;11:278–282.

125. Newman AS, Bertelson AD. Sexual dysfunction in diabetic women. J Behav Med 1986;9:261–270.

126. Bancroft J. Sexuality of diabetic women. Clinics in Endocrinology and Metabolism 1982;11:785–789.

127. Schreiner-Engel P, Schiavi RC, Vietorisz D, Smith H. The differential impact of diabetes type on female sexuality. J Psychosom Res 1987;31:23–33.

128. Yalla SV. Sexual dysfunction in the paraplegic and quadriplegic. In: Bennett AH, ed. Management of male impotence. Baltimore: Williams & Wilkins, 1994:181–191.

129. Comarr AE, Vigue M. Sexual counseling among male and female patients with spinal cord and/or cauda equina injury. Am J Phys Med 1978;57:215–227.

130. Berard EJJ. The sexuality of spinal cord injured women: physiology and pathophysiology: a review. Paraplegia 1989;27:99–112.

131. Rose SS. An investigation into sterility after lumbar ganglionectomy. Br Med J 1953;1:247–250.

132. Schover LR, Von Eschbach AC. Sexual and marital relationships after treatment for nonseminomatous testicular cancer. Urology 1985;25:251–255.

133. Aso R, Yasutom M. Urinary and sexual disturbances following radical surgery for rectal cancer and pudendal nerve block as a countermeasure for urinary disturbance. American Journal of Proctology 1974;25:60–74.

134. Hellstrom P. Urinary and sexual dysfunction after rectosigmoid surgery. Ann Chir Gynaecol 1988;77:51–56.

135. May AG, DeWeese J, Rob CG. Changes in sexual function following operation of the abdominal aorta. Surgery 1969;65:41–47.

136. Ohshiro T, Kosaki G. Sexual function after aorto-iliac vascular reconstruction. J Cardiovasc Surg 1984;25:47–50.

137. Hargreave TB, Stephenson TP. Potency and prostatectomy. Br J Urol 1977;49:683–688.

138. Segraves RT, Segraves KB. Medical aspects of orgasm disorders. In: O'Donohue W, Geer JH, eds. Handbook of sexual dysfunctions: assessment and treatment. Boston: Allyn & Bacon, 1993:225–252.

139. Morrell MJ. Sexual dysfunction in epilepsy. Epilepsia 1991;32 (Suppl 6):S38–S45.

140. Inthaler S, Donati F, Pavlincova E, Vassella F, Staldemann C. Partial complex epileptic seizures with ictal urogenital manifestations in a child. Neurology 1991;31:212–215.

141. Remillard GM, Andermann F, Testa GF, et al. Sexual ictal manifestations predominate in women with temporal lobe epilepsy: a finding suggesting sexual dimorphism in the human brain. Neurology 1983;33:323–330.

142. Backman DS, Rossel CW. Orgasmic epilepsy. Neurology 1984;34:559–560.

143. Warneke LB. A case of temporal lobe epilepsy with an orgasmic component. Canadian Psychiatric Association Journal 1976;21:319–324.

144. Blumer D. Hypersexual episodes in temporal lobe epilepsy. Am J Psychiatry 1970;126:1099–1106.

145. Kolarsky A, Freund K, Machek J, Polak O. Male sexual deviation: association with early temporal lobe damage. Arch Gen Psychiatry 1967;17:735–743.

146. Mitchell W, Falconer MA, Hill D. Epilepsy with fetishism relieved by temporal lobectomy. Lancet 1954;2:626–630.

147. Davies BM, Morgenstern FS. A case of cysticercosis, temporal lobe epilepsy, and transvestism. J Neurol Neurosurg Psychiatry 1960;23:247–249.

148. Taylor DC. Appetitive inadequacy in the sex behavior of temporal lobe epileptics. Journal of Neurovisceral Relations 1971; (Suppl 10):486–490.

149. Hierons R. Impotence in temporal lobe lesions. Journal of Neurovisceral Relations 1971; (Suppl 10):477–481.

150. Hierons R, Saunders M. Impotence in patients with temporal-lobe lesions. Lancet 1966;2:761–764.

151. Shukla GD, Srivastava ON, Katiyar BC. Sexual disturbances in temporal lobe epilepsy: a controlled study. Br J Psychiatry 1979;134:288–292.

152. Saunders M, Rawson M. Sexuality in male epileptics. J Neurol Sci 1970;10:577–583.

153. Toone BK, Edem J, Nanjee MN, Wheeler M. Hyposexuality and epilepsy: a community survey of hormonal and behavioral changes in male epileptics. Psychol Med 1989;19:937–943.

154. Demerdash A, Shaalan M, Midani A, Kamel F, Bahri M. Sexual behavior of a sample of females with epilepsy. Epilepsia 1991;32:82–85.

155. Mancall EL, Alonso RJ, Marlowe WB. Sexual dysfunction in neurological disease. In: Segraves RT, Schoenberg HW, eds. Diagnosis and treatment of erectile disturbances. New York: Plenum, 1985:65–86.

156. Herzog AG. Reproductive endocrine considerations and hormonal therapy for men with epilepsy. Epilepsia 1991;32 (Suppl 6):534–537.

157. Ramsay RE, Slater JD. Effects of antiepileptic drugs on hormones. Epilepsia 1991; 32 (Suppl 6):560–567.

158. Brown RG, Jahan Shahi M, Quinn N, Marsden CD. Sexual function in patients with Parkinson's disease and their partners. J Neurol Neurosurg Psychiatry 1990;53:480–486.

159. Esibill N. Impact of Parkinson's disease on sexuality. Sexuality and Disability 1983;6:120–125.
160. Lipe H, Longstreth WT, Bird TD, Linde M. Sexual function in married men with Parkinson's disease compared to married men with arthritis. Neurology 1990;40:1347–1349.
161. Uiti R, Tanner CM, Rajput AH, Goetz CG, Klawans HL, Thiessen B. Hypersexuality with antiparkinsonian therapy. Neuropharmacology 1989;12:375–383.
162. Kalliomaki JL, Markkanen TK, Mustonen VA. Sexual behavior after cerebral vascular accident. Fertil Steril 1961;12:156–158.
163. Ford AB, Orfirer AP. Sexual behavior and the chronically ill patient. Medical Aspects of Human Sexuality 1967;1:51–61.
164. Goddess ED, Wagner NN, Silverman DR. Post-stroke sexual activity of CVA patients. Medical Aspects of Human Sexuality 1979;13:16–30.
165. Hawton K. Sexual adjustment of men who have had strokes. J Psychosom Res 1984;28:243–249.
166. Monga TN, Lawson JS, Inglis J. Sexual dysfunction in stroke patients. Arch Phys Med Rehabil 1986;67:19–22.
167. Bray GP, DeFrank RS, Wolfe TL. Sexual functioning in stroke patients. Arch Phys Med Rehabil 1981;62:286–288.
168. Sjogren K, Fugl-Meyer AR. Adjustment to life after stroke with special reference to sexual intercourse and leisure. J Psychosom Res 1982;26:409–417.
169. Monga TN, Monga M, Raina MS, Hardjasudarma M. Hypersexuality in stroke. Arch Phys Med Rehabil 1986;67:415–417.
170. Kreutzer JS, Zasler ND. Psychosexual consequences of traumatic brain injury: methodology and preliminary findings. Brain Injury 1989;3:177–186.
171. Lusk MD, Kott JA. Effects of head injury on libido. Medical Aspects of Human Sexuality 1982;16:22–30.
172. Isern RD. Family violence and the Kluven-Bucy syndrome. South Med J 1987;80:373–377.
173. Gorman DG. Hypersexuality following septal injury. Arch Neurol 1992;49:308–310.
174. Lundberg PO. Sexual dysfunction in patients with neurological disorders. In: Gemme R, Wheeler CC, eds. Progress in sexuality. New York: Plenum, 1977:129–139.
175. Zeiss AM, Davies HD, Wood M, Tinklenberg JR. The incidence and correlates of erectile problems in patients with Alzheimer's disease. Arch Sex Behav 1990;19:325–331.
176. Janati A. Kluver-Bucy syndrome in Huntington's chorea. J Nerv Ment Dis 1985;173:632–635.
177. Offit AK. Psychiatric disorders and sexual functioning. In: Karasu TB, ed. Treatments of psychiatric disorders. Washington, DC: American Psychiatric Association, 1989 (vol 3):2253–2263.
178. Mathew RJ, Weinman ML. Sexual dysfunctions in depression. Arch Sex Behav 1982;11:323–328.
179. Casper RC, Redmond E, Katz MM, Schaffer CB, Davis JM, Koslow SH. Somatic symptoms in primary affective disorder. Arch Gen Psychiatry 1985;42:1098–1104.
180. Tamburello A, Seppecher MF. The effects of depression on sexual behavior: preliminary results of research. In: Gemme R, Wheeler CC, eds. Progress in sexology. New York: Plenum, 1977:107–128.
181. Kivela SL, Pahkala K, Eronen A. Depressive symptoms and signs that differentiate major and atypical depression from dysthymic disorder in elderly Finns. International Journal of Geriatric Psychiatry 1989;4:79–85.
182. Kivela SL, Pahkala K. Symptoms of depression in old people in Finland. Z Gerontol 1988;21:257–263.
183. Kivela SL, Pahkala K. Clinician-rated symptoms and signs of depression in aged Finns. Int J Soc Psychiatry 1988;34:274–284.
184. Roose SP, Glassman AH, Walsh BT, Cullen K. Reversible loss of nocturnal penile tumescence during depression: a preliminary report. Neuropsychobiology 1982;8:284–288.
185. Thase ME, Reynolds CF, Jennings JR, et al. Nocturnal penile tumescence diminished in depressed men. Biol Psychiatry 1988;24:33–46.
186. Schreiner-Engel P, Schiavi RC, Lifetime psychopathology in individuals with low sexual desire. J Nerv Ment Dis 1986;174:646–651.
187. Friedman S, Harrison G. Sexual histories, attitudes, and behavior of schizophrenic and normal women. Arch Sex Behav 1984;13:555–567.
188. Raboch J. The sexual development and life of female schizophrenic patients. Arch Sex Behav 1984;13:341–349.
189. Raboch J, Faltus F. Sexuality of women with anorexia nervosa. Acta Psychiatr Scand 1991;84:9–11.
190. Rosenheim E, Neumann M. Personality characteristics of sexually dysfunctional males and their wives. Journal of Sex Research 1981;17:124–138.
191. Schiavi RC. Psychological determinants of erectile disorders. Sexuality and Disability 1981;4:86–92.
192. Segraves KB, Segraves RT. Diagnosis of female arousal disorder. Sexual and Marital Therapy 1991;6:9–13.
193. Segraves KAB, Segraves RT. Differentation of biogenic and psychogenic impotence by sexual symptomatology. Arch Sex Behav 1987;16:125–137.
194. Segraves RT. Discrimination of psychogenic from organogenic impotence with psychometric instruments. Sexuality and Disability 1987;8:138–142.
195. Schiavi RC. Laboratory methods for evaluating erectile dysfunction. In: Rosen RC, Leiblum SR, eds. Erectile disorders: assessment and treatment. New York: Guilford, 1992:141–170.
196. Moore C. Evaluation of sexual disorders. In: Karasu TB, ed. Treatment of psychiatric disorders. Washington, DC: APA Press, 1989;3:2238–2247.
197. Melman A, Kaplan D, Redfield J. Evaluation of the first 70 patients in the Center for Male Sexual Dysfunction of Beth Israel Medical Center. J Urol 1984;131:53–55.
198. Buvat JJ, Lemaire A, Dehaene JL, Buvat-Herbaut M, Guien JD. Venous incompetence: critical study of the organic basis of high maintenance flow rates during artificial erection test. J Urol 1986;135:926–928.
199. Lue TF, Hricak H, Marich KW, Tanagho EA. Evaluation of vasculogenic impotence with high-resolution ultrasonography and pulse Doppler spectrum analysis. Radiology 1985;155:777–781.
200. Ertekin C, Reel F. Bulbocavernosus reflex in normal men and in patients with neurogenic bladder and/or impotence. J Neurol Sci 1976;28:1–15.
201. Segraves RT. Individual and couple therapy. In: Karasu TB, ed. Treatments of psychiatric disorders, volume 3. Washington, DC: APA Press, 1989:2334–2342.
202. Levine SB. Hypoactive sexual desire and other problems of sexual desire. In: Karasu TB, ed. Treatments of psychiatric disorders, volume 3. Washington, DC: APA Press, 1989:2264–2278.
203. Mellgren A. Treatment of ejaculation praecox with thioridazine. Psychother Psychosom 1967;15:454–460.
204. Singh H. Therapeutic use of thioridazine in premature ejaculation. Am J Psychiatry 1963;119:891.
205. Simpson GM, Blair JH, Amvsso D. Effect of antidepressants on genital urinary function. Diseases Nervous System 1965;26:787–789.
206. Eaton H. Clomipramine (Anafranil) in the treatment of premature ejaculation. J Int Med Res 1973;1:432–434.
207. Segraves RT, Saran A, Segraves K, Maguire E. Clomipramine vs. placebo in the treatment of premature ejaculation. Poster presented at New Clinical Drug Evaluation Unit Conference, Boca Raton, FL, May 26–29, 1992.
208. Segraves RT. Pharmacological enhancement of human sexual behavior. Journal of Sex Education and Therapy 1991;17:283–289.
209. Reid K, Morales A, Harris C. Double-blind trial of yohimbine in treatment of psychogenic impotence. Lancet 1987;2:421–423.
210. Riley AJ, Goodman RE, Kellet JM, Orr R. Double-blind trial of yohimbine hydrochloride in the treatment of erection inadequacy. Sexual and Marital Therapy 1989;4:17–26.

211. Susset JG, Tessier CD, Wincze J, Bansal S, Malhotra C, Schwacha MG. Effect of yohimbine hydrochloride on erectile impotence: a double-blind study. J Urol 1989;141:1360–1363.

212. Lal S, Ackman D, Thavundayil JX, Kiely ME, Etienne PC. Effect of apomorphine, a dopamine receptor agonist, on penile tumescence in normal subjects. Prog Neuropsychopharmacol Biol Psychiatry 1984; 8:695–699.

213. Danjov P, Alexandre L, Warot D, LaCombiez L, Puech AJ. Assessment of erectogenic properties of apomorphine and yohimbine in man. Br J Clin Pharmacol 1988;26:733–739.

214. Segraves RT, Bari M. Segraves K, Spirnak P. Effect of apomorphine on penile tumescence in men with psychogenic impotence. J Urol 1991;145:1174–1175.

215. Lal S. Apomorphine in the evaluation of dopaminergic function in man. Prog Neuropsychopharmacol Biol Psychiatry 1988;12: 117–164.

216. Benkert O, Crombach G, Kockott G. Effect of l-dopa on sexually impotent patients. Psychopharmacology 1972;23:91–95.

217. Pierini AA, Nusimovich B. Male diabetic sexual impotence: effect of dopaminergic agents. Arch Androl 1981;6:347–350.

218. Charney DS, Heninger GR. Alpha$_2$ adrenergic and opiate receptor blockage. Arch Gen Psychiatry 1986;43:1037–1041.

219. Fabbri A, Jannini EA, Gnessi L, et al. Endorphins in male impotence: evidence for naltrexone stimulation of erectile activity in patient therapy. Psychoneuroendocrinology 1989;14:103–111.

220. Byne W, Parsons B. Human sexual orientation: the biological theories reappraised. Arch Gen Psychiatry 1993;50:228–239.

221. Kraft-Ebing VR. Psychopathia sexualis. 12th (rev.) ed. New York: Physicians and Surgeons, 1925.

222. McCauley E, Urquiza AJ. Endocrine influences on human sexual behavior. In: JMA Sitsen, ed. Handbook of sexology, vol. 6. The pharmacology and endocrinology of sexual function. Amsterdam: Elsevier, 1988:352–387.

223. Gladve BA. Hormones in relationship to homosexual/bisexual/hetereosexual gender identify. In: JMA Sitsen, ed. Handbook of sexology, vol. 6. The pharmacology and endocrinology of sexual function. Amsterdam: Elsevier, 1988:388–409.

224. Gooren LJG. An appraisal of endocrine theories of homosexuality and gender dysphoria. In: JMA Sitsen, ed. Handbook of sexology, vol. 6. The pharmacology and endocrinology of sexual function. Amsterdam: Elsevier, 1988:410–424.

225. Money J, Dalery J. Iatrogenic homosexuality: gender identity in seven 46XX chromosomal females with hyperadnenocortical hermaphrodism born with a penis, three reared as boys, four reared as girls. J Homosex 1976;1:357–371.

226. Money J, Ehrhardt AA. Man and woman, boy and girl. Baltimore: Johns Hopkins University Press, 1972.

227. Donner G. Hormones and sexual differentiation of the brain. In: R Porter, J Whelan, eds. Sex, hormones, and behavior. Ciba Foundation Symposium 62 (new series). Amsterdam: Excerpta Medica, 1979:81–112.

228. Imperato-McGinley J, Peterson RE, Gautier T, Strurla E. Androgens and the evolution of male gender identity among male pseudohermaphrodites with 5 alpha-reductase deficiency. N Engl J Med 1979;300:1233–1237.

229. Meyer-Bahlburg HFL. Psychoendocrine research on sexual orientation. Current status and future option. Prog Brain Res 1984;61: 375–398.

230. Donovan BT. Humors, hormones and the mind. An approach to the understanding of behavior. New York: Stockton Press, 1988.

231. Bailey JM, Pillard RC. A genetic study of male sexual orientation. Arch Gen Psychiatry 1991;48:1089–1096.

232. Bailey JM, Pillard RC, Neale MC, Agyei Y. Heritable factors influence sexual orientation in women. Arch Gen Psychiatry 1993; 50:217–223.

233. Whitam FL, Diamond M, Martin J. Homosexual orientation in twins: a report on GI pairs and three triplet sets. Arch Sex Behav 1993;22:187–206.

234. Hamer DH, Hu S, Magnvson VL, Hu N, Pattatucci AML. A linkage between DNA markers on the X chromosome and male sexual orientation. Science 1993;261:321–327.

235. Gladue BA, Green R, Hellman RE. Neuroendocrine response to estrogen and sexual orientation. Science 1984;225:1496–1499.

236. Dorner G, Docke F. Gotz F, Rohde W, Stahl F, Tuonjes R. Sexual differentation of gonadotropin secretion, sexual orientation and gender role behavior. J Steroid Biochem Mol Biol 1987;27:1081–1087.

237. Gooren L, Fliers E, Courtney K. Biological determinants of sexual orientation. Annual Review of Sex Research 1990;1:175–196.

238. Levay S. A difference in hypothalamic structure between heterosexual and homosexual men. Science 1991;253:1034–1037.

239. Swaab DF, Hoffman MA. An enlarged suprachiasmatic nucleus in homosexual men. Brain Res 1990;537:141–148.

240. Allen LS, Gorski RA. Sexual orientation and the size of the anterior commissure in the human brain. Proc Natl Acad Sci 1992;89:7199–7202.

33

NEUROPSYCHIATRIC ASPECTS OF EPILEPSY

Michael R. Trimble, Howard A. Ring, and Bettina Schmitz

CLASSIFICATION OF EPILEPSY

Classifying epileptic seizures and epileptic syndromes has occupied epileptologists for centuries. Problems of terminology became obvious with increasing communication between international epileptologists in the middle of the 20th century. First outlines of international classifications of epileptic seizures (1) and epileptic syndromes (2) were published in 1970. The proposed classifications by the International League Against Epilepsy (ILAE) from 1981 and 1989 are based on agreements among international epileptologists and compromises between various viewpoints. They must not be regarded as definitive.

The changing role of psychiatric symptoms in relation to epilepsy in the last century is a good example of how much classification systems are determined by different approaches. In the middle of the 19th century, the epilepsy literature was dominated by psychiatrists who tried to categorize epilepsy based on their experiences with chronic patients in asylums. They spent more time on the psychopathological classification of psychiatric symptoms in epilepsy than on describing epileptic seizures (3–6). Specific psychiatric syndromes, especially short-lasting episodic psychoses and mood disorders, were considered diagnostically the same category as convulsions. In his classification of epilepsy from 1876, Samt distinguished 12 categories of epilepsy. Only three were characterized by epileptic seizures; the other nine categories were attributed to specific epileptic forms of insanity.

With the introduction of electroencephalography (EEG) in the 1930s, many episodic psychiatric states could be identified as nonepileptic in origin. Epileptic seizures, however, showed very different ictal EEG patterns. Since then, epileptologists have concentrated on the electroclinical differentiation of epileptic seizures.

Interestingly, the 1989 classification does not mention psychiatric criteria in the clinical definitions of epileptic syndromes. This neglect is remarkable because it is widely accepted that epilepsy is linked with certain psychiatric syndromes, which may be crucial in determining prognosis and quality of life. There are also recognized syndrome-related personality traits in juvenile myoclonic epilepsy (7) and temporal lobe epilepsy (8).

Classification of Seizures

Most authors in the 19th century (Table 33.1) simply differentiated seizures according to severity (petit mal, grand mal). Hughlings Jackson was the first to recognize the necessity of anatomical description, physiological delineation of disturbance of function, and pathological confirmation (9). In the 20th century, clinical events could be linked to ictal EEG findings. More detailed analyses of seizures became possible with simultaneous EEG-video monitoring and ictal neuropsychological testing. In the former, patients are monitored by video cameras and continuous EEG recordings for prolonged periods. The data are simultaneously displayed on a split-screen television monitor.

The International Classification of Epileptic Seizures (ICES) from 1981 is based on these improved intensive monitoring capabilities that have permitted accurate recognition of seizure symptoms and their longitudinal evolution. Presently, classification of seizures is weighted clinically and gives no clear definitions in terms of seizure origin. The ICES does not, however, reflect the most recent knowledge on the localizing significance of specific seizure symptoms. This approach has grown significantly since 1981 because of increased data from intensive monitoring and epilepsy surgery. Some parts of the ICES are thus outdated and in need of revision. Complex focal seizure types, for example, are not yet distinguished in the ICES according to a probable origin in the frontal or the temporal lobe.

The principal feature of the ICES is the distinction between seizures that are generalized from the beginning and those that are partial or focal at onset and may or may not evolve to secondary generalized seizures (Table 33.2). In generalized seizures there is initial involvement of both hemispheres. Consciousness may be impaired, and this impairment may be the initial manifestation. Motor manifestations are bilateral. The ictal EEG patterns initially are bilateral. Spikes, spike-wave compexes, and polyspike-wave complexes are all typical.

Partial seizures are those in which, in general, the first

clinical and EEG changes indicate initial activation of a system of neurons limited to part of one cerebral hemisphere. The other important feature of the ICES is the separation between simple and complex partial seizures, depending on whether there is preservation or impairment of consciousness.

Table 33.1. Fundamental Groups of Seizures

Focal or partial seizures
  Simple focal seizures
  Complex focal seizures
    With impairment of consciousness at onset
    Simple partial onset followed by impairment of consciousness
  Focal seizures evolving to generalized tonic-clonic seizures (GTC)
    Simple evolving to GTC
    Complex evolving to GTC (including those with simple partial onset)
Generalized seizures

Classification of Syndromes

"Epilepsy is the name for occasional sudden, excessive, rapid and local discharges of the grey matter." This simple definition was formulated by Jackson in 1866 long before the introduction of EEG (9). It has not lost its application for today. Recurrent epileptic seizures are pathognomonic

Table 33.2. International Classification of Epileptic Seizures (ILAE 1981)

Clinical Seizure Type	Ictal EEG
I. FOCAL (PARTIAL, LOCAL) SEIZURES	
A. Simple partial seizures	Local contralateral discharge starting over corresponding area of cortical representation (not always recorded on the scalp)
1. With motor symptoms	
a. Focal motor without march	
b. Focal motor with march (Jacksonian)	
c. Versive	
d. Postural	
e. Phonatory (vocalization or arrest of speech)	
2. With somatosensory or special-sensory symptoms (simple hallucinations, e.g., tingling, light flashes, buzzing)	
a. Somatosensory	
b. Visual	
c. Auditory	
d. Olfactory	
e. Gustatory	
f. Vertiginous	
3. With autonomic symptoms or signs (including epigastric sensation, pallor, sweating, flushing, piloerection, pupillary dilatation)	
4. With psychic symptoms (disturbance of higher cortical function). These symptoms rarely occur without impairment of consciousness and are much more commonly experienced as complex partial seizures.	
a. Dysphasic	
b. Dysmnesic (e.g., déja vu)	
c. Cognitive (e.g., dreamy states, distortions of time sense)	
d. Affective (fear, anger, etc.)	
e. Illusions (e.g., macropsia)	
f. Structured hallucinations (e.g., music, scenes)	
B. Complex focal seizures (with impairment of consciousness: may sometimes begin with simple symptomatology)	Unilateral or frequently bilateral discharge, diffuse or focal in temporal or frontotemporal regions
1. Simple partial onset followed by impairment of consciousness	
a. With simple partial features (as in A. 1–4) followed by impaired consciousness	
b. With automatisms	
2. With impairment of consciousness at onset	
a. With impairment of consciousness only	
b. With automatisms	
C. Focal seizures evolving to secondarily generalized seizures (this may be generalized tonic-clonic, tonic, or clonic)	Above discharge become secondarily and rapidly generalized
1. Simple partial seizures (A) evolving to generalized seizures	
2. Complex partial seizures (B) evolving to generalized seizures	
3. Simple focal seizures evolving to complex focal seizures evolving to	

Continued.

Table 33.2. *(Continued)*

Clinical Seizure Type	Ictal EEG
II. GENERALIZED SEIZURES	
A. 1. Absence seizures	Usually regular and symmetrical
a. Impairment of consciousness only	3 Hz but may be 2-4 Hz spike-and-
b. With mild clonic components	slow-wave complexes and may have
c. With atonic components	multiple spike-and-slow-wave-com-
d. With tonic components	plexes. Abnormalities are bilateral
e. With automatisms	
f. With autonomic components	
2. Atypical absence	EEG more heterogeneous; may include
May have:	irregular spike-and-slow-wave-com-
a. Changes in tone that are more pronounced than in A.1	plexes, fast activity, or other paroxys-
b. Onset and/or cessation that is not abrupt	mal activity. Abnormalities are bilat-
	eral but often irregular and asymetric
B. Myoclonic seizures	Polyspike and wave, or sometimes spike
Myoclonic jerks (single or multiple)	and wave or sharp and slow waves
C. Clonic seizures	Fast activity (10c/s or more) and slow
	waves; occasional spike-and-wave
	patterns
D. Tonic seizures	Low-voltage, fast activity or a fast rhythm
	of 9-10c/s or more decreasing in fre-
	quency and increasing in amplitude
E. Tonic-clonic seizures	Rhythm at 10 or more c/s decreasing in
	frequency and increasing in amplitude
	during tonic phase, interrupted by
	slow waves during the clonic phase
F. Atonic seizures	Polyspikes and wave or flattening or low-
	voltage fast activity

for all types of epilepsies (Table 33.3). The clinical spectrum of epilepsy, however, is much more complex, and an epileptic syndrome is characterized by a cluster of signs and syndromes customarily occurring together. These include such items as type of seizure, etiology, anatomy, precipitating factors, age of onset, severity, chronicity, diurnal and circadian cycling, and sometimes prognosis (10).

In contrast to a syndrome, a disease is characterized by a specific etiology and prognosis. Some recognized entities in the ICES are diseases; others are syndromes. Some of them may turn out to be diseases — a common etiology may still be discovered.

The ICES distinguishes generalized and localization-related (focal, local, partial) epilepsies. Generalized epilepsies are syndromes characterized by generalized seizures in which there is an involvement of both hemispheres from the beginning of the seizure. Seizures in localization-related epilepsies start in a circumscribed region of the brain. They may be simple or complex focal and may progress to secondary generalized tonic-clonic seizures.

The other important classification criterion refers to etiology. The ICES distinguishes idiopathic, symptomatic, and cryptogenic epilepsies. Idiopathic means that a disease is not preceded or occasioned by another. Symptomatic epilepsies and syndromes are considered the consequence of a known or suspected disorder of the central nervous system. In cryptogenic diseases, a cause is suspected but remains obscure, often due to limited sensitivity of diagnostic techniques.

Localization-Related Epilepsies and Syndromes

Seizure semiology and ictal EEG findings are the most important criteria for anatomical classification of localization-related epilepsies. As mentioned, the 1981 version of the ICES, with its emphasis on formal structures of seizures, is of limited benefit because it lacks the detailed localization incorporated into the ICES from 1989. The classification has been criticized because reliable localization often requires invasive EEG techniques. It is hoped that with more data from taxonomic studies, clinical symptoms or symptom clusters will be identified that eventually will allow classification on clinical grounds in most cases.

Temporal lobe epilepsies are divided into those with lateral temporal seizures with auditory hallucinations, language disorders (in cases of dominant hemisphere focus), or visual illusions and those with amygdala-hippocampal (mesio-basal limbic or rhinencephalic) seizures. The latter are characterized by simple seizure symptoms, such as rising epigastric discomfort, nausea, marked autonomic signs, and other symptoms, including borborygmi, belching, pallor, fullness of the face, flushing of the face, arrest of respiration, pupillary dilatation, fear, panic, and olfactory hallucinations. Complex focal seizures often begin with a motor arrest, typically followed by oroalimentary automatisms. The duration is typically over 1 minute, and consciousness recovers gradually.

Frontal lobe epilepsies are characterized by seizures of short duration, minimal or no postictal confusion, rapid

Table 33.3. International Classification of Epilepsies and Epileptic Syndromes (ILAE 1989)

1. Localization-related (focal, local, partial) epilepsies and syndromes
   1.1. Idiopathic (with age-related onset)
       At present, the following syndromes are established, but more may be identified in the future:
           Benign childhood epilepsy with centrotemporal spikes
           Childhood epilepsy with occipital paroxysms
           Primary reading epilepsy
   1.2. Symptomatic
       Chronic progressive epilepsia partialis continua of childhood (Kozhevnikov's syndrome)
       Syndromes characterized by seizures with specific modes of precipitation
       Temporal lobe epilepsy
           With amygdala-hippocampal seizures
           With lateral temporal seizures
       Frontal lobe epilepsy
           With supplementary motor seizures
           With cingulate seizures
           With seizures of the anterior frontopolar region
           With orbitofrontal seizures
           With dorsolateral seizures
           With opercular seizures
           With seizures of the motor cortex
       Parietal lobe epilepsies
       Occipital lobe epilepsies
2. Generalized epilepsies and syndromes
   2.1. Idiopathic, with age-related onset, listed in order of age
       Benign neonatal familial convulsions
       Benign neonatal convulsions
       Benign myoclonic epilepsy in infancy
       Childhood absence epilepsy (pyknolepsy)
       Juvenile absence epilepsy
       Juvenile myoclonic epilepsy (impuslive petit mal)
       Epilepsy with grand mal seizures (GTCS) on awakening
       Other generalized idiopathic epilepsies not defined above
       Epilepsies precipitated by specific modes of activation
   2.2. Cryptogenic or symptomatic (in order of age)
       West syndrome (infantile spasms, Blitz-Nick-Salaam Krämpfe)
       Lennox-Gastaut syndromes
       Epilepsy with myoclonic-astatic seizures
       Epilepsy with myoclonic absences
   2.3. Symptomatic
       2.3.1 Nonspecific etiology
           Early myoclonic encephalopathy
           Early infantile epileptic encephalopathy with suppression burst
           Other symptomatic generalized epilepsies not defined above
       2.3.2 Specific syndromes
           Epileptic seizures may complicate many disease states. Under this heading are included
           diseases in which seizures are presenting or predominant feature
3. Epilepsies and syndromes undetermined as to whether they are focal or generalized
   3.1. With both generalized and focal seizures
       Neonatal seizures
       Severe myoclonic epilepsy in infancy
       Epilepsy with continuous spike waves during slow-wave sleep
       Acquired epileptic aphasia (Landau-Kleffner syndrome)
       Other undetermined epilepsies not defined above
   3.2. Without unequivocal generalized or focal features

secondary generalization, prominent motor manifestations that are tonic or postural, complex gestural automatisms, and frequent falling. Ictal scalp EEGs may show bilateral or multilobar discharges. Accurate localization of frontal lobe epilepsies may be difficult.

Generalized Epilepsies and Syndromes

Idiopathic generalized epilepsies are characterized by an age-related onset (11). In general, patients are normal between seizures. Radiological investigations are negative. Frequently there is an overlap of idiopathic generalized epilepsies, especially of those manifesting in later childhood and adolescence.

Symptomatic generalized epilepsies and syndromes usually start in infancy or early childhood. In most children several seizure types occur. EEG discharges are less rhythmical and less synchronous than in idiopathic generalized epilepsies. There are neurological, neuropsychological, and radiological signs of diffuse encephalopathy. The only difference between cryptogenic and symptomatic syndromes is that in cryptogenic syndromes the presumed cause cannot be identified.

Epilepsies and Syndromes Undetermined as to Whether They Are Focal or Generalized

There are two groups of patients who cannot be classified as focal or generalized. The first group consists of patients with both generalized and focal seizures (e.g., patients with both focal seizures and absence seizures). The second group comprises patients without unequivocal generalized or focal features (e.g., patients with nocturnal grand mal).

Specific Syndromes

These are situation-related syndromes, such as febrile seizures, isolated seizures, and seizures occurring only when there is an acute metabolic or toxic event resulting from the effects of alcohol, drugs, eclampsia, and nonketotic hyperglycinemia.

EPIDEMIOLOGY OF EPILEPSY

Prevalence and Incidence

Epidemiological studies of epilepsy are often difficult to compare because of different study designs and definitions of epilepsy. Calculated incidence rates of epilepsy range between 20 and 70/100,000 per year. The incidence is age-dependent, with a maximum in early childhood and lowest rates in early adulthood (12). Incidence figures rise again in older age groups, probably because of the higher prevalence of cerebrovascular disease (13). The overall risk for epilepsy is slightly higher in males than in females. The point prevalence of active epilepsy is approximately 3–5/1000 (14). The cumulative lifetime prevalence has been estimated to be 3.5% (15).

There is thus a 10-fold difference between the point prevalence and the lifetime prevalence, suggesting that the disease remains active only in a small proportion of cases. The prevalence of epilepsy is higher in Third World countries, with prevalence rates of up to 37/1000 in Africa (16). This is probably related to a higher frequency of infectious diseases of the nervous system, such as neurocysticercosis and from perinatal complications.

Relative Frequency of Epileptic Syndromes

Research on the distribution of epileptic syndromes and epileptic seizures population studies have revealed conflicting results. In population-based studies, epilepsies with complex focal and focal seizures secondarily evolving to tonic-clonic seizures are most frequent, occurring in 69% of all patients. This is followed by primary generalized seizures in 30%, and absence or myoclonic seizures in less than 5% (15, 17).

PROGNOSIS OF EPILEPSY

Natural Course of Epilepsy

The natural course of untreated epilepsy is unknown. For ethical reasons no one has ever conducted a controlled study, and there are no systematic data from the days before antiepileptic drugs were introduced. Nineteenth century epileptologists emphasized the poor prognosis in epilepsy (18), but their experience was limited to institutionalized patients. Gowers (19) believed that seizures may beget seizures: "The tendency of the disease is to self-perpetuation, each attack facilitates the occurrence of another, by increasing the instability of nerve elements." Gowers studied the recurrence of seizures in 160 cases. A second seizure followed the first within 1 month in one-third of patients and within a year in two-thirds of patients.

Recurrence Risk After a First Seizure

It is methodologically extremely difficult to investigate the recurrence risk after an initial epileptic seizure (20). Figures in the literature range between 27 and 71%, depending on inclusion criteria, duration of follow-up, and whether or not patients are treated after a first seizure. The most important source of error has been the exclusion of patients with early recurrences of seizures before presentation. The longer the interval between first seizure and inclusion into the study, the lower is the recurrence rate (20).

The recurrence risk calculated from a population-based study in Rochester was 67% (21). English studies based on patients attending general practitioners have produced recurrence rates as high as 78% by 36 months (22) and 84% after variable length of follow-up (23).

Prognostic Studies

Recent prospective and population-based studies have challenged the older views that epilepsy is likely to be a chronic disease in as many as 80% of cases (24). In a population-based survey in Rochester, 20 years after the initial diagnosis of epilepsy, 70% of patients were in 5 years remission, and 50% of patients had successfully withdrawn medication (25). Goodridge and Shorvon (23) concluded from their study in Southeast England that 15 years after diagnosis, 81% of patients were seizure-free for at least 1 year.

From 104 patients who were followed after onset of treatment by Elwes et al. (26), 60% were in 1-year remission after a follow-up period of 24 months. By 8 years of follow-up, 92% had achieved a 1-year remission. It is recommended that antiepileptic drugs be withdrawn after a minimum seizure-free period of 2 years. Relapses occur in 12–72% after a 2-year remission and in 11–53% after a 3-year remission (27).

Approximately 5–10% of all epilepsies eventually include intractable seizures, despite optimal medication (28), most of them occurring in patients with complex partial seizures (29). Despite the overall favorable prognosis of epilepsy and

Table 33.4. Factors Affecting the Prognosis of Epilepsy

Negative Prognostic Factors
Diffuse encephalopathy
Psychiatric problems
Mental retardation
Early onset of epilepsy
Multiple seizure types
Simple and complex partial seizures
(Progressive) neurological symptoms
Long duration of active epilepsy
High number of seizures
High seizure frequency prior to treatment
Positive family history for epilepsy
Abnormal background EEG activity

the good response to treatment, the mortality of epilepsy is 2.3-fold higher than in the general population, being 3.8-fold higher in the first years of the illness (30). The incidence of sudden unexpected death in epilepsy has been estimated to be about 1/525 (31).

The prognosis of epilepsy largely depends on the syndromatic diagnosis. Idiopathic localization-related epilepsies, such as rolandic epilepsy, have an excellent prognosis in all respects. Prognosis in terms of seizure remission, social adjustment, and life expectancy, on the other hand, is extremely poor in symptomatic generalized epilepsies, such as West syndrome and in progressive myoclonus epilepsies.

Several studies have examined prognostic factors independent from the syndromatic diagnosis (Table 33.4). Most studies have consistently shown that diffuse encephalopathies, neurological, and cognitive deficits are associated with a poor outcome (22, 24).

There has been less agreement on the significance of other possible risk factors for poor prognosis, such as EEG features and a positive family history for epilepsy (26). Whether early treatment and medical prevention of seizures really improves the long-term prognosis—as suggested by Gowers and indicated by experimental data from animal epilepsy models—is still unclear and controversial.

BIOCHEMISTRY OF EPILEPSY

The cellular mechanisms responsible for epileptogenesis remain to be clarified. Much recent research into the biochemistry of epilepsy has focused on investigation of the effects of inhibitory and excitatory amino acid neurotransmitters on the excitability of neurons (32), together with the role of calcium in this process (33).

The major inhibitory neurotransmitter in the brain is γ-aminobutyric acid (GABA) (32), a monocarboxylic amino acid. It is distributed throughout the central nervous system and is a potent inhibitor of neuronal discharge. It may be used by as many as 40% of neurons (34). Two classes of GABA receptors have been characterized (35, 36), termed GABA$_A$ and GABA$_B$ and distinguished on the basis of their pharmacological characteristics (35). The GABA$_A$ receptor

is thought to be responsible for mediating CNS neuronal inhibition (37). In experimental epileptic foci in monkeys, it has been demonstrated that there are decreases in both the number of GABA receptors and in the levels of glutamate decarboxylase (GAD), a GABA-synthetic enzyme. It has further been shown in monkeys that following cortical injection of alumina gel to create a seizure focus, a selective loss of GAD-positive neuronal somata occurs before the animal starts to experience seizures (38).

The role of GABA-ergic mechanisms in epilepsy has been the focus of much pharmacological research into the treatment of the condition. In animal models of epilepsy, enhancing GABA-ergic neurotransmission has been shown to protect against seizures of various origins. However, this is not the case for GABA neurons in general but only for GABA systems—in particular, brain regions. Animal studies have demonstrated that increasing GABA-ergic activity in the substantia nigra controls both tonic and clonic seizures produced in the hindbrain, as well as clonic seizures originating in the forebrain (39). However, injections of the GABA agonist vigabatrin into other brain regions of rats, including the caudate, thalamus, and superior colliculus does not protect against experimental seizures (40).

Just as a deficit in inhibitory neurotransmitter activity has been implicated in generating seizure activity, so has an excess of excitatory activity. The excitatory amino acids glutamate and aspartate mediate the majority of excitatory transmission in the vertebrate nervous system. In a study using receptor autoradiography to investigate excitatory amino acid receptors in surgically excised temporal lobes from humans with epilepsy, it was observed that there was an increase in *N*-methyl-*D*-aspartate-sensitive glutamate and in kainic acid binding in the parahippocampal gyrus (41). The authors stated that it was not clear whether the observed changes resulted from or contributed to seizure activity. Nevertheless, their results suggested that vulnerability of the hippocampus in temporal lobe epilepsy may result, at least in part, from the presence of aberrant excitatory circuits in the parahippocampal gyrus.

Modulation of excitatory neurotransmission provides another avenue for pharmacological manipulation of seizure activity. Indeed, a new anticonvulsant, lamotrigine, most likely acts by inhibiting the release of excitatory amino acids (42).

Experimental models of epilepsy have demonstrated that calcium has an important role both in the induction of epilepsy and in the generation of seizures. The NMDA subtype of glutamate receptors constitutes an important route for influx of extracellular Ca^{2+} and functions as a receptor-operated channel (33). Studies in experimental models of epilepsy have demonstrated that there is a fall in extracellular Ca^{2+} at the time of seizure onset, probably because of increases in postsynaptic calcium uptake (43), mediated through NMDA-type glutamate receptors and voltage-operated calcium channels.

Calcium is central to neuronal function, and the increased excitation or diminished inhibition that underlie seizure activity are expressed through a variety of calcium systems (33). This central role for calcium has led to trials of calcium antagonists in the management of epilepsy. At the time of writing, however, this approach has not yet led to the development of any new antiepileptic drugs.

DIAGNOSIS OF EPILEPSY

Clinical Diagnosis and Differential Diagnosis

Epilepsy is a clinical diagnosis, defined by recurrent epileptic seizures. Most important for accurate syndromatic classification and optimal application of diagnostic techniques is the clinical interview. This should cover seizure-related information, such as subjective and objective ictal symptomatology, precipitation and frequency of seizures, history of seizures in first-degree relatives, and data relevant for etiology, such as complications during pregnancy and birth, early psychomotor development, history of brain injuries, and other disorders of the central nervous system. Other important information that should be obtained includes doses, side effects and efficacy of previous medical or nonmedical treatment, evidence for psychiatric complications in the past and psychosocial parameters, including educational and professional status, social independence, and psychosexual history.

The neurological examination may reveal signs of localized or diffuse brain damage. One should also look for skin abnormalities and minor stigmata suggestive of genetic diseases and dysontogenetic malformations. There may be signs of injuries caused by epileptic seizures, such as scars from recurrent falls, burns, and tongue-biting. Hirsutism, gingival hyperplasia, or acne vulgaris are indicative of side effects of long-term antiepileptic medication.

In most cases, a clinical interview together with a neurological examination are sufficient to distinguish between epilepsy and its wide spectrum of differential diagnoses (Table 33.5). There is, however, a substantial problem with pseudoseizures (see discussion that follows).

For correct interpretation of functional and structural diagnostic techniques, it is important to understand that in focal epilepsies different concepts of pathological cerebral regions have to be distinguished (44). The epileptogenic zone is defined as the region of the brain from which the patient's habitual seizures arise. Closely related but not necessarily anatomically identical are: (*a*) the irritative zone, defined as the region of cortex that generates interictal epileptiform discharges in the EEG; (*b*) the pacemaker zone, defined as the region of cortex from which the clinical seizures originate; (*c*) the epileptogenic lesion, defined as the structural lesion that is usually related to epilepsy; (*d*) the ictal symptomatic zone, defined as the region of cortex that generates the ictal seizure symptomatology; and (*e*) the functional deficit zone, defined as the region of cortex that in the interictal period is functioning abnormally. The diagnostic techniques applied in epilepsy are characterized by a selective specificity for these pathological regions (Table 33.6).

Electroencephalography

The interictal surface EEG is still the most important method in the diagnosis and assessment of all types of epilepsy. A routine EEG is recorded over 30 minutes during a relaxed condition, including photic stimulation procedures and 5 minutes of hyperventilation. Paroxysmal discharges strongly suggestive of epilepsy are spikes, spike waves, and sharp waves. These epileptiform patterns are, however, not epilepsy-specific. They may be observed in patients suffering from nonepileptic neurological diseases and even in a small proportion of normal subjects.

The sensitivity of the routine EEG is limited by restrictions of spatial and temporal sampling. About 50% of patients with epilepsy do not show paroxysmal epileptiform discharges on a single EEG recording (45). Their detection depends on the epileptic syndrome and the therapeutic status of the patient. In untreated childhood absence epilepsy, the EEG almost always shows generalized spike-wave complexes either occurring spontaneously or provoked by hyperventilation. In mild cryptogenic focal epilepsies, on the other hand, the interictal EEG is often negative. The temporal sensitivity can be increased by repeating the EEG or by carrying out long-term recordings with mobile EEGs. Paroxysmal discharges may furthermore be brought out by performing an EEG after sleep deprivation while the subject is asleep (Table 33.7). Simultaneous video EEG recordings

---

Table 33.5.   Differential Diagnosis of Epilepsy

Neurological disorders
   Transient ischemic attacks
   Migraine
   Paroxysmal dysfunction in multiple sclerosis
   Transient global amnesia
   Movement disorders (hyperexplexia, tics, myoclonus, dystonia, paroxysmal choreoathetosis)
   Drop attacks due to impaired CSF dynamics
Sleep disorders
   Physiological myoclonus
   Pavor nocturnus
   Somnabulism
   Enuresis
   Periodic movements in sleep
   Sleep-talking
   Bruxism
   Nightmares
   Sleep apnea
   Narcolepsy (cataplexy, automatic behavior, sleep attacks, hallucinations)
Psychiatric disorders
   ''Pseudoseizures''
   Anxiety attacks
   Hyperventilation syndrome
   Dissociative states, fugues
   Episodic dyscontrol, rage attacks
Medical disorders
   Cardiac arrhythmias
   Syncope (cardiac, orthostatic, reflex)
   Metabolic disorders (e.g., hypoglycemia)
   Hypertensive crisis
   Endocrine disorders (e.g., pheochromocytoma)

Table 33.6. Localization of Pathological Zones in Focal Epilepsies[a]

Epileptogenic zone	Ictal EEG with special electrode placements, functional imaging (SPECT, fMRI)
Irritative zone	Interictal EEG, MEG
Pacemaker zone	Ictal EEG with special electrode placements
Ictal symptomatic zone	Ictal EEG with special electrode placements
Epileptogenic lesion	CT, MRI
Functional deficit zone	Functional imaging (PET, SPECT, fMRI), neurological examination, neuropsychological testing, nonepileptiform interictal EEG abnormalities

[a]Adapted from Lüders HO, Awad I. Conceptual considerations. In: Lüders H, ed. Epilepsy surgery. New York: Raven Press, 1991:51–62.

of seizures are useful for differentiating between different types of epileptic seizures (Table 35.2) and nonepileptic seizures. Ictal EEGs are also required for exact localization of the epileptogenic focus when epilepsy surgery is considered.

Surface EEGs record only a portion of the underlying brain activity. Discharges that are restricted to deep structures or to small cortical regions may not be detected. The spatial resolution of the EEG can be improved by special electrode placements, such as pharyngeal and sphenoidal electrodes.

Invasive EEG methods with chronic intracranial electrode placement are necessary for complex analysis in cases with discordant or multifocal results of the ictal surface EEG and imaging techniques. These include foramen ovale electrodes positioned in the subdural space along the amygdala-hippocampal formation (46), epidural and subdural strip electrodes, and grids to study larger brain areas. Stereotactic depth electrodes provide excellent sensitivity to detect small areas of potentially epileptogenic tissue. The definition of exact location and boundaries of the epileptogenic region, however, is limited by the location and number of electrodes placed. Because of the limited coverage of implanted electrodes, it may be difficult to distinguish whether a seizure discharge originates from a pacemaker zone or represents spread from a distant focus. Complications, the most severe being intracerebral hemorrhages, occur in 4%.

Magnetoencephalography

Multichannel magnetoencephalography (MEG) has recently been introduced in the presurgical assessment as a supplementary method to EEG. The electric activity, which can be measured by EEG, produces a magnetic field perpendicular to the electric flow. This magnetic signal can be measured by MEG. In contrast to EEG, MEG is not influenced by intervening tissues with the advantage of noninvasive localization of deep electric sources. Disadvantages include high costs and the susceptibility to movement artifacts, making it extremely difficult to do ictal studies (47, 48).

Structural Imaging

Imaging studies should always be performed when a symptomatic etiology is suspected. Cranial computed tomography (CCT) is a quick, easy, and inexpensive technique. The sensitivity can be improved by scanning in the axis of the temporal lobe (in cases of temporal lobe epilepsy) and by using intravenous contrast enhancement. Except for a few pathologies, such as calcifications, magnetic resonance imaging (MRI) is superior to CCT in terms of sensitivity and specificity in detecting epilepsy-related lesions such as malformations, gliosis, and tumors. With optimized MRI technique (49), including T2-weighted images, inverse recovery sequences, coronal images perpendicular to the hippocampus and thin sections, the sensitivity in depicting mesial temporal sclerosis reaches 90% (50). Diagnosis of hippocampal pathology can be further improved by quantitative MR techniques such as T2-relaxometry (51) and volumetric studies (52).

MR spectroscopy (MRS) is a noninvasive method of measuring chemicals in the body. MRS does not produce images but instead generates numerical values for chemicals. With phosphate spectroscopy it is possible to study energy metabolism in relation to seizure activity (53). Proton MRS measures neuronal density, which has been found to be significantly decreased in the mesial temporal lobe of patients with mesial temporal sclerosis (54).

Functional Imaging

Single photon emission computed tomography (SPECT) in epilepsy has mainly been confined to the imaging of cerebral blood flow (rCBF) in focal epilepsy. The tracer most widely used nowadays is 99Tc-HMPAO. Interictally, there is localized hypoperfusion in an area extending beyond the epileptogenic region. Initially, there was considerable skepticism about the clinical value of the technique because the

Table 33.7. EEG Methods in the Diagnosis of Epilepsy

Interictal EEGs
  Routine surface EEG
  EEG after sleep withdrawl, during sleep
  Mobile long-term EEG
Ictal EEG
  Long-term video EEG
Special electrode placements (in the order of invasiveness)
  Nasopharyngeal electrodes
  Sphenoidal electrodes
  Formen-ovale electrodes
  Epidural electrodes (strips, grids)
  Subdural electrodes (strips, grids)
  Depth electrodes

early studies were of low resolution and the correlations with electroencephalographic findings were imprecise. Figures on the sensitivity of interictal focus detection of SPECT in the literature range from 40–80% (55, 56). In recent years there have been major technical developments in instrumentation. Using brain-dedicated multiheaded camera systems, the sensitivity of SPECT is comparable to FDG-PET (57). 99Tc-HMPAO is distributed within a few minutes after injection in the brain, where it remains fixed for about 2 hours. If the radioisotope is injected during or shortly after an epileptic seizure, scanning can be carried out postictally without problems from involuntary movements. Postictal and ictal SPECT are more sensitive than interictal SPECT and typically show hyperperfusion ipsilateral to the epileptogenic focus (58).

Compared with SPECT, positron emission tomography (PET) is superior with respect to spatial and contrast resolution. PET, however, is expensive and requires an on-site medical cyclotron. Ictal studies are difficult with PET because of the short half-life of positron-emitting radioisotopes. PET has mainly been used to study interictal bloodflow with ^{13}N labeled ammonia and oxygen-15, and glucose metabolism with 18F-fluordeoxyglucose (FDG) in focal epilepsy. Localized hypoperfusion and hypometabolism in the epileptogenic area as shown by PET are seen as a reliable confirmatory finding in the presurgical assessment of temporal lobe epilepsy (59). PET has also been used for imaging of benzodiazepine receptor binding (60) and opiate-receptor binding (61) in epilepsy.

Neuropsychology

Identification of neuropsychological deficits is important for optimizing education, professional training, and rehabilitation in patients with epilepsy. Another aim of neuropsychological testing is to establish the cognitive effects of antiepileptic drugs, seizure frequency, and "subclinical" EEG activity.

The presurgical assessment neuropsychological evaluation is used to identify localizable deficits that can be related to the epileptogenic lesion. Crucial for lateralizing temporal lobe epilepsies is the function of verbal and nonverbal memory (62). Another neuropsychological task in the presurgical assessment is forecasting postsurgical cognitive outcome, which sometimes requires the intracarotid sodium amylobarbital procedure (Wada test).

TREATMENT OF EPILEPSY

Once a diagnosis of epilepsy has been made, followed by the decision to treat, a number of options are available. Pharmacological, behavioral, and surgical approaches may be taken. The great majority of patients with epilepsy are treated with anticonvulsants. Recently there has also been renewed interest in attempts at behavioral and nonpharmacological approaches to the management of seizures. A minority of patients with drug-resistant epilepsy may proceed to have surgery.

The evaluation of the mental state in epilepsy is essentially the same as for any other patient. However, certain interesting and important features of the motor state and the psychopathology of some patients bear mention.

With regard to motor behavior, patients sometimes have a pattern of bradyphrenia, which may in some respects resemble a psychomotor retardation. In some patients this may be associated with ongoing, subclinical seizures. The latter may be revealed through subtle motor manifestations. These include paroxysms of rhythmic eye-blinking, mouth movements, or small frequent jerks of the hands, arms, or fingers, referred to as minipolymyoclonus.

The mental state may contain personality changes, including undue religiosity, altered sexual behavior, circumstantiality, rigidity of thinking, and an undertone of paranoia. Hypergraphia should always be asked about. This may be obvious only when, for example, a patient's diary is requested and read. The writing may be pedantic, repetitive, and mystical in content.

In patients with depression, there is often evidence of the underlying neurological condition. The mood swings may be rapid and severe, and may not last long. There is often much anxiety associated with the depression, and the presentation can be further influenced by the presence of an excessive anticonvulsant burden. Suicidal thoughts are frequent and should always be asked about.

Anxiety is also a common problem, and it can sometimes be very difficult, without EEG monitoring, to distinguish an aura of fear from a panic attack. The features can seem identical.

The delusions and hallucinations have varying themes, but mystical and religious themes are common. In postictal psychoses, complex visual hallucinations can occur with almost clear consciousness. In patients who present with a postictal twilight state, or a partial seizure status, careful testing of the cognitive state will reveal impairment of performance. This may fluctuate, and repeated testing may be necessary after a time.

Obviously, the patient's attitude toward his or her seizure disorder, and the way it has affected his or her life should be explored. This may lead into specific lines of psychosocial inquiry.

These approaches should not be viewed as being mutually exclusive. Hence, although in the discussion that follows these treatments are described separately, in practice, they may be combined. Indeed, if surgery is pursued, it is very likely that patients will be receiving antiepileptic medication both before and after the operation.

Antiepileptic Agents

Ideally, patients should be managed on a single drug. Approximately 75% of patients with epilepsy can be fully controlled on monotherapy (63), the choice of agent being determined by seizure type (Table 33.8). Carbamazepine and phenytoin are most effective for complex partial and generalized tonic-clonic seizures. For absence seizures,

Table 33.8. Antiepileptic Drugs

Seizure Type	First-line	Second-line
Partial	Carbamazepine	Valproic acid, clobazam, phenobarbital, acetazolamide,
	Phenytoin	clonazepam, vigabatrin, lamotrigine, gabapentin
Generalized	Carbamazepine	(Same as above)
	Phenytoin	
	Valproic acid	
Absence	Ethosuximide	
	Valproic acid	
Myoclonic	Clonazepam	
	Valproic acid	

ethosuxemide and sodium valproate are the most useful treatments. These drugs are generally thought of as the first-line treatments. Some patients with myoclonic epilepsy will respond well to sodium valproate, but others may require clonazepam. Of the remaining patients not controlled on monotherapy, addition of another first-line drug will gain control in a further 15%. However, some patients will go on to develop chronic seizures unrelieved by these treatments. In such circumstances, adjunctive therapies should be considered. A number of the more recently introduced anticonvulsants, often considered as second-line treatments, may be introduced, either alone or in combination with a first-line agent. Clobazam is efficacious in previously drug-resistant epilepsy, but its use is associated with a progressive loss of effect over the first 6 months of use. In one study the mean incidence of development of tolerance after 6 months of treatment was 45% (64). Three novel anticonvulsants, vigabatrin, gabapentin, and lamotrigine, have recently been introduced. Early efficacy studies have demonstrated that vigabatrin is associated with approximately a 50% reduction in seizure frequency in half the patients in whom it is used as add-on therapy. However, these agents appear to be associated with the occasional development of psychiatric side effects (65).

An important feature in the clinical use of the first-line treatments is therapeutic drug monitoring (TDR). It is appropriate for agents without unmeasured active metabolites and for which therapeutic response correlates with and depends on the serum concentration rather than the dose. For appropriate agents, indications for TDR include: (*a*) drug initiation or dose change, (*b*) investigation of absence of or change in therapeutic response, (*c*) investigation of suspected toxicity, and (*d*) situations in which pharmacokinetics may change, such as in renal or hepatic disease. Sampling should occur once a steady state has been achieved, 4–6 half-lives after treatment has been modified or introduced. TDR is particularly important for phenytoin because its hepatic metabolism is saturable. Thus, a small increase in dose can result in a disproportionate and unpredictable increase in serum concentration.

Behavioral Treatment

Pharmacological treatments of epilepsy are not uniformly successful in all patients. Even if good seizure control is obtained, many patients experience troublesome side effects of treatments that must be continued, often for many years. The need to take medication on a long-term basis has obvious implications for women wishing to become pregnant. In addition, many individuals describe feelings of oppression and an increased fear of being labeled as ill because of their ongoing need for regular drug taking. Surgical treatment is an option only for a minority of patients and is also not without physical and psychological sequelae. Not surprisingly, then, alternative treatment approaches should be sought.

It has been suggested that many patients with epilepsy have a mental mechanism they use to attempt to inhibit their seizures. In one study of 70 patients, 36% of them claimed that they could sometimes stop their seizures (66). A behavioral approach to the treatment of epilepsy is based on observations that epilepsy can be manipulated in a systematic way through environmental, psychological, and physical changes. The initial stage in this approach is a behavioral analysis of the ways in which environmental and behavioral factors interact with seizure occurrence (67).

Significant reductions in seizure frequency may be achieved by teaching patients a specific contingent relaxation technique that they must be able to employ rapidly when they identify a situation when they are at high risk of having a seizure (67). In a subsequent study of three children with intractable seizures, contingent relaxation alone did not significantly reduce seizures, but such a reduction was obtained following the addition of specific countermeasures aimed at changing the arousal level as it related to early seizure cues. For instance, the patient was instructed to suddenly jerk the head to the right when it would habitually move to the left with a feeling of drowsiness at the onset of a seizure (68). Other specific approaches to seizure inhibition have been reviewed by several authors (66, 69).

Some patients suffer from reflex seizures in that their seizures are precipitated by external stimuli. A number of people can identify specific environmental or affective triggers and may be able to develop specific strategies to abort or delay a seizure. These methods may involve motor or sensory activity, or they may be purely mental. However, in one study it was found that 50% of patients who inhibited their seizures at times had to "pay the price in subsequent discomfort" (70).

Primary seizure inhibition describes the direct inhibition

of seizures by an act of will. For example, a man whose seizures were precipitated by a feeling of unsteadiness tackled this problem by keeping his gaze fixed on a point when walking down an incline (66). The nature of the successful act varies from person to person, and this treatment approach will not be effective unless it is individually tailored, based on an analysis of each patient's seizures and any actions he or she may already have noticed that modify the seizures.

The term secondary inhibition is employed by Fenwick (66) to describe behavioral techniques that effect change in cortical activity in the partially damaged group 2 neurons around the focus, thereby reducing the risk both of a partial seizure discharge and of a generalized seizure discharge. The latter may otherwise follow recruitment of surrounding normal brain by group 2 neurons firing abnormally (71). An example of this is the act of maintaining alertness by a patient whose seizures appear in a state of drowsiness. Treatment in this case starts with trying to identify situations where the subject reliably tends to have seizures, or alternatively, to be free of them.

In addition to these seizure-related approaches, more general psychological strategies have been investigated. Several anecdotal reports have been published demonstrating benefit from a reward system that aims to reward seizure-free periods.

Based on the observation that some patients with olfactory auras can prevent progression of the seizure by applying a sudden, usually unpleasant olfactory counter-stimulus, Betts has explored the use of aromatherapy techniques in the control of epilepsy (72). So far, the relative differential contributions of specific olfactory stimuli as opposed to the general relaxation that are part of any treatment are not clear.

Specific biofeedback techniques have also been explored. Measurement of scalp electrical activity has demonstrated that there is an increase in surface-negative slow cortical potentials (SCPs) in the seconds before a seizure occurs. These SCPs represent the extent to which apical dendrites of cortical pyramidal cells are depolarized and hence indicate neuronal excitability (73). Studies using visual feedback of this effect have demonstrated that some patients are able to modulate cortical electrical activity with an associated decrease in seizure frequency (74). However, it appears that patients with epilepsy are less able than normal controls to regulate their cortical excitability. This impairment can be minimized by extending the amount of training received by those with epilepsy. In a study that gave 28 1-hour training sessions to 18 patients followed up for at least 1 year, six became seizure-free (73). However, not every patient who achieved reliable SCP control experienced a reduction in seizure frequency.

Nonspecific EEG biofeedback has been used to modulate cerebral electrical rhythms—for instance, to increase fast low-voltage activity and to supress slow-wave activity surrounding the epileptic focus (75).

A quite different biological approach that has been tried in some centers is that of vagal stimulation using an implanted stimulator. Among the drawbacks to this approach is that while the nerve is being stimulated—usually for 30 seconds every 5–10 minutes—the voice changes. More intense stimulation may be associated with throat pain or coughing. Nevertheless, in one series of 130 patients, mean seizure frequency decreased by 30% after 3 months and by 50% after 1 year of therapy. Altogether, 60–70% of the patients showed some response (76).

Ultimately, the teaching of any of these methods of self-control of seizures may increase morale, not only by reducing seizures, but also by providing patients with a sense of control over their epilepsy. An important aspect of many nonmedical treatments of epilepsy is that although they still have very limited proven benefit, they aim to consider seizures in the wider setting of the patient's life. In mainstream clinical management, it is sometimes easier to focus purely on seizure response to the latest change in anticonvulsant therapy.

Surgical Treatment

In patients with persistent epilepsy unrelieved by other treatments, surgical intervention should be considered. Surgery may be effective for three reasons (77):

1. It removes pathological tissue, including the primary focus;
2. It disconnects a focus from the rest of the brain when the primary focus is incompletely removed; and
3. It reduces the mass of neurons that behave abnormally.

Treatment centers that engage in routine surgical management of epilepsy generally have a standardized assessment process for patients being considered for such treatment. Although the program may vary a little from place to place, the general procedure is similar. Clinical history and examination focus on looking for etiological factors, evidence of localizing signs and symptoms, and a witnessed description of the seizures. In addition, psychosocial information must be gathered relating to education, employment, social support, and past and present mental state findings. All patients considered for surgery must undergo electroencephelographic (EEG) investigation. This may include several days of continuous video telemetry. The aim of telemetry is to obtain ictal recordings that give more valuable localizing information than interictal records. Recent advances in structural and functional neuroimaging have made invasive EEG recording less necessary. High-definition x-ray computed tomography (CT) of patients with focal epilepsy will reveal a lesion in 60–70% of cases (78). Magnetic resonance imaging (MRI) is now used routinely and will reveal local structural abnormalities not seen on CT (79). Current research programs are evaluating the relative benefits of functional imaging using SPECT compared with more invasive methods of seizure localization (80–82).

All patients being considered for epilepsy surgery should

have a neuropsychological assessment. This is important both to detect focal brain dysfunction and to predict the results of surgery, especially temporal lobe surgery (72). The intelligence quotient (IQ) may be measured using the Wechsler Adult Intelligence Scale. In some centers a score of less than 75 has been taken as evidence of diffuse neurological disorder, and hence as a relative contraindication to surgery. Before proceeding to surgery, it is important to investigate the hemispheric localization of language and memory. This is generally performed using the Wada test. Sodium amylobarbitone is injected into one internal carotid artery, and when that hemisphere is briefly supressed, language and memory tests are performed. The procedure is then repeated for the other hemisphere.

A number of surgical procedures have been developed. The most frequent is the removal of neocortical structures together with deep structures (77). The nature of potential perioperative complications and postsurgical neurological, cognitive, and psychiatric sequelae depend in part on the site of surgery, as discussed later in this chapter.

ROLE OF THE LIMBIC SYSTEM

Although definitions of the limbic system vary, most agree that central components include the amygdala, hippocampus, and their outflow pathways. The latter include, importantly, the limbic forebrain structures, such as the dopamine-rich nucleus accumbens and surrounding nuclei of the ventral striatum, and pathways to the hypothalamus, thalamus, and their connections down to the midbrain tegmentum. A recent description of some of these areas uses the concept of the extended amygdala, noting the close anatomical and neurochemical links between medial temporal structures and limbic forebrain structures (83).

To understand the role of the limbic system structures in epilepsy and in the behavior disorders of epilepsy, keep in mind that the limbic system modulates both behavior and emotion. In the 1930s, Papez (84) was first to suggest that a limbic circuit, which comprised the hippocampus, the mammillary body of the thalamus, the anterior thalamus, the cingulate gyrus, and a loop back to the hippocampus, was a neural substrate for the emotions.

The concept of the limbic system was developed further by MacLean (85). Basing his ideas on comparative anatomy, he introduced the "triune brain." Essentially, he pointed out how human brains contain a neocortex, a paleocortex, and a reptilian brain. The essential concept was that the limbic system (the paleocortex) was only developed in a very rudimentary way prior to the rise of mammals and is very poorly represented in reptiles. As MacLean reflected: "The history of the evolution of the limbic system is the history of the evolution of the mammals, while the history of the evolution of the mammals is the history of the development of a family way of life."

In other words, with the development of infant maternal bonding and the evolution of complex social behaviors, there

Table 33.9. Medical Differential Diagnosis of Seizures

Hypoglycemia
Vasovagal
Cardiac (TIA)
Migraine
Vestibular disorders
Narcolepsy
Dystonias, tics, stimulus-sensitive myoclonus
Sleep disorders
  Parasomnias
    REM
      Nightmares
      Sleep behavior disorder
    Non-REM
      Somnambulism
      Night terrors
  Hypersomnias
    Cataplexy
    Narcoleptic automatic behavior
    Sleep drunkenness

has been a parallel development of the neuroanatomical and arrangements of limbic structures.

The neuropathological changes in epilepsy are varied, but it has been known for a number of years that a specific form of pathology is found in many patients, particularly those with localization-related temporal lobe epilepsy. Mesial temporal sclerosis is a specific pathological lesion affecting largely hippocampal structures, particularly subfields within the hippocampus, such as CA1. It is known to occur secondary to early anoxic brain damage. A key history in many patients with this pathology is an early febrile convulsion, particularly one that has been prolonged or complicated. Patients may then be seizure-free for several years, developing simple or complex partial seizures in their adolescence.

Other pathologies found in the temporal lobes that affect limbic system structures often reflect developmental abnormalities. These include the hamartomas, a heterogeneous group of pathologies that are benign but arise in the brain during fetal development. Again, patients with such pathologies often remain seizure-free for many years, the first seizures erupting in late childhood or early adulthood.

It is common to loosely speak of "temporal lobe epilepsy." However, neuroanatomically, neurochemically, and neurophysiologically, there are clearly a number of subdivisions of the temporal lobes, as there are, for example, of the frontal lobes. One such subdivision is the limbic portion, the medial temporal structures—in particular, the amygdala, hippocampus, and parahippocampal gyrus. Thus, some authors have now more clearly distinguished a medial temporal syndrome, which may be referred to as limbic epilepsy. This syndrome's characteristics are shown in Table 33.9. Significantly, behavior disorders appear to be an integral part of the medial temporal syndrome, confirming the central role of limbic system structures in the development of emotions and behaviors.

In clinical practice, patients with temporal lobe epilepsy are often the most refractory to treat, often find themselves on several anticonvulsant drugs, and probably attend a chronic epilepsy clinic. Limbic epilepsy may therefore be defined as a form of seizure disorder with pathology in limbic system structures—usually arising during an early developmental period—in which patients have little relief from seizures and often present with behavior disorders. Knowing that the limbic system modulates emotional expression, we should not be surprised that a lesion there would have a profound effect on behavior during crucial periods of psychosocial development.

It is important to recognize the relationship of the anatomical structures of the limbic system and the outflow pathways from the hippocampus and amygdala. Thus, there are significant monosynaptic tracts linking the medial temporal structures to the dopamine-rich limbic forebrain. The latter are thought to be related to the development of psychosis in such conditions as schizophrenia. This finding must be relevant to the development of behavior disorders in patients with temporal lobe epilepsy.

As noted previously, the clinical phenomenology of the psychoses associated with temporal lobe epilepsy are often indistinguishable from schizophrenia in the absence of epilepsy. This may reflect the underlying anatomical homologies.

Finally, numerous neuropathological studies of schizophrenia reveal that where abnormalities of the hippocampus or parahippocampal gyrus are sought, they are invariably found (see Chapter 15). The pathological picture differs from that of classic mesial temporal sclerosis, in particular by the absence of a gliosis. Nevertheless, the neuronal disarray that is so frequently reported, which probably reflects abnormal neuronal migration during fetal development, is thought to be interlinked with the development of the schizophrenia syndrome. The relevance of the limbic system, therefore, is that this neuronal circuitry underlying the development of emotion and behavior is disrupted in patients who develop schizophrenia, as well as in patients with one form of epilepsy, namely temporal lobe or limbic system epilepsy. These patients are most likely to develop psychopathology resembling schizophrenia—hence the term "the schizophrenia-like psychoses of epilepsy," adopted by Slater (168).

PERSONALITY AND BEHAVIOR DISORDER IN EPILEPSY

The relationship between epilepsy and personality disturbances has been a controversial one. This is true despite the fact that reference to behavior problems in patients with epilepsy originates with the early history of the subject. European researchers in the mid-19th century began the first systematic observations and investigations of behavior within the asylum system, as more patients with chronic epilepsy became confined. Perhaps most applicable to our current dilemma are the writings of Morel (3), Falret (4), and Samt (6). Falret recognized both peri-ictal disorders and interictal problems defining patients who entered a prolonged abnormal mental state, "folie épileptique," in which slight epileptic paroxysms could be unrecognized or were substituted for by the abnormal mental state. Samt, in his classification, used the term epileptic equivalents. These were psychiatric presentations, recognized from their clinical form to be a manifestation of epilepsy, and described outbreaks of abnormal behavior, including episodes of violence, ecstasy, delirium, and stupor (86).

Morel is probably responsible for the development of the concept of the epileptic character. He noted, "Il est dans la nature des maladies nerveuses d'imprimer à l'idiosyncrasie physique et morale des malades un cachet tout à fait particulier" (Translation: "It is in the nature of nervous illnesses to imprint their own idiosyncratic physical and moral stamp.") (87). From these ideas grew the concept of larval or masked epilepsy, and it followed that the concept of epilepsy occurring without seizures was identified by behavioral features only. This legacy is still manifest in clinical practice, with concepts such as episodic dyscontrol.

Many studies have attempted to assess whether patients with epilepsy, when tested on personality rating scales, show different profiles from those of patients without epilepsy. Generally, the results support the hypothesis that patients with epilepsy have abnormal personalities. However, this outcome may be attributed to many factors. These include biological variables, for example, head injury following recurrent seizures, or the prescription of long-term anticonvulsant drugs, which may lead to behavioral change. Also, it may relate to psychosocial variables, such as stigmatization, and a low expectancy of achievement by the family or by teachers.

One crucial concept linked psychiatric disturbance in epilepsy with abnormalities of the temporal lobe. This idea arose at times when the biological basis of behavior was being explored through the understanding of the limbic system. Behavioral problems such as the Klüver-Bucy syndrome, occurring after bilateral extirpation of the amygdala, were described. Also, an integrated neuronal circuit that helped modulate emotions was recognized. With regard to epilepsy, the view that best summarized this approach was put forward by Gibbs and Stamps (88). They noted: "The patient's emotional reactions to his seizures, his family and his social situation are less important determinants of psychiatric disorder than the site and type of the epileptic discharge."

These views were based on observations that anterior temporal foci were common in patients with epilepsy who had an associated psychiatric disorder, the latter including not only psychosis but also personality change.

The rating scale most commonly used for scientific investigations has been the Minnesota Multiphasic Personality Inventory (MMPI). By and large, results using this scale have been mixed, although the scales that tend to be reported as most abnormal are the depression scale (D), the paranoia scale (Pa), the schizophrenia scale (Sc), and the psychesthenia scale (Pt). Hermann et al. (89) noted an association between adolescent age of onset of seizures and a high frequency of reporting on these psychotic subscales. In a separate study (90), these authors noted that patients with an aura of ictal fear scored higher on the MMPI profiles of paranoia, psychesthenia, schizophrenia, and psychopathic deviation.

The link of abnormal profiles to an aura of fear is interesting in that the latter suggests a site of seizure focus in the periamygdaloid region of the limbic system.

The controversial Bear-Fedio scale was developed by bringing together characteristics described in prior clinical reports of personality in epilepsy. In their original paper, now much criticized, Bear and Fedio (91) compared patients with unilateral temporal lobe epilepsy to normal subjects and a group with neuromuscular disorders. They noted that the epileptic patients had abnormal profiles, as predicted, particularly highlighting such features as humorlessness, dependence, circumstantiality, and an increased sense of personal destiny. Further, some laterality differences were noted; patients with left temporal lobe epilepsy describing more anger, paranoia, and dependence, while those with right temporal foci reported more elation. Several authors have argued that the scale does no more than assess nonspecific psychopathology. A further criticism is that the Bear-Fedio Inventory fails to confirm that all patients with temporal lobe epilepsy suffer from a distinctive personality profile. This, however, would seem an unrealistic expectation, and although Bear and Fedio (91) did refer to a consistent profile of changes, it was never claimed that this would be seen in all patients at all times.

The view that there is indeed an interictal behavior syndrome of epilepsy, associated largely with temporal lobe epilepsy, was most strongly supported by the writings of Geschwind and colleagues (92). Earlier reports of similar features were defined by Gastaut et al. (93). These reports highlighted changes in sexual behavior, hypergraphia (a tendency to compulsive and extensive writing), and religiosity. These reports also mentioned "stickiness" or viscosity, patients showing a striking preoccupation with detail and concerns over moral or ethical issues. Estimates of the frequency with which such a profile occurs, from cluster analysis studies using MMPI and other clinical variables, vary from 7% (94) to 21% (95).

Disagreement over the association between epilepsy and personality disorder persists, but those dealing with patients with chronic epilepsy are quite familiar with these personality changes. Sometimes these personality traits dominate the clinical picture interictally to the extent that patients' lives are compromised. In other cases, the features are found in creative people, (an artistic example may be Van Gogh; literary examples may be Flaubert or Dostoyevsky). In still other cases, the underlying tone of the personality is suggestive of these traits, but the features erupt more fully at times of seizures and seizure clusters. The evidence support-

ing the view that these abnormalities are more common in patients with temporal lobe epilepsy is not conclusive, but the number of positive studies outweigh the negative ones by far, and more recent studies confirm this theory.

EPILEPSY AND DEPRESSION

Depression is a clinically important concomitant of epilepsy. A link between the two states was described by Hippocrates: "Melancholics ordinarily become epileptics, and epileptics melancholics: of these two states what determines the preference is the direction the malady takes; if it bears upon the body, epilepsy, if upon the intelligence, melancholy" (96). This association has continued to intrigue observers down through the ages (97). In his textbook on epilepsy written in 1861, at the beginning of the scientific approach of the treatment to epilepsy, Reynolds (98) discussed the interactions between mental state and seizures. More recently a number of reviews have documented the nature of the association between depression and epilepsy (99–104).

Prevalence

Although most authors acknowledge that depression is more often seen in epilepsy than in the larger population, the significance of the association depends on the population studied. Very few studies have investigated the absolute prevalence of psychiatric morbidity in epilepsy in the community. Two studies in England assessed all the patients with epilepsy registered with a number of primary care physicians. In a sample of 218 patients, Pond et al. (105) recorded psychological difficulties in 29%. In half of these the difficulties were "neurotic" in nature. Fifteen years later, Edeh and Toone (106), in a similar community-based survey of 88 patients, recorded neurotic depression in 22% of their sample. Hence, psychiatric disturbances are often seen in epilepsy, but in the absence of a similarly assessed community control population, the significance of this frequency is difficult to interpret.

In a study of patients with temporal lobe epilepsy, 19% were found to have clinically apparent anxiety, while 11% were depressed (107).

The importance of understanding depression in epilepsy is highlighted when the frequency of suicide/parasuicide in this population is considered. Having reviewed 11 previous studies, Barraclough (99) reported a suicide rate five times that in the general population. Mathews and Barabas (108), analyzed eight studies and noted a suicide rate in epilepsy of 5% compared with 1.4% in control populations. In patients with temporal lobe epilepsy, the relative risk is even greater. There is also an increased risk of parasuicide, among these patients, particularly of overdoses.

Mania is rarely associated with epilepsy. Williams (109) described elation in just three of 2000 patients. The few cases reported in the literature are in the form of anecdotal accounts of individual cases (110, 111).

Table 33.10. Associations of Depression in Epilepsy[a]

Association	Number of Studies Finding Association	Number of Studies Finding No Association
Seizure characteristics		
seizure type	1	4
temporal focus	3	1
left focus	3	7
seizure frequency	1	4
seizure duration	1	4
Treatment-related		
polypharmacy	3	3
phenobarbitone	3	
low serum folate	3	
Personal factors		
male preponderance	2	3
loss of control	1	1
family depression history	1	1

[a]Adapted from Ring HA, Trimble MR. Depression in epilepsy. In: Depression in Neurological Disease. Eds: Starkstein SE & Robinson RG. Johns Hopkins University Press pp 63-83.

Etiology of Depression in Epilepsy

There are no clearly established mechanisms by which epilepsy may bring about clinical depression. Just as depression is a heterogeneous condition, so it is likely that various factors unique to each patient with epilepsy combine to generate specific forms of associated depressive illness. However, based on clinical and experimental observations, it is possible to explore possible etiological elements common across patients.

Unfortunately, although a number of studies have examined depression in epilepsy, the data from these investigations are not entirely comparable. Patients were recruited from various sources, ranging from the community to specialist neuropsychiatric clinics. Some were well controlled on antiepileptic medication, while others were being considered for surgical treatment following a long period of limited response to drug management. In addition, numerous assessment techniques were utilized, including clinical examination, structured interviews, and self-completed questionnaires. Likewise, the information obtained was interpreted using different diagnostic criteria and groupings. However, when evaluating these studies with a broader view, some tentative conclusions may be drawn (Table 33.10).

PSYCHOLOGICAL FACTORS

The social sequalae of having epilepsy were relevant more than 2000 years ago when Hippocrates referred to the condition as the "sacred disease." Since that time much has been written on the social stigmatization of those with epilepsy. Even in our own more enlightened times, there is evidence that this stigmatization persists (112). The most powerful means of reducing this prejudice is through educating the patients, their families, and the public about epilepsy.

The adverse effects of stigma, discrimination, vocational difficulties, and attendant strains of often unpredictable losses of consciousness were investigated by Hermann and Wyler (113), using the psychological construct of locus of control. In a population of patients awaiting temporal lobe surgery for epilepsy, it was concluded that there was a significant association between an external locus of control, indicating a feeling of loss of personal control over life, and depression.

In addition, for many patients there will be more general social difficulties associated with problems of living with a chronic and, at times, disabling illness. Turner and Beiser (114), in a controlled study, interviewed more than 700 people chronically disabled by various conditions, most frequently, heart disease or arthritis. They found that the disabled group suffered several disadvantages, regardless of their precise diagnosis. They were more likely to have a lower income and to be depressed. The authors explained the increased depression as a reaction to chronic stress associated with the difficulties of chronic illness. Quite likely these nonspecific factors also apply to individuals with epilepsy, even though they generally have fewer physical difficulties than some of the patients studied by Turner and Beiser (114).

The following review of potential biological mechanisms of depression illustrates that psychosocial factors may be critical in determining which of those patients with a particular biological state will go on to develop depression.

SEIZURE-RELATED FACTORS

The findings of several studies, summarized in Table 35.12, suggest that neither specific seizure types, (complex partial with or without secondary generalization or primary generalized seizures) nor frequency, nor duration of epilepsy are usually associated with depression. A majority of the studies that have addressed the issue report an association between interictal depression and a temporal lobe epilepsy. However, the situation is more equivocal regarding the laterality of the epileptic focus. A number of studies in the neurological literature have demonstrated that major depression is more often associated with left-, as opposed to right-hemisphere lesions, for example, after a cerebral vascular accident (CVA). However, poststroke mania is strongly associated with a right-hemisphere lesion in a limbic-connected area (115). In epilepsy there is also a link to the left hemisphere with depression (101), and cases of hypomania following seizures derived from the right temporal lobes have been reported (110, 115). In two cases religiosity was a prominent part of the mental state. Interestingly, all patients were male and had experienced a preceding flurry of seizures.

A study by Hermann et al. (113) suggests a possible complex association between temporal lobe epilepsy and the presence of depression. These authors observed that in their patients with left (but not right) temporal lobe epilepsy, there was a significant correlation between the degree of frontal lobe dysfunction, measured using a frontal lobe cognitive task, the Wisconsin Card Sorting Test, and the presence of a self-reported dysphoric mood state. Although acknowledging the limited value of self-reported ratings of mental states and the relatively mild nature of the mood disturbance, the authors concluded that their results suggested that the presence of concomitant frontal lobe dysfunction was important in the etiology of affective disturbance associated with temporal lobe epilepsy. This theory is compatible with observations from imaging studies of depression and with the literature on poststroke depression.

The role of the temporal lobes in the generation of affective states may also be investigated by considering the effects of temporal lobe surgery performed for the control of epilepsy. Apparently, in a minority of patients with chronic epilepsy, depression has worsened or developed de novo after temporal lobectomy (104). Should this occur, there is some evidence that it will do so acutely. Of 72 patients followed postsurgically for 1–2 years, there were six who made suicide attempts, and in every case this was in the first month after the operation (116). An increase in depression following anterior temporal lobectomy was also described by Bruton (117) in an analysis of the Falconer series of patients from the Maudsley Hospital. In this group of 249 patients, only one was considered depressed at the time of surgery, but during postsurgical follow-up, the incidence of depression rose to 10%, and six patients committed suicide. The mechanism of this effect is unknown, although the postsurgical increase in depression may in part be an artifact of comparing rates at a single point in time with those obtained over a prolonged follow-up period. It may also be a reflection of "forced normalization" (see discussion that follows) in some cases. This concept refers to patients who develop psychopathology when their seizures are brought under control, and their EEG becomes "more normal" than before, when they were psychiatrically well.

BIOCHEMICAL FACTORS

Biochemical links between epilepsy and depression remain to be established. However, several avenues have been explored. Animal studies have suggested that limbic seizures may alter the functioning of cerebral corticotrophin-releasing hormone (CRH) pathways. It has been suggested that these changes may increase vulnerability to stress-precipitated psychopathology (118). However, there is currently no evidence in humans to support this suggestion, and as yet there are no treatment implications.

Another potential biochemical mechanism that is based on human studies is that of folate depletion. This has been observed in patients on polytherapy (119), and a relationship between mental illness and folate deficiency was reported by Carney (120). Phenytoin and barbiturates may both lead to falls in serum, red blood cell (RBC), and cerebrospinal fluid (CSF) folate. In epilepsy a link between low folate and depression has been noticed in several patient groups (121, 122). Edeh and Toone (106) examined serum and RBC folate levels in a community sample of epileptic patients on monotherapy or polytherapy. They found that there were significantly lower folate concentrations in those on polytherapy and in those achieving psychiatric "caseness" using the Clinical Interview Schedule. This was true for the depressive neurosis subgroup but not for the anxiety subgroup. However, the authors emphasize that association does not imply causality, and the links between folate deficiency and mood change are not clear. In addition, therapeutic trials of folate have not been effective in treating depression, although some methyl donors, such *s*-adenosyl methionine, may be more promising.

Diagnosis of Depression in Epilepsy

Because an epileptic seizure is an event defined in time, many authors have used temporal definitions to characterize different associations between epilepsy and affective disturbance. The most common temporal separation is into prodromal, peri-ictal and interictal periods. The peri-ictal period includes the aura, the ictus itself, and the immediately postictal period.

PRODROMAL PHENOMENA

The prodrome, occurring hours to days before a seizure, was investigated by Blanchet and Frommer (123). They reported a prospective study in which 27 patients with epilepsy self-rated their moods using Personal Feelings Scales, and recorded life events on a daily basis for at least 56 days. During this time, 13 patients had at least one seizure. The authors observed that in these patients the mean ratings of mood on eight of the 10 scales showed a decline on the day(s) preceding the seizure and an increase after the seizure.

In four patients the mean Depression Scale rating on the day preceding the seizure was significantly lower than the mean rating on normal days. Although an increase in negative life events was reported by patients whose mood fell before seizures, this correlation was not significant.

There are several possible explanations for the association between lowered mood ratings and the subsequent occurrence of seizures. Lower mood may be a symptom of the prodromal phase of seizure activity, initiated by the same biological processes that bring about the seizure. Alternatively, perhaps the mood change itself precipitates a seizure. The authors discuss these possibilities but conclude that the question remains without a definitive answer because in their study the relationship of life events and mood to seizures apparently was independent.

PERI-ICTAL PHENOMENA

The aura is the earliest stage of subjective awareness of seizure activity. Many different sensations have been recorded (124). Taylor and Lochery (125) investigated 215 aura experiences in 88 patients with temporal lobe epilepsy. They recorded details of auras of various complexities and types, but remarkably, although there were 24 experiences of "epigastric fear," there were no reports of any other affective states.

Williams (109) investigated emotional phenomena in 2000 patients with epilepsy and found that 100 of them reported an emotion as part of the "epileptic experience." As in the study by Taylor and Lochery (125), the most commonly reported emotion was fear, occurring in Williams's sample in 61% of the 100 patients with emotional phenomena. On some occasions this fear was quite pervasive, with psychic and somatic features. In contrast to this, depression was reported less often, in just 21% (i.e., in 1% of the whole group). However, Williams observed that when depression did occur it tended to last far longer than the other peri-ictal phenomena, persisting for up to several days after the ictus. This was interpreted as being akin to naturally occurring depression, which tends to be self-sustaining.

Although of short duration, postictal depression may be severe, at times including suicidal ideation. Case descriptions give a clear impression that the depressive phase is more than purely an emotional reaction to the advent of a seizure, suggesting instead a biological link with the seizure process (126).

Thus peri-ictal depression, though it does occur, is not common but is characterized by a greater persistence than other postictal emotional phenomena. It is interesting to note that depressive auras appear to be particularly rare, whereas fear is more common.

INTERICTAL PHENOMENA

Recently several studies have investigated the phenomenology of interictal depression. Mendez et al. (127) compared 20 depressed epileptic inpatients to 20 nonepi-

Table 33.11. Categories of Epilepsies[a]

Doubtful epileptic (epileptoid) seizures
Major epileptic seizures
Minor epileptic seizures (petit mal)
Minor psychic-epileptic equivalents (petit mal)
Postepileptic insanity
Simple psychic-epileptic equivalents
Recurrent psychic-epileptic equivalents
Protracted epileptic insanity
Doubtful-epileptic (epileptoid) insanity
Circular epileptic insanity
Epilepsy with dementia
Habitual epileptic personality
Hysteroepileptic insanity (exclusively in females)

[a]From Samt P. Epileptishe irreseinsformen. Archiv für Psychiatric and Nervenkrankheiten 1876; 6:110–216.

leptic depressed subjects. Both groups met DSM III criteria for major depression. All the patients had endogenous features of depression—anergia, anhedonia, appetite, and sleep disturbance—but the authors concluded that there were other major distinguishing characteristics of the depressed patients with epilepsy compared with those of the nonepileptic group. These factors included a chronic dysthymic background, a relative lack of neurotic traits, such as somatization or self-pity, and a history of periods of agitated peri-ictal psychotic behavior.

The depressive characteristics of a larger group of epileptic patients meeting Research Diagnostic Criteria for major depressive disorder were described by Robertson et al. (122). These authors assessed 66 patients using clinical examination and a number of standardized rating scales. In this study patients obtained very high state and trait anxiety scores. The authors suggested that the high level of state anxiety may have been due to the depression, considering that it decreased significantly during a 6-week double-blind placebo-controlled trial of an antidepressant (128).

EPILEPSY AND PSYCHOSIS

In the middle of the 19th century, European psychiatrists noted the high incidence of psychotic episodes in institutionalized patients with epilepsy. Several authors described the specific psychopathology of psychiatric complications occurring in the context of epilepsy, using terms like "epilepsie larvee" (3), "grand mal intellectuel" (4), "epileptoid states" (5), and "epileptic equivalents" (129). Samt (6) introduced the idea that the pathophysiology of certain psychoses occurring in the context of epilepsy, especially episodic twilight states, was identical to the pathophysiology of motor seizures. He suggested that in the absence of true seizures, such epileptic equivalents were sufficient for a diagnosis of epilepsy (Table 33.11).

Some authors in the 19th century explicitly noted the rarity of chronic paranoia or true madness in patients with epilepsy. These observations resulted in intensive discussions on the nature of the relationship between epilepsy and

Table 33.12. Frequency of Mixed Psychoses in Epilepsy (Europe, Japan, U.S.)

Source of Patients	Author	Year	Prevalence (%)
Field study	Gudmundsson	1966	7
	Zielinski	1974	2
General practices	Edeh and Toone	1987	5
Neurological departments	Roger et al.	1956	9
	Standage and Fenton	1975	8
Epileptological departments	Bruens	1973	6
	Sengoku et al.	1983	6
	Schmitz	1988	4
Psychiatric departments	Roger et al.	1956	41
	Betts	1974	21
	Bash and Mahnig	1984	60

schizophrenia, a subject frequently chosen in theoretical disputes on definitions of terms like disease and symptom complex in psychiatry at the beginning of the 20th century (as others)(130, 131).

In cases of combined seizures and schizophrenia-like symptoms, these were preferably interpreted as either symptomatic seizures secondary to cerebral sequelae of insanity, e.g., brain edema in catatonia, or symptomatic psychoses due to seizures or the epileptic process (as others) (132, 133). In cases without an obvious temporal relationship between epileptic seizures and psychotic symptoms, it was speculated that both were not directly linked but caused by the same underlying brain pathology (134, 135). Ganter (137), Krapf (133), and Glaus (137) published a clinical case series with a prevalence rate of combinations lower than expected. These studies, together with observations of an alternation between periods with seizures and seizure free periods with psychosis in some patients, and the improvement of psychotic symptoms after spontaneous seizures in others, led to the theory of functional dependency and biological antagonism of schizophrenic and epileptic symptoms. This concept influenced von Meduna (138) to introduce iatrogenic convulsions into the treatment of schizophrenia.

With progress in the diagnosis and treatment in epilepsy, the disease became the realm of neurologists. Psychiatric aspects were neglected until they were "rediscovered" in the 1950s and 1960s (139–141). American and British authors reported an excess of schizophrenia-like psychoses in epilepsy patients, especially in those suffering from temporal lobe epilepsy (142–144).

Slater and his colleagues published a detailed analysis of 69 patients from two London hospitals who suffered from epilepsy and interictal psychoses. On the basis of this case series, the authors challenged the antagonism theory and postulated a positive link between epilepsy and schizophrenia. Although Slater was criticized for drawing conclusions on the basis of insufficient statistics (145), the temporal lobe hypothesis soon became broadly accepted and stimulated extensive research into the role of temporal lobe pathology in schizophrenia. The use of epileptic psychoses as a biological model or "mock-up" of schizophrenia (146) is largely based on Gibbs's, and Slater's work.

The possible impact of research of epileptic psychosis on the understanding of the pathophysiology of endogenous psychoses explains the bias in the literature toward study of interictal schizophrenia-like psychoses. The spectrum of psychotic syndromes in epilepsy is, however, much more complex, and psychotic complications are not restricted to patients with temporal lobe epilepsy.

Epidemiology

There are only four population-based studies on the frequency of mixed psychoses in epilepsy. Krohn (147), in a population-based survey in Norway, found a 2% prevalence of psychoses with epilepsy. In a field study of the Warsaw population, Zielinski (148) found prevalence rates for psychoses in epilepsy of 2–3%. In a field study of 2635 registered epilepsy patients in a district in Poland, only 0.5% were diagnosed with schizophrenia, but 19.5% suffered from postictal twilight states (149). Gudmundsson (150), in a study on the frequency of mixed psychoses in epilepsy in the population of Iceland, found prevalence rates for males of 6% and for females of 9%. These figures can be compared with findings of an earlier study by Helgason, who determined the risk of psychosis in the general population of Iceland using the same diagnostic criteria as Gudmundsson. Helgason found prevalence rates of 7% for males and 5% for females. The comparison of Helgason's and Gudmundsson's results suggests a similar risk for psychoses in people with and without epilepsy, being only slightly higher in females but slightly lower in males with epilepsy.

Most figures in the literature on the freuqency of psychosis in epilepsy derive from clinical case series and are therefore likely to be biased by unknown selection mechanisms. They cannot be regarded as representative of epilepsy in general. Table 33.12 presents prevalence rates as a function of the source of patients. The table suggests that psychoses are highly overrepresented in specialized centers.

There is thus no evidence from epidemiological studies for an excess of psychosis in people with epilepsy. However, clinical case series clearly indicate that psychosis is a significant problem in patients attending specialized centers. This finding suggests that there are risk factors for the development of psychosis related to complicated epilepsy and chronic illness.

Classification

There is no internationally accepted syndromic classification of psychoses in epilepsy. Psychiatric aspects are not considered in the international classification of epilepsies, and the use of operational diagnostic systems for psychiatric disorders such as the DSM-IV (151) is limited because, if applied strictly, a diagnosis of functional psychosis is not allowed in the context of epilepsy.

Most of previously proposed classification systems for psychosis in epilepsy (152–155) are based on a combination of psychopathological, etiological, longitudinal, and EEG parameters. Unfortunately, lacking taxonomic studies, our knowledge about regular syndromic associations is still limited. It seems, however, that in epileptic psychoses, diagnostic criteria are not strictly intercorrelated. Dongier (156) concluded from her detailed analysis of 536 psychotic episodes in 516 patients that it was not possible to deduce from the type of psychosis the type of epilepsy or vice versa. "Atypical" syndromes are not unusual, such as ictal and postictal psychoses in clear consciousness (157). Variations of phenomenology and precipitating factors can also be seen within individual patients who experience recurrent psychotic episodes (158,159). In addition, there is also some evidence for an etiological overlap between syndromes (160). Simplified classifications on doubtful hypothetical grounds seem inappropriate. For the time being, patients with epilepsy and psychoses should probably receive two separate diagnoses according to both the ICE and the DSM-IV. In addition, the relation between onset of psychosis and seizure activity, antiepileptic therapy and changes of EEG findings should be noted.

For pragmatic reasons, psychoses in epilepsy are grouped here according to their temporal relationship to seizures. Nevertheless, such a classification does not necessarily imply fundamental differences in terms of pathophysiology. Table 33.13 provides a comparative list of the syndromes described in more detail in the sections that follow.

SYNDROMES OF PSYCHOSES IN RELATION TO SEIZURE ACTIVITY

Ictal Psychoses

Prolonged focal and generalized nonconvulsive epileptic activity (occurring for several hours or days) may present with psychotic symptoms. Generalized nonconvulsive status, also called absence status, petit mal status, or spike-wave stupor (161), is characterized by altered or narrowed consciousness. Patients are disoriented and apathetic. Contact with the environment is partially preserved, and patients are often able to perform simple tasks. Positive psychotic symptoms, such as delusions and hallucinations, occur only in some patients.

The EEG shows generalized bilateral synchronous spike-wave complexes of variable frequency between 1 Hz and 4 Hz. In prolonged generalized status, however, the EEG patterns may become more irregular and lose their symmetric synchrony, making it difficult or impossible to distinguish complex focal status. The status may be terminated by spontaneous generalized tonic-clonic seizures.

Absence status typically occurs in patients with a known history of generalized epilepsy, but "atypical absence status" may occur as a first manifestation of epilepsy, especially in later life (162).

Two types of complex focal status (synonyms: status psychomotoricus, epileptic twilight state) have been distinguished: (a) a continuous form and (b) a discontinuous or cyclic form. The latter consists of frequently recurring complex partial seizures. Between seizures, patients may or may not experience simple focal seizure symptoms, and consciousness may recover to nearly normal states.

Noncyclic forms of complex partial status consist of prolonged confusional episodes or psychotic behavior. The EEG during complex partial status shows focal or bilateral epileptiform patterns and slowed background activity. Subtle rudiments of motor seizure symptoms, such as lid-fluttering and bursts of myoclonic jerks in absence status or mild oral activity automatisms in continuous complex partial status, may point to the underlying epileptic activity. Mutism and paucity of speech—or even speech arrest—occurs in both absence and complex partial status.

Table 33.13. Clinical Characteristics of Psychoses in Relation to Seizure Activity

	Ictal Pyschosis	Postictal Psychosis	Peri-ictal Psychosis	Alternative Psychosis	Interictal Psychosis
Consciousness	Impaired	Impaired or normal	Impaired	Normal	Normal
Duration	Hours to days	Days to weeks	Days to weeks	Days and weeks	Months
EEG	Status epilepticus	Increased epileptic and slow activity	Increased epileptic and slow activity	Normalized	Unchanged
Treatment	Antiepileptic drugs (IV)	Spontaneous recovery in many cases	Improvement of seizure control	Reduction of antiepileptic drugs	Neuroleptic drug

Complex partial status may arise from any part of the brain. In discontinuous complex partial status, understanding the seizure patterns may help for localization of the focal origin in the mesial or lateral temporal lobe or extratemporally. Continuous complex partial status is more often of frontal or extratemporal origin than cyclic status (164). Nonconvulsive status epilepticus requires immediate treatment with intravenous antiepileptic drugs.

Simple focal status or aura continua may cause complex hallucinations, thought disorders, and affective symptoms. The continuous epileptic activity is restricted and may escape scalp EEG recordings. Insight is usually maintained, and true psychoses emerging from such a state have not been described.

The presentation of these states may be subtle, and examination of the mental state, especially for mild confusion is necessary. Sometimes patients with partial status resemble schizophrenics very closely, and without knowledge of a history of epilepsy—for example in the emergency room—the ictal origin may be overlooked. Any suspicion of epilepsy should lead to a request for an EEG. If this is unavailable, an IV injection of a benzodiazepine may help to resolve the diagnosis.

Postictal Psychoses

Most postictal psychoses are precipitated by a series of generalized tonic-clonic seizures. More rarely, psychoses occur after single grand mal seizures or following a series of complex partial seizures (163). Postictal psychoses account for approximately 25% of psychoses in epilepsy (155, 164).

The relation to the type of epilepsy is not clear. Dongier (156) described a preponderance of generalized epilepsies, while Logsdail and Toone (165) noted a higher frequency of postictal psychosis in patients with focal epilepsies and complex focal seizures.

In most patients there is a characteristic lucid interval lasting from 1–6 days between the epileptic seizures and onset of psychosis (135), which may lead to an incorrect diagnosis.

The psychopathology of postictal psychosis is polymorphic, but most patients present with abnormal mood and paranoid delusions (166). Some patients are confused throughout the episode; others present with fluctuating impairment of consciousness and orientation. Sometimes there is no confusion whatsoever.

The EEG during postictal psychosis is deteriorated with increased epileptic as well as slow wave activity.

Psychotic symptoms spontaneously remit within days or weeks, often without need for additional neuroleptic treatment. However, in some cases chronic psychoses develop from recurrent and even a single postictal psychosis (157, 163). The pathophysiology is not known. Savard et al. (163) noted the clinical analogy of psychoses following complex partial seizures to other postictal phenomena, such as Todd's paresis or postictal memory loss. Logsdail and Toone

hypothesized that postictal psychosis results from increased postsynaptic dopamine sensitivity (167).

Peri-ictal Psychosis

Most authors do not distinguish peri-ictal from postictal psychoses. In peri-ictal psychosis, psychotic symptoms develop gradually and parallel to increases in seizure frequency. The relation to seizures is easily overlooked if seizure frequency is not carefully documented over prolonged periods. More rapid development of peri-ictal psychoses can be seen, especially during the presurgical assessment of patients with intractable epilepsy when a series of epileptic seizures may be provoked by withdrawal of antiepileptic drugs. Impairment of consciousness is more frequent than in postictal psychosis. Treatment of peri-ictal psychoses requires improvement of seizure control.

Interictal Psychoses

Interictal psychoses occur between seizures and cannot be linked directly to the ictus. They are less frequent than peri-ictal psychoses and account for 10–30% of diagnoses in unselected case series (157, 166). Interictal psychoses are, however, clinically more significant in terms of severity and duration than peri-ictal psychoses, which usually are short-lasting and often self-limiting (Table 35.15).

Slater stated that in the absence of epilepsy, the psychoses in their study group would have been diagnosed as schizophrenia (166). But they also mentioned distinct differences between process schizophrenia and the schizophrenia-like psychoses associated with epilepsy. They highlighted the preservation of warm affect and a high frequency of delusions and religious mystical experiences.

Other authors stressed the rarity of negative symptoms and the absence of formal thought disorder and catatonic states (169). McKenna et al. pointed out that visual hallucinations were more prominent than auditory hallucinations. Tellenbach (141) stated that delusions were less well organized, and Sherwin (158) remarked that neuroleptic treatment was less frequently necessary. There have been other authors, however, who denied any psychopathological diffrences between epileptic psychosis and schizophrenia (167, 168).

Using the Present State Examination and the CATEGO computer program, which is a semistandardized and validated method for quantifying psychopathology, it has been possible to compare the presentation of psychosis in epilepsy with process schizophrenia. Very few significant differences emerged from such studies (169, 170), suggesting that, assuming the patients were representative, a significant number will have a schizophrenia-like presentation indistinguishable from schizophrenia in the absence of epilepsy.

RISK FACTORS

The pathogenesis of psychotic episodes in epilepsy is likely to be heterogeneous. In most patients a multitude of

Table 33.14.   Risk Factors Associated with Interictal Psychoses of Epilepsy[a]

Sex	Bias to females
Age of onset	Early adolescence
Interval	Onset of seizures to onset of psychosis: 14 years
Epileptic syndrome	Temporal lobe epilepsy
Seizure type	Complex focal
Seizure frequency	Low, diminished
Neurological findings	Sinistrality
Pathology	Gangliogliomas, hamartomas
EEG	Mediobasal focus, especially left-sided

[a]From Trimble MR. The psychoses of epilepsy. New York: Raven Press, 1991, pp137.

chronic and acute factors can be identified that are potentially responsible for the development of a psychiatric disorder. These factors are difficult to investigate in retrospect, and whether or not the interpretation is causally related or simply interrelated is arguable.

The literature on risk factors is highly controversial; studies are difficult to compare because of varying definitions of the epilepsy, the psychiatric disorder, and the investigated risk factors. Most studies are restricted to interictal psychoses. Table 33.14 summarizes factors that have frequently been correlated with psychosis in epilepsy (171).

Genetic Predisposition

With few exceptions, most authors do not find any evidence for an increased rate of psychiatric disorders in relatives of epilepsy patients with psychoses (172).

Sex Distribution

There has been a bias toward female sex in several case series (173), which has not been confirmed in controlled studies (174, 175).

Duration of Epilepsy

The interval between age at onset of epilepsy and age at first manifestation of psychosis has been remarkably homogeneous in many series, ranging from 11–15 years. This interval has been used to postulate the etiological significance of the seizure disorder and a kindling-like mechanism. Some authors (152) have argued that the supposedly specific interval represents an artifact. They noted a wide range, being significantly shorter in patients with later onset of epilepsy. They also pointed out that persons whose psychosis did not succeed their epilepsy were excluded in most series, and that there is a tendency in the general population for the age of onset of epilepsy to peak at an earlier age than that of schizophrenia.

Type of Epilepsy

There is a clear excess of temporal lobe epilepsy in almost all case series of patients with epilepsy and psychosis.

Summarizing the data of 10 studies, 217—or 76%—of 287 patients suffered from temporal lobe epilepsy. The preponderance of this type of epilepsy is, however, not a uniform finding; in Gudmundsson's epidemiological study, for example, only 7% suffered from "psychomotor" epilepsy.

The nature of a possible link of psychoses to temporal lobe epilepsy is not entirely clear (176) partly because of ambiguities in the definition of TLE in the literature, either based on seizure symptomatology (psychomotor epilepsy), involvement of specific functional systems (limbic epilepsy), or on anatomical localization as detected by depth EEG or neuroimaging (amygdalo-hippocampal epilepsy). Unfortunately, most authors have not sufficiently differentiated frontal and temporal lobe epilepsy.

The temporal lobe hypothesis, although widely accepted, has been criticized for being based on uncontrolled case series, such as in the studies by Gibbs (142) and Slater and Beard (166). It was argued that temporal lobe epilepsy is the most frequent type of epilepsy in the general population and that there is a disproportionate number of patients with this type of epilepsy who present at specialized centers. There is a general consensus that psychoses are very rare in patients with neocortical extratemporal epilepsies (177, 178).

The findings are similar regarding rates of psychosis in TLE and generalized epilepsies. In fact, with only three exceptions (178–180), the majority of controlled studies failed to establish significant differences in the frequency of psychoses in generalized vs. temporal lobe epilepsy (180-184). However, many patients with generalized epilepsy show pathology of temporal structures, making classification difficult.

Several studies demonstrate that psychoses in generalized epilepsies differ from psychoses in TLE. The former are more likely to be short-lasting and confusional (183). Psychoses that are develop in generalized epilepsy are usually relatively mild and often remit before paranoid-hallucinatory symptoms are seen. Schneiderian first-rank symptoms and chronicity are more frequent in patients with temporal lobe epilepsy (185). This has considerable significance for psychiatrists attempting to unravel the underlying "neurology" of schizophrenia.

Type of Seizures

There is evidence from several studies that focal seizure symptoms that indicate ictal mesial temporal or limbic involvement are overrepresented in patients with psychosis. Hermann and Chabria (186) noted a relationship between ictal fear and high scores on paranoia and schizophrenia scales of the Multiphasic Personality Inventory (MMPI). Kristensen and Sindrup (176, 177) found an excess of dysmnesic and epigastric auras in their psychotic group. They also reported a higher rate of ictal amnesia.

Severity of Epilepsy

The strongest risk factors for psychosis in epilepsy are those that correlate with severity of epilepsy. These include long duration of active epilepsy, multiple seizure types (187-189), history of status epilepticus (166), and poor response to drug treatment. Seizure frequency, however, is reported by most authors to be lower in psychotic epilepsy patients than in nonpsychotic patients (190, 191). It is unclear if seizure frequency was low before or during the psychotic episode. This may represent a variant of forced normalization.

Laterality

Left lateralization of temporal lobe dysfunction or temporal lobe pathology as a risk factor for schizophreniform psychosis was originally suggested by Flor-Henry (174). Studies supporting the laterality hypothesis have been made using computed tomography (CT), neuropathology (193), neuropsychology, and PET (194).

Forced Normalization

A full understanding of the relationships between epilepsy and psychosis must consider the concept of forced normalization.

Earlier this century reports appeared that suggested there was some kind of antagonism between epilepsy and psychosis. Accordingly, von Meduna introduced convulsive therapy for the treatment of schizophrenia. In the 1950s Landolt (195) published a series of papers on patients who had epilepsy who became psychotic when their seizures were under control. He defined forced normalization as follows:

> Forced normalisation is the phenomenon characterised by the fact that, with the recurrence of psychotic states, the EEG becomes more normal, or entirely normal as compared with previous and subsequent EEG findings.

Forced normalization was thus essentially an EEG phenomenon. The clinical counterpart of patients becoming psychotic when their seizures were under control, and their psychosis resolving with return of seizures, was referred to as alternative psychoses by Tellenbach (141).

These phenomena have now been well documented clinically. The following are points important to note, however. First, the EEG does not need to become "normal," but the interictal disturbances decrease and in some cases disappear. Second, the clinical presentation need not necessarily be a psychosis, but sometimes is. In childhood, or in patients with mental handicaps, aggression and agitation are common. Other manifestations include pseudoseizures or other conversion symptoms, depression, mania, and anxiety states. Third, the psychotic episodes may last days or weeks. They may be terminated by a seizure, and the EEG abnormalities may then return. Finally, Landolt originally associated this phenomenon with focal epilepsies, but with the introduction of the succinimide drugs, he noted an association with the generalized epilepsies. Clearly, forced normalization may be provoked by the administration of anticonvulsants, and has been reported with barbiturates, benzodiazepines, ethosuximide, and vigabatrin.

The literature on antagonism between epilepsy and psychosis has been considered incompatible with the suggestions just outlined, regarding an increased association between epilepsy and psychosis. This disagreement has been resolved by more careful understanding of the original literature (196). Thus, within the association, namely of a link between psychosis and epilepsy, there may be an antagonism of symptoms, namely between seizures and the symptoms of psychosis—for example, hallucinations and delusions.

It is often denied that forced normalization occurs, probably with good reason. Thus, it is certainly rarer than Landolt contends, and studies are limited. It is difficult to document cases precisely, EEG recordings being difficult to obtain at the right times. However, other less enlightened reasons to ignore such findings relate to the fact that the concept brings psychiatry uncomfortably close to neurology, revealing a close biological link between seizures and psychosis. It also affects treatment. Thus, if in some patients, suppression of seizures provokes psychopathology, it means that seizures and epilepsy are not synonymous and that an understanding of the epileptic process and its treatment goes far beyond the control of seizures. In clinical practice it is important to recognize that some patients may indeed manifest these problems, which can lead to the continuation of severe behavior disturbances. Failure to treat the epilepsy appropriately can lead to considerable social disruption.

PSEUDOSEIZURES

The term pseudoseizure is a misnomer. Patients can present with pseudoepileptic seizures, or nonepileptic attack disorder, nonepileptic seizures. However, the seizures in these patients are very real, both to patients, third-party observers, and their physicians. Indeed, nearly 20% of patients attending chronic epilepsy clinics do not have epilepsy but have some form of nonepileptic disorder (197). Alternative terms, including hysterical seizures, and psychogenic seizures, are also inadequate, the former being pejorative, the latter defining a different kind of seizure altogether. Thus, psychogenic seizure should logically be used only to imply a form of reflex seizure induced by mental activities (198).

In the differential diagnosis of nonepileptic attacks, various psychiatric and other medical conditions should be considered. To limit the investigation exclusively to the neurological features of such patients—ignoring the rest of the differential diagnosis—is totally inappropriate. This approach leads to misdiagnosis and condemnation of the patient to taking anticonvulsant drugs, often unnecessarily, for many years.

Conversion symptoms are common in medical practice. In the stable form of hysteria, Briquet's hysteria (see below), it is estimated that nonepileptic seizures occur in 12% of patients.

It is important to note that although patients with established epilepsy may have pseudoseizures, the latter

Table 33.15. Psychiatric Differential Diagnosis of Seizures

Anxiety
  GAD
  Panic disorder (hyperventilation; depersonalization)
Depression (fugues)
Schizophrenia
Conversion disorder
Somatization disorder
Episodic dyscontrol
Malingering

GAD = Generalized Anxiety Disorder.

frequently occur in the absence of epilepsy, and it is usually unnecessary to entertain both diagnoses in the same patient. Lesser (203), after a review of the literature, cautioned against making a double diagnosis, noting definite epilepsy in only 12% and possible epilepsy in only 24% of over 300 reported cases of pseudoseizures.

Differential Diagnosis of Nonepileptic Attacks or Pseudoseizures

The medical and psychiatric conditions to be considered are shown in Tables 35.9 and 33.15. Obvious cardiological causes, for example, vasovagal attacks, frequently present in adolescence and often herald the development of pseudoseizures. It is important that they are not retrospectively thought to be epileptic seizures, making the whole clinical history mistaken. Metabolic conditions, for example, hypoglycemia, should always be considered in the differential diagnosis, and attempts made to rule out other common medical conditions should be listed.

One of the most common areas of misdiagnosis is with the sleep disorders. Both rapid eye movement (REM) and non-REM disorders can be misdiagnosed as epilepsy, as can some of the hypersomnolent conditions. Night terrors arise out of stage-four sleep, as opposed to the nightmares of REM sleep. They are associated with the sudden onset of restless motor activity, sometimes with a vocalization of fear.

REM behavior disorder, which occurs in patients who have subtle brain stem damage and no longer have the characteristic REM muscle paralysis, can present with kicking around, self-injury, and aggression. Cataplexy, if the other elements of Gélineau's triad (narcolepsy, sleep paralysis, and either hypnagogic or hypnopompic hallucinations) are absent, can look deceptively like an epileptic drop attack, although the crucial history of the precipitation by emotional events should be solicited by the physician.

Of the psychiatric conditions, the anxiety-related disorders are the most commonly misdiagnosed as epilepsy. In particular, panic attacks, especially if associated with episodes of déja vu, depersonalization, or autoscopy, are deceptive. The onset of the panic may be sudden, not obviously triggered by environmental events, and it may last only for a short time. Some patients have all of the autonomic elements of a panic attack without the subjective sense of fear—panic sine panic.

Clues in the history include past episodes of an anxiety-related condition, the environmental triggers, associated agoraphobia, and the classic nature of the panic attack, which rarely occurs as a manifestation of an epileptic seizure. Panic involves palpitations, sweating, rising apprehension and fear, and difficulty in breathing. Many patients reach a point at which they black out and experience amnesia for the episode.

Less severe anxiety disorders can also present with paroxysmal episodes of sensory or motor change, which to the uninformed may be thought of as epileptic.

A depressive illness often underlies a diagnosis of pseudoseizures. Clues in the history include a past history of depression, recent significant life events, for example a bereavement that might have precipitated a depressive illness, and the central features of a depression, which, unless they are asked for, may not be volunteered by a patient. These features include appetite and sleep changes, anhedonia, suicidal thoughts, and social withdrawal.

The importance of recognizing a depressive illness is obvious, since it is a readily treatable cause of pseudoseizures, and it is usually not treated effectively by antiepileptic drugs.

Schizophrenia rarely presents in the form of pseudoseizures, but the occasional patient may be seen with catatonic outbursts of motor activity, which are misinterpreted as paroxysmal epileptic events. These episodes were well described in the older textbooks but are seen less frequently today. Clinical observation of such attacks will reveal their nature, but occasionally videotelemetry is required.

Conversion disorder, presenting either as dissociative symptoms or as conversion hysteria, is still seen quite frequently in specialist practice, and must always be considered. While elements of secondary gain may be obvious, this may be a trap for the unwary clinician, and the diagnosis of conversion hysteria should be made on more solid ground. In particular, a past history of conversion phenomena, and associated clinical findings such as hemianesthetic areas and visual field defects with corkscrew patterns should be noted. See Dr. Ron's chapter in this book (Chapter 28) for more discussion.

Conversion epilepsy involves the mechanism of dissociation, which means patients will be amnesic for their attack. Patients who seem to know absolutely nothing about their seizures, especially after a several-year history of frequent episodes, rarely have epilepsy. Sexual abuse quite possibly may have occurred, and has important treatment implications.

Briquet's hysteria, or somatization disorder, is another condition where patients with pseudoseizures are seen. Such patients are often female and polysymptomatic. They characteristically have a history of an excessive number of surgeries and hospitalizations and present with numerous somatic complaints. Sociopathic personality traits and alcoholism may be noted in these patients' families.

The condition typically starts in early childhood and by definition is chronic. It is estimated that some 1–2% of consecutive female patients attending hospital for investigations and up to 10% of psychiatric inpatients have Briquet's hysteria. It is only by careful history taking and noting the potential abnormal illness behavior in the patient's background that the diagnosis can be secured.

In the differential diagnosis of pseudoseizures it is essential to take an adequate history, taking note of both psychiatric and neurological background features. In addition, information regarding such obvious factors as seizure-precipitating events should be sought, paying particular attention to the setting and timing of the very first attack. Seizures occurring many times a day in the presence of a normal interictal EEG are likely to be nonepileptic. In addition, talking, screaming, and displays of emotional behavior immediately after the attack are likely to lead to a similar conclusion.

The presence of paroxysmal abnormalities on the EEG does not necessarily mean a diagnosis of epilepsy. There are several patterns of EEG abnormality seen in psychiatric patients that may be reported as epileptiform. This can be very misleading. These patterns include small sharp spikes, which may be temporal in distribution, and are seen with affective disorder, and rhythmic midtemporal discharges, which arise in drowsiness and may be mistaken for bitemporal θ. Further, θ waves, sometimes paroxysmal, and even sharp waves, are often seen in patients with extreme anxiety disorders and schizophrenia. The diagnosis of epilepsy should never be based on a reporting of "epileptiform features" on an electroencephalogram.

It is often mistakenly believed that self-injury does not occur in pseudoseizures. In fact, self-injury is common, more so than in epileptic seizures. The environment of the self-injury is often different, and in particular, carpet burns, derived as the patient rubs his or her skin on the floor, may commonly be seen on the elbows or face. Patients with pseudoseizures sometimes even break bones.

Pseudostatus epilepticus also occurs. In fact, if patients present with status epilepticus, and their EEG is normal, including interictal EEGs, it is highly unlikely that they have epilepsy. Patients with pseudostatus are at particular risk for further morbidity, including respiratory depression from the excessive amount of medications given, which in some cases leads to surgical interventions with tracheostomy or artificial ventilation.

Measurement of prolactin can be helpful in the differential diagnosis of seizures. Significant elevations of this neurohormone occur, maximally between 15–20 minutes, after a generalized convulsion. It is less reliable in patients with complex partial seizures or frontal seizures, and not reliable in patients with simple partial seizures or in patients who have status epilepticus. The prolactin elevation needs to be a significant one (probably over 1,000 IU/L to be sure of an epileptic seizure) in the setting of a normal baseline (198). Although other neurohormones have been examined, including argenine vasopressin, luteinizing hormone (LH), and follicle-stimulating hormone (FSH), prolactin has remained the most reliable in this setting.

IMPAIRMENT OF COGNITIVE FUNCTION AND MEMORY IN EPILEPSY

Impairment of cognitive abilities and a decline of intellectual function have been described as a complication of epilepsy for many years. As with the behavioral problems noted earlier, the literature started to accumulate in the mid- to late 19th century. In recent years some of the factors underlying neuropsychological deficits, as well as the type of psychological deficits associated with varying seizure types, have been further clarified.

Several investigators have noted that patients with symptomatic epilepsy are more likely to have impaired intellect than those with epilepsy of no known cause (199). Preexisting brain damage, while an important variable, does not entirely explain the neuropsychological deficit. There appears to be some "epilepsy factor" that contributes to cognitive change in addition to the structural lesion (200).

Of the seizure variables, age of onset, duration of epilepsy, seizure type, and seizure frequency have been examined. Most investigators report an early age of onset to have a poorer prognosis with regard to intellectual abilities. Patients with generalized seizures tend to show more deficits of attention and concentration compared to patients with focal seizures. The latter, particularly with seizures arising from the temporal lobes, are more likely to show memory impairments. Patients with generalized absence seizures show impaired cognitive function for the duration of the EEG spike-wave abnormality, although generally, patients with this form of seizure show minimal interictal dysfunction. If absences are frequent, impaired performance in the classroom setting may lead to educational underachievement. Binnie (201) and his colleagues have pointed out how subclinical focal discharges may also have clinical significance, showing transient cognitive impairment (TCI) on selective tasks correlating with brief interictal EEG focal discharges.

Seidenberg et al. (202) compared a group of patients whose seizure frequency decreased during a test retest interval on psychological tests, with another group where it remained unchanged or was increased. Those with a decreasing seizure frequency showed improvements in intellectual quotients. Dodrill (203) also examined the long-term effect of seizures on psychological tasks and noted that a lifelong history of more than 100 individual convulsions is associated with decreased functioning in a variety of areas.

In some patients it is reasonable to consider a dementia of epilepsy. These patients show a cognitive deterioration, which is thus an acquired intellectual deficit, though this is not progressive in the way that parenchymatous degenerative dementias are. Patients halt or arrest in the progression of the intellectual decline. Identifying these patients prospectively is currently impossible, but retrospective studies (204) have suggested that generalized tonic-clonic seizures with recurrent head injury, and the prescription of certain anticonvulsant drugs—notably phenytoin and primidone—are somehow associated with this clinical picture.

The role of phenytoin in provoking an encephalopathy has been discussed for some time, since the early descriptions of dilantin dementia by Rosen (205). This picture affects only a minority of patients, and the possibility that it may be intertwined with metabolic disturbances, for example, folate deficiency. It seems that certain patients, particularly those with mental handicaps, severe intractable epilepsy, and recurrent head injuries may be most susceptible to this kind of encephalopathy, which may be partially reversible on removing either polytherapy or the phenytoin.

The effects of antiepileptic drugs on cognitive function have been an area of intense investigation in recent years. Extensive reviews are available (206), but here only a brief summary is given. In patients on polytherapy, rationalization with a diminished burden of anticonvulsant prescriptions improves cognitive function over a wide range of cognitive abilities (207).

There has been a debate regarding possible differences between individual antiepileptic drugs. Generally data favor the newer AEDs, carbamazepine, sodium valproate, and vigabatrin, and emphasize more cognitive impairments with phenytoin and phenobarbital (208–211). A controversy that has recently emerged is whether the cognitive impairments associated with anticonvulsant drugs reflect only motor impairments, or if there is some effect on higher cognitive function. Data regarding this issue are available in the literature (212) and support the view that most AEDs may bring about some motor slowing, which is reflected in cognitive tasks. However, differences can be discerned, particularly between carbamazepine and phenytoin in terms of higher cognitive tasks, the evidence favoring carbamazepine.

Several new antiepileptic drugs have recently been introduced to clinical practice, but information on their cognitive effects is rather limited. The only drug to have been investigated in any detail is vigabatrin, and several studies suggest that it appears to have no significant influence on cognitive abilities. If a trend can be detected, it is toward a psychotropic effect with some improvements (213). Further work with this drug and other new AEDs in the area of cognitive function is urgently needed.

Patients with epilepsy frequently complain of memory difficulties. While often this is related to problems of concentration and attention, and indeed may therefore not be a memory defect per se, it is clear that memory may be affected, particularly in patients with temporal lobe abnormalities. Most of the work in this area has been undertaken on patients undergoing temporal lobectomy, where careful testing of memory function prior to surgery is mandatory, and deficits may occur following removal of the offending temporal lobe. In other patients, however, memory function is usually improved by improving control of seizures. The role of antiepileptic drugs in exacerbating memory problems has yet to be clearly defined because the impairments associated with AEDs tend to affect concentration, attention, and psychomotor abilities, rather than memory function per se.

PSYCHIATRIC DISORDERS SECONDARY TO ANTIEPILEPTIC TREATMENTS

It has been known for a long time that antiepileptic drugs influence the mental state. These drugs can be broken down into those that have adverse effects and those that have beneficial effects. However, the behavioral toxicity profile of most drugs is not simple. A particular drug may influence one aspect of behavior positively and another negatively. The physician needs to be aware of these distinctions, and also to be aware that suppressing seizures at the expense of deterioration in the patient's behavior is not necessarily appropriate clinically and can provoke a great deal of havoc for the patient, both within their families and also vocationally.

The main adverse effect to note is the link between antiepileptic drugs and depression. Robertson et al. (122), studying epileptic patients on polytherapy presenting with a depressive illness, noted that patients on phenobarbitone were judged to be significantly more depressed than those not receiving the drug. This was in contrast to patients treated with carbamazepine who were less depressed and had lower anxiety scores than patients on other AEDs.

Further evidence that AEDs may be interlinked with mood come from the studies of Brent and colleagues (214). They had noted the high frequency with which adolescents with epilepsy presented to an emergency room, having taken an overdose of barbiturates. They then evaluated psychopathology in a group of adolescents on monotherapy with phenobarbital compared with a group on carbamazepine. Using DSM-IV-R, major depressive disorder was noted in 40% of the former and in only 4% of the latter. Figures for the reporting of suicidal ideation were 47% and 4% respectively. Further, when patients were changed from phenobarbitone to carbamazepine, depressive symptoms improved.

Another drug recently linked with depression is vigabatrin. Idiosyncratic responses are described in a group of patients given the drug as add-on therapy (213). The depression is in some cases related to control of seizure frequency (an example of forced normalization) and is more common in patients with a past history of affective disorder.

The effects of phenobarbitone are in contrast with the positive effects of carbamazepine on mood. This has been shown in several studies of patients with epilepsy, including that of Robertson et al. (122) and in the studies of Andrewes et al. (212). Post et al. (215) also provide data showing an effect of carbamazepine in acute depression and, while not as powerful as that of conventional antidepressants, it does provide evidence of antidepressant propensity in some patients.

Other AEDs that have been used to regulate mood in nonpsychiatric patients include valproic acid (216) and clonazepam (217).

Adverse effects of antiepileptic drugs are often seen in children. Essentially these include the provocation of conduct disorder, or the development of hyperactivity syndrome, clinically similar to attention-deficit-hyperactivity-disorder (ADHD). The drug most frequently implicated is phenobarbital, but similar responses have been shown following the use of some benzodiazepines (for example, clonazepam) and vigabatrin. Interestingly, all of these drugs have some action at the GABA-benzodiazepine receptor. Some underlying biological mechanism may be suggested, which requires further investigation.

The contribution of AEDs to the personality disturbances described in epilepsy is unclear. Certainly the original reports suggesting a psychotropic effect of carbamazepine (218) noted an effect on personality characteristics in patients with epilepsy. An interesting recent contribution is that of Rodin and Schmaltz (219). They used the Bear-Fedio Personality Inventory to examine 148 patients with epilepsy, 36 of whom had temporal lobe EEG abnormalities. They examined relationships between serum AED levels and scores on the rating scale and found no relationships for any AEDs except for carbamazepine. A significant inverse correlation was noted with total sum, elation, philosophical interests, sense of destiny, altered sexuality, and hypergraphia. These data suggest that some positive effect on the interictal personality syndrome may occur when patients on alternative medications are prescribed carbamazepine, although in the absence of further studies it is difficult to be dogmatic.

Throughout the literature on the effects of antiepileptic drugs on the mental state, two other features are noteworthy. First, patients with polytherapy do worse than patients on monotherapy. This is true with regard to personality problems and cognitive function. Polytherapy is also associated with depression. The reader should remember that a number of elements of mood, for example, irritability, can effect a personality change. Conversion of these patients to monotherapy particularly with drugs that have psychotropic properties, would seem important where this can be achieved.

Fischer et al. (220) and Roger et al. (221) described episodes of psychoses during ethosuximide treatment, the EEG often reverting to normal. In the majority of cases, no previous psychotic episodes were documented. Wolf (222, 223) has reemphasised the importance of both generalized seizures and drugs in the development of these psychoses. He has suggested that several clinical pictures may evolve, not all psychotic, and noted that the development of psychotic symptomatology was preceded by premonitory symptoms, especially insomnia, anxiety, and withdrawal. He noted an association between generalized idiopathic epilepsies, forced normalization, and the prescription of ethosuximide. In his series, sodium valproate was not involved. However, in another study (224) seven patients were described with no previous psychiatric histories, whose behavior problems emerged shortly after starting or altering antiepileptic drugs. Their EEGs, abnormal before change, normalized during these psychotic episodes. All patients had temporal lobe abnormalities, and only two were on succinimides.

Why AEDs should have adverse or beneficial effects on mood and behavior is unclear, but they do differ structurally, and therefore can be postulated to have markedly differing neurophysiological and neurochemical effects. Carbamazepine is related to the tricyclic drugs, and both carbamazepine and valproic acid powerfully suppress limbic-kindled seizures (213). These data suggest that they have a different effect at an anatomical level from, for example, phenytoin or phenobarbital.

Several AEDs, particularly those that appear to be associated with adverse effects, such as phenobarbital and phenytoin, lower serum folate levels. Folic acid is a crucial CNS factor in various enzymes that interlink, among other things, with the metabolism of monoamines. Clearly, patients with more severe psychopathology have the lowest folate levels when this is measured.

Psychiatric Disorders Following Surgery

Temporal lobectomy is an ever-increasing treatment for patients with intractable epilepsy. Ever since the early series, the possibility that surgery itself may be associated with the development of psychiatric disturbance, in particular psychosis, has been discussed. Some of the best evidence comes from the Maudsley series, initially described by Taylor (225) and more recently by Bruton (117). Most surgeons have stopped operating on floridly psychotic patients, based on the observation that psychoses generally do not improve with the operation. Few surgical groups, however, regularly include psychiatric screening as part of their preoperative assessment, and postoperative psychiatric follow-up is often nonexistent. Assessment of psychosocial adjustment is rarely performed, in contrast to the often scrupulous recording of neuropsychological deficits.

The Maudsley series show that some patients develop new psychosis postoperatively, and there is an increased reporting of depression. Suicide was reported in 2.4% of the sample, but accounted for 22% of the postoperative deaths.

The most notable improvement of behavior throughout several series concerns aggression.

Bruton has suggested that the development of postoperative psychoses may be more common with certain pathologies (gangliogliomas), and patients with right-sided temporal lobectomies may be more prone to these psychiatric disturbances. In some cases, the sudden relief of seizures that occurs following surgery may suggest a mechanism similar to forced normalization, although no persistent clear relationship emerges between the success of operation and the development of psychotic postoperative states. In the unpublished series from the National Hospitals, analysis of 50 patients assessed psychiatrically preoperatively and then followed for at least 3 months postoperatively, revealed that 16% developed depression, requiring psychiatric intervention. One patient became psychotic. With potential suicide rates up to 5%, these data emphasize the need for continuing psychiatric observations in patients who have received temporal lobectomy.

TREATMENT OF DEPRESSION IN EPILEPSY

Multiple factors may contribute to the development of depression in epilepsy, and any treatment approach should address all these areas. Initially, a clinical assessment of the severity of depression should be made because there is an increased risk of suicide. Subsequent actions will be determined by the result of this assessment. In addition, epilepsy, anticonvulsant, and psychosocial variables should be examined.

Seizure Status

Seizure control should be optimized. In addition, any change in the nature of seizures should be considered. For instance, a recent increase in seizure frequency or the development of secondarily generalized seizures in a patient with a focal epilepsy may be associated with the development of depression by virtue of the increased disruption to the daily life of the patient. Alternatively, depression may lead to increased seizures by such mechanisms as sleep deprivation or failure of compliance.

Antiepileptic Drug Use

Polypharmacy has been associated with depression by some authors, although others have failed to show this connection. As described before, the use of phenobarbital and vigabatrin have been linked to the development of depression.

The introduction of carbamazepine, structurally related to the tricyclic antidepressants, may have antidepressant effects. Dalby (218) compiled evidence that it was associated with an improvement in affective state. Carbamazepine has also been demonstrated to be antidepressant in nonepileptic depressed patients (215). In addition, it has a role as a prophylactic agent in the control of manic-depressive illness.

Hence, guidelines for the treatment of depression in patients with epilepsy depend on the severity of the depression and the epilepsy, and several strategies may be instituted before or together with the use of specific antidepressant medications. Attempts should be made to reduce polytherapy, and if patients are receiving phenobarbital or vigabatrin, consideration may be given to reducing these and introducing carbamazepine. Some antiepileptic drugs, particularly carbamazepine, but also probably valproic acid, appear to have psychotropic properties in their own right.

Specific Antidepressant Treatments

Clinical practice varies, but successful treatment of depression with antidepressants in patients with epilepsy has been reported by several authors (128). It is important to remember the possibility of drug interactions between antidepressants and antiepileptics (226).

A potential difficulty in giving antidepressants to patients with epilepsy is that these drugs may lower the seizure threshold. However, there is little evidence that the use of monoamine-uptake inhibitors is associated with the occurrence of seizures (101). Although seizures have often been reported in depressed patients taking therapeutic doses of tricyclic antidepressants, a causal relationship is difficult to establish. In part, this may occur because a small proportion of any large sample of people studied over time will probably have a seizure because of the onset of epilepsy during this time (226).

A prospective study of the incidence of antidepressant-induced seizures found that seizures requiring treatment with an AED occurred in less than one case in 1000 (227). All these observations were made in patients without epilepsy, and the implications for those who have the condition are not clear. Although Edwards (228) suggested that a family history of epilepsy is relevant, Blumer (103) concluded that a lowering of the seizure threshold with modest doses of a tricyclic antidepressant was rarely of clinical significance. In our practice we are cautious in giving tricylic agents to patients with epilepsy.

Although there is limited experience with electroconvulsive therapy for epilepsy, Betts (229) reports that it causes no problems and points out that in severe drug-resistant depression, with the attendant risk of suicide, it may be life-saving.

In light of the interplay of psychosocial and biological factors in the genesis of depression, several authors have pointed out the value of including the appropriate type of psychotherapy within the overall management plan (101, 103).

TREATMENT OF PSYCHOSES OF EPILEPSY

Essentially, management of psychiatric problems in patients with epilepsy is similar to that in patients without epilepsy, with a few caveats. Nonmedical treatments are always available and should be considered in individual cases.

Patients with psychoses should be treated with neuroleptic medications, although these, like most antidepressants, can lower the seizure threshold. To date, all known neuroleptics have this potential, although some more than others. Of the neuroleptics, phenothiazines are more likely to provoke seizures than the butyrophones, and of the available drugs, pimozide is perhaps the least likely to precipitate seizures. Patients most likely to have their seizure control disturbed are those with overt cerebral damage and patients given large initial doses or changes of dose that occur suddenly. Lithium also has a proconvulsant potential.

Ictal psychoses may occasionally require neuroleptic drugs, although they usually settle rapidly. The more important factor is to prevent patients from damaging themselves or causing harm to others, but a drug such as haloperiodol or pimozide at regular intervals may control behavior satisfactorily. Interictally, the paranoid or schizophrenia-like states need to be evaluated in terms of their relationship to seizure frequency. Thus, in patients who stop having seizures in association with the onset of psychosis, a neuroleptic that lowers the seizure threshold is the most logical prescription, for example, chlorpromazine.

When patients with epilepsy have no alteration of the seizure frequency, or the psychosis is occurring in the setting of increased seizure frequency, a neuroleptic less likely to precipitate seizures—such as haloperidol or pimozide—is logical. Sulpiride appears to be a reasonable alternative.

It should be recalled that patients on AEDs that increase hepatic metabolism will show lower serum levels of neuroleptics and may therefore require somewhat higher doses than patients not on these medications to achieve a similar clinical effect. Occasionally the addition of an antidepressant or a neuroleptic to a patient's prescription may lead to increases in serum AED levels. Although the addition of carbamazepine or sodium valproate to the regime of psychotic patients does not appear to resolve the psychosis, it may have psychotropic potential in patients who have epilepsy and behavior disturbances. Again, barbiturates and polytherapy should be avoided in these cases.

As with all psychiatric problems, psychopharmacological management alone is not sufficient. It is important to acknowledge that epileptic patients with psychosis bear the burden of epilepsy in addition to their psychosis. Patients with intermittent psychotic states are often perplexed and embarrassed about what has happened to them while psychotic. They also fear further continuing bouts, with a descent into insanity. Patients with continuous psychosis require the skills of paramedical intervention, and the full resources of community care may be needed to help them rehabilitate and to assist their families in coping with their difficulties. In many patients with chronic psychoses of epilepsy, the preservation of affect and lack of personality disintegration over years allow them to live in their communities, with their families, and even to marry. Maintaining them and bringing such support to them is important, sustaining them in the community and preventing their recurrent admission into the hospital. Further, in a good family environment with adequate medical facilities and follow-up care, patient compliance tends to be good.

OPTIMIZATION OF PSYCHOSOCIAL POTENTIAL

The concept of quality of life (QOL) has gained popularity in recent years, although its definition is problematic. To date there is little research on QOL in epilepsy. However, it is important to recognize that epilepsy involves more than seizures. Improving these patients' psychosocial potential requires attention to the many aspects of their lives; their own internal concept of their QOL has thus become an important management goal.

The World Health Organization (230) proposed three levels at which disease can affect an individual: impairment, disability, and handicap. Impairment relates more to abnormalities of body structure and organ systems, and disability is seen as the impact of the illness on a person's functional abilities and activity levels. It is the definition of handicap that most closely relates to quality of life, defining disadvantage due to disease or treatment that individuals experience in relationship to their peers and others. See Dr. Shapiro's and Dr. Wong's chapter (Chapter 43) in this book for more discussion.

A review of the literature on QOL reveals several life domains or areas thought essential to determining QOL in epilepsy (231), covering physical, cognitive, affective, social and economic aspirations of patients. The word "aspiration" is here used to emphasize an important concept in QOL research. Thus, future expectations are a major component of perceived quality of life, actual abilities being less important than a discrepancy between the patients' position as they are now, and their expected situation.

The diagnosis of epilepsy brings with it many psychosocial problems, including stigmatization, social isolation, psychological problems, and education and employment difficulties (232). Societal attitudes play a major role in determining QOL of patients with epilepsy. Discrimination and nonacceptance of patients, unfortunately, are still quite common. There are obvious ways to enhance these patients' psychosocial adjustment. At the outset, when patients are diagnosed, they should explore the concept of epilepsy and discuss their fears and myths about the condition. It is important to provide constant support from known individuals who will look after them as they learn to live with epilepsy.

Measuring QOL and the scientific study of improvements of QOL with various treatments (for example, monotherapy vs. polytherapy, or surgery, or even the introduction of new drugs) is in its infancy. There is a lack of appropriate measures for patients with epilepsy, existing QOL scales being developed for people with other specific physical illnesses, such as cancer.

Using a recently developed QOL schedule, based on repertory grid techniques, MacGuire and Trimble (233) have explored discrepancies between the way patients view their world now, and how they would like to live. This is a measure of the discrepancy between their current situation and aspirations, which is central to our concept of QOL. We have found, using such techniques that apparently, while seizures are undeniably significant to some patients in determining QOL, this is not true for many others. Cognitive and emotional factors rate highly, as do social isolation and lack of friendships. These data highlight the need for a broader management of epilepsy, again recognizing that the condition involves much more than having seizures.

References

1. Gastaut H. Clinical and electroencephalographic classification of epileptic seizures. Epilepsia 1970;11:102–113.
2. Merlis JK. Proposal for an international classification of the epilepsies. Epilepsia 1970;11:114–119.
3. Commission on Classification and Terminology of the International

League Against Epilepsy. 1989 proposal for revised classification of epilepsies and epileptic syndromes. Epilepsia 1989;30:389–399.

4. Morel B. D'une forme de delire, suite d'une surexcitation nerveuse se rattachent a une variete non encore d'ecrite d'epilepsie. Gaz Hebd Med Chir 1860;7:773-775.

5. Falret J. De l'etat mental des epileptiques. Archives Generales de Medicine 1860;16:661–679.

6. Griesinger W. Über einige epileptoide Zustände. Archiv Psychiatrie und Nervenkrankheiten 1868;1:320–333.

7. Samt P. Epileptische Irreseinsformen. Arch Psychiatr 1875;5: 393–444.

8. Geschwind N. Behavioural changes in temporal lobe epilepsy. Psychol Med 1978;9:217–219.

9. Taylor J Selected writings of John Hughlings Jackson. vol 2. London: Staples Press, 1958.

10. Commission on Classification and Terminology of the International League Against Epilepsy. 1981 proposal for revised clinical and electroencephalographic classification of epileptic seizures. Epilepsia 1981; 22:489–501.

11. Roger J, Bureau M, Dravet CH, Dreifuss FE, Perret A, Wolf P Epileptic syndromes in infancy, childhood and adolescence. London: John Libbey, 1992.

12. Shorvon SD. Epidemiology, classification, natural course and genetics of epilepsy. Lancet 1990;336:93–96.

13. Sander JWAS, Hart YM, Johnson AL, Shorvon SD. National general practice study of epilepsy: newly diagnosed epileptic seizures in a general population. Lancet 1992;336:1267–1271.

14. Zielinski JJ. Epidemiology. In: Laidlaw J, Richens A, eds. A textbook of epilepsy. Edinburgh: Churchill Livingstone, 1982:16–33.

15. Hauser WA, Kurland LT (1975) The epidemiology of epilepsy in Rochester, Minnesota, 1935 through 1967. Epilepsia 1975;16:1–66.

16. Danesi MA. African aspects. In: Dam M, Gram L, eds. Comprehensive epileptology. New York: Raven Press, 1990:795–805.

17. Juul-Jensen P, Foldsprang A. Natural history of epileptic seizures. Epilepsia 1983;24:297-312.

18. Esquirol J. Mental maladies: a treatise on insanity. Translated by E K Hunt. Philadelphia: Lea & Blanchard, 1845.

19. Gowers WR. Epilepsy and other chronic convulsive diseases. New York: William Wood & Co, 1885.

20. Elwes RDC, Reynolds EH. First seizure in adult life. Lancet II:1988;36.

21. Hauser W. Anderson VE, Loewnson RB, McRoberts EM. Seizure recurrence after a first unprovoked seizure. N Engl J Med 1982;307: 522–528.

22. Hart YM, Sander JWAS, Johnson AL, Shorvon SD. National general practice study of epilepsy: recurrence after a first seizure. Lancet 1992;336:1271–1274.

23. Goodridge DMG, Shorvon SD. Epileptic seizures in a population of 6000. I. Demographiy, diagnosis and classification, and role of the hospital services. Br Med J 1983;287:641–644.

24. Rodin E. The prognosis of patients with epilepsy. Springfield IL: Charles C Thomas, 1968.

25. Annegers JF, Hauser WA, Elveback LR. Remission of seizures and relapse in patients with epilepsy. Epilepsia 1979;20:729–737.

26. Elwes RDC, Johnson AL, Shorvon SD, Reynolds EH. The prognosis for seizure control in newly diagnosed epilepsy. N Engl J Med 1984;311:944–947.

27. Ehrhardt P, Forsythe WI 1989. Prognosis after grand mal seizures: a study of 187 children with three year remissions. Dev Med Child Neurol 1989;31:633–639.

28. Hauser WA The natural history of drug-resistant epilepsy: epidemiologic considerations. Bethesda, MD: NIH Consensus Development Conference on Surgery for Epilepsy, 1990:33–35.

29. Juul-Jensen P. Epidemiology of intractable epilepsy. In: Schmidt D, Morselli P, eds. Intractable epilepsy. New York: 5-11.

30. Hauser WA, Annegers JF, Elveback LR. Mortality in patients with epilepsy. Epilepsia 1980;21:399–412.

31. Leestma JE, Walcak T, Huges JR, Kalelkar MB, Teas SS. A prospective study on sudden unexpected death in epilepsy. Ann Neurol 1989;26:195–203.

32. Meldrum BS. Anatomy, physiology, and pathology of epilepsy. Lancet 1990;336:231–234.

33. Perlin JB, DeLorenzo RJ. Recent advances in epilepsy. In: Pedley TA, Meldrum BS, eds. Edinburgh: Churchill Livingstone, 1992: 15-36.

34. Guidotti I, Corda MG, Wise BC. GABAergic synapses: supramolecular organization and biochemical regulation. Neuropharmacology 1983;22:1471–1479.

35. Bormann J. Electrophysiology of GABA-A and GABA-B receptor subtypes. Trends Neurosci 1988;11:112–116.

36. Sivilotti L, Nistri A. GABA receptor mechanisms in the central nervous system. Prog Neurobiol 1991;36:35–92.

37. Holland KD, McKeon AC, Canney DJ, Covey DF, Ferrendelli JA. Relative anticonvulsant effects of GABAmimetic and GABA modulatory agents. Epilepsia 1992;33:981-986.

38. Ribak CE, Joubran C, Kesslak JP, Bakay RAE. A selective decrease in the number of GABAergic somata occurs in pre-seizing monkeys with alumina gel granuloma. Epilepsy Res 1989;4:126–138.

39. Gale K. GABA in epilepsy: the pharmacologic basis. Epilepsia 1989;30(suppl 3):S1–S11.

40. Iadarola MJ, Gale K. Substantia nigra: site of anticonvulsant activity mediated by gamma-aminobutyric acid. Science 1982;218:1237–1240.

41. Geddes JW, Cahan LD, Cooper SM, Kim RC, Choi BH, Cotman CW. Altered distribution of excitatory amino acid receptors in temporal lobe epilepsy. Exp Neurol 1990;108:214–220.

42. Richens A. Recent advances in epilepsy. In: Pedley TA, Meldrum BS, eds. Edinburgh: Churchill Livingstone, 1992:197–210.

43. Pumain R, Heinemann U. Stimulus- and amino acid-induced calcium and potassium changes in rat cortex. J Neurophysiol 1985;53:1–16.

44. Lüders HO, Awad I. Conceptual considerations. In: Lüders H, ed. Epilepsy surgery. New York: Raven Press, 1991:51–62.

45. Binnie CD. Electroencephalography. In: Laidlaw J, Richens A, Oxley J, eds. A textbook of epilepsy. Edinburgh: Churchill Livingstone, 1988:236–306.

46. Wieser HG, Elger CE, Stodieck SRG. The "foramen ovale electrode": a new recording method for the preoperative evaluation of patients suffering from mesio-basal temporal lobe epilepsy. Electroencephalogr Clin Neurophysiol 1985;661:314–322.

47. Stefan H. Multichannel magnetencephalography: recordings of epileptiform discharges. In: Lüders H, ed. Epilepsy surgery. New York; Raven Press, 1991:423–428.

48. Ricci GB. Magnetencephalography. In: Dam M, Gram L, eds. Comprehensive epileptology. New York: Raven Press, 1990: 405–421.

49. Jackson GD, Bercovic SF, Duncan JS, Connelly A. Optimizing the diagnosis of hippocampal sclerosis using magnetic resonance imaging. Am J Neur 1993;14(3):753-62.

50. Jackson GD, Bercovic SF, Tress BM, Kalnins RM, Fabinyi G, Bladin PF. Hippocampal sclerosis can be reliably detected by magnetic resonance imaging. Neurology 1990;40:1869–1875.

51. Jackson GD, Connelly A, Duncan JS, Grünewald RA, Gadian DG. Detection of hippocampal pathology in intractable partial epilepsy: increased sensitivity with quantitative magnetic resonance T2 relaxometry. Neurology 1993;43(9):1793-9.

52. Cook MJ, Fish DR, Shorvon SD, Straughan K, Stevens JM. Hippocampal volumetric and morphometric studies in frontal and temporal lobe epilepsy. Brain 1990;115:1001–1015.

53. Younkin DP, Deliveria-Papadopoulos M, Maris J, Donlon E, Clancy R, Chance B. Cerebral metabolic effects of neonatal seizures measured with in vivo P-31 NMR spectroscopy. Ann Neurol 1986;20: 513–519.

54. Connelly A, Jackson GD, Duncan JD, et al. 1H MRS in the investigation of temporal lobe epilepsy. Neurology 1994;44,850.

55. Rowe CC, Bercovic SF, Austin M, McKay WJ, Bladin PF. Visual and quantitative analysis of interictal SPECT with 99Tc-HMPAOm-

HMPAO in temporal lobe epilepsy. J Nucl Med 1991;32(9): 1688-94.

56. Biersack HJ, Reichmann K, Winkler C, et al. ^{99}Tc-labelled hexa-methylprpyleneamine oxime photon emission scans in epilepsy. Lancet 1985;2:1436–1437.

57. Andersen AR. Single photon computerized tomography in temporal lobe epilepsy. In: Dam M, Gram L, eds. Comprehensive epileptology. New York: Raven Press, 1990:375–383.

58. Rowe CC, Bercovic SF, Austin M, McKay WJ, Bladin PF, Patterns of postictal blood flow in temporal lobe epilepsy: qualitative and quantitative analysis. Neurology 1991;41(7):1096-1103.

59. Engel J, Kuhl DE, Phelps ME, Maziotta JC. Interictal cerebral glucose metabolism in partial epilepsy and its relation to EEG changes. Ann Neurol 1982;12:529–537.

60. Savic I, Persson A, Roland P, Pauli S, Sedvall G, Widen L In vivo demonstration of reduced benzodiazepine-receptor binding in human epileptic foci. Lancet 1988;8616:863–866.

61. Frost JJ, Mayberg HS, Fisher RS, et al. μ-opiate receptors measured by positron emission tomography are increased in temporal lobe epilepsy. Ann Neurol 1988;23:231–237.

62. Jones-Gotman M. Presurgical neuropsychological evaluation for localization and lateralization of seizure focus. In: Lüders H, Epilepsy surgery. ed. New York: Raven Press, 1991:469–476.

63. Reynolds EH, Shorvon SD. Monotherapy or polytherapy for epilepsy? Epilepsia 1982;22:1–10.

64. Heller AJ, Ring HA, Reynolds EH. Factors relating to the dramatic response to clobazam therapy in refactory epilepsy. Epilepsy Res 1988;2:276–280.

65. Ring HA, Reynolds EH. Vigabatrin. In: Pedley T, Meldrum BS, eds. Recent advances in epilepsy 5. London: Churchill Livingstone, 1991:177–195.

66. Fenwick P. Evocation and inhibition of seizures: behavioral treatment. In: Neurobehavioral problems in epilepsy (Advances in Neurology, vol. 55), eds. Smith D, Treiman D & Trimble M, New York: Raven Press, 1991:163–183.

67. Dahl J, Melin L, Lund L. Effects of a contingent relaxation program on adults with refractory epileptic seizures. Epilepsia 1987;28: 125–132.

68. Dahl A, Melin L, Leissner P. Effects of a behavioral intervention on epileptic seizure behavior and paroxysmal activity: a systematic replication of three cases of children with intractable epilepsy. Epilepsia 1988;29:172–183.

69. Mostofsky D, Balaschak BA. Psychobiological control of seizures. Psychol Bull 1977;84:723–750.

70. Antebi D, Bird J. The facilitation and evocation of seizures. Br J Psychiatry 1992;160:154–164.

71. Lockard JS. A primate model of clinical epilepsy: mechanisms of action through quantification of theraputic effects. In: Lockard JS, Ward AA, eds. Epilepsy: a window to brain mechanisms. New York: Raven Press, 1980:11–49.

72. Betts T, Boden S. Use of olfactory stimuli (aromatherapy) [Abstract]. Seizure 1(Suppl A): S25/3.

73. Rockstroh B, Elbert T, Birbaumer N, et al. Cortical self-regulation in patients with epilepsies. Epilepsy Res 1993;14:63–72.

74. Birbaumer N. Application of learnt cortical control to seizure behavior [Abstract]. Seizure 1(Suppl A): 25/4.

75. Whyler AR, Lockard JS, Ward AA, Finch CA. Condition EEG desynchronisation and seizure occurrence in patients. Electroencephalogr Clin Neurophysiol 1976;41:501–512.

76. Ben-Menachem E. Vagal stimulation for treatment of refractory partial epilepsy: an overview of clinical results [Abstract]. Seizure 1(Suppl A): S21/4.

77. Polkey CE. Surgical treatment of chronic epilepsy. In: Trimble MR, ed. Chronic epilepsy, its prognosis and management. New York: John Wiley & Sons, 1989:189–207.

78. Kendall B. Neuroradiology. In: Laidlaw J, Richens A, Oxley J, eds. A textbook of epilepsy. Edinburgh: Churchill Livingstone, 1988: 307–349.

79. Duncan R, Patterson J, Hadley DM, et al. CT, MR and SPECT imaging in temporal lobe epilepsy. J Neurol Neurosurg Psychiatry 53:11–15.

80. Hajek M, Siegel AM, Haldemann R, von Schulthess GK, Wieser HG (1991) Value of HM-PAO SPECT in selective temporal lobe surgery for epilepsy. Journal of Epilepsy 1991;4:43–51.

81. Dierckx RA, Vandevivere J, Dom L, et al. Single photon emission computed tomography using perfusion tracers in seizure disorders. Epilepsy Research 1992;12:131–139.

82. Devous MD. Single photon emission computed tomography in epilepsy. Semin Neurol 1990;20:325–341.

83. Alheid SF, Heimer L. New perspectives in basal forebrain organisation of special relevance for neuropsychiatric disorders Neuroscience 1988;27:1–39.

84. Papez JW. A proposed mechanism of emotion. 1937 Arch Neurol Psychiatry 1937;38:725–733.

85. MacLean PD. The triune brain: New York: Plenum, 1990.

86. Schmitz B, Trimble MR Epileptic equivalents - some 19th century views. Acta Neurol Scand 1992;140(suppl):122-126.

87. Reynolds JR Epilepsy. Churchill: London, 1861.

88. Gibbs FA, Stamps FW. Epilepsy handbook. Springfield: Charles C Thomas, 1953.

89. Hermann BP, Schwartz MS, Karnes WE, Valdat P. Psychopathology in epilepsy: relationship of seizure type to age of onset. Epilepsia 1980;21:15–23.

90. Hermann BP, Dikmen S, Schwartz MS, Karnes WE. Psychopathology in patients with ictal fear: a quantitative investigation. Neurology 1982;32:7–11.

91. Bear DM, Fedio P. Quantitative analysis of interictal behaviour in temporal lobe epilepsy. Arch Neurol 1977;34:454–467.

92. Waxman SG, Geschwind N. The interictal behaviour syndromes of temporal lobe epilepsy. Arch Gen Psychiatry 1975;32:1580–1586.

93. Gastaut H, Roger J, Lefevre N. Différenciation psychologique des épileptiques en fonction des formes électrocliniques de leur maladie. Revue Psychologique 1953;3:237-249.

94. Rodin E, Schmaltz S. The Bear-Fedio personality inventory. Neurology 1984;34:591–596.

95. Mungas DM. Behavioural syndromes of epilepsy. In: Bennett TL, ed. the neuropsychology of epilepsy. New York: Plenum, 1992.

96. Lewis AJ. Melancholia: a historical review. Journal of Mental Science 1934;80:1–42.

97. Temkin O. The falling sickness. Baltimore: Johns Hopkins University Press, 1971.

98. Reynolds J. Epilepsy: its symptoms, treatment and relation to other chronic convulsive diseases. London: John Churchill, 1861.

99. Barraclough B. Suicide and epilepsy. In: Reynolds EH, Trimble MR, eds. Epilepsy and pyschiatry. Edinburgh: Churchill Livingstone, 1981:72–76.

100. Dodrill CB, Batzel LW. Interictal behavioural features of patients with epilepsy. Epilepsia 1986;27(Suppl 2):S64–S76.

101. Robertson MM. Depression in patients with epilepsy reconsidered. In: Pedley TA, Meldrum BS, eds. Recent advances in epilepsy, vol 4. Edinburgh: Churchill Livingstone, 1988:205–240.

102. Robertson MM. The organic contribution to depressive illness in patients with epilepsy. J Epilepsy 1989;2:189–230.

103. Blumer D. Epilepsy and disorders of mood. In: Smith D, Treiman D, Trimble M, eds. Advances in neurology, vol. 55. New York: Raven Press, 1991:185–195.

104. Devinsky O, Bear DM. Varieties of depression in epilepsy. Neuropsychiatry, Neuropsychology and Behavioural Neurology 1991;4: 49–61.

105. Pond D, Bidwell B, Stein L. A survey of 14 general practices. Part 1: medical and demographic data. Psychiatr Neurol Neurochirurg 1960;63:217–236.

106. Edeh J, Toone BK. Antiepileptic therapy, folate deficiency, and psychiatric morbidity: a general practice survey. Epilepsia 1985;26: 434–440.

107. Currie S, Heathfield KWG, Henson RA, Scott DF. Clinical course

and prognosis of temporal lobe epilepsy. Brain 1971;94:173–190.

108. Mathews WS, Barabas G. Suicide and epilepsy: a review of the literature. Psychosomatics 1981;22:515–524.

109. Williams D. The structure of emotions reflected in epileptic experiences. Brain 1956;79:29–67.

110. Barczak P, Edmunds E, Betts T. Hypomania following complex partial seizures. Br J Psychiatry 1988;152:137–139.

111. Hurwitz TA, Wada JA, Kosaka BD, Strauss EH. Cerebral organization of affect suggested by temporal lobe seizures. Neurology 1985;35:1335–1337.

112. Betts TA. Psychiatry and epilepsy. In: Laidlaw J, Richens A, eds. A textbook of epilepsy. Edinburgh: Churchill Livingstone, 1982: 227–270.

113. Hermann BP, Seidenberg M, Haltiner A, Wyler AR. Mood state in unilateral temporal lobe epilepsy. Biol Psychiatry 1991;30:1205–1218.

114. Turner RJ, Beiser M. Major depression and depressive symptomatology among the physically disabled. J Nerv Ment Dis 178:343–350.

115. Byrne A. Hypomania following increased epileptic activity. Br J Psychiatry 1988;153:573–574.

116. Jensen I, Larsen JK. Mental aspects of temporal lobe epilepsy. J Neurol Neurosurg Psychiatry 1979;42:256–265.

117. Bruton CJ. The neuropathology of temporal lobe epilepsy. In: Maudsley Monograph No. 31, Oxford: Oxford University Press, 1988:

118. Adamec RE. Corticotrophin releasing factor – a peptide link between stress and psychopathology associated with epilepsy? Journal of Psychopharmacology 1991;5:96–104.

119. Reynolds EH. Interictal psychiatric disorders. Neurochemical aspects. In: Smith D, Treiman D, Trimble M, eds. In: Advances in neurology, vol. 55. New York: Raven Press, 1991:47–58.

120. Carney MWP. Serum folate values in 423 psychiatric patients. Br Med J 1967;4:512–516.

121. Trimble MR, Corbett JA, Donaldson D. Folic acid and mental symptoms in children with epilepsy. J Neurol Neurosurg and Psychiatry 1980;43:1030–1034.

122. Robertson MM, Trimble MR, Towmsend HRA. Phenomenology of depression in epilepsy. Epilepsia 1987;28:364–372.

123. Blanchet P, Frommer GP. Mood change preceding epileptic seizures. J Nerv Ment Dis 1986;174:471–476.

124. Lennox WG, Cobb S. Epilepsy. XIII. Aura in epilepsy: A statistical review of 1359 cases. Arch Neurol Psychiatry 1933;30:374–387.

125. Taylor DC, Lochery M. Temporal lobe epilepsy; origin and significance of simple and complex auras. J Neurol Neurosurg Psychiatry 1987;50:673–681.

126. Blumer D. Postictal depression: significance for the treatment of the neurobehavioral disorder of epilepsy. Journal of Epilepsy 1992;5: 214–219.

127. Mendez MF, Cummings JL, Benson F. Depression in epilepsy: significance and phenomenology. Arch Neurol 1986;43:766–770.

128. Robertson MM, Trimble MR. The treatment of depression in patients with epilepsy. a double-blind trial. J Affect Disord 1985;9:127–136.

129. Hoffmann F. Über die Eintheilung der Nervenkrankheiten in Siegburg. Allg Zschr Psychiatr 1872;19:367–391.

130. Kraepelin E. Psychiatrie. Leipzig: J.A. Barth, 1903.

131. Gurewitsch M. Zur differentialdiagnose des epileptischen Irreseins. Zugleich ein Beitrag zur Lehre von den kombinierten Psychosen. Z Ges Neurol Psychiatr 1912;9:359–390.

132. Lachmund Ueber vereinzelt auftretende Halluzinationen bei Epleptikern. Mschr Psychiatr Neurol 1904;15:434–444.

133. Krapf E. Epilepsie und Schizophrenie. Archiv fuer Psychiatrie und Nervenheilkunde 1928;83:547–586.

134. Sommer W. Postepileptisches irresein. Arch Psychiatr Nervenkr 1881;11:549-612.

135. Pohl Ueber das Zusammenvorkommen von Epilepsie und originärer Paranoia. Prager Med Wochenschr 1880;35.

136. Ganter R. Ein mit Schizophrenie kombinierter Fall von Epilepsie. Arch Psychiatr Nervenkr 1925;74:829–837.

137. Glaus A. Über Kombinationen von Schizophrenie und Epilepsie. Z Ges Neurol Psychiatr 1931;135:450–500.

138. Meduna L von. Versuche ueber die biogische Beeinglussung des Ablaufes der Schizophrenie. I. Campher- und Cadiazolkraempfe. Z Gesamte Neurol Psychiatr 1935;152:235–262.

139. Landolt H. Some clinical EEG correlations in epileptic psychoses (twilight states). Electroencephalogr Clin Neurophysiol 1953;5: 121.

140. Gastaut H. Colloque de Marseille. 15-19 Octobre 1956. Compte rendu du colloque sur l'etude electroclinique des episodes psychotiques qui survennient chez les epileptiques en dehors des crises cliniques. Rev Neurol 1956;95:587–616.

141. Tellenbach H. Epilepsie als Anfallsleiden und als Psychose. Ueber alternative Psychosen paranoider praegung bei "forcierter Normalisierung" (Landolt) des Elektroencephalogramms Epileptischer. Nervenarzt 1965;36:190–202.

142. Gibbs FA. Ictal and non-ictal psychiatric disorders in temporal lobe epilepsy. J Nerv Ment Dis 1951;113:522–528.

143. Pond DA. Discussion Remark. Proc. R Soc Lond [Med] 1962; 55:316.

144. Slater E, Beard AW, Glithero E. The schizophrenia-like psychoses of epilepsy. V. Discussion and conclusions. Brit J Psychiatry 1963;109: 95–150.

145. Stevens JR. Psychiatric implications of psychomotor epilepsy. Arch Gen Psychiatry 1966;14:461–471.

146. Roberts GW, Done DJ, Bruton C, Crow TJ. A "mock up" of schizophrenia: temporal lobe epilepsy and schizophrenia-like psychosis. Biol Psychiatry 1990;28:127–143.

147. Krohn W. A study of epilepsy in Northern norway, its frequency and character. Acta Psychiatr Scand 1961;150(suppl):215–225.

148. Zielinski JJ. Epidemiology and medical-social problems of epilepsy in Warsaw. (final report on research program No. 19-P-58325-F-01 DHEW. social and rehabilitation services). Washington, DC: U.S. Governement Printing Office, 1974.

149. Bilikiewicz A, Matkowski K, Przybysz K, Dabkowski M, Ksiazkiewicz-Cuwinska J, Jakubowska M. Untersuchungen zur Epidemiologie und Psychopathologie der zwischen 1976 und 1980 in der Woiwoidschaft Bydgoscz registrierten Epileptiker. Psychiatr Neurol Med Psychol (Leipzig) 1988;40:9–15.

150. Gudmundsson G. Epilepsy in iceland. Acta Neurol Scand 1966; 43(suppl):E1–124.

151. American Psychiatric Association. DSM-IV Diagnostic and statistical manual of mental disorders. (4th ed., Washington, DC, 1994.

152. Bruens JH. Psychoses in epilepsy. In: Vinken PJ, Bruyn GW, eds. Handbook of clinical neurology, vol. 15. Amsterdam: North Holland, 1974:593–610.

153. Köhler GK. Zur Einteilung der Psychosen bei Epilepsie. Zum Begriff "Psychosen bei Epoilepsie" bzw. "epileptische Psychosen". In: Wolf P, Köhler GK, eds. Psychopathologische und pathogenetische Probleme psychotischer Syndrome bei Epilepsie. Bern: Huber, 1980: 11–18.

154. Fenton GJ. Psychiatric disorders of epilepsy: classification and phenomenology. In: Reynolds EH, Trimble MR, eds. Epilepsy and psychiatry. Edinburgh: Churchill Livingstone, 1981:12–26.

155. Trimble M. The psychoses of epilepsy. New York: Raven Press, 1991.

156. Dongier S. Statistical study of clinical and electroencephalographic manifestations of 536 psychotic episodes occurring in 516 epileptics between clinical seizures. Epilepsia 1959;1:117–142.

157. Wolf P. Psychosen bei Epilepsie. Ihre Bedingungen und Wechselbeziehungen zu Anfaellen. Habilitationsschrift, Freie Universitaet Berlin, 1976.

158. Sherwin I. Differential psychiatric features in epilepsy; relationship to lesion laterality. Acta Psychiatr Scand (suppl 313) 1984;69:92–103.

159. Bash KW, Mahnig P. Epileptiker in der psychiatrischen Klinik. Von der Daemmerattacke zur Psychose. Eur Arch Psychiatr Neurol Sci 1984;234:237–249.

160. Wolf P. Classification of syndromes. In: Dam M, Gram L, eds. Comprehensive epileptology. New York: Raven Press, 1991:87–97.

161. Lee SI. Nonconvulsive status epilepticus. Arch Neurol 1985;42: 778–781.
162. Delgado-Escueta AV. Status epilepticus. In: Dam M, Gram L, eds. Comprehensive epileptology. New York: Raven Press, 1990: 375–383.
163. Savard G, Andermann F, Olivier A, Remillard GM. Postictal psychosis after partial complex seizures: a multiple case study. Epilepsia 1991;32:225–231.
164. Schmitz B. Psychosen bei Epilepsie. Eine epidemiologische Untersuchung. Thesis, FU Berlin, 1988.
165. Logsdail SJ, Toone BK. Postictal psychoses. A clinical and phenomenological description. Br J Psychiatry 1988;152:246–252.
166. Slater E, Beard AW. The schizophrenia-like psychoses of epilepsy. V. Discussion and conclusions. Br J Psychiatry 1963;109:143–150.
167. Köhler GK. Epileptische Psychosen - Klassifikationsversuche und EEG-Verlaufsbeobachtungen. Fortschr Neurol Psychiatry 1975;43: 99–153.
168. Helmchen H. Zerebrale Bedingungkonstellationen psychopathologischer Syndrome bei Epileptikern. In: Helmchen H, Hippius H, eds. Entwicklungstendenzen biologischer Psychiatrie. Stuttgart: Georg Thieme, 1975:125–148.
169. Kraft AM, Price TRP, Peltier D. Complex partial seizures and schizophrenia. Compr Psychiatry 1984;25:113-124.
170. Perez MM, Trimble MR. Epileptic psychosis–diagnostic comparison with process schizophrenia. Br J Psychiatry 1980;137:245–249.
171. Toone B. Psychoses of epilepsy. In: Reynolds EH, Trimble MR, eds. Epilepsy and psychiatry. Edinburgh: Churchill Livingstone, 1981: 113–137.
172. Glithero E, Slater E. The schizophrenia-like psychoses of epilepsy. IV. Follow-up record and outcome. Br J Psychiatry 1963;109:134-142.
173. Trimble MR. Interictal psychoses of epilepsy. In: Smith D, Treiman D, Trimble M, eds. Advances in neurology, vol. 55. New York: Raven Press, 1991:143–152.
174. Flor Henry P. Psychosis and Temporal Lobe Epilepsy. a controlled investigation. Epilepsia 1969;10:363–395.
175. Taylor DC. Ontogenesis of chronic epileptic psychoses. A reanalysis. Psychol Med 1971;1:247–253.
176. Kristensen O, Sindrup HH Psychomotor Epilepsy and Psychosis. I. Physical aspects. Acta Neurol Scand 1978a;57:361–369.
177. Kristensen O, Sindrup HH. Psychomotor epilepsy and psychosis. II. Electroencephalographic findings. Acta Neurol Scand 1987b;57: 370–379.
178. Schmitz B. Psychosis and epilepsy. The link to the temporal lobe. In: Trimble MR, Bolwig TG, eds. The temporal lobes and the limbic system. Wrightson: Biomedical Publishing 1992:149-167.
179. Onuma T. Limbic lobe epilepsy with paranoid symptoms: analysis of clinical features and psychological tests. Folia Psychiatr Neurol Jpn 1983;37:253–258.
180. Sengoku A, Yagi K, Seino M, Wada T. Risks of occurrence of psychoses in relation to the types of epilepsies and epileptic seizures. Folia Psychiatr Neurol Jpn 1983;37:221–226.
181. Gureje O. Interictal psychopathology in epilepsy—prevalence and pattern in a Nigerian clinic. Br J Psychiatry 1991;158:700–705.
182. Shukla GD, Srivastava ON, Katiyar BC, et al. Psychiatric manifestations in temporal lobe epilepsy. A controlled study. Br J Psychiatry 1979;135:411–417.
183. Small JG, Milstein V, Stevens JR. Are psychomotor epileptics different? Are psychomotor epileptpics different? Arch Neurol 1962; 7:187–194.
184. Mignone RJ, Donnelly EF, Sadowsky D. Psychological and neurological comparisons of psychomotor and non-psychomotor epileptic patients. Epilepsia 1970;11:345–359.
185. Bruens JH. Psychoses in epilesy. Psychiatria Neurologia Neurochirurgia 1971;74:174–192.
186. Hermann BP, Chabria S. Interictal psychopathology in patients with ictal fear. Arch Neurol 1980;37:667–668.
187. Standage KF, Fenton GW. Psychiatric symptom profiles of patients with epilepsy: a controlled investigation. Psychol Med 1975;5: 152–160.
188. Trimble MR, Perez MM. The phenomenolgy of the chronic psychoses of epilepsy. In: Koella WP, Trimble MR, eds. Temporal lobe epilepsy, mania and schizophrenia and the limbic system. Basel: Karger, 1982;98–105.
189. Ounsted C. Aggression and epilepsy. Rage in children with temporal lobe epilepsy. J Psychosomat Res 1969;13:237–242.
190. Rodin EA, Collomb H, Pache D. Differences between patients with temporal lobe seizures and those with other forms of epileptic attacks. Epilepsia 1976;17:313–320.
191. Lindsay J, Ounsted C, Richards P. Long-term outcome in children with temporal lobe seizures. II. Psychiatric aspects in childhood and adult life. Devel Med Child Neurol 1979;21:630-636.
192. Toone B, Dawson J, Driver MV. Psychoses of epilepsy. A radiological evaluation. Br J Psychiatry 1982;140:244–248.
193. Taylor DC. Mental state and temporal lobe epilepsy. A correlative account of 100 patients treated surgically. Epilepsia 1972;13: 727–765.
194. Trimble MR. PET-scanning in epilepsy. In: Trimble MR, Bolwig TG, eds. Aspects of epilepsy and psychiatry. New York: John Wiley & Sons, 1986:147–162.
195. Landolt H. Serial electroencephalographic investigations during psychotic episodes in epileptic patients and during schizophrenic attacks. In: Lorentz de Haas AM, ed. Lectures on epilepsy. Amsterdam: Elsevier, 1958;91-133.
196. Wolf P, Trimble MR. Biological antagonism and epileptic psychosis. Br J Psychiatry 1985;146:272–276.
197. Lesser RP. Psychogenic seizures. In: Pedley T, Meldrum BS, eds. Recent advances in epilepsy, vol. 2. Edinburgh: Churchill Livingstone, 1985.
198. Fenwick P. Precipitation and inhibition of seizures. In: Reynolds EH, Trimble MR, eds. Epilepsy and psychiatry. Edinburgh: Churchill Livingstone, 1981:306–321.
199. Bourgeois BFD, Presnky AL, Palkes HS, Talent BK, Busch SG. Intelligence in epilepsy: a prospective study in children. Ann Neurol 1983;14:438–444.
200. Kløve H, Matthews CG. Psychometric and adaptive abilities in epilepsy with different aetiology. Epilepsia 1966;7:330–338.
201. Binnie CD. Monitoring seizures. In: Trimble MR, Reynolds EH, eds. What is epilepsy? Edinburgh: Churchill Livingstone, 1986:82–87.
202. Seidenberg M, O'Leary DS, Berent S, Boll T. Changes in seizure frequency and test re-test scores on the WAIS. Epilepsia 1981;22: 75–83.
203. Dodrill C. Correlates of generalised tonic-clonic seizures with intelectual, neuropsychological, emotional and social function in patients with epilepsy. Epilepsia 1986;27:191–197.
204. Trimble MR. Cognitive hazards of seizure disorders, In: Trimble MR, ed. Chronic epilepsy its prognosis and management. New York: John Wiley & Sons, 1989.
205. Rosen JA. Dilantin dementia. Trans Am Neurol Assoc. 1966; 93:273.
206. Trimble MR, Thompson PJ. Neuropsychological aspects of epilepsy. In: Grant I, Adams KM, eds. Neuropsychological assessment of neuropsychiatric disorders. New York; Oxford University Press, 1986:321–346.
207. Thompson PJ, Trimble MR. Anticonvulsant drugs and cognitive functions. Epilepsia 1982a;23:531–544.
208. Thompson PJ, Huppert F, Trimble MR. Phenytoin and cognitive functions; effects on normal volunteers and implications for epilepsy. Br J Clin Psychol 1981;20:151–162.
209. Thompson PJ, Trimble MR. Comparative effects of anticonvulsant drugs on cognitive functioning. Br J Clin Pract 1982b;18 (suppl): 154–156.
210. Smith DB. Cognitive effects of antiepileptic drugs. In: Smith DB, Treiman DM, Trimble MR. Advances in neurology. New York: Raven Press, 1991:197–224.

211. Duncan JS, Sharvon SD, Trimble MR. Effects of removal of phenytoin, carbamazepine and valproate on cognitive function. Epilepsia 1990b;31:584–591.
212. Andrewes DG, Bullen JG, Tomlinson L, Elwes RDC, Reynolds EH. A comparative study of cognitive effects of phenytoin and carbamazepine in new referrals with epilepsy. Epilepsia 1986;26:128–134.
213. McGuire A, Duncan JS, Trimble MR. Effects of Vigabatrin on cognitive function and mood when used as add-on therapy in patients with intractable epilepsy. Epilepasia 1992;33:128–134.
214. Brent DA, Crumrine PK, Varma RR, Allan M, Allman C. Phenobarbital treatment and major depressive disorder in children with epilepsy. Pediatrics 1987;80:909–917.
215. Post RM, Uhde TW, Roy-Byrne PP, Joffe RT. Antidepressant effects of carbamazepine. Am J Psychiatry 1986;143:29–34.
216. McElroy SL, Keck PE Jr, Pope HG Jr, et al. Valproate in treatment of rapid-cycling disorder. J Clin Psychopharmacol 1988;8:275–279.
217. Chovinard G, Young SN, Annable L. Antimanic effect of clonazepam. Biolo Psychiatry 1983;18:451–466.
218. Dalby MA. Behavioural effects of carbamazepine. In: Penry JK, Daly DD, eds. Complex partial seizures and their treatment. New York: Raven Press, 1975:331–344.
219. Rodin E, Schmaltz S, Twitty G. What does the Bear-Fedio Inventory measure? In: Porter RJ, Mattson RH, Ward JR AA, Dam M, eds. The XVth Epilepsy International Symposium. New York: Raven Press, 1984;551–555.
220. Fischer M, Korskjeer G, Pederson E. Psychotic episodes with Zaronder treatment Epilepsia 1965;6:325–334.
221. Roger J, Grangeon H, Grey J, Lob H. Incidences psychiatriques et psychologiques du traitement par l'étho succimide chez les épileptiques. L'éncephale 1968;57:407–438.
222. Wolf P. The clinical syndromes of forced normalization. Folia Psychiatr Neurol Jpn 1984;38:137-192.
223. Wolf P. Acute behavioral symptomatology at disappearance of epileptiform EEG abnormality. Paradoxical or "forced" normalisation. In: Smith DB, Treiman D, Trimble MR, eds. Neurobehavioral problems in epilepsy. New York: Raven Press, 1991.
224. Palkanis A, Drake ME, Kuruvilla J, Blake K. Forced normalisation Arch Neurol 1987;44:289–292.
225. Taylor DC. Factors influencing the occurrence of schizophrenia-like psychosis in patients with temporal lobe epilepsy. Psychol Med 1975;5:249–254.
226. Richen A, Nawishy S, Trimble M. Antidepressant drugs, convulsions and epilepsy. Br J Clin Pharmacol 1983;15:295–298.
227. Jick H, Dinan BJ, Hunter JR, et al. Tricyclic antidepressants and convulsions. J Clin Psychopharmacol 1983;3, 182-185.
228. Edwards JG. Antidepressants and seizures: epidemiological and clinical aspects. In: Trimble MR, ed. psychopharmacology of epilepsy. Chichester: John Wiley & Sons, 1985:119–139.
229. Betts TA. Depression, anxiety and epilepsy. In: Reynolds EH, Trimble MR, eds. Epilepsy and Psychiatry. Edinburgh: Churchill Livingstone, 1981:60–71.
230. World Health Organization. International Classification of impairments, disabilities and handicaps. World Health Organization, Geneva, 1980.
231. Kendrick AM, Trimble MR. Repertory grid in the assessment of quality of life in epilepsy. In: Trimble MR, Dodson E, eds. Epilepsy and quality of life. New York: Raven Press, 1994:151-164.
232. Thompson P, Oxley J. Socio-economic accompaniments of severe epilepsy. Epilepsia 1988;29;S9(suppl):518.
233. McGuire A, Trimble MR (in press).

34

BASAL GANGLIA DISEASES

Mary Sano, Karen Marder, and George Dooneief

The most common features of diseases of the basal ganglia (BG) are movement disorders, psychiatric syndromes, and cognitive impairment. The movement disorder usually is the most prominent as well as the presenting and defining feature. These movement disorders, which reflect disturbances of the extrapyramidal motor system, range from subtle findings, such as asymptomatic rigidity, apparent only with facilitating maneuvers, to disabling impairments of posture, gait, and purposeful limb movement. The range of psychiatric manifestations in these diseases includes depression, psychosis, hallucinations, delusions, personality change, anxiety, agitation, paranoia, mania, and hyperactivity. Cognitive dysfunction can be subtle or frank: dementia is common in Parkinson's disease (PD), Lewy body disease, and Huntington's disease (HD). Table 34.1 lists many of the diseases affecting the BG. This chapter describes the neuropathology in the BG, including its motor signs and symptoms, which are often accompanied by psychiatric or cognitive manifestations. In some, the etiology remains obscure.

SUBCORTICAL DEMENTIA

Over the past two decades, discussion of cognitive change in BG disease has been shaped by the concept of "subcortical dementia." The term, originally proposed by Martin Albert, arose from the clinical description of patients with PD, HD, and progressive supranuclear palsy (PSP) (1–3). Albert's original paper focused on describing how the cognitive deficits in these conditions differed from those typical of Alzheimer's Disease (AD) and other cortical degenerations. However, although PD, AD, and PSP predominantly involve subcortical structures, both neuropathological and biochemical evidence suggests that varying degrees of cortical pathology also occur. Tasks that are thought to be especially sensitive to "subcortical" dysfunctions are those that require timed responses, rapid retrieval, and mental manipulation of known information. Multistaged planning tasks, often labeled as executive functions, have also been described as subcortical, with the understanding that these tasks also require frontal lobe function and connections to the frontal lobes from deeper structures involving the BG.

Although some authors have included personality changes, depression, and apathy in the description of "subcortical" dementia, these might better be classified as psychiatric manifestations (albeit with cognitive consequences) rather than as cognitive disturbances. In general, subcortical tasks are not modality-specific. Rather, deficits have been reported in language tasks, such as verbal fluency and naming, timed attentional tasks, visuospatial, constructional, and tracking tasks (4). Subcortical deficits in various combinations can be demonstrated in patients with BG disorders of a wide range of disease severity, including those with only mild motor disturbance. The particular value of the subcortical dementia concept is not in its localizing implication, but in the observation that subcortical cognitive deficits often can be ameliorated with medication or compensating strategies. Many treatable or reversible deficits have subcortical features.

However, it should be emphasized that a collection of subcortical cognitive deficits does not necessarily constitute a dementia. From our standpoint, dementia requires multiple cognitive deficits not attributable to a single focal deficit. For example, impaired planning, even in several modalities, does not constitute a constellation of deficits. Second, dementia requires that cognitive impairment be severe enough to have meaningful impact on social and occupational functioning. This may be difficult to determine in the face of physical impairment caused by the motor features of BG disease. Finally, cognitive impairment is not due to confusion or other states with altered consciousness. Given these criteria, it is not clear that subcortical dementia exists. As the impact of cognitive impairment increases in BG diseases, there is often neuropathological and neurochemical evidence of accompanying limbic and cortical involvement. When a dementia syndrome does occur in PD, it is often associated with significant evidence of cortical neuropathology. In contrast, in PSP, an entity with little evidence of cortical pathology, the cognitive deficit is usually described as mild, even as the motor manifestations become debilitating. Furthermore, the noncognitive manifestations of BG diseases often contribute to the functional impairment, making it difficult to asses the impact of the cognitive deficit. In HD and diffuse Lewy body disease (DLBD), for example, the psychiatric manifestations may

Table 34.1.　Summary of Motor, Cognitive, and Psychiatric Manifestations of Selected Basal Ganglia Diseases

Disease	Age of Onset	Motor Disturbance	Cognitive Deficits	Psychiatric Manifestations
Parkinson's disease	4th–6th decade; mean age: 65	rigidity; tremor; masked face; brady-kinesia; shuffling gait	executive functions; memory; fluency; visuospatial and construc-tion abilities; dementia	depression; anxiety; mania; psychosis
MPTP toxicity	depends on age at exposure	full range of PD features	executive function; motor sequenc-ing, construction; may occur in asymptomatics	depression ?
Huntington's disease	1st–8th decade	chorea; gait impairment; abnormal eye movement; impaired alternat-ing movements	executive functions; memory; motor sequencing; dementia	depression; apathy; irritability; mania
Progressive supranuclear palsy	4th–7th decade; mean age: 63 years	supranuclear gaze palsy; axial rigidity; dysarthria; bradykinesia	subcortical dementia; frontal lobe-like syndrome	personality change; emotional incon-tinence
Hallevorden-Spatz disease	1st or 2nd decade; late onset after 20	gait disturbance; rigidity; dystonia; dysarthria; pyramidal dysfunction; mutism	slowing of thought processes deficits of variable frequency and severity	impulsivity; aggressiveness; mood dis-turbance (generally infrequent)
Wilson's disease	2nd–3rd decade	tremor; bradykinesia; dysarthria; dys-phagia; chorea; dystonic posturing; rigidity	psychomotor deficits of variable fre-quency and severity	anxiety; depression; suicide; psychosis 25–33% have symptoms early; 50% have symptoms at some point
Tourette's syndrome	before age 20	multiple tics; vocalization	attention; concept formation; planning; executive functions	attention deficit disorder; obsessive compulsive disorder; depression
Diffuse Lewy body disease	5th–7th decade	rigidity; bradykinesia; gait disturbance; frequent falls; tremor (less common)	mild memory deficit to dementia; visuospatial abilities	confusion; hallucinations; delusions; agitation; depression

often be debilitating early, making it difficult to evaluate the contribution of cognitive deficits to functional loss.

For these reasons, we do not use the term "subcortical dementia," although we acknowledge the value of determining subcortical cognitive deficit. These topics are summarized in Table 34.1, and the issues are revisited as each clinical syndrome is described. An attempt has been made to describe the prominence, severity, and order of appearance of motor, psychiatric, and cognitive disturbances and to assess the degree to which a symptom is attributable to BG disease itself, to connected neuroanatomical or neurochemical systems or to other causes such as developmental and psychosocial factors.

PARKINSON'S DISEASE

Parkinson's disease (PD) is characterized by tremor, muscular rigidity, bradykinesia and loss of postural reflexes. The age of onset is typically between 50–65 years (5). Genetic and environmental factors have been implicated in its etiology, though the cause remains unknown. Neuropathologically, PD is characterized by neuronal loss and depigmentation in the substantia nigra and locus ceruleus. Pathological findings also include the presence of Lewy bodies in these areas. The principal biochemical deficit, a depletion of dopamine in the nigrostriatal tract, accounts for much of the clinical picture (6).

Although cognitive and psychiatric disturbances are common in PD, they are not requisite features of the diagnosis. In fact, cardinal features of the disease (bradykinesia, postural instability, rigidity, and tremor) can cloud the assessment of the behavioral manifestations, particularly depression. Historically, there has been considerable debate about whether depression is an intrinsic part of the same underlying disease or if it represents a reaction to neurological disability.

Psychiatric Manifestations

The most common psychiatric disturbance in PD is depression. A review of the literature reveals prevalence rates ranging from 12–90% (7). Much of this variation probably relates to methodological differences (e.g., different criteria for the diagnosis of depression, different source populations). Few studies have used population-based sampling techniques.

Theoretically, the assessment of depression may be complicated by the overlap in symptomatology between PD and depression. But Starkstein et al. (8) and Levin et al. (9) have demonstrated that the somatic items of the Beck Depression Inventory are associated with depression and mood disturbance rather than with the motor manifestations of PD. Similar patterns have been described using the Hamilton Depression Rating Scale (10). Because the earliest motor manifestations of PD (loss of agility, loss of facial expression, and a sense of slowness interpreted as psycho-

motor retardation) may lead an observer to suspect depression, the diagnosis of an affective disturbance must be confirmed by establishing the presence of depressed mood and anhedonia (11).

Using these criteria, estimates of prevalence of depression in PD have been 51% in clinic/hospital-based studies and 32% in population-based studies (12, 13). There is no relationship between age, age at onset, or duration of illness and the presence of depression in PD. The course of depression varies and may differ from that of primary depressive illness. About 22% of patients with PD and mood symptoms experience fluctuations in depressive symptoms (14). In a longitudinal study of patients with PD and the syndrome major depression or dysthymia, the remission rate was low over a 2.5-year follow-up period (15). Cummings (7) summarized these findings by suggesting that two groups of patients can be identified: those with persistent major affective disturbances and those with mood fluctuations.

The profile of depressive features in PD has been examined. Using the Beck Depression Inventory, several authors have noted elevated levels of dysphoria, and pessimism about the future, irritability, sadness and suicidal ideation, but overall little guilt, self-blame, or feelings of failure or punishment. This profile represents emotional complaints not attributable to PD symptoms and is consistent with the pattern seen in other depressions associated with chronic medical diseases (8–10).

Depletion of serotonin appears to play a role in major depression in PD because cerebrospinal fluid (CSF) concentrations of 5-hydroxyindoleacetic acid (5HIAA), a serotonin metabolite, are decreased in depressed patients with PD compared to both age-matched controls and PD patients without depression (16). However, PD patients without depression have levels of 5HIAA intermediate between those of depressed patients with PD and controls (17). Platelet imipramine binding, a peripheral marker of serotonin, follows the same pattern. In comparison with controls, patients with PD have decreased imipramine binding; and in those with both PD and depression, imipramine binding is even lower. These studies have been interpreted as evidence of a possible predisposition to depression in PD, rather than evidence of a biological marker of depression in PD, because there is inadequate specificity (18).

Although dopamine depletion is a characteristic of PD, it does not appear to play a causal role in major depression in PD. There is no association between the severity of PD and the presence or severity of depression, nor is there an association between CSF levels of the dopamine metabolite homovanilic acid (HVA) and depression (17). However, pharmacological evidence suggests that dopamine may play a role in mood swings in PD. Transient improvement in mood may accompany initiation of levodopa treatment, particularly in patients who do not meet criteria for major depression (19); stimulation of the dopamine system with methylphenidate causes euphoria in patients with PD who are not depressed, but does not improve mood in patients with PD and depression (19, 20).

Dopamine depletion, the source of the motor disturbance, plays a role in the functional disability of the patient. Several authors have found a modest correlation between functional disability and mood disturbances (7, 14, 21, 22). Some mood disturbances are at least partly a reaction to disability; depression, however, can aggravate disability. Studies of patients who experience severe on/off phenomena and dyskinesias have shown greater depression, anxiety, and other negative symptoms during akinetic periods, when dopamine levels are low (23). However, Lees (24) examined patients who experienced dyskinesias as well as on/off phenomena and found that the negative symptoms reappeared during the dyskinetic phase, presumably when dopamine levels are high.

Atypical depression with anxiety has also been reported in PD (25). Stein and colleagues (26) found nine of 24 patients with PD had a clinically significant current anxiety disorder, and in most cases (78%) this occurred after the diagnosis of PD. This study found that anxiety occurred most often in younger individuals and early in the course of PD. Also, the anxiety was not associated with either exposure to levodopa or the degree of disability. An imbalance in dopamine and norepinephrine concentration in the locus ceruleus has been implicated in anxiety in PD (27). Anxiety has also been reported in relation to dopamine replacement therapy. Up to 20% of patients who initiate dopaminergic drug treatment may experience anxiety, which is usually reduced when drug dosage is lowered.

Mania is rare in PD and is usually associated with excessive dopaminergic treatment. Euphoria can occur in up to 10% of patients taking levodopa (28), and hypomania has been reported in patients taking dopamine agonists (bromocriptine and pergolide) (29, 30). Studies with large numbers of patients suggest that the rate of hypomania is close to 2% (31). In general, these symptoms are reversible with reduction of the dose of dopamine agonists.

Psychosis can also occur in PD, and is usually characterized by paranoid delusions, hallucinations, and confusion. Historically, these symptoms were reported before the advent of significant levodopa treatment. However, with current use of both direct and indirect dopaminergic stimulation, 20–30% of patients with PD experience these symptoms (30, 31). The presence of dementia or a preexisting history of psychiatric problems increases the risk of these side effects. Although psychotic symptoms can occur after an increase in anti-Parkinson medication, it can also occur in the presence of a maintenance dose suggesting an intrinsic and progressive change in receptor status.

Treatment of Psychiatric Manifestations

Because psychosis can be the result of dopaminergic stimulation, when possible, reduction of antiparkinson medication is the first course of action. Often PD patients, during a confusional state will be much less parkinsonian, to the amazement of the caregivers. Therefore, they can tolerate a significant reduction in medication. On the other hand,

this course of action may have a serious deleterious effect on mobility and may increase disability. Traditional neuroleptics have been used, but they can further increase parkinsonian symptoms.

Clozapine, a dibenzodiazepine derivative, an atypical antipsychotic, has been used with success. Small, open-trial studies have found improvement in psychotic symptoms with no deterioration in parkinsonian symptoms. Some reports suggest that doses as small as 12.5 mg/day given in the evening may be efficacious, and few serious side effects have been noted with doses of up to 100 mg/day administered for several months (33, 34). Although clozapine may not be free of extrapyramidal side effects, it is usually used concomitantly with levodopa, thereby maximizing mobility and reducing parkinsonian disability. The most commonly reported side effect is sedation, which can often be managed by administering clozapine in the evening, adjusting the dose or using an alternating day treatment regimen. More serious though infrequent side effects, namely, agranulocytosis and leukopenia, require monitoring of the white blood cell count weekly.

With treatment periods longer than a year, there may be a diminution of the beneficial effects of clozapine on psychotic symptoms and deterioration in motor function (35). This trend is often accompanied by a worsening cognition, suggesting that disease progression may be responsible for the loss of efficacy.

Clozapine in low doses (12.5–37.5 mg/day) has been reported to be clinically useful in the treatment of tremor in PD, although the effect was not statistically significant (36). Clozapine at much higher doses (100–200 mg/day) may suppress dyskinesias, but in this dose range significant sedation can occur (37). In summary, there are no controlled clinical trials in PD, but evidence from case and anecdotal reports and open trials suggest that clozapine is beneficial in psychosis and offers significant advantages over other antipsychotics. Psychosis in patients with dementia and severe parkinsonian disability presents a management dilemma for which clozapine can play an important role.

Treatment of Depression

Double-blind studies have demonstrated that tricyclic antidepressants, which primarily increase noradrenergic function, are effective in the treatment of depression in PD (39–40); nortriptyline improved mood with no change in parkinsonian symptoms. Bupropion, an antidepressant with indirect dopaminergic activity, was minimally effective against depression in a subset of patients with PD and produced some improvement in the parkinsonian features (41).

In an open-label study, the serotonergic precursor 5-hydroxytryptophan produced clinical improvement in depressed patients with PD (15). Although the study was small, it indicates that the serotonergic neurotransmitter system may be targeted in the treatment of depression. The new antidepressants (selective serotonergic reuptake inhibitor antidepressants [SSRIs]) may be reasonable treatment choices

(42), although no clinical studies have been reported in depressed PD patients. However, they can in some cases aggravate parkinsonian symptoms by reducing dopamine turnover. Case studies indicating exacerbation of tremor, bradykinesia, gait disturbance, and rigidity have been reported with both fluoxetine and paroxetine (43–44). Both reports indicate reversal of these effects with cessation of the antidepressant. The combination of SSRIs and selegiline (a relatively selective MAO-B inhibitor, which may slow the disability of PD) has recently been associated with a wide range of adverse events, including serotonergic reactions and extrapyramidal signs (EPS). While some clinicians have used the two together safely, these have led to new warnings and the relabeling of compounds to warn against this combination. The wide range of adverse events and the fact that many occurred in patients receiving multiple medications make it difficult to assess the adverse effects. One problem in the interpretation of single case studies and regulatory surveillance reports is the potential for ascertainment bias. In two studies that used a standardized chart review of patients with PD, the incidence of increased EPS or disability was low and not serious, and in one report there was an equal rate of improvement in EPS (45, 46). The true risk of this combination cannot be assessed without a population-based review of the concomitant use of these medications in PD.

Electroconvulsive therapy (ECT) has been used with depressed patients with PD and benefits in both the motor and depressive symptoms have been reported, although some reports have suggested benefit in one area but not the other (47–49). Usually improvement in motor symptoms occurs after one or two treatments and before there is improvement in mood. The motor symptoms return soon after ECT is completed, although some patients remain improved for several weeks to months. ECT has also been used in the treatment of psychosis, psychotic depression, and mania, with reports of adverse reactions, including interictal delusion and cognitive impairment (50–52), suggesting this treatment is not useful in the presence of these symptoms. The advent of the new antidepressants and of clozapine may reduce the use of ECT, a trend which will make it difficult to assess the risk/benefit ratio of this treatment, because ECT will be used in cases which have failed other treatments.

Cognitive Impairment and Dementia

A range of cognitive deficit syndromes can be seen in PD. Most common restrictive deficits are in executive function, visuospatial function, and memory (53–55); these have been repeatedly demonstrated in samples of nondemented patients with PD. The more subtle cognitive findings associated with PD do not appear to be related to the severity of the motor disturbance. These deficits are often referred to as the subcortical dementia of PD. Patients with longer duration of illness have a greater likelihood of cognitive impairment.

Studies of dementia in PD provide estimates of the prevalence ranging from 6–81%; however, studies using strict diagnostic criteria for both dementia and PD yield lower rates. Brown and Marsden (56) reviewed 17 studies with a total of 2530 patients with PD and estimated an overall prevalence of dementia to be 35.1%. They argued that even this number may be an overestimate and suggested that the number may be closer to 15%. Rajput et al. reported the cumulative risk of dementia in PD to be 21.1%, while the risk in controls was only 5.1% (57). Overall, the prevalence of dementia in PD is higher than in the general population, but it is not possible yet to accurately estimate how much higher.

Dementia is more common with late-onset PD (58, 59). Several studies have demonstrated that the rate of dementia in those with onset after age 70 is nearly twice that of those with onset before age 60 (60). The rate of mortality in patients with PD and dementia is higher than in nondemented PD patients (60, 61). Patients with PD and dementia have a poor response to dopamine replacement therapy (62, 63).

The cause of the cognitive impairment in PD has been disputed. Disagreements partly reflect the heterogeneity of cognitive deficits found. Isolated deficits are generally attributed to a disturbance of subcortical systems. One common isolated deficit is executive dysfunction. Executive function deficits have been described in PD patients without other cognitive problems. Cools and his colleagues reported that patients with PD had difficulty switching between repetitive motor sequences (53). Tracking difficulties have been reported by several researchers (54, 55, 64) and an inability to plan and use predictive strategies has been postulated as the cause of the deficit.

In a community-based study, using a series of neuropsychological tests to compare nondemented patients with PD to community-dwelling elderly, performance in the PD group was significantly worse in tests of list learning, orientation, verbal fluency, drawing, and the timed aspects of attentional tests. There were no differences between the PD and control groups in tests of reasoning, comprehension, naming, or accuracy in target detection (65). In a comparison of mildly impaired, nondemented patients with PD, matched for performance on a mental status test to a group of patients with mild AD, Stern et al. found that the PD group performed more poorly on tests of verbal fluency and construction, but better on tests of both immediate and delayed memory (66). When PD patients with memory impairment were matched on immediate memory performance to patients with AD, the PD group performed more poorly in verbal fluency, but better on delayed recall. Overall, these cognitive findings suggest that at least two types of cognitive deficit can be identified in PD: a mild or focal deficit that parallels the description of subcortical deficits, and a more severe and global impairment consistent with dementia and having a pattern of both cortical and subcortical deficits. The presence of substantive memory impairment distinguishes the group with dementia.

Biochemical findings also support the notion that the range of cognitive findings in PD must involve both cortical and subcortical deficits. Early, specific cognitive deficits are related to dopaminergic systems and striatal neuronal degeneration. Cognitive slowing with impact on attentional mechanisms has been associated with noradrenergic deficits, particularly interruption of the locus ceruleus pathways to cortical areas (59, 67). Cholinergic denervation has also been demonstrated in patients with PD and dementia. In summary, there is great heterogeneity of cognitive impairment in PD, associated with varying combination of putative pathophysiological impairments.

MPTP TOXICITY

In 1979, Davis et al. reported the development of parkinsonism apparently resulting from an injection of a self-prepared meperidine analog, 1-methyl-4-phenyl-propionoxypiperidine (MPPP) (68). The clinical syndrome was attributed to the by-product, MPTP, which resulted from shortcuts taken in the synthesis of MPPP. The patient responded to standard antiparkinsonian therapy but died and was found at autopsy to have neuropathological changes (depletion of the dopamine-containing pigmented neurons of the pars compacta of the substantia nigra) characteristic of PD, but without Lewy bodies or degeneration of the locus ceruleus.

In 1982, Langston and colleagues identified a series of seven similar cases and approximately 400 other intravenous drug users exposed to MPTP. Examination of a number of exposed individuals revealed that some remained asymptomatic; others had subtle symptoms of PD; and still others had mild parkinsonism, suggesting that MPTP could produce a full range of disease stages comparable to PD (69).

In primates, experimental injection of MPTP produces akinesia, tremor, and difficulty in initiating movement. It also produces cognitive change, even in animals with few motor signs: (*a*) an object retrieval-detour task revealed response perseveration and deficits in response initiation, fine motor control, planning, and visuospatial ability; (*b*) the severity of the changes was dependent on the degree of motor and cognitive complexity inherent in the components of the task (70, 71); (*c*) decline in performance was seen on delayed response and delayed alternation tasks; perseverative errors were seen on these tasks as well, while visual discrimination performance was unimpaired (72); (*d*) delayed matching to sample, object retrieval, and visual pattern discrimination reversal deficits were seen in the absence of impaired visual pattern discrimination (73). These findings are consistent with compromise of the frontal-striatal axis, and are similar to deficits seen in humans with PD, further supporting the extent to which MPTP toxicity in primates models PD in humans.

Stern and Langston, in a study comparing cognitive performance in patients with MPTP-induced parkinsonism to age- and education-matched controls with a similar history of drug abuse, found general intellectual function, construction, category naming, and frontal lobe function to be worse in patients, although other aspects of performance (reaction time, attention, memory, and language function)

were comparable (74). Because this pattern of deficits is similar to that seen in PD, the authors suggest that the intellectual changes seen in MPTP-induced parkinsonism were due to dopamine deficiency. In a follow-up to this paper, they also assessed MPTP-exposed but relatively asymptomatic subjects (75). MPTP-exposed subjects performed similarly to patients with MPTP-induced parkinsonism on tests of construction and category naming. The MPTP-exposed subjects performed at a level between patients and controls on a test of executive function. The similarity of the pattern of intellectual deficit seen in MPTP-exposed individuals to patients with MPTP-induced parkinsonism and to patients with PD provides evidence that the dopamine system mediates a specific set of cognitive functions, and that changes in these functions can occur even in the absence of overt motor signs. Evidence from these and other studies of patients with PD and other diseases affecting the basal ganglia support the notion that performance on executive, constructional, and motor sequencing tasks are mediated by dopaminergic systems in the basal ganglia.

HUNTINGTON'S DISEASE

Huntington's disease (HD) is an autosomal-dominant disorder with complete penetrance, characterized by a triad of symptoms and signs: movement disorder, cognitive impairment, and psychiatric features. Though in adult-onset cases, chorea is the most recognizable feature, it is rarely the most functionally disabling aspect of the disease. The movement disorder of HD includes involuntary movements such as chorea, dystonia, athetosis, and motor restlessness in the classic form of the disease, and tremor and myoclonus in the juvenile (early-onset) variant. There are also abnormalities of voluntary movement, such as ocular disturbances (defective saccadic pursuit and tracking), abnormalities of gait, rapid alternating movement, and speech. The abnormalities of *voluntary* movement, which can often be elicited only by formal examination early in the disease, correlate best with the duration of illness (76). The severity of chorea generally plateaus after about 10 years, while the abnormalities of voluntary movement continue to worsen. The patient develops rigidity and pyramidal tract dysfunction in the terminal stages of illness.

Despite the characteristic picture of this genetic movement disorder, misdiagnosis is possible. In a survey of 212 patients with diagnoses of HD in a Maryland sample, 15% did not meet criteria for HD when examined by the study's physicians. The most common true diagnosis for these patients was tardive dyskinesia, together with schizophrenia, AD, or another psychiatric disorder that had been treated with neuroleptics. Eleven percent of the patients who actually had HD had initially been given other diagnoses, including alcoholism, posttraumatic movement disorder, or schizophrenia. The authors suggest that a detailed family history and familiarity with the characteristic profile of the disease, (particularly the presence of *voluntary* movement abnormalities) might improve diagnostic accuracy even early in the disease (77).

Although there are many phenotypic presentations, the disease has been identified as an unstable nucleotide repeat (CAG)n in a gene, IT15, on chromosome 4p16.3 (78). The CAG trinucleotide expansion (ranging from 36 to 121 repeats in HD patients) has been found to be both highly sensitive (98.8%) and highly specific with normal controls (99.1%) and controls with other neuropsychiatric disorders (100%) in a study of 1007 patients from 565 families worldwide (79). Repeat length of the CAG expansion has been found to correlate inversely (r = .7) with age of onset, particularly for those with repeat lengths over 60. Overall, repeat length accounts for 50% of the variance in age of onset (80). Juvenile cases tend to have the longest number of repeats. It was also found that sibling pairs tended to have highly correlated trinucleotide expansions, while parent-child pairs did not. When there was a great discrepancy between repeat length in parents and children, the parent was always the father, suggesting that CAG repeats inherited through the male germ line might be more likely to expand. The particular instability of the HD trinucleotide repeat during male gametogenesis has been confirmed by others (81). Repeat length has also been significantly correlated with age at death. No association between specific clinical features (movement disorder, psychosis, or cognitive impairment) and repeat length has been established (80).

Psychiatric Impairment

A wide spectrum of psychiatric disorders has been described in HD, including mood disorders (major depression and bipolar illness), dysthymia, schizophrenia, and personality disorders such as obsessive compulsive disorder (OCD).

In 1872, George Huntington noted that the "tendency to insanity, and sometimes to that form of insanity which leads to suicide is marked." Depression in HD is extremely common. In the first population-based investigation, using a study sample of 164 patients meeting criteria for HD in Maryland on April 1, 1980, major depressive disorder was found in 32% of the subjects. DSM-III diagnostic criteria for depression were used, except that the length of time for a depressive episode was extended to 1 month from 2 weeks. Nine percent of the subjects met criteria for bipolar disorder. The lifetime prevalence rate for mood disorder in this sample was 41% (82). Because this survey used multiple case-finding methods, did not depend solely on hospitalized patients or those with psychiatric admissions, and because it was population-based, it is probably a better estimate of the prevalence of mood disorder in HD than individual case reports. In anecdotal reports (83-85), depression occurred 5–10 years prior to the onset of chorea in HD. In the study by Folstein et al., affective symptoms preceded chorea or dementia in 23 of 34 cases from 2–20 years (average of 5.1 years) (82). The onset of affective disorder was concurrent with the onset of chorea in six cases and followed it in five. The fact that mood disorder preceded chorea is inconsistent

with the idea that it is solely a reaction to the illness, because some of the patients were not even aware that they were at risk for HD. These patients met criteria for major depression, which would probably be unlikely if this were just a depressive reaction. In addition, mania would not be an expected response to knowledge of affliction with a degenerative disease. In addition to the case series, Folstein et al. (82) examined the families of patients with and without a proband with major affective illness. They found that relatives of probands with HD and major mood disorder were significantly more likely to have a major mood disorder than relatives of probands without a mood disorder. When affective disorder was diagnosed in relatives, the lifetime prevalence was 2% for spouses and in-laws of probands but, in contrast, was 28% in the at-risk or affected family members. It is clear that there are families in which HD and major affective disorder co-occur at a greater-than-chance level. Although there are no other distinguishing characteristics between HD patients with and without mood disorder, this may reflect genetic heterogeneity.

As expected, suicide is more common among HD patients with affective disorder. Suicide tends to occur in patients in the early stages of the disease. In a large study, more than half of the suicides occurred in patients not yet diagnosed. The odds ratio for suicide increases with age from 1.3 (10–50 years) to 8.2 (50–70 years) (86).

Mania, although also reported, is less common than depression. Manic episodes with typical symptoms of elation, expansiveness, and self-importance may follow periods of depression. The manic state may last for weeks or may resolve spontaneously with a return to depression (77). Periods of hypomania are much more common than frank mania. They may be very brief, sometimes lasting only a few days, and are present in up to 10% of patients.

Apathy and irritability are very common, troublesome symptoms to patients and families. Apathy is believed to be a distinguishing feature between cortical and subcortical dementias (87). Apathy can be defined as a loss of emotion and may either be an internal feeling or a state of behavioral inaction. Caine and Shoulson (88) extended this concept to situational apathy, which is defined as a state of inactivity and lack of spontaneous expression that can be modified by the active participation of others. In 30 patients, situational apathy increased with increasing severity of illness. Four of 10 mildly affected individuals were situationally apathetic in contrast to all five of the severely disabled patients. In a study in which 26 HD patients were compared to 31 AD patients, there was no overall difference in the frequency of patients reporting apathy. When only demented HD patients were considered, the HD group was relatively more apathetic, suggesting that dementia further increases the level of apathy in these patients (89).

Irritability is "a feeling state characterized by reduced control of the temper which usually results in irascible verbal or behavioral outbursts but can be present without observed manifestations" (90). Irritability may be related to premorbid "bad temper," because among 26 HD patients, irritability correlated positively with "bad temper" (r = .59) when the patient's premorbid traits were rated by an informant on a 5-point scale (89).

Treatment

Major depression associated with HD can be treated in the same way as idiopathic major mood disorder. HD patients may respond to a tricyclic antidepressant, although it may be important to start at a very low dose, especially in the elderly or in those with dementia. Other options include serotonin reuptake blockers such as fluoxetine or sertraline. The SSRIs may be particularly useful for irritability without major depression.

Although lithium is usually employed in the treatment of mania, there may be an increased likelihood of lithium toxicity in HD because these patients are prone to dehydration. Therefore, carbamazepine may be a more effective first-line treatment (90).

There is no established pharmacological treatment for apathy. However, the use of haloperidol for movement disorder should be minimized in apathetic patients. This is because the functional impairment due to apathy exceeds the impairment due to chorea. Atypical neuroleptics (e.g., risperidone) may find a role in treating psychosis in the patient with HD. If behavioral strategies are ineffective in treating irritability, fluoxetine, sertraline, clomipramine, and clonazepam have been effective in some cases (90).

Neuropsychological Impairment

Neuropsychological deficits, progressing to dementia, are seen in HD. There is little debate as to the importance of cognitive impairment. It appears early, and is a major factor in reducing functional capacity. Mayeux et al. studied 33 patients followed longitudinally over an 8-year period and determined the relationship between a cognitive screening tool, the modified Mini-Mental State Examination (MMSE), and the Shoulson-Fahn Functional Capacity Score. They found a significant correlation between MMSE score and total functional capacity, not accounted for by depression or motor disability. Intellectual impairment and depression correlated significantly, but when the somatic symptoms were removed from the analysis, the relationship of depression to functional capacity was no longer significant (91).

Several studies have examined the earliest changes in cognitive function. Butters et al. (92) compared 22 patients with HD (mean duration = 5.5 years) with a group of six recently diagnosed HD patients (mean duration = 4.5 months). The recently diagnosed patients were significantly younger but had a similar level of education. The advanced HD patients showed a nonfocal pattern of deficits, with severe decrease on full-scale, verbal, and performance IQ scores, memory tests, and a test of verbal fluency. Only naming was intact. In contrast, the recently diagnosed HD patients had memory impairment, out of proportion to performance on IQ testing. The most impaired aspects of memory were paragraph recall and associative word learning, which are tests that involve the acquisition of new knowledge. Butters et al. (92) concluded that the memory impairment was present early and might implicate involvement of the hippocampus, dorsal medial nucleus of the thalamus, and the basal ganglia, prior to the cortical association areas.

Two studies have used different screening tests to determine whether there are specific cognitive patterns on screening tests that can be used to differentiate AD and HD. Brandt et al. (93) matched subsamples of AD and HD patients by performance on the Mini-Mental State Examination. Within each subsample, AD patients were significantly older and had a shorter disease duration. In general, HD patients had significantly impaired ability to perform serial subtraction, while AD patients had trouble with recall of three items. A linear discriminant function analysis using these tasks yielded correct classification of 83% of the AD and 84% of the HD cases. Salmon et al. (94) precisely matched 23 AD patients with 23 HD patients on an overall measure of dementia severity. Specific profiles emerged for the AD and HD patients. AD patients performed more poorly than the HD patients on memory tests, while the HD patients performed more poorly than the AD patients on tests of initiation and attention. Memory performance was notable for greater impairment on recall and orientation in the AD group compared with the HD group. This may reflect an impairment in consolidation among AD patients that remains relatively intact in HD. The initiation subtests particularly impaired in the HD patients were the verbal repetition and double alternating movements; both are involved in the programming of motor sequences. Salmon, like Brandt, suggests that these brief mental status tests can be useful in determining patterns of dementia. A linear discriminant function using these profiles correctly classified 82% of the AD patients and 91% of the HD patients. Severity of dementia made it very difficult to classify certain patients. Certainly early in the disease, these patterns are apparent. Whether the concept of subcortical dementia is useful remains unclear. Undoubtedly, damage to subcortical structures such as the caudate nucleus contributes to the cognitive profile seen in HD.

Bamford et al. (95) examined pathological correlates of cognitive impairment using imaging studies. She correlated four factors (psychomotor/executive, verbal memory, visuospatial, and general knowledge) derived from a principal-components factor analysis with computerized tomography (CT) measures of intercaudate (CC) and outer-table (OT) distances. All patients were in the relatively mild stages of HD; 34 were in stage I, with a mean total functional capacity (TFC) score of 11–13, and 26 were in stage II, with mean TFC of 7–10. The CT index that most strongly correlated with cognitive function (particularly the psychomotor factor) was the ratio of CC to OT. The tests comprising the psychomotor factor were highly correlated with the mean TFC (r = .56; p < .001). The psychomotor factor and the visuospatial factor clearly differentiated stage I from stage II patients. The authors reasoned that organizational and sequential planning skills were early cognitive impairments in HD because they discriminated between stage I and stage II and because striatal atrophy was highly correlated with neurological and behavioral manifestations of disease progression. However, the CC/OT ratio accounted for only 30% of the variance, suggesting that the measure was not sensitive enough to detect early abnormality (95).

To determine the clinical correlates of cognitive impairment, but not dementia, Girotti et al. (97) compared 20 nondemented HD patients with 44 controls with respect to motor and cognitive performance. Reaction time (RT) and movement time (MT) were correlated with performance on perceptual-motor and attention tasks. The slowing in RT and MT, believed to be indicative of bradykinesia, correlated with mental decline, while hyperkinesia did not show any significant relationship with cognitive impairment (96).

Although in any individual the cognitive, motor, and behavioral manifestations might contribute to disease severity, functional impairment is far more likely to be secondary to the psychiatric and cognitive problems than to the more obvious chorea.

PROGRESSIVE SUPRANUCLEAR PALSY

Progressive supranuclear palsy (PSP) was probably first described by Posey in 1904 as a case of upgaze paralysis, neck rigidity, pseudobulbar palsy, and dementia. Several similar descriptions of single cases appeared over the succeeding years until Steele, Richardson, and Olszewski published their seminal paper in *Archives of Neurology* in 1964 (97). They described the clinicopathological features of nine patients with a progressive neurological disorder characterized by (a) supranuclear ophthalmoplegia (especially vertical gaze palsy); (b) pseudobulbar palsy with prominent dysarthria; and (c) dystonic rigidity of the neck and upper trunk. There were four basic pathological findings:

1. Neurofibrillary tangles (NFT);
2. Granulovacuolar degeneration of nerve cells;
3. Loss of nerve cells; and
4. Gliosis.

They occurred in a characteristic distribution involving the basal ganglia (globus pallidus, substantia nigra, subthalamic nucleus), red nucleus, superior colliculi, pontine tegmentum, periaqueductal grey matter, and the dentate nucleus. Remarkably, the cerebral cortex, white matter, and inferior colliculi were normal. There were NFTs in the oculomotor nerve nuclei. The reticular formation was shrunken with neuronal loss and NFTs, and there were rare NFTs in the spinal cord. No senile plaques were seen, and the NFTs were unique—they possessed a different ultrastructure from NFTs seen in AD, postencephalitic PD, and the Guamanian Parkinson's-dementia complex (98). The ophthalmoplegia and pseudobulbar palsy are most likely correlated with the changes in the brainstem tegmentum and nuclei, while the akinesia and parkinsonian signs and

symptoms are probably related to changes in the substantia nigra and striatonigral degeneration (98). Similar reports followed, broadening the clinical spectrum, but the etiology has remained obscure.

Golbe et al. (99) reported a prevalence of 1.4 per 100,000 and an adjusted prevalence for the population over 55 of seven per 100,000. In comparison, the reported prevalence for PD is 90–100 per 100,000. Mean age at onset in their series was 63 (range 44–75). The most common presenting symptoms were gait change or fall (62%) and mental changes (22%). Median survival was 9.7 years. In a case-control study of risk factors for PSP, higher education and residence as an adult in an area with a population under 10,000 occurred significantly more frequently in cases than in controls. No other factors (including use of pesticides, use of well water, smoking, prior stroke, hypertension, and head trauma) were associated with PSP.

Clinical Features

The clinical description by Steele, Richardson, and Olszewski (97) was that of a disorder insidious in onset, beginning with subtle changes in personality, altered facies, unsteady gait, or visual or speech problems. Cognitive impairment, though noted early, remained mild. They described a paucity of expression and prominent jaw jerk but noted that blinking remained present. Dysarthria was generally severe and invariably progressive, with dysphagia sometimes appearing late in the course of disease. They did not observe emotional incontinence in any of their initial nine patients. There was rigidity of the axial neck and upper trunk musculature, producing extensor posturing and an inability to look down, which later progressed to more widespread rigidity. The gait was slow, and groping secondary to the inability to look down. Cerebellar and pyramidal findings were inconstant and often late in appearance, and few involuntary movements were observed. They thought that the most striking feature of the disorder was the ophthalmoplegia. Typically, this was a loss of voluntary vertical gaze, affecting downgaze more than upgaze, in the presence of normal vestibulo-ocular and caloric responses. Hence, they favored the term PSP for this disorder.

Since their paper, descriptions of other abnormal ocular phenomena have added tremendously to the list of eye findings in this disease: loss of willed and pursuit eye movements, apraxia of eye opening or closure, square wave jerks, hypometric saccades, gradual deficit of lateral gaze, internuclear ophthalmoplegia (unilateral or bilateral), loss of convergence, subjective complaints of poor near vision (probably a result of diminished convergence), diplopia (especially near diplopia, again related to poor convergence), disruption of optticokinetic nystagmus, loss of the fast component of nystagmus, blepharospasm, loss of Bell's phenomenon, retraction of the upper eyelids, ocular immobility producing a staring quality, and centrally fixed eyes late in the course with absent vestibulo-ocular response (100).

Other motor signs and symptoms associated with PSP have been: mild rest tremor (though generally not present), features of parkinsonism - bradykinesia and masked facies, frequent falls (especially early in the course), cerebellar and pyramidal tract signs (hyperreflexia and extensor plantar responses). Abnormal sleep patterns and sleep apnea have been noted. The clinical hallmark in all cases, however, is the supranuclear gaze palsy, and it is this finding that generally leads to the diagnosis.

Steele, Richardson, and Olszewski (97) observed a characteristic pattern of progression in their cases: (*a*) downgaze defect, rigid neck extension, and masked facies; (*b*) dysarthria; and (*c*) diffuse rigidity. Retrospective analysis has since revealed that the initial symptoms are usually vague unsteadiness with falls followed by vague disturbances in vision—patients are usually unaware of their inability to look down. As the disease progresses, there are more falls, neck rigidity, and paralysis of downgaze, which progresses to gross akinesia involving ocular, bulbar, axial, and finally limb structures. Drugs do not seem to slow the progression to complete immobility, cachexia, and death from infection (most commonly recurrent aspiration pneumonia or sepsis from decubitus ulcers). The diagnosis is usually made between 1–5 years from the onset and the median duration of disease until death is about 6 years.

There have been reports of patients with atypical presentations found to have the characteristic pathology at autopsy. Davis (101) reported a series of four cases without the classic ophthalmoplegia but with the classic pathology. Two presented with severe dementia and two had predominantly parkinsonian features, but without tremor, with normal arm swing and with a poor response to carbidopa/levodopa. Two had some difficulty with upgaze, and one had a rigid extended neck. All had gait problems early and frequent falls. Kleinschmidt-DeMasters et al. (102) reported a series of three cases with dementia, disordered gait, and some dysarthria, but without oculomotor deficits that were found at autopsy, to have classic PSP pathological findings. The implication of these atypical cases is that the hallmark (gaze palsy) may not be the earliest feature. Thus, PSP should be considered in the differential diagnosis of patients with dementia, gait disorder, dysarthria, or features of PD.

Laboratory evaluation is of little value in making the diagnosis. Occasionally there will be a slight increase in CSF protein or nonspecific EEG changes. CT and magnetic resonance imaging (MRI) usually reveal atrophy, which may be especially pronounced in the brainstem, and positron emission tomography (PET) demonstrates decreased glucose consumption in the frontal cortex. A definitive diagnosis, however, depends on the characteristic neuropathology.

Psychiatric Manifestations

PSP is often first manifest by vague changes in personality, and the triad of personality change, gait disturbance, and dysarthria often characterizes the early stages of this disorder. The personality changes, per se, have been poorly described in the literature. They are often considered mild and felt to possibly reflect mental slowing, bradyphrenia, or early dementia. However, the range of mental changes reported in PSP includes outbursts (emotional incontinence or pseudobulbar affect), delirium, hallucinations, and depression.

COGNITIVE IMPAIRMENT AND DEMENTIA

The dementia of PSP was characterized by Albert et al. in 1974 (103). According to these researchers, the four main facets of the disease are:

1. Forgetfulness;
2. Slowing of thought processes;
3. Emotional/personality changes (apathy or depression with occasional outbursts of irritability); and
4. Impaired ability to manipulate acquired knowledge.

They felt that this pattern of impairment was similar to that seen in other neurological diseases associated with subcortical pathology and classified it as a subcortical dementia. They remarked on the dichotomy of excessive time delay in carrying out intellectual functions but, if given sufficient time to respond, mostly intact verbal and perceptual/motor capacities. They contrasted this performance with cortical dementias, which have a predominance of language dependent dysfunction, perceptual problems, or perceptuomotor dysfunction.

In 1981, Kimura et al. (104) reported impairment in tasks requiring visual scanning and intellectual impairment only on tests requiring visual search or scanning, suggesting that the eye-movement disorder might be responsible for much of the observed cognitive impairment noted in earlier studies. In 1982, Fisk (105) noted similar impairment on psychological tests requiring visual scanning but reported that the IQ of patients with PSP was in the normal range and concluded that dementia was not a salient feature of PSP. In the midst of this controversy, Maher et al. in 1985 (106), reported a decrease in verbal and performance IQ when compared with premorbid testing and confirmed the findings of Albert et al. of a subcortical dementia without dysphasia, agnosia, or perceptual abnormalities and with especially poor performance on tests of frontal lobe function. Pillon et al. (107) noted dementia in 26 of 45 patients with PSP and found particular difficulty in tests of attention, lexical fluency, and imitation behavior, again suggesting frontal lobe dysfunction or disconnection. PET scan results demonstrating decreased glucose utilization in the frontal cortex support the notion that these deficits reflect frontal lobe dysfunction and may result from disconnection secondary to subcortical lesions. Additional clinical evidence of executive or frontal deficits were reported by Litvan et al. (108) who noted several types of impaired memory processes, including abnormally rapid forgetting, increased sensitivity to interference, and difficulty in using strategic long-term memory search processes. Dubois et al. (109) found central processing time to be increased in patients with PSP when compared to either patients with PD or to controls. This increase was associated with impairment in tests of frontal lobe function. In a study comparing the severity and specificity of cognitive impairment in AD, HD, PD, and PSP, Pillon et al. (110) noted that PSP was characterized by predominant "subcorticofrontal" cognitive and behavioral impairment at all stages. They noted that disturbances of "instrumental" functions like memory and language were characteristic of dementia of the Alzheimer type, while more "fundamental" functions such as attention and regulation of behavior were disrupted in the "subcortical" dementias. Furthermore, they noted that the frontal-lobe-like syndrome seen in PSP could be differentiated from the concentration-acquisition difficulties seen in HD. They concluded that the subcorticofrontal symptomatology of PSP was compatible with a "frontal deafferentation."

TREATMENT

In general, dopaminergic, cholinergic, and serotonergic agents have been ineffective in attempts to improve function in PSP. Noradrenergic agents have been tried in an attempt to specifically improve cognitive function, also without success. Furthermore, given the manifest differences in the neuropathology of PSP and AD, it is unlikely that currently approved treatment for dementia of the Alzheimer type would be of benefit in PSP.

HALLERVORDEN-SPATZ DISEASE

Hallervorden-Spatz disease (HSD) is a rare disorder characterized by extrapyramidal signs, other motor system dysfunction, and progressive mental deterioration. The etiology is unknown, but the disease follows a pattern suggestive of autosomal-recessive inheritance. Possible mechanisms implicated in the pathogenesis of HSD are lipid peroxidation, deficiency of fatty acid membrane components, and abnormalities of cyclic guanosine monophosphate metabolism (111). The neuropathological findings consist of lesions of the globus pallidus and the pars reticulata of the substantia nigra, accumulations of pigment, primarily iron, in these regions, and widespread neuroaxonal spheroids (112).

Disease onset is typically in the first or second decade of life, with gait difficulties or posture impairment, progressing to extrapyramidal dysfunction (rigidity, dystonia, and abnormal movements—usually choreoathetosis or tremor) as well as corticospinal tract involvement (spasticity, hyperreflexia, or extensor plantar responses). Dysarthria is universal and may be associated with dysphagia, hypophonia, or oromandibular dystonia and generally becomes increasingly severe, leading to mutism and feeding difficulty.

Psychiatric Manifestations and Cognitive Impairment

Intellectual retardation or decline is present in most patients. The clinical course varies from rapid deterioration

over 1–2 years to slow progression or even plateaus for many years (113). Because there is no biochemical marker for the disease, diagnosis often depends on autopsy. However, typical clinical findings in the presence of peripherally hypointense but centrally hyperintense lesions in the globus pallidus (known as "eye of the tiger" sign) on T2-weighted MRI support the diagnosis (114).

A late onset form has been described with onset after 20 years of age. In these cases parkinsonian manifestations may predominate rather than dystonic or choreic features (115). Other atypical presentations may include behavioral disturbances characterized by impulsiveness or aggressiveness, mood disorders, visual changes (either eye-movement abnormalities or retinal degeneration), and seizures.

Impaired cognitive function, often beginning with slowness of thought and disturbances in conceptual ability, progressively worsens to dementia. Neuropsychological studies have revealed a general loss of intellectual ability. Impairment was seen in those verbal tests requiring conceptual and analytic strategies (similarities, arithmetic), whereas performance test scores were all low and were worse than verbal test scores. This mental deterioration has been considered a form of subcortical dementia (116).

Treatment

Trihexyphenidyl and levodopa/carbidopa have been effective in treating the motor aspects, especially dystonia. However, no therapy for the intellectual deterioration has been of value.

WILSON'S DISEASE

Wilson's disease (WD), also known as hepatolenticular degeneration, is an autosomal-recessive inherited disorder of copper metabolism. The prevalence of WD is about 30 per million population (117). The gene for WD has been localized to chromosome 13 (118) and, while the exact biochemical abnormality remains unknown, excretion of copper by the liver is impaired. Excess copper accumulates, first in the liver and then in the brain and other organs. It is this accumulation of copper that is thought to be responsible for the clinical manifestations of WD (119).

Patients generally present in the second or third decade of life. The initial manifestations may include neurological, psychiatric, hepatic, ocular, renal, or articular abnormalities. Hepatic disease may take the form of an asymptomatic rise in liver enzymes, hepatitis, jaundice, or cirrhosis. Kayser-Fleischer rings (golden brown corneal rings) are generally visible by slit-lamp exam once neurological signs are present and are pathognomonic for the disorder. The initial neurological features are usually tremor, slowness of movement, dysarthria, dysphagia, choreic movements, or dystonic posturing. As the disease progresses, rigidity, fixed facies, "wing-beating" tremor and worsening bradykinesia may supervene.

Diagnosis

Low serum ceruloplasmin (less than 20 mg/dl), low serum copper (less than 80 μg/dl) and increased urinary copper excretion (more than 100 μg/24 hr) confirm the diagnosis. Early in the course, a high copper content in a liver biopsy or failure to incorporate ^{64}Cu into ceruloplasmin may be more sensitive. Basal ganglia lesions, generalized atrophy and ventricular dilation are commonly seen in both CT and MRI scans. With treatment, the radiological changes may reverse.

Pathology

The pathological changes involve, primarily, though not exclusively, the lenticular nuclei. Changes in the caudate, thalamus, cerebellar nuclei, subthalamic nuclei, pontine nuclei, and the surrounding white matter have all been described. These changes take the form of shrinking and discoloration, which may progress to cystic degeneration or cavitary necrosis. Cortical atrophy and vascular changes have also been noted. Presumably, the excess copper or ischemia (or both) is responsible for these effects (120).

Psychiatric Symptoms

There is a broad spectrum of psychiatric manifestations of WD. Reports have included cognitive impairment, confusional states, dementia, mental retardation or poor school performance, anxiety, irritability, emotional lability, "neurosis," psychosis, schizophrenia-like states, "incongruous behavior" (described as a "dissociation between environmental cues and behavior"), anorexia nervosa, alcohol abuse, criminality, affective disorders, and suicide. WD may present with psychiatric symptoms in 10–65% of cases. Most series report a figure in the 25–35% range. Behavioral symptoms, personality change, and mood disturbance seem to be the most frequent psychiatric manifestations, although the nature of these changes is often not specified. Psychosis is relatively infrequent. In their series of 195 cases, Dening and Berrios (121) noted that more than half of their sample displayed some form of psychological or behavioral disorder and that 20% of these patients were seen by a psychiatrist before the diagnosis of WD was made. In the follow-up to this report (122), they noted that the most common psychiatric symptoms were incongruous behavior, irritability, depression, and cognitive impairment and that significant improvement was seen only in incongruous behavior and cognitive impairment. Persistent psychiatric disturbance was associated with more dysarthria, incongruous behavior, and hepatic symptoms.

Cognitive Impairment

Variable degrees of dementia or other cognitive deficits have been observed in WD. WD has been considered an example of subcortical dementia characterized by memory loss, impairment of manipulation of acquired knowledge, personality changes, and slowness of mentation without aphasia, apraxia, or agnosia (123). In WD patients with a history of neurological involvement, mild cognitive deficits were reported by Medalia et al. (124). They noted that these patients were impaired in their ability to complete timed visuomotor tasks because of interference with their motor functioning, and they noted mild memory impairment on standardized tests. Lang et al. (123) devised a battery of neuropsychological tests that did not depend on manual dexterity. They found that the WD patient group means were within 1 standard deviation of controls and might thus still be considered psychometrically normal. However, the WD means were lower than controls on most tests. A global difference was seen when examining individual scores that exceeded 1 standard deviation of the test norms (125). They noted a significant difference on a perceptual speed task that did not require manual dexterity. Furthermore, they found that WD patients with neurological signs performed worse on a test of reasoning. The basal ganglia, in addition to their involvement in motor control, also have a role in the flow of information during cognitive processes and interact with the supplementary motor areas as an integration center for sensorimotor information (126). The psychomotor impairment in WD patients may result from the impaired interaction of the basal ganglia and cortical areas (127).

Treatment

Therapy in WD is based on decreasing the body's copper burden with the chelating agent D-penicillamine (1–2 g/day). In the patient unable to tolerate penicillamine, zinc acetate (50 mg zinc five times daily) or trientene (1–1.5 g/day) may be substituted. Daily lifelong treatment will prevent the occurrence of symptoms in patients identified in the presymptomatic stage (e.g., an apparently unaffected relative of a person with WD, diagnosed by abnormal laboratory tests). Treatment will generally improve (often to normal) most of the signs and symptoms in patients with WD (117). Improvement in measures of general intelligence and memory have been seen with treatment and have been more marked with longer duration of therapy (125). Discontinuation of therapy will usually be followed by death in about 3 years (128). When hepatic failure is evident, therapy is ineffective, with the possible exception of liver transplantation (129). In addition to decoppering, restriction of dietary copper is recommended. Anticholinergic medication has been of some benefit in patients with dystonia (127). Neuroleptics should be avoided in WP patients because of their potential to exacerbate the extrapyramidal syndrome (130).

DIFFUSE LEWY BODY DISEASE

Diffuse Lewy body disease (DLBD) is characterized neuropathologically by the presence of Lewy bodies (the primary pathological feature associated with PD) and clinically by dementia, parkinsonism, and psychosis. In DLBD, Lewy bodies are found in the brainstem, as they are in PD, and also in cortical areas (131). A transitional form has also been identified in which Lewy bodies are found in subcortical and diencephalic areas (131). Cortical Lewy bodies have been noted in deep small neurons of the temporofrontal lobes and in the cingulate, insular, and entorrhinal cortex (132, 133).

DLBD can co-occur with the pathological features of AD. In an autopsy series of patients with dementia, brains with neuritic plaques and few neurofibrillary tangles were more likely to have Lewy bodies (75%) than those with a preponderance of tangles (25%) (134). Such cases have been labelled the Lewy body variant (LBV) of AD. Several reports have suggested that DLBD has a younger age of onset than the LBV, but this is not a consistent finding. Recent reports indicate that the apolipoprotein E4 allele, which is overrepresented in AD, is also highly associated with LBV but is not evident in DLBD, suggesting a genetic difference between these entities (135). In addition to these distinctions, other nomenclatures describing similar entities appear in the literature and have been well summarized by Hansen and Galasko (136). There is considerable overlap in the clinical features of AD, LBV, and DLBD, with some differences stemming primarily from the order of appearance of symptoms.

Clinical Presentation

Most clinicopathological series suggest that DLBD patients usually present with dementia or extrapyramidal features and therefore typically carry an initial diagnosis of either AD or PD (Table 34.2). Several reports estimate that between 12–22% (132, 137) of those who initially present with dementia or extrapyramidal symptoms will have DLBD or LBV. Onset of illness is typically after age 65, though Kosaka has reported a series with a number of cases with onset before age 60. Gait disturbance is a commonly reported feature. Crystal reported that impaired gait occurred very early in four of six patients with DLBD (138), and others report frequent falling (139). Other common extrapyramidal features are bradykinesia, rigidity, and masked facies. Tremor is less commonly reported. Motor signs are common as an early feature in DLBD and as a late sign of the LBV of AD.

Psychiatric Manifestation, Cognitive Impairment, and Dementia

Dementia is a hallmark of the clinical syndrome, regardless of the coexistence of AD-like neuropathological changes. The specific cognitive impairments include memory deficits, apraxia, aphasia and dyscalculia, as well as impairments in subcortical cognitive functions such as fluency, visuospatial, and constructional abilities (137, 140). In a clinical pathological series of DLBD patients matched to a group of patients with AD for overall level of dementia,

patients with DLBD had equivalent memory and naming impairment but significantly more visual/spatial, constructional, and verbal fluency deficits (141). Sahgal et al. (142) reported greater impairment on a delayed visual matching task in a group of patients with DLBD than in a group of AD patients of equivalent severity, but there was no pathological verification of the patient groups (142).

The onset of cognitive deficit and dementia may be later when DLBD is the only pathology. Byrne described 15 cases in which only nine presented with dementia and only three had neurofibrillary tangles (137). All eventually developed dementia. Conversely, dementia is usually the presenting sign in the combination of DLBD and AD (138).

Psychiatric disturbances are very common in DLBD, with reports of hallucinations, delusions, anxiety, and depression. In a series of patients with DLBD and AD pathology, McKeith (139) reported that nearly 50% of patients presented with delusions, but others report minimal psychiatric symptomatology (141, 143). Psychiatric disturbances occur more often in DLBD (and LBV) than in "pure" AD. However, it is unclear if there are differences in the frequency of psychiatric manifestations between patients with DLBD and those with LBV.

The biochemical basis for the frequent psychotic symptoms seen in DLBD is uncertain, but a postmortem pathological series of patients with DLBD described by Perry et al. found significantly lower levels of choline acetyltransferase activity in frontal, temporal, and parietal cortex in those patients with hallucinations (144). Furthermore, it has been suggested that serotonergic hyperactivity may be associated with hallucinations, based on a twofold increase in the CSF levels of a serotonin metabolite in this group.

A fluctuating course has been described by several authors. Changes in cognition, occurring over short intervals, have been identified as a hallmark of this disease (144). McKeith and colleagues have proposed that fluctuations in cognitive testing and daily living skills are a defining feature. They report that the fluctuations may include episodic confusion interspersed with lucid intervals (139). Many other authors have reported similar fluctuations but comment that nearly 20% of patients do not demonstrate these fluctuations (137, 138, 140). Given the high prevalence of psychiatric symptoms in DLBD, it is difficult to determine if fluctuating cognition is due to the intermittent presence of psychotic symptoms.

Treatment

There are no systematic studies of treatment for cognitive, psychiatric, or motor disturbances in the disease. It has been suggested that individuals with parkinsonian syndromes other than idiopathic PD do not respond well to levodopa; thus, this line of treatment is often not pursued. Case reports of levodopa therapy have demonstrated mixed results with some reporting a benefit (132, 145), others reporting no benefit (146–148) and one reporting a transient response

Table 34.2. Summary of Clinicopathological Series of Cases with Diffuse Lewy Body Disease[a]

First Author	N	Pathology	Features	Fluctuations	Levodopa Response	Neuroleptic Response	Comment
Crystal (139)	6	3 cLB,scLB 3 cLB,scLB+nP,nT	67% EPS 100% dementia 83% psychsym	NA	0/1 improved	3/3 EPS++	fewer nT than in pure AD
Lippa (144)	12	5 cLB,scLB 7 cLB,scLB+nP,nT	8% EPS 83% dementia 8% psychsym	NA	NA	NA	
Byrne (128)	15	15 cLB,scLB	60% EPS 60% dementia 87% psychsym	80%	10/11 improved	EPS++	AD pathology not described
Hansen (142)	13 9*	13 cLB;12 scLB 13 nP and/or nT	100% EPS 77% dementia no psychsym	NA	NA	NA	clinical data for 9 of 13 cases
McKeith (140)	21	21 cLB, scLB, 21 nP, nT	71% EPS 60% dementia 81% psychsym	81%	1/1	5/14 EPS+ 8/14 EPS++	fewer nT than AD 10% initially, 62% after first visit less impaired than AD EPS: 33% severe, 53% mild
Dickson (134)	6	2 cLB, scLB 3 cLB, scLB, nP 1 cLB, scLB, nP, nT	83% EPS 100% dementia 67% psychsym	NA	NA	NA	
Forestl (141)	8	8 cLB, scLB, nP, nT	62% EPS 100% dementia 75% psychsym	38%	NA	NA	fewer nT than in AD described as intermittent confusion

[a]Key: cortical lewy bodies (cLB); subcortical lewy bodies (scLB); neuritic placques (nP); neurofibrilary tangles (nT); extrapyramidal signs including gait disturbance (EPS); psychiatric symptoms including hallucinations, delusions, agitation, depression (psychsym); mild to moderate (+); severe (++); not assessed (NA); Alzheimer's disease (AD).

(149). Mark et al. described two patients with akinetic parkinsonian features and gait disturbance who were not responsive to treatment with levodopa (148). These individuals had Lewy bodies in subcortical and diencephalic areas in a pattern consistent with the transitional form of DLBD. In a series of 15 patients, 11 were treated with levodopa; 10 had a definite benefit and one had a probable benefit. Of note, six of the 10 treated patients had initially presented with motor signs only (137). The overall impression from these reports is that a benefit from levodopa therapy may be apparent at the earliest stage, particularly if motor symptoms are a primary problem.

Reports of (standard) neuroleptic use in LBD and DLBD are more uniform and indicate dramatic deterioration of gait (138), other extrapyramidal signs (137) and, in a minority of cases, acute neuroleptic malignant syndrome (139) with little evidence of improvement in psychiatric symptoms. Although no systematic studies exist, it has been reported that depression responds to conventional tricyclic antidepressants (137).

TOURETTE'S SYNDROME AND OTHER TIC DISORDERS

Both transient and chronic tic disorders may be part of a continuum that share similar behavioral and psychiatric manifestations. Tourettes' syndrome (TS), initially characterized as a psychiatric disorder, has been reclassified as a movement disorder with presumed basal ganglia involvement and is perhaps the most widely studied tic disorder. Criteria for the diagnosis of TS (150) require onset before age 21, the presence of multiple tics and at least one vocalization. The type of tic may fluctuate with progression of tics following a rostral to caudal pattern. Although phenomenologically coprolalia is highly associated with this entity, large-scale studies suggest that it occurs in only one-third of the patients.

Studies support the notion that TS is a familial disease, and a single genetic locus has been suggested. However, the pattern of inheritance is unclear. Autosomal-dominant transmission with sex-specific penetrance has been hypothesized (151). Alternatively, Commings (152) has described semidominant, semirecessive inheritance. This hypothesis suggests that a wide range of other behaviors may also be manifestations of the same gene. Major difficulties in evaluating these two hypotheses are the relatively high prevalence of co-morbid conditions and the high prevalence of tic-like disorders in the general population. OCD and attention deficit disorder (ADD), with and without hyperactivity, are frequent co-morbid conditions.

A growing body of neuroimaging and postmortem evidence implicates the basal ganglia in TS and related disorders. PET studies have shown increased glucose utilization in the basal ganglia in TS compared to controls and no difference in glucose utilization in cortical regions. Increased glucose utilization in the caudate and left orbital gyrus have been seen in patients with OCD (153-154). Postmortem studies describe neuronal hypoplasia in the caudate and putamen with few changes in the cortex in TS (155, 156). Balthazar reported decreases in the size and density of cells in the striatum in the absence of gliosis (157). The left lenticular (caudate, putamen, and globus pallidus) region in TS is reduced in volume compared with controls. Neurons of this region are inhibitory, and a deficiency in these nuclei might be expected to lead to exaggerated behavior in TS.

Clinical Course

Although there are very few prospective longitudinal data available, several studies have suggested that the tic disturbance ameliorates with age. Patients tend to find their symptoms are worse in the first decade after diagnosis, and then gradually improve with each succeeding decade (158-160). Shapiro and Shapiro have reported improvement in adulthood in 35% of their patients, with 5–8% demonstrating complete recovery (161). Demographic studies suggest that the prevalence of TS decreases by about one-quarter in adulthood (162). Ascertainment bias may account for this impression. First, most of the patient survey studies were done through convenience samples retrospectively identified. Follow-up is traditionally higher among those who recover. Also, given the multiplicity of concomitant symptoms, it is possible that other diagnoses obscure TS. In a study of 58 adults with TS, Goetz and colleagues retrospectively examined associations between clinical features in childhood and adulthood (163). In this group, moderate to severe tics were reported by 28% of the cohort in childhood. Sixty percent reported moderate to severe tics during the time of worst functioning. The only predictor of mild tic severity in adulthood was mild tic severity during early and late adolescence. Peak childhood tic severity did not predict adult tic severity. Of note is the relative absence of disability in adults with TS and minimal intrusion into private and professional life. These findings suggest that the psychosocial and cognitive impact of TS may be manifest as developmental delay rather than permanent disability.

Psychiatric Manifestations

There is a wide range of psychiatric symptoms in TS. In children, behavioral disturbance usually precedes tics. In a study of 250 consecutive cases, 62% had ADD and 48.8% had ADD with hyperactivity (164). Most began with a history of ADD, 2–3 years prior to the development of tics. OCD is also a common finding in this group, with about half of those with TS having significant symptoms of OCD. These symptoms are more common in the most severe cases of TS. OCD symptoms occur after the onset of tics, appear to worsen with age, and are most pronounced around the age of 15 (150, 165, 166).

Cognitive Impairment

Much of the work examining cognition in TS has been done in children and adolescents. Several methodological issues are worthy of discussion. In a review of cognitive function in TS, Como (167) points out that many studies use small samples and do not adequately distinguish between TS and ADD with and without hyperactivity. Apparently, there is little evidence of intellectual impairment or focal neuropsychological deficits in individuals with pure TS. However, because comorbidity is very common, it is important to consider the cognitive profile of patients with both TS and ADD. Concept formation, visual scanning, and planning deficits have been reported in clinical samples with features of both diagnoses (168). Psychomotor speed and visual-perceptual ability also appear to be impaired in this group (169). This study also identified features of the tic disorder associated with poor performance on a concept formation task, tactile memory, and graphesthesia. The presence of complex tics was associated with impaired performance on visuomotor sequencing and fine motor skills. Many of these findings could be summarized as evidence of executive function deficits. On the other hand, these studies may simply reflect delayed development rather than true disability. Support for this hypothesis comes from a longitudinal study by Erenberg et al. (159). Although 63% of the patients in this cohort reported that learning disabilities interfered with their lives at the time of the first assessment, only 19% reported such problems on follow-up. A similar trend was reported by Goetz et al., who found that 67% of patients with TS received failing grades in school and 22% had entered special education programs. However, as adults, 98% were high school graduates and 90% were working full time or were full-time students (163).

Mild executive function deficits are reported in adults. Typically, they complain of disorganization at work and in personal affairs, such as bill paying, keeping appointments, and correspondence. They have difficulty completing tasks and trouble returning to tasks if interrupted. Deficits in formal testing of vigilance, sustained, and focused attention and impulsivity may also be evident in adulthood (167, 170). One conclusion from these findings is that true executive function deficits do exist as would be predicted in a disease of the basal ganglia. The age-dependent manifestations may reflect a differential rate of development of compensatory mechanisms as well as different age-specific social and occupational demands. However, unlike many of the other BG diseases, there is no evidence of progression of neuropathology or psychopathology.

Treatment

Treatment in TS must be guided by evaluating (*a*) the degree of disability caused by the tics; (*b*) the presence of ADD; and (*c*) the presence of OCD. Perhaps the oldest treatment modality was the use of neuroleptics, most commonly, the butyrophenone, haloperidol. There is ample evidence that this agent reduces tic frequency and severity, however, the side effects are significant and include sedation, dysphoria (often leading to noncompliance), acute dystonic reactions and akathisia, poor school performance, and school phobia (171–173).

Other neuroleptic drugs have been used in TS, including pimozide and fluphenazine, but whether they offer any improvement over haloperidol is unclear. Pimozide can prolong the Q-T interval on the electrocardiogram and should be avoided when this abnormality is noted before treatment initiation (172). A recent report suggests that botulinum toxin may ameliorate the intensity and frequency of tics and lesson the premonitory urges that can precede these involuntary movements (174). However, double-blind studies have not been conducted.

The presence of ADD with TS should direct treatment away from the neuroleptics. The most common treatment choice for this comorbid state is clonidine. This agent is an α_2-adrenergic agonist that blocks the presynaptic release of norepinephrine. Several reports suggest that the initial claims of improvement in up to 70% of cases may be overly optimistic (175), but its efficacy is generally accepted, particularly in those with mild to moderate tics. Although psychostimulants are not generally advisable in the combination of TS and ADD, tricyclic antidepressants, including desipramine (176, 177) and nortriptyline (178) have been found to improve both motor and behavioral symptoms. Recently, the selective MAO-B inhibitor selegiline has been reported to be beneficial in patients with these co-morbid conditions. In an open trial, Jancovic reported clinical improvement in ADD symptoms in 90% of those treated with selegiline (mean dose 8.1 mg/day) for 3 to 15 months (179). There were no serious adverse side effects, and only two of 29 patients experienced an increase in tics.

When TS occurs with disabling OCD, treatment regimens may focus on the use of selective serotonin reuptake inhibitors (SSRI). These agents have demonstrated efficacy in OCD and have proven beneficial in patients with TS and obsessive-compulsive symptoms (180, 181), although the addition of dopamine antagonist may be required (182). When the SSRIs fail, the addition of agents to increase serotonergic transmission (e.g., tricyclics) does not prove beneficial. Behavioral treatments have also been proposed in TS. Peterson and Azrin (183) report a reduction in tics with techniques such as habit reversal, self-monitoring, and relaxation training. However, others have warned that conditioning techniques may tend to focus attention on TS symptomatology, potentially leading to an increase in tic frequency and intensity (184) and suggest that it is most appropriate in the presence of obvious environmental stressors.

CONCLUSION

The diseases described in this chapter demonstrate the broad range of cognitive and psychiatric disorders that are associated with BG pathology. Some of these deficits result from the direct impact of damage to the basal ganglia and to the associated neurochemical systems. Other findings are related to projection areas innervated by the BG, especially the frontal cortex. It is important to characterize the full range of clinical findings both for diagnostic reasons and for management. There is a wide range of efficacy of treatments for the movement disorders described here. In some diseases (PSP, HSD, DLBD), limited efficacy is expected at best; in others (PD, HD and TS), relatively good efficacy is expected; and in one (WD), complete reversal can be achieved. In general, the efficacy of treatment for mood disorders is similar among patients with and without BG diseases. However, treatment of psychosis is problematic because neuroleptics usually exacerbate motor disturbances in patients with BG diseases and impair voluntary purposeful motor function, even when they suppress involuntary movements. Atypical neuroleptics, such as clozapine and risperidone, offer the hope of better treatment, but these have not been tested apart from the use of clozapine in PD. There are few treatments for cognitive impairment in any condition and, to complicate matters further, in BG disease, treatment for either behavioral or motor symptoms can worsen cognitive function. Clearly, the treatment of one problem can lead to exacerbation of another. For each symptom, it is necessary to weigh the degree of disability it produces, the likelihood of benefit with a given treatment and the probability of exacerbating other symptoms with such treatment in order to choose the best therapeutic approach.

Acknowledgments

This work was supported by the Charles S. Robertson Memorial Gift for Alzheimers Disease Research and by Federal Grants AG02802, AG07232, AG0737 and RROO654.

References

1. Albert ML. Subcortical dementia In Alzheimer's disease. In: Katzman R, Terry RD, Bick KL, eds. Senile dementia and related disorders. New York: Raven Press, 1979:173–180.
2. McHugh PR, Folstein MF. Psychiatric syndromes of Huntington's chorea: a clinical and phenomenologic study. In: Benson DF, Blumer D. Psychiatric aspects of neurologic disease. New York: Grune & Stratton, 1975:267–285.
3. Albert ML, Feldman RG, Willis AL. The subcortical dementia of supranuclear palsy. J Neurol Neurosurg Psychiatry 1974;37:121–130.
4. Brown RG, Marsden CD. "Subcortical dementia": the neuropsychological evidence. Neuroscience 1988;25:363–387.
5. Yahr MD. Parkinsonism. In: Rowland LP ed. Merritt's textbook of neurology, 8th ed. Philadelphia: Lea & Febiger, 1989;658–671.
6. Jellinger K. Overview of morphological changes in Parkinson's disease. In: Yahr M, Bergmann KJ, eds. Advances in neurology, vol 45. Parkinson's disease. New York: Raven Press;1986:1–18.
7. Cummings JL. Depression and Parkinson's disease: a review. Am J Psychiatry 1992;149:443–454.
8. Starkstein SE, Preziosi TJ, Forrester AW, Robinson RB. Specificity of affective and autonomic symptoms in depression and Parkinson's disease. J Neurol Neurosurg Psychiatry 1990;53:869–873.
9. Levin BE, Llabre MM, Weiner WJ. Parkinson's disease and depression: psychometric properties of the Beck Depression Inventory. J Neurol Neurosurg Psychiatry 1988;51:1401–1404.
10. Sano M. The basal ganglia and depression. Neuropsychiatry, Neuropsychology, Behavioral Neurology. 1991;4:41–48.
11. American Psychiatric Association, Diagnostic and statistical manual of mental disorders. 3rd ed., revised. Washington, DC, 1987.
12. Sano M, Stern Y, Williams JBW, Cote L, Rosenstein R, Mayeux R. Coexisting dementia and depression in Parkinson's disease. Arch Neurol 1989;46:1284–1286.
13. Hoen MM, Yahr MD. Parkinsonism: onset, progression and mortality. Neurology 1967;17:427–442.
14. Brown RC, MacCarthy B, Gotham AM, Dre GJ, Marsden CD. Depression and disability in Parkinson's disease: a follow-up of 132 cases. Psychol Med 1988;18:49–55.
15. Mayeux R, Stern Y, Sano M, Williams JBW, Cote L. The relationship of serotonin to depression in Parkinson's disease. Mov Disord 1988;3:237–244.
16. Kostic VS, Djuricic BM, Covickovic-Sternis N, Bumbasirevic L, Mrsulja BB. Depression and Parkinson's Disease: possible role of serotonergic mechanisms. J Neurol 1987;234:94–96.
17. Mayeux R, Stern Y, Williams JBW. Clinical and biochemical features of depression in Parkinson's disease. Am J Psychiatry 1986; 143:756–759.
18. Sano M, Stanley M, Lawton A, et al. ^{3}H-imipramine binding as a peripheral measure of serotonin in Parkinson's disease. Arch Neurol 1991;48:1052–1054.
19. Cantello R, Gilli M, Riccio A, Bergamasco B. Mood changes associated with "end-of-dose deterioration" in Parkinson's disease: a controlled study. J Neurol Neurosurg Psychiatry 1986;49:1182–1192.
20. Cantello R, Aguggia M, Gilli M, et al. Major depression in Parkinson's disease and the mood response to intravenous methylphenidate: possible role of the "hedonic" dopamine system. J Neurol Neurosurg Psychiatry 1989;52:724–731.
21. Gotham AM, Brown RG, Marsden CD. Depression in Parkinson's disease: a quantitative and qualitative analysis. J Neurol Neurosurg Psychiatry 1986;49:381–389.
22. Ehmann TS, Beninger RJ, Gawel MJ, Riopelle RJ. Depressive symptoms in Parkinson's disease: a comparison with disabled control subjects. J Geriatr Psychiatry Neurol 1990;2:3–9.
23. Menza M, Sage J, Marshall E, Cody R, Duvousin R. Mood changes and "on-off" phenomena in Parkinson's disease. Mov Disord 1990; 5:148–151.
24. Lees AJ. The on-off phenomenon. J Neurol Neurosurg Psychiatry 1989;51(Suppl):29–38.
25. Schiffer RB, Kurlan R, Rubin A, Boer S. Evidence for atypical depression in Parkinson's disease. Am J Psychiatry 1988;145:1020–1022.
26. Stein MB, Heuser IJ, Juncos JL, Uhde TE. Anxiety disorders in patients with Parkinson's disease. Am J Psychiatry 1990; 147:217–220.
27. Iruela LM, Ibanez-Rojo V, Palanca I, Caballero L. Anxiety disorders and Parkinson's disease [Letter]. Am J Psychiatry 1992;149: 719–720.
28. Celesia GG, Barr AN. Psychosis and other psychiatric manifestations of levodopa therapy. Arch Neurol 1970;23:193–200.
29. Jouvent R, Abensour P, Bonnet AM, et al. Antiparkinsonian and antidepressant effects of high doses of bromocriptine. Biol Psychiatry 1983;5:141–145.
30. Lang AE, Quinn N, Brincat S, et al. Pergolide in late-stage Parkinson's disease. Ann Neurol 1982;12:243–247.
31. Goodwin FK. Psychiatric side effects of levodopa in man. JAMA 1971;218:1915–1920.
32. Factor SA, Brown D. Clozapine prevents recurrence of psychosis in Parkinson's disease. Mov Disord 1992;7:125–131.
33. Wolk SI, Douglas CJ. Clozapine treatment of psychosis in Parkinson's disease: a report of five consecutive cases. J Clin Psychiatry 1992;53: 373–376.

34. Friedman JH, Lannon MC. Clozapine in the treatment of psychosis in Parkinson's disease. Neurology 1989;39:1219–1221.

35. Factor SA, Brown D, Molho ES, Podskalny GD. Clozapine: a 2-year open trial in Parkinson's disease patients with psychosis. Neurology 1994;44:544–546.

36. Friedman JH, Lannon MC. Clozapine-responsive Tremor in Parkinson's disease. Mov Disord 1990;5:225–229.

37. Bennett JP, Landow ER, Schuh LA. Suppression of dyskinesias in advanced Parkinson's disease. II. Increasing daily clozapine doses suppress dyskinesias and improve parkinsonism symptoms. Neurology 1993;43:1551–1555.

38. Strang RR. Imipramine in treatment of parkinsonism: a double blind placebo study. Br Med J 1965;2:33–34.

39. Andersen J, Aabro E, Gulmann N, Hjelmsted A, Pedersen HE. Antidepressant treatment in Parkinson's disease: a controlled trial of the effect of nortriptyline in patients with Parkinson's disease treated with L-dopa. Acta Neurol Scand 1980;62:210–219.

40. Laitinen L. Desipramine in treatment of Parkinson's disease. Acta Neurol Scand 1969;45:109–113.

41. Goetz CG, Tanner CM, Klawans HL. Bupropion in Parkinson's disease. Neurology 1984;34:1092–1094.

42. McCance-Katz EF, Marek KL, Price LH. Serotonergic dysfunction in depression associated with Parkinson's disease. Neurology 1992;42:1813–1814.

43. Steur EN. Increase of Parkinson disability after fluoxetine medication. Neurology 1993;43:211–213.

44. Jimenez-Jimenez, Tejeiro J, Martinez-Junquera G, Cabrera-Valdivia F, Alarcon J, Garcia-Albea E. Parkinsonism exacerbated by paroxetine. Neurology 1994;44:2406.

45. Caley CF, Friedman JH. Does fluoxetine exacerbate Parkinson's disease? J Clin Psychiatry 1992;53:278–282.

46. Waters CH. Fluoxetine and selegiline—lack of significant interaction. Can J Neurol Sci 1994;21:259–261.

47. Yudofsky SC. Parkinson's disease, depression, and electroconvulsive therapy: a clinical and neurobiologic synthesis. Compr Psychiatry 1979;20:579–581.

48. Young RC, Alexopoulos GS, Shamoian CA. Dissociation of motor response from mood and cognition in a parkinsonian patient treated with ECT. Biol Psychiatry 1985;20:566–569.

49. Burke WJ, Peterson J, Rubin EH: Electroconvulsive therapy in the treatment of combined depression and Parkinson's disease. Psychosomatics 1988;29:341–346.

50. Hurwitz TA, Calne DB, Waterman K. Treatment of dopaminomimetic psychosis in Parkinson's disease with electroconvulsive therapy. Can J Neurol Sci 1988;15:32–34.

51. Oh JJ, Rummans TA, O'Connor MK, Ahlskog JE. Cognitive impairment after ECT in patients with Parkinson's disease and psychiatric illness [Letter]. Am J Psychiatry 1992;149:271.

52. Figiel GS, Hassen MA, Zorumski C, et al. ECT-induced delirium in depressed patients with Parkinson's disease. Journal of Neuropsychiatry & Clinical Neurosciences 1991;3:405–11.

53. Cools AR, Van Den Berken JHL, Horstink MWI, Van Spaendonck KPM, Berger HJC. Cognitive and motor shifting aptitude disorder in Parkinson's disease. J Neurol Neurosurg Psychiatry 1984;47:443–453.

54. Flowers K. Lack of prediction in the motor behaviour of parkinsonism. Brain 1978;101:35–52.

55. Stern Y, Mayeux R, Rosen J. Contribution of perceptual motor dysfunction to construction and tracing disturbances in Parkinson's disease. J Neurol Neurosurg Psychiatry 1984;47:983–989.

56. Brown RG, Marsden CD. How common is dementia in Parkinson's disease? Lancet 1984;1:1262–1265.

57. Rajput AH, Offord KP, Beard CM, Kurland LT. A case-control study of smoking habits, dementia and other illnesses in idiopathic Parkinson's disease. Neurology 1987;37:226–232.

58. Lieberman AN, Dziatolowski M, Kupersmith M, et al. Dementia in Parkinson's Disease. Ann Neurol 1979;6:355–359.

59. DuBois B, Pillon B, Sternic N, et al. Age induced cognitive disturbances in Parkinson's disease. Neurology 1990;40:38–41.

60. Mindham RHS, Ahmed SWA, Clough CG. A controlled study of dementia in Parkinson's disease. J Neurol Neurosurg Psychiatry 1982; 45:969–974.

61. Marder K, Leung D, Tang M, et al. Are demented patients with Parkinson's disease accurately reflected in prevalence surveys? A survival analysis. Neurology 1991;41:1240–1243.

62. Mayeux R, Stern Y, Rosenstein R, et al. An estimate of the prevalence of dementia in idiopathic Parkinson's disease. Arch Neurol 1988;45:260–263.

63. Hietanen M, Teravainen H. The effect of age of disease onset on neuropsychological performance in Parkinson's disease. J Neurol Neurosurg Psychiatry 1988;51:244–249.

64. Richards M, Cote L, Stern Y. The relationship between visuomotor ability and perceptual motor function in Parkinson's disease. J Neurol Neurosurg Psychiatry 1993;56:400–406.

65. Richards M, Stern Y, Marder K, Cote L, Mayeux R. Relationships between extrapyramidal signs and cognitive function in a community-dwelling cohort of patients with Parkinson's disease and normal elderly individuals. Ann Neurol 1993;33:267–274.

66. Stern Y, Richards M, Sano M, Mayeux R. Comparison of cognitive changes in Alzheimer's and Parkinson's Disease patients. Arch Neurol 1993;50:1040–1045.

67. Mann DMA, Yates PO, Hawkes J. The pathology of the human locus coeruleus. Clin Neuropathol 1983;2:1–7.

68. Davis GC, Williams AC, Markey SP, et al. Chronic parkinsonism secondary to injection of meperidine analogues. Psychiatr Res 1979;1:249–254.

69. Ruttenber AT, Garbe PL, Kalter HD, et al. Meperidine analog exposure in California narcotics abusers: initial epidemiologic findings. In: Markey SP, Castagnoli N, Trevor AJ, Kopin IJ, eds. MPTP: a neurotoxin producing a parkinsonism syndrome. New York: Academic Press, 1986:339–353.

70. Taylor JR, Elsworth JD, Roth RH, Sladek JR Jr, Redmond DE Jr. Cognitive and motor deficits in the acquisition of an object retrieval/detour task in MPTP-treated monkey. Brain 1990;113 (Pt 3):617–637.

71. Taylor JR, Roth RH, Sladek JR Jr, Redmond DE Jr. Cognitive and motor deficits in the performance of an object retrieval task with a barrier-detour in monkeys (Ceropithecus aethiops sabaeus) treated with MPTP: long-term performance and effect of transparency of the barrier. Behav Neurosci 1990;104:564–576.

72. Schneider JS, Kovelowski CJ 2d. Chronic exposure to low doses of MPTP. I. Cognitive deficits in motor asymptomatic monkeys. Brain Res 1990;519:122–128.

73. Schneider JS, Roeltgen DP. Delayed matching-to-sample, object retrieval, and discrimination reversal deficits in chronic low dose MPTP-treated monkeys. Brain Res 1993;615:351–354.

74. Stern Y, Langston JW. Intellectual changes in patients with MPTP-induced Parkinsonism. Neurology 1985;35:1506–1507.

75. Stern Y, Tetrud JW, Martin WR, Kutner SJ, Langston JW. Cognitive change following MPTP exposure. Neurology 1990;40:261–264.

76. Folstein SE. Huntington's disease: a disorder of families. Baltimore: Johns Hopkins University Press, 1989.

77. Folstein ES, Leigh RJ, Parhad MI, Folstein FM. The diagnosis of Huntington's disease. Neurology 1986;36:1279–1283.

78. The Huntington's Disease Collaborative Research Group. A novel gene containing a trinucleotide repeat that is expanded and unstable on Huntington's disease chromosomes. Cell 1993;72:9971–9983.

79. Kremer B., Goldberg P, Andrew S, et al. A worldwide study of the Huntington's disease mutation; the sensitivity and specificity of measuring CAG repeats. N Engl J Med 1994;330:1401–1406.

80. Andrew S, Goldberg P, Kremer B, Telenius H, et al. The relationship between trinucleotide (CAG) repeat length and clinical features of Huntington's disease. Nature Genetics 1993;4:398–403.

81. Duyao M, Ambrose C, Myers R, Novelletto A, et al. Trinucleotide repeat length instability and age of onset in Huntington's disease. Nature Genetics 1993;4:387–392.

82. Folstein ES, Abbott HM, Chase AG, Jensen AB, Folstein FM. The

association of affective disorder with Huntington's Disease in a case series and in families. Psychol Med 1983;13:537–542.

83. Bolt JM. Huntington's chorea in the west of Scotland. Brit J Psychol 1970;116:259–270.

84. Dewhurst K, Olliver J, Trick KL, McKnight A. Neuro-psychiatric aspects of Huntington's disease. Confinia Neurologia 1969;31:258–268.

85. Mattson B. Huntington's chorea in Sweden II. Social and clinical data. Acta Psychiatr Scand 1974;255(Suppl):221–235.

86. Schoenfeld M, Myers R, Cupples A, Berkman B, Sax D, Clark E. Increased rate of suicide among patients with Huntington's disease. J Neurol Neurosurg Psychiatry 1984;47:1283–1287.

87. McHugh RP, Folstein FM. Psychiatric syndromes of Huntington's chorea: a clinical and phenomenologic study. In: Benson DF, Blumer D, eds. Psychiatric aspects of neurologic disease. New York: Grune & Stratton, 1975.

88. Caine DE, Shoulson I. Psychiatric syndrome in Huntington's disease. Am J Psychiatry 1983;140:6.

89. Burns A, Folstein ES, Brandt J, Folstein FM. Clinical assessment of irritability, aggression, and apathy in Huntington and Alzheimer disease. J Nerv Ment Dis 1990;178:20–26.

90. Ranen N, Peyser C, Folstein S. A physicians guide to the management of Huntington's disease. Baltimore: Huntington's Disease Society of America, 1993.

91. Mayeux R, Stern Y, Herman A, Greenbaum L, Fahn S. Correlates of early disability in Huntington's disease. Ann Neurol 1986;20:727–731.

92. Butters N, Sax D, Montgomery K, Tarlow S. Comparison of the neuropsychological deficits associated with early and advanced Huntington's disease. Arch Neurol 1978;35:585–589.

93. Brandt J, Folstein ES, Folstein FM. Differential cognitive impairment in Alzheimer's disease and Huntington's disease. Ann Neurol 1988;23:555–561.

94. Salmon PD, Kwo-on-Yuen FP, Heindal CW, Butters N, Thal JL. Differentiation of Alzheimer's disease and Huntington's disease with the Dementia Rating Scale. Arch Neurol 1989;46:1204–1208.

95. Bamford KA, Caine ED, Kido DK, Plassche WM, Shoulson I. Clinical-pathologic correlation in Huntington's disease: a neuropsychological and computed tomography study. Neurology 1989;39:796–801.

96. Girotti F, Marano R, Soliveri P, Geminiani G, Scigliano G. Relationship between motor and cognitive disorders in Huntington's disease. J Neurol 1988;235:454–457.

97. Steele J, Richardson J, Olszewski J. Progressive supranuclear palsy. Arch Neurol 1964;10:333–359.

98. Jellinger K, Riederer P, Tomonaga M. Progressive supranuclear palsy: clinico-pathological and biochemical studies. J Neural Transm 1980;16(Suppl):111–128.

99. Golbe L, Davis P, Schoenberg B, Duvoisin R. Prevalence and natural history of progressive supranuclear palsy. Neurology 1988;38:1031–1034.

100. Maher E, Lees A. The clinical features and natural history of the Steele-Richardson-Olszewski syndrone. Neurology 1986;36:1005–1008.

101. Davis P, Bergeron C, McLachlan D. Atypical presentation of progressive supranuclear palsy. Ann Neurol 1985;17:37–43.

102. Kleinschmidt-DeMasters BK. Early progressive supranuclear palsy: pathology and clinical presentation. Clin Neuropathol 1989;8:79–84.

103. Albert M, Feldman R, Willis A. The "subcortical dementia" of progressive supranuclear palsy. J Neurol Neurosurg Psychiatry 1974;37:121–130.

104. Kimura D, Barnett H, Burkhart G. The psychological test pattern in progressive supranuclear palsy. Neuropsychologia 1981;19:301–306.

105. Fisk J, Goodale M, Burkhart G, Barnett H. Progressive supranuclear palsy: the relationship between ocularmotor dysfunction and psychological test performance. Neurology 1982;32:698–705.

106. Maher E, Smith E, Lees A. Cognition deficit in the Steele-Richardson-Olszewski syndrome. J Neurol Neurosurg Psychiatry 1985;48:1234–1239.

107. Pillon B, Dubois B, Plosha A, Agid Y. Severity and specificity of cognitive impairment in Alzheimer's disease, Huntington's disease and progressive supranuclear palsy. Neurology 1991;41:634–643.

108. Litvan I, Grafman J, Gomez C, Chase T. Memory impairment in patients with progressive supranuclear palsy. Arch Neurol 1989;46:765–767.

109. Dubois B, Pillon B, Legault F, Agid Y, Lhermitte F. Slowing of cognitive processing in progressive supranuclear palsy. Arch Neurol 1988;45:1194–1199.

110. Pillon B, Dubois B, Agid Y. Severity and specificity of cognitive impairment in Alzheimer's, Huntington's, and Parkinson's diseases and progressive supranuclear palsy. Ann N Y Acad Sci 1991;640:224–227.

111. Tripathi RC, Tripathi BJ, Bauserman SC, Park JK. Clinicopathologic correlation and pathogenesis of ocular and central nervous system manifestations in Hallervorden-Spatz syndrome. Acta Neuropathol (Berl) 1992;83:113–119.

112. Swaiman KF. Hallervorden-Spatz syndrome and brain iron metabolism. Arch Neurol 1991;48:1285–1293.

113. Dooling E, Schoene W, Richardson E. Hallervorden-Spatz syndrome. Arch Neurol 1974;30:70–83.

114. Sethi K, Adams R, Loring D, ElGammal T. Hallervorden-Spatz syndrome: clinical and magnetic resource imaging correlations. Ann Neurol 1988;24:692–694.

115. Alberca R, Rafel E, Chinchon I, Vadillo J, Navarro A. Late onset parkinsonian syndrome in Hallervorden-Spatz disease. J Neurol Neurosurg Psychiatry 1987;50:1665–1668.

116. Angelini L, Nardocci N, Rumi V, Zorzi C, Strada L, Savoiardo M. Hallervorden-Spatz disease: clinical and MRI study of 11 cases diagnosed in life. J Neurol 1992;239:417–425.

117. Scheinberg I, Sternlieb I. Wilson's disease. Philadelphia: WB Saunders 1984:86–91.

118. Frydman M, Bonne-Tamir B, Farrar L, et al. Assignment of the gene for Wilson's disease to chromosome 13. Proc Natl Acad Sci 1984;82:1819–1821.

119. Wilson S. Progressive lenticular degeneration: a familial nervous disease associated with cirrhosis of the liver. Brain 1912;34:295–309.

120. Starosta-Rubinstein S, Young AB, Kluin K, et al. Clinical assessment of 31 patients with Wilson's disease. Correlations with structural changes on magnetic resonance imaging. Arch Neurol 1987;44:365–370.

121. Dening TR, Berrios GE. Wilson's disease. Psychiatric symptoms in 195 cases. Arch Gen Psychiatry 1989;46:1126–1134.

122. Dening T, Berrios G. Wilson's disease: a longitudinal study of psychiatric symptoms. Biol Psychiatry 1990;28:255–265.

123. Lang C, Muller D, Claus D, Druschky KF. Neuropsychological findings in treated Wilson's disease. Acta Neurol Scand 1990;81:75–81.

124. Medalia A, Isaacs-Glagerman K, Scheinberg IH. Neuropsychological impairment in Wilson's disease. Arch Neurol 1988;45:502–504.

125. Lang C. Is Wilson's disease a dementing condition?. J Clin Exp Neuropsychol 1989;11:569–570.

126. Benecke R, Rothwell J, Day B, Marsden C. Disturbance of sequential movements in patients with Parkinson's disease. Brain 1987;110:361–379.

127. Hefter H, Arendt G, Stremmel W, Freund HJ. Motor impairment in Wilson's disease, I: slowness of voluntary limb movement. Acta Neurol Scand 1993;87:133–147.

128. Scheinberg I, Jaffe M, Sternlieb I. The use of trientine in preventing the effects of interrupting penicillamine therapy in Wilson's disease. N Engl J Med 1987;317:209–213.

129. Sternlieb I. Wilson's disease: indications for liver transplants. Hepatology 1984;4 (Suppl):15s–17s.

130. Akil M, Schwartz JA, Dutchak D, Yuzbasiyan-Gurkan V, Brewer GJ. The psychiatric presentations of Wilson's disease. J Neuropsychiatry Clin Neurosci 1991;3:377–382.

131. Kosaka K, Tsuchiya K, Yoshimur M. Lewy body disease with and

without dementia: a clinicopathological study of 35 cases. Clin Neuropathol 1988;7:299–305.

132. Gibb WRG, Mountjoy CQ, Mann DMA, Lees AJ. A pathological study of the association between Lewy body disease and Alzheimer's disease. J Neurol Neurosurg Psychiatry 1989;52:701–708.

133. Dickson DW, Davies P, Mayeux R, et al. Diffuse Lewy body disease: neuropathological and biochemical studies of six patients. Acta Neuropathol (Berl) 1987;75:8–15.

134. Hansen AL, Masliah E, Galasko D, Terry DR. Plaque-only Alzheimer's disease is usually the Lewy body variant, and vice versa. J Neuropathol Exp Neurol 1993;52:648–654.

135. Galasko D, Saitoh T, Xia y, Thal L, Katzman R, Hill LR, Hansen L. Apolipoprotein E allele e4 is overrepresented in Lewy body variant of Alzheimer's disease. Neurology 1994;44:1950–1951.

136. Hansen LA, Galasko D. Lewy body disease. Current Opinion in Neurology and Neurosurgery 1992;5:889–894.

137. Byrne EJ, Lennox G, Lowe J, Godwin-Austen BR. Diffuse Lewy body disease: clinical features in 15 cases. J Neurol Neurosurg Psychiatry 1989;52:709–717.

138. Crystal HA, Dickson DW, Lizardi JE, Davies P, Wolfson LI. Antemortem diagnosis of diffuse Lewy body disease. Neurology 1990;40:1523–1528.

139. McKeith IG, Perry RH, Fairbairn SJ, Perry EK. Operational criteria for senile dementia of Lewy body type (SDLT). Psychol Med 1992;22:911–922.

140. Forstl H, Burns A, Luthert P, Cairns N, Levy R. The Lewy-body variant of Alzheimer's disease: clinical and pathological findings. Br J Psychiatry 1993;162:385–392.

141. Hansen L, Salmon D, Galasko D, et al. The Lewy body variant of Alzheimer's disease: a clinical pathologic entity. Neurology 1990;40:1–8.

142. Sahgal A, Galloway HP, McKeith GI, et al. Matching to sample deficits in patients with senile dementias of the Alzheimer and Lewy body types. Arch Neurol 1992;49:1043–1046.

143. Lippa CF, Smith W, Swearer JM. Alzheimer's disease and Lewy body disease: a comparative clinicopathological study. Ann Neurol 1994;35:81–88.

144. Perry EK, McKeith I, Thompson E, et al. Topography, extent and clinical relevance of neurochemical deficits in dementia of Lewy body type, Parkinson's disease and Alzheimer's disease. Ann N Y Acad Sci 1986;640:197–202.

145. Ikeda K, Ikeda S, Yoshimura T, et al. Idiopathic parkinsonism with Lewy type inclusions in the cerebral cortex: a case report. Acta Neuropathol 1978;41:165–168.

146. Sima AAF, Clark AW, Sternberger NA, Sternberger LA. Lewy body dementia without Alzheimer changes. Can J Neurol Sci 1986;13:490–497.

147. Mitsuyama Y, Fukanaga H, Yamashita M. Alzheimer's disease with widespread presence of Lewy bodies. Folia Psychiatr Neurol Jpn 1984;38:81–88.

148. Mark MH, Sage JI, Dickson DW, Schwarz KO, Duvoisin RC. Levodopa-responsive Lewy body parkinsonism: clinicopathologic study of 2 cases. Neurology 1992;42:1323–1327.

149. Yoshimura M. Cortical changes in parkinsonian brain: a contribution to the delineation of "diffuse Lewy body disease." J Neurol 1993;229:17–32.

150. Kurlan R. Tourette's syndrome: current concepts. Neurology 1989;39:1625–1630.

151. Pauls DL, Leckman JF. The inheritance of Gilles de la Tourette's syndrome and associated behaviors: evidence for autosomal dominant transmission. N Engl J Med 1986;315:993–997.

152. Comings DE. A controlled study of Tourette's syndrome. VII. Summary: a common genetic disorder causing disinhibition of the limbic system. Am J Hum Genet 1987;41:839–866.

153. Singer HS, Reiss AL, Brown JE, Aylward EH, Shih B. Volumetric MRI changes in basal ganglia of children with Tourette's syndrome. Neurology 1993;43:950–956.

154. Peterson B, Riddle MA, Cohen DJ, Katz LD, Smith JC. Reduced basal ganglia volumes in Tourette's syndrome using three-dimensional reconstruction techniques from magnetic resonance images. Neurology 1993;43:941–949.

155. Haber SN, Kowall NW, Vonsattel JP, Bird ED, Richardson EP. Gilles de la Tourette's syndrome: a postmortem neuropathological and immunohistochemical study. J Neurol Sci 1986;75:225–241.

156. Richardson EP. Neuropathological studies of Tourette's syndrome. In: Friedhoff AJ, Chase TN, eds. Gilla de la Tourette's syndrome. New York: Raven Press, 1982:83–87.

157. Balthazar K. Uber das anatomishe substrat der generalisierten tic-krankeit (maladie des tics, Gilles de la Tourette): Entwicklung-shemmung des corpus striatum. Arch Psychiatr Nervenkr 1956;195:531–549.

158. Dowling BR, Budman LC. The natural history of Gilles de la Tourette syndrome. In: Kurlan R, ed. Handbook of Tourette's syndrome and related tic and behavioral disorders. New York: Marcel Dekker, 1993:27–39.

159. Erenberg G, Cruse RP, Rothner AD. The natural history of Tourette syndrome: a follow-up study. Ann Neurol 1987;22:383–385.

160. Nee LE, Polinsky RJ, Ebert MH. Tourette syndrome: Clinical and family studies. In: Friedhoff AJ, Chase TN, eds. Gilles de la Tourette syndrome. New York: Raven Press, 1982:291–295.

161. Shapiro ES, Shapiro AK. Gilles de la Tourette Syndrome and tic disorders. Harvard Medical School Mental Health Letter 1989;5(11).

162. Burd L, Kerbeshian J, Wilkenheiser M, Fisher W. Prevalence of Gilles de la Tourette syndrome in North Dakota adults. Am J Psychiatry 1986;143:787–788.

163. Goetz, CG, Tanner CM, Stebbins GT, Leipzig G, Carr WC. Adult tics in Gilles de la Tourette's syndrome. Neurology 1992;42:784–788.

164. Comings DE, Coming BG. Tourette syndrome: clinical and psychological aspects of 250 cases. Am J Hum Genet 1985;37:435–450.

165. Bruun RD, Budman CL. The natural history of Gilles de la Tourette syndrome. In: Kurlan R, ed. Handbook of Tourette's syndrome and related tic and behavioral disorders. New York: Marcel Dekker, 1993:27–42.

166. Musisi S, Sandor P, Lang A, Moldofsky H. Gilles de la Tourette's syndrome: a follow-up study. J Clin Psychopharmacol 1990;3:197–199.

167. Como GP. Neurological testing. In: Kurlan R, ed. Handbook of Tourette's syndrome and related tic and behavioral disorders. New York: Marcel Dekker, 1993:221–242.

168. Bornstein RA. Neuropsychological performance in children with Tourette's syndrome. Psychiatry Res 1990;33:73–81.

169. Bornstein RA. Neuropsychological correlates of obsessive characteristics in Tourette syndrome. J Neuropsychiatr Clin Neurosci 1991;3:157–162.

170. Denckla MB, Reader MJ. Education and psychosocial interventions: executive dysfunction and its consequences. In: Kurlan R, ed. Handbook of Tourette's syndrome and related tic and behavioral disorders. New York: Marcel Dekker, 1993:431–451.

171. Bruun RD, Subtle and underrecognized side effects of neuroleptic treatment in children with Tourette's disorder. Am J Psychiatry 1988;145:621–624.

172. Singer HS, Walkup JT. Tourette syndrome and other tic disorders. Diagnosis, pathophysiology and treatment. Medicine 1991;70:15–32.

173. Sandor P, Musisi S, Moldofsky H, Lang A. Tourette syndrome: a follow-up study. J Clin Psychopharmacology 1990;10:197–199.

174. Jankovic J. Botulinum toxin in the treatment of dystonic tics. Move Disord 1994;9:347–349.

175. Goetz, CG, Tanner CM, Wilson RS, Carroll VS, Como PG, Shannon KN. Clonidine and Gilles de la Tourette syndrome: double blind study using objective rating methods. Ann Neurol 1987;21:307–310.

176. Riddle MA, Hardin MT, Cho SC, Woolston JL, Leckman JF. Desipramine treatment of boys with attention deficit disorder and tics: preliminary clinical experience. J Am Acad Child Adolesc Psychiatry 1988;27:811–814.

177. Spencer T, Biederman J, Kerman K, Steingard R, Wilens T. Desipramine treatment of children with attention-deficit hyperactivity disorder and tic disorder or Tourette's syndrome. J Am Acad Child Adolesc Psychiatry 1993;32:354–360.
178. Spencer T, Biederman J, Wilens T, Steingard R, Geist D. Nortriptyline treatment of children with attention-deficit hyperactivity disorder and tic disorder or Tourette's syndrome. J Am Acad Child Adolesc Psychiatry 1993;32:205–210.
179. Jancovic J. Deprenyl in attention deficit associated with Tourette's syndrome. Arch Neurol 1993;50:286–288.
180. Kurlan R, Como PG, Deeley C, McDermott M, McDermott MP. A pilot controlled study of fluoxetine for obsessive-compulsive symptoms in children with Tourette's syndrome. Clin Neuropharmacol 1993;16:167–172.
181. Riddle MA, Hardin MT, King R, Scahill L, Woolston JL. Fluoxetine treatment of children and adolescents with Tourette's and obsessive compulsive disorders: preliminary clinical experience. J Am Acad Child Adolesc Psychiatry 1990;29:45–48.
182. McDougle CJ, Goodman WK, Leckman JF, Price LH. The psychopharmacology of obsessive compulsive disorder. Implications for treatment and pathogenesis. Psychiatr Clin North Am 1993;16:749–766.
183. Peterson AL, Azrin NH. An evaluation of behavioral treatments for Tourette syndrome. Behav Res Ther 1992;30:167–174.
184. Burd L, Kerbeshian J. Treatment-generated problems associated with behavior modification in Tourette disorder. Dev Med Child Neurol 1987;29:831–833.

35

GILLES DE LA TOURETTE SYNDROME AND OBSESSIVE-COMPULSIVE DISORDER

Mary M. Robertson and Jessica Yakeley

Undeniably, there is a connection between Gilles de la Tourette syndrome (GTS) and obsessive-compulsive disorder (OCD). Their relationship is, however, complex and can be debated from several perspectives. To explore this relationship thoroughly, we first describe GTS and OCD separately, followed by a discussion about how they overlap.

GILLES DE LA TOURETTE SYNDROME

Definition and Diagnostic Criteria

The generally accepted diagnostic criteria for GTS are those included in *Diagnostic and Statistical Manual of Mental Disorders,* 4th edition (DSM-IV) of the American Psychiatric Association (APA) (1) and the 10th Edition of The International Statistical Classification of Diseases and Related Health Problems (World Health Organization [WHO]). These include both multiple motor and one or more vocal tics, which do not necessarily present concurrently, occur many times a day (usually in bouts), and last more than 1 year; the anatomical location, number and frequency, complexity and severity of the tics classically change over time (1, 2).

Although the current diagnostic criteria in DSM-IV (1) include age at onset before 18 years, DSM-III (3) originally required that symptoms began before the age of 15 years and the International Classification of Diseases (ICD 10) (2) has no such age restrictions. In this context, at least two reports in the literature have appeared in which GTS symptoms commenced at the ages of 35 (4) and 45 (5) in otherwise apparently normal persons. In addition, we have seen several such cases in clinical practice (Eapen et al.—in preparation), although one had OC symptoms beginning at the age of 10. The age stipulation may, therefore, be somewhat arbitrary.

Robertson (6) reviewed the literature on GTS thoroughly in 1989 and, when appropriate in this text, that work is cited. However, both controversial areas and more recent investigations are discussed in detail.

History

The first clear medical description of GTS was made in 1825, when Itard (7) reported the case of a French noblewoman, the Marquise de Dampierre, who developed the first symptoms of GTS at the age of 7. Sometime later the prominent French neuropsychiatrist and pupil of Charcot, Georges Gilles de la Tourette (8), described nine cases of GTS, which earned him eponymous fame, emphasizing the triad of multiple tics, coprolalia, and echolalia. The first reported case of GTS in the United Kingdom (U.K.) may possibly have been Mary Hall of Gadsden, who was reported in 1663 by William Drage (9). Also, Dr. Samuel Johnson, the prominent 18th-century literary figure and genius, was most likely also afflicted with GTS (10, 11), while others have suggested that Mozart likewise had GTS (12–14), although this has been disputed (15, 16).

Prevalence

The exact prevalence of GTS is unknown, but a currently accepted figure is 0.5/1000 (17); this will probably, however, prove to be an underestimate. This disorder was once considered a rarity, but is now being more widely recognized and diagnosed. In an international registry published in 1973 (18), as few as 174 patients were identified in the United States (U.S.), and 53 in the U.K.

The prevalence of GTS depends, at least in part, on the definition of GTS, the type of ascertainment method, and the type of epidemiological investigation undertaken (6, 19). Eight epidemiological studies in GTS have been conducted, with the majority being in the U.S. (*n* = 4), others being in France (*n* = 2), England (*n* = 1), and Israel (*n* = 1) (19). The generally accepted figure of 0.5/1,000 (5/10,000) means approximately 110,000 patients in the U.S. and 25,000 in the U.K., but rates range from 0.77/10,000 for males and 0.22/10,000 for females (20), to 2.87/10,000 (21), and finally, 105.05/10,000 for boys and 13.18/10,000 for girls (22). A recent population-based study in Israel reported a prevalence estimate of 4.28/10,000 (sex-specific prevalences were 4.90/10,000 for boys and 3.10/10,000 for girls) (23).

Apart from definition and ascertainment method, there are other reasons for the exact numbers of people with GTS being unknown, including misdiagnosis and the reluctance of relatives to divulge family histories, as suggested by the case reports of Hajal and Leach (24). The apparent increase in the number of patients in recent years may also be partly explained by the fact that many cases now being diagnosed tend to be those with milder symptoms. Most of the figures given are thought to be underestimates because, in family studies, many mild GTS cases who have never consulted a doctor for their symptomatology have been identified (25–28). Some suggest that in special school populations GTS is very common (29), being as prevalent as 1,200/10,000 (22). In conclusion, the exact prevalence of GTS is unknown, and currently accepted figures are almost definitely underestimates. However, undoubtedly, more cases are coming to medical attention either through clinical or research sources, and with more epidemiological studies, the true prevalence rates will become clearer.

Epidemiology

GTS is found in all cultures and racial groups, but is rare among the American black population, which has been represented in varying but small proportions in a number of studies, ranging from 0.5–8.7% (30, 31). Most large reports have come from the U.S. (30–37), but significant numbers of patients have also been reported from Europe including the U.K. (9, 38–40), Germany (18, 41), the Netherlands (42), Denmark (43), and France (44), as well as New Zealand (45), Canada (46), the former Soviet Union (47–49), Japan (50, 51), Korea (52), Hong Kong (53), China (54, 55), and India (56, 57). These studies, plus case reports from Ceylon, Puerto Rico, Australia, (for details, see reference 6), India (58), Finland (59), South America (60), Malta (61) and the Middle East (62, 63), highlight the worldwide distribution of the disorder.

Some early studies found an unexpectedly large proportion of their GTS subjects to have an Eastern European/Ashkenazic-Jewish background (30, 64, 65), although this finding has not been reported by other investigators (9, 33, 37, 38, 66-70). It should be noted that two of the three studies reporting such a preponderance were from metropolitan New York (30, 64), which has a large Jewish population.

Demography

The majority of studies indicate that GTS occurs three to four times more commonly in males than in females (30, 31, 35, 38, 42, 43, 45, 66, 71-74). The syndrome is found in all social classes (8, 30, 33, 66), although two studies (30, 33) found a clustering in social class three. Asam (41) and Robertson et al. (38) reported respectively that 63% of 16

GTS patients and 61% of 59 (classified according to the Registrar General's classification) failed to attain their parental social class; this suggests that patients with GTS may well underachieve socially.

Clinical Characteristics

The clinical characteristics of patients with GTS seem independent of culture, as they occur with some degree of uniformity irrespective of the country of origin. The age at onset of symptoms ranges from 2–15 years, with a mean of 7 years being most common, and the most frequent initial symptoms involving the eyes (e.g., eye-blinking, eye-rolling). Although often referred to as a tic disorder, patients with GTS usually demonstrate a variety of complicated movements, including licking, hitting, jumping, smelling, squatting, abnormalities of gait, and forced touching (6). Licking as a motor tic is exhibited by some 20% of patients (43), while spitting is found in 9% (38).

The onset of vocalizations is usually later than that of the motor tics, with a mean age of onset at 11 years, with throat-clearing, sniffing, grunting, coughing, barking, snorting, humming, clicking, colloquial emotional exclamations, low- and high-pitched noises, and inarticulate sounds being the usual utterances (6). Vocalizations have been reported as initial symptoms in some 12–37% of subjects, of which the most frequent was repeated throat-clearing (43, 70). Many GTS individuals also describe premonitory "sensory" experiences that are distinct from the actual motor or vocal tic (75).

Coprolalia (the inappropriate and involuntary uttering of obscenities) occurs in less than one-third of clinic patient populations (76), but in very few children (37) or mildly affected cases, such as affected relatives of a proband, where it is encountered in only 2–4% (27, 77). Coprolalia, reported in 22% of GTS individuals in an epidemiological study (21), usually has a mean age of onset of 13–14 years, disappearing later in up to a third of cases (6). There is some suggestion that it may be culturally determined because only 4% have true coprolalia in Japan (78) but 26% do in Denmark (43). Some have noted that coprophenomena are infrequent in certain GTS patients from middle-class and strict religious backgrounds (79), while coprolalia has been shown to be more frequent in those with moderate or severe GTS symptoms (37). Copropraxia (involuntary and inappropriate obscene gestures) is reported in 1–21% of clinic samples (6).

Echolalia (the imitation of sounds or words of others) and echopraxia (the imitation of movements or actions of others) occur in 11–44% of patients. Palilalia (the repetition of the last word or phrase in a sentence or the last syllable of a word uttered by the patient) occurs in 6–15% of patients (6). It has been pointed out that these symptoms are common as GTS develops into its fullest form, while other subjective symptoms, such as sensory tics, mental coprolalia, coprographia, and mental palilalia are only discovered when inquired about directly (76). While these clinical features are not essential to make the diagnosis of GTS, the presence of any of these behaviors would increase the clinician's diagnostic confidence.

Tics and vocalizations are invariably aggravated by anxiety, stress, boredom, fatigue, and excitement, while sleep, alcohol, orgasm, fever, relaxation, or concentrating on an enjoyable task usually lead to temporary disappearance of symptoms (6). Premenstrual stress and exogenous stimulants, such as caffeine, methylphenidate, and amphetamines, have been implicated in tic exacerbation (76, 80). Characteristically, the course of GTS over the person's lifetime is punctuated by the appearance of new tics and the disappearance of older ones (6). During adolescence the symptoms tend to be more unpredictable from day to day, and it is estimated that in a third of patients the tic symptoms will remit completely by late adolescence. An additional third will show significant improvement in symptoms, while the remaining third will continue to be symptomatic during adulthood (76). Spontaneous remissions have been reported in 3–5% (18, 30) of patients followed up for about 6 months to 3 years.

Abuzzahab and Anderson (18) reported some significant cross-cultural symptom differences between France, Italy, the U.K., and the U.S., such as fewer eye and neck tics and more echokinesis in France; more eye tics in Italy; less echophenomena in the U.K., and more neck tics, coprolalia, and a younger age of onset in the U.S. A German sample, on the other hand, did not differ significantly from any others. Many reported differences, however, have not been replicated in later studies (9, 30).

It was once thought that movements disappeared during sleep, but this has now been shown not to be the case (81, 82). Apparently, tics of the eyes, face, and head are often quite persistent and remain the most refractory of pharmacological interventions (83).

A problematic area for parents, teachers, and some physicians is the idea that GTS is a so-called "involuntary" disorder of movement, and yet the patients are able to suppress symptoms during an interview or while involved in certain tasks, for example, while at school or while playing a sport (79).

Psychopathology, Associated Features, and Behaviors

There has recently been much interest in the types of psychopathology and associated behaviors encountered in GTS, but there is some disagreement as to the frequency and exact relationship between these and GTS (6, 76). The issues that have attracted most interest and agreement have been in the area of psychopathology, with some consensus on obsessive-compulsive behaviors (OCB), OCD, depression and anxiety disorders, attention deficit and hyperactivity disorder (ADHD), and self-injurious behaviors (SIB). Some types of behavior, such as OCB, are intimately linked to GTS both from a phenomenological and genetic standpoint and thus represent an integral part of the syndrome. Others, such as ADHD, are associated with GTS, although the precise

nature of the relationship is unclear. A variety of other disturbances, on the other hand, occur in a substantial proportion of clinic patients. Often, however, these symptoms—for which the patient is referred to a physician—represent referral bias.

Thus, antisocial behavior (33, 84), inappropriate sexual activity (33, 38, 66), and exhibitionism (70) occur in clinic GTS populations but to varying degrees (e.g., 6–16%; (70). Aggressive behavior has been reported in patients with GTS (66, 73, 84, 85), in proportions as high as 21% of one sample (42), and 31% of another (38). Comings and Comings (70) noted that discipline problems occur in 41% of females and 45% of males, being one of the main recurrent themes elicited when interviewing GTS families. These authors also found anger and violence common in GTS (42%), with similar frequency in males and females. In 22% of the sample, the violence did not result in destruction of property or physical attacks on other persons, but in 19% there was destruction of property, injury of people, or killing of animals, and in 1% the violence resulted in legal problems. Those patients who were hyperactive demonstrated more violence (70).

In a seven-part study, Comings and Comings (86) presented their data on the associated features of GTS, including ADHD, learning disorders, school problems, conduct disorder, schizoid behaviors, sleep problems, and affective disorder. They compared 246 patients with GTS, 47 random normal controls, 17 patients with Attention deficit disorder (ADD), and 15 with "ADD secondary to a GTS gene" using a locally devised 425-item questionnaire based on the Diagnostic Interview Schedule and the DSM-III. All patients and/or their parents were seen. In brief, it was found that GTS patients were significantly different from controls for symptoms of inattention, impulsivity, hyperactivity, a variety of conduct problems (lying, stealing, starting fires, vandalism, fighting, aggression, short temper, problems with drugs and alcohol), and "schizoid" symptoms (thinking that people were looking at them or plotting against them, and having hallucinations) (86).

Despite these findings, is the extreme antisocial behavior just described truly increased in GTS? From the authors' experience in both clinical (38, 40) and pedigree (27, 28) settings, and from data of epidemiological surveys (21), apparently very few GTS subjects in the community exhibit antisocial behavior. Thus, documentation of such behavior may reflect an artifact of referral, as GTS patients with more severe problems are more likely to be referred to specialists. In this context it should be noted that in one study, 12 out of 50 (24%) children with GTS were referred to their clinic for reasons other than simple motor or vocal tics, examples for the reasons being conduct and/or learning disorders, sleep disturbances, stuttering, hyperactivity, and/or difficulty with interpersonal relationships (87). Most significantly, the behavioral symptoms of GTS are subject to the same waxing and waning as the motor and vocal symptoms, and can even persist after the characteristic tics and sounds have largely disappeared (83).

Sleep disturbances in GTS subjects are common, and the account that follows is based on several studies (21, 33, 66, 84, 86, 88). The abnormalities of sleep frequently reported include insomnia (initial, middle, and delayed), sleep-talking, nightmares, night terrors, somnambulism, enuresis, bruxism, general restlessness, and inability to take afternoon naps. There has, however, been some debate as to whether or not the sleep disturbances are indicative of a disorder of arousal. Thus, Mendelson et al. (89) noted that intermittent waking time was substantially longer and non-REM sleep time was significantly shorter in GTS patients when compared with controls. When the patients were given haloperidol, there was a marked increase in δ sleep time and percentage, with values similar to those for volunteers (89). Barabas et al. (90, 91) reported somnambulism and night terrors in 19 (33%) of their 57 patients, which was a significantly higher rate than that found in children with seizure disorders (3%) or learning disabilities (8%). This finding also suggests that GTS is, therefore, a disorder of arousal. Erenberg (92) reported nightmares and insomnia in 22% of GTS subjects, but as there was neither somnambulism nor enuresis in their cohort, they concluded that it was not a disorder of arousal. Barabas et al. (92a), pointed out that the average age of the latter group was much higher than that of their group and that this might partly explain the discrepancy in findings. They also noted that disorders of arousal tended to occur in younger children and disappear with age. Others (93) have also argued against GTS being a disorder of arousal, based on results of physiological and neurophysiological testing on GTS patients and controls.

Barabas et al. (94) reported migraine in 26.6% of a cohort of 60 patients with GTS (ages 6–21 years), which was significantly higher than the figures for 72 children with seizure disorders (11.3%) and learning disabilities (8.0%), and the figure which was quoted for the general population (4.0–7.4%). These authors suggested that in a group of children with GTS, migraine and GTS may coexist, reflecting a similar abnormality of serotonin metabolism underlying both disorders. Van de Wetering et al. (42) found a similar percentage of migraine sufferers (20%) in a sample of 66 GTS patients. A generally accepted figure for the prevalence of migraine in the general population is taken from large community studies in Wales by Waters and colleagues, and in the U.S. by Markush and colleagues, and is given as 23.2% for women of 21 and over, and 14.9% for men (95). Considering the data from these studies, the prevalence of migraine in GTS does not appear to be increased.

PSYCHOPATHOLOGY

It is perhaps no coincidence that some of the first comments on the psychopathology of GTS patients were made by Georges Gilles de la Tourette himself in 1899 (96), when he commented on the anxieties and phobias of his patients. In that paper he noted the ideas of Guinon (97), who suggested that "tiqueurs" nearly always had associated psychiatric disorders characterized by multiple phobias,

arithmomania, and agoraphobia. Robertson and Reinstein (98) have translated and documented the original accounts of psychopathology associated with GTS by the early French physicians Georges Gilles de la Tourette, Grasset, and Guinon. Meige and Feindel (99), in "the confessions of a victim to tic," described the psychopathology of their tic patient, who almost certainly had GTS, drawing attention to "the fundamental importance of the psychical element that precedes the motor reaction."

From 1900–1965 the GTS literature was predominantly psychoanalytical, with many classic descriptions by early writers (100–106). Although some investigators, such as Shapiro and colleagues (30, 106, 107), claimed that no specific psychopathology is found in association with GTS, they (30) did , however, report that only one patient of their cohort of 34 was free from psychiatric illness, the majority being diagnosed as having various types of "personality disorders." They pointed out that there may be a subgroup of GTS patients who have a great deal of difficulty with compulsive ritualistic behaviors.

Others, such as the Comings' (108–111), suggest that GTS is associated with a wide variety of psychopathology, including learning disorders, dyslexia, conduct disorder, phobias, panic attacks, mania and manic depressive disorder, schizoid behaviors, alcoholism, drug abuse, and pathological gambling. Most investigators report and agree that the psychopathology is more specific, however, and it is generally accepted that OCB, anxiety, depression, ADHD, and SIB are found in a large number of GTS patients.

Several studies have found GTS patients to be more depressed than control groups (40, 42, 109), while others suggest that the depression is related to the duration of the GTS (38). This might be attributable to the stress of having a chronic, socially disabling and stigmatizing disease (6). GTS patients have demonstrated more anxiety than controls (40), although Coffey et al. (112) suggest that there may be a subgroup of GTS patients with non-OCD pure anxiety disorders. Depression and anxiety are certainly associated with GTS, but we maintain that they are likely to be secondary phenomena.

The relationship between GTS and ADHD has been studied extensively by the Comings (109, 110) and reviewed recently by Robertson and Eapen (80) and Towbin and Riddle (113). Evidently, ADHD occurs in a substantial proportion of GTS patients, ranging from 21–90% of GTS clinic populations, but the precise relationship between the two disorders is complex and remains unclear (80, 113). There have been suggestions that GTS and ADHD are genetically related (109, 111, 114–116), followed by refutations (117) and debate (118). A recent study by Pauls et al. (119) found that the rates of ADD were not significantly increased among relatives of GTS when compared to controls. However, results also suggest that there may be two types of individuals with GTS and ADD: one in whom the ADD is independent of GTS and the second in whom the ADD is secondary to the GTS. Thus, the relationship between the disorders is complex and merits further study.

An association between some types of SIB and GTS has been suggested (39), although the exact nature of this is unclear (for reviews, see 120, 121). Remarkably, however, even individuals with mild GTS, encountered in epidemiological (21) and pedigree (27) studies, have exhibited SIB, suggesting that it may be integral in some individuals with GTS, and not necessarily associated with severity of GTS or referral bias. SIB does, however, seem to be related to psychopathology, especially hostility and obsessionality (39).

There is no association between psychosis and GTS, apart from a few case reports: these include mania (122), bipolar disorder (123), schizophreniform psychosis (27, 124, 125), and psychosis in the setting of learning disability (126). There have been two reports (127, 128) of children with visual impairment, Ganser syndrome, and GTS, and the authors note that a number of their patients (all children) with GTS have experienced "brief auditory hallucinations" that varied between true hallucinations and intense eidetic auditory imagery. The authors (129) later described "schizophreni-form" symptoms in 11 cases of GTS (although only two were typical and uncomplicated), demonstrating how childhood schizophrenia can be misdiagnosed; all of the children actually had GTS. Six cases of concurrent GTS and Asperger's syndrome have been reported by the same group (130). Robertson et al. (38) reported no psychotic patients in a cohort of 90, although three exhibited ideas of reference.

There is now impressive evidence that GTS and obsessionality are related, and this is discussed in detail later.

In conclusion, it appears that patients with GTS are especially prone to depression, which may be related to the duration of the GTS, partly connected to the reality that GTS sufferers have a chronic, socially disabling, and stigmatizing disease. Anxiety is also high in patients with GTS, but some of this could be accounted for by the depression. ADHD and SIB occur in a substantial number of GTS individuals, but the precise relationship between them are unclear. There is no generally accepted association between GTS and psychosis.

FAMILY PSYCHOPATHOLOGY

If, indeed, psychopathology is an important and distinctive feature of GTS, a positive family history of psychiatric illness might be expected, but this aspect has not received much attention. Gilles de la Tourette himself, in 1899 (96), had already noted that the family history of patients with GTS was almost invariably "loaded for nervous disorder." Samuel Johnson's father, Michael, clearly suffered from depression, "a general sensation of gloomy wretchedness," and it is from him that his famous son "inherited . . . a vile melancholy" (131). Comings (110) asserts that a wide variety of psychopathologies are found in relatives of GTS probands. Other than Comings, only case reports and small studies have noted a positive family history of psychopathology (53, 72, 132–134). Corbett and colleagues (132)

studied the parents of tiqueurs (individuals with tics or GTS) and found that 57 of 184 children (31%) of tiquers had one or both parents who were psychosomatically ill; over half of these were mothers with affective illness. This was a significantly higher number when compared to a out of clinic sample and a psychiatric hospital population (132). Montgomery et al. (135) specifically addressed the question and found that 70% of 30 first-degree relatives of 15 GTS patients satisfied Feighner criteria for psychiatric illness, the most common diagnoses being unipolar depression, obsessive-compulsive illness and panic disorder. Robertson et al. (38) reported that 48% of 90 probands had a positive family history of psychiatric illness, of which the most common disorders were depression, schizophrenia, and obsessional disorder. Robertson and Gourdie (27) reported a wide range of psychopathology in 85 family members of a GTS proband. Individuals completed standardized psychiatric rating scales and, with the exception of the Leyton Obsessional Trait Inventory, there were no statistical differences between cases and noncases. All individuals were also diagnosed using the Schedule for Affective Disorders and Schizophrenia-Lifetime version (SADS-L), and 21 family members had shown psychiatric illness at some time, but these were not in excess of the lifetime risks for major psychiatric illness, such as major depressive disorder, alcohol abuse, schizophrenia, and other "neurotic" disorders (27).

Pauls et al. (136) have specifically tested the Comings' hypothesis. They examined the relationship between GTS and psychopathology in 338 biological first-degree relatives (FDRs) of 86 GTS probands, 92 biological FDRs of 27 unaffected control probands, and 21 nonbiological FDRs of 6 adopted GTS probands, mostly by direct interview. Results showed that anxiety, panic disorder, phobias, affective disorders, substance abuse, and psychotic disorders are not genetically related to GTS.

Etiology — Evidence from the Neurosciences

NEUROPHYSIOLOGICAL EVIDENCE

Shapiro et al. (30) reviewed the literature on electroencephalographic (EEG) findings in GTS in 11 studies; of 127 patients reported, 66% were said to have abnormal EEGs. In their own cohort of 79 patients, 47% had EEG abnormalities, this being more common in children (71%) than in adults (25%). Other investigations have reported lower rates, with some degree of consistency. Abnormalities have been found in 12.5% (137), 13% (9), 17% (138, 139), 20% (140), and 37% (38) of GTS clinic patient populations. Abnormalities detected are, however, nonspecific, and, in particular, there is no evidence of any paroxysmal activity time-locked to the tics (139). In summary, EEG findings in GTS are mostly normal, with abnormalities being minor and nonspecific. It has been suggested that among GTS patients who are more psychologically impaired and who have more learning disabilities, there are more dysrythmias on the EEG (141), but this was based on a small number of patients.

In view of the wide spectrum of clinical manifestations of the tics of GTS, it is not surprising to find an equally wide variation in electromyogram (EMG) patterns recorded from muscles. One study has addressed the subject comprehensively (139). In EMG recordings of simple tics, cocontraction of prime mover and antagonist muscles was seen more frequently, and more complex tics were associated with a variety of EMG patterns. The same investigators reported that the buildup of a negative potential over the half-second or so before EMG activation of an involved muscle (the premovement, readiness, or Bereitschafts potential, and probably representing the summed activity of changing firing patterns in cortical neurons in preparation for a voluntary movement) was absent in six cases of GTS. This suggests that the simple tics of GTS are not generated through the normal cortical motor pathways utilized for willed human movements.

Visual and sensory evoked potentials have been investigated in GTS by Obeso et al. (139) and Krumholz et al. (137), but no consistent abnormalities have been demonstrated. Late components of the event-related auditory evoked potentials were investigated in a controlled study (142). It was concluded that GTS subjects have no abnormalities in early or late components, but that the components in the range 90–280 msec are affected, and may reflect specific attentional deficits that can occur in some patients with GTS.

Tolosa et al. (143) evaluated neuronal excitability in 23 GTS patients by studying the effect of a conditioning stimulus on the blink reflexes. Studies were repeated during maximal voluntary tic inhibition. Results indicated that there is increased brainstem interneuron excitability in GTS, with reduction of this excitability during voluntary tic inhibition.

NEURORADIOLOGICAL EVIDENCE
Structural Evidence

Structural abnormalities of the brain in GTS have been sought by a variety of neuroimaging techniques, including computerized tomography (CT) and magnetic resonance imaging (MRI). To date, although abnormalities have been few and only small numbers of patients have been examined, there are implications that abnormalities of the basal ganglia are found in GTS.

In investigations using CT scans, only 22 of 176 (13%) documented CT scans have been abnormal, and only some of the abnormalities appear to be of possible etiological significance. Robertson et al. (38) documented 71 of 73 GTS patients to have normal CT scans (both abnormalities were cavum septum pellucidum cavities in patients who head-banged). In a controlled study (144), CT scans were performed on 19 patients with GTS and compared with those of patients with infantile autism, ADD, and a language disorder, and a control group of 20 medical patients. No significant differences were found between groups or

controls with respect to total ventricular volume, right: left ventricular volume ratio, ventricular asymmetries, ventricle: brain ratios, or brain density. Regeur et al. (43) reported 47 of 53 CT scans in GTS patients to be normal. Abnormalities included a small arachnoid cyst in the occipital region, a suprasellar epidermoid, a large defect in the right temporo-parietal region, slight cortical atrophy, and two that showed asymmetry of the ventricles. In contrast to the findings of these studies, Caparulo et al. (145) reported abnormalities, such as mild ventricular dilatation, prominent sylvian fissures, or cortical sulci in 38% of patients (6 of 16). Chase et al. (146) reported 7 of 9 normal CT scans; abnormalities were mild ventricular dilatation and mild, diffuse cortical atrophy. Others have reported markedly enlarged occipital horns of the lateral ventricles bilaterally (147), a large porencephalic cyst in the right hemisphere involving the right basal ganglia, as well as contrast enhancement in the region of the lef basal ganglia (148). Other CT reports have included that of Yeragani et al. (149) who documented a mild increase in the density of the caudate nuclei thought to be due to calcification, while Lakke and Wilmink (150) reported a pineal tumor. Vieregge et al. (151) reported twins concordant for GTS who also had ventricular asymmetry on CT scan.

MRI scans in GTS suggest minor abnormalities in the basal ganglia. Some, however, have been normal even when GTS subjects are compared with controls (63, 146, 152), but these studies are limited, however, because of the small numbers involved (n = 13) and lack of quantitative analysis. A few abnormalities on MRI that have been described include that of Sandyk (153), who reported a 7-year-old boy whose MRI revealed asymmetric cerebral peduncles, Robertson et al. (154), who reported a case of severe GTS who necessitated psychosurgery (limbic leukotomy) and who had a high-signal lesion in the right globus pallidus on MRI, and Demeter (152), who documented two patients who showed focal abnormalities involving the basal ganglia. Two recent controlled MRI studies involving 51 GTS patients and 32 controls indicate that the basal ganglia are abnormal in GTS (155, 156). In particular, the lenticular region in the left hemisphere is reduced in volume compared with controls. Likewise, there is an attenuation in GTS patients of the left side prominence relative to the right side observed in control groups (157).

In conclusion, despite the relatively small numbers involved, more abnormalities in brain structure in GTS are being reported using MRI than CT technique. This probably reflects the diagnostic accuracy of MRI and the ability to detect subtle abnormalities. Most likely, the next phase of research into structure will use quantitative MRI.

Functional Evidence

Functional imaging using positron emission tomography (PET) and single photon emission computerized tomography (SPECT) have yielded interesting abnormalities, especially considering the abnormalities found in OCD.

One study using PET showed abnormalities in five GTS patients when compared with controls (158). In the GTS patients there was a fairly close positive association between metabolism in the basal ganglia (particularly the corpus striatum) and metabolism throughout the cerebral cortex. Regional glucose metabolism seemed to also have a close inverse association with the severity of vocal tics in the middle and inferior parts of the frontal lobes bilaterally, extending posteriorly from the frontal poles to the central gyrus. Coprolalia, in contrast, was inversely correlated with hypometabolism in the left parasylvian region (158). Continuing their work in the area, Chase et al. (146) assessed 12 untreated GTS patients with matched normal controls using an improved PET scanner, with higher resolution and sensitivity than the former scanner. At horizontal levels from 8.4–8.8 cm caudal to the vertex, nonnormalized glucose utilization rates were approximately 15% below control values in the region of the frontal cingulate and possibly insular cortex and in the inferior corpus striatum ($p < 0.01$). In a controlled study, Stoetter et al. (159) examined 18 GTS patients and found that GTS patients had lower relative metabolic rates in inferior, limbic regions of the cortex, striatum and subcortical limbic structures, and higher relative metabolic rates in superior, sensorimotor cortices.

SPECT imaging has shown hypoperfusion in the basal ganglia, thalamus, and frontal and temporal cortical areas (160), as well as elevated frontal cortex blood flow (relative to basal ganglia, inclusive of caudate nucleus and putamen) in GTS patients (161). Moriarty et al. (162) examined 50 GTS patients and 20 controls using HMPAO SPECT. Patients differed from controls on measures of relative blood flow to the left caudate, anterior cingulate cortex, and the left dorsolateral prefrontal cortex. Severity of tics was related to hypoperfusion of the left caudate and cingulate and the left medial temporal region. Hypoperfusion in the left dorsolateral prefrontal region was related to mood. The authors related their findings to known functions of the frontal lobe and striatum. A wide range of perfusion patterns was seen, however, and no characteristic patterns for behavioral subgroups has been documented using HMPAO SPECT (162). Riddle et al. (163) found hypoperfusion in basal ganglia and frontal areas, reaching statistical significance in the left putamen-globus pallidus (relative Technetium-99m-hexamethyl propylene amine oxime [HMPAO] uptake 4% lower in GTS when compared to controls).

George et al (164) performed single slice dynamic SPECT with ^{123}I-iodo-6-methoxybentamide (^{123}I-IBZM) in 15 GTS patients (eight unmedicated) and six healthy volunteers. Unmedicated GTS patients showed no differences from control subjects, while GTS patients taking D_2-blocking medications had significantly decreased ^{123}I-IBZM binding compared with normal control subjects in both right and left basal ganglia. These results suggest that D_2-receptor availability, as measured by ^{123}I-IBZM SPECT is not abnormal in GTS.

In summary, despite the small numbers, functional imaging using PET and SPECT have demonstrated metabolic and perfusion abnormalities in the basal ganglia and frontotemporal areas, with special reference to the putamen (146, 158, 165). We, however, suggest that the basal ganglia abnormalities are specific, whereas the hypofrontality may well be a nonspecific finding, also found in depression and schizophrenia (166–168). D_2-receptors, however, appear to be normal in GTS apart from medication effects.

NEUROPATHOLOGICAL POST-MORTEM EVIDENCE

In the first case of "idiopathic" GTS to be carefully studied postmortem (PM), no abnormalities were found (169). Balthasar (170) subsequently suggested that there was pathological development of the striatum after a careful cell count of the brain of a patient with GTS, which showed that the number of small striatal cells matched the cell count in a 1-year old child. Richardson (171), reviewing the two, concluded that there were no distinctive histopathological abnormalities.

More recently, PM investigations have suggested decreased 5HT and glutamate (especially in the subthalamus) in many areas of the basal ganglia (172), as well as a reduction in the second messenger cyclic AMP and an increased number of dopamine uptake carrier sites in the striatum (173). Haber and colleagues (174, 175) reported detailed neuropathological and immunohistochemical PM examinations on five GTS patients and found a reduction of dynorphin-like immunoreactivity in the globus pallidum. These findings excite much interest, but require replication, and clearly, more PM studies with satisfactory controls are necessary for any more definitive statements to be made.

BIOCHEMICAL EVIDENCE

Dopaminergic System

The neurochemical basis for GTS is, as yet, not known. A thorough review (176) examines the evidence for biochemical abnormalities, and the main hypothesis is of an imbalance of central nervous system neurotransmitter agents. Dopamine has received the most support, because haloperidol and other dopamine antagonists reduce the symptoms in a large number of patients, while stimulants such as pemoline and methylphenidate exacerbate the symptoms. In addition, homovanillic acid has been found to be decreased in the CSF of some GTS patients, although the methods involved have been criticized (176). Friedhoff (177) addressed the possible role of D_1 and D_2 receptors in GTS, highlighting a distinction between the two. Thus, the D_2 system, unlike the D_1, is sensitive to "adaptive unregulation." When blocked by D_2 antagonists, such as haloperidol or pimozide, it increases the number of receptors, which serves to overcome the blockade. A similar phenomenon does not occur in the

D_1 system unless there are very long periods of blockade. The implications of this difference and its relevance to GTS are discussed in detail by Friedhoff, including such issues as epigenetic transmission and the male-to-female ratio (177). The eye-blink rate, a supposed correlate of central dopamine activity, has been found by some (100, 178) but not others (179) to be increased in patients with GTS.

Other Transmitter Mechanisms

Investigations implicating noradrenergic systems and acetylcholine have been equivocal, and there is little support for the involvement of serotonin or γ-aminobutyric acid in the pathophysiology of GTS (176). Others (180) have suggested an underactivity of the endogenous opioid system.

With no one transmitter convincingly implicated to date, the importance of animal models and further PM studies is stressed. Cohen et al. (181) have stated that GTS reflects the interaction among genetic, neurophysiological, behavioral, and environmental factors. Eldridge and Denckla (182) suggest that a complex interaction of androgenic and immunological factors are involved in susceptibility to neurodevelopmental disability and, therefore, GTS. They further note that, when viewed in this context, the observation of Balthasar (170) of an increased number of neurons in the caudate and putamen, suggesting the persistence of an immature neuronal pattern, may be more understandable (182). Moreover, it has been hypothesized that the brain regions involved in GTS are those that participate in primitive reproductive behavior and whose development are under sex hormone control (183).

Bonnet (178) addressed the anatomical localization of GTS and concluded that the biochemical structure of the limbic forebrain structures, particularly the anterior cingulate cortex, and their interrelationships with other specific nuclei suggest they are the anatomical site for GTS. Trimble and Robertson agreed (184). Others have suggested that pathology in the periaqueductal gray matter and midbrain tegmentum (150, 185) and in the amygdaloid complex (186) may be implicated in GTS.

OTHER BIOCHEMICAL EVIDENCE

Robertson et al. (187) reported that 10 of 80 GTS patients had an abnormally low serum copper level. Two of the 10 were investigated in detail with copper radioisotope studies. Both exhibited abnormalities of copper handling, in that there was fast disappearance of copper from the plasma, slow uptake by the liver, and low incorporation of copper into ceruloplasmin. Wilson's disease was excluded in all 80 subjects on the basis of detailed clinical examination. The abnormalities found, however, carried no etiological or treatment implications.

GENETIC EVIDENCE

In the quest for finding an etiological factor for GTS, the interest in the genetics of the disorder has mushroomed in the recent past, and many groups and laboratories have become involved. A number of recent investigations have addressed the question of a genetic predisposition in GTS, but the precise genetics are unclear (188), as it can be sporadic (189), and 50% of the human genome has now been excluded (190). At present, nevertheless, the evidence is mostly in support of a major autosomal-dominant gene.

Convincing evidence for a genetic factor comes from twin data in which monozygotic (MZ) twins have been concordant for GTS (30, 65, 151, 191–193). However, a male GTS whose MZ twin was discordant has been reported (194). Also, the large twin study of Price et al. (195) involving 43 pairs of same-sex twins, in which concordance rates were only 77% and 23% for MZ and dizygotic (DZ) pairs respectively, suggests that nongenetic factors also play a role in the expression of GTS. The original data from the large study (195) were reexamined, and it was found that in each case of discordant twins, the unaffected co-twin had a higher birth weight than the affected twin (196). It was therefore speculated that some prenatal events or exposures, such as maternal stress, antiemetic medication, or other unknown agents may lead to changes in the sensitivity of some dopaminergic receptors, and this could partially determine the eventual severity of expression of the GTS diathesis (196).

In addition, numerous family studies provide stronger evidence for the genetic factors involved in GTS, as many relatives of probands with GTS may present with either GTS or motor or vocal tics only (24, 33, 34, 64, 67, 197, 198). Several large multiply affected families have also been reported (25–27, 199, 200), and in all there is an increased incidence of tics (simple or chronic) and GTS in the relatives of probands with GTS.

Recent studies using complex segregation analysis on independent samples (28, 36, 201, 202, 203) and on large families (204, 205) suggest the presence of a major autosomal-dominant gene with varying but usually high penetrance. Some have shown that OCB is a phenotypic variation of the putative GTS gene (28).

Genetic linkage studies are underway in several centers in the U.S. and Europe. A range of chromosomal anomalies in GTS has been reported (for review, see 206), which have led to investigations for linkage. Reports have tentatively assigned the gene to chromosomes 3 (207), 11 ([D_2 receptors] (177)), and 18 (208, 209), and the dopamine D_3 receptor gene (210), but there has been much debate (211–213). Chromosomes 7 and 18 (214), 11 (215), and the D_1-dopamine receptor (216) have been excluded. Notably, Robertson and Trimble (206) reported that 65 of 68 (96%) consecutive GTS patients had entirely normal chromosomes. Their findings, plus a review of the literature, suggest that currently no one chromosomal abnormality can be said to be absolutely characteristic of GTS. Bilineality (i.e., affected individuals on both maternal and paternal sides of index cases) has been reported (216a) which suggests that homozygosity is not uncommon in GTS and might further explain difficulties in localizing the gene defect by linkage analysis.

Two studies (217, 218) have analyzed HLA typing in GTS, and both found no association between GTS and HLA-A or HLA-B antigens or haplotypes. The latter authors also found no association between GTS and HLA-C or HLA-DR antigens.

In conclusion, GTS is probably inherited by autosomal-dominant transmission with incomplete, but high penetrance, and at least some types of OCB may be phenotypical expressions of the putative GTS gene(s). It has also been suggested, however, that some prenatal events or exposures, such as maternal stress, antiemetic medication or other unknown agents may lead to changes in the sensitivity of some dopaminergic receptors. This could partially determine the eventual severity of expression of the GTS diathesis. Further studies on the mechanism of inheritance may well be assisted by more precise definition of the phenotypes involved. Future studies quite likely will show that the mechanism is more complicated than a single gene, because previous studies have not entirely ruled out the possibility of other alleles, multifactorial inheritance, or genetic heterogeneity.

EVIDENCE FROM ALLERGY

There is a widely held belief among both the lay public and GTS patients that GTS symptoms are associated with allergy. In addition, Bruun (17), reviewing 300 patients with GTS, stated that although there is no evidence that allergies cause GTS, her clinical experience has shown that symptom exacerbation is often associated with seasonal allergy responses and the ingestion of allergens in food, as well as by the drugs used to treat allergies. Although others (219, 220) also report exacerbation of symptoms on exposure to allergens, there has been little scientific evidence for the involvement of allergy in GTS (221). A recent controlled study indicates that GTS individuals do not have more allergies than controls, but do have more hyperactivity (Robertson, Kalali, and Brostoff—in preparation).

Diagnostic Evaluation

As with all neuropsychiatric patients, the clinician must take a full and detailed medical and psychiatric history, examine the mental state, and perform thorough physical and neurological examinations. However, there are also methods or aspects of assessment that require special mention.

ASSESSMENT AND RATING OF TIC SEVERITY

Both clinicians and researchers need to first make an accurate description and measure the severity of GTS. To this end, there are several schedules currently in use. The problems in rating tic severity, statistical considerations for quantitative assessment of tics, and an in-depth discussion of available instruments has been elegantly reviewed by Kurlan and McDermott (222).

Briefly, the precise measurement of tic frequency nearly always poses a problem, because the severity is often variable and dependent on several factors. Recently an attempt to overcome some of the difficulties has been made by using video recordings; in addition, recordings of patients' movements while performing prescribed tasks have been made using the large-scale integrated (LSI) motor-activity monitor, which looks like and is worn as a wristwatch (223).

There are three self-report schedules that are used in the evaluation of GTS. The Tourette Syndrome Questionnaire (TSQ) (35), is a structured parental and/or self-report schedule that was originally developed for an epidemiological survey and offers a systematic way of obtaining relevant information, such as personal and demographic data, developmental history, family history, general medical and treatment history, the course of tic behaviors, and the impact of GTS on the person's life. A second parent and/or self-report instrument was developed for a needs assessment survey conducted for the Tourette Syndrome association of Ohio by Stefl and colleagues (cited in 222). The final schedule, the Tourette Syndrome Symptom Checklist (TSSL), was devised by Cohen and co-workers (224) to assist parents in making daily or weekly ratings of tic severity. The schedule, which takes into account the frequency and disruption of both tics and behavioral symptoms, has been used successfully to monitor the longitudinal course of GTS and to document changes during medication trials (225).

There are also several clinician or observer schedules available for the assessment of tics and GTS. Tanner et al. (226) developed a scale that enables an observer to count the patient's tics under several different conditions that are videotaped (patient alone, with the examiner, sitting quietly, and performing a task). The Tourette Syndrome Severity Scale (TSSS) was developed by Shapiro and colleagues (32, 227, 228) for use in a clinical trial evaluating pimozide in the treatment of GTS. It includes a composite rating of severity composed of five items or factors, the scores of which are totaled and converted to a global severity rating. The items are as follows: (a) the degree to which tics are noticeable to observers, (b) whether the tics elicit comments or curiosity, (c) whether others consider the patient odd or bizarre, (d) whether the tics interfere with functioning, and (e) whether the patient is incapacitated or hospitalized because of the tics. The Tourette Syndrome Global Scale (TSGS), which combines a variety of ratings for tic symptoms and social functioning into an overall global score for severity, was developed by Cohen and his colleagues (229). The section on tics rates frequency and disruption for both simple and complex motor and vocal tics, which are combined in a complicated mathematical formula. Social functioning includes ratings of behavior, restlessness, learning, school, and occupational problems. Problems with the TSGS, however, include social functioning tending to be underweighted because of the multiplication of frequency by disruption scores (230).

The Yale Global Tic Severity Rating Scale (GTSS) was developed to refine measurement of GTS symptoms, building on the developers' experience with the TSGS (230). When using the GTSS, examiners rate the number, frequency, intensity, complexity, and interference of both motor and vocal tics, generating a total tic score, an overall impairment rating, and a global severity score. The Yale group (230) has also produced a Global Clinical Impression Scale (GCIS) for tics. It is a 7-point ordinal scale ranging from "normal" to "extremely severe" for a rating of the impact of GTS symptoms on daily functioning.

Goetz et al. (231) devised a scale for examiners to rate patient videotaped sessions recorded under standardized conditions in three settings (seated quietly with the examiner in the room; reading aloud with the examiner in the room; seated quietly without the examiner in the room). The videotapes are then reviewed, and examiners assess various body regions, rating both motor and vocal tic severity (based on a 0–5 scale) as well as counting both motor and vocal tics.

Shapiro and colleagues (32) devised the Shapiro TS Severity Scale (STSSS) and also use videotaped recordings under three conditions.

1. Computation condition—during which the subjects are asked to add up numbers for 2.5 minutes;
2. Reading condition—subject reads three paragraphs for 2.5 minutes; and
3. No-stimulus condition—subject is seated alone after the examiner has left the room.

After the videotape session, examiners again rate tic number, type, and severity.

A schedule that is widely used internationally for research is The Schedule for Tourette's syndrome and other behavioral syndromes. Developed at Yale by Pauls and Hurst (232) it is comprehensive and allows collection of information (tics and behaviors) about both the patient and family members, taking approximately 4 hours to complete. Robertson and Eapen (in preparation) have developed a similar schedule (the TQ) at the National Hospital for Neurology and Neurosurgery Queen Square in the U.K., which takes about 1½ hours to administer and which has been widely used in the U.K. studies. It has been shown to be both reliable and valid.

NEUROLOGICAL EXAMINATION

In a group of patients examined by Shapiro et al. (30), subtle neurological deficits were found in 57%, and 20% were left-handed or ambidextrous, from which the authors argued an organic etiology. Most (78%) had minor motor asymmetry, while 20% had chorea or choreoathetoid movements. In contrast, Lees et al. (9), using a standardized handedness questionnaire (233), found 87% of their sample of 53 patients to be right-handed, and other investigators have reported only minor nonspecific neurological abnormalities in a few patients (9, 21, 37, 38, 43). Abnormalities reported have included chorea, dystonia, torticollis, dysphonia, dysdiadochokinesis, postural abnormalities, reflex asymmetry, motor incoordination, nystagmus, and unilateral Babinski reflexes.

NEUROPSYCHOLOGICAL EVALUATION

Early neuropsychological studies have been reviewed by Golden (31) and Robertson (6), who note an average IQ in GTS patient cohorts, with verbal/performance discrepancies of 15 points (performance being the lower), specific deficits in reading, writing, and arithmetic, and dysfunction on the Halstead-Reitan Neuropsychological Assessment Battery. Language skills appear to be largely unimpaired, while consistent deficits in visuopractic performance have been documented by a number of authors. Recent controlled studies have suggested that the Intention Editor is impaired in GTS (234). This editor, a key mechanism that underlies the will and which begins to function in early childhood, is triggered whenever there are several intentions competing in parallel with each other and is hypothesized to be a subcomponent of the Supervisory Attentional System, which serves inhibition and is subserved by frontal circuits (234). There also appears to be deficits in attention, especially on more complex tasks, including serial addition, block-sequence span (forward), the trail-making test, and letter cancellation vigilance tasks (235). Because subject GTS and controls did not differ significantly in IQ (which was in the normal range), it was suggested that these findings represented selective deficits rather than global impairments in functioning for the GTS group (235).

Many have investigated the effects of medication on cognitive function in patients with GTS. Apparently, haloperidol has no consistent global effect on performance (31). One study, however, indicated that GTS patients receiving medication, especially butyrophenones, had lower IQ scores (38). It still remains to be shown, however, that individual patients are not impaired and that there is not a deleterious effect on specific areas of cognitive function (31).

Specific learning problems were found in 36% of 200 children with GTS (37). Learning disability and GTS have been reported to coexist in some individuals (126, 236), the combination being reported in 10% of one GTS cohort (68).

DIFFERENTIAL DIAGNOSIS

Most of the conditions that should be considered in the differential diagnosis of GTS are described in detail by Bruun and Shapiro (237), Sacks (238), and Robertson (6), and include the athetoid type of cerebral palsy, seen quite commonly among learning-disabled populations with an age at onset between birth and 3 years. These patients have evident neurological deficits, and a static course after the age of 3. Dystonia musculorum deformans, usually presenting with a torsion dystonia often in the legs, is usually progressive, with a crippling state resulting 10–15 years after the onset; remissions are rare. Encephalitis lethargica, in its chronic form, and the more rare klazomania, an acute postencephalitic state, may mimic the symptoms of GTS, but there is usually other evidence or history of encephalitis and parkinsonian symptoms are associated with these. Huntington's chorea usually begins in the 3rd–5th decade, but 1% of cases have an onset in early childhood. However, a positive family history of the disorder, with attendant dementia and progression to death within 10–20 years is the norm.

A condition similar to GTS has been reported following both short-term (239) and long-term (240-245) use of neuroleptics. Sacks (238) distinguishes GTS from cases of "acquired Tourettism," in which symptoms identical to those of GTS are seen in the setting of an acute or chronic cerebral insult, occurring most commonly in postencephalitic patients, but also found after head trauma (246) and carbon monoxide poisoning (247), and "tardive Tourette Syndrome," coined by Stahl (241), and occurring in patients treated with long-term neuroleptic drugs, either arising as an elaboration of lower-level dyskinesia, or de novo.

One of the most difficult differential diagnoses is that of tics of childhood, which commence between the ages of 5–10 years, but many remit spontaneously and usually improve with age. For a review of the diagnostic criteria for transient tic disorder, chronic motor tic disorder, and GTS, see Woody and Laney (248) or DSM-IV (1).

Spasmodic torticollis usually presents between ages 30–50 years, although it can commence at any age. It is a form of focal torsion dystonia that may be associated with more widespread disease and spastic speech. Approximately half of the cases are progressive; some remit spontaneously, while others remain static. Sydenham's chorea occurs more frequently in females, and 75% of cases are associated with rheumatic fever, eosinophilia, and ECG abnormalities. The choreiform movements are usually self-limiting. Wilson's disease usually presents between the ages of 10–25 years, and the classic signs are Kayser-Fleischer rings, cirrhosis or hepatitis, dementia, and associated copper abnormalities in the serum and urine. It is usually progressive and fatal if untreated within several years. Once neurological signs, for example, abnormal movements, are present, Kayser-Fleischer rings are almost always detectable (6).

Uncommon disorders, such as Hallervorden-Spatz disease, Pelizaeus-Merzbacher disease, status dysmyelinatus, and Jakob-Creutzfeldt disease should also be considered in the differential diagnosis of GTS, but most of these have distinctive clinical features, classical courses, and characteristic types of movements that usually make it possible to differentiate them from GTS (237). Other conditions to be excluded are hypoparathyroidism and epilepsy, especially myoclonus epilepsy.

Comings and Comings (70) stress that wrong diagnoses of GTS are common, and suggest the main reasons for this include unfamiliarity with the syndrome, suppressibility of the symptoms, and the erroneous belief that coprolalia must

be present. It is noteworthy, however, that despite the usually typical presentation of GTS, diagnostic difficulties do occur (249, 250).

Management

Successful management of the person with GTS, requires both psychosocial measures and pharmacological intervention for the individual, as well as various strategies for dealing with the patient's family. For many adults with mild GTS, explanation and reassurance are often sufficient for their peace of mind. Several such patients have an initial appointment and require only one or two immediate follow-up sessions to be given feedback about investigations that are routinely performed, information about self-help groups, and booklets for relatives and general practitioners. In a similar way, parents of mildly affected children can often be reassured by the diagnosis, explanation about the nature of the disorder, information about self-help groups, and booklets for teachers. For the moderate to severely afflicted patient, who may have the associated features of OCB, ADHD, SIB, and possibly antisocial behavior, the management is more complex.

DRUG THERAPY

Drug therapy is, at present, the mainstay of treatment for the motor and vocal symptoms as well as some of the associated behaviors of GTS, and the medications most commonly used are dopamine antagonists. Other medications, however, are also useful in the treatment of both the motor and vocal tics as well as the associated behaviors.

The butyrophenone haloperidol was first used successfully for GTS by Seignot in 1961 (251). Since then, dopamine antagonists such as haloperidol, pimozide (252, 253), and sulpiride (254) have been widely and successfully used. Doses are relatively small, beginning with, for example, in the case of haloperidol, 0.25–0.5 mg daily and increasing by 0.5 mg per week, often with 2–3 mg daily being sufficient (31). Extrapyramidal side effects, sedation, and dysphoric states are common with haloperidol (255, 256), but less so with pimozide (257). In some patients the sleepiness associated with the haloperidol was thought to adversely affect behavioral manifestations of GTS (258). School phobia and avoidance have also been reported as unwanted side effects of haloperidol (259) and pimozide, which were successfully reversed by the addition of a tricyclic antidepressant (260). Butyrophenones may also impair concentration and scholastic achievement (261), may be associated with lower IQ's on formal testing (38), and may cause tardive dyskinesia (262). Electrocardiogram (ECG) changes (significantly prolonged QT_c interval) during treatment with pimozide have been reported (263). Accordingly, some clinicians find it prudent to monitor patients receiving pimozide with an ECG.

Sulpiride causes fewer extrapyramidal problems, including tardive dyskinesia and dystonia, as well as less cognitive and sedative side effects when compared with haloperidol and pimozide. However, gynecomastia, galactorrhea, menstrual irregularities, and possible depression have been reported (254, 264). Tiapride, with a similar profile to sulpiride, has also been used (265).

Bruun (17) notes that GTS patients can be very sensitive to side effects from neuroleptic agents, mainly because GTS patients (including children) developed tardive dyskinesia when treated with neuroleptics (266, 267), especially when a family history of movement disorders, including GTS, was present (268). Jeste et al. (245) suggest low-dose bromocriptine for the treatment of dyskinesias secondary to neuroleptics in GTS. Recently tardive dyskinesia has been reported in a case of GTS who was receiving sulpiride (269). A cautionary note to the prescribing of neuroleptics in children has been made by Silverstein and Johnston (270), who reported that although these drugs were indicated at times, they were not without problems. In fact, syndromes similar to tardive dyskinesia were found in 140 of 410 (35%) of children with a variety of psychiatric disorders whom these researchers treated.

Uhr et al. (271) successfully treated four patients with GTS with piquindone, which preferentially blocks dopamine receptors in the mesolimbic system rather than the nigrostriatal system, and also selectively blocks D_2 receptors; motor tics responded to lower doses than vocal tics.

Clonidine has also been used successfully in GTS patients (17, 107, 272, 273). Bruun (17) noted that some 15% of patients had a better response to a combination of clonidine and haloperidol than they had to haloperidol alone. Clonidine may well be the agent of choice if a child has GTS and associated ADHD (80).

Specific serotonin reuptake inhibitors (SSRIs) (e.g., fluoxetine; (274) can be used to treat the OC aspects of GTS, and augmentation of these antiobsessional effects of SSRIs (e.g., fluvoxamine) by neuroleptics (e.g., pimozide) has been reported in patients with OCD and GTS (275, 276).

Mesulam and Petersen (277) reviewed the pharmacological treatment of 58 patients treated over an 8-year period. They noted that differences in response patterns were common and thus required individualized tailoring of management. Generally, dopamine-blocking neuroleptics were the mainstay of therapy, but frequently midcourse alterations were required because previously successful drugs stopped working or their side effects became intolerable. Clonidine proved inferior to neuroleptics in the treatment of motor and vocal tics, but they suggested it may have a role in some patients with prominent OC symptomatology. Interestingly, tardive dyskinesia never occurred in their cohort (277).

Other drugs that have been tried with varying success are neuroleptics such as fluphenazine, penfluridol, the antidepressant clomipramine, the anticonvulsant clonazepam, the calcium antagonists nifedipine and verapamil, naloxone, lithium carbonate, tetrabenazine, progabide, and physostigmine (for details, see reference 6). Because the acetylcholine system has been implicated in GTS, oral lecithin has been tried in the treatment of GTS, but without success (278).

PSYCHOSOCIAL MANAGEMENT

For the most part, formal psychodynamic psychotherapy and psychoanalysis have little place in treating the symptoms of GTS. Massed practice—over rehearsal of the target tic (279, 280)—and other forms of behavior therapy (281) can sometimes be helpful, but in general, behavioral approaches have limited value (282). Tansey (283) reported the successful response of a patient with GTS to EEG sensorimotor rhythm biofeedback training.

What is vitally important is supportive psychotherapy, counseling, and advice to both the patient and family, as the illness can be disabling to not only the affected individual, but also distressing to relatives. Support in helping the patient and family to cope are important, as is guidance to teachers (284). In many instances, as the doctors in charge of the patient, we write letters to teachers and principals informing them about GTS and its associated behaviors (especially ADHD, which may simultaneously affect concentration and disrupt a class). We may also suggest individual tuition, extra explanation, extra time in examinations, allowing the use of word processors or computers in the classroom, or stating that the child is unlikely to be of danger to others in, for example, a chemistry class or swimming pool.

For the severely affected patient, who may have the associated features of ADHD, SIB, and aggressive behavior, the management is complex. It is best handled by doctors and health professionals who are well acquainted with the disorder. In these cases, management includes counseling, regular assessment of mood and danger to the individual (depression and SIB), and often the prescribing of more than one medication e.g., an SSRI and sulpiride. When the GTS symptomatology and associated behaviors are very severe and life-threatening, although not common, neurosurgical treatment has been used (154, 285).

Prognosis

There have been no substantial long-term follow-up studies to document the exact course of the syndrome. However, from the literature of case reports and from clinical experience, it is clear that it is usually a lifelong illness. Adolescence, difficult in the lives of most people, is a time of both emotional and physical unpredictability. It is associated with growth spurts, hormonal changes, and the development of secondary sexual characteristics. Not surprisingly, tics and associated TS symptoms seem to become worse and more problematic at this time. There is some evidence that temper tantrums, aggression, and explosiveness appear in the preadolescent period, become severe in teenage years, and gradually recede thereafter; the tic symptomatology of GTS also ameliorates with age (286). The earliest illustration of this was the Marquise de Dampierre, originally described by Itard in 1825 (7) and again by Gilles de la Tourette himself in 1885 (8): her symptoms began at the age of 7 years, and she continued to exhibit them until she died at the age of 85. There have been occasional reports of complete remission (287, 288), but this is the exception. Abduzzahab and Anderson (18) report that 3.3% of patients spontaneously remit, while Shapiro et al. (30) note that coprolalia remits in 19% of subjects.

GTS Conclusions

GTS is no longer the rarity it was once thought to be, and both case reports and large cohorts have been reported worldwide. The clinical characteristics and are well established, and the core symptomatology is uniform and genetically determined (motor and vocal tics); the associated symptoms are variable (SIB, ADHD) and are likely to be the result of a variety of genetic and environmental factors in predisposed individuals. An important aspect of GTS is OCB, which may well be a phenotype of the putative GTS gene(s). Genetic studies suggest that GTS is inherited via autosomal-dominant transmission with high penetrance. Although more than 50% of the genome has already been excluded, this is likely the result of imprecise definition of the clinical phenotypes or genetic heterogeneity. Future research therefore will emphasize genetics and more precise definition of the phenotype. Once genetic linkage is established, it will be possible to identify the actual gene and its causative mutations, followed by prenatal diagnosis and genetic counseling as well as development of new treatments based on a knowledge of the disease pathways.

PM and neuroimaging studies suggest both structural changes and functional abnormalities in the basal ganglia, cingulum, and frontal areas, although the specificity of the latter finding is questioned. MRI studies might shed light on subtle structural changes, which may, in turn, correlate with changes in function assessed by SPECT and fMRI, among other tests.

The identification of an endophenotype would spark much interest and may well be found using a combination of genetic and neuroimaging techniques.

From the reviewers' clinical practice, allergy may have an effect on many GTS patients, making their symptoms worse. Dietary manipulation may well be an area worth pursuing in the future, especially in the case of children, where one is hesitant to use medication unless absolutely necessary. There are no controlled trials of sulpiride vs. haloperidol or pimozide, and these also would be useful.

OBSESSIVE-COMPULSIVE DISORDER

Definition

The currently accepted definition of OCD appears in the American Psychiatric Association DSM-IV (1). OCD is characterized by recurrent obsessions or compulsions sufficiently severe to cause marked distress, that are time-consuming, or significantly interfere with the person's normal routine, functioning, social activities, or relationships. Obsessions are recurrent ideas, thoughts, images, or impulses that enter the mind and are persistent, intrusive, and unwelcome. Attempts are made to ignore or suppress these thoughts, or to neutralize them with some other thought or action. The individual recognizes them as a product of his or her own mind. Compulsions are repetitive, purposeful behaviors performed in response to an obsession, and are designed to neutralize or prevent discomfort or some dreaded event or situation. However, the activity is excessive, or not connected realistically with what it is designed to prevent. The affected person recognizes that his or her behavior is unreasonable.

History

OCD has been described by authors for centuries, and since the Medieval period, Latin terms such as obsession, compulsion, and impulsion appear in the European medical literature to describe OCD-like behavior and phenomena. In his comprehensive review of the conceptual history of OCD during the 19th century, Berrios (289) focuses on French psychiatrists, who were instrumental in the development of its classification through insanity, neurosis, and psychosis to the final position as part of the new class of neuroses. Formally recognized in the 1830s as a cluster of related symptoms, over the next 40 years the components of OCD were differentiated and defined, separating the terms obsession from delusion, and compulsion from impulsion. Magnan, between 1835 and 1916 (290), reinforced the view that OCD occurred only in subjects affected by degeneration, which encouraged the idea of the OCD sufferer as having a pathological personality. By the turn of the century between 1859-1947, Janet (291) had confirmed the natural history of OCD and included it in the category of psychasthenia, along with anxiety and tic disorders. OCD was considered to be a manifestation of distorted or pathological emotions, a concept that influenced Freud's subsequent theories.

During the first half of the 20th century the etiology of OCD was based on the Freudian psychodynamic theories of defense and hidden conflict. OCD was one of the illnesses most frequently cited to illustrate the fundamental principles of psychoanalysis. Based on his successful analysis of the famous case of the Rat Man, a young man who was tormented by thoughts of rats eating their way through his anus, Freud (292) suggested that obsessions occurred as a result of regression to the anal stage of psychosexual development, and warned against punitive or overly restrictive parenting practices. Obsessions were seen as the guilty manifestations of repressed aggressive and sexual impulses, which explained why the content of many of the obsessions of OCD patients involved issues of excretion, contamination, or sexual fantasy.

Psychoanalysis and psychotherapy were largely abandoned as effective treatments for OCD in favor of behavioral therapy in the 1960s and 1970s. However, with the advent of new imaging techniques and the discovery of novel drug treatments, OCD is no longer considered to be a psychological disorder, and it now represents a model neuropsychiatric illness.

Clinical Characteristics

OCD is classified as an anxiety disorder in DSM-IV (1), characterized by obsessive thinking and compulsive behavior. Obsessions and compulsions can take various forms. Obsessional thoughts are intrusive words, ideas, and beliefs that are often upsetting and unwelcome, even though the person recognizes them to be a product of his or her own mind. Obsessional doubts by these patients involve excessive and inappropriate concern about previous actions and their consequences. For example, they might fixate on the possibility that they left their front door open, allowing a burglar to enter, even though they can clearly remember locking up the house. Obsessional fears are feelings of uneasiness and dread about imagined events that might happen, which may be highly improbable or unreasonable, such as the death of a friend or that the person will be unfairly blamed for something. They may also be concerned with the fear of harming oneself or others. Obsessional ruminations are recurring thoughts of a complex nature, such as the ending of the world. Obsessional images are unwelcome mental pictures that often suddenly intrude upon the mind, often of an unacceptable nature, possibly involving violent or sexual scenes. Obsessional impulses are urges to carry out an act that is usually socially unacceptable, which the patient does not want to do and which he or she will resist, such as shouting obscenities, or carrying out a crime such as shoplifting or stabbing, or causing self-harm.

Compulsions (also called obsessional rituals) are repeated and meaningless rituals performed in a purposeful and stereotyped way that may be performed to neutralize an obsessional thought that precedes them. For example, the repeated washing of hands may be an action to allay obsessional fears of contamination with germs, or the obsessional doubt of failing to turn off the gas may lead to compulsive checking. Although the compulsion may seem to reduce the anxiety resulting from the obsession and produce a tension release in its performance, the person strongly resists carrying out the ritual and does not derive pleasure from it. The compulsion may occasionally have no apparent connection with an obsession, except for an obsessional urge to carry out the act, such as ordering things in a particular way. Patients will often go to great lengths to hide their compulsive acts and rituals because of embarrassment and fear of being considered mad. This often leads to a delay in diagnosis.

Most obsessions and compulsions involve issues of cleanliness and contamination, safety and aggression, order, sex, and religion. In a survey (293) reporting the obsessions and compulsions of 70 child and adolescent patients with OCD, 43% had obsessions involving disgust with bodily wastes or secretions, dirt, germs, chemical and environmental contamination; 24% had obsessional fears that something terrible might happen; and 17% had obsessions of symmetry and exactness, such as the way things should be arranged or organized. Thirteen percent had obsessions of a religious nature; and 4% had forbidden or perverse sexual thoughts, images, or impulses, for example, involving bestiality, pedophilia, incest, or homosexuality. Other obsessions (294) may involve seemingly neutral images, colors with special significance, and intrusive sounds, words, or music. Somatic obsessions involve preoccupations with parts of the body, such as the shape of one's nose.

Compulsions mostly take the form of cleaning, checking, repeating, counting, and ordering. In the same study (293), 85% of subjects had rituals of excessive hand washing, bathing, showering, tooth brushing, or grooming; 51% had repeated rituals, such as going in and out of doors, or getting up and down from a chair; 46% had compulsions of checking doors, stoves, car brakes etc.; 23% had cleaning rituals involving contact with contaminants; 20% had rituals involving the need to touch; 18% had counting rituals; and 17% had ordering and arranging compulsions, such as rearranging drawers or packing and unpacking suitcases. Other compulsions involve hoarding and collecting, the need to tell, ask, or confess, and a special way of dressing.

Epidemiology

Until a decade ago, OCD was thought to be a rare condition, with one of the earliest psychiatric community surveys in 1943 reporting a prevalence of only 0.3% in a Tennessee community (295). In the 1950s and 1960s, a series of retrospective chart review studies recording the frequency of OCD found in psychiatric patients allowed investigators to calculate that the prevalence of OCD in the general population was about 5 in 10,000 (296–299). Concurrent "second generation" psychiatric community surveys based on methods developed for screening American military for nonspecific psychiatric disorder during World War II were scarcely more sophisticated than the earlier surveys and usually included any OCD findings in the much larger category of neurosis.

It is only since the refinement of the diagnostic criteria for OCD and the development of more accurate interviewing techniques that we have been able to gain a more accurate picture of the epidemiology of this disorder. The Diagnostic Interview Survey (DIS) has been suggested as a good instrument for determining the prevalence of OCD, and has been used in the Epidemiological Catchment Area (ECA) studies (300), nine of which have been performed, including five in the U.S. This survey was designed to determine the prevalence of DSM-III Axis I psychiatric disorders in the general population. Eight of the surveys have given figures for lifetime prevalence of OCD ranging from 1.9–3.2% (301–311).

These studies revealed that OCD was 50–100 times more common than previously thought, and that it was the most common psychiatric illness after the phobias, substance abuse, and depression. Despite the questionable validity of these findings, based on criticism of some of the methods involved in the ECA surveys, subsequent epidemiological studies have given similar figures for such high rates of prevalence. Data from these studies also suggest reasons why the prevalence of OCD was underestimated for so long.

Many patients with OCD are embarrassed about their symptoms, and they are kept a secret. They may thus never come to the attention of health professionals. One family study revealed that often siblings are unaware that anything is abnormal with the OC brother or sister who hides his or her symptoms (312). Others may present in medical settings other than psychiatric, such as the dermatology clinic for chapped hands from excessive washing (313), the dentist for gum lesions from overbrushing, the oncologist or infectious disease specialist for obsessions with HIV and AIDS, and the plastic surgeon for obsessions with body image. These medical specialists may be unfamiliar with the features of the disorder and hence fail to make the diagnosis. Sufferers may seek care from outside of the medical profession and may turn to a family member, friend, or religious leader instead.

OCD is reported to occur worldwide. Surveys, including DIS studies, in Canada, Puerto Rico, and New Zealand—as part of integrated research with the ECA American studies—and others in diverse cultures such as Europe and Africa have given consistently similar prevalence rates as those in the U.S. The only exception is the DIS study in Taiwan, which gave very much lower lifetime prevalence figures of 0.3% in rural areas and 0.9% in Taipei. This may be because the Chinese suffer from lower rates of psychiatric illness, or that different methods of analysis were used in interpretation of the data (314).

OCD occurs in all social classes, and although some studies show an association with above-average class and intelligence, this may have been related to bias in the design of the studies (315). Patients with OCD are more likely to be celibate, divorced, or socially isolated (296–298, 316).

The age at onset is often early, with an estimated 60% of persons with OCD reporting their first symptoms before the age of 25 years, and 30% experiencing the onset of obsessions and compulsions between the ages of 5–15 (317). Although earlier studies suggested parity between the sexes (315), the DIS studies found that overall OCD was more common in women by a ratio of about 1.5:1. The mean age at onset of first symptoms was 21.4 years for men and 19.6 years for women. The disorder is, however, being increasingly recognized in children and adolescents. The studies also looked at how the prevalence of OCD varied with age, and found that in women there is a peak between ages 25–34, and in men between ages 35–54 for 6-month prevalence. Caution must be used in interpreting the differences found in age of lifetime prevalence. With the exception of Puerto Rico, lifetime prevalence was highest in the 25–44 age group and falls off with increasing age. This could be a cohort effect in that patients with later birthdates are more susceptible to developing OCD, or these results may be simply due to older probands forgetting the symptoms from which they suffered earlier in their life (300). The lifetime morbid risk of developing OCD within a normal life span was calculated to be 5.4%, from the data obtained from the study in Edmonton, Canada (307).

Early follow-up studies of adult patients with OCD revealed the chronic or episodic course of the disorder

Table 35.1. Comorbid Conditions Associated with OCD

Affective Disorders
  Major depressive disorder
  Dysthymia
Anxiety Disorders
  Separation anxiety disorder
  Panic disorder
  Agoraphobia
  Generalized anxiety disorder
  Simple phobia
  Social phobia
Tourette Syndrome and Other Tic Disorders
  Eating disorders
  Anorexia nervosa
  Bulimia nervosa
OC (Anankastic) Personality Disorder
Habit Disorder
  Trichotillomania
  Onychophagia
Body Dysmorphic Disorder
Neurological Disorders
  Epilepsy
  Sydenham's chorea
  Postencephalitic Parkinson's disease

(296–299, 318, 319), with only 12–32% (318, 319), of subjects recovering completely. However, up to 50% spontaneously improved (297), and severe disability was rare (296, 298), with most being able to continue in employment (31, 319). Although some of these studies involved large groups of patients, the length of follow-up time varied enormously, diagnostic criteria were not consistent, and it is unclear what treatment, if any, the patients studied had received. More recent prospective follow-up studies of children and adolescents with OCD apply more stringent methodology (320, 321) but continue to stress the unfavorable long-term outcome of many patients. This problem does not seem to have been solved by the availability of behavioral therapy or drug treatment (322, 323). Data from the ECA studies in Edmonton (Canada) and Christchurch (New Zealand) found that the 1-year-recovered rates or proportion of cases who met criteria for OCD at some time in the past, but not in the year preceding interview, was as low as 39% and 50% respectively (300), indicating that for the majority, OCD is a persistent disorder. The ECA studies found that only one-third of patients experience spontaneous remission, sometimes after years of illness, and in 10% their illness runs a continuous deteriorating course (324).

Psychopathology and Associated Disorders (Table 35.1)

The wide range of psychiatric and neurological disorders found in association with OCD is summarized in Table 35.1. The high rates of comorbidity of such conditions in patients with OCD may lead to diagnostic confusion and has challenged traditional concepts of the classification of OCD in relation to other psychiatric disorders. Evidence emerging from epidemiological, genetic and family, phenomenological, and treatment studies demonstrates significant overlap in the clinical characteristics of many of these disorders, and suggests etiological relationships between them. The heterogeneity of OCD and its relationship to comorbid symptoms has been examined by some authors, who have categorized OCD patients according to three core features of the disorder: abnormal risk assessment, pathological doubt, and incompleteness (312). They observed that patients with abnormalities in risk assessment had higher levels of anxiety associated with their symptoms and were more likely to suffer from a comorbid anxiety disorder. On the other hand, patients with incompleteness had lower levels of anxiety but were more likely to have compulsive personality features and to have associated multiple tics or habit disorders.

The relationship of OCD to individual associated disorders is discussed in more detail as follows.

MOOD DISORDERS

Symptoms of depression are extremely common in patients with OCD. Up to 80% have dysphoric moods (325), two-thirds have a lifetime history of a major depression, and one-third have a major depression at the time of diagnosis (326). There has been controversy as to whether these depressive symptoms are from a separate secondary disorder, or whether they are integral to OCD. An association between depressive illness and obsessional illness has been documented in the literature as early as 1934 (327), and confirmed over the years (296, 328–330). As recently as 1980, it was speculated that obsessional symptoms are coping devices that defend against depression (331).

OC symptoms are seen in 23–28% of depressed patients (332), but these are usually related to depressive symptomatology in their content, such as obsessive thoughts of guilt. Some authors attempt to distinguish whether depression or OCD is the primary illness by the temporal relationship between the two, diagnosing OCD only if it occurs first (325). Thus, it has been found that the majority (85%) of these patients have an affective disorder secondary to their OCD, while the remainder have a coexisting primary unipolar recurrent depression (326).

Other investigators, however, prefer to regard OCD as a distinct illness with associated depressive symptomatology (333). They cite recent evidence from treatment studies showing that the symptoms of depression in OCD respond to serotonergic drugs, corresponding to improvement in the obsessions and compulsions (334–337). One of these studies (337) showed that the response of the depressive symptoms of the OCD patients to these drugs was more rapid than that seen in depression, with a response time course of 2 weeks, consistent with that of OCD. Other evidence to suggest that OCD is a separate entity from depression comes from studies that show a low response rate of the depressive symptoms of OCD to placebo, whereas in depression a placebo response rate of 30–50% is commonly

reported (338, 339). It also seems that the depressive symptomatology in OCD does not respond to antidepressants that are ineffective in OCD, OCD responding only to serotonergic drugs (333). Other evidence contributing to the distinction of OCD from major depression is the different sex distribution and time course of the two disorders. The ratio of women to men in depression is 2:1, whereas in OCD there is a more equal sex distribution. Depression characteristically has an episodic course with periods of remission, while OCD has a waxing and waning course.

ANXIETY DISORDERS

OCD is classified as an anxiety disorder and has a significant overlap with other anxiety disorders. The ECA epidemiological studies found that 22% of OCD patients had a lifetime history of simple phobia, 18% had social phobia, 12% had panic disorder, and 2% had separation anxiety disorder. Other associated anxiety states include generalized anxiety disorder and agoraphobia. As with OCD and depression, it may be diagnostically difficult to distinguish OCD from these other anxiety disorders. For example, 60% of OCD patients experience panic attacks (326), but these are usually secondary to the obsessive fears of the patient, such as the fear of harming someone. These secondary fears do not constitute a diagnosis of panic disorder, in which spontaneous panic attacks occur. OC symptoms in panic disorder are less frequent than panic symptoms in OCD, with one study finding that 27% of patients with panic disorder had OC symptoms.

OCD patients with extreme avoidance behavior may be erroneously diagnosed as suffering from one of the phobic disorders. For instance, an OCD patient who suffers from cleanliness obsession to the extent that he or she cannot leave the house for fear of contamination, may be diagnosed wrongly as having agoraphobia. In contrast to the OCD patient, an agoraphobic can obtain relief by staying at home, whereas the OCD sufferer will still be afraid of being contaminated by the air, food, or people with whom he or she remains in contact.

EATING DISORDERS

Many mental health workers have noted similarities in the clinical features of OCD and anorexia nervosa and bulimia nervosa (340–342). The extreme preoccupations with food, weight, and body image that are characteristic of eating disorders can be viewed as obsessions similar to those occurring in OCD. Likewise, ruminative calorie counting and ritualistic behavior regarding food may resemble the rituals and compulsions of OCD. Neurobiological similarities also exist between OCD and the eating disorders. Abnormalities in serotonin metabolism and regulation are implicated in both types of these disorders (343, 344), and neuroimaging techniques, such as PET, have demonstrated increased metabolic activity in the caudate nucleus in both illnesses.

Several studies have investigated the prevalence of eating disorders among patients with OCD and vice versa, and have demonstrated significant comorbidity. One retrospective study of a series of 280 patients with OCD found that 10.6% of the women had a history highly suggestive of anorexia nervosa (340). Conversely, a study in which bulimia patients were directly interviewed revealed that 33% of those with active bulimia and 32% of those with inactive bulimia had met DSM-III criteria for OCD at some time in their lives (345).

The overlap in symptoms of the two types of disorder has been demonstrated in a study in which self-rating scale, the Eating Disorder Inventory, was administered to 59 OCD clinic patients and 60 normal controls (346). Scores obtained from these patients were compared to 32 female inpatients with anorexia nervosa or bulimia nervosa. The patients with OCD scored significantly higher than the controls on all aspects of the Inventory, including drive for thinness, bulimia, body dissatisfaction, perfectionism, interpersonal distrust, and maturity fears. Interestingly, the male patients with OCD, compared with the healthy male controls, had more symptoms than the women with OCD. This finding contrasts with the much greater incidence and prevalence of eating disorders in women than men in the general population. The female patients in this study obtained scores that were halfway between those of the women with eating disorders and the normal women.

The aforementioned studies thus suggest a link between OCD and eating disorders. It has even been proposed that eating disorders represent a variant of OCD, starting with the adolescent period (347). Further research is needed to determine the exact diagnostic and etiological relationship between OCD and eating disorders.

OC PERSONALITY DISORDER

The relationship between OCD and OC personality disorder is controversial. Psychoanalytic theories imply that the two disorders form part of a continuous spectrum, with a normal type of personality with obsessive or compulsive traits at one end and the most severe form of OCD at the other, with OC personality disorder somewhere in the middle. Several studies have suggested that this personality disorder is more common in patients with OCD than would be expected in the normal population (296, 348, 349). Others, however, have found that the disorders are not related (350–352). One investigation evaluated personality dysfunction in 23 patients with primary OCD and an age- and sex-matched group of patents with major depressive disorder. They found no significant difference in frequency or type of personality disorder diagnosis between the two groups. The most common personality disorder observed in the OCD group of patients was a mixed type with avoidant, dependent, and passive-aggressive features. Interestingly, the frequency of compulsive personality disorder, as well as schizoid personality disorder, was very low in both groups (350).

Perhaps differences in opinion as to whether OCD and OC personality disorder are related—as well as differences in the differential diagnosis of OCD—may partly depend on the nosological scheme used to classify the personality disorders (312). The American concept of OC personality disorder as defined by DSM-IV criteria (1) is based on Freudian psychoanalytic theory of anal-compulsive symptoms. The classic distinction between this personality disorder and OCD is that in the former, obsessions and compulsions are considered ego-syntonic, i.e., they cause no distress to the individual concerned, whereas in OCD, the symptoms are ego-dystonic. The European equivalent to the OC personality disorder is termed anankastic personality disorder as defined in ICD 10 (2), and makes no distinction between ego-syntonic and ego-dystonic symptoms. This type of personality disorder is found in a much higher percentage of patients with OCD than is the DSM-IV (1) OCD.

HABIT DISORDERS, DYSMORPHOPHOBIA, AND OTHER DISORDERS

The so-called habit disorders, such as trichotillomania, characterized by chronic severe hair pulling, and onychophagia, or severe nail biting, are abnormal behaviors that bear some resemblance to the compulsions seen in OCD in that they are repetitive, purposeful, stereotyped, and anxiety-relieving. These similarities and the evidence that trichotillomania and onychophagia, like OCD, respond to serotonergic uptake inhibitors such as clomipramine (353, 354) and fluoxetine (355, 356) have led to the theory that these disorders are variants of OCD. However, other researchers have indicated that this class of drugs is not as effective for hair pulling as previously thought. A placebo-controlled double-blind cross-over 18-week study to investigate the efficacy of fluoxetine in 21 adult patients with trichotillomania showed no significant short-term benefit (357). There have also been reports that relapse may occur in the chronic treatment of trichotillomania with clomipramine (358). Other evidence that trichotillomania is a distinct disorder from OCD comes from neuroimaging studies and studies of the clinical features of the two conditions. PET studies have shown a different pattern of regional cerebral glucose metabolism in women with trichotillomania from that seen in patients with OCD (359). Furthermore, comparison of the clinical features between a group of eight trichotillomania and 13 OCD patients showed that the former group experienced a greater degree of pleasure in hair pulling than the OCD patients did in enacting their compulsions, and that the two groups differed in terms of associated depression, anxiety, and personality characteristics (360).

Body dysmorphic disorder is a somatoform disorder in which a normal-appearing person has a nondelusional preoccupation with an imagined defect in appearance. The patient's concerns are excessive, distressing, persistent, and disruptive to his or her life-style, and are thus similar to the obsessions of OCD. There have been reports in the literature illustrating the diagnostic overlap between OCD and body dysmorphic syndrome (361, 362), and response of the latter disorder to treatment with SSRIs (363).

Trichotillomania, onychophagia, and dysmorphophobia are included in a group of associated disorders that resemble OCD, which have been called the OC spectrum disorders (312). Other conditions that comprise this group are hypochondriasis, GTS, eating disorders, and impulse-control disorders such as kleptomania, compulsive gambling, pyromania, and the paraphilias (364). Many clinicians have empirically treated these OC spectrum disorders with SSRIs without firm evidence that these agents are effective, lacking controlled trials. Further phenomenological, family, biological, and treatment studies are needed to determine whether these disorders are actual variants of OCD, comorbid conditions, or separate syndromes with overlapping characteristics that complicate the differential diagnosis.

OCD AND NEUROLOGICAL DISORDERS

OC symptoms can occur in a number of neurological conditions, which should be excluded before a diagnosis of primary OCD is made. Such cases of "secondary OCD," however, represent only a small proportion of the total number of patients with OCD, the majority of whom have no neurological history (365).

As early as 1924 it was observed that OC symptoms occurred in patients with postencephalitic parkinsonism (366), a finding that was confirmed by subsequent investigators in the years following the pandemic of encephalitis lethargica after the First World War (365–367). OC traits but not symptoms are common in Parkinson's disease (368), although paradoxically, oral levodopa in the treatment of parkinsonism can occasionally cause obsessions and compulsions (74). OC symptoms can occur following head trauma, either at birth (369), or as a result of accidents (370). Up to one-third of patients with Sydenham's chorea have OC symptoms (371, 372), which has also been reported in patients with Huntington's chorea (373) and rarely in diabetes insipidus (374). OC symptoms have been noted to develop in cases of epilepsy, notably Napoleon, who was epileptic and who had a compulsive ritual of counting the number of windows in the buildings that he passed (365). There are a number of case reports of OC symptoms occurring in patients with petit mal (375), grand mal (376), and temporal lobe epilepsy (365), and as part of the epileptic aura (377, 378). However, because both OCD and epilepsy are common conditions, the observed association between the two disorders may not be significant (379).

Childhood OCD

EPIDEMIOLOGY

Although Janet commented on obsessions occurring in childhood as early as 1903 (382), and retrospective reports of OCD patients revealed that one-third to one-half of adults with OCD first experienced OC symptoms in childhood or

adolescence (296–299, 349), the condition was until recently considered a rarity in pediatric psychiatry. The early descriptions of childhood OCD were based on single case reports or small clinical series (381–385). Subsequent epidemiological studies have been based on populations of child psychiatric patients and found that OCD was present in only 0.2–1.33% (320, 386, 387). The only epidemiological study to date of OCD in an unselected population of adolescents (388) gave a lifetime prevalence rate of 1.9%, much higher than previous clinical estimates but in concordance with the rates found in adults from the ECA studies. This study used the diagnostic criteria of DSM-III (3), and subjects were directly interviewed by experienced child psychiatrists familiar with OCD. The previous underestimation of prevalence may have been due to underdiagnosis of OCD or because of the clinician's unwillingness to diagnose a child as having a disease thought to have a poor prognosis (387).

COURSE AND PROGNOSIS

There have been few prospective follow-up studies of childhood OCD, but they all concluded that long-term outcome was poor, with around half of the subjects reporting no improvement on follow-up at 1–7 years since diagnosis (320, 321, 389). Follow-up of the 20 adolescents identified with OCD in an entire high school population of 5596 students at 2 years showed that all continued to suffer from persistent OCD or other psychiatric disorders with OC features (390). The availability of drug treatment seems not to have improved this poor prognosis. In a recent prospective study of children treated with clomipramine, 50% still fulfilled diagnostic criteria for OCD 2–5 years later, even in those children with a positive initial response to the drug (323). A subsequent follow-up study of 54 OCD children and adolescents who had been treated more aggressively with behavioral and drug therapy found slightly less than half had no improvement 2–7 years later (391–393). These studies confirm the seemingly malignant nature of the disorder, with spontaneous remission occurring in only one-third of patients, and 10% following a deteriorating course (394).

CLINICAL FEATURES

Clinical features of OCD in children tend to be similar to those seen in adults, although different subgroups may be identified. The most frequent symptoms reported are repeated washing and contamination obsessions, checking rituals, and concerns with ordering and arranging. Retrospective analysis of the case notes of 44 consecutive OCD patients referred to an adolescent unit in Oxford between 1974 and 1984 (395) showed that 73% of patients had checking rituals, 64% had washing rituals, with 50% having both. The sex ratio in that study was roughly equal. In a National Institute of Mental Health (NIMH) sample of 70 children and adolescents with OCD seen between 1977 and 1987, rituals were the most common presenting complaint, and of these washing and cleaning were the most common, occurring in 85% of patients at some time during the course of their illness (396). Children who performed rituals in the absence of obsessions were more common than "pure" obsessives, although most commonly, subjects expressed both. This refutes earlier findings that compulsions and obsessions are inseparable (397). Boys predominated in this series by a ratio of 2:1. The mean age at onset was 10 years, but eight of the patients had symptoms before the age of 7. This subset was predominantly male, and it was suggested that early-onset OCD may have a genetic basis and be related to GTS.

Similarities in the phenomenology of children with OCD studied in countries as diverse as Denmark, India, and Japan reveal there are few cultural differences in the content of obsessional thoughts, with the most frequent obsessions concerning dirt and contamination (387, 398, 399).

Early theories that the obsessions and compulsions of OCD are extreme variants of the superstitions, ritualistic play, and behavioral patterns of normal children (400), were explored in a recent comparative study as part of the NIMH research, in which children with severe OCD, normal children, and their respective parents were interviewed about the children's early developmental rituals and their current superstitious beliefs. Both sets of children reported the same frequency of superstitions, although the parents of the OCD children recalled more pronounced early ritualized behavior than the parents of the normal controls. These results could have one of three sources. First, this may represent differential recall of the parents in a manner biased toward the current state of their child. In other words, the parents of a child with OCD are more likely to recall earlier similar manifestations to those the child has currently, than the parents of a child who is well. Second, OCD may begin subclinically as short-lived episodes of repetitive behavior, retrospectively labeled as rituals. Finally, continuity may exist between normal development ritualistic behavior and childhood OCD, with exaggerated rituals being markers of those children who would subsequently develop OCD. Prospective studies are needed to elucidate these issues.

ASSOCIATED DISORDERS

Like OCD in adults, childhood OCD has a wide range of comorbidity, the associated disorders being similar to those seen in adults, with the exception of GTS and developmental disorders. In the NIMH study, only 26% of children had OCD as the single diagnosis. Depression and anxiety are particularly common and may occur before or after the onset of OCD. Another study (401) of 21 clinically referred children and adolescents with OCD found 38% had an anxiety disorder, such as separation anxiety or overanxious disorder, and 29% had a mood disorder, such as major depression or dysthymia. This may be because affective and anxiety symptoms are associated features of OCD, or that obsessions and compulsions are features of mood and anxiety disorders.

Other disorders found to be associated with OCD in children are alcohol and substance abuse, conduct disorders, and ADHD (396, 402, 401). One study of 44 adolescents with OCD (395) found that temper outbursts and disruptive behavior occurred in over half, and that many had poor peer relationships often predating the reported onset of OCD symptoms. This could be interpreted in two different ways. Perhaps previously secret or minor symptoms of OCD prevented the child from making adequate social relationships. Alternatively, children with social maladjustment for other reasons may predispose to the development of such symptoms. In another study (274), the parents of children with OCD completed a Child Behavioral Checklist (CBCL), a standardized questionnaire designed to categorize the behavioral problems and competencies of children ages 4–16. The parents reported high levels of behavioral problems in their children but felt that these interfered more with social functioning rather than academics and activities, where they reported normal levels of achievement.

In the NIMH study, 30% of the children had chronic motor tics, which were more often seen in younger patients, males, and those with acute illness. The author proposed that this subgroup may represent an alternative form of GTS. In another study, tics were observed in 24% of 21 children and adolescents with OCD, even though children with GTS had been excluded from the study. The relationship between tics, GTS, and OCD, and the evidence for a common etiology, is discussed in more detail later in this chapter.

Eating disorders, such as bulimia and anorexia, have also been found to be associated with childhood OCD (403). It has been suggested that several unwanted repetitive behaviors of childhood such as eating disorder, trichotillomania, and onychophagia may be variants of OCD (394). This has been based on family studies suggesting a common genetic basis (404) and treatment studies that suggest that these disorders respond to SSRIs (353, 354).

As in adults, OCD has been observed in children with neurological diseases, including epilepsy (405), Sydenham's chorea (372, 406) Huntington's Chorea, Wilson's disease and Segawa's dystonia (394). The association between these basal ganglia diseases, as well as GTS and childhood OCD, suggests that basal ganglia pathology may be present in this disorder.

FAMILY HISTORY

Several studies have looked for OCD and other psychiatric disorders in the families of children with OCD. In one family study (407), 145 FDRs of 46 children and adolescents with severe primary OCD were interviewed. Thirty percent of probands had at least one FDR with OCD: 25% of fathers and 9% of mothers received a diagnosis of OCD. Forty-five percent of fathers and 65% of mothers were diagnosed as having some other psychiatric disorder, most commonly an affective disorder. Five percent of the siblings had a diagnosis of definite OCD, and 4% with subclinical OCD. The increased familial rate of OCD over that expected in the general population, and the observation that the presenting OCD symptoms of probands and their parents were usually dissimilar suggest a genetic basis to OCD rather than simply social or cultural transmission. Another study found that 4 of 21 (19%) children and adolescents with OCD had a parent with OCD and 11 (52%) had a parent with OC symptoms (274). These results are consistent with a much earlier study that reported 71% of the families studied had a positive family history of obsessions and compulsions.

In summary, recent research has shown that OCD in children is more common than previously thought, and emphasizes the need for greater awareness among pediatricians and child psychiatrists of this disorder. Similarities in phenomenology, epidemiology, sex ratio, comorbidity, and family history suggest a continuity between childhood and adolescent OCD, and that seen in adults. Onset of OCD in childhood, however, seems to be more frequently associated with a poor prognosis. Some authors have proposed an ethological model for OCD, suggesting that OCD and associated disorders, such as trichotillomania and nail biting, are inappropriately released grooming behaviors (394, 408, 409). Further research and prospective studies of large cohorts of children with OCD are needed to understand the etiology, pathophysiology, and natural history of childhood OCD.

Etiology

Until very recently obsessions and compulsions were thought to be products of intrapsychic conflict, and psychodynamic theories have dominated the etiological hypotheses of OCD for most of this century. However, in the past decade evidence from brain imaging, psychopharmacological studies, and advances in treatment have challenged these concepts. OCD is now viewed as a model neuropsychiatric illness. The neuroanatomical basis of OCD has been inferred from the results of new radiological techniques, neuropsychological and electrophysiological studies in people with OCD, and the occurrence of OC behavior in patients with certain brain lesions or neurological disorders. At a molecular level, the biochemical mechanisms underlying the disorder are being elucidated by investigating abnormalities of neurotransmission in OCD patients, which has led to the so-called serotonin hypothesis of OCD. The evidence for this and the involvement of other neurotransmitter systems in the modulation of OC behavior are reviewed in more detail in the following sections.

STRUCTURAL AND FUNCTIONAL ABNORMALITIES

Neuroradiological Evidence

Structural abnormalities of the brain in OCD have been sought by using various brain imaging techniques, but as yet results have been inconsistent. Using CT scans, Insel et al. (410) found no significant anatomical differences compared with normal controls, whereas others have found that adolescent patients with OCD had a significantly higher mean ventricular brain ratio than controls (411). More recently, Luxenberg et al. suggested involvement of the basal ganglia in the pathogenesis of OCD as CT scanning of young male patients showed reduced caudate volumes (412). Furthermore, there have been several reports of patients showing compulsive stereotypical behavior. Two cases followed carbon monoxide poisoning, one after a wasp sting (413), and one of unknown etiology (414), who had CT scans that showed bilateral cavitation of the basal ganglia. The association of OCD symptoms with some cases of neurological disease that involve dysfunction of the basal ganglia, such as postencephalitic parkinsonism (365–367) and Sydenham's chorea (371, 372), is further evidence to support the involvement of this part of the brain in OCD.

MRI studies have given similar results. Kellner et al. could detect no consistent gross brain anatomical abnormalities on MRI in 12 patients with OCD (415). Garber et al. also found no structural abnormality unique to OCD but observed regional tissue abnormalities, particularly in the orbital frontal cortex, which correlated strongly with symptom severity in patients with OCD (416).

Neuroimaging techniques such as PET, which allow functional rather than anatomical assessment of the brain, have extended the findings of neuroanatomical studies by indicating that orbitofrontal-basal circuitry may mediate OC behavior. PET studies of cerebral glucose metabolism in patients with OCD have found increased rates in the caudate nuclei and left orbital gyri (417, 418); in the left orbitofrontal, right sensorimotor, and bilateral prefrontal and anterior cingulate regions (419); and in both orbital gyri (420). The patients in the latter study who had not been on medication were rescanned after treatment with clomipramine (421). Symptomatic improvement coincided with a return in glucose metabolism to more normal levels in orbital frontal regions as well as the basal ganglia, compared with normal controls. Moreover, those patients who had responded well to treatment showed more marked changes in cerebral glucose metabolism than those who responded poorly.

Neuropsychological Evidence

Encouraged by these neuroradiological findings, researchers have looked for correlating neuropsychological deficits in frontal lobe, basal ganglia, or limbic system functioning in patients with OCD. Earlier studies gave inconsistent results but were methodologically flawed by small sample size, questionable selection criteria for both patients and controls, and choice of test instruments. Neuropsychological testing of OCD patients has detected frontal lobe dysfunction (411, 422–424), memory impairment (423, 425), and reduction of visual-spatial skills, performance IQ, and motor functioning, which are predominantly right-sided activities (410, 422, 423, 426). Recent studies designed to avoid the methodological problems encountered previously found cognitive deficits consistent with basal ganglia or right-hemisphere disturbance but no frontal lobe dysfunction. Boone et al. (427)

revealed subtle visual-spatial and visual-memory deficits in 20 nondepressed OCD patients. These were most pronounced in those with a family history of OCD, but the researchers documented no difference in frontal lobe functioning, verbal memory, attention, or intelligence compared with matched normal controls. Zielinski et al. (428) also noted visual-spatial and nonverbal processing deficits consistent with subcortical or right-hemisphere pathology in 21 patients with OCD, who actually scored equal or better than normal controls on frontal lobe tasks.

Christensen et al. (429) did not find a significant decrease in visual-spatial performance on neuropsychological testing of 18 nondepressed OCD patients compared with 18 nondepressed controls, but did identify a recent nonverbal memory deficit correlating to abnormalities of the limbic and paralimbic areas of the right hemisphere.

The variations in frontal lobe performance between these recent studies and previously reported evidence for frontal lobe impairment in OCD may be due to the inclusion in earlier studies of depressed OCD subjects who may perform poorly on frontal lobe tests. However, quite possibly the frontal lobe tests employed were not sufficiently sensitive to detect abnormalities within specific regions of the frontal lobes, such as the orbital frontal area, in which abnormalities have been detected on radiological studies (416, 419, 420).

Electrophysiological Evidence

Electrophysiological studies of patients with OCD have not been conclusive. Abnormalities in EEG in OC states have been noted from as early as 1944 (375), but they are not present in all patients, and the findings are neither consistent nor pathognomonic. Jenike (430) found that four of 12 patients with OCD had EEG abnormalities over the temporal lobes, but only one improved with antiepileptic medication. Insel et al. (410) found that two of 18 OCD patients had abnormal EEGs, but no difference was detected on their CT brain scans compared with normal controls. Abnormalities in somatosensory and auditory evoked potentials have also been discovered in some OCD patients (431–433), but these have been difficult to interpret. Finally, selective electrical stimulation of the cingulum can produce stereotypical movements (434), but these do not approach the complexity or sophistication of the obsessions and compulsions of OCD.

In summary, these electrophysiological, brain imaging, and neuropsychological studies have yielded somewhat conflicting results. Still, the overall evidence points toward the orbitofrontal and anterior cingulate-basal ganglia-thalamocortical circuits as representing the neuroanatomical substrate for OCD.

BIOCHEMICAL ABNORMALITIES

The Serotonin Hypothesis

The neurotransmitter serotonin or 5-hydroxytryptamine (5-HT) has been implicated to play an important role in the pathogenesis of OCD. Convincing evidence from several different lines of research has led to a serotonergic neurochemical hypothesis for OCD. The studies to date that have investigated such a role for serotonin can be grouped under three main separate headings (435): (a) drug treatment studies, (b) peripheral markers of 5-HT function, and (c) pharmacological challenge studies.

Drug treatment studies. The most impressive evidence for serotonergic involvement in this disorder arises from the numerous drug response studies demonstrating the efficacy of drugs that inhibit neuronal uptake of 5-HT in ameliorating the obsessions and compulsions of OCD. It was first noted in the 1960s that the tricyclic antidepressant clomipramine had antiobsessional properties, even when evidence of an underlying depressive illness was lacking (436–438). Since 1980, clomipramine has been found to be a superior drug in its antiobsessive effects to placebo. Unlike antidepressive drugs, such as amitriptyline, desipramine or clorgyline, which preferentially block uptake of norepinephrine over serotonin, clomipramine has been confirmed in double-blind placebo-controlled trials (322, 334, 339, 439, 440–444). Its efficacy has also been proven in a large recent multicenter trial in the treatment of patients with OCD (445). Although conventional norepinephrine reuptake inhibitor antidepressants are without significant antiobsessional effect (445), the pharmacologically active metabolite of clomipramine, desmethylclomipramine, has noradrenergic reuptake properties, which casts doubt on the belief that serotonin is essential in clomipramine's mechanism of action in the therapy of OCD. One study demonstrated a positive correlation between levels of this metabolite and improvement on symptoms (446), but other researchers have refuted this (334, 447).

Additional evidence for the role of serotonin in OCD came with the development of more selective and potent 5-HT uptake inhibitors. Various studies confirmed their effectiveness in OCD. Thus, double-blind, placebo-controlled clinical trials of fluvoxamine (335–337), fluoxetine (448), and sertraline (449) have confirmed their antiobsessional action and their superiority to desipramine (450). Zimeldine and trazodone, a serotonin 5-HT$_2$ antagonist (451, 452), may also have antiobsessional properties.

The mechanism by which these drugs produce their therapeutic effects in OCD and their interaction with the brain's 5-HT system have not been fully elucidated. Significant reuptake inhibition of 5-HT can be detected after a single administration of a 5-HT reuptake inhibitor, yet it takes several weeks for their antiobsessional therapeutic action to become clinically apparent. There is ample evidence that the long-term administration of 5-HT uptake inhibitors produces changes in 5-HT function, but there is dispute over the direction of such changes. Thus, electrophysiological studies in animals show enhanced postsynaptic 5-HT neurotransmission with the chronic administration of such drugs (453, 454). The drugs appear to inhibit presynaptic autoreceptor 5-HT release. Conversely, down-regulation of the 5-HT$_2$ receptor subtype has been demonstrated after long-term administration of 5-HT uptake inhibitors (455,

456), suggesting that they cause an overall decrease in serotonergic transmission. These differences may be explained by representing a differential action on separate subtypes of 5-HT receptor, of which there are at least eight (457), some of which possess reciprocal functional interaction. Furthermore, these drugs may, by their serotonergic action, induce compensatory alterations in other neurotransmitter systems that are more directly involved in the pathogenesis of OCD (435).

Peripheral markers. The peripheral measurement of serotonin and its metabolites may reflect central nervous system 5-HT neurotransmission. Hence, abnormalities of putative peripheral markers of 5-HT, including whole blood (458, 459) and platelet serotonin concentration (460), imipramine binding in platelets (461–466), and cerebrospinal fluid (CSF) levels of the 5-HT metabolite 5-hydroxyindoleacetic acid (5-HIAA) (440, 461, 467, 468), have been sought in OCD. Although in general no coherent differences have emerged from these peripheral marker studies between patient groups and controls, some subgroups of OCD patients showed evidence of abnormal 5-HT turnover. In one study, OCD patients with a family history of OCD had significantly higher blood 5-HT levels than either those with no family history or normal controls (459). This finding suggests that increased serotonergic activity occurs in this subset. On the other hand, very low levels of the 5-HT metabolite, 5-HIAA have been detected in the CSF of patients with recurrent violent obsessions, implying a decrease in 5-HT turnover (469).

Pharmacological challenge studies. A more direct approach to the investigation of 5-HT receptor function disturbance in OCD was anticipated with the introduction of neuroendocrine probe research. In pharmacological challenge studies, the neuroendocrine, physiological, or behavioral responses to selective serotonergic agents can be interpreted as a measure of the integrity of the hypothalamic serotonergic system. For example, the relative rise or fall in plasma levels of pituitary hormones or cortisol after the administration of such a probe can be monitored, and the observed blunting or enhancement of the normal neuroendocrine response can be interpreted as representing under- or overactivity of 5-HT transmission respectively. Similarly, the exacerbation or amelioration of OC symptoms in patients with OCD, as well as in healthy controls, after serotonergic pharmacological challenge can be viewed as behavioral markers of changes in central 5-HT activity.

Unfortunately, the results of such studies have been confusing and inconclusive. The most frequently used serotonergic probe is a metabolite of trazodone, called *m*-chlorphenylpiperazine (mCPP), which acts as an agonist for certain 5-HT receptor subtypes and may act as an antagonist for others. Administration of this agent reliably causes increases in body temperature and levels of serum prolactin and cortisol in laboratory animals (470) and produces behavioral responses akin to anxiety seen in humans. Nevertheless, mCPP has been given to normal volunteers and patients with OCD with variable results.

Some studies in untreated OCD patients found a blunting of the normal prolactin response but no change in the cortisol response (471, 472), suggesting hyposensitivity of some 5-HT receptors. Another investigator found a blunting of the cortisol rather than the prolactin response (473) and no change in these responses in patients whose symptoms had remitted with SSRI treatment (474). However, another study found enhancement of the cortisol response after treatment.

The discovery that mCPP was not as selective a 5-HT probe as originally thought, having action at noradrenergic, dopaminergic and muscarinic receptors, as well as serotonergic receptors, has led researchers to examine the clinical effects of putative, more selective 5-HT agonists and antagonists. Studies using the 5-HT$_{1A}$ agonist, ipsapirone (475) and the serotonin agonist and reuptake inhibitor fenfluramine (471, 476) showed no difference in prolactin and cortisol between OCD patients and controls. An increase in the prolactin response, however, was observed with intravenous L-tryptophan (472), which is a 5-HT precursor, but it may also alter dopamine transmission (477).

The results of pharmacological challenge studies examining the behavioral responses of OCD patients and normal controls have been equally inconsistent. Thus, the mCPP given to OCD patients induced exacerbations of OC symptoms in some studies (471, 473) but not in others (435, 472). On the other hand, differential anxiety-related responses between subject populations after mCPP challenge that distinguishes OCD from panic disorder have been more consistently observed. In these cases, mCPP failed to produce heightened anxiety in OCD patients (471, 472) but caused panic attacks in patients with panic disorders (478, 479). L-tryptophan fenfluramine, and ipsapirone shown to produce negligible behavioral effects in OCD patients (471, 472, 475, 476). Metergoline, a 5-HT$_1$ and 5-HT$_2$ receptor antagonist, apparently improved obsessional symptoms in untreated patients when given as a single dose (473). But when administered in repeated doses, it reversed the therapeutic effect of clomipramine in OCD patients (480), although these latter results may not have been significant.

The lack of consensus arising from these serotonergic challenge studies may in some part be due to inherent methodological flaws in their design. The symptomatology measured in the studies after a single dose of the pharmacological probe may bear little resemblance to the obsessions and compulsions seen in the clinical setting of OCD, where response to intervention is observed over a much longer period of days or weeks. Furthermore, the behavioral responses observed may have been influenced by environmental triggers, which may be difficult to control. Other variables, such as menstrual cycle or seasonal changes, may alter 5-HT function. Results of earlier neuroendocrine and behavioral challenge studies should be reinterpreted in light of more advanced understanding of the complexity of brain 5-HT pathways and its multiple subsystems and receptors. Barr et al. (435) have tried to reconcile the disparate findings of these studies by proposing that OCD is characterized by neuroendocrine hyposensitivity linked with behavioral hypersensitivity to serotonergic stimulation. Baldwin et al. (481) observed an enhanced prolactin and growth hormone response to L-tryptophan. They hypothesized that dysfunction of 5-HT receptors may be important in the pathogenesis of OCD. Future double-blind placebo-controlled studies using more selective test compounds are required to delineate the precise serotonin deficit underlying this disorder.

Difficulties in the interpretation of the studies implicating 5HT in the pathophysiology of OCD must be due to, at least in part, the fact that there are many 5-HT receptor subtypes ($5\text{-HT}_{1A\text{-}E}$, 5-HT_2, 5-HT_3, 5-HT_4) (435). It has been stated that the ongoing identification of new subtypes of 5-HT receptors makes conclusions based on the specificity of a particular challenge agent problematic (435). We would extend that cautioning to any treatment studies and investigations of peripheral 5-HT receptors.

Dopamine and Other Neurotransmitters

Alternatively, other neurotransmitter systems may be more directly involved in OCD. Challenge studies of the noradrenergic agents clonidine (482, 484) and yohimbine (485) give no firm evidence that significant dysfunction of the noradrenergic system occurs in OCD. However, there is some evidence that the clinically relevant action of SSRIs in OCD is related to the down-regulation of α-adrenergic receptors (486, 488). Exacerbated obsessions and compulsions in two patients with the opiate antagonist naloxone (489) has promoted speculation that opiate receptors may be operational in OC symptomatology.

A more convincing case has been made for the role of dopamine in some forms of OCD following the results of preclinical studies (490). Animal studies have shown that some dopaminergic agents such as L-dopa, bromocryptine, and the stimulant amphetamine, produce stereotypical behavior analogous to the compulsive rituals seen in patients with OCD (491–494). Moreover, the use of such stimulants in humans has been documented to induce purposeful and repetitive actions in previously healthy subjects that closely resemble the compulsions occurring in OCD (495–499). The basal ganglia, an area richly innervated by dopamine-containing and 5-HT-containing neurons, has been implicated as forming part of the neuroanatomical substrate for OCD as a result of the brain imaging and neuropsychological studies just reviewed. Similarly, dopamine neurotransmission is probably affected in both OCD and GTS. GTS is a disorder considered to be due in part to disturbed dopamine metabolism, and the presence obsessions and compulsions in some neurological diseases involving the basal ganglia, support the notion that dopamine neurotransmission is affected in OCD.

Drug response data have strengthened a dopamine-serotonin hypothesis of OCD. SSRIs have been shown to have dopamine-blocking activity (500), which may contribute to their antiobsessional effect. In addition, there are reports that neuroleptic dopamine antagonists have been successfully used in conjunction with a 5-HT uptake inhibitor in the treatment of some cases of GTS concomitant with OCD (274), and OCD unresponsive to the 5-HT uptake inhibitor alone (276). Fluoxetine has been associated with extrapyramidal symptoms similar to those seen with neuroleptic treatment (501–504), and decreased CSF levels of the principal dopamine metabolite homovanillic acid (HVA) have been found following fluoxetine treatment (505). These findings have been interpreted as fluoxetine-facilitating serotonergic inhibition of striatal dopamine neurons. However, clomipramine administration has been associated with increased levels of HVA in the CSF (440). A recent study of CSF neurochemistry in children and adolescents with OCD showed that CSF HVA levels did not correlate with OCD symptoms (506). These conflicting results may be explained by the existence of several forms of OCD, some of which may involve dysregulation of dopamine neurotransmission. The reader is referred to Chapter 9 for a review of neurochemical anatomy.

Family and Genetic Evidence

The few studies that have looked for evidence of a genetic basis to OCD have involved only small numbers of patients, as well as using different methods and diagnostic criteria, so the results have been difficult to interpret. Nevertheless, the data obtained are in favor of an underlying genetic defect in OCD. Twin studies have revealed higher concordance rates for OCD among monozygotic twins than for dizygotic twins (507, 508), as well as OC traits among twins (509–511). In no cases, however, did concordance approach unity, indicating that expression of OCD is probably influenced by nongenetic factors. Most family studies have shown that there is a significantly higher incidence of OCD among FDRs of patients with OCD than in the general population (296, 318, 512–515). Two recent studies, although uncontrolled, employed stricter diagnostic criteria and more stringent methodology than in previous studies by directly interviewing all FDRs of OCD patients (516, 407). The rates of OCD in the parents of such patients were significantly greater than those obtained in the ECA studies that determined the prevalence of OCD in the general population (302). Presenting OC symptoms of probands and their parents were usually dissimilar, arguing against any simple social or cultural transmission.

There is convincing evidence that GTS and OCD share a genetic etiology, but that not all cases of OCD are associated with GTS. The findings from these genetic studies and data described earlier in this chapter suggest that OCD can be divided into at least three categories: (*a*) sporadic (no family history), (*b*) familial (positive family history), and (*c*) OCD associated with a family history of tics or GTS (86). This challenges traditional assumptions of etiological homogeneity in OCD.

Although genetic linkage studies are currently being

conducted in GTS to try to establish a relationship between a marker and the hypothetical gene for the disorder, this methodology has not been used to date in OCD. It is hoped that these techniques will be applied to future research, but until biological markers are identified, the family history of OCD is the strongest evidence suggesting a genetic foundation underlying at least some forms of OCD.

ETIOLOGICAL CONCLUSIONS

Until recently OCD has been the subject of etiological controversy. It is now widely accepted that OCD is a neurobiological entity, and that psychodynamic or cognitive theories of etiology have been unfounded. Brain imaging studies, neuropsychological testing, and the association with some neurological diseases, as well as improvement of OC symptoms after prefrontal leukotomy and cingulotomy, implicate anatomical and functional abnormalities of the orbitofrontal and basal ganglia areas of the brain in OCD patients. The biochemical basis of OCD is being deduced from the success of new drug treatments, neuroendocrine and behavioral data from pharmacological challenge studies, and CSF examination in OCD patients. Despite somewhat conflicting evidence, the dysregulation of cerebral neurotransmitter systems involving serotonin and dopamine is strongly implicated in the pathophysiology of this disorder. In time, the anatomical, functional and biochemical findings may be consolidated, and become more clear, as neuroradiological techniques such as PET and SPECT are refined. Radioligands selective for specific neurotransmitter receptor subtypes can also be applied to examine changes in brain metabolism under different conditions in the living brain. Finally, it appears that OCD is probably not one but several related conditions, and that some cases are inherited.

Diagnosis of OCD

Because of the secretive nature of the disease and the reluctance of sufferers to reveal their symptoms, OCD can be difficult to recognize and diagnose by even the most experienced physicians. Two simple screening questions have been designed to isolate symptoms of the disorder. These questions can be asked routinely in suspected cases, while taking a history, as follows: "Are you bothered by thoughts coming into your mind that make you anxious and that you are unable to get rid of?" "Are there certain behaviors that you do over and over that may seem silly to you or to others but that you feel you just have to do?" (517).

If the answers to these questions are affirmative, the clinician can proceed to inquire further about the nature, frequency, onset, duration, and severity of the obsessions and compulsions expressed by the patient. A thorough assessment of both the psychological and physical status of the patient is desirable in view of the manifold presentation of OCD. Physical symptoms may include skin problems in obsessive hand washers, respiratory and gastrointestinal allergies in obsessive hoarders, hair loss in patients with

trichotillomania, and poor personal hygiene or nutritional status in patients with a fear of contamination of poisoning (518). An accurate evaluation of these patients' psychological status will reveal the presence of comorbid disorders such as depression and anxiety, the symptoms of which may be the presenting features.

A number of standardized inventories or rating scales have been constructed to assess OCD. These have been used both in clinical settings and for research purposes, and in particular to document treatment response. The Leyton Obsessional Inventory (LOI) (519) was the first rating scale to quantify subjective reports of obsessive feelings and behavior. The original inventory consisted of 69 questions and was designed as a supervised card-sorting procedure that gives information about feelings of resistance and interference with other activities, in addition to the straightforward answers to the questions. It has been subsequently administered as a questionnaire (520). Scores differentiate well between obsessional patients and normal volunteer subjects, although it has been criticized for its lack of reliability and validity data, and also because it was originally designed to study houseproud housewives (excessively concerned with cleaning and tidying their homes), and not for OC patients (74). The LOI in its card-sorting form has been adapted for use in the assessment of childhood OCD and is termed the LOI – Child Version. It has been found to reliably distinguish OCD adolescents from normal controls and from other psychiatric patients with severe OC symptoms. It can be also used as a valid instrument in treatment studies (521).

Other rating scales that have been used to tap OC symptomatology are the Sandler-Hazari Scale (522), the Obsessive-Compulsive Check List (523), and Maudsley-Obsessive Comprehensive Inventory (524). Recently the Yale-Brown Obsessive Compulsive Scale (Y-BOCS) has been designed to provide a specific measure of the severity of OCD symptoms independent of the particular type of obsession or compulsion present (525, 526). The Y-BOCS consists of a scale of 10 items, each rated from 0 (no symptoms) to 4 (extreme symptoms), with separate subtotals for severity of obsessions and compulsions. Being a clinician-rated instrument, it avoids the problems of self-assessment, such as resistance to changing self-ratings over a period of time (439). The Y-BOCS has been assessed as a valid instrument suitable for use as an outcome measure in drug trials of OCD (337).

The differential diagnosis of OCD is large and includes all of the associated psychiatric and neurological conditions, such as the other anxiety disorders, depression, GTS, eating disorders, trichotillomania, body dysmorphic syndrome, and personality disorders discussed previously. Misdiagnosis is common because of the overlapping characteristics of OCD and these comorbid conditions. For example, the morbid preoccupations and depressive ruminations that can occur in major depression may be confused with the obsessional thoughts of OCD. The former, however, are seen to be related to depressive symptomatology, such as thoughts of guilt, and there are few attempts to suppress them, in contrast with the obsessions seen in OCD. Likewise, anxiety disorders can be distinguished from OCD by the content of the anxious thoughts being realistic to patients with anxiety and irrational to patients with OCD. The extreme avoidance behavior of some patients with OCD differs from that of the phobic patient in being less effective in providing relief. Other disorders, however, may be more difficult to differentiate from OCD. The complex tics of GTS, for instance, may be identical to compulsions seen in OCD, such as the need to touch or the need for symmetry. Diagnostic accuracy may be paramount in distinguishing whether a GTS patient with complex tics also has comorbid OCD, as recent evidence suggests that such patients who are resistant to treatment with SSRIs alone may respond to a combination of fluvoxamine and a neuroleptic (312, 276).

The diagnosis of OCD is currently an area of confusion and controversy, and the present diagnostic criteria are under review (527). Recent research has led investigators to question the traditional views that obsessions are cognitive and compulsions are behavioral, that obsessions and compulsions can occur independently of each other, that they are always ego-dystonic, and that the sufferer always recognizes that they are senseless. A functional model has been proposed in which a dynamic relationship exists between obsessions and compulsions in which compulsions always occur with obsessions they are designed to neutralize. These compulsions may be thoughts that are formulated to neutralize other thoughts or obsessions, and are thus termed "cognitive compulsions." The other main area of concern is how to establish precise definitions that distinguish OCD accurately from the many conditions that are associated with it. This task cannot be satisfactorily completed until the relationships between OCD and these disorders are fully understood. Most likely, in the future OCD will be regarded as a heterogeneous disorder with separate phenomenological subgroups that require different treatment.

Treatment

There is little evidence that psychoanalysis and dynamic psychotherapy are effective (528, 529) in managing OCD, and these approaches to the treatment of this disorder have largely been abandoned. Advances in behavioral theories and techniques, and more recently in pharmacotherapy, have led to rational and integrated psychopharmacological treatment regimes for a condition that was until a decade ago considered mainly treatment-resistant. Psychosurgery is now reserved as a final option for only the most refractory cases.

BEHAVIOR THERAPY

Meyer was the first to demonstrate that exposure and response prevention was a successful treatment for OCD inpatients (530), and in the past two decades many studies have confirmed the efficacy of behavioral treatments for OCD as well as highlighting their limitations. The most widely evaluated and useful techniques are exposure and response prevention (531). Exposure in-vivo therapy requires the patient to maintain contact with the stimuli that provoke the obsessions or compulsions, until habituation occurs. Response prevention instructs the patients to refrain from ritualistic behavior, despite often overwhelming urges to do so. For example, patients with contamination fears or compulsive washing may be exposed in real life to dirt, blood, or excrement, and prevented from washing. When the anticipated dreaded consequences fail to materialize, the patient's anxiety and symptomatology improve. More recently, exposure in fantasy, or imaginal exposure, in which the patient is asked to think about the feared stimulus without being exposed to it in reality, has been added to reinforce the gains achieved with exposure in vivo, particularly for those patients with catastrophic thinking.

Several follow-up studies have demonstrated significant improvements in OCD symptomatology following exposure therapy after various periods of time, ranging from 1–6 years, depending on the study (446, 532–534). Foa et al. (534) found that 90% of a group of patients treated with exposure and response prevention therapy intensively for 3 weeks experienced some immediate symptomatic improvement, with 80% continuing these benefits after 1 year. Marks reported improvement persisting in up to 75% of patients 2–4½ years after completion of such therapy (315). O'Sullivan et al. (533) showed lasting gains 6 years after the treatment course, and that the best predictor of long-term outcome was improvement at the end of treatment. Moreover, they demonstrated that exposure periods of long duration were more effective than short sessions, with those patients who had had 6 weeks of therapy experiencing more longlasting improvement than those who were subjected to it for only 3 weeks. The treatment period can also be effective with limited therapist contact time.

These encouraging results, however, disguise the fact that a substantial proportion of patients with OCD (up to 30%) refuse or fail to complete behavior therapy because of its arduous time-consuming and often frightening tasks. The high response rates reported in the aforementioned studies reflect the outcome of the most motivated patients. Poor response to behavior therapy is most often seen in those patients with concomitant depression, those who use CNS-depressing drugs, and patients who are obsessional ruminators with no obvious compulsive behaviors (535). Cognitive therapy has been advocated by some authors to use as an adjunct to existing behavioral techniques in the treatment of OCD, based on theories that obsessions and compulsions originate in thoughts (536, 537), but to date, controlled trials are lacking.

Recent studies have shown that the combination of behavior and drug therapies may be the optimum management strategy for OCD. Although O'Sullivan et al. (533) found no benefit of clomipramine over placebo in the long-term outcome of OCD patients who had also been treated with exposure therapy, others have found that clomipramine and behavior techniques have additive effects, at least early on (441, 538). Preliminary findings of trials combining the newer SSRI agents fluvoxamine and fluoxetine with behavioral therapy suggest that one treatment enhances the effectiveness of the other (539, 540).

DRUG THERAPY

Numerous psychotropic drugs have been tried in the past 25 years to control the symptoms of OCD, but only the potent SSRIs have consistently proven beneficial. The tricyclic antidepressant clomipramine was first reported in the 1960s as an effective drug for some patients with obsessional symptoms (436). During the next decade, a number of uncontrolled studies confirmed that it was useful in the treatment of patients with primary OCD (541, 542). Since then, many controlled double-blind studies have demonstrated the superiority of clomipramine over placebo (334, 339, 441, 440, 444). In two recent large multicenter double-blind placebo-controlled studies, involving over 500 outpatients with OCD at 21 different centers in North America (445), clomipramine was found to be significantly superior to placebo on all measures of OC symptom severity. There have been fewer studies that compare the efficacy of clomipramine in the treatment of OCD to that of other drugs classed as antidepressants, but the trend emerges that agents with less potent serotonin reuptake blocking activity are ineffective for reducing obsessions and compulsions.

Thus, double-blind drug treatment studies have demonstrated that clomipramine is superior in its antiobsessional effect to nortriptyline (440), amitryptyline (442), clorgyline (439), imipramine (543), and desipramine (393). These studies also explored the issue that success with clomipramine in patients with OCD could simply reflect an antidepressant effect rather than specific antiobsessional and anticompulsive effects. Ultimately, the findings demonstrated that clomipramine ameliorated OC symptomatology in nondepressed patients (334, 439, 440, 442, 444, 543).

The antiobsessional effect of clomipramine could be the result of its alteration of serotonin transmission. With this theory in mind, in the past 5 years, researchers have experimented with other nontricyclic serotonin reuptake inhibitors that would not (unlike clomipramine) lose their selectivity for blocking serotonin reuptake in vivo, and lack significant activity for histaminic, cholinergic and α-adrenergic receptors. The most rigorously studied has been fluvoxamine, which was shown in a single-blind study (544) and in subsequent double-blind studies (335, 337, 540, 545) to be more effective than placebo in OCD patients. Studies reporting beneficial treatment with fluoxetine have been less rigorously controlled, involving for the most part open trials (546–549).

Few studies directly compare the efficacies of the different SSRIs in OCD. In one controlled comparative study (447), the therapeutic effect of fluoxetine was found to be equivalent to that of clomipramine in OCD patients. In another multicenter double-blind study (550), sertraline was more effective than placebo in reducing OC symptoms, but its drug effect was not as large as that observed in studies of clomipramine and fluvoxamine. Comparing the response rates in independent trials of clomipramine, fluvoxamine, and fluoxetine in OCD patients, no drug emerges as significantly superior in efficacy. Clinician choice therefore depends more on matching the patient with the anticipated side-effect profile than on drug efficacy. Clomipramine, like other tricyclic antidepressants, has anticholinergic side effects, such as weight gain, dry mouth, blurred vision, nausea, and constipation, which may be troublesome. These side effects are less often encountered with the newer SSRIs, although nausea is common with fluvoxamine (335, 337, 545), and insomnia and weight loss can occur with fluoxetine (551).

The empirical use of higher doses of antidepressant drugs in OCD than in depression is common, but there is little evidence that this is necessary. A recent 10-week study showed no advantage for the administration of a daily dose of 40 or 60 mg doses over 20 mg of fluoxetine in OCD patients (552). The antiobsessional effect of these drugs tends to take longer to emerge than the antidepressant effect observed in the treatment of depression, with the initial response sometimes not seen until 4–6 weeks after starting medication (337, 440, 553). A trial of therapy should therefore continue for at least 10 weeks. It is unclear how long maintenance therapy should be continued. One double-blind placebo-controlled study of clomipramine found a 90% rate of relapse within 2 months of discontinuing treatment regardless of whether the duration had been for 4–8 months, 8–12 months, or over 12 months (554). Most clinicians would treat for a period of 6–12 months and then gradually taper the dose, but in view of these high reported relapse rates, patients may need medication indefinitely. There is emerging evidence that treatment with lower doses than those used initially to produce a response may be effective in maintaining OCD patients free of symptoms (555).

Although SSRIs can be very successful in improving the symptoms of some OCD patients, 40–60% of patients exhibit minimal to no change after treatment with an adequate trial of an SSRI alone. These treatment-refractory patients therefore represent a large proportion of the population of OCD sufferers, and a number of different biological therapeutic strategies have been advocated for this group of patients. Although debatable, there may be some value in substituting one SSRI for another if the patient fails to respond to an adequate trial of the first. Combination therapies have also been recommended (553). If a purely antiobsessional regimen is ineffective, several different augmenting agents have been used, mostly based on anecdotal reports of their use in patients who did not respond to more conventional treatment.

Thus, other agents that also modify serotonergic function, such as the amino acid precursor of serotonin tryptophan (556, 557), the serotonin releaser and reuptake blocker fenfluramine (558), and the serotonin type 1A agonist buspirone (415, 420, 423, 559) have been added to ongoing SSRI therapy with variable success. There are also individual case reports and small open case studies that document improvement in OC symptoms when lithium is added to chronic treatment with SSRIs (560-563). Nevertheless, two double-blind trials of lithium addition to ongoing clomipramine (564) and fluvoxamine (565) treatment have failed to show significant benefit. In light of new evidence that brain dopamine transmission may also be involved in the mediation of OC manifestations of some patients with OCD—in particular those with a personal or family history of tics—the role of neuroleptics in the treatment of OCD has been reevaluated. Neuroleptics alone do not seem to be effective, but combination therapy involving treatment with SSRIs and low-dose dopamine-blocking agents may be of use (276), although the hazards of long-term treatment with the latter must be appreciated.

Although OCD is classified as an anxiety disorder there have been only a few reports of idiosyncratic response to anxiolytics such as clonazepam (566, 567) and alprazolam (568, 569) in OCD patients. No systematic studies of their role as augmenting agents exist, but their use in conjunction with SSRIs is quite common, despite the risks of producing dependency with long-term administration. A few uncontrolled studies have reported improvement in OCD symptoms after treatment with monoamine oxidase inhibitors (MAOIs) (570). But a more recent controlled study comparing clomipramine and the selective MAOI clorgyline in OCD patients failed to find any difference between the two groups (439). Trazodone (452), clonidine (571), and antiandrogens (567) have also been described in a few case reports as producing a positive response in patients with OCD, but these results must be considered with caution. Until well-designed controlled studies involving large numbers of patients are undertaken, the use of drugs other than SSRIs in the treatment of OCD remains speculative.

NEUROSURGICAL TREATMENT

Nonpharmacological biological treatments of OCD have included ECT, phototherapy, and psychosurgery. ECT is not generally effective in ameliorating obsessions and compulsions but may be indicated for the treatment of severe depressive or suicidal symptoms in the medication-refractory OCD patient (553). Treatment with bright light therapy in a recent study investigating the role of seasonal symptomatic variation in a small group of OCD patients had no significant effect on symptoms (572).

Neurosurgery is reserved for the minority of patients who fail to respond to behavior therapy and SSRIs and have chronic, unremitting illness for at least 2 years with severe life disruption. Very few "psychosurgical" procedures are now performed, following their unjustifiable overuse with often disastrous consequences in the 1940s and 1950s. Also, it is impossible to perform double-blind controlled trials.

Still, follow-up studies show that of all the disorders treated by neurosurgery, OCD consistently responds best (573). With a greater understanding of functional neuroanatomy, and the development of more precise and accurate techniques, such as stereotactic cryosurgery, thermocoagulation, and multifocal leukocoagulation, adverse effects, such as epilepsy, cognitive deficits, or personality change are rare, and mortality approaches zero. Procedures that interrupt the pathways from the frontal cortex to the basal ganglia, such as cingulotomy, anterior capsulotomy, and orbital frontal leukotomy, are most effective in ameliorating disabling OC symptoms in such patients (574). Follow-up studies show that at least two-thirds of patients improve following psychosurgery (541, 542). The most extensive such study interviewed at a mean of 12-year follow-up 90 patients with OCD who had been operated on between 1960–1974 (573). Thirty percent had completely recovered with no symptoms and required no treatment; 38% were well with mild residual symptoms; 26% had improved but still had significant interfering symptoms; and only 6% remained unchanged, and one was worse. Postoperative epilepsy occurred in only one case; no personality change was detectable to themselves or others in 85% of cases; and operative morbidity was minimal and lasted only a few days after surgery. Relapse was rare unless recurrent depression was also present. These results confirm the efficacy of neurosurgery in chronic, intractable cases of OCD, as well as providing further research data for a neuroanatomical model of this condition.

Summary

The mainstay of treatment of OCD is an 8–12 week trial of pharmacotherapy with one of the SSRIs, which have been shown in double-blind controlled trials to be superior to placebo in improving the symptoms of OCD. There is no convincing evidence to suggest that one SSRI has more efficacy than another, so clinician choice depends on side-effect profile, availability, and patient preference. The duration of treatment should be at least 6 months and often longer, considering the high rates of relapse following cessation of treatment. Although published controlled research support for combination treatments is scanty, augmentation of SSRI treatment with agents such as lithium, buspirone, or a neuroleptic may be useful for the patient who has failed to respond to an SSRI alone, particularly if there is concurrent depression, anxiety disorder, or tics. Neurosurgery is reserved for the most severe refractory cases. Recent evidence suggests that behavior therapy and SSRIs are complementary, and this combination may be the optimum treatment available for the OCD patient. Finally, the importance of education, reassurance, and self-help must not be underestimated. Family therapy and helping the OCD patient to cope at work or school may be as crucial to the outcome for the patient as pharmacobehavioral intervention.

GILLES DE LA TOURETTE SYNDROME AND OBSESSIVE-COMPULSIVE DISORDER—THE LINKS

That GTS and OCD are linked is undisputed, but the precise relationship is complex. Evidence for the connection continues to grow. The link can be viewed from several perspectives, including historical, epidemiological, phenomenological, genetic, and neurochemical, which we consider in detail as follows.

Historical Evidence

The first documentation of GTS was by Itard in 1825 (7) when he described the Marquise de Dampierre. Many years later Charcot saw the Marquise, and his observations were recorded by his student Georges Gilles de la Tourette in 1885. In this account Gilles de la Tourette described the obsessive thoughts that plagued her, as well as her motor tics and vocalizations (575). Charcot, however, was the first neurologist to identify the involuntary "impulsive" ideas, such as doubting mania, double-checking, touching, and arithmomania (an obsession with counting and numbers) as part of GTS and to link these to the impulsive movements (30). Some of these "impulsions" would now be classified as compulsions (current definitions specify that execution of an impulsive deed gives the patient some form of pleasure, satisfaction, or excitement; on the other hand, the patient derives only relief from tension from carrying out the compulsive activity. Thus, impulsive acts are ego-syntonic, whereas compulsive acts are ego-dystonic) (576).

Following Charcot and Gilles de la Tourette's studies, several other 19th century neurologists and physicians became interested in the relationship between these psychological aspects of GTS and its motor and vocal manifestations. Later, in 1899, Gilles de la Tourette (96) documented the anxieties and phobias of his patients, acknowledging the ideas of Guinon (97), who suggested that "tiqueurs" nearly always had associated psychiatric problems characterized by multiple phobias and agoraphobia. Soon after, Grasset in 1890 (577), also referred to the obsessions and phobias of patients, which were to him an accompaniment of the tic disorder, representing psychical tics. Recently, Robertson and Reinstein (98) translated these writings of Gilles de la Tourette, Guinon, and Grasset, illustrating how they described the psychopathology of people with "compulsive tic disorder" with particular reference to OCD, including checking rituals, arithmomania, folie du doute, delire de toucher (forced touching), folie du pourqoui (the irresistible habit of seeking explanations for the most commonplace, insignificant facts by asking perpetual questions) and "mania" for order.

Meige and Feindel (99), in their classic text, "confessions of a victim to tic," described a patient whom they considered to be the prototype of a tic patient. It is now clear that this patient had GTS. He had motor tics that began at the age of 11 years, echophenomena (copying behaviors), a vocal tic

("tic of phonation dating back to his 15th year") and coprolalia ("an impulse to use slang"). He was also impulsive, had suicidal tendencies and OCB. Meige and Feindel (99) stated: "the frequency with which obsessions, or at least a proclivity for them, and tics are associated, cannot be a simple coincidence." They described case histories of their tic patients who had typical features of OCD, including the relief of anxiety, which accompanied the carrying out of a particular motor act. They also noted that often there was no direct connection between a patient's obsessions and the tics, the former occurring in the form of extraordinary scrupulousness, phobias, and excessive punctiliousness in their actions. They mentioned in particular, arithmomania, onomatomania (the dread of uttering a forbidden word or the impulse to intercollate another) and folie du pourquoi.

Kinnear-Wilson (578) also acknowledged a relationship between tics and OCD: "no feature is more prominent in tics than its irresistibility...The element of compulsion links the condition intimately to the vast group of obsessions and fixed ideas." Later, Ascher (579) reported that all of the five GTS patients he reported had obsessive personalities, while Bockner (287) noted that the majority of GTS cases described in the literature had OC neurosis.

Epidemiological Evidence

These historical findings and speculations were based primarily on anecdotal descriptions of single case studies to reveal a more definite link between OC symptomatology and GTS. Shapiro et al. (30) divided the history of GTS into seven periods, starting in 1825 with the first description. The fourth period, called "Epidemiology and Reviews," commenced in 1954 with the retrospective studies of Zausmer (580), but it was not until 1962 that Torup (581) documented the frequency of obsessional symptoms, traits, or illness in a population of GTS patients. In a study of 237 children treated for tics between 1946–1947 in Denmark, 12% were judged to have a compulsive behavior pattern (581). Since that investigation, many epidemiological studies have revealed significant percentages of GTS and tic patient populations experiencing some form of OC phenomena. These reported rates have, in general, tended to increase in recent years. Thus, Kelman in 1965 (71), Fernando in 1967 (72) and Corbett et al. in 1969 (73) reported figures of 11%, 31%, and 12.5% respectively, whereas by the 1970s and 1980s, some investigators recorded rates reaching far higher figures, for example, 32% (70), 33% (18), 38% (41), and even some as high as 60% (88), 66% (135), 68% (33), 71% (134), 74% (84), and 80% (85). The earlier lower figures may have resulted from a variety of causes, including the use of less specific measures to assess OCD, differences in the definition of OCD, or an unusually high frequency of OCD in control studies (30).

It should be noted, however, that the Shapiros (107, 582, 583) have consistently failed to observe an association between GTS and any specific psychiatric syndrome or psychodynamic factors. In a controlled study employing the Minnesota Multiphasic Personality Inventory (MMPI), a group of GTS patients failed to differ significantly from general psychiatric outpatients on factors such as overt and underlying psychosis, OC traits, inhibition of hostility, hysteria, and general maladjustment (30). They also found OC traits in 12.8% of GTS patients and in 14.6% of controls (30). They did acknowledge, however, that only one GTS patient of 34 was free from psychiatric illness, the majority being diagnosed as having various types of "personality disorders." They pointed out, in addition, that there may be a subgroup of GTS patients who have substantial difficulty with OC rituals (30).

Lifetime prevalence of OCD ranges from 1.9% to 3.2%, despite problems with the definition of OCD and its differentiation from other psychiatric diagnoses (especially anxiety disorders and depression). Apparently, the prevalence of OCD in patients with GTS is much greater than would be expected by chance alone. In this context, since 1987, the diagnoses of OCD and GTS are no longer mutually exclusive according to accepted diagnostic conventions. Thus, in its definition of OCD, DSM-III in 1980 stated that the obsessions or compulsions must not be due to another mental disorder, such as GTS, schizophrenia, major depression, or organic mental disorder (3), whereas the current DSM-IV published in 1994 states that in some people with GTS, an associated diagnosis is OCD (1).

More recent investigations have employed specially designed inventories to assess the incidence of OCD among GTS patients and normal controls. Thus, Frankel and colleagues (584) used a questionnaire derived from the LOI in their controlled study of British and American patients with GTS, American patients with OCD, and normal control American subjects, reporting that 47% of GTS males and 86% of GTS females met diagnostic criteria for OCD. Green and Pitman (585) also found more OC problems in GTS patients compared with controls. Caine et al. (21) reported that 49% of the 41 patients in their epidemiological study of Monroe County (New York) school children had obsessional ideas or associated ritualistic behavior, although only three were significantly impaired to warrant a diagnosis of OCD; this study was limited in that it included only children.

Van de Wetering et al. (42) in a controlled study, used a Dutch version of the LOI on 66 Dutch GTS patients and reported that 47% admitted to obsessive rituals, 18% to obsessive thoughts, and 4% to obsessive imaging. Robertson and colleagues (38) used both the LOI and the obsessional scale of the Crown Crisp Experiential Index (CCEI, previously known as the Middlesex Hospital Questionnaire) and found that 37% of 90 GTS patients in the U.K. reported OCB. In this study, coprolalia and echophenomena were significantly associated with OC phenomena. However, the use of different questionnaires or scales in these studies, the varying sample sizes, and cultural differences may all contribute to the diversity of figures obtained.

There have been far fewer investigations demonstrating the occurrence of tics and other associated features of GTS, such as coprolalia, echophenomena, and ADD in OCD patients. Rasmussen and Tsuang (586) reported a prevalence of 5% of GTS in OCD patients, which is still greater than the generally accepted figure of 0.5/1000 for GTS in the general population (17). Pitman et al. (587), in their study of 16 GTS outpatients, 16 OCD outpatients, and 16 normal controls, reported that 37% (six patients) of the OCD group satisfied criteria for any tic disorder (only one patient met criteria for GTS), compared with only one subject in their control group. Ten patients (63%) in the GTS group, however, met criteria for OCD. These figures suggest that although OCD might now be considered an integral part of GTS (6), the majority of OCD subjects do not suffer from a tic disorder, and may represent a separate etiological group. Rappoport (293) suggests that some 20% of OCD patients have tics.

Phenomenological Evidence

This area has not been extensively explored, although recent studies have attempted to define the precise phenomenology of the OC thoughts and behaviors that occur in GTS patients, to relate these to other variables, and to compare them to the symptomatology that occurs in OCD patients without a tic disorder. Pitman et al. (587) reported that certain kinds of compulsive behaviors, such as touching and symmetry behaviors ("evening-up" rituals to ensure that the body is symmetrical or balanced), occurred more often in the GTS patients than in an OCD group, although some GTS patients exhibited compulsions such as checking, washing, and counting. Similarly, the types of tics occurring in those OCD patients suffering from a tic disorder were not unlike those commonly experienced by GTS patients, such as eye-blinking, and noises, such as humming, sniffing, and throat-clearing. They also noted other phenomena that occurred at much higher rates in both the GTS and OCD groups than in the control sample, such as pathological doubt, slowness, and depersonalization. Both groups also shared high rates of unipolar depressive illness and generalized anxiety disorder compared with the controls. These results led the authors to propose "the notion of a symptomatic continuum from simple tic to complex tic to compulsion" (587). However, despite the large symptomatic overlap, the two conditions were not phenomenologically identical. Echophenomena, a history of ADD, and SIB occurred frequently in GTS but not in OCD patients, whereas phobic and panic disorders were much more common in the OCD group (587).

An overlap in the type of OC symptoms experienced by GTS and non-GTS OCD patients (including checking and fear of contamination) was also reported by Frankel et al. (584). In addition, they documented that symptomatology changed with age in GTS patients, with younger individuals exhibiting compulsive behaviors related to impulse control, and older patients manifesting behaviors more classically associated with OCD, such as checking, arranging, and fear of contamination (584).

George et al. (588) studied prospectively 10 subjects with OCD and 15 with OCD and comorbid GTS using the Y-BOCS, the LOI and a new questionnaire designed to emphasize the differences in symptoms between these two groups. Results showed that subjects with comorbid OCD and GTS had significantly more violent, sexual, and symmetrical obsessions and more touching, blinking, counting, and self-damaging compulsions. The group with OCD alone had more obsessions concerning dirt or germs and more cleaning compulsions. The subjects who had both disorders reported that their compulsions arose spontaneously, whereas the subjects with OCD alone reported that their compulsions were frequently preceded by cognitions (588).

Leckman et al. (589) examined OC symptoms in 177 patients with OCD, of whom 56 were tic-related and 121 had non-tic-related OCD. Patients with tic-related OCD reported more OC symptoms, including more aggressive, religious, and sexual obsessions, as well as checking, counting, ordering, touching and hoarding compulsions than did patients with non-tic-related OCD.

Eapen, Pauls, and Robertson (in preparation) also examined patients with primary GTS and compared them with patients with GTS and OCD. Patients with OCD had significantly more obsessions to do with dirt, germs, contamination, and fear of something bad happening, and compulsions concerned with washing and cleaning.

Others have suggested that the frequency of OC symptoms increases with the duration of GTS (135). However, Robertson et al. (38) failed to demonstrate a significant relationship of OC symptoms with either age or duration of GTS. Robertson et al. (38) compared adults with GTS with depressed adults and normal controls on questionnaires measuring obsessionality, depression, and anxiety. The GTS and depressed groups both scored significantly higher than the normal controls on all measures. The GTS subjects, however, had similar scores on measures of obsessionality to those of the depressed subjects but significantly lower scores on measures of depression and anxiety. This suggests that obsessionality is a prominent feature of GTS, and that the psychopathological profile is different from that of patients with major depressive disorder.

Coprolalia, on the other hand, has rarely been described in OCD patients. Pitman and Jenike (590), however, presented a single case history of a man who fulfilled DSM-III-R (200) criteria for OCD, who had manifested coprolalia since the age of 6, but otherwise did not satisfy criteria for a diagnosis of GTS. They emphasized that this case further blurred the phenomenological distinction between the two disorders, and remind us that both Janet (380), and Meige and Feindel (99) also observed an association between coprolalia and obsessions almost a century ago.

Others have also observed that GTS and OCD share clinical features, such as waxing and waning of symptoms, early age at onset, lifelong course, ego-dystonic behavior, worsening with depression, and anxiety, and their occurrence in the same families (33, 591).

Evidence from Family and Genetic Studies

As noted previously, researchers have suggested that genetic factors are involved in GTS and possibly OCD. Having established that they are inherited disorders, these investigations went on to look for a genetic relationship between GTS and OCD.

Among the studies that reported concordant monozygotic (MZ) twin sets was the work of Jenkins and Ashby (192). In that study, both twins were described as obsessional. A triplet study in which the triplets were reared apart showed 100% concordance for GTS but not OCD (592).

In several family studies of GTS, relatives with OCB but without tics or GTS have been reported (25, 27, 86, 593). As part of a large family study of GTS, Pauls et al. (594) interviewed 90% of all FDRs of 32 GTS probands, as well as obtaining family history reports about each family member from all available data obtained. Although the authors acknowledge the difficulties in making an accurate diagnosis of OCD, they found the frequency of OCD diagnoses among these FDRs significantly higher (nine to 13 times) than the frequency of OCD estimated in the general population from the ECA study in which similar methodology was employed (302). Furthermore, the rates of GTS and OCD were practically the same in families of GTS probands with OCD as in families of GTS probands without OCD. In addition, the frequency of OCD without GTS among FDRs was significantly elevated, particularly among the female relatives, in both groups of families. Subsequent segregation analysis performed on these results gave further support to the autosomal-dominant model for GTS, but also indicated that in at least a proportion of cases, GTS and OCD constitute alternate expressions of the same autosomal-dominant gene, and that this expression may be sex-specific (593).

Eapen et al. (28) performed complex segregation analyses on families ascertained through 40 unselected consecutive GTS patients (168 FDRs, all of whom were directly interviewed). Results were consistent with an autosomal-dominant gene with high penetrance. Moreover, their results showed that OCB was an integral part of the expression of GTS, whereas within the families, motor tics (chronic or transient) may not always be etiologically or genetically related to GTS.

In summary, twin, family and, more importantly, complex segregation analysis studies strongly suggest that a genetic relationship exists between GTS and OCB.

Neurochemical and Neuroanatomical Evidence

The evidence presented thus far would suggest that GTS and OCD share some common neurochemical and neuroanatomical bases. As stated earlier, in GTS patients, PM and neuroimaging studies suggest structural and functional abnormalities in the basal ganglia, cingulum, and frontal areas. Also, the absence of premovement potentials prior to the tics indicates that the movements are subcortical in origin

(139). In OCD, similar studies suggest orbitofrontal, anterior cingulate-basal ganglia-thalamocortical circuits as the neuroanatomical substrate.

Unfortunately, to date, direct evidence to support this hypothesis is scarce. So far, a unique neurochemical abnormality has not been established in either condition. Dopamine is, however, thought to be the main neurotransmitter involved in GTS, while serotonin, not dopamine, is considered the major neurotransmitter involved in OCD. But results from recent treatment and electrophysiological studies do not exclude the possibility that dopamine abnormalities may also be involved in OCD (595). Although OCD responds poorly to dopamine antagonist drugs alone, McDougle et al. (596) found that in an open trial, nine of 17 fluvoxamine-resistant OCD patients responded to combined fluvoxamine-dopamine antagonist treatment. Several studies are underway examining the efficacy of combined SSRIs and dopamine antagonists in the treatment of OCD. Quite possibly, the OCD patients who respond to such combined treatment could represent the subgroup proposed above that is associated with a family history of GTS.

Although researchers on the whole have not concluded that serotonin is involved in the pathophysiology of GTS (176), others (74) suggest that it may be a hyposerotonergic condition. In addition, recent reports (551) have shown the successful treatment of OC symptoms in GTS patients with both clomipramine and fluoxetine, the latter drug also decreasing the severity of tics in one patient. The use of other forms of treatment of GTS and OCD also highlights the similarities and differences between the two conditions.

Formal psychoanalytic psychotherapy is now widely considered to have little place in the treatment of either disorder (597). Behavioral therapy has been the first line of treatment in OCD for over 20 years. This is still the case, despite a 25% failure rate, high rates of refusal, and dropout among otherwise suitable patients, and recent evidence that combining exposure therapy with SSRIs may be more effective than exposure alone (333, 537, 540). By contrast, behavioral therapy is no longer thought to be effective in ameliorating the tics and vocalizations of GTS, and this practice has largely been abandoned (6). Thus, combined drug therapy and behavior therapy would appear to be the treatment of choice for OCD with GTS.

To summarize, despite differences in the effectiveness of pharmacological treatment in the two disorders, the tics, vocalizations, and OCD in GTS patients and their relatives may be products of common neurophysiological disturbances. The striatum and limbic system receive extensive projections from both dopamine and serotonin transmitter systems. Disturbances in these parts of the brain could be responsible for dopamine-mediated tics and vocalizations, and serotonin-medicated obsessions and compulsions in these patients.

OCD and GTS Conclusions

The evidence we have presented suggests that both GTS and OCD have a genetic basis, which in some cases is linked and results in common neurochemical abnormalities. The phenotype of the anticipated GTS gene(s) may be expressed as a spectrum of symptoms with chronic multiple tics (CMTs) or GTS alone at one end, and some types of OCD at the other. This GTS-associated OCD appears to represent a separate subcategory of the DSM-III-R defined OCD, indicating that OCD in its entirety may be comprised of a heterogeneous group of conditions of different etiology. If so, it would be necessary to reevaluate both the classification and treatment of OCD. Future studies are needed to confirm these conclusions, and the results from the ongoing genetic linkage studies and the combined treatment studies are eagerly awaited.

In conclusion, therefore, at least some types of OCD (e.g., OCB) are probably an integral part of GTS. In this context, it is interesting to note that Pierre Janet in 1903 (380), in his treatise *Les Obsessions et la Psychasthenie*, described three stages of psychasthenic illness: the first was the "psychasthenic state," the second "forced agitations," which included motor tics, while the third was obsessions and compulsions (598).

References

1. American Psychiatric Association. Diagnostic and Statistical Manual of Mental Disorders. 4th ed. Washington, D.C.: American Psychiatric Association, 1994.
2. World Health Organization. International classification of diseases and health related problems. 10th revision. Geneva, Switzerland: World Health Organization, 1992.
3. American Psychiatric Association. Diagnostic and statistical manual of mental disorders. 3rd ed. Washington, D.C.: American Psychiatric Association, 1980.
4. Araneta E, Magen J, Musci MN, et al. Gilles de la Tourette's syndrome symptom onset at age 35. Child Psychiatry Hum Dev 1975;5:224–230.
5. Marneros A. Adult onset of Tourette's syndrome: a case report. Am J Psychiatry 1983;140:924–925.
6. Robertson MM. The Gilles de la Tourette syndrome: the current status. Br J Psychiatry 1989;154:147–169.
7. Itard JMG. Memoire sur quelques fonctions involuntaires des appareils de la locomotion de la prehension et de la voix. Arch Gen Med 1825;8:385–407.
8. Gilles de la Tourette G. Etude sur une affection nerveuse caracterisee par de l'incoordination motrice accompagnee d-echolalie et de copralalie. Arch Neurol 1885;9:19-24,158–200.
9. Lees AJ, Robertson MM, Trimble MR, et al. A clinical study of Gilles de la Tourette syndrome in the United Kingdom. J Neurol Neurosurg Psychiatry 1984;47:1–8.
10. McHenry LC Jr. Samuel Johnson's tics and gesticulations. J Hist Med Allied Sci 1967;22:152–168.
11. Murray TJ. Dr. Samuel Johnson's movement disorders. Br Med J 1979;i:1610–1614.
12. Fog R, Regeur L. Did WA Mozart suffer from Tourette's syndrome? World Congress of Psychiatry Abstracts VII 1983;F401:342.
13. Gunne L. Hade Mozart Tourette's syndrome? Lakartingen 1991;66:4325–4326.
14. Simkin B. Mozart's scatological disorder. Br Med J 1992;305:1563–1567.
15. Davies PJ. Mozart's scatological disorder. Br Med J 1993;306:521–522.
16. Karhausen LR. Mozart's scatological disorder. Br Med J 1993;306:522.
17. Bruun RD. Gilles de la Tourette's syndrome: an overview of clinical experience. J Am Acad Child Adolesc Psychiatry 1984;23:126–133.
18. Abuzzahab FE, Anderson FO. Gilles de la Tourette's syndrome. Minn Med 1973;56:492–496.

19. Tanner CM. Epidemiology. In: Kurlan R, ed. Handbook of Tourettes and related tic disorders. New York: Marcel Dekker, 1993:337–344.

20. Burd L, Kerbeshian J, Wikenheiser M, et al. Prevalence of Gilles de la Tourette's syndrome in North Dakota adults. Am J Psychiatry 1986;143:787–788.

21. Caine ED, McBride MC, Chiverton P, Bamford KA, Rediess S, Shiao J. Tourette syndrome in Monroe County school children. Neurology 1988;38:472–475.

22. Comings DE, Himes JA, Comings BG. An epidemiologic study of Tourette's syndrome in a single school district. J Clin Psych 1990;51:463–469.

23. Apter A, Pauls DL, Bleich A, et al. A population based epidemiological study of Tourette's syndrome among adolescents in Israel. In: Chase TN, Friedhoff AJ, Cohen DJ, eds. Advances in neurology, vol 58. Tourette syndrome; genetics, neurobiology and treatment. New York: Raven Press, 1992:62–66.

24. Hajal F, Leach AM. Familial aspects of Gilles de la Tourette syndrome. Am J Psych 1981;138:90–92.

25. Kurlan R, Behr J, Medved L, et al. Familial Tourette's syndrome: report of a large pedigree and potential for linkage analysis. Neurology 1986;36:772–776.

26. Kurlan R, Behr J, Medved L, et al. Severity of Tourette's syndrome in one large kindred: implication for determination of disease prevalence rate. Neurology 1987;44:268–269.

27. Robertson MM, Gourdie A. Familial Tourette's syndrome in a large British pedigree: associated psychopathology, severity and potential for linkage analysis. Br J Psychiatry 1990;156:515–521.

28. Eapen V, Pauls DL, Robertson MM. Evidence of autosomal dominant transmission in Tourette's syndrome. United Kingdom cohort study. Br J Psychiatry 1993;162:593–596.

29. Kurlan R. Tourette's syndrome in a special education population. Hypotheses. Adv Neurol 1992a;58:75–81.

30. Shapiro AK, Shapiro E, Bruun RD, Sweet RD. Gilles de la Tourette syndrome. New York: Raven Press, 1978.

31. Golden GS. Psychologic and neuropsychologic aspects of Tourette's syndrome. Neurol Clin 1984;21:91–102.

32. Shapiro AK, Shapiro ES, Young JG, Fineberg TE. Gilles de la Tourette syndrome. New York: Raven Press, 1988.

33. Nee LE, Caine ED, Polinsky RJ, Edlridge R, Ebert MH. Gilles de la Tourette syndrome: clinical and family study of 50 cases. Ann Neurol 1980;7:41–49.

34. Kidd KK, Prusoff BA, Cohen DJ. The familial pattern of Tourette syndrome. Arch Gen Psychiatry 1980;37:1336–1339.

35. Jagger J, Prusoff BA, Cohen DJ, Kidd KK, Carbonari CM, John K. The epidemiology of Tourette's syndrome: a pilot study. Schizoph Bull 1982;8:267–278.

36. Comings DE, Devor EJ, Cloninger CR. Detection of a major gene for Gilles de la Tourette syndrome. Am J Hum Genet 1984;36:586–600.

37. Erenberger G, Cruse RP, Rothner AD. Tourette syndrome: an analysis of 200 pediatric and adolescent cases. Clev Clin J Med 1986;53:127–131.

38. Robertson MM, Trimble MR, Lees AJ. The psychopathology of Gilles de la Tourette syndrome: a phenomenological analysis. Br J Psychiatry 1988;152:383–390.

39. Robertson MM, Trimble MR, Lees AJ. Self-injurious behavior and the Gilles de la Tourette syndrome. A clinical study and review of the literature. Psychol Med 1989;19:611–625.

40. Robertson MM, Channon S, Baker J, Flynn D. The psychopathology of Gilles de la Tourette's syndrome: a controlled study. Br J Psychiatry 1993;162:114–117.

41. Asam U. A follow-up study of Tourette syndrome. In: Friedhoff AJ, Chase TN, eds. Gilles de la Tourette syndrome. Advances in neurology, vol 35. New York: Raven Press, 1982:225–232.

42. Van de Wetering BJM, Cohen AP, Minderaa RB, et al. Het syndroom van Gilles de la Tourette: Klinische Bevindigen. Ned Tijdschr Geneeskd 1988;132:21–25.

43. Regeur L, Pakkenberg B, Fog R, et al. Clinical features and long-term treatment with pimozide in 65 patients with Gilles de la Tourette's syndrome. J Neurol Neurosurg Psychiatry 1986;49:791–795.

44. Debray-Ritzen P, Dubois H. Maladies des tics de l'enfant. Rev Neurol 1980;136:15–18.

45. Robertson MM, Verrill M, Mercer M, James B, Pauls DL. The Gilles de la Tourette syndrome in New Zealand. A postal survey. Br J Psychiatry 1994;164:263–266.

46. Wand RR, Fulton WA, Shady GA, et al. Tourette syndrome and medical treatment in Canada. Neurosci Biobehav Rev 1988;12:229–231.

47. Morkovkin AV, Chekhonin VP, Kammenykh LN. Immunoenzyme method of determining the specific cerebral alpha 2-globulin in the blood serum of children with Tourette syndrome. Zh Nevropatol Psikhiatrii 1986;86:1474–1476.

48. Pushkov VV. Treatment of Tourette syndrome. Zh Nevropatol Psikhiatrii 1986;86:1476–1479.

49. Schelkunov El, Kenunen OG, Pushkov VV, et al. Heart rate, blood pressure regulation and neurotransmitter balance in Tourette's syndrome. J Am Acad Child Adolesc Psychiatry 1986;25:645–652.

50. Kondo K, Nomura Y. Tourette syndrome in Japan: etiologic considerations based on associated factors and familial clustering. In: Friedhoff AJ, Chase TN, eds. Gilles de la Tourette syndrome. Advances in neurology, vol 35. New York: Raven Press, 1982:271–276.

51. Nomura Y, Segawa M. Tourette syndrome in the Chinese: a follow up of 15 cases. In: Friedhoff AJ, Chase TN, eds. Gilles de la Tourette syndrome. Advances in Neurology, vol 35. New York: Raven Press, 1992:277–280.

52. Min SK, Lee H. A clinical study of Gilles de la Tourette syndrome in Korea. Br J Psychiatry 1986;149:644–647.

53. Lieh Mak F, Chung SY, Lee P, Chen S, eds. Tourette syndrome in the Chinese: a follow up of fifteen cases. Adv Neurol 1982;35:281–284.

54. Bai CH, Han-Quin LF. Tourette's syndrome; report of nineteen cases. Chin Med J 1983;96:45–48.

55. Chen HB, Lu Fei HQ. Tourette syndrome. Report of nineteen cases. Chin Med J 1983;96:45–50.

56. Menawat AS, Singh HB, Panwar RB, et al. Gilles de la Tourette's disease (report of a family). J Assoc Physicians India 1980;28:241–244.

57. Eapen V, Srinath S. Descriptive study of tic disorders in children. Indian Journal of Psychology and Medicine 1990;83–92.

58. Eapen V, Srinath S. Gilles de la Tourette syndrome in India—two cases. Psychol Rep 1992;70:1–2.

59. Salmi K. Gilles de la Tourette's disease. The report of a case and its treatment. Acta Psychiatr Scand 1961;36:156–162.

60. Eapen V, Robertson MM. Gilles de la Tourette syndrome—a case report from Guyana in South America. Behav Neurol 1992;5;39–41.

61. Eapen V, Robertson MM. Gilles de la Tourette Syndrome in Malta—psychopathology in a multiply affected pedigree. Arab J Psychiatry 1995;6:113–118.

62. El-Assra A. A case of Gilles de la Tourette's syndrome in Saudi Arabia. Br J Psychiatry 1987;151:397–398.

63. Robertson M, Trimble MR. Gilles de la Tourette syndrome in the Middle East. Report of a cohort and a multiply affected pedigree. Br J Psychiatry 1991;158:416–419.

64. Eldridge R, Sweet R, Lake CR, Shapiro AK. Gilles de la Tourette's syndrome: clinical, genetic, psychologic, and biochemical aspects in 21 selected families. Neurology 1977;27:115–124.

65. Wassman ER, Eldridge R, Abuzzahab IS Sr, Nee L. Gilles de la Tourette syndrome: clinical and genetic studies in a mid western city. Neurology (Minneap) 1978;28:304–307.

66. Moldofsky H, Tullis C, Lamon R. Multiple tics syndrome (Gilles de la Tourette's syndrome). J Nerv Ment Dis 1974;15:282–292.

67. Erenberger G, Rothner AD. Tourette syndrome: a childhood disorder. Clev Clin J Med 1978;45:207–212.

68. Golden GS, Hood OJ. Tics and tremors. Pediatr Clin North Am 1982;29:95–103.

69. Lucas AR, Beard CM, Rajput AH, et al. Tourette syndrome in Rochester, Minnesota, 1968–1979. In: Friedhoff AJ, Chase TM, eds. Gilles de la Tourette syndrome. Advances in Neurology, vol 35. New York: Raven Press, 1982:267–269.

70. Comings DE, Comings BG. Tourette syndrome: clinical and psychological aspects of 250 cases. Am J Hum Genet 1985;37:435–450.

71. Kelman DH. Gilles de la Tourette's disease in children: a review of the literature. J Child Psychol Psychiatry 1965;6:219–226.

72. Fernando SJM. Gilles de la Tourette's syndrome: a report on four cases and a review of published case reports. Br J Psychiatry 1967;113:607–617.

73. Corbett JA, Matthews AM, Connell PH. Tics and Gilles de la Tourette's syndrome: a follow-up study and critical review. Br J Psychiatry 1969;115:1229–1241.

74. Yaryura-Tobias JA, Neziroglu F. Obsessive compulsive disorders: pathogenesis, diagnosis, and treatment. New York: Marcel Dekker, 1983.

75. Lang AE. Premonitory ("sensory") experiences. In: Kurlan R, ed. Handbook of Tourette's and related disorders. New York: Marcel Dekker, 1993:17–26.

76. Bruun RD, Budman CL. The natural history of Tourette's syndrome. In: Chase TN, Friedhoff AJ, Cohen DJ, eds. Tourette's syndrome: genetics, neurobiology and treatment. Advances in Neurology, vol 58. New York: Raven Press, 1992:1–6.

77. McMahon WM, Leppert M, Filloux F, et al. Tourette's syndrome in 161 related family members. Adv Neurol 1992;58:159–165.

78. Nomura Y, Segawa M. Tourette syndrome in Oriental children: clinical and pathophysiological considerations. Adv Neurol 1982;36:277–280.

79. Butler IJ. Tourette's syndrome. Some new concepts. Neurol Clin 1984;2:571–580.

80. Robertson MM, Eapen V. Pharmacologic Controversy of CNS stimulants in Gilles de la Tourette syndrome. Clin Neuropharmacol 1992;15, 5:408–425.

81. Glaze DG, Jankovic J, Frost JD. Sleep in Gilles de la Tourette syndrome: disorder of arousal. Neurology 1982;32:586–592.

82. Incagnoli T, Kane R. Developmental perspective of the Gilles de la Tourette syndrome. Percept Mot Skills 1983;57:1271–1281.

83. Leckman JF, Cohen DJ. Recent advances in Gilles de la Tourette syndrome: implications for clinical practice and future research. Psychiatric Developments 1983;3:301–316.

84. Stefl ME. Mental health needs associated with Tourette syndrome. Am J Public Health 1984;74:1310–1313.

85. Yaryura-Tobias JA, Neziroglu F, Howard S, et al. Clinical aspects of Gilles de la Tourette syndrome. Journal of Orthomolecular Psychiatry 1981;10:263–268.

86. Comings DE, Comings BG. Hereditary agoraphobia and obsessive-compulsive behavior in relatives of patients with Gilles de la Tourette's syndrome. Br J Psychiatry 1987;151:195–199.

87. Minderaa RB, Van Gemert TM, Van De Wetering BJM. Onverwachte presentatiewijzen van het symdroom van Gilles de la Tourette. Tijdschrift voor Psychiatrie 1988;30:246–254.

88. Hagin RA, Beecher R, Pagano G, et al. Effects of Tourette syndrome on learning. In: Friedhoff AJ, Chase TN, eds. Gilles de la Tourette syndrome. Advances in neurology, vol. 35. New York: Raven Press, 1982.

89. Mendelson WB, Caine ED, Goyer P, et al. Sleep in Gilles de la Tourette syndrome. Biol Psychiatry 1980;15:339–343.

90. Barabas G, Matthews WS, Ferrari M. Somnambulism in children with Tourette syndrome. Dev Med Child Neurol 1984;26:457–460.

91. Barabas G, Matthews WS, Ferrari M. Disorders of arousal in Gilles de la Tourette's syndrome. Neurology 1984;34:815–817.

92. Erenberg G. Sleep disorders in Gilles de la Tourette syndrome. Neurology 1985;35:1397.

92a. Barabas G, Matthews WS, Ferrari M. Sleep disorders in Gilles de la Tourette's syndrome. Neurology 1985;35:1397.

93. Bock R, Goldberger L. Tonic, phasic and cortical arousal in Gilles de

94. Barabas G, Matthews WS, Ferrari M. Tourette's syndrome and migraine. Arch Neurol 1984;41:871–872.

95. Smith RA. Inheritance and epidemiology of headache. In: Dalessio DJ, ed. Wolff's headache and other head pain. 4th ed. Oxford University Press, 1980:339–344.

96. Gilles de la Tourette G. La maladie des tics convulsifs. La Sem Med 1899;19:153–156.

97. Guinon G. Sur la maladie des tics convulsifs. Rev Med 1886;6:50–80.

98. Robertson MM, Reinstein DZ. Convulsive Tic Disorder Georges Gilles de la Tourette, Guinon and Grasset on the phenomenology and psychopathology of Gilles de la Tourette syndrome. Behavioral Neurology 1991;4:29–56.

99. Meige H, Feindel E. Tics and their treatment. Translated and edited by SAK Wilson. New York: William Wood and Co., 1907.

100. Ferenczi S. Psycho-analytic observations on tic. Int J Psychoanal 1921;2:1–30.

101. Mahler MS, Rangell L. A Psychosomatic study of maladie des tics (Gilles de la Tourette's disease). Psychiatry Q 1943;17:579–603.

102. Mahler MS. Tics and impulsions in children: a study of motility. Psychoanal 1944;13:430–444.

103. Mahler MS, Luke JA, Daltroff W. Clinical and follow up study of the tic syndrome in children. Am J Orthopsychiatry 1945;15:631–647.

104. Mahler MS, Luke JA. Outcome of the tic syndrome. J Nerv Ment Dis 1946;103:433–445.

105. Fenichel O. The psychoanalytic theory of neurosis. New York: Norton and Company, 1945.

106. Heuscher JE. Intermediate states of consciousness in patients with generalized tics. J Nerv Ment Dis 1953;117:29–38.

107. Shapiro AK, Shapiro ES. Tourette syndrome; history and present status. In: Friedhoff AJ, Chase TN, eds. The Gilles de la Tourette syndrome. Advances in neurology, vol 35. New York: Raven Press, 1982:17–23.

108. Comings DE. A controlled study of Tourette syndrome. VII. Summary. A common genetic disorder due to disinhibition of the limbic system. Am J Hum Genet 1987;41:839–836.

109. Comings DE, Comings BG. A controlled study of Tourette syndrome, I-VII. Am J Hum Gen 1987;41:701–866.

110. Comings De. Tourette syndrome and human behavior. Duarte California: Hope Press, 1990.

111. Comings DE, Comings BG. Comorbid behavioral disorders. In: Kurlan R, ed. Handbook of Tourette's syndrome and related tic and behavioral disorders. New York: Marcel Dekker, 1993:111–150.

112. Coffey B, Frazier J, Chen S. Comorbidity, Tourette's syndrome and anxiety disorders. In: Chase TN, Friedhoff AJ, Cohen DJ, eds. Advances in neurology, vol 58. New York: Raven Press, 1992; 95–104.

113. Towbin KE, Riddle MA. Attention deficit hyperactivity disorder. In: Kurlan R, ed. Handbook of Tourette syndrome and related tic disorders. New York: Marcel Dekker, 1993:89–110.

114. Comings DE, Comings BG. Tourette's syndrome and attention deficit disorder with hyperactivity: are they genetically related? J Am Acad Child Psychiatry 1984;23:138–146.

115. Comings DE, Comings BG. A controlled family history study of Tourette's syndrome, I: attention deficit hyperactivity disorder and learning disorders. J Clin Psychiatry 1990;51:275–280.

116. Knell E, Comings D. The sex ratio for tics, and attention deficit disorder (ADD) in persons with tics, is approximately 1:1 in relatives of Tourette's syndrome (TS) probands. 41st Annual Meeting of American Society of Human Genetics. Clin Gen 1990; Abstract (0244):1. 126.

117. Pauls DL, Cohen DJ, Kidd KK, et al. The Gilles de la Tourette syndrome [Letter to the editor]. Am J Hum Genet 1988;43:206–209.

118. Comings DE, Comings BG. Tourette's syndrome and attention deficit disorder. In: Cohen DJ, Bruun RD, Leckman JF, eds.

Tourette's syndrome and tic disorders; clinical understanding andtreatment. New York: John Wiley & Sons, 1988:119–135.

119. Pauls DL, Leckman JF, Cohen DJ. The familial relationship between Gilles de la Tourette syndrome, attention deficit disorder, learning disabilities, speech disorders and stuttering. J Am Acad Child Adolesc Psychiatry 1993;32:1044–1050.

120. Robertson MM. Self injurious behavior and Tourette syndrome. In: Chase TN, Friedhoff AJ, Cohen DJ, eds. Advances in neurology, vol 58. New York: Raven Press, 1992:105–114.

121. Robertson MM, Yakeley JW. Obsessive-compulsive disorder and self-injurious behavior. In: Kurlan R, ed. Handbook of Tourette's syndrome and related tic and behavioral disorders. New York: Marcel Dekker, 1993:45–87.

122. Bleich A, Bernout E, Apter A, et al. Gilles de la Tourette syndrome and mania in an adolescent. Br J Psychiatry 1985;146:664–665.

123. Burd L, Kerbeshian J. Gilles de la Tourette's syndrome and bipolar disorder. Arch Neurol 1984;41:1236.

124. Caine ED, Margolin DI, Brown GL, Ebert MH. Gilles de la Tourette's syndrome, tardive dyskinesia and psychosis in an adolescent. Am J Psychiatry 1978;135:241–243.

125. Takevchi K, Yamashita M, Morikiyo M, et al. Gilles de la Tourette's syndrome and schizophrenia. J Nerv Ment Dis 1986:174–248.

126. Reid AH. Gilles de la Tourette syndrome in mental handicap. Journal of Medical Deficiency Research 1984;28:81–83.

127. Burd L, Kerbeshian J. Tourette syndrome, atypical pervasive developmental disorder and Ganser syndrome in a 15 year old, visually impaired, mentally retarded boy. Can J Psychiatry 1985;30:74–76.

128. Kerbeshian J, Burd L. A second visually impaired, mentally retarded male with pervasive developmental disorder, Tourette disorder Ganser's syndrome: diagnostic classification and treatment. Int J Psychiatry Med 1986;6:67–75.

129. Kerbeshian J, Burd L. Are schizophreniform symptoms present in attenuated form in children with Tourette disorder and other developmental disorders? Can J Psychiatry 1987;32:123–135.

130. Kerbeshian J, Burd L. Asperger's syndrome and Tourette syndrome: the case of the pinball wizard. Br J Psychiatry 1986;148:731–736.

131. Boswell J. The life of Samuel Johnson LLD. London: George Routledge & Sons, 1867.

132. Corbett JA, Mathews AM, Connell PH, Shapiro DA. Tics and Gilles de la Tourette's syndrome: A follow-up study and critical review. Br J Psychiatry 1969;115:1229–1241.

133. Field JR, Corbin KB, Goldstein NP, Klass DW. Gilles de la Tourette syndrome. Neurology (Minneap) 1966;16:453–462.

134. Morphew JA, Sim M. Gilles de la Tourette's syndrome: a clinical and psychopathological study. Br J Med Psychol 1969;42:293–301.

135. Montgomery MA, Clayton PJ, Friedhoff AJ. Psychiatric illness in Tourette syndrome patients and first-degree relatives. In: Friedhoff AJ, Chase TN, eds. Gilles de la Tourette Syndrome. Advances in neurology, vol 35. New York: Raven Press, 1982:335–339.

136. Pauls DL, Leckman JF, Cohen DJ. Evidence against a genetic relationship between Gilles de la Tourette syndrome and anxiety, depression, panic and phobic disorders. Br J Psychiatry 1994;164:215–221.

137. Krumholz A, Singer HS, Niedermeyer E, et al. Electrophysiological studies in Tourette's syndrome. Ann Neurol 1983;14:638–641.

138. Bergen D, Tanner CM, Wilson R. The electroencephalogram in Tourette syndrome. Ann Neurol 1981;11:382–383.

139. Obeso JA, Rothwell JC, Marsden CD. The neurophysiology of Tourette's syndrome. In: Friedhoff AJ, Chase TN, eds. Gilles de la Tourette syndrome. Advances in neurology, vol 35. New York: Raven Press, 1982:105–114.

140. Verma NP, Syrigou-Papavasiliou A, Lewitt PA. Electroencephalographic findings in unmedicated, neurologically and intellectually intact Tourette syndrome patients. Electroencephalogr Clin Neurophysiol 1986;64:12–20.

141. Lucas AR, Rodin EA. Electroencephalogram in Gilles de la Tourette's disease. Mexico City: Fifth World Congress of Psychiatry, 1973: 85–89.

142. Van de Wetering BJM, Martens CMC, Fortgens C, et al. Late components of the auditory evoked potentials in Gilles de la Tourette syndrome. Clin Neurol Neurosurg 1985;87:181–186.

143. Tolosa ES, Montserrat L, Bayes A. Reduction of brainstem interneuron excitability during voluntary tic inhibition in Tourette's syndrome. Neurology 1986;36(Suppl):118–119.

144. Harcherik DF, Cohen DJ, Ort S, et al. Computed tomographic brain scanning in four neuropsychiatric disorders of childhood. Am J Psychiatry 1985;142:731–734.

145. Caparulo BK, Cohen DJ, Rothman SL, et al. Computed tomographic brain scanning in children with developmental neuropsychiatric disorders. J Am Acad Child Psychiatry 1981;20:338–357.

146. Chase TN, Geoffrey V, Gillespie M, et al. Structural and functional studies of Gilles de la Tourette syndrome. Rev Neurol (Paris) 1986;142:851–855.

147. Shaenboen MJ, Nigro MA, Martocci RJ. Colpocephali and Gilles de la Tourette's syndrome. Arch Neurol 1984;41:1023.

148. Kjaer M, Boris P, Hansen LG. Abnormal CT scan in a patient with Gilles de la Tourette syndrome. Neuroradiology 1986;28:362–363.

149. Yeragani VK, Blackman M, Barker GB. Biological and psychological aspects of a case of Gilles de la Tourette syndrome. J Clin Psych 1983;44:27–29.

150. Lakke JPWF, Wilmink JT. A case of Gilles de la Tourette's syndrome with midbrain involvement. J Neurol Neurosurg Psychiatry 1985; 48:1293–1296.

151. Vieregge P. Gilles de la Tourette syndrome in monozygotic twins. J Neurol Neurosurg Psychiatry 1987;50:1554–1556.

152. Demeter S. Structural imaging in Tourette's syndrome. In: Chase TN, Friedhoff AJ, Cohen DJ, eds. Adv Neurol, vol 58. New York: Raven Press, 1992:201–206.

153. Sandyk R. A case of Tourette syndrome with midbrain involvement. Int J Neurosci 1988;43:171–175.

154. Robertson M, Doran M, Trimble M, Lees AJ. The treatment of Gilles de la Tourette syndrome by limbic leucotomy. J Neurol Neurosurg Psychiatry 1990;53:691–694.

155. Peterson B, Riddle MA, Cohen DJ, et al. Reduced basal ganglia volumes in Tourette's syndrome using three-dimensional reconstruction techniques from magnetic resonance images. Neurology 1993; 43:941–949.

156. Singer HS, Reiss AL, Brown JE, et al. Volumetric MRI changes in basal ganglia of children with Tourette's syndrome. Neurology 1993;43:950–956.

157. Witelson SF. Clinical neurology as data for basic neuroscience: Tourette's syndrome and the human motor system. Neurology 1993;43:859–861.

158. Chase TN, Foster NL, Fedio P, et al. Gilles de la Tourette syndrome: studies with the fluorine-18-labelled fluorodeoxyglucose positron emission tomographic method. Ann Neurol 1984;15(Suppl):S175.

159. Stoetter B, Braun AR, Randolph C, et al. Functional neuroanatomy of Tourette syndrome: limbic motor interactions studied with FDG PET. Adv Neurol 1992;58:213–226.

160. Hall M, Costa DC, Shields J, Heavens J, Robertson M, Ell PJ. Brain perfusion patterns with 99Tcm-HMPAO/SPET in patients with Gilles de la Tourette syndrome - short report. Nuclear Medicine 1990;27(Suppl):243–245.

161. George MS, Trimble MR, Costa DC, et al. Elevated frontal cerebral blood flow in Gilles de la Tourette syndrome A 99Tcm-HMPAO SPECT study. Psychiatry Res 1992;45:143–151.

162. Moriarty J, Costa DC, Schmitz B, Trimble MR, Ell PJ, Robertson MM. Brain perfusion abnormalities in Gilles de la Tourette syndrome. Br J Psychiatry 1995;167:249–254.

163. Riddle M, Rasmussen AM, Woods SW, Hoffer PB. SPECT imaging of cerebral blood flow in Tourettes syndrome. Adv Neurol 1992;58: 207–212.

164. George MS, Robertson MM, Costa DC, Ell PJ, Trimble MR, Pilowsky L, Verhoeff MPLG. Dopamine receptor availability in Tourette's syndrome. Psychiatry Research: Neuroimaging 1994;55: 193–203.

165. Baxter LR, Guze BH. Neuro-imaging. In: Kurlan R, ed. Handbook

of Tourette's syndrome and related tic and behavioral disorders. New York: Marcel Dekker, 1993:289–304.

166. Baxter LR Jr, Schwartz JM, Phelps ME, et al. Reduction of prefrontal cortex glucose metabolism is common to three types of depression. Arch Gen Psychiatry 1989;46:243–250.

167. Deutsch G. The non-specificity of frontal dysfunction in disease and altered states: cortical blood flow evidence. Behav Neurol 1992;5: 301–307.

168. Berman KF, Doran AR, Pickar D, Weinberger DR. Is the mechanism of prefrontal hypofunction in depression the same as in schizophrenia? Regional cerebral blood flow during cognitive activation. Br J Psychiatry 1993;162:183–192.

169. Dewulf A, Van Bogaert L. Etudes anatomo-cliniques de syndromes hypercinetiques complexes - Partie 3. Une observation anatomo-clinique de maladie des tics (Gilles de la Tourette). Monatsschrift fur Psychiatrie und Neurologie 1941;104:53–61.

170. Balthasar K. Uber das anatomische substrat der generalisierten Tic-Krankheit (maladie des tics, Gilles de la Tourette): Entwicklung-shemmung des corpus striatum. Archiv fur Psychiatrie und Nerven-krankheiten (Berlin) 1957;195:531–549.

171. Richardson EP. Neuropathological studies of Tourette syndrome. In: Friedhoff AJ, Chase TN, eds. Gilles de la Tourette syndrome. Advances in neurology, vol 35. New York: Raven Press, 1982:83–87.

172. Anderson GM, Pollak ES, Chatterjee D. Brain monamines and amino acids in Gilles de la Tourette syndrome: a preliminary study of subcortical regions (letter). Arch Gen Psychiatry 1992;49:584–586.

173. Singer HS. Neurochemical analysis of post-mortem cortical and striatal brain tissue in patients with Tourette syndrome. Adv Neurol 1992;58:135–144.

174. Haber SN, Kowall NW, Vonsattel JP, et al. Gilles de la Tourette's syndrome: a postmortem neuropathological and immunohistochemical study. J Neurol Sci 1986;75:225–241.

175. Haber SN, Wolfer D. Basal ganglia peptidergic staining in Tourette's syndrome: a follow up study. In: Chase TN, Friedhoff AJ, Cohen DJ, eds. Tourette's syndrome; genetics, neurobiology and treatment. Advances in neurology, vol 58. New York: Raven Press, 1992: 145–150.

176. Caine ED. Gilles de la Tourette's syndrome: a review of clinical and research studies and consideration of future directions for investigation. Arch Neurol 1985;42:393–397.

177. Friedhoff AJ. Insights into the pathophysiology and pathogenesis of Gilles de la Tourette syndrome. Rev Neurol (Paris) 1986;142: 860–864.

178. Bonnet KA. Neurobiological dissection of Tourette syndrome: a neurochemical focus on a human neuroanatomical model. In: Advances of neurology, vol 35. New York: Raven Press, 1982:77–82.

179. Karson CN, Kaufmann CA, Shapiro AK, et al. Eye-blink rate in Tourette's syndrome. J Nerv Ment Dis 1985;173:566–568.

180. Merikangas JR, Merikangas KR, Kopp U, et al. Blood choline and response to clonazepam and haloperidol in Tourette's syndrome. Acta Psychiatr Scand 1985;72:395–399.

181. Cohen DJ, Detlor J, Shaywitz B, et al. Interaction of biological and psychological factors in the natural history of Tourette syndrome: a paradigm for childhood neuropsychiatric disorders. In: Friedhoff AJ, Chase TN, eds. Gilles de la Tourette syndrome. Advances in neurology, vol 35. New York: Raven Press, 1982:31–40.

182. Eldridge R, Denckla MB. The inheritance of Gilles de la Tourette's syndrome. N Engl J Med 1987;317:1346–1347.

183. Kurlan R. The pathogenesis of Tourette's syndrome. A possible role of hormonal and excitatory neurotransmitter influences in brain development. Arch Neurol 1992b;49:874–876.

184. Trimble MR, Robertson MM. The psychopathology of tics. In: Marsden CD, Fahn S. Modern trends in neurology. Movement disorders, vol 2. London: Butterworths, 1987:406–422.

185. Devinsky O. Neuroanatomy of Gilles de la Tourette's syndrome: possible midbrain involvement. Arch Neurol 1983;40:508–514.

186. Jadresic D. The role of the amygdaloid complex in Gilles de la Tourette syndrome. Brit J Psychiatry 1992;161:532–534.

187. Robertson M, Evans K, Robins A, et al. Abnormalities of copper in Gilles de la Tourette syndrome. Biol Psychiatry 1987;22 968–978.

188. Zausmer DM, Dewey ME. Tics and heredity. Br J Psychiatry 1987;150:628–634.

189. Baraitser M. The genetics of neurological disorders. London: Oxford University Press, 1982.

190. Pakstis AJ, Heutink P, Pauls DL, et al. Progress in the search for genetic linkage with Tourette syndrome: an exclusion map covering more than 50% of the autosomal genome. Am J Hum Genet 1991;48:281–294.

191. Escalar G, Majeron MA, Finavera L, et al. Contributo alla conoscenza della sindrome Gilles de la Tourette. Minerva Med 1972;63:3517–3522.

192. Jenkins RL, Ashby HB. Gilles de la Tourette syndrome in identical twins. Arch Neurol 1983;40:249–251.

193. Waserman J, Lal S, Gauthier S. Gilles de la Tourette syndrome in monozygotic twins. J Neurol Neurosurg Psychiatry 1983;46:75–77.

194. Ellison RM. Gilles de la Tourette syndrome. Med J Aust 1964;1: 153–155.

195. Price RA, Kidd KK, Cohen DJ, et al. A twin study of Tourette syndrome. Arch Gen Psychiatry 1985;42:815–820.

196. Leckman JF, Price RV, Walkup JT, et al. Nongenetic factors in Gilles de la Tourette's syndrome. Arch Gen Psychiatry 1987;44:100.

197. Dunlap JR. A case of Gilles de la Tourette's disease (Maladie des tics): a study of the intrafamily dynamics. J Nerv Ment Dis 1960;130: 340–344.

198. Friel PB. Familial incidence of Gilles de la Tourette's disease, with observations on aetiology and treatment. Brit J Psychiatry 1963;122: 655–658.

199. Guggenheim MA. Familial Tourette syndrome. Ann Neurol 1979; 5:104.

200. American Psychiatric Association. Diagnostic and statistical manual of mental disorders. 3rd Ed. Revised. Washington, DC. American Psychiatric Association. 1987.

201. Devor EJ. Complex segregation analysis of Gilles de la Tourette syndrome: further evidence for a major locus mode of transmission. Am J Human Genet 1984;36:704–709.

202. Price RA, Pauls DL, Caine ED. Pedigree and segregation analysis of clinically defined subgroups of Tourette syndrome. Am J Hum Genet 1984;36:178.

203. Pauls DL, Leckman JF. The inheritance of Gilles de la Tourette syndrome and associated behaviors. Evidence for autosomal dominant transmission. N Engl J Med 1986;315:993–997.

204. Pauls DL, Pakstis AJ, Kurlan R, et al. Segregation and linkage analyses of Tourette's syndrome and related disorders. J Am Acad Child Adolesc Psychiatry 1990;29:195–203.

205. Curtis D, Robertson MM, Gurling HMD. Autosomal dominant gene transmission in a large kindred with Gilles de la Tourette syndrome. Br J Psychiatry 1992;160:845–849.

206. Robertson MM, Trimble MR. Normal chromosomal findings in Gilles de la Tourette syndrome. Psychiatric Genetics 1993;3: 95–99.

207. Brett P, Curtis D, Gourdie A, et al. Possible linkage of Tourette syndrome to markers on short arm of chromosome 3 (C3p21-14). Lancet 1990;336:1076.

208. Comings DE, Comings BG, Dietz G, et al. Evidence of the Tourette syndrome gene is at 18 g 22.1. Abstracts. Berlin: 7th International Congress of Human Genetics, 1986: Abstract M, 11, 23:620.

209. Donnai D. Gene localization in Tourette's syndrome. Lancet 1987; i:627.

210. Comings DE, Muhleman D, Dibtz G, et al. Association between Tourette's syndrome and homozygosity at the dopamine D3 receptor gene. Lancet 1993;341:906.

211. Heutink P, Sandkuyl LA, van de Wetering BJM, et al. Linkage and Tourette syndrome. Lancet 1991;337:122–123.

212. Brett P, Schneiden V, Jackson G, et al. Chromosome markers in Tourette's syndrome. Lancet 1991;337:184–185.

213. Brett P, Robertson MM, Gurling HMD, Curtis D. Failure to find

linkage and increased homozygosity for the dopamine D3 receptor gene in Tourette's syndrome. Lancet 1993;341:1225.

214. Heutink P, van de Wetering BJM, Breedveld GJ, et al. No evidence for genetic linkage of Gilles de la Tourette syndrome on chromosomes 7 and 18. J Med Genet 1990;27:433–436.

215. Devor EJ, Grandy DK, Civelli O, et al. Genetic linkage is excluded for the D2-dopamine receptor lambda HD2G1 and flanking loci on chromosome 11q22-q23 in Tourette syndrome. Hum Hered 1990; 40:105–108.

216. Gerlenter J, Kennedy JL, Grandy GK, et al. Exclusion of close linkage of Tourette's syndrome to D1 dopamine receptor. Am J Psychiatry 1993;150:449–453.

216a. Kurlan R, Eapen V, Stern J, McDermott MP, Robertson MM. Bilineal transmission in Tourette's syndrome families. Neurology 1994;44:2336–2342.

217. Comings DE, Gursey B, Hecht T, et al. HLA typing in Tourette syndrome. In: Friedhoff AJ, Chase TN, eds. Gilles de la Tourette syndrome. Advances in neurology, vol 35. New York: Raven Press, 1982:251–253.

218. Caine ED, Lowell RW, Chiverton P, et al. Tourette syndrome and HLA. J Neurol Sci 1985;69:201–206.

219. Rapp DJ. Allergy and Tourette's syndrome. Ann Allergy 1986; 56:507.

220. Mandell M. Allergy and Tourette's syndrome. Ann Allergy 1986;56: 507–508.

221. Finegold I. Allergy and Tourette's syndrome. Ann Allergy 1985;55: 119–121.

222. Kurlan R, McDermott M. Rating tic severity. In: Kurlan R, ed. Handbook of Tourette's and related disorders. New York: Marcel Dekker, 1993:199–220.

223. Gillies D, Forsythe W. Treatment of multiple tics and the Tourette syndrome. Dev Med Child Neurol 1984;26:822–833.

224. Cohen DJ, Leckman JF. Tourette syndrome: advances in treatment and research. J Am Acad Child Adolesc Psychiatry 1984;23: 123–125.

225. Cohen DJ, Detlor J, Young JG, Shaywitz BA. Clonidine ameliorates Gilles de la Tourette syndrome. Arch Gen Psychiatry 1980;37:1350–1357.

226. Tanner CM, Goetz CG, Klawans HL. Cholinergic mechanisms in Tourette syndrome. Neurology (NY) 1982;32:1315–1317.

227. Shapiro AK, Wayne HL, Eisenkraft G. Semiology, nosology and criteria for tic disorders. Rev Neurol (Paris) 1983;142:824–832.

228. Shapiro AK, Shapiro ES. Controlled study of pimozide versus placebo in Tourette's syndrome. J Am Acad Child Adolesc Psychiatry 1984;23:161–173.

229. Harcherik D, Leckman J, Detlor J, Cohen DF. A new instrument for clinical studies of Tourette's syndrome. J Am Acad Child Adolesc Psychiatry 1984;23(2):153–160.

230. Leckman JF, Riddle MA, Pradin MT, et al. The Yale Global Tic Severity Scale: initial testing of clinician rated scale of tic severity. J Am Acad Child Adolesc Psychiatry 1989;28:566–573.

231. Goetz CG, Tanner CM, Wilson RS, et al. Clonidine and Gilles de la Tourette syndrome: double blind study using objective rating methods. Ann Neurol 1987;21:307–310.

232. Pauls DL, Hurst CR. Schedule for Tourette and other behavioral syndromes. New Haven, CT: Child Study Center, Yale University of Medicine, 1981.

233. Annett M. A classification of hand preferences by association analysis. Br J Psychol 1970;61:303–321.

234. Baron-Cohen S, Cross P, Crowson M, Robertson MM. Can children with Gilles de la Tourette syndrome edit their intentions? Psychol Med 1994;24:29–40.

235. Channon S, Flynn D, Robertson MM. Attentional deficits in Gilles de la Tourette syndrome. Neuropsychiatry Neuropsychol Behav Neurol 1992;5:170–177.

236. Golden GS, Greenhill L. Tourette syndrome in mentally retarded children. Ment Retard 1981;19:17.

237. Bruun RD, Shapiro AK. Differential diagnosis of Gilles de la Tourette's syndrome. J Nerv Ment Dis 1972;155:328–332.

238. Sacks OW. Acquired Tourettism in adult life. In: Friedhoff AJ, Chase TN, eds. Gilles de la Tourette syndrome. Advances in neurology, vol 35. New York: Raven Press, 1982:89–92.

239. Lal S, Alansari E. Tourette-like syndrome following low dose short-term neuroleptic treatment. Journal Canadienes Sciences Neurologiques 1986;13:125–128.

240. Klawans HL, Falk AK, Nausieda PA, Weiner WJ. Gilles de la Tourette syndrome after long-term chlorpromazine therapy. Neurology (NY) 1978; 28:1064–1068.

241. Stahl SM. Tardive Tourette syndrome in an autistic patient after long-term neuroleptic administration. Am J Psychiatry 1980;137: 1267–1269.

242. Seeman MV, Patel J, Pyke J. Tardive dyskinesia with Tourette-like syndrome. J Clin Psychiatry 1981;42:357–358.

243. Fog R, Pakkenberg H, Regeur L, et al. "Tardive" Tourette syndrome in relation to long term neuroleptic treatment of multiple tics. In: Friedhoff AJ, Chase TN, eds. Gilles de la Tourette syndrome. Advances in Neurology. Vol 35. New York: Raven Press, 1982: 419–421.

244. Mueller J, Aminoff MJ. Tourette-like syndrome after long-term neuroleptic drug treatment. Br J Psychiatry 1982;141:191–193.

245. Jeste DV, Cutler NR, Kaufmann CA, et al. Low-dose apomorphine and bromocriptine in neuroleptic-induced movement disorders. Biol Psychiatry 1983;18:1085–1091.

246. Fahn S. A case of post-traumatic tic syndrome. In: Friedhoff AJ, Chase TN, eds. Gilles de la Tourette syndrome. Advances in neurology, vol 35. New York: Raven Press, 1982:349–350.

247. Pulst SM, Walshe TM, Romero JA. Carbon monoxide poisoning with features of Gilles de la Tourette syndrome. Arch Neurol 1983;40:443–444.

248. Woody RC, Laney M. Tics and Tourette's syndrome: a review. J Arkansas Med Soc 1986;83:53–55.

249. Feinberg TE, Shapiro AK, Shapiro E. Paroxysmal myoclonic dystonia with vocalizations: new entity of variant of preexisting syndromes? J Neurol Neurosurg Psychiatry 1986;49:52–57.

250. Fahn S. Paroxysmal myoclonic dystonia with vocalizations. J Neurol Neurosurg Psychiatry 1987;50:117–118.

251. Seignot MJN. Un cas de maladie des tics de Gilles de la Tourette gueri par le R 1625. Ann Med Psychol (Paris) 1961; 119:578–579.

252. Shapiro AK, Shapiro E, Fulop G. Pimozide treatment of tic and Tourette disorders. Pediatrics 1987;79:1032–1039.

253. Shapiro E, Shapiro AK, Fulop G, et al. Controlled study of haloperidol, pimozide and placebo for the treatment of Gilles de la Tourette syndrome. Arch Gen Psychiatry 1989;46:722–730.

254. Robertson MM, Schnieden V, Lees AJ. Management of Gilles de la Tourette syndrome using sulpiride. Clin Neuropharmacol 1990;13: 229–235.

255. Caine ED, Polinsky RJ. Haloperidol-induced dysphoria in patients with Tourette syndrome. Am J Psychiatry 1979;136:1216–1217.

256. Bruun RD. Dysphoric phenomena associated with haloperidol treatment of Tourette syndrome. In: Friedhoff AJ, Chase TN, eds. Gilles de la Tourette syndrome. Advances in neurology, vol 35. New York: Raven Press, 1982:433–436.

257. Ross MS, Moldofsky H. A comparison of pimozide and haloperidol in the treatment of Gilles de la Tourette's syndrome. Am J Psychiatry 1978;135:585–587.

258. O'Quinn AN, Thompson RJ. Tourette's syndrome: an expanded view. Pediatrics 1980;66:420–424.

259. Mikkelsen EJ, Detlor J, Cohen DJ. School avoidance and social phobia triggered by haloperidol in patients with Tourette's disorder. Am J Psychiatry 1981;138:1572–1575.

260. Linet LS. Tourette syndrome, pimozide and school phobia: the neuroleptic separation anxiety syndrome. Am J Psychiatry 1985;142: 613–615.

261. Bruun RD. The natural history of Tourette's syndrome. In: Cohen

DJ, Bruun RD, Leckman JF, eds. Tourette's syndrome and tic disorders: clinical understanding and treatment. New York: John Wiley & Sons, 1988:21–39.

262. Korczyn AD. Pathophysiology of drug induced dyskinesias. Neuropharmacology 1972;11:601–607.

263. Fulop G, Phillips RA, Shapiro AK, et al. ECG changes during haloperidol and pimozide treatment of Tourette's disorder. Am J Psychiatry 1987;144:673–675.

264. Gerlach J, Casey DE. Sulpiride in tardive dyskinesia. Acta Psychiatr Scand 1984; 69 (Suppl 311):93–102.

265. Eggers C, Rothenberger A, Berghaus V. Clinical and neurobiological findings in children suffering from tic disease following treatment with tiapride. Eur Arch Psychiatr Neurol Sci 1988;237:223–229.

266. Mizrahi EM, Holtzman D, Tharp B. Haloperidol-induced tardive dyskinesia in a child with Gilles de la Tourette's disease. Arch Neurol 1980;37:380.

267. Caine ED, Polinsky RJ. Tardive dyskinesia in persons with Gilles de la Tourette's disease. Arch Neurol 1981;38:471–472.

268. Golden GS. Tardive dyskinesia in Tourette syndrome. Pediatr Neurol 1985;1:192–194.

269. Eapen V, Katona CLE, Barnes TRE, Robertson MM. Sulpiride-induced tardive dyskinesia in a person with Gilles de la Tourette syndrome. J Psychopharmacol 1993;7:290–292.

270. Silverstein F, Johnston MV. Risks of neuroleptic drugs in children. J Child Neurol 1987;2:41–43.

271. Uhr SB, Pruitt B, Berger PA, et al. Improvement of symptoms in Tourette syndrome by piquindone, a novel dopamine-2 receptor antagonist. Int Clin Psychopharmacol 1986;1:216–220.

272. Leckman JF, Detlor J, Harcherik DF, et al. Short and long term treatment of Tourette's syndrome with clonidine: a clinical perspective. Neurology 1985;35:343–351.

273. Singer HS, Gammon K, Quaskey S. Haloperidol, fluphenazine and clonidine in Tourette syndrome: controversies in treatment. Pediatr Neurosci 1986;12:71–74.

274. Riddle MA, Hardin MT, King R, et al. Fluoxetine treatment of children and adolescents with Tourette's and obsessive-compulsive disorders: preliminary clinical experience. J Am Acad Child Adolesc Psychiatry 1990;29:45–48.

275. Delgado PL, Goodman WK, Price LH, et al. Fluvoxamine/pimozide treatment of concurrent Tourette's and obsessive compulsive disorder. Br J Psychiatry 1990;157:762–765.

276. McDougle CJ, Goodman WK, Price LH, et al. Neuroleptic addition in fluvoxamine-refractory obsessive-compulsive disorder. Am J Psychiatry 1990;147:652–654.

277. Mesulam MM, Petersen RC. Treatment of Gilles de la Tourette's syndrome: eight-year, practice-based experience in a predominantly adult population. Neurology 1987;37:1828–1833.

278. Moldofsky H, Sandor P. Lecithin in the treatment of Gilles de la Tourette's syndrome. Am J Psychiatry 1983;140:1627–1629.

279. Clark DF. Behavior therapy of Gilles de la Tourette syndrome. Brit J Psychiatry 1966;112:771–778.

280. Storms L. Massed negative practice as a behavioral treatment for Gilles de la Tourette's syndrome. Am J Psychother 1985;39:277–281.

281. Doleys DM, Kurtz PS. A behavioral treatment programme for the Gilles de la Tourette syndrome. Psychol Rep 1974;35:43–48.

282. Savicki V, Carlin AS. Behavioral treatment of Gilles de la Tourette syndrome. Int J Child Psychother 1972;1:97–109.

283. Tansey MA. A simple and complex tic (Gilles de la Tourette's syndrome): their response to EEG sensorimotor rhythm biofeedback training. Int J Psychophysiol 1986.

284. Stefl ME, Rubin M. Tourette syndrome in the classroom: special problems, special needs. J Sch Health 1985;55:72–75.

285. Kurlan R, Kersun J, Ballantine HT Jr, Caine ED. Neurosurgical treatment of severe obsessive compulsive disorder associated with Tourette's syndrome. Mov Disord 1990;5:152–155.

286. Bruun RD, Budman CL. The National History of Gilles de la

Tourette syndrome. In: Handbook of Tourette's syndrome and Related Tic and Behavioral Disorders. Ed. Kurlan R., Marcel Dekker: New York, 1993:27–42.

287. Bockner S. Gilles de la Tourette's disease. J Ment Sci 1959;105:1078–1081.

288. Fernando SJM. Six cases of Gilles de la Tourette's syndrome. Br J Psychiatry 1976;128:436–441.

289. Berrios GE. Obsessive-compulsive disorder: its conceptual history in France during the 19th century. Compr Psychiatry 1989;30:283–295.

290. Magnan V. Considerations generales sur la folie (des hereditaires ou degeneres). Prog Med 14:1089–1090.

291. Janet P. L'automatisme psychologique. Paris: Alcan, 1889.

292. Freud S. Three case histories. Translated by Rieff. New York: Macmillan, 1973:15–102.

293. Rapoport JL. The neurology of obsessive-compulsive disorder. JAMA 1988;260:2888–2890.

294. Rapoport JL. The boy who couldn't stop washing. Collins, 1990.

295. Roth WF, Luton FH. The mental health program in Tennessee. Am J Psychiatry 1942;99:662–675.

296. Kringlen E. Obsessional neurotics: a long-term follow-up. Br J Psychiatry 1965;111:709–722.

297. Lo WH. A follow-up study of obsessional neurotics in Hong Kong Chinese. Br J Psychiatry 1967;113:823–832.

298. Ingram E. Obsessional illness in mental hospital patients. J Ment Sci 1961;107:382–402.

299. Pollitt J. Natural history of obsessional states. Br Med J (Clin Res) 1957;1:194–198.

300. Bebbington P. The prevalence of OCD in the community. Current Approaches "Obsessive Compulsive Disorder." Duphar Medical Relations 1990:7–19.

301. Myers JK, Weissman MM, Tischler GL, et al. Six month prevalence of psychiatric disorders in three communities: 1980–1982. Arch Gen Psychiatry 1984;41:959–967.

302. Robins LN, Helzer JE, Weissman MM, et al. Lifetime prevalence of specific disorders in three sites. Arch Gen Psychiatry 1984;41:949–958.

303. Karno M, Hough RL, Burnham MA, et al. Lifetime prevalence of specific psychiatric disorders among Mexican Americans and non-Hispanic whites in Los Angeles. Arch Gen Psychiatry 1987;44:695–701.

304. Burnham MA, Hough RL, Escobar JI, et al. Six month prevalence of specific psychiatric disorders among Mexican Americans and non-Hispanic whites in Los Angeles. Arch Gen Psychiatry 1987;44:687–694.

305. Blazer D, George LK, Landerman R, et al. Psychiatric disorders: a rural/urban comparison. Arch Gen Psychiatry 1985;42:651–656.

306. Canino GJ, Bird HR, Shrout PE, et al. The prevalence of specific psychiatric disorders in Puerto Rico. Arch Gen Psychiatry 1987;44:727–735.

307. Bland RC, Newman SC, Orn H. Epidemiology of psychiatric disorders in Edmonton. Acta Psychiatr Scand 1988; 77 (Suppl):338.

308. Reiger DA, Boyd JH, Burke JD, et al. One month prevalence of mental disorders in the United States. Arch Gen Psychiatry 1988;45:977–986.

309. Weissman MM, Leaf PJ, Tischler GL, et al. Affective disorders in five United States communities. Psychol Med 1988;18:141–154.

310. Oakley-Browne MA, Joyce PR, Well JE, Bushnell JA, Hornblow AR. Christchurch psychiatric epidemiology study, Part I: six month and other period prevalences of specific psychiatric disorders. Aust N Z J Psychiatry 1989;23:315–326.

311. Wells JE, Bushnell JA, Hornblow AR, Joyce PR, Oakley-Browne MA. Christchurch psychiatric epidemiology study: methodology and lifetime prevalence for specific psychiatric disorders. Aust N Z J Psychiatry 1989;23:327–340.

312. Rasmusen SA, Eisen JL. The epidemiology and differential diagno-

sis of obsessive compulsive disorder. J Clin Psychiatry 1992; 53 (Suppl 4):4–10.

313. Rasmussen SA. Obsessive-compulsive disorder in dermatologic practice. J Am Acad Dermatol 1985;13:965–967.

314. Hwu HG, Yeh EK, Chang LY. Prevalence of psychiatric disorders in Taiwan defined by the Chinese Diagnostic Interview Schedule. Acta Psychiatr Scand 1989;79:136–147.

315. Marks IM. Fears, phobias, and rituals: panic, anxiety, and their disorders. New York: Oxford University Press, 1987:497–498.

316. Karno M, Golding JM, Sorenson SB, Burnham MA. The epidemiology of obsessive-compulsive disorder in five US communities. Arch Gen Psychiatry 1988;45:1094–1099.

317. Perse T. Obsessive-compulsive disorder: a treatment review. J Clin Psychiatry 1988;49:48–55.

318. Lewis A. Problems of obsessional illness. Proc R Soc Lond 1935;29:325–336.

319. Rudin E. Ein Beitrag zur Frage der Zwangskrankheit, insbesondere ihrer herediataren Beziehungen. Archiv fur Psychiatrie und Zeitschrift gesmter neurologisher Psychiatrie 1953;191:14–54.

320. Hollingsworth CE, Tangnay PE, Grossman L, Pabst P. Long-term outcome of obsessive compulsive disorder in childhood. J Am Acad Child Adolesc Psychiatry 1980;19:134–144.

321. Zeitlin H. The natural history of psychiatric disorder in children. Oxford: Oxford University Press, 1986.

322. Leonard H, Swedo SE, Rapoport J, et al. Treatment of obsessive-compulsive disorder with clomipramine and desipramine in children and adolescents. A double blind crossover comparison. Arch Gen Psychiatry 1989;46:1088–1092.

323. Flament MF, Koby FE, Rapoport JL, et al. Childhood obsessive-compulsive disorder: a prospective follow-up study. J Child Psychol Psychiatry 1990;31:363–380.

324. Karno M, Golding JM. Obsessive compulsive disorder. In: Robins LN, Reiger DA, eds. Psychiatric disorders in America. Epidemiologic catchment area study. New York: Free Press, 1991.

325. Black JL. Obsessive compulsive disorder: a clinical update. Mayo Clin Proc 1992;67:266–275.

326. Rasmussen SA, Eisen JL. Clinical and epidemiologic findings of significance to neuropharmacologic trials in OCD. Psychopharmacol Bull 1988;24:466–470.

327. Lewis AJ. Melancholia: a clinical survey of depressive states. J Ment Sci 1934;80:277–278.

328. Stengel E. A study of some clinical aspects of the relationship between obsessional neurosis and psychotic reaction types. J Ment Sci 1945;91: 166–187.

329. Kendall R, Discipio W. Obsessional symptoms and obsessional personality traits in patients with depressive illness. Psychol Med 1970;1:65–72.

330. Coryell W. Obsessive compulsive disorder in primary unipolar depression. J Nerv Ment Dis 1981;169:220–224.

331. Miller DE. A repertory grid of obsessionality. Br J Med Psychol 1980;53:59–66.

332. Black DW, Noyes R Jr. Comorbidity and obsessive-compulsive disorder. In: Maser JD, Cloninger CR, eds. Comorbidity of mood and anxiety disorders. Washington, DC: American Psychiatric Press, 1990:305–316.

333. Montgomery SA. Is obsessive compulsive disorder diagnostically independent of both anxiety and depression? In: Montgomery SA, Goodman WK, Goeting N, eds. Obsessive compulsive disorder. Current approaches: Duphar Medical Relations, Ashford Colour Press: Gosport, Hants, 1990:1–6.

334. Flament MF, Rapoport JL, Berg CJ, et al. Clomipramine treatment of childhood obsessive-compulsive disorder. A double-blind controlled study. Arch Gen Psychiatry 1985;42:977–983.

335. Perse TL, Greist JH, Jefferson JW. Fluvoxamine treatment of obsessive compulsive disorder. Am J Psychiatry 1987;144:1543–1548.

336. Cottraux J, Mollard E, Bouvard M. A controlled study of fluvoxamine and exposure in obsessive compulsive disorder. Arch Gen Psychiatry 1990;46:36–44.

337. Goodman WK, Price LH, Rasmussen SA. Efficacy of fluvoxamine in obsessive compulsive disorder. Arch Gen Psychiatry 1989a;46: 36–44.

338. Montgomery SA. Clomipramine in obsessional neurosis: a placebo-controlled trial. Pharm Med 1980;1:189–192.

339. de Veaugh Geiss J, Landau P, Katz R. Treatment of obsessive compulsive disorder with clomipramine. Psychiatr Ann 1989;19: 97–101.

340. Kasvikis YG, Tsakiris F, Marks IM, Basaglu M, Nashirvani HF. Past history of anorexia nervosa in women with obsessive-compulsive disorder. International Journal of Eating Disorders 1986:1069–1075.

341. Rothenberg A. Eating disorders as a modern obsessive-compulsive syndrome. Psychiatry 1986;49:45–53.

342. Solyom L, Freeman RJ, Miles JE. A comparative psychometric study of anorexia nervosa and obsessive neurosis. Can J Psychiatry 1982;27:282–286.

343. Kaye WH, Ebert MH, Gwirtsman HE, Weiss SR. Differences in brain serotonergic metabolism between nonbulimic and bulimic patients with anorexia nervosa. Am J Psychiatry 1984; 141: 1598–1601.

344. Murphy DL, Pigott TA. A comparative examination of a role for serotonin in obsessive-compulsive disorder, panic disorder, and anxiety. J Clin Psychiatry 1990; 51 (Suppl):53–58.

345. Hudson JI, Pope HG Jr, Yurgelun-Todd D, Jonas JM, Frankenburg FR. A controlled study of lifetime prevalence of affective and other psychiatric disorders in bulimic outpatients. Am J Psychiatry 1987; 144:1283–1287.

346. Pigott TA, Altemus M, Rubenstein CS, et al. Symptoms of eating disorders in patients with obsessive-compulsive disorder. Am J Psychiatry 1991;148:1552–1557.

347. Rothenberg A. Adolescence and eating disorder: the obsessive-compulsive syndrome. Psychiatr Clin North Am 1990;13:469–488.

348. Rosenberg CM. Familial aspects of obsessional neurosis. Br J Psychiatry 1967;113:405–413.

349. Black A. The natural history of obsessional neurosis. In: Beech HR, ed. Obsessional states. London: Methuen and Co., 1974: 19–54.

350. Joffe RT, Swinson RP, Regan JJ. Personality features of obsessive-compulsive disorder. Am J Psychiatry 1988;145:1127–1129.

351. Mavissakalian M, Hammann MS, Jones B. Correlates of DSM-III personality disorder in obsessive compulsive disorder. Compr Psychiatry 1990;31:481–489.

352. Sciuto G, Diaferia G, Battaglia M, et al. DSM-III-R personality disorders in panic and obsessive-compulsive disorder: a comparison study. Compr Psychiatry 1991;32:450–457.

353. Swedo SE, Leonard HL, Rapoport JL, et al. A double-blind comparison of clomipramine and desipramine in the treatment of trichotillomania (hair-pulling). N Engl J Med 1989;321: 497–501.

354. Leonard HL, Lenane M, Swedo S, et al. A double-blind comparison of clomipramine and desipramine treatment of severe onychophagia (nail biting). Arch Gen Psychiatry 1991;48:821–827.

355. Winchel RM, Stanley B, Guido J, et al. An open trial of fluoxetine for trichotillomania (hair pulling). Maui, Hawaii: Presented at the 28th annual meeting of the American College of Neuropsychopharmacology, December 13, 1989.

356. Stanley MA, Bowers TC, Taylor DJ. Treatment of trichotillomania with fluoxetine (letter). J Clin Psychiatry 1991;52:282.

357. Christenson GA, Popkin MK, Mackenzie TB, Realmuto GM. Lithium treatment of chronic hair pulling. J Clin Psychiatry 1991; 52:116–120.

358. Pollard CA, Ibe O, Krojanker DN, Kitchen AD, Bronson SS, Flynn TM. Clomipramine treatment of trichotillomania: a follow-up report on four cases. J Clin Psychiatry 1991;52:128–130.

359. Swedo SE, Rapoport JL, Leonard HL, et al. Regional cerebral glucose metabolism of women with trichotillomania. Arch Gen Psychiatry 1991;48:828–833.

360. Stanley MA, Swann AC, Bowers TC, et al. A comparison of clinical feature in trichotillomania and obsessive-compulsive disorder. Behav Res Ther 1992;30:39–44.

361. Brady KT, Austin L, Lydiard RB. Body dysmorphic disorder: the relationship to obsessive-compulsive disorder. J Nerv Ment Dis 1990;178:538–540.

362. Hollander E, Neville D, Frankel M, et al. Body dysmorphic disorder. Diagnostic issues and related disorders. Psychosomatics 1992;33:156–165.

363. Hollander E, Liebowitz MR, Winchel R, et al. Treatment of body dysmorphic disorder with serotonin reuptake blockers. Am J Psychiatry 1989;145:786–770.

364. McElroy SL, Hudson JI, Pope H Jr, et al. The DSM-III-R impulse control disorders not elsewhere classified: clinical characteristics and relationship to other psychiatric disorders. Am J Psychiatry 1992;149:318–327.

365. Kettl PA, Marks IM. Neurological factors in obsessive-compulsive disorder. Two case reports and a review of the literature. Br J Psychiatry 1986;149:315–319.

366. Mayer-Gross W, Steiner G. Z. ges. Neurol Psychiatr 1921;73:283.

367. Von Economo C. Encephalitis lethargica, its sequellae and treatment. Newman KO, translator. New York: Oxford University Press, 1931.

368. Trimble MR. Neuropsychiatry. London: John Wiley & Sons, 1981.

369. Capstick N, Seldrup U. Obsessional states: a study in the relationship between abnormalities occurring at birth and subsequent development of obsessional symptoms. Acta Psychiatr Scand 1977;56:427–439.

370. McKeon J, McGuffin P, Robinson P. Obsessive-compulsive neurosis following head injury: a report of 4 cases. Br J Psychiatry 1984;144:190–192.

371. Freeman J, Aron A, Collard D. The emotional correlates of Sydenham's chorea. Pediatrics 1965;35:42–49.

372. Swedo SE, Rapoport JL, Cheslow DL. High prevalence of obsessive-compulsive symptoms in patients with Sydenham's chorea. Am J Psychiatry 1989;146:246–249.

373. Jenike M. Update on obsessive-compulsive disorder. Curr Affect III 1990;9:5–12.

374. Barton R. Diabetes insipidus and obsessional neurosis: a syndrome. Lancet 1965;1:133–135.

375. Pacella BL, Polatin P, Nagle SH. Clinical and EEG studies in obsessive compulsive states. Am J Psychiatry 1944;100:830–838.

376. Garmany G. Obsessional states in epileptics. J Ment Sci 1947;93:639–643.

377. Brickner RM. A human cortical area producing repetitive phenomena when stimulated. J Neurophysiol 1940;3:128–130.

378. Penfield W, Jasper H. Epilepsy and the functional anatomy of the human brain. London: Churchill Livingstone, 1954.

379. Guerrant J, Anderson W, Fischer A, Weinstein M, Jaros RM. Personality of epilepsy. Springfield, IL: Charles C Thomas, 1962:43–54.

380. Janet P. Les obsessions et al psychiasthenie, vol 1. Paris: Felix Alcan, 1903.

381. Hall MB. Obsessive-compulsive states in childhood: their treatment. Arch Dis Child 1935;10:49–59.

382. Kanner L. Child psychiatry. Springfield, IL: Charles C Thomas, 1935:450–457.

383. Berman L. Obsessive, compulsive neurosis in children. J Nerv Ment Dis 1942;95:26–39.

384. Despert LJ. Differential diagnosis between obsessive-compulsive neurosis and schizophrenia in children. In: Hoch PH, Zubin J, eds. Psychopathology of childhood. New York: Grune & Stratton, 1955:240–253.

385. Regner E. Obsessive compulsive neuroses in children. Acta Psychiatr Neurol Scand 1959;34:110–125.

386. Judd LL. Obsessive compulsive neurosis in children. Arch Gen Psychiatry 1965;12:136–143.

387. Thomsen PH, Mikkelsen HU. Children and adolescent with obsessive-compulsive disorder: the demographic and diagnostic characteristics of 61 Danish patients. Acta Psychiatr Scand 1991;83:262–266.

388. Flament M, Whitaker A, Rapoport JL, et al. Obsessive compulsive disorder in adolescence: an epidemiological study. J Am Acad Child Adolesc Psychiatry 1988;27:764–771.

389. Warren W. Some relationships between the psychiatry of children and of adults. J Ment Science 1960;106:815–826.

390. Berg CZ, Rapoport JL, Whitaker A, et al. Childhood obsessive compulsive disorder: a two-year prospective follow-up of a community sample. J Am Acad Child Adolesc Psychiatry 1989;28:528–533.

391. Leonard H, Swedo S, Coffey M. Clomipramine vs desipramine in childhood obsessive-compulsive disorder. Psychopharmacol Bull 1988;24:43–45.

392. Leonard H, Swedo S, Rapoport J, Coffey M, Cheslow D. Treatment of obsessive compulsive disorder with clomipramine and desmethylimipramine: a double blind crossover comparison. Psychopharmacol Bull 1988;24:252–266.

393. Leonard H, Swedo SE, Rapoport J, et al. Treatment of child obsessive compulsive disorder with clorimipramine and desipramine: a double blind crossover comparison. Psychopharmacol Bull 1988;24:93–95.

394. Rapoport JL, Swedo SE, Leonard HL. Childhood obsessive compulsive disorder. J Clin Psychiatry 1992; 53 (Suppl 4):11–17.

395. Allsopp M, Verduyn C. Adolescents with obsessive-compulsive disorder: a case note review of consecutive patients referred to a provincial regional adolescent psychiatry unit. J Adolesc 1990;13:157–169.

396. Swedo SE, Rapoport JL, Leonard JL, et al. Obsessive-compulsive disorder in children and adolescents. Clinical phenomenology of 70 consecutive cases. Arch Gen Psychiatry 1989;46:33–341.

397. Goodwin DW, Guze SB, Robins E. Follow-up studies in obsessional neurosis. Arch Gen Psychiatry 1969;20:182–187.

398. Honjo S, Hirano C, Murase S, et al. Obsessive compulsive symptoms in childhood and adolescence. Acta Psychiatr Scand 1989;80:83–91.

399. Khanna S, Srinath S. Childhood obsessive-compulsive disorder. Psychopathology 1988;21:254–258.

400. Peller L. Libidinal phases, ego development and play. Psychoanalytic Study of the Child 1954;10:178–199.

401. Riddle MA, Scahill L, King R, et al. Obsessive compulsive disorder in children and adolescent. Phenomenology and Family History 1990;29:766–772.

402. Bolton D, Turner T. Obsessive compulsive neurosis with conduct disorder: a report of two cases. J Child Psychol Psychiatry 1984;25:133–139.

403. Whitaker A, Johnson J, Schaffer D, et al. Uncommon troubles in young people: prevalence estimates of selected psychiatric disorders in a non-referred adolescent population. Arch Gen Psychiatry 1990;47:487–496.

404. Lenane M, Swedo SE, Rapoport JL. Rates of obsessive compulsive disorder for first-degree relatives of patients with trichotillomania: a research note. J Child Psychol Psychiatry 1992;33:925–933.

405. Levin B, Duchowny M. Childhood obsessive-compulsive disorder and cingulate epilepsy. Biol Psychiatry 1991;30:1049–1055.

406. Chapman AH, Pilkey L, Gibbons MJ. A psychosomatic study of eight children with Sydenham's chorea. Pediatrics 1958;21:582–595.

407. Lenane MC, Swedo SE, Leonard H, Pauls DL, Sceery W, Rapoport JL. Psychiatric disorders in first degree relatives of children and adolescents with obsessive compulsive disorders. J Am Acad Child Adolesc Psychiatry 1990;29:407–412.

408. Swedo S. Rituals and releasers: an ethological model of OCD. In: Rapoport JL, ed. Obsessive compulsive disorder in children and adolescents. Washington, DC: American Psychiatric Press, 1989:269–288.

409. Winslow J. Neuroethology of obsessive-compulsive behavior. In:

Zohar J, Rasmussen S, Insel T, eds. Psychobiology of obsessive compulsive disorder. New York: Springer-Verlag 1989.

410. Insel TR, Donnelly EF, Lalakea ML, et al. Neurological and Neuropsychological studies of patients with obsessive-compulsive disorder. Biol Psychiatry 1983;18:741–751.

411. Behar D, Rapoport JL, Berg MA, et al. Computerized tomography and neuropsychological test measures in adolescents with obsessive-compulsive disorder. Am J Psychiatry 1984;141:363–369.

412. Luxenberg JS, Swedo SE, Flament MF, et al. Neuroanatomical abnormalities in obsessive-compulsive disorder detected with quantitative x-ray computed tomography. Am J Psychiatry 1988;145:1089–1093.

413. Laplane D, Baulac M, Widlocher D, Dubois B. Pure psychi akinesia with bilateral lesions of basal ganglia. J Neurol Neurosurg Psychiatry 1984;47:377–385.

414. Williams AC, Owen C, Heath DA. A compulsive movement disorder with cavitation of caudate nucleus. J Neurol Neurosurg Psychiatry 1988;51:447–448.

415. Kellner CH, Jolley RR, Holgate RC, et al. Brain MRI in obsessive-compulsive disorder. Psychiatry Res 1991;36:45–49.

416. Garber HJ, Ananth JV, Chiu LC, et al. Nuclear magnetic resonance study of obsessive-compulsive disorder. Am J Psychiatry 1989;146:1001–1005.

417. Baxter LR, Phelps ME, Mazziotta JC, et al. Local cerebral glucose metabolic rates in obsessive-compulsive disorder. A comparison with rates in unipolar depression and in normal controls. Arch Gen Psychiatry 1987;44:211–218.

418. Baxter LR Jr, Schwartz JM, Phelps ME, et al. Cerebral glucose metabolic rates in nondepressed patients with obsessive-compulsive disorder. Am J Psychiatry 1988;145:1560–1563.

419. Swedo SE, Schapiro MB, Grady CL, et al. Cerebral glucose metabolism in childhood-onset obsessive-compulsive disorder. Arch Gen Psychiatry 1989;46:518–523.

420. Nordahal T, Benkelfat C, Semple W. Cerebral glucose metabolic rates in obsessive-compulsive disorder. Neuropsychopharmacology 1989;2:23–28.

421. Benkelfat C, Nordahal TE, Semple WE, et al. Local cerebral glucose metabolic rates in obsessive-compulsive disorder. Patients treated with clomipramine. Arch Gen Psychiatry 1990;47:840–848.

422. Head D, Bolton D, Hymas N. Deficit in cognitive shifting ability in patients with obsessive-compulsive disorder. Biol Psychiatry 1989;25:929–937.

423. Cox CS, Fedio P, Rapoport JL. Neuropsychological testing of obsessive-compulsive adolescents. In: Rapoport JL, ed. Obsessive-compulsive disorder in children and adolescents. Washington, DC: American Psychiatric Press, 1989:73–85.

424. Malloy P. Frontal lobe dysfunction in obsessive-compulsive disorder. In: Perecman E, ed. The frontal lobes revisited. New York: The IRBN Press, 1987:207–223.

425. Sher KJ, Frost RO, Kushner M, Crews TM, Alexander JE. Memory deficits in compulsive checkers: replication and extension in a clinical sample. Behav Res Ther 1989;27:65–69.

426. Hollander E, Schiffman E, Cohen B, et al. Signs of central nervous system dysfunction in obsessive-compulsive disorder. Arch Gen Psychiatry 1990;47:27–32.

427. Boone KB, Ananth J, Philpott L, Kaur A, Djenderedjian A. Neuropsychological characteristics of nondepressed adults with obsessive-compulsive disorder. Neuropsychiatry, Neuropsychology, and Behavioral Neurology 1991;4:96–109.

428. Zielinski CM, Taylor MA, Juzwin KR. Neuropsychological deficits in obsessive-compulsive disorder. Neuropsychiatry, Neuropsychology, and Behavioral Neurology 1991;4:110–126.

429. Christensen GA, Mackenzie TB, Mitchell JE, Callies AL. A placebo-controlled, double-blind crossover study of fluoxetine in trichotillomania. Am J Psychiatry 1991;148:1566–1571.

430. Jenike MA, Brotman. The EEG in obsessive-compulsive disorder. J Clin Psychiatry 1984;46:122–124.

431. Beech HR, Ciesielski KT, Gordon PK. Further observations of evoked potentials in obsessional patients. Br J Psychiatry 1983;142:605–609.

432. Shagass C, Roemer RA, Straumanis JJ, Josiassen RC. Distinctive somatosensory evoked potential features in obsessive-compulsive disorder. Biol Psychiatry 1984;19:1507–1524.

433. Towey J, Bruder G, Hollander E, et al. Endogenous event-related potentials in obsessive-compulsive disorder. Biol Psychiatry 1990;28:92–98.

434. Talairach J, Bancard J, Geiver S, et al. The cingulate gyrus and human behavior. Electroencephalogr Clin Neurophysiol 1973;34:45–52.

435. Barr LC, Goodman WK, Price LH, McDougle CJ, Charney DS. The serotonin hypothesis of obsessive compulsive disorder: implications of pharmacologic challenge studies. J Clin Psychiatry 1992;53(Suppl 4):17–28.

436. Fernandez CE, Lopez Ibor AJ. La monoclorimipramina en enfermos psiquiatricos resistentes a otros tratamientos. Actas Luso Esp Neurol Psiquiat 1969;26:119–147.

437. Van Renynghe-de-Voxvrie G. Use of anafranil (G34586) in obsessive neuroses. Acta Neurol Psychiatr Belg 1968;68:787–792.

438. Capstick N. Chlorimipramine in obsessional states. Psychosomatics 1971;12:332–335.

439. Insel TR, Murphy DL, Cohen RM, Alterman I, Kilts C, Linnoila M. A double-blind trial of clomipramine and clorgyline. Arch Gen Psychiatry 1983;40:605–612.

440. Thoren R, Asberg M, Cronholm B, Jonertedt L, Traskman L. Clomipramine treatment of obsessive-compulsive disorder: I. A controlled study. Arch Gen Psychiatry 1980;37:1281–1285.

441. Marks IM, Stern RS, Mawson D, Cobb J, McDonald R. Clomipramine and exposure for obsessive compulsive rituals: I. Br J Psychiatry 1980;136:1–25.

442. Ananth J, Pecknold JC, Van Den Steen N, et al. Double-blind comparative study of clomipramine and amitriptyline in obsessive neurosis. Biol Psychiatry 1981;5:257–262.

443. Zohar J, Insel T. Obsessive-compulsive disorder: psychobiological approaches to diagnosis, treatment and pathophysiology. Biol Psychiatry 1987;22:667–687.

444. Mavissakalian M, Turner SM, Michelson L, Jacob R. Tricyclic antidepressants in obsessive-compulsive disorder: antiobsessional or antidepressant agents? II. Am J Psychiatry 1985;142:572–576.

445. Clomipramine Collaborative Study Group. Clomipramine in the treatment of patients with obsessive-compulsive disorder. Arch Gen Psychiatry 1991;48:730–738.

446. Kasvikis Y, Marks IM: Clomipramine in obsessive-compulsive ritualizers treated with exposure therapy: relations between dose, plasma levels outcome and side effects. Psychopharmacology 1988;95:113–118.

447. Stern RS, Marks IM, Wright J, et al. Clomipramine: plasma levels, side effects and outcome in obsessive compulsive neurosis. Postgrad Med J 1980;56(1 Suppl):134–139.

448. Pigott TA, Pato MT, Bernstein SE, et al. Controlled comparisons of clomipramine and fluoxetine in the treatment of obsessive-compulsive disorder. Behavioral and biological results. Arch Gen Psychiatry 1990;47:926–932.

449. Chouinard G, Goodman WK, Greist J, et al. Results of a double-blind placebo controlled trial of a new serotonin uptake inhibitor, sertraline, in the treatment of obsessive-compulsive disorder. Psychopharmacol Bull 1990;26:279–284.

450. Goodman WK, Price LH, Delgado PL, et al. Specificity of serotonin reuptake inhibitors in the treatment of obsessive-compulsive disorder. Comparison of fluvoxamine and desipramine (see comments). Arch Gen Psychiatry 1990b;47:577–585.

451. Kahn RS, Westenberg HG, Jolles J. Zimeldine treatment of obsessive-compulsive disorder. Biological and neuropsychological aspects. Acta Psychiatr Scand 1984;69:259–261.

452. Prasad, AJ. Obsessive-compulsive disorder and traxodone (Letter). Am J Psychiatry 1984;141:612–613.

453. Blier P, Chaput Y, de Montigny C. Long-term 5-HT reuptake blockade, but not monoamine oxidase inhibition, decreases the function of terminal 5-HT autoreceptors: an electrophysiological study in the rat brain. Naunyn Schmiedebergs Arch Pharmacol 1988;337:246–254.

454. Blier P, de Montigny C, Chaput Y. A role for the serotonin system in the mechanism of action of antidepressant treatments: preclinical evidence. J Clin Psychiatry 1990;51(Suppl 4):14–20.

455. Peroutka SJ, Snyder SH. Chronic antidepressant treatment decreases spiroperidol-labeled serotonin receptor binding. Science 1980;210:88–90.

456. Zohar J, Murphy DL, Zohar-Kadouch RC, et al. Serotonin in major psychiatric disorders. Washington, DC: American Psychiatric Press, 1990.

457. Drugs affecting 5-hydroxytryptamine function. Drug Ther Bull 1993;37:25–26.

458. Yaryura-Tobias JA, Bebirian RJ, Neziroglu FA, Bhagavan HN. Obsessive-compulsive disorders as a serotonergic defect. Res Commun Psychol Psychiatry Behav 1977;2:279–286.

459. Hanna GL, Yuwiler A, Cantwell DP. Whole blood serotonin in juvenile obsessive-compulsive disorder. Biol Psychiatry 1991;29:738–744.

460. Flament MF, Rapoport JL, Murphy DL, et al. Biochemical changes during clomipramine treatment of childhood obsessive-compulsive disorder (published erratum appears in Arch Gen Psychiatry 1987;44:548). Arch Gen Psychiatry 1987;44:219–225.

461. Insel TR, Mueller EA, Alterman I, et al. Obsessive-compulsive disorder and serotonin: is there a connection? Biol Psychiatry 1985;20:1174–1188.

462. Weizman A, Carmi M, Hermesh H, et al. High affinity imipramine binding and serotonin uptake in platelets of eight adolescent and ten adult obsessive-compulsive patients. Am J Psychiatry 1986;143:335–359.

463. Black DW, Kelly M, Myers C, Noyes R Jr. Tritiated imipramine binding in obsessive-compulsive volunteers and psychiatrically normal controls. Biol Psychiatry 1990;27:319–327.

464. Bastani B, Arora RC, Meltzer HY. Serotonin uptake and imipramine binding in the blood platelets of obsessive-compulsive disorder patients. Biol Psychiatry 1991;30:131–139.

465. Vitello BH, Shimon H, Behar D, et al. Platelet imipramine binding and serotonin uptake in obsessive-compulsive patients. Acta Psychiatr Scand 1991;84:29–32.

466. Kim SW, Dysken MW, Pandey GN, Davis JM. Platelet ^{3}H-imipramine binding sites in obsessive-compulsive behavior. Biol Psychiatry 1991;30:467–474.

467. Kruesi MJ, Rapoport JL, Hamburger S, et al. Cerebrospinal fluid monoamine metabolites, aggression, and impulsivity in disruptive behavior disorders of children and adolescents. Arch Gen Psychiatry 1990;47:419–426.

468. Lydiard RB, Ballenger JC, Ellinwood E, et al. CSF monoamine metabolites in obsessive-compulsive disorder. New York: Presented at the 143rd annual meeting of the American Psychiatric Association, 1990. Cited in Barr LC, Goodman WK, Price LH, McDougle CJ, Charney DS. The serotonin hypothesis of obsessive compulsive disorder: Implications of pharmacologic challenge studies. J Clin Psychiatry 1992;53(4 Suppl) 17–28.

469. Leckman JF, Goodman WK, Riddle MA, et al. Low CSF 5HIAA and obsessions of violence: report of two cases. Psychiatry Res 1990;35:95–99.

470. Aloi JA, Insel TR, Mueller EA, et al. Neuroendocrine and behavioral effects of m-chlorophenylpiperazine administration in rhesus monkeys. Life Sci 1984;43:1325–1331.

471. Hollander E, DeCaria CM, Nitescu A, et al. Serotonergic function in obsessive-compulsive disorder: behavioral and neuroendocrine responses to oral m-chlorophenypiperazine and fenfluramine in patients and healthy volunteers. Arch Gen Psychiatry 1992;49:21–28.

472. Charney DS, Goodman WK, Price LH, et al. Serotonin function in obsessive-compulsive disorder. A comparison of the effects of tryptophan and m-chlorophenylpiperazine in patients and healthy subjects. Arch Gen Psychiatry 1988;45:177–185.

473. Zohar J, Mueller A, Insel TR, et al. Serotonergic responsivity in obsessive-compulsive disorder. Comparison of patients and healthy controls. Arch Gen Psychiatry 1987;44:946–951.

474. Zohar J, Insel TR, Zohar-Kadouch RC, Hill JL, Murphy DL. Serotonergic responsivity in obsessive-compulsive disorder. Effects of chronic clomipramine treatment. Arch Gen Psychiatry 1988;46:167–172.

475. Lesch KP, Hoh A, Disselkamp-Tietze J, et al. 5-hydroxytryptamine receptor responsivity in obsessive-compulsive disorder: comparison of patients and controls. Arch Gen Psychiatry 1991;48:540–547.

476. McBridge PA, DeMeo MD, Sweeney JA, et al. Neuroendocrine and behavioral responses to challenge with the indirect serotonin agonist DL-fenfluramine in adults with obsessive-compulsive disorder. Biol Psychiatry 1992;31:19–34.

477. Van Praag HM, Lemus C, Kahn R. Hormonal probes of central serotonergic activity: do they really exist? Biol Psychiatry 1987;22:86–98.

478. Kahn RS, Wetzler S, Van Praag HM, et al. Behavioral indications for serotonin receptor hypersensitivity in panic disorder. Psychiatry Res 1988;25:101–104.

479. Charney DS, Woods SW, Goodman WK, et al. Serotonin function in anxiety. II: effects of the serotonin agonist, MCPP, in panic disorder patients and healthy subjects. Psychopharmacology 1987;92:14–24.

480. Benkelfat C, Murphy DL, Zohar J, et al. Clomipramine in obsessive-compulsive disorder. Further evidence for a serotonergic mechanism of action. Arch Gen Psychiatry 1989;46:23–28.

481. Baldwin D, Fineberg N, Bullock T, Montgomery S. Serotonin 1A receptors and obsessive-compulsive disorder. In: Gastpar M, et al, ed. Serotonin 1A receptors in depression and anxiety. New York: Raven Press, 1992:193–200.

482. Siever LJ, Insel TR, Jumerson DC, et al. Growth hormone response to clonidine in obsessive-compulsive patients. Br J Psychiatry 1983;142:184–187.

483. Lee MA, Cameron OG, Gurguis GN, et al. Alpha 2-adrenoreceptor status in obsessive-compulsive disorder. Biol Psychiatry 1990;27:1983–1093.

484. Hollander E, DeCaria C, Nitescu A, et al. Noradrenergic function in obsessive-compulsive disorder: behavioral and neuroendocrine responses to clonidine and comparison to healthy controls. Psychiatry Res 1991;37:161–177.

485. Rasmussen SA, Goodman WK, Woods SW, et al. Effects of yohimbine in obsessive compulsive disorder. Psychopharmacology 1987;93:308–313.

486. Janowsky A, Okada F, Manier DH, Applegate GD, Sulser F. Role of serotonergic input in the regulation of the B-adrenergic receptor-coupled adenylate cyclase system. Science 1982;219:900–901.

487. Blier P, de Montigny C, Chaput Y. Modifications of the serotonin system by anti-depressant treatments: implications for the therapeutic response in major depression. J Clin Psychopharmacol 1987;7:24S–35S.

488. Racagni G, Bradford D. Florence, Italy: Proceedings of the 14th Collegium Internationale Neuro-Psychopharmacologicum Congress, 1984:733.

489. Insel TR, Pickar D. Naloxone administration in obsessive-compulsive disorder: report of two cases. Am J Psychiatry 1983;140:1219–1220.

490. Goodman WK, McDougle CJ, Price LH, et al. Beyond the serotonin hypothesis: a role for dopamine in some forms of obsessive-compulsive disorder. J Clin Psychiatry 1990a;51(Suppl):36–43, 55–58.

491. Creese I, Iversen SD. The role of forebrain dopamine systems in amphetamine induced stereotyped behavior in the rat. Psychopharmacologia 1974;39:345–357.

492. Loew DM, Vigouret J-M, Jaton A. Neuropharmacology of bro-

mocriptine and dihydroergotoxine (Hydergine). In: Goldstein M, ed. Ergot compounds and brain function: neuroendocrine and neuropsychiatric aspects. New York: Raven Press, 1980:63–74.

493. Wallach MB, Gershon S. A neuropsychopharmacological comparison of d-amphetamine, L-dopa and cocaine. Neuropharmacology 1971; 10:743–752.

494. Willner JH, Samach M, Angrist BM, et al. Drug-induced stereotyped behavior and and its antagonism in dogs. Comm Behav Biol 1970;5:135–142.

495. Randrup A, Munkvad HM. Stereotyped activities produced by amphetamine in several animal species and man. Psychopharmacologia 1967;11:300–310.

496. Koizumi HM. Obsessive-compulsive symptoms following stimulants. Biol Psychiatry 1985;20:1332–1337.

497. Frye PE, Arnold LE. Persistent amphetamine-induced compulsive rituals: response to pyridoxine (B6). Biol Psychiatry 1981;16: 583–587.

498. Leonard HL, Rapoport JL. Relief of obsessive-compulsive symptoms following stimulants. Biol Psychiatry 1987;20:1332–1337.

499. McDougle CJ, Goodman WK, Delgado PL, et al. Pathophysiology of obsessive compulsive disorder (Letter). Am J Psychiatry 1989;146: 1350–1351.

500. Austin LS, Lydiard RB, Ballenger JC, et al. Dopamine blocking activity of clomipramine in patients with obsessive-compulsive disorder. Biol Psychiatry 1991;30:225–232.

501. Lipinski JF Jr, Mallya G, Zimmerman P, et al. Fluoxetine-induced akathisia: clinical and theoretical implications. J Clin Psychiatry 1989;50:339–342.

502. Tate JL. Extrapyramidal symptoms in a patient taking haloperidol and fluoxetine. Am J Psychiatry 1989;146:399–400.

503. Bouchard RH, Pourcher E, Vincent P. Fluoxetine and extrapyramidal side effects. Am J Psychiatry 1989;146:1352–1353.

504. Brod TM. Fluoxetine and extrapyramidal side effects. Am J Psychiatry 1989;146:1353.

505. Meltzer HY, Young M, Metz J, Frang VS, Schyve PM, Arora RC. Extrapyramidal side effects and increased serum prolactin following fluoxetine, a new antidepressant. J Neural Transm 1979; 45:165–175.

506. Swedo SE, Leonard HL, Kruesi MJP, et al. Cerebrospinal fluid neurochemistry in children and adolescents with obsessive-compulsive disorder. Arch Gen Psychiatry 1992;49:29–36.

507. Inouye E. Similar and dissimilar manifestations of obsessive-compulsive neurosis in monozygotic twins. Am J Psychiatry 1965; 121:1171–1175.

508. McKeon J, McGuffin P, Robinson P. Obsessive-compulsive neurosis following head injury: a report of 4 cases. Br J Psychiatry 1984;144: 190–192.

509. Torgerson S. Genetic factors in anxiety disorders. Arch Gen Psychiatry 1983;40:1085–1089.

510. Carey G, Gottesman I. Twin and family studies of anxiety, phobic and obsessive disorders. In: Klein DF, Rabin JG. Anxiety: new research and current concepts. New York: Raven Press, 1981.

511. Clifford CA, Murray RM, Fulker DW. Genetic and environmental influences on obsessional traits and symptoms. Psychol Med 1984; 14:791–800.

512. Luxenberger H. Hereditat und Familientypus der Zwangsneurotiker. Archiv fur Psychiatrie 1930;91:590–594.

513. Brown FW. Heredity in the psychoneuroses (summary). Proc R Soc Lond 1942;35:785–790.

514. Cohen ME, Badal DW, Kilpatrick A, Reed EW, White PD. The high familial prevalence of neurocirculatory asthenia (anxiety neurosis, effort syndrome). Am J Hum Genet 1951;3:126–158.

515. Carey G. A clinical genetic twin study of obsessive and phobic states [Ph.D. Thesis]. Minnesota: University of Minnesota, 1978.

516. Pauls DL, Raymond CL, Hurst CR, Rasmussen S, Goodman W, Leckman JF. Transmission of obsessive compulsive disorder and associated behaviors. Montreal, Canada: Proceedings of the 43rd Meeting of the Society of Biological Psychiatry, 1988b.

517. Rasmussen SA, Eisen JL. Clinical features and phenomenology of obsessive-compulsive disorder. Psychiatr Ann 1989;19:67–73.

518. Alarcon RD. How to recognize obsessive-compulsive disorder. Postgrad Med 1991;90:131–143.

519. Cooper J. The Leyton Obsessional Inventory. Psychol Med 1970;1: 46–64.

520. Snowdon J. A comparison of written and postbox forms of the Leyton Obsessional Inventory. Psychol Med 1980;10:165–170.

521. Berg CJ, Rapoport JL, Flament M. The Leyton Obsessional Inventory-child version. J Am Acad Child Adolesc Psychiatry 1986;25(1):84–91.

522. Mears R. Obsessionality: the Sandler-Hazari scale and spasmodic torticollis. Br J Med Psychol 1971;44:181–182.

523. Philpot R. Recent advances in the behavioral measurement of obsessional illness. Scott Med J 1975;20 (Suppl 1):33–40.

524. Rackman C, Hodgson R. Obsessions and compulsions. Engelwood Cliffs, NJ: Prentice-Hall, 1980.

525. Goodman WK, Price LH, Rasmussen SA, et al. The Yale-Brown Obsessive-Compulsive Scale. II. Validity. Arch Gen Psychiatry 1989;46:1012–1016.

526. Goodman WK, Price LH, Rasmussen SA, et al. The Yale-Brown Obsessive-Compulsive Scale. I. Development, use, and reliability. Arch Gen Psychiatry 1989;46:1006–1011.

527. Foa EB, Kozak MJ. Diagnostic criteria for obsessive-compulsive disorder. Hosp Comm Psychiatry 1991;42:679–680, 684.

528. Greist JH. Treatment of obsessive compulsive disorder psychotherapies, drugs, and other somatic treatment. J Clin Psychiatry 1990;51 (Suppl):44–50.

529. Malan DH. Individual psychotherapy and the science of psychodynamics. London: Butterworths, 1979:218–219.

530. Meyer V. Modification of expectations in cases with obsessive rituals. Behav Res Ther 1966;4:270–280.

531. Piacentini J, Jaffer M, Gitow A, et al. Psychopharmacologic treatment of child and adolescent obsessive compulsive disorder. Pediatric Psychopharmacology 1992;15:87–107.

532. Robertson J. A controlled investigation of the treatment of obsessive-compulsive disorders [MD dissertation]. London: Middlesex Hospital, 1979.

533. O'Sullivan G, Noshirvani H, Marks I, Monteiro W, Lelliott P. Six-year follow-up after exposure and clomipramine therapy for obsessive compulsive disorder. J Clin Psychiatry 1991;52:150–155.

534. Foa E, Steketee G, Grayson JB, et al. Deliberate exposure and blocking of obsessive compulsive rituals: immediate and long-term effects. Beh Ther 1984;15:450–472.

535. Greist JH. An integrated approach to treatment of obsessive compulsive disorder. J Clin Psychiatry 1992;53 (Suppl 4):38–41.

536. Emmelkamp MG, Beens H. Cognitive therapy with obsessive-compulsive disorder: A comparative evaluation. Behav Res Ther 1991;29:293–300.

537. Salkovikis PM. Cognitive factors in obsessive-compulsive disorder. Current approaches. Obsessive Compulsive Disorder. Montgomery SA, Goodman WK, Goeting N, Eds. Ashford Colonial Press, Gosport, Hants: Duphar Medical Relations 1990:26–37.

538. Marks I, Lelliott P, Basoglu M, et al. Clomipramine, self-exposure and therapist aided exposure in obsessive-compulsive ritualizers. Br J Psychiatry 1988;152:522–534.

539. Turner SM, Beidel DC, Stanley MA, et al. A comparison of fluoxetine, flooding and response prevention in the treatment of obsessive compulsive disorder. Journal of Anxiety Disorders 1988; 2:219–225.

540. Cottraux J, Mollard E, Bouvard M, et al. A controlled study of fluvoxamine and exposure in obsessive compulsive disorder. Int Clin Psychopharmacol 1990;5:17–30.

541. Ananth J. Treatment of obsessive compulsive neurosis: pharmacological approach. Psychosomatics 1976;17:180–184.

542. Rack PH. Clinical experience in the treatment of obsessional states. J Int Med Res 1977;5:81–96.

543. Volavka JF, Neziroglu, Yaryura-Tobias JA. Clomipramine and

imipramine in obsessive-compulsive disorder. Psychiatry Res 1985; 14:85–93.

544. Price L, Goodman W, Charney D, Rasmussen S, Heninger G. Treatment of severe obsessive-compulsive disorder with fluvoxamine. Am J Psychiatry 1987;144:1059–1061.

545. Jenike MA, Hyman S, Baer L, et al. A controlled trial of fluvoxamine in obsessive-compulsive disorder: implications for a serotonergic theory. Am J Psychiatry 1990;147:1209–1215.

546. Turner SM, Jacob RG, Beidel DC, Himmelhoch J. Fluoxetine treatment of obsessive compulsive disorder. J Clin Psychopharmacol 1985;5:207–212.

547. Fontaine R, Chouinard G. An open clinical trial of fluoxetine in the treatment of obsessive-compulsive disorder. J Clin Psychopharmacol 1986;6:98–101.

548. Jenike MA, Buttolph L, Baer L, Ricciardi J, Holland A. Open trial of fluoxetine in obsessive-compulsive disorder. Am J Psychiatry 1989; 146:909–911.

549. Liebowitz MR, Hollander E, Schneier F. Fluoxetine treatment of obsessive-compulsive disorder: an open clinical trial. J Clin Psychopharmacol 1989;9:423–427.

550. Chouinard G, Goodman W, Greist J, et al. Results of a double-blind placebo controlled trial of a new serotonin uptake inhibitor, sertraline, in the treatment of obsessive-compulsive disorder. Psychopharmacol Bull 1990;26:279–284.

551. Riddle MA, Leckman JF, Hardin MT, Anderson GM, Cohen DJ. Fluoxetine treatment of obsessions and compulsions in patients with Tourette's syndrome (Letter). Am J Psychiatry 1988;145: 1173–1174.

552. Wheadon DE. Placebo controlled multi-center trial of fluoxetine in OCD. Florence, Italy: Presented at the 5th World Congress of Biological Psychiatry, 1991. Cited in Barr CL, Goodman WK, Price LH et al. The serotonin hypothesis of obsessive compulsive disorder: Implications of Pharmacologic challenge studies J Clin Psychiatry 1992;56(4 Suppl)17–28.

553. Zohar J, Zohar-Kadouch RC, Kindler. Current concepts in the pharmacological treatment of obsessive compulsive disorder. Practical Therapeutics and Drugs 1992;43:210–218.

554. Pato MT, Zohar KR, Zohar J, Murphy DL. Return of symptoms after discontinuation of clomipramine in patients with obsessive-compulsive disorder. Am J Psychiatry 1988;145:1521–1525.

555. Pato MT, Hill JL, Murphy DL. A clomipramine dosage reduction study in the course of long-term treatment of obsessive-compulsive disorder patients. Psychopharmacol Bull 1990;26:211–214.

556. Rasmussen SA. Lithium and tryptophan augmentation in clomipramine-resistant obsessive-compulsive disorder. Am J Psychiatry 1984;141:1283–1285.

557. Mattes JA. A pilot study of combined trazodone and tryptophan in obsessive-compulsive disorder. Int Clin Psychopharmacol 1986;1: 170–173.

558. Hollander E, DeCariar CM, Schneier FR, et al. Fenfluramine augmentation of serotonin reuptake blockade antiobsessional treatment. J Clin psychiatry 1990;51:119–123.

559. Markovitz PJ, Stagno SJ, Calabrese JR. Buspirone augmentation of fluoxetine in obsessive-compulsive disorder. Am J Psychiatry 1990; 147:798–800.

560. Stern TA, Jenike MA. Treatment of obsessive-compulsive disorder with lithium carbonate. Psychosomatics 1983;24:671–673.

561. Golden RN, Morris JE, Sack DA. Combined lithium-tricyclic treatment of obsessive-compulsive disorder. Biol Psychiatry 1988; 23:181–185.

562. Eisenberg L, Asnis G. Lithium as an adjunct treatment in obsessive-compulsive disorder (Letter). Am J Psychiatry 1986;142.

563. Ruegg RG, Evans DL, Comer WS, et al. Lithium plus fluoxetine treatment of obsessive compulsive disorder [Abstract]. In: New Research Program and Abstracts of the 143rd annual meeting of the American Psychiatric Association. New York: American Psychiatric Association, 1990:NR 92.

564. Pigott TA, Pato MT, L'Heureux F, et al. A controlled comparison of

565. McDougle CJ, Price LH, Goodman WK, et al. A controlled trial of lithium augmentation in fluvoxamine-refractory obsessive-compulsive disorder: lack of efficacy. J Clin Psychopharmacol 1991;11: 175–184.

566. Bodkin JA, White K. Clonazepam in the treatment of obsessive compulsive disorder associated with panic disorder in one patient. J Clin Psychiatry 1989;50:265–266.

567. Hewlett WA, Vinogradov S, Agras WS. Clonazepam treatment of obsessions and compulsions. J Clin Psychiatry 1990;51:158–161.

568. Tesar GE, Jenike MA. Alpraxolam as treatment for a case of obsessive compulsive disorder. Am J Psychiatry 1984;141:689–690.

569. Tollefson G. Alprazolam in the treatment of obsessive symptoms. J Clin Psychopharmacol 1985;5:39–42.

570. Jenike MA. Rapid response of severe obsessive compulsive disorder to tranylcypromine. Am J Psychiatry 1981;138:1249–1250.

571. Knesevich JW. Successful treatment of obsessive compulsive disorder with clonidine hydrochloride. Am J Psychiatry 1982;139:364–365.

572. Yoney TH, Pigott TA, L'Heureux F, Rosenthal NE. Seasonal variation in obsessive compulsive disorder: preliminary experience with light treatment. Am J Psychiatry 1991;148:1727–1729.

573. Bird JM, Crow CD. Psychosurgery in obsessional-compulsive disorder: old techniques and new data. Current approaches. Obsessive compulsive disorder. Montgomery SA, Goodman WK, Goeting N, Eds. Ashford Colonial Press, Gosport Harris Duphar Medical Relations 1990:82–92.

574. Mindus P. Capsulotomy in anxiety disorders: a multidisciplinary study. Stockholm, Sweden: Kongl Carolinska Medico Chirurgiska Institute, 1991. Cited in Goodman WK, McDougle CJ, Price LH. Pharmacotherapy of obsessive compulsive disorder. J Clin Psychiatry 1992;53(4 Suppl)29–37.

575. Stevens H. The syndrome of Gilles de la Tourette and its treatment. Med Ann DC 1964;33:277–279.

576. Hoogduin K. On the diagnosis of obsessive-compulsive disorder. Am J Psychother 1986;40:36–51.

577. Grasset J. Lecons sur un cas de maladie des tics et un cas de tremblement singulier de la tete et des membres gauches. Arch Neurol 1890;20:27-45, 187–211.

578. Kinnear-Wilson SAK. Tics and allied conditions. J Neurol Psychopathol 1927;8:93–109.

579. Ascher E. Psychodynamic consideration in Gilles de la Tourette's disease (maladie des tics): with a report of five cases and discussion of the literature. Am J Psychiatry 1948;105:267–276.

580. Zausmer DM. The treatment of tics in childhood: a review and follow-up study. Arch Dis Child 1954;29:537–542.

581. Torup E. A follow-up study of children with tics. Acta Pediatr Scand 1962;51:261–268.

582. Shapiro AK, Shapiro E, Wayne H, Clarkin J. The psychopathology of Gilles de la Tourette's syndrome. Am J Psychiatry 1972;129: 87–94.

583. Shapiro E, Shapiro AK, Clarkin J. Clinical psychological testing in Tourette's syndrome. J Pers Assess 1974;38:464–478.

584. Frankel M, Cummings JL, Robertson MM, et al. Obsessions and compulsions in Gilles de la Tourette's syndrome. Neurology 1986; 36:378–382.

585. Green RC, Pitman RK. Tourette syndrome and obsessive-compulsive disorder. In: Jenike MA, Baer L, Minichiello WO, eds. Obsessive-compulsive disorder: theory and management. Littleton, MA: PSGP Publishing, 1986.

586. Rasmussen SA, Tsuang MT. Clinical characteristics and family history in DSM III obsessive-compulsive disorder. Am J Psychiatry 1986; 143:317–322.

587. Pitman RK, Green RC, Jenike MA, Mesulam MM. Clinical comparison of Tourette's disorder and obsessive-compulsive disorder. Am J Psychiatry 1987;144:1166–1171.

588. George MS, Trimble MR, Ring HA, et al. Obsessions in obsessive-

compulsive disorder with and without Gilles de la Tourette's syndrome. Am J Psychiatry 1993;150:93–97.

589. Leckman JF, Grice DE, Barr LC, de Vries ALC, Martin C, Cohen DJ, McDougle CJ, Goodman WK, Rasmussen SA. Tic-related vs. non-tic-related obsessive compulsive disorder. *Anxiety* 1995 (in press).

590. Pitman RK, Jenike MA. Coprolalia in obsessive-compulsive disorder: a missing link. J Nerv Ment Dis 1988;176:311–313.

591. Cummings JL, Frankel M. Gilles de la Tourette syndrome and the neurological basis of obsessions and compulsions. Biol Psychiatry 1985;20:1117–1126.

592. Segal NL, Dysken MW, Bouchard TJ Jr, Pedersen NL, Eckert ED, Heston LL. Tourette's disorder in a set of reared apart triplets: genetic and environmental influences. Am J Psychiatry 1990; 147:196–199.

593. Pauls DL, Leckman J, Towbin KE, et al. A possible genetic relationship exists between Tourette's syndrome and obsessive-compulsive disorder. Psychopharmacol Bull 1986a;22:730–733.

594. Pauls DL, Towbin KE, Leckman JF, et al. Gilles de la Tourette's syndrome and obsessive compulsive disorder. Evidence supporting a genetic relationship. Arch Gen Psychiatry 1986;43:1180–1182.

595. Crespi F, Martin KF, Marsden C. Simultaneous in vivo voltammetric measurement of striatal extracellular DOPAC and 5-HIAA levels: effect of electrical stimulation of DA and 5HT neuronal pathways. Neuroscience Lett 1988;90:285–291.

596. McDougle CJ, Goodman WK, Price LH, et al. Neuroleptic addition in fluvoxamine refractory OCD [Abstract]. Am Psychiatr Assoc New Res Abstracts, 1989:NR 350.

597. Rapoport JL. Childhood obsessive compulsive disorder. J Child Psychol Psychiatry 1986;27:289–295.

598. Pitman RK. Pierre Janet on obsessive compulsive disorder (1903). Arch Gen Psychiatry 1987;44:226–232.

36
CORTICAL DEMENTIA

Charles E. Wells and Peter J. Whitehouse

Alzheimer's disease (AD) is the most common degenerative dementia and is characterized clinically by progressive loss of abilities in a number of cognitive and behavioral domains. The term degenerative implies progressive decline in the number of neurons in the central nervous system. In the first part of this chapter we initially review the systems neuroscience approach to the understanding of AD, namely the characterization of the populations of neurons affected and their associated neurotransmitters. In the second section we review the cytoskeletal and extracellular abnormalities associated with this neuronal loss. And, finally, we consider clues to its etiology, which lie primarily in the area of molecular biology and especially genetics.

None of the biological markers of AD that we discuss here can be measured adequately in life without a brain biopsy, which is rarely performed because it usually has few therapeutic implications. Therefore, AD remains a clinical impression that needs to be confirmed by analysis of tissue obtained at autopsy. Even with the examination of necropsy material, however, diagnostic dilemmas remain. For example, it is still not clear whether there are qualitative as well as quantitative differences in the neuronal loss and cellular changes found in AD when compared with normal aging. Moreover, the clinical heterogeneity has a biological basis. For example, the relationships between Lewy body dementia and AD are controversial. The term AD itself may well encompass several processes or diseases. Perhaps some of the biological changes we review represent the final common pathway of a number of etiological events.

SYSTEMS NEUROSCIENCE
Neocortex

Neuronal loss occurs in a number of brain areas in patients with AD (1, 2) although the pathological changes were originally observed by Alois Alzheimer in the neocortex. Gross cortical atrophy is accompanied by loss of neurons and synapses, with associated astrogliosis. Neurofibrillary tangles (NFT) and senile plaques (SP) are observed in the cortex, primarily in association areas. White matter may also be involved, perhaps partly due to the loss of neurons.

Alterations in blood vessels also occur, including deposition of amyloid (amyloid angiopathy) as well as neurotransmitter receptor and other neurochemical changes.

The cortical neurons that are affected in AD use a number of neurotransmitters, including excitatory amino acids such as glutamate, as well as neuropeptides, corticotrophin releasing factor, and somatostatin (3, 4). Variable changes occur in other neuromodulators, such as substance P and neuropeptide Y.

Hippocampus and Hippocampal-Associated Circuits

Prominent pathology occurs in the hippocampus and may underlie some of the significant memory problems that occur in the disorder (5). Loss of pyramidal cells is greatest in CA1, CA2, and the entorhinal cortex. Granulovacular degeneration is often commonly seen in the hippocampus. Pathology also occurs in associated structures such as the amygdala.

Basal Forebrain Cholinergic Systems

Loss of cells in the cholinergic basal forebrain, which includes the nucleus basalis of Meynert, the nucleus of diagonal band, and medial septum, is also a consistent feature of AD (6). This abnormality has attracted particular attention because the reductions in choline acetyltransferase associated with the loss of neurons in the basal forebrain have been most strongly associated with the cognitive impairment (7). Moreover, tacrine, a cholinesterase inhibitor that increases levels of acetylcholine in the brain of patients with AD, has recently been recommended for approval by the Food and Drug Administration. In association with the loss of cholinergic neurons, there is also loss of specific neurotransmitters, including muscarinic receptors (particularly M_2), and nicotinic receptors (8).

Cholinergic neurons in the basal forebrain express nerve growth factor (NGF) receptors, and in animal models NGF has been shown to rescue neurons with experimentally induced damage in this structure. In Sweden two patients have already been given intraventricular NGF to try to

Figure 36.1. Low-power view showing numerous neurofibrillary tangles and extracellular neuritic plaques.

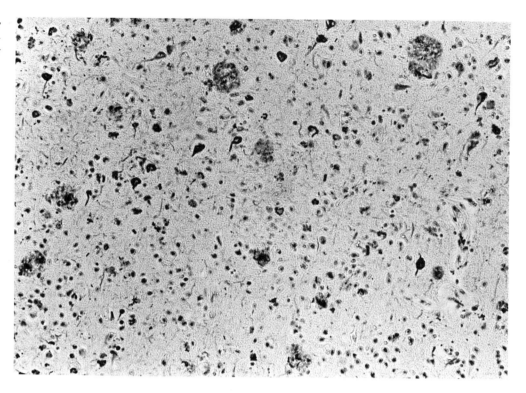

enhance the viability of these cell populations and to slow the progression of disease.

Brainstem Monoaminergic Systems

Loss of cells in the noradrenergic locus ceruleus (9) and serotonergic raphe nucleus (10) also occur in AD, although perhaps less consistently than in some of the other areas already discussed. Dysfunction in cells in these populations may be associated with some of the noncognitive symptoms found in the disorder, such as depression and psychosis (10).

Conclusion

AD is a multisystem disorder involving a large number of different neuronal populations. Claims have been made for pathology in many other areas of brain besides those just described. Some findings are not consistently reported (e.g., retina) and others show considerable variability across individual patients (e.g., hypothalamus). The challenge for the future is to understand which populations are affected and how to develop drugs to either prevent the damage in the first place or treat symptoms that result from the loss of specific populations of neurons and their synapses.

CELLULAR NEUROSCIENCE

Neurofibrillary Tangles

In 1907 Alzheimer was the first to describe neurofibrillary tangles (NFT), although the association between dementia and senile plaques had been described previously. NFTs are perhaps most strongly associated with specific neuronal loss

because they occur in populations of neurons in which cell dysfunction and eventual death occur. NFTs are composed of 15-nm straight filaments and 10-nm paired helical filaments (2, 11). Immunocytochemically the NFTs have been found to have several associated cellular constitutents, including microtubular-associated proteins, such as tau and ubiquitin (11). Many believe that tau or a modification of tau forms the core of the NFT (12). Abnormalities in phosphorylation may also occur. Others claim that there are abnormalities in certain growth-associated proteins in NFTs and that the cytoskeletal changes represent abnormal attempts at regeneration (Fig. 36.1).

Senile Plaques

Senile plaques (SP) occur in high frequency in amygdala, hippocampus, and neocortex (1). They are spherical structures that have three principal components, abnormal neurites and glia cells surrounding a central core of amyloid. The main constituent of the core of amyloid is a protein referred to as the β-A4 peptide. This approximately 42-amino-acid peptide is part of a much larger precursor protein, the amyloid precursor protein (APP) (13). Various forms of APP of different molecular weights exist. Whether or not the amyloid protein itself is neurotoxic is controversial (14), but great efforts are under way to understand the processing of amyloid, i.e., how β-A4 forms from APP in the brain and how the process is altered in AD. As recent genetic studies described in the next section demonstrate, mutations in the gene for the APP located on chromosome 21 can cause AD.

The origin of the amyloid is unclear, some believing that it is bloodborne and others believing it is derived from neurons or glia. A major unsolved part of the amyloid process is how the β-A4 protein, a small peptide, forms the β-pleated sheet, a configuration that is amyloidogenic. These SPs and NFTs have been claimed to be associated with the severity of clinically apparent dementia. It is more likely that the loss of neurons, synapses, and neurotransmitter elements is a more direct cause of the cognitive impairment.

MOLECULAR NEUROSCIENCE

Major advances have been made recently in understanding the molecular pathogenesis of AD. Much of it has been focused on the formation of SP motivated by genetic discoveries of abnormalities in the gene for APP (15) in rare families. It has been known since the 1930s that some cases of AD are familial and that some pedigrees demonstrate autosomal-dominant inheritance. In the 1940s an association between AD and Down syndrome was discovered (16). Individuals with trisomy 21 invariably develop SPs and NFTs after about the age of 35, and some develop dementia superimposed on the preexisting mental retardation. An explosion of knowledge has occurred recently in which linkage studies have identified other possible genetic abnormalities on chromosomes 14 and 19 as well as 21.

Specific genetic mutations have been described in the APP, which is known to be located on the 21st chromosome. On chromosome 21 these mutations occur at two locations, involving several different possible amino acid substitutions. Their existence strongly suggests that at least one cause of AD is an abnormality in the APP.

How these mutations affect the processing of the protein and result in the accumulation in SPs is not known. Several different enzymes have been described that are involved in the processing of amyloid, and two major routes of metabolism have been described. Hopes have been raised that, if enough could be understood about the processing of amyloid, drugs could be developed to interfere with the basic pathogenic mechanism that leads to neuronal death. For example, the so-called Swedish mutation on chromosome 21 appears in cell culture to affect the endolysosomal processing pathway (17).

Most of the work on familial AD has focused on early-onset disease, in which patients begin to suffer the disorder in their 40s. However, a linkage exists between chromosome 19 and late-onset disease. Specifically, apolipoprotein E, a lipid-processing protein, has been associated with both late-onset and sporadic disease (18). This finding has particularly important implications because this risk factor (specifically homozygosity for E4 allele) may be associated with a large number of cases of AD. These genetic approaches may not only lead to the development of more effective therapies but also to diagnostic tests. In fact it is now possible in the early-onset families to perform pre-symptomatic testing, which of course raises complicated ethical issues.

Other factors that may contribute to the development of AD include metals and other environmental toxins. Claims have been made, for example, that aluminum is found in NFTs and SPs. Although some studies have observed this association, it is not clear that the aluminum is more than a secondary effect after a primary pathogenetic event has occurred (1). Epidemiological studies have contributed a number of interesting observations, including the possibility that head injury and cardiovascular disease are risk factors for AD. Both insults might affect blood-brain barrier and the deposition of amyloid in brain. Other studies have also shown that higher education can lower the risk of AD, possibly through a mechanism of increased functional brain reserve (19). Also, some epidemiological studies have suggested that smoking may be protective in AD; this observation is particularly interesting given the consistently reported reductions of nicotinic cholinergic receptors in cortical specimens from patients with AD and the fact that smoking increases nicotinic receptors (2, 8).

Conclusion

The study of AD remains one of the most active areas of molecular, cellular, and systems neuroscience. The major challenge ahead is to bridge the gap between a molecular characterization of the genetic abnormalities in the disease and the clinical symptoms that we see in patients so that we can more effectively develop both diagnostic tests and therapeutic interventions.

CARE OF THE DEMENTED PATIENT

The ultimate aim in all of medicine is to apply knowledge of basic pathophysiological mechanisms of disease to the treatment of diseased patients. It is indeed unfortunate that, so far, there are virtually no connecting bridges between what is known of the basic pathophysiology of dementia and the care of patients with dementia. As detailed previously, an understanding of the basic processes underlying AD has grown at an astonishing rate over the past several years. At the same time, investigations of multi-infarct dementia, the dementia of Parkinson's disease, and of Pick's disease are growing, but not quite as fast as the AD research pace. Yet, except for attempts to improve memory by increasing the brain's supply of acetylcholine, nothing learned about basic disease processes so far has enhanced the treatment of patients with dementia. Knowledge about the care of demented patients—and a great deal *is* known about caring for these patients—remains almost entirely experiential and symptom-dominated.

Meanwhile, neurologists, neuropsychiatrists, and psychiatrists are facing constantly increasing demands that they devote their skills to the care of demented patients. These demands will continue to grow at least for the next 20 years, during which time the total number of physicians devoting themselves to these three specialties is expected to increase little if at all, and during a time when the federal government is desperately trying to prevent increased spending on medical care for the elderly. Complicating the situation further, medical care for demented patients is one of the most labor intensive of all the medical specialties. These are frightening realities as we strive for improved quality of care for people with dementia.

The very notion that physicians should provide care for the demented patient is something of a late 20th century phenomenon. Through much of recorded history, dementia was a diagnosis made more often by the family than by the physician, and families assumed, quite rightly in most instances, that physicians had nothing to offer. Medical intervention was considered appropriate only in those most advanced cases with severe behavioral complications. Even in these cases, medical intervention was usually limited to confining the patient to a state mental hospital (an asylum) for the remainder of his or her life. If one consults medical textbooks (internal medicine, neurology, or psychiatry) of earlier years, one seldom finds any mention of the medical care of the demented patient before the early 1970s. Demented patients simply were not brought to physicians because of their dementia. If the diagnosis was made at all, it was usually almost as an afterthought of the internist or general practitioner, made when the patient was brought for some other medical problem, and recorded as, "family also mentions that patient is becoming senile," after which the dementia received no further attention.

Many experienced neurologists can recall seeing few patients diagnosed with AD during their early training. Similarly, many psychiatrists of the same generations recall that patients with "organic brain disease" were then deemed unsuitable for treatment or hospitalization in many psychiatric institutions. Dementia surely existed then, though not in the numbers now affected, but it was a silent and invisible disease, one seldom mentioned on death certificates even as a contributory cause of death.

The world is now very different. Thanks to the aging of the population in economically advanced countries and to the work of the Alzheimer's Disease and Related Disorders Association, AD is now on the tip of everyone's tongue. Yet in many ways, "the more things change, the more they stay the same." In most communities, large and small, often even in those with prestigious medical institutions, families still must search for a physician willing to try to provide continuous care for their demented family member. Although AD and related disorders have become "hot" areas in medical research, the medical profession as a whole has remained wary of providing care for these patients. In many communities there may not be even one physician willing to be identified publicly as a "dementia doctor."

The reasons for this are clear. First, the care of the patient with dementia often fails to provide the physician with the usual gratification and satisfaction that come with the care of persons with other disorders. It is rare—extremely rare—that the physician does not have to tell the patient and the family that the patient has an incurable illness. Moreover, because so many demented patients are unaware of their functional loss and thus of their need for medical attention, the ties that bind patient to physician are often not only weak

but nonexistent. Such patients may regard the physician as an adversary rather than a friend and view medical help as punishment rather than succor. Second, the care of the demented patient requires totally different clinical skills from those needed in other areas of medicine, and these skills are not taught in most medical schools or residency training programs. Most physicians who do a good job caring for these patients and their families have had to train themselves, often with more help from nursing and social work professionals than from physician mentors. Third, although caring for demented patients is both labor- and time-intensive, payment for these services is poor compared with that deemed appropriate for other medical services. Moreover, the system of payment is fragmented, chaotic, and unpredictable. Not surprisingly, medical students choose procedure-intensive specialties rather than caring for dementia patients while Medicare, the primary insurer for most of these patients, not only reduces fees paid for services on a yearly basis but also annually narrows the list of services that are covered.

This section deals with the needs of patients, families, and those professionals who seek to care for patients with AD and other dementing disorders. Examples of problems encountered in clinical practice supplement these discussions.

DIAGNOSIS

In the early days of this dementia era, accurate diagnosis was thought to give new hope to physicians caring for these patients. Studies began appearing in the late 1960s and early 1970s suggesting that perhaps as many as 15% of patients with dementia (or appearing to be demented) were suffering from treatable and thus potentially reversible disorders (20). Normal pressure hydrocephalus, vitamin B_{12} deficiency, hypothyroidism, depression, and a host of other medical, neurological, and psychiatric disorders were sought, and appropriately so, in every patient thought to be demented. There was hope that a sizable number of these patients might be treatable, and for a while this seemed to be the case.

Over the years, however, the yield from such diagnostic persistence seems to have dwindled, at least among those patients seen by neuropsychiatrists. In part this may result from the wide dissemination of these early studies, so that internists and general physicians now often routinely search for treatable causes in patients with dementia whom they see. In part this also may be because early studies often included a larger portion of patients in the presenium than are usually encountered in clinical practice today. In part, too, this may be because correction of the so-called treatable causes for dementia does not often result in a gratifying improvement in the dementia. For example, neuropsychiatrists continue to see demented patients who have low vitamin B_{12} levels, whether due to absorptive or nutritional causes, but only rarely do they encounter a demented patient in whom replacement of B_{12} results either in significant cognitive or functional improvement or in an appreciable slackening in the progression of the dementing process.

Such observations must not be allowed to lead neuropsychiatrists to the neglect of the niceties of the diagnostic process. At the same time, neuropsychiatrists must recognize that the diagnostic process per se is a fairly unimportant part of the overall medical care of the person with dementia. It should not be the focus of professional ministrations. Although one must still strive for an accurate syndrome (dementia) and disease (e.g., AD) diagnosis, at this stage of our knowledge, one seldom sees a demented patient in whom accurate disease diagnosis has any appreciable influence on the treatment of the person being cared for or on the ultimate outcome.

In this area of medicine, diagnosis is always a two-step process in which the physician seeks to answer two questions sequentially:

1. Does the patient have dementia?
2. If so, what is the disease causing the dementia?

Most patients who come or are brought to neuropsychiatrists with clinical presentations suggesting dementia seek answers to these two questions or, perhaps more often, another opinion concerning answers that have been offered by earlier examining physicians. Fortunately or unfortunately, ancillary diagnostic measures alone seldom permit an unequivocal diagnosis of dementia. Even more rarely do they allow a definite diagnosis of the two most common diseases (AD and multi-infarct dementia) causing dementia. These diagnoses still depend on the physician's skill and acumen. Overreliance on codified diagnostic criteria or on ancillary tests often leads to diagnostic error. It is comforting to the physician that in the best study published to date, accuracy in the diagnosis of AD was superior when based on clinical judgment than when based on any of three frequently used lists of "diagnostic criteria" for AD (21).

Syndrome Diagnosis

The criteria for the diagnosis of dementia are set out clearly and explicitly in the *Diagnostic and Statistical Manual of Mental Disorders (Fourth Edition),* published by the American Psychiatric Association (22). To summarize, the diagnosis of dementia can be made whenever a patient demonstrates impaired memory plus defects in at least one other area of cognition or changes in personality; when this impairment interferes with work, social activities, or relationships with others; when this is not due to delirium; and when "the disturbance cannot be accounted for by any nonorganic mental disorder." According to these criteria, the diagnosis of dementia is straightforward, even simple, save for the last criterion. The core problem is that all the other diagnostic criteria can be met in all the major "nonorganic mental" disorders as well, i.e., in those mental disorders for which no specific neurochemical or neuropathological basis has yet been identified.

In truth, most patients with dementia present in a straightforward manner, and with a careful history and clinical examination, the diagnosis is seldom in doubt. When there is doubt, though, the neuropsychiatrist is likely to be the specialist who must confront the problem, and it is at this level that the diagnostic dilemma is considered here. When all of these criteria are met, except for the last, what features should cause the clinician to doubt the diagnosis of dementia? Several factors come immediately to mind: a history of recent onset and rapid progression of symptoms; *marked* inconsistency in performance on cognitive testing from one examination to another; persistent clinical manifestations of either hypomania or depression; a lack of fit or congruence between various elements in the history, clinical examination, and results of ancillary diagnostic testing; a sense on clinical examination that the patient is dissimilar, in some precise or imprecise way, from most other demented patients for whom one has cared. Although any one or all of these features can raise doubts about the diagnosis of dementia, none rules it out. How does the neuropsychiatrist proceed?

In most medical specialties, the consultant turns to ancillary diagnostic procedures, and so does the neuropsychiatrist. For the neuropsychiatrist, however, none of the ancillary diagnostic instruments available to the neuropsychiatrist is as reliable diagnostically as are those possessed by most other specialties. To put it simply, when the diagnosis of dementia is questioned on the basis of any of the features just listed, there is no ancillary diagnostic procedure that can *with certainty* establish the diagnosis. Depressed and hypomanic elderly patients evincing cognitive impairment may have modest electroencephalographic (EEG) abnormalities, abnormalities on neuropsychological testing, and abnormalities on computerized tomography (CT) or magnetic resonance imaging (MRI) examination of the brain and yet still not have dementia. Similarly, patients may have significant dementia in the absence of any demonstrable abnormality on the EEG, CT, or MRI examination of the brain, and neurological examination. Among the readily available ancillary diagnostic procedures, only neuropsychological testing possesses the sensitivity to rule out dementia. Unfortunately, though, when there is cognitive impairment on clinical examination, neuropsychological testing always reveals abnormalities. Thus, its utility is severely limited in the sort of diagnostic dilemma under consideration here.

Patients and their families are now much better informed about dementia than they were only a few years ago, and many of them have learned and have hoped that on occasion, depression may mimic dementia. In fact, among those patients who are seen for diagnostic purposes, the question asked most often is, "Couldn't all these changes be due to depression and not dementia?" Sadly enough, the answer almost always is, "No."

Although dementia *may* mimic depression, it seldom (if ever) does so very accurately or convincingly. The neuropsychiatrist is much more likely to encounter two other categories of patients about whom diagnostic questions are raised: (*a*) elderly patients with depression alone but with definite cognitive defects; and (*b*) elderly patients with both depression and dementia.

In the first group it must be acknowledged at the outset that patients with depression alone, especially among the elderly, often present defects in memory and in other cognitive functions. These are manifested most prominently by a failure to keep up with the details of everyday life (perhaps due to impaired attention and concentration), problems with names, slowness in thinking, and usually a striking awareness of the defects and of the effort required to answer questions and to commit new facts to memory. At the same time, these patients often demonstrate no difficulty in carrying out activities that require memory, usually show no circumstantiality, perseveration, or tangentiality in their speech, and when not prodded by questions often demonstrate a clear recollection of events both recent and remote. It is in patients such as these that a formal mental status examination is likely to lead the examiner astray.

For these patients the examiner must seek to create a relaxed atmosphere in which the patient does not feel pressure. Then the examiner must encourage the patient to talk spontaneously about events in the recent and remote past and must listen carefully for problems with memory, disorganization in thought processes, difficulty with names, trouble fitting past events into correct temporal sequence, blurring of descriptive details, and impaired logic. It is only through such indirect observational techniques that the examiner will be able to evaluate and measure the patient's level of cognitive functioning. Essentially, the examiner must create an atmosphere in which patients unconsciously demonstrate how well they can function rather than consciously demonstrating their defects when required to respond to specific questions. It is through such techniques that the examiner obtains a "sense" that the patient is somehow different from most patients with dementia.

It is vitally important for the patient's well being that the neuropsychiatrist determine, in the first visit if possible, that the depressed patient with cognitive impairment is *not* demented. Most of these patients who seek help are convinced that they have AD or multiple strokes, the usual helplessness and hopelessness of depression being compounded by their perceptions of cognitive failure. It is well established that a sizable percentage of patients who are demented also satisfy the diagnostic criteria for a coexisting major depression. Most likely, clinicians are seeing such patients more frequently now, because depression is generally considered an understandable reaction to the loss of cognitive functions. Unfortunately, the mistaken assumption that depression is often misdiagnosed as dementia has shattered many hopes. When a patient presents with clinical features of depression as well as dementia (even if the evidence for dementia is modest), effective treatment of the depression is not likely to result in clinically significant improvement in the dementia and most certainly will not slow the progressive course of the dementing illness. This does not mean, of course, that depression in the demented patient should not be treated and treated vigorously. By and large depression in the elderly demented patient can be treated just as effectively as in the elderly nondemented

patient. Nevertheless, certain problems arise. All of the antidepressants have the capacity to cause cognitive impairment, and this is much more likely to occur when the brain is diseased. Thus, it is not unusual to see the dementia paradoxically worsen as the depressive symptomatology resolves.

Disease Diagnosis

For the most part, once the syndrome of dementia is diagnosed, disease diagnosis is stereotyped and routine. It does not require the clinical skills that the diagnosis of dementia itself requires. From a practical standpoint, the single most important requirement for disease diagnosis is to be sure that one does not overlook a treatable cause for dementia (23-28). Again, neuropsychiatrists now seldom identify a potentially treatable cause for dementia, much less actually bring about improvement in the cognitive dysfunction per se. It is almost certainly a tribute to the improved skills of internists and general physicians that few demented patients now arrive at neuropsychiatrists' offices for consultation requiring any diagnostic procedures to establish a diagnosis. Most patients who come now for diagnostic purposes have already had thorough medical evaluations including physical examination, urinalysis, and chemistry profile, often with thyroid function studies, B_{12} and folate levels as well. What else is left to be done to establish a disease diagnosis?

Diagnostic Studies

As neuropsychiatrists see more patients with dementia and hone their clinical skills accordingly, they usually find that these patients require fewer diagnostic instruments other than the history and clinical interview. This section describes the usefulness of each available diagnostic aid in this context.

Patients often come on referral from other physicians along with some historical data, either from conversations with the referring physicians or through medical records supplied by them. Other patients come through the insistence of their families, who often telephone in dire need of help. When families call, they are often asked to come in for an initial visit with an associate social worker or nurse specialist who then can provide a full history before the patient actually comes for evaluation. A sizable portion of patients still arrive for initial evaluation without our having any knowledge of their problems or their previous medical, neurological, or psychiatric history. Whether or not any background information about the patient is available, the patient should almost invariably be interviewed alone and in private before the physician talks with family members or other caretakers. One almost never encounters a patient who is so disorganized or so agitated that this practice must be foregone. To do otherwise is potentially degrading and demeaning to the patient.

In this initial evaluative interview, the physician should strive to create an atmosphere in which the patient can feel at ease. To this end, it helps to provide an examining room that resembles a sitting room, rather than an office, with soft lights and comfortable chairs. It may also help for the examiner to pull his or her chair close to the patient (unless the patient seems suspicious). The basic objective of the interview is to create a situation in which the patient can demonstrate how well he or she can function. Not that one pays no attention to the patient's losses and limitations, but the examiner should try never to give the impression that it is these that are of primary interest. To this end, some physicians seldom perform a formal mental status examination though they almost constantly interpolate various of its aspects into the conversation. Most of the examiner's initial comments should be nondirective ("Tell me about," rather than "What is?") with requests for precise data evolving in a natural way out of the patient's verbalizations. Such an interview must be slow-paced, nonhurried, and nonthreatening. The mental status examination as it is often performed may come across as an assault on the patient. If the neuropsychiatrist cannot make a diagnosis of dementia on the basis of a diagnostic interview without a formal mental status examination, he or she probably should not be in the practice of neuropsychiatry. One does not want the patient to emerge from this initial encounter with the physician with a sense of failure but with dignity and self-esteem intact. If this is not achieved, the interview has failed.

Even when no historical data about the patient are available, and even when the patient is too impaired to provide any relevant history of the present illness, it is always best to deal with the patient privately first. With patients who often are seeing every vestige of independence and self-sufficiency being stripped away from them, it is important, at least symbolically, to deal with them as competent and independent persons.

At this initial encounter, one may or may not carry out a neurological examination. One does so, of course, if there are features that suggest a focal brain lesion or lesions, or the examination can be done later if additional information strengthens the suspicion. In patients seen primarily because of symptoms of dementia, the neurological examination per se seldom yields new information that is decisive either in diagnosis or in therapy.

The interview with family members or other caretakers usually follows this initial patient encounter. This "family interview" (usually without the patient) has two basic objectives: (a) to obtain a fuller history than the patient may be able to provide; and (b) to determine exactly what it is that the patient and family may be seeking. The examiner begins by requesting a thorough description of the onset and the course of the illness. At the same time, the examiner can, on the basis of the earlier visit with the patient, assess how well or how poorly the family appreciates the magnitude of the patient's impairment. The history of the dementia itself is usually presented with an astounding sameness, and for the most part the examiner listens, seeking for clues or symptoms that suggest opportunities for therapeutic intervention. These might include a history of subacute progression;

the differential points on Hachinski's scale (29); a remitting course that might suggest recurrent delirium; early urinary incontinence and ataxia that raise the possibility of normal pressure hydrocephalus; use of medications that might seriously compromise brain function; presence of pervasive depressive symptoms or prominent somatization; unusual historical features, such as recurrent severe headaches or syncope. In short, the examiner is attentive to details beyond the usual history of dementia that might indicate a diagnosis other than AD or another disorder superimposed on AD.

At this point in the evaluation, the diagnosis is usually obvious, if not certain. Most often, the patient will have AD, multi-infarct dementia, or the dementia associated with Parkinson's disease. When there are unusual features, either by history or on clinical examination and when the diagnosis remains uncertain, the neuropsychiatrist usually has little problem setting forth a schedule of ancillary diagnostic procedures aimed at achieving an accurate disease diagnosis. When the diagnosis seems obvious, though, how far should the physician proceed with ancillary diagnostic studies?

Ancillary diagnostic studies. As the clinician's experience grows, fewer and fewer ancillary diagnostic studies appear to be truly helpful (23). If the patient has not had a recent medical evaluation, the physician should usually order a chemistry profile, vitamin B_{12} level and folate levels, and thyroid function studies (usually T4 and TSH), and then refer the patient for full medical evaluation. These studies are done more because it is basic to good medical practice than because one expects this to be of much assistance in caring for the patient's dementia. The cost is not high, even though the yield (in terms of new and additional diagnoses) is low. If the patient has had a recent medical evaluation, but B_{12} and folate levels and thyroid function studies were not done, these should be ordered. The process thus far seems reasonably simple and straightforward.

There is much less certainty about the next step because most other diagnostic procedures are costly and capable of distressing the patient. At this point in the diagnostic process, decisions regarding further studies may be based less on medical necessity than on the family's understanding of the disease process and their purpose in seeking assistance. For example, if a family is insistent that a patient can function at a level above that which the clinician knows to be possible, neuropsychological testing or even an occupational therapy consultation may be requested, primarily to seek collateral data to support the clinical conclusions. Or if a family is especially hesitant to accept a diagnosis of AD, one may order more ancillary diagnostic procedures than usual so that the family can be convinced that other diagnoses have been excluded. For the family that comes seeking reassurance that "everything has been done," the physician may order additional tests to fulfill that request. Finally, when one fears that patients or their families are not psychologically prepared to accept a diagnosis of AD or another dementing disorder, additional diagnostic tests may serve as a way to slow the momentum of the diagnostic process, to allow time to help them prepare for the diagnosis.

Table 36.1.   Criteria for Clinical Diagnosis of Probable and Possible Alzheimer's Disease[a]

Criteria for clinical diagnosis of *probable* Alzheimer's disease
  Dementia demonstrated by clinical examination
  Deficits in two or more cognitive functions
  Slowly progressive worsening of cognitive functions
  Consciousness unimpaired
  Onset between ages 40–90
  Absence of systemic or other brain disorders that could account for the clinical dysfunction
Criteria for clinical diagnosis of *possible* Alzheimer's disease
  Presence of dementia in the absence of systemic or other brain disorders that might account for the dementia, even when certain features in onset, presentation, or clinical course are unusual
  Other systemic or brain disorders may be present but are not considered to be the cause for the dementia

[a]Modified from McKhann G, Drachman D, Folstein M, Katzman R, Price D, Stadlan EM. Clinical diagnosis of Alzheimer's disease: report of the NINCDS-ADRDA work group under the auspices of Department of Health and Human Services Task Force on Alzheimer's disease. Neurology 1984; 34:939-944.

The demented patient's interests are not best served by the use of a standard battery of diagnostic procedures for each patient (although this may be necessary in the research setting). The physician should be cautious and sparing in the use of diagnostic procedures, both because of their cost and because of the often fragile nature of these patients' adjustment (e.g., neuropsychological testing can result in catastrophic reactions, and MRI may be terrifying for an uncomprehending subject). A procedure should be ordered only if the physician is seeking an answer to an essential and specific question or to serve a vital purpose in the patient's care.

Thus, an EEG may serve this patient population when there is uncertainty about the existence of a physical brain disease, when one suspects a delirium may be superimposed on a dementing illness (when sequential EEGs may help in following its course), or when some clinical feature suggests the possibility of a subclinical seizure disorder. Unless there is a specific reason to suspect a disorder other than AD or multi-infarct dementia, a CT scan or MRI of the brain may be of little value except for cases in which the family needs these for reassurance that the patient has no intracranial tumor (30). These procedures are expensive, however, and again, MRI may be quite upsetting. Most important, though, their yield (in terms of therapeutic interventions) in "routine" cases is virtually nil.

There is likewise no justification for routine examination of the spinal fluid. When dementia is the salient clinical feature, cerebrospinal fluid (CSF) examination seldom contributes significantly to either diagnosis or plans for patient care.

Psychological and neuropsychological testing should be employed sparingly, in part because of their costs and in part because neuropsychological testing is especially stressful for many patients, even in the hands of the most sensitive neuropsychologist. Neuropsychological testing is most helpful in two groups of patients: those who fear they are demented but clearly are not (in whom negative findings can be used to bolster the diagnosis of "no dementia") and those suspected to have an early dementia but whose performance in interview does not demonstrate definite defects (in whom testing will usually demonstrate performance still within the normal range but at a lower level than would have been predicted from education and occupation). More sensitive tests continue to be developed to aid in recognition of the second group (31,32).

A third less frequent indication for neuropsychological testing is to establish quantitatively the severity of a patient's cognitive loss for a family caught up in denial. Psychological testing per se can be especially helpful in two clinical situations: (*a*) to establish the severity and pervasiveness of depression in the patient with dementia plus depression (33); (*b*) to document the presence of psychotic thought processes in demented patients whose statements are somewhat bizarre but not clearly psychotic in the context of cognitive impairment compounded by confabulation.

Positron emission tomography (PET) and single photon emission computed tomography (SPECT) are the most recent arrivals on the diagnostic scene. While each of these may yield information of clinical interest and value in the patients with dementia, so far there is no convincing evidence that they are of great value in patients whose diagnosis is uncertain on clinical grounds.

For the long run, the accurate diagnosis of AD rests on clinical expertise. The more skillful the clinician, the fewer ancillary diagnostic instruments he or she will need to employ. This does not mean that the skilled clinician overlooks the accepted diagnostic criteria for the diagnosis of AD. Rather, the clinician should use discretion about the extent ancillary diagnostic procedures should be used to satisfy these criteria.

The most commonly used criteria for the diagnosis of AD are those proposed by the NINCDS-ADRDA Work Group (34). The criteria proposed by the NINCDS-ADRDA Work Group can be seen in Table 36.1. The American Psychiatric Association's criteria (22) include all the criteria for the diagnosis of dementia (see earlier discussion) plus an "insidious onset with a generally progressive deteriorating course" and "exclusion of all other specific causes of Dementia by history, physical examination, and laboratory tests."

In the dementing disorders, the process of disease diagnosis should be regarded not only as a search to identify a disease but also as a quest for opportunities for therapeutic intervention. Too often patients and their families have been left to face the diagnosis of AD alone, dismissed by the physician's preemptory statement that "of course, we have no treatment for that." Patient care has often received scant attention even in textbooks that focus on dementia and geriatric psychiatry (35–38). The next section emphasizes some of the therapeutic opportunities that these patients present.

Treatment

AD and other dementing diseases have been viewed too narrowly as disorders of cognition. Recently disordered affect and behavior have been recognized as major parts of the clinical manifestations of these disorders — just as patients with major affective disorders often present with cognitive and behavioral dysfunction, patients with AD often have significant affective and behavioral problems. Indeed, these dimensions of the disease may come to dominate the clinical picture far more than cognitive failure.

COGNITIVE PROBLEMS

Ever since the discovery that acetylcholine is reduced in the brains of patients with AD (39), efforts have been made to use pharmacological agents to increase the brain's supply of acetylcholine, in hopes that this might improve memory and other cognitive functions. This approach was eminently reasonable because anticholinergic agents had long been known to impair these functions.

Efforts have centered chiefly on increasing the supply of acetylcholine precursors available to the brain (by increasing blood levels of choline and/or lecithin) and the manipulation of enzyme functions to increase the levels of acetylcholine at neurotransmitter sites. There is general agreement that augmenting supplies of acetylcholine precursors has been of no value in AD, and virtually no efforts are continuing to utilize this route of treatment.

Although there are endless ways by which enzyme function might be altered with a possible increase in acetylcholine resulting, anticholinesterase agents have been most widely studied. There is no unanimity of opinion regarding the effectiveness of anticholinesterase agents, and recently reported well-designed and well-executed studies have not resolved the problem (40–43). Tacrine (1,2,3,4-tetrahydro-9-acridinamine monohydrochloride monohydrate) is the agent most thoroughly studied, but in studies involving AD patients selected for showing some initial improvement on cognitive testing with the administration of tacrine, the results have been far from impressive. When tacrine is administered over time, improvement in cognitive test results is not unusual. Seldom, however, is this improvement accompanied by impressive gain in performance of the activities of daily living or in the quality of the patient's life. Also, the use of this agent is not without problems and possible dangers. Impaired liver function is a frequent side effect, not only requiring liver function studies to be performed on a regular basis throughout the period of treatment, but also limiting dosage of the drug in some patients and requiring that it be discontinued in others.

Tacrine has recently been approved by the Food and Drug Administration for general use in the treatment of cognitive dysfunction due to AD. Thus, physicians are now debating whether or not they should recommend its use in their patients. Most will probably solve this dilemma by presenting both the pros and the cons, then leaving the decision to the patients and their families. The availability of this drug is especially welcome for those patients and families who insist that "something must be done" often accompanied by "we'll try anything."

It does not appear worthwhile to review here all the efforts made to treat the cognitive impairment of AD with these and similar agents. To date, therapeutic efforts have focused on trying in one way or another to increase the supply of acetylcholine available in the brain. The results can be summed up in a single statement: If a patient diagnosed with AD shows striking cognitive or behavioral improvement when treated with any agent now available, the patient almost certainly does not have AD.

DEPRESSION

Depression is a frequent companion of AD (and probably other dementing disorders as well, although it has been less well studied in other disorders), especially in its not too far advanced stages (26, 27). Indeed, it is depression that so often leads to diagnostic uncertainty early in the course of AD. In these instances, when a patient appears clearly to be depressed and less clearly to be demented, the physician is often hesitant to diagnose a dementia, maintaining hope that effective treatment of the depression will erase the suspicions of dementia. More commonly in these cases, successful treatment of depression serves to make clear the manifestations of underlying dementia. The rates of depressive disorders in AD have been reported between 0–86%, although most well-researched series report rates between 17–29%. With a frequency this high, depression in AD offers the neuropsychiatrist a promising window for therapeutic intervention, for it can often be treated with remarkable effectiveness. Indeed, adequate treatment of depression in AD is probably the single most effective therapeutic intervention that the physician has to offer the patient.

Usually the diagnosis of depression in AD presents no problems, for it most often appears much like depression in nondemented elderly persons. There are, however, a few special guidelines for this patient population. Demented patients with depression do not always complain of depression or even perceive themselves to be depressed. Thus, the physician often must depend on the statements of caretakers and on behavioral observations rather than on what the patient says. In attending to the caretaker's history and to observations, one must be sure that the manifestations of depression are persistent and not situation-determined and be careful not to misinterpret emotional incontinence as depression. Since it has become general knowledge that depression can mimic dementia and since depression is now widely regarded as a treatable illness, the family's story of depression often reflects pure wishful thinking, and the physician must be guided by clinical observations. Even when the demented patient denies feelings of depression, chronic irritability and irascibility and/or a plethora of ill-defined somatic complaints should alert the examiner to the possibility.

Although patients with dementia plus depression do not always appear sad and forlorn, they always appear to be miserable human beings, and the misery may take many guises — chronic anger and negativism, endless complaints of somatic distress for which no cause can be established, withdrawal with refusal to eat or take any responsibility for daily care, recurrent delusions and hallucinations of death and suffering.

The treatment of depression in the patient with AD or other dementing disorders is basically the same as in depressed patients without dementia (44), and it rests on a combination of pharmacotherapy plus supportive psychotherapy, both tailored to meet the special needs of the dementia patient. As yet, there is no "antidepressant of choice" in the treatment of demented patients with depression. As is the case for depressive illnesses in general, the choice is often based on the wish to avoid or to utilize a recognized side effect of a specific antidepressant rather than on differences in antidepressant effectiveness per se.

With the growth of available antidepressants, neuropsychiatrists have increasingly used the newer, selective serotonin reuptake inhibitors (fluoxetine, sertraline, and paroxetine) in an effort to avoid the anticholinergic side effects of the tricyclic antidepressants. The new medications are not, of course, without side effects themselves, and they seem especially prone to accentuate anxiety and restlessness and/or psychotic manifestations in the susceptible patient. Although one should obey the admonition to begin treatment in the demented (and usually elderly) patient with doses of psychotropic medications lower than those used in the nondemented patient, they often require as much medication to achieve an effective result as do nondemented patients.

Pharmacological therapy may be effective by itself, but the physician should not neglect the use of psychotherapeutic tools as well. Virtually every study of treatment for depression has shown better results when psychotherapy is combined with pharmacological treatment, although there are no well-controlled studies for depression in dementia. In addition, psychotherapy offers the physician an opportunity to mold a therapeutic relationship with patient and family that may be difficult to achieve otherwise. Clearly, psychotherapeutic techniques differ in these patients, often coming down simply to spending time with the patient, showing genuine and unhurried concern about his or her present and past life and problems, providing simple guidance and

understanding. In treating patients such as these, the physician comes to realize that time is both the physician's most expensive and most valuable commodity.

In patients with AD, it is also important to consider the possibility that severe behavioral problems may be a manifestation of superimposed depression. This is an easy consideration, of course, when the patient talks of wanting to die or threatens suicide, but the possibility of depression should be considered even when the manifestations are chiefly agitation, disgruntlement, and hostility. The physician should also recall that electroconvulsive therapy (ECT) may occasionally be effective even in patients with far-advanced AD when other treatment measures are ineffective.

In summary, depression is a common, treatable accompaniment of AD and other dementing disorders. Although it may be disguised in some patients by behavioral manifestations such as agitation, assaultiveness, or persistent screaming, it can usually be recognized and diagnosed easily. Depression in dementia offers the neuropsychiatrist an excellent best opportunity for gratifying therapeutic intervention in the demented patient.

DELUSIONAL IDEATION AND BEHAVIOR

Delusions and the resulting behavioral abnormalities are frequent reasons for patients with AD and other dementing disorders to be brought to physicians. There is some evidence suggesting that delusions become less common as the dementia becomes more severe, though certainly they may occur at any stage of the disease. The delusions occur in many forms. Some can be understood as remotely possible consequences of cognitive failure. For example, although it is inaccurate, it is not totally illogical for the demented person who is constantly misplacing objects to believe that they are being stolen. Most, however, cannot be so easily explained, e.g., the patient's belief that he or she is being poisoned, or the belief that the patient's husband is selling the home and moving back with her to a city where they lived long ago. Equally mysterious is the not infrequent belief of the patient that his wife is not his wife, and the rarer belief that his wife is an imposter, a double (Capgras' syndrome).

From a diagnostic and therapeutic standpoint, the most essential element is that the physician not mistake confabulations for delusions. In practice, the two are often confused by the unwary, and even the cautious person sometimes finds their separation difficult. Confabulations are "false stories" rather than "false beliefs," and the demented person seldom sticks with the same story for very long. A distinction must also be made between delusions and illusions, which are misperceptions or misinterpretations of real events. For example, it is an illusion, not a delusion, when an incontinent person interprets a nurse's attempt to clean him as a threat and a danger rather than a service. These distinctions are important from a therapeutic standpoint because we possess no therapeutic measures likely to reduce confabulation and none except calm reassurance likely to influence illusions.

Other treatment measures probably do more harm than good.

Among the many manifestations of dementia, delusions are among those most amenable to treatment. Before beginning to treat a demented patient's delusions, however, it is important to determine—whenever possible—that the delusions are not a manifestation of delirium or depression. In delirium, treatment aimed specifically at reducing the delusions may appreciably worsen the delirium; in depression, treatment of delusions alone may leave the patient only half-treated, i.e., the depression goes along unchanged. In some patients, though, resolution of delusions seems to lead to a lifting of the depression as well.

Treatment for delusions in the demented patient is basically no different from treatment of delusions in nondemented patients: it rests primarily on pharmacological intervention, though behavioral approaches may play important supplemental roles. Among the many antipsychotic drugs available, no one agent has been proved more effective than another in the demented patient. As in the nondemented patient, choice is usually based on the desire to utilize side effects therapeutically (e.g., to give a sedating antipsychotic to the patient who is sleeping poorly) or to avoid a potentially undesirable side effect (e.g., to choose one having relatively few peripheral cardiovascular side effects in the demented patient with diabetes). In the demented patient, doses chosen to initiate therapy are usually smaller than in nondemented patients, though the demented eventually may require comparable doses to achieve adequate control. All of the antipsychotics may, of course, not only worsen the cognitive dysfunction but also precipitate delirium or produce other undesirable side effects. As with all pharmacological therapy, the physician must constantly weigh the pros and cons.

Although behavioral techniques seldom play a major role, they may nevertheless be very helpful. Reassurance is, of course, the most basic behavioral tool, and it should be applied freely whenever the patient is anxious and fearful. Equally important, though more difficult for most caretakers, is the technique of benign disinterest. As a general rule, once the presence of delusions is established, the less said about them, the less attention accorded them, the better. It is not therapeutic to question patients repeatedly about their delusions or to discuss them at length with them. Behavioral measures can help even in cases in whom antipsychotics appear to be ineffective.

HALLUCINATIONS

Except as a manifestation of delirium, hallucinations are relatively rare in AD and other dementing illnesses. When they occur, they are more likely to be visual than otherwise, but any sensory modality may be involved. As is the case for delusions, hallucinations must be distinguished from illusions. The person who misinterprets bright lights outside a window at night as a fire or the sounds of calm voices in the room next door as a fight is experiencing illusions, not hallucinations. As already written, we have no effective treatment for illusions, but if the patient can be helped by whatever means to become less anxious and fearful, the illusion may be reduced in frequency or at least become less threatening.

In the occasional patient with AD, however, hallucinations may come to dominate the clinical picture and be the chief cause for problems in care. The following case studies illustrate this phenomenon.

The patient was an 85-year-old widow, in good physical health, with a well-established diagnosis of AD. Nevertheless, she still lived alone in her own home next door to her daughter, took care of her own daily needs, and participated in family and church activities. She began to experience visual hallucinations in which she perceived a circus being set up on the vacant lot across the street. Initially she was bemused, even entertained by the activity, and she would sit on her porch for long periods watching. Gradually, however, the performances grew more dangerous and frightening to her, and she began staying inside and drawing the curtains so that she wouldn't have to see them. Although initially she recognized the hallucinations as such and would even joke about them to her family, gradually they became more real and she no longer could acknowledge them to be imaginary. When not experiencing hallucinations, she showed no signs of distress or depression. Treatment with a variety of antipsychotic and anxiolytic agents to levels tolerated by the patient had little success. Her anxiety and fearfulness concerning the hallucinations lessened somewhat, but the hallucinations themselves continued.

Another patient, a woman in her late 70s with diagnosed AD, Stage 3 on Reisberg's scale (45), lived alone in her own apartment in a retirement complex, taking care of all her daily needs, including cooking. In the evening, she began to observe "little people" gathering outside her living room window, peering inside in a friendly fashion. Since she lived on a high floor of the building, initially she recognized that she was hallucinating and enjoyed the hallucinations rather than being frightened by them. Gradually the numbers of little people increased and began coming into the room and sitting on various pieces of furniture. Their numbers increased, their appearance grew less benign, and they began to fill the room, so that the patient grew frightened. Soon the patient no longer recognized them as hallucinations and began to call the emergency 911 number for help, which led to her seeing a neuropsychiatrist. On examination, the signs of dementia were obvious, but she showed neither anxiety or depression in the office setting. In talking of the experiences, she would sometimes call them hallucinations but at other times talked of the "little people" as real. Once again, multiple efforts at therapy were disappointing.

In patients with Alzheimer's disease in whom visual hallucinations have come to dominate the clinical picture, the hallucinations are almost uniformly poorly responsive to the treatment modalities now available. Indeed, when such a patient is seen for the first time, it is wise to inform the family (and the patient when appropriate) that the prognosis for effectively controlling the hallucinations is poor.

BEHAVIORAL PROBLEMS

Although behavioral abnormalities have always been a problem in AD and other dementias, until recently they received little attention from either clinicians or investigators (46–49). They are probably the leading cause for families and caretakers seeking help from neuropsychiatrists, and they are unquestionably the chief cause for hospitalizing patients who have AD. Yet neither DSM-IV (3) nor ICD-9-CM (50) contains a diagnostic classification appropriate for the patient with AD who also has severe behavior problems. Under the restrictions imposed by these manuals, the best that can be done is to diagnose patients with AD with severe behavioral problems as having "senile dementia with delusional features," accepting the disordered behavior as clear evidence of a distorted perception of reality, even though the "delusions" themselves may be difficult to specify. This is a disagreeable compromise, however, for the neuropsychiatrist is likely to see far more AD patients with behavioral aberrations than with true delusions.

For the most part, behavioral disturbances have, in the past, simply been lumped together, and there is still no generally accepted classification for the various forms taken in the context of "behavioral problems." Table 36.2 provides a classification culled in part from several recent publications.

Distressing Repetitive Behaviors

Although seldom the primary reason for the family or other caretaker to seek medical help, repetitive bizarre behaviors are often among the most stressful for the caretaker to endure. Repetitive behaviors take many forms. Some patients cling to their caretakers, never wanting them out of their sight, following them from room to room, often even into the bathroom if the door is not locked. Often this is associated with incessant questioning, usually the same question repeated continuously. Others occupy themselves taking objects out of closets, drawers, or kitchen cabinets, then replacing them, though never in the accepted order. Another patient may ceaselessly pack and unpack a suitcase or purse. Others hoard, repetitively hiding food, money, or specific objects—often so that they cannot be found. One patient's husband had even given up the household cleaning service because his wife had hidden so much money over the years that he was fearful it could be stolen without his ever knowing it.

Most of the time no effective intervention will be found to modify any of these behaviors. It has been said that if the behavior is ignored, it may gradually diminish, or that if it arises from anxiety, measures to reduce anxiety may help. Neither of these measures really helps in most cases. Ignoring the behavior may, of course, ease the plight of the caretaker even without modifying the behavior; and anxiolytics may reduce the separation anxiety when the patient is locked out of the bathroom, but the basic problem remains unchanged. Distraction may, of course, occupy the patients for a period, but once the alternative is terminated, the distressing behavior usually is promptly resumed.

Table 36.2. Classification of Behavioral Problems in Dementia

Distressing repetitive behaviors
Dangerous, careless behaviors
Restless, agitated, hostile, assaultive behaviors
Overelated, overactive, intrusive behaviors
Insomnia and diurnal rhythm reversals
Repetitive screaming and crying out
Inappropriate sexual behaviors
General regression, refusal to eat

Dangerous, Careless Behaviors

As is true for the repetitive behaviors, dangerous and careless behaviors may take many forms, and it is as impossible that they all be listed here as that any demented patient can be protected from them all. It would have been impossible to predict, for example, that one patient would use a screwdriver in an effort to disconnect an electric appliance plug that seemed to be stuck. There are three behaviors, though, about which the neuropsychiatrist is most likely to be consulted: (*a*) unsafe driving, (*b*) unsafe use of mechanical equipment (especially stoves and motorized lawn mowers), and (*c*) wandering. In truth, physicians can only rarely be helpful in putting a stop to any of these dangerous behaviors. Occasionally the physician's authority may be sufficient to get the demented patient to agree to give up driving or cooking or mowing (although usually it is insufficient). Even so, the patient may forget that he or she has agreed to any such thing, and carry on as before. The simple truth is that the only certain way for the patient to be protected from these activities is for the automobile, stove, or mower to be made inoperative or for the keys to be safely hidden. Anxiolytic or antipsychotic agents may help reduce the hostility and frustration that often occurs following these prohibitions, but they do little to alter the attempted behavior itself.

Wandering falls into the same category of dangerous behaviors, but it is often even more distressing to caretakers and more difficult to control. It is often the prime reason for a patient's institutionalization. Caretakers grow fearful even to let the patient out of sight for fear they may wander off and come to harm. Sleep may grow virtually impossible because the patient may wake and walk outside at almost any moment. Although wandering seems most difficult to control in the home setting, it remains a serious problem in many institutionalized patients as well.

Unless the family or caretaker is willing for the patient to be locked up at home or in a unit in an institution, we have no good measures to stop wandering. Anxiolytics or antipsychotics may reduce restless and exploratory behavior, but they seldom control it entirely, and most patients who are so inclined continue occasionally to wander, though their attempts may be less frequent. Anxiolytics or antipsychotics may also be of great value in reducing patients' frustrations (sometimes even catastrophic reactions) when they find they cannot get out of a locked door. Occasionally, daily vigorous exercise seems to lessen a patient's proclivity to escape.

Nursing homes are especially easy places for patients to wander, because safety regulations often prohibit their exit doors being locked. In such situations, other measures sometimes help. The wandering patient should, for example, always be placed on an upper floor to decrease the likelihood he or she will be able to figure out how to get to the first floor, where it may be easy to leave. Similarly, if there is a unit from which access is especially complicated, that is the best unit for the wanderer. Other simple measures may help, such as having wandering patients wear distinctive identification badges or armbands that might alert staff seeing them near a building exit. Newer electronic devices are available, such as wrist or ankle bands, that trigger an alarm if the patient goes beyond a certain line, but these devices are expensive and are thus seldom used.

Restless, Agitated, Hostile, Assaultive Behavior

These are probably the most frequent behavioral problems for which the neuropsychiatrist is consulted. Although all these behaviors may be manifestations of the dementing disease itself, the physician should always seek other explanations. Is the patient taking some medication that might be causing such behavior? Is the patient slipping into and out of delirium? Is the patient experiencing pain that he or she cannot describe but which results in such behaviors? Is the patient delusional and acting on the basis of the delusions? Most often, these inquiries will not yield positive answers, but they should always be made.

Treatment of these problem behaviors usually requires both behavioral and pharmacological measures. From a practical standpoint, behavioral measures are usually difficult to utilize in the home setting, and pharmacological management is usually the cornerstone of treatment there. Various agents have been used and are discussed more fully in the sections that follow. Management of these behavioral problems is usually difficult and especially so in the outpatient setting. If the problems are severe and the patient remains in the home, treatment usually cannot succeed without the collaborative efforts of the physician, caretakers, visiting nurse, and social worker.

Even though behavioral techniques are essential in the management of these patients, pharmacological measures remain the definitive treatment when no specific inciting cause for the agitation and hostility can be found (46–49, 51, 52). Having said that, little more can be stated, because the use of neuropharmacological agents for these behaviors is almost entirely a matter of trial and error, and families need to know this during the initial meeting. At the same time, they should be told that even if medications can effectively control the target symptoms, often this cannot be achieved without producing some clearly undesirable side effects, whether that be sedation, stiffness, or even further reduction in cognitive capacities. Effective control of severe agitation or assaultiveness with medications thus often exacts a price.

Almost every agent known to affect the central nervous system (with the possible exception of the antiparkinsonian agents) has been tried in these patients, and almost every agent has appeared to be effective at one time or another in one or more patients (53–60). Antipsychotics and anxiolytics are the agents most frequently employed, but the process of trial and error often expands to include antidepressants, mood stabilizers, and anticonvulsants. Indeed, the spectrum of drugs that may be tried in difficult situations is limited only by the physician's creativity.

There are virtually no hard research data to guide the physician to answer the question, "Which drug should I choose first?" In practice, the choice is always influenced by a host of factors, the first being the general medical condition of the patient. For example, the physician recognizes that certain medicines are to be avoided, initially at any rate, in the patient with impaired cardiac conduction or with an unstable peripheral vasculature; others especially to be avoided in the patient with unsteady gait and a history of falls. Beyond that, the physician's choice usually rests upon a consideration of possible side effects, which are especially to be avoided and which might be utilized therapeutically in the specific patient under consideration. In these days of increased general knowledge of drugs, one cannot forget that families also often have very specific ideas about which drugs are acceptable and which are not.

The choice for an initial pharmacological agent is usually between an antipsychotic or an anxiolytic drug, and even in this initial decision, firm guidelines are lacking, much less firm guidelines to the choice of a specific agent. Since these patients are usually elderly, are often frail and unsteady on their feet (many with a history of falls), and often are already receiving a number of medicines for various other medical disorders, even this initial choice is seldom easy. The two side effects that figure most prominently in the physician's deliberations are sedation and extrapyramidal motility disturbances. In most agitated patients, one cannot deal effectively with the agitation without encountering at least one of these side effects. In practice, it is often easier to deal with sedation than with stiffness and immobility. Obviously this does not lead immediately to a choice between an antipsychotic and anxiolytic, but it does mean that the choice for an initial pharmacological agent in the agitated patient with dementia is likely to be one of the lower potency antipsychotic agents or a benzodiazepine with a midrange half-life. In practice, this means that initial considerations usually include chlorpromazine, thioridazine, loxapine or molindone, and lorazepam or clonazepam. An additional consideration at this point may be the availability of the drug in an injectable form, because many of these patients refuse to accept oral medications initially. Although one usually begins with small doses of psychotropic medicines, especially in elderly patients with diagnosed brain disease, small doses are often remarkably ineffective in highly agitated demented patients. In many patients the dangers of prolonged agitation outweigh the dangers of short-term oversedation.

Beyond the antipsychotic and benzodiazepine anxiolytics, a wide variety of psychopharmacological agents has been reported to be effective in quelling agitation in some patients. These include lithium, carbamazepine, propranolol, buspirone, antidepressants (especially trazodone and fluoxetine), and meprobamate. As a practical matter, these are seldom the initial drugs of choice, and the physician usually turns to them when the antipsychotic and/or benzodiazepines have been either ineffective or have caused unacceptable side effects. A case might be made for choosing lithium or carbamazepine initially if the agitation is accompanied by euphoria or great pressure of speech. Although both propranolol and buspirone have been reported quite useful (and desirable because of their relative absence of side effects), the long delay before the onset of their effectiveness often rules out their prescription for the severely agitated person.

For the agitated demented patient, hospitalization may be not only desirable but essential for the dangerous behavior to be brought under control. Hospitalization offers several distinct advantages: (*a*) an opportunity to observe the patient's behavior in a new, structured environment; (*b*) an opportunity to observe the effectiveness of behavioral treatment techniques put into use by well-trained and experienced staff; (*c*) an opportunity to modify pharmacological agents on a daily basis based on observations of the physician and those of a well-trained nursing staff; (*d*) an opportunity to use medications in combinations and dosages that would be avoided were the patient not under constant medical observation; (*e*) breathing space for the family to consider their options for the patient's continued care after discharge.

The dividends of hospitalization will be greatest if the patient can be hospitalized on a psychiatric unit devoted to the care of demented patients. Such units should be small (a unit designed for 10–15 patients is probably ideal), and the staff-to-patient ratio must be high. The nursing staff must be not only well trained but also comfortable with both medical and psychiatric nursing, because many of the patients will have major medical problems that require aggressive medical treatment. Strong internal medical support is essential. Social work and activities therapy must be readily available and of the highest quality. Above all, the entire staff must be devoted to the care of this population of patients, because their care is usually difficult and demanding, and the outcomes are often disappointing.

Threatening and assaultive behaviors are always very stressful for families and caretakers alike. The physician should inform the family that such behaviors are usually transient, as are so many of the behavioral manifestations of dementia, and that it is unlikely they will remain a dominant clinical feature. Thus, paradoxically, as the disease grows worse, behavioral problems may lessen. Because of this, medications require periodic reassessment; those that are virtually essential for one period may not even be needed in another.

OVERELATED, OVERACTIVE, INTRUSIVE BEHAVIORS

The dividing line between these behaviors and the agitated and hostile behaviors just described is not always clear. Indeed, these patients may also become irritable and angry when their wishes are thwarted. Usually, however, in this group irritability and anger do not dominate the scene, and their behavior is usually marked more by a sense of energy and hypomanic excitement, at times even accompanied by inappropriate jocularity or a trace of grandiosity. Usually these patients rather quickly become favorites of the staff, until their incessant activity begins to wear thin. Often there is a history that suggests a preexisting cyclothymic personality, occasionally even a bipolar disorder.

Rarely can these behaviors be controlled by any measures other than psychopharmacological ones. Neuroleptics and benzodiazepines are the drugs of choice, but when these are ineffective or cause unacceptable side effects, there is probably more reason to try lithium, carbamazepine, or valproate in this group than in any other. Lithium, carbamazepine, or valproate alone may be effective, but the need for monitoring of blood levels makes their long-term maintenance difficult.

INSOMNIA AND DIURNAL RHYTHM REVERSALS

These symptoms are frequent in demented patients, often accompanied by pacing and restlessness, and they are usually difficult to treat. They are also often major stresses for the family, whose sleep disturbance may equal that of the patient as they are kept awake by noise and by their fears about what may befall the patient in his or her nocturnal wanderings. One inquires, of course, about possible medical causes for the insomnia (urinary tract infection, arthritic pain, reflex esophagitis), especially because patients may complain little about them as they seldom complain about or even deny the insomnia itself. Sometimes relieving such physical distress helps the insomnia, but rarely does it solve the problem.

Most medical publications dealing with insomnia emphasize the importance of the obvious—keeping the patient awake during the daytime if possible, a program of daily exercise as tolerated, and regular toileting. In fact, the physician seldom sees a patient with insomnia whose family has not already exhausted themselves trying these measures, and these approaches rarely help very much, even in the better-controlled hospital setting.

In practice, effective treatment of insomnia in the demented patient depends upon the pharmacological management. In these patients, most of whom already have far-advanced dementia, there is no reason for hesitation because of scruples about possible dependence or habituation. Caution is advised with regard to the side effects that these medications often but not inevitably produce, but these can usually be managed by selection and careful dosage titration.

Sometimes, when the insomnia is not too severe, sleep can be improved by bedtime doses of aspirin, acetaminophen, or an antihistamine (such as promethazine). Of course, families have often already tried these without success, and patients are rarely seen because of "not too severe" insomnia. A wide variety of agents may be used to promote sleep, including not only the recognized hypnotics but also antidepressants, anxiolytics, and sometimes even the more sedating neuroleptics. In fact, an antidepressant, specifically trazodone, may be used first, in part because it can foster nighttime sleep without excessive daytime sedation, and because it may also reduce daytime restlessness. Small doses of amitriptyline may also be quite effective and well tolerated. As for the hypnotics, chloral hydrate is often a first choice, because even in doses of 1 gram or more, it is often tolerated in the elderly demented patient without daytime drowsiness or hangover ensuing. Temazepam too is often surprisingly well tolerated, even for prolonged periods of time. When patients have sleep problems and also require daytime anxiolytics or antipsychotics because of restlessness and agitation, the insomnia often can be handled effectively simply by giving a larger dose of the anxiolytic or neuroleptic agent at bedtime. Paradoxical reactions and ineffectiveness are not unusual, but neither should cause the physician to stop trying to help.

Chronic, severe insomnia should be regarded as a major problem in this group of patients, and it should be treated aggressively. Conscientious primary care physicians often hesitate to do so. However, the dangers of inadequate treatment exceed those of overtreatment, provided the patient has a reliable caretaker who will keep the physician informed of any untoward changes that might be attributed to the medication.

REPETITIVE SCREAMING AND CRYING OUT

Repetitive unprovoked screaming and crying out are among the most distressing symptoms encountered in patients with dementia and among those most difficult to treat effectively (61–63). These symptoms may overwhelm the family and can stretch the tolerance of even the most devoted staff in nursing homes or hospitals. Screaming can always be stopped, of course, by giving the patient enough medicine to produce deep somnolence, but in most instances this is not an acceptable treatment option—with good reason—and especially not over the long term.

In these patients one should always seek a nonpharmacological remedy first. Does the screaming result from some unsuspected pain or discomfort (a collapsed vertebral body, urinary retention, fecal impaction)? Even when one or more of these can be identified, their relief seldom leads to a cessation of the screaming, but they should not be overlooked. Can the screaming be stopped by some environmental intervention (isolation in a quiet spot, placement among a group of active people, one-to-one personal attention, soothing music)? Although these may end the screaming briefly, they too are seldom effective for very long.

Invariably the physician will have to turn to pharmacological measures, and these too are often ineffective, individually or in combination. The response of the screaming patient to pharmacological intervention is so unpredictable that a reasonable protocol as to how the physician should proceed cannot even be offered. Anxiolytics, antipsychotics, antidepressants, sedatives, lithium, and antiepileptic drugs all seem to have been helpful periodically but most often have been ineffective. This is a situation where trial and error prevail, without any guidelines as to what should be tried first. Success seems to be entirely a matter of chance, and the physician who chances upon an effective agent is lucky. Some of the problems are illustrated by the following case report.

The patient was a 79-year-old married woman with a long history of dementia associated with paranoid delusions, wandering, agitation, and combativeness. On admission she was severely demented, highly agitated, strikingly malnourished, and had almost certainly been physically abused by her husband. She had no history of earlier psychiatric problems and was not found to have any serious medical problems other than malnutrition and probable AD. A CT of the brain revealed cortical and ventricular atrophy, and the EEG manifested diffuse slow activity.

Once in the hospital, her combativeness disappeared, she began to eat better, and she became cooperative within the limits of her capabilities. Nevertheless, she remained restless and at times agitated, and she began to scream out loudly and constantly during her waking hours (and she often slept poorly). Her screaming could be interrupted at times by her eating or responding briefly to questions, to which she always answered that she was in no discomfort and had no idea why she was screaming.

The screaming continued, loud and almost incessant, for over a month in the hospital, despite multiple attempts using behavioral techniques and pharmacological therapy (including thioridazine, chlorpromazine, perphenazine, loxapine, lorazepam, diazepam, trazodone, fluoxetine, nortriptyline, desipramine, and carbamazepine). She responded little—if at all—to any behavioral or pharmacological measures, and thus it was impossible to transfer her to a nursing home for long-term care. Finally, in desperation, she was given ECT. Her screaming began to abate after the first treatment, and after a total of five bilateral treatments she remained calm, cooperative, apparently comfortable and content, and without any screaming. With her continued improvement, she was transferred to a long-term care facility without difficulty.

INAPPROPRIATE SEXUAL BEHAVIOR

These behaviors are among those most distressing to families and caretakers (including the professional caretaking staff), although these behaviors seldom pose any serious threats to others. They occur most often in men. The most common problems include inappropriate fondling or touching, offensive sexual verbalizations, and masturbation that can be observed by others. Occasionally it takes the form of continued insistence by the demented patient on sexual congress with the spouse or other convenient sexual object.

Most of the first group of behaviors can be dealt with effectively by behavioral techniques. Calm, quiet, firm statements (made without any sign of irritability or embarrassment) that such behavior is inappropriate and will not be tolerated will usually stop troublesome fondling, touching, or verbalizations, but occasionally the caretaker may have to leave the patient alone for a while to prove that it truly will not be tolerated. In the patient with severe memory impairment, the caretaker must repeat this behavior repeatedly, because the patient will not recall the incidents. This usually does not stop the patients from trying, but it does generally abbreviate the undesirable activity. Masturbation within the view of others is best handled by providing the patient adequate opportunities for masturbation in private. This behavior seems to surface more often in the patient cared for in an institution than in the patient cared for at home, perhaps because most institutions make no provision for the individual's privacy.

When behavioral techniques are ineffective, hormonal therapy should be tried. In men, conjugated estrogens given on a daily basis may be adequate to reduce these unacceptable behaviors. When this is not effective or if the patient refuses oral medications, regular injections of medroxyprogesterone are often effective.

INCONTINENCE

Frequent incontinence (especially fecal incontinence), along with aggressive behavior, are probably the most common causes for patients with AD and other dementias to be institutionalized. Urinary incontinence usually precedes fecal incontinence in the progression of these diseases and can often be managed effectively. When urinary incontinence begins in the demented patient, the physician should first consider the possibility of a urinary tract infection. If there is no evidence for infection, and if the patient is still capable of recognizing the urge to urinate and can still find the bathroom, the patient should probably be referred for urological consultation. For the patient with advanced dementia, escorting the patient to the bathroom on a regular schedule (approximately every 2 hours during waking hours) is often surprisingly effective. Nocturnal incontinence can often be controlled by waking the patient on schedule once or twice nightly for trips to the bathroom.

In the patient with beginning fecal incontinence, the physician should first be certain that the patient does not have a fecal impaction, a frequent problem in the elderly population. If not, fecal incontinence can often be avoided with a regular toileting schedule as described above, especially when this is combined with a daily regimen of stool softener plus fiber additives, augmented as needed by judicious use of laxatives.

GENERAL REGRESSION AND REFUSAL TO EAT

Therapeutic intervention is seldom effective when these distressing behaviors occur as manifestations of far-advanced dementias. Rarely these may be the major manifestations of a superimposed depressive illness, in which case the patient will usually appear sad and miserable as well. When regressed behavior and refusal to eat occur simply as additional symptoms in the gradually unfolding presentation of dementia, patients usually seem comfortable, at ease, and in no distress. Insistence that one take action to slow the course of the disease usually worsens rather than helps the situation. Occasionally, stimulant medications (such as methylphenidate) seem to help a little in reversing the regression, and regular feeding of nutritional supplements may slow the progressing inanition. Such interventions help the patient little, but may relieve the anxieties of the family.

If they live long enough for the disease to progress to very advanced stages, almost all demented patients eventually lose their appetite and quit eating. No remedy is known. At this point, each family confronts a serious problem, one in which all choices appear bad. They must choose either to let the disease take its natural course or to begin artificial feeding (by nasogastric tube, gastrostomy, or total parenteral nutrition). In most nursing facilities, parenteral feeding once begun may be stopped only in the most exceptional circumstances. Unfortunately, many institutions will not allow patients to remain and be cared for unless artificial feeding is begun.

Family Needs

The physician who cares for the patient with dementia must assume responsibility for the care of that patient's family as well. Their needs may even seem much greater than those of the patient, but families often are ashamed and hesitant even to acknowledge any needs, much less to ask for help directly. From the very first encounter, physicians should try to make it clear that their concern for the family almost equals that for the patient. Sometime during those early encounters, it should almost always be stated that the physician regards both the identified patient and the family equally as patients. Few stresses in life are more costly, mentally and physically, than caring over a period of years for a patient with AD or some other slowly progressing dementia. The physician should be especially concerned about those families that boast about their self-sufficiency.

The physician should always seek to make the family's daily care of the patient as simple and easy as possible. One of the most useful tasks the physician can perform is to simplify and unify the patient's care as much as feasible, to be a bulwark against the fragmentation of medical care in which these patients and their families so often find themselves. When neuropsychiatrists are more willing to identify themselves as the team leaders in the patient's medical care, they will serve patients and families to the best of their abilities. Few internists and general physicians are equipped to provide the kind of care needed, although physicians now being trained specifically in geriatric medicine may be successful.

Except in unusual circumstances, the physician should always spend time privately with the family, as many as are present, at the time of the first patient visit. After the examination of the patient in private, the physician sits down with the family in private, usually beginning with an open-ended question such as, "Tell me what sort of worries or problems you have about Mr. _____ ." Thus, in this initial visit with the family, the physician seeks to learn not only the essential facts about the patient's medical-neuropsychiatric history but about the problems the family may be having dealing with the likely diagnosis and with the patient's daily care, about their fears both for the patient and for themselves, about the family dynamics, with special attention to cohesiveness or divisiveness, and about the strengths and weaknesses of the support system (both social and financial) available to the patient. Obviously all this data cannot be obtained in an initial interview, but all these facets can at least be touched upon.

DISCUSSING THE DIAGNOSIS

Whenever the physician sits down with patient and/or family to discuss diagnosis, two things must be explained. First, they need to be told in some detail about how a diagnosis is reached, i.e., how the various elements in history, clinical examination, and ancillary diagnostic testing are utilized and the importance of ruling out the treatable cause for dementia before reaching a diagnosis of AD or multi-infarct dementia. With families that are especially skeptical or with those who tend to minimize the extent of the patient's cognitive loss, examples may be offered from the earlier clinical examination of the patient, e.g., that even though the family reported that "the problems aren't too bad," the patient was unable to state the month and year or the names and relationships of family members sitting in the waiting room. Second, it should be emphasized, especially if this discussion of the diagnosis includes the patient, that there is no way to make a diagnosis of AD on clinical grounds with *absolute* certainty, so that the physician does not permanently abolish any hope for better things. This should be done in such a way that the family understands that this lack of absolute certainty is a function of the limitations of our available diagnostic procedures and not a personal limitation, so that the patient and family do not begin a process of doctor shopping in search of a more desirable diagnosis.

Whenever one must make a diagnosis of AD, which virtually everyone now knows to be a disease for which we lack any specific treatment, one should also try to spend some time emphasizing what we as neuropsychiatrists do have to offer patients and family, emphasizing our availability and our wish to continue to help with problems, whatever their nature, that will arise.

EDUCATING THE FAMILY

The physician plays a second major role with the family, that of teacher—about the disease itself, of what has happened, and what is to come. Teaching involves, of course, more than just teaching about Alzheimer's disease

or another dementing disorder itself, about its course and what to expect. It should focus, even in its early stages, on how the disease is likely to progress and especially on the demands that will be made of caretakers. Contrary to newspaper reports, most families remain committed to the care of their kin and insistent that they will provide it. When feasible, it is best to have as many family members as possible involved in this learning process, not only for their edification but to help them unite into a caretaking team, so that no one family member takes on the caretaking responsibilities alone. At the same time, the physician tries to encourage openness and honesty between family members in confronting the extent of the patient's disability. Too often spouses try to hide from their children and others just how impaired the patient has become, thus taking on an even heavier and at times debilitating burden. At the same time, spouses often leave other family members with a heavy load of guilt once the extent of the care required comes to light. Thus, the physician should emphasize from the very beginning that good care needs more than a single caretaker and that the person who seizes all these responsibilities is likely to break down and bring chaos upon the whole caretaking system.

The physician is not, of course, the only teacher for the families. Often they have already studied the subject at length before coming. Even so, the family should be advised to read and learn as much as they can about these diseases and what happens to persons who have them. Two excellent manuals for families that can be recommended are Nancy L. Mace's and Pater Rabins' *The 36-Hour Day* (64) or *The Loss of Self,* by Donna Cohen and Carl Eisdorfer (65).

Most family members are fearful about whether AD is inherited, and even though they may not ask about this directly, the physician usually should bring up the subject and try to teach them what is known about the genetic aspects of this disorder. The aim is to help them understand that although the risk of their developing AD is greater than that for the general population, the risk (except in a very few families) is not so great that it warrants their living in constant apprehension. Discussion of this topic also offers an opportunity to talk with the family about the importance of a tissue diagnosis and to set in motion the consideration of an eventual autopsy.

PROVIDING SUPPORT

Caring for a relative with AD is usually a thankless task for the family member who takes on that responsibility. Ideally other family members should be the caretaker's chief source of support, and this is indeed often the case, but not always. Sometimes those who are closest and, therefore, most expected to provide this support simply cannot face the patient's deterioration and so begin to shun both patient and caretaker alike. Sometimes there is dissension, some family members thinking the patient should already have been put into a nursing home, or conversely, others thinking the patient already in a nursing home should have been kept longer at home. Other family members might complain that the caretaker is doing either too much or too little to assist the patient. The most capable caretakers often fail to escape criticism.

Even when family and friends are unfailingly supportive, however, caregivers need support from professionals, along with continued guidance. Physicians, social workers, nurses, and even the office receptionist play roles in providing this support, and its provision cannot be assigned to any single individual. The broader this network of support can be extended, the better for the caretaker. It is not unusual to find beyond the physician that the caregiver's support system includes hospital nurses, visiting nurses, hospital social workers, social workers from the outpatient clinic, receptionists, ministers, and counselors from the local Alzheimer's Disease Association and Mental Health Association. Often the caretaker has learned which professional is most helpful with the different problems as they arise. A good support system conveys to the caretaker that it is all right to call for help whenever and as often as it is needed. If the calls become too frequent or too trivial, this problem can be dealt with directly, because it is usually a sign that the caretaker is becoming overwhelmed.

Formal support groups, such as those that may be provided by the ADRDA and the local Mental Health Association, may be of great benefit to caretakers. Such support groups are now widely available even in small cities. For a variety of reasons, families are often hesitant to join such groups, but even when they have reservations, it is best to urge them to go at least once or twice before deciding they are not for them. Leaders of these groups often provide another valuable service for patients and families alike, steering those who have found the medical profession unresponsive to their needs to clinics and physicians they know are sure to respond. Such support groups are not for everyone; for some caregivers, any public disclosure of need or grief is too much, too painful. The physician must take care not to push too strongly for group participation for such individuals.

Support groups deal mainly with the daily problems involved in care—for the patient and for the caretaker. They cannot deal with the deeper, even more painful problems, especially those concerning guilt, anger, and conflict that so often beset the caretaker under stress. Sometimes these problems can be dealt with effectively in special psychotherapy groups. For example, a psychotherapy group organized especially for the spouses of younger patients with AD may be especially helpful. Not infrequently, AD in a spouse or parent seems to trigger emotional problems that caretakers have long repressed but never dealt with effectively. These caretakers should be urged to involve themselves in individual psychotherapy.

CONTINUED CARE OF PATIENT NEEDS

The neuropsychiatrist who *cares for* patients with dementia, as contrasted with serving as a consultant to them, must be willing to function as the physician to whom the family turns first when problems in care arise. This involves the physician in caring for or telling the family how to care for a variety of medical problems outside the bounds of neuropsychiatry as a specialty. This means, for example, that when a husband calls and tells the neuropsychiatrist that his wife with AD has another urinary tract infection, which was treated successfully 6 weeks ago with a sulfa drug, the neuropsychiatrist ought to prescribe that sulfa drug again and send her to her internist only if the drug is ineffective. Or, as in a recent instance, when a wife calls and reports that her husband, already bedridden, has a cough and fever of 102.6° F, she was told to contact her internist immediately. This may even involve making occasional house calls, when a patient refuses to come to the office or the problems of transporting the patient are overwhelming.

The caretaker's burden often can be lightened appreciably by visits from social workers, nurses, or home care assistants, either on a regular basis or when specific problems arise. Many of the services provided by these professionals now are covered by Medicare and other insurance programs. Even when they are not and when the cost must be absorbed by the family, they are frequently effective means for reducing the overall costs of medical care, both by cutting the need for frequent physician visits and by helping the family to continue care for the patient at home instead of in an institution. The bonds forged between family and these visiting caretakers not surprisingly sometimes hold the entire support system together.

RESPITE NEEDS

From the very beginning, the physician should emphasize the caretakers' need for rest and respite from their caretaking responsibilities. As with so much advice, it often goes unheeded, but one should always try. Whenever possible, it is best to begin providing the caretaker with regular periods of relief early in the course of the disease, so that it becomes a part of the patient's scheduled care plan. As patients become more and more incapacitated, and, therefore, more and more dependent on their caretakers, they often begin to want the caretaker in their sight every waking moment, although they may simultaneously declare that they need no one to "look after" them. Once this stage is reached, it is much more difficult for both patient and caretaker to adjust to regular periods of separation.

Respite can be provided either in the home or away from home. At home it is usually not too difficult to set up a plan whereby the principal caretaker is provided regular relief by other family members, close friends, or paid attendants. The principal caretaker is often, perhaps even usually, unwilling to ask directly for such help, and the physician and others must take the lead in providing it. Sometimes volunteer agencies are also available to provide these services and a variety of other supports.

In most larger cities, a variety of respite services are also available outside the home. When the disease is not too far advanced, senior citizens' centers often offer a number of scheduled activities in which the patient can still participate without special supervision. As the disease advances, thought should be given to placing the patient, for one or several days each week, in an adult day care program. Such programs, often designed especially for persons with AD or other dementias, are now available in most larger cities. A recent development has been the establishment of work programs adapted to the particular needs of patients with dementia. Such programs may be especially valuable for younger patients whom dementia has forced into early retirement and indolence, with resulting feelings of worthlessness.

GIVING ADVICE

Everything a physician does may, of course, be considered advice, but there are several specific areas of concern where the physician can anticipate that the family will need advice. Almost every family considers, for example, even if only to reject it, placement of the patient in a nursing home or other institutional setting. Understandably, this possibility is often rejected immediately in the early phases of the dementing disease, but as the disease continues to eradicate the patient's faculties, as the patient's needs for care multiply, and especially as the years of caregiving erode the family's strengths, the possibility of placement almost always resurfaces. The physician's skill and sensitivity are possibly of greater importance in this than in any of the other services provided to the family.

Before the family begins seriously to consider institutional placement, the physician should assess the patient's suitability for care in a day care program and possibly advise this as a means of postponing or avoiding full-time placement outside the home. There is often a surprising reluctance on the part of family members to commit their affected kin to regular participation in these day programs despite what appears to be their obvious benefits. In some ways it is harder to overcome this hurdle than to recommend full-time institutional placement. Many patients benefit tremendously from day programs, and it is unfortunate that they are not more fully utilized.

Should the patient be placed in an institution? If so, when and where? Clearly the physician cannot provide unequivocal answers to these questions. Even in cases in which the physician believes the choice is unequivocal, he or she must take pains to remember that the physician does not make these decisions—the physician only advises. The choice always rests with the family, and the family must not be put in the position of believing they are opposing the physician, whatever the choice may be. This is most likely to happen when it seems that by all reasonable criteria the patient should be removed from the home, yet the family cannot bring itself to take this step. The family must feel that the physician's support will continue, even when they do not accept the physician's advice.

In the experience of most neuropsychiatrists, families move patients with AD and other dementing disorders to nursing homes with great reluctance, and in most cases only when they believe they have no other choice. The truth is, though, that almost every patient with AD will ultimately require institutional placement unless they are fortunate enough to have another illness to cause their death earlier or unless the family possesses unusual resources. One family managed to keep their mother at home with the children, fortunately numerous, taking 24-hour caretaking shifts, year after year. Another husband, obviously wealthy, maintained his wife with AD at home in a comatose state for over 6 years, but it required a staff of 10 full- or part-time employees. But these are clearly exceptions, and for most, the question will be not "if," but "when." As a still-working husband with no family to help said recently, "I know I can't keep her at home forever, but how do I know when?"

Placement outside the home may reasonably be advised when (a) there is reason to believe the patient is not receiving good care at home (usually because the caretaker is too disabled to provide it); (b) the patient's behavior becomes dangerous to the caregiver(s) and cannot be controlled by behavioral or pharmacological means; (c) the patient is no longer aware where he or she is or misperceives the caregiver and other family members; (d) the caregiver's mental or physical health appears to be at the breaking point because of the continuing stress of responding to the patient's needs. Even in these circumstances, it is surprising how often caretakers insist on continuing the patient's stay at home "just a little longer."

Advice does not end, of course, with the recommendation for placement but must embrace recommendations regarding the level of care required, the availability of the care needed, and when possible advice as to which facilities are most likely to suit the patient's particular needs. Families tend to believe that the only alternative to home care is the nursing home and are often surprised at other options—special boarding homes, assisted living in retirement complexes, intermediate nursing home care, nursing home care in special AD units. Even when the level of care needed can be easily established, there may be a wide variability between the care offered, so that it may require considerable skill to match a patient with a specific institution. One facility may, for example, work skillfully with the irritable and complaining patient, while another may provide good care only for the pleasant and cooperative one. The physician must rely heavily on the social worker who specializes in the care of demented patients. This individual frequently visits and stays in touch with staff at the facilities in the area to assist caretakers in these important details of placement. The social worker is also invaluable in advising these families regarding the complexities of payment for care, insurance, governmental support available, and similar concerns.

The physician also must frequently take the lead in advising patients and/or families to seek legal advice regarding such matters as powers of attorney for health care, living wills, conservatorship, and guardianship. Families often believe that a simple power of attorney will be enough to carry them through, but this is not the case. The aim of such plans should be very simple—for the patient to give to a trusted caretaker or caretakers the widest possible latitude to make decisions for the patient (financial, medical, psychiatric, domiciliary) once the patient becomes disabled. Ideally these steps should be taken when the disease process is not too far advanced, when the patient is still competent legally, so that the adversarial process involved in the granting of conservatorship of guardianship can be avoided. If the patient has no relative or close friend willing to assume these responsibilities, public guardians are usually available and often serve faithfully.

Whether or not patients and families have planned ahead and negotiated these legal mazes, physicians must often thrust upon them questions regarding artificial life supports, especially treatment of life-threatening intercurrent infections, involuntary feeding, resuscitation, and life maintenance by artificial measures such as intubation and mechanical ventilation. Families should be urged to address these issues before a crisis arises, and whenever possible to make these family decisions rather than leaving the choice by default to the single family member having legal responsibility. Usually family members find it fairly easy to make a choice against resuscitation and mechanical ventilation. Even so, the physician must remain sensitive to the family's needs and take care to avoid becoming an advocate for his or her personal views. In other words, advice can be offered but should never be pushed. This was brought home to one of us (CEW) forcefully recently when an elderly, childless woman complained. Her elderly husband, bedridden with far-advanced dementia, had been hospitalized because of pneumonia, and she had been pushed vigorously by the pulmonologist to accept a "do not resuscitate" order that she had refused. "He just doesn't understand," she said. "I want him with me every minute I can have him, no matter what."

Families often have more trouble reaching decisions about involuntary feeding and treatment of intercurrent infections in patients with late-stage dementia. Both seem on the surface so humane that caregivers fail to think the issues through. Nutrition almost invariably suffers in very late-stage AD and sometimes becomes a focus of the family's concern. The physician should try to help the family come to regard this as a loss of hunger rather than as an act of refusal to eat. These patients never appear hungry, and no treatment measure restores their hunger. Before making decisions, families need to be aware that feeding through nasogastric tube or gastrostomy can preserve the patient in a vegetative state for years. With regard to treatment of intercurrent infections such as pneumonias, families must recognize that, unless they have a very firm agreement to the contrary with their internist, any call for assistance and especially any visit to a hospital emergency room will almost certainly result in the patient's being treated aggressively with antibiotics. Families should be helped to make the distinction between treatment to relieve distress and treatment for a specific condition, however serious, causing no apparent distress.

BEYOND SUPPORT

As stated earlier, caring for a patient with AD is often a thankless task; it is also one that seldom fails to evoke a criticism at one time or another. The patient being cared for is not typically gracious and may even be hostile and abusive. Family and friends are frequently openly disapproving, seeing the care either as inadequate or too restrictive. Even the advice of professionals can be interpreted as a reflection of the caretaker's inadequacy. The task of caretaking is not only perpetually lonely, but it can become one in which the caretaker comes to feel he or she is a prisoner who can do no right.

Thus, over the years physicians who care for these patients have expanded their role, going beyond the ordinary boundaries of support as most neuropsychiatrists might define it. Caretakers need from the physician a sense that they are genuinely liked and openly approved by their physicians as friends. In most instances there is no difficulty in personally liking and approving the efforts of the caretakers. Indeed, most physicians are often in awe of the sacrifices they make, sometimes for years on end, and of their unselfishness. It may be difficult, though, to go beyond this recognition to its open expression.

In all encounters with families, physicians should make a conscious effort to openly acknowledge the caregivers' tireless efforts and struggles. Whenever possible this should go even beyond the life of the patient, sometimes to include visits to the family when the patient has died. When death occurs, letters to the family should express not only sympathy but recognition of the family's difficult but impressive job of caring for the deceased.

Physician Needs

Those physicians who truly care for patients with AD and other dementias must develop a set of skills and a style of practice that differ in many ways from those of the typical neurologist and psychiatrist. Neurologists and psychiatrists who wish to serve only as consultants to those who take on primary care responsibilities for these patients have, in fact, little of value to offer. To serve patients with dementia, neuropsychiatrists must be willing to assume responsibility for the immediate and continued care of these patients, to be the one the family turns to first for help when problems arise. Thus, the physician who cares for demented patients assumes a role much more like that of the general practitioner or pediatrician than that of the specialist consultant.

To provide the best care for the demented patient, a team of caregivers is required. The physician practicing alone is at a distinct disadvantage. The team does not have to be large—a physician and social worker acting together may be able to provide excellent care, but independently, each is inadequate. The team may be expanded to include a nurse, psychologist, and primary care physician. Whether they work as full-time members of the team or not, the lead physician must have free and easy access to social worker, nurse, psychologist, and primary care physician to make certain that all facets of patient care are properly addressed.

As the head of the treatment team, the physician must also work with those who extend medical care outside the hospital and outpatient setting—home health agencies, visiting nurses, and social workers, day care centers, retirement homes, nursing homes, government agencies, the legal system. The physician must learn to use these extended team members not only to provide care for the patient but to serve as his or her eyes and ears when office visits are too difficult or fail to reveal the patient's true needs.

Although neuropsychiatrists taking responsibility for the care of demented patients must have ready access to the patients' primary care physicians, they must also be willing to assume some of the responsibilities usually borne by the primary care physician. Most of these patients have medical problems unrelated to the dementia, and they cannot be expected to shuttle between the neuropsychiatrist and primary care physician for every problem that arises. Thus, the neuropsychiatrist must be willing and able to deal with some of the minor medical problems common to such patients. These include indigestion, constipation, urinary tract infections, upper respiratory infections, allergies, degenerative arthritis, among others. The neuropsychiatrist may not take responsibility for these problems when they are complex or severe, but the patient cannot be sent to another physician with every routine but bothersome medical problem.

Perhaps the most striking difference between caring for these patients and for others is the enormous amount of time and attention required by their families. Family needs often far exceed those usually regarded as medically necessary as they apply to patient care—explanation of diagnosis and pathology, explanation of treatment programs, direction in patient care, help in planning for future care. These families present the physician with unusually high levels of tension, stress, and conflict. Families sometimes find it difficult to reach a consensus on diagnosis, severity of impairment, care needs, and how they will be provided. Denial is frequently blatant. Role reversals almost always cause dissension. The dissolution of the matriarch or patriarch often leads to a reemergence of long-buried sibling rivalries. The physician must try to deal with all this while not losing sight of the primary objective, which is the care of the patient. Family conflicts sometimes too complex for human understanding must be dealt with on an almost daily basis. This requires not only sensitivity, tact, and understanding, but at times blunt talk and limit-setting.

A practice dominated by patients with dementia is often also a practice focused on crisis—in the patient, in the family, in the environment. The neuropsychiatrist often is not consulted until the moment when "something must be done." Thus, the physician is often denied the niceties of careful planning and contemplation. For example, virtually all patients hospitalized with dementia enter as emergencies, and at least half the new patients seen in the outpatient setting fit the same criteria, at least as defined by their caretakers.

The physicians caring for these patients must also learn to deal with death, in a close and intimate way to which many neurologists and psychiatrists are unaccustomed. He or she must help families deal not only with the inevitability of the patient's death but frequently with how far to postpone it. Should the patient's nutrition be artificially maintained? Should an intercurrent infection be treated? Should the patient be resuscitated? Prearranged legal directives guide the physician only so far; in the end it is the family, with the help of the physician, that makes the decision.

Thus, any practice that includes a significant portion of patients with dementia is stressful. This is true not only because of the demands made on the practitioner as just enumerated, but because the prognosis in every patient with AD and similar dementias is hopeless. Even the oncologist, to whom the most difficult cancer problems are referred, sees more remissions and cures than does the dementiologist.

Why then should any physician choose such a practice? The answers are few and simple: first, because the need is great. Physicians often shun these patients when their care requires more than a quick diagnostic appraisal. In turn, these patients are shunted from one medical specialist to another, none being willing to be the patient's true physician. Second, the needs of these families are great, and their appreciation for help is very gratifying. Even the most difficult families usually acknowledge their gratitude at finally having found a physician willing to at least try to fulfill their needs. Lastly, it is the physician's duty not only to cure but also to comfort and care for those for whom there is no cure. Fulfilling this responsibility is curiously satisfying to those trained and willing to grasp the opportunity.

References

1. Koo EH, Price DL. The neurobiology of dementia. In: Whitehouse PJ, ed. Dementia. Philadelphia: FA Davis, 1993:55–91.
2. Whitehouse PJ, Landreth G, Younkin S. Molecular biology of Alzheimer's disease. In: Molecular genetic medicine, vol 3. New York: Academic Press, Inc., 1993 (in press).
3. Davies P, Katzman R, Terry RD. Reduced somatostatin-like immunoreactivity in cerebral cortex from cases of Alzheimer's disease and Alzheimer senile dementia. Nature 1980;288:279–280.
4. DeSouza EB, Whitehouse PJ, Kuhar MJ, Price DL, Vale WW. Reciprocal changes in corticotropin-releasing factor (CRF)-like immunoreactivity and CRF receptors in cerebral cortex of Alzheimer's disease. Nature 1986;319:593–595.
5. Ball MJ, Fisman M, Hachinski V, et al. A new definition of Alzheimer's disease: a hippocampal dementia. Lancet 1985;1:14–16.
6. Whitehouse PJ, Price DL, Struble RG, Clark AW, Coyle JT, DeLong MR. Alzheimer's disease and senile dementia: loss of neurons in the basal forebrain. Science 1982;215:1237–1239.
7. Bartus RT, Dean RL III, Beer B, Lippa AS. The cholinergic hypothesis of geriatric memory dysfunction. Science 1982;217:408–417.
8. Whitehouse PJ, Martino AM, Antuono PG, et al. Nicotinic acetylcholine binding sites in Alzheimer's disease. Brain Res 1986;371:146–151.
9. Perry EK, Tomlinson BE, Blessed G, et al. Neuropathological and

biochemical observations on the noradrenergic system in Alzheimer's disease. J Neurol Sci 1981;51:279–287.

10. Zweig RM, Ross CA, Hedreen JC, et al. The neuropathology of aminergic nuclei in Alzheimer's disease. Ann Neurol 1988;24:233–242.

11. Perry G, Friedman R, Shaw G, Chau V. Ubiquitin is detected in neurofibrillary tangles and senile plaque neurites of Alzheimer's disease brains. Proc Natl Acad Sci USA 1987;84:3033–3036.

12. Wischik CM, Novak M, Edwards PC, Klug A, Tichelaar W, Crowther RA. Structural characterization of the core of the paired helical filament of Alzheimer's disease. Proc Natl Acad Sci USA 1988;85:4884–4888.

13. Glenner GG, Wong CW. Alzheimer's disease: initial report of purification and characterization of a novel cerebrovascular amyloid protein. Biochem Biophys Res Commun 1984:120:885–890.

14. Yankner BA, Duffy LK, Kirschner DA. Neurotrophic and neurotoxic effects of amyloid β protein: reversal by tachykinin neuropeptides. Science 1990;250:279–282.

15. Goate A, Chartier-Harlin M-C, Mullan M, et al. Segregation of a missense mutation in the amyloid precursor protein gene with familial Alzheimer's disease. Nature 1991;349:704–706.

16. Oliver C, Holland AJ. Down's syndrome and Alzheimer's disease: a review. Psychol Med 1986;16:307–322.

17. Shoji M, Golde TE, Ghiso J, et al. Production of the Alzheimer amyloid β protein by normal proteolytic processing. Science 1992;258:126–129.

18. Strittmatter WJ, Saunders AM, Schmechel D, et al. Apolipoprotein E: high-avidity binding to β-amyloid and increased frequency of type 4 allele in late-onset familial Alzheimer's disease. Proc Natl Acad Sci USA 1993;90:1977–1981.

19. Hill LR, Klauber MR, Salmon DP, et al. Functional status, education, and the diagnosis of dementia in the Shanghai survey. Neurology 1993;43:138–145.

20. Wells CE. Chronic brain disease: an overview. Am J Psychiatry 1978;135:1–12.

21. Kekull WA, Larson EB, Reifler BV, Lampe TH, Yerby MS, Hughes JP. The validity of 3 clinical diagnostic criteria for Alzheimer's disease. Neurology 1990;40:1364–1369.

22. American Psychiatric Association. Diagnostic and statistical manual of mental disorders. 4th edition, revised. Washington, DC: American Psychiatric Association, 1994.

23. Wells CE. The differential diagnosis of psychiatric disorders in the elderly. In: Cole JO, Barrett JE, eds. Psychopathology in the aged. New York: Raven Press, 1980:19–31.

24. Wells CE. Pseudodementia. Am J Psychiatry 1979;136:895–900.

25. Rabins PV, Merchant A, Nestadt G. Criteria for diagnosing reversible dementia caused by depression: validation by 2-year follow-up. Br J Psychiatry 1984;144:488–492.

26. Teri L, Wagner AW. Assessment of depression in patients with Alzheimer's disease: concordance among informants. Psychol Aging 1991;6:280–285.

27. Teri L, Wagner A. Alzheimer's disease and depression. J Consult Clin Psychol 1992;60:379–391.

28. Consensus Conference. Differential diagnosis of dementing diseases. JAMA 1987;258:3411–3416.

29. Hachinski VC, Iliff LD, Zilhka E, et al. Cerebral blood flow in dementia. Arch Neurol 1975;32:632–637.

30. MacInness WD, Rysavy JA, McGill JE, et al. The usefulness and limitations of CT scans in the diagnosis of Alzheimer's disease. J Clin Neuropsychol 1990;12:127–130.

31. Sands LP, Katz IR, Doyle S. Detecting subclinical changes in cognitive functioning in older adults. Part I: Explication of the method. American Journal of Geriatric Psychiatry 1993;1:185–196.

32. Sands LP, Katz IR, Doyle S. Detecting subclinical changes in cognitive functioning in older adults. Part II: Initial validation of the method. American Journal of Geriatric Psychiatry 1993;1:275–287.

33. Alexopoulos GS, Abrams RC, Young RC, Shamoian CA. Cornell scale for depression in dementia. Biol Psychiatry 1988;23:271–284.

34. McKhann G, Drachman D, Folstein M, Katzman R, Price D, Stadlan EM. Clinical diagnosis of Alzheimer's disease: report of the NINCDS-ADRDA work group under the auspices of Department of Health and Human Services Task Force on Alzheimer's disease. Neurology 1984;34:939–944.

35. Cummings JL, Benson DF. Dementia. A clinical approach. 2nd. ed. Boston: Butterworth-Heinemann, 1992.

36. Foster JR. Alzheimer's disease and related disorders. In: Lazarus LW, Jarvik LF, Foster JR, Lieff JD, Mershon SR. Essentials of geriatric psychiatry. A guide for health professionals. New York: Springer-Verlag 1988:1138–1146.

37. Katzman R. Diagnosis and management of dementia. In: Katzman R, Rowe JW, eds. Principles of geriatric neurology. Philadelphia: FA Davis, 1992:165–206.

38. Wells CE, ed. Dementia. 2nd. ed. Philadelphia: FA Davis, 1977.

39. Sims NR, Bowen DM, Smith CCT. Glucose metabolism and acetylcholine systhesis in relation to neuronal activity in Alzheimer's disease. Lancet 1980;1:333–336.

40. Farlow M, Gracon SI, Hershey LA, Lewis KW, Sadowsky CH, Dolan-Ureno J. A controlled trial of tacrine in Alzheimer's disease. JAMA 1992;268:2523–2529.

41. Small GW. Tacrine for treating Alzheimer's disease [Editorial]. JAMA 1992;2564–2565.

42. Davis KL, Thal LJ, Gamzu ER, et al. A double-blind, placebo-controlled multicenter study of tacrine for Alzheimer's disease. N Engl J Med 1992;327:1253–1259.

43. Growdon JH. Treatment for Alzheimer's disease? [Editorial]. N Engl J Med 1992;327:1306–1308.

44. Preskorn SH. Recent pharmacologic advances in antidepressant therapy for the elderly. Am J Med 1993;94 (Suppl 5A):5–11.

45. Reisberg B, Ferris SH, deLeon MJ, et al. The Global Deterioration Scale (GDS): an instrument for the assessment of primary degenerative dementia. Am J Psychiatry 1982;139:1136–1139.

46. Howell T, Watts DT. Behavioral complications of dementia: a clinical approach for the general internist. J Gen Intern Med 1990;5:431–437.

47. Maletta GJ. Management of behavioral problems in elderly patients with Alzheimer's disease and other dementias. Clin Geriatric Med 1988;4:719–747.

48. Reisberg B, Borenstein J, Franssen E, Shulman E, Steinberg G, Ferris SH. Remediable behavioral symptomatology in Alzheimer's disease. Hosp Community Psychiatry 1986;37:1199–1201.

49. Wragg RE, Jeste DV. Neuroleptic and alternative treatments: management of behavioral symptoms and psychosis in Alzheimer's disease and related conditions. Psychiatr Clin North Am 1988;11:195–213.

50. International Classification of Diseases, 9th revision, Clinical modification, 4th ed. Los Angeles: Practice Management Information Corp., 1993.

51. Colenda CC, Hamer RM. Antecedents and interventions for aggressive behavior of patients at a geropsychiatric state hospital. Hosp Comm Psychiatry 1991;42:292–297.

52. Spira N, Dysken MW, Davis JM, Salzman C. Treatment of agitation and psychosis. In: Salzman C, ed. Clinical geriatric psychopharmacology. New York: McGraw-Hill, 1984:49–76.

53. Colenda CC. Buspirone in treatment of agitated demented patient. Lancet 1988;1:1169.

54. Helms PM. Efficacy of antipsychotics in the treatment of behavioral complications of dementia: a review of the literature. J Am Geriatr Soc 1985;33:206–209.

55. Lovett WC, Stokes DK, Taylor LB, Young ML, Free SM, Phelan DG. Management of behavioral symptoms in disturbed elderly patients: comparison of trifluoperazine and haloperidol. J Clin Psychiatry 1987;48:234–236.

56. Risse SC, Barnes R. Pharmacologic treatment of agitation associated with dementia. J Am Geriatr Soc 1986;34:368–376.

57. Simpson DM, Foster D. Improvement in organically disturbed behavior with trazodone treatment. J Clin Psychiatry 1986;47:191–193.

58. Steele C, Lucas MJ, Tune L. Haloperidol versus thioridazine in the

treatment of behavioral symptoms in senile dementia of the Alzheimer's type: preliminary findings. J Clin Psychiatry 1986;47:310–312.

59. Stotsky B. Multicenter study comparing thioridazine with diazepam and placebo in elderly, nonpsychotic patients with emotional and behavioral disorders. Clin Ther 1984;6:446–459.

60. Yudofsky SC, Silver JM, Hales RE. Pharmacologic management of aggression in the elderly. J Clin Psychiatry 1990;51 (Suppl 10):22–28.

61. Carlyle W, Killick L, Ancill R. ECT: an effective treatment in the screaming demented patient. J Am Geriatr Soc 1991;39:637–639.

62. Cohen-Mansfield J, Werner P, Marx MS. Screaming in nursing home residents. J Am Geriatr Soc 1990;38:785–792.

63. Greenwald BS, Marin DB, Silverman SM. Serotonergic treatment of screaming and banging in dementia. Lancet 1986;2:1464–1465.

64. Mace NL, Rabins PV. The 36-hour day. Baltimore: Johns Hopkins University Press, 1981.

65. Cohen D, Eisdorfer C. The loss of self. New York: New American Library, 1986.

37

NEUROBEHAVIORAL FEATURES OF CEREBROVASCULAR DISEASE

John R. Absher and James F. Toole

This chapter reviews the behavioral components of cerebrovascular disease (CVD), including common vascular syndromes; lesion localization, with an emphasis on arterial distribution; clinical diagnosis of focal neurobehavioral syndromes, including vascular dementia; and management considerations.

CVD is a leading cause of mortality in the U.S. Alterations in behavior resulting from CVD produce substantial morbidity in the elderly population. As more people survive strokes, behavioral problems secondary to CVD become increasingly common.

Strokes can result from cardiac abnormalities, carotid or vertebral arterial disease, atherosclerosis of the aortic arch, extracranial or intracranial arterial disease, and even venous thrombosis, which can embolize to the brain through a patent foramen ovale. Abnormalities of the blood constituents, such as polycythemia, macroglobulinemia, elevations of blood lipids, sickle cell disease, other hypercoagulable states, and connective tissue disorder, can result in stroke, and subsequently, dementia or neurobehavioral abnormalities on a vascular basis.

The diverse etiologies produce many different syndromes. For example, ischemic disease (e.g., Binswanger's disease) may be gradually progressive, and hemorrhagic disease (e.g., subarachnoid hemorrhage) may be rapidly fatal. CVD may be clinically "silent," despite extreme disease, or may be obscured by its overlap with other brain diseases (e.g., degenerative dementias). Discrete lesions may produce both focal and generalized neuropsychological impairments (1).

Although individual symptoms may indicate the precise site (and even the type) of brain damage, or provide clues to its underlying pathophysiology, clinical syndromes often defy attempts at "localization" (e.g., vascular dementias). Many behavioral and cognitive symptoms may be manifest in a single patient, even when the symptoms suggest "focal"

neurobehavioral syndromes, such as Broca's aphasia or Gerstmann syndrome. Complex assortments of deficits often suggest the diagnosis of a vascular dementia syndrome. This diagnostic process is reviewed later in this chapter.

BACKGROUND

The neurobehavioral syndromes of CVD have been elucidated by laborious clinical pathological correlation, painstakingly accumulated over the past century. The dramatic advent of computerized tomography (CT) and magnetic resonance imaging (MRI) allowed in vivo correlations. In addition, longitudinal studies led to an explosion of information regarding the neurobehavioral consequences of stroke.

Stroke is a particularly apt disorder for behavioral study because of its defined limits, sudden onset with abrupt change in behavior, and because of the usual survival of the patient so that the evolution of the process over time can be evaluated. Initially, only clinical pathological correlations related the neuroanatomical damage to specific clinical phenomena. These anatomical studies can now be coupled with functional mapping by positron emission tomography (PET) and single photon emission computerized tomography (SPECT) so that functional changes occurring at the site of the lesion and at distantly interconnected regions can be evaluated and defined anatomically. Functional neuroimaging has been particularly valuable because behavioral disturbances may occur without an abnormal neurological examination, yet changes may be seen on MR, PET, SPECT, and specialized cognitive or neurobehavioral tests. Many of these specialized "bedside examination" techniques are discussed here. When possible, the neurobehavioral features of CVD are described on a vessel-by-vessel basis, to illustrate their potential localizing value.

Figure 37.1. Overview of arterial domain. (Reprinted with permission from Toole JF. Cerebrovascular disorders. 4th ed. New York: Raven Press; 1990, 81.)

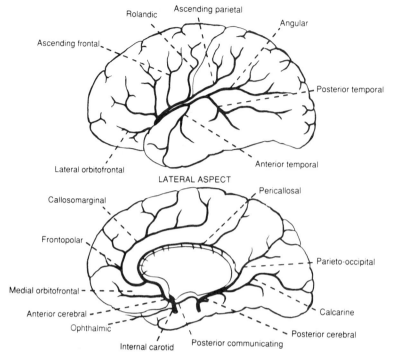

LATERAL ASPECT

MEDIAN SAGITTAL ASPECT

SYNDROMES OF SIGNIFICANCE: CLASSIFIED BY ARTERIAL TERRITORY

The brain is supplied by the two carotids and, in general, by the two vertebral arteries. Most neurobehavioral deficits result from lesions in the distribution of the carotid artery, left hemisphere strokes being slightly more likely to produce noticeable deficits than right hemisphere strokes, due largely to left hemisphere dominance for language. Neurobehavioral deficits also result from strokes within the vertebral basilar distribution, particularly the posterior cerebral artery territory. The neurobehavioral disorders, therefore, can be divided into carotid or vertebrobasilar syndromes with subdivisions into large surface-conducting arteries, boundary zone (or watershed) disorders, and arteriolar and capillary disorders. The vascular dementias are discussed separately. See Figure 37.1 for an overview of arterial domains.

Internal Carotid Artery and Branches

Neurobehavioral disorders may result from CVD in most branches of the internal carotid artery. Even ophthalmic artery infarction (or optic nerve damage) can produce, rarely, a classical neurobehavioral disorder: Anton's syndrome, or the denial of blindness (2).

ANTERIOR CHOROIDAL ARTERY

The anterior choroidal artery supplies a portion of the thalamus, globus pallidus, and internal capsule. The anterior choroidal artery syndrome generally results from occlusion due to atherosclerosis and can produce unilateral or bilateral thalamic lesions. Left-hemisphere infarcts can produce a thalamic aphasia characterized by relatively preserved repetition and comprehension ability, with impaired language output (3). This variety of thalamic aphasia resolves rapidly and has a favorable prognosis compared with most other aphasias. The bilateral anterior choroidal artery syndrome may produce acute pseudobulbar palsy, mutism, abulia, and inappropriate laughter (4).

ANTERIOR CEREBRAL ARTERY

The anterior cerebral artery supplies the medial aspects of frontal and parietal lobes and the anterior two-thirds of the corpus callosum. This artery joins its opposite through the anterior communicating artery. Its loss, either unilaterally or bilaterally, can result in lesions of the corpus callosum, cingulate gyri, supplementary motor area, or other medial structures.

Callosal infarction can produce a callosal disconnection syndrome. This syndrome includes three essential features: (*a*) left limb tactile anomia, (*b*) left-limb apraxia, and (*c*) left-limb agraphia (5). These deficits result from disconnection of the left hemisphere centers for language from the right hemisphere. Such deficits may easily escape detection on routine neurological examinations, and this fact illustrates why the importance of callosal pathways was poorly appreciated until the middle of this century (6).

Lesions of the cingulate gyri may cause profound behavioral alterations. Strokes within anterior cerebral artery territory may lead to infarction of the opposite hemisphere through propagation of clot through the anterior communicating artery or because one anterior cerebral artery is "dominant" for blood supply to the other hemisphere. Although unilateral strokes in the cingulate region may not produce substantial behavioral compromise, bilateral damage often leads to akinetic mutism. Akinetic mutism is "a state of unresponsiveness to the environment with extreme reluctance to perform even elementary motor activities. The patient lies quietly in bed, immobile, sometimes sleepy but often open-eyed and seemingly alert. On occasion his gaze may follow the examiner, but he will not react to the examiner's presence or to any stimuli except painful ones. . . . Akinesia and mutism appear without paralysis or gross motor and sensory alterations and with an intact neopallium" (7). The cingulate gyrus has long been recognized as a typical location for damage in patients with akinetic mutism (Fig. 37.2) (7).

Most patients with cingulate strokes remain vigilant, unlike those with the "paramedian thalamic syndrome" resulting from mesencephalic artery infarction, which disconnects the ascending reticular activation system from its thalamic and cortical targets, impairing basic arousal (8, 9). Cingulate damage leaves these pathways for basic arousal intact in akinetic mutism and selectively impairs the will to interact with one's surroundings.

Supplementary motor area strokes in the left hemisphere can produce a transcortical motor aphasia, characterized by preserved repetition, despite naming and verbal fluency deficits (10). This type of aphasia sometimes is accompanied by failure to initiate motor programs for language (motor neglect), as many of these patients are mute at presentation;

bilateral lesions in the region of the supplementary motor area can produce akinetic mutism.

MIDDLE CEREBRAL ARTERY

The middle cerebral artery supplies vast areas of the cerebral hemisphere. There are usually two major branches of the middle cerebral—an anterior or frontal branch and a posterior branch. Deep nuclei, such as the caudate, putamen, and globus pallidus, and deep white matter (internal capsule and corona radiata) receive blood supply via this critical arterial system. Vast areas of the brain may be affected by disease within the middle cerebral distribution, but the occipital lobe, cerebellum, and brainstem are typically spared.

In the left hemisphere, the middle cerebral artery supplies important functional centers for motor behaviors such as language output. The left hemisphere is usually dominant for language, even in nonright-handed persons. Executive functions and praxis, language comprehension, reading, and writing are important functions of the dominant left hemisphere. Working memory is probably a dominant function of the left dorsolateral convexity (11). The left middle cerebral territory is arguably the most important vascular distribution, because neurobehavioral deficits within this territory can be devastating. For example, a left middle cerebral artery infarction of its entire territory produces grossly impaired language comprehension, inability to produce meaningful written or spoken language or gestures (global aphasia), and right hemiplegia.

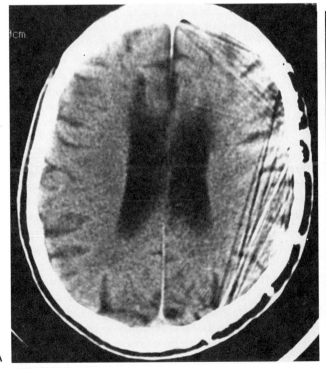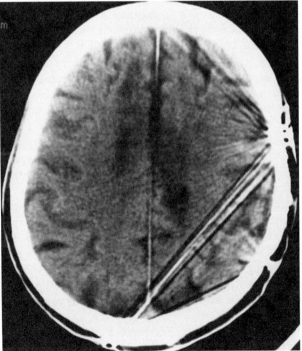

A   B

Figure 37.2.   CT of a 60-year-old man who became acutely mute and immobile. During his hospitalization, bilateral anterior cerebral artery infarctions were identified. Note the lesion in the right anterior cingulate region, and the larger lucency in the left anterior cerebral artery territory. He has remained essentially akinetic, but is now able to speak in soft, short phrases.

The anterior branch of the middle cerebral artery supplies the dorsolateral frontal lobe. Broca's aphasia results from damage to the left inferior and posterior frontal lobe premotor cortices responsible for coordinating complex linguistic motor activities of the mouth, tongue, palate, and lips. Basic coordination and praxis may be normal, despite language output abnormality, or a facial apraxia may be found in association with the Broca's aphasia (12). The left premotor association area is important for the integration of language and motor behaviors, and strokes in this same brain area may lead to ideomotor apraxia, where the left hand is unable to follow verbal commands, despite adequate strength, coordination, and sensory function (sympathetic apraxia). In some cases there is preserved ability to perform the same maneuvers spontaneously. The left hand is apraxic because of disconnection of the right hemisphere from verbal commands that are normally processed in the left superior temporal gyrus and inferior parietal lobule, transferred to the left motor association areas, and then interpreted transcallosally by the right motor association area (6).

Left frontal convexity strokes may impair other complex aspects of executive ability, the ability to shift or divide attentional resources, or reason. Depression may result from left dorsolateral frontal lobe strokes (13), while right-sided strokes may produce aprosodias. The anatomical basis and clinical features of the aprosodias are similar to the aphasias (e.g., motor, conduction, and transcortical varieties have been described) (14). Damage to the orbital frontal lobe often produces severe personality alterations and an acquired sociopathy, manifested either as inappropriate social behaviors or an incapacity to perform meaningful planning and organizational tasks (15). Judgment and reasoning are severely affected, and patients demonstrate little concern for the effect their behaviors may have on others.

The posterior branch of the middle cerebral arterial territory supplies a large portion of primary sensory and sensory association areas (including parietal, temporal, and occipital association areas), insula, and deep white and gray matter. Strokes within this territory can produce a number of classical neurobehavioral syndromes such as alexia *with* agraphia, Gerstmann syndrome, conduction aphasia, parietal apraxia, transcortical sensory aphasia, hemi-inattention or neglect, and Wernicke's aphasia.

Alexia with agraphia occurs with occlusions of the posterior branches of the left middle cerebral artery that destroy the angular gyrus in the critical brain area for translating written symbols into meaning and vice versa, and for instructing the left motor association areas important for the mechanics of writing (16, 17). Dejerine identified this syndrome, as well as pure alexia, in the last part of the 19th century (18).

The Gerstmann syndrome consists of agraphia, acalculia, finger agnosia, and right-left disorientation, and typically results from left angular gyrus lesions (19). Rarely, a right-sided lesion may produce this syndrome if the right hemisphere is dominant for language (20). Damage to the

angular gyrus of the left inferior parietal lobule or nearby regions produces these symptoms. Partial syndromes are common. Taken as a whole, there are no other sites in the nervous system to which damage can produce all four of the cardinal signs, and this fact supports the localizing value of the Gerstmann syndrome.

Conduction aphasia typically results from disconnection lesions situated between Wernicke's area and Broca's area (21). Patients cannot repeat, but comprehension and verbal fluency are preserved. The anatomical basis of conduction aphasia has become a controversial topic (22).

Parietal apraxia is a bilateral apraxia without hemiparesis (23–25). Damage in the parietal lobe (especially on the left) may disrupt "visuokinesthetic engrams" leading to bilateral apraxia (24, 26). Parietal apraxia is similar in its pathogenesis to the agraphia and constructional disturbances seen in Gerstmann syndrome in that the mechanisms for these syndromes probably relate to faulty communications between posterior language areas and the left frontal motor association cortex, which is responsible for relaying verbal commands to the right hemisphere. Patients with transcortical sensory aphasia follow commands poorly with both hands, but comprehension testing documents severe deficits to simple yes/no questions, and often inability to name objects (27, 28). Preserved repetition allows these patients to repeat commands or questions verbatim (echolalia). Both of these disorders result from damage within the inferior parietal lobule. Lesions deep to the supramarginal gyrus have been associated with parietal apraxia, (16, 17, 25), while damage to angular gyrus and adjacent (more posterior) heteromodal association cortex produces transcortical sensory aphasia (27, 28). Either the watershed zone or the posterior cerebral artery territory may be involved (28).

Hemi-inattention and neglect may occur with left middle cerebral territory strokes, particularly the posterior branch, but right-hemisphere damage is probably more likely to produce left hemi-neglect than the reverse. These attentional disturbances are further described below.

Wernicke's aphasia results from temporal lobe infarction in the posterior third of the superior temporal gyrus and in small portions of the inferior parietal lobule. The exact boundaries of Wernicke's area vary among individuals (e.g., as with right-hemispheric language dominance). Patients with damage in this region cannot comprehend spoken or written language, have rapid and paraphasic speech output, and cannot repeat (29–31). Paranoia or violence are occasional manifestations of this aphasia.

A rare vascular syndrome that results from bilateral strokes in this region is pure word deafness or auditory verbal agnosia (32, 33). The primary auditory cortices or nearby first-order association areas of both temporal lobes are destroyed (32). Patients complain about being unable to understand anything spoken, as if others are speaking a foreign language. The meaning of familiar sounds (e.g., doorbell) is typically preserved in such patients, and reading, writing, and spontaneous speech are preserved (32).

Vertebrobasilar Circulation

The vertebral arteries ascend through the transverse foramina of the cervical vertebrae and join to form the basilar artery. There are several branches of the vertebrobasilar system, but most neurobehavioral disturbances due to CVD in the vertebrobasilar (or "posterior") circulation are caused by disease within the posterior cerebral arteries. Thalamoperforating vessels are also important for disturbances such as the paramedian thalamic syndrome, thalamic amnesia, thalamic aphasia, and thalamic neglect. Strokes within small penetrating vessels to the midbrain and pons can also produce neurobehavioral syndromes such as the mesencephalic form of akinetic mutism, peduncular hallucinosis, and amnesia.

BASILAR ARTERY

A large midbrain and pontile infarct may result from CVD of the basilar artery, producing the locked-in syndrome: the loss of all motor functions other than eyelid or eye movements (4). Persons with the locked-in syndrome lack the capacity to communicate except through blinking or moving the eyes, although such movements may indicate intact cortical functions such as language comprehension. These patients, in theory, have normal intellect, normal feelings, and normal emotions. A cursory neurological examination may fail to uncover signs of consciousness, and such individuals may be inappropriately declared comatose.

A milder deficit from damage within this arterial system is the mesencephalic form of the akinetic mute state (7), which probably should be viewed as a locked-in state with preservation of some limb or head movements. Arousal is generally impaired, in contrast to akinetic mutism from cingulate damage.

Small lesions within the cerebral peduncles, specifically the pars reticulata of the substantia nigra, may rarely produce hallucinosis (34). Micropsia and kaleidoscopic, highly patterned visual hallucinations occur. Fortunately, this syndrome is extremely rare.

Lesions of the small arteries and arterioles that supply the hypothalamus, the region of the mammillary bodies, and the medial thalamus may result in a devastating amnestic syndrome called thalamic amnesia (35, 36). There is almost always some damage to hypothalamus, mammillary bodies, or fornices.

POSTERIOR CEREBRAL ARTERY

Posterior cerebral artery infarction can result in parietal and occipital damage. Four classical neurobehavioral syndromes occur with strokes in the posterior cerebral artery territory: achromatopsia, prosopagnosia, pure alexia, and Anton's syndrome.

Achromatopsia occurs with damage to the ventral visual association areas, especially on the left (37). Often there is an associated visual field defect, so that part or all of the contralateral visual field cannot be tested. Right-sided lesions

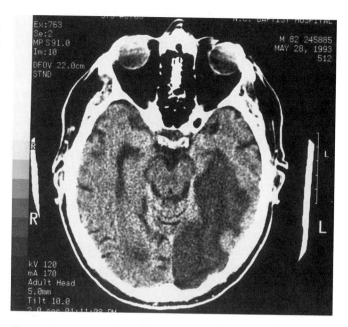

Figure 37.3. CT of a 70-year-old man who was admitted for slight right-sided weakness and numbness. He was noted on exam to have a right homonymous hemianopsia, hemi-inattention to tactile stimuli on the right (despite only minimally impaired sensory function), and decreased exploratory head and eye movements into the right hemispace. In addition, he could not read but was able to write. A complete left posterior cerebral artery territory stroke prevented linguistic interpretation of visual material perceived by the right hemisphere.

tend to produce only contralateral achromatopsia, while left-sided lesions may affect the whole visual field.

Prosopagnosia occurs with damage to both inferior visual association areas (37, 38) and rarely with unilateral right-sided lesions (39, 40). This disorder is characterized by normal ability to match, sort, or draw faces, as well as preserved ability to recognize gender and emotional facial expressions (41). What is lacking is the ability to connect this normal visual perception with its meaning. Patients are unable to recognize any familiar face, although other clues (voice, characteristic gait, a distinguishing trait such as facial hair) may lead to correct identification.

Alexia without agraphia may occur following complete left posterior cerebral artery infarction (Fig. 37.3).

All left-hemisphere visual input is disrupted, and right-hemisphere visual input is disconnected from the left-hemisphere center for language (18). The result is a visual anomia and alexia. Writing is preserved because the posterior and anterior language areas of the left hemisphere are intact.

Anton's syndrome is a denial of blindness or lack of insight into the fact that one is unable to see. In such cases, the patients may hallucinate and imagine scenes that they describe and, based upon hearing and previous experience, act as if they can see. Bilateral occipital lobe infarcts that produce bilateral homonymous hemianopsias (cortical blindness) are often found in patients with Anton's syndrome (42).

Boundary Zone (Watershed Area)

The major conducting arteries on the surface of the brain result in large infarctions in their vascular distribution. In certain instances these are confined to the watershed distribution between the major arteries, where there are insufficient collaterals or reduced perfusion pressure in both arteries. This boundary or watershed zone extends in a C-shaped pattern from the anterior polar frontal lobe, parasagitally a few centimeters from midline to the posterior parietal-occipital visual association areas. A boundary zone probably also exists in the deep parenchyma, but the term watershed infarction is typically reserved for cortical damage. Frontal lobe damage in the boundary zone may produce a transcortical motor aphasia, and transcortical sensory aphasia can result from damage within the posterior cerebral artery territory, or the posterior boundary zone (28). An isolation aphasia (mixed transcortical aphasia) can result when both the anterior and posterior boundary zones are damaged, or when there is a "double disconnection" affecting both anterior and posterior speech areas (43, 44). When the most posterior aspects of these boundary zones are damaged bilaterally, the Balint's syndrome may result.

Transcortical motor aphasia and transcortical sensory aphasia were discussed earlier in reference to middle cerebral artery infarctions. The mixed transcortical aphasias are a combination of the language output problems of the transcortical motor aphasias and the language comprehension problems of the transcortical sensory aphasias. Patients with this disorder can repeat very well and, in fact, may have echolalia as their major speech output. There may be a remarkable preservation of naming ability in some patients with mixed transcortical or atypical aphasias (Fig. 37.4) (43, 44). This observation raises the argument that such disorders should be considered disconnection syndromes rather than aphasias (44), because naming is impaired in virtually all aphasias.

Balint's syndrome consists of three unique visual/spatial deficits: (a) inability to direct gaze upon command (apraxia of gaze or ocular apraxia), (b) inability to simultaneously perceive all elements of a visual scene (simultananagnosia), and (c) paradoxical ability to direct hand movements better without than with visual guidance (optic ataxia) (45).

Arteriolar-Capillary Infarctions

The penetrating arterioles have no anastomoses between them. As a consequence, each arteriolar capillary is isolated (46). Small infarctions within those vessels can result in micro-infarctions, which, until the advent of MRI often went undetected. Now one can see the results of chronic ischemia or abnormalities in the capillaries as leukoaraiotic changes and/or lacunar infarctions. The distinction between these two syndromes is traditional but may be artificial. Lacunar infarctions are due to the loss of an arteriole and result in spherical infarctions no larger than 1–2 cm. In leukoaraiosis, the extreme example being Binswanger's disease (see below), diffuse damage occurs deep within the substance of the brain near the ventricles (47). Lacunar infarcts traditionally involve gray matter in the basal ganglia or brainstem, while leukoaraiosis affects the white matter. Most of the lacunar syndromes (pure motor hemiparesis, pure sensory stroke, clumsy hand dysarthria, etc.) are not further discussed. Leukoaraiosis is discussed below, in the context of the vascular dementias.

SYNDROMES OF SIGNIFICANCE: BY SYMPTOMS OR SIGNS

The discussion of vascular syndromes must begin with a definition of terms. There are many types of vascular dementia, each of which fulfills the essential criteria for a dementia syndrome. Two common definitions of dementia are used clinically. The DSM-III-R (or DSM-IV) definition requires impairment in memory and at least one other cognitive domain (48). Cummings and Benson advocate a slightly different definition of dementia that allows patients without memory impairment to be labeled as demented, but three cognitive domains must be impaired to fulfill the criteria (49). No confusional state can be present that could account for the symptoms, confusion being a reflection of grossly disturbed attention. The description and classification of the vascular dementia syndromes may be based on analyses of cognitive domains, or vascular mechanisms. Most often, mechanistic classification terms are preferred (e.g., multi-infarct dementia, lacunar state, and hypoxic-ischemic encephalopathy), and cognitive domains are analyzed to verify the required number of deficits.

This section is divided into two parts. First, each cognitive domain is explored to provide an overview of the many types of deficits that can result from CVD. Second, the topic of vascular dementia is briefly reviewed.

Cognitive Domains Affected by Cerebrovascular Disease

Deficits that are "circumscribed" (i.e., focal; discrete; isolated to a single domain) often provide clues to neural organization and brain function. Although few deficits are completely circumscribed, those that are the most nearly circumscribed are of considerable interest. Careful attention to the possibility of circumscribed deficits increases sensitivity to deficits in each major domain and thereby enhances the capacity to identify vascular dementia in its earliest stages, when it may be most susceptible to intervention. Such focal deficits also serve to differentiate vascular from degenerative dementias.

All major spheres (or domains) of higher mental ability may be individually affected by CVD: attention, language, memory, visual-spatial ability, and executive ability. These domains of mental functioning represent "cognitive" abilities, while mood or affective disorder, personality change, hallucinations, delusions, and anxiety are examples of psychiatric alterations. CVD may produce circumscribed cognitive and psychiatric behavioral alterations.

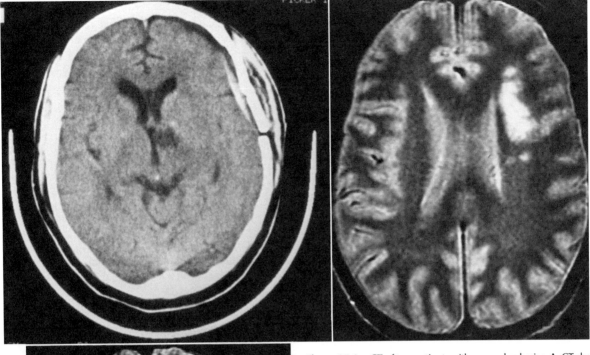

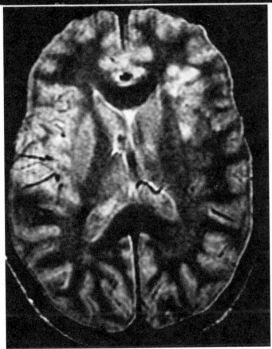

Figure 37.4. CT of two patients with unusual aphasias. **A,** CT showing the brain of a 54-year-old man who developed a halting, paraphasic, nonfluent aphasia (with largely preserved repetition), echolalia, and palilalia after a left anterior thalamic infarction. **B** and **C,** CT showing a left anterior insula and deep subcortical frontal lesion in a 54-year-old left-handed man. He demonstrated paraphasias, impaired comprehension, poor category list generation, and a mixed aprosodia. There was no evidence of apraxia. This case suggests "crossed global aprosodia," atypical aphasia, and right-hemisphere dominance for praxis.

The major behavioral syndromes related to CVD are listed in Table 37.1 and are discussed in the following sections.

ATTENTIONAL DISTURBANCES

Immediate Attention

Immediate attention, or attention span, is a basic cognitive process that influences many brain functions. Attention may be disturbed in the acute period following injury from CVD. Mesulam et al. noted impaired attention (i.e., "acute confusional state") due to right middle cerebral artery infarction (50), and a similar syndrome may follow left-hemisphere stroke (51). Even when immediate attention (i.e., forward digit span, or word span) is intact, the ability to direct, shift, and sustain attention can be impaired. Strokes can impair any one of these aspects of attention, without affecting other attentional processes. Attention can be impaired at the input, processing, or output stages of cognition.

Table 37.1. Neurobehavioral Syndromes of Significance Associated with Cerebrovascular Disease

Categorized by Arterial Supply	Categorized by Symptom or Sign
Anterior choroidal artery	Attentional disturbances
thalamic/subcortical aphasia	acute confusion
acute pseudobulbar palsy, mutism, abulia,	inattention
inappropriate laughter	neglect
Anterior cerebral artery	motor neglect
callosal disconnection syndrome	anosognosia
akinetic mutism	Language disturbances
transcortical motor aphasia	dysarthria
Middle cerebral artery	dysfluency
all aphasia types	comprehension defect
all aprosodia types	impaired repetition
personality change	anomia
alexia with agraphia	reading/writing disturbance
Gerstmann syndrome	Memory disturbances
sympathetic and parietal apraxias	transient global amnesia
neglect and inattention	procedural memory impairment
pure word deafness	category-specific amnesias
Basilar artery	Visuospatial dysfunction
locked-in syndrome	Executive dysfunction
peduncular hallucinosis	Emotional/affective disturbances
amnesia	pseudobulbar affect
Posterior cerebral artery	aprosodia
achromatopsia	mania
prosopagnosia	depression
pure alexia	anxiety
Anton's syndrome	Hallucinations/delusions
Boundary zone (watershed)	Personality changes
transcortical aphasias	Vascular dementia syndromes
Balint syndrome	multi-infarct dementia
Arteriolar-capillary infarction	Binswanger's disease
leukoaraiosis	Angular gyrus syndrome
vascular dementia syndromes	Amnesia

Inattention

Inattention is a condition in which a patient fails to report or respond to stimuli presented to one side of his or her body. Visual, tactile, and auditory stimuli are most commonly tested. The involvement of several modalities, the improvement in performance when the patient is asked to attend to the defective side, and "extinction" to double simultaneous stimulation (failure to acknowledge two simultaneous stimuli, although both stimuli, presented individually, are correctly acknowledged) are all suggestive of inattention. Inattention is a partial neglect syndrome in that the patient can be aided to recognize the affected side. Attention to perceptual signals or inputs is disrupted in inattention.

Neglect

Neglect denies relatively normal percepts access to consciousness and is characterized by defective attention to stimuli originating in the spatial environment contralateral to a brain lesion (hemispace). As with inattention, neglect should not be attributable to a primary sensory or perceptual impairment, although minor abnormality is common. Denial of clinical deficits (asomatagnosia, or anosognosia) is relatively common, and may affect one-half of the body

(Figs. 37.4 and 37.5). It may be impossible to verify intact sensory ability on the neglected side. Clinically, there appears to be a continuum from mild hemi-inattention to severe hemineglect and hemianosognosia (hemisomatagnosia).

In addition to its influence on perceptual or input functions, neglect can occur during the processing stages between input and output. For example, "mental representational" aspects of neglect have been proposed, manifested by patients who neglect half of remembered places (52). Two stroke patients were asked to recall (from two opposite perspectives) a familiar square in Milan, Italy; they enumerated objects only on the right side of the internal mental representation of the square.

Motor Neglect

Motor neglect is also called inattention or intentional neglect, defined as the impaired ability to initiate a movement that cannot be attributed to paresis or abnormalities of tone (53, 54). It is distinguished from apraxia by the normal performance seen when the patient finally initiates the maneuver. It is distinguished from bradykinesia by the relatively normal speed of movement, once initiated. Thus, it is best conceptualized as a subtle form of motor initiation disturbance, with psychomotor retardation and akinesia being extreme forms. Motor neglect can occur as an isolated manifestation of stroke (55).

Thus, input, processing, and output "attentional" processes may all be selectively disrupted by CVD, but combined syndromes are common (53). Heilman and co-workers suggest a complex circuit for attention involving the mesencephalic reticular formation, several nonspecific nuclei of the thalamus, portions of the inferior parietal lobule, the frontal lobe, and cingulate gyrus (56). Mesulam recently proposed a cortical network theory for directed attention, language, and memory (57). Dysfunction of the network for attention affects many brain areas, and this may explain the tendency for attentional disturbances to produce impairments in many cognitive and noncognitive functions.

The presence of gross impairment in immediate attention must raise suspicion that one is dealing with an acute (or chronic) confusional state, or reversible encephalopathy, rather than a dementia syndrome. Bedside testing of attention and language, and close observation for fluctuating levels of alertness are usually necessary to identify confusional states.

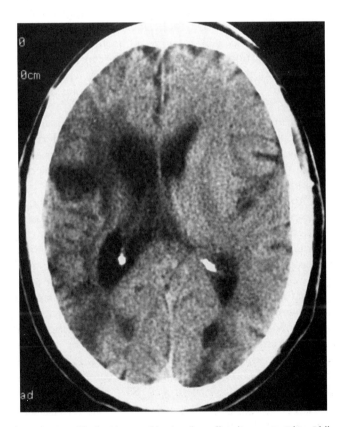

Figure 37.5. CT of a 68-year-old man who suffered an acute right middle cerebral artery infarction. A prior left occipital infarction had left him with a right hemianopsia. The acute infarct ablated most vision on his "good" left hemi-field. Thus, he was essentially cortically blind, and barely had light perception in a small portion of his right visual field. Nevertheless, he did not mention this finding until specifically asked by the examiners. Also, he denied being touched or pinched on his left side, even while withdrawing the left arm and leg from the pain. When his own left arm was held up to the side of his face, he still guessed that the hand touching him must be the examiner's.

Anosognosia

When attentional impairments eliminate awareness of one's own impairments (e.g., hemiparesis), the hemineglect involves some degree of denial or 'anosognosia," the lack of knowledge of deficits (58). Somatagnosia is not uncommon, and may be detected in patients with hemineglect who deny ownership of the paralyzed limb when asked, "Whose hand is this?" as the hand is shown to them and stroked against the intact side of the face or body. Patients may develop anosognosia for blindness (Anton's syndrome), aphasia (59), hemichorea-hemiballism (60), prosopagnosia (61), and apraxia (62). Thus, lesions in a multitude of different brain areas may produce anosognosia, but the right hemisphere is most often damaged (63). Anosognosia, like agnosia, thus seems capable of domain specificity.

LANGUAGE DISTURBANCES

Speech and Language

It is clinically convenient to conceptualize communication disorders as speech or language problems. Speech disorders consist of defective phonation (sound or "phoneme" generation) or defective articulation (the ability to modify sounds using the tongue, palate, lips, and respiratory musculature). For example, in the syndrome of clumsy-hand dysarthria, oral, facial, and lingual articulatory functions are disrupted, usually by infarction of the basis pontis (64). Medullary infarcts may selectively impair phonation, when lower cranial nerves are affected. Thus, speech impairments occur in the presence of intact language ability, or interfere with language evaluation.

Speech may be entirely spared in the presence of severe language disorders. Language is acquired communication ability based on written symbols (graphemes), auditory/verbal symbols (phonemes), or gestures (i.e., as in sign languages) that are combined (e.g., through grammar and syntax) to convey meaning. Aphasias are acquired behavioral syndromes characterized by specific patterns of language abnormality. The aphasias are classified based on the pattern of impairments in naming, repetition, comprehension, and fluency (65). Reading, writing, pragmatics (the normal give and take of dialogue), discourse (the overall plan or story line), and prosody (the ability to understand and express emotion by alterations in the melody or intonation of speech) may also be impaired in the aphasias (Fig. 39.4).

Each language function can be selectively affected by CVD. Table 37.2 lists examples of major language functions along with reported instances of selective impairment due to stroke. Identifying the components of language disorder provides valuable clues to lesion localization.

Fluency

Fluency is a term used to describe the ease of language production. Persons who hesitate when speaking, truncate sentences, produce language output slowly (usually less than 50 words per minute), exhibit many grammatical errors, and

Table 37.2.   Language Disturbances and Focal Brain Damage

Function	Condition	Damaged Sites	References
Naming	anomia, proper names only	left temporal lobe	85
Repetition	conduction aphasia	left peri-sylvian zone	21, 22, 25
Comprehension	transcortical sensory aphasia	left temporal, parietal, occipital lobes, or thalamus	27, 28
Fluency	transcortical motor aphasia	left frontal lobe, thalamus	10, 28
Reading	alexia	left occipital lobe	18
Writing	agraphia	left frontal lobe	119
Prosody	aprosodia	right hemisphere	14, 96
Gesture	pantomime agnosia	left occipital	120

who seem to struggle to produce each word are described as nonfluent. Fluent speech flows easily and effortlessly such that many words are produced (e.g., often over 200 words per minute). Fluent language disorders are far more likely to arise from damage posterior to the central sulcus (or inferior to the sylvian fissure) than from frontal lobe damage, which typically produces nonfluent aphasias.

Comprehension

Comprehension deficits are more likely to result from posterior temporoparietal brain damage than from frontal lobe damage, although frontal lobe injury can impair comprehension as well (66). Simple commands and yes/no questions test basic comprehension, but more complex commands and questions are necessary to identify minor abnormalities of comprehension.

Repetition

The ability to repeat words, phrases, or sentences is mediated by cortical regions surrounding the sylvian fissure, and damage almost anywhere within this large zone may impair repetition ability. Outside this perisylvian zone, cerebral damage usually spares repetition ability.

Naming

Naming requires neural structures that retrieve meaning and mechanisms to translate meaning into "motor programs" that drive the speech apparatus for communication. Anterior and posterior sites of damage may impair naming ability; some degree of anomia is almost always present in aphasia, with rare exceptions in some cases of transcortical or atypical aphasia (Fig. 37.4) (43, 67). Access to the knowledge of word meaning may be compromised by visual, auditory, or tactile disorders that may be mistaken for naming impairment. To verify that naming disturbance is present, both written and spoken language production and comprehension should be checked, since a patient with visual impairment may be able to name an object only if it is held or described verbally.

Figure 37.6 depicts a simplified classification scheme for the aphasias (atypical, jargon, and subcortical aphasias are not included). By testing naming, fluency, repetition, and

comprehension, excellent localizing information is gained during the neurological examination.

MEMORY DISTURBANCES

Memory impairments can result from brain damage following hypoxic-ischemic injury (e.g., cardiac arrest) (68), hemorrhage (69), or infarction (e.g., bilateral posterior cerebral artery occlusion) (70–73). Transient global amnesia may follow a similar process (i.e., a TIA with true amnesia as its hallmark) (74–76), although other etiologic possibilities, such as seizures, have not been excluded (77). Selective memory problems (78) may result from stroke and be limited in duration, or limited to specific types of information. Detection of memory impairments is enhanced by attention to each remarkable facet of this complex cognitive domain.

Neuropsychological aspects of memory include semantic versus episodic memory; immediate, recent, and remote memory; verbal versus nonverbal memory; procedural versus declarative memory; and generic versus specific memory. Episodic memories are those that require "time-tags" to be associated with specific knowledge. Damasio has demonstrated that strokes can specifically impair this aspect of memory in some patients with amnesia (79). This disorder of "time-tagging" may be limited to new learning (anterograde) impairment (80). Isolated retrograde amnesia has rarely been reported (81), but stroke is seldom the cause. Isolated retrograde amnesia suggests psychogenic amnesia more often than CVD-related amnesia (82). New learning is commonly impaired by strokes, while remote memories are often spared. Verbal memory is disrupted by left-sided lesions (e.g., thalamic, fornix, and temporal lobe infarcts) (73). Nonverbal memory deficits more commonly emerge after right- than left-sided strokes (83).

Inability to access specific semantic categories of knowledge can occur after stroke. For example, van Lancker and Klein noted dissociation of common and proper noun recognition following stroke (84). Warrington and McCarthy describe in detail one stroke patient's category-specific semantic memory performance (85). Damasio et al. suggest that damaged neural systems (e.g., the visual or somatosensory systems), not the conceptual category (e.g., animals), determine apparent category specificity (86, 87).

Procedural memory is stored knowledge of motor acts or procedures, such as riding a bicycle or walking. Focal strokes can disrupt procedural memory mechanisms, leading to an impairment in ability to learn new motor skills. Defective procedural memory is an "anterograde" problem, demonstrated by failure to acquire skill at a normal rate, while apraxia reflects inability to demonstrate motor skills that have already been learned. It is tempting to speculate that retrograde procedural amnesia is the same thing as ideational apraxia. Ideomotor apraxia would then be a failure to access procedural memories (motor programs) on the basis of auditory or visual commands.

The specific vs. generic memory distinction relates to the difference between unique and categorical identification. What something is (e.g., a woman) represents generic memory; specific memory permits the unique identification of an object (e.g., my wife.) to be stated. Focal disturbances of specific memory are agnosias (i.e., prosopagnosia, in the example given), and the latter terminology is typically used to describe these impairments. Patients with prosopagnosia can tell that a face is a face, and can determine gender, age, and emotional expressions, despite their inability to verbalize knowledge of unique identity (41). When generic memory is impaired, specific memory is not possible.

The ambiguity of the term agnosia is most plainly illustrated by comparing the two classical varieties of agnosia (associative and apperceptive) to the specific and generic functions of memory. In apperceptive agnosia, general ideas about the identity of an object are not evoked by the usual stimulus (e.g., they see but cannot perceive) (88). Patients may be able to spontaneously describe the same object in piecemeal fashion. In the associative agnosias such as prosopagnosia, intact perceptions can be described in generic terms, but unique identification (specific memory) cannot be evoked by the visual stimulus.

All of these facets of memory clearly cannot be carefully screened at the bedside; a straightforward approach that tests learning, recall, and recognition of words and pictures is sufficient to identify most patients with recent memory

impairment. Typically, the patient is read a list of eight to 10 words, three or four times. After each presentation, the patient attempts to recall all the words, and the examiner keeps track of his responses. Most normal people learn nine or 10 words after four tries. About 5–10 minutes later, the patient is again asked to provide the words. If recall is impaired (i.e., less than seven to eight words were recalled), recognition memory should be tested. One way to do this is simply to provide a category clue for each word. Multiple choice lists should be presented if the category clue does not lead to a correct response. Alternatively, a long list of words, including those on the original list of words and an equal or greater number of foils, can be read to the patient, who must provide a yes or no response indicating recognition of each word. A similar procedure may be used for visual spatial memory. Patients are shown a series of figures, then asked to draw them from memory. A delayed picture recall is also useful, as is having the patient circle one of several figures in a multiple choice array to see if he/she can recognize previously drawn pictures that could not be spontaneously recalled. Nonverbal memory can also be tested by hiding objects in the room while the patient observes. Later, the patient is asked to state the names of the objects and where each has been hidden.

Long-term memory testing requires knowledge of several facts about the patient's past. Birthdate, schools attended, years of military service, family members and personal data (Social Security number, phone number, address, etc.) are convenient examples of such facts that may be readily verified. Patients are also asked to name the current president and recent presidents. Most normal adults can name at least the last four to five presidents. These simple bedside memory tests identify most patients with clinically significant memory disturbances.

PERCEPTUAL DEFICITS

There is a continuum of cognitive function between sensation and memory. Sensory impressions blend into percepts. Bits and pieces of a single object may be perceived separately (Balint syndrome), indicating that some "assembly" or synthesis of individual percepts is required for normal perception. The failure of prosopagnosic patients to access knowledge relevant to correctly perceived faces indicates that access to long-term memories is also necessary for recognition of percepts. This also suggests that recognition requires some sort of emotional or covert recognition that may be either impaired or spared in prosopagnosia (89, 90). By keeping these elements of the sensory and amnestic continuum in mind during the evaluation, one can often uncover evidence of perceptual disturbances.

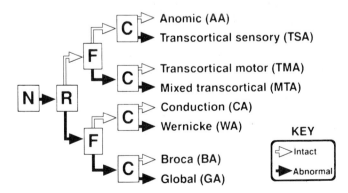

Figure 37.6. A simplified scheme for classifying most aphasic disorders, based on performance on naming (N), repetition (R), comprehension (C), and fluency (F) tests. Eight aphasia types result, as shown, by applying this simple scheme. Atypical aphasias are not included.

VISUOSPATIAL DYSFUNCTION

Visuospatial abilities encompass a large number of complex brain functions, many of which may be disturbed

Table 37.3. Five Classification Schemes for Memory[a]

Classification	Dimensions	Examples	Important Structures
Semantic vs. episodic	Time dependency	name of an item; what one did yesterday	highly distributed orbitofrontal cortex (highly distributed)
Immediate vs. recent vs. remote	Interval before access	seconds; minutes to days; weeks to years	prefrontal cortex medial temporal lobes (highly distributed)
Verbal vs. nonverbal	Linguistic relevance	word recall; figure recall	left hemisphere right hemisphere
Procedural vs. declarative	Conscious awareness	riding a bicycle; a recipe	subcortical nuclei left hemisphere
Generic vs. specific	Uniqueness	''That's a woman''; ''That's my wife''	highly distributed anterior temporal lobes (highly distributed)

[a]Time dependency means that the memory only makes sense in temporal context with other memories. The time interval is not the only important feature distinguishing immediate from recent memory, or recent from remote. For example, distraction is very important in distinguishing immediate from recent memory, and the shift from recent to remote probably relates to memory consolidation. Linguistic relevance refers to the symbols of language such as written or spoken words, sentences, or sign language. Nonverbal materials are other things such as drawings, visual scenes, music or sounds, gestures or movements. Conscious awareness (and the ability to describe in words what is remembered) distinguishes procedural from declarative memory. Uniqueness relates to the number of members in a category. Examples are given. The neuroanatomy is complex, and many structures contribute to each type of memory process. The most clinically relevant brain areas are listed; damage to these sites can markedly impair the memory processes indicated.

by CVD. Visuomotor abilities are those skills related to eye-hand coordination, praxis, and constructional ability. Visuoverbal skills relate to language tasks such as reading, or naming or describing things perceived visually.

Naming and reading are typically assessed as part of the language evaluation. Visuomotor ability is continually probed by having the patient copy simple or complex two-dimensional figures. Memory for the drawings can be checked by asking the subject to draw the figures from memory after a 5–30 minute delay. Recognition is checked by slowing the subject clusters of three to five similar drawings and asking him/her to identify the one that he/she drew previously. These simple bedside tests will identify many patients with visuospatial deficits (Table 37.3).

FRONTAL-SUBCORTICAL (EXECUTIVE) DISTURBANCES

Complex motor behaviors require intact strength, coordination, and praxis. When planning, sequencing, timing, and other integrative functions are required for complex behavior, executive ability is required (91). Because subcortical-cortical circuits interconnecting the frontal lobe, thalamus, and basal ganglia are probably involved with some of these higher abilities, the term frontal-subcortical functions seems an appropriate synonym for executive functions (92).

Frontal-subcortical circuit impairments may result from CVD. An excellent example of a highly integrated executive ability is the ability to play a musical instrument; there are several reported instances of specific musical deficits following stroke. For example, one subject continued to read, write, and play music, despite alexia for words (93). Musical execution and appreciation require many frontal-subcortical circuits that play important roles in normal cognition (92). The playing of music is generally a bihemispheric activity (93), and the ability to plan, create, and execute motor behaviors to achieve anticipated social and emotional

musical goals undoubtedly requires the temporal lobes (94) and several other brain areas. Neurobehavioral tests such as the serial hand sequences test of Luria, the multiple loops, the alternating/reciprocal programs, and the go-no-go tasks are used to explore frontal/executive skills at the bedside (49). The ability to sing (94) reproduce a rhythmic series of finger taps (95), and speak with normal melody and prosody (14, 96) are related frontal/executive skills that likely have a right frontal lobe localization (97).

Psychiatric Types of Behavioral Alteration in Cerebrovascular Disease

EMOTIONAL OR AFFECTIVE DISTURBANCES

Pseudobulbar Affect

Mood is an internal experience of emotion that usually corresponds to outward appearance, or affect. Occasionally, CVD produces dissociations between mood and affect so that appearances do not correspond to internal emotional experience. When bilateral brain damage is present, particularly in the frontal operculum, corticobulbar tracts, or basal ganglia, pseudobulbar palsy may result (98). This disorder is characterized by dysarthria, brisk jaw jerk, and stereotypical emotional facial expressions (e.g., crying, smiling) that are not accompanied by an appropriate degree of mood change.

The right hemisphere may be organized for emotional aspects of language, and its organization partially parallels that of the left hemisphere (96). Patients with right frontal lobe damage may be unable to modify language output (or facial expression or gesture) to reflect deeply felt emotions (96). Comprehension of the emotional qualities of speech (e.g., an angry voice, a sad voice) may be selectively impaired by right posterior temporal-parietal damage (96). There may be an emotional language disorder corresponding to each major aphasia type. Emotional comprehension, expression, and affect all appear to be dissociable in some subjects with CVD (Fig. 37.4).

Robinson and co-workers investigated poststroke mood disturbances such as mania and depression (99). Their work indicates that the experience of emotion may also be selectively altered by CVD: either depression or mania may result from stroke, depending on predisposing factors and lesion localization (13). Depression may occur without an appropriately sad affective expression, but it is doubtful that mania can be diagnosed in the absence of affective alteration (euphoric or happy, or occasionally irritable and anxious). Affect and emotion are partially circumscribed domains of higher brain function. Emotional and affective brain functions may be selectively perturbed by CVD.

Mania

Mania is more likely to occur in persons with a family history of bipolar illness who suffer a right-hemispheric infarction. (13, 100) Lesions within several right-hemispheric structures have been reported in association with mania: the right frontal lobe, the right thalamus, the right caudate, and the right temporal lobe. (13, 100–102) Occasionally, left-hemispheric strokes may precipitate mania (100). This issue is discussed further in Chapter 13, where poststroke depression is also discussed.

Depression

Left frontal lobe damage predisposes to major depressive disorder, with higher risks as the lesion approaches the frontal pole (99). Right-hemispheric strokes can also predispose to dysthymic mood, or minor depression, and this has been most often found in association with posterior damage (99). Subcortical strokes, such as within the left thalamus and caudate, can also produce depression (99). The degree of functional impairment does not predict risk for depressed mood, but depressed mood seems to impair functional recovery (103).

Anxiety

Anxiety is a feeling of worry or concern, usually without obvious cause. It is differentiated from phobic disorders because the latter result from identifiable precipitants (e.g., snakes, closed spaces). Anxiety may be a direct consequence of a focal brain injury, often accompanies other mood disturbances such as depression, and usually occurs when there is cortical infarction rather than isolated subcortical damage (104). Anxiety is relatively common among patients with vascular dementia, affecting 30–40% of patients. Orbital frontal lobe structures are likely anatomical sites where metabolic abnormalities occur in obsessive-compulsive disorder (105), and damage in this area may cause some cases of organic anxiety or obsessive-compulsive behavior.

HALLUCINATIONS AND DELUSIONS

Hallucinations are sensory/perceptual experiences that do not result from tactile, visual, olfactory, gustatory, or auditory stimuli. Illusions are partly based on real sensory impressions, but these stimuli evoke an aberrant perception or interpretation (e.g., one sees a snake when looking at an electrical cord). Delusions are false beliefs that are qualitatively or quantitatively beyond the realm of accepted culturally distinctive religious or metaphysical beliefs. Delusions may or may not be associated with perceptual abnormalities such as illusions or hallucinations. Delusions are the hallmark of psychosis; hallucinations and illusions may occur without psychosis, as in the visual hallucinations associated with classical migraine.

Visual hallucinations may follow occipital, parietal, or temporal lobe infarctions (106). Although right-sided temporal, parietal, and occipital strokes have been described in association with visual hallucinations (107), the site of damage producing hallucinations may be left-sided or subcortical (106). An accumulation of lesions, as in multi-infarct dementia (MID), leads to increasing risk for organic hallucinosis due to CVD. Psychosis often accompanies the hallucinations in such patients.

PERSONALITY CHANGES

Personality reflects deeply ingrained, chronic qualities of behavior, some of which may be genetically determined. Many facets of cognitive and behavioral function contribute to personality, perhaps because the term subsumes so many aspects of behavior. Cerebrovascular damage can dramatically alter personality (Figs. 37.4 and 37.7).

Vascular Dementia Syndromes

Multiple infarcts scattered through a variety of locations within the central nervous system, each presumably with a definite effect upon brain function, can combine into a syndrome of deficits that exceeds that of individual infarcts (e.g., MID). A critical exercise in making this diagnosis is identifying the focal deficits that result from the scattered infarcts. Enhanced sensitivity to focal deficits can be achieved by increasing the sophistication of the neurological examination to include the neurobehavioral examination of cognitive and behavioral functions, as briefly described earlier. Certain clinical clues may also suggest a MID diagnosis.

Among the generally accepted characteristics of MID are its sudden onset (in contrast to the slow decline that is characteristic of Alzheimer's disease), and often stepwise or fluctuating course. Patients with MID often have preserved insight into their deficits, whereas those with Alzheimer's disease generally do not. As a rule, there is a history of one or more strokes in the past, and because of the male propensity to cerebral infarction, the disease tends to be a masculine disorder.

Multiple infarcts are not the only cause of vascular dementia. On occasion, extracranial arterial disease, particularly in the carotid and vertebral arteries, may constrict cerebral blood flow and perfusion pressure so that a global cerebral ischemic syndrome can result. Chronic or repeated hypotension can also lead to an hypoxic-ischemic encephalopathy (108). Global hypoperfusion may result from arteriolar narrowing from chronic hypertension or from hypotension, producing ischemic demyelination and lacunar infarction. When vast areas of the subcortical white matter surrounding the ventricles become damaged by this process, the patient has Binswanger's disease, a slowly progressive or stepwise form of vascular dementia that is usually severe. Binswanger's disease patients typically have a subcortical dementia syndrome (i.e., a dementia syndrome with subcortical behavioral features such as dysarthria, mood disturbance, a retrieval deficit on memory testing, and slow movements), and hypertension (109, 110), or other vascular risk factors (111). Patients with this disorder may have a variety of neurological signs such as motor deficits, clumsiness, incoordination of limb movements, vertiginous episodes, gait abnormalities, convulsions, and hemianopic or quadrantanopic defects in vision. They frequently develop pseudobulbar affect, depression, apathy, and psychomotor retardation (112, 113). In addition, they develop deficits in judgment with lack of insight and, occasionally, hallucinatory episodes and paranoid ideation (114).

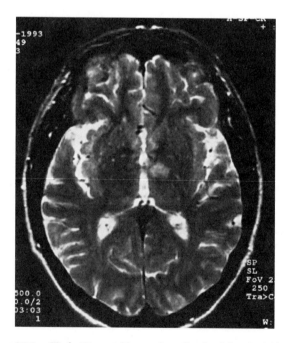

Figure 37.7. CT of a 72-year-old man who suffered an infarction within the left subthalamus and inferior portion of the thalamus. He acutely developed severe hemiballismus, leg greater than arm, on the right. In addition, his personality changed completely. He became sexually inappropriate, and propositioned no fewer than six nurses during his hospitalization. He suddenly exposed his genitals during rounds, in front of four family members and eight medical staff. He touched his groin while others were in his hospital room, and he cursed vociferously. All of these behaviors were completely out of character, based on his premorbid personality.

Focal strokes or reductions in blood flow can result in brain abnormalities that appear to be diagnostic of dementia. The angular gyrus syndrome is an example of a focal stroke syndrome masquerading as a dementia syndrome (i.e., Alzheimer's disease) (115). Patients with this syndrome have severe language disturbances (transcortical sensory aphasia being most typical) that impair comprehension of words, despite intact repetition and fluent speech output (a pattern commonly seen in Alzheimer's disease). Verbal memory is also defective, and constructional ability is usually disturbed as well. Amnesic syndromes may also resemble vascular dementia, but other behavioral functions (besides memory) remain largely intact. Unless each cognitive domain is specifically examined, through neuropsychological assessment or bedside neurobehavioral examination, such individuals may be presumed to suffer from a dementia syndrome.

Nearly identical neurobehavioral syndromes can result from damage in widely separated brain regions, and this has led to the tendency to describe vascular dementia syndromes in terms of their associated neurobehavioral features, rather than on the basis of specific vascular abnormalities. Although the vascular-anatomical approach works well for many focal syndromes, it fails in the classification of the vascular dementias. Even for some types of discrete lesions (e.g., those producing amnesia), the anatomical classification is ambiguous. For example, amnesia has been reported as a vertebrobasilar arterial syndrome due to bilateral hippocampal lesions, resulting from either bilateral posterior cerebral artery infarctions (70) or, in some instances, bilateral anterior choroidal artery infarctions. The mammillothalamic artery, arising from the top of the basilar artery, can result in destruction of the mammillary bodies, mammillothalamic tract, and medial thalamic nuclei, destroying the capacity to store new memories (73). Thus, widely separated anatomical sites within different vascular systems result in remarkably similar amnestic syndromes. These disparities can be explained by damage to separate sites in a memory network or circuit.

DIAGNOSTIC EVALUATION

The diagnostic evaluation of individuals for vascular dementia includes an appropriate history to determine whether there is a progressive, acquired cognitive impairment fulfilling the diagnosis of dementia, and vascular risk factors such as hypertension. The Hachinski ischemic score (HIS), or the modified HIS should be considered (Table 37.4) as a gauge to the probability that the dementia results from CVD (116, 117). The diagnostic evaluation to determine the source of the problem causing vascular dementia includes a full cardiac evaluation of the heart, the extracranial arteries, and the intracranial vessels down to and including the capillary circulation. Acceptable studies would include cardiovascular examination with palpation and auscultation, inspection of the retinal vascular system for disease of the arterioles, a search for cardiac sources for

Table 37.4. Hachinski Ischemic Score

Symptom/Sign	Points
Abrupt onset of dementia	2
Stepwise deterioration	1
Fluctuating course	2
Nocturnal confusion	1
Relative preservation of personality	1
Depression	1
Somatic complaints	1
Emotional lability	1
Hypertension	2
History of stroke	2
Focal neurological symptoms	2
Focal neurological signs	2
Other signs of arteriosclerosis	1

emboli and constrictions of the outflow tracts. This would include echocardiography, duplex ultrasound of the carotid bifurcations, imaging, preferably with MR—but CT if the former is unavailable—complete blood count, lipid profile, platelet count, and differential, and studies of blood oxygenation. One must exclude the possibility of hypothyroidism, B_{12} deficiency, toxic encephalopathy, and drug or medication reaction.

PET and SPECT techniques can demonstrate the patchy pattern of functional impairment that is characteristic of CVD. Dysfunction at sites distant from a single lesion may be identified, and the subcortical effects of microcirculatory disorders (e.g., Binswanger's disease) can also be demonstrated.

MANAGEMENT

Primary and Secondary Stroke Prevention

The best way to preserve brain functioning is to prevent neuronal damage. The neurochemistry of neuronal injury and death may reveal clues to "neuroprotective" therapies. For example, calcium-mediated release of excitatory amino acid neurotransmitters may promote neuronal injury. Levels of aspartate and glutamate increase in response to neuronal injury, and these excitotoxins are known to activate specific receptors that mediate cell death. Because calcium transport is mediated by these receptors, their activation can result in calcium accumulation. The extra calcium potentiates lysosomal activity, further excitatory amino acid release, and neuronal injury and death. Inhibitors of NMDA receptors, calcium channel blockers, and other related strategies are being explored as potential "neuroprotective" therapies. The ultimate goal of this research is to develop specific drug treatments that can be administered within minutes of stroke onset to salvage or protect portions of the brain that might otherwise die.

Having suffered an initial infarction, all effective means for reducing subsequent infarction must be initiated by addressing the modifiable risk factors. Patients are counseled regarding cessation of tobacco or alcohol abuse, normalization of blood constituents (e.g., cholesterol, platelets, red blood cells) and blood pressure, and the initiation of regular exercise to keep the blood circulating properly and the heart in good condition. For those who have had an initial cerebral infarction, the daily use of aspirin in appropriate dosage is a necessary concomitant to therapy. For those who are aspirin-resistant, ticlopidine adds an extra measure of risk reduction. Patients with presumed embolic infarction (e.g., due to cardiac arrhythmia), hypercoagulability, or continued strokes on aspirin or ticlopidine typically receive warfarin. Hemorrheologic agents such as pentoxifylline can be used as well.

Management of Behavioral Complications

In general, psychotropic agents are used to control the various behavioral complications of CVD. Neuroseptic agents such as haloperidol or chlorpromazine may be used for hallucinations and delusions. Antidepressants such as the tricyclic agents, serotonin reuptake inhibitors (e.g., fluoxetine), stimulants (e.g., methylphenidate), or tetracyclic agents (e.g., trazodone) may sometimes be helpful for depression, psychomotor retardation, agitation, sleep disturbance, and episodic aggressiveness. Benzodiazepines (e.g., oxazepam, temazepam), lithium, and propranolol may occasionally be useful for anxiety, agitation, episodic violence, and aggressiveness. Antiepileptics are also useful in some patients with aggressiveness (e.g., carbamazepine), or mood disturbance (e.g., valproic acid).

Basic pharmacological guidelines for managing patients with CVD should note that pharmacokinetics, pharmacodynamics, and physiological responsiveness to the effects of psychotherapeutic drugs are likely to be different in patients with CVD than in usual psychiatric settings. Therefore, low doses should be used at first and all increases monitored carefully for evidence of deleterious side effects. The minimum number of drugs necessary to control symptoms should be used. This requires clear discussion with the patient and family about the extent of "control" that is necessary. Drug management must coincide with consultation to caregivers so that they consider advanced directives, alternative living arrangements for the patient, and other nonpharmacological means of support such as day care centers and support groups.

References

1. Hom J. Contributions of the Halstead-Reitan battery in the neuropsychological investigation of stroke. In: Bornstein RA, Brown G, eds. Neurobehavioral aspects of cerebrovascular disease. New York: Oxford University Press, 1991:165–181.
2. McDaniel KD, McDaniel LD. Anton's syndrome in a patient with posttraumatic optic neuropathy and bifrontal contusions. Arch Neurol 1991;48:101–105.
3. McFarling D, Rothi LJ, Heilman KM. Transcortical aphasia from ischaemic infarcts of the thalamus: a report of two cases. J Neurol Neurosurg Psychiatry 1982;45:107–112.

4. Toole JF. Cerebrovascular disorders. 4th ed. New York: Raven Press; 1990:86.

5. Watson RT, Heilman KM. Callosal apraxia. Brain 1983;106: 391–403.

6. Absher JR, Benson DF. Disconnection syndromes: an overview of Geschwind's contributions. Neurology 1993;43:862–867.

7. Segarra JM, Angelo JN. In: Benton AL, ed. Behavioral change in cerebrovascular disease. New York: Harper & Row, 1970:3–14.

8. Guberman A. The syndrome of bilateral paramedian thalamic infarction. Neurology 1983;33:540–546.

9. Gentilini M, De Renzi E, Crisi G. Bilateral paramedian thalamic artery infarcts: report of eight cases. J Neurol Neurosurg Psychiatry 1987;50:900–909.

10. Bogousslavsky J, Regli F. Anterior cerebral artery territory infarction in the Lausanne Stroke Registry. Clinical and etiologic patterns. Arch Neurol 1990;47:144–150.

11. Petrides M, Alivisatos B, Meyer E, Evans AC. Functional activity of the human frontal cortex during the performance of verbal working memory tasks. Proc Natl Acad Sci USA 1993;90:878–882.

12. Kertesz A, Hooper P. Praxis and language: the extent and variety of apraxia in aphasia. Neuropsychologia 1982;20:275–286.

13. Robinson RG, Boston JD, Starkstein SE, Price TR. Comparison of mania and depression after brain injury: causal factors. Am J Psychiatry 1988;145:172–178.

14. Gorelick PB, Ross ED. The aprosodias: further functional-anatomical evidence for the organization of affective language in the right hemisphere. J Neurol Neurosurg Psychiatry 1987;50:553–560.

15. Damasio AR, Tranel D, Damasio H. Individuals with sociopathic behavior caused by frontal damage fail to respond autonomically to social stimuli. Behav Brain Res 1990;41:81–94.

16. Geschwind N. Disconnexion syndromes in animals and man. II. Brain 1965;88:585–644.

17. Geschwind N. Disconnexion syndromes in animals and man. I. Brain 1965;88:237–294.

18. Damasio AR, Damasio H. The anatomic basis of pure alexia. Neurology 1983;33:1573–1583.

19. Roeltgen DP, Sevush S, Heilman KM. Pure Gerstmann's syndrome from a focal lesion. Arch Neurol 1983;40:46–47.

20. Moore MR, Saver JL, Johnson KA, Romero JA. Right parietal stroke with Gerstmann's syndrome. Appearance on computed tomography, magnetic resonance imaging, and single-photon emission computed tomography. Arch Neurol 1991;48:432–435.

21. Benson DF, Sheremata WA, Bouchard R, Segarra JM, Price D, Geschwind N. Conduction aphasia. A clinicopathological study. Arch Neurol 1973;28:339–346.

22. Damasio H, Damasio AR. The anatomical basis of conduction aphasia. Brain 1980;103:337–350.

23. Heilman KM, Rothi LG, Mack L, Feinberg T, Watson RT. Apraxia after a superior parietal lesion. Cortex 1986;22:141–150.

24. Heilman KM, Rothi LJ, Valenstein E. Two forms of ideomotor apraxia. Neurology 1982;32:342–346.

25. Poncet M, Habib M, Robillard A. Deep left parietal lobe syndrome: conduction aphasia and other neurobehavioral disorders due to a small subcortical lesion. J Neurol Neurosurg Psychiatry 1987;50: 709–713.

26. De Renzi E, Lucchelli F. Ideational apraxia. Brain 1988;111:1173–1185.

27. Coslett HB, Roeltgen DP, Gonzalez Rothi L, Heilman KM. Transcortical sensory aphasia: evidence for subtypes. Brain Lang 1987;32:362–378.

28. Kertesz A, Sheppard A, MacKenzie R. Localization in transcortical sensory aphasia. Arch Neurol 1982;39:475–478.

29. Damasio AR, Geschwind N. The neural basis of language. Annu Rev Neurosci 1984;7:127–147.

30. Galaburda AM, Geschwind N. The human language areas and cerebral asymmetries. Rev Med Suisse Romande 1980;100:119–128.

31. Basso A, Bracchi M, Capitani E, Laiacona M, Zanobio ME. Age and evolution of language area functions. A study on adult stroke patients. Cortex 1987;23:475–483.

32. Coslett HB, Brashear HR, Heilman KM. Pure word deafness after bilateral primary auditory cortex infarcts. Neurology 1984;34: 347–352.

33. Mendez MF, Geehan GR, Jr. Cortical auditory disorders: clinical and psychoacoustic features. J Neurol Neurosurg Psychiatry 1988; 51:1–9.

34. McKee AC, Levine DN, Kowall NW, Richardson EP Jr. Peduncular hallucinosis associated with isolated infarction of the substantia nigra pars reticulata. Ann Neurol 1990;27:500–504.

35. McEntee WJ, Biber MP, Perl DP, Benson DF. Diencephalic amnesia: a reappraisal. J Neurol Neurosurg Psychiatry 1976;39:436–441.

36. Squire LR, Amaral DG, Zola-Morgan S, Kritchevsky M, Press G. Description of brain injury in the amnesic patient N.A. based on magnetic resonance imaging. Exp Neurol 1989;105:23–35.

37. Damasio A, Yamada T, Damasio H, Corbett J, McKee J. Central achromatopsia: behavioral, anatomic, and physiologic aspects. Neurology 1980;30:1064–1071.

38. Damasio AR, Damasio H, Van Hoesen GW. Prosopagnosia: anatomic basis and behavioral mechanisms. Neurology 1982;32: 331–341.

39. Landis T, Cummings JL, Christen L, Bogen JE, Imhof HG. Are unilateral right posterior cerebral lesions sufficient to cause prosopagnosia? Clinical and radiological findings in six additional patients. Cortex. 1986;22:243–252.

40. Benton A. Facial recognition 1990. Cortex 1990;26:491–499.

41. Tranel D, Damasio AR, Damasio H. Intact recognition of facial expression, gender, and age in patients with impaired recognition of face identity. Neurology 1988;38:690–696.

42. Della Sala S, Spinnler H. Anton's (Redlich-Babinski's) syndrome associated with Dide-Botcazo's syndrome: a case report of denial of cortical blindness and amnesia. Schweiz Arch Neurol Psychiatr 1988;139:5–15.

43. Heilman KM, Tucker DM, Valenstein E. A case of mixed transcortical aphasia with intact naming. Brain 1976;99:415–426.

44. Pirozzolo FJ, Kerr KL, Obrzut JE, Morley GK, Haxby JV, Lundgren S. Neurolinguistic analysis of the language abilities of a patient with a "double disconnection syndrome:" a case of subangular alexia in the presence of mixed transcortical aphasia. J Neurol Neurosurg Psychiatry 1981;44:152–155.

45. Ruessmann K, Sondag HD, Beneicke U. Visuospatial disorders and related lesions of the brain. Int J Neurosci 1989;46:123–126.

46. Moody DM, Bell MA, Challa V.R. Features of the cerebral vascular pattern that predict vulnerability to perfusion or oxygenation deficiency: an anatomic study. Am J Neuroradiol 1990;11:431–439.

47. Román GC. Senile dementia of the Binswanger type. A vascular form of dementia in the elderly. JAMA 1987;258:1782–1788.

48. American Psychiatric Association. Diagnostic and statistical manual of mental disorders, third edition revised 3rd ed. Washington, DC: American Psychiatric Association; 1987:78.

49. Cummings JL, Benson DF. Dementia: a clinical approach. 2nd ed. Boston: Butterworth-Heinemann; 1993:1.

50. Mesulam MM, Waxman SG, Geschwind N, Sabin TD. Acute confusional states with right middle cerebral artery infarctions. J Neurol Neurosurg Psychiatry 1976;39:84–89.

51. Devinsky O, Bear D, Volpe BT. Confusional states following posterior cerebral artery infarction. Arch Neurol 1988;45: 160–163.

52. Bisiach E. Unilateral neglect, representational schema and consciousness. Brain 1979;102:609–618.

53. Butter CM, Rapcsak S, Watson RT, Heilman KM. Changes in sensory inattention, directional motor neglect and "release" of the fixation reflex following a unilateral frontal lesion: a case report. Neuropsychologia 1988;26:533–545.

54. Meador KJ, Watson RT, Bowers D, Heilman KM. Hypometria with hemispatial and limb motor neglect. Brain 1986;109:293–305.

55. Valenstein E, Heilman KM. Unilateral hypokinesia and motor extinction. Neurology 1981;31:445–448.
56. Heilman KM, Valenstein E. Mechanisms underlying hemispatial neglect. Ann Neurol 1979;5:166–170XXX.
57. Mesulam MM. Large-scale neurocognitive networks and distributed processing for attention, language, and memory. Ann Neurol 1990;28:597–613.
58. Levine DN, Calvanio R, Rinn WE. The pathogenesis of anosognosia for hemiplegia. Neurology 1991;41:1770–1781.
59. Lebrun Y. Anosognosia in aphasics. Cortex 1987;23:251–263.
60. Lazzarino LG, Nicolai A. Hemichorea-hemiballism and anosognosia following a contralateral infarction of the caudate nucleus and anterior limb of the internal capsule. Riv Neurol 1991;61:9–11.
61. Young AW, de Haan EH, Newcombe F. Unawareness of impaired face recognition. Brain Cogn 1990;14:1–18.
62. Selnes OA, Pestronk A, Hart J, Gordon B. Limb apraxia without aphasia from a left sided lesion in a right handed patient. J Neurol Neurosurg Psychiatry 1991;54:734–737.
63. Schacter DL. Toward a cognitive neuropsychology of awareness: implicit knowledge and anosognosia. J Clin Exp Neuropsychol 1990;12:155–178.
64. Glass JD, Levey AI, Rothstein JD. The dysarthria-clumsy hand syndrome: a distinct clinical entity related to pontine infarction. Ann Neurol 1990;27:487–494.
65. Damasio AR, Geschwind N. The neural basis of language. Ann Rev Neurosci 1984;7:127–147.
66. Samuels JA, Benson DF. Some aspects of language comprehension in anterior aphasia. Brain Lang 1979;8:275–286.
67. Heilman KM, Rothi L, McFarling D, Rottmann AL. Transcortical sensory aphasia with relatively spared spontaneous speech and naming. Arch Neurol 1981;38:236–239.
68. Cummings JL, Tomiyasu U, Read S, Benson DF. Amnesia with hippocampal lesions after cardiopulmonary arrest. Neurology 1984;34:679–681.
69. Valenstein E, Bowers D, Verfaellie M, Heilman KM, Day A, Watson RT. Retrosplenial amnesia. Brain 1987;110:1631–1646.
70. Benson DF, Marsden CD, Meadows JC. The amnesic syndrome of posterior cerebral artery occlusion. Acta Neurol Scand 1974;50:133–145.
71. Kooistra CA, Heilman KM. Memory loss from a subcortical white matter infarct. J Neurol Neurosurg Psychiatry 1988;51:866–869.
72. Benke T. Visual agnosia and amnesia from a left unilateral lesion. Eur Neurol 1988;28:236–239.
73. Akiguchi I, Ino T, Nabatame H, et al. Acute-onset amnestic syndrome with localized infarct on the dominant side—comparison between anteromedial thalamic lesion and posterior cerebral artery territory lesion. Jpn J Med 1987;26:15–20.
74. Milandre L, Donnet A, Rumeau C, Cherif AA, Khalil R. Transient global amnesia followed by vertebrobasilar ischemia in a case of dolichoectatic basilar artery. Acta Neurol Belg 1990;90:248–253.
75. Stillhard G, Landis T, Schiess R, Regard M, Sialer G. Bitemporal hypoperfusion in transient global amnesia: 99m-Tc-HM-PAO SPECT and neuropsychological findings during and after an attack. J Neurol Neurosurg Psychiatry 1990;53:339–342.
76. Gorelick PB, Amico LL, Ganellen R, Benevento LA. Transient global amnesia and thalamic infarction. Neurology 1988;38:496–499.
77. Feuer D, Weinberger J. Extracranial carotid artery in patients with transient global amnesia: evaluation by real-time B-mode ultrasonography with duplex Doppler flow. Stroke 1987;18:951–953.
78. Damasio AR, Graff-Radford NR, Damasio H. Transient partial amnesia. Arch Neurol 1983;40:656–657.
79. Damasio AR, Graff-Radford NR, Eslinger PJ, Damasio H, Kassell N. Amnesia following basal forebrain lesions. Arch Neurol 1985;42:263–271.
80. Bowers D, Verfaellie M, Valenstein E, Heilman KM. Impaired acquisition of temporal information in retrosplenial amnesia. Brain Cogn 1988;8:47–66.
81. Stuss DT, Guzman DA. Severe remote memory loss with minimal anterograde amnesia: a clinical note. Brain Cogn 1988;8:21–30.
82. Benson DF. Amnesia. South Med J 1978;71:1221–1227, 1231.
83. Ross ED. Sensory-specific and fractional disorders of recent memory in man. I Isolated loss of visual recent memory. Arch Neurol 1980;37:193–200.
84. van Lancker D, Klein K. Preserved recognition of familiar personal names in global aphasia. Brain Lang 1990;39:511–529.
85. Warrington EK, McCarthy RA. Categories of knowledge: further fractionation and an attempted integration. Brain 1987;110:1273–1296.
86. Damasio AR. Category-related recognition defects as a clue to the neural substrates of knowledge. Trends Neurosci 1990;13:95–98.
87. Damasio AR, Damasio H, Tranel D, Brandt JP. Neural regionalization of knowledge access: preliminary evidence. Cold Spring Harbor Symp Quant Biol 1990;55:1039–1047.
88. Warrington EK, James M. Visual apperceptive agnosia: a clinico-anatomical study of three cases. Cortex 1988;24:13–32.
89. McNeil JE, Warrington EK. Prosopagnosia: a reclassification. Q J Exp Psychol [A] 1991;43:267–287.
90. Tranel D, Damasio AR. Knowledge without awareness: an autonomic index of facial recognition by prosopagnosics. Science 1985;228:1453–1454.
91. Stuss DT, Benson DF. Executive system. In: Stuss DT, Benson DF, eds. The frontal lobes. New York: Raven Press; 1986:204–216.
92. Cummings JL. Frontal-subcortical circuits and human behavior. Arch Neurol 1993;50:873–880.
93. Judd T, Gardner H, Geschwind N. Alexia without agraphia in a composer. Brain 1983;106:435–457.
94. Takeda K, Bandou M, Nishimura Y. [Motor amusia following a right temporal lobe hemorrhage--a case report]. Rinsho Shinkeigaku 1990;30:78–83.
95. Lang W, Obrig H, Lindinger G, Cheyne D, Deecke L. Supplementary motor area activation while tapping bimanually different rhythms in musicians. Exp Brain Res 1990;79:504–514.
96. Ross ED, Mesulam MM. Dominant language functions of the right hemisphere? Prosody and emotional gesturing. Arch Neurol 1979;36:144–148.
97. Joseph R. The right cerebral hemisphere: emotion, music, visual-spatial skills, body-image, dreams, and awareness. J Clin Psychol 1988;44:630–673.
98. Besson G, Bogousslavsky J, Regli F, Maeder P. Acute pseudobulbar or suprabulbar palsy. Arch Neurol 1991;48:501–507.
99. Parikh RM, Lipsey JR, Robinson RG, Price TR. A two year longitudinal study of poststroke mood disorders: prognostic factors related to one and two year outcome. Int J Psychiatry Med 1988;18:45–56.
100. Starkstein SE, Boston JD, Robinson RG. Mechanisms of mania after brain injury. 12 case reports and review of the literature. J Nerv Ment Dis 1988;176:87–100.
101. Starkstein SE, Robinson RG. Affective disorders and cerebral vascular disease. Br J Psychiatry 1989;154:170–182.
102. Starkstein SE, Mayberg HS, Berthier ML, et al. Mania after brain injury: neuroradiological and metabolic findings. Ann Neurol 1990;27:652–659.
103. Parikh RM, Robinson RG, Lipsey JR, Starkstein SE, Fedoroff JP, Price TR. The impact of poststroke depression on recovery in activities of daily living over a 2-year follow-up. Arch Neurol 1990;47:785–789.
104. Starkstein SE, Cohen BS, Fedoroff P, Parikh RM, Price TR, Robinson RG. Relationship between anxiety disorders and depressive disorders in patients with cerebrovascular injury. Arch Gen Psychiatry 1990;47:246–251.
105. Baxter LR, Jr, Phelps ME, Mazziotta JC, Guze BH, Schwartz JM, Selin CE. Local cerebral glucose metabolic rates in obsessive-compulsive disorder. A comparison with rates in unipolar depression and in normal controls [published erratum appears in

Arch Gen Psychiatry 1987;44:800]. Arch Gen Psychiatry 1987;44:211–218.

106. Berthier M, Starkstein S. Acute atypical psychosis following a right hemisphere stroke. Acta Neurol Belg 1987;87:125–131.

107. Peroutka SJ, Sohmer BH, Kumar AJ, Folstein M, Robinson RG. Hallucinations and delusions following a right temporoparietooccipital infarction. Johns Hopkins Med J 1982;151:181–185.

108. Sulkava R, Erkinjuntti T. Vascular dementia due to cardiac arrhythmias and systemic hypotension. Acta Neurol Scand 1987;76:123–128.

109. Tohgi H, Chiba K, Kimura M. Twenty-four-hour variation of blood pressure in vascular dementia of the Binswanger type. Stroke 1991;22:603–608.

110. Forette F, Boller F. Hypertension and the risk of dementia in the elderly. Am J Med 1991;90:14S–19S.

111. Bennett DA, Wilson RS, Gilley DW, Fox JH. Clinical diagnosis of Binswanger's disease. J Neurol Neurosurg Psychiatry 1990;53:961–965.

112. Erkinjuntti T. Types of multi-infarct dementia. Acta Neurol Scand 1987;75:391–399.

113. Bogucki A, Janczewska E, Koszewska I, Chmielowski M, Szymanska R. Evaluation of dementia in subcortical arteriosclerotic encephalopathy (Binswanger's disease). Eur Arch Psychiatry Clin Neurosci 1991;241:91–97.

114. Turkington D, Geddes J. Delusional depression responding to clomipramine in Binswanger's disease. J Nerv Ment Dis 1990;178:459–460.

115. Benson DF, Cummings JL. Angular gyrus syndrome simulating Alzheimer's disease. Arch Neurol 1982;39:616–620.

116. Hachinski VC, Iliff LD, Zilhka E, et al. Cerebral blood flow in dementia. Arch Neurol 1975;32:632–637.

117. Rosen WG, Terry RD, Fuld PA, et al. Pathological verification of ischemic score in differentiation of dementias. Ann Neurol 1980;7:486–488.

38

NEUROBEHAVIORAL ASPECTS OF CEREBRAL WHITE MATTER DISORDERS

Christopher M. Filley

Disorders of human behavior constitute an extremely diverse and challenging group of conditions that involves neurology, psychiatry, and several related disciplines. These disorders have been recognized in some fashion since antiquity, but the past 150 years have witnessed an expansion of biomedical inquiry into the description of these frequently disabling illnesses. Advances in psychology and the basic neurosciences have also proceeded at a rapid pace, providing additional information on neurobehavioral disorders and the phenomena of normal human behavior. At the source of all such investigation is an abiding fascination in the origin of the extraordinary range of behavior that can be designated as uniquely human.

A textbook on neuropsychiatry is an attempt to conjoin the clinical disciplines of neurology and psychiatry into a unifying synthesis, addressing the various disorders of human behavior. Such an ambitious goal is increasingly appropriate in light of mounting evidence that neurological disease has frequent behavioral manifestations, and, conversely, that psychiatric disorders may have their origin in neurological dysfunction. As this knowledge accumulates, there is a growing need for clinicians who are familiar with both specialties and who can deal effectively with the complex behavioral problems with which patients frequently present. The emerging interest in neuropsychiatry indicates a welcome emphasis on significant clinical problems that have too often not found a comfortable position in either neurology or psychiatry (1, 2).

One discipline that contributes to neuropsychiatry is behavioral neurology (3), the subspecialty of neurology concerned with the effects of demonstrable brain disease or injury on behavior. This approach adopts as its foundation the convincing demonstration of brain lesions, and proceeds to the precise correlation of anatomical destruction with behavioral observations. The advantage of this focus on brain-behavior relationships is the opportunity to explore both human disease and health by attempting to understand the neuroanatomical basis of behavior. If all behavior is mediated by the brain, a position adopted empirically and

with much success by neuroscientists, then it becomes possible to consider behavior in neuroanatomical terms.

Behavioral neurology has traditionally concerned itself primarily with the cerebral cortex and the many syndromes related to cortical damage. The phrase "higher cortical function" is often used to describe the behavioral neurologist's area of interest (4), and even the substantial literature on cerebral disconnection from the 1960s (5) did little to divert attention from the cortex. In recent years, however, it has been repeatedly demonstrated that higher functions depend on many more structures than the cortex alone, and a broader view is required. A number of diseases, for example, are now thought to alter behavior by their effects on subcortical structures such as the basal ganglia and thalamus, and the concept of subcortical dementia has recently become popular (6). In light of this information, it is most appropriate to consider the cerebral hemispheres as the essential site of the mind's activities, and the term "higher cerebral function" best describes the interests of the behavioral neurologist.

This chapter addresses an area that has been insufficiently discussed in the examination of brain-behavior relationships: the cerebral white matter. Gray matter—cortical and then later subcortical—has been studied in considerable detail, but white matter has been regarded as making a relatively minor contribution to behavior. Despite the fact that white matter comprises a large component of cerebral volume, and that it is often selectively damaged by pathology, strong evidence relating neurobehavioral dysfunction to white matter involvement has been lacking. The advent of magnetic resonance imaging (MRI) in recent years, and its excellent demonstration of cerebral white matter (7), has played a major role in highlighting this area. In addition, neuropsychological studies have contributed significant information pertaining to the behavioral associations of cerebral white matter. As the various afflictions of cerebral white matter are reviewed, it will become clear that neurobehavioral disorders are frequent in these conditions. Accordingly, it is possible to construct tentative hypotheses about the role of white matter in the genesis of human behavior.

NEUROBIOLOGY OF CEREBRAL WHITE MATTER

The central nervous system (CNS) is made up of two grossly distinguishable forms of tissue: gray matter and white matter. Gray matter is darker than white matter on freshly cut brain sections, the latter having a glistening white hue owing to the presence of lipid-rich myelin. There are approximately 100 billion (10^{11}) neurons in the human brain (8), and gray matter structures, including the cerebral cortex and the subcortical nuclei, contain the cell bodies of these neurons. The great majority of the brain's neurons (99% or more) are interneurons, so that most of the brain's activity is concerned with various forms of processing that take place between sensory input and motor output. The white matter is made up of axons surrounded by myelin, and most myelinated cerebral neurons are also classified as interneurons. Vast numbers of myelinated axons serve to interconnect billions of cortical and subcortical neurons within and between the cerebral hemispheres. Normal brain function depends critically on the integrity of cerebral white matter, which facilitates continuous and efficient intercellular communication. This review begins with a brief discussion of the microscopic and gross anatomy of cerebral white matter, and then considers pertinent aspects of its physiology.

Anatomy

White matter makes up slightly less than one-half of the volume of the mature human brain (9). Its characteristic structural feature is myelin, a complex mixture of lipids (70%) and protein (30%) that encases axons. Myelin is laid down in a concentric fashion around axons by oligodendrocytes, cells of glial origin that serve to myelinate CNS axons in a manner analogous to the Schwann cells of the peripheral nervous system. The myelination of axons proceeds in such a way that leaves short segments of the axonal membrane unmyelinated. These segments, called nodes of Ranvier, have special relevance to the speed of impulse propagation.

Myelination of the brain is a gradual process in development that occurs primarily after neuronal differentiation is complete. All of the brain's neurons are formed by the end of the sixth fetal month, and myelination begins in the third month and continues well into postnatal life (10). CNS structures show great variability as to their myelination, some areas maturing in utero or shortly after birth and some not becoming fully myelinated until the second or third decade of life (10). There is a strong likelihood that, in general, myelination parallels functional maturity, so that cerebral areas attain their maximal capabilities only when myelination is complete (11). This characteristic of white matter has important neurobehavioral implications. In particular, axons in the cerebral commissures and association areas are quite late to myelinate (10), a fact that probably

relates to the continuing processes of social and intellectual maturation that occur into adolescence and beyond. In support of this notion, recent MRI studies of hydrocephalic infants and children have established a strong correlation between the extent of cerebral myelination and psychomotor development (12, 13).

In later life, data exist to show that white matter volume declines to a greater extent than that of gray matter: there is an increase in the hemispheric gray to white ratio from 1.1 at age 50 to 1.5 at age 100 (9). This deterioration may be due to changes in the chemical composition of myelin (14), to ischemia in the white matter from a number of causes (15), or other factors. It is likely that the seemingly ubiquitous designation "cerebral atrophy" that is applied to brain imaging studies in the normal elderly may, in many cases, refer more to degeneration of white matter than to cortical cell loss.

In terms of gross anatomy, the large central core of white matter that lies between the lateral ventricles and the cortex is known as the centrum semiovale. Within this mass of tissue, three types of cerebral white matter fibers can be identified: projection fibers, which convey impulses to the cortex from distant sites or vice versa; association fibers, which interconnect regions of the same hemisphere; and commissural fibers, which connect homologous regions in the two hemispheres.

The most important projection fiber systems are the corticofugal bundles, which convey motor impulses to effector regions of the neuraxis, and the corticopetal bundles, which carry incoming sensory information to the primary sensory cortices. The major corticofugal tracts lie in the internal capsule, which contains upper motor neuron fibers destined for the brainstem and spinal cord. The primary corticopetal bundles are the optic radiations, which project visual information to the occipital lobes; the auditory radiations to the temporal lobes; and the thalamocortical radiations, which relay somatosensory information to the parietal lobes.

Association systems are of major importance for the interaction of neocortical areas that are critical to higher functions. These systems include the short association fibers, also known as arcuate or U fibers, which connect adjacent cortical gyri, and five long association fiber systems. The long tracts are the arcuate (superior longitudinal) fasciculus, the superior occipitofrontal fasciculus, the inferior occipitofrontal fasciculus, the cingulum, and the uncinate fasciculus. On close inspection, it is evident that these fiber systems provide the basis for extensive communication between the frontal lobes and the temporal, parietal, and occipital lobes. A high concentration of white matter underlies the frontal lobes (16), and there is no lobe of the brain that does not have strong bidirectional connections with the frontal lobes (Table 38.1).

Important neurobehavioral implications can again be drawn from these anatomical data. The patterns of connectivity are consistent with the primacy of the frontal lobes in the organization of human behavior. The frontal lobes are the largest and most recently evolved areas of the brain, and

Table 38.1. Long Association Fibers

Tract	Lobes Connected
Arcuate (superior longitudinal) fasciculus	Frontal, parietal, temporal, occipital
Superior occipitofrontal fasciculus	Frontal, parietal, occipital
Inferior occipitofrontal fasciculus	Frontal, temporal, occipital
Cingulum	Frontal, parietal, temporal
Uncinate fasciculus	Frontal, temporal

their connections via white matter pathways to other cerebral regions enable the integration of all aspects of cerebral function that are unique to humans. The ability of the frontal lobes to connect to the rest of the brain implies that white matter disorders can be positioned to disrupt the executive functions by which behavior is regulated.

Commissural fibers run primarily in the massive corpus callosum, a broad, dense structure of some 300 million myelinated axons that crosses the midline and connects all zones of the cortex on both sides. Smaller commissural connections are made by the anterior commissure, the hippocampal commissure, and, in some brains, a bundle connecting the thalami, known as the massa intermedia.

Other fiber systems that deserve comment are the ascending neuronal pathways from the brainstem and basal forebrain that project to widespread areas of the cerebral hemispheres. The reticular formation of the brainstem plays a vital role in the maintenance of arousal and alertness (17). Of equal importance because of their participation in mood, motivation, and memory are the major neurotransmitter systems that innervate the cortex: the noradrenergic fibers originating in the locus ceruleus of the rostral pons, the serotonergic tracts arising from the raphe nuclei of the brainstem, the dopaminergic systems projecting rostrally from the midbrain ventral tegmental area, and the cholinergic fibers from the nucleus basalis of Meynert. These neuropharmacological systems course rostrally in the deep subcortical white matter—most notably the median forebrain bundle—to reach their destinations in the cortical mantle (18). In addition, important cholinergic fiber systems travel within the fornix and the external capsule (19). These systems are all vulnerable to white matter lesions because of the long trajectories between their sites of origin and their final destinations.

A final anatomical feature of interest is the observation that the ratio of white matter to gray matter is higher in the right than the left hemisphere (20). The implications of this asymmetry are as yet uncertain, but it is plausible that a pathological process that affects white matter diffusely will have a disproportionate effect on the right hemisphere and its functions.

Physiology

Nervous and muscular tissues are intrinsically excitable, and this property forms the basis for the functioning of the nervous and muscular systems. Axons in the CNS and peripheral nervous system are designed to propagate an electrical event known as an action potential. This phenomenon, which involves a depolarization of the cell membrane, is the fundamental activity of neural tissue, and white matter plays a critical role in the effective conduction of this electrical signal. Communication between neurons ultimately depends, of course, on synaptic transmission, an area of major neuroscientific interest, but in order for the nerve impulse to reach the synapse at all, axonal conduction is required.

When a cerebral neuron is not conducting an impulse, its axonal membrane has an electrical charge and a resting potential, by virtue of which the inside of the neuron is negative (about -70 mV) with respect to the outside of the cell. Under these conditions the neuron is said to be polarized. The resting potential is maintained by the action of the sodium-potassium pump, a membrane-bound molecule that transports sodium outside the cell at the expense of energy derived from adenosine triphosphate (ATP). When an impulse is to be propagated, there is a large and sudden influx of sodium ions through specific voltage-gated sodium channels in the membrane. This influx of positively charged ions transiently reverses the polarity of the membrane, resulting in a depolarization of the axon. Repolarization is then quickly restored by the efflux of potassium ions, following the passage of the action potential. After a refractory period during which no impulse can be generated, another action potential can be propagated.

The speed of impulse conduction is quite significantly influenced by the presence of myelin around the axon. Large myelinated fibers conduct impulses as much as 100 times faster than small unmyelinated axons (21). This capacity is made possible in part by the nodes of Ranvier, which allow for a "jump" of the impulse from node to node in a process known as saltatory conduction. In contrast, conduction in unmyelinated fibers is much slower because the action potential travels in a continuous fashion over the entire length of the axon. Another advantage conferred by myelin is that axonal conduction is much more efficient in terms of energy expenditure; there is less need for ATP to restore the membrane's resting potential if ion conductance takes place only at the widely separated nodes of Ranvier.

Normal impulse conduction in the brain is dependent on the proper functioning of myelin. Rapid axonal impulse conduction, in turn, undoubtedly contributes to the normal physiology of the brain as a whole. Dysfunction of myelin, whether it be from pathological states or from changes related to the developmental stage of the brain, can lead to neurobehavioral alterations that reflect a general slowing of neuronal communication. Interestingly, aged laboratory animals show a slowing of conduction velocity between the basal forebrain and the neocortex, an observation that may reflect an age-related decrement in subcortical myelin (22). It is conceivable that some of the neurobehavioral alterations of normal aging in humans—cognitive slowing, impaired vigilance, forgetfulness, and the like—may be partly due to changes in cerebral white matter.

Clinical assessment of cerebral white matter can be assisted by the use of in vivo neurophysiological techniques.

In recent years, the emergence of evoked potentials (EPs) has allowed for the measurement of conduction time across certain well-defined CNS white matter tracts (23). EPs involve the application of a sensory stimulus (visual, auditory, or somatosensory) in a standardized manner, and the subsequent recording of the electrical response as it occurs along the appropriate CNS pathway. As such, EPs are most useful in the assessment of primary sensory systems that may be damaged by white matter illnesses. Demyelinative disorders have witnessed the greatest use of EP technology to date. By identifying and localizing areas of white matter dysfunction in the CNS, EPs have improved the detection of many CNS white matter lesions that impair primary sensory function.

The application of EP principles to neurobehavioral disorders has been more difficult. The neurophysiology of cognition and emotion is clearly more complex than primary sensory or motor function. In theory, demonstration of white matter dysfunction in neurobehavioral syndromes should be possible, but there is still too little understanding of the role of white matter in higher function. Long-latency event-related potentials such as the P300 may hold promise in this regard, as they involve the evaluation of neurophysiological function in white matter areas more concerned with cognition (24).

CEREBRAL WHITE MATTER DISORDERS

In attempting to address the neurobehavioral consequences of cerebral white matter disorders, two problems immediately arise. First, the identification of a cerebral white matter disorder is often difficult. Many illnesses that are known to damage hemispheric white matter, such as Binswanger's disease, also have lesser effects on other structures such as the basal ganglia, and even multiple sclerosis, the classic CNS demyelinative disease, can damage the cortex because there is some myelin within the cortical gray matter. Second, clinical data describing neurobehavioral impairment in white matter diseases are often quite fragmentary or even completely lacking. Because of a long-standing assumption that higher function depends on cortical gray matter, diseases of white matter have been regarded as having at most a minor effect on behavior, and attention to cognitive and emotional changes in clinical reports may be minimal or absent.

In this account, we consider cerebral white matter disorders to be those diseases or injuries that primarily, though perhaps not exclusively, damage the white matter of the brain. This criterion requires a degree of judgment as to which entities should be included, but the decision is always based on valid neuropathological information. Inclusion of conditions that affect behavior are based on clinical reports that offer enough data to indicate a definite or probable association of white matter dysfunction with neurobehavioral impairment. Further study may disprove some of these associations, but a broadly inclusive approach is adopted here in the interest of stimulating interest in this neglected

Table 38.2. Adult Cerebral White Matter Disorders

Demyelinative	Multiple sclerosis
Vascular	Binswanger's disease
	Stroke
Toxic	Toluene dementia
	Alcoholic dementia
	Radiation
	Chemotherapy
Metabolic	Cobalamin deficiency
	Hypoxia
	Marchiafava-Bignami disease
	Central pontine myelinolysis
Infectious	Acquired immune deficiency syndrome
	Progressive multifocal leukoencephalopathy
Traumatic	Traumatic brain injury
	Corpus callosotomy
Hydrocephalic	Normal pressure hydrocephalus
Neoplastic	Gliomatosis cerebri
	Solitary tumors

area. Remarkably, all of these conditions can be related to some variety of neurobehavioral deficit.

The following section describes cerebral white matter disorders that commonly affect adults (Table 38.2) and those that affect infants and children (Table 38.3). Some disorders are appropriately included in both categories. In previous accounts of CNS white matter disease, the custom has been to classify diseases based on demyelination (myelinoclasis) vs. dysmyelination (the leukodystrophies), the former being acquired and the latter hereditary. Whereas this distinction is still useful neuropathologically, other types of CNS white matter disorders are now recognized, including a variety of vascular, toxic, metabolic, infectious, traumatic, congenital, hydrocephalic, and neoplastic causes. The disorders affecting infants and children are discussed in part to provide further evidence of the neurobehavioral importance of cerebral white matter. In addition, these disorders are noteworthy because some afflicted individuals survive into or even present in adolescence or adulthood.

As the discussion proceeds, it will become apparent that dementia is the syndrome dominating the available data regarding neurobehavioral sequelae of cerebral white matter involvement (25). Affective disorders (26) and psychoses (27) are also recognized, despite little formal and systematic study. Focal neurobehavioral syndromes (5) are uncommon in these conditions, but a growing literature has provided documentation of amnesia, aphasia, and other discrete syndromes due to white matter disease.

Adult Disorders

DEMYELINATIVE DISEASES

This group of illnesses, the most significant of which is multiple sclerosis (MS), has been known for many years to be capable of significant morbidity, but only recently has its impact on neurobehavioral function been more adequately recognized. It is now well documented that demyelinative cerebral disease can manifest neurobehavioral signs and symptoms as initial or most prominent features of the illness. To the many distressing aspects of MS and related diseases that are already known can now be added frequent cognitive and emotional disturbances.

MS is certainly the most common of the demyelinative diseases, and the one subjected to the most detailed neurobehavioral analysis. Before reviewing the growing literature on cognitive and emotional features of MS, it is useful to mention the other demyelinative diseases briefly. These have been little studied in neurobehavioral terms, in part because of their rarity, but also because other features dominate the clinical picture. The problematic entity of Schilder's disease persists in many textbooks and requires explanation; Schilder originally suggested that this "diffuse cerebral sclerosis" was a variant of MS (28). Despite the labeling of various leukodystrophies as Schilder's disease over the years, inclusion of this entity within the category of severe MS seems most appropriate. A clinically similar illness is the concentric sclerosis of Balo, the distinguishing feature of which is the presence of alternating bands of myelin preservation and destruction in concentric rings (29). The variant of MS known as neuromyelitis optica or Devic's disease specifically attacks spinal cord and optic nerves and typically has few neurobehavioral manifestations (30). For clinical purposes, knowledge of MS and its sequelae is clearly a priority.

Despite the fact that Charcot did recognize an "enfeeblement of the memory" when he made his detailed observations of MS in the late 19th century (31), little appreciation of such complications was apparent until a century later. Recent studies have supported and amplified Charcot's comments, however, and memory is indeed impaired in many MS patients (32). There is evidence that the memory problem is more related to retrieval than encoding or storage, because free recall tasks are more difficult for MS patients than recognition tasks (33).

Attentional function has been examined in some detail, and deficits of sustained attention, also known as vigilance, have been documented (34). Studies using the Paced Auditory Serial Addition Test (PASAT) (35) and the Trail Making Test (32) also demonstrate attentional deficits in MS patients. These disturbances are closely allied with slowing of information processing, a feature also noted to be prominent in the subcortical dementias (6). Impairments in attention and vigilance may play a key role in the functional limitations experienced by many patients with MS, especially as they contribute to memory dysfunction.

Deficits in other areas are also well documented, and a substantial number of individuals with MS have impairments that clearly indicate the presence of dementia. In a landmark study, Heaton and colleagues studied 100 patients with MS using a comprehensive neuropsychological battery and found that, compared with 100 normal subjects, the MS patients had significant cognitive impairment on a variety of measures (32). Patients were divided into those with the chronic-progressive form of the illness (n = 43) and those with the relapsing-remitting form (n = 57); the former group had a higher prevalence of cognitive impairment (98%) than the latter (68%), and had significantly greater impairment as well (32).

Subsequently, other investigators demonstrated that the total lesion area of cerebral MS plaques on MRI is significantly correlated with cognitive impairment (36, 37). It has also been proposed that cerebral white matter involvement (Fig. 38.1) may cause cognitive impairment when a "threshold" level of demyelination is reached (37). Furthermore, deficits on the Wisconsin Card Sorting Test have been found in MS patients to correlate with frontal lobe demyelination, suggesting that focal lesion areas can cause specific impairments (38). These studies cast doubt on the commonly held view that cerebral MS plaques are often clinically "silent." It is likely, in fact, that cognitive and emotional dysfunction are frequently overlooked, because even routine screening tests of mental status, such as the Mini-Mental State Examination (39), are insensitive to the deficits of many MS patients (36). The emerging understanding of the effects of demyelinative disease on cognitive function has led to MS being variously termed a subcortical (40) or a white matter dementia (25).

Emotional disorders are also common in MS. Again, it was Charcot who first made reference to disorders of affect, noting among other changes a "foolish laughter without cause" (41). This phenomenon, which has come to be known as euphoria, has long been recognized as a particularly striking feature (42), but in actuality it is a rather uncommon late sequel that occurs in severe disease (43). More frequent are the mood disorders; depression and bipolar disorder both appear to occur with greater than expected frequency in MS. Another notable syndrome is emotional dysregulation, or pseudobulbar affect, characterized by laughter and weeping without sufficient emotional stimulation, and resulting from disinhibition of the facial musculature.

Depression would not be surprising, of course, in a

Table 38.3. Childhood Cerebral White Matter Disorders

Leukodystrophies	Metachromatic leukodystrophy
	Adrenoleukodystrophy
	Krabbe's disease
	Pelizaeus-Merzbacher disease
	Canavan's disease
	Alexander's disease
Amino acidopathies	Phenylketonuria
	Maple syrup urine disease
Congenital	Hydrocephalus
	Callosal agenesis
Vascular	Periventricular leukomalacia
Infectious	Postinfectious encephalomyelitis
	Acute hemorrhagic leukoencephalitis
Traumatic	Traumatic brain injury
Toxic	Radiation
	Chemotherapy

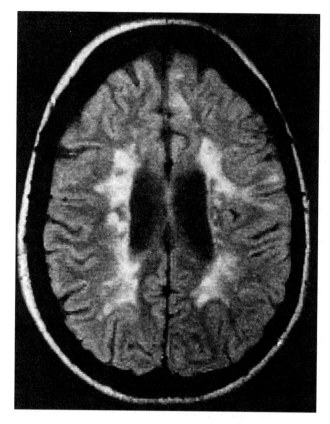

Figure 38.1. T2-weighted axial MRI scan of a demented patient with MS. (Reproduced with permission from Filley CM, Franklin GM, Heaton RK, Rosenberg NL. White matter dementia: clinical disorders and implications. Neuropsychiatry Neuropsychol Behav Neurol 1989;1:239–254.)

patient diagnosed with a chronic and potentially disabling illness such as MS, and it is not possible as yet to exclude a reactive cause for a depressive disorder in this setting. However, considerable evidence indicates that the presence of cerebral demyelination is associated with depression. Minden and colleagues found that scores on the Beck Depression Inventory were higher in MS patients than in most patients with other medical conditions (44). Schiffer and Babigian noted that MS patients were more often diagnosed as depressed by psychiatric clinicians than were patients with temporal lobe epilepsy and amyotrophic lateral sclerosis (45). Schiffer and colleagues also found that MS patients with cerebral disease were more likely to have a history of depressive episodes than those with primarily spinal involvement (46). The neuroanatomical locus of white matter disease resulting in this manifestation is unclear, although one MRI study implicating involvement of the temporal lobes has appeared (47).

Bipolar disorder is less common than depression in MS, but it is similarly less common in the general population. Some data suggest that bipolar disorder may also be associated with cerebral demyelination. There appears to be a significantly higher lifetime risk for bipolar disorder in MS patients than in comparable populations without neurological disease (48). Demyelination of the temporal lobes has also been implicated in this context (47).

Euphoria is characterized by the striking appearance of elated unconcern in the presence of severe neurological disability. Extensive frontal lobe demyelination has been suggested to account for this clinical feature (49). Emotional dysregulation is a related phenomenon, and is better known to neurologists as pseudobulbar affect. Bilateral lesions of the corticobulbar tracts that disinhibit brainstem motor nuclei are thought to be responsible (49); patients report that laughter and weeping occur with emotional provocation that would not typically evoke these reactions, and that the affective display is more dramatic than that which is suggested by their actual mood at the time (49).

VASCULAR DISEASE

Much of behavioral neurology has been built on careful studies of syndromes following cerebral infarction. Cerebrovascular disease remains an important clinical problem from many points of view. Although classical stroke syndromes tend to reflect cortical dysfunction, white matter can also be preferentially or even uniquely damaged. A number of older reports describing cerebral white matter disconnections are pertinent in this context, and a growing body of information is documenting both diffuse and focal syndromes as a result of vascular white matter disease of the brain. In addition, there is growing interest in frequently noted white matter changes in the brains of elderly individuals that probably reflect more subtle vascular abnormalities as well.

Binswanger's disease (BD) is the term given to an old clinical entity (50) that has recently been studied with renewed interest because of the availability of MRI. Originally described neuropathologically as a condition with demyelination of the cerebral white matter, usually with scattered lacunar infarctions, BD is also known as subcortical arteriosclerotic encephalopathy (51). The disease is thought to be caused by chronic cerebral ischemia that is most pronounced in the subcortical periventricular white matter (51). As such, BD is a form of vascular dementia, a term preferred by some to indicate cognitive impairment due to cerebral ischemia of any sort (52). Others adhere to the term BD to distinguish this predominantly subcortical condition from the entity involving more widespread cerebral infarcts known as multi-infarct dementia (51). The exact mechanisms leading to the development of BD are still not entirely clear, but possibilities include cerebral atherosclerosis secondary to hypertension (51), repeated hypotensive episodes in patients with long-standing hypertension (53), and ischemia related to cerebral amyloid angiopathy (54). The clinical course is one of slowly progressive dementia, accompanied by variable degrees of psychosis, motor signs, and gait disorder; abrupt changes in neurological status that imply an episode of infarction can be observed (51). The disease is rarely encountered in the absence of hypertension (55). Aphasia and movement disorder are uncommon (25).

The relationship between BD and the frequent appearance of white matter changes on the MRI scans of elderly patients is of considerable interest. These "unidentified bright objects" or "UBOs" (56) were initially unexplained, and even now their pathophysiological origin and neurobehavioral significance are debated. The alterations take the form of focal, sometimes confluent areas of white matter change that are best seen on T2-weighted images (56). At first somewhat loosely termed BD by early observers (57), it was soon appreciated that many individuals with these white matter hyperintensities (WMH) are cognitively intact, and that some WMH are apparently insignificant in neurobehavioral terms (58). The term "leukoaraiosis" has also been applied to these findings, in an effort to use a purely descriptive label in the absence of a secure neurobiological explanation (59). Recent studies in healthy elderly subjects suggest that there may be a threshold effect relating WMH and cognitive dysfunction; as is postulated with MS (37), the greater the white matter area involved, the greater the likelihood of cognitive impairment (60). It is noteworthy that neuropsychological studies have documented subtle deficits in attention among asymptomatic hypertensive men (61), and that even in neuropsychologically normal hypertensive men, MRI studies have shown ventricular enlargement, suggesting white matter loss (62). Moreover, cognitive deficits in elderly hypertensive individuals have been associated with the degree of white matter change on MRI (63). It is increasingly plausible that hypertension and other atherosclerotic risk factors contribute to a spectrum of alterations ranging from asymptomatic white matter change to leukoaraiosis to frank dementia in BD.

There have been other observations revolving around the appearance of WMH on MRI scans. Studies of elderly patients presenting to psychiatric hospitals have suggested a relationship between white matter lesions and syndromes of depression (64) and paranoid psychosis (65). The nature of these associations is not clear, but vascular abnormalities may play a role in the pathogenesis of the emotional disorders. Much more work needs to be done on these issues to determine if WMH contribute to psychiatric states or whether they are simply age-related phenomena that appear incidentally. If there is a clear association between WMH and psychiatric disease, a critical issue would be to define the cerebral areas that are responsible.

Stroke syndromes have also been reported that document the occurrence of focal deficits with discrete white matter infarcts. Classic studies have described syndromes such as conduction aphasia and ideomotor apraxia from lesions of the left arcuate fasciculus (5), and apraxia of the left hand from a lesion of the anterior corpus callosum is well known (66). Pure word deafness, due to a lesion in the left auditory radiation (5), pure alexia, from a lesion of the splenium of the corpus callosum and left occipital cortex (5), and associative visual agnosia, following bilateral lesions of the inferior occipitofrontal fasciculus (5) are also recognized. In recent years, aphasia with white matter infarction has been more carefully analyzed. Alexander and colleagues presented a large series of patients with left-hemisphere white matter lesions, and proposed a model to explain the various features

of aphasia by the disconnections of areas within the left-hemisphere language zone (67). Kooistra and Heilman reported a case of verbal memory deficit due to an infarct of the posterior limb of the left internal capsule (68). Bogousslavsky and colleagues documented one autopsy-verified case of neglect from an infarct confined to the posterior limb of the right internal capsule (69), and Hublet and Demeurisse described a similar case manifesting topographical disorientation from a vascular lesion in the same location (70). Nighoghossian and colleagues presented a case of spatial delirium, also known as reduplicative paramnesia, consequent to an infarct in the subcortical white matter of the right frontal lobe (71). All of these syndromes have also been reported as a result of cortical damage, and the white matter location of the lesions in these cases indicates that white matter structures contribute to cerebral networks subserving neurobehavioral functions.

TOXIC DISORDERS

The nervous system is vulnerable to a wide variety of toxic insults, and the pathogenesis of toxic syndromes is quite diverse. Many toxins are presumed to act on neuronal cell bodies, axonal processes, neurotransmitter systems, and synaptic function. There are, however, a small number of toxins that exert their main effect on the white matter of the brain. These intoxications are still incompletely understood, as observations have been made primarily with MRI, and there have been few neuropathological investigations. Preliminary data on white matter pathology are beginning to appear, but basic myelinotoxic mechanisms remain obscure.

Toluene is a widely used organic solvent that is now conclusively associated with cerebral white matter damage (72). Convincing cases first came to medical attention because of the unfortunate practice of solvent vapor abuse, which involves extraordinary exposure of the CNS to daily inhalation of toluene, found in commonly available spray paints (73). Dementia has been noted in patients with prolonged exposure, in addition to ataxia, eye movement disorders, and anosmia (74). MRI has disclosed diffuse white matter rarefaction with cerebral atrophy (75). A careful postmortem study of one demented long-term abuser disclosed cerebral and cerebellar myelin loss (72). Finally, the severity of dementia has been shown to correlate well with the degree of cerebral white matter change, as displayed by MRI (76) (Fig. 38.2).

Alcohol (ethanol, ethyl alcohol) is a more common intoxicant that has a long history but still unsettled effect on the CNS (77). The best known syndrome consequent to the long-term problem of alcoholism is the Wernicke-Korsakoff syndrome, a combination of acute encephalopathy and chronic amnesia due to dietary deficiency of thiamine (78). This disorder does not have a striking tendency to affect myelin, and in contrast, numerous gray matter nuclei in the diencephalon and brainstem are affected (78). Alcoholic dementia, however, is more strongly associated with white matter damage.

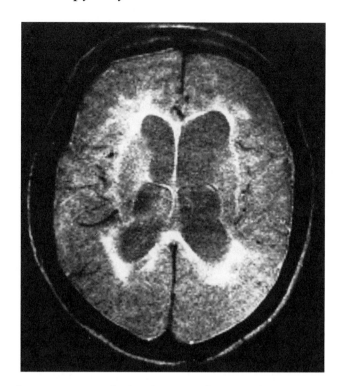

Figure 38.2. T2-weighted axial MRI scan of a severely demented toluene abuser. (Reproduced with permission from Filley CM, Heaton RK, Rosenberg NL. White matter dementia in chronic toluene abuse. Neurology 1990;40: 532–534.)

Dementia in alcoholics, which must be differentiated from the more restricted amnesia seen in Korsakoff's psychosis (25, 77), has an uncertain basis, but increasing evidence from computerized tomography (CT) (79), MRI (80), animal studies (81), and neuropathological investigations (16, 82) has demonstrated disproportionate atrophy of white matter. Dementia in alcoholics is, in addition, potentially reversible (83), suggesting further that white matter, not gray matter, is primarily involved. There is also evidence that CT scans can show improvement—decrease in size of lateral ventricular volume—with abstinence (79), again indicating that white matter may be the primary target of alcohol (25).

Cancer chemotherapeutic agents comprise another category of cerebral white matter toxins. Toxic effects of chemotherapeutic agents on the brain were first recognized with CT, but MRI greatly improved the imaging of these effects because they take the form of leukoencephalopathy (84). The most frequently encountered drug in this regard is methotrexate (MTX), a folic acid antagonist that causes either an insidious dementia, or, less often, an acute confusional state (85). Diffuse white matter involvement has been documented neuropathologically (84). Another agent capable of causing similar leukoencephalopathy is 1,3-bis (2-chloromethyl)-1-nitrosourea (BCNU) (86). Drugs that are infrequently associated with these changes are arabinosyl cytosine (Ara-C) (87), thiotepa (88), 5-fluorouracil (5-FU) and its derivatives (89), and cisplatin (90).

Finally, another toxic insult to the cerebral white matter is cranial irradiation (91). This effect is most often noted 1–2 years after radiation, and generally requires 5000 cGy or more (92). A dementia syndrome resembling subcortical dementia has been described and is presumably caused by leukoencephalopathy that spares the cortex and subcortical gray matter (92).

METABOLIC DISORDERS

Included in this category are four syndromes in which white matter pathology is firmly documented. Cobalamin (vitamin B_{12}) is an essential nutrient of the nervous system that has long been associated with pernicious anemia and subacute combined degeneration of the spinal cord. In addition to myelopathy, however, cerebral white matter changes are also pathologically verified (93), and dementia (94) and psychosis (95) have both been attributed to cobalamin deficiency. Some investigators maintain that undetected cobalamin deficiency is a frequent cause of numerous neuropsychiatric disorders (96). This area is under active investigation, and it seems plausible that cerebral white matter disease is responsible for the neurobehavioral manifestations of cobalamin deficiency. Folate, another vitamin routinely assessed in this setting, can be deficient in a manner clinically similar to that of cobalamin deficiency, and a reversible dementia has occasionally been documented (97). No neuropathological data on folate deficiency are available, however, and the question of whether this condition damages white matter cannot presently be answered.

Anoxia is a well-known neurological syndrome in its usual manifestations. These include acute encephalopathy, coma, persistent vegetative state, and death, and the pathology typically affects gray matter areas such as cerebral cortex, hippocampus, and basal ganglia (98). An unusual sequel, however, is a demyelinative encephalopathy that supervenes days after an apparent recovery from an anoxic episode (94). The pathogenesis of postanoxic demyelination is unknown, but dementia and motor abnormalities are common if the individual survives (99).

Marchiafava-Bignami disease (MBD) is a poorly understood disorder often associated with alcoholism, in which the corpus callosum is severely damaged (100). Originally described in Italian drinkers of red wine, it is now evident that MBD is not confined to Italians or even to alcoholics (78). Although the condition is rare, a variety of neurobehavioral features have been described, and dementia may occur (100).

Central pontine myelinolysis (CPM) is another white matter disorder in alcoholism, probably caused by overly rapid correction of hyponatremia (101). Acute confusional state due to CPM has been observed and attributed to the pontine lesion interrupting the ascending neurotransmitter systems responsible for the maintenance of arousal and attention (102). Myelinolysis in the hemispheric white matter has also been observed (103).

INFECTIOUS DISEASES

Many infectious diseases attack the cerebrum, but relatively few have their primary effect on the white matter. The dementia associated with the acquired immune deficiency syndrome (AIDS), known as the AIDS-dementia complex (ADC), is the best example of a cerebral white matter infection, and the opportunistic infection progressive multifocal leukoencephalopathy (PML) is the other entity in this group. AIDS is now well recognized to be a disease with frequent CNS involvement (104), and direct viral invasion of the brain is typical of the illness. The brunt of the pathology appears to involve the white matter of the hemispheres, with multinucleated giant cells and myelin pallor; the basal ganglia, brainstem, and cortex are less affected (105). Concomitant with these findings, MRI scans demonstrate diffuse white matter hyperintensity (106), and the dementia syndrome itself has features suggestive of subcortical dementia (104). It is noteworthy, however, that movement disorder is uncommon in ADC, as in other white matter dementias (25).

PML is an uncommon viral infection that has come to increased prominence as a result of the AIDS epidemic but which also occurs in patients with malignancies such as leukemia and lymphoma, chronic steroid therapy, systemic lupus erythematosus, and other illnesses. The disease is caused by an infection of oligodendrocytes in cerebral white matter, originating with a member of the papovavirus group known as the JC virus. In contrast to the diffuse nature of the ADC, PML is a multifocal infection of the white matter (107). Neurological deficits and neurobehavioral features are those associated with the areas of white matter involved (107).

TRAUMATIC DISORDERS

The investigation of CNS trauma has recently shed new light on mechanisms of brain injury, and increasing evidence is accumulating to indicate that cerebral white matter is significantly involved. The cortex can clearly be damaged as well, as in the case of cortical contusion or in hypoxic-ischemic injury (108), but the entity of diffuse axonal injury has been gaining increasing acceptance as the most common sequel of traumatic brain injury (TBI) (109).

Clinical and experimental studies of TBI have demonstrated that diffuse axonal injury commonly occurs in nonpenetrating head injury (108, 109). This widespread injury to cerebral white matter involves both myelin and axons, and leaves the cortex essentially spared. Depending on the severity of the impact, the clinical picture may be one of concussion, defined as a traumatically induced alteration of the mental state (110), or of loss of consciousness, with prolonged coma and severe long-term disability (111). Neurobehavioral deficits in TBI survivors are frequent, and range from inattention and memory disturbance in the postconcussion syndrome (112) to severe dementia or persistent vegetative state following severe TBI (113).

Imaging studies, particularly MRI, document the frequent occurrence of white matter lesions (114). Associated cortical damage often results in superimposed neurobehavioral impairments.

Lesions of the corpus callosum (CC) are not often encountered as isolated neuropathological findings, but an extensive literature exists on surgically induced CC lesions. These patients are of considerable interest in view of the still mysterious role of the this commissure in the processes of interhemispheric communication. Corpus callosotomy has been performed frequently for the relief of intractable seizure disorders, and studies of neurobehavioral function after callosotomy have indicated that deficits are relatively subtle (115). However, the striking phenomenon of intermanual conflict can be seen acutely after callosotomy (115), and apraxia (66), agraphia (115), and tactile agnosia (116) of the left hand can also be demonstrated.

HYDROCEPHALIC DISORDERS

Normal pressure hydrocephalus (NPH) is considered a reversible dementia syndrome of adults (117). The cause of the illness remains unexplained in many patients, although cases are known to follow TBI, meningitis, and subarachnoid hemorrhage. In any event, NPH presents with the well-known triad of dementia, incontinence, and gait disorder, and some cases respond favorably to shunting procedures (117). The major neuropathology is in the periventricular white matter (118), and the dementia syndrome is quite similar to other disorders of white matter in that there is a subcortical pattern to the neurobehavioral disturbance and there is no movement disorder (25).

NEOPLASTIC DISORDERS

Neoplasms of the brain typically involve widespread areas of the cerebrum or posterior fossa and do not as a rule confine themselves to gray or white matter selectively. In addition, mass effects from a tumor and the often significant edema associated with malignancy add further to the diffuse nature of brain involvement. There is, however, the unusual condition of gliomatosis cerebri, in which cerebral white matter is diffusely invaded by a tumor of the glioma category (119). This rare neoplasm is characterized clinically by changes in personality and memory loss. Other signs and symptoms such as hemiparesis, ataxia, papilledema, headache, and seizures are seen less often (120).

A more specific disorder of memory has been reported by Heilman and Sypert in a patient with spongioblastoma unipolare who developed a profound deficit in recent memory related to bilateral destruction of the posterior fornix (121). This neoplastic amnestic syndrome involved damage to the most important white matter structure of the medial temporal and limbic memory system.

Childhood Disorders

LEUKODYSTROPHIES

This group of hereditary diseases of myelin has been the subject of much biochemical and genetic study (122), but detailed knowledge of neurobehavioral features is not as available. In part, this is because unfortunately, there is often a fatal outcome from these diseases in early life. Nevertheless, these disorders offer dramatic evidence that deficiencies in the development of normal mentation can be due to abnormalities in cerebral white matter, and consideration of brain-behavior relationships in these conditions is instructive. Moreover, there are occasional examples of these diseases presenting in later life or even adulthood (122), and an appreciation of the potential of genetic diseases to have a delayed onset is increasingly important.

Metachromatic leukodystrophy (MLD) is the best known and most clinically relevant member of this group because of its well-characterized biochemical pathology, relative frequency, and presentation with adult and juvenile as well as infantile neurobehavioral syndromes. MLD is an autosomal recessive disorder of central and peripheral myelin that is caused by a deficiency in the enzyme arylsulfatase A (123). Typically the onset is between the first and fourth years of life with delayed mental and motor development; the combination of dysmyelination of central white matter and dysmyelinating peripheral neuropathy results in a variable mixture of upper and lower motor neuron signs. Onset in childhood and adult life has been well described, and psychosis resembling schizophrenia is frequent (124). Dementia is also well recognized (125) and often supervenes after a long period of psychosis (27). MRI scans show diffuse white matter hyperintensity in the cerebrum (Fig. 38.3) that correlates well with widespread white matter changes at autopsy (126).

Adrenoleukodystrophy (ALD) is similar to MLD in many respects, but is accompanied by adrenocortical insufficiency (127). Two forms of the disease are recognized, an X-linked form presenting in boys and rarely in adolescence or adult life, and an autosomal recessive type that occurs in the neonatal period (127). Both varieties are characterized by an inability to degrade very-long-chain fatty acids, and the diagnosis depends on the demonstration of these fatty acids in the blood (127). Treatment of adrenal insufficiency does not correct the neurological features of the illness. Dementia and psychosis are prominent in this disorder (128), and MRI scans demonstrate diffuse white matter disease (129).

Four other white matter diseases are usually listed as uncontroversial members of the leukodystrophy group. Krabbe's disease, or globoid cell leukodystrophy, affects infants most often, and usually causes death within 2 years. Onset of dementia in adolescence and survival into adulthood have been observed (130). An autosomal recessive disease, this condition is caused by a deficiency of galacto-cerebrosidase, and cerebral dysmyelination is extensive (131). Pelizaeus-Merzbacher disease very rarely presents in adulthood, and patients may show dementia and psychosis

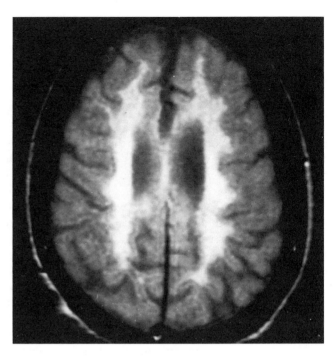

Figure 38.3. T2-weighted axial MRI scan of a patient with MLD who had psychosis followed later by dementia. (Reproduced with permission from Erratum. Psychosis with cerebral white matter disease. Neuropsychiatry Neuropsychol Behav Neurol 1993;6:142.)

(132). Islands of intact myelin appear amid abnormal white matter, giving a tigroid pattern in the hemispheres (133). Canavan's disease, also known as spongy degeneration of the white matter, usually begins in early infancy with macrocephaly and arrested development, but onset after age 15 has been noted (134). Alexander's disease typically presents with developmental delay before age 2, but adult onset cases have been reported to resemble MS (135).

AMINO ACIDOPATHIES

These metabolic disorders of infancy are, in general, of little relevance to the behavioral neurologist and of greater interest to the pediatric neurologist and biochemist. However, phenylketonuria (PKU) and its rarer relative maple syrup urine disease (MSUD) are marked by striking changes in the cerebral white matter that are likely to account for the neurobehavioral sequelae of these diseases. PKU is the most common of the aminoacidurias and is inherited as an autosomal recessive trait. The fundamental biochemical lesion is a deficiency of the hepatic enzyme phenylalanine hydroxylase, which results in severe white matter pathology in the cerebrum and mental retardation if untreated with dietary restriction of phenylalanine (136). MSUD is a less common affliction that is also inherited as an autosomal recessive trait. Treatment with dietary restriction of branched-chain amino acids may permit normal development by presumably preventing the white matter changes in the cerebrum that have been documented (137).

CONGENITAL DISORDERS

Hydrocephalus falls into the congenital category and can be a result of aqueductal stenosis, the Arnold-Chiari malformation, the Dandy-Walker syndrome, germinal matrix hemorrhage, or perinatal infection (138). Mental retardation is common in untreated cases (139), although language is relatively spared (140). Also in this category is callosal agenesis, in which the CC does not develop normally. Neurobehavioral signs are typically minimal, mainly because of the preservation of noncallosal commissures in this condition (115, 141).

VASCULAR DISORDERS

An important neonatal disease of cerebral white matter is periventricular leukomalacia. This disorder, encountered in newborns who are premature and in cardiorespiratory distress, involves bilateral destruction of periventricular white matter; despite some uncertainty as to pathogenesis, the condition appears to result from circulatory insufficiency (142). There seems to be a selective vulnerability of the developing white matter to hypoperfusion, so that gray matter is spared (143); this situation parallels that of adult BD, in which considerable evidence suggests that the cerebral white matter is also selectively damaged by hypotension. Survivors often have significant mental retardation (142).

INFECTIOUS DISORDERS

Although postinfectious encephalomyelitis is not, strictly speaking, a white matter infection, it nearly always follows acute infection with measles, mumps, rubella, varicella, or other viruses (144). The disease may also occur after vaccination (145). Mental changes, particularly acute confusional states, are common during the illness, and mental retardation occurs in some survivors (146). The cerebral white matter is significantly demyelinated, and MRI is sensitive to these lesions (147). The disorder is assumed to be a virus-induced immune-mediated condition, and the term acute disseminated encephalomyelitis is an alternate designation.

Acute hemorrhagic leukoencephalitis is a more severe form of postinfectious encephalomyelitis (144). This is a fulminant illness that also follows viral infection, and is frequently fatal (148). Survivors may have severe mental retardation.

TRAUMATIC DISORDERS

TBI in children is unfortunately common, caused not only by accidents but from nonaccidental trauma as well (149). Diffuse axonal injury is again the most consistent pathology, and deficits in cognitive and emotional behavior may be devastating (111). In particular, impulse control and comportment may be severely disturbed at a time in social development when they are critically needed (111).

TOXIC DISORDERS

Toxic insults to the brain from radiation and chemotherapy in children are increasingly recognized (150). Radiation appears to have especially severe effects on neurobehavioral function through its propensity to damage cerebral white matter (151). Younger children are more vulnerable to both these insults, and nonlanguage skills appear to be more frequently impaired (150).

PROGNOSIS AND TREATMENT

A summary of the prognosis and treatment of cerebral white matter disorders presents difficulties because of the impressive variety of pathological processes involved. The severity of these conditions ranges from mild to catastrophic, and therapy varies greatly, depending on such factors as the type of white matter disorder, the extent of functional disability, and the age of the patient. However, some general principles of white matter structure and function in health and illness may shed light on these poorly understood questions.

It is well known that neurons in the human nervous system do not develop after birth, and it has been assumed that neurons lost from disease or injury do not regenerate. Recent advances in the understanding of neurotrophic factors such as nerve growth factor are raising hopes that damaged neurons may indeed be recoverable (152), but for clinical purposes this idea is not yet a reality. Gray matter areas of the brain may still be regarded as regions that, once destroyed, do not recover. Clinical improvement must result from other areas assuming functions they did not subserve previously, or to the use of compensatory strategies to overcome the deficit. White matter, however, may not be so irrevocably damaged; there is mounting evidence that spontaneous recovery may be surprisingly robust, and that a number of interventions can potentially enhance the process of recovery. The basis for this more optimistic view is that white matter lesions, even if diffuse, do not primarily injure neuronal cell bodies, and therefore the cellular sites of neurobehavioral function remain intact. Even those white matter lesions that damage axons in addition to myelin—such as severe MS plaques, ischemic infarcts, and diffuse axonal injury—may not involve such lasting dysfunction as lesions in which the major target is the neuronal cell body.

Spontaneous Recovery

The question of whether recovery follows the withdrawal of the pathological insult in the cerebral white matter has not been resolved, but a substantial body of evidence suggests that myelin can regenerate and restore normal function if the pathology is not overwhelmingly severe. Most of the literature concerns demyelinative diseases, but insights from other illnesses are also able to shed light on this intriguing problem.

It is a common clinical observation that MS patients typically have a waxing and waning course, and indeed the subtype of relapsing-remitting MS is defined by this fluctuation. Clearly the disease is intermittent in its intensity, and recovery must be taking place from time to time. One factor contributing to this pattern is the inherent variability of MS, reasons for which are presently unknown. There is also, however, growing evidence that remyelination can occur in the CNS (153, 154). Other information now becoming available suggests that even in axonal segments that remain demyelinated, functional recovery may proceed as a result of an increase in the membrane density of sodium channels (155). Both of these mechanisms would indicate that specific interventions might be designed that could enhance natural recovery processes.

Another likely mechanism of recovery, most relevant in white matter infarction, would be the assumption of a lost ability by another cerebral area, similar to the recovery that follows cortical lesions (156). An interesting report of anterior commissure hypertrophy in callosal agenesis suggests that functional compensation may occur by structural modification of white matter tracts (157).

There are other encouraging data in the realm of spontaneous recovery that come from studies on alcoholism. As reviewed earlier, alcohol abusers who are abstinent can often show neuropsychological improvement (83), and imaging studies of the brain demonstrate reversal of cerebral atrophy (79). There is good reason to believe that the white matter is selectively damaged in alcoholism (81, 82), and that improvement on CT or MRI is due to a restitution of white matter that eventually results in clinical recovery of neurobehavioral function (25). Recovery from other toxic disorders, notably dementia from toluene, chemotherapeutic agents, and cranial irradiation, has not been as evident; these observations may imply heavier exposure to the toxin or a different mode of white matter toxicity. Nevertheless, it is plausible that white matter may possess a resiliency that can be exploited for clinical purposes.

Pharmacotherapy

A detailed discussion of pharmacotherapy is beyond the scope of this review, but it is clear that some of the cerebral white matter syndromes, such as depression, bipolar disorder, and psychosis, can be approached with established psychopharmacological modalities. This section focuses on selected drug treatments, with specific application to disorders of white matter. Effective treatment will ultimately depend on the elucidation of a wide variety of neuropathological processes that are incompletely understood as yet.

Pharmacological treatment of cerebral white matter disorders could take one of three forms: prevention, restitution of function in damaged areas, and stimulant therapy for bolstering the function of intact cerebral regions. Prevention would be most pertinent in the case of cerebrovascular disease, where an evolving body of data is accumulating to clarify the value of antiplatelet aggregation drugs, such as aspirin and ticlopidine, and the standard anticoagulants, heparin and warfarin (158). With the same intent, careful control of arterial blood pressure and other risk factors has an established prophylactic effect for vascular disease (159). Avoidance of alcohol and solvent vapor abuse has clearly beneficial effects, and TBI is preventable with certain precautions. Restitution of function in diseased areas is exemplified by the ongoing efforts to find an effective immune treatment for MS (160), cobalamin treatment for vitamin B_{12} deficiency (161), antiviral drugs for ADC (162) and dietary adjustment for PKU (163) and MSUD (164). The enhancement of cerebral regions left undamaged by the disease or injury involves consideration of CNS stimulants or other agents designed to improve some form of compensation in view of the primary deficit. Methylphenidate, dextroamphetamine, amantadine, and bromocriptine have been explored in a range of CNS disorders; these drugs have effects on catecholaminergic systems that travel through white matter tracts. Preliminary studies in MS (165), AIDS-related complex (166), and TBI (167) have been encouraging.

Surgical Treatment

Surgical treatment in cerebral white matter diseases has a fairly limited role. Two instances where surgery may prove valuable are shunting procedures, ventriculoperitoneal or lumboperitoneal, in NPH (168), and the bone marrow transplantation procedure being explored in MLD (169). Shunting for NPH is an established technique but remains controversial because criteria for patient selection are uncertain (168). A single case of MLD has been reported to be arrested by bone marrow transplantation (169).

Cognitive Rehabilitation

This approach to therapy, only recently subjected to any critical evaluation, attempts to improve functional ability in neurobehavioral conditions through various combinations of cognitive retraining (with or without computers), psychotherapy, and vocational counseling (170). The greatest use thus far for cognitive rehabilitation has been in TBI. There are many theories as to why such intervention might be efficacious, but knowledge of this area is very limited. Few data exist as well on outcome (171), and it is best to adopt a skeptical attitude until more compelling information appears.

ROLE OF CEREBRAL WHITE MATTER IN HUMAN BEHAVIOR

Having reviewed the neurobiology of cerebral white matter and the many disorders to which it is vulnerable, we now examine how this sizable portion of the cerebral hemispheres participates in neurobehavioral function. A number of converging lines of evidence are considered to characterize the role of cerebral white matter in cognition and emotion.

Maturation and Aging of the Brain

Before summarizing the effects of white matter destruction on neurobehavioral function, a review of the normal developmental stages of white matter in the brain is in order. As mentioned previously, myelination in the brain occurs predominantly after neuronal cell bodies and axons are formed. Furthermore, it proceeds in a sequential manner, so that regions lower in the neuraxis myelinate first and more rostral areas much later. In adulthood, after the mature configuration of white matter is attained, there is little neuronal attrition or change in white matter, and the organism maintains its adult effectiveness at a high level. In later life, the proportion of white matter in the brain shows a significant decline, a surprising fact in view of the emphasis placed upon changes in gray matter that has preoccupied investigators in this field. Even though the white matter attrition may be secondary to cortical cell loss in aging, the fact that white matter volume diminishes more than that of gray matter cannot be avoided. In a sense, the brain reverts to a composition more reminiscent of its early life, with a relative paucity of white matter in comparison to gray matter.

The importance of this sequence is not entirely clear, but it seems evident that cerebral white matter plays an important role in neurobehavioral capacities at all ages. Myelination of the association areas of the hemispheres, especially the frontal lobes, is essential for the development of normal adult behavior, with all the integration and regulation of higher function that are implicit in that concept. Conversely, gradual loss of myelin in the elderly brain may well play a role in the subtle neurobehavioral changes of aging that are being increasingly documented. Between these extremes, the mature architecture of the brain mediates adult cognitive and emotional processing by the interaction of gray and white matter structures. Failure to take into account the role of cerebral white matter in normal and abnormal neurobehavioral function at all ages would seem to be a perilous omission.

Subcortical Dementia

By way of introduction to the behavioral neurology of cerebral white matter, a consideration of the term "subcortical dementia" is helpful. This idea was popularized two decades ago (172, 173), and has fueled much debate and useful investigation (6). The notion that a relatively specific profile of neurobehavioral signs and symptoms could be ascribed to diseases of the subcortical gray matter heralded a shift in thinking that considered the contributions of noncortical structures to higher function (174). Although not without its critics (175, 176), the concept appears to be established as a legitimate entity that is useful in the elucidation of distinctly different syndromes within the general category of dementia (177, 178).

Subcortical dementia was first described in patients with progressive supranuclear palsy (172) and Huntington's disease (173), and later came to be associated with the dementia syndromes of Parkinson's disease (179), Wilson's disease (180), spinocerebellar degeneration (181), the lacunar state (182), depression (183), and even tardive dyskinesia (184). A distinct profile of forgetfulness, slowness of thought processes, emotional changes, and an inability to manipulate acquired knowledge was observed, in the presence of a movement disorder and without aphasia, apraxia, and agnosia (172). Other investigators have used terms such as a "dilapidation" of cognition, apathy, and inertia (173). Because the subcortical dementias are typically associated with diseases of the basal ganglia, skeptics have argued that the only difference between subcortical and cortical dementias is the presence or absence of a movement disorder. Subsequent research, however, has shown that these dementia syndromes do show measurable neurobehavioral differences from the cortically based dementia of Alzheimer's disease (AD), in which amnesia, aphasia, apraxia, and agnosia may all be prominent (185).

It has been recognized (174) that many clinical features of subcortical dementia—in particular forgetfulness, cognitive slowing, emotional changes, and impaired abstracting ability—resemble the manifestations of frontal lobe disease (186). Moreover, many of the subcortical diseases have secondary effects on the frontal lobes (187) because of the strong anatomical relationships between basal ganglia and thalamus and the frontal cortex (188). These similarities have led some to propose alternative designations such as "frontal systems dementia" and "frontosubcortical dementia," but the popularity of the term subcortical dementia seems secure at present.

Another useful concept that has arisen from a consideration of subcortical dementia is the distinction between "fundamental" and "instrumental" functions (174). Fundamental functions are those that provide for the timing and activation of intrinsic cortical processes, and include arousal, attention, motivation, and mood (174). Instrumental functions are more specific and describe the discrete abilities of memory, language, praxis, and perception, which are primarily associated with the neocortex (174). Mesulam has referred to these two classes of higher functions in a slightly different manner, using the terms "state-dependent" and "channel-dependent" functions (189), but the contrast is similar. Subcortical systems, especially the ascending reticular activating system, the major neurotransmitter nuclei in the brainstem and basal forebrain, the limbic system, and the basal ganglia, subserve the fundamental functions, while neocortical areas carry out the instrumental activities. The dichotomy so outlined serves to organize a current conceptual framework of brain-behavior relationships.

In the last decade, further inquiry into non-AD dementias has extended the list of subcortical dementias. Entries to the list now include MS, BD, and the ADC. An extensive literature on MS in particular has evolved (40), and a neuropsychological distinction of MS dementia from the dementia of AD has been reported (190). The ADC has also been subjected to considerable study (104) as part of the widespread assault on the ominous problem of AIDS.

Behavioral Neurology of Cerebral White Matter

White matter, of course, qualifies as another subcortical structure, but, at first glance, it is not immediately apparent that it should have any significant role in higher function. Myelin, after all, may be irrelevant to the synaptic events that occur in the gray matter and contribute to learning, memory, and complex cognitive and emotional processes. Undoubtedly the extraordinary activities of the cortex play a preeminent role in the elaboration of the human behavioral repertoire. An understanding of this region alone, however, will not suffice to address the many issues of brain-behavior relationships. The vast connectivity of the brain should serve as a clue to the interdependence of cortical and other cerebral regions, and white matter, of course, is responsible for the majority of these connections. White matter pathways figure prominently in the multiple computations that produce the final output that is observable as human behavior. Probably all of these tracts can be affected by pathological processes attacking white matter. Neuronal function is intimately dependent on intact myelin; dramatic slowing of conduction velocity and even conduction block, seen typically in demyelinating peripheral neuropathy, are also thought to result from white matter lesions in the CNS (191). Although it is too simplistic to suppose that slowed central conduction in these disorders is solely responsible for neurobehavioral impairments, it is undoubtedly the case that certain aspects of cognitive and emotional processing can be rendered less efficient by a primary disturbance of cerebral white matter.

At this point, a consideration of the notion of disconnection in behavioral neurology is pertinent (5, 66). In this scheme, lesions that affect the cerebral connections between areas concerned with specific functions act to disconnect these zones from each other and cause identifiable neurobehavioral syndromes. These disconnections may be in either cortical or white matter regions. Recent studies using positron emission tomography (PET) scans of deep white matter infarction have demonstrated metabolic abnormalities in cortical regions anatomically connected but pathologically intact (192). Event-related potential studies in MS patients have disclosed P300 abnormalities that correlate with MRI changes and cognitive impairment (24). These observations indicate that white matter has an important integrative role in the activities of the cortex. Neurobehavioral syndromes resulting from white matter lesions occur because of disruption of pathways between relevant cerebral areas, both cortical and subcortical (67). Disconnections such as these, therefore, illustrate the contributions of white matter systems to normal behavior, although many details remain obscure. The old concept of diaschisis (193), which refers to the remote effects of a focal cerebral lesion, is also illuminated by these considerations; cerebral dysfunction in

Table 38.4. Diffuse Neurobehavioral Syndromes of Cerebral White Matter

Syndrome	Structures Involved
Dementia	Hemispheric white matter
Mental retardation	Hemispheric white matter
Depression	Ascending catecholaminergic fibers
Bipolar disorder	Ascending catecholaminergic fibers
Euphoria	Frontal lobe white matter
Psychosis	Frontal-limbic connections

areas other than the site of the primary pathology must surely implicate white matter pathways.

Obviously, the anatomical complexity of the cerebral white matter, as it participates in vast networks of cerebral neurons, is extraordinary. Incomplete knowledge of the details of white matter connections in the brain precludes a complete summary of their role in higher function, and only the broad outlines of this topic can presently be sketched. However, it is useful to summarize the clinical manifestations of disorders of cerebral white matter and attempt to delineate a profile of consistent features. Tables 38.4 and 38.5 list the major neurobehavioral syndromes that have been described.

The most frequent neurobehavioral presentation of cerebral white matter disorder is dementia. In children, the related syndrome of mental retardation is also very common. Diseases and injuries of white matter tend to involve diffuse and widespread areas of the cerebral hemispheres, and the lesions disrupt many different networks to produce the multidimensional impairments of dementia. Involvement of frontal lobe white matter is very common, and manifestations of frontal lobe dysfunction frequently contribute to the dementia syndrome. In general, the white matter dementias resemble the subcortical dementias in that inattention, forgetfulness, emotional changes, and absence of aphasia are typical (25). One key distinction, however, is that movement disorders are not prominent in the white matter dementias (25). This feature is not universal but consistent enough to be clinically useful as a guideline. The subcortical dementias are associated primarily with diseases of the basal ganglia, and it is not surprising that disorders of movement are common.

Emotional disorders are recognized as additional complications of the cerebral white matter disorders. Depression, bipolar disorder, euphoria, and emotional dysregulation are all well described, particularly in MS. It is likely that these manifestations are more common than currently believed, since there is an understandable tendency to ascribe mood disorder, especially depression, to a psychological reaction to the diagnosis of a serious neurological disease. Nevertheless, evidence favoring the neurological basis for mood disorder is steadily accumulating, and further studies using clinical measures, combined with MRI and other techniques, will be of great value. Disruption of the ascending catecholaminergic systems from the brainstem to the cortex appears to be the most plausible explanation for depression and bipolar disorder, and bifrontal white matter disease seems to play a role in the genesis of euphoria.

Psychosis is another recognized feature of the cerebral white matter disorders, and is particularly striking in MLD (124). A better appreciation of psychosis would likely develop if careful description of psychotic changes in known white matter disease was undertaken, and if individuals with psychotic illness were evaluated more thoroughly for white matter diseases. Apparently, psychosis occurs earlier than dementia in these conditions, sometimes preceding memory or other cognitive impairment by many years (27, 124). One possibility for this sequence is that psychosis occurs at an early stage in the illness when a "thought disorder" is plausible because of intact cortical systems and at least partially preserved intracerebral communication; later, when more extensive white matter damage has supervened, there is further disturbance of these systems that results in dementia, or an inability even to generate a thought disorder (27). The localization of white matter areas associated with psychosis is uncertain, but disruption of frontal-limbic connections has been postulated (27, 47, 124).

Finally, focal syndromes form another category of neurobehavioral affiliations of the cerebral white matter (5, 67). Some classic syndromes are well known, and others are being described; clinical observation coupled with MRI studies will surely disclose more of these. It is probable, in fact, that all of the classic neurobehavioral syndromes (194) will be seen with white matter lesions. Because interactions of cortical and subcortical structures very likely provide the basis for all neurobehavioral activity, and white matter pathways provide the connections within these circuits, lesions of white matter are certain to disrupt neurobehavioral functions, depending on their location (195).

Although focal syndromes are apparent in the white matter disorders that involve limited areas of pathology, diffuse impairment affecting arousal, attention, motivation, and mood is more common. As a general rule, fundamental functions are more affected by white matter pathology than instrumental functions. Focal syndromes occur by virtue of discrete damage to association, commissural, or projection fibers, and cause instrumental deficits such as aphasia, whereas long ascending fibers and multiple intracortical tracts are diffusely affected in a widespread fashion to result in disturbances of fundamental functions such as dementia, mood disorder, and psychosis.

Table 38.5. Focal Neurobehavioral Syndromes of Cerebral White Matter

Syndrome	Structures Involved
Amnesia	Fornix
Conduction aphasia	Left arcuate fasciculus
Sympathetic apraxia	Anterior corpus callosum
Ideomotor apraxia	Left arcuate fasciculus
Pure word deafness	Left auditory radiation
Pure alexia	Splenium of corpus callosum[a]
Associative visual agnosia	Bilateral inferior occipitofrontal fasciculus

[a]Left occipital cortex is also damaged.

Neuropsychological Aspects

Systematic investigation of neuropsychological status in patients with cerebral white matter disorders has only begun. These studies have concentrated for the most part on the dementias. In general, the results of these investigations have confirmed that the white matter disorders resemble the subcortical diseases quite closely. Memory is frequently impaired, and the deficit appears to involve retrieval more than encoding because recognition memory is normal or less impaired than retrieval (33). Language is typically spared, although dysarthria may be present (51, 74, 104, 196). Visuospatial abilities have not been carefully studied but appear to be impaired (32, 150). Complex cognitive tasks such as reasoning and concept formation are often affected, and perseveration can be seen (32, 40). Alterations in mood, affect, and personality have been frequently noted (40, 51, 74, 104).

One area that deserves particular consideration is attention. This important neuropsychological domain has been the subject of much discussion since the time of William James (197), and has more recently been referred to as a "frontier in neuropsychology" by Geschwind (198). Unfortunately, the concept is difficult to define, and use of the term differs considerably among authors. In general, attention may be considered to be the ability to focus mental effort on selected material while simultaneously excluding competing but inessential input (198). Clinical deficits in attention and vigilance are notable in the white matter disorders, and may well relate to the damage in connecting pathways of neural systems devoted to the maintenance of attention (25). These fiber systems include the ascending reticular activating system, numerous neurotransmitter systems originating in the brainstem and basal forebrain and terminating in the cortex, and the extensive white matter tracts coursing caudally from the frontal lobes to posterior cerebral regions. The right hemisphere may be dominant for some aspects of attention, particularly directed attention to the left hemispace (199), and the larger amount of white matter in the right hemisphere (20) may be relevant in this regard. As is the case with any neurobehavioral domain, there is thus a large-scale neuronal network that subserves the function (200). This network may be damaged at many sites by lesions of the white matter.

The cerebral white matter disorders may offer a productive opportunity to explore further the cerebral basis of attention and its alterations with developmental changes and pathology. Of great importance, for example, is a better understanding of neurobehavioral changes in the elderly. Quite possibly, certain aspects of attentional function that are impaired in aging, such as speed of information processing (201) and "effortful" processing (202), are selectively affected because of the deterioration of white matter that is characteristic of this age group (9). In white matter diseases such as MS, sustained attention or vigilance is often impaired (190), and slowed information processing, as measured by tests such as the PASAT (35), is a common finding. In this regard, white matter disorders appear to simulate the effects of normal aging, where similar defects have been found (203). Indeed, a recent study of neuropsychological performance in ADC and normal aging found a remarkable similarity between these groups (204). There is also evidence that WMH in the elderly brain are related to impairments in the speed of information processing, again suggesting that attentional systems may be preferentially affected by white matter damage (205). These intriguing ideas clearly require much more systematic study.

In children, an interesting entity called the "nonverbal learning disabilities syndrome" (NLD syndrome) has been presented by Rourke to characterize the neuropsychological deficits resulting from dysfunction of cerebral white matter (206). The NLD syndrome is defined as deficits in visuospatial abilities, complex problem solving, and emotional adjustment in the presence of well-developed language skills. The syndrome has been seen in children with a variety of white matter disorders, and the preponderance of right-hemisphere defects has been linked to the evidence that a higher proportion of hemispheric volume is white matter in the right when compared with the left (20). More investigation is needed to assess the validity of this concept.

Distributed Neurobehavioral Networks

In recent years, advances in many areas of clinical and basic neuroscience have led to a conceptualization of higher cognitive functions being carried out by large-scale neurobehavioral networks (200). In this scheme, vast arrays of interconnected neurons, numbering perhaps in the millions (207), interact to subserve neurobehavioral functions (200). Attention, memory, language, visuospatial ability, cognition, and emotional competence are all organized in this manner. This formulation represents a modification of localizationist theories of the 19th century in that multiple cortical, white matter, and subcortical areas participate in the production of neurobehavioral activities (208). On the other hand, the idea of equipotentiality, which holds that all areas of the cerebrum are equally capable of performing neurobehavioral tasks (209), is misleading. An intermediate position has now become well defined and accepted. It is clear from PET studies that not all brain areas take part in a specific task, but that, for example, in the case of memory, a selective network of anatomically related brain regions is critical for new learning to occur (210). Thus, there is a growing consensus that distributed networks, details of which are still incomplete, mediate higher functions, both cognitive and emotional. As a result of a new sophistication in understanding the cerebral basis of the mind, it can now be stated that neurobehavioral activities are both localized and distributed (200).

Cerebral white matter forms an essential component of the anatomical systems in the brain that underlie specific neurobehavioral functions. There is no cognitive or emotional domain that does not involve an integrated network of cortical and subcortical structures working in conjunction to perform the mental act. White matter, by virtue of its extensive distribution throughout the brain, participates in all these networks. There is now an empirical as well as an intuitive basis for this view.

FUTURE DIRECTIONS

The task of defining the role of cerebral white matter in neurobehavioral function is an enormous one. Little systematic effort has been devoted to this inquiry, reflecting a bias in favor of "higher *cortical* function." Despite the abundance of opportunities to explore these intriguing relationships, research has been remarkably limited. Without minimizing the importance of cortical and subcortical gray matter structures in behavioral neurology, it is appropriate to focus directly on the substantial contributions of the cerebral white matter.

The most pressing need is for greater emphasis on correlation of clinical phenomenology with various measures of white matter pathology. The traditional lesion method of behavioral neurology, based on careful clinical observation and supplemented by detailed neuropsychological evaluation, can be equally well applied to the white matter disorders of the brain, particularly now that MRI provides an elegant and noninvasive means of viewing the areas of interest. In parallel with these clinical studies, a more precise understanding of the neuroanatomy of cerebral white matter as it participates in neurobehavioral circuitry will be crucial. The insights gained from PET and single photon emission computed tomography (SPECT) promise to be of additional utility in delineating the unique contributions of white matter (211). Correlation of clinical with neuropathological data will provide important information, as there is much variability among the many causes and sites of white matter dysfunction. Promising information is also beginning to appear from clinical neurophysiology, and the measurement of long-latency event-related potentials may be a useful way to measure the role of white matter tracts in neurobehavioral function. Finally, neuropharmacologists will doubtless make a contribution to the neurochemical aspects of these disorders and their treatment.

The study of clinical brain-behavior relationships continues to grow as a vital component of the many disciplines concerned with human behavior in all its variety. Neurologists and psychiatrists will assume primary responsibility for the care of patients with such disorders, and will play a central role in clinical research as well. In the cerebral white matter disorders, as in other areas of neurobehavioral investigation, it becomes ever more crucial to follow a path that avoids both a "mindless neurology" and a "brainless psychiatry" (212).

Acknowledgments

The author is grateful to James P. Kelly, M.D., B.K. Kleinschmidt-DeMasters, M.D., and Michele Ferguson, M.D., for their helpful comments on this work. Linda Baldwin provided expert secretarial assistance.

References

1. Cummings JL, Hegarty A. Neurology, psychiatry, and neuropsychiatry. Neurology 1994; 44:209–213.
2. Yudofsky SC, Hales RE. The reemergence of neuropsychiatry: definition and direction. J Neuropsychiatry 1989;1:1–6.
3. Damasio AR. Behavioral neurology: research and practice. Semin Neurol 1984;4:117–119.
4. Luria AR. Higher cortical functions in man. New York: Basic Books, 1980.
5. Geschwind N. Disconnexion syndromes in animals and man. Brain 1965;88:237–294, 585–644.
6. Cummings JL, Benson DF. Subcortical dementia. Review of an emerging concept. Arch Neurol 1984;41:874–879.
7. Council on Scientific Affairs Report of the Panel on Magnetic Resonance Imaging. Magnetic resonance imaging of the central nervous system. JAMA 1988;259:1211–1222.
8. Kandel ER. Nerve cells and behavior. In: Kandel ER, Schwartz JH, Jessell TM. Principles of neural science. 3rd ed. New York: Elsevier, 1991:18.
9. Miller AKH, Alston RL, Corsellis JAN. Variation with age in the volumes of grey and white matter in the cerebral hemispheres of man: measurements with an image analyzer. Neuropathol Appl Neurobiol 1980;6:119–132.
10. Yakovlev PI, Lecours AR. The myelogenetic cycles of regional maturation in the brain. In: Minkowski A, ed. Regional development of the brain in early life. Oxford: Blackwell, 1967:3–70.
11. Flechsig P. Developmental (myelogenetic) localization of the cerebral cortex in the human subject. Lancet 1901;2:1027–1029.
12. van der Knapp MS, Valk J, Bakker CJ, et al. Myelination as an expression of the functional maturity of the brain. Dev Med Child Neurol 1991;33:849–857.
13. Fletcher JM, Bohan TP, Brandt ME, et al. Cerebral white matter and cognition in hydrocephalic children. Arch Neurol 1992;49:818–824.
14. Malone MJ, Szoke MC. Neurochemical changes in white matter. Aged human brain and Alzheimer's disease. Arch Neurol 1985;42:1063–1066.
15. Awad IA, Johnson PC, Spetzler RF, Hodak JA. Incidental subcortical lesions identified on magnetic resonance imaging in the elderly. II. Postmortem pathologic correlations. Stroke 1986;17:1090–1097.
16. Harper CG, Kril JJ, Holloway RL. Brain shrinkage in chronic alcoholics: a pathological study. Br Med J 1985;290:501–505.
17. Plum F, Posner JB. Diagnosis of stupor and coma. Philadelphia: FA Davis, 1982:11–15.
18. Nauta WJH, Fiertag M. Fundamental neuroanatomy. New York: WH Freeman, 1986:126.
19. Saper CB. Diffuse cortical projection systems: anatomical organization and role in cortical function. In: Mountcastle VB, Plum F, Geiger SR, eds. Handbook of physiology. Bethesda: American Physiological Society, 1987:176–178.
20. Gur RC, Packer IK, Hungerbuhler JP, et al. Differences in the distribution of gray and white matter in the human cerebral hemispheres. Science 1980;207:1226–1228.
21. Martin JH, Jessell TM. Modality coding in the somatic sensory system. In: Kandel ER, Schwartz JH, Jessell TM. Principles of neural science. 3rd ed. New York: Elsevier, 1991:351.
22. Aston-Jones G, Rogers J, Shaver RD, Dinan TG, Moss DE. Age-impaired impulse flow from nucleus basalis to cortex. Nature 1985;318:462–464.
23. Chiappa KH. Pattern shift visual, brainstem auditory, and short-latency somatosensory evoked potentials in multiple sclerosis. Neurology 1980;30:110–123.
24. Honig LS, Ramsey RE, Sheremata WA. Event-related potential P300 in multiple sclerosis. Relation to magnetic resonance imaging and cognitive impairment. Arch Neurol 1992;49:44–50.
25. Filley CM, Franklin GM, Heaton RK, Rosenberg NL. White matter dementia: clinical disorders and implications. Neuropsychiatry Neuropsychol Behav Neurol 1989;1:239–254.
26. Trimble MR, Grant I. Psychiatric aspects of multiple sclerosis. In: Benson DF, Blumer D, eds. Psychiatric aspects of neurologic disease, vol. 2. New York: Grune & Stratton, 1982:279–298.
27. Filley CM, Gross KF. Psychosis with cerebral white matter disease. Neuropsychiatry Neuropsychol Behav Neurol 1992;5:119–125.
28. Schilder P. Zur Kenntniss der sogennanten diffusen Sklerose. Z Gesamte Neurol Psychiatr 1912;10:1–60.
29. Adams RD, Victor M. Principles of neurology. 5th ed. New York: McGraw-Hill, 1993:791–792.
30. Filley CM, Sternberg PE, Norenberg MD. Neuromyelitis optica in the elderly. Arch Neurol 1984;41:670–673.
31. Charcot JM. Lectures on the diseases of the nervous system delivered at La Salpetriere. London: New Sydenham Society, 1877.
32. Heaton RK, Nelson LM, Thompson DS, Burks JS, Franklin GM. Neuropsychological findings in relapsing-remitting and chronic-progressive multiple sclerosis. J Consult Clin Psychol 1985;53:103–110.
33. Rao SM, Hammeke TA, McQuillen MP, Khatri BO, Lloyd D. Memory disturbance in chronic progressive multiple sclerosis. Arch Neurol 1984;41:625–631.
34. Grafman J, Rao SM, Litvan I. Disorders of memory. In: Rao S, ed. Neurobehavioral aspects of multiple sclerosis. New York: Oxford, 1990:102–117.
35. Litvan I, Grafman J, Vendrell P, Martinez JM. Slowed information processing in multiple sclerosis. Arch Neurol 1988;45:281–285.
36. Franklin GM, Heaton RK, Nelson LM, Filley CM, Seibert C. Correlation of neuropsychological and magnetic resonance imaging findings in chronic/progressive multiple sclerosis. Neurology 1988;38:1826–1829.
37. Rao SM, Leo GJ, Haughton VM, St. Aubin-Faubert P, Bernardin L. Correlation of magnetic resonance imaging with neuropsychological testing in multiple sclerosis. Neurology 1989;39:161–166.
38. Arnett PA, Rao SM, Bernardin L, et al. Relationship between frontal lobe lesions and Wisconsin Card Sorting Test performance in patients with multiple sclerosis. Neurology 1994;44:420–425.
39. Folstein MF, Folstein SE, McHugh PR. "Mini-mental state." A practical method for grading the cognitive state of patients for the clinician. J Psychiatr Res 1975;12:189–198.
40. Rao SM. Neuropsychology of multiple sclerosis. A critical review. J Clin Exp Neuropsychol 1986;8:503–542.
41. Charcot JM. Lectures on the diseases of the nervous system delivered at La Salpetriere. London: New Sydenham Society, 1873.
42. Surridge D. An investigation into some psychiatric aspects of multiple sclerosis. Br J Psychiatry 1969;115:749–764.
43. Rabins PV, Brooks BR, O'Donnell P, et al. Structural brain correlates of emotional disorder in multiple sclerosis. Brain 1986;109:585–597.
44. Minden SL, Orav J, Reich P. Depression in multiple sclerosis. Gen Hosp Psychiatry 1987;9:426–434.
45. Schiffer RB, Babigian HM. Behavioral disorders in multiple sclerosis, temporal lobe epilepsy, and amyotrophic lateral sclerosis. An epidemiologic study. Arch Neurol 1984;41:1067–1069.
46. Schiffer RB, Caine ED, Bamford KA, Levy S. Depressive episodes in patients with multiple sclerosis. Am J Psychiatry 1983;140:1498–1500.
47. Honer WG, Hurwitz T, Li DKB, Palmer M, Paty DW. Temporal lobe involvement in multiple sclerosis patients with psychiatric disorders. Arch Neurol 1987;44:187–190.
48. Schiffer RB, Wineman NM, Weitkamp LR. Association between bipolar affective disorder and multiple sclerosis. Am J Psychiatry 1986;143:94–95.
49. Rabins PV. Euphoria in multiple sclerosis. In: Rao SM, ed. Neurobehavioral aspects of multiple sclerosis. New York: Oxford, 1990:180–185.
50. Binswanger O. Die Abgrenzung der allgemeinen progressiven Paralyse. Berl Klin Wochenschr 1894;31:1102–1105, 1137–1139, 1180–1186.

51. Babikian V, Ropper AH. Binswanger's disease: a review. Stroke 1987;18:2–12.
52. Garcia JH, Brown GG. Vascular dementia: neuropathologic alterations and metabolic brain changes. J Neurol Sci 1992;109:121–131.
53. Brun A, Englund E. A white matter degeneration in dementia of the Alzheimer type: a pathoanatomical study. Ann Neurol 1986;19: 253–262.
54. Gray F, Dubas F, Roullet E, Escourolle R. Leukoencephalopathy in diffuse hemorrhagic cerebral amyloid angiopathy. Ann Neurol 1985;18:54–59.
55. Ma K-C, Lundberg PO, Lilja A, Olsson Y. Binswanger's disease in the absence of chronic arterial hypertension. Acta Neuropathol 1992;83: 434–439.
56. Kertesz A, Black SE, Tokar G, Benke T, Carr T, Nicholson L. Periventricular and subcortical hyperintensities on magnetic resonance imaging: "rims, caps, and unidentified bright objects." Arch Neurol 1988;45:404–408.
57. Kinkel WR, Jacobs L, Polachini I, Bates V, Heffner RR. Subcortical arteriosclerotic encephalopathy (Binswanger's disease). Computed tomographic, nuclear magnetic resonance, and clinical correlations. Arch Neurol 1985;42:951–959.
58. Filley CM, Davis KA, Schmitz SP, et al. Neuropsychological performance and magnetic resonance imaging in Alzheimer's disease and normal aging. Neuropsychiatry Neuropsychol Behav Neurol 1989;2:81–91.
59. Hachinski VC, Potter P, Merskey H. Leuko-araiosis. Arch Neurol 1987;44:21–23.
60. Boone KB, Miller BL, Lesser IM, et al. Neuropsychological correlates of white-matter lesions in healthy elderly subjects. Arch Neurol 1992;49:549–554.
61. Boller F, Vrtunski PB, Mack JL, Kim Y. Neuropsychological correlates of hypertension. Arch Neurol 1977;34:701–705.
62. Salerno JA, Murphy DGM, Horwitz B, et al. Brain atrophy in hypertension. Hypertension 1992;20:340–348.
63. van Swieten JC, Geyskes GG, Derix MMA, et al. Hypertension in the elderly is associated with white matter lesions and cognitive decline. Ann Neurol 1991;30:825–830.
64. Coffey CE, Figiel GS, Djang WT, Saunders WB, Weiner RD. White matter hyperintensity on magnetic resonance imaging: clinical and neuroanatomic correlates in the depressed elderly. J Neuropsychiatry 1989;1:135–144.
65. Breitner JCS, Husain MM, Figiel GS, Krishnan KRR, Boyko OB. Cerebral white matter disease in late-onset paranoid psychosis. Biol Psychiatry 1990;28:266–274.
66. Geschwind N, Kaplan E. A human cerebral deconnection syndrome. Neurology 1962;12:675–685.
67. Alexander MP, Naeser MA, Palumbo CL. Correlations of subcortical CT lesion sites and aphasia profiles. Brain 1987;110:961–991.
68. Kooistra CA, Heilman KM. Memory loss from a subcortical white matter infarct. J Neurol Neurosurg Psychiatry 1988;51:866–869.
69. Bogousslavsky J, Miklossy J, Regli F, Deruaz J-P, Assal G, Delaloye B. Subcortical neglect: neuropsychological, SPECT, and neuropathological correlations with anterior choroidal artery territory infarctions. Ann Neurol 1988;23:448–452.
70. Hublet C, Demeurisse G. Pure topographical disorientation due to a deep-seated lesion with cortical remote effects. Cortex 1992;28: 123–128.
71. Nighoghossian N, Trouillas P, Vighetto A, Phillipon B. Spatial delirium following a right subcortical infarct with frontal deactivation. J Neurol Neurosurg Psychiatry 1992;55:334–335.
72. Rosenberg NL, Kleinschmidt-DeMasters BK, Davis KA, Dreisbach JN, Hormes JT, Filley CM. Toluene abuse causes diffuse central nervous system white matter changes. Ann Neurol 1988;23: 611–614.
73. Knox JW, Nelson JR. Permanent encephalopathy from toluene intoxication. N Engl J Med 1966;275:1494–1496.
74. Hormes JT, Filley CM, Rosenberg NL. Neurologic sequelae of chronic solvent vapor abuse. Neurology 1986;36:698–702.
75. Rosenberg NL, Spitz MC, Filley CM, Davis KA, Schaumburg HH. Central nervous system effects of chronic toluene abuse—clinical, brainstem evoked response and magnetic resonance imaging studies. Neurotoxicol Teratol 1988;10:489–495.
76. Filley CM, Heaton RK, Rosenberg NL. White matter dementia in chronic toluene abuse. Neurology 1990;40:532–534.
77. Lishman WA. Cerebral disorder in alcoholism. Syndromes of impairment. Brain 1981;104:1–20.
78. Victor M, Adams RD, Collins GH. The Wernicke-Korsakoff syndrome. 2nd ed. Philadelphia: FA Davis, 1989.
79. Carlen PL, Wortzman G, Holgate RC, Wilkinson DA, Rankin JG. Reversible cerebral atrophy in recently abstinent chronic alcoholics measured by computed tomography scans. Science 1978;200:1076–1078.
80. Gallucci M, Amicarelli I, Rossi A, et al. MR imaging of white matter lesions in uncomplicated chronic alcoholism. J Comput Assist Tomogr 1989;13:395–398.
81. Hansen LA, Natelson BH, Lemere C, et al. Alcohol-induced brain changes in dogs. Arch Neurol 1991;48:939–942.
82. de la Monte SM. Disproportionate atrophy of cerebral white matter in chronic alcoholics. Arch Neurol 1988;45:990–992.
83. Ron MA. Brain damage in chronic alcoholism: a neuropathological, neuroradiological and psychological review. Psychol Med 1977;7: 103–112.
84. Lee Y-Y, Nauert C, Glass JP. Treatment-related white matter changes in cancer patients. Cancer 1986;57:1473–1482.
85. Shapiro WR, Chernik NL, Posner JB. Necrotizing encephalopathy following intraventricular instillation of methotrexate. Arch Neurol 1973;28:96–102.
86. Madajewicz S, West GR, Park HC, et al. Phase II study-intraarterial BCNU therapy for metastatic brain tumors. Cancer 1981;47: 653–657.
87. Wang JJ, Pratt CB. Intrathecal arabinosyl cytosine in meningeal leukemia. Cancer 1970; 25:531–534.
88. Gutin PH, Levi JA, Wiernik PH, Walker MD. Treatment of malignant meningeal disease with intrathecal thioTEPA: a phase II study. Cancer Treat Rep 1977;61:885–887.
89. Kuzuhara S, Ohkoshi N, Kanemaru K, Hashimoto H, Nakanishi T, Tokoyura Y. Subacute leukoencephalopathy induced by carmofur, a 5-fluorouracil derivative. J Neurol 1987;234:365–370.
90. Feun LG, Wallace S, Stewart DJ, et al. Intracarotid infusion of cisdiaminedichloroplatinum in the treatment of recurrent malignant brain tumors. Cancer 1984;54:794–799.
91. Valk PE, Dillon WP. Radiation injury of the brain. AJNR 1991;12: 45–62.
92. DeAngelis LM, Delattre J-Y, Posner JB. Radiation-induced dementia in patients cured of brain metastases. Neurology 1989;39:789–796.
93. Adams RD, Kubik CS. Subacute degeneration of the brain in pernicious anemia. N Engl J Med 1944;231:1–9.
94. Strachan RW, Henderson JG. Psychiatric syndromes due to avitaminosis B12 with normal blood and marrow. Q J Med 1965:34: 303–317.
95. Smith ADM. Megaloblastic madness. Br Med J 1960;2:1840–1845.
96. Lindenbaum J, Healton EB, Savage DG, et al. Neuropsychiatric disorders caused by cobalamin deficiency in the absence of anemia or macrocytosis. N Engl J Med 1988;318:1720–1728.
97. Pincus JH, Reynolds EH, Glaser GH. Subacute combined system degeneration with folate deficiency. JAMA 1972;221:496–497.
98. Richardson JC, Chambers RA, Heywood PM. Encephalopathies of anoxia and hypoglycemia. Arch Neurol 1959;1:178–190.
99. Plum F, Posner JB, Hain RF. Delayed neurological deterioration after anoxia. Arch Intern Med 1962;110:18–25.
100. Merritt HH, Weisman AD. Primary degeneration of the corpus callosum (Marchiafava-Bignami's disease). J Neuropathol Exp Neurol 1945;4:155–163.
101. Norenberg MD, Leslie KO, Robertson AS. Association between rise of serum sodium and central pontine myelinolysis. Ann Neurol 1982;11:128–135.

102. Price BH, Mesulam M-M. Behavioral manifestations of central pontine myelinolysis. Arch Neurol 1987;44:671–673.

103. Thompson DS, Hutton JT, Stears JC, Sung JH, Norenberg M. Computerized tomography in the diagnosis of central and extrapontine myelinolysis. Arch Neurol 1981;38:243–246.

104. Navia BA, Jordan BD, Price RW. The AIDS dementia complex: I. Clinical features. Ann Neurol 1986;19:517–524.

105. Sharer L. Pathology of HIV-1 infection of the central nervous system. A review. J Neuropathol Exp Neurol 1992;51:3–11.

106. Olsen WL, Longo FM, Mills CM, Norman D. White matter disease in AIDS: findings at MR imaging. Neuroradiology 1988;169:445–448.

107. Krupp LB, Lipton RB, Swerdlow ML, Leeds NE, Llena J. Progressive multifocal leukoencephalopathy: clinical and radiographic features. Ann Neurol 1985;17:344–349.

108. Alexander MP. Traumatic brain injury. In: Benson DF, Blumer D, eds. Psychiatric aspects of neurologic disease, vol. 2. New York: Grune & Stratton, 1982:219–248.

109. Adams JH, Graham DI, Murray LS, Scott G. Diffuse axonal injury due to nonmissile head injury in humans: an analysis of 45 cases. Ann Neurol 1982;12:557–563.

110. Kelly JP, Nichols JS, Filley CM, Lillehei KO, Rubinstein D, Kleinschmidt-DeMasters BK. Concussion in sports: guidelines for the prevention of catastrophic outcome. JAMA 1991;266:2867–2869.

111. Filley CM, Cranberg LD, Alexander MP, Hart EJ. Neurobehavioral outcome after closed head injury in childhood and adolescence. Arch Neurol 1987;44:194–198.

112. Rimel RW, Giordani B, Barth JT, Boll TJ, Jane JA. Disability caused by minor head injury. Neurosurgery 1981;9:221–228.

113. Jennett B, Bond M. Assessment of outcome after severe brain damage. Lancet 1975;1:480–484.

114. Levin HS, Amparo EG, Eisenberg HM, et al. Magnetic resonance imaging and computerized tomography in relation to the neurobehavioral sequelae of mild and moderate head injuries. J Neurosurg 1987;66:706–713.

115. Bogen JE. The callosal syndromes. In: Heilman KM, Valenstein E, eds. Clinical neuropsychology. 3rd ed. New York: Oxford, 1993:337–407.

116. Gazzaniga MS, Risse GL, Springer SP, Clark E, Wilson DH. Psychologic and neurologic consequences of partial and complete cerebral commissurotomy. Neurology 1975;25:10–15.

117. Adams RD, Fisher CM, Hakim S, Ojemann RG, Sweet WH. Symptomatic occult hydrocephalus with "normal" cerebrospinal fluid pressure. N Engl J Med 1965;273:117–126.

118. DelBigio MR. Neuropathological changes caused by hydrocephalus. Acta Neuropathol 1993;85:573–585.

119. Sarhaddi S, Bravo E, Cyrus AE. Gliomatosis cerebri: a case report and review of the literature. South Med J 1973;66:883–888.

120. Couch JR, Weiss SA. Gliomatosis cerebri. Report of four cases and review of the literature. Neurology 1974;24:504–511.

121. Heilman KM, Sypert GW. Korsakoff's syndrome resulting from bilateral fornix lesions. Neurology 1977;27:490–493.

122. Menkes JH. The leukodystrophies. N Engl J Med 1990;322:54–55.

123. Austin J, Armstrong D, Fouch S, et al. Metachromatic leukodystrophy (MLD). VIII. MLD in adults; diagnosis and pathogenesis. Arch Neurol 1968;18:225–240.

124. Hyde TM, Ziegler JC, Weinberger DR. Psychiatric disturbances in metachromatic leukodystrophy. Insights into the neurobiology of psychosis. Arch Neurol 1992;49:401–406.

125. Shapiro EG, Lockman LA, Knopman D, Krivit W. Characteristics of the dementia in late-onset metachromatic leukodystrophy. Neurology 1994;44:662–665.

126. Waltz G, Harik SI, Kaufman B. Adult metachromatic leukodystrophy. Value of computed tomographic scanning and magnetic resonance imaging of the brain. Arch Neurol 1987;44:225–227.

127. Moser HW, Moser AE, Singh I, O'Neill BP. Adrenoleukodystrophy: survey of 300 cases: biochemistry, diagnosis, and therapy. Ann Neurol 1984;16:628–641.

128. Powell H, Tindall R, Schultz P, Paa D, O'Brien J, Lampert P. Adrenoleukodystrophy. Electron microscopic findings. Arch Neurol 1975;32:250–260.

129. Kumar AJ, Rosenbaum AE, Naidu S, et al. Adrenoleukodystrophy: correlating MR imaging with CT. Radiology 1987;165:497–504.

130. Crome L, Hanefeld F, Patrick D, Wilson J. Late onset globoid cell leucodystrophy. Brain 1973;96:841–848.

131. Norman RM, Oppenheimer DR, Tingey AH. Histological and chemical findings in Krabbe's leucodystrophy. J Neurol Neurosurg Psychiatry 1961;24:223–232.

132. Seitelberger F. Pelizaeus-Merzbacher disease. In: Vinken PJ, Bruyn GW, eds. Handbook of clinical neurology, vol. 10. New York: Elsevier, 1970:150–202.

133. Lowenberg K, Hill TS. Diffuse sclerosis with preserved myelin islands. Arch Neurol Psychiatry 1933;29:1232–1245.

134. Adachi M, Schneck L, Cara J, Volk BW. Spongy degeneration of the central nervous system (van Bogaert and Bertrand type; Canavan's disease). Hum Pathol 1973;4:331–347.

135. Russo LS, Aron A, Anderson PJ. Alexander's disease: a report and reappraisal. Neurology 1976;26:607–614.

136. Malamud N. Neuropathology of phenylketonuria. J Neuropathol Exp Neurol 1966;25:254–268.

137. Silberman J, Dancis J, Feigin I. Neuropathological observations in maple syrup urine disease. Arch Neurol 1961;5:21–33.

138. Adams RD, Victor M. Principles of neurology. 5th ed. New York: McGraw-Hill, 1993:545.

139. Laurence KM. Neurological and intellectual sequelae of hydrocephalus. Arch Neurol 1969;20:73–81.

140. Dennis M, Hendrick EB, Hoffman HJ, Humphreys RP. Language of hydrocephalic children and adolescents. J Clin Exp Neuropsychol 1987;9:593–621.

141. Chiarello C. A house divided? Cognitive functioning with callosal agenesis. Brain Lang 1980;11:128–158.

142. DeReuck J, Chatta AS, Richardson EP. Pathogenesis and evolution of periventricular leukomalacia in infancy. Arch Neurol 1972;27:229–236.

143. Young RSK, Hernandez MJ, Yagel SK. Selective reduction of blood flow to white matter during hypotension in newborn dogs: a possible mechanism of periventricular leukomalacia. Ann Neurol 1982;12:445–448.

144. Johnson RT, Griffin DE, Gendelman HE. Postinfectious encephalomyelitis. Semin Neurol 1985;5:180–190.

145. Fenichel GM. Neurological complications of immunization. Ann Neurol 1982;12:119–128.

146. Johnson RT, Griffin DE, Hirsch RL, et al. Measles encephalomyelitis—clinical and immunological studies. N Engl J Med 1984;310:137–141.

147. Epperson LW, Whitaker JN, Kapila A. Cranial MRI in acute disseminated encephalomyelitis. Neurology 1988;38:332–333.

148. Coxe WS, Luxe SA. Acute hemorrhagic leukoencephalitis. J Neurosurg 1963;20:584–596.

149. Billmire ME, Meyers PA. Serious head injury in infants: accident or abuse? Pediatrics 1985;75:340–342.

150. Fletcher JM, Copeland DR. Neurobehavioral effects of central nervous system prophylactic treatment of cancer in children. J Clin Exp Neuropsychol 1988;10:495–538.

151. Price R, Jamieson P. The central nervous system in childhood leukemia II. Subacute leukoencephalopathy. Cancer 1975;35:306–318.

152. Snider WD, Johnson EM. Neurotrophic molecules. Ann Neurol 1989;26:489–506.

153. Prineas JW, Connell F. Remyelination in multiple sclerosis. Ann Neurol 1979;5:22–31.

154. Ghatak NR, Leshner RT, Price AC, Felton WL. Remyelination in the human central nervous system. J Neuropathol Exp Neurol 1989;48:507–518.

155. Moll C, Mourre C, Lazdunski M, Ulrich J. Increase of sodium

channels in demyelinated lesions in multiple sclerosis. Brain Res 1991;556:311–316.

156. Kinsbourne M. The minor cerebral hemisphere as a source of aphasic speech. Arch Neurol 1971;25:302–306.

157. Fischer M, Ryan SB, Dobyns WB. Mechanisms of interhemispheric transfer and patterns of cognitive function in acallosal patients of normal intelligence. Arch Neurol 1992;49:271–277.

158. Grotta JC. Current medical and surgical therapy for cerebrovascular disease. N Engl J Med 1987;317:1505–1516.

159. Garraway WM, Whisnant JP, Furlan AJ, Phillips LH, Kurland LT, O'Fallon WM. The declining incidence of stroke. N Engl J Med 1979;300:449–452.

160. Weiner HL, Hafler DA. Immunotherapy of multiple sclerosis. Ann Neurol 1988;23:211–222.

161. Beck WS. Cobalamin and the nervous system. N Engl J Med 1988;318:1752–1754.

162. Schmitt FA, Bigley JW, McKinnis R, et al. Neuropsychological outcome of zidovudine (AZT) treatment of patients with AIDS and AIDS-related complex. N Engl J Med 1988;319:1573–1578.

163. Centerwall WR, Centerwall SA, Armon V, Mann LB. Phenylketonuria. II. Results of treatment of infants and young children. J Pediatr 1961;59:102–118.

164. Committee on Nutrition, American Academy of Pediatrics. Special diets for infants with inborn errors of amino acid metabolism. Pediatrics 1976;57:783–792.

165. Murray TJ. Amantadine therapy for fatigue in multiple sclerosis. Can J Neurol Sci 1985;12:251–254.

166. Holmes VF, Fernandez F, Levy JK. Psychostimulant response in AIDS-related complex patients. J Clin Psychiatry 1989;50:5–8.

167. Gualtieri T, Chandler M, Coons TB, Brown LT. Amantadine: a new clinical profile for traumatic brain injury. Clin Neuropharmacol 1989;4:258–270.

168. Graff-Radford NR, Godersky JC, Jones MP. Variables predicting surgical outcome in symptomatic hydrocephalus in the elderly. Neurology 1989;39:1601–1604.

169. Shapiro EG, Lipton ME, Krivit W. White matter dysfunction and its neuropsychological correlates: a longitudinal study of a case of metachromatic leukodystrophy treated with bone marrow transplant. J Clin Exp Neuropsychol 1992;14:610–624.

170. Prigatano GP, Fordyce DJ, Zeiner HK, Roueche JR, Pepping M, Word BC. Neuropsychological rehabilitation after closed head injury in young adults. J Neurol Neurosurg Psychiatry 1984;47:505–513.

171. Thompson LL, Filley CM. A preliminary study of outcome after cognitive rehabilitation. Journal of Neurologic Rehabilitation 1989;3:117–127.

172. Albert ML, Feldman RG, Willis AL. The "subcortical dementia" of progressive supranuclear palsy. J Neurol Neurosurg Psychiatry 1974;37:121–130.

173. HcHugh PR, Folstein MF. Psychiatric syndromes of Huntington's chorea: a clinical and phenomenological study. In: Benson DF, Blumer D, eds. Psychiatric aspects of neurologic disease, vol. 1. Orlando: Grune & Stratton, 1975:267–285.

174. Albert ML. Subcortical dementia. In: Katzman R, Terry RD, Bick KL, eds. Alzheimer's disease: senile dementia and related disorders. New York: Raven, 1978:173–180.

175. Mayeux R, Stern Y, Rosen J, Benson DF. Is subcortical dementia a recognizable clinical entity? Ann Neurol 1983;14:278–283.

176. Whitehouse PJ. The concept of subcortical and cortical dementia: another look. Ann Neurol 1986;19:1–6.

177. Pillon B, Dubois B, Lhermitte F, Agid Y. Heterogeneity of cognitive impairment in progressive supranuclear palsy, Parkinson's disease, and Alzheimer's disease, Neurology 1986;36:1179–1185.

178. Huber SJ, Shuttleworth EC, Freidenberg DL. Neuropsychological differences between the dementias of Alzheimer's and Parkinson's disease. Arch Neurol 1989;46:1287–1291.

179. Cummings JL. Intellectual impairment in Parkinson's disease: clinical, pathologic, and biochemical correlates. J Geriatr Psychiatry Neurol 1988;1:24–36.

180. Medalia A, Isaacs-Glaberman K, Scheinberg IH. Neuropsychological impairment in Wilson's disease. Arch Neurol 1988;45:502–504.

181. Skre H. Spino-cerebellar ataxia in western Norway. Clin Genet 1974;6:265–288.

182. Ishii N, Nishahara Y, Imamura T. Why do frontal lobe symptoms predominate in vascular dementia with lacunes? Neurology 1986;36:340–345.

183. Caine ED. Pseudodementia: current concepts and future directions. Arch Gen Psychiatry 1981;38:1359–1364.

184. Famuyiwa OO, Eccleston D, Donalson AA, Garside RF. Tardive dyskinesia and dementia. Br J Psychiatry 1979;135:500–504.

185. Katzman R. Alzheimer's disease. N Engl J Med 1986;314: 964–973.

186. Hecaen H, Albert ML. Human neuropsychology. New York:John Wiley & Sons, 1978:354–378.

187. Cummings JL, Benson DF. Subcortical mechanisms and human thought. In: Cummings JL, ed. Subcortical dementia. New York: Oxford University Press 1990:251–259.

188. Alexander GE, DeLong MR, Strick PL. Parallel organization of functionally segregated circuits linking basal ganglia and cortex. Annu Rev Neurosci 1986;9:357–381.

189. Mesulam M-M. Attention, confusional states, and neglect. In: Mesulam M-M, ed. Principles of behavioral neurology. Philadelphia: FA Davis, 1985:125–168.

190. Filley CM, Heaton RK, Nelson LM, Burks JS, Franklin GM. A comparison of dementia in Alzheimer's disease and multiple sclerosis. Arch Neurol 1989;46:157–161.

191. Waxman SG. Conduction in myelinated, unmyelinated, and demyelinated fibers. Arch Neurol 1977;34:585–589.

192. Metter EJ, Mazziotta JC, Itabashi HH, Mankovich NJ, Phelps ME, Kuhl DE. Comparison of glucose metabolism, x-ray CT, and post-mortem data in a patient with multiple cerebral infarcts. Neurology 1985;35:1695–1701.

193. Feeney DM, Baron J-C. Diaschisis. Stroke 1986;17:817–830.

194. Kirshner H. Behavioral neurology: a practical approach. New York: Churchill Livingstone, 1986.

195. Filley CM, Kelly JP. Neurobehavioral effects of focal subcortical lesions. In: Cummings JL, ed. Subcortical dementia. New York: Oxford University Press, 1990:59–70.

196. Olmos-Lau N, Ginsberg MD, Geller JB. Aphasia in multiple sclerosis. Neurology 1977;27:623–626.

197. James W. The principles of psychology, vol. 2. New York: Holt, Rinehart & Winston, 1890.

198. Geschwind N. Disorders of attention: a frontier in neuropsychology. Philos Trans R Soc Lond 1982;298:173–185.

199. Mesulam M-M. A cortical network for directed attention and unilateral neglect. Ann Neurol 1981;10:309–325.

200. Mesulam M-M. Large-scale neurocognitive networks and distributed processing for attention, language, and memory. Ann Neurol 1990;28:597–613.

201. Craik FIM, Byrd M. Aging and cognitive deficits. The role of attentional resources. In: Craik FIM, Trehub S, eds. Aging and cognitive processes. New York: Plenum, 1982:191–211.

202. Hasher L, Zacks RT. Automatic and effortful processes in memory. J Exp Psychol [Gen] 1979;108:356–388.

203. Jacewicz MM, Hartley AA. Age differences in the speed of cognitive operations: resolution of inconsistent findings. J Gerontol 1987;42: 86–88.

204. van Gorp WG, Mitrushina M, Cummings JL, Satz P, Modesitt J. Normal aging and the subcortical encephalopathy of AIDS. Neuropsychiatry Neuropsychol Behav Neurol 1989;2:5–20.

205. Junque C, Pujol J, Vendrell P, et al. Leuko-araiosis on magnetic resonance imaging and speed of mental processing. Arch Neurol 1990;47:151–156.

206. Rourke BP. Syndrome of nonverbal learning disabilities: the final

common pathway of white-matter disease/dysfunction? Clin Neuropsychol 1987;1:209–234.

207. John ER, Tang Y, Brill AB, Young R, Ono K. Double-labeled metabolic maps of memory. Science 1986;233:1167–1175.

208. Damasio H, Damasio A. Lesion analysis in neuropsychology. New York: Oxford, 1989.

209. Lashley KS. Brain mechanisms and intelligence. Chicago: University of Chicago Press, 1929.

210. Fazio F, Perani D, Gilardi MC, et al. Metabolic impairment in human amnesia: a PET study of memory networks. J Cereb Blood Flow Metab 1992;12:353–358.

211. Prichard JW, Brass LM. New anatomical and functional imaging methods. Ann Neurol 1992;32:395–400.

212. Cummings JL. Clinical neuropsychiatry. Orlando: Grune & Stratton, 1985:1–4.

39

TRAUMATIC BRAIN INJURY

Jordan Grafman and Andres Salazar

Traumatic brain injury (TBI) is the leading cause of death and disability in young adults today; every 5 minutes one person dies and another is permanently disabled from TBI (1). Largely because it affects the young, the total economic cost of TBI has been estimated at over $25 billion per year. The incidence of TBI requiring hospitalization is about 200/100,000. Yet, it has been generally ignored by psychiatrists and neurologists, perhaps as no other subject in these specialties (relative to its incidence). So little is known about the short- and long-term neurobehavioral consequences of TBI that the entire field is a fertile ground for basic, pharmacological, acute clinical, behavioral, and neurorehabilitation research. Although basic laboratory, acute clinical, and prevention research may be more likely to lead to long-term solutions, the need for immediate practical clinical research into the behavioral and rehabilitation problems of TBI patients is particularly pressing at this time, for both economic and humanitarian reasons. Additionally, head-injured patients with focal lesions (due to either gunshot/fragment wounds or contusions/bleeds) continue to offer unique opportunities for studying specific aspects of brain function.

In this chapter, we review the current understanding of the pathogenesis of TBI and its neurobehavioral consequences, and then outline a practical management approach to the TBI patient based on that knowledge.

PATHOPHYSIOLOGY OF TBI

TBI is a dynamic process. Not only does the pathological picture continue to evolve over the first few hours and days after trauma, often with devastating secondary injury, but the physiological and clinical aspects of the recovery process itself can continue for a period of years. Thus, the notion of a "dynamic prognosis" requiring intermittent revision is especially relevant to the head-injured patient, both because of the long period of recovery, and because the many poorly understood variables involved still make outcome prediction as much of an art as a science.

In addition, the TBI victim often manifests a multitude of systemic abnormalities, not only as consequence of concomitant trauma elsewhere in the body, but secondary to the brain injury itself. Changes in nutrition (2), cardiopulmonary status (3, 4), circulating catecholamines (5), and coagulation (6) are among those described.

Pathology

The pathology of closed head injury (CHI) can be reduced to a four-component classification (7). Three parallel components were initially identified: (*a*) focal injury, (*b*) diffuse axonal injury (DAI), and (*c*) superimposed hypoxia/ischemia. Later, diffuse microvascular injury with loss of autoregulation was implicated as playing an important role in the acute stage of moderate and severe head injury. All of these pathological features have been reproduced in animal models of angular acceleration without impact (8).

FOCAL INJURY

Focal contusions often occur under the site of impact and thus result in focal neurological deficits referable to that area (e.g., aphasia, hemiparesis). The most common location for contusions after acceleration/deceleration injury is in the orbitofrontal and anterior temporal lobes, where brain tissue lies next to bony edges. Thus, a relatively typical pathological picture is often seen in CHI, and the most troubling clinical sequelae are behavioral and cognitive abnormalities that may be referable to the frontal and temporal lobe injury. Subdural hematomas are common occurrences, with rapid decelerations such as occur with impact after a fall, especially in the aged, and are usually due to rupture of bridging veins. Recent studies suggest that delays longer than 4 hours in the surgical management of hematomas significantly worsens prognosis. Delayed hematomas as well as bleeding into contusions are particularly important in the so-called "talk and die" patient, who may initially appear to be at low risk but then deteriorates unexpectedly (9).

DIFFUSE AXONAL INJURY

Diffuse axonal injury (DAI) is one of the most important causes of persistent severe neurological deficit in CHI. Originally described as a "shearing" injury of axons, it was characterized by axonal "retraction" balls microscopically in the hemispheric white matter, corpus callosum, and brainstem (10, 11). Recent work with *mild to moderate* fluid-percussion injury in animal models has shown that the typical light microscopic histopathology of DAI may not emerge until 12–24 hours postinjury. The only early abnormality is a relatively subtle focal intra-axonal disruption seen on electron microscopy, with an intact axon sheath. This leads to a disturbance of axonal flow, accumulation of transport material with axonal ballooning proximal to the injury, and then eventual *delayed* severing of axons several hours later (12, 13). The role of alterations in calcium metabolism at the injured site on the axon may be particularly important. One obvious clinical implication of these findings is that there may be a potential 12–24 hour window of therapeutic opportunity postinjury during which future treatments may prevent total axonal disruption. Another important conclusion from these studies is that DAI can be demonstrated after "minor" head injury, and occurs even in the absence of morphopathological change in any other vascular, neural, or glial elements. This confirms earlier uncontrolled pathological studies in humans and makes such axonal damage the most likely organic basis for the "postconcussion syndrome" and for the cumulative effects of repeated concussion, as seen in some boxers (14, 15).

Interestingly, one major feature of the pathology of dementia pugilistica is the presence of neurofibrillary tangles (NFT), but not Alzheimer plaques. NFT in Alzheimer's disease, and in other conditions such as Guamanian amyotrophic lateral sclerosis (ALS), have been postulated to result from abnormalities in axonal flow, in the latter case probably related to aberrant calcium metabolism (16). Thus, some of the challenges posed in these seemingly disparate areas of neuropsychiatry may eventually find common ground and similar solutions.

HYPOXIA-ISCHEMIA

The classic pathology of hypoxia-ischemia, involving mainly the hippocampus and the vascular border zones of the brain, is all too often superimposed on the other pathological features that are more specific for TBI. The traumatized brain is particularly sensitive to hypoxia-ischemia, and the relationship is probably more than just additive. When present, such pathology, including the concomitant brain swelling, can become a major determinant of ultimate clinical outcome; the most significant improvements in the management of the TBI patient have resulted from recognition of the importance of this component and its prevention.

DIFFUSE MICROVASCULAR DAMAGE

This finding has also been implicated as a major component of both closed and penetrating TBI (17, 18). Diffuse perivascular damage with astrocytic footplate swelling is a prominent feature at both the light and electron microscopic

levels within minutes of high-velocity gunshot wound in nonhuman primates. In CHI the vascular response appears to be biphasic. Depending on the severity of the trauma, early changes include an initial transient systemic hypertension (probably related to release of catecholamines), an early loss of cerebrovascular autoregulation, with a decreased response to changes in CO_2, and a transient breakdown of the blood-brain barrier (BBB), probably because of endothelial changes (although endothelial tight junctions may remain intact early). The loss of autoregulation makes the brain particularly susceptible to fluctuations in systemic blood pressure. For example, systemic hypertension can increase the risk of hyperemia and brain swelling, more commonly seen in younger patients. The early dysfunction of the BBB results in rapid swelling of perivascular astrocytes, which peaks at about 1 hour postinjury but begins to recover by 6 hours. Later endothelial changes include formation of intraluminal microvilli or blebs and craters, which peak at about 6 hours postinjury but can persist as long as 6 days.

Although the clinical significance of these changes is still not known, they are probably related to the loss of autoregulation, to the altered vascular sensitivity to circulating neurotransmitters, and to cerebral edema. Importantly, very similar endothelial changes can be induced in nontraumatized animals by applying various superoxide radical generators to the intact pial surface. Both cyclo-oxygenase inhibitors such as indomethacin and oxygen-free-radical scavengers such as superoxide dismutase will prevent or reverse these arteriolar changes experimentally in trauma models, suggesting that such drugs may eventually play a role in the management of TBI (19).

Mechanisms of Secondary Tissue Injury

Over the past decade, *delayed* secondary injury at the cellular level has come to be recognized as a major contributor to the accumulated tissue loss after TBI. As alluded to earlier, a cascade of physiological, vascular, and biochemical events is set in motion in injured tissue. This includes changes in arachidonic acid metabolites such as the prostaglandins and the leukotrienes (20), the formation of oxygen-free radicals (21), changes in neuropeptides (22), electrolytes such as calcium and magnesium (23), excitatory neurotransmitters such as glutamate or acetylcholine (24), lymphokines such as interleukin-1, or lactic acid (25) (Table 39.1). These products can result in progressive secondary injury to otherwise viable brain tissue through a number of mechanisms: e.g., by producing further ischemia or altering vascular reactivity, by producing brain swelling (edema or hyperemia), by injuring neurons and glia directly or activating macrophages that result in such injury, or by establishing conditions favorable to secondary infection. In other words, much of the ultimate brain loss after TBI may not be due to the injury itself, but to an uncontrolled vicious cycle of biochemical events set in motion by the trauma.

Table 39.1. Secondary Injury in TBI

Hypoxia/ischemia
Mass effect
   Delayed hematoma
  Brain swelling
    Cerebral edema
    Hyperemia
  Hydrocephalus
Infection
Potential cellular mechanisms
  Phospholipid metabolism
    Lipid peroxidation (arachidonic acid chain)
    Prostaglandins, leukotrienes
    Platelet-activating factor (PAF)
  Oxygen-free radicals
    Free iron catalysis
  Excitotoxic mechanisms
    Glutamate (NMDA) receptors
    Acetylcholine
  Neuropeptides
    Endorphins (dynorphin)
    Thyrotropin-releasing hormone (TRH)
  Calcium and magnesium metabolism abnormalities
  CNS lactic acidosis
  Axonal flow abnormalities

The control of this complex series of cellular events remains one of the most important challenges in the acute management of head injury today. These events constitute a potential window of opportunity during which brain swelling and nerve cell death could be prevented by pharmacological or other intervention in the first few hours after an injury.

ARACHIDONIC ACID METABOLITES

As one of the breakdown products of phospholipids, arachidonic acid (AA) is particularly plentiful in the brain, and its metabolites are likely to play a role in secondary brain injury. AA is metabolized through two major pathways, the cyclooxygenase path, leading to the formation of prostaglandins, and the lipoxygenase path, leading to the formation of leukotrienes. Both pathways may play a role, but the cyclooxygenase pathway appears to be the most important in TBI; among the metabolites that may be most active are prostaglandin E_2 and thromboxane. Various animal studies have demonstated marked elevations in cerebrospinal fluid (CSF) and brain prostaglandins within minutes of injury (26, 27). Theoretically, these metabolites could produce secondary injury by inducing vasospasm, thrombosis, and/or edema. However, therapeutic trials using cyclooxygenase inhibitors in animals have been disappointing, particularly when they are administered more than a few minutes after the injury (19, 28).

OXYGEN-FREE RADICALS

Oxygen-free radicals are also very active species biologically, and have been shown to be produced early in ischemic and traumatic tissue injury, both in the CNS and elsewhere (21). The superoxide radical (O^*) is formed through a variety of mechanisms, including both the xanthine oxidase and the cyclooxygenase pathways, and results in tissue injury in its own right by combining directly with cellular elements. However, when combined with its own breakdown product, hydrogen peroxide, in the presence of free iron it forms the hydroxyl radical, OH^*, which is even more destructive. The hydroxyl radical's affinity for the abundant lipids in brain results in lipid peroxidation, with further release of arachidonic acid. A vicious cycle ensues in which more free radicals are produced through the cyclooxygenase pathway, along with prostaglandins, overwhelming natural superoxide scavenging mechanisms. The continued presence of free iron is essential for this vicious cycle, thus providing one likely explanation for the toxicity of free blood in TBI patients, including its possible relationship to posttraumatic epilepsy.

Pharmacological intervention to reduce the formation of such radicals and/or to scavenge those already formed would be expected to reduce ultimate tissue injury, and the complexity of the biochemical events involved provides several potential therapeutic avenues. Animal models have confirmed this potential benefit in several systems. These include the use of steroids (especially the nonglucocorticoid 21-aminosteroids or "lazaroids") to inhibit lipid peroxidation and the release of arachidonate (29); cyclooxygenase inhibitors to block prostaglandin formation; xanthine oxidase inhibitors such as allopurinol; iron chelators such as desferroxamine (30); enzymes such as superoxide dismutase and catalase (19); and various other free radical scavengers such as mannitol and tocopherol.

Excitotoxins

Another potential mechanism of secondary injury that has received increasing attention, particularly in the stroke and ischemia literature, is the role of excitotoxins, and especially of agonists of the NMDA subclass of glutamate receptors (24). Theoretically, the sustained release of excess amounts of such naturally occurring neurotransmitters after an injury can lead to eventual neuronal death. The mechanisms for this effect are not yet clear, but they may involve alterations in calcium and magnesium metabolism and activation of various enzyme systems. Among these might be phospholipase A, with consequent release of arachidonic acid and activation of the superoxide cycle discussed earlier. Experimental therapeutic interventions aimed at the excitotoxin mechanism include NMDA receptor antagonists such as dextromethorphan or MK-801 and acetylcholine antagonists such as scopolamine (31).

Other endogenous agents that have received attention in recent years are various neuropeptides such as the endorphins (particularly dynorphin) and TRH. However, both animal and clinical studies of opiate antagonists such as naloxone and its analogues, have been disappointing, although TRH and its analogues still hold some promise (22, 32).

MANAGEMENT

Acute Cases

INITIAL EVALUATION AND RESUSCITATION IN SEVERE TBI

Acute management of TBI is primarily directed at the prevention of secondary injury, especially that related to hypoxia/ischemia or to expanding mass lesions. An organized team approach is essential to accomplish this goal, from pre-hospital, through intensive care unit (ICU) and postacute care. The cornerstone of early neuropsychiatric evaluation is the use of the Glasgow coma scale score (GCS), along with checks of lateralization, brainstem function, and pupillary response; a system for easily recording sequential changes in these and other vital parameters is an integral part of trauma care (33). Although the GCS has been criticized for its simplicity, it has proved to be very reproducible across individual examiners and institutions. Accordingly, it serves as a solid basis for evaluation of potential deterioration over time. More detailed neuropsychiatric examinations are probably not warranted until the patient is well stabilized in the ICU. A history from witnesses, particularly with regard to the onset of coma, is important not only for decisions on acute care, but for long-term prognosis. For example, the presence of an initial "lucid" or "semi-lucid" interval in a now-comatose patient suggests a possible hematoma requiring prompt surgery. At the same time, it makes severe diffuse axonal injury unlikely and points to a relatively favorable prognosis, provided there is no further secondary damage.

The importance of cardiopulmonary resuscitation (CPR) and management in TBI care cannot be overstated; airway and shock management should be the top priority in any trauma patient. Superimposed hypoxia/ischemia can be the single most important determinant of ultimate outcome in severely head-injured patients. We know from animal experiments that the traumatized brain is particularly sensitive to hypoxia/ischemia. In addition, levels of hypercarbia tolerated by the normal brain can lead to critical marginal increases in intracranial pressure (ICP) after TBI. As noted previously, among the most important improvements in TBI patient care over the past decade has been the introduction of emergency care and transport systems that include paramedic training in early, on-site fluid resuscitation and intubation.

The comatose TBI patient is often hypoxic or hypercarbic, even though he or she may appear to be ventilating normally. Patients in coma (GCS < 8) should thus be intubated and hyperventilated, if possible, to a pCO_2 of 25–30 (but preferably not below that level for more than brief periods). Sedation with morphine 4–12 mg IV every 2–4 hours to prevent systemic hypertension; or paralysis with pancuronium bromide 4 mg every 2–4 hours should be used as needed. The stomach should be emptied to prevent aspiration. Immobilization of the head in the plane of the body is advisable, not only because of the possibility of associated cervical fracture (about 5%), but for airway maintenance and prevention of venous occlusion, which might raise ICP. Elevation of the head will further facilitate cranial venous return.

Shock should suggest the possibility of hemorrhage elsewhere in the body. Fluid resuscitation should rely on normal saline or Ringer's lactate solution, but TBI patients should not be overly hydrated; central venous pressure monitoring can be helpful in this regard. Dextrose and water should be avoided, not only because it is hypotonic, but because of the potential for increased lactic acidosis and cerebral necrosis in the hypoxic/ischemic patient with elevated blood sugars (34). Although formal studies have not been done on this latter issue in head-injured patients, we prefer to avoid maintenance with any dextrose solutions in the early acute phase. In addition to standard laboratory tests, evaluation for coagulopathies with platelet count, PT/PTT, thrombin time, fibrinogen, and fibrinogen split products may also be indicated (6).

RADIOLOGIC EXAMINATION

Computerized tomography (CT) has become standard in the management of mass lesions in the head-injured patient and should be utilized when available in all patients with GCS less than 12 ("does not obey commands") or when focal signs accompany a mild head injury. This should be done as soon as possible after the patient has been resuscitated and stabilized. As noted before, delays of more than 4 hours postinjury in evacuation of hematomas have been associated with significant deterioration in outcome. Comatose patients, however, must remain accompanied by a physician or critical care nurse; quite often a "stabilized" patient arrests or suffers irreversible brain damage because of a simple airway problem in the elevator on the way to the CT suite. The usefulness of magnetic resonance imaging (MRI) in the acute situation is limited in part by the difficulty of managing the comatose patient in most scanners.

In conscious patients with mild confusion and no lateralizing signs, a skull x-ray and observation may be sufficient. However, a fracture on x-ray markedly increases the risk of a surgical lesion and is indication for a CT scan even in the alert TBI patient. In any case, a high index of suspicion for delayed hematomas is imperative. One study found that the large differences in mortality of TBI patients found across a variety of hospitals with different resources was accounted for not by the high-risk ICU patient, but by deterioration of patients initially obeying commands and considered to be at "low" risk (35).

INTENSIVE CARE UNIT

Once a surgical mass lesion has been treated or excluded, the comatose patient should be managed in the intensive care unit. The avoidance of secondary insults to the brain remains the principal goal of therapy. The same principles of care and treatment just given for earlier stages of care are generally continued, and, as before, organization, training, and adherence to fairly simple principles are the mainstay of care.

INTRACRANIAL PRESSURE MONITORING

Although many physicians, particularly neurologists, may be reluctant to give up the neurological examination as the principal measure of patient progress, recent studies suggest that the ICP, which is one determinant of cerebral perfusion pressure, is a more sensitive parameter. For example, the classic Cushing triad has been shown to occur less than 25% of the time in patients with ICP > 30 mm Hg, a level that almost invariably proves fatal if not controlled (36). Yet it is much easier to prevent a rise to that level by treating when the patient is at 15 mm Hg, than it is to bring ICP down from a level of 25-30 mm Hg. ICP has repeatedly been shown to correlate significantly with outcome, and its monitoring is increasingly used in the care of the comatose TBI patient. In one recent study, survival was 92% for patients with their ICP controlled, as opposed to 17% for those without their ICP controlled (37). The particular monitoring technique used is determined by the neurosurgeon and the facilities available. Choices include an intraventricular catheter, a subarachnoid screw, or fiberoptic epidural transducers.

A relatively simple algorithm in use for treating ICP elevations is the therapeutic intensity level (TIL). It has the advantage of also providing a standard measure of severity of ICP elevations in TBI patients. The TIL outlines an orderly increase in therapeutic vigor from simple sedation through barbiturate coma. Although treatment is always individualized for each patient, a new level of therapy is generally instituted when the previous level has failed to control ICP below 20 mm Hg. Each specific therapy is assigned a point value; the TIL score at a specific time is the sum of points for the interventions in use at that time. Thus, a patient with an ICP of 15 at a TIL of 12 is quite different from a patient with the same ICP at a TIL of 3. It should be emphasized, however, that using the TIL algorithm must not replace entertaining the possibility that progressive ICP elevations may also occur because of surgical lesions such as delayed hematoma, or hydrocephalus. Similarly, seizures, hyponatremia, and airway problems will raise the ICP.

Barbiturate coma is the last step in the recommended nonsurgical control of ICP, and has recently been confirmed to improve outcome in patients with otherwise uncontrolled ICP. In a recent large controlled study, patients under age 45 who were randomized to barbiturate were almost twice as likely to have ICP controlled; in the absence of cardiovascular risks, barbiturate therapy was over five times as likely to control ICP as was nonbarbiturate therapy (37). Barbiturate coma is induced with pentobarbital at an initial loading dose of of 10 mg/kg IV over 30 minutes. An additional 5 mg/kg is then given every hour for three doses, always with close monitoring of blood pressure. Serum levels should then be maintained at 3–4 mg/100 mL with doses of about 1 mg/kg/hr.

MEDICAL THERAPY FOR PREVENTION OF SECONDARY INJURY

Specific medical therapy aimed at minimizing secondary injury is still in its infancy. Ideally, in this context active clinical research begs to be integrated with clinical care. Such treatments should generally be started as soon as possible after the injury, preferably even before the patient goes to surgery or the ICU. Mannitol is the most valuable of the agents presently available, perhaps because in addition to its osmotic effects, it is also an oxygen-free radical scavenger. The usual initial dose is 1 g/kg in the adult. Patients are then maintained on .25 g boluses every 4 hours as necessary to control ICP (see above) as long as serum osmolarity is under 310. Some surgeons advocate the continued use of low-dose mannitol. Other diuretics such as furosemide are still used by some practitioners in specific situations.

Corticosteroids for acute TBI are still overprescribed; about 42% of over 1000 neurosurgeons responding to a recent U.S. Army survey report using steroids routinely in head-injured patients. Nevertheless, several recent, well-conducted, controlled studies have failed to show any benefit of steroids at various doses, and other studies have shown a deleterious effect on the metabolism of the TBI patient (38). Consequently, we do *not* recommend the use of steroids in these patients. However, nonglucocorticoid steroids (the "lazaroids") currently under investigation may offer a useful approach in the near future. Other experimental agents discussed earlier may enter the therapeutic armamentarium in the near future.

POSTTRAUMATIC EPILEPSY

The overall risk of epilepsy in patients with closed head injury is relatively small: 2–5% overall, and about 11% for patients with severe CHI (39). Some studies, however, have shown a higher incidence in patients with depressed skull fracture (15%), hematoma (31%), or penetrating brain wounds (50%) (33, 40). In all cases, the risk decreases markedly as time passes. Although the relative risk of developing epilepsy after penetrating head injury (PHI) is still 25 times higher than the normal age-matched population at 10–15 years postinjury, most patients with PHI can be 95% certain of remaining seizure-free if they have no seizures for the first 3 years postinjury (41).

The ongoing debate over the use of prophylactic antiepileptic drugs in head-injured patients must be separated into two questions: (*a*) Are AEDs indicated in a patient with posttraumatic epilepsy (PTE)?; and (*b*) Do prophylactic AEDs prevent the onset of PTE? In light of data suggesting that most patients with one posttraumatic seizure will have recurrent seizures for some time, most clinicians reply yes to the first question. The use of prophylactic anticonvulsants to prevent the onset of PTE is the more controversial issue. AED prophylaxis has been based on several uncontrolled studies over the past 4 decades. However, one recent large uncontrolled study and three recent controlled, randomized studies have shown that phenytoin, even when given under carefully monitored conditions with maintenance of adequate blood levels, does not prevent the development of PTE beyond the first week after injury (40, 42–44).

Prophylactic phenobarbital is theoretically preferable because of its suppressant effect on the kindling phenomenon and its reported superoxide radical scavenging effect. Although the clinical data on its potential value remain equivocal, it is the agent of choice in much of Europe (45). Further controlled studies of this and other agents are clearly needed. In any case, in light of the sensitivity of the acutely traumatized brain to the secondary insult of a grand mal seizure, we recommend routine acute use of phenytoin or phenobarbital in high-risk CHI and in PHI patients for a period of 2–4 weeks only. Because of the sometimes subtle cognitive effects of phenytoin and phenobarbital, however, carbamazepine may be the agent of choice for longer-term therapy in patients who have manifested PTE with one or more seizures.

ASSESSING THE SEVERITY OF A HEAD INJURY

Kraus and Sorenson (46) have described a variety of approaches to classify the severity of a traumatic CHI injury (as illustrated in Table 1.1 of their chapter). Most commonly, severity of injury is defined on the basis of a patient's GCS score on entrance to an emergency room. Typically, on the GCS, a *mild* head injury is defined by a score that falls into the 13–15 range; a *moderate* head injury falls into the 9–12 range; and a *severe* head injury falls into the 0–8 range. The GCS is used most frequently to record the severity of a head injury because it tends to be a relatively objective scale, whereas other indices of head injury severity, such as duration of loss of consciousness or posttraumatic amnesia, may be more difficult to document. Greater severity of head injury, as measured by the GCS score, correlates well with a poorer outcome as measured by global scales such as the Glasgow Outcome Scale or more detailed neuropsychological tests.

Post-Acute and Long-Term Rehabilitation

With the greater involvement of patient advocate groups and insurers, the field of TBI rehabilitation has grown exponentially (47). Multiple therapies, including coma stimulation, reality orientation, cognitive rehabilitation, speech therapy, occupational therapy, recreation therapy, among others, have been applied to the TBI patient. Yet their use has been largely empirical, and there has been a paucity of scientific validation for these sometimes expensive interventions (including comparison with minimal care, supportive models). If progress is to be made in this area, rehabilitation modalities must be subject to the same scrutiny for indications, dosage, duration of treatment and

efficacy as are other medical treatments, such as drugs. The most pressing challenge in the field is the development of reproducible, universally accepted measures of function and ultimate outcome with which to compare the value of various interventions (48, 49).

One of the most encouraging aspects of TBI rehabilitation is the amazing ability of the young adult brain to *compensate* for many aspects of injury naturally. This is particularly apparent in head injury naturally. This is particularly apparent in head injury, as opposed to progressive conditions such as MS, or even stroke in older individuals. Disabilities such as hemiparesis, seizures, and certain language disorders may appear more dramatic initially, but the most devastating long-term impairments are the cognitive and especially the attentional and behavioral deficits that often persist following TBI. The goal of therapy should be the independence and community reintegration of the patient within his or her limits, rather than the specialized treatment of specific deficits simply because "they are there." Unfortunately, scarce resources available to the patient are often used up in the early acute and postacute phases on evaluation and therapy of deficits that will improve anyway or that have little effect on the ultimate goal of independence. Some therapies may actually be counterproductive by fostering continued dependence. Interventions that may be more cost-effective, like training in specific community reintegration skills such as decision making and certain forms of behavioral modification, may end up being omitted for lack of funds.

Rehabilitation facilities and the medical insurance industry are increasingly turning to the use of "case managers" or "care managers" in this field. The care manager should be a physician or health care professional who is responsible for the integration of various modalities of care and the allocation of resources for the head-injured patient. A principal role of the neurologist, psychiatrist, or neurosurgeon should be to help place the entire rehabilitation process on a firm footing by providing care managers with an accurate pathological diagnosis (i.e., focal contusions, DAI, hypoxia/ischemia). There should also be an *ongoing* assessment of status and prognosis in terms that are useful to the entire rehabilitation team (47). No less important is the identification of neurological complications, such as delayed hematoma or hydrocephalus, and the monitoring of other medical conditions and medications that may be impeding recovery.

MRI may be especially useful at this stage in identifying clinically significant focal contusions, but electrophysiological studies such as EEG and evoked responses have not proven to be particularly helpful. Evaluation at this stage should include particular attention to input from family and attendants who spend considerable time with the patient. Neuropsychological testing is an important part of the evaluation, but is of very limited value in the confused patient. When performed, these tests should focus on measurement of expected deficits for guiding therapy and evaluating progress (attentional deficits, posttraumatic amnesia) rather than on standard batteries that seek to confirm anatomical deficits already identified on MRI or CT, or which investigate in detail cognitive domains of limited practical interest to the case.

The use of pharmacologic agents (and particularly psychotropic medications) in TBI rehabilitation continues to hold much promise, but treatment still remains largely empirical. Properly controlled therapeutic trials are lacking, again largely because of the difficulty of defining patient groups and measuring outcomes. The sensitivity of the traumatized brain or the confused patient to medication must always be considered, and treatment must be tailored to each individual. Overmedication with AEDs, sedatives, or stimulants is a frequent problem; paradoxical responses to sedation in confused patients are especially common. Nevertheless, judicious use of adequate sedation can help reestablish sleep-wake cycles; and methylphenidate, dextroamphetamine, or bromocryptine may be useful as adjuncts in the management of the lethargic or apathetic patient. Carbamazepine is also beginning to emerge as a possible useful adjunct in the management of certain behavioral problems.

Recent unconfirmed clinical and animal studies have suggested that the combination of dextroamphetamine with physical therapy in the early phases of rehabilitation can permanently improve ultimate motor scores (50). The most interesting feature of these studies is that it is the combination of the two modalities that is crucial for the effect; it is not just an additive phenomenon. These findings have given new life to the study of the role of neurotransmitters in structural neural recovery. Another promising area of neural recovery research concerns the interaction of various trophic factors, such as nerve growth factor, glial growth factors, and interleukin-1 (IL-1) in the process of axonal sprouting and reinnervation (10).

Outcome

A surprisingly good overall outcome can be seen in many young, moderately severe to severely injured patients, a finding which probably reflects compensation for lost functions more so than recovery of the injured tissue itself. Thus, "floating" or dynamic endpoints can be identified in the post-TBI course: resolution of coma, return to orientation, resolution of posttraumatic amnesia, resolution and stable duration of retrograde amnesia, number of significant deficits identified on initial neuropsychological testing, number of significant deficits identified on the last neuropsychological evaluation, and the steepness of the recovery slopes. Nevertheless, an important milestone yet to be reached in the TBI field is the development of reproducible, universally accepted measures of function and long-term outcome with which to compare the value of various interventions (1). Final outcome is a composite of a number of elements, including preinjury, neurological, cognitive, behavioral, and psychosocial function, all of which may interact differently in each individual patient.

When evaluating efficacy of a given therapy, one must study all of these elements in the context of outcome as a whole; any evaluation battery should thus include at least some measure of each. It is misleading, for example, to use improvement in a particular overlearned memory task as a measure of outcome. On the other hand, one must maintain some level of flexibility of endpoints between TBI therapeutic trials; that is, one must be prepared to learn from each trial and modify endpoints appropriately for the next.

Although there may not be any ideal surrogate or summary measure for "outcome," return to gainful employment may be a practical one in most TBI populations. We have had the opportunity to study the disabilities that affect return to work in a large cohort (N = 520) of head injured Vietnam veterans. A 1-week, standardized multidisciplinary outcome evaluation was completed on each of them. Some 15 years postinjury, 56% of these men were gainfully employed, compared to 82% of a physically uninjured Vietnam War veteran control group (51). The occupational distribution of those who were working was essentially no different from that of normal uninjured young American males (52). After exclusion of severe aphasic or triplegic patients, none of whom worked, a multistage statistical analysis of these data, including factor and multiple logistic regression analyses, identified seven specifically defined disabilities that strongly influenced return to work. These were: posttraumatic epilepsy, hemiparesis, visual field loss, verbal memory loss, visual memory loss, psychological problems, and violent behavior. Interestingly, these seven items were found to be almost equally influential, so that a simple sum of the items could yield a "disability score" that predicted return to work. Patients were able to compensate fairly well for up to any three impairments, but beyond that there was a sharp drop in work rates. Other factors contributing significantly to return to work included preinjury intelligence, total brain volume loss on CT scan, and education postinjury (53, 54). This experience is yet another reminder of the importance of considering "outcome" as dependent on a set of functional skills, rather than identifying one or two disabilities as the only target of experimental therapies.

COGNITIVE AND BEHAVIORAL ASPECTS OF OUTCOME

Given the mix of pathologies that could affect outcome in TBI, it may seem surprising that a typical syndrome of cognitive and behavioral change can be described. Some TBI patients may present striking deficits in language, perception, and visual-spatial processing, but the more typical picture post-TBI emphasizes deficits in memory, attention, personality, and social cognition.

Memory problems include a notable loss of explicit retrieval of new information presented postinjury (posttraumatic amnesia), along with a more modest period of retrograde amnesia for events preceding the injury (55). However, immediate recall and older memories are generally intact, as are implicit or automatic memory processes. Temporal order judgment may be affected. The deficit thus appears to be primarily in the encoding and "consolidation" of new episodic memories and may reflect hippocampal, reticular, thalamic, or even basal forebrain (see below) damage. In the case of story recall, head injury patients may have difficulty not only in recalling the story but in conceptualizing its thematic elements. This may give them particular difficulty in selectively recalling the most important story elements. Head injury patients may be able to utilize semantic information in encoding and retrieving information, but they are less successful at this than controls. Of course, the longer the duration of posttraumatic amnesia and the more severe the initial head injury as judged by the emergency room GCS score, the more likely the patient will experience persistent memory problems. These same predictive factors appear important for predicting other persistent cognitive deficits.

Memory problems may be accompanied by slowed information processing (identified by slowed response times or increased latencies in the late event-related brain potentials such as the P300 or N400). This slowing of information processing may be due to a combination of diffuse axonal shearing, damage to projection systems from the brainstem, and focal frontal lesions. Slowed information processing can affect the quality of memory encoding and rehearsal as well as fluency and response times independent of motor control deficits. Often access to a source of knowledge is slowed even though the search through the semantic network where that knowledge is stored may be normal. Dramatically slowed information processing usually recovers after several months, except in the case of the most severely injured patient.

Attentional deficits are frequently reported after CHI, and they usually take the form of a deficit in sustained effortful attention. The patient may also have difficulty refocusing his or her attention after a period of delay. This deficit may not be as apparent if the task is of short duration. It is not always clear if the subject is distracted by other stimuli on the screen, in the room, or internalized thought. It is usually characterized by omitted responses and increased variance in response times to targets. Patients may also have difficulty inhibiting responses to previously associated stimuli—even when the association is currently irrelevant. These deficits are associated with damage to the prefrontal cortex. Attentional control deficits may also result in a diminished ability to divide available cognitive resources to handle a multifaceted task.

A deficit in concept formation is frequently reported by head-injured patients and their families. This problem is usually coupled with an inability to shift mental set, manifested by perseveration on tasks such as the Wisconsin Card Sorting Test (WCST). Patients may appear to use concrete problem-solving strategies. They may also have trouble initiating any problem-solving strategies unless they are encouraged to do so by the environment or another person. These deficits in executive functions almost always follow prefrontal lobe lesions (most frequently with dor-

solateral lesions) but may even appear after reticular thalamic lesions. Patients may demonstrate reasonably intact memory, perception, language, and even attention, yet still have major executive function deficits. A subtler form of this problem may even appear after so-called minor closed head injury. The nature of these deficits have been reviewed by Grafman. (56).

Perhaps the most impressive problem in TBI patients (usually reported by family members) is a change in mood and personality (57, 58). The patient may be disinhibited, behave irrationally, have mood swings, ignore social convention, and not care about the future consequences of his or her current actions. A few may also manifest aggressive or even violent behavior for months or years after the injury. This aggressive behavior can be either directed or nondirected, and may be accompanied by an often explosive autonomic and emotional response. Some of these "episodic dyscontrol" events are thought by some to be a subtle form of temporal lobe epilepsy, particularly because they often appear to respond to antiepileptic drugs such as carbamazepine. The most likely neuropathological basis for these social cognitive and behavioral disorders is damage to the prefrontal cortex, including the orbitofrontal region (59). Improved neuropsychiatric clinical assessment of these problems in conjunction with therapeutic management is sorely needed. Furthermore, family members may also benefit from neuropsychiatric intervention. Early in the course of recovery, family members may appear relieved simply to be told that the patient will survive and recover. However, as time passes, significant others can become overwhelmed in their effort to adjust to the permanent neurobehavioral changes in a loved one.

In addition, damage to the basal forebrain (BFB) in the proximal orbitofrontal lobe may contribute to the episodic memory and attentional deficits. In our long-term study of head-injured Vietnam War veterans, we have found that BFB-injured men differed from their non-BFB injured matches only in having a longer loss of consciousness postinjury, episodic memory deficits, and poorer performance on the WCS (60, 61). The basal forebrain lesions alone, however, were not sufficient to produce a generalized dementia (as had been suggested by prior research with patients suffering from Alzheimer's disease).

NEUROPSYCHOLOGICAL ASSESSMENT

The neuropsychological assessment of TBI can begin at a very early stage. The Galveston Orientation and Amnesia Test (GOAT) can be used with the disoriented patient and is designed for repeated administration (55). It allows the investigator to evaluate the duration and severity of posttraumatic amnesia as well as the duration of retrograde amnesia. This evaluation is important because the duration of posttraumatic amnesia is a powerful predictor of eventual outcome. A more detailed retrograde amnesia test can supplement the GOAT. Other tests that make minimal demands on the patient, such as simple and choice response time tasks (to measure speed of information processing), picture naming (to measure visual recognition/name retrieval), verbal fluency (to measure strategic memory search/name retrieval), and letter cancellation (to measure spatial attention) can aid the investigator in establishing the acute recovery slope (over days/weeks early in the course of recovery) and in determining when more extensive neuropsychological testing can be attempted.

The more formal neuropsychological evaluation should incorporate standard clinical measures such as the Wechsler Adult Intelligence Scale-Revised, Wechsler Memory Scale-Revised, and the neurobehavioral rating scale. Other, more experimental, tests of memory, attention, personality, and social cognition are used in TBI, but none has emerged as specific for TBI, and a full review is beyond the scope of this chapter (62). The specific battery used in a given hospital is often dependent on the particular interests of the attending neuropsychologist (55, 62–64).

TBI patients are usually evaluated at least three times in the postacute recovery period. To chart the slope of cognitive recovery, it is important to include some repeatable tests in the evaluation that are relatively resistant to test–retest or "practice" artifact. Repeatable tests may be clinical tests that have different versions equated for difficulty or information processing tests on which stimuli can be randomly selected for presentation. In these tests, the dependent measure reflects the subject strategy rather than the particular stimuli used. Examples are various versions of the selective reminding test and of choice reaction-time tests.

Long-term recovery is usually assessed by evaluating the rate of improvement, preferably with at least three testing points and over at least 1 year postinjury. In addition to the neuropsychological measures, other indices of recovery, such as functional independence in activities of daily living, employability, school performance, family and community adjustment, and other social functions, become more important at this stage.

Besides the clinical utility of neuropsychological evaluations, the study of TBI patients may provide insights into basic mechanisms of attention, memory, and social cognition. For example, acute retrograde amnesias can be ideally studied in TBI, and the frequency of frontal lobe injury also makes TBI a good population to use in the study of executive function deficits. Modern brain-imaging techniques lend a particularly exciting dimension to such studies.

"Minor" Head Injury

A group of patients that has been frequently mismanaged in the past is that with so-called "minor" head injury (64). Not only has axonal damage been demonstrated in animal models of concussion, but MRI as well as positron emission tomography (PET) have repeatedly shown structural and metabolic changes in humans with minor head injury as well. The most important element in the management of these cases is the recognition that there is usually an organic, pathological basis for their complaints, at least in the early,

postinjury period, and that it usually resolves over a few months. If mishandled, however, these patients often develop an overlying neurosis which makes evaluation and management infinitely more difficult.

There is nothing more frustrating to the intelligent minor head injury victim than to be told there is "nothing wrong" by his physician, his family, and his employer. Proper counseling should thus include not only the patient, but also the family, school, or employer. MRI, auditory evoked potentials, and specific neuropsychological tests such as choice reaction time early in the course can help delineate the deficits (65, 66). One important research challenge in this area is better defining the anatomical, physiological, and behavioral criteria for recognizing and measuring the severity of minor head injury (64).

The basic elements of the postconcussion syndrome are cognitive, somatic, and affective. Clinically significant neuropsychological impairments have been documented repeatedly even after minor "dings" without loss of consciousness (67). The most frequent somatic complaints in one large recent study were headache (71%), decreased energy or "fatigue" (60%), and dizziness (53%); these had all markedly improved at 3 months (63). The proper management of the "fatigue" element (which may relate to orbitofrontal injury) is a major factor in recovery, and requires the cooperation of the school or employer (68). We suggest a graded return to full work load over a period of 4–8 weeks.

CONCLUSIONS

Head trauma is a common cause of neuropsychiatric impairment. The development of therapeutic agents that can reduce the severity of the pathological changes caused by the trauma should have a major effect on survival rates and the quality of that survival. The neuropsychiatric sequelae of head trauma include deficits in attention, executive functions, social cognition and personality, and memory. Moderate and severe head injuries are likely to lead to persistent problems in these areas. Mild head injury can often result in subtle but significant cognitive impairment that is often difficult to discriminate from a neurotic reaction to an experience of trauma. Although rehabilitation techniques may be of benefit to patients recovering from TBI, there are few controlled studies that can reliably document these benefits. The neuropsychiatrist, who has traditionally been absent from the TBI evaluation and treatment team, should be encouraged to assume an important new role in contributing to the evaluation and management of the cognitive and social-personality problems that emerge following TBI (69).

References

1. Department of Health and Human Services. Interagency head injury task force report. Washington, DC: Department of Health and Human Services, 1989.
2. Gadisseaux P. Nutrition and CNS trauma. In: Becker D, Povlishock J, eds. Central nervous system trauma status report. Bethesda, MD:

National Institute of Neurological and Communicative Disorders and Stroke (NINCDS), National Institutes of Health (NIH), 1985; 207–216.

3. Clifton G, Robertson C, Grossman R. Management of the cardiovascular and metabolic responses to severe head injury. In: Becker D, Povlishock J, eds. Central nervous system trauma status report. Bethesda, MD: National Institute of Neurological and Communicative Disorders and Stroke (NINCDS), National Institutes of Health (NIH), 1985;139–159.

4. Gildenberg P, Frost, E. Respiratory care in head injury. In: Becker D, Povlishock J, eds. Central nervous system trauma status report. Bethesda, MD: National Institute of Neurological and Communicative Disorders and Stroke (NINCDS), National Institutes of Health (NIH), 1985;161–176.

5. Woolf P, Hamil R, Lee L, Cox C, McDonald J. The predictive value of catecholamines in assessing outcome in traumatic brain injury. J Neurol Surg 1987;66:875–882.

6. Kaufman H, Mattson J. Coagulopathy in head injury. In: Becker D, Povlishock J, eds. Central nervous system trauma status report. Bethesda, MD: National Institute of Neurological and Communicative Disorders and Stroke (NINCDS), National Institutes of Health (NIH), 1985;187–206.

7. Hume Adams J, Graham DI, Gennarelli TA. Contemporary neuropathological considerations regarding brain damage in head injury. In: Becker D, Povlishock J, eds. Central nervous system trauma status report. Bethesda, MD: National Institute of Neurological and Communicative Disorders and Stroke (NINCDS), National Institutes of Health (NIH), 1985;65–77.

8. Gennarelli T, Thibault L. Biological models of head injury. In: Becker D, Povlishock J, eds. Central nervous system trauma status report. Bethesda, MD: National Institute of Neurological and Communicative Disorders and Stroke (NINCDS), National Institutes of Health (NIH), 1985:391–404.

9. Marshall L, Toole B, Bowers S. The national traumatic coma data bank. II: Patients who talk and deteriorate: implications for treatment. J Neurosurg 1983;59:285–288.

10. Gennarelli T, Thibault L, Adams J, Graham D, Thompson C, Marcinin R. Diffuse axonal injury and traumatic coma in the primate. Ann Neurol, 1982;12:564–574.

11. Strich S. The pathology of brain damage due to blunt head injuries. In: Walker A, Caveness W, Critchley M, eds. The late effects of head injury. Springfield, IL: Charles C Thomas, 1969:501–526.

12. Povlishock J. The morphopathologic responses to head injuries of varying severity. In: Becker D, Povlishock J, eds. Central nervous system trauma status report. Bethesda, MD: National Institute of Neurological and Communicative Disorders and Stroke (NINCDS), National Institutes of Health (NIH), 1985;443–452.

13. Povlishock J, Coburn T. Morphopathological change associated with mild head injury. In: Levin H, Eisenberg H, Benton A, eds. Mild head injury. New York: Oxford University Press, 1989;37–53.

14. Jordan B. Boxing. Arch Neurol 1987;44:453–459.

15. Oppenheimer D. Microscopic lesions in the brain following head injury. J Neurol Neurosurg Psychiatry, 1968;31:299–306.

16. Gajdusek D. Hypothesis: Interference with axonal transport of neurofilament as a common pathogenic mechanism in certain diseases of the central nervous system. N Engl J Med 1985;312:714–719.

17. Allen I, Kirk J, Maynard R, Cooper G, Scott R, Crockard A. An ultrastructural study of experimental high velocity penetration head injury. Acta Neuropathol 1983;59:277–282.

18. Maxwell W, Irvine A, Adams J, Graham D, Gennarelli T. Response of cerebral microvasculature to brain injury. J Pathol 1988;155:327–335.

19. Wei E, Kontos H, Dietrich W, Povlishock J, Ellis E. Inhibition by free radical scavengers and by cyclooxygenase inhibitors of pial arteriolar abnormalities from concussive brain injury in cats. Circ Res 1981;48: 95–103.

20. Ellis E, Wright K, Wei E. Cyclooxygenase products of arachdonic acid metabolism in cat cerebral cortex after experimental concussive brain injury. J Neurochem 1981;37:892–896.

21. Kontos H, Wei E. Superoxide production in experimental brain injury. J Neurosurg 1986;64:803–807.

22. Faden A. Neuropeptides and CNS injury. Arch Neurol 1986;43: 501–504.

23. McIntosh T, Faden A, Yamakami I, Vink R. Magnesium deficiency exacerbates and pretreatment improves outcome following traumatic brain injury in rats. J Neural Trauma 1988;5:17–31.

24. Faden A, Demediuk P, Panter S, Vink R. The role of excitatory amino acids and NMDA receptors in traumatic brain injury. Science 1989;244:798–800.

25. Suguru I, Marmarou A, Clarke G, Andersen B, Fatouros P, Young H. Production and clearance of lactate from brain tissue, CSF, and serum following experimental brain injury. J Neurosurg 1988;69:736–744.

26. Carey M. An experimental brain missile wound; ascertaining pathophysiology and evaluating treatments to lower mortality and morbidity. U.S. Army Medical Research and Development Command, 1987.

27. Shohami E, Shapira Y, Sidi A, Cotev S. Head injury induces increased prostaglandin synthesis in rat brain. J Cereb Blood Flow Metab 1987;7:58–63.

28. Shapira Y, Davidson E, Weindenfeld Y. Dexamethasone and indomethacin do not affect brain edema following head injury in rats. J Cereb Blood Flow Metab 1988;8:395–402.

29. Hall E. Effects of the 21-aminosteroid U-74006F on posttraumatic spinal cord ischemia. J Neurosurg 1988;68:462–465.

30. Panter SS, McSwigan JD, Sheppard JR, Emory CR, Frey WHD. Glial fibrillary acidic protein and Alzheimer's disease. Neurochem Res 1985;10:1567–1576.

31. Hayes R. Neurochemical mechanisms of mild and moderate head injury: implications for treatment. In: Levin H, Eisenberg H, Benton A, eds. Mild head injury. New York: Oxford University Press, 1989:54–79.

32. Faden A, Jacobs T, Smith M, Holaday J. Comparison of TRH, naloxone, and dexamethasone treatments in experimental spinal injury. Neurology 1983;33:673–678.

33. Jennett B, Teasdale G. Management of head injuries. Philadelphia: FA Davis, 1981.

34. Plum F. What causes infarction in ischemic brain: the Robert Wartenberg lecture. Neurology 1983;33:222–233.

35. Cohen WA. Neuroradiological imaging of head trauma. In: Greenberg J, ed. Handbook of head and spine trauma. New York: Marcel Dekker, 1993:77–111.

36. Marshall L. Closed head injury. In: Annual course #104. Head injuries. New Orleans: American Academy of Neurology, 1986.

37. Eisenberg H, Frankowski R, Contant C, Marshall L, Walker M. High-dose barbiturate control of elevated intracranial pressure in patients with severe head injury. J Neurosurg 1988;69:15–23.

38. Deardeu M, Gibson J, McDowall D. Effect of high dose dexamethasone on outcome from severe head injury. J Neurosurg 1986;64: 81–88.

39. Annegers J, Grabow J, Groover R, Laws EJ, Elveback L, Kurland L. Seizures after head trauma: a population study. Neurology 1980;30: 683–689.

40. Salazar A, Jabbari B, Vance S, Grafman J, Amin D, Dillon J. Epilepsy after penetrating head injury. I: Clinical correlates. Neurology 1985; 35:1406–1414.

41. Weiss G, Salazar A, Vance S, Grafman J, Jabbari B. Predicting posttraumatic epilepsy in penetrating head injury. Arch Neurol 1986;43:771–773.

42. Penry J, White B, Brackett C. A controlled prospective trial study of the pharmacologic prophylaxis of posttraumatic epilepsy. Neurology 1979;29(Suppl):600.

43. Tempkin NR, Dikman S, Wilensky AJ, Keihm J, Chabel S, Winn H. A randomized double-blinded study of phenytoin for the prevention of post-traumatic seizures. NEJN 1990;323:497–502.

44. Young B, Rapp R, Norton A. Failure of prophylactically administered phenytoin to prevent early posttraumatic seizures. J Neurosurg 1983;58:231–241.

45. Parenti G, Arrigo A, Rossi G, Canaticchi R, Murri L. Phenobarbital in

the prophylaxis of late post-traumatic epilepsy. In: Murri L, Parenti G, Annegers JF, eds. Pharmacological prophylaxis for posttraumatic epilepsy, Pisa, Italy: Pacini Editore, 1991:43–58.

46. Kraus JF, Sorenson SB. Epidemiology. In: Silver JM, Yudofsky SC, Hales RE, eds. Neuropsychiatry of traumatic brain injury. Washington, DC: American Psychiatric Press, 1994:3–42.

47. Alexander M. Diagnosis and long-term management of severe head injury. In: Annual Course #420. Head injury. Chicago, IL: American Academy of Neurology, 1989.

48. Prigitano GS, ed. Rehabilitation interventions after traumatic brain injury. In: Bach-Y-Rita P, ed. Traumatic brain injury. New York: Demos, 1989.

49. Bach-Y-Rita P. A conceptual approach to neural recovery. In: Bach-Y-Rita P, ed. Traumatic brain injury. New York: Demos, 1989.

50. Feeney D, Gonzalez A, Law W. Amphetamine, haloperidol and experience interact to affect rate of recovery after motor cortex injury. Science 1982;217:855–857.

51. Schwab K, Grafman J, Salazar A, Kraft J. Residual impairments and work status fifteen years after head injury: a report of the Vietnam head injury study. Neurology 1992;43:95–103.

52. Kraft J, Schwab K, Salazar A, Brown R. Occupational and educational achievements of head injured Vietnam veterans. Arch Phys Med Rehabil 1993;74:596–601.

53. Grafman J, Salazar A, Weingartner H, Vance S, Amin D. The relationship of brain-tissue loss volume and lesion location to cognitive deficit. J Neurosci 1986;6:301–307.

54. Grafman J, Jonas B, Martin A, et al. Intellectual function following penetrating head injury in Vietnam veterans. Brain 1988;111:169–184.

55. Levin H, Goldstein F. Neurobehavioral aspects of traumatic brain injury. In: Bach-Y-Rita P, ed. Traumatic brain injury. New York: Demos, 1989:53–72.

56. Grafman J. Alternative frameworks for the conceptualization of prefrontal lobe functions. In: Boller F, Grafman J, eds. Handbook of neuropsychology, vol 9. Amsterdam: Elsevier Science Publishers, 1994:187–202.

57. Brooks N, Campsie L, Symington C, Beattie A, McKinlay W. The five year outcome of severe blunt head injury: A relative's view. J Neurol Neurosurg Psychiatry 1986;49:764–770.

58. Lezak M. Living with the characterologically altered brain injured patient. J Clin Psychol 1978;39:592–598.

59. Grafman J, Vance S, Weingartner H, Salazar A, Amin D. The effects of lateralized frontal lesions on mood regulation. Brain 1986;109:1127–1148.

60. Salazar A, Grafman J, Vance S, Weingartner H, Dillon J, Ludlow C. Unconsciousness and amnesia following penetrating head injury: neurology and anatomy. 1986;36:178–187.

61. Salazar A, Grafman J, Schlesselman S, Vance S, Mohr JP, Carpenter M, Pevsner P, Ludlow C, Weingartner H. Penetrating war injuries of the basal forebrain: neurology and cognition. Neurology 1986;36:459–465.

62. Levin H, Grafman J, Eisenberg H, eds. Neurobehavioral recovery from head injury. New York: Oxford University Press, 1987.

63. Levin H, Mattis S, Ruff R, et al. Neurobehavioral outcome following minor head injury: a three-center study. J Neurosurg 1987;66:234–243.

64. Levin HS, Eisenberg HM, Benton AL, eds. Mild head injury. New York: Oxford University Press, 1989.

65. Eisenberg H. Mild to moderate brain injury clinical diagnosis. In: Levin H, Eisenberg H, Benton A, eds. Mild head injury. Cambridge: Blackwell, 1989:95–105.

66. Gentilini M, Nichelli P, Schoenhuber R. Assessment of attention in mild head injury. In: Levin HS, Eisenberg HM, Benton AL, eds. Mild head injury. New York: Oxford University Press, 1989:163–175.

67. Barth JT, Alves WM, Ryan TV, et al. Mild head injury in sports: neuropsychological sequelae and recovery of function. In: Levin HS, Eisenberg HM, Benton AL, eds. Mild head injury. New York: Oxford University Press, 1989:257–275.

68. Wrightson P. Management of disability and rehabilitation services after mild head injury. In: Levin H, Eisenberg H, Benton A, eds. Mild head injury. New York: Oxford University Press, 1989:245–256.

69. Silver JM, Yudofsky SC, Hales RE. Neuropsychiatry of traumatic brain injury. Washington, DC: American Psychiatric Press, 1994.

40

NEUROMUSCULAR DISEASES

Ghislaine Savard and Angela Genge

The development of a neuropsychiatric syndrome is not generally expected in neuromuscular diseases, which by definition must include predominant muscle and nerve symptomatology. However, there are noteworthy exceptions. First, in myotonic dystrophy (MD) and in Duchenne muscular dystrophy (DMD), intellectual deterioration can occur with or without behavioral disorders. Second, in postpolio syndrome (PPS), peripheral fatigue can be accompanied by mental fatigue and cognitive difficulties. Third, in myasthenia gravis (MG), memory loss can occur. Fourth, in amyotrophic lateral sclerosis (ALS), a dementia of a frontal type can develop. And perhaps fifth, the chronic fatigue syndrome (CFS), with its combination of neuromuscular and psychiatric symptoms, could be considered here.

Neuropsychiatric features of interest in this chapter are an integral part of the primary neuromuscular disease process. Thus, it is implied that they are not caused by any other confounding factors such as the use of drugs with neuropsychiatric side effects of their own, or emotional difficulties adjusting to physical handicap.

Neuromuscular diseases may well represent the last frontier for neuropsychiatry. A pioneering effort and a high degree of clinical suspicion are needed to detect more extensively the neuropsychiatric features of neuromuscular diseases. This chapter is not exhaustive but will focus on the above-mentioned neuromuscular diseases. There are additional primary neuromuscular diseases in which cerebral involvement occurs, such as carnitine deficiency and mitochondrial diseases, and many secondary neuromuscular syndromes in which cerebral dysfunction and myopathy both result from a common etiology (AIDS myalgia, thyroid disease myopathy, alcoholic myopathy, and others). Those are not addressed here.

MYOTONIC DYSTROPHY

Myotonic dystrophy (MD) is an autosomal-dominant neuromuscular disease with an incidence of at least 1:8,000 (1). It is the most common form of muscular dystrophy in adults. Although mainly considered a disease of muscle characterized by progressive weakness, wasting and myotonia, MD is truly a multisystem disease. Patients with MD

often suffer from cardiac conduction defects, smooth muscle dysfunction, cataracts, abnormal glucose response, and in males, premature balding and testicular atrophy; sometimes patients are treated for many years for those problems before the diagnosis of MD is entertained.

Biomedical studies have failed to identify the defective protein in MD, although a defect in a protein kinase has long been suspected (2). The MD gene region has been localized to the long arm of chromosome 19, and recently, specific DNA markers have been identified (3–5). An abnormal expansion of a trinucleotide repeat, cytosine thymidine guanine (CTG), has been implicated: although the normal CTG repeat varies between 5 and 30 repeats, it exceeds 50 repeats in MD (6–8). The length of this "MD segment" can vary in size between patients and even between siblings within the same family. This may explain the striking phenotypic variability in MD both within and between families. The size of MD segment has also been shown to increase in successive generations and to correlate directly with an increased severity and earlier onset of disease. This reflects the phenomenon of genetic anticipation, whereby affected children have a more severe phenotype than their parents (9).

Clinically, MD patients are subdivided in three groups according to age of onset and clinical syndrome (10, 11). In the mildest form, which can go undetected, onset is typically in middle or old age. Characteristic findings are cataracts, minimal or no muscle abnormality, and infrequent central nervous system (CNS) disturbances. In the classical form, onset is in adolescence or in early adult life. Major findings include myotonia and muscle weakness of the face, forearms, and feet. Muscles most frequently involved include facial muscles, elevators of the eyelids, temporalis and masseter muscles, sternocleidomastoid muscles, distal muscles of the forearm, and dorsiflexors of the feet. Other muscular groups may become involved, including quadriceps, diaphragm, and intercostal muscles, intrinsic muscles of the hands and feet, palatal and pharyngeal muscles, tongue, and extraocular muscles. Patients with the classical form can become quite disabled secondary to respiratory muscle weakness, congestive heart failure or heart block, or pharyngeal and laryngeal weakness. The most severe form of MD occurs congenitally and is associated with generalized muscular hypoplasia and mental retardation. Neonatal mortality is high; survivors go on to develop the classical form of MD. Congenital MD is exclusively maternally transmitted; the reason for this is not known.

From a neuropsychological point of view, mental retardation (MR) has long been known to occur in MD (12, 13).

Estimates of the frequency of cognitive deficits in MD patients generally range from 36–60% (14–19). In a well-controlled study, MD patients were administered the Wechsler Adult Intelligence Scale (WAIS) (20) and the Mini-Mental State Examination (MMSE) (18, 21). Of the 27 MD patients in that series, borderline mental functioning (intellectual quotient [IQ] between 71 and 84) was present in 15 (55%). Six of the 27 (22%) had an IQ lower than 70, indicating MR. Six MD patients had a score of less than 23 on MMSE. Curiously, in both male and female patients with MD, more severe cognitive dysfunction seems associated with a maternal inheritance pattern. Although there are exceptions, and normal intellectual function is compatible with MD, this association bears mention at times of genetic counseling.

Cognitive dysfunction in MD can be worsened, transiently or chronically, by secondarily acquired cerebral dysfunction from cardiac, respiratory, or other organ failure. This was illustrated by Roche in a case report of a 39-year-old MD patient of low average intelligence who developed heart block and hypotension resulting in a cardiogenic dementia. The cardiogenic dementia was substantially reversed by cardiac pacing (22).

Mental illness has also been known to occur in MD. Maas described a characteristic temperament that was cheerful and condescending, and which remained morbidly so in the face of eventual pitiable physical state and an often dreary psychosocial downward course (13). Psychopathology (schizoid, paranoid, epileptoid, hypomanic, or hysteroid in type) was thought to be reactive and the product of social deterioration seen in families with MD.

In one uncontrolled study, personality profiles were assessed carefully by interview and with the Minnesota Multiple Personality Inventory (MMPI) (23) in 25 MD patients (15). Forty-four percent had unremarkable personality, 24% had mild personality difficulties, and 32% had prominent personality abnormalities. Serious personality difficulties were mostly encountered in patients with lower cognitive ability and advanced physical handicap. Again, personality variables were thought to reflect coping efforts in reaction to poor health.

Brumback emphasized that personality disturbance and cognitive symptoms in MD might be caused by depression (17). He reported on 16 MD patients who had major depression, according to criteria of the *Diagnostic and Statistical Manual of Mental Disorders* (DSM-III) (24) and based on scores on the Hamilton Scale (25). He found their depression responsive to treatment with the tricyclic antidepressant imipramine in doses up to 150 mg a day. Follow-up extended to a mean of 26 weeks. Unexpectedly,

the indolence of these patients was ameliorated, and in the opinion of families, the patients' personalities were improved in a gratifying manner. Brumback remarked that poor social aptitude, personality, and cognitive deterioration can occur secondarily to depression and can be reversible. Perhaps in MD the basic genetic defect results in an abnormality of aminergic receptors of etiological relevance to a mood disorder. Mental illness in MD is no longer seen as situational, but as a neuropsychiatric syndrome, with affective manifestations as well as personality and cognitive deterioration (26). Brumback's conclusion that depression is a major finding in MD has not been generally accepted (27).

Cerebral involvement in MD has been documented by magnetic resonance imaging (MRI). Ventricles are enlarged, and a lumpy or thick pattern of periventricular hyperintensity has been described (28). Distinctive white matter changes in the anterior temporal lobes have been reported (19, 29).

In one MD patient who died after presenting mental deterioration, apathy, hypersomnolence, and an end-stage delirium, the postmortem pathological examination of the brain showed neurofibrillary changes similar to that seen in Alzheimer's disease. Other changes included gliosis and neuronal atrophy in the thalamus (30). The relevance of this is not clear, but a concentration of neurofibrillary changes in the limbic system certainly could influence the psychic manifestations of MD.

Management of patients with MD currently involves identification of the disease and of the affected individuals within a family. Psychometric testing and neuropsychiatric consultation are considered as valuable investigations to delineate possible dysfunction, and also to determine preserved strengths. This will assist in promoting optimal psychological adjustment to the disease and will facilitate social, school, and vocational integration.

DUCHENNE MUSCULAR DYSTROPHY

Duchenne muscular dystrophy (DMD) is an X-linked genetic disorder causing a severe myopathy with multi-organ system involvement. It is caused by a deletion in the 2.5 Mb gene at locus X p21 on the short arm of the X chromosome, which encodes for a protein product named dystrophin (31). Dystrophin is a component of the sarcolemmal membrane of normal skeletal muscle, but is absent from the skeletal muscle of people with DMD. The amino acid sequence of dystrophin, which has been deduced from the DMD gene of cDNA sequence, suggests that dystrophin is a membrane-associated cytoskeletal protein involved in the anchoring of the sarcolemmal proteins to the cytoskeleton. Dystrophin is part of a large complex referred to as the dystrophin-glycoprotein complex. The loss of associated proteins as a result of the lack of dystrophin may initiate the degenerative cascade of muscular dystrophy (32). Dystrophin is also found in the brain, specifically in the cortex, the hippocampus, and the Purkinje cells of the cerebellum (33). However, the dystrophin isoforms of the brain are different from those in muscle, and their role in the brain and in the neuropathology of DMD are unknown.

Typically, DMD presents in a young boy whose walking is delayed. Proximal muscle weakness causing difficulty climbing stairs and rising from the floor becomes manifest by 3 or 5 years of age. Lumbar lordosis causing distortion of posture develops. Weakness of the shoulder girdle later appears. Calves are noticeably enlarged in most patients. Loss of ambulation occurs by ages 9–12. Contractures and scoliosis are frequent problems, while cardiac myopathy is rarer. Death from respiratory failure occurs in early adulthood. Serum creatine kinase is 40 times normal. Electromyography and muscle biopsy show characteristic changes. Curently, antibodies to different parts of the dystrophin molecule can be used to identify the abnormality on muscle tissue. DNA analysis can also be used to identify truncated dystrophin or its absence.

Mental subnormality is found in DMD. Studies have shown a fairly consistent picture of an average IQ of 85 for children afflicted with DMD, i.e., approximately one standard deviation (1 SD) below the mean. The presence of intellectual impairment is not correlated with age or degree of physical handicap. Little is known of the emotional development of these children. Leibowitz studied 57 children between 3–13 years old, using standard intelligence tests, a reading test, and the Rutter behavior questionnaire (34, 35). Intelligence scores were about 1 SD below the mean, with higher functioning on performance than on verbal tasks, in line with accepted thinking. The majority of children did well on the Rutter, although, in nearly a third, scores above a cutoff point were indicative of some measure of emotional disturbance that did not directly correlate with low IQ. The Rutter questionnaire rates how parents and teachers perceive the child's behavior; pathological scores are categorized as neurotic, antisocial, or undifferentiated. The children's perceptions of their own behavior are not rated. Etiological factors proposed for the pathological scores included overrepresentation of the male sex in this sample, cerebral dysfunction, expectancy of short life span, and poor integration in the school.

Neuropsychiatric assessment of the child with DMD is needed. Special attention should be directed at personality and mood disorders of the type generally associated with mental retardation. Inability to develop social interpersonal graces, lack of empathy, behavioral rigidity, impulsiveness, labile mood, and poor frustration tolerance may require therapeutic interventions with milieu therapy, behavioral modification, and psychopharmacology.

BECKER DYSTROPHY

Becker dystrophy (BD), is a distinct entity sometimes erroneously referred to as the benign form of DMD. The genetic locus of BD is separate and far removed from that of DMD, although both are on the same chromosome. Symptoms and signs are reminiscent of DMD, but age of onset is later, at 5–15 years of age, and progression is slower.

The presenting feature is usually weakness of the pelvic girdle and proximal leg muscles, with ensuing difficulty in running and climbing stairs. Calves are enlarged. Inability to walk is expected to occur around the age of 27 years. Death from respiratory failure is likely to occur by age 55. The activity of serum creatinine kinase during the earlier stages of BD can be increased as much as in DMD. In muscle biopsies, the presence of nuclear clumps, numerous internal nuclei and split fibers, and the relative lack of adipose cell replacement may help distinguish BD from DMD (36). Muscle dystrophin is decreased in amount and in size, as it is in DMD.

Mental retardation is known to occur in BD, but its behavioral correlates have not been studied extensively.

POSTPOLIO SYNDROME

The postpolio syndrome (PPS) refers to the now well-defined and stereotypic features that present in patients previously affected by acute poliomyelitis (AP). Of all AP survivors, 25–40% could develop PPS (37). Typically, it occurs 28–35 years after the initial attack of polio and at a time when functional stability has been achieved and present for at least 15 years (38). Clinical features include new-onset fatigability, weakness, loss of muscle bulk, and muscle and joint pain. Respiratory difficulties and increased deformity can occur. Cold intolerance, sleep difficulties, and cognitive difficulties are sometimes present. The muscle atrophy is assymetric and is usually most prominent in those muscles that were originally most severely affected; however, it may also involve previously subclinically affected muscles, including bulbar muscles (38, 39). The weakness is slowly progressive. Fortunately, patients do not return to the state of disability present at the time of AP (39).

In AP the polio virus causes an acute febrile illness, followed 7–14 days later by acute paralysis. It is expected that less than 1% of those infected develop symptoms and that 30–60% of symptomatic patients go on to develop neurological deficit. In paralyzed limbs, roughly 50% of motor neurons are destroyed. In normal or near-normal limbs, up to 20% of neurons die as well. Most, if not all, of the originally involved motor units are affected in PPS. Following the recovery process of resprouting and continuous remodeling of the postpolio motor unit, many postpolio motor units will be larger than normal (38). These larger motor units might become vulnerable to degeneration again later in life. Such degeneration may underly the development of PPS.

Although PPS is a clinical diagnosis that lacks pathognomonic laboratory criteria, electromyographic studies can be useful to confirm chronic and ongoing denervation. But both symptomatic PPS patients and controls (those with a history of paralytic polio and residual deficit but without PPS) have abnormalities on electromyography (EMG). These consist of spontaneous activity in the form of fibrillations and positive sharp waves as well as large-amplitude polyphasic voluntary motor unit potentials. The former are suggestive of active denervation, and the latter provide evidence of previous paralytic polio. Muscle biopsies, single-fiber EMG, or macro-EMG are research tools rather than clinical investigations. Single-fiber EMG revealed increased jitter and blocking in PPS patients and in above-defined controls, suggesting a neuromuscular junction transmission defect. Studies with stimulation single-fiber EMG with different frequencies in symptomatic PPS patients show that jitter decreases with intramuscular (or intravenous) edrophonium injection, indicating correction (improvement) of the neuromuscular defect in many PPS patients. In an uncontrolled open trial of oral administration to PPS patients of the anticholinesterase pyridostigmine, Trojan et al. reported improvement in fatigue in 60% of patients, pointing to the possibility that muscular fatigue may be caused by a presynaptic acetylcholinesterase responsive neuromuscular defect (40, 41). Such a defect cannot be directly linked to an occurrence going back to acute AP, or to an occurrence coincident with PPS.

Muscle biopsies in PPS show fiber type grouping and nuclear bag fibers, as well as angular atrophic fibers. There is a known correlation between ongoing denervation and high grades of fiber grouping and increased fiber density, suggesting that motor units most enlarged by previous sprouting are most likely to become unstable later in life. Also, positive immunohistochemical staining for neural cell adhesion molecule (NCAM) supports the EMG findings of ongoing denervation. The problem is that all of these findings are consistent with either a past history of AP or new-onset PPS. So far, the etiology of PPS is unknown, but research developments are attracting greater interest (42).

Competing theories include premature aging of affected motor neurons (43), genetic factors (44), abnormal energy metabolism of affected muscle fibers (45), persistent ongoing denervation, persistent viral activity (46–48), and a dysimmune reaction (49).

From a neuropsychiatric point of view, PPS is intriguing mainly because of its presentation with fatigue. Fatigue has been reported as a problem in about 89% of PPS patients (50). It is usually defined as a sense of exhaustion after routine physical exertion. Physical activity must be interrupted sooner than before because of a markedly lower endurance.

To measure fatigue's impact on the quality of life, Packer administered a fatigue severity rating scale (FSS) (51) to 12 PPS patients (52). In this small series, patients with PPS had higher scores on FFS than are known for nondisabled populations, but had comparable scores to subjects diagnosed with multiple sclerosis or with systemic lupus erythematosus. Despite the return of strength with rest, eventual disengagement from various activities occurs, and quality of life suffers.

In a series of 86 PPS fatigued patients who were compared to 20 healthy controls, 23% of PPS patients scored 14 or higher on the Beck Depression Inventory (53), indicating mild to moderate depression (37). No significant differences were found between depressed and nondepressed PPS patients on the progression of fatigue severity in the

previous 6 months or on the variation of fatigue with time of day. Depression was not a major contributing variable to the prevalence or description of fatigue in PPS patients.

Another hypothesis is that fatigue is an expression of the psychology of some AP survivors. Bruno believes that there is something unique about the AP experience that predisposes to the development of maladaptive personality traits (54). The experience of AP was often emotionally overwhelming, especially if emotional deprivation and abuse could not be prevented. Paralysis meant loss of control and dependency on others; hospitalization meant separation from loved ones and often painful treatments, including multiple surgeries. The behavior of AP survivors who ceaselessly thrive for normality and attempt to become unduly accomplished despite the real limitations posed by handicap, may represent an attempt to overcome the trauma of AP. This disordered personality profile makes it difficult to adjust to the necessary life changes that the development of PPS entails.

Bruno also considered the fact that between 70–96% of polio survivors with fatigue report concomitant problems with concentration, memory, attention, word finding, maintaining wakefulness, and thinking clearly (55). Bruno reported on six carefully selected PPS patients who were studied with neuropsychological tests that assess attention and other higher-level cognitive processes (56). In his admittedly small series, he found an association between an impaired ability to maintain attention and to process complex information rapidly and severe subjective fatigue. Incidentally, he also found evidence of an impairment of delayed recall of nonverbal information unrelated to the degree of fatigue, as reported also by Freidenberg (57). Bruno concluded that small but objective decrements in cognitive functioning are likely to be felt as subjectively very significant by fatigued PPS patients who, by temperament, value normality to the utmost. The question arises whether mental fatigue, like other PPS features, can be attributed to the degeneration later in life of cerebral nervous pathways that have been damaged at the time of AP. Dysfunction of the reticular activating system, sleep maintenance mechanisms, and respiratory centers have been proposed to underlie central fatigue in PPS.

So far, the mainstay of treatment is focused on preventing or limiting muscle fatigue by applying the general principle of energy conservation with work simplification skills, frequent daily rests, and prescription of mobility aids. Neuropsychiatric consultation seems warranted when the presence of fatigue, chronic pain, and sleep disorder become problematic. It is important to rule out major affective disorder, depression—if concomitant—and to treat it properly, preferably with nonsedating antidepressant drugs, such as selective serotonin reuptake blockers like fluoxetine, in full therapeutic dosage. The management of fatigue, chronic pain, and sleep disorder is more challenging to the psychiatrist when depression is not present. In these cases, a symptomatic approach is best. The use of a sedative serotoninergic tricyclic antidepressant such as amitriptyline in small doses (e.g., 25–75 mg at bedtime) may help with pain control and sleep regulation. Amantadine does not appear to be significantly superior to placebo in reducing fatigue (58). Pyridostigmine is being administered only under a research protocol and is not yet approved for clinical use (40).

MYASTHENIA GRAVIS

Myasthenia gravis (MG) is a nonhereditary disease that affects mainly adults, although a juvenile onset can occur. MG is believed to be an autoimmune disease in which the presence of autoantibodies to skeletal muscle acetylcholine receptors (AChRs) renders AChRs nonfunctional at the level of the neuromuscular junction. The result is an impairment of transmission across the neuromuscular junction. These anti-AChR antibodies can be detected in the serum of up to 95% of MG patients. Loss of receptors may be attributed to accelerated degradation caused by antibody attachment and complement-mediated destruction.

Clinical and immunological heterogeneity in MG is well known. In mild cases, fatigue of the muscular system, marked by progressive paralysis of the muscle without sensory changes or atrophy, is produced upon exercising. In more severe cases, muscular weakness is present at rest. Extraocular muscles are typically affected, but any muscle, including respiratory muscles, can be attacked. Thymic hyperplasia (or a frank thymoma) is a frequent accompanying feature. The disease develops over a few days or weeks and may advance irregularly or remain at the same level of severity for years. Remissions occur and relapses are unpredictable as to time of occurrence and severity. The life of a MG patient is endangered by the progression of paralysis. Respiratory insufficiency, which may come on quite abruptly or progress insidiously, is a fatal complication in some 5–10% of cases (59).

Diagnosis is made from the characteristic finding on EMG studies of a decremental response to repeated stimulation, and from the disappearance of weakness following the intravenous administration of edrophonium chloride (Tensilon test).

Although the peripheral manifestations of MG have been well documented, there have been sporadic reports that suggest central nervous system (CNS) involvement as well (60). The presence of anti-AChR antibodies in cerebrospinal fluid (CSF) may result from passive diffusion from serum, especially if the blood-brain barrier is inflamed, or from local synthesis within the CNS.

In a study of 44 MG patients, Muller reported on the immunological abnormalities found in CSF: 50% of patients had a lymphoid reaction in their CSF, and in 15 of 40 patients, serum and CSF immunoglobulin G (IgG) and anti-AChR antibody analysis suggested local synthesis of anti-AChR antibodies within the CNS (60).

A direct effect of anti-AChR antibodies on central cholinergic pathways has been suggested as underlying memory difficulties in MG patients. Nicotinic AChRs are found in the central as well as in the peripheral nervous system, particularly in the hippocampus, hypothalamus, and the cerebral cortex. Nicotinic AChRs have an important role in higher cognitive processes, especially memory.

In a controlled study, Davidov-Lustig et al. administered the revised Wechsler Memory scale (20) and attempted to correlate the results with several disease parameters. A positive correlation was obtained between the severity of forgetfulness and the inability to memorize and retain learned material and the severity of peripheral myasthenic signs (61).

Earlier studies have documented cognitive impairment, which is reversible with plasma exchange. Plasma exchange is a technique whereby anti-AChR autoantibodies are removed from sera as well as from CSF to some degree.

Tucker studied the performance on a battery of cognitive tasks of 12 MG patients compared with 10 healthy control subjects and 10 medical control subjects with chronic disease of a nonneurological nature (62). The myasthenic group was significantly impaired relative to both control groups on performance on the Wechsler Memory Scale (Logical and Design Reproduction) (20). In one MG patient, memory impaired prior to plasmapheresis improved with plasmapheresis on two separate occasions.

Aarli reported a case of a thymectomized woman with MG receiving prednisone who developed amnesia for recent events during a benign acute febrile illness (63). Improvement in mnemonic function occurred when 9 months later plasma exchange was performed.

In another small series of 5 MG patients, the Zung self-rating depression scale (64) was added to cognitive tests, which included the Mini-Mental State Examination (MMSE) (21) and a logical memory test (65). No patient was found to be clinically depressed pre- or post-plasma exchange, but all five had significantly worse scores as compared with normal controls on all the tests before plasma exchange. Following plasma exchange, which brought about improvement in motor function in all, mean scores on the Zung, the MMSE, and on the logical memory test improved significantly.

However, Lewis found no cognitive deficits in his MG patients, either compared to controls or to their own performance after plasma exchange, based on memory tests before and after plasma exchange (66).

From a neuropsychiatric point of view, the potential for behavioral sequelae of the central manifestations of MG is only beginning to be addressed. Traditionally, psychopathology, if present, was understood as reactive to the stress of an uncertain clinical course and to the nature of physical symptoms that characterize MG. In a series of 20 MG patients compared to 15 patients with polymyositis/dermatomyositis, significantly more patients with MG (40%) than controls (7%) were diagnosed with panic disorder (67). It is not known whether this high prevalence of an anxiety disorder stems from the psychological sense of a loss of control in patients with MG, or, if possibly, it can be related to the central cholinergic effects of MG.

Table 40.1. Case Definition Criteria for CFS

A case of CFS must fulfill both major and minor criteria.

Major criteria

   A. New onset of persistent or relapsing, debilitating fatigue in a person with no previous history of such symptoms that does not resolve with bedrest and that is severe enough to reduce or impair average daily activity to less than 50% of the patient's premorbid activity level, for at least 6 months.

   B. Fatigue that is not explained by the presence of other obvious medical or psychiatric illness.

Minor criteria

   At least six symptoms plus at least two signs, or at least eight symptoms from the list below: Symptoms: mild fever or chills, sore throat, painful lymph nodes, generalized muscle weakness, myalgia, prolonged generalized fatigue after exercise, headaches, migratory arthralgia without swelling or redness, neuropsychological complaints, sleep disturbance, symptom complex developing over a few hours to a few days; Physical signs: low-grade fever, nonexudative pharyngitis, palpable or tender anterior or posterior, cervical, or axillary lymph nodes.

The management of MG patients is divided into two parts: the treatment of the acute episodes of severe paralysis and the long-term management. Neostigmine is the drug of choice for the treatment of acute attacks. Special attention to the prevention of respiratory problems is essential. In the long term, no treatment may be necessary between attacks in the milder cases. In more severe cases, neostigmine remains the most useful drug. If the patient becomes resistant to neostigmine, pyridostigmine may be substituted. In the chronic and disabling MG, thymectomy and immunotherapy, including corticosteroid therapy, are utilized. If psychiatric complications develop, avoidance of psychotropic medications with significant anticholinergic side effects—such as tricyclic antidepressants or certain neuroleptics—avoids memory dysfunction as well as aggravation of weakness.

AMYOTROPHIC LATERAL SCLEROSIS

Amyotrophic lateral sclerosis (ALS) is the most common of a group of syndromes called motor system diseases. Motor system diseases are characterized by a progressive degenerative disorder of motor neurons in the cerebral cortex, brainstem, and spinal cord, manifested clinically by muscular weakness and wasting without sensory changes, and by spasticity with exaggeration of tendon reflexes.

Classical ALS is a disease of middle life, generally appearing in the fifth or sixth decade. It is usually a sporadic disease, but a family history of a similar disease can be elicited in 5–10% of cases. Onset is insidious. Weakness can be asymmetric early on, but eventually muscle wasting becomes symmetric, widespread, and accompanied by visible fascicular twitchings of groups of muscle fibers. Dysarthria and impairment of chewing and swallowing result from involvement of muscles supplied by the brainstem. Manifestations of pseudobulbar palsy—such as involuntary and explosive weeping or laughter—result from involvement of corticobulbar fibers. Progression is unhalting and leads to extensive paralysis, with death from respiratory weakness or aspiration pneumonia, generally within 2–5 years from onset.

Classical ALS is widely regarded as an illness confined to the voluntary motor system, with intelligence and cognitive function preserved. But dementia, parkinsonism, and sensory changes can occur in association with ALS: it is not known whether these combined entities represent variants of classical ALS or are separate entities altogether.

Psychosis most often in the form of delirium has been reported (68). Dementia is estimated to occur in 2% of cases of sporadic ALS, according to Jokelainen (69). In familial ALS, dementia has been reported in up to 15% of families (70). Neuropathological findings are widespread in the brain of ALS patients; the severity of the cerebral lesions in different structures may vary from case to case, from clinically silent cerebral atrophy to dementia of the frontal lobe type with marked neuron loss and gliosis in the frontal and temporal lobes.

The effects of newly-developed treatments for ALS on patients' mental status have not yet been studied.

CHRONIC FATIGUE SYNDROME

Chronic fatigue syndrome (CFS) is a diagnosis of exclusion. It is given consideration once familiar medical conditions have been ruled out, including infections, malignancy, autoimmune, inflammatory, endocrine, hematological, toxic, neurological, and psychiatric diseases (71). Historically, it resembles febricula, neurasthenia, DaCosta's syndrome (72), chronic brucellosis (73), chronic Epstein-Barr virus syndrome (74), Royal Free disease (75), and myalgic encephalomyelitis (76).

The Centers for Disease Control (CDC) has proposed a case definition that is rigorous and research oriented (77). It may well exclude milder forms of the syndrome. There are two major and 11 minor criteria. There are also three physical signs. A case of CFS must fulfill both major criteria and at least six minor symptoms plus at least two signs, or at least eight symptoms (Table 40.1).

Further clarifications of this definition were accepted following an NIH proposal (78). Mainly, certain psychiatric diagnoses were excluded from CFS, such as schizophrenia, bipolar affective disorder, psychotic depression, and substance abuse. The following additional disorders were allowed, provided that onset and response to psychiatric therapy are mentioned: nonpsychotic depression: if concurrent, 1 month post onset or 6 months or more before onset, recurrent or nonrecurrent; anxiety disorders (generalized or panic disorder), and somatoform disorders (conversion, psychogenic pain, or psychological factors complicating physical disease).

Current theories of the etiology of this disorder include infection, dysimmune process, or a variant of a mental illness. A disorder of sleep regulation, namely an α-rhythm disturbance (7.5–11 Hz) in the EEG during nonrapid eye movement, accompanied by increased nocturnal vigilance and nonrestorative sleep, has also been considered (79). A neuroendocrine etiology implicating a hypothalamic dysfunction with a functional deficit of corticotropin releasing factor has also been studied (80).

The typical picture of acute onset of symptoms following a respiratory or gastrointestinal infection supports an infectious etiology (81). The Epstein-Barr virus (EBV) was implicated when patients with the typical symptoms were found to have an abnormal reactivated pattern of antibodies to EBV, suggesting chronic EBV infection (82, 83). However, not all patients with CFS have evidence of EBV infection (84); controls without CFS also have the reactivation pattern, and patients with CFS have elevated titers of antibodies to other viruses such as herpes simplex, measles, and cytomegalovirus.

Human herpes virus type 6 (HHV-6) is the cause of *roseola infantum,* a common childhood illness. Antibodies to HHV-6 have been found in the sera of 60–90% of the general population and 80–100% of patients with CFS (85–87). Active replication of HHV-6 in mononuclear cells has been demonstrated in up to 81% of patients with CFS (88). HHV-6 may be the cause of viral symptoms in CFS, or the high titers may be the result of nonspecific polyclonal stimulation.

Other pathogens implicated have been human T-lymphotrophic virus type 2, a retrovirus (HTLV-2) (89), cytomegalovirus, hepatitis A (90), influenza and rubella (91), brucella (73), *Borrelia burgdorferi* (92), *Clostridium jejuni* (93), and others. No single agent has been found to be the cause.

Multiple immune system alterations have been found in patients with CFS. The most consistent immunological abnormality detected has been low natural killer cell cytotoxicity (94). NK cells are increased in number but decreased in cytotoxicity compared with controls. Investigators have also found diminished in vitro production of major natural killer (NK) cell activators, γ-interferon and interleukin-2, by cultured lymphocytes (95). Other changes observed include alterations in CD4 and CD8 cells; however, these have not been consistent. As well, the humoral response of patients with CFS has been abnormal, including mild IgA deficiency, elevated immune complexes, the presence of cold agglutinins, positive antinuclear antibodies, and false-positive serology for syphilis (94). These results have provided circumstantial support for the hypothesis that CFS is a dysimmune disorder; however, the role of psychological factors such as comorbid depression and their effect on the immune system also needs to be taken into account.

Fatigue and the role of muscle disease has been carefully examined. Strength testing in multiple situations is normal (96, 97). 31p-magnetic resonance spectroscopy shows no consistent abnormality of skeletal muscle metabolic patterns (98–101). Muscle histopathology is normal (102). EMG changes may be normal or abnormal but do not account for the fatigue (103). Therefore, no significant myopathy is present.

Finally, the role of mental illness is unclear. In the Royal Free epidemic that occurred in 1955 among nursing and medical staff at the Royal Free Hospital in London, chronic fatigue was initially believed to represent viral encephalomyelitis, but was later found more compatible with mass hysteria (75). A follow-up study from 1968–1969 demonstrated that the affected nurses, when compared with matched controls, had higher neuroticism, and that in the 13 years following the epidemic, many had faked symptoms for secondary gains, which is compatible with the diagnosis of malingering (104). There were two suicides; two became chronic invalids; and five became permanently disabled.

Contemporary research studies have shown that the majority of patients with the CFS (*a*) are white middle-aged women, (*b*) have abnormal personality traits, (*c*) firmly believe that their fatigue has a physical cause. Current major depression and somatization disorder are common. Depressive symptoms have been reported in 35–70% of CFS patients (105, 106). Reports on the temporal relation of the onset of depression and the onset of CFS are inconsistent.

Wessely and Powell reported on patients presenting to a neurological center with unexplained chronic fatigue of a minimum 6-month duration (107). In a prospective study, these patients were compared with fatigued patients admitted to a psychiatric hospital and diagnosed with major depression, and fatigued patients with known neuromuscular disease. Seventy-two percent of the CFS patients were found to meet criteria for a mental disorder, using diagnostic criteria that excluded fatigue as a symptom, compared with 36% of the neuromuscular group. There was no difference in subjective complaints of physical fatigue between all groups. Mental fatigue was equally common in CFS and depressed patients, but occurred only in those neuromuscular patients who were also diagnosed with psychiatric disorder. Twenty-eight percent of the CFS patients had mental and physical fatigue but no psychiatric diagnosis. The major difference between the CFS patients and psychiatric patients was in the patients' attribution of symptoms: the CFS patients attributed their symptoms to a viral illness, while the psychiatric patients blamed a wealth of psychic factors in the genesis of their fatigue and abnormal mood.

These findings are consistent with two often-quoted studies of the mental health of patients who present with a chief complaint of fatigue. Manu prospectively evaluated 100 adults with a chief complaint of fatigue in an internal medicine outpatient clinic (108). Using the Diagnostic Interview Schedule, a highly comprehensive and reliable instrument, it was found that 66 patients had one or more mental disorders that were considered a major cause of their chronic fatigue (mood disorder, 47 patients; somatization disorder, 15 patients; anxiety disorder, 9 patients). Five had medical conditions explaining their fatigue, and in 31, fatigue remained of unknown origin. In the other study, among the 1159 consecutive patients surveyed in a primary care clinic, 276 (24%) indicated that fatigue was a major problem. Of 102 patients in whom screening psychometric instruments, including the Beck Inventory (53), were administered, 82 (80%) had marked depression or somatic anxiety. After 1 year of follow-up, only 29 (28%) had improved.

Studies using formal neuropsychological testing have not revealed unequivocal abnormalities in attention and memory (80, 109–111).

Management with antidepressant drugs has been proposed (105), and results from small series are becoming available (112).

Nortriptyline, a tricyclic antidepressant with a well-defined therapeutic plasma level in major depression (50–150 ng/ml) was tested in a single-case, double-blind, placebo-controlled study for the treatment of CFS (113). The patient, a 35-year-old woman with a diagnosis of CFS, according to CDC criteria, also carried a diagnosis of major depression. Objective measures of change were obtained using the Beck Inventory of Depression (53) and the CFS Checklist, which measures the severity of Holmes criteria for CFS (77). The design of the trial was A-B-A-B (drug-placebo-drug-placebo). Maximal doses of 60 mg a day were used and well tolerated by the patient. Significant but incomplete relief of affective and physical symptoms with decreases in fever and lymphadenopathy occurred with treatment with nortriptyline. It is generally accepted that the analgesic effect of tricyclic antidepressant occurs separately and at lower doses than the antidepressant effect. It is not known if this patient's functional recovery was due to an analgesic effect of nortriptyline or if it was due to an anti-fatigue or immunological effect of the drug.

Encouraging results have also been reported in the treatment of CFS using fluoxetine 20 mg a day (114), sertraline 50 mg/day (115), phenelzine 15–30 mg/day (116), and buproprion (115).

Clearly, the administration of antidepressant medication in CFS is not without controversy, especially in those patients with CFS who do not have a concurrent mental disorder that would warrant in itself the use of such pharmacotherapy). Thus, an immunological profile should be determined before and at regular intervals during drug treatment. Immunological benefit has been tentatively ascribed to antidepressant drug use, and an attempt to document responses from the point of view of fatigue, affect, and immunological profile appears clinically worthwhile. Psychopharmacology should be initiated only after a therapeutic alliance has been established, because patients with CFS appear to be highly critical of psychotropic medication and intolerant of side effects. Explanation of the deconditioning phenomenon that unavoidably accompanies inactivity must be repeatedly provided, and encouragement to participate in a graded exercise program is

crucial. Also, undue validation of the sick role must be tactfully avoided.

Among immunological approaches to the treatment of CFS, immunoglobins, essential fatty acids, immune modifiers, and ion flow treatments are encouraging, even if results are preliminary (116). Use of acyclovir has proven disappointing. Amantadine has not yet been used in a controlled trial in CFS related disorders.

Acknowledgments

The authors thank Dr. Neil Cashman (Department of Neurology, Montreal Neurological Hospital, McGill University) for his help in the preparation of this chapter.

References

1. Harper PS. Myotonic dystrophy. Philadelphia: WB Saunders, 1989:384.
2. Roses AD, Appel SH. Muscle membrane protein kinase in myotonic muscular dystrophy. Nature 1974;250:245–247.
3. Aslanidis C, Jansen G, Amemiya C, et al. Cloning of the essential myotonic dystrophic region and mapping of the putative defect. Nature (London) 1992;355:548–551.
4. Buxton J, Shelbourne P, Davies J, et al. Detection of an unstable fragment of DNA specific to individuals with myotonic dystrophy. Nature (London) 1992;355:547–548.
5. Harley HG, Brook JD, Rundle SA, et al. Expansion of an unstable DNA region and phenotypic variation in myotonic dystrophy. Nature (London) 1992;355:545–546.
6. Brook JD, McCurrach ME, Harley HG, et al. Molecular basis of myotonic dystrophy: expansion of a trinucleotide(CTG) repeat at the 3* end of a transcript encoding a protein kinase family member. Cell 1992;68:799–808.
7. Fu YH, Pizzuti A, Fenwick Jr RG, et al. An unstable triplet repeat in a gene related to myotonic muscular dystrophy. Science 1992;255:1256–1258.
8. Mahadevan M, Tsilfidis C, Sabourin L, et al. Myotonic dystrophy mutation: an unstable CTG repeat in the 3*untranslated region of the gene. Science 1992;255:1253–1255.
9. Howeler CJ, Busch HFM, Geraedts JPM, Niermeijer MF, Staal A. Anticipation in myotonic dystrophy. Fact or fiction. Brain 1989;112:779–797.
10. Dyken PR. The changing syndromes of dystrophia myotonia. Neurology 1969;19:292.
11. Dyken PR, Harper PS. Congenital dystrophia myotonica. Neurology 1973;23:465–473.
12. Adie WJ, Greenfield JG. Dystrophia myotonica (myotonia atrophica). Brain 1923;46:73–127.
13. Maas O, Paterson AS. Mental change in families affected by dystrophia myotonica. Lancet 1937;1:21–23.
14. Woodward JB III, Heaton RK, Simon DB, Ringel SP. Neuropsychological findings in myotonic dystrophy. J Clin Neuropsychol 1982;4:335–342.
15. Bird TD, Follet C, Griep E. Cognitive and personality function in myotonic muscular dystrophy. J Neurol Neurosurg Psychiatry 1983;46:971–980.
16. Portwood MM, Wicks JJ, Lieberman JS, et al. Intellectual and cognitive function in adults with myotonic muscular dystrophy. Arch Phys Med Rehabil 1986;67:299–303.
17. Brumback RA. Disturbed personality and psychosocial adjustment in myotonic dystrophy: relationship to intellectual cognitive function and underlying affective disorder (depression). Psychol Rep 1987;60:70:783–796.

18. Perini GI, Columbo G, Armani M, et al. Intellectual impairment and cognitive evoked potentials in myotonic dystrophy. J Nerv Ment Dis 1989;177:750–754.

19. Huber SJ, Kissel JT, Shuttleworth EC, Chakeres DW, Clapp LE, Brogan MA. Magnetic resonance imaging and clinical correlates of intellectual impairment in myotonic dystrophy. Arch Neurol 1989; 46:536–540.

20. Wechsler D. Manual-Wechsler Adult Intelligence Scale (Revised). New York: Psychological Corporation 1981.

21. Folstein M, Folstein S, McHugh P. Mini-mental State. A practical method for grading the cognitive state of patients for the clinician. J Psychiatry Res 1975;12:189–198.

22. Roche SW, Schwarz A, Lane RJM, Bridges LR. Reversal of cognitive deficit by cardiac pacing in a young man with dystrophia myotonica. J Roy Soc Med 1991;84:625–626.

23. Good PKE, Branter JP. A practical guide to the MMPI. Minneapolis: Univ. of Minn. Press, 1974.

24. American Psychiatric Association Task Force on Nomenclature. Diagnostic and statistical manual of mental disorders. 3rd ed., (DSM-III). Washington, DC: American Psychiatric Association, 1980;205–224.

25. Hamilton M. A rating scale for depression. J Neurol Neurosurg Psychiatry 1960;23:56–62.

26. Brumback RA. Magnetic resonance imaging and clinical correlates of intellectual impairment in myotonic dystrophic. Arch Neurol 1990; 47:253–254.

27. Duveneck MJ, Portwood MM, Wicks JJ, Lieberman JS. Depression in myotonic muscular dystrophy. Arch Phys Med Rehabil 1986;67: 875–877.

28. Glantz RH, Wright RB, Huckman MS, Garron DC, Siegel IM. Central nervous system magnetic resonance imaging findings in myotonic dystrophy. Arch Neurol 1988;45:36–37.

29. Damian MS, Bachmann G, Herrmann D, Dornof W. Magnetic resonance imaging of muscle and brain in myotonic dystrophy. J Neurol 1993;240:8–12.

30. Yoshimura N, Otake M, Igarashi K, Matsunaga M, Takebe K, Kudo H. Topography of Alzheimer's neurofibrillary change distribution in myotonic dystrophy. Clin Neuropathol 1990;9:234–239.

31. Hoffman EP, Brown RH Jr, Kunkel LM. Dystrophin: the protein product of the Duchenne muscular dystrophy locus. Cell 1987;51: 919–928.

32. Ervasti JM, Campbell KP. Membrane organization of the dystrophin-glycoprotein complex. Cell 1991;66:1121–1131.

33. Rossiter BJF, Stirpe NS, Caskey CT. Report of the MDA gene therapy conference, Tucson, Arizona, September 27–28, 1991. Neurology 1992;42:1413–1418.

34. Rutter M. A children's behaviour questionnaire for completion by teachers: preliminary findings. J Child Psychol Psychiatry 1967; 8:1–11.

35. Leibowitz D, Dubowitz V. Intellect and behavior in Duchenne muscular dystrophy. Dev Med Child Neurol 1981;23:577–590.

36. Carpenter S, Karpati G. Becker dystrophy. In: Carpenter S, Karpati G, eds. Pathology of skeletal muscle. New York: Churchill Livingstone 1984;420–421.

37. Berlly MH, Strauser WW, Hall KM. Fatigue in postpolio syndrome. Arch Phys Med Rehabil 1991;72:115–118.

38. Dalakas M. Postpolio syndrome. Curr Opin Rheum 1990;2: 901–907.

39. Munsat TL. Poliomyelitis--new problems with an old disease. N En J Med 1991;324:1206–1207.

40. Trojan DA, Gendron D, Cashman NR. Anticholinesterase-responsive neuromuscular junction transmission defects in post-poliomyelitis fatigue. J Neurol Sci 1993;114:170–177.

41. Trojan DA, Gendron D, Cashman NR. Stimulation frequency-dependent neuromuscular junction transmission defects in patients with prior poliomyelitis. J Neurol Sci 1993;118:150–157.

42. Stone R. Post-Polio Syndrome: remembrance of viruses past. Science 1994;264:909.

43. Wiechers DO, Hubbell SL. Late changes in the motor unit after acute poliomyelitis. Muscle Nerve 1981;4:524–528.

44. Nee L, Dambrosia J, Bern E, et al. Paralytic polio: a 45 year follow-up of 46 twin pairs (POSTER #17). The post-polio syndrome: advances in the pathogenesis and treatment. Ann N Y Acad Sci Apr 27-30, 1994.

45. Sivakumar K, Sinnwell T, Yildiz E, et al. Study of fatigue in muscles of patients with post-polio syndrome by in vivo 31p magnetic resonance spectroscopy: a metabolic cause for fatigue (POSTER #18). The post-polio syndrome: advances in the pathogenesis and treatment, Ann N Y Acad Sci Apr 27-30, 1994.

46. Sharief MK, Hentges R, Ciardi M. Intrathecal immune response in patients with the post-polio syndrome. N Engl J Med 1991;325: 749–755.

47. Muir P, Nicholson F, Sharieff MK, et al. Evidence for persistent enterovirus infection of the central nervous system in patients with previous paralytic poliomyelitis and post-polio syndrome. [Abstract]. The post-polio syndrome: advances in the pathogenesis and treatment. Ann N Y Acad Sci Apr 27-30, 1994.

48. Leparc I, Kopecka H, Fuchs F, et al. Search for poliovirus in specimens from patients with the post-polio syndrome. [Abstract]. The post-polio syndrome: advances in the pathogenesis and treatment. Ann N Y Acad Sci Apr 27-30, 1994.

49. Monzon M, Dalakas MC. Virological studies in blood, serum and spinal fluid in patients with post-polio syndrome (PPS). [Abstract]. The post-polio syndrome: advances in the pathogenesis and treatment. Ann NY Acad Sci Apr 27-30, 1994.

50. Halstead LS, Rossi CD. Post-polio syndrome: clinical experience with 132 consecutive outpatients. In: Halstead LS, Weichers DO eds. Research and clinical aspects of the late effects of poliomyelitis. White Plains, NY: March of Dimes Birth Defects Foundation, 1987:13–26.

51. Krupp LB, La Rocca NG, Muir-Nash RN, et al. The fatigue severity scale: application to patients with multiple sclerosis and systemic lupus erythematosus. Arch Neurol 1989;48:1121–1123.

52. Packer TL, Martins I, Krefting L, Brouwer B. Activity and post-polio fatigue. Orthopedics 1991;14:1223–1226.

53. Beck AT, Ward CH, Mendelson M, Mock J, Erbaugh J. An inventory for measuring depression. Arch Gen Psychiatry 1961;4:561–571.

54. Bruno RL, Frick NM. The psychology of polio as prelude to post-polio sequelae: behavior modification and psychotherapy. Orthopedics 1991;14:1185-1193.

55. Bruno RL, Frick NM, Cohen J. Polioencephalitis, stress, and the etiology of post-polio sequelae. Orthopaedics 1991;14:1269–1276.

56. Bruno RL, Galski T, DeLuca J. The neuropsychology of post-polio fatigue. Arch Phys Med Rehabil 1993;74:1061–1065.

57. Freidenberg DL, Freeman D, Huber SJ, et al. Postpoliomyelitis syndrome: assessment of behavioral features. Neuropsychiatry Neuropsychol Behav Neurol 1989;2:272–281.

58. Stein DP, Dambrosia J, Dalakas M. Treatment of fatigue in post-polio syndrome (PPS) using amantadine: a double-blind placebo controlled study [Abstract]. The Post-polio syndrome: advances in the pathogenesis and treatment. Ann N Y Acad Sci Apr 27-30, 1994.

59. Adams RD, Victor MJ. Myasthenia gravis and episodic forms of muscular weakness. In: Adams RD, Victor M eds. Principles of neurology. New York: McGraw-Hill, 1989: 1150–1167.

60. Muller KMI, Taskinen E, Lefvert AK, et al. Immunoactivation in the central nervous system in myasthenia gravis. J Neurol Sci 1987;80: 13–23.

61. Davidov-Lustig M, Klinghoffer V, Kaplan-Dinur A, et al. Memory abnormalities in myasthenia gravis: possible fatigue of central nervous system cholinergic circuits. Autoimmunity 1992;14:85–86.

62. Tucker DM, Roeltgen DP, Wann PD, Wertheimer RI. Memory dysfunction in myasthenia gravis: evidence for central cholinergic effects. Neurology 1988;38:1173–1177.

63. Aarli JA, Gilhus NE, Thorlacius S, Johnsen HJ. Recovery from global amnesia during plasma exchange in myasthenia gravis: report of a case. Acta Neurol Scand 1989;80:351–353.

64. Zung WWK. A self-rating depression scale. Arch Gen Psychiatry 1965;12:63–70.

65. Iwasaki Y, Kinoshita M, Ikeda K, Shiojima T, Kurihara T. Neuropsychological function before and after plasma exchange in myasthenia gravis. J Neurol Sci 1993;114:223–226.

66. Lewis SW, Ron MA, Newsom-Davis J. Absence of central functional cholinergic deficits in myasthenia gravis. J Neurol Neurosurg Psychiatry 1989;52:258–261.

67. Paradis CM, Friedman S, Lazar RM, Kula RW. Anxiety disorders in a neuromuscular clinic. Am J Psychiatry 1993;150:1102–1104.

68. Ziegler LH. Psychotic and emotional phenomena associated with amyotrophic lateral sclerosis. Arch Neurol Psychiat 1930;24: 930–936.

69. Jokelainen M. Amyotrophic lateral sclerosis in Finland. 1. an epidemiologic study. Acta Neurol Scand 1977;56:185–193.

70. Hudson AJ. Amyotrophic lateral sclerosis and its association with dementia, parkinsonism and other neurological disorders: a review. Brain 1981;104:217–247.

71. Kroenke K, Wood DR, Mangelsdorff AD, Meier NJ, Powell JB. Chronic fatigue in primary care. JAMA 1988;260:929–934.

72. Straus SE. History of chronic fatigue syndrome. Rev Infect Dis 1991;13(Suppl 1):S2–S7.

73. Evans AC. Brucellosis in the United States. Am J Public Health 1947;37:139–151.

74. Holmes GP, Kaplan JE, Stewart JA, Hunt B, Pinsky PF, Schonberger LB. A cluster of patients with a chronic mononucleosis-like syndrome: is Epstein-Barr virus the cause? JAMA 1987;257:2297–2302.

75. Medical Staff of the Royal Free Hospital. An outbreak of encephalomyelitis in the Royal Free Hospital group, London, in 1955. Br Med J 1957;ii:895–904.

76. McEvedy CP, Beard AW. Concept of benign myalgic encephalomyelitis. Br Med J 1970;1:11–15.

77. Holmes GP, Kaplan JE, Gantz NM, et al. Chronic fatigue syndrome: a working case definition. Ann Intern Med 1988;108:387–389.

78. Schluederberg A, Strauss SE, Peterson P, et al. Chronic fatigue syndrome research-definition and medical outcome assessment. Ann Intern Med 1992;117:325–331.

79. Moldofsky H. Fibromyalgia, sleep disorder and chronic fatigue syndrome. In: Bock GR, Whelan J, eds. Ciba Foundation symposium 173:Chronic fatigue syndrome. Chichester: John Wiley & Sons, 1993: 262–279.

80. Wessely S. The neuropsychiatry of chronic fatigue syndrome. In: Bock GR, Whelan J, eds. Ciba Foundation symposium 173: Chronic fatigue syndrome. Chichester: John Wiley & Sons, 1993:212–237.

81. Straus SE, Dale JK, Wright R, Metcalfe DD. Allergy and the chronic fatigue syndrome. J Allergy Clin Immunol 1988;81:791–795.

82. Jones JF, Ray CG, Minnich LL, Hicks MJ, Kibler R, Lucas DO. Evidence for active Epstein-Barr virus infection in patients with persistent, unexplained illness:elevated anti-early antigen antibodies. Ann Intern Med 1985;102:1–7.

83. Straus SE, Tosato G, Armstrong G, et al. Persisting illness and fatigue in adults with evidence of Epstein-Barr virus infection. Ann Intern Med 1985;102:7–16.

84. Sumaya CV. Serologic and virologic epidemiology of Epstein-Barr virus: relevance to chronic fatigue syndrome. Rev Infect Dis 1991;13(Suppl):S19–S25.

85. Gold D, Bowden R, Sixbey J, et al. Chronic fatigue: a prospective clinical and virologic study. JAMA 1990;264:48–53.

86. Landay AL, Jessop C, Lennette ET, Levy JA. Chronic fatigue syndrome: clinical condition associated with immune activation. Lancet 1991;338:707–712.

87. Daugherty SA, Henry BE, Peterson DL, Swarts RL, Bastien S, Thomas RS. Chronic fatigue syndrome in northern Nevada. Rev Infect Dis 1991;(Suppl 1):S39–S44.

88. Buchwald D, Cheney PR, Peterson DL, et al. A chronic illness characterized by fatigue, neurologic and immunologic disorders, and active human herpes virus type 6 infection. Ann Intern Med 1992; 116:103–113.

89. DeFreitas E, Hilliard B, Cheney PR, et al. Retroviral sequences related to human T-lymphotropic virus type II in patients with chronic fatigue immune dysfunction syndrome. Proc Natl Acad Sci 1991;88: 2922–2926.

90. Salit IE. Sporadic postinfectious neuromyasthenia. Can Med Assoc J 1985;133:659–663.

91. Bell EJ, McCartney RA, Riding MH. Coxsackie B viruses and myalgic encephalomyelitis. J Roy Soc Med 1988;81:329–331.

92. Krupp LB, Mendelson WB, Friedman R. An overview of chronic fatigue syndrome. J Clin Psychiatry 1991;52:403–410.

93. Peterson PK, Schenck CK, Sherman R. Chronic fatigue syndrome in Minnesota. Minn Med 1991;74:21–26.

94. Klimas NG, Salvato FR, Morgan R, Fletcher MA. Immunologic abnormalities in chronic fatigue syndrome. J Clin Microbiol 1990; 28:1403–1410.

95. Kibler R, Lucas DD, Hicks MJ, Poulos BT, Jones JF. Immune function in chronic active Epstein-Barr virus infection. J Clin Immunol 1985;5:46–54.

96. Stokes MJ, Cooper RG, Edwards RHT. Normal muscle strength and fatigability in patients with effort syndromes. Br Med J 1988;297: 1014–1017.

97. Gibson H, Carroll N, Coakley J, Edwards RHT. Recovery from maximal exercise in chronic fatigue states. Eur J Clin Invest 1990;20:A29.

98. Arnold DL, Bore PJ, Radda GK, Styles P, Taylor DJ. Excessive intracellular acidosis of skeletal muscle on exercise in a patient with a post-viral exhaustion fatigue syndrome. A 31P nuclear magnetic study. Lancet 1984;1367–1369.

99. Jamal GA, Miller RG. Neurophysiology of postviral fatigue syndrome. Br Med Bull 1991;47:815–825.

100. Wong R, Lopaschuk G, Zhu G, et al. Skeletal muscle metabolism in the chronic fatigue syndrome. In vivo assessment by 31P nuclear magnetic resonance spectroscopy. Chest 1992;102:1716–1722.

101. Barnes PR, Taylor DJ, Kemp GJ, Radda GK. Skeletal muscle bioenergetics in the chronic fatigue syndrome. J Neurol Neurosurg Psychiatry 1993;56:679–683.

102. Behan PO, Behan WMH, Bell EJ. The postviral fatigue syndrome—an analysis of the findings in 50 cases. J Infect Dis 1985;10:211–222.

103. Jamal GA, Hansen S. Electrophysiological studies in the post-viral fatigue syndrome. J Neurol Neurosurg Psychiatry 1985;48:691–694.

104. McEvedy CP, Beard AW. Royal Free Epidemic of 1955: a reconsideration. Br Med J 1970;1:7–11.

105. Abbey SE, Garfinkel PE. Chronic fatigue syndrome and the psychiatrist. Can J Psychiatry 1990; 35:625–633.

106. Brickman AL, Fins AI. Psychological and cognitive aspects of chronic fatigue syndrome. In: Goodnick PJ, Klimas NG eds. Chronic fatigue and related immune deficiency syndromes. Washington, DC: American Psychiatric Press, 1993;67–94.

107. Wessely S, Powell R. Fatigue syndromes: a comparison of chronic postviral fatigue with neuromuscular and affective disorders. J Neurol Neurosurgery Psychiatry 1989;52:940–948.

108. Manu P, Matthews DA, Lane TJ. The mental health of patients with a chief complaint of chronic fatigue. Arch Intern Med 1988;148: 2213–2217.

109. Million C, Salvato F, Beaney N, et al. A psychological assessment of chronic fatigue syndrome/chronic Epstein-Barr virus patients. Psychol Health 1989;131–141.

110. Altay HT, Abbey SE, Toner BB, et al. The neuropsychological dimensions of postinfectious neuromyasthenia (chronic fatigue syndrome):a preliminary report. Int J Psychol Med 1990; 20:141–149.

111. Sandman CA, Barron JL, Nackoul K, Goldstein J, Fidler F. Memory deficits associated with chronic fatigue immune dysfunction syndrome. Biol Psychiatry 1993;33:618–623.

112. Goodnick PJ, Sandoval R. Treatment of chronic fatigue syndrome and related disorders: psychotropic agents. In: Goodnick PJ, Klimas NG, eds. Chronic fatigue and related immune deficiency syndromes. Washington, DC: American Psychiatric Press, 1993;131–159.

113. Gracious B, Wisner KL. Nortriptyline in chronic fatigue syndrome:a

double-blind, placebo controlled single case study. Biol Psychiatry 1991;30:405–408.

114. Klimas NG, Morgan R, Van Riel F, Fletcher MA. Observations regarding use of an antidepressant, fluoxetine, in chronic fatigue syndrome. In: Goodnick PJ, Klimas NG, eds. Chronic fatigue and related immune deficiency syndromes. Washington, DC: American Psychiatric Press, 1993;95–108.

115. Goodnick PJ, Sandoval R. Treatment of chronic fatigue syndrome and related disorders: immunological approaches. In: Goodnick PJ, Klimas NG, eds. Chronic fatigue and related immune deficiency syndromes. Washington, DC: American Psychiatric Press, 1993; 109–129.

116. Gantz NM, Holmes GP. Treatment of patients with chronic fatigue syndrome. Drugs 1989;38:855–862.

41

BEHAVIORAL SYNDROMES IN NEUROTOXICOLOGY

Roberta F. White, Robert G. Feldman, and Susan P. Proctor

Exposure to neurotoxicants often produces effects on cerebral structures and functions. Acute exposure may manifest obvious symptoms. Insidious and chronic exposures result in long-standing, undiagnosed toxic states, often characterized by more subtle and often permanent functional impairments. Attention has been focused on the need for earliest detection of these "subclinical" toxic states, especially those behavioral syndromes associated with exposure to particular neurotoxicants (1–4).

This chapter describes an approach to the evaluation of toxin-related neurological dysfunction and clinical differential diagnosis. Emphasis is given to methods of assessing behavioral syndromes associated with neurotoxic exposures.

NEUROLOGICAL EVALUATION AND DIAGNOSIS

Diagnosis of neurological abnormalities secondary to exposure requires evaluation to ascertain that abnormal observed findings are not due to any other primary neurological disease and can be attributed only to the exposure (5). Many neurological symptoms and examination findings are similar in toxic encephalopathy and other disorders. For example, headache secondary to migraine, a mass, or unruptured aneurysm must be differentiated from symptomatic headache associated with exposure to carbon monoxide, carbon disulfide, lead, zinc, or nitrates. Dementia due to Alzheimer's disease or arteriosclerosis, and the dementia syndrome of depression must be differentiated from encephalopathy caused by exposure to organic solvents, styrene, lead, and certain insecticides. Epilepsy, distinguished by transient disturbances in awareness with or without movements, must be recognized as a primary diagnosis separate from disturbances of consciousness due to intoxications, which also may result in diminished consciousness or even convulsions. Symptoms of Parkinson's disease must be differentiated from the disturbances of posture that result from

a reaction to phenothiazine medications or exposure to carbon disulfide, carbon monoxide, or manganese. Findings of white matter disease, suggestive of the diagnosis of multiple sclerosis, must be differentiated from the effects of exposure to certain toxicants (e.g., leptophos, aminopropionitrile, triorthorcresyl). Muscle weakness and atrophy symptomatic of peripheral neuropathy or primary anterior horn cell disease may be a result of that exposure to heavy metals, which can produce a similar neuromuscular picture.

The strategies used to reach a diagnosis in occupational and environmental neurology include both a detailed exposure history and symptom review, a careful neurological examination, and the use of selected sensitive neurophysiological and neuropsychological test batteries. To properly evaluate alterations in central nervous system functioning and to identify structural versus functional disturbances, certain laboratory tests are useful:

1. Computerized axial tomography (CT) can indicate ventricular size, symmetry, and presence of mass lesions. Experience with certain toxic exposures suggests that they are sometimes associated with the finding of cortical atrophy on CT scan.
2. Magnetic resonance imaging (MRI) provides essentially the same information as the CT scan except that white and gray matter can be differentiated more clearly. Our experience with MRI in toxicant-exposed patients also suggests that atrophy is a consistent finding. In addition, we are seeing evidence of small white matter lesions in some patients (6), some of whom seem to improve in the absence of exposure. Other investigators have reported seeing white matter lesions following toluene exposure (7–9).
3. Electroencephalography (EEG) records the electrical activity of the brain during waking and sleeping. It is useful in demonstrating asymmetries of electrical activity due to mass lesions, identifying focal disturbances, showing epileptic tendencies, and demonstrating slowing due to toxic or metabolic conditions.

NEUROPSYCHOLOGICAL TESTING

Although behavior may be assessed through descriptions of observed changes provided by at-risk subjects and other persons familiar with them, formal neuropsychological testing offers reliable, standardized procedures for objectively evaluating specific aspects of change in cognitive function (3, 10, 11). There are specific, standardized rules for administering and scoring these tests. Results may be analyzed objectively through published normative data on the expected ranges of scores based on age, sex, and education. In addition, the tests have been validated in both research and clinical settings on patients with known brain damage, allowing clear interpretation of results by independent neuropsychologists. Reliability of the tests (test-retest) is often established. Finally, the tests are used widely, and results from them may be applied in many diagnostic and treatment settings. (See Chapter 42 for further discussion.)

Batteries of tests may be designed for clinical diagnosis of encephalopathy in individual patients (clinical batteries) as well as for screening large groups of hazard-exposed subjects (epidemiological batteries) (11). Skill areas assessed by these tests include the broad area of attention (including vigilance, as well as ability to hold and manipulate information), motor skills and reaction time, concept formation (reasoning), language, and visuospatial abilities. Mood and personality are also assessed. The most commonly used criterion for inclusion of a test in a battery is its confirmed sensitivity to particular neurotoxicants as previously documented in the research literature. Because the mean differences between data obtained from exposed vs. nonexposed groups in research populations may be quite small, it is often impossible to directly apply norms from epidemiological studies to the clinical assessment of individual patients.

In clinical situations it is generally more appropriate to select neuropsychological tests that will assess as many functions as possible to provide a profile of abilities and deficits in a given individual. Perhaps the most difficult situation arises with respect to estimating the severity of past exposure. Evaluation of deficits often occurs after exposure has ceased, at a time when the body burden of suspected substances is no longer elevated or environmental levels can no longer be ascertained. Obtaining an occupational/environmental history to estimate the extent of exposure (duration and intensity) is of the utmost importance. Essential to this inquiry are questions about the patient's current and previous occupations, job tasks, places of residence and employment, and hobbies (12). To elicit information about exposures to known neurotoxic substances, a checklist of neurotoxicants can be used for patient response.

An extensive neuropsychological test battery for clinical assessment has evolved (4, 13, 14). The battery (Table 41.1) is designed to cover a wide range of functions and to analyze as many manifestations of neurotoxicant-induced encephalopathy as possible. The battery is extensive enough to allow localization of cerebral dysfunction in cases with specific constellations of deficits, and aid in the differen-

tial diagnosis of toxic encephalopathy versus other neuropsychiatric disorders if cognitive deficits are observed. Although it is quite clear that certain functional areas—short-term memory, attention, mood, visuospatial skills, reasoning, and motor abilities—are particularly sensitive to the effects of these substances in adults, others are relatively resistant to the effects of exposure (language skills, remote memory) (13), the need to differentiate specific patterns of dysfunction associated with the varying exposures is obvious.

BEHAVIORAL EFFECTS OF EXPOSURE TO NEUROTOXICANTS

Metals

INORGANIC LEAD

Lead neurotoxicity has been associated with signs of encephalopathy such as restlessness, irritability, tremor, poor memory, drowsiness, and stupor, progressing to seizures, coma, and death in severe forms of lead poisoning. As cases of severe acute toxicity have become less frequent, increasing attention has been focused on the milder, "subclinical" manifestations of lead exposure. In particular, the behavioral effects of exposure to inorganic lead have received increased attention (15–18). Evidence suggests that changes in behavioral and cognitive functioning are observable in patients with blood lead levels < 70 mg/100 dl. Although results in studies of adults have not always been consistent (19), there is good reason to suggest that lead exposure can lead to impairments in affect, attention, psychomotor function, verbal concept formation, short-term memory, and visuospatial abilities (20–25).

In a study of lead-exposed factory workers, a neuropsychological test battery was administered annually over 3 years (20, 21). The test battery included the Profile of Mood States (POMS), Continuous Performance Testing (CPT), Santa Ana Dexterity Test, Wechsler Memory Scale, and several WAIS-R subtests (Vocabulary, Similarities, Block Design, and Digit Symbol). The POMS was found to be especially sensitive to changes in blood lead level on the day of testing. As blood levels rose above 40 mg/100 dl, the reported rates of depression, confusion, fatigue, and anger increased significantly. In addition, verbal short-term memory skills were found to be consistently impaired as lead levels rose.

In lead-exposed workers evaluated in our Environmental and Occupational Neurology program, we have observed dysfunction in affect, attention and cognitive tracking, short-term memory verbal reasoning and concept formation, as well as loss of motor coordination and speed and visuospatial abilities. Blood-lead levels in such patients are generally highly elevated (60–90 mg/100 dl).

Mood disorders are common, with subjective complaints of apathy, irritability, and diminished ability to control anger. The POMS has consistently revealed an increased score on the fatigue scale. Attentional deficits may be

Table 41.1. Neuropsychological Assessment of Possible Toxic Encephalopathy[a]

Domain	Description	Implications
General Intellect		
Wechsler IQ tests (WAIS-R, WISC, WPPSI)	IQ measures	Overall level of cognitive function compared with population norms
Peabody Picture Vocabulary Test	Single word comprehension	Measure of verbal intelligence in adults; can be sensitive to exposure in children
Stanford-Binet	IQ measure	Similar to Wechsler tests
Wide Range Achievement Test	Academic skills in arithmetic, spelling, reading	Estimate of premorbid ability patterns in adults; can be sensitive to exposure in children
Attention, Executive Functioning		
Digit Span (WAIS-R)	Digits forward and backward	Measures simple attention and cognitive tracking
Arithmetic (Wechsler tests)	Oral calculations	Assesses attention, tracking, and calculation
Trail Making Test	Connect-a-dot task requiring sequencing and alternating sequences	Measures attention, sequencing, visual scanning, speed of processing
Continuous Performance Test	Acknowledgment of occurrence of critical stimuli in a series of orally or visually presented stimuli	Assesses attention
Paced Auditory Serial Addition	Serial calculation test	Sensitive measure of attention and tracking speed
Wisconsin Card Sorting Test	Requires subject to infer decision-making rules	Tests ability to think flexibly
Verbal, Language		
Information (Wechsler tests)	Information usually learned in school	Estimate of native abilities in adults
Vocabulary (Wechsler tests)	Verbal vocabulary definitions	Estimate of verbal intelligence; sensitive to concreteness associated with brain damage (including toxic encephalopathy)
Comprehension (Wechsler tests)	Proverb definitions, social judgment, problem solving	Sensitive to reasoning skills; can be impaired after exposure to neurotoxicants
Similarities (Wechsler tests)	Inference of similarities between nominative words	Sensitive to reasoning skills; can be impaired after exposure to neurotoxicants
Controlled Oral Word Association	Word list generation within alphabetical or semantic categories	Assesses flexibility, planning, arousal, processing speed, ability to generate strategies, somewhat sensitive to exposure
Boston Naming Test	Naming of objects depicted in line drawings	Sensitive to aphasia; also sensitive to native verbal processing deficits or those acquired through childhood exposure
Reading Comprehension (Boston Diagnostic Aphasia Exam)	A direct screening test of simple reading comprehension	Sensitive to moderate-to-severe dyslexia, usually insensitive to toxic exposure in adults
Writing Sample	Patient writes to dictation or describes a picture	Assesses graphomotor skills, spelling
Visuospatial, Visuomotor		
Picture Completion (Wechsler tests)	Identification of missing details in line drawing	Measures perceptual analysis
Santa Ana Formboard Test	Knobs in a formboard are turned 180° with each hand individually and both hands together	Measures motor speed and coordination
Finger tapping	Speed of tapping with each index finger	Sensitive to lateralized manual motor speed

Continued.

Table 41.1. *(Continued)*

Domain	Description	Implications
Memory		
Logical Memories-Immediate and Delayed Recall (IR, DR) (Wechsler Memory Scales)	Recall of paragraph information read orally on an immediate and 20-minute delayed recall	Sensitive to new learning and retention of newly learned information
Verbal Paired Associate Learning DR (Wechsler Memory Scales)	Two paired words are presented in a list of pairs; subject must recall second word; test is presented on immediate and delayed recall	Measures abstract verbal list IR, learning, retention
Figural Memory (Wechsler Memory Scales)	Multiple choice recognition of using recognition (not recall) performance measures	Assesses visual recognition memory
Digit Symbol (Wechsler tests)	Coding task requiring matching symbols to digits	Complex task assessing motor speed, visual scanning, working memory
Picture Arrangement (Wechsler tests)	Sequencing of cartoon frames to represent meaningful stories	Measures visual sequencing, ability to infer relationships from visuospatial/social stimuli
Block Design (Wechsler tests)	Assembly of 3-D blocks to replicate 2-D representation of designs	Assesses abstract visual construction ability and planning
Object Assembly (Wechsler tests)	Assembly of puzzles	Measure of concrete visual construction skills, Gestalt recognition
Boston Visuospatial Quantitative Battery	Drawings of common objects spontaneously and to copy	Measures constructional abilities, motor functioning
Hooper Visual Organization Test	Identification of correct outline of drawings of cut up objects	Sensitive to Gestalt integration processing
Rey-Osterreith Complex Figure (copy condition)	Drawing of a complicated abstract visual design	Sensitive to deficits in visuospatial planning and construction
Visual Paired Associate Learning, IR, DR (Wechsler Memory Scales)	Six visual designs are paired with six colors; recognition memory is tested immediately after the six are presented on learning trials and at delayed recall	Test of abstract visual learning using recognition (not recall) performance measures
Visual Reproductions, IR, DR (Wechsler Memory Scales)	Visual designs are drawn immediately after presentation and on delayed recall	Measures visual learning and retention
Delayed Recognition Span Test	Based on delayed nonmatching to sample paradigm, discs are moved about on a board to assess recognition memory for words, color, spatial locations	Assesses new learning
Peterson Task	Words or consonants are presented and must be recalled after a period of distraction	Measures sensitivity to interference in new learning
California Verbal Learning Test	Subject is presented with list of 16 words (which can be semantically related) over multiple learning trials and with an interference list	Provides multiple measures of new learning, recall, recognition memory, use of strategies and sensitivity to interference
Rey-Osterreith (IR, DR)	Complex design is drawn from IR immediately after it has been copied and at a 20-minute delayed recall	Assesses memory for visual information which is difficult to encode verbally
Personality, Mood		
Profile of Mood states	65 single word descriptors of affective symptoms are endorsed by degree of severity on six scales	Sensitive to clinical mood disturbance and to affective changes secondary to toxicant exposure
Minnesota Multiphasic Personality Inventory (R)	True-false responses provided on personality inventory summarized on multiple clinical dimensions	Provides description of current personality function; some scales sensitive to exposure; screening for inconsistency and malingering

ªModified from White RF, Proctor SP. Research and clinical criteria for the development of neurobehavioral test batteries. J Occup Med 1992; 34:140–148.

observed on simple tasks such as the Continuous Performance Test (CPT) and on repeating digits forward. These deficits become even more pronounced on tasks requiring holding and manipulating information (reciting digits backward, counting by 3s beginning with the number 1) and sequencing of material. Difficulties in accurately completing oral arithmetic problems are common among lead-exposed patients and appear to reflect attention deficits. Tendencies to respond impulsively are sometimes noted during testing sessions.

The effects of lead on short-term memory are well documented and are consistently evident in the testing of lead-exposed patients. This is observed in recall of verbal narrative material, paired associate learning, drawings of visual designs under conditions of immediate recall, and recognition of visual stimuli (designs, unfamiliar faces) with multiple-choice formats. Frequently, disproportionate loss of information is observed when delayed recall of newly learned information is assessed relative to immediate recall, especially when recall (not recognition memory) paradigms are used. This effect is particularly evident when large amounts of information are presented or the material is difficult to master. Both the extent of the memory impairment and the loss of information from memory on delays suggest that lead-related memory disorders are not entirely attentional.

The ability to respond to complex verbal reasoning tasks requiring abstraction, application of principles of social knowledge or judgment, proverb interpretation (e.g., Wechsler Adult Intelligence Scale—Revised [WAIS-R] Comprehension subtest), and ability to deduce similarities (WAIS-R Similarities subtest) appear to be diminished following lead exposure. Impaired ability to define vocabulary words abstractly is also typical of this group (WAIS-R Vocabulary subtest) (20). In our testing, significant slowing and inefficiency are commonly evident in tests of motor control and speed when patients are asked to draw symbols under digits to match a code (Digit Symbol subtest, WAIS-R) or to turn pegs 90° in a form board (Santa Ana Test). Lastly, visuospatial problems may be noted, with difficulties in organizing visual material (e.g., Block Designs on the WAIS-R).

Despite the aforementioned areas of dysfunction, certain well-retained abilities are apparent in *adult* patients with lead levels of less than 90 mg/100 dl. Language skills, long-term memory, recall of information learned in school, and reading appear to be unaffected in the adults tested. This is not true in children, however (17, 26).

Results of earlier studies carried out in children have been contradictory. Although neuropsychological deficits in children with "moderate" lead exposure were identified by Landrigan and co-authors (27) and others (28–31), these were not observed by Baloh et al. (32) or Lansdowne and co-authors (33). Needleman et al. (15), controlling for several sources of error that may have contributed to these discrepancies, found significant impairment in neuropsychological test function in children whose teeth had the highest dentin lead levels. Other studies have also demonstrated

significant effects of lead exposure on test performance in children (34–36). Again, deficits were observed in the areas of psychomotor speed, verbal concept formation, visuospatial abilities, and attention.

MERCURY

Elemental and inorganic mercury compounds are used in industry, agriculture, and medicine. Organic mercury compounds are also found in fungicides, preservatives, denaturants for ethyl alcohol, antiseptics, and herbicides (37).

Accidental absorption of organic mercury occurs as a result of inhalation, percutaneous absorption, or ingestion. Acute intoxication has reportedly resulted in abdominal pain, nausea, vomiting, diarrhea, headaches, and chills. Behavioral disturbances manifested by mood changes, depression, irritability, and changes in personality may result from chronic mercury intoxication (38). Behavioral effects of mercurialism have been classified into three major areas: (*a*) disturbances of the motor system, manifested by fine muscle tremor; (*b*) deterioration of intellectual capacities (memory, concentration, and logical reasoning); and (*c*) alterations of emotional state with associated symptoms of depression, fatigue, listlessness, irritability, and social sensitivity (23).

Kurland and co-authors (39) described massive destruction of cerebellum, calcarine cortex, and basal ganglia that resulted from the ingestion of methyl mercury-containing fish by people and animals living in the vicinity of Minamata Bay, Japan. The onset of illness in this outbreak began with a progressive peripheral neuropathy, followed by ataxia, dysarthria, deafness, blindness, the development of spasticity, and intellectual impairment.

In contrast to these severe neurological effects, subtle changes, such as those seen in "micromercurialism," may be the result of chronic low-level exposure. Similar to the effect of other environmental and industrial toxicants, the effects of mercury depend upon the level and duration of exposure as well as individual susceptibility and rate of absorption. Changes in motor function (as assessed by tapping performance) and in reaction time were reported in chloraldehyde workers exposed to mercury (40). Impaired motor performance was confirmed in a study by Langolf et al. (41), who also found decrements in cortical tracking associated with increased urine mercury levels. Mercury exposure has also been related to impaired visual memory (42–44).

Affective symptomatology of anxiety and depression, as measured by the Minnesota Multiphasic Personality Inventory, was identified in thermometer factory workers exposed to mercury (45). In addition, motor and visuospatial deficits were noted. Language and naming functions were normal in these workers.

We observed similar findings on extensive neuropsychological screening of nine workers whose jobs involved replacing regulators that contained mercury. The mean duration of time at this task was 16 years. Tests of memory, verbal reasoning, sequencing, and visuospatial and visuomotor tasks were adversely affected among subjects who had urine levels of mercury ranging from 133–328 mg/L. Short-term memory problems on moderately difficult visual tasks were seen. These included the ability to recognize faces on delayed recall memory testing (Milner Test), ability to draw visual designs from memory (Wechsler Memory Scale visual reproductions), and multiple-choice recall of visual designs (Benton Test). Difficulties were also observed on vigilance as assessed by Continuous Performance Testing, showing occasional omission errors, incorrect responses, and mildly varying response times. Performance on the Santa Ana Form Board Test was below expectation, based on norms developed using nonexposed factory control workers in a previous study (20). One subgroup of workers employed from 11–24 years (mean of 20 years) had particularly consistent evidence of mild encephalopathy, manifested by the aforementioned deficits and impaired visuospatial organization. Also noted in this group were problems in matching previously unfamiliar faces (Milner Test), replicating visual designs made of red and white blocks (Block Design subtest, WAIS-R), and assembling puzzles (Object Assembly subtest, WAIS-R). In addition, attentional deficits were more pronounced in this group. Thus, they had difficulty with the mental control subtest of the Wechsler Memory Scale (counting backward from 20, and counting by 3s, beginning with the number 1), as well as on Digit Span and Oral Arithmetic Testing (WAIS-R subtests). A statistical analysis relating the period of exposure to mercury with test performance yielded significant correlation between the impaired ability to draw visual designs under conditions of delayed recall (Wechsler Memory Scale, Visual Reproductions, Delayed Condition) and with impaired ability to recall previously unfamiliar faces after short delays under multiple-choice conditions (Milner Facial Recognition Test) (Pearson correlation coefficient, p < 0.05).

ARSENIC

Arsenic, a constituent of numerous minerals, is found in soil, water, and in foods, particularly seafood (46). This element exists in various chemical states, each of which has its own toxicological potential. Arsenic trioxide is recovered as a by-product from smelting copper-, lead- and gold-bearing ores (37). Arsenic compounds are used in insecticides, herbicides, and wood preservatives, in solder and steel as an alloying ingredient, as oxidizing and refining agents in glass manufacture, as preservatives in tanning and taxidermy, and as a component of semiconductors.

Inhalation and ingestion are the main routes of entry of arsenic into the body. Once absorbed, arsenic is widely distributed in the tissues, including the liver, abdominal viscera, bone, skin, hair, and nails. Remarkably, arsenic can be detected in hair and nails months after it has disappeared from urine and feces (37). Both peripheral nervous system and central nervous system effects have been documented following acute and chronic exposures to arsenic. Electro-physiological studies have provided objective quantification of functional impairment in the peripheral nervous system, including both sensory and motor dysfunction, following exposure to arsenic.

However, few reports exist, except in case documentation, linking chronic arsenic intoxication to specific neurobehavioral effects (47, 48). A feeling of weakness, lassitude, dizzy spells, and fatigability was reported by most men of a battalion of 170 soldiers chronically exposed to arsenic (49). A feeling of progressive anxiety, along with nausea, vomiting, diarrhea, and hot flashes, has been observed in cases of chronic arsenicalism (50). A case of a 56-year-old woman with arsenic poisoning who later manifested signs of a permanent organic psychosis characterized by agitation, paranoid-delusional thinking, and progressive disturbance of judgment and self-care functions was reported (51). Lastly, a symptom complex of malaise, emotional lability, insomnia, and depression was identified in six patients with arsenic poisoning (52).

MANGANESE

Manganese is especially known for its alloying properties with both ferrous and nonferrous metals. In the form of manganese oxide, it is utilized in the manufacture of paints, disinfectants, fertilizers, varnishes, pyrotechnics, and as a depolarizer in cell batteries. Principal sources of industrial exposure occur in mining, transporting, crushing, and sieving of ore (37). Exposure primarily results from inhalation of metal dust or fumes and can occur in industrial workers as well as in people living in the areas surrounding manganese smelters.

The effects of manganese intoxication vary from person to person. Many cases go unrecognized or unreported, since not every exposed individual is affected or experiences symptoms (53). Although severe manganese intoxication is clearly recognizable, manifestations of low-level manganese intoxication require formal neuropsychological testing to document cognitive disorders (53). In a group of 30 foundry workers exposed to manganese at low levels (0.25 mg/m^3) for a mean of 9.9 years, inferior performance on Simple Reaction Time, Digit Span and Finger Tapping were noted (54, 55).

The patterns of neurological deficit in severe manganese intoxication are quite characteristic and are marked by a behavioral and postural (dystonic) syndrome. The neurotoxicity of manganese was first recognized after the appearance of neurological disorders in manganese miners in Chile and India (56, 57). Early neurological patterns were suggestive of an acute disorder and included irritability, nervousness, and emotional instability. For some, visual and auditory hallucinations appeared in addition to compulsive, repetitive, uncontrollable actions. Symptoms in six men exposed while working in a manganese ore crushing plant typified the course of chronic manganese intoxication as insidious and progressive, beginning with complaints of asthenia, anorexia, apathy, and insomnia (58). The initial phase concurred with the earlier descriptions of this "manganese madness" reported by Mena and co-authors (56).

Two cases of manganese intoxication were reported in workers involved in a process of cleaning manganese steel casting in which metal fumes were generated. In both individuals, there were personality changes and problems with memory (59).

The second stage of manganese intoxication, sometimes referred to as "Mn psychosis," may, after months of continued exposure, progress into a stage characterized by speech disorder, gait disturbance, slowness and clumsiness of movement, and postural imbalance. Signs of dystonia appear in the third stage. These signs include an awkward high-stepping gait ("cock walk"), as well as tremor and chorea (60).

Solvents

CARBON DISULFIDE

Carbon disulfide, a heavy volatile liquid, is a solvent for lipids, sulfur, rubber, oils, waxes, industrial chemicals, phosphorus, and resins. Primarily, it is used in the agricultural industry in various insecticides, in the rubber industry, and in the rayon industry, where it is used for the preparation of rayon viscose fibers. Inhalation of the vapor is the major route of entry, although percutaneous absorption of both liquid or vapor may also occur. Perhaps the best-known manifestation of advanced carbon disulfide intoxication is polyneuropathy.

One hundred cases of carbon disulfide intoxication were identified among workers in two large viscose rayon plants who were exposed to hazardous conditions during World War II (61). In addition to peripheral neuropathy, the workers presented with headache, vertigo, diminished sexual function, psychosis, and extrapyramidal disturbances. In a later report, the same author reported on 43 workers from four other viscose rayon plants in whom he found chronic encephalopathy, pseudobulbar paralysis with mental deterioration, frequent extrapyramidal involvement, and focal signs of cerebral infarction due to thrombosis (62). For three patients, necropsy was done and revealed a generalized diffuse vascular sclerosis of small arteries and capillaries of the brain and spinal medulla. Seppalainen and Tolonen (63) performed EEGs on 54 male viscose rayon workers exposed for several years to carbon disulfide and compared them to 50 control subjects. Among the carbon disulfide workers, 21 EEGs were abnormal as compared with six in the control group. The types of EEG abnormalities were compatible with toxic encephalopathy. The findings of earlier reports were corroborated in a later study of 250 workers exposed to carbon disulfide (64). A high incidence of abnormal EEG tracings was found in the workers exposed to carbon disulfide. It was postulated that the observed abnormality could be the manifestation of diffuse toxic cerebral changes, the effect on the smallest diameter vessels in carbon disulfide vasculoencephalopathy, or a combination of the two mecha-

nisms. Parkinsonism has also been described following carbon disulfide exposure (65) as have CT scan abnormalities (66).

Hanninen et al. (67, 68) demonstrated a broad range of psychological effects that could be differentiated in acute and latent carbon disulfide poisoning. These authors employed a battery of tests that included WAIS Digit Span, Similarities, Block Design, Picture Completion, and Digit Symbol; Bourdon-Wiersma Vigilance Test; Santa Ana Dexterity Test; Symmetry Drawing; Benton Visual Retention Test; Rorschach; and Mira Test. This was accomplished by analyzing three groups of 50 subjects: unexposed workers, those with long histories of exposure but no manifest symptoms, and workers with clinical poisoning. The poisoned workers showed disturbances in speech, psychomotor functioning, dexterity, alertness, and intellectual processes requiring visualization. They were less spontaneous. The other exposed group showed motor disturbances and impaired visualization, but were normal in their speech. Tuttle et al. (69) employed a similar battery of neuropsychological tests with similar results.

Most investigations of the effects of carbon disulfide have focused on visuomotor function, attention, and intelligence, which are motor and cognitive processes primarily dependent on the integrity of the central nervous system. Other behavioral disturbances, called "psychoneurasthenic" difficulties, have also been related to carbon disulfide exposure (70). These difficulties may represent an organic affective disturbance and include changes in mood or personality; excessive irritability; increased physical complaints such as headache, dizziness, weakness, and fatigue; and memory loss. These complaints usually precede the onset of more obvious neurological involvement, i.e., peripheral neuropathy. Frequently, depressive symptoms have been reported.

Similar complaints were described in workers exposed to concentrations of CS$_2$ varying from 4.3–129 ppm (71). General fatigue, insomnia, paresthesias, and headache were found to be prominent clinical complaints of chronically exposed workers in whom central and peripheral nervous system lesions were found (63).

We have examined a 28-year-old man, an electrician in a rayon manufacturing facility, who developed symptoms that were difficult to characterize until neuropsychological tests were done. His history between July and September of 1976 included extensive exposure of up to 7 days a week working in the solution room and around extruder machines. During a 2-week period, when he was involved in the installation of a carbon disulfide monitor, this patient was doused by carbon disulfide leaking from pipes around which he worked. His shirt disintegrated where the liquid had soaked the cloth. After 2 to 3 months, his family began to note changes in his personality. He was irritable, forgetful, and appeared depressed. He had difficulty remembering names of people he should have known, his mind wandered, and he had difficulty following conversations. There was a loss of interest in his favorite recreational activities. While driving a car, he noted that his mind wandered. He had poor attention and concentration. At that time, the patient had developed a tremor that interfered with his ability to hold his tools steadily.

Psychometric studies showed constructional deficits (Block Design and Object Assembly, WAIS-R.) The Shipley-Hartford Conceptional Quotient was depressed, suggesting impaired intellectual efficiency and poor verbal abstract function. The ability for sustained attention was reduced on vigilance testing. Memory testing revealed difficulty in acquiring new information. There was poor performance on Smith's Symbol Digit Modalities test, reflecting inefficiency in perceptual motor speed, new learning, and sequential analysis.

The difficulties in perceptual motor and sequential analysis functions on testing, combined with the poor attention span and memory, were consistent with subacute encephalopathy due to toxic exposure to carbon disulfide. Very little improvement in performance was seen on reexamination 2 years after the cessation of exposure. Although he was less irritable and his attention seemed slightly better, he was unable to work because of a general attitude of disorganization as well as his tremor.

Carbon disulfide has been shown convincingly to cause impaired psychomotor function, especially affecting dexterity and speed. Tests that measure these changes reliably include the Santa Ana Dexterity Test and tests of simple reaction time. Higher cortical functions, especially visuomotor abilities and concentration, are also affected by carbon disulfide exposure and may be assessed by utilizing the Block Design, Digit Symbol, and Digit Span subtests of the WAIS-R. Subtle symptoms such as mood changes, irritability, and increased systemic complaints may precede overt neurological illness from carbon disulfide exposure and can be assessed by the use of standard interview questionnaires.

TRICHLOROETHYLENE

Trichloroethylene (TCE), a colorless aliphatic hydrocarbon liquid, is a widely used industrial solvent, particularly in metal degreasing and extraction processes. It is also used in many chemical processes, the cleaning of optical lenses and photographic plates, in painting and enameling, and as an adhesive in the shoe industry. In these processes, TCE may be heated and is easily volatilized, increasing the danger of inhalation, the most significant route of exposure. In the presence of light, flame, or alkaline substances, TCE can produce decomposition products, namely dichloroacetylene, chlorine, hydrochloric acid, carbon monoxide, and phosgene (37).

The toxicology of TCE has been extensively described (72–74). Occurrences of undesirable effects following exposure to TCE are frequent in industrial settings, with central nervous system (CNS) depression as the predominant physiological response to exposure. Typical manifestations include visual disturbances, mental confusion, fatigue, and impaired concentration. Of particular note is TCE's predilection for selective neurotoxic action on the trigemi-

nal nerve and the lasting depression following significant exposure.

The behavioral aspects of TCE intoxication in workers have often been overlooked. This may be partly because of the paucity of populations with exposure to TCE only; it is often used with other solvents or neurotoxicants. Acute exposure studies of TCE in nonoccupational populations have produced contradictory results. Although Salvani et al. (75) showed effects on reaction time, motor dexterity, and reaction time, these findings have not been replicated by other workers. Johnson et al. (76), reviewing studies of acute exposure to TCE, suggested that 300 ppm was the necessary dose to affect behavioral function.

One of the subjects, whom we have previously described (77, 78), demonstrated complex behavioral changes associated with exposure to TCE. An owner of a carburetor cleaning plant, the patient had been acutely intoxicated by vapors of TCE. He recovered from acute confusion, headache, and dizziness, but peripheral neuropathy became evident after 7–10 days. His symptoms of distal numbness and muscle cramps in extremities persisted for almost 2 years after exposure. The patient's difficulty in solving sequential problems and poor memory affecting acquisition of new information interfered with his ability to work successfully. He also exhibited a change in personality. Follow-up 16 years after the exposure (79) showed persistence in his difficulties in solving multiple-step problems and in making business decisions. Moreover, there was evidence of moderate depression on the Minnesota Multiphasic Personality Inventory as well as attentional, visuospatial, and short-term memory deficits.

The results of neuropsychological tests on eight adult patients with TCE exposure evaluated in our program and diagnosed with encephalopathy are summarized here. In five patients, TCE was one of multisubstance exposures; in three cases, TCE was the only apparent source of exposure. All of these patients exhibited signs of encephalopathy, which was moderate to severe in degree. Of particular importance was the consistent finding of a severe agitated depression. At times, this was accompanied by violent tendencies directed toward others and themselves. The patients reported severe agitation and an inability to function following exposure. Information gleaned from their observers concurred with these reported behavioral changes.

In addition, neuropsychological testing revealed memory deficits that were especially pronounced when comparing immediate recall of new information to delayed recall on both visual and verbal tasks. Expressive recall of visual designs (Visual Reproduction subtest, Wechsler Memory Scale), recall of narrative material presented in two paragraphs (Logical Memory subtest, Wechsler Memory Scale), and recall of very difficult paired associates (Verbal Paired Associate Learning) were consistently impaired. Less consistent memory deficits were observed in delayed recall under multiple-choice conditions of faces (Milner Facial Recognition Test) and a simpler paired associate learning test

(Wechsler Memory Scale subtest). Moderate to severe visuospatial deficits were also frequently seen in these patients, as evidenced by the performance subtests of the WAIS. Visuoconstruction tasks involving puzzles, block designs, and sequencing of stories (Object Assembly, Picture Arrangement, and Block Design subtests of the WAIS-R) were especially affected.

TOLUENE

Toluene, a colorless liquid derived from coal tar, is used as a solvent and thinner in the printing, rubber, lumber, furniture, and chemical industries. It is a basic component in many glues, lacquers, inks, cleaning liquids, paints, and adhesives. Atmospheric toluene largely results from motor vehicle vapor emissions because toluene is a constituent of gasoline (37). As with other solvents, inhalation is a major route of entry and, to a lesser extent, percutaneous absorption occurs. Exposure to intensely high levels may occur through accidental inhalation at the workplace or intentional inhalation as in the case of glue sniffing for "recreational" purposes.

The principal health effect of toluene is on the central nervous system. Low levels produce reduced performance and perceptions of fatigue and dizziness, whereas higher levels have excitatory effects such as euphoria, exhilaration, and agitation. Although the inhaled vapors usually induce a temporary euphoria, addiction can result, leading to serious damage to the nervous system (80). Caution must be used in generalization of results from epidemiological studies because exact exposure levels and knowledge of other concomitant exposures are not always known and toluene is often used in combination with other solvents. As a result, it is impossible to identify one single causative factor except in the cases of toluene sniffing. Several case reports exist describing a constellation of symptoms for toluene abusers. These include mental confusion, inappropriate laughter, suicidal tendencies, dyscoordination, and emotional lability (81). In addition, neurobehavioral deficits have been described in groups of toluene-exposed workers (82). Toluene has been associated with cerebellar dysfunction (7, 8, 80) and with lesions in cerebral white matter (7), with associated neuropsychological deficits (9).

PERCHLOROETHYLENE

Perchloroethylene (PCE, tetrachloroethylene), a colorless liquid, is another major solvent used particularly in dry cleaning, fabric finishing, metal degreasing, and other applications (83). Exposure to PCE may occur as a result of inhalation of vapors and secondarily through direct skin contact. Symptoms attributable to CNS depression have been reported and include vertigo, impaired memory, confusion, fatigue, drowsiness, irritability, loss of appetite, and uncoordination.

In a study of dry-cleaning workers, Tuttle and co-authors (84), using the Santa Ana Dexterity Test, Wechsler Digit Span and Digit Symbol, the Neisser letter search, and simple and choice reaction time, could not demonstrate deleterious behavioral effects of exposure to PCE. However, differences in performance were found between morning and afternoon testing. Mean 8-hour time-weighted average (TWA) exposure was 1 ppm over a 5-day test.

One patient seen in our clinic after PCE exposure was tested on two occasions. Initial testing was done within a few weeks after she stopped working in a dry-cleaning establishment, where she had noticed memory and mood difficulties. This testing confirmed problems in motor skills, impulse control, mood (fatigue and confusion), short-term memory, and attention. Testing was later repeated 21 months after initial testing. Marked improvements were observed in memory, attention, visual organization, mood, and, to a lesser degree, reasoning. The improvement in memory was quite dramatic (22 points on the WMS). Despite these findings, scores on certain tests remained below expectation. These included the ability to replicate visual block designs (WAIS-R), attention on Continuous Performance Testing, and two short-term memory tests (Logical Memory subtest, WMS; Auxiliary Difficult Paired Associate Learning Task).

Insecticides

CHLORDANE

Chlordane, a multicomponent organochlorine insecticide, is well known for its use in the control of termites and carpenter ants. Chlordane is absorbed through the skin, but more readily via the lungs and from the gastrointestinal tract. It is retained primarily in adipose tissue.

There is a dearth of literature on the behavioral effects associated with chlordane exposure. Comments here, then, will be limited to a discussion of cases evaluated in our program. A family of five members with chronic exposure to chlordane was examined in our clinic after chlordane had permeated the air of their home. Two children with histories of learning disabilities, ages 8 and 11 years, were tested at school prior to their exposure. Postexposure testing was completed in our clinic and revealed consistent, significant changes in test scores on verbal concept formation. This occurred in both children when they were asked to deduce similarities and to define words (Similarities and Vocabulary subtests, WISC-R). In addition, a higher-order visuospatial reasoning task was also significantly impaired relative to preexposure performance (Block Design subtest, WISC-R). Unfortunately, changes in short-term memory and motor skills could not be assessed because these functions were not evaluated at preexposure testing. Attentional deficits and mood disturbances of a severe degree were observed in both children. However, these were difficult to interpret reliably, given the history of attentional deficits and the recent death of their mother. A third child (age 5 years) was examined without comparison testing available. He also evidenced attentional deficits and hyperactivity of such an extent that reliability of the test scores was questionable. Again, the etiology of these behavioral symptoms was unclear.

Two adults from the family were tested—the father, who was consistently in the home because of a physical disability, and a family friend, who frequently visited. Both showed short-term memory deficits, especially characterized by loss of information on delays for complex verbal and visual material. This was observed on recall of narrative material and visual designs (WMS) as well as a difficult paired associate learning test. In addition, a mood disorder with complaints of fatigue, anger, and clinical depression was seen on testing (Profile of Mood States, Minnesota Multiphasic Personality Inventory) and interview with both patients. Moderate visual organizational difficulties were also observed. In the father, mild attentional deficits were seen in the test results (particularly on Continuous Performance Testing).

DISCUSSION

In 1983, a Joint World Health Organization and National Institute for Occupational Safety and Health Workshop on Neurotoxic Illness (85) addressed the importance of international collaboration in the development, validation, and application of neurobehavioral tests for detecting neurotoxic illness (76). In developing neuropsychological test batteries to assess occupational exposures for both research and clinical settings, we have used the following guidelines: (*a*) examination of a broad range of cognitive functions; (*b*) inclusion of tests that are ecologically valid, i.e., tests that will generate predictions about the patient's functioning in daily life; (*c*) administration of tests known to be sensitive to neurotoxicant exposures; (*d*) inclusion of tests with demonstrated clinical utility in other settings, i.e., tests available and familiar to practicing clinicians; and (*e*) inclusion of tests that have been validated on patients with specific types of brain damage (11).

Although the test battery actually administered to a patient or used in research projects may vary, the battery of tests we have found useful has been derived from those commonly used in testing for toxic encephalopathies (Table 41.1).

Research Populations

In completing occupational studies, we have found it necessary to edit carefully the test battery because of the limited time that is usually available for testing. Thus, in addition to the guidelines just listed, we consider brevity of testing as essential. In the third year of a 3-year lead study (21), for example, we used a battery that was sensitive to low-level exposures, which required about 45 minutes to administer.

Another critical consideration for research testing is that of acceptability of tasks to workers, because cooperation can be highly variable during testing in these settings.

Clinical Patients

Test batteries for clinical patients with suspected neurotoxicant-related encephalopathy can generally include greater numbers of tests and time spent in testing. In addition, the patient is usually self-motivated to participate fully and attentively in the testing process. However, several problems are encountered in working with these patients.

One such problem is that of *hypochondriacal response to* occupational or environmental exposures. We have tested a number of patients who are convinced that they have suffered intellectual changes and memory disturbances as a result of exposures to toxicants. These claims are not verifiable on formal cognitive testing. When no encephalopathy is identified with intellectual testing, the use of the personality tests (e.g., MMPI—see Table 41.1), qualitative data, and interview responses may be necessary to form alternative psychiatric and social hypotheses.

Another problem frequently mentioned in occupational settings is that of *malingering*. However, in our population, we have found many fewer instances of malingering than we have of *hysterical* or *somatoform disorders*. Malingering tends to show up in a large battery of tests as highly uneven and inconsistent test performance, with exaggeration of subjective symptoms on interview.

Other areas of difficulty in neuropsychological testing involve background patient characteristics. Again, *psychiatric disorders*, manifesting typically as somatoform responses to occupational disorder, are frequent. In addition, a patient may have a long-term psychiatric disorder upon which neurotoxicant exposure is superimposed. Psychological testing and a psychiatric interview are included to assess these factors. Many patients with occupational or environmental exposures have histories of *learning disability*, and many of them are unaware of this fact. Very rarely do they have prior testing or prior diagnostic information that is helpful in differentiating the effects of neurotoxicant exposure versus that of early "minimal brain dysfunction." However, with sufficiently broad testing of cognitive and academic skills, the patterns associated with learning disability often can be identified and taken into account when other diagnoses are being considered.

Another area of difficulty is *cultural background* of patients. Frequently, patients whose second language is English are tested; in these cases, greater emphasis is placed on the motor, visuospatial, visual memory, and mood tests than on language and other highly culturally bound tasks for diagnostic purposes. We have, through interpreters, used translation in completing testing, but still find that less language-dependent tests are the most reliable.

Finally, a patient may have concurrent *neurologically based impairments* arising from head injuries, alcohol abuse, or other primary neurological disorders. These are assessed by including tests known to be sensitive to the patient's neurological disorder, though differentiation of etiologies can become quite difficult.

The differentiation of cognitive deficits arising from

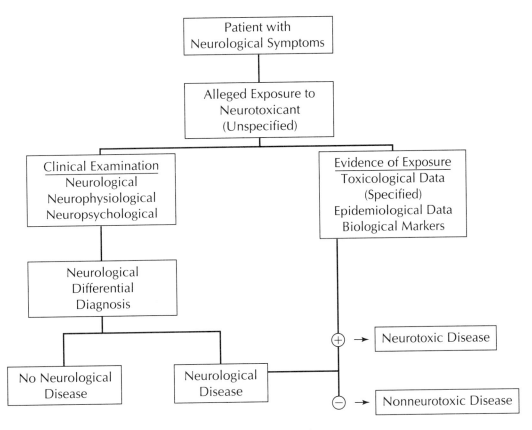

Figure 41.1. Approach to diagnosis.

exposures versus those arising from *depression* alone is another area of great difficulty in the neuropsychological diagnosis of neurotoxicant exposure. It is well known that cognitive deficits are associated with depression alone (86). This becomes particularly problematic in the area of neurotoxicant exposure, because organic depression is commonly concomitant with exposure to these substances. As a result, it is at times difficult to determine if the depression being observed on personality and mood tests is causing the cognitive deficits elicited or if the entire pattern of deficits suggests neurotoxicant exposure. This is handled in our clinic by examining past history, evaluating the pattern of difficulties observed on cognitive tests (whether impaired tests are those commonly observed with specific neurotoxicant exposures), and by looking at the nature of the depression. For example, depression in patients with significant toxic encephalopathy predominantly involves feelings of fatigue and apathy; but with certain substances, there is significant agitation as well.

Given the complexity of individual testing and the sometimes subtle nature of psychological changes accompanying toxicant exposures, one must be thorough when making an evaluation. Distinguishing the effects of exposure from other mitigating factors is obviously required but remains a challenge.

Often the clinical manifestations occur in the presence of an unknown neurotoxicant or when the identified substance is not previously known to be neurotoxic (Fig. 41.1). The high level of suspicion concerning the possible effects of alleged neurotoxicant exposure may lead to a diagnosis of neurotoxicant encephalopathy. However, it is necessary to fully assess all other possible causes for the clinical manifestations observed. Such an approach requires detailed occupational and environmental information, to be obtained by questionnaire, interview, medical and neurological examinations, and neurophysiological studies of peripheral nerve function, as well as the use of standardized neuropsychological testing.

References

1. Hernberg S. Neurotoxic effects of long-term exposure to organic hydrocarbon solvents: epidemiologic aspects. In: Holmstedt B, Lauwerys R, Mercier M, Roberfroid M, eds. Mechanisms of toxicity and hazard evaluation. Amsterdam: Elsevier, 1980:307–317.
2. Baker EL, White RF, Murawski B. Clinical evaluation of the neurobehavioral effects of occupational exposure to organic solvents and lead. International Journal of Mental Health 1988:14:135–138.
3. White RF. The role of the neuropsychologist in the evaluation of toxic central nervous system disorders. Semin Occup Med 1986;1:191–196.
4. White RF. Feldman RG. Neuropsychologic assessment of toxic encephalopathy. Am J Indust Med 1987;11:395–398.
5. Feldman RG, Auerbach S, Babikian V, et al. Neurology in family practice. In Rakel RE, ed. Textbook of family practice. 4th ed. Philadelphia: WB Saunders, 1990:1426–1473.

6. White RF, Feldman RG, Moss MB, Proctor SP. Magnetic resonance imaging (MRI), neurobehavioral testing, and toxic encephalopathy: two cases. Environ Res 1993b;61:117–123.

7. Rosenberg NL, Kleinschmidt-DeMasters BK, Davis KA, Dreisbach JN, Hormes JT, Filley CM. Toluene abuse causes diffuse central nervous system white matter changes. Ann Neurol 1988a;23:611–614.

8. Rosenberg NL, Spitz MC, Filley CM, David K, Schaumberg HH. Central nervous system effects of chronic toluene abuse-clinical, brainstem worked response on magnetic resonance imaging studies. Neurotoxicol Teratol 1988b;10:489–495.

9. Filley CM, Heaton RK, Rosenberg NL. White matter dementia in chronic toluene abuse. Neurology 1990;40:532–534.

10. White RF. The role of neuropsychological testing in the assessment of solvent exposure. Occupational and Environmental Medicine Report 1988;2:54–56.

11. White RF, Proctor SP. Research and clinical criteria for the development of neurobehavioral test batteries. J Occup Med 1992;34:140–148.

12. Feldman RG, Travers PH. Environmental and occupational neurology. In: Feldman RG, ed. Neurology: the physician's guide. New York: Thieme-Stratton, 1984:191–212.

13. White RF, Feldman RG, Proctor SP. Neurobehavioral effects of toxic chemicals. In: White RF, ed. Clinical syndromes in adult neuropsychology. New York: Elsevier, 1992:1–51.

14. Feldman RG, White RF, Eriator II, Jabre JF, Feldman ES, Niles CA. Neurotoxic effects of trichloroethylene in drinking water: approach to diagnosis. In: Isaacson RI, Jensen KF, eds. The vulnerable brain and environmental risks, vol. 3. New York: Plenum, 1994:3–23.

15. Needleman HL, Gunnoe C, Leviton A, et al. Deficits in psychological and classroom performance of children with elevated dentine lead levels. N Engl J Med 1979;300:689–695.

16. Feldman RG, Ricks NL, Baker EL. Neuropsychological effects of industrial toxins: a review. Am J Indust Med 1980;1:211–227.

17. Feldman RG, White RF. Lead neurotoxicity and disorders of learning and attention. J Child Neurol 1992;7:354–359.

18. Boey KW, Jeyaratnan J. A discriminant function analysis of neuropsychological effects of low lead level. Toxicology 1988;49:309–314.

19. Ryan CM, Morrow L, Parkinson D, Bromet E. Low level lead exposure and neuropsychological functioning in blue collar workers. Int J Neurosci 1987;36:29–39.

20. Baker EL, Feldman RG, White RF, et al. Occupational lead neurotoxicity: a behavioral and electrophysiological evaluation. Study design and year one results. Brit J Indust Med 1984;41:352–361.

21. Baker EL, White RF, Pothier LJ, et al. Occupational lead neurotoxicity: improvement in behavioral effects following exposure reduction. Brit J Indust Med 1985;42:507–516.

22. Grandjean P, Arnvig E, Beckmann J. Psychological dysfunction in lead-exposed workers: relation to biological parameters of exposure. Scand J Work Environ Health 1978;4:295–303.

23. Hanninen H. Behavioral effects of occupational exposure to mercury and lead. Acta Neurol Scand 1982;66(Suppl 92):167–175.

24. Valciukas JA, Lilis R, Rischbein A, Selikoff IJ. Central nervous system dysfunction due to lead exposure. Science 1978;201:465–467.

25. Jeyaratnan J, Boey KW, Ong CN, Chia CB, Phoon WO. Neuropsychological studies of lead workers in Singapore. Brit J Indust Med 1986;43:626–629.

26. White RF, Diamond R, Proctor SP, Morey C, Hu H. Residual cognitive deficits 50 years after childhood lead poisoning. Brit J Ind Med 1993a;50:613–622.

27. Landrigan PJ, Baker EL, Feldman RG, et al. Increased lead absorption with anemia and slowed nerve conduction in children near lead smelter. J Pediatr 1976;89:904–910.

28. de la Burde B, Choate MS. Early asymptomatic lead exposure and development at school age. J Pediatr 1975;87:638–642.

29. Wigg NR, Vimpani GU, McMichael PJ, Baghurst PA, Robertson EF, Roberts AJ. Port Pirie cohort study. J Epidemiol Comm Health 1988;42:213–219.

30. Winneke G, Beginn U, Ewert T, et al. Comparing the effects of

31. perinatal and later childhood lead exposure on neuropsychological outcome. Environ Res 1985;38:155–167.

31. Benetou-Marantidou A, Wakou S, Micheloyannis J. Neurobehavioral estimation of children with life-long increased lead exposure. Arch Environ Health 1988;43:392–396.

32. Baloh RW, Sturm R, Green B, Gleser G. Neurophysiological effects of chronic asymptomatic increased lead absorption: a controlled study. Arch Neurol 1975;32:326–330.

33. Lansdowne RG, Shepherd J, Clayton BE, Delves HT, Graham PJ, Turner WC. Blood lead levels, behavior and intelligence: a population study. Lancet 1974;1:538–541.

34. Needleman HL, Schell A, Bellinger D, et al. The long-term effects of exposure to low doses of lead in childhood. N Engl J Med 1990;322:83–88.

35. McMichael AJ, Baghurst PA, Wigg NR, et al. Port Prairie cohort study: environmental exposure to lead and children's abilities at the age of four years. N Engl J Med 1988;319:1037–1043.

36. Dietrich KN, Succop PA, Berger OG, et al. Lead exposure and the cognitive development of urban preschool children: the Cincinnati lead study cohort at age 4 years. Neurotoxicol Teratol 1991;13:203–211.

37. Clayton GD, Clayton FE, eds. Patty's industrial hygiene and toxicology, vols. 2A, 2B, and 2C. New York: John Wiley & Sons, 1981.

38. Feldman RG. Neurological manifestations of mercury intoxication. Acta Neurol Scand 1982;66:201–209.

39. Kurland LT, Faro SN, Siedler H. Minamata disease. World Neurology 1960;1:370–391.

40. Miller JM, Chaffin DB, Smith RG. Subclinical psychomotor and neuromuscular changes in workers exposed to inorganic mercury. Am Ind Hyg Assoc J 1975;36:725–733.

41. Langolf GD, Chaffin DB, Henderson R, Whittle HP. Evaluation of workers exposed to elemental mercury using quantitative tests of tremor and neuromuscular functions. Am Ind Hyg Assoc J 1978;39:976–725–733.

42. Angotzi G, Cassitto MG, Camerino D, et al. Rapporti tra esposizione a mercurio e condizioni di salute in un gruppo di lavaroti addetti alla dritillazione di mercurio. Med Lav 1980;71:463–480.

43. Forzi M, Cassitto MG, Bulgheroni C, Foa V. Psychological measures in workers occupationally exposed to mercury vapors: a validation study. In: Horvath M, ed. Adverse effects of environmental chemicals and psychotropic drugs, vol. 2. Amsterdam: Elsevier, 1976:165–171.

44. Piikivi L, Hanninen H. Psychological performance and long-term exposure to mercury vapor. In: Hernberg S, Kahn H, eds. Proceedings of the Second Finnish-Estonian Symposium on early effects of toxic substances. Helsinki: Institute of Occupational Health, 1981:165–169.

45. Vroom FG, Greer M. Mercury vapor intoxication. Brain 1972;95:305–318.

46. U.S. Department of HEW, Public Health Service, CDC. Criteria for a recommended standard. Occupational exposure to inorganic arsenic: new criteria. NIOSH Publication No. 75-149. Washington, DC: Government Printing Office, 1975.

47. Bolla-Wilson K, Bleecker ML. Neuropsychological impairment following inorganic arsenic exposure. J Occup Med 1987;29:500–503.

48. Morton WE, Caron GA. Encephalopathy: an uncommon manifestation of workplace arsenic poisoning? Am J Ind Med 1989;15:1–5.

49. Zettel H. The effects of chronic arsenic damage on heart and blood vessels. Z Klin Med 1943;142:689.

50. McCutchen JJ, Utterback RA. Chronic arsenic poisoning resembling muscular dystrophy. South Med J 1966;59:1139–1145.

51. Schenk VW, Stolk PJ. Psychosis following arsenic (possibly thallium) poisoning. Psychology, Neurology and Neurochemistry 1967;70:31–37.

52. Frank G. Neurologische und psychiatriche folgesymptome vei akuter Arsen-Wasserstoff-Vergiftung. J Neurol 1976;213:59–70.

53. Feldman RG. Manganese. In: de Wolff FA, ed. Handbook of clinical neurology, vol. 20(64). Intoxications of the nervous system, part I. Amsterdam: Elsevier, 1994:1–20.

54. Iregren A. Psychological test performance in foundry workers exposed

to low levels of manganese. Neurotoxicol Tetrol 1990;12:673–675.

55. Wennberg A, Iregren A, Struwe G, Cizinsky G, Hagman M, Johansson L. Manganese exposure in steel smelters; a health hazard to the nervous system. Scand J Work Environ Health 1991;17:255–262.

56. Mena I, Marin O, Fuenzalida S, Cotzias GC. Chronic manganese poisoning: clinical picture and manganese turnover. Neurology 1967;17:128–136.

57. Chandra SV, Seth PK, Mankeshwar JK. Manganese poisoning: clinical and biochemical observations. Environ Res 1974;7:373–380.

58. Cook DG, Fahn S, Brait KA. Chronic manganese intoxications. Arch Neurol 1974;30:59–64.

59. Whitlock CM, Amuso SJ, Bittendender JB. Chronic neurological disease in two manganese steel workers. Am Ind Hyg Assoc J 1966;27:454–459.

60. Chandra SV. Neurological consequences of manganese imbalance. In: Dreosti IE, Smith RM, eds. Neurobiology of the trace elements, vol. 2. Neurotoxicology and neuropharmacology. Clifton, NJ: Humana Press, 1983:167–196.

61. Vigliani EC. Clinical observations on carbon disulfide intoxication in Italy. Industrial Medicine and Surgery 1950;19:240-2.

62. Vigliani EC. Carbon disulfide poisoning in viscose rayon factories. Brit J Ind Med 1954;11:235–244.

63. Seppalainen AM, Tolonen M. Neurotoxicity of long-term exposure to carbon disulfide in the viscose rayon industry: a neurophysiological study. J Work Environ Health 1974;11:145–153.

64. Styblova V. Electroencephalography in diagnosis of early cerebral changes due to carbon disulfide. Int Arch Occup Environ Health 1977;38:263–282.

65. Peters HA, Levine LL, Matthews CG, Chapman LJ. Extrapyramidal and other neurologic manifestations associated with carbon disulfide fumigant exposure. Arch Neurol 1988;45:537–540.

66. Aaserud O, Gjerstad L, Nakstad P, et al. Neurological examination, computerized tomography, cerebral blood flow and neuropsychological examination in workers with long-term exposure to carbon disulfide. Toxicology 1988;49:277–282.

67. Hanninen H. Behavioral study of the effects of carbon disulphide. In: Xintaras C, Johnson BL, de Groot I, eds. Behavioral toxicology: early detection of occupational hazards. NIOSH Publication No. 74-126. Washington, DC: Government Printing Office, 1974:73–80.

68. Hanninen H, Nurminen M, Tolonen M, Martelin T. Psychological tests as indicators of excessive exposure to carbon disulfide. Scand J Psychiatry 1978;19:163–174.

69. Tuttle TC, Wood GC, Grether CB. Behavioral and neurological evaluation of workers exposed to carbon disulfide. NIOSH Publications No. 77-128. Washington, DC: Government Printing Office, 1976.

70. Lilis R. Behavioral effects of occupational carbon disulfide exposure. In: Xintaras C, Johnson BL, de Groot I, eds. Behavioral toxicology: early detection of occupational hazards. NIOSH Publication No. 74-126. Washington, DC: Government Printing Office, 1974:51–59.

71. Tuttle TC, Reed DE, Grether CB. Behavioral, neurological and physiological effects of carbon disulfide exposure: review and evaluation. Interim report for NIOSH Contract HSM-99-73-35, Westinghouse Behavioral Safety Center, Columbia, MD, 1973.

72. Defalque RJ. Pharmacology and toxicology of trichloroethylene. Clin Pharmacol Ther 1961;2:665–688.

73. Feldman RG. Trichloroethylene. In: Vinken PJ, Bruyn GW, eds. Handbook of clinical neurology. Amsterdam: North-Holland 1979: 457–464.

74. Huff JE. New evidence on the old problems of trichloroethylene. Industrial Medicine 1971;40:25–33.

75. Salvani M, Binaschi S, Riva M. Evaluation of the psychophysiological functions in humans exposed to trichloroethylene. Brit J Ind Med 1971;28:293–295.

76. Johnson B, ed. Prevention of neurotoxic illness in working populations. New York: John Wiley & Sons, 1987.

77. Feldman RG, Lessell S. Neuro-ophthalmalogic aspects of trichloroethylene exposure. In: Burnett J, Barbeau A, eds. Progress in neuro-ophthalmology. Amsterdam: Excerpta Medica, 1969:281–286.

78. Feldman RG, Mayer RM, Taub A. Evidence for peripheral neurotoxic effect of trichloroethylene. Neurology 1970;20:599–606.

79. Feldman RG, White RF, Currie JN, Travers PH, Lessell S. Long-term follow-up after single exposure to trichloroethylene. Am J Ind Med 1985;8:119–126.

80. Bor JW, Hurtig HI. Persistent cerebellar ataxia after exposure to toluene. Ann Neurol 1977;2:440–442.

81. Grabski DA. Toluene sniffing producing cerebellar degeneration. Am J Psychiatry 1961;118:461–462.

82. Cherry N, Hutchins H, Pace T, Waldron HA. Neurobehavioral effects of repeated occupational exposure to toluene and paints. Br J Ind Med 1985;42:291–300.

83. Parker JC, Bahlman LJ, Leidel NA, et al. Tetrachloroethylene (perchloroethylene). Am Ind Hyg Assoc J 1978;39:A23.

84. Tuttle RC, Wood GC, Grether CB, Johnson BL, Xintaras C. A behavioral and neurological evaluation of dry cleaners exposed to perchloroethylene. Part 2 of NIOSH Contract HSM-99-73-35, Division of Biomedical and Behavioral Science, Cincinnati, OH, 1977.

85. WHO/NIOSH Workshop Final Report. Workshop on the prevention of neurotoxic illness in working populations. Cincinnati, OH, May 23–26, 1983.

86. Lezak MD. Neuropsychological assessment. Oxford: Oxford University Press, Inc., 1983.

42

ASSESSMENT OF BRAIN INJURIES IN LEGAL CASES: NEUROPSYCHOLOGICAL AND NEUROPSYCHIATRIC CONSIDERATIONS[a]

David Faust

Although there is no guarantee of fairness in courtroom disputes over brain injury, poor preparation on the part of experts decreases the odds of a just outcome. The purpose of this chapter is not to debate the merits of psychiatrists', psychologists', or neuropsychiatrists' *courtroom* involvement, although it should be acknowledged that the author does hold negative views on many such activities (1, 2) Rather, recognizing the extent to which courtroom activities do occur and influence human lives, my intent is to provide information and suggestions that might improve the quality of legal assessments. Given the state of the art, various shortcomings need to be discussed, but awareness of problems can help one identify or develop better alternatives, and in a number of instances it is possible to provide positive suggestions.

The bulk of this chapter directly addresses neuropsychology and neuropsychological assessment, but much of the material also pertains to psychiatric and neuropsychiatric assessment. In brain damage cases, many of the diagnostic and assessment tasks are similar across these disciplines, especially when objective methods fail to yield hard evidence of dysfunction. For example, both the neuropsychologist and the neuropsychiatrist attempt to ascertain cognitive and affective status. Furthermore, literature on such matters as the effects of mild head injury or depression on cognitive performance is relevant to both groups, and both also often face the same types of courtroom challenges or lines of cross-examination. Thus, although reference is generally made to "neuropsychology" and "neuropsychologists," this is often a convenience to avoid the cumbersome practice of repeatedly listing the disciplines and their respective practitioners.

In the subsequent material, I provide a brief overview of neuropsychology and avenues for challenging neuropsychological and neuropsychiatric evidence. Some of these areas of potential challenge are then examined in detail, followed by a discussion of neuropsychological test batteries and mild head injury.

NEUROPSYCHOLOGY

Overview of Neuropsychology

Neuropsychology is dedicated to the study of brain-behavior relationships, with an emphasis on higher cortical functions. Some neuropsychologists engage solely in research or clinical activities, and others divide their time between the two areas. Clinical activities within neuropsychology may involve assessment, or the provision of therapeutic services to such groups as patients with brain impairments. Assessment activities are the primary focus here.

The aims of neuropsychological assessment vary, depending on the practitioner's orientation and approach. Assessment may be used to aid in determining the presence of brain damage or the effects of brain damage on behavioral and cognitive functioning. Neuropsychologists' involvement in the legal arena seems to occur most frequently in personal injury and workers' compensation cases. Practitioners do participate in a range of other cases, such as those involving an individual's competence to manage his or her own affairs, criminal responsibility, and child custody. Many cases involve head injury or claims of head injury, or, increasingly, exposure to neurotoxins.

Neuropsychological examination usually is far more detailed and comprehensive than the typical mental status examination of neurologists and other physicians, and it usually allows for quantification of results and comparison to

[a]This chapter is adopted in part from Faust (1995), which appears in the 5th edition of J. Ziskin's text, Coping with Psychiatric and Psychological Testimony, (131). Los Angeles, Law and Psychology Press.

normative groups or expectations. An attempt to provide a standard description of neuropsychological assessment techniques is complicated by the considerable diversity in the field. Indeed, differences in examination techniques can be so broad that two neuropsychologists examining the same person may employ tests with little or no overlap in specific content. Various surveys (3, 4) suggest, in fact, that the "standard" in neuropsychology, at least if this is defined by frequency of use or popularity, is that *there is no standard approach to neuropsychological assessment*. Thus, no matter what approach or battery a practitioner may employ, whether this is one of the set batteries, such as the Halstead-Reitan (H-R), or some type of more flexible approach (see below), the practitioner is still within a minority. Consequently, lawyers can establish that no matter what approach a particular neuropsychologist has used, most members of the profession employ a different overall approach. The results obtained on neuropsychological assessment can differ, depending on the specific measures employed, which creates uncertainty about the extent to which the ultimate conclusions reflect the examinee's status as opposed to the measures utilized. (For a more detailed description of neuropsychological assessment procedures, see Fogel and Faust [5], and Chapter 3 of this volume.)

STRATEGIES FOR CHALLENGING NEUROPSYCHOLOGICAL AND NEUROPSYCHIATRIC EVIDENCE

There are at least five basic strategies for challenging neuropsychological evidence. First, questions can be raised about the expert's credentials. Second, the attorney can point out flaws in the conduct of the examination, and in particular errors of omission and commission. Third, the lawyer can attempt to establish the presence of bias; errors of omission and commission serve as one potentially potent means for doing so. For example, repeated failure to accord credit that is due on test items can easily create the perception that the expert lacks objectivity. Fourth, the lawyer can challenge the underlying scientific bases of the expert's work. Finally, the lawyer can try to show that the expert's assumptions and conclusions are faulty. For example, the attorney may introduce contrary facts or attempt to establish flaws in the expert's reasoning. Most attorneys will stick to familiar territory and hesitate to venture into scientific research, although others become remarkably versed in the literature and are very well prepared to challenge the expert's knowledge and methodology. In the materials that follow, three of these areas of challenge are examined in greater detail: credentials, scientific bases, and errors of omission and commission.

It is a mistake to assume that the competent cross-examiner will try to challenge the expert point by point, or even try to follow the contour or content of the direct testimony. The attorney's task is to compromise the expert's credibility and, if possible, to put on affirmative elements of his or her case. For example, if the lawyer can show that the expert was biased in considering facts, even those that have little direct bearing on the final opinion, the task is usually

accomplished. Furthermore, once the expert's testimony is compromised or the witness weakened, the attorney may then introduce evidence favoring his or her side of the case, such as that suggesting good functional capacities, which a credible witness could easily negate. Therefore, the expert who tries to do too much, stretches a bit too far, or allows weak or tenuous elements or procedures to enter into his or her work, creates openings that a lawyer can exploit.

Neuropsychologists' Education, Training, and Credentials

Currently, there are no formal restrictions on who can call himself/herself a neuropsychologist. However, professional organizations within neuropsychology have issued various education and training guidelines. In many cases, experts will fail to meet some, or even many, of these guidelines. Detailed recommendations for training and education have been provided in a document entitled, *Reports of the INS-Division 40 Task Force on Education, Accreditation, and Credentialing* (16). The International Neuropsychological Society (INS) and Division 40 of the American Psychological Association, at the time of this writing, are the largest professional organizations in neuropsychology. Many experts who present themselves as clinical neuropsychologists will belong to one or both of these organizations. Hence, it would be difficult for them to claim that the recommendations of these organizations are of no relevance to them.

There is no licensure examination in neuropsychology, and neuropsychologists complete the same generic licensing examination for general practice as do other psychologists. The examination contains limited content directly related to neuropsychology, and its successful completion clearly does not ensure that a neuropsychologist is competent. Different organizations, in particular the American Board of Clinical Neuropsychology in conjunction with the American Board of Professional Psychology, offer a diplomate in clinical neuropsychology. To date, only a fairly small percentage of practitioners have pursued such certification. Furthermore, even if the clinician received extensive education and training in neuropsychology, and obtained a diplomate in clinical neuropsychology, there is a lack of research to suggest that such credentials demonstrate or prove competence in clinical decision making. For example, there is a paucity of published research demonstrating that those who have successfully completed the diplomate examination achieve greater diagnostic or predictive accuracy. There are, however, dozens of studies within clinical psychology and psychiatry in general (see Chapter 8 of Ziskin and Faust, [7]), and a number of studies within neuropsychology (8–13) that fail to demonstrate a relationship between training, experience, and judgmental accuracy. For an overview of this research, see Wedding and Faust (14) and Faust et al. (2).

Limits in Scientific Knowledge

An attack on underlying science and scientific methodology can be either broad or specific. The lawyer may try to attack the expert's field in general, pointing out, for example, the relative standing of psychiatry or neuropsychology in comparison to more advanced sciences. In addition or alternatively, the lawyer may attack the particular methods used in the case at hand. When selecting and defending methods, or when determining whether assessment methods are sufficient to become involved in a particular legal dispute in the first place, it is important to consider the differences that can exist between clinical and legal questions.

Suppose some method of psychological assessment is of demonstrated validity for some particular purpose. Perhaps neuropsychological battery X is correct in Y percentage of cases in identifying brain damage among certain types of individuals with certain types of conditions. An expert may assert that this level of accuracy also applies to the case at hand, or indicate that the method is helpful in answering other types of questions, such as whether the individual can return to his or her former employment. However, claims or demonstrations of clinical utility often do not establish that the method or clinician is able to answer legal questions with reasonable accuracy or validity, or is capable of aiding the trier of fact (7).

A clinical diagnosis may not relate in any clear way to the alleged consequences of an injury or event. For example, the diagnosis of brain damage may relate minimally to a legal issue, such as the individual's everyday functioning or mental competency. As Reitan (15) states, "It is meaningful to label only if the label has some significance. The label of 'brain damage' has little specific significance, considering the great variability among individuals who fall in this category" (p. 13). Along related lines, scientific knowledge and research may relate minimally to questions of legal interest. In the subsequent discussion, particular attention is given to four areas in which the gap between neuropsychology and law seems central: the identification of "subtle" brain damage, the assessment of everyday functional capacities, the apportionment of cause, and the appraisal of prior functioning. Because of space limitations, it is not possible to address other areas that can greatly complicate neuropsychological and neuropsychiatric assessment, such as limitations in norms or standards for intact functioning and the application of methods to special populations, including the young, the elderly, and ethnic and cultural minorities. (Treatment of these topics can be found in Faust [1]; and Faust et al. [2].)

Obvious Versus Subtle Cases

In a range of legal disputes, particularly those involving mild head injury or exposure to toxins, there frequently is no hard evidence of brain damage. In these cases, the lawyer often presents neuropsychological evidence to try to establish the presence of brain injury. The expert might be able to cite some impressive-sounding literature about the accuracy of her procedures in accomplishing this task. Although a considerable portion of the research in applied clinical neuropsychology does involve the accuracy with which tests and methods identify or localize brain damage, most of it has minimal application to the legal context.

Many studies on the accuracy of neuropsychological methods involve individuals for whom brain damage has been established with virtual or near certainty by some other method, such as MRI. In these types of cases, the courts do not need the neuropsychologist's assistance in identifying brain damage, for when brain damage can be identified with virtual certainty through some other means, the trier of fact does not need the neuropsychologist to indicate what is already known.

In contrast, when the courts need help in determining whether brain damage is present because other methods do not provide clear evidence, the neuropsychologist is generally reduced to speculation and guesswork. One reason is that the field has thus far developed only limited methodology for evaluating the accuracy of neuropsychological assessment techniques when other methods cannot identify brain damage with relative certainty, and does not have scientifically-established assessment procedures for making such determinations. Also, although many studies demonstrate reasonable accuracy in identifying obvious or gross disorder, which can usually be detected through other methods anyway, various studies show lower or poor accuracy when neuropsychological methods are applied to less obvious cases (16–20). The latter studies might involve cases in which brain damage still can be established with a high degree of accuracy through other means, such as CT. As Golden (21) indicates, various interpretive techniques in neuropsychology evolved around clear-cut cases of brain damage, such as major strokes. He observes that "these techniques become questionable when they are taken from such evaluations to the more subtle and difficult forensic evaluations" (p. 12).

If neuropsychological assessment methods are of questionable accuracy in cases that are subtle but for which it is still possible to obtain independent verification of brain damage through other methods, such reservations would seem to be even greater in cases in which independent verification is not available, especially absent the needed research. Furthermore, much of the research on more subtle discriminations involves the H-R battery and suggests decreased accuracy in such cases. If the practitioner has used the H-R, the implications are clear. If the practitioner has used some other battery, there is likely to be little or no formal research on the accuracy of the method with subtle cases, in the face of other research that suggests that neuropsychological methods lose accuracy as cases become less obvious or gross.

Assessment of Everyday Functioning

In many courtroom cases, a key issue is how the individual is functioning in everyday life and is likely to function in the future. The implications of a brain injury are much different, for example, if it is associated with minimal versus substantial impairment in everyday functioning. Unfortunately, the neuropsychologist's attempt to link test or observational data to everyday functioning is greatly hampered by insufficient knowledge and methodology. Commentators have been noting these limits for years, and studies examining the relation between performance on neuropsychological tests and everyday functioning, which were quite limited in number until more recently, have yielded mixed results at best (3, 22–35).

In 1983, Costa (25) described neuropsychologists' attempts to answer questions about everyday functioning as follows:

> To the extent that we rely on tests, we tend to load our batteries, which contain assessment techniques put there for other reasons, namely, to diagnose brain damage or explicate behavior relations, and go by the seat of our pants. Our patients deserve better than this. They deserve decisions and recommendations that are founded increasingly upon empirical validation (p. 7).

More recently, Guilmette et al. (3) noted, "Assessment of capacity to work or to perform other everyday tasks of independent living begs for more research on the 'external validity' of our measures and the development of other means to assess such crucial functioning" (p. 390). In 1992, Puente (32) stated that "few studies have addressed the ability of neuropsychological tests to predict everyday functioning or activities of daily living and vocational performance" (p. 301). And in 1995, Binder and Thompson (24) observed that "relatively little is known" (p. 33) about the capacity of neuropsychological assessment methods to determine (predict) current or future behavior.

A few examples of research on neuropsychological test performance and everyday functioning can be provided. Dodrill and Clemmons (26) related H-R performance among a group of adolescents with seizure disorder to their functional status 3–11 years later. Most of the H-R tests were not useful in predicting vocational adjustment or independence in living. Even the few variables or tests that showed statistically significant relations to functioning were of limited practical utility. Use of these variables to predict vocational adjustment and independent living produced respective improvements of 19% and 4% over the level of accuracy expected by chance. Greater improvement over chance level was attained in predicting results on an index of overall adjustment, although the authors noted that only gross distinctions were possible. For example, it was not possible to differentiate those classified on this index as nonfunctioning versus partially functioning.

Dunn et al. (28) obtained modest relations between neuropsychological test performance and results on a measure designed to assess everyday functioning among geriatric patients. The authors indicated that cross-validation of their results was needed, and that even the modest associations they obtained may have been inflated. Even disregarding this possibility, the authors note that given such modest relations, individuals who perform poorly on neuropsychological tests may show adequate everyday living skills, and vice versa. They also note that the relations they obtained between test performance and various facets of everyday functioning did not necessarily align with previously described, clinically-based guidelines (or what might be considered clinical lore). They likewise note that in their study, neuropsychological test results, while globally related to overall functioning, did not show more specific relations with particular functional capacities. They state, "A clear pattern of specific neuropsychological functions meaningfully associated with specific daily living skills did not emerge in this study. Therefore, while the two domains appear to be moderately related, prediction of a patient's daily functioning in a particular area from neuropsychological test data is not supported by the results of this study" (p. 115).

Partly in response to the limitations of traditional neuropsychological methods for assessing everyday functioning, efforts have been made to design questionnaires that aid in such determinations. These questionnaires typically have various items referring to the capacity to perform one or another everyday task (e.g., "I have trouble remembering appointments"). The questionnaires may be completed by the examinee, by an informant, or by both. Some of these questionnaires are analyzed informally. For others, quantitative scores or indices are derived. Many of the questionnaires focus on memory functioning. In addition to or in lieu of such questionnaires, the clinician may simply ask the examinee or informants interview questions about everyday functioning.

Research suggests, however, that self-reports of everyday functioning often show limited correspondence to either performance on neuropsychological tests or more direct measures of everyday functioning (1, 2, 36–40), with errors occurring in both directions. As is well known, for example, some brain injuries damage self-appraisal capacities and lead to denial of serious impairments. Other individuals are aware of deficits but are hesitant to admit to them. In contrast, other individuals overreport problems. Such errors may be inadvertent and stem from normal human limits in self-insight or self-appraisal capacities. Research also suggests that depression leads individuals to overreport or overperceive cognitive and functional difficulties (36, 37, 41). Additionally, of course, individuals may purposely overstate their problems. The litigation context complicates all of these matters. For example, an individual with serious brain impairment may be inadequately compensated due to a neurologically-based, false denial of problems. Alternatively, an individual may have strong incentives to exaggerate or misrepresent problems and thus may obtain unwarranted compensation.

A neuropsychologist may assert that inaccurate self-reports are due to brain damage, not to purposeful error or to inadvertent error of the type that is nonpathological or common to the general population, such as simple forgetting or difficulties perceiving oneself objectively. The assertion certainly can be correct, but sometimes this is something of a "heads I win; tails you lose" proposition. If the plaintiff agrees with the neuropsychologist's conclusions about dysfunction in one or another area, the plaintiff has insight; if the plaintiff disagrees, he or she lacks insight. This leaves no room for the possibility that the examiner's conclusions are wrong. Particularly in cases in which it is assumed that brain damage has impaired self-appraisal capacities, it is incumbent upon the clinician to obtain collateral or outside sources of information on matters that extend beyond the evaluation setting (see further discussion below).

If the clinician notes inconsistencies between his own impressions (or collateral information) and the individual's self-report, and if these inconsistencies are attributed to brain dysfunction, the question becomes whether the clinician can tell the difference between purposely erroneous reports, inadvertent errors in self-reports secondary to brain damage, inadvertent errors secondary to nonpathological factors, and instances in which the patient is correct and the examiner is not. The query posed here is not meant to apply to cases involving severe brain damage, but rather to the type of situation in which the presence or severity of brain damage is in dispute and the neuropsychologist describes problems in one or another area that the individual denies or does not report (at least initially). For example, the clinician might describe problems in reading and mild to moderate problems in recall, but the person says there is no notable difference when reading the morning paper and that he or she remembers as well (or as badly) as always.

Despite what may be confident pronouncements about the ability to distinguish the presence, or causes, of erroneous self-reports or lack of insight, the professional literature contains articles describing the lack of scientific underpinnings for such efforts. When discussing assessment of patients' insight into, or awareness of, their problems, Prigatano et al. (38) state, "No measurement technique has emerged to deal with this important clinical phenomenon" (p. 42, 163). According to McGlynn and Schacter (1989), there is a paucity of objective or quantitative measures for assessing lack of awareness. They note that such methods as rating scales and questionnaires designed for this purpose have various methodological problems. They further observe that lack of insight or awareness may be seen in conditions other than brain damage, and indicate that "no firm criteria have yet been developed" (p. 192) to distinguish between alternate causes for lack of awareness.

Apportionment of Cause

In tort law, monetary compensation rests on a determination that the event in question fully or partly caused some sort of damage. For example, if a plaintiff did indeed suffer brain injury but it was due to birth trauma rather than the recent car accident, the defendant is off the hook. In cases of purported brain injury, causal determinations can become complex. For example, there may be agreement about the outcome (i.e., brain dysfunction), but not its determinants. Alternatively, there may be dispute about what condition the plaintiff has, which in turn may affect causal attributions. For example, if the plaintiff does not have diffuse but rather localized brain damage, then it may not be a closed head injury suffered in a fall at work, but rather a benign cyst that accounts for his problems. Alternatively, if the plaintiff does not have brain damage but rather a psychiatric disorder, then

it may not have been a neurosurgeon's slip but instead a bitter divorce that is to blame. Finally, if there are multiple causative agents, the court may need to determine the extent to which the event in question contributed to the negative outcome.

The court's need to determine and apportion cause may create serious difficulties for the neuropsychologist. Many factors can impair cognitive processes or lower scores on neuropsychological tests. Furthermore, many of the factors or variables that influence test performance have similar manifestations, thereby making differential diagnosis, or the correct identification of etiology, problematic. For example, both alcohol abuse and mild head injury can result in decreased memory and learning, diminished speed of mental operations, and reduced capacities for problem solving (43).

Alternatively, the particular effects of one or another agent may not be well documented or understood, or may be highly variable. For example, little is known about the specific effects of many neurotoxins, and for some chemical agents research has yielded contrary findings. Finally, even should knowledge about one or another factor be fairly sound, there is often little known about the combined or interactive effects of multiple agents. In some cases, over a dozen factors can be identified that may have altered test results or cognitive functions.

Some experts make little attempt to identify alternate causes for lowered test performance. Others will make the effort, but limitations in knowledge can make it very difficult to determine whether, to what extent, and in just what manner such factors have influenced results. In addition, practitioners frequently use batteries for which there is little or no research involving the particular factors in question. For example, although there have been numerous studies on alcohol and test performance involving the H-R, it is not clear how useful this information is to the practitioner who has put together his or her own idiosyncratic battery. Consequently, lawyers can sometimes make considerable headway with questions directed at the potential influence of alternate factors, their overlap with the problems claimed in the case at hand, and the limited or nonexistent scientific methodology or knowledge needed to differentiate their contribution to the observed difficulties.

In some cases, it will be possible to establish alternate causes, such as depression or alcohol abuse, as the most likely explanation for the observed difficulties. This will sometimes lead to the conclusion that the accident or event in question did not cause the plaintiff's difficulties. In other cases, alternate causes for lowered test performance may still be blamed on the accident. For example, the low scores may be due to depression, but the jury may decide that the accident set off a chain of events that culminated in this disorder. Whatever the jury decides, it is to be hoped that compensation is based on what really ails the individual, and proper treatment is offered based on an accurate identification of etiology. Unfortunately, in too many cases, examiners are quick to jump to conclusions, resulting in poor clinical management. For example, the clinician may be so geared toward looking for brain damage that routine cases of depression are missed and individuals suffer needlessly until, and unless, the correct diagnosis is eventually made.

Affective and mood states, such as anxiety or depression, are among the more common alternative explanations for decreased neuropsychological test performance (44–52). Although research outcomes have differed, likely due to such factors as definitional and measurement variance, some studies suggest sizeable effects. For example, in Dean et al.'s (45) study, depressed psychiatric patients obtained mean Performance IQ scores 20 points below that of matched controls. Differences of this magnitude can change IQ classification by two or three categories, such as from average to borderline or deficient.

Abuse of alcohol or other psychoactive substances also needs to be considered. Short of permanent and severe brain dysfunction, alcohol abuse can lead to less obvious but permanent effects, or significant dysfunction that may last for years. Studies that examine individuals who have stopped drinking for months to years generally show superior cognitive functioning to that of recently detoxified alcoholics (43, 53). The evidence is mixed, however, on whether the cognitive functioning of abstainers returns to normal in all areas. In a number of the studies, improvement occurs to the point that alcoholics who remain abstinent eventually perform similarly to nonalcoholic controls, although this may require as long as 2–3 years.

Lack of sleep and fatigue can also decrease attention and concentration, and thus secondarily affect various other cognitive functions. Some practitioners perform 8 hours of interviewing and testing in 1 day. As Benton (54) notes, "Too many neuropsychologists are not sufficiently sensitive to the physical condition and affective status of their patients. They are seemingly unaware that the performances which they are eliciting are also determined by a variety of nonneurological factors of a physical, emotional, and motivational nature (particularly fatigue and sagging motivation but also distrust and hostility) that interact with the condition of the brain" (p. 414).

Preexisting intellectual weaknesses or learning disabilities may also account for lowered test scores. Research suggests that learning difficulties or disabilities may persist in part, or wholly, into adulthood (55–59). (For more detailed discussion of these and other alternative causes, see Faust [1, 2]).

Problems Determining Prior Functioning

To determine whether an injury has led to a decrease in functioning, one needs to know what the individual's baseline was initially, or prior to the injury or event in question. As Boll (60) states, "In attempting to appreciate the neurocognitive sequelae of any event, one must understand the abilities that the patient has brought to that event, and the abilities which are likely to remain once the event has transpired. There is simply no sense in expecting someone to 'recover' to a position which they had not attained initially"

(p. 480). Lezak (50) indicates that in certain areas of functioning, or in cases of gross deficit, one can draw inferences regarding brain damage or decline without knowing prior functioning. She indicates that in most cases, however, "A first step in measuring intellectual deficit in an adult is to establish—or estimate, when direct information is not available—the patient's premorbid performance level for all of the functions and abilities being assessed" (p. 90).

Different methods have been applied to the task of determining prior functioning, none of which has approached a high level of accuracy and a number of which have produced poor results (61–67). These methods include the use of sociodemographic predictors, comparison of performance on Wechsler Intelligence Scale subtests that supposedly are and are not sensitive to brain damage, the use of reading recognition tasks, and the "best performance method" (68). In the best performance method, one presumes that the highest score or scores across a neuropsychological profile represent areas of preserved functioning and thereby provide an estimate of prior overall functioning. Both theoretical analysis that considers the wide variation in functioning that individuals commonly display, and empirical study (69) suggest that this method often leads to gross overestimates of prior abilities, and thus false conclusions about the presence or extent of loss.

The use of sight-reading measures, such as the National Adult Reading Test (NART-R), has recently gained increasing attention. The basic rationale is that word identification tends to be unaffected by brain damage. Wiens et al. (67) reviewed research on the NART-R and comment that a number of investigations have yielded promising results. However, in their study, the NART-R demonstrated only limited power in predicting intellectual functioning, and there was a decided tendency toward misestimation, sometimes to an extreme degree, among the more and less intelligent. They state that "for the present sample as a whole, NART-R performance provided a modest estimate of current WAIS-R FSIQ [Full-Scale IQ] that was similar to findings of other recent studies. As a reliable and sensitive estimate of intelligence for individuals at other than average levels of ability, however, it appears of questionable value" (p. 83).

Studies examining the use of sociodemographic predictors, such as education and occupation, also show increased error among individuals of high or low intellectual levels. It is in cases of high or low prior intelligence that it is especially crucial to determine previous functioning, because interpretive procedures often have to be adjusted the most. For example, low average cognitive performance may reflect no change for someone who started at this level, but gross change for someone who started with superior intellectual ability.

The great bulk of research has been aimed at developing methods for estimating prior IQ scores or intellectual functioning. Ironically, for many conditions, such as mild head injury, neuropsychologists will assert that IQ scores usually are not affected, and rather that other particular functions (e.g. executive functions) are far more likely to be impaired. How useful can a method be for determining whether change in functioning has occurred if it is designed to measure a function that purportedly should not change when the condition of interest occurs?

The relative failure to develop accurate methods for estimating prior functioning in the most intensively researched area—overall intellectual functioning—raises substantial doubt about the accuracy of estimations involving less well-researched areas. Neuropsychological assessments often cover a range of functions, including various facets of memory, language, and visual-motor skills. Many of these functions are minimally covered by IQ tests, which is a primary reason for using neuropsychological batteries. In most cases, there is essentially no scientific information on the success achieved in estimating prior functioning in the areas covered on neuropsychological batteries, even when there are standard methods for forming these estimates in the first place.

Although acknowledging the limits of methods, some authors (63, 65) note that at least some of them, such as those based on demographic variables, are still preferable to the subjective or impressionistic methods that are sometimes used. Given the shortcomings of available methods, the clinician frequently needs to seek out concrete evidence about prior functioning (e.g., school records, occupational records) and information from collateral sources (preferably neutral ones). Failure to do so can easily lead to false conclusions about prior functioning, which can have an overwhelming impact on a case witness should the lawyer be prepared to present counterfactual evidence. I have consulted in numerous cases in which postinjury test results presumed to reflect substantial losses seemed perfectly consistent with preinjury data, such as school achievement and group intelligence testing.

Summary and Elaboration

Whatever the status of clinical neuropsychology, the field shows a lack of validated scientific methods or demonstrated capacities to address a number of key legal questions or needs, such as the identification of brain damage in "subtle" cases. These limits are most evident in the neuropsychologist's attempts to describe or predict everyday functioning. As the foregoing research suggests, performance on neuropsychological tests often shows limited or minimal relation to everyday functioning. Perhaps in recognition of this deficiency, many clinicians also obtain some type of self-report data. However, examinee's self-reports also fail to show a dependable relation with everyday functioning because of such potential factors as falsification or inadvertent error. Although the expert may claim some special capacity to distinguish between accurate and inaccurate self-reports, such claims lack a supportive body of scientific research. Lacking consistent or dependable relations between everyday functioning, neuropsychological test results, and self-report, these latter two data sources cannot substi-

tute for the direct observation of everyday functioning. Indeed, it is everyday functioning that is often of greatest relevance in legal cases. Without an established scientific basis from which to formulate descriptions of current everyday functioning or to predict future functioning, such judgments often rest primarily on guesswork and speculation.

Errors of Commission and Omission

Although I have no way of knowing how representative my experience might be, in the cases I review as a legal consultant, I am consistently impressed with the frequency of errors of commission and omission in the conduct of examinations. Such errors offer attorneys for the opposing side a way to destroy an expert's credibility. The expert should assume that lawyers can gain access to their complete file on the examinee, and that lawyers may have other experts review the materials.

One of the most common errors of commission I have found is the mis-scoring of psychological tests. I have reviewed Wechsler Intelligence Scales with 20 or 30 scoring errors, including repeated failures to add numbers correctly. It is rather embarrassing for the expert when it can be shown that he or she committed the same kind of errors used to diagnose brain dysfunction.

I also find that experts frequently violate standard procedures for test administration. For example, the expert might terminate a test or subtest prematurely, or before the discontinuation rule is met. In one case in which a child obtained somewhat low scores, an expert prematurely discontinued half of the subtests on the Wechsler Intelligence Scale for Children—Revised and never mentioned it in the report. This same expert had also written an article discussing the importance of following standardized test procedures exactly. Violations of standard procedures also occur in the use of structured interviews.

Experts frequently use inferior methods when better methods are available. They may depend on interview procedures, tests, test norms, or interpretive rules that research shows are not as strong as other available techniques. For example, neuropsychiatrists may incorporate psychometrically weak items into their mental status examinations, or might evaluate the performance of an elderly individual using standards derived from research on middle-aged subjects.

Overdiagnosis seems to be a common problem. Experts may overestimate prior functioning due to sole reliance on a plaintiff's self-report or the use of flawed procedures, such as the best performance method. Obviously, if prior functioning is overestimated, the result can be a false impression about loss or the extent of loss. Other bases for overdiagnosis include insufficient appreciation of normal variation in functioning, or the fact that most individuals have at least some cognitive weaknesses, failure to recognize the extent of overlap between normal and abnormal populations, and the use of inappropriate performance or normative standards. Each of these factors can also work in the opposite direction. For example, the use of overly lenient normative standards can lead to false-negative errors.

Common errors of omission include the failure to adequately assess for malingering, incomplete consideration of alternative explanations of etiology, and, perhaps most importantly, failure to obtain and review collateral information. Collateral sources, such as prior school and work records and interviews with individuals who knew the person well both pre- and postinjury, can help in addressing four issues that are almost always germane in legal cases: *(a)* past functioning, *(b)* current functioning, *(c)* cause of the presenting difficulties, and *(d)* the examinee's honesty and accuracy as an informant.

It is hard to overstate the importance of obtaining collateral information. Many experts have found themselves horribly compromised because of a failure to do so. The psychiatrist who claims that the plaintiff's obsession with his spouse's fidelity represents paranoia may be confronted with testimony from three admitted lovers. The neuropsychologist who claims that the Full Scale IQ of 92 represents a huge loss may be confronted with results on this same test administered pre-injury, which produced a score of 91. And the neuropsychiatrist who indicates that a plaintiff seemed forthright in providing information may be asked whether he or she is aware of the plaintiff's prior crimes, his three previous head injuries, and his repeated failure to complete treatment for cocaine addiction.

Even should the expert believe, correctly, that factors that come to light at trial have no impact on his or her conclusions, the jury may well think otherwise. Once it appears that the expert was careless, a juror may simply think, "That's not the kind of doctor I'd want to see," and give no credence to the expert's testimony. Furthermore, a poor impression can result when the cross-examining lawyer seems to know more about the plaintiff than the expert.

There are many sources of information about an individual's past and present functioning. In obtaining and reviewing records, experts might try to keep a dual perspective in mind. First, records can provide direct facts relating to the individual's functioning. For example, school records often contain results on achievement and aptitude tests. Second, many types of records may provide direct or indirect samples of cognitive abilities or competencies, although not intended or designed for such purposes. For example, although the past work file provides facts about employment, it may also contain forms that the individual completed, thereby offering a sample of preinjury writing abilities.

Potential sources of information about past functioning include school, military, and employment records. With such types of information, there may be multiple files at the same setting or institution. For example, college records may include not only the transcript, but application materials that are kept elsewhere, and student health clinic records. One should also try to obtain all past medical and mental health records, if applicable.

Information about current functioning can also come from school or work records, if the individual is currently engaged in such endeavors. Other possible sources of information include driving records, job applications, home videos, diaries, other assessments (e.g., vocational rehabilitation evaluations), treatment records, and the plaintiff's deposition. For example, a driving record may indicate that the same individual who is purported to be too spatially disordered to operate a vehicle safely put 20,000 miles on an old Chevy, had no accidents, received no tickets, and routinely handled the rush hour in downtown Boston.

Home videos may show the examinee engaged in activities that would not seem possible based on self-report. In one case in which I consulted, a plaintiff who complained bitterly about back and shoulder problems was able to drag a buck through the snow to his Jeep, with the moment immortalized on video tape. Treatment records may make reference to activities the plaintiff denied being able to perform. Depositions with the plaintiff may show language comprehension and attentional abilities that seem far beyond those demonstrated on examination. Careful review of background records can not only help avoid situations in which the clinician might otherwise be fooled, but can greatly strengthen testimony in cases of legitimately injured individuals.

TEST BATTERIES/ASSESSMENT METHODS

This section focuses on more commonly used neuropsychological test batteries and approaches to assessment, such as the H-R. It should be stated from the outset, however, that many clinicians do *not* use standardized batteries that have received adequate scientific evaluation, but rather construct their own combination of tests or procedures (3). Similarly, many clinicians also alter their assessment methods or test selection across examinees, or even during the process of an assessment as the initial data come in, an approach often referred to as "flexible" or "tailored."

Whenever a practitioner uses a personal compilation of tests or procedures, whether the compilation remains consistent or is altered across examinees, the "battery" or particular combination usually is idiosyncratic to that clinician. A lawyer can therefore ask the expert to produce studies in peer-reviewed journals (as opposed to impressionistic or anecdotal evidence) that demonstrate the validity of his or her procedure. An expert may argue that there is validation research on some or all of the tests within his or her battery. However, one needs to know about validation research for the use of the tests together. Whatever the accuracy level obtained by one or another test, the accuracy attained when the tests are combined may differ. For example, one test may correctly indicate normal status, but a second test may falsely indicate otherwise, perhaps leading to a mistaken conclusion that would have been avoided had the second test been omitted.

Many studies on neuropsychological assessment techniques examine accuracy in identifying or localizing brain damage. Research outcomes are highly variable, with some studies showing low accuracy rates and others showing much better results. However, studies cannot necessarily be taken at face value and may not apply to the case at hand. For example, some research includes patients with major psychiatric disorders who have been minimally worked up for organic brain conditions, and assumes that all errors on tests are due to the psychiatric disorder. Other studies have produced overestimates of diagnostic accuracy. For example, as noted, inflated accuracy rates can be created by the use of extreme groups or the elimination of equivocal cases. In contrast, in the legal arena, neuropsychologists often evaluate cases in which the evidence for brain damage is equivocal, or in which difficult discriminations must be made. The central question then is how well neuropsychological assessment methods do when applied to comparable cases in a comparable manner, and when addressing comparable questions. For example, it matters little how well or how poorly a procedure might prove in discriminating brain damage from normality when the issue is everyday functioning, or when the practitioner does not use the method as designed.

Structured Batteries: The Halstead-Reitan Neuropsychological Battery

This discussion focuses on the adult version of the H-R, although there are other versions for individuals below age 15 (70). The battery for adults includes a core set of five tests (Category Test, Tactual Performance Test, Seashore Rhythm Test, Speech-Sounds Perception Test, and Finger Tapping [or Oscillation] Test), from which seven scores are derived that are used in calculating the Impairment Index. Tests administered in addition to Halstead's five core measures generally include the Trail Making Test, Strength of Grip (Hand Dynamometer), the Aphasia Screening Test, and procedures for examining sensory perception. Other tests, which are not formally part of the H-R, are also frequently used, in particular the Minnesota Multiphasic Personality Inventory (MMPI) and the WAIS-R. (For a detailed description of the H-R battery and allied procedures, see Reitan and Wolfson, [717]).

To compute the Impairment Index, one divides the number of scores that fall outside a cutoff point by the total number of scores. Reitan advises that scores at or above .5 be classified as indicative of brain damage (71). Research suggests that this cutoff point can lead to frequent misdiagnoses of brain damage among certain groups, especially those who are older or less educated (72). Even so, many clinicians use cutoff lower than .5, which, of course tends to exacerbate this problem with overdiagnosis.

Parenthetically, even if one ignores the concern that normal individuals commonly exceed Reitan's upper limit for the Impairment Index, it is still evident that with a cutoff point of .5, individuals can perform abnormally on as many as three of the seven components of the Impairment Index and still be classified as normal (at least on this basis). Experts may pick out deviant results on one or two of the component tests, or from one or a few other tests among a battery, and claim that they establish brain damage. In such circumstances, a lawyer can bring out the fact that normal

individuals may perform "abnormally" on a certain percentage of tests. Heaton et al.'s (72) updated norms for the H-R suggest that the unusual result is for individuals to complete a neuropsychological battery *without* obtaining some low or "abnormal" scores. The same point can apply to the neuropsychiatrist who observes difficulties on one or two isolated parts of mental status testing.

VARIATIONS IN H-R PROCEDURES

Although, in theory, the H-R is a standardized procedure, the test instructions and methods that clinicians use when administering the battery can vary considerably. Such variation may be due in part to the circulation of different H-R manuals. Snow (73) indicates that variations in the administration of the H-R may have a considerable impact on testing results. Examiners may also use materials or equipment that deviate from those Reitan has specified, or may use shortened versions of tests. For example, rather than using the standard equipment for the Category Test, which involves a projection system and levers that are pressed to signal responses, the clinician may use a paper-and-pencil format.

Reitan has published detailed instructions for the administration of his battery and seems to take a very dim view of such alterations in standardized methods and equipment (71), warning that they typically have not gained sufficient validation. He states that "such validation is *absolutely necessary* to provide reliable and meaningful data for interpretation" (p. 121, italics added). He states further, "Over the years we have made a determined effort to maintain standardization of each test, down to the last detail, so that the published research results and clinical interpretations may serve validly" (p. 121).

VARIATIONS IN H-R NORMATIVE STUDIES

The "traditional" or "standard" norms that are commonly used for the H-R often misidentify normal individuals as abnormal, which has led to various attempts to develop more adequate normative data. The results of these studies have sometimes differed considerably. Some of these differences can be attributed to such factors as the age or education of subjects, but in other cases, there are no obvious explanations for discrepancies in results, nor clear-cut guides or methodological features that would allow one to select one study over another. The potential discrepancies among narrative studies are well illustrated by Fromm-Auch and Yeudall's (74) review of such investigations. For example, 50 or more errors on the Category Test is the "traditional" cutoff point for identifying abnormal performance. However, if one uses the common criterion of two standard deviations beyond the mean as the cutting point, then according to some studies that Fromm-Auch and Yeudall summarize, 60, 70, or even more than 100 errors falls within the normal range.

A considerable advance was made with the publication of Heaton et al.'s (72) normative system for the H-R. Heaton et al. divide their subjects by age, education, and gender. Especially with older and less educated individuals, the contrasts between the results obtained using traditional norms and Heaton et al.'s norms are sometimes dramatic. For example, assume that a 70-year-old male with an 8th grade education obtains a score of .7 on the Impairment Index, or a result that clearly exceeds the traditional cutoff of .5 used to identify brain damage. When analyzed with the Heaton et al. system, this level of performance is found to be as good as or better than nearly seven of 10 *normal* men from the same reference group.

RESEARCH AND COMMENTARY ON THE H-R

Discussing potential limits in the H-R battery, especially when used for legal purposes, is in no way intended to diminish Halstead and Reitan's magnificent contributions to neuropsychology. A number of these problems have already been covered and are only briefly reiterated here. In fact, much of the research on such matters as reduced accuracy in subtle cases and limitations in determining everyday functioning have involved the H-R. This is largely because the H-R has been by far the most thoroughly researched battery in neuropsychology, and its strengths and limitations are much better known than are those of other batteries. Thus, often it is not that scientific research has shown that other batteries or approaches are better, but rather that many critical areas have been subjected to little or no study.

Subtle Cases

As noted, in comparison to studies focusing on more obvious or gross cases, studies involving more subtle cases have produced lower, or much lower, accuracy rates. According to Klesges et al. (17), studies on the H-R have yielded hit rates ranging from 94% to less than 43%. In their study, accuracy in distinguishing brain-damaged from normal subjects barely exceeded the level that could have been achieved by disregarding the testing entirely and simply assuming that all subjects were brain damaged. Results of studies such as those conducted by Sherer et al. (19) and Mutchnick et al. (18) also stand in contrast to the impressive figures commonly reported in studies involving less demanding discriminations. Of course, none of these studies answers the question or issue that is often first and foremost in legal cases: How accurate is the H-R (or other neuropsychological methods) in cases in which there is no independent, trustworthy means for identifying brain damage? While the scientific community awaits a clear answer and struggles to create adequate methodology to address the issue, some experts do not find such "academic" concerns inhibiting and readily take the stand and testify as if these matters were already known to them.

Everyday Functioning

There is no need to review the materials already provided on the limitations of neuropsychological assessment techniques for determining everyday functioning. Much of this research has involved the H-R. It should further be obvious that if methods lack precision for determining current everyday functioning, they are likely to be an even weaker determinant of past or future functioning. Assessment of past functioning is often needed to ascertain whether a change has occurred, and future functioning is often the major consideration in assigning damages.

Overdiagnosis

Many studies suggest that the traditional norms for the H-R lead to overdiagnosis, especially among those who are older, less well-educated, or come from different ethnic or cultural groups (72, 75–81). For example, Heaton et al. (82) report on the performance of 500 normal individuals or controls on the H-R in relation to such subject variables as age and education. They examined commonly used norms or cutoff points for various H-R tests or subtests and found that a number of these measures frequently led to the misidentification of abnormality. For subjects at or above 60 years of age, various H-R indices or tests led to the erroneous identification of abnormality in 21–91% of the cases. The frequency of false-positive errors was lower among the subjects from 40–50 years of age, although the rates were as high as about 72%. For individuals below age 40, false-positive rates ranged as high as about 46%. Particularly high rates of misdiagnosis were obtained among those who were both older and less educated.

Other Limitations

Research raises other concerns about the H-R battery, such as the adequacy of test-retest reliability (83) and its use with special populations or cultural minority groups (1). Also, as might be expected given ongoing controversies about basic approaches to neuropsychological assessment, proponents of flexible strategies often criticize the structured or set approaches that characterize such batteries as the H-R. For example, Heilman and Valenstein (84) state, "We support a flexible approach to the study of brain-behavior relationships . . . . Inflexible test batteries, although necessary for obtaining normative data, limit our view of the nervous system if used exclusively" (pp. 15–16). Benton (54), while acknowledging certain advantages of structured approaches, also points out limitations and proposes a rather radical shift away from traditional fixed batteries. Others suggest that the H-R, or standardized test batteries or measures in general, often fail to pinpoint neuropsychological difficulties (85, 86).

Structured Batteries: The Luria-Nebraska Neuropsychological Battery

The Luria-Nebraska Neuropsychological Battery (LNNB) (87) is a shorter procedure than the H-R. The LNNB items and scales are intended to tap a variety of areas, such as memory, verbal functions, motor coordination, and reasoning. The LNNB is an attempt to quantify the essentially qualitative diagnostic approach of the great Russian neuropsychologist Alexander Luria, an enterprise that many neuropsychologists reject on first principles. The

LNNB has been the subject of heated controversy, almost from its inception, and recent surveys suggest that few practitioners align themselves with its underlying approach to neuropsychological assessment. In the Guilmette et al. (3) survey, less than 20% of the respondents indicated that they use the LNNB regularly or more often. In addition, using this battery is not necessarily the same as adopting the basic philosophy or strategy of assessment advocated by its creators. Stated differently, those using the battery can use it in their own way. In fact, in Guilmette et al.'s survey, only 6% of the respondents identified themselves as adopting the LNNB approach to neuropsychological assessment, or holding this basic orientation, a figure similar to that which Putnam and DeLuca (4) obtained.

Research on the LNNB has produced mixed outcomes. It has been noted that some of the more positive studies were published by Golden and associates, and some of the more negative studies by independent investigators. Lezak (50) states:

> A considerable gap separates the evaluations of this battery made by Golden and his colleagues from those by neuropsychologists who are not affiliated with them. Golden and his group, without exception, offer data supporting their claims that this battery is a diagnostically efficient instrument. Other neuropsychologists have concluded that the battery is diagnostically unreliable. In evaluating the literature on this instrument, it is important to know the nature of the data on which such differing conclusions have been based. (p. 570)

Lezak reiterates these points in the 1995 update of her book. In fact, attempts to replicate promising investigative results with the LNNB have sometimes yielded very negative outcomes (88, 89).

Various criticisms of the battery have also been raised, such as shortcomings in its assessment of language disorders (90) and memory functions (91). More generally, the validity and utility of the LNNB have been a topic of intense, if not vehement, dispute. For example, Reynolds (92) notes that the LNNB has been the subject of major controversy, and that it "has been criticized on the basis of inadequate reliability, validity, item content, administration and scoring procedures, and as a bastardization of Luria's own methods." Adams (93) referring to the LNNB, states, "Never before in the history of clinical neuropsychology has so much controversy centered around one instrument" (p. 878). Mapou (94) observes that "neither the entire scale nor any subscale [of the LNNB] has been adequately shown to be a valid measure of any specific cognitive function" (p. 275), and Spiers (95) contends that the LNNB "does not adequately or comprehensively assess any major neuropsychological function."

Flexible and Process/Qualitative Approaches

FLEXIBLE BATTERY APPROACHES

Many neuropsychologists vary the combination of tests used in assessment (3, 4, 96). Muriel Lezak (50, 68, 97) is perhaps the most prominent spokesperson for this "flexible battery" or "individualized approach" to neuropsychological assessment. According to Lezak, the approach involves tailoring assessment not only in relation to the referral question, but often also in relation to initial testing results. For example, should the examinee show problems in certain areas, one might add additional tests to further assess that area. Lezak (97) states, "Few if any examinations conducted within this framework can be identical in the instruments used, the extent to which limits are tested, or the amount of effort expended in interviewing and history-taking" (p. 30). She further notes, "Together, the uniqueness of each patient with known or suspected brain damage and the variety of reasons for examining these patients call for flexibility, common sense, and inventiveness in the conduct of an examination adapted to the patient" (p. 30). Many neuropsychologists rely on Lezak's work or employ approaches that incorporate the type of flexibility that she describes.

Just as there are many supporters and opponents to set or standardized batteries, there are also considerable numbers of professionals on either side of the arguments about the flexible approach. Russell (98) argues that the neuropsychologist who depends solely on a flexible approach is limited to evaluating suspicions or hypotheses about problem areas. Furthermore, although advocates of the flexible approach may emphasize the integration of data or configural analysis, Russell states flatly that "accurate pattern analysis is only possible when a set rather than a flexible battery of tests is utilized" (p. 50). Hartman (99), Costa (100), and Benton (54), have also criticized various aspects of the flexible approach.

Whatever the potential merits of the flexible approach within the clinical context, it creates major problems when applied to legal assessments. First, such an approach seems to represent nearly an ultimate form of eclecticism. There is not *a* flexible battery shared by clinicians, but rather different clinicians use different flexible batteries, and even the same clinician may alter his or her battery substantially when assessing different examinees. As such, various practitioners have essentially designed their own idiosyncratic batteries, and may reinvent them nearly each time a new examinee is seen. A lawyer can ask the expert to produce formal validity data on his or her invention or particular battery. Of course, it is unlikely that such scientific data exist, and if a different procedure is used with most or all patients, there will be little or no validity evidence because those specific procedures will rarely if ever have been previously used in that particular combination.

Practitioners utilizing a flexible battery not only start with differing combinations of tests, but also may alter standard methods of test administration. To the extent that alterations occur, it is doubtful that the norms and interpretive guidelines that are based on routine administration of these tests can be used validly. The *Standards for Educational and Psychological Testing* (101), a joint publication of the American Psychological Association, American Educational Research Association, and the National Council on Measurement in Education, is clear on these matters, stating, for example, that "when a test user makes a substantial change in test format, mode of administration, instructions, language, or content, the user should revalidate the use of the test for the changed conditions or have a rationale supporting the claim that additional validation is not necessary or possible" (p. 41). A clinician's mere belief that the changes "work" would hardly seem adequate for asserting that formal validity research is unnecessary. As such, lawyers may question experts very closely about alterations in standard instructions or administration procedures. Some examiners attempt to substitute "clinical judgment" or "experience" for formal normative data, a strategy that has many shortcomings (2, 13).

The flexible approach also makes it extraordinarily difficult to conduct research. If virtually every examinee receives a different form of assessment or set of tests, how does one determine effectiveness or accuracy across cases? One has essentially performed a unique set of procedures with every individual, and must conduct a separate "experiment" for every case seen. This practice is not unlike attempting to determine the effects of different classes of medications, when nearly every patient is given a unique medication or combination of medications and dosages. Given these extraordinary methodological complications, it is not surprising that scant formal scientific research has been conducted on the accuracy of the flexible approach to neuropsychological assessment. Accordingly, particularly for courtroom application, it must be considered experimental.

PROCESS/QUALITATIVE APPROACHES

Many of the criticisms and limitations that apply to the flexible battery approach also pertain to what are often termed "process" or "process/qualitative" methods of neuropsychological assessment. The process approach places decreased emphasis on quantitative scores and increased emphasis on qualitative features of performance, such as the strategies examinees use in approaching test items. The process approach has been championed by such individuals as Edith Kaplan. Milberg, Hebben, and Kaplan (86) describe one version of this approach. However, it is important to realize that other neuropsychologists who follow the process approach may use specific tests or procedures that show limited overlap with those that Milberg et al. discuss. Thus, different neuropsychologists who describe their approach as process or process/qualitative may share little more than a set of strategies and assumptions, and may employ substantially different test batteries. In this sense, there is no specific set of procedures that can be identified as representing the "standard" process method of neuropsychological assessment.

Milberg et al. (86) indicate that although their approach incorporates a core set of tests, exact procedures vary with each patient and are quite flexible. As the authors state, "The only limits to the procedures that are employed (beyond the patient's tolerance and limitations) are the examiner's knowledge of available tests of cognitive function and his ingenuity in creating new measures for particular deficit areas" (p. 67). They further state, "It has been necessary to modify many original test measures to facilitate the collec-

tion of data about individual cognitive strategies . . . . Most of the modifications involved techniques of data collection rather than changes in the test procedures themselves" (p. 68). They note that such an approach allows one to calculate standard scores in the standard manner, while also gathering additional information. They do indicate, however, that "other procedural modifications involve adding new components to published tests so that the functions of interest are measured more comprehensively" (p. 69).

According to the description of these authors, the process approach shares the flexibility and individual tailoring that characterize Lezak's method, and as such it is prone to many of the same criticisms. Another point of similarity is the paucity of scientific research on validity, especially for such batteries as a whole (rather than for one or another test or procedure that might be included in one or another practitioner's battery). This limited research grounding is exemplified by Kaplan et al.'s (102) manual describing their modified procedures for the administration and interpretation of the WAIS–R. In the last chapter of the manual, the authors encourage investigators to study the clinical observations they have presented. They also discuss the need to develop normative data on the changes they have made to the original WAIS-R. They note that some of problems in test performance they present as possible indicators of brain dysfunction may occur occasionally with normal individuals, and they then state that "it is important for future research to provide normative data for the varieties of error types described in the manual. (p. 107). They note that research is also needed on the reliability of test scores and observations, and on the validity of the interpretations of testing performance they have outlined.

Major publications on tests and measurement, such as Anastasi's (103) text and the *Standards for Educational and Psychological Testing* (101), describe such steps as obtaining normative data and appraising reliability as very basic, preliminary stages in test development. In fact, these are often considered prepublication requirements, not something to find out about later, perhaps after many serious, incorrect decisions have been made. For example, if a test has significant problems with reliability, it will very likely lead to frequent errors, and a major overhaul, if feasible, may well be needed.

None of the foregoing discussion is meant to denigrate Dr. Kaplan and her colleagues, or their major contributions to the field. Although the process approach may be clinically warranted, it remains mainly in an experimental and yet-to-be-validated stage of development. Given the limitations described, its use in the forensic context seems highly questionable.

HEAD INJURY

Overview and Definition

This discussion deals mainly with mild head injury. There is no universally accepted definition for mild head injury, and criteria have sometimes differed considerably. Common definitions, however, limit loss of consciousness (LOC) to about 20 minutes and post-traumatic amnesia (PTA) to about 24 hours. Mild head injury has also been defined as a score of 13–15 on the Glasgow Coma Scale (104) at some point in time following the event, such as when the person is first seen at the hospital (despite the variation in times between injury and first assessment).

Whether or not PTA is preceded by LOC, individuals often describe the end of PTA as when they awoke. Of course, if a person has no memory of prior events for some time period, he or she might well conclude that he or she had been unconscious. In some circumstances, other individuals who were with the injured party can confirm or deny the subjective impression of LOC. In other situations there are no witnesses, or witnesses arrive after the person has cleared, and it may never be possible to determine what portion of this unremembered period of time, if any, was spent unconscious. All of this affects efforts to appraise injury severity. According to most definitions, the maximal periods of time at which head injuries exceed boundaries for classification at lower levels of severity are much shorter for LOC than PTA.

Even if an individual falls within the previously noted parameters for mild head injury, complications can shift the classification upward. For example, if CT or magnetic resonance imaging (MRI) demonstrates intracerebral bleeding, the designation of mild head injury becomes questionable (105). However, there is disagreement about how skull fractures, by themselves, should alter classification. For example, in an otherwise mild head injury, many would not change the classification with a basilar fracture, and some would not do so even with a depressed fracture (104, 105).

As may be evident from this discussion, the division of head injuries into such categories as mild, moderate, and severe, is somewhat arbitrary. However, many injuries clearly fall into one or another category, and the purpose of constructing explicit definitions is so that when conducting or analyzing research, one can determine just what type of injury is involved. It then becomes possible to compare an injured individual to others with like injuries in order to formulate judgments about such matters as likely course and outcome.

It can also be asked at what point none of the categories apply and rather the individual did not experience a head (brain) injury. Many definitions of mild head injury specify outer limits but are silent on minimal requirements. First, it is important to differentiate between *head* and *brain* injuries. Obviously, individuals can suffer injuries to the face or head without suffering brain injuries. Second, it is crucial to consider causal mechanisms. In particular, a distinction must be made between events, such as blows to the head, that can generate significant acceleration/deceleration forces, and other processes that can cause brain injury, such as diseases or slow crushing injuries. Most of the discussion in this section, and many courtroom cases, involve acceleration/

deceleration injuries, and the classification systems discussed here refer only to these types of events.

Almost all definitions of mild head injury require, at minimum, some *alteration* in consciousness. This may be something less than frank LOC, and rather the individual may be stunned or dazed. Distinctions can be difficult because emotional reactions to accidents can cause mental alterations, such as dissociative states, and other mechanisms, such as hyperventilation, can cause lightheadedness. Rather, one is referring to an alteration in consciousness secondary to a physically caused disruption in brain functioning. These individuals often look stunned and are obviously confused, having difficulty remembering events from moment to moment (their being in the midst of PTA). A distinction also needs to be made between such symptoms of head trauma, which usually have an immediate onset, and the possible effects of medications that may be administered shortly after the accident. Also, given the association between substance abuse and accidents, alterations in consciousness may merely or mainly reflect the effects of these agents. Toxic screens or statements by the injured party or observers may help to clarify the issue. Finally, although it is unusual, some individuals are lucid initially and then show a rapid or gradual onset of neurologic symptoms, often because of intra- or extracerebral bleeding.

If there is no alteration in consciousness (and in the absence of secondary complications), then there are usually strong grounds to conclude that the individual did not experience a clinically relevant brain event. Information about LOC and PTA is often available, although it may require some digging. Ambulance run sheets and initial statements to police, the rescue squad, and ER personnel can be useful. For example, an individual may have told the EMT and the ER nurse that he or she experienced no LOC. Such information is usually given in the context of immediate medical concerns, well before a lawsuit may have come to the forefront, and may contradict statements given months or years later. Witnesses may also be able to provide critical information. For example, a witness may report that the individual engaged in a series of coherent actions immediately following the accident (e.g., called the police, provided directions to the location, and exchanged information with the other driver). Statements to the insurance company, items on accident forms, and deposition responses can also be informative. For example, on deposition, the plaintiff may give a very detailed description (which may be corroborated by others) of the events before, during, and after the accident.

Finally, a question that often arises in legal cases is whether an individual must hit his or her head against an object in order to suffer a brain injury. For example, in some cases, claims of brain damage arise from low-impact car accidents in which the person is restrained and does not strike his or her head. Complete coverage of this issue is not possible, but a few basic points can be made.

There is no doubt that brain injury can occur without the head striking an object. For example, brain damage can result from rapid and repeated shaking of babies. In one line of experimental studies, animals were subjected to acceleration/deceleration forces under conditions in which their heads were not allowed to strike objects. Given sufficient forces, brain injuries resulted (106–108). The level of forces required to injure the brain or alter brain functions must be considered, however. For example, in Ommaya and Gennarelli's research, absent rotational forces, peak positive accelerations of over 1000 times the force of gravity (i.e. 1000 g's) did not necessarily produce concussions.

There are complications in applying these types of animal studies to human events. Although it is clear that considerably lower forces may be sufficient to cause brain injury in humans (108), one certainly is not talking about fender-benders. Some claims of brain damage are ludicrous given the accident at issue, which may have involved forces to the head that were no greater than those resulting from a jump off a 6-inch ledge.

Research and Commentary on Mild Head Injury

In the early 1980s, some studies on mild head injury suggested that serious, lasting deficits were common. Many of these persisting problems were classified under the rubric of post-concussion syndrome (PCS). Although descriptions of PCS often differ somewhat, one commonly finds reference to various cognitive, emotional, and medical complaints or symptoms. For example, many lists include such symptoms as decreased attention and concentration, memory problems, reduced speed or efficiency of mental operations, irritability, fatigability, dizziness, and hypersensitivity to noise and light.

These earlier studies were problematic in a number of ways, perhaps most importantly because they included a disproportionate number of individuals who tend to do poorly on neuropsychological tests even absent a head injury, such as those who are socially disadvantaged or less well educated. Also, head injuries are frequently associated with alcohol problems and other prior difficulties, including psychiatric and learning problems (109). Consequently, studies of mild head injury should include a carefully matched control group.

In the last decade, studies with proper control groups suggest that a substantial number of individuals do experience difficulties in the initial period following a mild head injury. However, within about 1–3 months, most of these individuals show good recovery and are often statistically indistinguishable from matched controls on neuropsychological tests (109–113).

This same research also shows that some individuals have more persistent problems or complaints. Documentation is often limited to subjective reports of symptoms, which themselves may involve only isolated problems, such as headaches. Estimates of the frequency of persistent problems differ considerably, and as Dikmen and Levin (109) note, "There are no reliable estimates of late symptom rates" (p. 31). There is, however, agreement among many authors that any difficulties that may persist, at least those based on brain factors, are usually subtle or minor (109, 110, 114–116). Of course, with certain activities or occupations (e.g., air traffic controller), subtle problems may be a serious matter.

The etiology of persistent complaints has been vigorously argued (109, 117–119), and it is very unlikely that a single explanation will cover all cases. In the sections that follow, six proposed causes or explanations are reviewed: organic factors, psychiatric factors, malingering/litigation, base rates, iatrogenic disorder, and preexisting problems.

ORGANIC/BRAIN CAUSES

Some individuals presumed to have experienced a mild head injury have had more serious or complicated injuries (105, 109). Computed tomography (CT) or MRI, especially if obtained around the time of injury, may detect structural abnormalities that are otherwise missed. Williams et al. (105) found that in comparison to individuals with uncomplicated mild head injury, almost all of whom were reported to show good recovery, about 25% of those with complicated injuries did not achieve such positive outcomes. For some individuals, such as those who abuse alcohol, traumatic injury is superimposed on an already vulnerable or damaged brain. However, the topic of vulnerability is beyond the scope of this chapter, and given the limited research, most conclusions about such matters are speculative.

FUNCTIONAL FACTORS

One of the most common explanations for persisting symptoms is the preexistence or development of psychiatric reactions or disorder (109, 114, 120–122). For example, individuals with long-standing hypochondriacal tendencies may misinterpret benign physical sensations or intellectual shortcomings as indicative of brain damage. Such a person may be convinced that forgetting a few items at the shopping mall demonstrates a serious loss of capacity. Alternatively, as noted earlier, affective states and mood disorder can impede performance on neuropsychological tests and can also lead to the exaggeration of cognitive difficulties. In fact, problems attributed to brain damage, such as impaired attention and concentration, decreased motivation, and reduced speed of mental operations, may overlap completely with depressive symptomatology.

MALINGERING/LITIGATION

Much literature acknowledges the potential role of malingering and litigation in the perpetuation of symptoms or complaints (109, 121, 123, 124). Estimates of frequency vary widely, and it is hard to imagine how the issue can be resolved when there is often no way to determine with certainty whether an individual is or is not malingering.

Some clinicians believe that lay individuals are uninformed about the symptoms of mild head injury. However, a number of studies in which individuals are asked to simulate the self-reports of persons with mild head injury or to describe such symptoms show that lay persons often achieve a reasonable approximation (119, 124). (For further information on malingering and methods of detection, see Faust [125] and Rogers [126].)

BASE RATES

Recent studies suggest that many of the symptoms reported after mild head injury occur with similar frequency among the general population. As such, if one looks for symptoms of mild head injury, one often will be able to find some confirming evidence, even if the head injury itself has caused no deficits. The obvious result can be a false-positive diagnosis of brain damage or PCS. Also, researchers may attribute or overattribute observed problems to head injury if they are unaware of the frequency with which such problems occur among the general population. Other research (119) suggests that retrospective accounts or recollections of preinjury problems may underestimate their frequency and thereby lead to false conclusions about whether, or the extent to which, a change in functioning has occurred. All of this implies that a thorough review of background records may well turn up evidence that the problems blamed on the head injury predated the event.

Gouvier et al. (127) obtained self-reports and relatives' reports of various problems among a group of college graduates and compared the results to those obtained in prior studies examining patients with head injuries that produced PTA of 24 hours or more. In comparing self-reports across these presumably normal college students and subjects with head injuries, no significant differences were found on items addressing memory problems, problems becoming interested in things, loss of temper, irritability, fatigue, or impatience. The only significant differences were obtained on items addressing concentration, difficulties with reading, and restlessness. In comparing relatives' reports, no significant differences were found on items assessing loss of temper, visual problems, irritability, restlessness, fatigue, and impatience. In fact, only one significant difference was found — this on an item addressing difficulties remembering things.

The frequency with which a number of these symptoms were reported for presumably normal individuals is also impressive. For example, relatives' reports for the college students showed the following rates of endorsement for these items: "often impatient" — 49%; "often irritable" — 43%. Endorsement rates for other items included: "often loses temper" — 38%; "often restless" — 33%; and "tires easily" — 35%. On self-report, about one-third of these college students endorsed the items, "difficulty becoming interested" and "often loses temper." Almost 28% indicated that they tire easily, and over 40% indicated that they are often impatient. Thus, at least among this group of college students, the base rates for a number of these complaints were considerable, and many of the students described themselves, or were described by relatives, as displaying

more than one such "symptom." Clinicians may interpret complaints about even a few of these "symptoms" as strong evidence of PCS. Additional studies by Gouvier et al. (128), Mittenberg et al. (119), and Wong et al. (124) also show that symptoms and complaints that have been associated with mild head injury seem to be common among normal individuals.

IATROGENIC DISORDER/EXPECTATION

A number of authors suggest that persistent problems following head injury can be caused by iatrogenic factors (118, 119, 129). Mittenberg et al. (119) describe individuals who had *not* experienced a head injury rate the frequency with which they had *previously* experienced PCS-like symptoms, such as forgetfulness, difficulties concentrating, and negative emotional states. These researchers then had individuals who *had* experienced head injury do the same thing. The reader might keep in mind research suggesting that, if anything, those who experience head injuries have a greater prevalence of preexisting problems than the general population. Mittenberg et al. found that the head-injured group provided significantly lower estimates of prior problems than the noninjured group. They interpret these results to mean that head-injured individuals are susceptible to forming unrealistically positive beliefs about their past functioning, and thus to reinterpreting preexisting difficulties as new problems caused by the accident.

Mittenberg et al. also note that lay individuals often seem to have a fairly good idea about symptoms that might follow from a head injury. They further emphasize that supposed symptoms of mild head injury are very common among the general population. They discuss the process by which individuals may come to reinterpret prior failings as new symptoms stemming from head injury. They indicate that medical students often reinterpret benign and common bodily experiences as signs of serious disorder, and observe that "like medical students' disease, PCS symptoms occur frequently in the normal population" (p. 203). They suggest that the cause of both "syndromes" may revolve around expectancy. It should also be clear that problems with overdiagnosis, discussed previously, could contribute to a plaintiff's false beliefs about abnormality.

PREEXISTING DIFFICULTIES

Again, many factors can lower scores on neuropsychological tests. Head-injured individuals are also not representative of the population as a whole and have a greater frequency of preexisting difficulties. One such example is a markedly increased frequency of alcohol problems, which might be expected given the association between car accidents, head injuries, and alcohol abuse.

In cases involving alcohol abuse, it may be claimed, correctly or not, that it is not the alcohol use, or the alcohol use alone, that accounts for cognitive difficulties, and rather that the head injury makes the major contribution. Alterman et al. (130) found that a group of diagnosed alcoholics did show difficulties on certain neuropsychological tests, but that among the alcoholic group, no differences in test performance were obtained between those with and without a history of mild head injury. Alterman et al. interpret their results as showing that difficulties seen on testing were a product of prior alcohol intake, not mild head trauma.

CONCLUSION

The existing state of scientific knowledge on the neuropsychological assessment of people with subtle cognitive or behavioral problems warrants caution in making diagnoses based primarily on test results. Comprehensive multimodal clinical assessment may yield more credible opinions, but it must be subject to reasonable limits on causal attribution and prediction of the future as outlined in this chapter.

References

1. Faust D. Neuropsychological (brain damage) assessment. In: Ziskin J, Coping with psychiatric and psychological testimony, ed. 5, vols. 1–3, Los Angeles: Law & Psychology Press, 1995.
2. Faust D, Ziskin J, Hiers JB, Jr. Brain damage claims: coping with neuropsychological evidence, vols. 1 & 2. Los Angeles, CA: Law and Psychology Press, 1991.
3. Guilmette TJ, Faust D, Hart K, Arkes HR. A national survey of psychologists who offer neuropsychological services. Arch Clin Neuropsychol 1990;5:373–392.
4. Putnam SH, DeLuca JW. The TCN professional practice survey: Part II: An analysis of the fees of neuropsychologists by practice demographics. Clin Neuropsychol 1991;5:103–124.
5. Fogel BS, Faust D. Neurologic assessment, neurodiagnostic tests, and neuropsychology in medical psychiatry. In: Stoudemire A, Fogel BS, eds. Psychiatric care of the medical patient. New York: Oxford University Press, 1993:367–413.
6. Reports of the INS-Division 40 Task Force on Education, Accreditation, and Credentialing. Clin Neuropsychol 1987;1:29–34.
7. Ziskin J, & Faust D. Coping with psychiatric and psychological testimony, 4th ed. vols. 1–3. Los Angeles: Law & Psychology Press, 1988.
8. Faust D, Guilmette TJ, Hart K, Arkes HR, Fishburne FJ, Davey L. Neuropsychologists' training, experience, and judgment accuracy. Arch Clin Neuropsychol 1988;3:145–163.
9. Goldberg LR. The effectiveness of clinicians' judgments: The diagnosis of organic brain damage from the Bender-Gestalt Test. J Consult Clin Psychol, 1959;23:28–33.
10. Lacks PB, Newport K. A comparison of scoring systems and level of scorer experience on the Bender-Gestalt Test. J Pers Assess 1980;44: 351–357.
11. Leli DA, Filskov SB. Clinical-actuarial detection and description of brain impairment with the W-B form 1. J Clin Psychol 1981;37: 623–629.
12. Leli DA, Filskov SB. Clinical detection of intellectual deterioration associated with brain damage. J Clin Psychol 1984;40:1435–1441.
13. Wedding D. Clinical and statistical prediction in neuropsychology. Clin Neuropsychol 1983;5:49–55.
14. Wedding D, & Faust D. Clinical judgment and decision making in neuropsychology. Arch Clin Neuropsychol 1989;4:233–265.
15. Reitan RM. Theoretical and methodological bases of the Halstead-Reitan Neuropsychological Battery. In: Grant G, Adams KM, eds., Neuropsychological assessment of neuropsychiatric disorders. New York: Oxford University Press, 1986:3–29.
16. Boake C, Adams RL. Clinical utility of the Background Interference Procedure for the Bender-Gestalt Test. J Clin Psychol 1982;38: 627–631.
17. Klesges RC, Fisher L, Pheley A, Boschee P, Vasey M. A major validational study of the Halstead-Reitan in the prediction of CAT-scan assessed brain damage in adults. Int J Clin Neuropsychol 1984;6:29–34.
18. Mutchnick MG, Ross LK, Long CJ. Decision strategies for cerebral dysfunction IV: determination of cerebral dysfunction. Arch Clin Neuropsychol 1991;6:259–270.
19. Sherer M, Scott JG, Parsons OA, Adams RL. Relative sensitivity of the WAIS-R subtests and selected HRNB measures to the effects of brain damage. Arch Clin Neuropsychol 1994;9:427–436.
20. Sweet JJ, Osmon DC, Rozensky RH, Tovian SM. Comparison of the decision-tree and standard methods of the Luria-Nebraska neuropsychological battery. J Consult Clin Psychol 1985;53:185–188.
21. Golden CJ. Forensic neuropsychology: Introduction and overview. In: Golden CJ, Strider MA, eds. Forensic neuropsychology. New York: Plenum Press, 1986:1–47.
22. Baird AD, Adams KM, Ausman JI, Diaz FG. Medical, neuropsychological, and quality-of-life correlates of cerebrovascular disease. Rehabilitation Psychology 1985;30:145–155.
23. Baird AD, Brown GG, Adams KM, et al. Neuropsychological deficits and real-world dysfunction in cerebral revascularization candidates. J Clin Exp Neuropsychol 1987;9:407–422.
24. Binder LM, & Thompson LL. The ethics code and neuropsychological assessment practices. Arch Clin Neuropsychol 1995;10:27–46.
25. Costa L. Clinical neuropsychology: a discipline in evolution. J Clin Neuropsychol 1983;5:1–11.
26. Dodrill CB, Clemmons D. Use of neuropsychological tests to identify high school students with epilepsy who later demonstrate inadequate performances in life. J Consult Clin Psychol 1984;52:520–527.
27. Donovan DM, Kivlahan DR, Walker RD. Clinical limitations of neuropsychological testing in predicting treatment outcome among alcoholics. Alcohol Clin Exp Res 1984;8:470–475.
28. Dunn EJ, Searight HR, Grisso T, Margolis RB, Gibbons JL. The relation of the Halstead-Reitan Neuropsychological Battery to functional daily living skills in geriatric patients. Arch Clin Neuropsychol 1990;5:103–117.
29. Heaton RK, Pendleton MG. Use of neuropsychological tests to predict adult patients' everyday functioning. J Consult Clin Psychol 1981;49:807–821.
30. Osmon DC. The use of test batteries in clinical neuropsychology. In CJ Golden, P. Vicente eds. Foundations of Clinical Neuropsychology, New York: Plenum Press, 1983:113–141.
31. Pfeffer RI, Kurosaki TT, Harrah CH Jr., Chance JM, Filos S. Measurement of functional activities in older adults in the community. J Gerontol 1982;37:323–329.
32. Puente AE. The status of clinical neuropsychology. Arch Clin Neuropsychol 1992;7:297–312.
33. Shelton MD, Parsons OA. Alcoholics' self-assessment of their neuropsychological functioning in everyday life. J Clin Psychol 1987;43:395–403.
34. Skurla E, Rogers JC, Sunderland T. Direct assessment of activities of daily living in Alzheimer's Disease. A controlled study. J Am Geriatr Soc 1988;36:97–103.
35. Tupper DE, Cicerone KD, eds. The neuropsychology of everyday life: assessment and basic competencies. Boston: Kluwer Academic Publishers, 1990.
36. Gass CS, Russell EW, Hamilton RA. Accuracy of MMPI-based inferences regarding memory and concentration in closed-head-trauma patients. Psychological Assessment: A Journal of Consulting and Clinical Psychology 1990;2:175–178.
37. Larrabee GJ, West RL, Crook TH. The association of memory

complaint with computer-simulated everyday memory performance. J Clin Exp Neuropsychol 1991;13:466–478.

38. Prigatano GP, Altman IM, O'Brien KP. Behavioral limitations that traumatic-brain-injured patients tend to underestimate. Clin Neuropsychol 1990;4:163–176.

39. Ryan JJ, & Lewis CV. Comparison of normal controls and recently detoxified alcoholics on the Wechsler Memory Scale-Revised. Clin Neuropsychol 1988;2:173–180.

40. Weissman HN. Distortions and deceptions in self presentation: effects of protracted litigation in personal injury cases. Behavioral Sciences & the Law, 1990;8:67–74.

41. Otto MW, Bruder GE, Fava M, Delis DC, Quitkin FM, Rosenbaum JF. Norms for depressed patients for the California Verbal Learning Test: Associations with depression severity and self-report of cognitive difficulties. Arch Clin Neuropsychol 1994;9:81–88.

42. McGlynn SM, Schacter DL. Unawareness of deficits in neuropsychological syndromes. J Clin Exp Neuropsychol 1989;11:143–205.

43. Parsons OA. Determinants of cognitive deficits in alcoholics: The search continues. Clin Neuropsychol 1994;8:39–58.

44. Buckelew SP, Hannay HJ. Relationships among anxiety, defensiveness, sex, task difficulty, and performance on various neuropsychological tasks. Percept Mot Skills 1986;63:711–718.

45. Dean RS, Gray JW, Seretny ML. Cognitive aspects of schizophrenia and primary affective depression. Int J Clin Neuropsychol 1987a;9:33–36.

46. Deptula D, Manevitz A, Yozawitz A. Asymmetry of recall in depression. J Clin Exp Neuropsychol 1991;13:854–870.

47. Fogel BS, Sparadeo FR. Single case study: Focal cognitive deficits accentuated by depression. J Nerv Ment Dis 1985;173:120–124.

48. Hart RP, Kwentus JA, Wade JB, Hamer RM. Digit Symbol performance in mild dementia and depression. J Consult Clin Psychol 1987;55:236–238.

49. King DA, Caine ED, Cox C. Influence of depression and age on selected cognitive functions. Clin Neuropsychol 1993;7:443–453.

50. Lezak MD. Neuropsychological assessment, 2nd, ed. New York: Oxford University Press, 1983.

51. Newman PJ, Sweet JJ. The effects of clinical depression on the Luria-Nebraska Neuropsychological Battery. Int J Clin Neuropsychol 1986;8:109–114.

52. Sackeim HA, Freeman J, McElhiney M, Coleman E, Prudic J, Devanand DP. Effects of major depression on estimates of intelligence. J Clin Exp Neuropsychol 1992;14:268–288.

53. Grant I. Alcohol and the brain: neuropsychological correlates. J Consult Clin Psychol 1987;55:310–324.

54. Benton A. Clinical neuropsychology: 1960-1990. J Clin Exp Neuropsychol 1992;14:407–417.

55. Lambert NM. Adolescent outcomes for hyperactive children. Am Psychol 1988;43:786–799.

56. McCue PM, Shelly C, Goldstein G. Intellectual, academic and neuropsychological performance levels in learning disabled adults. Journal of Learning Disabilities, 1986;19:233–236.

57. Rourke BP, Young GC, Strang JD, Russell DL. Adult outcomes of childhood central processing deficiencies. In: Grant I & Adams KM, eds. Neuropsychological assessment of neuropsychiatric disorders, New York: Oxford University Press, 1986:244–267.

58. Spreen O. Prognosis of learning disability. J Consult Clin Psychol 1988;56:836–842.

59. American Psychiatric Association. Diagnostic and statistical manual of mental disorders. 4th ed. Washington, D.C., 1994.

60. Boll TJ. Developing issues in clinical neuropsychology. J Clin Exp Neuropsychol 1985;7:473–485.

61. Bolter J, Gouvier W, Veneklasen J, Long CJ. Using demographic information to predict premorbid IQ: A test of clinical validity with head trauma patients. Clin Neuropsychol 1982;4:171–174.

62. Goldstein FC, Gary HE Jr, Levin HS. Assessment of the accuracy of regression equations proposed for estimating premorbid intellectual functioning on the Wechsler Adult Intelligence Scale. J Clin Exp Neuropsychol 1986;8:405–412.

63. Kareken DA, Williams JM. Human judgment and estimation of premorbid intellectual function. Psychological Assessment 1994;6:83–91.

64. Klesges RC, Fisher L, Vasey M, Pheley A. Predicting adult premorbid functioning levels: Another look. Int J Clin Neuropsychol 1985;7:1–3.

65. Reynolds CR, Kaufman AS. Clinical assessment of children's intelligence with the Wechsler Scales. In: Wolman BB, ed. Handbook of intelligence, New York: John Wiley and Sons 1985:601–661.

66. Silverstein AB. Accuracy of estimates of premorbid intelligence based on demographic variables. J Clin Psychol 1987;43:493–495.

67. Wiens AN, Bryan JE, Crossen JR. Estimating WAIS-R FSIQ from the National Adult Reading Test – Revised in normal subjects. Clin Neuropsychol 1993;7:70–84.

68. Lezak MD. Neuropsychological assessment, 3rd. ed. New York, NY: Oxford University Press, 1995:29–49.

69. Mortensen EL, Gade A, Reinisch JM. A critical note on Lezak's "best performance method" in clinical neuropsychology. J Clin Exp Neuropsychol 1991;13:361–371.

70. Boll TJ. The Halstead-Reitan Neuropsychology Battery. In SB Filskov, TJ Boll eds., Handbook of Clinical Neuropsychology New York: John Wiley & Sons, 1981;577–607.

71. Reitan RM, & Wolfson D. The Halstead-Reitan neuropsychological battery. Theory and clinical interpretation (2nd ed.). Tucson, AZ: Neuropsychology Press, 1993.

72. Heaton RK, Grant I, Matthews CG. Comprehensive norms for an expanded Halstead-Reitan battery. Odessa, Florida: Psychological Assesment Resources, 1991.

73. Snow WG. Standardization of test administration and scoring criteria: some shortcomings of current practice with the Halstead-Reitan Test Battery. Clin Neuropsychol 1987;1:250–262.

74. Fromm-Auch D, Yeudall LT. Normative data for the Halstead-Reitan Neuropsychological Tests. J Clin Neuropsychol 1983;5:221–238.

75. Bornstein RA. Classification rates obtained with "standard" cut-off scores on selected neuropsychological measures. J Clin Exp Neuropsychol 1986;8:413–420.

76. Bornstein RA, Paniak CG, O'Brien W. Preliminary data on classification of normal and brain-damaged elderly subjects. The Clin Neuropsychol 1987;1:315–323.

77. Chavez EL, Schwartz MM, Brandon A. Effects of sex of subject and method of block presentation on the Tactile Performance Test. J Consult Clin Psychol 1982;50:600–601.

78. Gordon NG, O'Dell JW, Bozeman N. Variation in neuropsychological performance as a function of sex. J Psychol 1981;109:127–131.

79. Long CJ, Klein K. Decision strategies in neuropsychology II: determination of age effects on neuropsychological performance. Arch Clin Neuropsychol 1990;5:335-345.

80. Naugle RI, Cullum CM, Bigler ED. Evaluation of intellectual and memory function among dementia patients who were intellectually superior. The Clinical Neuropsychologist, 1990;4:355–374.

81. Steinmeyer CH. A meta-analysis of Halstead-Reitan test performances of non-brain damaged subjects. Arch Clin Neuropsychol 1986;1:301–307.

82. Heaton RK, Grant I, Matthews CG. Differences in neuropsychological test performance associated with age, education, and sex. In: Grant I, Adams KM, eds. Neuropsychological Assessment of neuropsychiatric disorders. New York: Oxford University Press, 1986:100–120.

83. Hannay HJ. Some issues and concerns in neuropsychological research: an introduction. In: Hannay HJ, ed. Experimental Techniques in human neuropsychology. New York: Oxford University Press, 1986:3–14.

84. Heilman KM, Valenstein E, 2nd. eds. Clinical neuropsychology, 2nd ed. New York: Oxford University Press, 1985.

85. Bond JA, & Buchtel HA. Comparison of the Wisconsin Card Sorting Test and the Halstead Category Test. J Clin Psychol 1984;40:1251–1255.

86. Milberg WP, Hebben N, Kaplan E. The Boston process approach to neuropsychological assessment. In: Grant I, Adams KM, eds. Neuropsychological assessment of neuropsychiatric disorders. New York: Oxford University Press, 1986:65-86.

87. Golden CJ, Purisch AD, Hammeke TA. Manual for the Luria-Nebraska neuropsychological battery: forms I and II. Los Angeles: Western Psychological Services, 1985.

88. Hermann BP, & Melyn M. Identification of neuropsychological deficits in epilepsy using the Luria-Nebraska Neuropsychological Battery: a replication attempt. J Clin Exp Neuropsychol 1985;7: 305–313.

89. Stanley B, Howe JG. Identification of Multiple Sclerosis using double discrimination scales derived from the Luria-Nebraska Neuropsychological Battery: an attempt at cross-validation. J Consult Clin Psychol 1983;51:420–423.

90. Mittenberg W, Kasprisin A. Localization and diagnosis in aphasia with the Luria-Nebraska Neuropsychological Battery. J Consult Clin Psychol 1985;53:386–392.

91. Larrabee GJ, Kane RL, Schuck JR, Francis DJ. Construct validity of various memory testing procedures. J Clin Exp Neuropsychol 1985;7:239–250.

92. Reynolds CR. Determining statistically reliable strengths and weaknesses in the performance of single individuals on the Luria Nebraska Neuropsychological Battery. J Consult Clin Psychol 1982;50: 525–529.

93. Adams RL. Review of the Luria-Nebraska Neuropsychological Battery. In: Mitchell JV Jr, ed. The ninth mental measurements yearbook. Lincoln, NE: University of Nebraska Press, 1985:878-881.

94. Mapou RL. Testing to detect brain damage: An alternative to what may no longer be useful. J Clin Exp Neuropsychol 1988;10:271–278.

95. Spiers PA. Have they come to praise Luria or to bury him?: The Luria-Nebraska controversy. J Consult Clin Psychol 1981;49: 331–341.

96. McCaffrey RJ, Malloy PF, Brief DJ. Internship opportunities in clinical neuropsychology emphasizing recent INS training certificate. Professional Psychology: Research and Practice, 1985;16:236–252.

97. Lezak MD. An individualized approach to neuropsychological assessment. In: Logue PE, Schear JM, eds. Clinical neuropsychology: a multidisciplinary approach. Springfield, IL: Charles C Thomas, 1984:29–49.

98. Russell EW. Theory and development of pattern analysis methods related to the Halstead-Reitan Battery. In: Logue PE, Schear JM, eds. Clinical neuropsychology. A multidisciplinary approach. Springfield, Illinois: Charles C Thomas, 1984:50–98.

99. Hartman DE. Book review [Understanding brain damage: A primer of neuropsychological evaluation, Walsh KM. New York: Churchill Livingstone, 1985]. Arch Clin Neuropsychol 1986;1:31–33.

100. Costa L. Clinical neuropsychology: problems and prospects. The Clinical Neuropsychologist 1988;2:3–11.

101. American Psychological Association. Standards for educational and psychological testing. Washington, DC, 1988.

102. Alexander MP. Traumatic brain injury. In. Benson DF, Blumer D, eds. Psychiatric aspects of neurological disease, vol. 2. New York: Grune & Stratton, 1982.

103. Kaplan E, Fein D, Morris R, Delis DC. Manual for the WAIS-R NI (WAIS-R as a neuropsychological instrument). New York: The Psychological Corporation, 1991.

104. Anastasi A. Psychological Testing 6th ed. New York: Macmillan, 1988.

105. Jennett B, Teasdale G. Management of head injuries. Philadelphia: FA Davis Company.

106. Williams DH, Levin HS, Eisenberg HM. Mild head injury classification. Neurosurgery 1990;27:422–428.

107. Gennarelli TA, Thibault LE, Adams JH, Graham DI, Thompson CJ, Marcincin RP. Diffuse axonal injury and traumatic coma in the primate. Ann Neurol 1982;12:564–574.

108. Ommaya AK, Gennarelli TA. Cerebral concussion and traumatic unconsciousness. Brain 1974;97:633–654.

109. Thibault L, Gennerelli T, & Margulies S. Animal, physical, and analytic models for use in the development of improved head injury critria (Report Number: DOT HS 807 481; Date: 3-15-89). National Highway Traffic Safety Administration. Available from the National Technical Information Service, Springfield, VA 22161.

110. Dikmen SS, Levin HS. Methodological issues in the study of mild head injury. Journal of head trauma rehabilitation 1993;8:30–37.

111. Alves W, Macciocchi SN, Barth JT. Postconcussive symptoms after uncomplicated mild head injury. J of head trauma rehabilitation 1993;8:48–59.

112. Gentilini M, Nichelli P, Schoenhuber R, et al. Neuropsychological evaluation of mild head injury. Journal of Neurology, Neurosurgery, and Psychiatry 1985;48:137–140.

113. Levin HS, Mattis S, Ruff RM, et al. Neurobehavioral outcome following minor head injury: a three-center study. J Neurosurg 1987;66:234–243.

114. Levin HS, Eisenberg HM, Benton AL, eds. Mild head injury. New York: Oxford University Press.

115. Dikmen SS, Temkin N, Armsden G. Neuropsychological recovery: relationship to psychosocial functioning and postconcussional complaints. In: Levin HS, Eisenberg HM, Benton AL, eds. Mild head injury. New York: Oxford University Press, 1989:229-241.

116. Gronwall D. Cumulative and persisting effects of concussion on attention and cognition. In: Levin HS, Eisenberg HM, Benton AL, eds. Mild head injury. New York: Oxford University Press.

117. Ruff RM, Levin HS, Mattis S, et al. Recovery of memory after mild head injury: A three-center study. In: Levin HS, Eisenberg HM, Benton AL, eds. Mild head injury. New York: Oxford University Press 1989:176–188.

118. Binder LM. Persisting symptoms after mild head injury: A review of the postconcussive syndrome. J Clin Exp Neuropsychol 1986;8: 323–346.

119. Colohan ART, Dacey RG Jr, Alves WM, Rimel RW, Jane JA. Neurologic and neurosurgical implications of mild head injury. Journal of Head Trauma Rehabilitation 1986;1:13–21.

120. Mittenberg W, DiGiulio DV, Perrin S, & Bass AE. Symptoms following mild head injury: expectation as aetiology. J Neurol Neurosurg Psychiatry 1992;55:200–204.

121. Alexander MP. Neuropsychiatric correlates of persistent postconcussive syndrome. Journal of Head Trauma Rehabilitation 1992;7: 60–69.

122. Capruso DX, Levin HS. Cognitive impairment following closed head injury. Neurol Clin 1992;10:879–893.

123. Binder LM. Malingering following minor head trauma. Clin Neuropsychol 1990;4:25–36.

124. Wong JL, Regennitter RP, Barrios F. Base rate and simulated symptoms of mild head injury among normals. Arch Clin Neuropsychol 1994;9:411–425.

125. Faust D. The detection of deception. Neurol Clin 1995;13:255–265.

126. Rogers R, ed. Clinical assessment of malingering and deception. New York: Guilford Press, 1988.

127. Gouvier WD, Uddo-Crane M, Brown LM. Base rates for postconcussional symptoms. Arch Clin Neuropsychol 1988;3:273–278.

128. Gouvier WD, Cubic B, Jones G, Brantley P, Cutlip Q. Postconcussion symptoms and daily stress in normal and head-injured college populations. Arch Clin Neuropsychol 1992;7:193–211.

129. Modlin HC, Sargent J. Neuropsychological assessment in a head injury case. Bull Menninger Clin 1986;50:50–57.

130. Alterman AI, Goldstein G, Shelly C, Bober B, Tarter RE. The impact of mild head injury on neuropsychological capacity in chronic alcoholics. Int J Neurosci 1985;28:155–162.

131. Ziskin J. Coping with psychiatric and psychological testimony, 5th ed, vols. 1–3. Los Angeles: Law and Psychology Press, 1995.

43

NEUROPSYCHIATRY OF DISABILITY AND REHABILITATION

Randall T. Schapiro and Tony M. Wong

The neuropsychiatry of disability and rehabilitation requires an understanding of certain terms. The World Health Organization (WHO) has defined an "impairment" as "caused by the underlying disorder resulting in clinical signs and symptoms" (1). "Disability" is defined as "reflecting the personal limitations imposed upon the activities of daily living (ADLs)" (1). Thus, disability revolves around ADLs: dressing, eating, toileting. "Handicap" reflects the environmental situation that limits the person with a disability from achieving an optimal social role, and it results from a combination of disability, impairment, and a number of other factors, including resources, intelligence, and psychological status (1). That is, handicap is the role of a person with a disability in society (Table 43.1).

Many people with disabilities are not handicapped, and some people with handicaps have little disability and/or impairment. The man who is quadriplegic yet totally runs his company, uses computers for assistance, and is quite independent, would not be considered handicapped, although he clearly has a disability.

Disability also refers to the medicolegal status of an individual who is unable to return to gainful employment; thus, financial compensation is awarded in accordance with the assessed level of incapacity.

Neurologists are trained to diagnose diseases of the nervous system. They should be capable of managing both the acute and long-term manifestations of neurological disease, including those of rehabilitation. Physiatrists are specialists in physical medicine and rehabilitation and provide rehabilitative services for people with diseases of many varying etiologies.

Over time, it has become clearer that diseases often present with cultural, social, and ideological influences. Early distinctions between nervous diseases and diseases of the nervous system became blurred. It was not until the 19th and 20th centuries that localized abnormalities of the nervous system could consistently be traced to abnormalities in function, with disability leading to handicap (2).

Neurologists, psychiatrists, physiatrists have all become specialized rehabilitation physicians. Each specialty has a different historical perspective, but each is interested in anatomy, physiology, and *functional* outcomes. The neurologist may emphasize impairment, but all emphasize handicap.

The scope of rehabilitation may be broad, but it relates to function, disability, and handicap. Thus, emphasis is placed on efficiency and accuracy of performance of daily living activities. Therapists work with patients to achieve this efficiency. Physical therapists, occupational therapists, speech pathologists, and nurses all work to improve the whole person. The neurorehabilitation specialists evaluate not only how a disease can be managed but also whether a person with a disability can be trained to function at a higher level of performance.

For example, to ascertain the rehabilitative capacity of a person, the clinician must know whether the person is cognitively intact to assimilate instructions and apply the rehabilitative modalities. There must be realistic goal-setting to improve the person's disability, which leads to less handicap. In addition, these goals should be placed in an appropriate framework of time. Thus, the clinical practice of neurorehabilitation is a complex, ongoing process, which involves not only coordination and cooperation within the professional interdisciplinary team, but between the patient and this team.

GENERAL CLINICAL CONSIDERATIONS

Bringing an impairment closer to its original, premorbid function is called "restorative" rehabilitation. This is what is practiced in most rehabilitation units and is particularly goal-oriented. Clearly, this is also what many patients and their families expect when initiating a course of rehabilitation. However, people with chronic neurological impairments or even progressive neurological disease may benefit from rehabilitative modalities with goals of maintaining the status quo for as long as possible (3). This is called "maintenance"

Table 43.1. The World Health Organization's Definition of Terms

Impairment—the neurological examination
Disability—the activities of daily living
Handicap—the function in society

Table 43.2. The Rehabilitation Team

Neurology
Physiatry
Psychiatry/neuropsychiatry
Clinical nursing
Physical therapy
Occupational therapy
Speech pathology
Neuropsychology/clinical psychology
Psychiatry
Social services
Clergy
Nutrition services
Therapeutic recreation
Orthotics

rehabilitation. In fact, a person's neurological impairment may worsen while his/her ability to perform a task (disability) may remain static or improve if successful rehabilitation occurs. To avoid undue disappointment and misunderstanding, it is crucial that the distinction between restorative and maintenance rehabilitation for any given patient be clarified to both the patient and the family, and definitely within the treatment team.

Cognitive rehabilitation, which has been defined as a "systematic, functionally oriented service of therapeutic cognitive activities, based on an assessment and understanding of the person's brain-behavioral deficits," (4) has been a growing practice in recent years, and its efficacy has been the subject of wide debate in the literature (5–9). The underlying, and disputable, assumption behind most cognitive remediation techniques and programs is that neuronal growth or regeneration can be actively facilitated by the exercise of the appropriate neuronal circuits. At issue, then, is whether specific cognitive rehabilitation/remediation is more effective than general rehabilitation. An important corollary is whether the specific effects of cognitive rehabilitation are generalizable. Unfortunately, part of the problem is that there has been a paucity of outcome studies examining the effectiveness of cognitive remediation programs (10). Existing reviews of research on cognitive remediation strategies are mixed at best. For example, Benedict (11), reviewing 40 studies of cognitive remediation with traumatically brain-injured patients, found that although performance on selective attention and speed of processing tasks can be enhanced with practice, direct remediation of self-regulation deficits and memory disorders was less successful. Interested practitioners might find the recently published guidelines for cognitive rehabilitation by the Head Injury Interdisciplinary Special Group of the American Congress of Rehabilitation Medicine helpful (4).

Cognitive remediation techniques might be questionable in terms of their actual efficacy, but they should not be confused with compensatory strategies, which are directed more at the level of handicap as opposed to impairment. That is, environmental and behavioral interventions are utilized to take advantage of residual areas of strength or unimpaired functions, and to compensate for the patient's impairment(s). An example of this would be the use of memory books, appointment books, electronic alarms, or other cues to help the patient with a memory disorder who is otherwise relatively cognitively unimpaired.

Many structural problems within the nervous system are amenable to pharmacological approaches. Spasticity, spasms, rigidity, some tremors, bladder/bowel dysfunction, and pain are among those most commonly managed by medical approaches.

The most important goal for a rehabilitation program is the development of a life management plan. This plan should be a blueprint that allows a person with a disability to function at the highest possible level. The plan should have input from the therapists involved in the individual's management. Many professionals are involved in the development of this overall strategy, each with a distinct and an overlapping role (Table 43.2). The physician oversees the medical process leading to the production of the blueprint. The physical therapist sets goals directing physical improvement in the function of body parts. The occupational therapist emphasizes daily living activities. The speech pathologist works with language, communication, swallowing, and cognition. Nursing reinforces all that is done by others and initiates bladder and bowel training regimens. Neuropsychologists evaluate and generate plans for improving behavior and cognitive deviations. Social workers evaluate the person's general role in society. Obviously, it is essential for all these professionals to work together to generate a rehabilitative plan for life management strategies.

Rehabilitation generally emphasizes function; dysfunction often follows destruction of anatomical structures. Clearly, anatomically specific lesions of the brain cause consistent patterns of dysfunction. Thus, lesions of the motor strip into the internal capsule cause a contralateral hemiplegia. Abnormalities of regions of the parietal and frontotemporal lobes may result in aphasia, apraxia, and agnosia. These three higher cortical functions may be the critical factors in determining a person's eventual handicap, and often complicate the process of rehabilitation.

Communication is essential to the development of a rehabilitation plan. Unfortunately, many neurorehabilitation patients have, in addition to their physical impairments, deficits in their language/communication systems. Whatever classification scheme is used in describing aphasia, language impairment when present becomes a major target for rehabilitation. In addition, it can be an impediment to rehabilitation if not diagnosed and dealt with properly. It is far more disabling and thus much harder to rehabilitate a person who has a receptive impairment and does not understand instructions. Even more challenging and complicated is the global aphasic, who has difficulty both with understanding and expressing language. Patients with a non-fluent or motor aphasia understand instructions but have trouble with oral and written output. Communication becomes frustrating and depressing. The neurorehabilitative professional must attempt to discover ways of communication for the aphasic individual. Without innovation in this area, the prognosis for rehabilitation is poor. On the neurorehabilitation team, the speech pathologist and the neuropsychologist can help by providing diagnostic information as well as by providing practical suggestions by which communication with the aphasic patient can be facilitated. In addition to the obvious issues that arise with the aphasic patient during the more acute phases of rehabilitation, the neurorehabilitation professional also needs to be mindful of the long-term issues that are likely to be prominent. For example, Benson (12) described various psychosocial consequences of aphasia, including potential changes in life-style, economic status, social position, family position, physical status, recreational activity, and sexual function.

Another complicating factor in neurorehabilitation is apraxia, which can be described as the motor system's equivalent of aphasia. It is the inability to execute learned or skilled movements that cannot be accounted for by weakness, problems with sensation or coordination, poor comprehension, intellectual deterioration, or uncooperativeness. Apraxia is thought to result from either faulty integration or disconnection of motor with sensory and language centers (13). Because almost all cases of apraxia are associated with left-hemispheric lesions in right-handers, apraxia is commonly associated with aphasia (14). During clinical examination, patients with apraxia are unable to perform a particular movement upon command. However, they might be able to perform the same movement as an automatic action apart from the examination. Although several varieties of apraxia have been described in the literature (14), the most easily and commonly observed in neurorehabilitative practice are *buccofacial* and *limb apraxias*. In buccofacial apraxia, which often accompanies a nonfluent aphasia, patients have great difficulty moving their lips, tongues, or cheeks in response to command. With limb apraxia, patients cannot move the limbs on either side of the body to perform simple actions on command. These as well as other apraxias can often complicate the course of rehabilitation, as efforts of the physical and occupational therapists (and other members of the team) may be hampered by their manifestations. However, one common principle to remember is that apraxic patients typically perform better when cues are supplied or when requested to imitate the examiner, rather than when a verbal request or command is given in isolation.

Another symptom that can result from a left-hemisphere lesion, albeit posterior, is *agnosia,* an impairment in recognition that cannot be attributed to a primary sensory defect. *Visual agnosia* occurs in lesions of the visual association regions. The patient cannot recognize objects and, at times, surroundings. The inability to recognize one's own fingers is *finger agnosia.* Tactile agnosia is called *astereognosis.* It is the

inability to recognize a simple object by palpation, despite the presence of reasonable sensory capabilities. *Autotop/agnosia* is a loss of the ability to identify a whole body part. This may be a whole side of the body, and it is a parietal lobe problem. *Anosognosia,* which is discussed in more detail later, describes a lack of recognition of one's own impairment. *Auditory agnosia* is the inability to perceive the meaning of sound despite the absence of deafness.

Apraxia and agnosia may lead to significant disability, despite a potential lack of weakness. Unfortunately, because an impairment of the patient's conscious understanding of the deficit often accompanies these problems, rehabilitation becomes very difficult.

Neurological disease may be divided into several categories, listed in Table 43.3.

Each of these processes may lead to disability, but each has a different degree of rehabilitative potential.

Selecting a Patient for Rehabilitation

In selecting a patient for rehabilitation of a neurological problem, certain criteria must be fulfilled. Rehabilitation is not easy, and great physical and mental work are necessary for complete success. Thus, the patient must be able to physically withstand the significant time commitment. Most rehabilitation programs require 2–4 hours of solid rehabilitative therapies each day. A patient who is not capable of being up that long from bed each day, or who does not have that prospect in the near future, is not appropriate for a formal rehabilitation setting.

Cognition also plays a major role in determining eligibility (15). Although many neurological patients have cognitive difficulties, some have such extensive problems that their capacity to learn and store new information is severely impaired. Excluding these patients thus becomes essential because the prognosis for effective rehabilitation under these conditions is poor (15).

Neuropsychological screening with a battery of psychological tests or procedures to determine the patient's cognitive/behavioral status may lead to decisions on the timing of the neurorehabilitation process (16, 17). It may be necessary to simply wait for the brain to "settle down" to obtain the most from the rehabilitative process. Although the Halstead-Reitan and the Luria-Nebraska neuropsychological batteries have been popular methods of diagnostically

Table 43.3. Forms of Neurological Disease

Traumatic disease of the nervous system:
  Disease of the brain: traumatic brain injury (TBI)
  Disease of the spinal cord: spinal cord injury (SCI)
Acquired nontraumatic neurological disease:
  Vascular: cerebrovascular disease (stroke)
  Neoplastic
  Toxic-metabolic
  Infectious
  Degenerative: Alzheimer's disease, multiple sclerosis (MS)
Congenital neurological disease

dissecting the functional brain (18), there are other satisfactory methods of neuropsychological assessment (19, 20). Whatever the battery or approach, an adequate assessment usually addresses the major categories of neuropsychological functioning, including: attention/concentration; memory; speech/language; visuospatial/visuomotor skills; and the so-called "executive" functions.

The patient's extent of awareness with regard to his/her impairments must also be examined critically, because this may be a significant factor that will impede rehabilitative progress. The term anosognosia was first used by Babinski in 1914 (21) in describing patients who demonstrate a disturbance in awareness of left hemiplegia following acute brain insult, but it is now commonly used to describe a variety of forms of altered self-awareness that are presumed to be secondary to neurological disturbance. Disturbances of awareness secondary to psychological processes, or denial, can also be expected with patients who have acquired a significant disability (22). Although the difference between a neurologically based vs. a psychologically based unawareness deficit is often difficult to distinguish (23), in either case the prognosis of the patient is less than optimal unless the issue is addressed and/or treated.

It is very important to identify alcohol and other drug problems prior to admission. Besides altering the physical capabilities of the patient, the addiction may also alter the attitudes and motivation. Thus, directive management is essential. Numerous patients with neurological trauma use alcohol or other mind-altering drugs to some extent. These individuals must be screened carefully (24).

PRACTICE HINTS: THE NEUROREHABILITATIVE PATIENT

Medically stable with a disease process that is rehabilitative. It is essential that the time spent on rehabilitation be actually spent on rehabilitation as opposed to management of primary medical problems. The patient must be able to focus his/her attention to the business of rehabilitation. Although progressive neurological disease may be rehabilitated, there should be some hope that the efforts will result in some period of increased functioning.

Physically capable of learning. Reality testing of the therapy situation is necessary to assess the likelihood of rehabilitating a particular person. Time is literally money, and decisions regarding practicality of rehabilitation for the severely disabled may be important.

Cognitively capable of learning. To be efficiently rehabilitated, the patient must have the potential to learn or in some way assimilate the skills. This may mean a period of time to allow the brain to reach a stage of healing that would bring about efficiency. At the same time, immobility can be devastating. Thus, skills teaching must be adjusted for each situation.

Behaviorally tolerable. Despite significant cognitive capability, if behaviors are out of control, no efficient rehabilitation will take place. The judicious use of medication to control impulses or to deal with anger and/or

depression in an individual might be considered. Or, if appropriate, a behavioral management program might be useful in attenuating the undesired behaviors. This may indeed be preferable, especially because many antidepressants and other medications have anticholinergic properties that will retard or inhibit cognitive recovery. Behavioral problems may delay the beginning of a particular sequence of rehabilitation.

SPECIFIC CLINICAL ISSUES

In this section, important and common clinical issues that are encountered in neurorehabilitative practice are discussed. The topics covered are by no means exhaustive, but they do reflect the comprehensive nature of neurorehabilitation in that syndromes, symptoms, and issues are addressed.

Depression

Neurological illness may lead to frank depression without cognitive or behavioral deficits (25). This may be reactive or secondary to brain disease. Symptoms of depressive illness are apparent in three areas: affective regulation, somatic concerns, and cognition (26). Typically there is withdrawal, poor concentration, and feelings of hopelessness. This may be accompanied by fatigue, constipation, decreased appetite, early-morning awakenings, and decreased libido. The reader should review the chapter on mood disorders in this volume for a fuller discussion of this syndrome.

Effective rehabilitation ideally requires maximal effort, motivation, and cooperation by the patient. Therefore, because depression is one of the most common clinical problems encountered by neuropsychiatrists, accurate diagnosis and management of this syndrome are critical to the successful rehabilitation of the patient.

Recognizing depression in the patient who has neurological disease may be very challenging. Often the vegetative signs of depression—decreased appetite, sleep dysfunction, and expression of depression—are masked by the effects of the neurological disorder. Sometimes the physical lesion will neurochemically contribute to the depression process.

The clinician must be alert to changes in behavior of the patient with neurological impairments. He/she needs to listen to the therapist's and family's description of the behavioral changes not only during therapy sessions but also throughout the day. Although the vegetative depression signs may be masked, they often are expressed to some degree and may be the key to the diagnosis (27).

Administration of objective standard psychological tests for depression may helpful. Unfortunately, however, interpretation of these tests may be complicated because somatic concerns and certain vegetative signs that may be typically pathognomonic in nonmedical, nonhospitalized patients may be real manifestations of the medical disease itself.

Simply being admitted to a rehabilitation unit and discovering major losses may lead to a reactive depression or a temporary adjustment reaction. It is not unusual to see patients angry, fearful, anxious, grieving, and having coping difficulties. Recognition and/or acknowledgment of these symptoms and signs can be helpful in leading the patient through this difficult time in his/her life.

Patients with prior histories of depression may develop neurological problems (25). These may include the complications of the psychotropic medications, including decreased concentration, nystagmus, ataxia, decreased language function, and decreased memory, along with their primary neurological problem.

Neurological illness may cause symptoms that appear to be secondary to depression but are actually secondary to the neurological process. These include inertia, decreased initiative, reclusiveness, and decreased spontaneous speech. This syndrome of apathy occurs with lesions in the frontal lobe, caudate nucleus, and thalamus (25).

Fisher described the syndrome "abulia" (28). In its most severe form, this is a degree of akinetic mutism—lack of movement and speech. These people are slow and have difficulty completing tasks. Lesions of the frontal lobe (stroke, demyelination, Alzheimer's disease, tumors) often cause this problem. The basal ganglia, thalamus, and substantia nigra also play a role in inertia behavior (29, 30).

To differentiate abulia from depression, attention should be paid to past history. Most patients who develop severe depression had symptoms of a similar sort prior to the neurological loss. Cognitive testing may be helpful in the differentiation by revealing frontal system signs.

The cognitive and motor effects of depression can make the neurological process appear worse. Attention to the neuroanatomy of the process, premorbid conditions, and cognitive testing may be helpful in identifying the contribution of depression.

Sometimes drugs that are used to treat a neurological disease and/or other medical conditions may actually cause or exacerbate the depression. For example, the use of barbiturates or phenytoin to treat seizures, the use of centrally acting hypertensive agents, the use of antiarrhythmic drugs, and the use of corticosteroids may contribute to a rehabilitative patient's depression (31). Thus, care must be taken to use drugs with lesser side effects whenever feasible.

Following accurate diagnosis, the treatment of depression and/or depressive symptoms in a rehabilitative context can also be complicated, and a number of factors must be considered. At times management is empirical. Obviously, if the patient is verbal and shows minimal cognitive or language processing problems, counseling/psychotherapy may be valuable. However, if the depression is so severe that cooperation is an issue and rehabilitation is therefore hampered, many patients will benefit from a trial of antidepressants. Tricyclic antidepressants (e.g., amitriptyline, desipramine, doxepin, imipramine, and nortriptyline) are very often the pharmacological treatment of choice for depressive illness, their common mechanism being the blockade of reuptake of serotonin and catecholamines (26). However, in a rehabilitative context, consideration of secondary pharmacological actions of a particular tricyclic is especially important. For example, drugs that are highly anticholinergic should be avoided, as they may result in impairing new learning and memory, or even lead to an anticholinergic delirium. Obviously, a drug-induced impairment in cognition in a patient who may already be suffering from cognitive sequelae of a stroke or other brain injury may severely attenuate any potential rehabilitative gains. For this reason, tricyclics that are fairly high on the anticholinergic continuum (e.g., amitriptyline) should probably be avoided in this context. It is especially important to consider the other secondary effects of the tricyclics—such as their antihistaminergic and α-receptor blockade properties—when determining drug choice. More recently, the use of second-generation antidepressants such as sertraline and fluoxetine have become more popular because of their more benign side-effect profile. Nevertheless, each of these agents has unique side effects that may complicate treatment; e.g., the SSRIs may aggravate ataxia or tremors.

PRACTICE HINTS: DEPRESSION

Note changes from previous behavior patterns. Comparison of the patient's mood before and after the neurologic illness is important in determining the possibility of depression. Sometimes a behavioral pattern that is not necessarily abnormal by many standards is clearly abnormal for a specific individual. Deviation from previous baseline behavior can be an indicator of a depression that could inhibit the rehabilitative process if not treated.

Obtain psychological testing/evaluation. Sometimes the only way to determine depression is to test for it. The testing is most helpful if it includes neuropsychological as well as routine psychological testing. The Beck Depression Inventory and the Hamilton Rating Scale are examples of brief measures that are fairly reliable. The Minnesota Multiphasic Personality Inventory (MMPI) is surprisingly useful and accurate in identifying an underlying depression in a person who may deny it, but it is also a very lengthy and time-consuming procedure that many patients are unable to tolerate or to complete.

Allow intervention through individual and/or group therapy. Counseling and/or psychotherapy can be very effective in treating depression. It may even be the preferred mode in the rehabilitative setting because many antidepressants have adverse effects on cognition. The processing of or the ventilation of one's feelings related to depression is often helpful. However, unless the therapy is professionally supervised and directed, the ventilation may turn into increased and undirected anger, which is counterproductive.

If the patient is agitated, consider a sedating antidepressant. If significant agitation is present, such that the course of rehabilitation is threatened, the use of sedating antidepressants may be helpful and necessary. Treatment of agitated depression with medication usually is necessary prior to talking therapy.

If patient is withdrawing from society, utilize an energizing antidepressant. With withdrawal, rehabilitation becomes impossible. Newer, energizing antidepressants (fluoxetine, sertraline, paroxetine) are very useful to break through the retarded depression of disability. Stimulants may have a role in selected patients.

Multiple Sclerosis

Multiple sclerosis (MS) is a disease of the myelin in the central nervous system. It is immunologically based and leads to spotty demyelination and plaque formation (gliosis). It is a very unpredictable process that may develop into significant disability in one-third of the people who contract it (32). Although there is a genetic predisposition (10–20% have it in the family), it is generally considered sporadic. Epidemiologically it is more often a disease of women (1.8:1), Caucasians, and higher socioeconomic groups (33). It is a disease of young adults beginning most often in the 15–50 age group (34).

Characteristically it is episodic, occurring with exacerbations, and then settles down with remissions. Some symptoms attenuate, while others progress.

Neuropsychiatrically this process is extremely important because the disease affects many people in the family. It is not unusual for the person with MS to already be married and have children. Economically it often leads to family tragedy.

Loss of motor function may be obvious in people with MS. Less obvious, but very important, may be cognitive dysfunction (35, 36). In recent years there has been stronger evidence of cognitive problems in many patients with MS, and in some these are significant deficits. Despite decades of ignorance regarding the effect of MS on cognition, recent studies indicate that as many as 65% of people with MS have some cognitive dysfunction (35). The dementia appears to be subcortical in origin. This distinguishes it from Alzheimer's disease. It is characterized by deficits in recent memory, sustained attention, conceptual reasoning, and information processing. Speech and intellect are preserved. Cognitive decline is not uniform in MS. There appears to be a transmission problem–transmitting material to storage or from storage. Because the person with MS may look well and, in fact, may show little other disability, large and unrealistic expectations for performance may remain. Added to this may be demyelination in the limbic system, leading to a decrease in biogenic amines and depression. These issues are discussed in greater detail in Chapter 40 of this volume.

Despite its prevalence, cognitive rehabilitative techniques for MS are rather crude. Compensatory strategies utilizing notebooks, word associations, tape recorders, and other devices are helpful. Unfortunately, major efforts to enhance the cognitive rehabilitation of MS are lacking. Much more time has been devoted to traumatic brain injury rehabilitation. Speech pathologists, occupational therapists, and neuropsychologists continue to delve into retraining techniques.

As more demyelination occurs multifocally, bilaterally in the cerebral hemispheres, a pseudobulbar picture of hyperemotionality (laughing, weeping), increased impulsivity, and gait apraxia accompany the mental impairment. In any one person there may be an emphasis on any one of these clinical signs or symptoms.

If disability continues, the family structure becomes jeopardized. Role reversal is common. If the husband (father) is afflicted with MS, the wife (mother) may become the single wage-earner in the family without surrendering any of the maternal roles. If the wife (mother) is affected, the husband (father) may need to become the homemaker, caretaker, and wage-earner of the family. The stress this puts on the family structure is obvious. Children are often assigned roles that are usually reserved for mature adults. There is often rebellion with these new positions. The patient may feel helpless and feel the frustration and pain within the family. This guilt can worsen the situation because secondary depression leads to further dysfunction. All of these factors may be compounded if there is a significant loss of intellectual function. Abuse, both adult and child, may arise from the stress.

Early recognition of these scenarios is essential for successful management. Social agencies may provide significant help. Counseling is essential. To resolve potential problems, there has to be a change in the family response to the stresses.

At the same time, it is critical to determine the neuropsychological status of the patient. This is necessary not only to understand the deficits but also to grasp the strengths and capabilities of the patient. Neuropsychology, occupational therapy, and speech pathology all contribute to a better understanding of the patient. Specific ideas that will allow the disabled person to help him/herself are sought. Whether the disability is in dressing or thinking, appropriate independence is ideal. For example, if the person is having problems with verbal memory, written cue cards may be used (37).

Social isolation may be one of the biggest psychological factors in cognitive decline (38). As the person with MS becomes less capable, there often is a social withdrawal from friends and family. This leads to a decrease in social skills and starts a cycle that is self destructive. Day programs that force participation may renew these social skills. This renewal may decrease the stress within the family structure. We believe it is essential to seek outside activities for the patient with MS.

Supportive relationships protect people who experience physical decline. Relationships may exist between chronic illness and suicide. Age, race, sex, income, and functional limitation have not been found by some to show significant correlation with suicidal ideations. Others have related disability to these thoughts. Progression of disease, fear of dying, and fear of consciousness when dead have slight correlation. Hopelessness, fear of premature death, and fear of the unknown can negatively affect suicidal tendencies. On the other hand, religious orthodoxy, self-perceived religiosity, belief in a supreme being, and family and friend support can mitigate suicidal thoughts. These findings have been documented (39, 40).

PRACTICE HINTS: MULTIPLE SCLEROSIS

Explain the diagnosis carefully and completely. At the outset, a clear explanation of MS is very important. It is essential for the patient to understand what MS is and what it is not. It is vital to communicate that a diagnosis of MS is not an automatic prescription for a wheelchair. Education may allow for a certain amount of empowerment for the patient.

Group therapy for the newly diagnosed is recommended, with a goal of adjusting to the diagnosis. After the diagnosis is explained from a neurological standpoint, adjustment must take place. This is eased with professional psychological help. Group therapy for newly diagnosed, not for patients with significant disabilities, is very helpful. If disabilities are too mixed, too much comparison and the shock of MS problems detracts from the therapeutic atmosphere.

If cognitive decline is suspected, confirm with neuropsychological evaluation. If cognitive decline is noted, obtaining baseline studies with a goal of teaching compensatory techniques is helpful. If full neuropsychological testing is not indicated, a screening evaluation may be simply performed at much less expense. If job survival is at hand, the full testing is necessary.

Teach compensatory techniques. Compensation (e.g., computer aids, notebooks) may be useful for many of the disabilities of MS, including the neuropsychiatric ones.

Continue to stimulate intellectually (do not isolate). If cognitive problems surface, there is a tendency for the patient to withdraw. Every effort should be given to prevent this by mainstreaming, use of day care, and continuing to include the patient in day-to-day activities. However, denial of the cognitive problems will only cause exasperation for all involved.

If the patient is depressed, utilize an appropriate antidepressant and counseling. Depression needs to be treated actively with whatever means is appropriate for the situation. This may require drugs, talking, or both kinds of therapy.

Give hope and schedule return appointments. Acting pessimistic and giving up does no one good. Patients need to know the real situation, but fairly. Return appointments allow for the following of patients and also assure them that they are not being abandoned. This is important in any chronic disease.

Chronic Fatigue Syndrome

A potential new arena for combining neurology with psychiatry involves the study of fatigue. Fatigue is a major disabling factor and can be symptomatic of many different diseases. However, in recent years, it has become the focus of a possible distinct syndrome. Under the name chronic fatigue syndrome, chronic Epstein-Barr virus, chronic mononucleosis, the "yuppie disease," postviral fatigue syndrome, and myalgic encephalomyelitis, fatigue is likened to the "neurasthenia" of the psychiatric literature of the past (41, 42).

A presumed disease complex that has no widely accepted etiology, chronic fatigue syndrome (CFS) has remained a controversial topic in both the academic and the clinical arenas, mainly because of its elusive diagnosis and/or case definition. One commonly used definition was developed by the Centers for Disease Control (CDC) in 1988, which involved two major criteria and 14 minor criteria (43). According to this definition, a patient must meet both of two major criteria and either eight of the 11 symptom criteria or six of the 11 symptom criteria and two of three physical criteria. The two major criteria that must be met are: (*a*) new onset of persistent or relapsing, debilitating fatigue or easy fatigability in a patient with no previous history of similar symptoms, which does not resolve with bedrest, with the fatigue severe enough that the patient's average daily activity is reduced to below 50% of premorbid levels for at least 6 months; and (*b*) other clinical conditions that may produce similar symptoms must be excluded by thorough evaluation. The interested reader should refer to Chapter 40 of this volume for a listing and description of the remaining criteria, which includes symptoms such as mild fever, sore throat, painful lymph nodes, muscle weakness, and myalgia. Although complaints of fatigue are commonly encountered in primary care practice, a recent study (44) suggests that the actual occurrence of CFS when using the CDC criteria may be quite low (0.3% point prevalence).

In addition to difficulties with reliable diagnosis of CFS, there has been considerable debate as to its underlying cause or etiology (45, 46), although most would probably agree that multiple medical and psychological factors are involved. Recent studies have demonstrated difficulties in information processing efficiency similar to those of MS (see earlier discussion), although they also indicate more problems than can be accounted for by depression alone. Rather, a selective impairment in information processing efficiency is implicated (47). Further neuropsychiatric research is necessary to uncover the pathophysiology and management of this complex problem.

PRACTICE HINTS: CHRONIC FATIGUE SYNDROME

Do not prejudge and treat as a primary mental health disorder. In reality, patients with this syndrome are often waiting for the professional to indicate that they have a mental health problem. They will then move on to another professional, adding the previous physician to their long list of failures. The best approach is to keep an open mind.

Manage somatization as it appears. Symptom management is essential to allow for a degree of comfort in an uncomfortable process. Pain should be managed without habit-forming medication. If depression is present, it should be treated as depression seen in other medical problems. Physical therapy may be useful for the management of weakness.

Utilize energizing antidepressants. The newer energizing antidepressants are very helpful, even if clinical depression is not obvious. Explaining to the patient that this is not labeling the whole process as psychiatric is essential prior to the acceptance of the therapy by the patient.

Follow cases with return appointments. As with other chronic processes, follow-up is necessary. This shows interest on the part of the professional as well as giving the patient reassurance.

Counsel as appropriate. Counseling from a professional may be helpful. This should be done in a supportive, nonpejorative manner. If psychiatric care is indicated, the topic should be broached in a careful manner, and the therapist should be selected carefully for a therapeutic relationship to develop. A recent study (48) suggests that a cognitive-behavioral approach aimed at reducing avoidance or learned helplessness in the CFS patient may be a helpful intervention.

Cerebrovascular Disease

The neuropsychiatric aspects of cerebrovascular disease (CVD) are determined by a number of interrelated factors. Whether the cerebrovascular process is hemorrhagic or ischemic, whether embolic or thrombotic, is less important than the neuroanatomical location of the insult. Prognostically, the hemorrhage may reabsorb, leaving viable brain tissue to function, but the disability that is left will be determined by the location of the cerebrovascular accident (CVA). See Abscher's and Toole's chapter on stroke elsewhere in this volume for a more thorough discussion of this topic.

Higher cortical functions become more important than paresis from a rehabilitation point of view (49). It is far easier to compensate for a plegic arm or leg than for an agnosia, apraxia, or most other neuropsychological disorders. Because CVD originates in the brain, cognition is typically involved to some degree (50). Impairments in attention/concentration, memory, language, visuomotor/visuoperceptual skills, and the so-called "executive" functions (e.g., maintenance of mental set, organization, response inhibition) may be present, depending on the location and/or type of stroke involved. Complicating rehabilitative efforts may be the presence of denial or unawareness of deficit syndromes in some patients. It is very difficult to teach around a disability that is not recognized by the person with the disability.

Adding to the complexity of rehabilitation are the various neurobehavioral problems that are often seen in the stroke patient. For example, patients with an executive dysfunction secondary to an anterior CVA may exhibit impulsivity or behavioral/emotional disinhibition. Thus, they may have difficulty controlling their frustration and may give up easily. Or, they may behave impulsively in ways that are counterproductive to their rehabilitative regimen and ultimately to their well-being (e.g., getting out of bed or out of their wheelchair without help). In some cases, they may lose patience so quickly that they are at risk of harming themselves or others. Prognostically, it is foreboding to see significant higher cortical involvement with accompanying impulsivity, as it is clearly easier to restore ADL skills to almost anyone who can participate actively and intelligently in the rehabilitation process. Other neurobehavioral problems may include emotional lability, confusion, anxiety, and others, which may compromise the patient's ability to cooperate or remain motivated toward rehabilitation. Although most stroke patients do not exhibit these specific problems, they are of practical significance for many.

Chronic, ongoing depression will sabotage any rehabilitation program. Depression frequently accompanies stroke and may be a primary or secondary sequel to the CVA. The vascular system serves both myelinated and nonmyelinated parts of the brain. As such it can involve primary affective structures, giving rise to primary or endogenous depression (51, 52). Obviously, many who are faced with increased disability will go through a reactive depression as well (53). If the disease is diffuse, multifocal, or bilateral, a hyperemotional syndrome results. This usually presents with slurred speech, dysphagia, and gait apraxia. Because of the appearance of brainstem abnormalities despite the lack of primary brainstem involvement, the term pseudobulbar palsy is utilized. The person may or may not be depressed, despite the frequent episodes of crying. Pharmacological intervention with tricyclic antidepressants or SSRIs may be helpful in this process (26). The interested reader can consult Robinson's and Travella's discussion (Chapter 14) in this volume for a more comprehensive description of poststroke depression.

The rehabilitation process for CVA is similar to others, with the involvement of a team of professionals, including a physician, physical therapist, occupational therapist, speech pathologist, neuropsychologist, and nurse. Neurobehavioral abnormalities or tendencies may be recognized by any or all involved. Time may solve some problems, whether it be weeks or months. Others will need intensive therapy. The therapy may be hampered because the stroke patient may be elderly and may lack stamina or may have complicating medical illnesses.

Because of the impairment of higher cortical function seen after many strokes, neuropsychological assessment should play a crucial role in the rehabilitation of these patients. Although neuropsychological evaluations have been historically (54) useful in diagnosing the presence and location of brain dysfunction, with the advent of sophisticated neuroradiological tools (i.e., CT and MRI scans), its primary role and importance have somewhat shifted. This is particularly true in the rehabilitation setting, where the neuropsychological exam can be very helpful for (*a*) determining the nature and extent of the cognitive and behavioral sequelae of the stroke; (*b*) assessing cognitive/behavioral strengths and weaknesses to assist in treatment planning; (*c*) establishing a cognitive baseline from which to assess the extent and speed of recovery; (*d*) providing information that will guide postdischarge planning or placement, and; (e) differentiating between psychological and neurological/medical etiologies underlying a neurobehavioral issue. Although impairments in higher cortical function may often be evident through clinical observation, the neuropsychological evaluation has the advantage — by its inclusion of psychometric assessment — of providing more detailed and objective documentation of deficits. In addition, subtle deficits that may not be evident by observation or detected by less sensitive procedures are more likely to be discovered in a comprehensive neuropsychological evaluation.

PRACTICE HINTS: CEREBROVASCULAR DISEASE

Treat underlying medical problems aggressively. Medical problems can interfere with the psychological functioning of the person with stroke. They can hide the psychological problems from view. An aggressive approach is necessary to make progress.

Undertake a thorough rehabilitative evaluation, using physical therapy, occupational therapy, speech therapy professionals. To understand the neuropsychiatric situation, data from the rehabilitation team are essential. No neuropsychiatric conclusions should be made until the full report of others is in the data bank.

Higher cortical function disturbances require innovative approaches of therapists, including weighting extremities, developing alternative sources of sensory inputs, patterning of movements, developing increased awareness. Higher cortical problems require solutions that must be developed on the scene. Reading about them in books, while helpful, is no substitute for first-hand experience. The team approach is necessary for these complex problems.

Assess for depression. Depression disorders can submerge and complicate rehabilitation attempts. Depression must be diagnosed and treated as quickly as possible. Be careful to distinguish a "minor" reactive depressive episode secondary to adjustment issues from a frank clinical depression.

Consider neuropsychological testing. If there is doubt as to the neuropsychological status of the patient, objective testing may be enlightening. This can allow for a more logical rehabilitative plan.

Parkinson's Disease

Parkinson's disease (PD) is a degenerative disease of the brain that has significant neurobehavioral ramifications. The cardinal features of PD include bradykinesia, tremor, and rigidity.

This progressive disease of dopamine production (55) also causes a primary, slowly progressive dementia (56, 57). The dementia is similar to Alzheimer's disease, but when coupled with the other disabling features of PD, it can be particularly devastating. Although PD usually occurs in the sixth and seventh decades, it may occur at younger ages. Depression commonly accompanies the progressive process

Table 43.4. Neuropsychiatric Symptoms of Parkinson's Disease

Delirium
Dementia
Depression

(58). Delirium, dementia, and depression are the most common psychiatric manifestations (Table 43.4). Depression occurs in over 50% of PD patients (59). Neuropsychological damage often includes the ventral tegmentum, hippocampus, and entorhinal cortex (60). The symptoms of depression are the typical ones of decreased activities, decreased appetite, fatigue, decreased libido, feelings of guilt, worthlessness, decreased concentration, hypersomnolence, or insomnia. Some medications used in PD also contribute to depression, including carbidopa/levodopa, bromocriptine, and amantadine (61). As with many of the other syndromes discussed in this chapter, the neurobehavioral features of this disease may have a significant impact upon rehabilitative efforts if they are not managed successfully. That is, the patient's lack of motivation, negative self-image, and hopelessness may undermine the otherwise effective interventions of the rehabilitation team.

Treatment of depression includes tricyclic antidepressants and occasionally electroconvulsive therapy (ECT). These may also help other Parkinson's symptoms.

The PD patient typically has a masking of the face, giving the impression of a very unhappy person with no sense of humor. That may be far from the case because the unhappy look is secondary to physical, not psychological, processes that prevent spontaneous movements of the face. The slow movements are also suggestive of slow thinking, giving the impression of more dementia than is actually present.

Significant dementia occurs in PD about 30% of the time. Neuropsychological deficits occur in up to 40% of those tested without obvious mental impairment. Frontal lobe dysfunction appears to be involved to some extent in the decreased cognition as well as in the depression of PD.

The rehabilitation of PD requires tremendous patience on the part of the therapists. Increasing mobility is a major goal. Stimulating the mobility of the mind should also be an aim of the rehabilitation team.

PRACTICE HINTS: PARKINSON'S DISEASE

If the patient is developing cognitive problems, review medications and attempt to readjust. Often, cognitive problems in PD are exacerbated by medication toxicity or side effects. Sometimes it is a no-win situation, where lowering the drug levels makes for worsening of the physical signs of the disease. A happy medium should be sought.

Be aware that most tranquilizers exacerbate PD symptoms. Phenothiazines and butyrophenones cause a worsening of PD symptoms. Thus, they should be avoided in the PD patient. At present, elozapine is the neuroleptic of choice in PD with psychosis.

Attempt to keep the environment as stable as possible. Changes in the environment may increase the confusion from the dementia of PD. Managing the environment can be helpful in minimizing behavioral aberrations.

Because of the progressive nature of PD, a skilled nursing home may eventually be necessary. Knowing the process may allow for a more smooth transition to a change in living situation. This may help both the patient and the family. There is no easy transition, but knowledge may help.

Neuromuscular/Skeletal Pain

One would think that degenerative diseases of the peripheral nervous system would not be very applicable to neuropsychiatry. However, because of society's trends, injuries of the neuromuscular-skeletal system do commonly bridge gaps between neurology and psychiatry. Low back pain is among the more costly injuries in America. The pain may be intolerable, but often there is little evidence on formal exam to indicate severity of the injury. Workers' compensation laws have encouraged the growth of a whole industry of disability determinations. To play the game, one needs to know the rules, and there are many. These are available from various rating sources, including: state workers' compensation offices, the Social Security Administration, specific insurance companies, and the American Medical Association.

Often these rules put the physician, whose lofty goal is to relieve the pain and suffering of his/her patient, in a most difficult position. If the physician rates the patient objectively, the patient may receive a very low percentage disability rating. In anger and protest, that patient may abandon the physician. This puts a significant stress on the patient-physician relationship.

Chronic pain is among the more disabling symptoms. It has strong implications in the neuropsychiatry of disability and rehabilitation. Despite major advances in pharmacological approaches to pain and advances in aggressive surgical procedures, there is no solution for the management of persistent pain. How patients respond to pain remains a mystery; some tolerate amazing amounts of stimulus, and others simply do not. The litigious society of today also adds to the confusion, providing incentives for ongoing work-related or personal injury pain.

Obviously, there can be psychological input into a legitimately painful process. Secondary gain is quite common. Depression, anxiety, and belief systems also contribute. Knowledge of the psychological background of patients with chronic pain can help in the management and goal-setting of treatments.

Table 43.5 lists common psychiatric diagnoses in patients with chronic pain (62, 63).

There have been a number of approaches to chronic pain based on neuropsychiatry. Some are physiologically based, with emphasis on exercise, surgery, and medications. Others

Table 43.5. Psychiatric Diagnoses of Pain

307.80	Somatoform pain disorder
301.51	Factitious disorder with physical symptoms
V65.20	Malingering
300.11	Conversion disorder
300.70	Hypochondriasis
316	Psychological factors affecting physical conditions
300.40	Dysthymia (depressive neurosis)
309.00	Adjustment disorder with depressed mood
309.82	Adjustment disorder with physical complaints

stress the psychology of pain, emphasizing the psychological makeups of individuals and their backgrounds. In these approaches, counseling, biofeedback, and nonmedical strategies are used.

Most pain management programs are multidisciplinary to some extent. They are obviously expensive, but the disability of chronic pain is expensive in itself.

There are three steps in the rehabilitation of pain patients:

1. Accurate physical and psychological diagnosis;
2. Establishment of reasonable goals; and
3. Selection and implementation of treatments.

The impact of pain on the patient and the family must be assessed. Pain may be seen as a solution to a problem rather than the problem itself. It may legitimize unacceptable behavior. Litigation may slow the rehabilitation process considerably.

Because of the large number of variables, it is very hard to adequately assess pain rehabilitation programs. However, pain remains a major disabler, and successful rehabilitation requires a rehabilitation program that is organized and eclectic.

PRACTICE HINTS: MUSCULOSKELETAL PAIN

A proper diagnosis is essential before commencing treatment. To treat the "whole" person with chronic pain, it is essential to have a real, correct diagnosis. Too often presumed diagnoses of discogenic, posttraumatic, muscle strains, and other muscoloskeletal pain lack confirmation.

Avoid habit-forming medication. Pain syndromes appear to be fertile ground for the development of chemical dependency. Opiates should be minimized in most cases of chronic pain.

Attempt aggressive physical and occupational therapies. Physical, occupational, and (if appropriate) vocational therapy will help in the neuropsychiatric management of patients with chronic pain. Without these interfacing, little progress will be made.

Eliminate litigation. Pending litigation will almost always sabotage any progress in a pain process. Even before initiating the treatment, litigation issues should be addressed.

Manage depression. Depression should be treated as in any other disorder. It may be masked behind the guise of anger.

Consider a specific type of pain program for a given personality. Different pain program approaches may be helpful for different types of individuals. The cause of the pain is less important when compared with the personality of the individual in this selection. Pain programs may be quite helpful if they are used appropriately, considering the individual patient.

Conversion Reactions

Chronic diseases and disabilities often lead to disability behavior that appears beyond that expected by the impairment. Thus, the disability and the handicap appear exaggerated. If this exaggeration is being feigned, the term "malingering" is utilized. The secondary gain is usually obvious and the disability performance may be dramatic. In a real sense there is criminal intent because the patient is perpetrating a known falsehood, a fraud. This is, in fact, stealing a disability.

Conversion reactions are different. They are as old as the history of neuropsychiatry. The patient who is undergoing a conversion reaction is unaware of the exaggeration of symptoms and findings beyond that expected from the physical impairment (63). The patient has displaced his/her anxiety or depression toward a physical symptom (64). This often results in the exhibition of no specific psychiatric symptoms. To imply to these individuals that there is a mental component is tantamount to calling them liars. They have no insight into their mental problems and usually desire none (65, 66).

The management of conversion reactions is fraught with difficulties not only because of the lack of psychological insight but also because of the presence of some physical problems that are often poorly understood. Thus, a patient with MS may have mild weakness but exhibits far more weakness because of fear of becoming weak in the future.

There is no standard way to approach this situation, but conflict usually yields poor results (67). Pointing out to the patient the discrepancy in behavior brings about a defensive posture that allows no therapeutic victory. It appears more appropriate to work with the patient physically while trying to help psychiatrically in a more subtle fashion (68). This is truly an amalgamation of neurology and psychiatry.

There is usually some secondary gain to be obtained from the exaggeration, and this must be limited or corrected to make progress. Often the reason for the disability (secondary gain) is no longer appropriate and an excuse to be relieved of the disability via timely rehabilitation may be of benefit.

PRACTICE HINTS: CONVERSION REACTION

There is no "right way" to manage.   Despite the long history of conversion reactions, no standards of successful management have been developed.

Calling the person a psychiatric problem dooms the treatment to failure.   Although no absolute tested guidelines are known, it is clear that this type of patient, more than any other, resents the psychiatric label and will not accept it. *After gaining the confidence of the patient, psychiatric*

intervention may be possible.   Neuropsychiatric counseling may become possible later in the management of the patient. If psychiatric counseling begins too early, long-term improvement will not occur. Often the patient will show short-term improvement if confronted. Then, after leaving the acute treatment situation, the patient regresses.

Usually behaviorally oriented treatment is most successful. These patients initially respond to cause-and-effect solutions. Later, more subtle psychological interventions may become helpful.

Traumatic Brain Injury

Traumatic brain injury (TBI) is the original manifestation of a neurological process that may be encompassed in the term, "neuropsychiatry." It is a major problem, with 50–75,000 people each year in the U.S. suffering severe head injury (69). Most injuries occur in young males who are otherwise healthy but because of brain trauma are almost never the same again.

Obviously, location of the injury determines what type of problems are likely to be forthcoming. These may encompass the entire range of apraxias, aphasias, agnosias, plegias and visual difficulties, along with other specific and general cognitive and personality/behavior problems.

Often at the time of injury the person looks quite different from a neuropsychiatric perspective than he/she will several months later. Time heals many of the wounds (12, 70–72). The initial edema subsides and the brain settles down. Although plasticity of nervous system is well known in children, the extent to which the adult brain is plastic following injury is uncertain (73, 74).

Despite the lack of good supportive literature, some clinicians believe that patterning of sequences can mold motor pathways in the adult brain. More often, however, compensatory techniques use existing capabilities, relying on preserved further development of talents.

There are three causes of abnormal behaviors in the TBI patient: (*a*) impaired cognition, (*b*) focal cortical injury, and (*c*) psychological inability to adapt to injury-related stressors (75). The patient with TBI has problems with higher cortical functions and concentration. Superimposed upon these may be a pseudobulbar emotional lability which, at times, can be annoying as well as dangerous and may be combined with impaired arousal and slow processing. Behavior modification techniques along with psychoactive medication may be necessary to control the outbursts of anger and inappropriate behavior that may occur (76–79). Agitation has been controlled with β-blockers as well as tranquilizing medications (80–82). A structured, controlled environment with a trained staff is essential.

Alongside the hyperemotionality may be a hypersexuality (83). This may be expressed with aggressiveness secondary to the brain damage. These complications should be managed without the severely pejorative approaches of the uninformed. Again, behavioral modification techniques may be helpful along with an attempt to educate the individual in other modes of expressing desires and emotions.

Seizures may complicate the problems, and these may be difficult to control. The seizures can be simple or complex (84). They can significantly alter the behavior of the patient. Medical management should be aggressive because even subclinical seizures may slow the rehabilitative process and decrease the attentiveness of the patient. Although monotherapy (single medication) is preferable, sometimes multiple anticonvulsants are necessary.

Measuring quality of life issues is extremely important in evaluating rehabilitation programs from a neuropsychiatric point of view (85, 86). This is a multidimensional problem. Neuropsychological measures are easily obtained and standardized, but they are not usually measured against real-life outcomes (87, 88). The preinjury status of individuals is difficult to measure in a standardized way postinjury. Separating the natural history of improvement from that brought by a rehabilitation program is also difficult.

Goals set for a typical cognitive rehabilitation program include living and managing at home (daily activities, medication administration, independent living, increased endurance, preparation of light meals); leisure activities (community recreation, fitness programs, group activities, public transport, telephone); community living (management of frustration, social situations, budget, safety, group discussions, driver's license); prevocational (vocational planning, complete multistep activities, increased endurance, being punctual) (86).

Although no controlled studies have been performed, cognitive rehabilitation programs appear to help with specific retraining of some cognitive functions (87, 89). Direct remediation of deficits in information processing and attention accompanied by counseling, improved information processing, interpersonal skills, and a decreased emotional disturbance are sought.

Specific cognitive skills include attention perception, information integration, retrieval, and executive control. The most effective approach involves paying attention to the person and working with him or her to set goals. The attention itself may be the stimulus to improvement rather than the detailed content of the program (9).

Models of cognitive rehabilitation programs fall into three categories: (*a*) functional adaptation, (*b*) general stimulation, and (*c*) the process-specific approach (90). The functional approach involves environmental manipulations or compensatory strategies. General stimulation uses tasks that encourage cognitive processing. A process-specific approach is oriented toward target remediation of deficits in specific cognitive areas.

Factors that influence the cognitive outcome from TBI include age, depth and duration of coma, CT abnormality, evoked potentials, and serum catecholamine levels. These appear to give an indication of the amount of brain damage that has occurred. Thus, an important approach to cognitive rehabilitation of the brain-injured patient is to limit damage as much as possible, with aggressive acute management of

hemorrhage, hypoxia, and medical complications. Objective research into outcomes of formal cognitive rehabilitation has shown conflicting results. There are issues of internal validity to these studies, and the testing is designed to show particular outcomes (91–93).

Coma stimulation programs have become more popular even though they have not been shown to change outcomes of individuals in coma. They may teach families a greater awareness of the potential for change in their family member, but that is not necessarily good. The Glasgow Coma Scale may, however, be insensitive to change because slight recoveries do occur.

Psychostimulants include dopamine agonists, methylphenidate, amphetamines, and some antidepressants.

Cognitive rehabilitation remains a controversial management tool, partially because of the lack of good controlled studies and because of the large cost in a society that is becoming more medically cost conscious. Thus far, there is little evidence that computers enhance cognitive performance, but there is a significant body of evidence that compensatory strategies can be taught. These strategies enrich lives and allow retraining for work. Cognitive rehabilitation programs generally include speech pathology, neuropsychology, and occupational therapy.

What becomes important in assessing these programs revolves around the definition of success. If changes on certain tests are considered success, all the programs appear to work, but if actual changes in the meshing into society are the goals, this approach may not be as clearly successful.

PRACTICE HINTS: TRAUMATIC BRAIN INJURY

Remember that time is a great healer. Often the worst neuropsychiatric problems in TBI are solved with time. The brain does heal and settle down to some degree with time. Patience is a virtue.

Neuropsychological evaluation is very helpful and should be repeated as necessary. Neuropsychological testing can help document objectively the progress that is being made with rehabilitation. As such it may give guidance as to the direction of the treatment. Because the TBI patient typically manifests problems with integrating or "pulling together" his/her cognitive abilities, it is important that a neuropsychological evaluation's assessment of discrete cognitive abilities is not confused with the patient's total functional presentation.

Medications should be used judiciously. Any medication must be used carefully in the TBI patient. Side effects of a behavioral nature may cloud the progress.

The staff must be very patient, especially with wild behavioral aberrations. Behavior problems are common with TBI. The staff needs to be aware of the process and avoid, if at all possible, methods involving physical restraint. Dangerous objects should be kept out of the patient's reach.

The family should be involved in the therapy. It's best to include the family when describing how to deal with a loved one who has TBI. Obviously there are exceptions to this, particularly when pre-existing relationship problems are present.

Spinal Cord Injury

Spinal cord injury (SCI) provides the basis of many dedicated rehabilitation units. Because of the recent lack of morbid wars, the use of seat belts, a 55-mile per hour speed limit, and other activities aimed at the preservation of health, the number of such injuries has been decreasing in America.

Nonetheless, SCI will affect 7,000–10,000 Americans each year, with a prevalence rate of 150,000–200,000 cases, most of whom will be young adults (94). Obviously a proportion of these will have concomitant head injuries.

A pure SCI spares the brain and the resulting secondary cognitive complications. However, it does not spare the self-image problems that accompany such a drastic injury. The typical pattern of SCI develops in a young "macho" male adult who suddenly moves from a strong image to a weak one (95). In addition to learning to live without the functional use of his legs and/or arms, he has to change his own self-image. The emotional trauma is immense. The stages of grief have been noted previously and apply here. No one with SCI adjusts quickly.

Sadness and grief must be distinguished from depression, which requires independent management. With appropriate encouragement and professional help, over time, adjustments can occur that allow individuals to live fruitful and fulfilling lives.

Sexuality is particularly an issue for both males and females with SCI. Body image alteration is very prominent, and sexual function is always altered. Alternative ways of expressing sexuality need to be discussed, along with exploration of different ways of approaching sexual performance. The use of penile vasodilating agents and penile vacuum devices to induce vascular engorgement may be useful in males.

All of this needs to take place in an emotional environment that may be quite different from that which was previously present. A reassessment of attitudes becomes essential.

PRACTICE HINTS: SPINAL CORD INJURY

Neuropsychological testing may help discover concomitant head injury. If progress is not being made in the rehabilitative process, testing may give the reason, and from those findings a new direction may be developed.

Counseling and antidepressant medications are probably necessary to manage the ensuing depression. Depression is always present following SCI. Management should be aggressive with all modalities.

Open discussion and counseling regarding body image are absolutely necessary: There is no substitute for open discussion and counseling about very difficult issues. This is especially true with SCI.

Aggressive physical and occupational therapy are essential. Needless to say, rehabilitation remains the mainstay of SCI. It is extremely important to have experienced, qualified personnel for these complex patients.

Stress what is possible, as opposed to what is not. Any rehabilitation program should stress the positive. Each therapist is, in reality, a psychotherapist and should have some understanding of the principles of psychotherapy.

Be open in discussing sexuality, using the language that is most familiar to the patient. Most of these patients are at an age where sexual functioning is most important. Thus, this needs to be discussed early in the rehabilitation process. Skilled therapists of all varieties with consistent messages are necessary.

Medicolegal Aspects of Disability

In addition to dealing with the challenging clinical issues among patients with disabilities, the rehabilitation professional is often expected to make decisions or determinations on vocational capacity that have legal implications. According to Rothstein (96), there are two primary reasons for the legal significance of such assessments:

1. Several forms of income replacement and benefits such as Social Security disability insurance, workers' compensation, and long-term disability insurance are based on the disabled person's projected lost earning capacity; and
2. State and federal laws prohibit employment discrimination against otherwise qualified individuals with handicaps.

Despite the frequent need for many physicians to make these decisions, the determination of disability may not be so clear-cut. In the American Medical Association's (AMA's) *Guides to the Evaluation of Permanent Impairment* (97), a distinction is made between "impairment," which refers to "an alteration of an individual's health status that is *assessed by medical means,*" and "disability," which describes "an alteration of an individual's capacity to meet personal, social, or occupational demands or statutory or regulatory requirements," and *"which is assessed by nonmedical means."* (italics ours). Unfortunately, this proposed differentiation between impairment and disability can be problematic in that it implies a dichotomy by which the rehabilitation professional simply needs to determine the level of impairment objectively and provides that information to others for the final judgment on disability. In practice, however, it is difficult to determine impairment without taking into account some of the very factors that the *Guides* would leave to be assessed by "nonmedical means." Still, when medical professionals do utilize social and vocational variables in determining impairment, low inter-rater reliability is demonstrated (98).

Although there are various resources available to physicians for determining level and extent of disability (e.g., the AMA's *Guides,* the Social Security Administration's publications/tables, and state workers' compensation regulations), many of these can be problematic in actual practice. For example, the Social Security Administration's grid system for determining vocational disability has been criticized as arbitrary, inaccurate, oversimplified, and inflexible (96). Because of the inherent difficulties involved in determining disability objectively, it is no surprise that medical professionals may differ in their conclusions on a particular patient, thus leading to an adversarial situation in which a non-medical professional (i.e., judge) decides which opinion is more valid.

In addition to Social Security disability and workers' compensation evaluations, other situations that may involve the rehabilitation physician's assessment include: personal injury litigation; expert witness testimony; return to work determinations (letter/note); Veterans' benefits; and impartial medical evaluations (IMEs). Evaluation in these contexts involves the understanding of issues that extend beyond the mere medical determination of impairment. In many cases, the use of consultations and/or evaluations by other rehabilitation professionals (e.g., neuropsychologists, psychologists, speech pathologists, physical therapists, occupational therapists) may be helpful in determining the resultant disability.

Adjustment to Disability

Adjustment to disability is never easy, and there is no standard approach that patients take to that end. There are many differing models of adjustment. Some of these models are quite intriguing and appear to fit a set of patients, but none fits all. It is popular to believe that patients will go through the stages of the grieving model made popular by a number of different authors. These well-known stages may include: shock, anger, denial, acceptance. Although this model is operational and often helpful, it does not necessarily apply even to a majority of rehabilitation patients.

There is a real question as to whether anybody with a major neurological disability ever really "accepts" the disability. The coping process really never ends. Thus, it is important for coping skills to be emphasized in rehabilitation. These include crisis intervention, education, competence building, problem solving, goal setting, and others.

The whole rehabilitation team should be prepared to become "counselors" during the rehabilitation process. The team meetings may become forums for discussion. Formal psychotherapy and psychotropic medications may become necessary.

With chronic disabilities, adjustment involves the patient's family. Family members typically are affected adversely after a neurolgical problem occurs. Coping with these problems leads to an increase of a psychosomatic nature and to increased drug use among families. This was particularly noted in TBI patients but is likely in other neurological processes. Finances, behavior, and uncertainty all contribute to the problem.

Immediately after neurological injury, families are often grateful for the survival of their member. This changes to bewilderment and confusion over time. It is hoped that

significant acceptance and adjustment follow to allow for adaptation to the situation. Related to this, follow-up care should include, in addition to the necessary medical/physical aspects of rehabilitation, the emotional adjustment issues that are sure to surface for many patients, especially for those who have persistent sequelae. Referral to appropriately trained and experienced mental health professionals should be considered seriously.

Family Issues in Neurorehabilitation

While treating a patient who is in neurorehabilitation, it is important not to ignore the family or significant others of the patient. Families are often highly involved in the rehabilitation setting. They are typically interested in a wide range of information pertaining to, and in addition to, the diagnosis and treatment of their loved one. For example, return to work/school, potential for independent self-care, need for continued rehabilitation, availability for supportive care, financial resources, and other discharge-related issues are fundamental concerns to most families. With certain diagnoses, such as TBI, personality and/or behavior change is a valid concern for the family. In addition to these more explicit issues, family members might also be dealing with a host of responses, including shock, confusion, grief, loss, fear, anger, depression and anxiety. Therefore, it is crucial that rehabilitation professionals are sensitive to these issues, and that they provide adequate education, support, and referral to appropriate resources to families of their patients.

It is also important for the clinician to understand that the family potentially plays a critical role in the successful rehabilitation of the patient. For example, in a study by Lehmann et al. (99) evaluating outcome and prediction in stroke rehabilitation, it was found that family involvement was a significant predictor of whether patients were ultimately discharged home or went to an institution, with higher family involvement related to a greater likelihood of the patient returning home. As Lehnmann et al. suggest, because family involvement can be influenced by the patient's treatment team, it is important to focus on this factor. Indeed, it may have the potential effect of maximizing outcome. Similarly, Evans et al. (100) examined the relationship between prestroke family function and interaction, and outcome at 6 months and 1 year poststroke. Significant among their findings was that family interaction variables accounted for 28% of the variance in time of rehospitalization, compared with 10% of the variance accounted for by predictors not related to family assessment (e.g., lesion location, age, length of initial hospital stay, dysphasia, mental status, and socioeconomic status). Especially noteworthy was their finding that a positive family factor, affective responsiveness (i.e., the ability to respond with the appropriate quality and quantity of feelings, predicted reduced rehospitalization time.

As indicated by the studies just described and others in the rehabilitation literature supporting the importance of family factors in positive rehabilitation outcome, interventions directed toward improving or increasing family involvement should be a necessary consideration in the treatment team's plans. Investment of time and other resources in family education and support will ultimately benefit the patient.

PRACTICE HINTS: FAMILY ISSUES

Invest time and other resources in family education. This should include not only formal family meetings with the treatment team, but also availability of each team member, including the physician, to family members to answer questions or to provide education and/or advice on a continuous basis. For many families, a simple invitation to "call me if there are any questions," may be polite, but impractical because medical personnel are often intimidating to lay persons. Instead, take some initiative and seek out family members periodically to ask them if there are any questions or concerns that need to be addressed.

Communicate with the family in a respectful but comfortable manner. Avoid professional jargon and overly sophisticated language that might only serve to confuse and distance the family. In other words, speak to them in terms that they understand, without being patronizing. Allow time for questions to clarify or to prevent misunderstanding.

Encourage family members to be responsive to the patient. Sometimes family members will, with good intentions, attempt to motivate the patient by pushing him/her to "work harder." Although it is important for the patient to be highly invested in the treatment regimen, the family should be reminded of their important role as a source of emotional support and understanding for their loved one. Thus, the need to "push" the patient should be balanced by an empathetic understanding of the patient's emotional struggles with the difficulties of adjustment to disability.

For families with problematic interactions, consider intervention. If the family is adjusting poorly to the patient's hospitalization, or if family interaction patterns are problematic, secondary to premorbid or other factors, some sensitive intervention might be needed. Formal family therapy, a caregiver's support group, or psychotherapy for individuals other than the patient may be helpful in such circumstances.

SUMMARY

Because the scope of this field is so large, this chapter has presented merely a cursory overview of some current issues in the neuropsychiatry of rehabilitation. This continues to be a developing specialty in which phenomenal growth has been reflected in many areas in recent years, including: the increase of rehabilitation hospitals and units with a neurobehavioral emphasis; the appearance of additional rehabilitation-oriented professional journals that encompass neuropsychiatric issues; and the development of professional organizations such as the American Society of Neurorehabilitation. Despite the tremendous advancement in interest and in the knowledge base, the efficacy of rehabilitation will improve as more reliable outcome studies are conducted, particularly in the area of cognitive remediation and rehabilitation.

References

1. World Health Organization. International Classification of Impairments, Disabilities, and Handicaps, World Health Organization, 1980.
2. Romberg M. A manual of nervous diseases of man. London: Sydenham, 1853.
3. Feigenson J, Scheinberg L, Catalano M, et al. The cost-effectiveness of multiple sclerosis rehabilitation: a model. Neurology 1981;31:1326–1322.
4. Harley JP, Allen C, Braciszeski TL, et al. Guidelines for cognitive rehabilitation. Neurorehabilitation 1992;2:62–67.
5. Berrol S. Issues in cognitive rehabilitation. Arch Neurol 1990;47:219–220.
6. Gordon WA, Hibbard MR. Critical issues in cognitive remediation. Neuropsychology 1992;6:361–370.
7. Hachinski V. Cognitive rehabilitation. Arch Neurol 1990;47:224.
8. Levin HS. Cognitive rehabilitation—unproved but promising. Arch Neurol 1990;47:223–224.
9. Volpe BT, McDowell FH. The efficacy of cognitive rehabilitation in patients with traumatic brain injury. Arch Neurol 1990;47:220–222.
10. Tupper DE. Rehabilitation of cognitive and neuropsychological deficit following stroke. In: Bornstein RA, Brown G, eds. Neurobehavioral aspects of cerebrovascular disease. New York: Oxford University Press, 1991:337–358.
11. Benedict RHB. The effectiveness of cognitive remediation strategies for victims of traumatic head-injury: a review of the literature. Clinical Psychology Review 1989;9:605–626.
12. Benson DF. Neuropsychiatric aspects of aphasia and related language impairments. In: Yudofsky SC, Hales RE, eds. The American Psychiatric Press textbook of neuropsychiatry. 2nd ed. Washington, DC: American Psychiatric Press, 1992;311–327.
13. Kaufman DM. Clinical neurology for psychiatrists. 3rd ed. Philadelphia: WB Saunders, 1990:156.
14. Heilman KM, Gonzalez Rothi LJ. Apraxia. In: Heilman KM, Valenstein E, eds. Clinical neuropsychology. 2nd ed. New York: Oxford University Press, 1985:131–150.
15. Michell J. The ninth mental measurements yearbook 1 and 2. Lincoln: University of Nebraska Press, 1985.
16. Caplan B. Neuropsychology in rehabilitation: its role in evaluation and intervention. Arch Phys Med Rehabil 1982;63:362–366.
17. Rohe D. Psychologic aspects of rehabilitation. In: DeLisa J, ed. Rehabilitation medicine principles and practice. Philadelphia: JB Lippincott, 1988.
18. Reitan R. Theoretical and methodological bases of the Halstead Reitan Neuropsychological Test Battery. In: Grant I, Adams K, eds. Neuropsychological assessment of neuropsychiatric disorders. New York: Oxford University Press, 1986:3–30.
19. Bigler ER. Diagnostic clinical neuropsychology. Rev. ed. Austin: University of Texas Press, 1988:31–82.
20. Howieson DB, Lezak MD. The neuropsychological evaluation. In: Yudofsky SC, Hales RE, eds. The American Psychiatric Press textbook of neuropsychiatry. 2nd ed. Washington, DC: American Psychiatric Press, 1992:127–150.
21. Prigatano GP, Schacter DL. Introduction. In: Prigatano GP, Schacter DL, eds. Awareness of deficit after brain injury. New York: Oxford University Press, 1991:3–16.
22. Caplan B, Schecter J. Denial and depression in disabling illness. In: Caplan B, ed. Rehabilitation psychology desk reference. Rockville, MD: Aspen Systems, 1987:133–170.
23. Schacter GP, Prigatano DL. Forms of unawareness. In: Prigatano GP, Schacter DL, eds. Awareness of deficit after brain injury. New York: Oxford University Press, 1991:258–262.

24. Hurt R, Morse R, Swanson W. Diagnosis of alcoholism with a self administered alcoholism screening test: results of 1,002 consecutive patients receiving general examinations. Mayo Clin Proc 1980;55: 365–370.

25. Caplan L, Ahmed I. Depression and neurological disease. Gen Hosp Psychiatry 1992;14:177–185.

26. Clothier J, Grotta J. Recognition and management of post stroke depression in the elderly. Clin Geriatr Med 1991;3:493–506.

27. Minot S. Depression, what does it mean? Am J Nurs 1986;86: 285–293.

28. Fisher C. Abulia minor versus agitated behavior. Clinical Neurology 1983;33:337–344.

29. Alexander G, DeLong M, Strick P. Parallel organization of functionally segregated circuits linking basal ganglia and cortex. Annu Rev Neurosci 1986;9:357–381.

30. Nauta W, Domesick V. Afferent and efferent relationships of the basal ganglia. In: Functions of the basal ganglia. Ciba Foundation Symposia 1984;107:3–29.

31. Fogel BS, Stone AB. Practical pathophysiology in neuropsychiatry: a clinical approach to depression and impulsive behavior in neurological patients. In: Yudofsky SC, Hales RE, eds. The American Psychiatric Press textbook of neuropsychiatry. 2nd ed. Washington, DC: American Psychiatric Press, 1992:329–344.

32. Kurtzke J, Beebe G, Nagler B, Kurland L, Auth T. Studies on the natural history of multiple sclerosis. Journal of Chronic Disease 1977;30:819–830.

33. Kurtzke J. Epidemiologic contributions to multiple sclerosis: an overview. Neurology 1980;30:61–79.

34. Dean G, Kurtzke J. On the risk of multiple sclerosis according to age of immigration to South Africa Br Med J 1971 Sept 25; 3(777): 725–9.

35. Rao S, Leo G, Bernardin L, Unverzagt F. Cognitive dysfunctions in multiple sclerosis I. Neurology 1991;41:685–691.

36. Rao S, Leo, G, Ellington C, Namertz T, Bernardin L, Unverzagt F. Cognitive dysfunctions in multiple sclerosis II. Neurology 1991;41: 692–696.

37. Schapiro R. Multiple sclerosis, a rehabilitative approach to management. New York: Demos, 1991. N.Y.

38. Schapiro R, Soderberg J, et al. The multiple sclerosis achievement center: a maintenance rehabilitation approach toward a chronic progressive form of disease. Journal of Neurorehabilitation 1988;2: 21–25.

39. Stenager E, Koch-Henriksen N, et al. Suicide and multiple sclerosis: an epidemiological investigation. J Neurol, Neurosurg Psychiatry 1991;155:543–545.

40. Sadovnick A, Eisen K, Ebers G, Paty D. Cause of death in patients attending multiple sclerosis clinics. Neurology 1991;41:1193–1196.

41. Greenberg D. Neurasthenia in the 1980's: chronic mononucleosis, chronic fatigue syndrome, and anxiety and depressive disorders. Psychosomatics 1990;31:129–137.

42. Wessely S. Old wine in new bottles: neurasthenia and "ME." Psychol Med 1990;20:35–53.

43. Holmes G, Kaplan J, Gantz N, et al. Chronic fatigue syndrome: guidelines for research. Ann Intern Med 1988;108:387–389.

44. Bates DW, Schmitt W, Buchwald D, et al. Prevalence of fatigue and chronic fatigue syndrome in a primary care practice. Arch Intern Med 1993;153:2759–2765.

45. Alexander EL, Kumar AJ, Kozachuk WE. The chronic fatigue syndrome controversy. Ann Intern Med 1992;117:343–344.

46. Swartz M. The chronic fatigue syndrome—one entity or many? N Engl J Med 1988;319:1726–1728.

47. DeLuca J, Johnson S, Natelson B. Information processing efficiency in chronic fatigue syndrome and multiple sclerosis. Arch Neurol 1993;50:301–304.

48. Butler S, Chalder T, Ron M, Wessely S. Cognitive behaviour therapy in chronic fatigue syndrome. J Neurol Neurosurg Psychiatry 1991; 54:153–158.

49. Adams G, Hurwitz L. Mental barriers to recovery from strokes. Lancet 1963;1:533–537.

50. Feigenson J, McDowell F, Meese P, et al. Factors influencing outcomes and length of stay in a stroke rehabilitation unit. 1. Analysis of 248 unscreened patients, medical and functional prognostic indicators. Stroke 1977;8:651.

51. Morris P, Robinson R, Raphael B, Samuels J, Mallory P. The relationship between risk factors for affective disorder and post stroke depression in hospitalized stroke patients. Austral N Z J Psychiatry 1992;20:208–217.

52. Starkstein S, Bryer J, Berthier M, et al. Depression after stroke: the importance of cerebral hemisphere assymetries. Journal of Neuropsychiatry and Clinical Neurosciences 1991;3:3:276-285.

53. Bruckbauer E. Recognizing post stroke depression. Rehabilitation Nursing 1991;16:1:34-36.

54. Mapou RL. Testing to detect brain damage; an alternative to what may no longer be useful. J Clin Exp Neuropsychol 1988;10:271–278.

55. Hoehn M, Yahr M. Parkinsonism: onset, progression, and mortality; Neurology 1967;17:427–442.

56. Huber S, Shuttleworth E, Paulson G. Dementia in Parkinson's disease. Arch Neurol 1986;43:987–990.

57. Cummings J. Intellectual impairment in Parkinson's disease: clinical, pathologic, and behavioral correlates. J Geriatr Psychiatry Neurol 1988;1:24–36.

58. Cummings J. Depression and Parkinson's disease: a review. Am J Psychiatry 1992;149:443–454.

59. Bunting L, Fitzsimmons B. Depression in Parkinson's disease. J Neurosci Nurs 1991;23:3:158–164.

60. Torach R, Morris J. The association of the ventral tegmental area histopathology with adult dementia. Arch Neurol 1988;45:497–501.

61. Jouvent R, Abensour P, Bennet A, Widscher D, Agid Y, Lhermitte F. Antiparkinsonian and antidepressant effects of high doses of bromocriptine: an independent comparison. J Affect Disord 1983;5: 141–145.

62. Turk D. Psychological assessment of patients with persistent pain I; Pain Management 1990;165–172,

63. American Psychiatric Association. Diagnostic and statistical manual of mental disorders. 4th ed. Washington, DC: American Psychiatric Association, 1994.

64. Jones M. Conversion reaction: anachronism or evolutionary form? A review of neurologic, behavioral, and psychoanalytic literature. Psychol Bull 1980;87:427–441.

65. Sullivan M, Buchanan D. The treatment of conversion disorders in a rehabilitation setting. Canadian Journal of Rehabilitation 1989;2:3: 175–180.

66. Stewart T. Hysterical conversion reactions: some patient characteristics and treatment team reactions. Arch Phys Med Rehabil 1983; 64:308–310.

67. Quality Assurance Project Treatment Outlines for the Management of Somatoform Disorders. Australi N Z J Psychiatry 1985;19: 397–407.

68. Blanchard E, Hansen M. Behavioral treatment of hysterical neurosis: symptom substitution and symptom return reconsidered. Psychiatry 1976;39:118–129.

69. Frankowski R. The demography of head injury in the United States. In: Miner, M, Wagner K, eds. Neurotrauma 1986;1:1–17. London: Butterworths.

70. Namerow N. Current concepts and advances in brain injury rehabilitation; Journal of Neurorehabilitation 1987;1:101–114.

71. Dikmen S, Tenkin N, McLean A, Wyler A, Machamer J. Memory and head injury severity. J Neurol Neurosurg Psychiatry 1987;50:1613–1618.

72. Kotsoris H, Volpe B. Clinical characteristics of delayed recovery from post traumatic ataxia. Journal of Neurorehabilitation 1987;2:73–78.

73. Bach-y-Rita P. Brain plasticity as a basis of sensory substitution. Journal of Neurorehabilitation 1987;1:67–71.

74. Boyeson M, Bach-y-Rita P. Determinants of brain plasticity. Journal of Neurorehabilitation 1989;3:35–57.

75. Namerow N. Current concepts and advances in brain injury rehabilitation. Journal of Neurorehabilitation 1987;1:101–114.

76. Bonke C. Medical complications related to traumatic brain injury. In: Horn L, Cope D, eds. Traumatic brain injury. Phil Hanley and Belfas: 1989:43–58.

77. Bonke C, Boake C. Traumatic brain injury rehabilitation. Neurosurg Clinics of North America 1991;2:473–482.

78. Burke W, Wesolowski M, Guth M. Comprehensive head injury rehabilitation: an outcome evaluation. Brain Inj 1988;2:313–322.

79. Kazdin A. Behavior modification in applied setting. Rev ed. Dorsey Press, Homewood, Illinois, 1980.

80. Brooke M, Patterson D, et al. The treatment of agitation during initial hospitalization after traumatic brain injury. Arch Phys Med Rehabil 1992;73:917–920.

81. Brooke M, Questad K, Patterson D, Bashak K. Agitation and restlessness after closed head injury: a prospective study of 100 consecutive admissions; Arch Phys Med Rehabil 1992;73:320–330.

82. Rao N, Jellinck H, Wollstrom D. Agitation in closed head injury: haloperidol effects on rehabilitation outcome. Arch Phys Med Rehabil 1985;66:30–34.

83. Oddy M, Coughlan T, Tyerman A, et al. Social adjustment after closed head injury: a further follow-up seven years after injury. J Neurol Neurosurg Psychiatry 1985;48:564–568.

84. Temkin N, Dikmen S, Wilensky A, et al. A randomized, double blind study of phenytoin for the prevention of post traumatic seizures. N Engl J Med 1990;323:497–502.

85. Rappaport M., Herrero-Backe, C., Rupport, M., et al: Head injury outcome up to ten years later; Archives of Phys Med and Rehab 70:885-892, 1989.

86. Mills V, Nesbeda T, Katz D, Alexander M. Outcomes for traumatically injured patients following post acute rehabilitation programmes. Brain Inj 1992;6:219–228.

87. Prignatano G, Fordyce C, Zamer H. Neuropsychological rehabilitation after closed head injury in young adults. J Neurol Neurosurg Psychiatry 1984;47:505–513.

88. Ponsford J, Kinsella G. Evaluation of a remedial program for attention deficits following closed-head trauma. J Clin Exp Neuropsychol 1988;10:693–708.

89. Sherzer B. Rehabilitation following severe head trauma. Arch Phys Med Rehabil 1986;67:366–374.

90. Sohlberg M, Mateer C. Effectiveness of an attention training program. J Clin Exp Neuropsychol 1987;9:117–130.

91. Ben-Yishay Y. Working approaches to remediation of cognitive deficits in brain damaged. Supplement to Eleventh Annual Workshop for Rehabilitation Professionals, New York, 1983.

92. Lincoln N, Whiting I, Cockburn J, Bhavnani G. An evaluation of perceptual retraining. Internal Rehabilitation Medicine 1985;7:99–101.

93. Butler R, Namerow N. Cognitive retraining in brain injury rehabilitation: a critical review. Journal of Neurorehabilitation 1988;2:97–101.

94. Judd F, Brown D, Burrows G. Depression, disease, and disability: application to patients with traumatic spinal cord injury. Paraplegia 1991;29:91–96.

95. Judd F, Stene J, Webber J, Brown D, Burrows G. Depression following spinal cord injury: a prospective inpatient study. Br J Psychiatry 1989;154:668–671.

96. Rothstein MA. The law-medicine interface in assessing vocational capacity. In: Scheer SJ, ed. Medical perspectives in vocational assessment of impaired workers. Gaithersburg, MD: Aspen Systems, 1991:407–422.

97. American Medical Association. Guides to the evaluation of permanent impairment. 3rd ed. Chicago: AMA, 1988.

98. Scheer SJ. The physician's responsibility in assessing vocational capacity. In: Scheer SJ, ed. Medical perspectives in vocational assessment of impaired workers. Gaithersburg, MD: Aspen Systems, 1991:1–33.

99. Lehmann JF, DeLateur BJ, Fowler RS, et al. Stroke rehabilitation: outcome and prediction. Arch Phys Med Rehabil 1975;56:383–389.

100. Evans RL, Bishop DS, Matlock A, Stranahan S, Halar EM, Noonan WC. Prestroke family interaction as a predictor of stroke outcome. Arch Phys Med Rehabil 1987;68:508–512.

44

CURRENT DIAGNOSTIC ISSUES IN NEUROPSYCHIATRY

Gary J. Tucker

The chronological span (1952–1994) of the American Psychiatric Association's *Diagnostic and Statistical Manuals* (DSM) truly mirrors the changing notions of the etiology and understanding of mental illness. DSM-IV, published in 1994, graphically highlights the resurgence of neuropsychiatry and the relationship of the central nervous system (CNS) dysfunctions to behavioral disorders (1). With all of the mental disorders, a descriptive historical chain can be traced dating back many centuries. The major symptoms of mental illness are unchanged. Only the precision of the symptomatic specifications of schizophrenia, affective disorders, and the "neurotic conditions," have changed with the advent of DSM-III and DSM-IV. DSM-III brought, for psychopathological syndromes, the use of explicit operationally-defined diagnostic criteria. Although DSM-I referred to schizophrenic reactions and DSM-II discussed schizophrenia as a disease entity, the symptoms and syndromes are still recognizable. However, with regard to the "Organic Conditions," the changes have been major and there is almost no relationship between the descriptions in DSM-I and II and those in DSM-III and IV.

All of the DSM definitions of "organicity" are based on symptoms first clearly delineated by Bleuler in 1924 as an "organic psycho-syndrome" (2). The symptoms of this syndrome included labile or shallow affect, defects in orientation, memory, intellectual functions, and judgment (2). To this day, they still stand as the major defining symptoms of CNS dysfunction. In DSM-I, conditions that manifested these symptoms were grouped into two major categories, "acute" and "chronic" organic syndromes (3). Although never stated, it was implied that an acute brain syndrome was probably delirium and defined by reversibility of these symptoms, whereas chronic disorders were permanent, irreversible, represented diffuse impairment, and implied a dementia. In 1968, DSM-II changed the term "organic disorder" to "organic syndrome," for reasons that are unclear (other than symmetry with the rest of the nomenclature), and made major new categorical distinctions for the organic conditions of "psychotic" and "nonpsy-

chotic" (4). Reversible and nonreversible distinctions were retained, but the major classification became dependent on the presence of psychosis. Whether these conceptualizations represented the influence of state hospital populations and the problems that caused patients to be placed in them, they certainly bore little resemblance to the common clinical entities of dementia, delirium, and amnestic disorders.

CHANGING TERMINOLOGY

In 1980, DSM-III represented a radical but more clinically relevant conceptual shift. We now see clear definitions of delirium, dementia, and amnestic syndromes. We also see the addition of four behavioral syndromes not primarily defined by the traditional "organic" symptoms outlined by Bleuler (2). These conditions mainly manifested behavioral symptoms rather than clinically evident cognitive dysfunctions. Specific conditions that were defined included an organic delusional syndrome, organic hallucinosis, organic affective syndrome, and organic personality syndrome. In 1987, DSM-III-R added organic anxiety disorders to this list (5). In part, these modifications probably reflected the changing clinical experience of psychiatrists. It was during this period that psychiatry became a presence in most general hospitals, and psychiatrists became exposed to patients who clearly had medical illnesses, seizure disorders, head trauma, and brain tumors and who also often had behavioral syndromes as their primary symptoms.

The DSM-IV process began in 1989, partly because of the impetus of the International Classification of Diseases' revision (6); but it was also a reflection of the many studies that had been done on the pathological entities described in DSM-III and DSM-III-R (7). DSM-IV reflects major changes in the conceptualization of psychiatric illnesses consistent with the increasing knowledge of how the CNS affects behavior. Although DSM-III seemed to reflect the changes and conceptualization of mental illness related to the development of psychiatry in general hospitals, DSM-IV most clearly represents the knowledge explosion in the neurosciences as related to behavior. The new imaging techniques, the great scientific and public interest in conditions such as Alzheimer's disease, as well as the increasing molecular and biochemical understanding of the CNS, have led to increased data and hope for further clarification of the role of the CNS in behavior (8). With this more enlightened approach to psychiatry, the conceptualization of all psychiatric illnesses has changed.

In the preliminary discussions for DSM-IV, a strong priority was to eliminate the arbitrary dichotomy in the DSM nomenclature between "organic" and "nonorganic" conditions (9, 10). The authors argued that the arbitrary distinctions between conditions that could be directly attributed to CNS dysfunction and conditions in which the etiology was, as yet, unknown resulted from a lack of knowledge rather than because of a real difference. Consequently, in DSM-IV the "organic" distinction no longer exists, and we have categories of disordered behavior that range from delirium, dementia, and amnestic disorder to other psychopathological conditions such as schizophrenia, mood disorders, and anxiety disorders. Thus, all etiological distinctions of one set of conditions are related to disorders of the CNS, and the other, either unknown or not related, has been removed. This represents more than a semantic breakthrough. It is a major conceptual shift (11–15). The other changes in DSM-IV have been previously well described (11, 13, 16–24) and consist mainly of the following points:

1. There were major changes in the diagnostic criteria for delirium. The major criterion for the diagnosis of delirium used in DSM-III, "impairment of consciousness" was restored. Also, the number of symptoms was reduced by using the global term "changes in cognition" for such specific symptoms as "disorganized thinking," "perceptual changes." Most of these changes were made because of the difficulty in evaluating specific symptoms in medically and surgically ill patients. It was also recognized that dementia is one of the major risk factors for delirium and as such, the terms, ". . . not better accounted for by a preexisting or evolving dementia" were added to the diagnostic criteria (18).
2. The dementia criteria were made more consistent with other widely used diagnostic schemes, e.g., the National Institute of Neurologic and Communicative Disorders and Stroke (NINCDS) and the Alzheimer's Disease and Related Disorders Association (ADRDA), by using terms such as "aphasia" and "apraxia." However, the major criterion still remains multiple cognitive deficits. An important addition is the ability to stipulate the major behavioral disturbances that frequently accompany dementias, e.g., delusions, depression, and agitation (21), which are some of the major reasons dementia patients are referred to psychiatrists.
3. The primary behavioral "organic" diagnoses, e.g., "Organic Mood Disorders," are now called "Mood Disorders Due to a General Medical Condition (specify condition)"

Table 44.1. Primary Areas Where Symptoms May Be Observed in Dysfunction of the Central Nervous System

Cognitive
  orientation
  affect modulation
  memory
  intelligence
  judgment
Behavioral
  arousal
  mood
  anxiety
  perception
  personality
  motor

and have been moved to the section on Mood Disorders. Thus, the nomenclature reflects more how a clinician thinks. For example, the clinician, when presented with a patient with a mood disorder, usually includes in the differential diagnosis the possible various causes of mood disorder—psychological or biological. This format is the same for anxiety disorders, psychotic conditions, and other disorders (16).

4. Several new categories, e.g., personality change, catatonic, sleep and sexual disorders, all due to "general medical conditions," were also added (20).
5. Several categories were recommended for inclusion in the Appendix (postconcussive and mild cognitive disorder), in response to the argument that more research and study were needed to better delineate these conditions. Age-Associated Memory Decline was included under the heading of "Conditions that May Be of Clinical Interest." Also included in this category were Medication-Induced Movement Disorders (19, 22, 23, 25).

These recommendations were based as much as possible upon the large amount of diagnostic descriptive data which became available following the publication of DSM-III and DSM-III-R (7). Still, the entire DSM-IV process raised many persistent theoretical and practical concerns about neuropsychiatric diagnoses that have yet to be answered and are very important for our field and for future nomenclatures.

PROBLEMS IN NEUROPSYCHIATRIC DIAGNOSIS

Remarkably, the extensive literature reviews concerning DSM-IV reveal a very limited number of behavioral symptoms (Table 44.1). It is apparent that any insult to the CNS causes a very limited number of symptoms. The classic organic psycho-syndrome symptoms (described by Bleuler) of labile and shallow affect, defects in orientation, memory, intellectual function, and judgment, are present to a varying degree in most CNS disturbances (2). The classic behavioral symptoms, whether due to psychological reasons or to insults to the CNS, are also limited in number, and usually fall into the following areas: disturbances of arousal, mood, anxiety, perception, personality, and motor activity. These behavioral symptoms, coupled with the intellectual changes just noted, constitute almost the entire possible range of psychopathology. When one looks at a wide range of CNS conditions, from head trauma to electroencephalographic (EEG) abnormalities, it is quite apparent that similar behavioral symptoms and syndromes recur repeatedly. For example, if we look at patients with mild head trauma, the prominent symptoms are headache, dizziness, fatigue, decreased concentration, decreased memory, irritability, and depression (26). In the same way, if we look at psychiatric inpatients with EEG abnormality without head trauma, we see a similar array of symptoms (27). Consequently, it must be concluded that because the CNS has a *limited number of ways of responding to stress,* the symptoms we observe may have very little to do with indicating *specific* etiologies. Patients may experience hallucinations from head trauma, a toxin in the blood, an endocrine disturbance, an infectious process, or sleep deprivation, but all we might see clinically is the symptom (28), even though the etiology may differ greatly. It would make sense to postulate that the same anatomical or biochemical network is being activated to produce the symptom, but it is still only a hypothesis in most cases.

Besides raising doubts about etiology, the limited number of symptoms has dramatic effect on syndrome criteria. For example, it is evident from the literature reviews that the symptoms we stipulate as being important diagnostically to a specific syndrome can have major effects on the inclusiveness of the diagnosis. Liptzin et al. (19) showed that when the DSM-III-R criteria for delirium were used, of 125 cases that met DSM-III criteria, 26 did not meet DSM-III-R criteria. Consequently, the simple change from making the criterion in DSM-III-R "reduced attention" rather than "clouding of consciousness," as stipulated in DSM-III, and the inclusion of "disorganized thinking," greatly restricted those being designated as "delirious." In a similar fashion, Fenton (29) noted that in using DSM-III criteria for schizophrenia, and then applying DSM-III-R criteria to the same patients, 10% of the sample was lost. This change was caused simply by eliminating the criteria "onset before age 45" and requiring prominent delusions or hallucinations.

Clearly, minor changes in diagnostic criteria and symptomatic definition can radically change the population we are attempting to describe. This not only highlights the arbitrary nature of the process, but raises questions about our attempts at creating syndromes and recognizing symptom patterns as diagnoses.

CRITERIA FOR DELINEATING BEHAVIORAL SYNDROMES

Also evident in the DSM-IV process is the constant dilemma of trying to generalize syndromes or relationships reported primarily from single case studies or small samples.

Much of the literature on behavioral changes associated with medical illnesses rests entirely on case reports. Because of the relative infrequency and unusual nature of many of these cases, they are often deemed worthy of reporting (16). Thus, syndromes and associations frequently become locked into the literature or are formulated prematurely. For example, the supposed interictal personality syndrome associated with seizure disorders was described by Waxman and Geschwind on the basis of three cases (30). The triad of symptoms they found in these patients included: hyposexuality, hypergraphia, and philosophical or religious preoccupations. However, when one looks at large samples of patients with seizure disorders, this limited triad of symptoms does not hold up (31, 32).

The behavioral changes in medical conditions that have received the most systematic study are the neurological disorders. There have been large-scale studies of patients with stroke, Parkinson's disease, and Huntington's disease (16). However, because of the difficulty in collecting large samples of these patients for behavioral study, much is written based on one or two large samples often coming from the same institution. For example, the studies of depression following stroke have been done in several large patient samples from the same institution (33). When a community sample is studied, the high correlations of stroke and depressive disorder do not seem to hold up (34).

One of the most difficult questions raised by the DSM-IV process was establishing criteria for the association between medical illness and behavioral disturbance. In the first place, most of the psychiatric diagnoses have exclusion criteria for the presence of medical illnesses, so there is no clear guideline on when this exclusion should be ignored. It is also evident that even in the primary psychiatric disorders, we are frequently dealing with a mixture of cognitive and behavioral symptoms. For example, it is quite clear that many affective disorders have a marked cognitive disturbance associated with them. Similarly, with regard to affective disturbances in stroke patients and patients with basal ganglia disorder, there is often an obvious affective disorder as well as cognitive disturbances. As a result, perhaps we are merely seeing variations on the same theme, and the clinician is the one who makes the distinction based on the aspect of the condition in which he/she is interested. The literature concerning the incidence of behavioral disturbance in general medical inpatients, regardless of the specific condition, reveals similar prevalence rates—between 10–30% of affective disturbances (35, 36). Similar ranges of percentages are reported for many neurological conditions, leaving the clinician to wonder if we are not dealing with a general severity factor associated with any illness, whether its primary site is the CNS or other anatomical locations, and if the behavioral disturbance represents a general severity factor rather than being specific to any condition (16).

As noted earlier, the inclusion and/or exclusion of various symptoms affects the ability to make a diagnosis of an illness in a particular patient. In a similar fashion, depending upon how we define many of the symptoms associated with either neurological or medical conditions, we may find a greater or lesser incidence of behavioral disturbance in the condition. In most cases, if the strict DSM-III-R or DSM-IV criteria are applied to a condition where there is a prominent neurological disorder, then it is very difficult to meet the diagnostic criteria for mood disorder. Generally, we opted, as part of the DSM-IV process, to have a "sounds like" criteria. In other words, if there were prominent mood disorder symptoms in the patient, these were deemed sufficient to have an association. But to establish an association, we also felt that some guidelines were necessary. We proposed consideration of the following criteria:

1. A previous definition of a specific psychopathological syndrome associated with the medical condition;
2. Delineation of other manifestations of the primary medical condition;
3. Demonstration of an active cerebral or systemic pathological process; and
4. Demonstration of an elevated prevalence rate between the proposed etiological disorder and the described psychopathological picture in the literature.

Currently many behavioral conditions cited as being related to a specific medical or neurological disorder do not reach the level of these criteria but rest more strongly upon anecdote and case report (16).

CENTRAL NERVOUS SYSTEM LOCALIZATION OF BEHAVIORAL DISORDERS

Historically one of the most interesting problems confronting physicians is the association between specific brain regions and specific psychopathology or symptomatology. We have been confronted with this debate as far back as the phrenologists in the 18th century, if not earlier. Many have tried to localize specific behavioral changes associated with a specific brain region (37). A review of the literature indicates clearly that lesions in different areas of the CNS cause similar symptomatology. For example, a recent study by Anderson on the Wisconsin Card Sort Test, which is supposed to be specific to frontal lobe damage, noted that some patients with extensive frontal lobe damage performed well on this test, and some subjects with damage outside the frontal lobe area failed (38). Consequently, linking a specific behavioral syndrome to a specific anatomical region with our current knowledge does not seem appropriate. Reviewing various supposed regional syndromes highlighted the fact that the anatomical designation of brain regions into frontal lobe, temporal lobe, and occipital lobe, among others, was probably a historical artifact, true mainly for gross motor and sensory functions.

In light of modern physiology with concepts of simultaneous distributive processing, the regional localization literature was fraught with extensive conflicts. The age-old debate between people such as Lashley (39) and Chapman and Wolfe (40), who believed it was the amount of tissue destroyed rather than the localization in the CNS of a

Table 44.2. Major Neuropsychiatric Syndromes Represented in DSM-IV and ICD-10[a]

	DSM-IV[b]	ICD-10[b]
Delirium	X	X
Dementia	X	X
Early	X	X
Late	X	X
Behavioral		
Stipulation (e.g., depressed, psychoses, etc.)		
Specific dementias (vascular, HIV, Parkinson's disease, etc.)	X	X
Amnestic disorders	X	X
Transient	X	
Chronic	X	
Behavioral syndromes		
Anxiety disorder	X	X
Affective disorder (including bipolar, manic, etc.)	X	X
Psychotic disorder	X	X
Catatonic disorder	X	X
Sexual disorder	X	
Sleep disorder	X	
Dissociative disorder		X
Specific disorders		
Age-associated cognitive decline	X	
Postconcussive syndrome[c]		X
Postencephalitic		X
Mild neurocognitive impairment[c]		X
Personality change		
Labile	X	
Dishinhibited	X	
Aggressive	X	
Apathetic	X	
Paranoid	X	

[a]Specifics of diagnostic criteria vary in each system, but in general, they are compatible.
[b]All DSM-IV and ICD-10 disorders can also be substance-related due to either intoxication or withdrawal.
[c]In DSM-IV Appendix for further study before inclusion.

lesion, has not been solved. As a result, we felt that in DSM-IV it was best to describe the syndromes seen with brain damage as an apathetic syndrome or a labile syndrome, rather than stipulating this as a frontal lobe-specific syndrome. Similarly, other disturbances in patients with brain injury were given descriptive labels, e.g., labile, disinhibited, aggressive, apathetic, or paranoid syndromes, rather than anatomical labels. An overview of the approximate relationship between the syndromes of DSM-IV and those of the International Classification of Diseases, 10th edition (ICD-10) is presented in Table 44.2.

CONCLUSION

Where does this leave us? First, it is apparent that we need very careful descriptions of patients. In this respect, we must attempt to make as reliable and reproducible as many of our symptom definitions as possible. A good, recent example is the attempt to operationalize the diagnostic criteria for delirium (41). It is also important to use symptom schedules in our evaluations so that we are aware of all the symptoms the patient has had (42). With the current diagnostic process, we are often aware of what symptoms may be present but are never assured of what symptoms the patient has that are not included in the diagnostic criteria. As a result, for many years we have ignored the combination of anxiety and depressive symptoms by focusing on the prominent symptom, highlighting that symptom as our diagnostic entity, and ignoring other symptoms.

We are especially interested in the role of CNS dysfunction and its causal relationship to behavioral changes. In this respect, both parts of the equation must be well defined. Both the neurological symptoms the patient manifests and the neurological diagnosis must be clear (43). Additionally, the symptoms on which the diagnosis is based must be clear, reliable, and reproducible. Good psychiatric diagnostic schedules and careful evaluations of cognitive and behavioral function with standardized measures must be used in large samples to determine these relationships (44, 45). Too often the schedules and symptoms that are examined are those that one postulates are present, and other symptoms and diagnoses are frequently ignored.

Although the many new imaging techniques are exciting, there has always been a question of the standardization of the interpretation of the results from different machines. For example, it is not clear how well standardized one positron emission tomography (PET) machine is when compared with another. In a similar manner, how standardized are the magnetic resonance imaging (MRI) techniques and interpretation of the results? Undoubtedly, the dynamic measures of MRI spectroscopy and single photon emission computed tomography (SPECT) analysis have raised questions concerning reproducibility and standardization of these techniques.

Perhaps rather than studying artificial syndromes such as schizophrenia, we should begin looking at specific symptoms (46). Hallucinations, for example, could be explored productively using a number of different techniques (47). For example, many of the studies of schizophrenia usually conclude by saying there are particular ventricular changes noted on MRI in a "subgroup of patients." This means that the findings are not present in all patients. This might also be interpreted as meaning that the group of patients selected for a study is heterogeneous due to the use of polythetic diagnostic criteria. Consequently, defining subjects by single or specific symptoms, or groups of specific symptoms, may be a more successful method of investigating disorders biologically (48).

Also needed in the fields of psychiatry and behavioral disorders are good longitudinal studies that follow symptoms and syndromes, not only over time, but also through autopsy and anatomical and biochemical analysis. Such studies would require a much closer working relationship between psychiatrists, neurosurgeons, neurologists, neuropsychologists, and neuroscientists than we have now. Perhaps the departmental organization that we all live in is as much an historical artifact as the gross anatomical lobular divisions of the brain. Ultimately it would be in our best

interests to work in more functional groups such as a department of clinical neuroscience. In the meantime, our efforts to further delineate syndromes by expert consensus will continue.

References

1. American Psychiatric Association. Diagnostic and Statistical Manual-IV. Washington, DC: American Psychiatric Press, 1994.
2. Bleuler E. Textbook of psychiatry. New York: MacMillan, 1924.
3. American Psychiatric Association. Diagnostic and Statistical Manual. Washington, DC: American Psychiatric Press, 1952.
4. American Psychiatric Association. Diagnostic and Statistical Manual-II. Washington, DC: American Psychiatric Press, 1968.
5. American Psychiatric Association. Diagnostic and Statistical Manual-III-R. Washington, DC: American Psychiatric Press, 1987.
6. The ICD-10 Classification of Mental and Behavioral Disorders. Geneva: World Health Organization, 1992.
7. Skodol AE, Spitzer RL, eds. An annotated bibliography of DSM-III. Washington, DC: American Psychiatric Press, 1987.
8. Coyle JT. Neuroscience and psychiatry. In: Talbott J, Hales R, Yudofsky S, eds. American Psychiatric Press textbook of psychiatry. Washington, DC: American Psychiatric Press, 1988:3–32.
9. Taylor MA. DSM-III organic mental disorders. In: Tischler G, ed. Diagnosis and classification in psychiatry. Cambridge, MA: Cambridge University Press, 1987.
10. Spitzer RL, Williams JBW, First M, et al. A proposal for DSM-IV: solving the "organic/nonorganic" problem. J Neuropsychiatry Clin Neurosci 1989;1:126–127.
11. Popkin MK, Tucker GJ, Caine E, et al. The fate of organic mental disorders in DSM-IV: a progress report. Psychosomatics 1989;30:438–441.
12. Lipowski ZJ. Is "organic" obsolete? Psychosomatics 1990;31:342–344.
13. Tucker GJ, Popkin MK, Caine ED, et al. Reorganizing the "organic" disorders. Hosp Community Psychiatry 1990;41:722–724.
14. Spitzer RL, First MB, Williams JBW, et al. Now is the time to retire the term "organic mental disorders." Am J Psychiatry 1992;149:240–244.
15. Tucker GJ, Caine E, Popkin MK. DSM-IV Source Book, vol 1. Washington, DC: American Psychiatric Press, 1994:185–194.
16. Tucker GJ, Caine ED, Popkin MK. Introduction to Section II, Delirium, dementia, and amnestic and other cognitive disorders. In: Widiger TA, Frances AJ, Pincus HA, et al., eds. DSM-IV source book, vol. 1. Washington, DC: American Psychiatric Association, 1994:185–198.
17. Popkin MK, Tucker GJ. "Secondary" and drug induced mood, anxiety, psychotic, catatonic and personality disorders: a review of the literature. J Neuropsychiatry 1992;4:369–385.
18. Tucker GJ, Caine E, Folstein M, et al. Introduction to background papers for the suggested changes to DSM IV: cognitive disorders. J Neuropsychiatry 1992;4:366–368.
19. Liptzin B, Levkoff S, Gottlieb F, Johnson J. Delirium. J Neuropsychiatry 1993;5:154–160.
20. Gutierrez R, Atkinson J, Grant I. Mild neurocognitive disorder. J Neuropsychiatry 1993;5:161–177.
21. Tucker GJ. Regional syndromes. J Neuropsychiatry 1993;5:260–264.
22. Rebok G, Folstein M. Dementia. J Neuropsychiatry 1993;5:265–276.
23. Caine E. Amnesic disorders. J Neuropsychiatry 1993;5:6–8.
24. Caine E. Should aging associated cognitive decline be included in DSM-IV. J Neuropsychiatry 1993;5:1–5.
25. Tucker GJ. DSM-IV background papers on cognitive disorders. J Neuropsychiatry 1994;6:14.
26. Brown S, Fann J, Grant I. Post-concussional disorders. J Neuropsychiatry 1994;6:15–22.
27. Tucker GJ, Detre T, Harrow M, Glosser G. Behavior and symptoms of

psychiatric patients and the electroencephalogram. Arch Gen Psychiatry 1965;12:278–286.

28. Pincus J, Tucker GJ. Behavioral neurology. 3rd ed. New York: Oxford University Press, 1985.

29. Fenton W, McGlashan T, Heinssen R. A comparison of DSM III and DSM-III-R schizophrenia. Am J Psychiatry 1988;145:1446–1449.

30. Waxman G, Geschwind N. The interictal behavioral syndrome of temporal lobe epilepsy. Arch Gen Psychiatry 1975;32:1580–1586.

31. Bear D, Fedio P. Quantitative analysis of interictal behavior in temporal lobe epilepsy. Arch Neurol 1977;34:454–467.

32. Mungas D. Interictal behavior abnormality in temporal lobe epilepsy. Arch Gen Psychiatry 1982;39:108–111.

33. Robinson RG, Balduc PL, Price TR. Two-year longitudinal study of post-stroke mood disorders. Stroke 1987;18:837–843.

34. House A, Dennis M, Warlow C, et al. Mood disorders after stroke and their relation to lesion location. Brain 1990;113:1113–1129.

35. Katon W, Schulberg H. Epidemiology of depression in primary care. Gen Hosp Psychiatry 1992;14:237–247.

36. Kroenke K, Arrington ME, Mangelsdorff AD. The prevalence of symptoms in medical outpatients and the adequacy of therapy. Arch Intern Med 1990;150:1685–1689.

37. Benson F. The history of behavioral neurology. Neurol Clin 1993;11:1–8.

38. Anderson S, Damasio H, Jones R, Tranel D. Wisconsin card sorting test performance as a measure of frontal lobe damage. J Clin Exp Neuropsychol 1991;13:909–922.

39. Lashley KS. Brain mechanisms and intelligence. Chicago: University of Chicago Press, 1929.

40. Chapman LF, Wolff HG. The cerebral hemispheres and the highest integrative functions of man. Arch Neurol 1959;1:357–424.

41. Tryepacz PT, Baker RW, Greenhouse J. A symptom rating scale for delirium. Psychiatry Rev 1988;23:89–97.

42. Andreasen N, Flower M, Arndt S. The comprehensive assessment of symptoms and history. Arch Gen Psychiatry 1992;49:615–623.

43. Menza R, Golbe L, Cody R, Forman N. Dopamine-related personality traits in Parkinson's disease. Neurology 1993;43:505–508.

44. Spitzer RL, Endicott J, Robins E. Research diagnostic criteria. New York: Biometrics Research Division, New York State Psychiatric Institute, 1975.

45. Endicott J, Spitzer RL. A diagnostic interview: the Schedule for Affective Disorders and Schizophrenia (SADS). Arch Gen Psychiatry 1978;35:837–844.

46. Carpenter WT Jr, Buchanan RW, Kirkpatrick B, Tamminga C, Wood F. Strong inference, theory testing, and the neuroanatomy of schizophrenia. Arch Gen Psychiatry 1993;50:825–831.

47. Barta P, Pearlson G, Powers R, et al. Auditory hallucinations and smaller bipolar temporal gyral volume in schizophrenia. Am J Psychiatry 1990;147:1457–1462.

48. Tamminga C, Thaker G, Buchanan R, et al. Limbic system abnormalities identified in schizophrenia using PET with fluorodeoxyglucose and neocortical alterations with deficit syndrome. Arch Gen Psychiatry 1992;49:522–530.

INDEX

Page numbers followed by an italic "f" denote figures; those followed by an italic "t" denote tables.